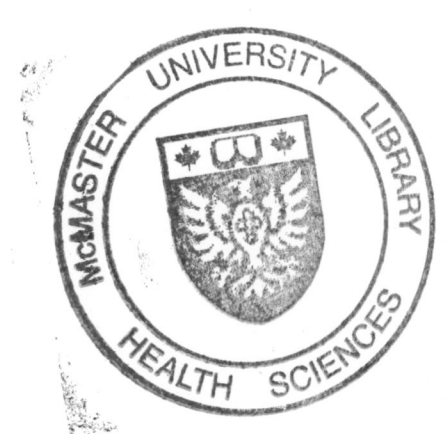

Practical Pulmonary Pathology

Practical Pulmonary Pathology
A Diagnostic Approach
SECOND EDITION

Kevin O. Leslie, MD
Professor and Chair
Division of Anatomic Pathology
Department of Laboratory Medicine and Pathology
Mayo Clinic Arizona
Scottsdale, Arizona

Mark R. Wick, MD
Professor of Pathology
Division of Surgical Pathology
University of Virginia Medical Center
Charlottesville, Virginia

ELSEVIER
SAUNDERS

ELSEVIER
SAUNDERS

1600 John F. Kennedy Blvd.
Ste. 1800
Philadelphia, PA 19103-2899

PRACTICAL PULMONARY PATHOLOGY:
A DIAGNOSTIC APPROACH

ISBN: 978-1-4160-5770-3

Notices

Knowledge and best practice in this field are constantly changing. As new research and experience broaden our understanding, changes in research methods, professional practices, or medical treatment may become necessary.

Practitioners and researchers must always rely on their own experience and knowledge in evaluating and using any information, methods, compounds, or experiments described herein. In using such information or methods they should be mindful of their own safety and the safety of others, including parties for whom they have a professional responsibility.

With respect to any drug or pharmaceutical products identified, readers are advised to check the most current information provided (i) on procedures featured or (ii) by the manufacturer of each product to be administered, to verify the recommended dose or formula, the method and duration of administration, and contraindications. It is the responsibility of practitioners, relying on their own experience and knowledge of their patients, to make diagnoses, to determine dosages and the best treatment for each individual patient, and to take all appropriate safety precautions.

To the fullest extent of the law, neither the Publisher nor the authors, contributors, or editors, assume any liability for any injury and/or damage to persons or property as a matter of products liability, negligence or otherwise, or from any use or operation of any methods, products, instructions, or ideas contained in the material herein.

ISBN: 978-1-4160-5770-3

Acquisitions Editor: William R. Schmitt
Publishing Services Manager: Pat Joiner-Myers
Project Manager: Marlene Weeks
Design Direction: Lou Forgione

Printed in China

Last digit is the print number: 9 8 7 6 5 4 3 2 1

Contributors

Timothy C. Allen, MD, JD
Professor and Chair
Department of Pathology
The University of Texas Health Science Center at Tyler
Tyler, Texas

Mattia Barbareschi, MD, PhD
Associate Director
Department of Surgical Pathology
S. Chiara Hospital
Trento, Italy

Mary Beth Beasley, MD
Associate Professor of Pathology
Department of Pathology
Mount Sinai Medical Center
New York, New York

Kelly J. Butnor, MD
Assistant Professor of Pathology
Department of Pathology
University of Vermont College of Medicine
Fletcher Allen Healthcare
Burlington, Vermont

Alberto Cavazza, MD
Unità Operativa di Anatomia Patologica
Ospedale S. Maria Nuova
Reggio Emilia, Italy

Oi-Yee Cheung, MD
Consultant
Department of Pathology
Queen Elizabeth Hospital
Hong Kong

Andrew Churg, MD
Professor of Pathology
Department of Pathology
University of British Columbia
Vancouver, Canada

Thomas V. Colby, MD
Professor and Chair
Department of Laboratory Medicine and Pathology
Mayo Clinic Arizona
Scottsdale, Arizona

Giorgia Dalpiaz, MD
Unit of Radiology
Bellaria Hospital
Bologna, Italy

Megan K. Dishop, MD
Department of Pathology
The Children's Hospital
Aurora, Colorado

Junya Fukuoka, MD, PhD
Clinical Professor
Laboratory of Pathology
Toyama University Hospital
Toyama, Japan

Paolo Graziano, MD
Consultant Pathologist
Unit of Pathology
C. Forlanini Hospital
A.O. San Camillo-Forlanini
Rome, Italy

Dawn E. Jaroszewski, MD
Consultant
Department of Thoracic Surgery
Mayo Clinic Arizona
Scottsdale Arizona

Kirk D. Jones, MD
Assistant Clinical Professor of Pathology
Department of Pathology
University of California
San Francisco, California

Andras Khoor, MD
Associate Professor and Chair
Department of Laboratory Medicine and Pathology
Mayo Clinic Jacksonville
Jacksonville, Florida

Madeleine D. Kraus, MD
Department of Pathology
St. Luke's Medical Center
St. Louis, Missouri

Kevin O. Leslie, MD
Professor and Chair
Division of Anatomic Pathology
Department of Laboratory Medicine and Pathology
Mayo Clinic Arizona
Scottsdale, Arizona

Mario Maffessanti, MD
Professor of Diagnostic Imaging
Istituto di Radiologia
Ospedale di Cattinara
Trieste, Italy

Osamu Matsubara, MD
Professor of Pathology
National Defense Medical College
Department of Pathology
Tokoworaza, Japan

Stacey E. Mills, MD
Professor of Pathology
Division of Surgical Pathology
University of Virginia Medical Center
Charlottesville, Virginia

Cesar A. Moran, MD
Professor of Pathology
Department of Pathology and Laboratory Medicine
University of Texas M. D. Anderson Cancer Center
Houston, Texas

Stephen S. Raab, MD
Professor and Vice Chair
Department of Pathology
University of Colorado Health Sciences Center
Aurora, Colorado

Jon H. Ritter, MD
Associate Professor
Department of Surgical Pathology
Washington University
St. Louis, Missouri

Victor L. Roggli, MD
Professor of Pathology
Duke University Medical Center
Durham, North Carolina

Louis A. Rosati, MD
Associate Pathologist
Department of Pathology
Banner Desert Medical Center
Mesa, Arizona

Mark H. Stoler, MD
Professor of Pathology and Clinical Gynecology
Associate Director of Surgical Pathology and Cytopathology
Department of Pathology
University of Virginia Health System
Charlottesville, Virginia

Henry D. Tazelaar, MD
Professor of Pathology
Department of Laboratory Medicine and Pathology
Mayo Clinic
Scottsdale, Arizona

William D. Travis, MD
Attending Thoracic Pathologist
Department of Pathology
Memorial Sloan Kettering Cancer Center
New York, New York

Robert W. Viggiano, MD
Consultant
Department of Pulmonary Medicine
Mayo Clinic Scottsdale
Scottsdale, Arizona

Mark R. Wick, MD
Professor of Pathology
Division of Surgical Pathology
University of Virginia Medical Center
Charlottesville, Virginia

Joanne L. Wright, MD
Professor of Pathology
Department of Pathology
University of British Columbia
Vancouver, Canada

Samuel A. Yousem, MD
Professor of Pathology
University of Pittsburgh Medical Center
Pittsburgh, Pennsylvania

Series Preface

It is often stated that anatomic pathologists come in two forms: "Gestalt"-based individuals, who recognize visual scenes as a whole, matching them unconsciously with memorialized archives; and criterion-oriented people, who work through images systematically in segments, tabulating the results—internally, mentally, and quickly—as they go along in examining a visual target. These approaches can be equally effective, and they are probably not as dissimilar as their descriptions would suggest. In reality, even "Gestaltists" subliminally examine details of an image, and, if asked specifically about particular features of it, they are able to say whether one characteristic or another is important diagnostically.

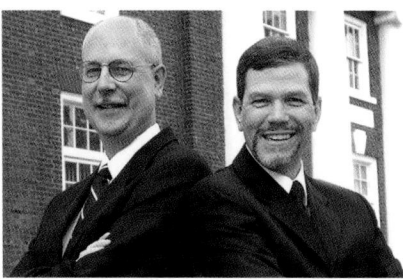

In accordance with these concepts, in 2004 we published a textbook entitled *Practical Pulmonary Pathology: A Diagnostic Approach* (PPPDA). That monograph was designed around a *pattern-based* method, wherein diseases of the lung were divided into six categories on the basis of their general image profiles. Using that technique, one can successfully segregate pathologic conditions into diagnostically and clinically useful groupings.

The merits of such a procedure have been validated empirically by the enthusiastic feedback we have received from users of our book. In addition, following the old adage that "imitation is the sincerest form of flattery," since our book came out, other publications and presentations have appeared in our specialty with the same approach.

After publication of the PPPDA text, representatives at Elsevier, most notably William Schmitt, were enthusiastic about building a *series* of texts around pattern-based diagnosis in pathology. To this end we have recruited a distinguished group of authors and editors to accomplish that task. Because a panoply of patterns is difficult to approach mentally from a practical perspective, we have asked our contributors to be complete and yet to discuss only principal interpretative images. Our goal is to eventually provide a series of monographs that, in combination with one another, will allow trainees and practitioners in pathology to use salient morphologic patterns to reach with confidence final diagnoses in all organ systems.

As stated in the introduction to the PPPDA text, the evaluation of dominant patterns is aided secondarily by the analysis of cellular composition and other distinctive findings. Therefore, within the context of each pattern, editors have been asked to use such data to refer the reader to appropriate specific chapters in their respective texts.

We have also stated previously that some overlap is expected between pathological patterns in any given anatomic site; in addition, specific disease states may potentially manifest themselves with more than one pattern. At first, those facts may seem to militate against the value of pattern-based interpretation. However, pragmatically, they do not. One often can narrow diagnostic possibilities to a very few entities using the pattern method, and sometimes a single interpretation will be obvious. Both of those outcomes are useful to clinical physicians caring for a given patient.

It is hoped that the expertise of our authors and editors, together with the high quality of morphologic images they present in this Elsevier series, will be beneficial to our reader-colleagues.

Kevin O. Leslie, MD
Mark R. Wick, MD

Preface

It has been 5 years since *Practical Pulmonary Pathology: A Diagnostic Approach* (PPPDA) was first published. We are happy to report that the original version of this book was warmly received, with a distribution of approximately 8000 copies. Readers seemed to find our pattern-based approach to be a useful one in the daily practice of anatomic pathology, judging by the direct feedback we received. We also were honored when PPPDA won the 2005 Textbook of the Year Award from the Royal Society of Medicine and Royal Society of Authors.

In light of these successes, and in view of the fact that hospital pathology continues to grow rapidly in scope and complexity, we decided to prepare a second edition of our book. Several features are new to this edition. These include inevitable additions to, and revisions of, the prior text because of advances in our understanding of the pertinent disease processes. Corresponding references have been added, and they are current through mid-2010. Moreover, many illustrative photomicrographs have been changed. In an effort to improve the visual presentation of the topics discussed. Finally, self-assessment questions tied to all the chapters in the current book have been compiled and are available online. It is hoped that these questions will be useful to pathologists in their maintenance of certification and as a reflection of their mastery of the information in the book.

As before, we begin with the general patterns of disease and then add key morphologic findings that assist the reader in focusing on appropriate sections of the book where similar findings are discussed. This approach is facilitated by a structural overlay that limits the patterns. We have found that six general patterns occur, and these are best appreciated at scanning magnification with the microscope. We could begin at an even lower "magnification" using the high-resolution computed tomogram (CT), and this is what our radiology colleagues commonly do as they assemble a differential diagnosis based on observed findings in this medium (see Chapter 3). In practice, the CT images may not be readily available to the pathologist at the time the biopsy is interpreted; so for our six pathology patterns, we begin with a tissue section mounted on a glass slide.

An overview of the six patterns is presented, and each pattern is then illustrated in the pages that follow. Most of the patterns were devised to navigate the "diffuse lung diseases" commonly referred to as *interstitial lung diseases* or *ILD*. Given the tumefactive nature of neoplasms, these are heavily represented in Pattern 5 (Nodules), but some non-neoplastic diseases, such as sarcoidosis, nodular infections, Wegener's granulomatosis, and certain neumoconioses, may also manifest as a nodular pattern. Rarely, neoplasms can present as diffuse "interstitial" lung disease clinically and radiologically.

A basic knowledge of the two-dimensional structure of the lung is essential for accurately assessing patterns of disease. We assume that the reader is familiar with basic lung anatomy by the time a diagnostic problem is being evaluated in the patient care setting, but a brief review is always helpful (see Chapter 1).

Once the overriding or dominant pattern is recognized, the diagnostician assesses the cellular composition and any other distinctive findings that accompany the pattern. In the case of a tumor forming a nodular mass, the presence of prominent spindled cells, or large granular cells, or clear cells provides a direction for creating a differential diagnosis. Within each pattern, we have attempted to use such qualifying elements to direct the reader to the appropriate chapter for further study, reasonably confident that the answer will lie within. For the unusual finding not identified in the list for a given pattern, the reader is directed to the appendix, where we have assembled a "visual encyclopedia" of distinctive findings and artifacts.

Naturally, overlap occurs between patterns, and this too can be a useful guide to the correct diagnosis. For example, some infections are both *nodular* and have *airspace filling* (e.g., botyromycosis, aspiration pneumonia), whereas others are characterized by *acute lung injury* and *diffuse airspace filling* (e.g., pneumoccocal pneumonia, pneumocystis pneumonia.) In fact, some diffuse inflammatory conditions in the lung may manifest five of the six patterns, in different areas of the same biopsy (e.g., rheumatoid lung). Nevertheless, as more and more information is accrued from the biopsy, the differential diagnosis becomes more limited. In some cases, it may be necessary to include several possibilities in the final diagnosis, especially for the non-neoplastic diseases, where the effect of ancillary data not available at the time of diagnosis may be very large.

Once again, we are grateful to all of the authors who generously and diligently updated their chapters in the second edition of PPPDA. In addition, many thanks are due to our colleagues at the Mayo Clinic and the University of Virginia for their strong support of this project. Finally, this work could not have reached fruition without the valuable help of our editor, William Schmitt of Elsevier, and the editorial and production expertise of Peggy Gordon and Clay Cansler.

Kevin O. Leslie, MD
Mark R. Wick, MD

Contents

Pattern-Based Approach to Diagnosis

A fundamental truth about medical textbooks is that they are often not read from beginning to end once a student of medicine has progressed beyond the basic medical school curriculum. In the practice of medicine, textbooks are more commonly used as references for learning about a disease or entity that a clinician suspects a patient may have based on history, physical findings, and imaging/laboratory data gleaned from an initial screening evaluation. The disease-based textbook is analogous to a dictionary or encyclopedia, both of which are much easier to use if a person already has a good idea of what he or she is investigating.

Today, the vast majority of diagnosis-oriented medical textbooks continue to exist as compendia of individual diseases, more or less grouped by the anatomical compartment or structure affected (e.g., brainstem diseases, bile duct diseases, glomerular diseases) or a common mechanism if one is discernible (e.g., inflammatory diseases, neoplastic diseases). Typically, the discussion of each disease begins with a historical introduction, continues with the characteristics of the disease, and ends with the treatment and prognosis. This book is no different, but the authors have added this introductory material as a tool to help navigate the contents. The approach is based on the premise that six primary histopathologic patterns exist for all lung diseases. Identifiable using the low-magnification microscope objective lens, these patterns serve as the introductory image of the disease process (in truth, chest imaging with high-resolution computed tomography is an even better place to begin—see Chapter 3). Once the primary pattern is recognized, the histopathologist must collect additional findings from the biopsy specimen. With the primary pattern and secondary attributes in hand, a cogent differential diagnosis can be proffered. This process is significantly enhanced by knowledge of the clinical presentation and imaging characteristics, but if these are not available when the slides are being examined, they still can be useful for narrowing the differential diagnosis after the histopathology has been evaluated. A detailed analysis on the use of clinical, radiologic, and histopathologic data in the evaluation of the diffuse medical lung diseases (often referred to as *interstitial lung diseases*, or *ILDs*) is available for the interested reader (open access file for download).* The Worksheet for the Pattern-Based Approach to Lung Disease, located on page xvi, is a printable form for organizing these data.

A basic knowledge of the two-dimensional structure of the lung is essential for accurately assessing patterns of disease. We assume that the reader is familiar with basic lung anatomy by the time a diagnostic problem is being evaluated in the patient care setting, but a brief review is always helpful (see Chapter 2). An overview of the six major patterns is provided (page xvii), followed by illustrations of each pattern. The pattern-based approach presented here was devised mainly to assist in the interpretation of the diffuse lung diseases, commonly referred to as *ILDs*. Given the tumefactive nature of neoplasms, these are heavily represented in Pattern 5 (Nodules), but some non-neoplastic diseases, such as sarcoidosis, nodular infections, Wegener granulomatosis, and certain pneumoconioses, may also manifest a nodular pattern. Rarely, neoplasms can present as diffuse ILD clinically and radiologically (e.g., lymphangitic carcinoma, intravascular lymphoma). Within each of the major patterns, the authors have provided the reader with the appropriate chapters and relevant pages in the book for further study, reasonably confident that the answer (or approach) to a particular diagnostic problem will be present. There are diagnostic considerations for which no specific chapter or page number is provided. Some of these may require reference to another source. For the distinctive or unusual finding not identified in the list for a given major pattern, the reader is directed to the Appendix, where the authors have assembled a "visual encyclopedia" of distinctive findings and artifacts encountered in the course of microscopic evaluation.

As every diagnostic pathologist knows, overlap occurs between diseases, and sometimes this overlap can be useful in establishing the correct diagnosis. For example, some infections are both nodular (Pattern 5) and have airspace filling (e.g., botryomycosis, aspiration pneumonia), whereas others are characterized by acute lung injury and diffuse airspace filling (e.g., pneumococcal pneumonia, pneumocystis pneumonia). In fact, some diffuse inflammatory conditions of the lung may manifest all of the six patterns, in different areas of the same biopsy (e.g., rheumatoid lung). In some cases, it may be necessary to include several possibilities in the final diagnosis, especially for the non-neoplastic diseases, where the effect of ancillary data not available at the time of diagnosis may be very large. The exposition begins with Pattern 1 (Acute Lung Injury), because this is the pattern that dominates all others and is most often the reason a biopsy was performed at all.

---

*See Leslie KO: My approach to interstitial lung disease using clinical, radiological and histopathologic patterns. *J Clin Pathol.* 2009;62(5):387–401.

Worksheet for the Pattern-Based Approach to Lung Disease

Patient Information

Age: _____   Gender: Male   Female

Disease Onset

Acute (hours to days)   Subacute (weeks to a few months)   Chronic (months to years)

Character of Infiltrate(s) on CT Scan

Nodular   Ground glass   Consolidation   Reticular   Honeycombing

Biopsy Information

Transbronchial biopsy   Cytology specimen   Surgical wedge biopsy

Lung Pathology Pattern

Pattern 1 (Acute Lung Injury)
With hyaline membranes (DAD)
With necrosis (infection)
With fibrin and organization only (infection, CVD, drug, EP)
With siderophages (infection, CVD, drug, EP)
With background fibrosis (acute on chr disease ddx)
With vasculitis (infection, DAH, CVD, drug, EP)
With eosinophils (infection, drug, EP)

Pattern 3 (Cellular Infiltrates)
With lymphocytes and plasma cells (NSIP ddx)
With neutrophils (infection, DAH, drug)
With fibrin and organization (infection, CVD, drug)
With granulomas (infection, HP, hot tub, drug, LIP ddx)
With background fibrosis (NSIP ddx, chr drug)
With vasculitis (infection, CVD, DAH)
With pleuritis (CVD)

Pattern 5 (Nodules)
With granulomas (infection, sarcoid, aspir)
With lymphoid cells (lymphoma, PLCH, WG)
With necrosis (infection, tumor, infarction)
With atypical cells (virus, tumor, EP)
With OP (infection, aspir, idiop nod OP)
With vasculitis (infection, WG)
With stellate scars (PLCH)

Pattern 2 (Fibrosis)
With temporal heterogeneity (UIP)
With diffuse septal fibrosis (NSIP ddx)
With granulomas (sarcoid, chr HP)
With acute lung injury (acute on chr disease ddx)
With honeycombing only (many causes)
With pleuritis (CVD)

Pattern 4 (Alveolar Filling)
With macrophages (EP, SRILD, aspir)
With granulomas (infection, hot tub, aspir)
With giant cells only (aspir, EP, hard metal)
With neutrophils (infection, aspir, DAH capil)
With eosinophilic material (PAP, PAM, edema)
With blood only (artifact)
With blood + siderophages (DAH, IPH, smoker)
With OP (infection, drug, CVD, COP)

Pattern 6 (Minimal Changes)
With small airways disease (OB)
With vascular disease (PHT, VOD)
With cysts (PLCH, LAM)
With no specific findings (sampling)

aspir, aspiration; chr, chronic; COP, cryptogenic organizing pneumonia; CVD, collagen vascular disease; DAD, diffuse alveolar damage; DAH, diffuse alveolar hemorrhage; DAH capill, diffuse alveolar hemorrhage with capillaritis; ddx, differential diagnosis; drug, drug toxicity; EP, eosinophilic pneumonia; hard metal, cobalt-associated hard metal disease; hot tub, "hot tub" lung; HP, hypersensitivity pneumonitis; idiop, idiopathic; IPH, idiopathic pulmonary hemosiderosis; LAM, lymphangioleiomyomatosis; LIP, lymphoid interstitial pneumonia; nod, nodular; NSIP, nonspecific interstitial pneumonia; OB, obliterative bronchiolitis (constrictive bronchiolitis); OP, organizing pneumonia; PAM, pulmonary alveolar microlithiasis; PAP, pulmonary alveolar proteinosis; PLCH, pulmonary Langerhans cell histiocytosis; UIP, usual interstitial pneumonia; smoker, changes related to cigarette smoking; SRILD, smoking-related interstitial lung disease; virus, viral infection; VOD, veno-occlusive disease; WG, Wegener granulomatosis.

Pattern	Diseases to Be Considered
Acute lung injury	Diffuse alveolar damage (DAD)
	Infection
	Eosinophilic pneumonia
	Drug toxicity
	Certain systemic connective tissue diseases
	Diffuse alveolar hemorrhage
	Irradiation injury
	Idiopathic (acute interstitial pneumonia)
	Acute hypersensitivity pneumonitis
	Acute pneumoconiosis
	Acute aspiration pneumonia
	Idiopathic acute fibrinous and organizing pneumonitis
Fibrosis	Usual interstitial pneumonia (UIP)
	Collagen vascular diseases
	Chronic eosinophilic pneumonia
	Chronic drug toxicity
	Chronic hypersensitivity pneumonitis
	Nonspecific interstitial pneumonia (NSIP)
	Smoking-related ILD/advanced Langerhans cell histiocytosis
	Sarcoidosis (advanced)
	Pneumoconioses
	Erdheim-Chester disease
	Hermansky-Pudlak syndrome
	Idiopathic pleuroparenchymal fibroelastosis
	Idiopathic airway-centered fibrosis
Chronic cellular infiltrates	Hypersensitivity pneumonitis
	Nonspecific interstitial pneumonia (NSIP)
	Systemic connective tissue diseases
	Certain chronic infections
	Certain drug toxicities
	Lymphocytic and lymphoid interstitial pneumonia
	Lymphomas and leukemias
	Lymphangitic carcinomatosis
Alveolar filling	Infections
	Airspace organization (organizing pneumonia)
	Diffuse alveolar hemorrhage
	Desquamative interstitial pneumonia (DIP)
	Respiratory bronchiolitis-associated ILD
	Alveolar proteinosis
	Dendriform (racemose) calcification
	Alveolar microlithiasis
	Mucostasis and mucinous tumors
Nodules	Infections (mycobacterial and fungal, primarily)
	Primary and metastatic neoplasms
	Wegener granulomatosis
	Sarcoidosis/berylliosis
	Aspiration pneumonia
	Pulmonary Langerhans cell histiocytosis
Nearly normal biopsy	Chronic small airways disease (as constrictive bronchiolitis)
	Vasculopathic diseases
	Lymphangioleiomyomatosis (LAM)
	Other rare cystic diseases

Pattern 1 Acute Lung Injury

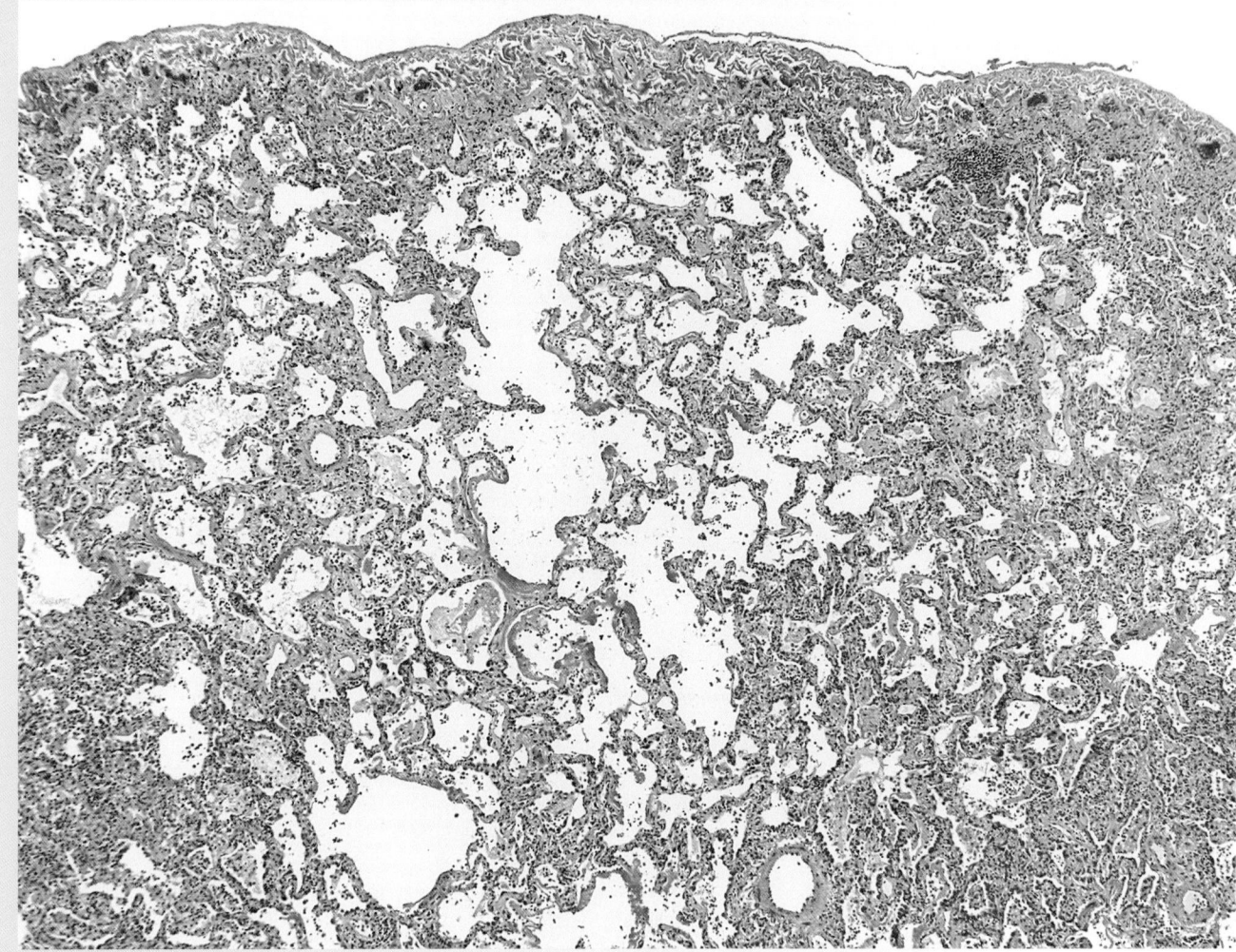

Elements of the pattern: The lung biopsy shows patchy or diffuse edema, fibrin, and reactive type 2 cell hyperplasia. The dominance of non-cellular, protein-rich material imparts an overall red or pink appearance to the biopsy at scanning magnification (in routine hematoxylin-eosin stained sections).

Special stains for organisms are required for all lung specimens that show acute injury.

Additional Findings	Diagnostic Consideration	Chapter:Page
Hyaline membranes	Diffuse alveolar damage	Ch. 5:117
Necrosis in parenchyma	Infection	Ch. 5:120
	Some tumors	Ch. 16:584
	Infarct	Ch. 10:363
Necrosis in bronchioles	Infections	Ch. 5:123; Ch. 8:287
	Acute aspiration	Ch. 8:284
Fibrin in alveoli	Diffuse alveolar damage	Ch. 5:120
	Drug toxicity	Ch. 5:128
	Connective tissue disease	Ch. 5:131
	Infection	Ch. 5:123; Ch. 6:192
Eosinophils in alveoli	Eosinophilic lung diseases	Ch. 5:129; Ch. 7:239
Siderophages in alveoli	Diffuse alveolar hemorrhage	Ch. 5:131; Ch. 10:366
	Drug toxicity	Ch. 10:367
	Infarct	Ch. 6:143; Ch. 10:363
Fibrinous pleuritis	Connective tissue diseases	Ch. 5:126
	Eosinophilic pneumonia	Ch. 5:129
	Pneumothorax	Ch. 7:260
Neutrophils	Infections	Ch. 5:133
	Capillaritis in diffuse alveolar hemorrhage	Ch. 10:370
Atypical cells	Acute lung injury	Ch. 5:133
	Viral infections	Ch. 5:134
	Leukemias	Ch. 15:508
	Intravascular lymphoma	Ch. 15:525
Fibrin + vacuolated macrophages	Infection	Ch. 6:163
	Drug toxicity	Ch. 5:128
	Connective tissue diseases	Ch. 5:128

Pattern 2 Fibrosis

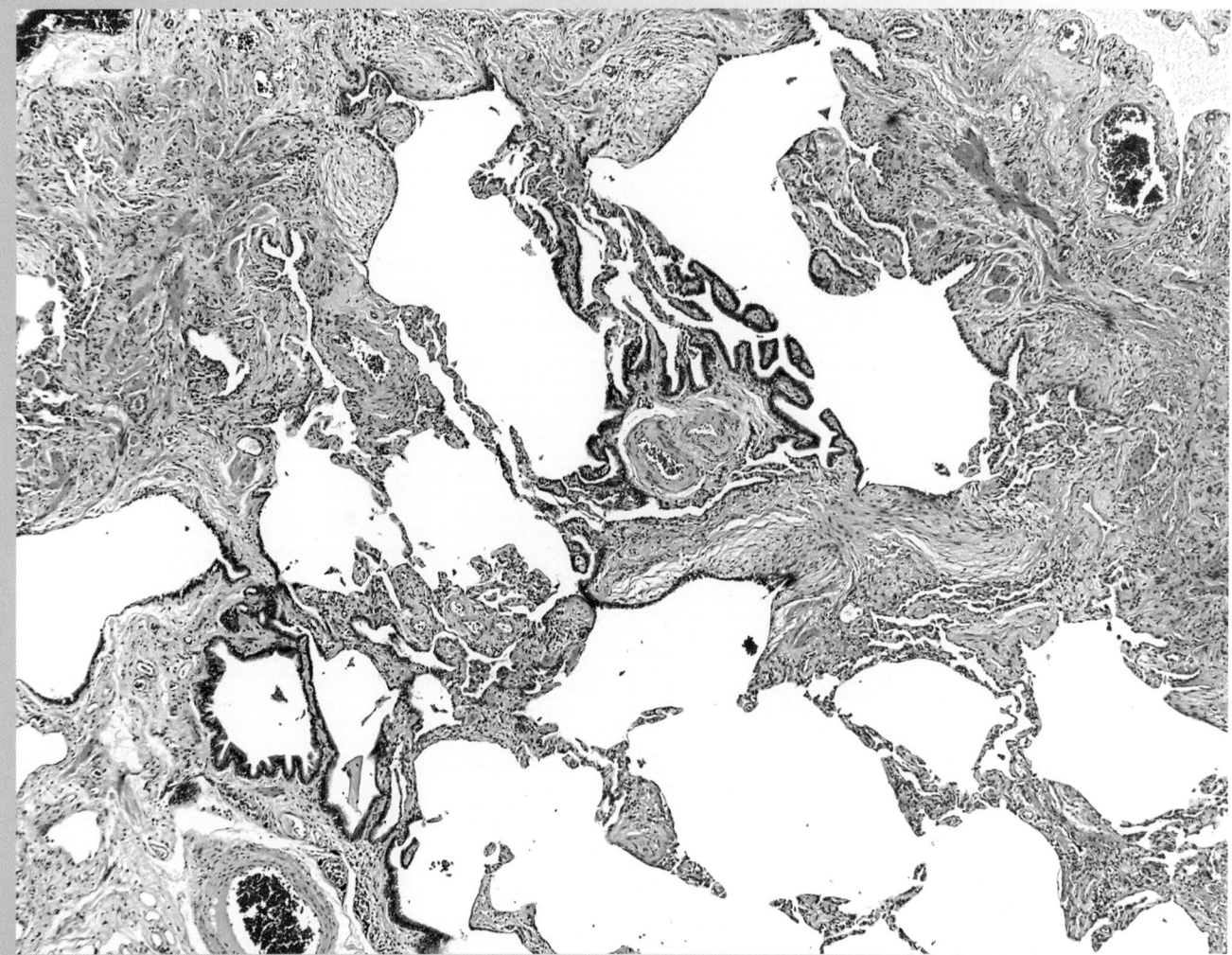

Elements of the pattern: The lung biopsy is involved by variable amounts of fibrosis. As in Pattern 1, the biopsy tends to be more pink than blue at scanning magnification, as a result of collagen deposition (in routine hematoxylin-eosin stained sections). Some fibrosis patterns are accompanied by chronic inflammation that may impart a blue tinge to the process, or even dark blue lymphoid aggregates.

Significant lung fibrosis is always associated with some degree of structural remodeling. Avoid diagnosing "fibrosis" on transbronchial biopsies.

Pattern 2 Fibrosis

Additional Findings	Diagnostic Consideration	Chapter:Page

Hyaline membranes	"Acute on chronic" disease
	    Infection on fibrosis
	    Drug toxicity on fibrosis
	    Connective tissue disease in "exacerbation"
	Acute exacerbation of idiopathic pulmonary fibrosis (IPF)
		Not specifically addressed
		
		Ch. 7:218

Microscopic honeycombing	Usual interstitial pneumonia (UIP) Hypersensitivity pneumonitis Connective tissue disease	Ch. 7:215 Ch. 7:252 Ch. 7:231
Prominent bronchiolization	Pulmonary Langerhans cell histiocytosis Respiratory bronchiolitis ILD Connective tissue diseases Chronic hypersensitivity pneumonitis Small airways disease Chronic aspiration	Ch. 7:257 Ch. 7:225 Ch. 7:231 Ch. 7:252 Ch. 8:296 Ch. 7:251; Ch. 8:287
Uniform alveolar septal fibrosis	Connective tissue diseases Postirradiation	Ch. 7:231 Not specifically addressed
Peripheral lobular fibrosis	UIP/IPF Erdheim Chester disease Rosai-Dorfman disease Chronic eosinophilic pneumonia	Ch. 7:215 Ch. 7:260 Ch. 18:252 Ch. 7:239
Siderophages in alveoli	Chronic cardiac congestion Chronic venous outflow obstruction Chronic hemorrhage in connective tissue disease Chronic hemorrhage in bronchiectasis Pneumoconiosis Pulmonary Langerhans cell histiocytosis Smoking-related interstitial lung disease Chronic renal dialysis Idiopathic pulmonary hemosiderosis	Not specifically addressed Not specifically addressed Ch. 7:235 Not specifically addressed Ch. 9:314 Ch. 7:257 Ch. 7:228 Not specifically addressed Ch. 10:370
Fibrinous pleuritis	Connective tissue disease Eosinophilic pleuritis in pneumothorax	Ch. 7:231 Ch. 7:260; Appendix:768
Prominent non-necrotizing granulomas	Sarcoidosis	Ch. 7:250
Many vacuolated cells	Chronic airway obstruction Drug toxicity Hermansky-Pudlak syndrome Genetic storage diseases	Not specifically addressed Not specifically addressed Ch. 7:263 Ch. 4:112
Prominent chronic inflammation	Nonspecific interstitial pneumonia (NSIP) Rheumatoid arthritis and other connective tissue diseases	Ch. 7:221 Ch. 7:231
Airway-centered scarring	Pulmonary Langerhans cell histiocytosis Pneumoconiosis Chronic hypersensitivity pneumonitis Connective tissue diseases Idiopathic airway-centered fibrosis Idiopathic pleuroparenchymal fibroelastosis Chronic aspiration	Ch. 7:257 Ch. 8:298 Ch. 7:252 Ch. 7:231 Not specifically addressed Ch. 7:268 Ch. 7:251; Ch. 8:287

Pattern 3 Chronic Cellular Infiltrates

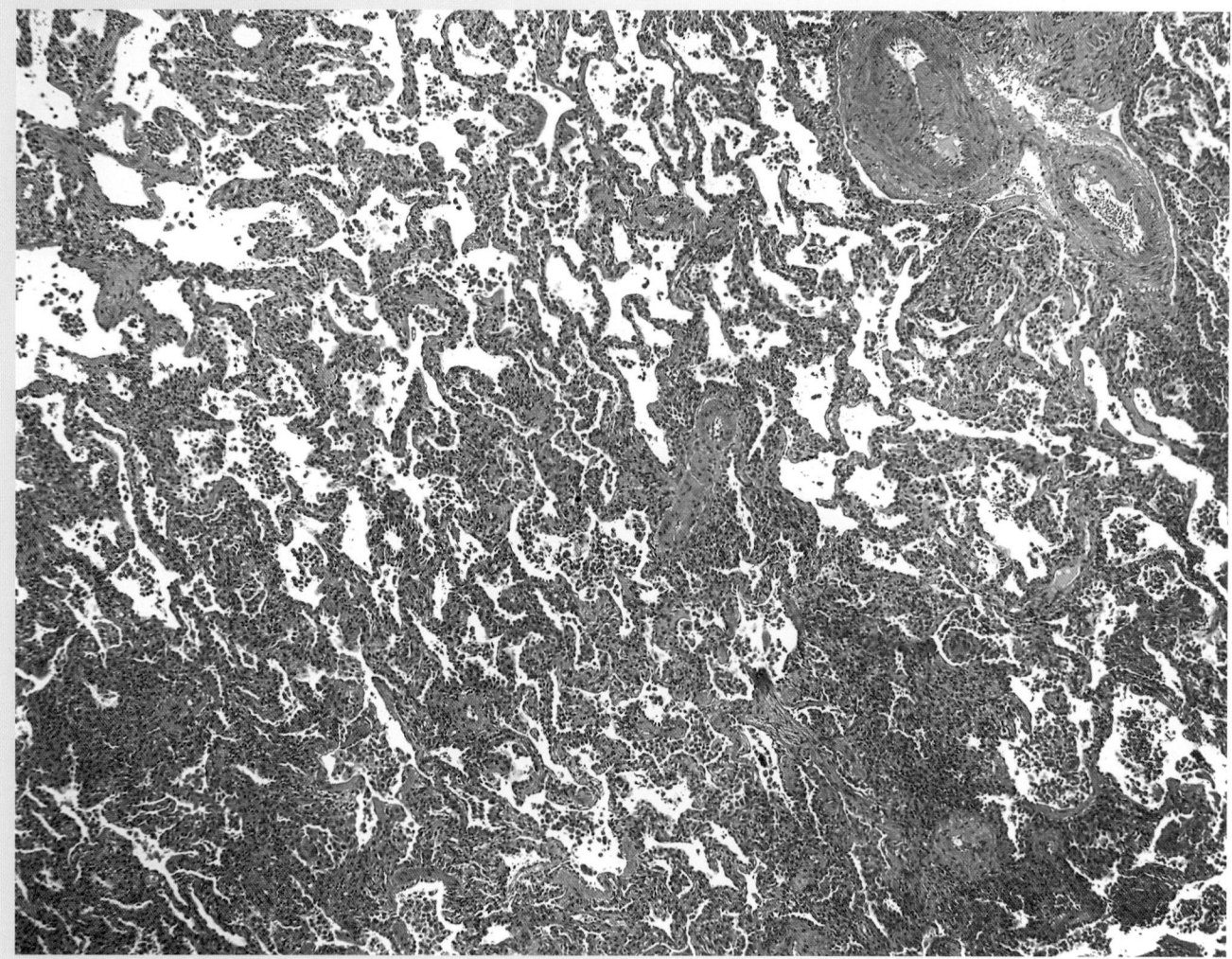

Elements of the pattern: The lung biopsy is dominated by interstitial chronic inflammation and variable reactive type 2 cell hyperplasia. The dominance of mononuclear infiltrates may impart an overall blue appearance to the biopsy at scanning magnification (in routine hematoxylin-eosin stained sections).

Pattern 3 Chronic Cellular Infiltrates

Additional Findings	Diagnostic Consideration	Chapter:Page
Hyaline membranes	"Acute on chronic" connective tissue disease	Ch. 5:126
	Drug toxicity	Ch. 5:128
	Diffuse alveolar hemorrhage	Ch. 10:366
Necrosis in parenchyma	Viral and fungal infections	Ch. 6:166, 187
	Aspiration	Ch. 6:150; Ch. 8:284
	Infarction in antiphospholipid syndrome	Ch. 7:236
Necrosis in bronchioles	Viral infections	Ch. 6:187
	Aspiration	Ch. 6:150; Ch. 8:284
Poorly formed granulomas (small and non-necrotizing)	Hypersensitivity pneumonitis (subacute)	Ch. 7:252
	Atypical mycobacterial infection	Ch. 7:254
	"Hot tub lung"	Ch. 6:164
	Lymphoid interstitial pneumonia	Ch. 7:229
	Drug toxicity	Ch. 7:242
Well formed necrotizing granulomas	Infections	Ch. 6:166
	Rare drug reactions	Not specifically addressed
	Necrotizing sarcoidosis	Ch. 10:357
	Middle lobe syndrome	Ch. 8:282
Eosinophils in alveoli	Eosinophilic lung diseases	Ch. 5:129; Ch. 7:239
	Smoking-related lung diseases	Ch. 7:228
Siderophages in alveoli	Diffuse alveolar hemorrhage	Ch. 10:366
	Chronic cardiac congestion	Not specifically addressed
	Drug toxicity	Ch. 7:242
Fibrinous/chronic pleuritis	Connective tissue diseases	Ch. 7:231
	Thoracic trauma/infection	Not specifically addressed
	Pancreatitis-associated pleuritis	Not specifically addressed
Patchy organizing pneumonia	Drug toxicity	Ch. 7:242
	Connective tissue diseases	Ch. 7:231
	Infections	Not specifically addressed
	Cryptogenic organizing pneumonia	Ch. 7:223
	Diffuse alveolar hemorrhage	Ch. 10:366
	Aspiration	Ch. 6:150; Ch. 8:284
Atypical cells	Viral infections	Ch. 6:187
	Lymphangitic carcinoma	Ch. 7:268
Multinucleated giant cells	Hard metal disease	Ch. 9:329
	Mica pneumoconiosis	Ch. 9:322
	Hypersensitivity pneumonitis	Ch. 7:252
	Intravenous drug abuse	Ch. 7:246
	Drug toxicity	Ch. 7:242
	Aspiration pneumonia	Ch. 6:150; Ch. 8:284
	Eosinophilic pneumonia	Ch. 5:129; Ch. 7:239
Dense mononuclear infiltration	Lymphomas	Ch. 15:520
	Lymphoid interstitial pneumonia	Ch. 7:229
	Connective tissue diseases	Ch. 7:231
	Hypersensitivity pneumonitis	Ch. 7:252
	Certain infections (the atypical pneumonias)	Ch. 6:151
Lymphoid aggregates/germinal centers	Connective tissue diseases	Ch. 7:231
	Diffuse lymphoid hyperplasia	Ch. 7:230; Ch. 15:516
	Lymphoid interstitial pneumonia	Ch. 7:229
	Follicular bronchiolitis	Ch. 8:285

Pattern 4 Alveolar Filling

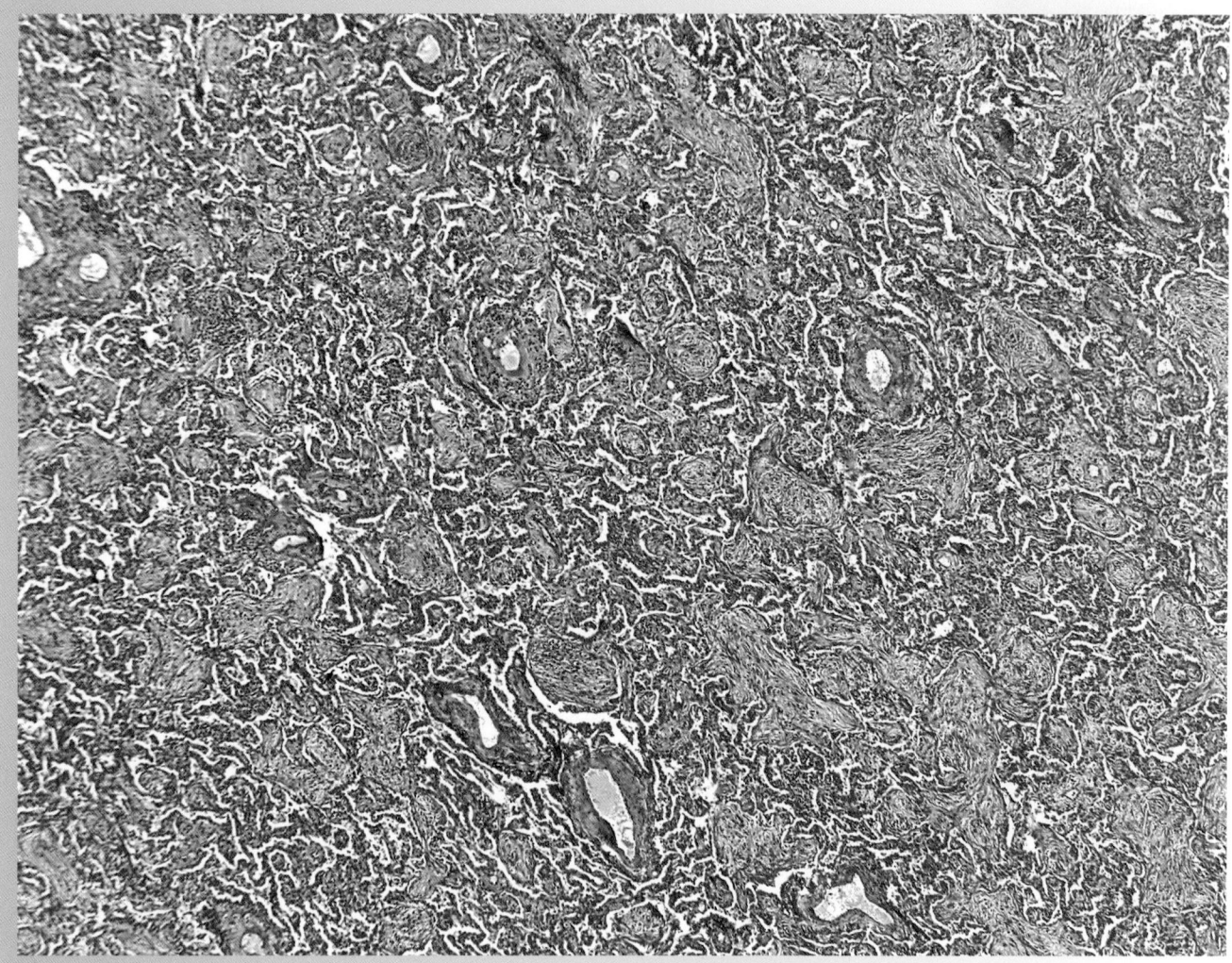

Elements of the pattern: The dominant finding is alveolar spaces filled with cells or noncellular elements.

Pattern 4 Alveolar Filling

Additional Findings	Diagnostic Consideration	Chapter:Page
Hyaline membranes and fibrin	Organizing diffuse alveolar damage	Ch. 5:117; Ch. 6:151
Necrosis and neutrophils	Bacterial infection Viral and fungal infection	Ch. 6:148 Ch. 6:166, 187
Organizing pneumonia	Organizing infection Drug toxicity Cryptogenic organizing pneumonia	Ch. 6:148 Ch. 7:242 Ch. 7:223
Fibrin and macrophages	Eosinophilic pneumonia, poststeroid Drug toxicity Connective tissue diseases Malakoplakia-like reaction	Ch. 5:129; Ch. 7:239 Ch. 7:242 Ch. 7:231 Ch. 6:143
Eosinophils and macrophages	Eosinophilic lung diseases	Ch. 5:129; Ch. 7:239
Siderophages and fibrin	Diffuse alveolar hemorrhage	Ch. 10:366
Mucin	Mucostasis in small airways disease Bronchioloalveolar carcinoma Cryptococcus infection	Ch. 8:293 Ch. 16:560 Ch. 6:171
Bone/calcification	Dendriform calcification Metastatic calcification Pulmonary alveolar microlithiasis	Ch. 7:225; Appendix:772 Appendix:772 Ch. 7:265
Atypical cells	Bronchioloalveolar carcinoma Herpesvirus infections Acute eosinophilic pneumonia Carcinomas and sarcomas	Ch. 16:560 Ch. 6:192 Ch. 5:129; Ch. 7:239 Not specifically addressed
Proteinaceous exudates	Edema Pulmonary alveolar proteinosis (PAP) PAP reactions Pneumocystis pneumonia	Not specifically addressed Ch. 7:266 Ch. 7:266 Ch. 6:177
Multinucleated giant cells	Hard metal disease Eosinophilic pneumonia Wegener granulomatosis Aspiration pneumonia	Ch. 9:329 Ch. 5:129; Ch. 7:239 Ch. 10:341 Ch.6:150; Ch. 8:284
Polypoid mesenchymal bodies resembling chorionic villi	Bullous placental transmogrification	Appendix:777

Pattern 5 Nodules

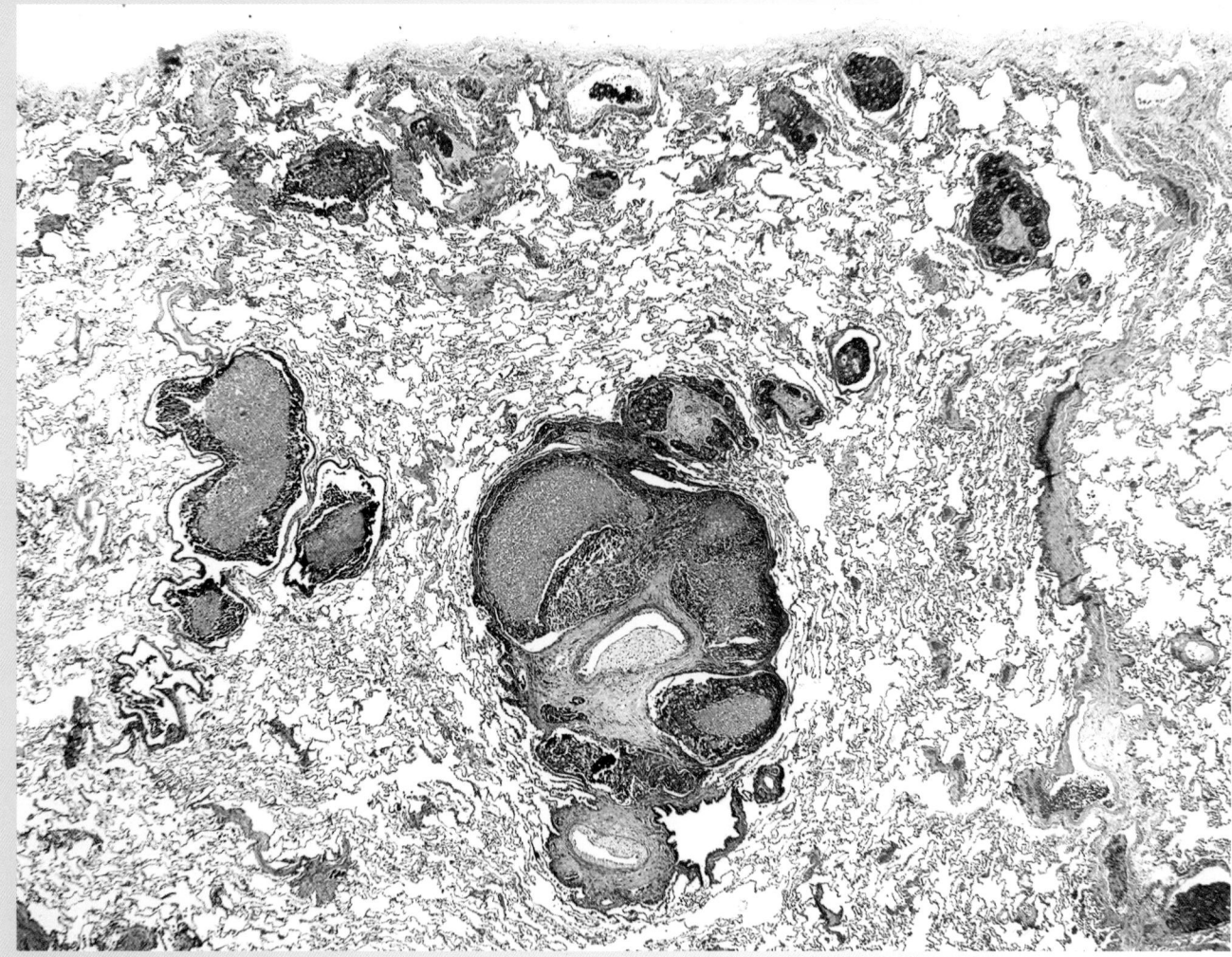

Elements of the pattern: One, or many, nodules of variable size and shape. An interface between the nodular lesion and more normal lung should be discernible. In the case of very large nodules encompassing the entire specimen, radiologic imaging can be used as part of the definition.

Pattern 5 Nodules

Additional Findings	Diagnostic Consideration	Chapter:Page
Large neoplastic lymphoid cells	Malignant lymphoma	Ch. 15:529
Small lymphoid cells without germ centers	MALT lymphoma, low grade	Ch. 15:520
Small lymphoid cells with germ centers	Follicular bronchiolitis	Ch. 15:511
	Diffuse lymphoid hyperplasia	Ch. 15:511
	Intraparenchymal lymph node	Not specifically addressed
Giant multinucleated neoplastic cells	Sarcomatoid carcinoma	Ch. 14:445
	Large cell undifferentiated carcinoma	Ch. 16:570
	Primary and metastatic sarcomas	Ch. 14:454
	Primary or metastatic pleomorphic carcinomas	Ch. 14:445
	Primary or metastatic melanoma	Ch. 14:478
	Giant cell tumor (primary or metastatic)	Not specifically addressed
Primitive small round neoplastic cells	Small cell carcinoma	Ch. 13:422
	Malignant lymphoma	Ch. 15:529
	Small cell squamous carcinoma	Ch. 15:552
	Metastatic tumors	Ch. 17:597
	Ewing sarcoma	Ch. 17:626
	Primitive neuroectodermal tumor	Ch. 13:433
	Small cell osteosarcoma	Ch. 17:622
	Neuroblastoma	Ch. 13:435
	Pleuropulmonary blastoma (with cysts)	Ch. 14:491
Spindled or fusiform neoplastic cells	Primary sarcomatoid carcinoma	Ch. 14:445
	Primary and metastatic sarcomas	Ch. 14:454
	Lymphangioleiomyomatosis (with cysts)	Ch. 7:261
	Inflammatory myofibroblastic tumor	Ch. 18:648; Ch. 19:691
	Benign metastasizing leiomyoma	Not specifically addressed
	Localized fibrous tumor	Ch. 14:463
	Extra-abdominal desmoid tumor	Ch. 19:702
Large pink epithelioid neoplastic cells	Poorly differentiated primary carcinomas	Ch. 16:570
	Large cell undifferentiated carcinoma	Ch. 16:570
	Metastatic carcinomas	Ch. 17:606
	Metastatic sarcomas	Ch. 17:616
	Epithelioid hemangioendothelioma	Ch. 14:460
	Melanoma (primary or metastatic)	Ch. 14:474
Large clear epithelioid neoplastic cells	Primary clear cell adenocarcinoma	Ch. 16:566
	Primary squamous carcinoma	Ch. 16:552
	Large cell carcinoma (primary)	Ch. 16:570
	Sugar tumor	Ch. 19:703
	Perivascular epithelioid cell tumor (PEComa)	Ch. 19:687
	Metastatic clear cell carcinoma	Ch. 17:609
	Metastatic clear cell sarcoma	Ch. 17:616

Continued

Additional Findings	Diagnostic Consideration	Chapter:Page
Large basophilic epithelial cells with peripheral palisade	Large cell undifferentiated carcinoma	Ch. 16:570
	Large cell neuroendocrine carcinoma	Ch. 13:425
	Basaloid large cell lung carcinoma	Ch. 16:557
	Basaloid squamous carcinoma	Ch. 16:557
	Certain metastatic tumors	Not specifically addressed
Glands or tubules, malignant	Primary adenocarcinoma	Ch. 16:556
	Metastatic adenocarcinoma	Ch. 17:605
	Carcinoid tumor (primary or metastatic)	Ch. 13:417
	Synovial sarcoma (primary or metastatic)	Ch. 14:469
	Fetal-type primary adenocarcinoma	Ch. 14:450
	Carcinosarcoma (primary or metastatic)	Ch. 14:445
Glands or tubules, benign or mild atypia	Alveolar adenoma	Ch. 19:679
	Adenoma of type II cells	Ch. 19:680
	Pulmonary sclerosing hemangioma	Ch. 19:694
	Hamartoma	Ch. 18:645
	Micronodular pneumocyte hyperplasia	Ch. 7:265
	Adenomatoid tumor	Ch. 19:688
Malignant heterologous elements (cartilage, bone, skeletal muscle)	Carcinosarcoma	Ch. 14:445
	Metastatic teratocarcinoma	Not specifically addressed
	Metastatic sarcoma	Not specifically addressed
Distinct keratinization	Primary squamous cell carcinoma	Ch. 15:552
	Squamous metaplasia of terminal airways	Ch. 5:118, 122
	Basaloid squamous cell carcinoma	Ch. 16:557
	Adenosquamous carcinoma	Ch. 16:570
	Metastatic squamous cell carcinoma	Not specifically addressed
Pigmented cells	Cellular phase of Langerhans cell histiocytosis	Ch. 7:257
	Primary or metastatic melanoma	Ch. 14:474
	Melanotic carcinoid tumor	Ch. 13:417
	Metastatic angiosarcoma (hemosiderin)	Not specifically addressed
Malignant with dominant necrosis	Small cell carcinoma	Ch. 13:422
	Sarcomatoid carcinoma (primary or metastatic)	Ch. 14:445
	High-grade malignant lymphoma	Ch. 15:529
Benign with necrosis	Necrotizing infections	Ch. 5:120, 123; Ch. 8:287
	Bacterial	
	Fungal	
	Mycobacterial	
	Viral	
	Wegener granulomatosis	Ch. 10:341
	Churg Strauss syndrome	Ch. 10:351
	Lung infarct	Not specifically addressed

Continued

Additional Findings	Diagnostic Consideration	Chapter:Page
Benign with dominant organizing pneumonia	Nodular organizing pneumonia	Not specifically addressed
	Aspiration pneumonia	Ch. 6:150; Ch. 8:284
Benign with well formed granulomas	Granulomatous infection	Ch. 6:166
	Fungal	
	Mycobacterial	
	Bacterial (botryomycosis)	
	Sarcoidosis/berylliosis	Ch. 6:250
	Certain pneumoconioses	Not specifically addressed
	Aspiration pneumonia	Ch. 6:150; Ch. 8:284
	Necrotizing sarcoidosis	Ch. 10:357
Benign with stellate airways centered lesions and variable fibrosis	Pulmonary Langerhans cell histiocytosis	Ch. 7:257
	Certain inhalational injuries	Not specifically addressed
	Pneumoconioses	Not specifically addressed

Pattern 6 Nearly Normal Lung

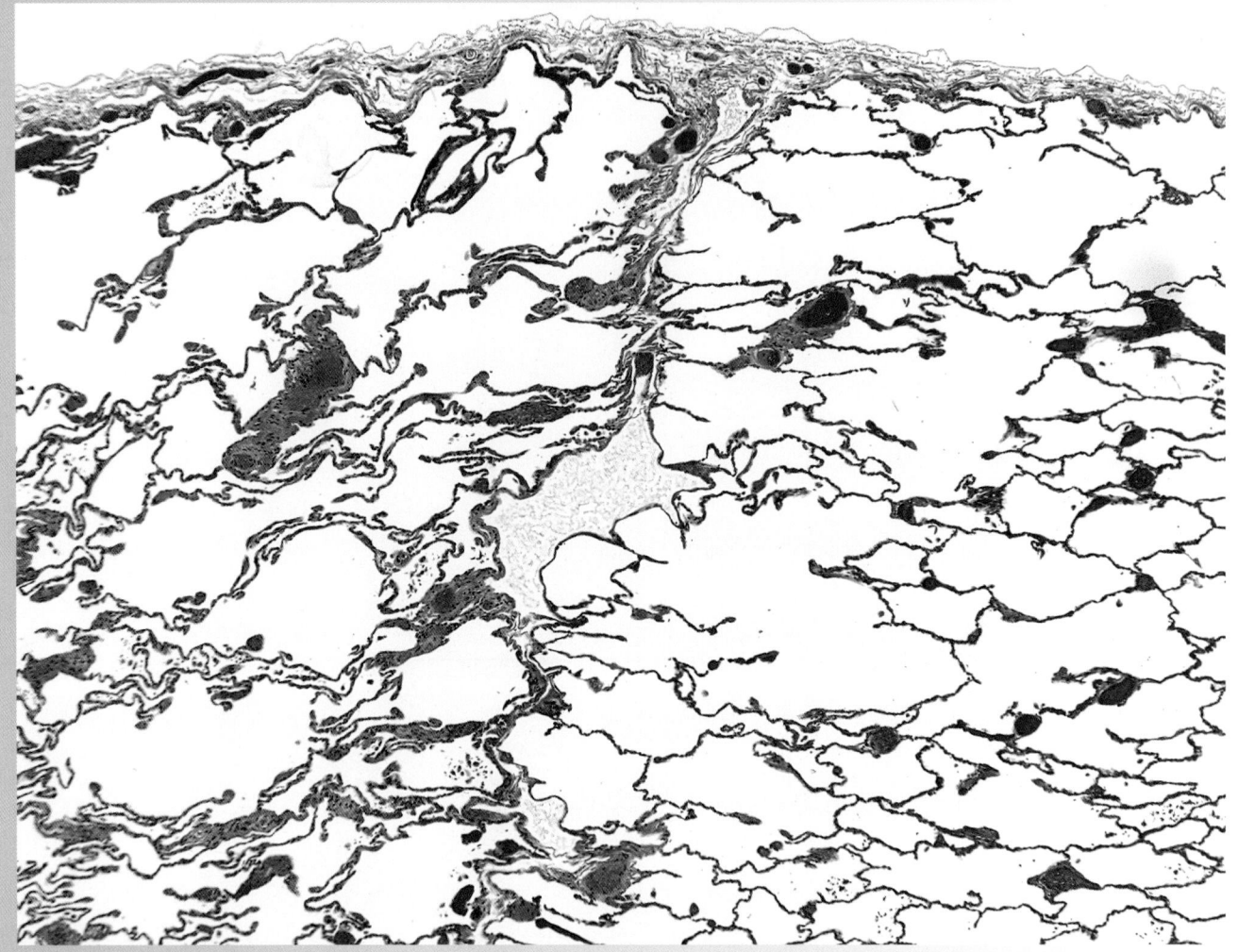

Elements of the pattern: The lung biopsy has little or no disease evident at scanning magnification.

Pattern 6 Nearly Normal Lung

Additional Findings	Diagnostic Consideration	Chapter:Page
Thick pulmonary arteries	Pulmonary hypertension	Ch. 11:377
	Chronic obstructive pulmonary disease	Ch. 8:304
Cysts	Lymphangioleiomyomatosis	Ch. 7:261
	Pulmonary Langerhans cell histiocytosis	Ch. 7:257
	Bullous emphysema	Not specifically addressed
Patchy hyaline membranes	Acute lung injury, early (may be subtle)	Not specifically addressed
Airway scarring	Constrictive bronchiolitis (CB)	Ch. 8:297
Bronchiolization (bronchiolar metaplasia)	Small airways disease with or without CB	Ch. 8:297
Dilated bronchioles	Small airways disease with or without CB	Ch. 8:297
Bronchioles absent, markedly decreased, or dilated	Constrictive bronchiolitis	Ch. 8:297
Prominent emphysema	Small airways disease with or without CB	Ch. 8:297
Atypical cells	Lymphangitic and intravascular carcinoma	Ch. 7:268

Lung Anatomy

Kevin O. Leslie, MD, and Mark R. Wick, MD

Development and Gross Anatomy

Airway Development

During early embryogenesis (at approximately day 21 after fertilization), the lungs begin as a groove in the ventral floor of the foregut (Fig. 1-1) This foregut depression becomes a diverticulum of endoderm, surrounded by an amorphous condensation of splanchnic mesoderm that lengthens caudally in the midline, anterior to the esophagus. By the fourth week of gestation, two lung buds form as distal outpouchings.[1,2] A series of repetitive nondichotomous branchings begins during week 5 and results in the formation of the primordial bronchial tree by the eighth week of gestation.

By 17 weeks, the rudimentary structure of the conducting airways has formed. This phase of lung development is referred to as the "pseudoglandular stage" because the fetal (postgestational week 7) lung is composed entirely of tubular elements that appear as circular gland-like structures in two-dimensional tissue sections (Fig. 1-2). The subsequent stages of development (canalicular, 13–25 weeks; terminal sac, 24 weeks to birth; and alveolar, late fetal to the age of 8–10 years)

are dedicated to the formation of the essential units of respiration, the acini[1-5] (Fig. 1-3). The postnatal lung continues to accrue alveoli until the age of approximately 10 years (Fig. 1-4).

The Pleura

Immediately after their formation, the lung buds grow into the medial walls of the pericardioperitoneal canals (splanchnic mesoderm) and in doing so become invested with a membrane that will be the visceral pleura (analogous to a fist being pushed into a balloon.) In this process, the lateral wall of the pericardioperitoneal canal becomes the parietal pleura, and the compressed space between becomes the pleural space (Fig. 1-5).

The Lung Lobes

By the end of gestation, five well-defined lung lobes are present, three on the right (upper, middle, and lower lobes) and two on the left (upper and lower lobes).[3,6,7] Each of the five primary lobar buds is invested with visceral pleura. Each lobe in turn is composed of one or more segments, resulting in a total of 10 segments per lung (Fig. 1-6). The presence of the heart leads to the formation of a rudimentary third lobe on the left side termed the lingula (more properly regarded as a part of the left upper lobe than as an independent structure). In fact, the right middle lobe and the lingula are analogous structures: Each has an excessively long and narrow bronchus, predisposing these lobes to the pathologic effects of bronchial compression by adjacent lymph nodes or other masses. When such compression occurs, the consequent chronic inflammatory changes in the respective lobe are referred to as "middle lobe syndrome."[8]

As gestation proceeds, airway branching continues to the level of the alveolar sacs, with a total of about 23 final subdivisions (20 of which occur proximal to the respiratory bronchioles). In successive order proceeding distally, the anatomic units formed are the lung segments, secondary and primary lobules (Fig. 1-7), and finally acini. With each successive division, the resulting airway branches are smaller than their predecessors, but each has a diameter greater than 50% of the airway parent. This phenomenon leads to a progressive increase in airway volume with each successive branching and a significant reduction in airway resistance in more distal lung. The acinus consists of a central respiratory bronchiole that leads to an alveolar duct and terminates in an alveolar sac, composed of many alveoli (Fig. 1-8).

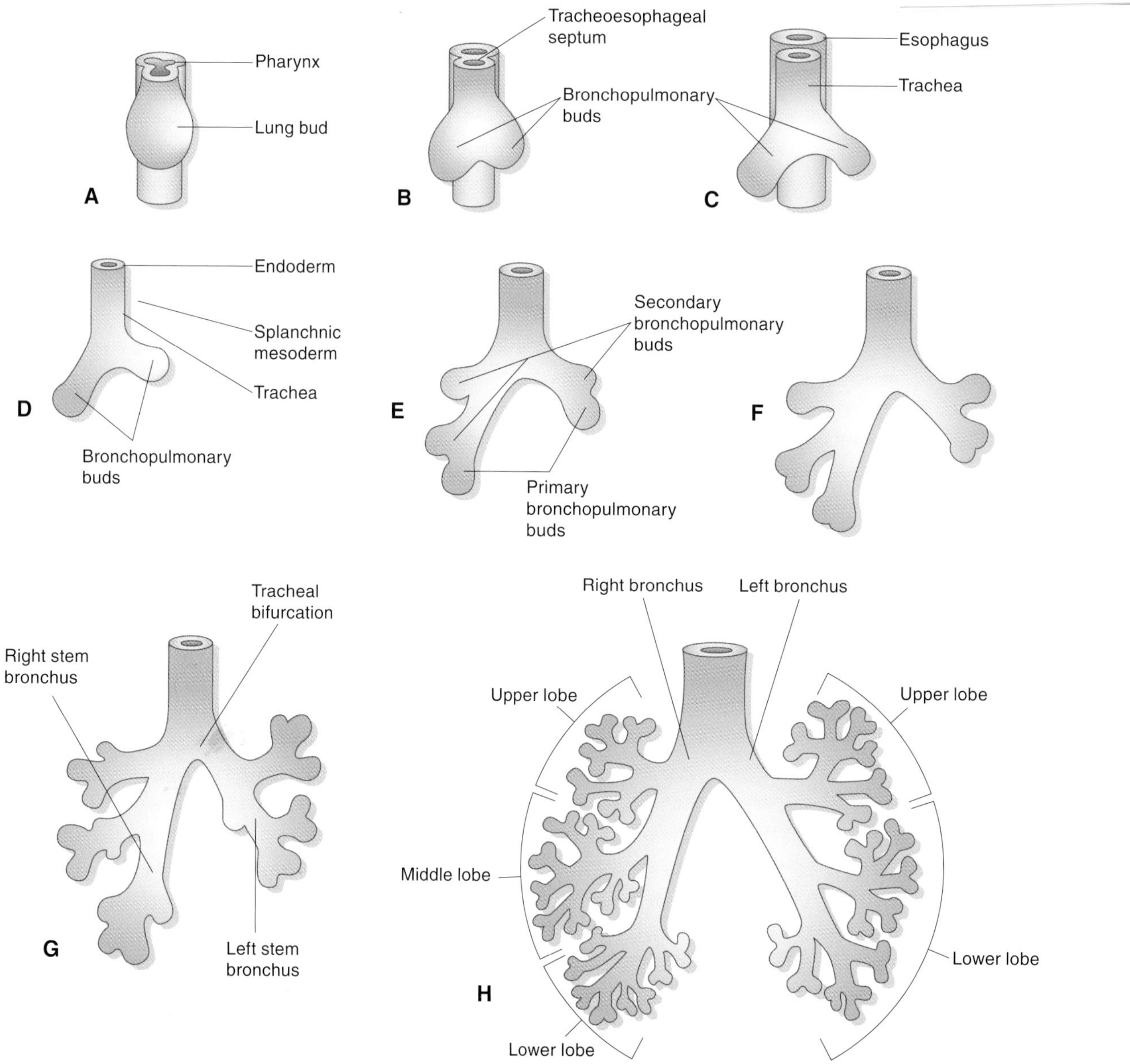

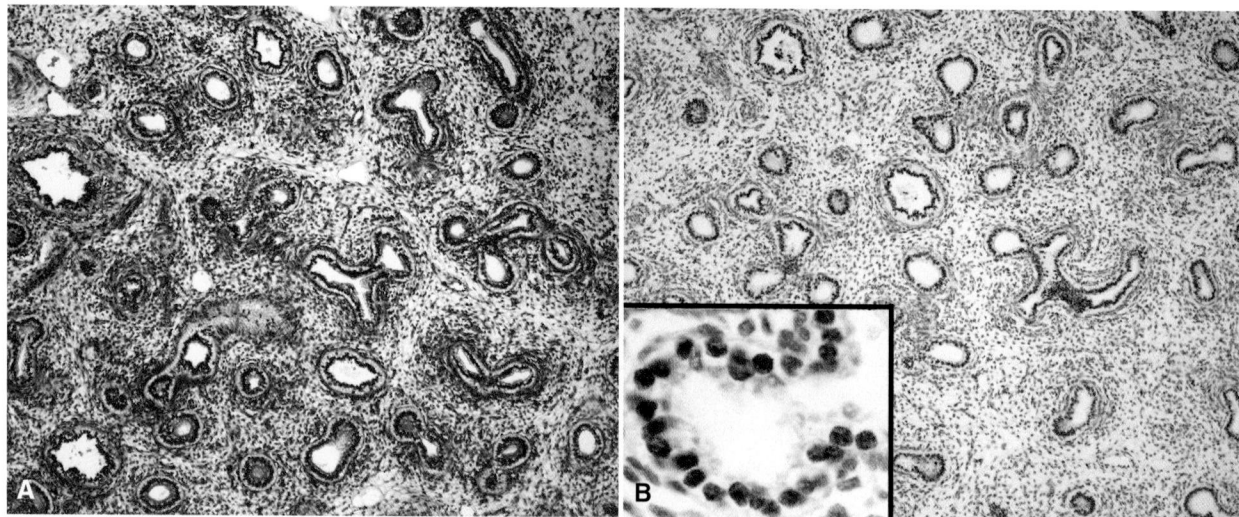

Figure 1-1. Diagrammatic representation of the successive stages in the development of the bronchi and lungs: **A** to **D,** 4 weeks; **E** and **F,** 5 weeks; **G,** 6 weeks; **H,** 8 weeks. (Reprinted with permission from Moore K. *The Developing Human*. Philadelphia: WB Saunders; 1973.)

Figure 1-2. A, In the early stage of lung development, the bronchi resemble tubular glands and are surrounded by undifferentiated mesenchyme. This stage is referred to as pseudoglandular because of this appearance (at 5–17 weeks of gestation.) **B,** Immunohistochemical staining for thyroid transcription factor-1 (brown chromogen, hematoxylin counterstain) is positive in the nuclei of the immature airway cells.

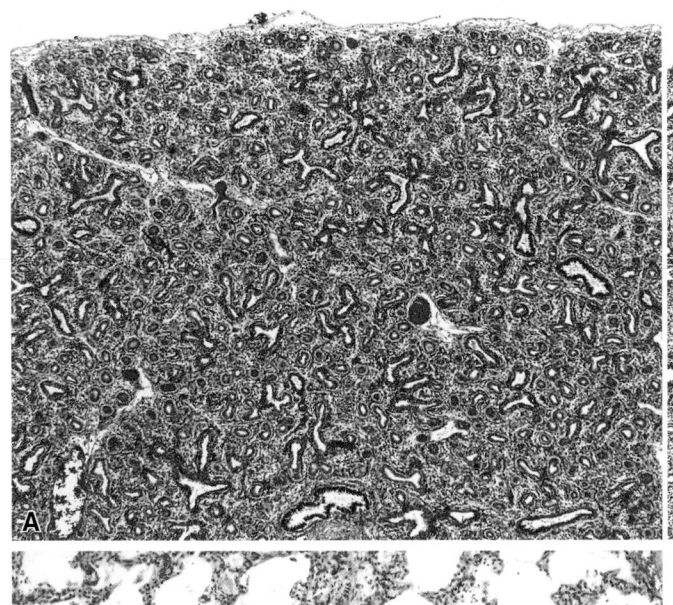

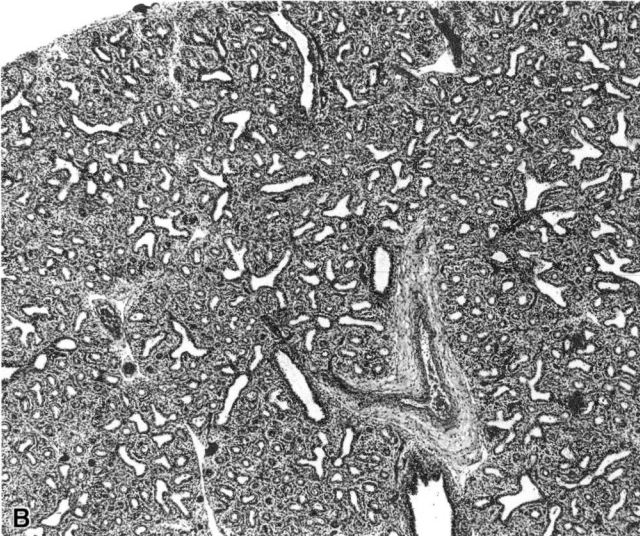

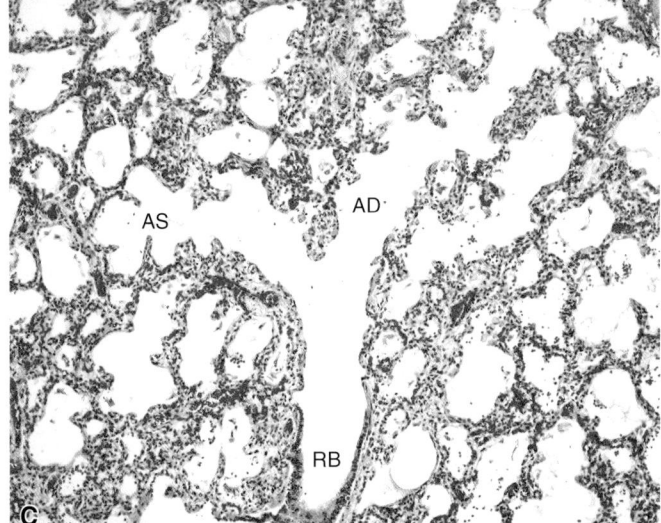

Figure 1-3. The remaining stages in lung development are illustrated here in tissue sections from developing human lung. **A,** The canalicular period occurs in the interval between 13 and 25 weeks after fertilization. Airway lumens become dilated and more prominent, and the mesenchymal tissue surrounding them becomes progressively vascularized. **B,** The terminal sac period occurs from 24 weeks to birth. The terminal buds of the airways at this juncture are referred to as *primitive alveoli*. **C,** The final phase of lung development is referred to as the alveolar period and crosses into childhood (extending from the late fetal stage to 10 years of age). New alveoli continue to form well after birth. AD, alveolar duct; AS, alveolar sac; RB, respiratory bronchiole.

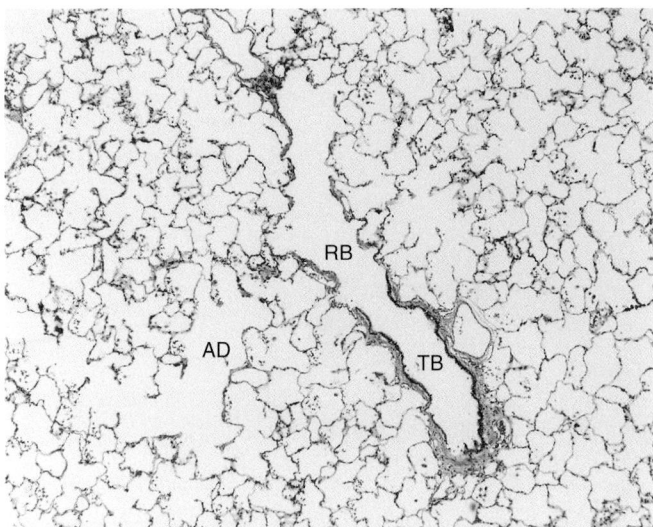

Figure 1-4. The mature lung lobule consists of terminal bronchioles with their respective respiratory bronchioles, alveolar ducts, and alveolar sacs. Here the Y-shaped division of the terminal bronchiole into respiratory bronchioles and alveolar ducts can be seen in the lung of a child. AD, alveolar duct; RB, respiratory bronchiole; TB, terminal bronchiole.

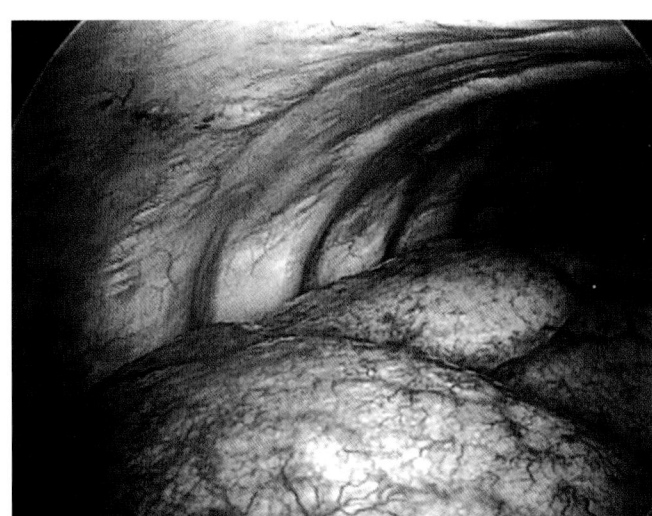

Figure 1-5. View of the collapsed lung during thoracoscopic surgery demonstrates the visceral and parietal pleural surfaces.

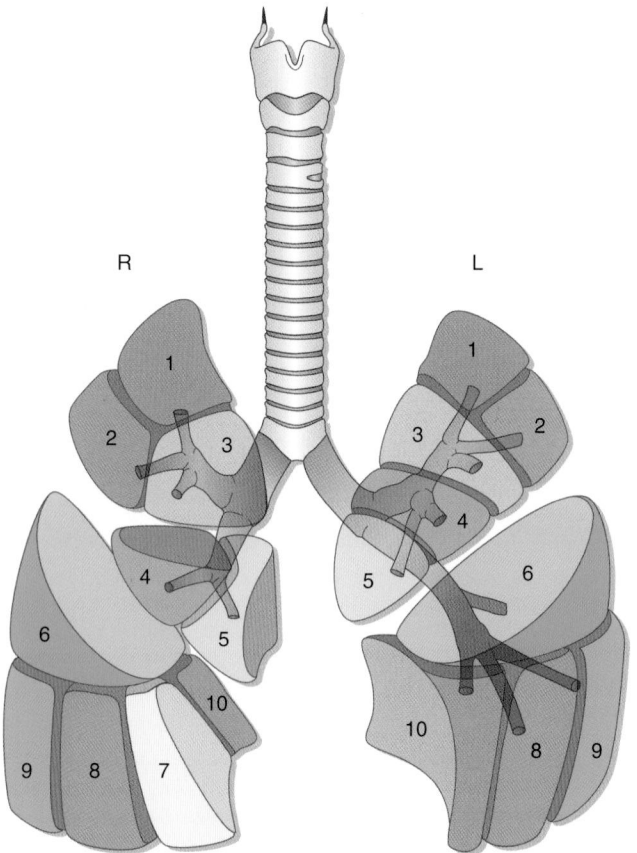

Figure 1-6. Ten distinct segments are present in each lung. (Reprinted with permission from Nagaishi C. *Functional Anatomy and Histology of the Lung*. Baltimore: University Park Press; 1972.)

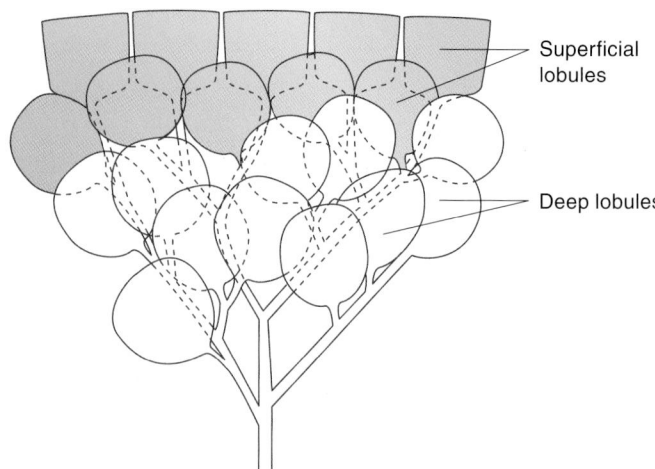

Figure 1-7. The pulmonary lobules are configured into two layers that probably play important roles in the physical dynamics of respiration. The superficial layer is 3 to 4 cm thick. (Reprinted with permission from Nagaishi C. *Functional Anatomy and Histology of the Lung*. Baltimore: University Park Press; 1972.)

Microscopic Anatomy

The microscopic lung structure relevant to this chapter begins with the trachea and conducting airways and ends with the alveolar gas exchange units. This overview is intended to refresh the surgical pathologist's existing knowledge of the normal lung. For the reader interested in greater detail, the comprehensive and authoritative review of gross and microscopic lung anatomy by Nagaishi is recommended.[4]

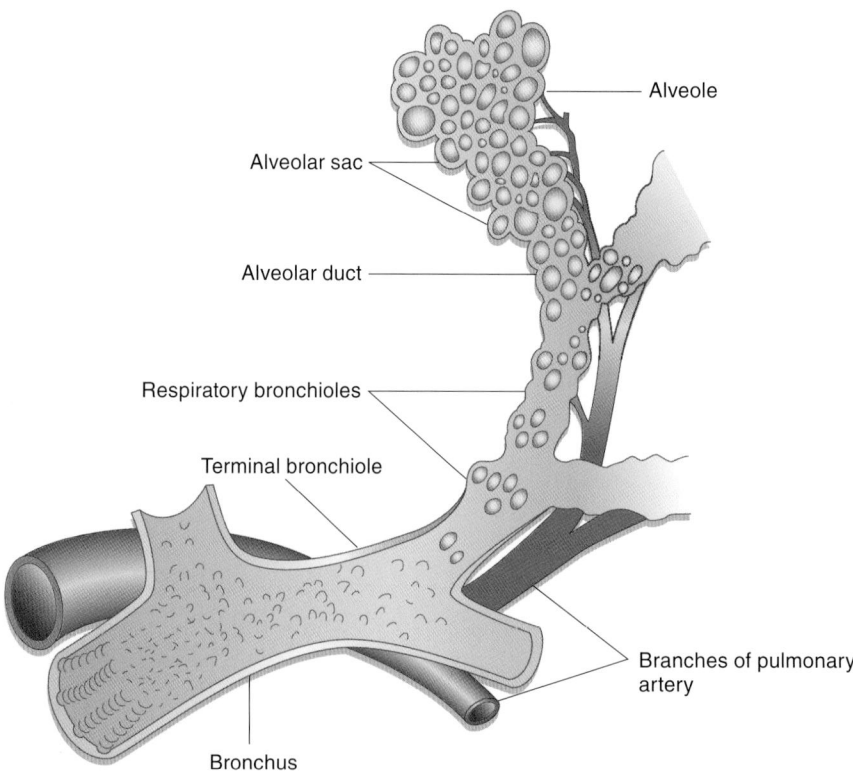

Figure 1-8. This three-dimensional schematic diagram demonstrates the relationship between pulmonary artery and airway and also illustrates the junction of a terminal bronchiole with the acinus. (Reprinted with permission from Nagaishi C. *Functional Anatomy and Histology of the Lung*. Baltimore: University Park Press; 1972.)

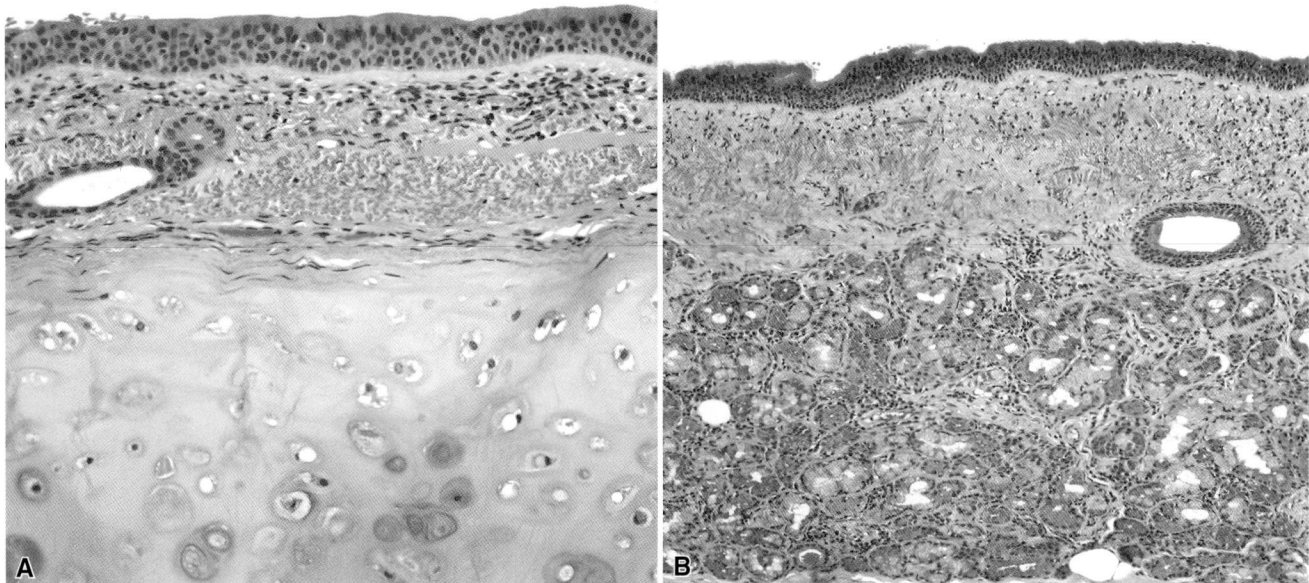

Figure 1-9. A, The tracheal mucosa is closely applied to the anterior cartilaginous portion, with scant subepithelial tissue. **B,** Posteriorly, cartilage is absent, tracheal glands are abundant, and muscle is prominent.

The Conducting Airways

Each of the major divisions of the tracheobronchial tree—trachea, bronchi, and bronchioles—has a specific role in lung function, as reflected in their respective microscopic anatomy.

The Trachea

The trachea is the gateway to the lung and is exposed to environmental factors in highest concentration. This rigid tube is designed for conducting gas, with rigid C-shaped cartilage rings that protect it from frontal injury and also prevent collapse during the negative changes in intrathoracic pressure that occur during respiration. The open side of the cartilage ring faces posteriorly, where the trachealis muscle completes the tracheal circumference. This arrangement allows the esophagus to abut the "soft" side of the trachea, down to the level of the carina. Respiratory epithelium (pseudostratified, ciliated, columnar-type), submucous glands, and smooth muscle combine to prepare inspired air for use in the lung by adding moisture and warmth (Fig. 1-9) while trapping dust particles and chemical vapor droplets before they can reach more delicate peripheral lung. For all of these reasons, when diseases affect the trachea, the potential for impact on general respiratory function is significant.

The Bronchi

The bronchi begin at the carina and extend into the substance of the lung. They are large conducting airways that have cartilage in their walls. As in the trachea, the cartilage of the primary bronchi is C-shaped, but this configuration changes to that of puzzle piece–like plates once the bronchus enters the lung parenchyma. Within the substance of the lung, the cartilage plates decrease in density progressively as the bronchial diameter decreases, resulting in increasing area between individual plates. Mucous glands are positioned just beneath the surface epithelium and may be seen in endobronchial biopsy specimens (Fig. 1-10).

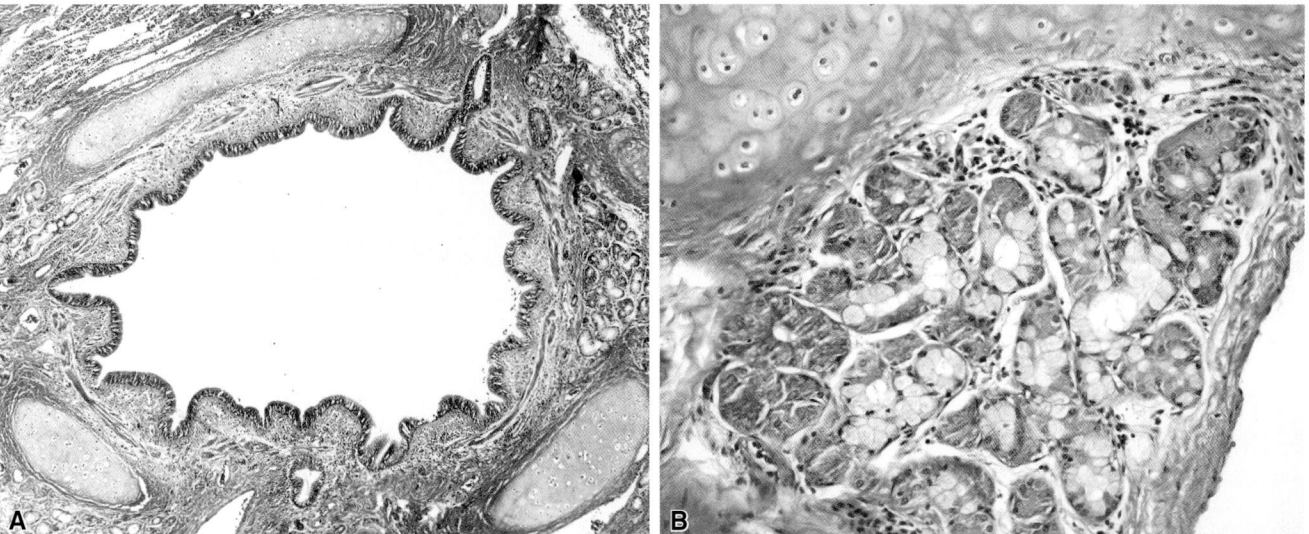

Figure 1-10. A, A segmental bronchus in cross section demonstrates the relationship of the structural elements of the cartilaginous airways. Discontinuous cartilage plates and a seromucous gland are evident (*center right*). **B,** The relationship between serous and mucous glands in this structure is better seen at higher magnification.

When inflamed or distorted by crush artifact, they may simulate granulomas or tumor. These glands connect to the airway lumen by a short duct. The bronchi divide and subdivide successively, becoming ever smaller on their way to the peripheral lung.

The Bronchioles

The bronchioles are the final air conductors and by definition lack cartilage altogether (and therefore sometimes are referred to as "membranous") (Fig. 1-11). The bronchioles have no alveoli; these are acquired more distally in the pulmonary acinus. The terminal bronchiole is the smallest conducting airway without alveoli in its walls. There are about 30,000 terminal bronchioles in the lungs, and each of these, in turn, directs air to approximately 10,000 alveoli. The cells that line the airways are columnar in shape and ciliated. Their nuclei are present at multiple levels in each cell—a phenomenon referred to as *pseudostratification* (Fig. 1-12).

Pseudostratified columnar epithelium typically is identifiable as far distal as the smallest terminal bronchioles, where the cells then rapidly become more cuboidal in shape and their nuclei more basally situated (Fig. 1-13). In the normal mucosa, mucus-secreting cells (goblet cells) typically are present in low numbers, most often as individual units. It may be quite difficult to identify any goblet cells in the epithelium of small bronchioles. When these cells are numerous, they may be distended with mucus; this finding should suggest the presence of underlying airway disease (Fig. 1-14).

Airway Mucosal Neuroendocrine Cells

Airway mucosal neuroendocrine cells typically present as single cells in the respiratory epithelium with clear cytoplasm (Fig. 1-15). Rarely, these cells may aggregate to form so-called neuroepithelial bodies. Immunohistochemical stains decorate these cells when addressed with antibodies directed against the common neuroendocrine markers chro-

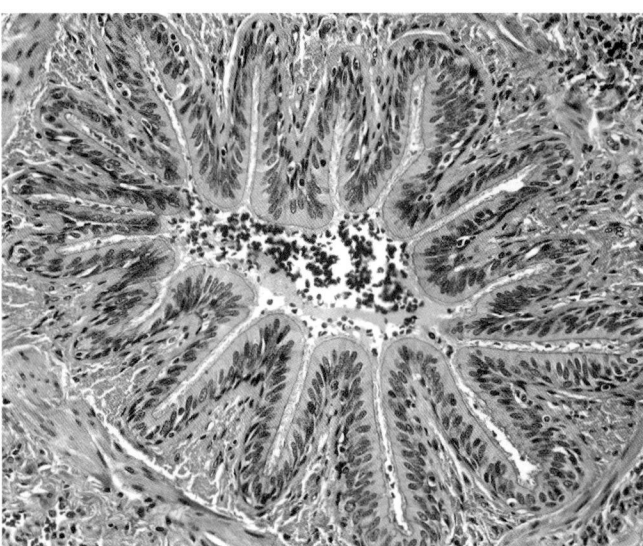

Figure 1-11. The membranous airways (bronchioles) lack cartilage in their walls but rather have prominent smooth muscle. The mucosa is respiratory in type, with uniform delicate cilia.

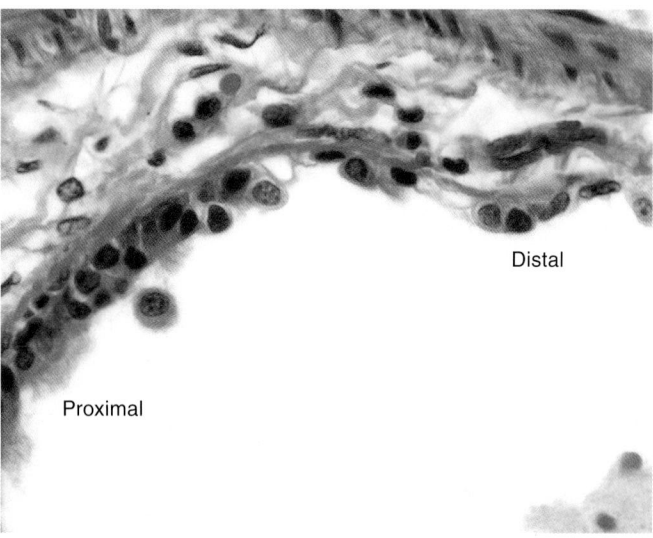

Figure 1-13. The transition from respiratory columnar epithelium to flattened alveolar lining cells is rather abrupt, with a recognized zone of cuboidal nonciliated cells present although difficult to identify with consistency in lung sections.

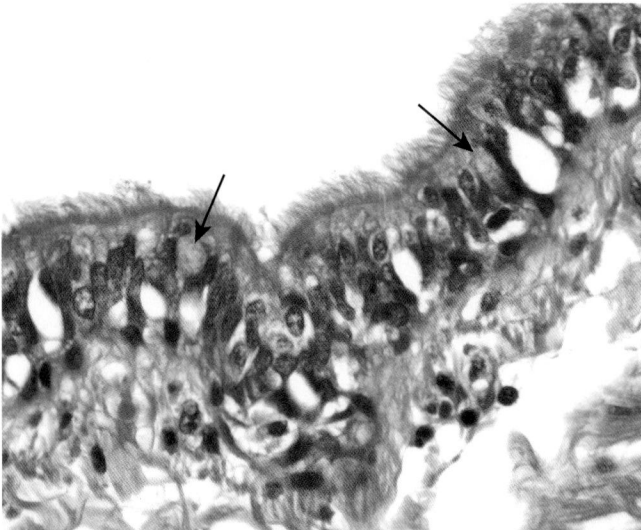

Figure 1-12. The respiratory epithelium is columnar, pseudostratified, and ciliated. Scattered goblet cells can be seen interspersed between ciliated columnar cells (*arrows*), and the nuclei of the columnar cells are present at varying levels within the cell. The subepithelial region is loose areolar tissue and a basal lamina beneath the epithelium is easily recognizable, although not overly distinct or thickened.

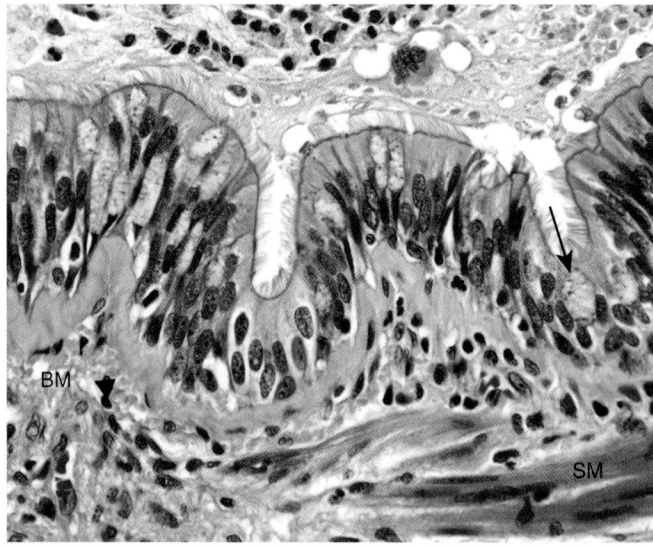

Figure 1-14. After irritation of the airway epithelium from any cause, goblet cell hyperplasia may occur (*arrow* on goblet cell). This finding is typical in patients with asthma, as is prominent thickening of the basement membrane (BM) (*arrowhead*) beneath the epithelium. SM, smooth muscle.

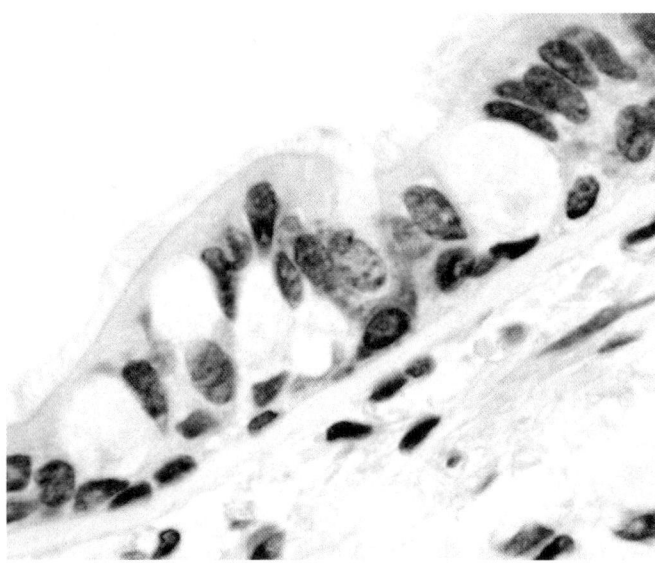

Figure 1-15. Very sparse (and rare) neuroendocrine cells are present in the normal lung. (Immunohistochemical stain for synaptophysin with red chromogen, hematoxylin counterstain.)

mogranin A and synaptophysin, as well as a number of more esoteric neuropeptides. The exact function of these cells is unknown. It has been suggested that lung neuroendocrine cells play a role in regulating ventilation-perfusion relationships and also may be important in airway morphogenesis.[9]

Airway-Associated Lymphoid Tissue

Airway-associated lymphoid tissue may be present in the normal lung, but in such instances it is very sparse and typically occurs at the bifurcation points of the airways (Fig. 1-16). This lung lymphoid tissue generally is referred to as *bronchus-associated lymphoid tissue* (BALT) and is believed to be analogous to the mucosa-associated lymphoid tissue (MALT) of the gastrointestinal tract.[10] The strategic localization of BALT at airway divisions may be a consequence of exposure to inhaled antigens and other airstream particles that are likely to strike these

areas.[11] BALT foci are associated with specialized epithelial cells in the mucosa, and the constituent lymphoid cells (mainly T lymphocytes) are admixed with macrophages and dendritic cells. The epithelial and dendritic cells of the BALT presumably play a role in the detection of inhaled allergens, viruses, and bacteria; accordingly, BALT is considered to be a critical component of the lung's immune defense system. The bronchial BALT may become hyperplastic, with follicular germinal center formation. Such germinal centers may be sampled at bronchoscopic biopsy, presenting a potential diagnostic challenge when crushed or cut in such a way that the follicular center lymphoid cells appear as a nodule or sheet in the specimen. BALT also may be important in diseases of immunologic origin that produce bronchiolitis, such as connective tissue diseases (e.g., Sjögren syndrome, rheumatoid arthritis), as well as graft-versus-host disease in organ transplantation, immunoglobulin deficiency states, and even inflammatory bowel disease.

Epithelial Basement Membrane

Epithelial basement membrane lies immediately beneath the airway epithelium and is routinely visible in association with an eosinophilic matrix of type III collagen. A fine layer of elastic tissue is present beneath the epithelial basement membrane. Collagen may come to separate this elastic tissue from the overlying basement membrane in airway injury associated with subepithelial fibrosis.

The Smooth Muscle of the Airways

The smooth muscle of the airways is arranged in a complex spiral pattern. The bronchovascular bundle encompasses the airway, the accompanying pulmonary artery, a network of lymphatic channels, a common adventitia, and a sheath of loose connective tissue. The connective tissue of the bronchovascular bundle diminishes progressively in the smallest bronchioles of the lung.

The Acinus

The acinus begins distal to the terminal bronchiole and is where most of the gas exchange occurs in the lungs. The acinus includes (in order proceeding distally) the respiratory bronchioles (primary and secondary), the alveolar ducts, and the alveolar sacs (Fig. 1-17). Respiratory

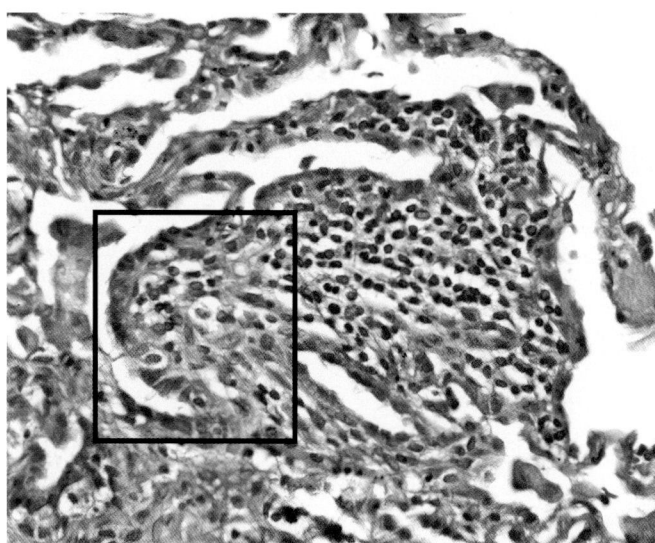

Figure 1-16. Bronchus-associated lymphoid tissue (BALT) is uncommon in normal lungs but may be increased in the lungs of smokers and in a number of other settings. These small aggregations of benign lymphoid cells are closely approximated to the airway epithelium (*boxed area*), typically with an intraepithelial component analogous to tonsillar epithelium.

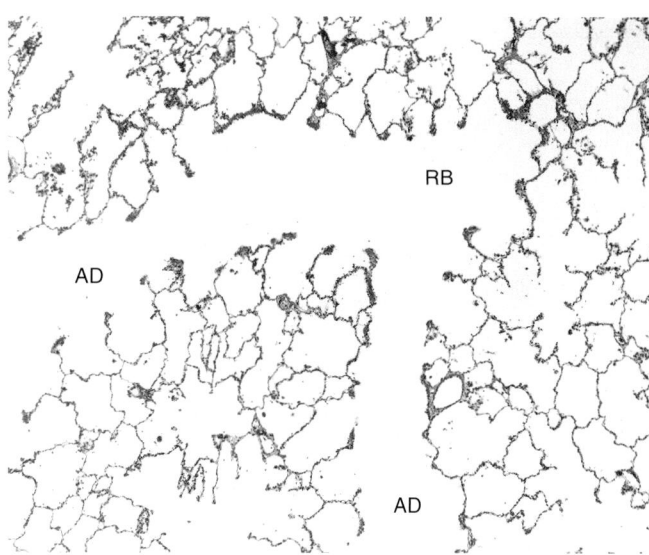

Figure 1-17. A scanning magnification view of the acinus. A branched respiratory bronchiole (RB) can be seen leading into two primary alveolar ducts (AD), fully lined by alveoli.

bronchioles have progressively more alveoli in their walls with successive distal generations. The last conducting structure, the alveolar duct, is entirely lined by alveoli. The alveolar ducts terminate in alveolar sacs, which are globular aggregations of adjacent alveoli. As the airways of the acinus branch and diminish in diameter progressively, an abrupt transition from cuboidal cells to flattened epithelium is seen.

The Alveoli

Most of the alveolar surface that faces the inspired air is covered by extremely flat type I epithelial cells that are not readily seen with the light microscope. These thin and flattened cells are well suited to gas exchange (Fig. 1-18). The type II epithelial cells are cuboidal in shape, and although they cover less surface area, they are greater in total number than the type I cells. They are present at the angular junctions of alveolar walls (the alveolus being more like a geodesic dome than a sphere). The surface of the type II cell facing the alveolar airspace has microvilli that can sometimes be appreciated on light microscopy as slight roughening. Type II cells contain large numbers of organelles and are responsible for the production of surfactant, a substance that lowers surface tension and is essential for preventing alveolar collapse at low intra-alveolar pressures. Type II cells are the progenitor cells of the

alveolar type I cells and, after an injury, divide and replace them. Type I and type II cells have tight junctions that present a physical barrier between the interstitial fluid and the alveolar air.

The Alveolar Walls

The alveolar walls are composed of a capillary net (Fig. 1-19), the extracellular matrix, and sparse cellular elements including mast cells, smooth muscle cells, pericytes, fibroblast-like cells, and occasional lymphocytes.[12] The mesenchymal cells of the interstitium have been the subject of considerable study. Unstimulated, they resemble fibroblasts and have few organelles. During the repair phase of an injury, actin and myosin appear in the cytoplasm and develop contractile properties that play an important role in lung repair.[13–15] Capillary endothelial cells within the acinus are joined by tight or semi-tight junctions. The semi-tight junctions exist to allow larger molecules to traverse the capillary wall.

Alveolar Macrophages

Alveolar macrophages play an essential role as phagocytes and, under appropriate stimulation, secrete soluble factors that are an essential part of the lung's immunologic defense and response to injury. As mobile

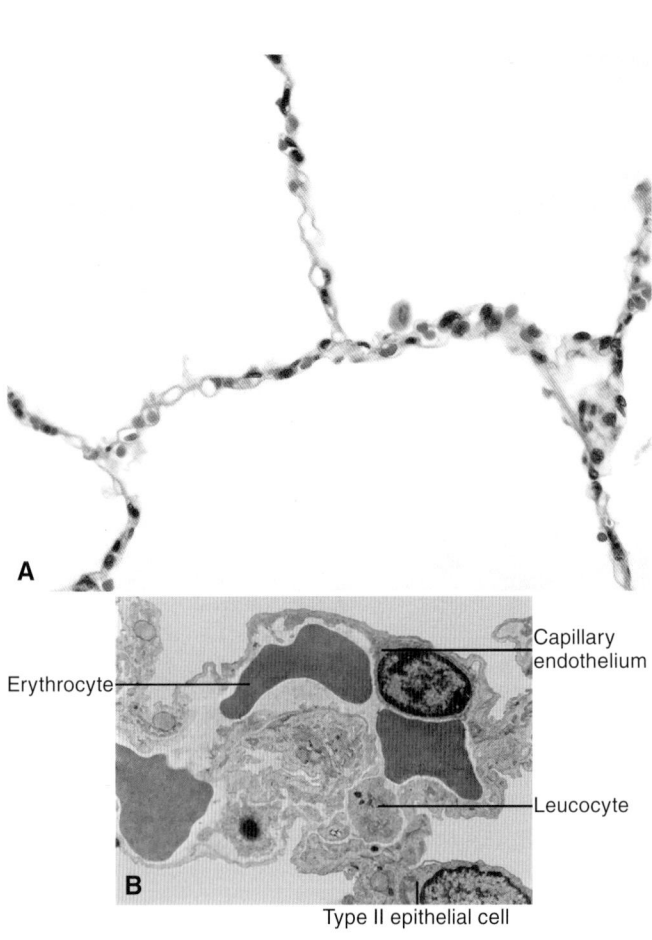

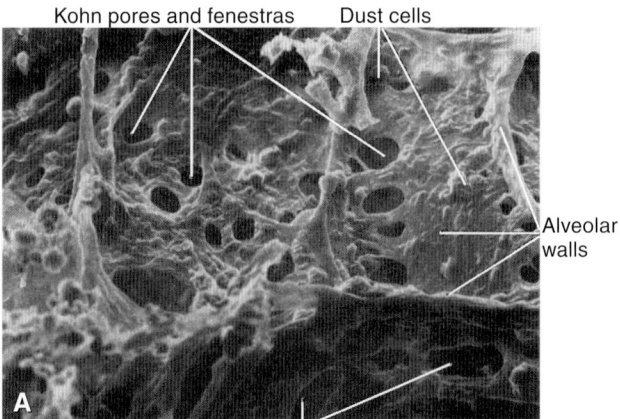

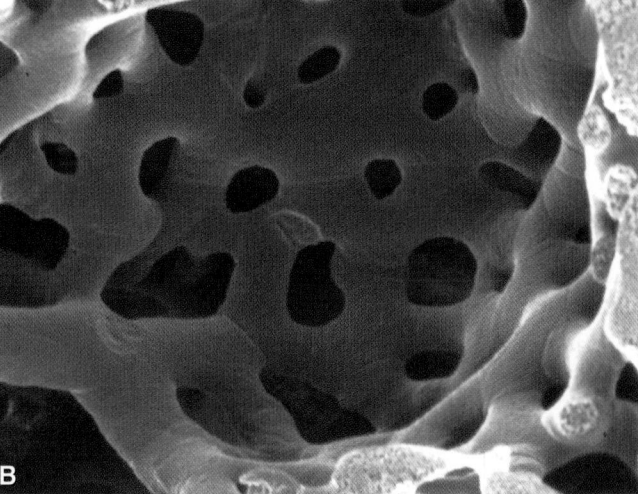

Figure 1-18. **A,** High-magnification view of five adjacent alveoli with delicate alveolar walls. Most of the visible nuclei in the normal alveolar wall belong to endothelial cells. **B,** Electron microscopy emphasizes this point: A prominent endothelial cell nucleus is seen adjacent to two red blood cells (RBCs). Note the extremely attenuated fusion of endothelial cytoplasm, basal laminae, and type I cell cytoplasm above these RBCs (not readily visible, even on ultrastructural examination). (Reprinted with permission from Nagaishi C. *Functional Anatomy and Histology of the Lung*. Baltimore: University Park Press; 1972.)

Figure 1-19. **A,** A scanning electron micrograph of adult human lung showing the internal aspect of the alveolus. The liberal communication between alveoli in adjacent alveolar sacs is made possible by the pores of Kohn. **B,** The capillary network of the alveolus is demonstrated in this scanning electron micrograph of a methacrylate vascular cast. (**A,** Reprinted with permission from Nagaishi C: *Functional Anatomy and Histology of the Lung*. Baltimore: University Park Press; 1972. **B,** Courtesy of A. Churg, MD, and J. Wright, MD, Vancouver, Canada.)

cellular elements, they are capable of removing engulfed particulates by migrating into the interstitium (and eventually, lymphatic channels) or ascending the mucociliary escalator of the airways.

The Pulmonary Arteries

The pulmonary arteries carry venous blood to the lungs for gas exchange with the inspired air in the alveolar spaces. The pulmonary circulation is a low-pressure system (with a mean systolic pressure of 14 mm Hg) and is considerably shorter in length than the systemic circulation.[16,17] Nevertheless, a doubling of the resting blood flow to the lung results in only a small increase (by approximately 5 mm Hg) in pressure.

The pulmonary arteries arise from the conus arteriosus of the right ventricle of the heart and run in parallel with the airways within the lung.[18,19] The main trunk of the pulmonary artery bifurcates into right and left main trunks at the fourth thoracic vertebral body. These trunks follow the right and left main bronchi into the lung (Fig. 1-20). The diameter of the pulmonary artery and that of the accompanying airway in cross section are roughly equal. The pulmonary arteries branch at a rate similar to that for the airways but also have a second distinctive branching pattern identifiable in peripheral lung, with right-angle origins for branches having significantly smaller caliber (Fig. 1-21) designed to supply peribronchiolar alveoli.

The pulmonary arteries are composed of three layers, the intima, the media, and the adventitia, similar to the systemic arteries; however, for arteries of the same diameter, systemic vessels have a significantly thicker muscular layer. In the adult, two or more elastic laminae are present in arteries larger than 1 mm in diameter. Arteries between 100 and 200 μm (between 0.1 and 0.2 mm) in diameter are muscular and have internal and external elastic laminae (Fig. 1-22). Smaller arteries may be muscular or nonmuscular. The two elastic laminae appear fused in smaller arteries as a result of progressive attenuation of smooth muscle. Where muscle is absent, a single fragmented elastic lamina is all that separates the intima from the adventitia. In the adult, arterial muscle extends down to the level of the alveoli. The ratio of arterial wall thickness to external arterial diameter often is a useful marker for abnormality. Nondistended muscular arteries have a medial thickness that should represent approximately 5% of external arterial diameter.

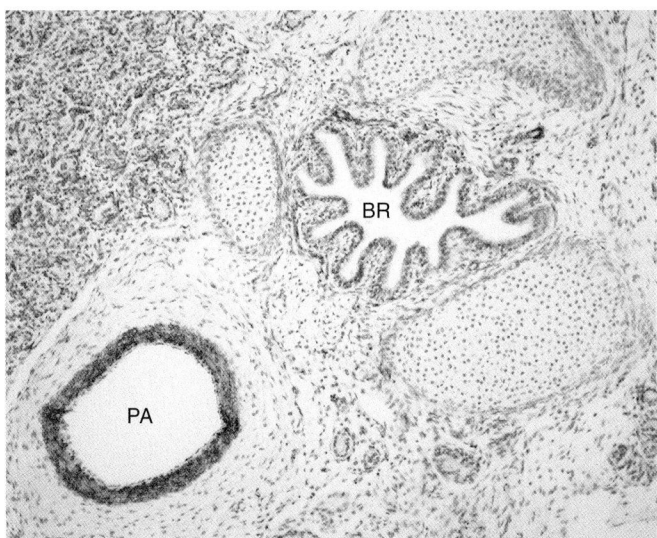

Figure 1-20. This microscopic section of fetal lung shows the characteristic early relationship of pulmonary artery branches to bronchi. The smooth muscle layer of each of these structures is outlined in *brown*. (Immunohistochemical stain for alpha smooth muscle actin, brown chromogen, hematoxylin counterstain.) BR, bronchus; PA, pulmonary artery.

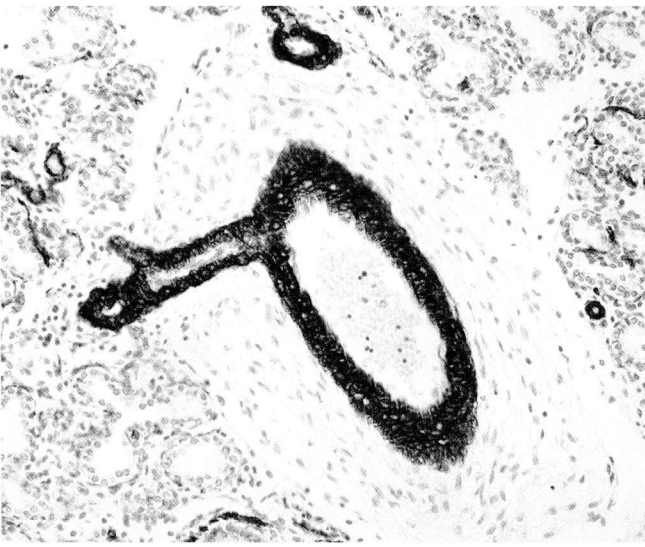

Figure 1-21. The distinctive pattern of pulmonary artery branching in the lung parenchyma is nicely illustrated in this fetal lung. (Immunohistochemical stain with monoclonal antibody directed against alpha smooth muscle actin, brown chromogen, hematoxylin counterstain).

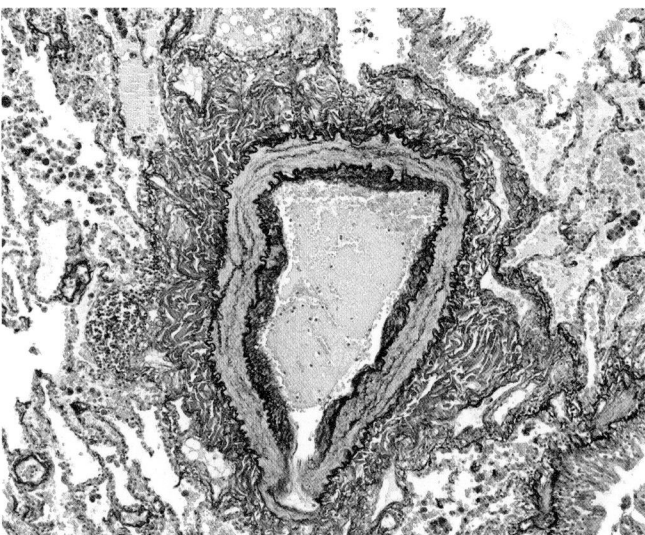

Figure 1-22. Pulmonary artery in peripheral lung showing internal and external elastic lamina. (Elastic van Gieson histochemical stain.)

The Pulmonary Veins

The pulmonary veins carry oxygenated blood back to the heart for systemic distribution. The large veins are present adjacent to the main arteries at the hilum, but the pulmonary veins within the lung parenchyma travel along a separate course within the interlobular septa, beginning on the venous side of the alveolar capillary bed. The intralobular pulmonary veins coalesce to form larger channels that join the interlobular septa at the periphery of the acinus (Fig. 1-23). The veins are indistinct structures in the lung and often are difficult to identify.[18,20] Most of the vascular structures identifiable at scanning magnification in tissue sections of lung are pulmonary arteries (with their adjacent airway). The most reliable method for locating a pulmonary vein in tissue sections is to find the junction of the pleura with an interlobular septum (Fig. 1-24). This is an important technique, because every lung biopsy for diffuse disease should be evaluated

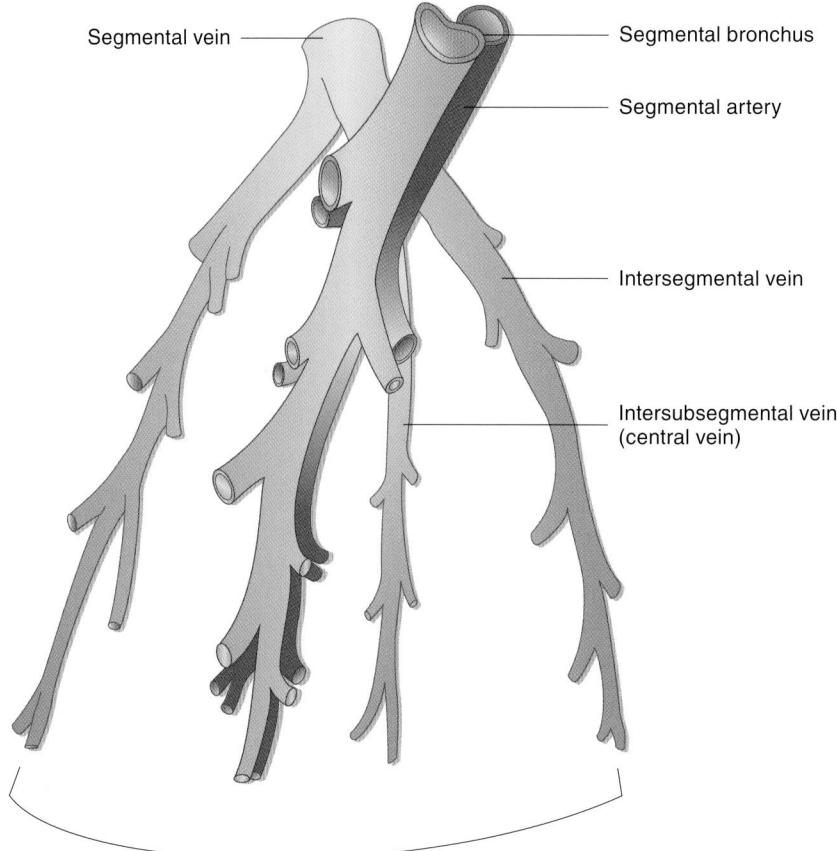

Figure 1-23. The lobular relationship of pulmonary arteries and veins is illustrated in this simplified diagram. (Reprinted with permission from Nagaishi C. *Functional Anatomy and Histology of the Lung*. Baltimore: University Park Press; 1972.)

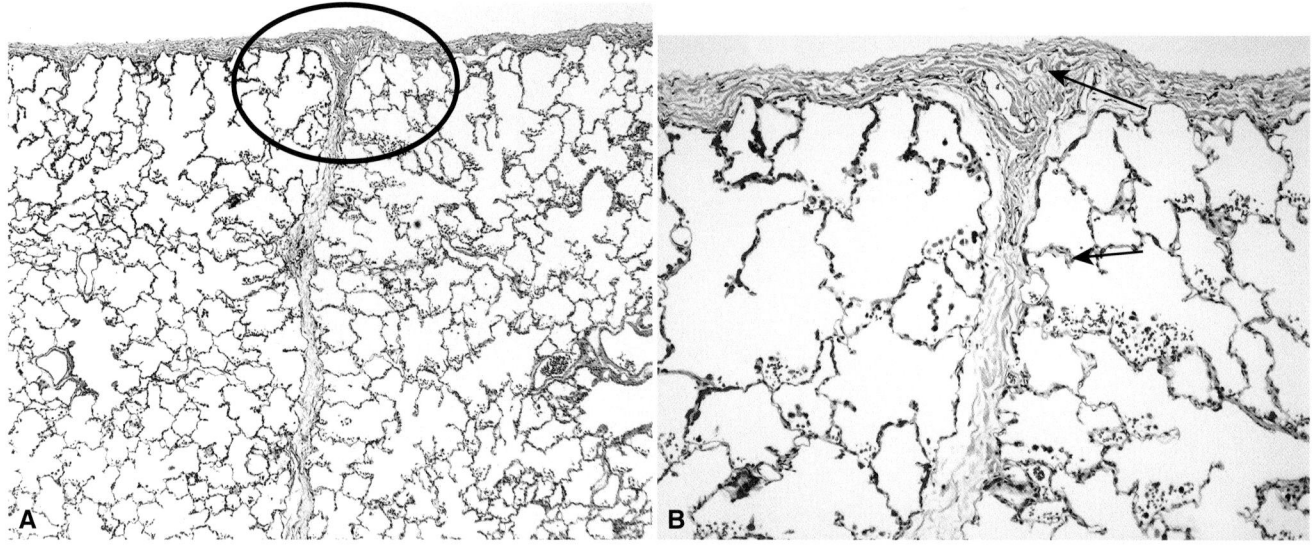

Figure 1-24. A, Study of the pulmonary veins and lymphatics is facilitated by finding junctions of pleura with interlobular septa. **B,** At higher magnification of the oval area in part A, the delicate vessels, with red blood cells (RBCs) in their lumens, are seen to be veins. The veins have slightly thicker walls than those of adjacent lymphatics. *Large arrow*, pleural vein; *small arrow*, peripheral lobular vein.

systematically in search of pathologic alterations in each of the main compartments (airways, arteries, veins, acinar structures, and pleura). The veins have a single elastic lamina (Fig. 1-25) and sparse smooth muscle.

The Bronchial Arteries

The bronchial arteries supply arterial blood to the lung and arise most commonly from the descending aorta, although a number of anomalous origins are described. The bronchial arteries run parallel to the airways within the bronchovascular sheath, where small branches supply capillary networks of the mucosa, airway smooth muscle, and adventitia.[20,21] The largest-diameter bronchial arteries can be seen in the adventitia of the airway. Submucosal branches are nearly imperceptible. On the venous side of the bronchial artery–supplied capillary net, bronchial veins within the lung eventually join pulmonary veins and return their blood to the left atrium.

1

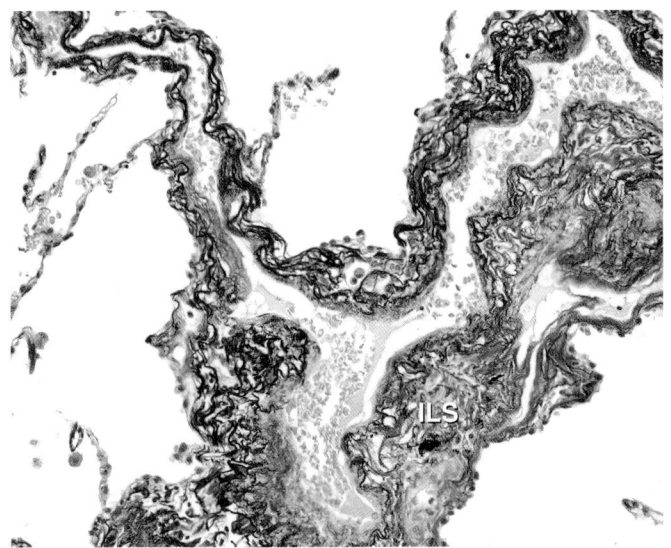

Figure 1-25. A larger pulmonary vein stained for elastic tissue shows a single elastic lamina. (Elastic van Gieson histochemical stain.) ILS, interlobular septum.

The Pulmonary Lymphatics

The lymphatic vessels of the peripheral lung begin at the outer edge of the acinus, draining along interlobular septa to coalesce finally at the hilum.[22] A separate centriacinar system is present in the bronchovascular sheaths, beginning around the level of the respiratory bronchiole.[23] No lymphatics are present in the alveolar sacs, where it is believed that the interstitial space serves the purpose of extracellular fluid collection and drainage to more proximal regions. The lymphatic net of the pulmonary arteries extends further distally in the acinus than does that associated with the terminal airways.[23] The lymphatic networks of the airways and pulmonary arteries anastomose freely during their course back to the hilum. The lymphatics (and veins) also are distributed over the surface of the lobes within the pleura. The relationship among airways, arteries, veins, and lymphatics is nicely illustrated by Okada,[23] in Figure 1-26. When affected by certain diseases such as diffuse lymphangiomatosis (Fig. 1-27A) or lymphangiectasis (see Fig. 1-27B), the distribution of the pulmonary lymphatics becomes much more apparent.

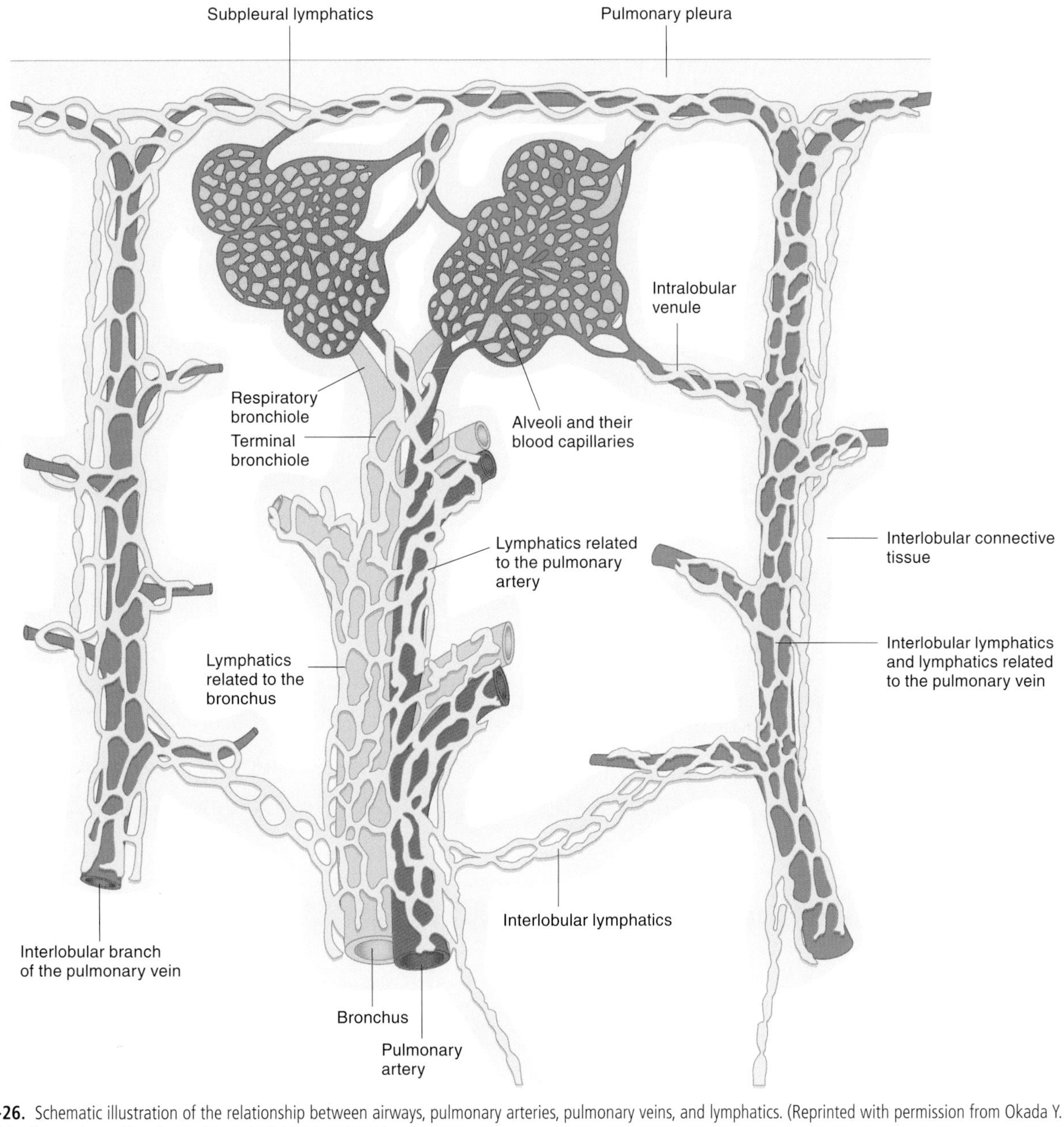

Subpleural lymphatics

Pulmonary pleura

Intralobular venule

Respiratory bronchiole

Terminal bronchiole

Alveoli and their blood capillaries

Lymphatics related to the pulmonary artery

Interlobular connective tissue

Interlobular lymphatics and lymphatics related to the pulmonary vein

Lymphatics related to the bronchus

Interlobular branch of the pulmonary vein

Interlobular lymphatics

Bronchus

Pulmonary artery

Figure 1-26. Schematic illustration of the relationship between airways, pulmonary arteries, pulmonary veins, and lymphatics. (Reprinted with permission from Okada Y. *Lymphatic System of the Human Lung*. Siga, Japan: Kinpodo Publishing; 1989.)

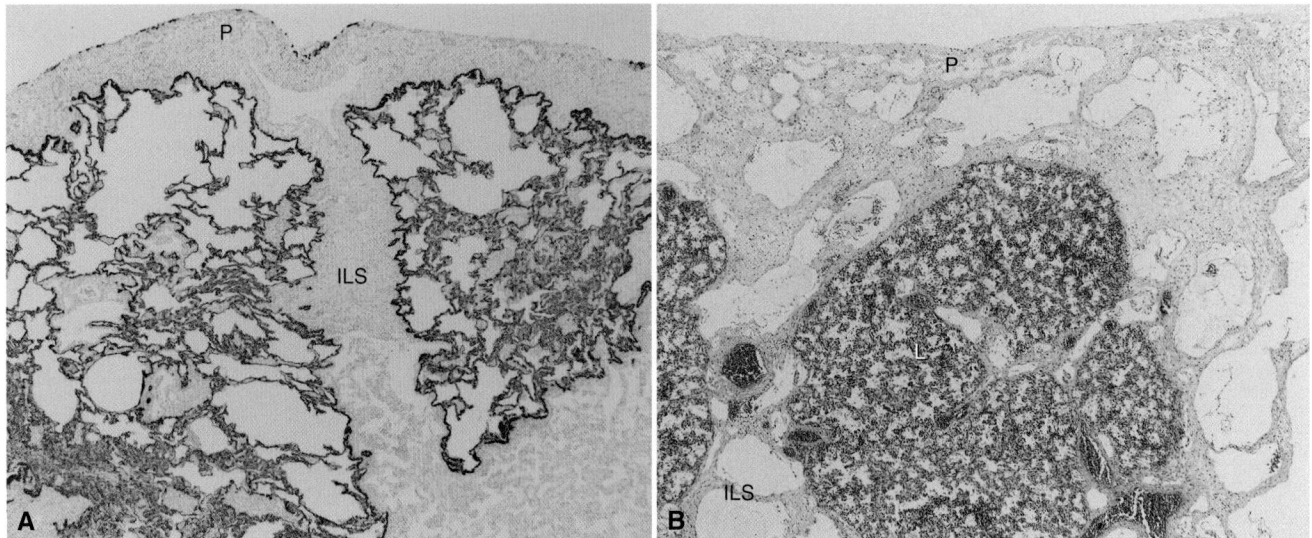

Figure 1-27. **A,** The pleural (P) and septal (ILS) distribution of lymphatics is dramatically accentuated in this example of the rare disorder known as diffuse pulmonary lymphangiomatosis. **B,** Similar accentuation is produced by lymphangiectasis. ILS, interlobular septum; L, lobule.

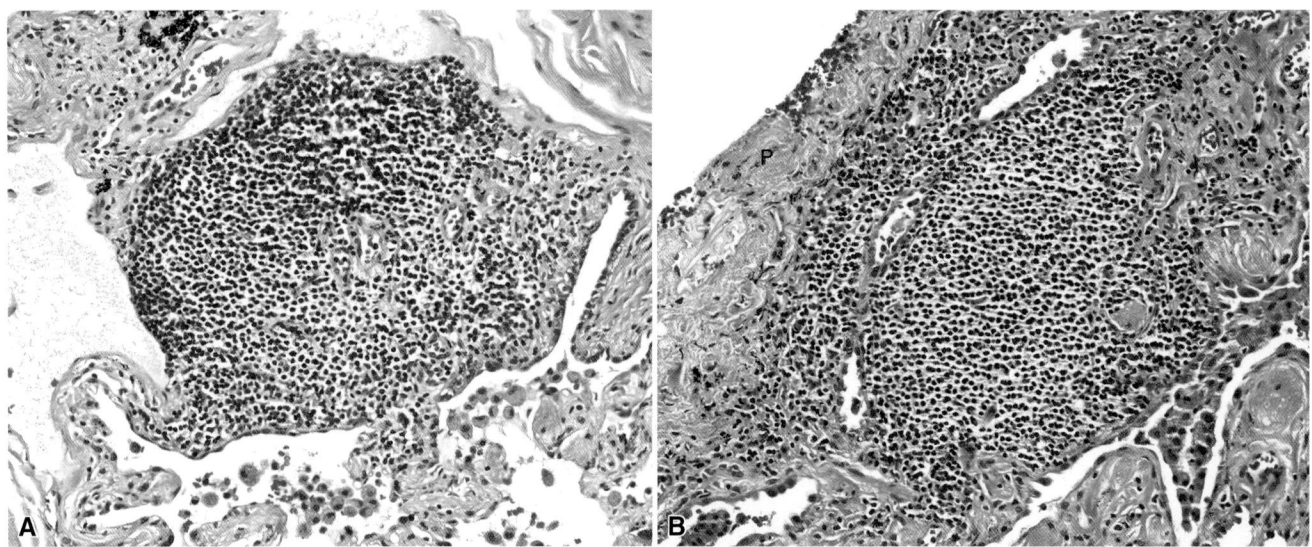

Figure 1-28. Lymphoid aggregates in the lung may occur along interlobular septa (**A**), and in the pleura (P), as seen in part **B**. Germinal centers may be evident.

Other Pulmonary Lymphoid Tissue

Lymphoid Aggregates

Lymphoid aggregates are uncommon in the lung under normal circumstances. They have no capsule and are composed of B cells, T cells, and dendritic cells. Lymphoid aggregates increase in the lungs of cigarette smokers[11,24] and may be present within interlobular septa or the pleura (Fig. 1-28) and in the subpleural connective tissue.[25] Lymphoid aggregates may be one of the sources for the condition known as diffuse lymphoid hyperplasia.

Dendritic Cells

Dendritic cells are antigen-presenting cells that function in concert with T lymphocytes to develop acquired immunity. Dendritic cells occur in the epithelium and subepithelial tissue of the airways. Their kidney-shaped nucleus is eccentrically placed, and they feature prominent cytoplasmic protrusions. Dendritic cells strongly express the major histocompatibility complex (MHC) antigens.[26] A subpopulation of dendritic cells carry the Langerhans cell marker[24] and contain Birbeck granules in their cytoplasm on ultrastructural examination.[27] Langerhans cells are increased in the lungs of smokers and can be identified by immunohistochemical techniques using antibodies directed against S100 protein and CD1a. The Langerhans cell is involved in the smoking-related disease known as *pulmonary Langerhans cell histiocytosis* (formerly known as pulmonary eosinophilic granuloma or histiocytosis X).

Self-assessment questions related to this chapter can be found online on the Expert Consult site for this title.

References

1. Moore K. *The Developing Human*. Philadelphia: WB Saunders; 1973.
2. Langeman J. *Medical Embryology*. 2nd ed. Baltimore: Williams & Wilkins; 1969.
3. Wells LJ, Boyden EA. The development of the bronchopulmonary segments in human embryos of horizons XVII to XIX. *Am J Anat*. 1954;95(2):163–201.
4. Nagaishi C. *Functional Anatomy and Histology of the Lung*. Baltimore: University Park Press; 1972.
5. Boyden EA. Development of the pulmonary airways. *Minn Med*. 1971;54(11):894–897.
6. Boyden EA. Observations on the anatomy and development of the lungs. *Lancet*. 1953;73(12):509–512.
7. Boyden EA. Observations on the history of the bronchopulmonary segments. *Minn Med*. 1955;38(9):597–598.

8. Kwon KY, Myers JL, Swensen SJ, Colby TV. Middle lobe syndrome: a clinicopathological study of 21 patients. *Hum Pathol.* 1995;26(3):302–307.

9. Aguayo S, Schuyler W, Murtagh J, et al. Regulation of branching morphogenesis by bombesin-like peptides and neutral endopeptidase. *Am J Respir Cell Mol Biol.* 1994;10:635–642.

10. Bienenstock J, Johnston N, Perey D. Bronchial lymphoid tissue I. Morphological characteristics. *Lab Invest.* 1973;28:686–692.

11. Richmond I, Pritchard G, Ashcroft T, et al. Bronchus associated lymphoid tissue (BALT) in human lung: its distribution in smokers and non-smokers. *Thorax.* 1993;48:1130–1134.

12. Thurlbeck W. Chronic airflow obstruction. In: Churg A, ed. *Pathology of the Lung.* 2nd ed. New York: Thieme Medical Publishers; 1995:739–825.

13. Fukuda Y, Ishizaki M, Masuda Y, et al. The role of intraalveolar fibrosis in the process of pulmonary structural remodeling in patients with diffuse alveolar damage. *Am J Pathol.* 1987;126(1):171–182.

14. Leslie K, King Jr TE, Low R. Smooth muscle actin is expressed by air space fibroblast-like cells in idiopathic pulmonary fibrosis and hypersensitivity pneumonitis. *Chest.* 1991;99(suppl 3):47S–48S.

15. Leslie KO, Mitchell J, Low R. Lung myofibroblasts. *Cell Motil Cytoskeleton.* 1992;22(2):92–98.

16. Parker JC, Cave CB, Ardell JL, et al. Vascular tree structure affects lung blood flow heterogeneity simulated in three dimensions. *J Appl Physiol.* 1997;83(4):1370–1382.

17. Li CW, Cheng HD. A nonlinear fluid model for pulmonary blood circulation. *J Biomech.* 1993;26(6):653–664.

18. Huang W, Yen RT, McLaurine M, Bledsoe G. Morphometry of the human pulmonary vasculature. *J Appl Physiol.* 1996;81(5):2123–2133.

19. Hislop AA. Airway and blood vessel interaction during lung development. *J Anat.* 2002;201(4):325–334.

20. Boyden EA. Human growth and development. *Am J Anat.* 1971;132(1):1–3.

21. Boyden EA. The developing bronchial arteries in a fetus of the twelfth week. *Am J Anat.* 1970;129(3):357–368.

22. Okada Y, Ito M, Nagaishi C. Anatomical study of the pulmonary lymphatics. *Lymphology.* 1979;12(3):118–124.

23. Okada Y. *Lymphatic System of the Human Lung.* Siga, Japan: Kinpodo Publishing; 1989.

24. van Haarst J, de Wit H, Drexhage H, Hoogsteden HC. Distribution and immunophenotype of mononuclear phagocytes and dendritic cells in the human lung. *Am J Respir Cell Mol Biol.* 1994;10(5):487–492.

25. Kradin R, Mark E. Benign lymphoid disorders of the lung, with a theory regarding their development. *Hum Pathol.* 1983;14:857–867.

26. Van Voorhis W, Hair L, Steinman R, Kaplan G. Human dendritic cells. Enrichment and purification from peripheral blood. *J Exp Med.* 1982;155(4):1172–1187.

27. Soler P, Moreau A, Basset F, Hance AJ. Cigarette smoking-induced changes in the number and differentiated state of pulmonary dendritic/Langerhans cells. *Am Rev Respir Dis.* 1989;139(5):1112–1117.

Optimal Processing of Diagnostic Lung Specimens

Dawn E. Jaroszewski, MD, Robert W. Viggiano, MD, and Kevin O. Leslie, MD

Optimal specimen handling is essential for the accurate interpretation of biopsies and cytologic preparations obtained in the course of evaluating the patient with lung disease.[1–9] The limited number of sampling techniques available can be divided into three general categories: bronchoscopy, transthoracic needle core biopsy or aspiration, and surgical wedge biopsy of peripheral lung through a transthoracic approach.[8,10–13]

The focus of this chapter is on these techniques and the specimens thereby obtained, with emphasis on how they should be prepared and handled in the laboratory. Once an appropriate sample of adequate quality has been obtained, the addition of pertinent clinical data and radiologic information greatly increases the likelihood of a meaningful and accurate diagnosis.[13–15] Even when the diagnostic goal is simply to rule out malignancy, the effect of other information may be substantial, especially when the sample is of marginal quality or size. In the case of diffuse non-neoplastic lung diseases (often referred to as "interstitial lung diseases"), a reasonable amount of clinical and radiologic information is essential for accurate interpretation. Without such information, even the experienced lung pathologist may need to resort to a purely descriptive diagnosis.[15]

In this chapter, specimen characteristics and processing steps are presented for each of the common lung samples taken in the course of clinical evaluation for pulmonary disease. Also, for each type of sample, the benefits and limitations are reviewed. Such a working knowledge of specimen handling for each procedure ensures the greatest likelihood of success in establishing a specific diagnosis and, in the end, a rational treatment plan. An overview of biopsy procedures and the specimens generated is presented in Table 2-1.

Specimens Obtained through the Flexible Bronchoscope

The flexible bronchoscope was introduced in the United States in the late 1960s, after successful use in Japan.[8] Despite several decades of experience with the rigid bronchoscope, the advent of the flexible bronchoscope (Fig. 2-1) allowed evaluation of the major conducting airways without use of general anesthesia and with less morbidity.[8,16] Furthermore, the flexible instrument has the advantage of providing better access to more distal and obliquely branched airways. The rigid bronchoscope still has major uses in certain settings, mainly those in which the device's larger bore is an advantage, but today pulmonary endoscopy is dominated by the flexible bronchoscope.

Endobronchial Biopsy

Modern flexible bronchoscopes allow the operator to accurately visualize the structural integrity of the bronchial tree and its mucosal surfaces, commonly as far distal as the sixth order bronchi[17,18] (Fig. 2-2). Biopsy of visualized mucosal lesions most commonly is performed using cupped forceps (Fig. 2-3A) introduced through the flexible shaft of the bronchoscope.[8] With this technique, the airway mucosa, lamina propria, and musculature are sampled with or without fragments of cartilage (see Fig. 2-3B). The closed forceps is extracted from the bronchoscope and the biopsy is dislodged from the cupped ends of the device and placed in fixative or other solution (see later discussion). A sterile needle or fine-tipped forceps (Fig. 2-4) is useful for removing the delicate tissue specimen. The tissue specimens obtained in this way average 2 to 3 mm in greatest dimension. The lymphovascular network of the peribronchial sheath often is included in these samples, making it possible to identify metastatic disease when present in lymphatic or vascular channels (Fig. 2-5).

Table 2-1. Diagnostic Sampling Techniques, Specimens Obtained, and Common Analyses Performed

Sampling Technique	Specimens/Common Analyses
Sputum expectoration	Cytologic smears and centrifuge preparations Fixed or air-dried, then stained for cytopathologic examination Microbiologic cultures performed as indicated
Bronchoscopy with: Washings	Cytologic smears and centrifuge preparations Fixed or air-dried, then stained for cytopathologic examination Microbiologic cultures performed as indicated
Brushings	Cytologic smears and centrifuge preparations Fixed or air-dried, then stained for cytopathologic examination Microbiologic cultures performed as indicated
Endobronchial biopsy	Forceps tissue biopsy specimen, 2–3 mm in size Fixed and processed for histopathologic examination Microbiologic cultures and other testing performed as indicated
Transbronchial biopsy	Forceps tissue biopsy specimen, 2–3 mm in size Processed for histopathologic examination Microbiologic cultures and other testing performed as indicated
Bronchoalveolar lavage (BAL)	Cytologic smears and centrifuge preparations Fixed or air-dried, then stained for cytopathologic examination and biochemical analysis Microbiologic cultures and other testing performed as indicated
Transbronchial fine needle aspiration	Cytologic smears and centrifuge preparations Fixed or air-dried, then stained for cytopathologic examination Microbiologic cultures and other testing performed as indicated
Surgical "wedge" lung biopsy (either video-assisted or open)	3- to 5-cm peripheral lung tissue sample including pleura and alveolar parenchyma Fixed and processed for histopathologic examination Microbiologic cultures and specialized testing performed as indicated
Transthoracic needle core biopsy and aspiration	Core biopsy fragment(s), cytologic smears and centrifuge preparations Smears and cellular preparations: fixed or air-dried, then stained for cytopathologic examination, with special stains for organisms and other specialized techniques as indicated Core tissue specimens: fixed and processed for histopathologic examination Microbiologic cultures and specialized assays performed as indicated
Thoracentesis	Cytologic centrifuge preparations Fixed or air-dried, then stained for cytopathologic examination Microbiologic cultures, biochemical analysis, and specialized assays performed as indicated

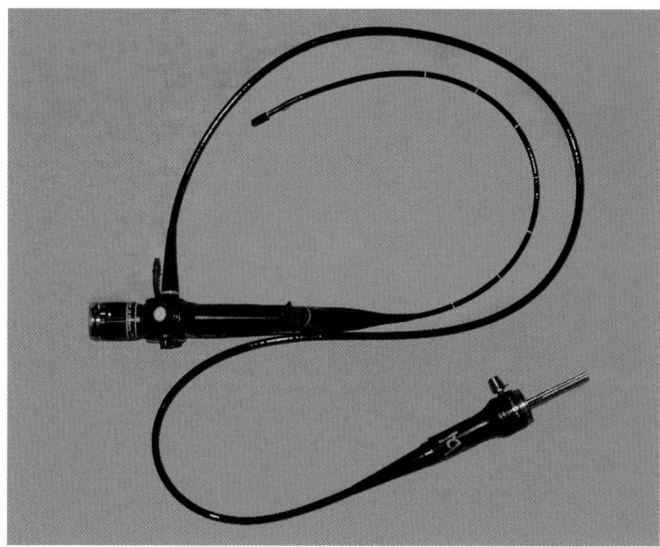

Figure 2-1. Bronchoscopy. The modern flexible bronchoscope.

or special studies (e.g., immunocytochemistry studies, molecular genetic analysis). When these solutions are not available in the bronchoscopy suite or at the bedside, specimens can be placed in a closed container on a sterile, saline-soaked, nonstick wound dressing pad and transferred to the laboratory for processing, after the bronchoscopy is completed. Gauze or mesh pads are not appropriate for transport because the tissue may become entwined in the mesh material, making extraction difficult and tissue damage likely. As with all small, freshly obtained biopsy specimens, caution must be exerted to avoid prolonged exposure to air, because drying artifact can render the specimen uninterpretable.

For tissue examination by light microscopy, the usual specimen fixation is accomplished using 10% neutral-buffered formalin (4% formaldehyde solution). Biopsies should be submersed in fixative, with an optimal fixative-to-specimen volume ratio of at least 10:1. For reasons of safety and disposal cost, some laboratories have replaced their formalin solutions with special non-aldehyde fixatives, most of which use alcohol as the primary fixing agent. Of note, all fixatives produce a certain degree of histologic artifact in tissues and cells, and these artifacts can influence the accuracy of the diagnosis. For this reason, it is essential that the pathologist responsible for interpreting the specimen be consulted regarding the type of fixative to be used. Despite some hazards in handling and disposal, 10% neutral-buffered formalin remains the standard agent for lung biopsy fixation.

For transferring bronchoscopic biopsy specimens from carrier or fixative solutions into cassettes for paraffin embedment, a useful device is a polystyrene pipette with the tip cut off with scissors (Fig. 2-6). This pipetting device allows the operator to transfer delicate specimens without tearing or crushing. Transferring of these specimens using forceps is to be avoided.

When infection is a consideration, bronchoscopic biopsy specimens can be transported directly to the microbiology laboratory for processing.[4,19,20] In most scenarios, biopsy samples are sent for histopathologic evaluation and microbiologic studies directly from the bronchoscopy suite or bedside. For endobronchial and transbronchial samples, the optimal number of biopsy specimens varies depending on the radiologic distribution of disease,[15,21–23] bronchoscopy findings,[8,11,16] and the specific diagnostic entities under consideration.[8,24,25] As a general guideline, if the patient is tolerating the procedure well, the greater the number of biopsy specimens, the greater the likelihood of establishing a definitive diagnosis.[8,23,25]

To avoid drying, specimens should be placed immediately into fixative solution or other transport medium. Immediate agitation of the samples in the solution vial helps reexpand any crush artifact induced by the biopsy procedure, and if done in a carrying medium, the supernatant can be aliquoted and sent for cytopathogic evaluation

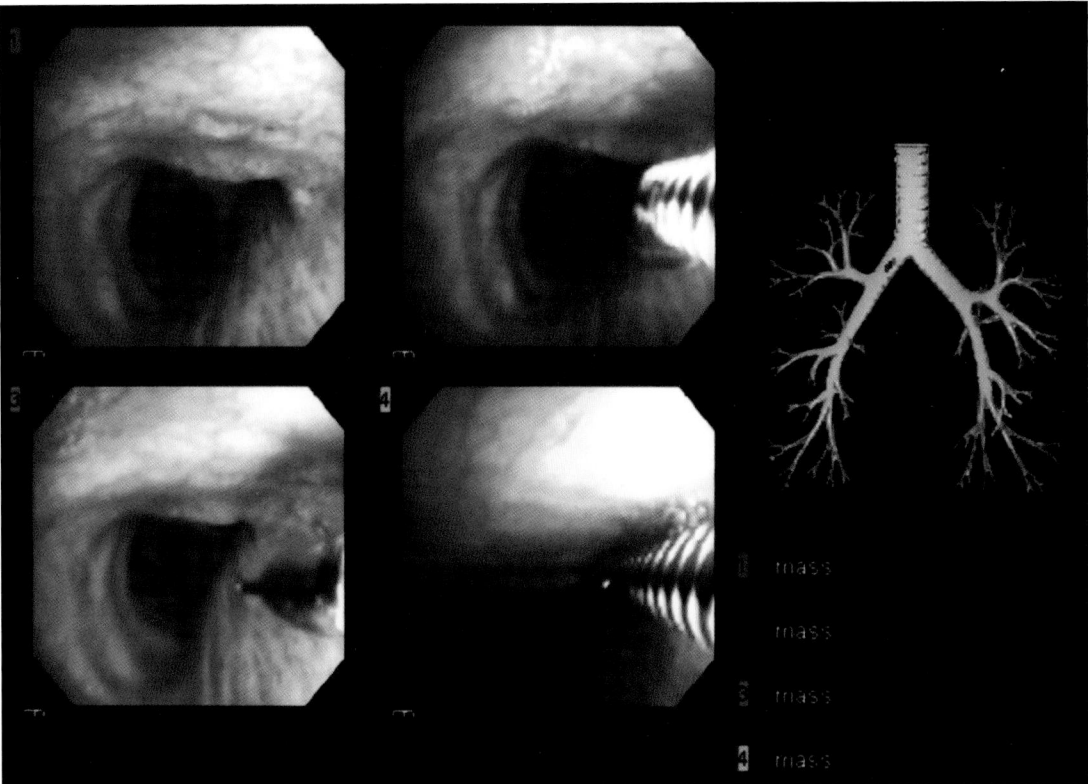

Figure 2-2. Bronchoscopy. Endoscopic view of right main bronchus with a needle biopsy device inserted (*right upper and lower images* and *left lower image*). Note the guide diagram (*extreme right*), with a *red dot* indicating the position of the bronchoscope tip.

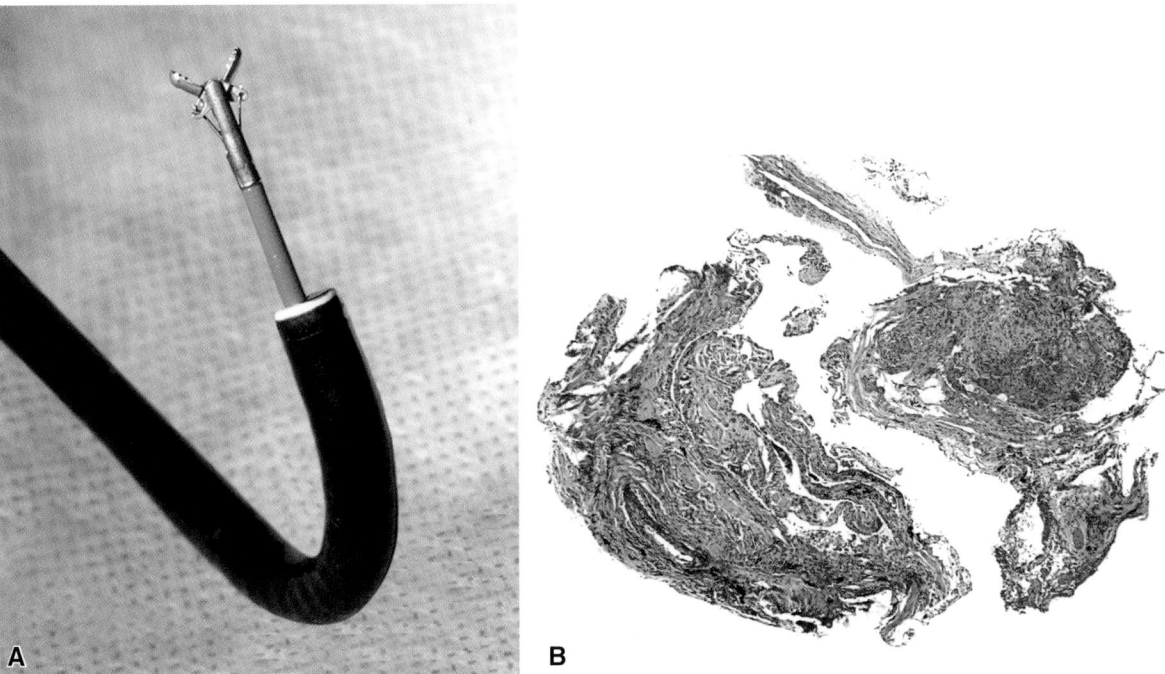

A **B**

Figure 2-3. Bronchoscopic biopsy. **A,** Cupped biopsy forceps. **B,** Bronchoscopic biopsy specimen. The airway epithelium, subepithelial tissue, and muscle wall are typically present with variable cartilage.

Transbronchial Biopsy

In contrast with endobronchial biopsy, the transbronchial biopsy technique is intended to sample alveolar lung parenchyma beyond the cartilaginous bronchi.[8,16,17,26] This technique uses either crocodile-style (Machida) forceps or cupped forceps manipulated by the operator

(Fig. 2-7). To obtain the biopsy specimen, the forceps is advanced with the jaws closed into a distal airway until resistance is met. The forceps is retracted slightly and then advanced slightly, with the jaws open. The jaws are then closed and the forceps is pulled out through the bronchoscope. Advancing the forceps at end-expiration can be helpful in

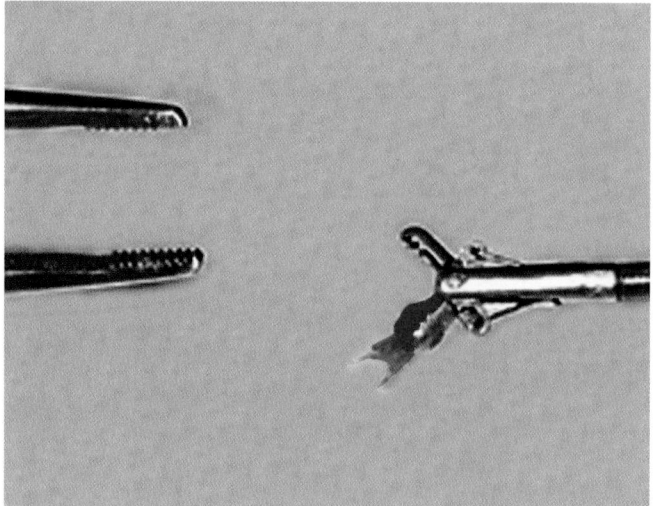

Figure 2-4. Bronchoscopic biopsy. Removing the specimen from the device with fine-tipped forceps is not advised. Alternatively, a sterile needle can be used.

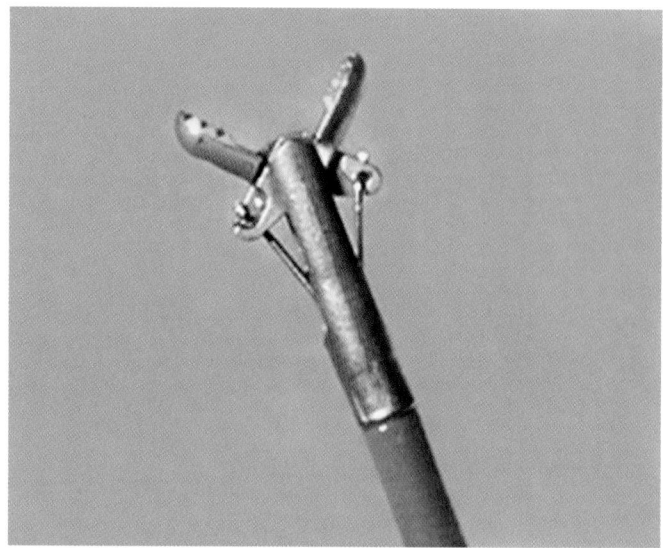

Figure 2-7. Transbronchial biopsy. The cupped biopsy forceps with open jaws is commonly used for transbronchial biopsy.

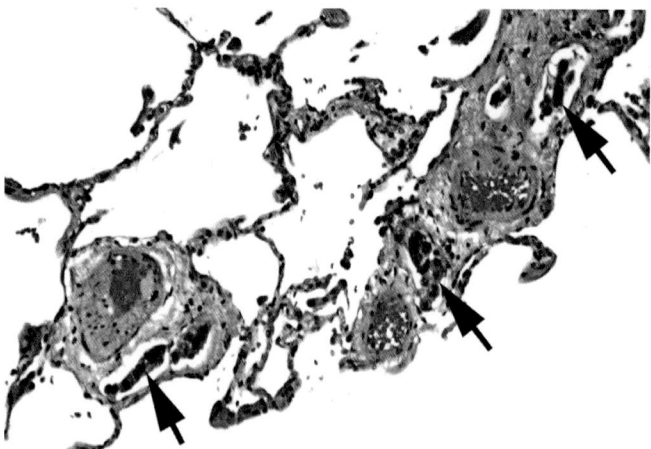

Figure 2-5. Lymphangitic carcinoma. Transbronchial biopsy specimen showing lymphangitic carcinoma (*arrows*) in dilated lymphatic channels included in the sample.

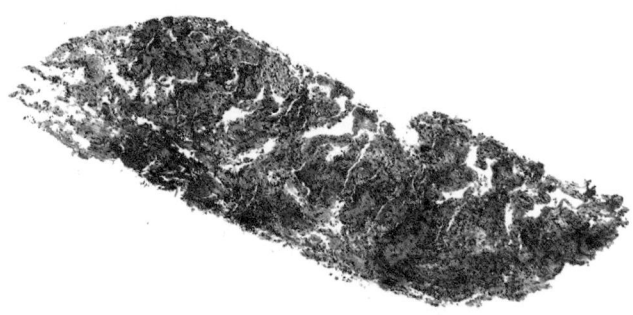

Figure 2-8. Transbronchial biopsy. Low-magnification image of a transbronchial biopsy specimen of generous size.

forcing the bronchiolar wall and peribronchiolar lung parenchyma into the mouth of the device. The successful parenchymal biopsy specimen appears finely ragged (Fig. 2-8) and usually measures between 2 and 3 mm in diameter.[26–28]

As with endobronchial samples, the transbronchial sample is teased from the forceps with a sterile needle, and the same precautions are advised to avoid damage during handling and transfer to fixative or other solution. The truncated pipette technique also is useful in this setting. Once processed, both types of biopsy specimens should be serially sectioned for thorough microscopic evaluation.[2]

Bronchial Brushings

Visualized lesions of the airway epithelium can be sampled for cytologic evaluation.[8,11,16] The technique involves the use of a conical bristle brush (Fig. 2-9). Under direct visualization, the brush is agitated against the mucosal surface of the airway, forcing cells into the interstices of the bristles (Fig. 2-10). The brush is removed from the bronchoscope and can be applied directly to glass slides. Cells and secretions smeared on slides can be immediately fixed for cytologic evaluation using the Papanicolaou staining method or air-dried for use with the Wright-Giemsa staining technique (this choice is best made in consultation with the pathologist). Immediate fixation of slides is best accomplished by direct immersion in 95% alcohol immediately after smearing of the sample on the slide. Each fixation and staining technique produces characteristic artifacts, and the use of one over the other depends on operator training and preference.

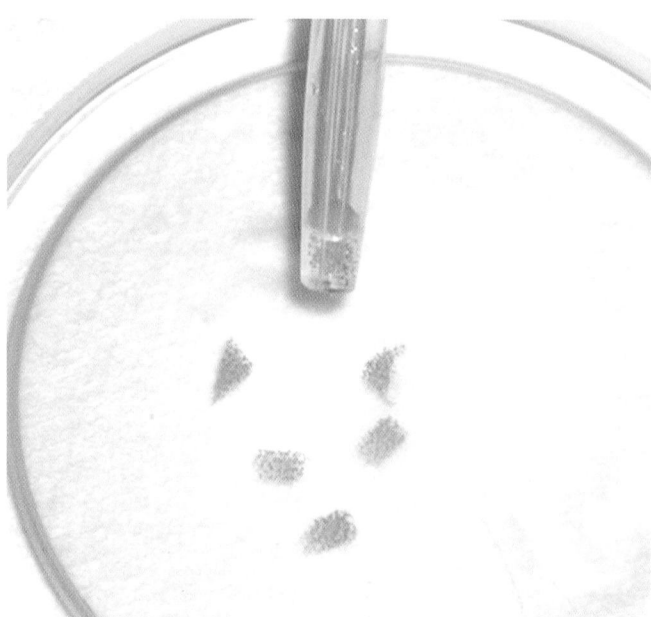

Figure 2-6. Transferring biopsy specimens. For the pipette transfer method, the pipette tip is cut off to provide a wider orifice.

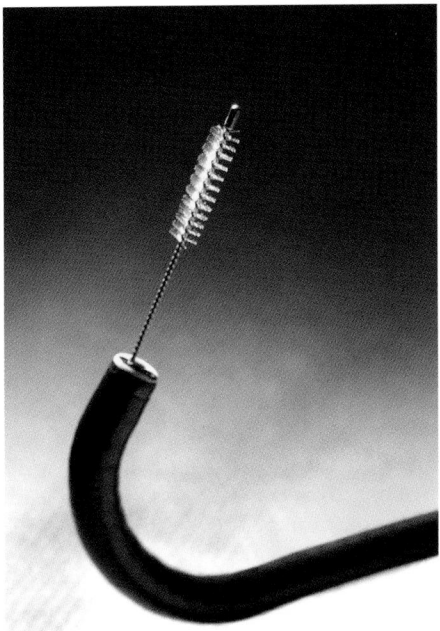

Figure 2-9. Bronchial brush. The conical bronchial bristle brush.

Bronchial Washings and Bronchoalveolar Lavage

Bronchial washings and bronchoalveolar lavage (BAL) specimens are less "lesion-directed" sampling techniques and rely on the presence of shed cells within the airways and more peripheral lung.[11,31-35] Bronchial washings are obtained by aspiration of sterile saline solution applied near the tip of the bronchoscope (Fig. 2-11). The washings consist of

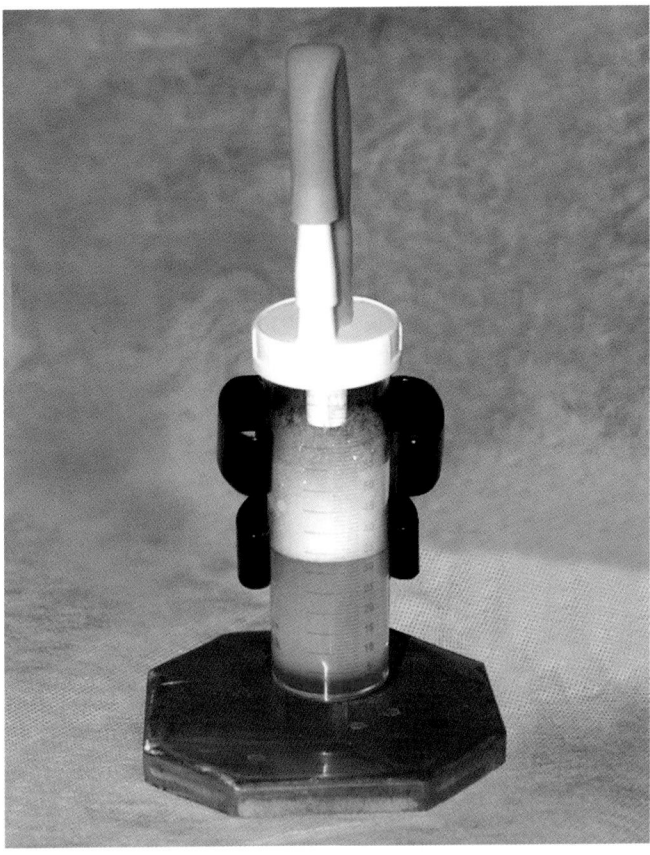

Figure 2-11. Bronchial washings. Bronchial washings are obtained by aspiration of sterile saline solution applied near the tip of the bronchoscope. The sample is limited in size and has a variably blood-tinged, frothy appearance.

If slides are not available for smear preparations, the brush can be cut off and placed directly into a small vial of sterile saline, which is then shaken vigorously to dislodge cells into the fluid. This fluid sample of suspended cells is sent to the laboratory for millipore filtration or cytocentrifuge-type application onto slides,[8,11,16,29,30] analogous to the handling of washings and lavage specimens, discussed next. With ever-increasing demands for molecular genetic information for use in patient management (typically in the setting of malignant tumor), aliquoting this liquid suspension of cells and saving a portion of it in collaboration with the local pathologist is advisable and may avoid the need for resampling of tumor in cases in which surgical tumor removal is not an option.

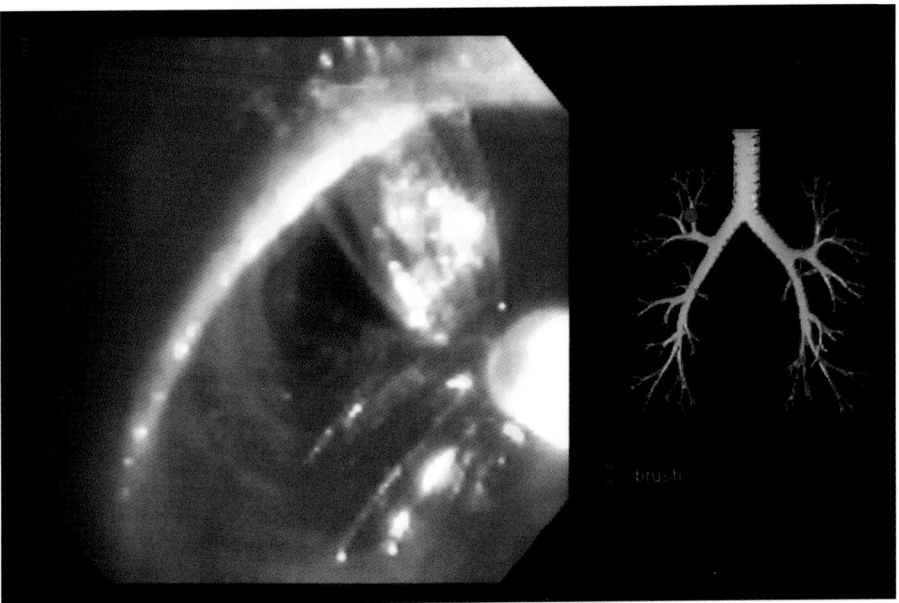

Figure 2-10. Bronchial brushing. Application of the brush to the airway mucosa.

a rather concentrated cellular preparation of bronchial epithelial cells and macrophages with variable amounts of inflammatory cells and mucus. Because of the relatively small sample volume (as with the bronchial brush sample when this is placed into solution), a limited number of assays can be performed on the bronchial washing specimen. Cytologic examination and cultures are the most commonly ordered tests on these samples. If a diagnosis of tumor is likely, saving an aliquot for special studies is prudent. If initial aliquots are judged to be nondiagnostic, the saved sample can be recruited.

BAL, by contrast, retrieves a large volume of saline that is injected into the airways, allowing more extensive sampling of lung parenchyma and airway luminal secretions. Cell density in the fluid typically is low, and centrifuge or filter techniques are required for microscopic examination.

The lavage procedure is performed by instilling multiple aliquots of sterile saline (20–50 mL), followed, after a variable dwell time, by subsequent aspiration of this fluid into a flask or syringe at the bedside. BAL fluid from normal lungs consists primarily of macrophages with a few inflammatory cells[34] (Fig. 2-12). A potential advantage of BAL over the bronchial washing technique is the capability to analyze noncellular elements included, such as surfactant content, serum proteins (e.g., albumin, immunoglobulins, enzymes), and mucus.[36,37] In current practice, the BAL technique is used primarily in the clinical setting for the diagnosis of infection in the immunocompromised host.[36,38–41] As a research tool in the study of interstitial lung diseases, however, BAL has been used extensively for quantitation of cellular components.[19,28,36,42–44]

In processing the BAL fluid, the operator must determine what types of analysis will be performed in advance. A typical sample might be divided into a number of aliquots, some of which would be sent to the cytopathology laboratory, whereas others would be handled by the general laboratory (microbiology, chemistry, hematology). For cytopathology evaluation, the bronchial washing smears and cytocentrifuge preparations can be air-dried for the Wright-Giemsa staining method. More commonly, in the United States, smears are fixed in an equal volume of either Saccomanno's fixative (2% Carbowax and 50% ethyl alcohol) or simply 50% (or greater) ethyl alcohol solution. These fixed smears are then stained using the Papanicolaou method or other staining techniques.

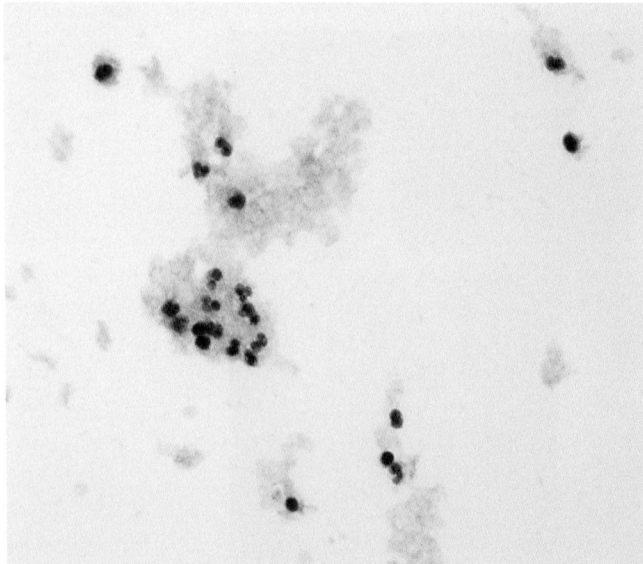

Figure 2-12. Bronchoalveolar lavage. A lavage fluid sample with macrophages and neutrophils. (ThinPrep, Papanicolaou stain.)

Transbronchial Fine-Needle Aspiration

Transbronchial fine-needle aspiration (TBNA) initially was introduced by Wang and Terry in 1983[45] as a staging tool in the evaluation of patients with lung cancer. The use of TBNA has expanded considerably since that time[46–48] for the diagnosis of both central and peripheral lung lesions, even in the absence of endobronchial abnormalities.[48] Endoscopic ultrasound imaging has increased the accuracy of TBNA in recent years and is becoming a standard part of the TBNA procedure in many settings.[49–51] The specimens generated by this technique are very small, sometimes no more than a drop or two, and when the target is solid tissue, these samples consist of thick cellular material. To prepare direct smear preparations for cytopathologic evaluation and rapid stains for organisms, the needle is removed from the syringe (or other aspiration device) and then reattached after air has been aspirated into the syringe. The air is then rapidly forced out through the needle tip, forcing the sample out of the needle hub and onto a slide. Alternatively, a drop can be expressed directly onto a slide (close to the label end) and smeared using a feathering technique (Fig. 2-13). The slide smear is then either air-dried or immediately fixed before staining. For microbiology cultures or fluid-based cytocentrifuge preparations, the needle is rinsed directly into culture or cytopathology fixative medium, respectively.

Rigid Bronchoscopy

Rigid bronchoscopy is a procedure that has been used for more than 125 years.[52,53] With the introduction of the flexible bronchoscope, use of rigid bronchoscopy has declined, but some lesions are more readily biopsied using this device, especially when larger quantities of tissue are required[53,54] (Fig. 2-14). The procedure requires use of general anesthesia and expertise in airway management. Large fragments of tumor (or foreign bodies) can be removed and cautery can be applied to control any bleeding encountered. For large, highly vascular, or mostly necrotic tumors, this may be the most prudent and useful procedure for obtaining diagnostic specimens.

Specimens Obtained by Transthoracic Needle Biopsy and Aspiration

Thoracentesis

Thoracentesis derives its greatest practical application in the evaluation of pleural effusion samples for cells and noncellular elements.[55–57] As with BAL fluid examination, a number of specific analyses typically are performed. If collected after hours, the sterile thoracentesis fluid can be stored unfixed at 4°C for processing the next day. The aliquoted thoracentesis fluid specimens are distributed to the appropriate laboratory for analysis (e.g., microbiology, chemistry, hematology). Chemical determinations of glucose, amylase, lactate dehydrogenase, and other analytes are compared with cellular composition determined by cytopathology evaluation. The cytocentrifuge or millipore filter also can be evaluated cytopathologically for the presence of malignant neoplasm. Rapid stains for microorganisms can be performed as indicated.

Closed Pleural Biopsy

Available pleural needle biopsy devices include the Cope, Abrams, and Tru-Cut needles that produce a very small biopsy sample (Fig. 2-15). Inflammatory, infectious, and neoplastic diseases of the pleura can be diagnosed using these devices, despite the limitations of biopsy size and somewhat randomness of sampling.[58] These small specimens should be handled in a fashion analogous to those obtained from bronchoscopic biopsy techniques (as described previously).

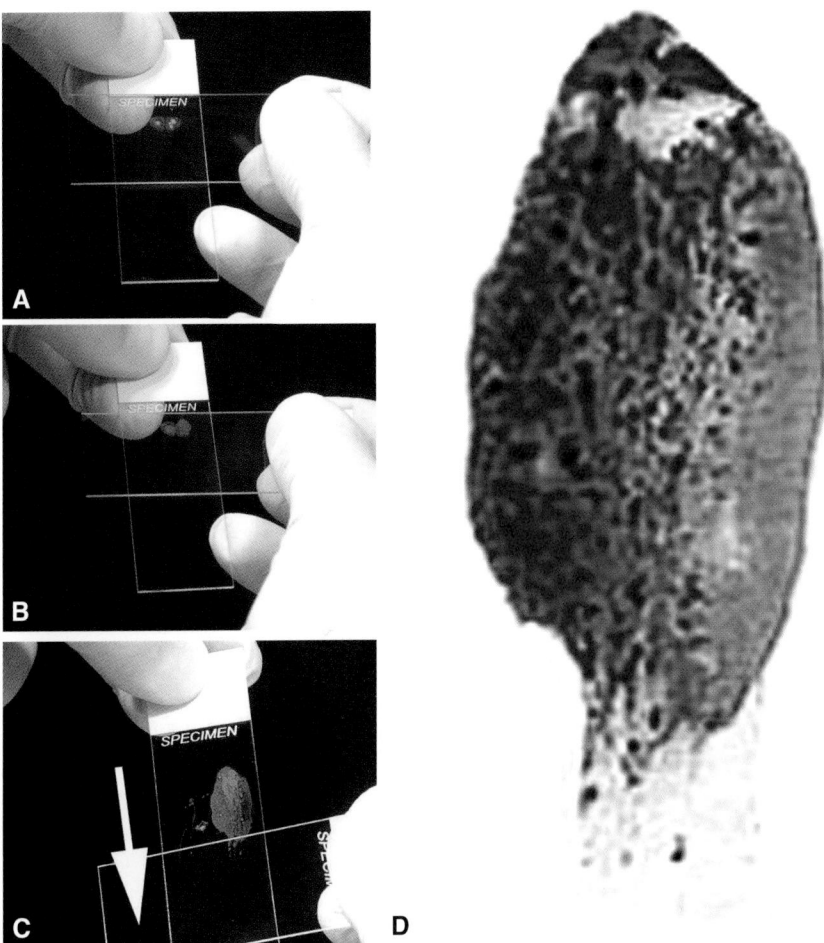

Figure 2-13. Preparing direct cytologic smears from small tissue or fluid samples. The optimal technique for making cytology smears from scrapings or needle aspiration is illustrated. **A,** A small amount of sample is placed on the slide near the specimen label end, and a second slide is brought up next to the sample at right angle to the sample slide. **B,** Once the sample is contacted by the right-angle slide, this "feathering" slide is flattened slightly while pulled forward in a smooth motion toward the operator, as seen in part **C.** The feathered smear can be fixed immediately or allowed to air-dry, depending on the staining technique chosen. **D,** The ideal smear is oval in shape. The specimen shown was stained with the toluidine blue rapid method. (Smear technique courtesy of Dr. Matthew Zarka, Mayo Clinic, Scottsdale, AZ.)

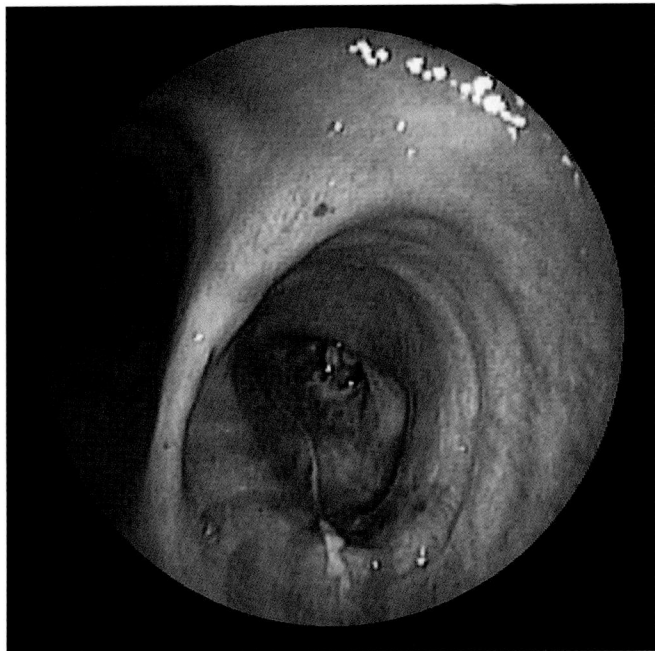

Figure 2-14. Rigid bronchoscopy. A large obstructing tumor mass is well visualized.

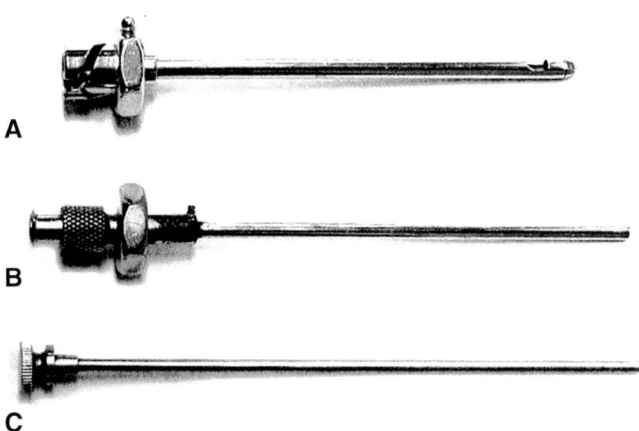

Figure 2-15. Pleural biopsy. **A,** The Abrams pleural biopsy needle consists of an outer trocar with a blunt tip and a side cutting port near the tip (right). The trocar is pulled across the parietal pleural edge, hooking this tissue into the side port. **B,** The inner cutting cannula is then forced across the cutting port from within, following along a spiral guide path seen on the left end of the outer sheath. **C,** The stylet keeps the needle channel closed during initial insertion into the pleural space thereby avoiding the creation of a pneumothorax.

Transthoracic Fine-Needle Core Aspiration and Biopsy of the Lung

In current practice, the use of transthoracic needle aspiration biopsy has become commonplace.[10,59–64] This procedure typically is performed in the radiology department, because biopsy by this method is always performed under radiologic guidance. Samples are similar to those obtained by transbronchial needle aspiration and should be handled accordingly (as discussed previously). Assistance from a cytotechnologist during the procedure is a cost-effective benefit to ensure adequacy of the specimen before termination of the procedure.[65] Recent advances in needle biopsy devices have allowed for better tissue samples and greater likelihood of accurate diagnosis.[66–69] If the technique generates a semiliquid sample, this should be handled as described for transbronchial needle aspiration specimens. If a core of tissue is generated (typically 1 mm in diameter), this can be processed like other needle core samples received in surgical pathology. In addition to routine hematoxylin and eosin–stained sections and any number of sectioning levels that typically are obtained for routine evaluation, the histology laboratory also should make four to six unstained sections (mounted on slides designed for immunohistochemical stains) at the time of initial sectioning in histology. Having these extra sections available saves time and avoids having to return to the tissue block later when special stains may be necessary, which can be a problem because block resurfacing between sectioning wastes a certain amount of tissue.

Specimens Obtained by Thoracoscopy

Surgical biopsy of lung parenchyma is indicated in several specific situations:

- A target judged to be too small to permit biopsy by interventional radiologic techniques[70,71]
- Peripheral lesions that have eluded endobronchial biopsy attempts[1,13]
- Suspected interstitial and inflammatory lung disease[14,15]

The introduction of a high-resolution video endoscopic system has changed the practice of elective thoracic surgery. With this procedure, smaller incisions are made and a thoracoscope with a video camera is introduced along with the instruments (Fig. 2-16). Video-assisted thoracic surgery (VATS) has become the standard of care for obtaining most surgical biopsy specimens. It has been used in the diagnosis and treatment of pulmonary diseases since the early 1990s.[72–75] The mortality rate is low, duration of hospital stay is decreased, and patient recovery is hastened in comparison with standard thoracotomy.[73] Specimens measuring 2 to 3 cm across and larger (Fig. 2-17) are easily obtained, and patients often can be discharged from the hospital less than 24 hours. With VATS, the same thoracic access ports also provide access for sampling ipsilateral lymph nodes that may contain neoplastic disease or other abnormalities.

Although it confers undeniable benefits, VATS usually requires the collapse of one lung, so all conditions that contradict this

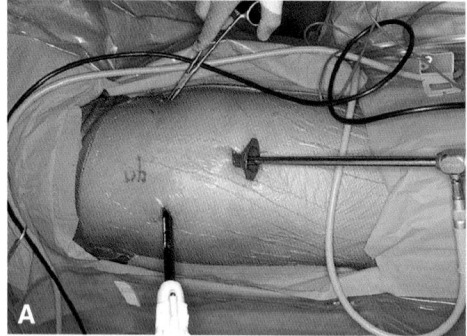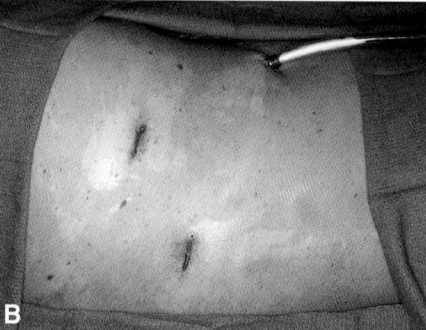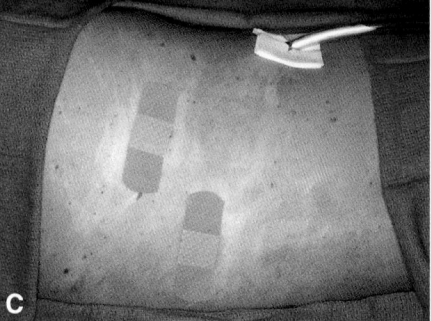

Figure 2-16. Video-assisted thoracoscopic surgery. **A,** Three incisions are made for instruments: video scope, stapler, and manipulator device. The sutured incisions are small (**B**) and require minimal dressing (**C**). The drain, seen at *upper right* in parts **B** and **C,** will be removed later.

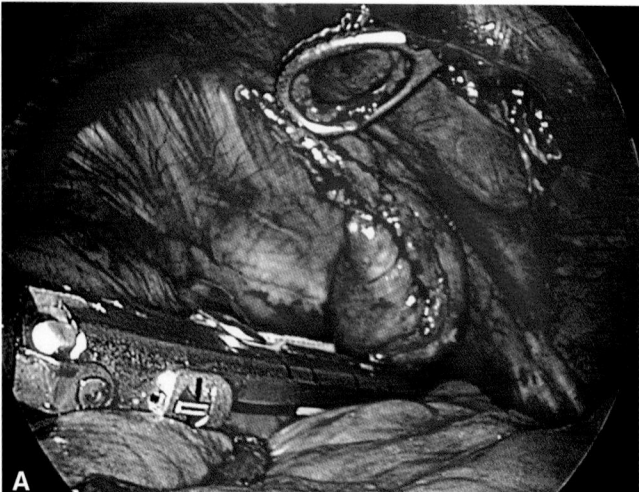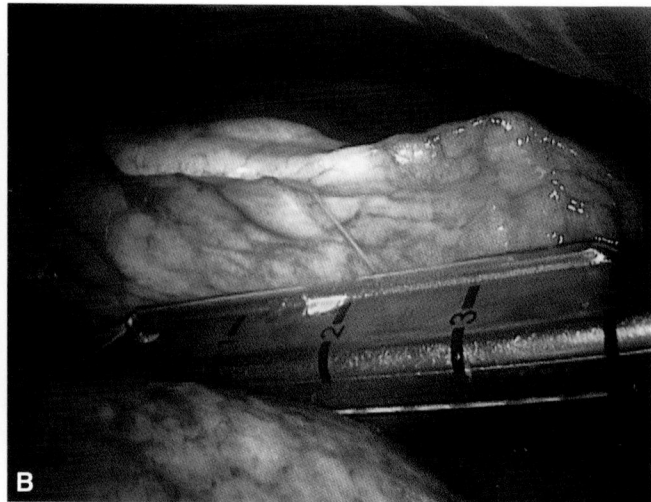

Figure 2-17. Video-assisted thoracoscopic surgery. **A,** Videoscopic view of lung and parietal chest wall, with the lung tissue selected for biopsy (*center*) held while the stapler isolates this tissue from surrounding lung. The double staple line produced allows safe surgical incision for removal. **B,** A closer view of the stapling process.

maneuver may prevent use of this approach. Tumor deposition and dissemination can be prevented by adherence to well-established oncologic surgical principles.[76,77] Meticulous technique is required to avoid laceration of tumor during excision and contamination of the distant pleura or lung by the instruments. The use of an impermeable "endocatch" bag for specimen retrieval is mandatory (Fig. 2-18). A sterile lavage of all port sites also is done at the conclusion of surgery.

Before any wedge lung biopsy is performed, consultation among the radiologist, chest physician, and thoracic surgeon is essential to ensure appropriate sampling and the identification of ideal locations for biopsy. These considerations are especially important for the investigation of interstitial lung disease, and in patients suspected of having idiopathic pulmonary fibrosis, in which disease tends to localize to the lower lobes. Retrieval of tissue from more than one biopsy site is necessary, preferably from widely separated areas or different lobes. In the ideal scenario, such determinations are based on best surgical judgment combined with the specific characteristics of the disease as identified on clinical and radiologic grounds.

Specimen Processing

Processing of the wedge lung biopsy specimen requires techniques different from those used in handling specimens from other organs. A typical surgical lung biopsy specimen as it is received from surgery is shown in Figure 2-19. If the wedge tissue sample is to be divided for different types of analysis (e.g., microbiological cultures, electron microscopy, molecular diagnostic studies), these portions can be separated before routine processing for morphologic assessment. Preparing frozen sections from air-filled lung tissue poses some special problems. Unfixed lung tissue is easily compressed, especially when attempts are made to slice it into thin (typically less than 5 mm) sections unfixed. Severe compression may result in artifactual atelectasis, thereby compounding the difficulty of histopathologic assessment. The simplest and most reliable technique for preparing frozen sections is to cut a 5- to 6-mm slab from the biopsy specimen using a fresh scalpel and freezing it without further preparation. For most lung diseases, the frozen sections generated this way are reasonably interpretable. Alternatively, some authors have recommended injecting the actual slab section (not the whole biopsy) with a stabilizing solution before freezing. To accomplish this, a dilute solution of embedding compound can be gently infused into the cut surface of the slab using a 21- to 23-gauge needle attached to a 5-mL syringe.

After any intraoperative consultation has been completed, the remainder of the specimen can be prepared for processing using a number of techniques, all designed to restore the normal inflated state of the tissue (VATS specimens are received deflated and stapled closed). We prefer a simple technique that is as good as either of the two more elaborate methods also described here and requires no special equipment or needles: After all staples have been removed from the sample, the specimen is vigorously shaken for 2 minutes in a container half-filled with fixative solution (appropriately sealed with paraffin film). This maneuver forces the sample repeatedly against the inner walls of the container and nicely distributes fixative within the elastic lung parenchyma. In most instances, atelectatic areas are fully restored. A second technique uses a small volume of carbonated water added to the fixative solution to assist in reexpansion of alveoli (no agitation required). Finally, some authors have proposed using a small-gauge needle and syringe to gently reinflate the sample with fixative. This procedure should be performed only after the staples have been removed from the sample to avoid overinflation. Injection into the cut lung surface is preferable to injecting through the pleural surface (Fig. 2-20A). After fixation of 1 to 2 hours, the specimen can be safely and easily sliced into 3- to 5-mm sections for final processing (see Fig. 2-20B).

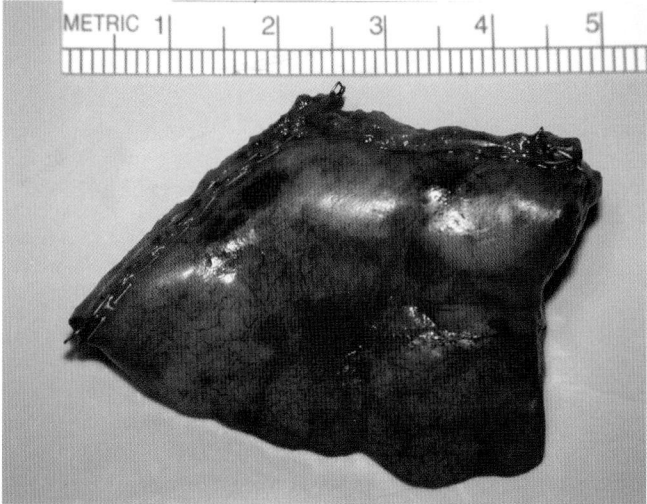

Figure 2-19. Optimal surgical lung biopsy. The surgical wedge specimen should measure 3–5 cm in length and 3 cm in depth (from pleural surface to the stapled edge at specimen midpoint).

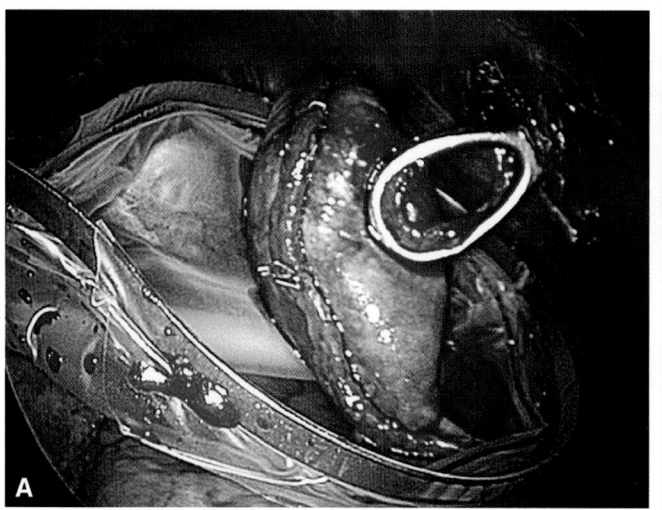
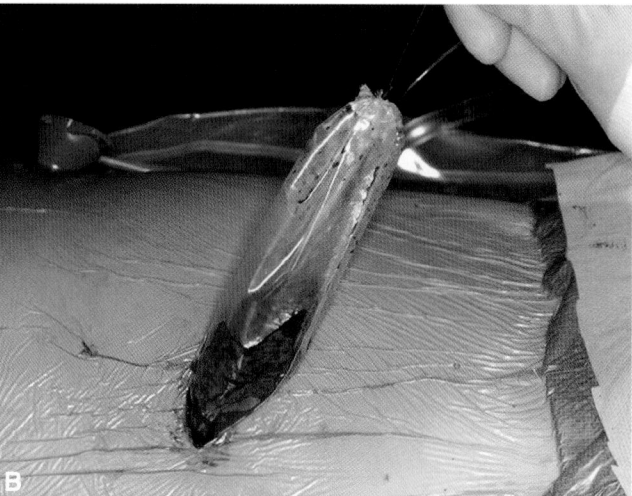

Figure 2-18. Video-assisted thoracoscopic surgery. The biopsy specimen is transferred into a specimen bag (**A**) for safe retrieval through the incision (**B**).

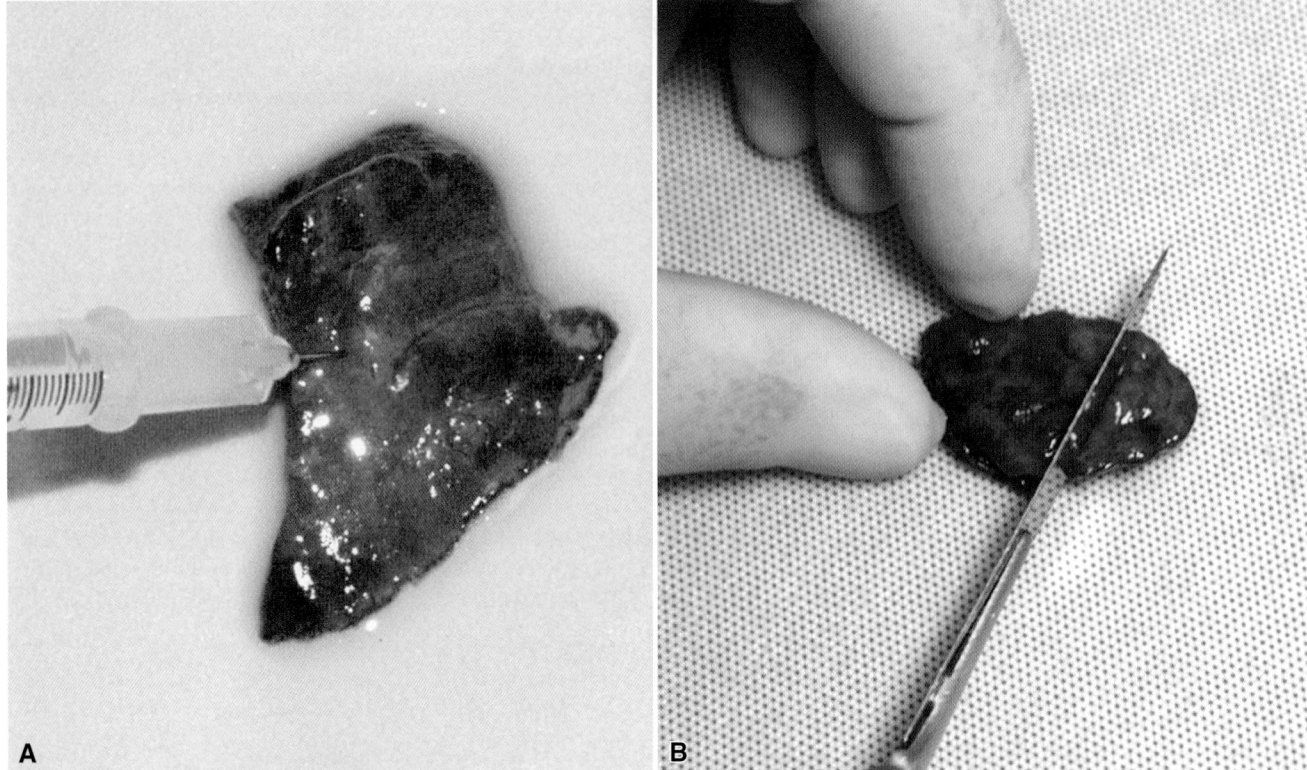

Figure 2-20. Fixation and sectioning of the surgical wedge biopsy specimen. **A,** A tuberculin syringe (with a 23- to 25-gauge needle) can be used for inflating lung wedge biopsy specimens through the cut lung surface after the surgical staples are removed. **B,** Once the specimen has been shaken in or injected with fixative, submersion in the fixative solution for an additional 1–2 hours improves gross section quality and avoids reintroducing atelectactic changes.

Conclusions

Liberal communication among the chest physician, radiologist, pathologist, and thoracic surgeon is strongly advised before embarking on any lung biopsy procedure, especially those associated with procurement of wedge biopsy specimens. Such a multidisciplinary approach is cost-effective and increases the likelihood of accurate results.

Self-assessment questions related to this chapter can be found online on the Expert Consult site for this title.

References

1. Mikel U, ed. *Advanced Laboratory Methods in Histology and Pathology.* Washington, DC: American Registry of Pathology; 1994.
2. Nagata N, Hirano H, Takayama K, et al. Step section preparation of transbronchial lung biopsy. Significance in the diagnosis of diffuse lung disease. *Chest.* 1991;100:959–962.
3. Bonetti F, Chiodera PL, Pea M, et al. Transbronchial biopsy in lymphangiomyomatosis of the lung. HMB45 for diagnosis. *Am J Surg Pathol.* 1993;17:1092–1102.
4. Chastre J, Fagon JY, Soler P, et al. Diagnosis of nosocomial bacterial pneumonia in intubated patients undergoing ventilation: comparison of the usefulness of bronchoalveolar lavage and the protected specimen brush. *Am J Med.* 1988;85:499–506.
5. Miller R, Nelems B, Müller NL, et al. Lingular and right middle lobe biopsy in the assessment of diffuse lung disease. *Ann Thorac Surg.* 1987;44:269–273.
6. Rosen P. Frozen section management of a lung biopsy for suspected *Pneumocystis* pneumonia. *Am J Surg Pathol.* 1977;1:79–82.
7. Travis W, Borok Z, Roum JH, et al. Pulmonary Langerhans cell granulomatosis (histiocytosis X). A clinicopathologic study of 48 cases. *Am J Surg Pathol.* 1993;17:971–986.
8. Zavala D. Diagnostic fiberoptic bronchoscopy: techniques and results of biopsy in 600 patients. *Chest.* 1975;68:12–19.
9. Churg A. An inflation procedure for open-lung biopsies. *Am J Surg Pathol.* 1983;7:69–71.
10. Yang P, Lee YC, Yu CJ, et al. Ultrasonographically guided biopsy of thoracic tumors. A comparison of large-bore cutting biopsy with fine-needle aspiration. *Cancer.* 1992;69:2553–2560.
11. Popp W, Rauscher H, Ritschka L, et al. Diagnostic sensitivity of different techniques in the diagnosis of lung tumors with the flexible fiberoptic bronchoscope. Comparison of brush biopsy, imprint cytology of forceps biopsy, and histology of forceps biopsy. *Cancer.* 1991;67:72–75.
12. Burt ME, Flye MW, Webber BL, Wesley RA. Prospective evaluation of aspiration needle, cutting needle, transbronchial and open lung biopsy in patients with pulmonary infiltrates. *Ann Thorac Surg.* 1981;32:146–153.
13. Leslie KO, Lanza LA, Helmers RA, Colby TV. Diagnostic sampling of lung tissues and cells. In: Davis G, Marcey T, Seward E, eds. *Medical Management of Pulmonary Diseases.* New York: Marcel Dekker; 1999:213–220.
14. Leslie K, Colby T. Classification and pathology of diffuse interstitial lung disease. *Semin Clin Immunol.* 1999;1:7–15.
15. Leslie K, Colby T, Swensen S. Anatomic distribution and histopathologic patterns in interstitial lung disease. In: Schwarz M, King TJ, eds. *Interstitial lung disease.* Hamilton: BC Decker; 2002:31–50.
16. Mitchell D, Emerson CJ, Collins JV, Stableforth DE. Transbronchial lung biopsy with the fibreoptic bronchoscope: analysis of results in 433 patients. *Br J Dis Chest.* 1981;75:258–262.
17. Kovnat DM, Rath GS, Anderson WM, Snider G. Maximal extent of visualization of bronchial tree by flexible fiberoptic bronchoscopy. *Am Rev Respir Dis.* 1974;110(1):88–90.
18. Joos L, Patuto N, Chhajed PN, Tamm M. Diagnostic yield of flexible bronchoscopy in current clinical practice. *Swiss Med Wkly.* 2006;136(9–10):155–159.
19. Haslam P, Turton CW, Heard B, et al. Bronchoalveolar lavage in pulmonary fibrosis: comparison of cells obtained with lung biopsy and clinical features. *Thorax.* 1980;35:9–18.
20. Delvenne P, Arrese JE, Thiry A, et al. Detection of cytomegalovirus, *Pneumocystis carinii,* and *Aspergillus* species in bronchoalveolar lavage fluid. A comparison of techniques. *Am J Clin Pathol.* 1993;100:414–418.
21. Guinee Jr DG, Feuerstein I, Koss MN, Travis WD. Pulmonary lymphangioleiomyomatosis. Diagnosis based on results of transbronchial biopsy and immunohistochemical studies and correlation with high-resolution computed tomography findings. *Arch Pathol Lab Med.* 1994;118:846–849.
22. Colby TV, Swensen SJ. Anatomic distribution and histopathologic patterns in diffuse lung disease: correlation with HRCT. *J Thorac Imaging.* 1996;11(1):1–26.
23. Popovich Jr J, Kvale PA, Eichenhorn MS, et al. Diagnostic accuracy of multiple biopsies from flexible fiberoptic bronchoscopy. A comparison of central versus peripheral carcinoma. *Am Rev Respir Dis.* 1982;125:521–523.
24. Gilman M, Wang K. Transbronchial lung biopsy in sarcoidosis: an approach to determine the optimal number of biopsies. *Am Rev Respir Dis.* 1980;122:721–724.

25. Flint A, Martinez FJ, Young ML, et al. Influence of sample number and biopsy site on the histologic diagnosis of diffuse lung disease. *Ann Thorac Surg.* 1995;60:1605–1607.

26. Andersen H. Transbronchoscopic lung biopsy for diffuse pulmonary diseases. Results in 939 patients. *Chest.* 1978;73(suppl 5):734–736.

27. Cazzadori A, Di Perri G, Todeschini G, et al. Transbronchial biopsy in the diagnosis of pulmonary infiltrates in immunocompromised patients. *Chest.* 1995;107(1):101–106.

28. Guilinger R, Paradis IL, Dauber JH, et al. The importance of bronchoscopy with transbronchial biopsy and bronchoalveolar lavage in the management of lung transplant recipients. *Am J Respir Crit Care Med.* 1995;152:2037–2043.

29. Willcox M, Kervitsky A, Watters LC, King Jr TE, et al. Quantification of cells recovered by bronchoalveolar lavage. Comparison of cytocentrifuge preparations with the filter method. *Am Rev Respir Dis.* 1988;138(1):74–80.

30. Robb J, Melello C, Odom C. Comparison of Cyto-Shuttle and cytocentrifuge as processing methods for nongynecologic cytology specimens. *Diagn Cytopathol.* 1996;14(4):305–309.

31. Poletti V, Romagna M, Allen KA, et al. Bronchoalveolar lavage in the diagnosis of disseminated lung tumors. *Acta Cytol.* 1995;39:472–477.

32. Winterbauer R, Lammert J, Selland M, et al. Bronchoalveolar lavage cell populations in the diagnosis of sarcoidosis. *Chest.* 1993;104:352–361.

33. The BAL Cooperative Steering Committee. Bronchoalveolar lavage constituents in healthy individuals, idiopathic pulmonary fibrosis, and selected comparison groups. *Am Rev Respir Dis.* 1990;141:S169–S202.

34. Merchant R, Schwartz DA, Helmers RA, et al. Bronchoalveolar lavage cellularity. The distribution in normal volunteers. *Am Rev Respir Dis.* 1992;146:448–453.

35. Cobben N, Jacobs JA, van Dieijen-Visser MP, et al. Diagnostic value of BAL fluid cellular profile and enzymes in infectious pulmonary disorders. *Eur Respir J.* 1999;14:496–502.

36. American Thoracic Society Statement. Clinical role of bronchoalveolar lavage in adults with pulmonary disease. *Am Rev Respir Dis.* 2001;142:481–486.

37. Reynolds HY, Fulmer JD, Kazmierowski JA, et al. Analysis of cellular and protein content of broncho-alveolar lavage fluid from patients with idiopathic pulmonary fibrosis and chronic hypersensitivity pneumonitis. *J Clin Invest.* 1977;59(1):165–175.

38. Abramson MJ, Stone CA, Holmes PW, Tai EH. The role of bronchoalveolar lavage in the diagnosis of suspected opportunistic pneumonia. *Aust N Z J Med.* 1987;17(4):407–412.

39. Bye M, Bernstein L, Shah K, et al. Diagnostic bronchoalveolar lavage in children with AIDS. *Pediatr Pulmonol.* 1987;3:425–428.

40. Kahn FW, Jones JM. Diagnosing bacterial respiratory infection by bronchoalveolar lavage. *J Infect Dis.* 1987;155:862–869.

41. Martin II WJ, Smith TF, Sanderson DR, et al. Role of bronchoalveolar lavage in the assessment of opportunistic pulmonary infections: utility and complications. *Mayo Clin Proc.* 1987;62:549–557.

42. Goldstein RA, Rohatgi PK, Bergofsky EH, et al. Clinical role of bronchoalveolar lavage in adults with pulmonary disease. *Am Rev Respir Dis.* 1990;142:481–486.

43. Hunninghake GW, et al. Inflammatory and immune processes in the human lung in health and disease: evaluation by bronchoalveolar lavage. *Am J Pathol.* 1979;97:149–206.

44. Kvale PA. Bronchoscopic biopsies and bronchoalveolar lavage. *Chest Surg Clin N Am.* 1996;6(2):205–222.

45. Wang K, Terry P. Transbronchial needle aspiration in the diagnosis and staging of bronchogenic carcinoma. *Am Rev Respir Dis.* 1983;127(3):344–347.

46. Rosenthal D, Wallace J. Fine-needle aspiration of pulmonary lesions via fiberoptic bronchoscopy. *Acta Cytol.* 1984;28:203–210.

47. Wagner ED, Ramzy I, Greenberg SD, Gonzalez JM. Transbronchial fine-needle aspiration. Reliability and limitations. *Am J Clin Pathol.* 1989;92:36–41.

48. Mehta AC, Kavuru MS, Meeker DP, et al. Transbronchial needle aspiration for histology specimens. *Chest.* 1989;96:1228–1232.

49. Eloubeidi MA. Endoscopic ultrasound-guided fine-needle aspiration in the staging and diagnosis of patients with lung cancer. *Semin Thorac Cardiovasc Surg.* 2007;19(3):206–211.

50. Vilmann P, Puri R. The complete "medical" mediastinoscopy (EUS-FNA + EBUS-TBNA). *Min Med.* 2007;98(4):331–338.

51. Zias N, Chroneou A, Gonzalez AV, et al. Changing patterns in interventional bronchoscopy. *Respirology.* 2009;14(4):595–600.

52. Helmers RA, Sanderson DR. Rigid bronchoscopy. The forgotten art. *Clin Chest Med.* 1995;16(3):393–399.

53. Melo N, Salero S, Fernandes G, et al. Rigid bronchoscopy—a 2.5 year experience. *Rev Port Pneumol.* 2006;6(suppl 1):30–31.

54. Chao YK, Liu YH, Hsieh MJ, et al. Controlling difficult airway by rigid bronchoscope—an old but effective method. *Interact Cardiovasc Thorac Surg.* 2005;4(3):175–179.

55. Berquist TH, Bailey PB, Cortese DA, Miller WE. Transthoracic needle biopsy: accuracy and complications in relation to location and type of lesion. *Mayo Clin Proc.* 1980;55(8):475–481.

56. Crosby JH, Hager B, Hoeg K. Transthoracic fine-needle aspiration. Experience in a cancer center. *Cancer.* 1985;56(10):2504–2507.

57. Larscheid RC, Thorpe PE, Scott WJ. Percutaneous transthoracic needle aspiration biopsy: a comprehensive review of its current role in the diagnosis and treatment of lung tumors. *Chest.* 1998;114(3):704–709.

58. Von Hoff DD, LiVolsi V. Diagnostic reliability of needle biopsy of the parietal pleura. A review of 272 biopsies. *Am J Clin Pathol.* 1975;64(2):200–203.

59. Sanders C. Transthoracic needle aspiration. *Clin Chest Med.* 1992;13(1):11–16.

60. Böcking A, Klose KC, Kyll HJ, Hauptmann S. Cytologic versus histologic evaluation of needle biopsy of the lung, hilum and mediastinum. Sensitivity, specificity and typing accuracy. *Acta Cytol.* 1995;39:463–471.

61. Milman N. Percutaneous lung biopsy with semi-automatic, spring-driven fine needle—preliminary results in 13 patients. *Respiration.* 1993;60:289–291.

62. Smyth R, Carty H, Thomas H, et al. Diagnosis of interstitial lung disease by a percutaneous lung biospy sample. *Arch Dis Child.* 1994;70:143–144.

63. Lohela P, Tikkakoski T, Ammälä K, et al. Diagnosis of diffuse lung disease by cutting needle biopsy. *Acta Radiol.* 1994;35:251–254.

64. Williams A, Santiago S, Lehrman S, Popper R. Transcutaneous needle aspiration of solitary pulmonary masses: how many passes? *Am Rev Respir Dis.* 1987;136:452–454.

65. Nasuti J, Gupta P, Baloch Z. Diagnostic value and cost-effectiveness of on-site evaluation of fine-needle aspiration specimens: review of 5,688 cases. *Diagn Cytopathol.* 2002;27(1):1–4.

66. Zavala DC, Bedell GN. Percutaneous lung biopsy with a cutting needle. An analysis of 40 cases and comparison with other biopsy techniques. *Am Rev Respir Dis.* 1972;106(2):186–193.

67. Zavala DC. The diagnosis of pulmonary disease by nonthoracotomy techniques. *Chest.* 1973;64(1):100–102.

68. Zavala DC, Rossi NP. Nonthoracotomy diagnostic techniques for pulmonary disease. *Arch Surg.* 1973;107(2):152–154.

69. Zavala DC. Pulmonary biopsy. *Adv Intern Med.* 1976;21:21–45.

70. Bernard A. Resection of pulmonary nodules using video-assisted thoracic surgery. The Thorax Group. *Ann Thorac Surg.* 1996;1:202–204, discussion 204–205.

71. Chang AC, Yee J, Orringer MB, Iannettoni MD. Diagnostic thoracoscopic lung biopsy: an outpatient experience. *Ann Thorac Surg.* 2002;74(6):1942–1946, discussion 46–47.

72. Allen MS, Deschamps C, Jones DM, et al. Video-assisted thoracic surgical procedures: the Mayo experience. *Mayo Clin Proc.* 1996;71(4):351–359.

73. Jaklitsch MT, DeCamp Jr MM, Liptay MJ, et al. Video-assisted thoracic surgery in the elderly. A review of 307 cases. *Chest.* 1996;110(3):751–758.

74. Rubin JW, Finney NR, Borders BM, Chauvin EJ. Intrathoracic biopsies, pulmonary wedge excision, and management of pleural disease: is video-assisted closed chest surgery the approach of choice? *Am Surg.* 1994;60(11):860–863.

75. Solaini L, Prusciano F, Bagioni P, et al. Video-assisted thoracic surgery (VATS) of the lung: analysis of intraoperative and postoperative complications over 15 years and review of the literature. *Surg Endosc.* 2008;22(2):298–310.

76. Ang KL, Tan C, Hsin M, Goldstraw P. Intrapleural tumor dissemination after video-assisted thoracoscopic surgery metastasectomy. *Ann Thorac Surg.* 2003;75(5):1643–1645.

77. Anraku M, Nakahara R, Matsuguma H, Yokoi K. Port site recurrence after video-assisted thoracoscopic resection of chest wall schwannoma. *Interact Cardiovasc Thorac Surg.* 2003;2(4):483–485.

Computed Tomography of Diffuse Lung Diseases and Solitary Pulmonary Nodules

Mario Maffessanti, MD, and Giorgia Dalpiaz, MD

Foundations

Living with X-Rays and Working with Computed Tomography

X-Rays and Computed Tomography

Radiology is the science of studying anatomy and pathology using x-rays—electromagnetic waves (like visible light, only with a much shorter wavelength) capable of penetrating the tissues. In computed tomography (CT), the widely recognized imaging standard of reference for assessment of most pulmonary abnormalities, a collimated fan beam of radiation is generated by an x-ray tube inside a gantry (Fig. 3-1).

The beam is quite homogeneous when entering the body (ingoing radiation) but, point by point, inhomogeneous when exiting (outgoing radiation) because of different attenuations produced by the tissues. The attenuation highly depends on the characteristics of the tissue, calcium being at the highest and air at the lowest end of a scale with soft tissue densities (e.g., organs, muscles, blood vessels, interstitium) and fat in between (see Fig. 3-1).

Always point by point, the outgoing radiation activates a matrix of tiny sensible elements (detectors) during a continuous spiral movement of the tube-detectors system around the body (scan), and the information acquired is stored in a computer. At the end of the process, the system contains a digital three-dimensional map of single unitary elements (voxels) composing the scanned volume (see Fig. 3-1).

Computed Tomography, Spiral Computed Tomography, and High-Resolution Computed Tomography

For viewing, CT is able to return the values of a two-dimensional matrix of voxels on a monitor over a scale of grays (gray-scale), where the brightest (white) spots represent the elements with higher attenuation and the darkest (black) the ones of lower attenuation. Although spiral CT is able to show images of equal quality along planes in any direction, the axial (transverse), frontal (coronal), and sagittal (lateral) views are used more commonly (Figs. 3-2 to 3-4). For each view, a stack of images may be seen in sequence simply by browsing at the workstation through the volumetric data set; at the end of the diagnostic process, the entire volume is investigated from multiple points of view.

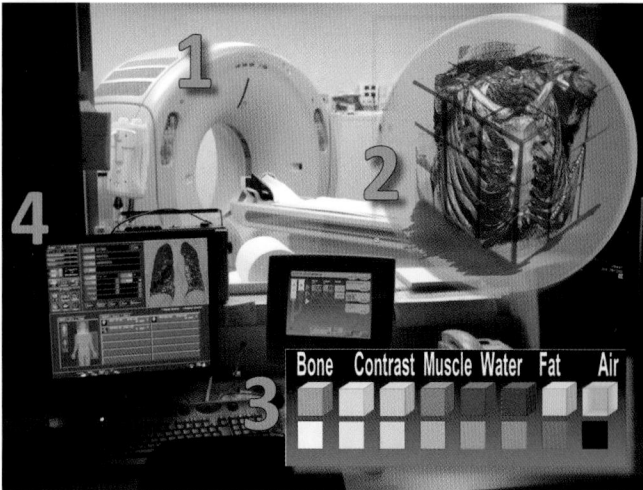

Figure 3-1. The figure summarizes conceptually the steps of a computed tomography examination, from the acquisition of the images in the gantry (1) to their displaying on a monitor (4). In the computer, the information about a set of volume units of body (voxels) (2) is rendered on the monitor on a scale of grays, according to their average attenuation (3).

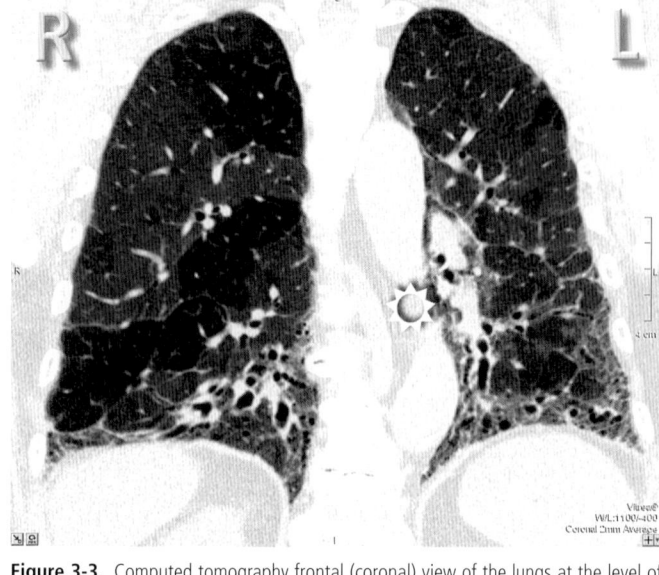

Figure 3-3. Computed tomography frontal (coronal) view of the lungs at the level of the descending aorta (*sun*) (case with lung pathology). Again, the right of the patient is to the left of the viewer. The patient is always seen vis-à-vis. R, right; L, left.

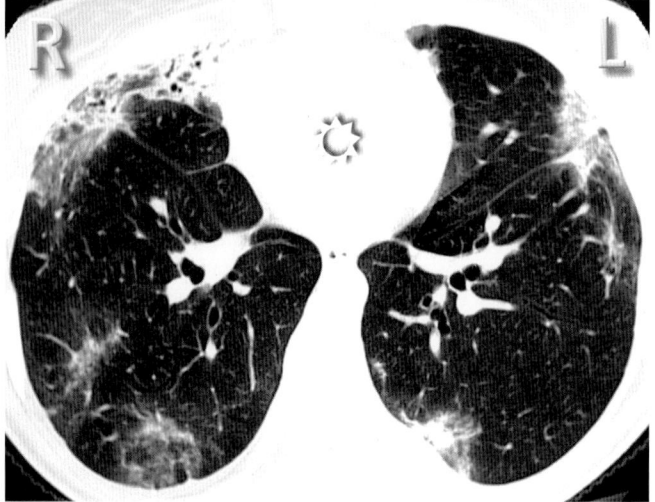

Figure 3-2. Computed tomography transverse (axial) view of the lungs at the level of the heart (*sun*) (case with lung pathology). In the axial images, it is as if the patient were seen from below. Consequently, the right lung is to the left of the viewer. R, right; L, left.

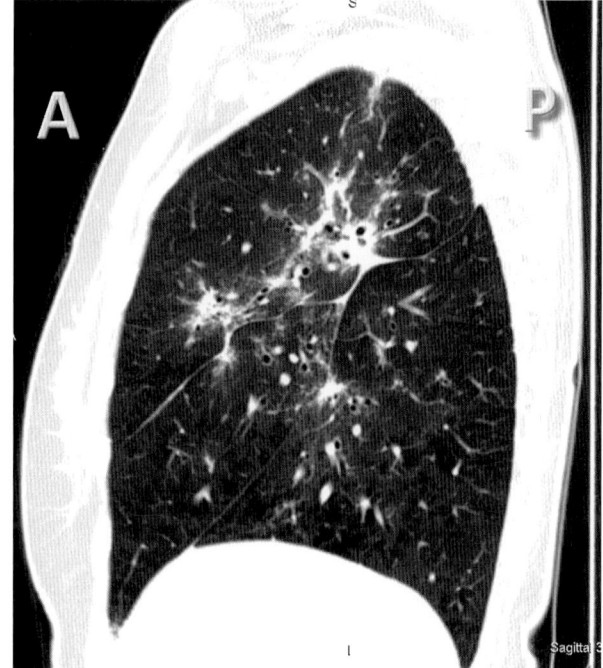

Figure 3-4. Computed tomography sagittal (lateral) view of the right lung (case with lung pathology). In the sagittal images, the anteroposterior and the craniocaudal directions are explored. A, anterior; P, posterior.

With a diffuse lung disease (DLD), the high-resolution option is used. An actual collimation of 0.5 to 2 mm and a high spatial frequency reconstruction algorithm (edge enhancing) generate the final images.[1] The narrow collimation reduces the voxel size, thereby minimizing the averaging of densities (attenuations) inside them, and this allows the rendering of subtle anatomical details (down to 0.1–0.2 mm in the most favorable conditions[1]). A limit is the noise of the image because of the reduced radiation penetrating such small voxels. However, at the pulmonary level, the difference of attenuation (contrast) between lung structures and air is high; thus, the signal is high, and the final signal-to-noise ratio remains adequate for diagnostic purposes.

Terminology

In general, the structures that attenuate more are whiter (thus, more opaque or dense or also hyperdense) than the structures that attenuate less (thus, more transparent or lucent or also hyperlucent). Therefore,

the concept of density/opacity/attenuation of an element is a relative one, and for the object of interest it should be expressed in comparison with a reference structure, usually the surrounding background. The mediastinal vessels, for example, are denser than the fat in which they are embedded, but in turn this fat is denser than the tracheal lumen containing air (Fig. 3-5).

In CT, the observed attenuations also can be described using a quantitative scale measured in Hounsfield units (HUs), where the zero value is given to water. Most common densities are air (−1000 HU),

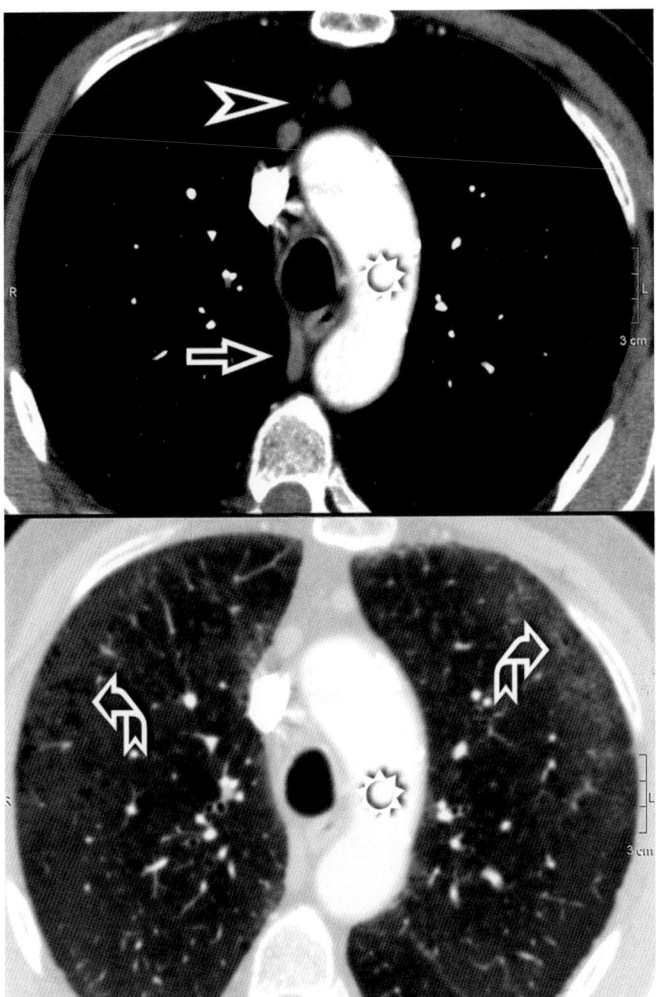

Figure 3-5. Effect of different window settings on the same image at the level of the aortic arch (*sun*). The *upper figure* has been documented with a mediastinal window that optimizes the contrast on the details at the soft tissue level. The azygos vein (*arrow*), for example, and a couple of small lymph nodes in the anterior mediastinum (*arrowhead*) are nicely seen. The lung window (*lower image*), on the contrary, optimizes the contrast at the lung level and allows recognition of small hyperlucencies (*curved arrows*) inside faint peripheral lung opacity.

fat (−120 HU), water (0 HU), muscle (+40 HU), radiologic contrast medium (+130 HU), and bone (+400 or more HU).

If a special iodinated substance (contrast medium) is injected intravenously before the examination, the visibility of the tissues is enhanced (contrast enhancement) because iodine is a powerful absorber of radiation (see Fig. 3-5). A contrast medium is used rarely in the studies performed for a suspected DLD but frequently when a mass or a vascular condition is under investigation.

The body structures are best observed on monitors or films where the brightness/contrast is optimized to bring out the details of the image. However, human eye limitations do not allow a real-time appreciation of these details over the entire dynamic range of chest attenuations. Fortunately, all pertinent data are available to the machine, and the operator needs only to press a button to switch, through a dedicated processing referred to as windowing and leveling, from a mediastinal window (where the details in the lung are squeezed down to the absolute blackness) to a lung window (where the soft tissues are leveled out but the lung structures stand out with maximal detail) (see Fig. 3-5).

Lung Anatomy

Arteries, Veins, and Bronchi

When examined using a lung window, the lungs appear as overall grayish structures delineated by the mediastinum and thoracic cage. Their shape depends on how they are cut by the plane of the section (see Figs. 3-2 to 3-4). The homogeneously whitish elements standing out over this background are blood vessels, which appear roundish or linear depending on the plane of section. Their size should be appropriate to their position within the lung (central versus peripheral) (Fig. 3-6). Each artery is joined by a companion airway, characterized longitudinally as a pair of tapering whitish lines separated by air, which branch regularly ("railway track" appearance). The airways appear as white rings when cut transversely (see Fig. 3-6). Actually, the visibility of bronchial structures within an aerated parenchyma is far below the visibility of companion vessels because of the mostly air-containing nature of the former. Consequently, when looking at a normal lung, the general feeling is of a predominance of blood vessels with only sporadic visibility of bronchioles within the outer third of the lungs.

The outer wall of the arteries and both the outer and inner surface of the bronchial walls should present a sharply defined interface with the surrounding parenchyma (Fig. 3-7). As a rule, bronchial walls in corresponding regions of both lungs should be similar in thickness. Moreover, coupled bronchi and arteries should present roughly the same diameter, and this in turn depends on their position (central or peripheral).[1] The arteries tend to divide dichotomously, whereas the veins often present a monopodial branching with several smaller branches flowing into a main collection drain. Arteries and veins also have a different course that becomes almost perpendicular at the level of the vein entrance into the mediastinum and right heart (see Fig. 3-7).

Mediastinal and thoracic pleura are invisible when normal. However, they can appear as subtle tiny linear opacities at the fissural level, where two layers fuse radiologically (see Fig. 3-7). When normal, lymphatics are not visible at any level, their size being inadequate to be perceptible radiologically.

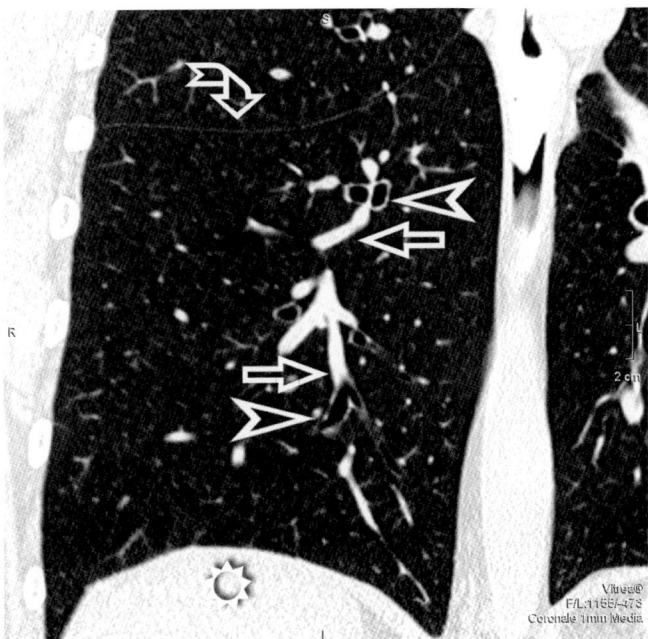

Figure 3-6. Frontal view of a normal right lung, inferiorly delimitated by the diaphragmatic dome (above the *sun*). White lines and dots within the pulmonary parenchyma are vessels (*arrows*). Black lines and rings are bronchi (*arrowheads*). The figure also shows a pleural fissure (*curved arrow*).

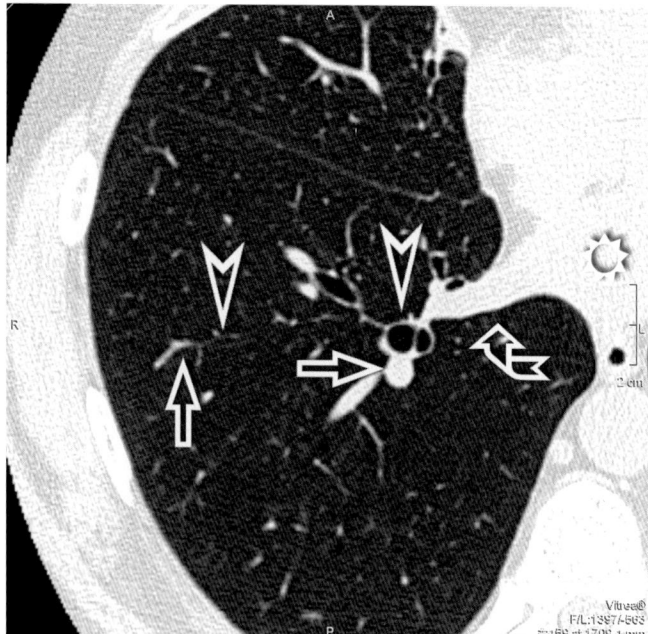

Figure 3-7. Arteries (*arrows*) and bronchi (*arrowheads*) run parallel to each other, and they are approximately the same size at every level. The right inferior pulmonary vein (*curved arrow*) enters the left atrium (*sun*).

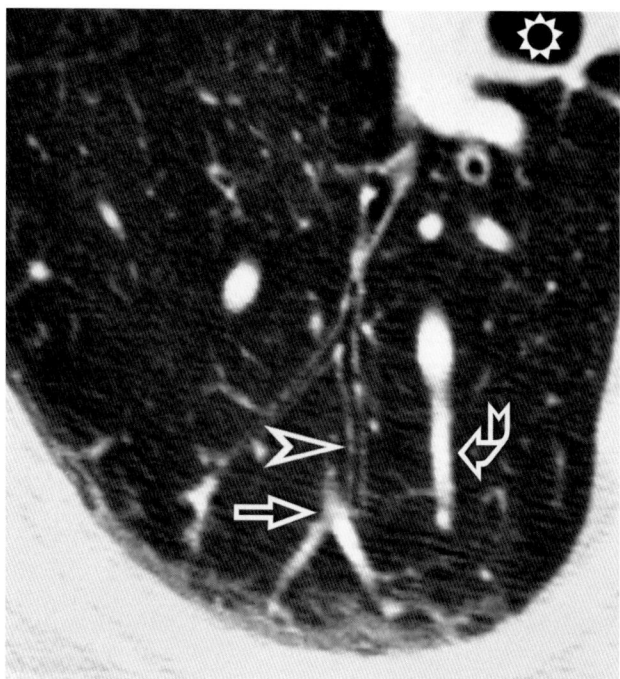

Figure 3-8. Close-up detail of the posterior portion of the right lung in an axial view at the level of the intermediate bronchus (*sun*). Here we are facing the lobular level, with the centrilobular artery (*arrow*) and bronchiole (*arrowhead*) and a perilobular vein (*curved arrow*).

Secondary Lobule

At the periphery of the lung, after 28 generations of arteries and 23 generations of bronchi,[2] arteries and bronchi become so small that they become invisible. As a consequence, the far peripheral pulmonary parenchyma should have no visible vessels, and the same and even more is true for the bronchi (see Figs. 3-6 and 3-7). Thus, the appreciation of vessels immediately below the pleural surface should point at an abnormality. However, exceptions are possible in the most dependent areas (Fig. 3-8), where the hydrostatic pressure is higher and the vessels larger.

The centrilobular bronchioles, in particular, should not be visible, and also, when normal, the interstitial framework at the lobular level should not be appreciable per se. Consequently, when an intralobular network of white lines and/or the walls of bronchioles become visible, this means that they are thickened and hence abnormal. In general, under normal circumstances, the lobular architecture is discernible only here and there when fragments of centrilobular arteries and perilobular veins are identified; this is more frequent in the dependent portions of the lung (see Fig. 3-8).

Special Techniques

Increasing Visibility

Multiplanar Reformation

The high-resolution computed tomography (HRCT) technique has existed since the end of the 1970s, but it was the development of the spiral multislice scanning machines in the early years of the 21st century that allowed the generation of consistent high-quality images in every spatial plane in nearly every patient (MPR). The first and most popular way to render the data is called averaged because, pixel by pixel, the images show the average attenuation of the tissues across the plane of section. The natural high contrast of lung tissue and thin collimation of the x-ray beam, coupled with a high frequency algorithm of reconstruction, guarantee sharp details of anatomical and pathologic elements down to well less than 1 mm in size (see Fig. 3-8).

Pathology that occurs in the central or peripheral regions of the lung is best studied in axial images (see Fig. 3-2). Diseases that show upper or lower lung prevalence benefit from visualization in coronal view (see Fig. 3-3). Finally, disorders that prevail in the parahilar regions or in the costophrenic angles are best depicted in the sagittal view (see Fig. 3-4). With the volumetric approach, the planes may be varied according to the needs of the operator and targeted on the suspected disease (Box 3-1).

Box 3-1. Lung Predominance in Specific Diffuse Lung Disease

Upper Lung
Hypersensitivity pneumonitis
Langerhans cell histiocytosis
Sarcoidosis
Cystic fibrosis
Pneumocystis jiroveci pneumonia

Lower Lung
Idiopathic usual interstitial pneumonia (UIP)
Nonspecific interstitial pneumonia (NSIP)
Asbestosis
Desquamative interstitial pneumonia

Central Lung
Pulmonary hemorrhage
Pulmonary alveolar proteinosis
Renal edema

Peripheral Lung
Chronic eosinophilic pneumonia
Idiopathic UIP
NSIP
Asbestosis
Organizing pneumonia

Curved Multiplanar Reformation

Having the entire volume available and working digitally makes it possible to reconstruct objects traveling in and out of a two-dimensional plane along curved reformatted images (curved MPR). This allows a structure to be traced and displayed as if it lay along a single plane. For example, an intuitive visualization of the entire course of a bronchus from a cavitated lesion to its origin can be achieved by displaying it along a manually or automatically generated centerline of the bronchial lumen (Fig. 3-9). The curved reformatted images are not real, but they are effective and easy to generate and therefore suitable for practical purposes (e.g., "virtual" bronchoscopy).

Increasing Ambience

Maximum Intensity Projection

When averaging, no information from the patient is lost, but averaging requires a millimetric slice thickness. Otherwise, the details of interest are lost because the operator averages them in with the background. However, in doing so the operator loses the ambience (e.g., where pathologic lesions exist in space, which is of extraordinary significance for the diagnostic process). Increasing the thickness of the slice lowers resolution and results in the superimposition of too many elements in the same image. For this reason, a number of techniques have been implemented.

The maximum intensity projection (MIP) technique renders only the voxels with higher attenuation in a thick slice (0.5–2 cm). The technique is suitable to render tridimensionally the vascular tree standing against a black background; moreover, with MIP, it is possible to obtain a comprehensive representation of the position of various lesions inside the lobular framework[3] (Fig. 3-10). In selected cases, MIP images are useful for distinguishing between vessels and nodules and, when nodules are present, to assess their profusion.

Minimum Intensity Projection

The minimum intensity projection (minIP) technique renders only the voxels with lower attenuation in a thick slice (0.5–2 cm). This technique is useful for improving the visualization of hyperlucent elements (bronchi, emphysema, bullae, honeycombing) and some opacities, allowing a more precise study of their attributes and distribution. The

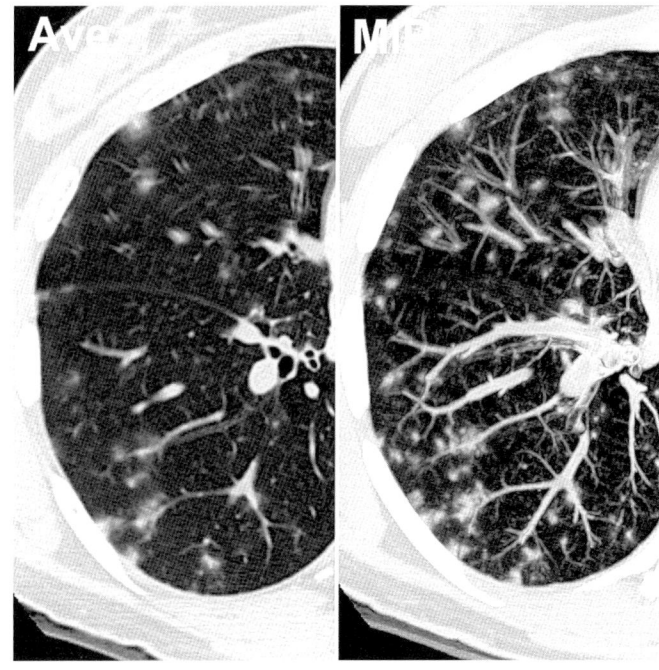

Figure 3-10. The image to the *left* (Ave.) is an axial view of the right lung in a patient with multiple nodular lesions. The maximum intensity projection (MIP) image to the *right* shows a thicker axial slab at the same level and in a way that the relationships between the lesions and the vessels are more easily appreciated, as in a tridimensional environment.

minIP technique is also ideal for investigating bronchial caliper and course, particularly within areas of increased density (Fig. 3-11).

Volume Rendering

Volume rendering (VR) techniques may be also used in the assessment of DLD. When implemented, the machine renders only the structures within a specific range of attenuations and contained within a chosen volume. Volume rendering may be useful for studying a volume of lung

Figure 3-9. Axial view (*left*) and curved reformatted image (*right*) of the right paramediastinal region in a patient with emphysema and a cavitary lesion of the lung. The axial image is in a plane. The right is artificially reconstructed along the drainage bronchus (*arrows*); however, it is effective in showing the bronchial ramifications from the hilum to the periphery. MPR, multiplanar reformation.

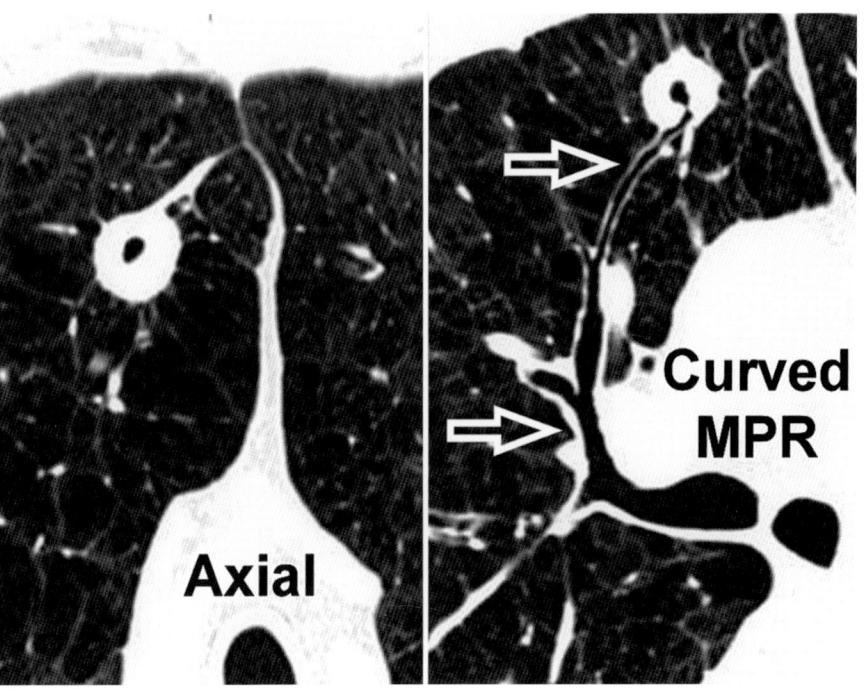

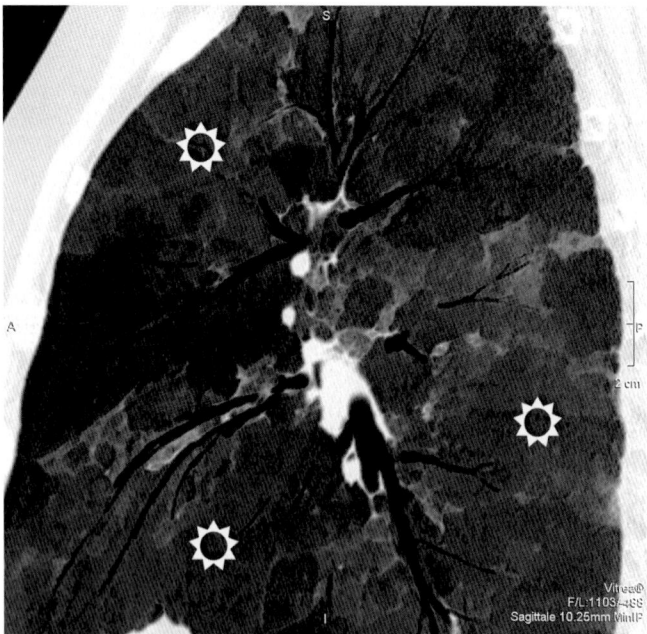

Figure 3-11. Sagittal view (minIP image) of a lung in a patient with patchy areas of increased opacity (*suns*). Note how easily the extension of the opacities is grasped with this technique and how precisely the bronchial elements inside them are depicted.

in three dimensions from within or for inspecting its surface from outside (external volume rendering) (Fig. 3-12). This is particularly useful for concisely looking at the pulmonary surface and its abnormalities and for helping to make medical decisions (e.g., determining the site of a surgical biopsy).

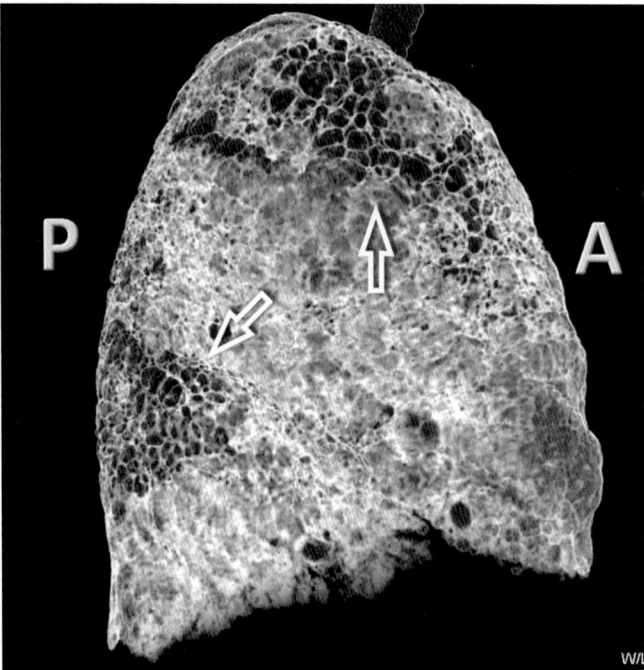

Figure 3-12. Tridimensional external lateral view of a lung in a patient with patchy hyperlucencies due to idiopathic UIP (*arrows*). With this technique (tridimensional volume rendering), it is possible to obtain synthetic and effective visions of both lung surfaces from different points of view. A, anterior; P, posterior.

Prone and Expiratory Computed Tomography

CT examinations are routinely performed on supine patients at the end of inspiration. Then, the higher content of air in the lungs allows better contrast (hence, better visibility) of anatomy and pathology.

However, in supine patients, some whiter atelectatic lung is frequently seen in the most dependent posterior areas (see Fig. 3-8), where it may simulate pathology or, alternatively, hide it. These normal densities disappear with prone positioning (Fig. 3-13), and indeed some experts suggest the routine use of prone scans when diseases under consideration characteristically involve posterior lung (e.g., asbestosis).[4]

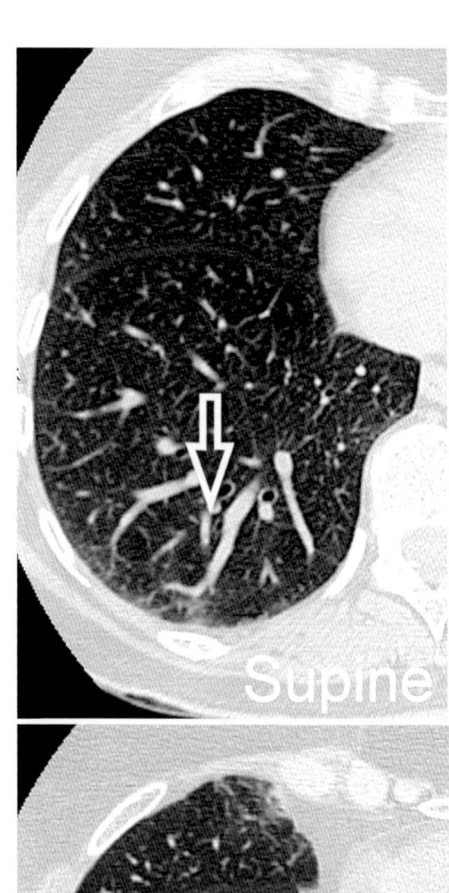

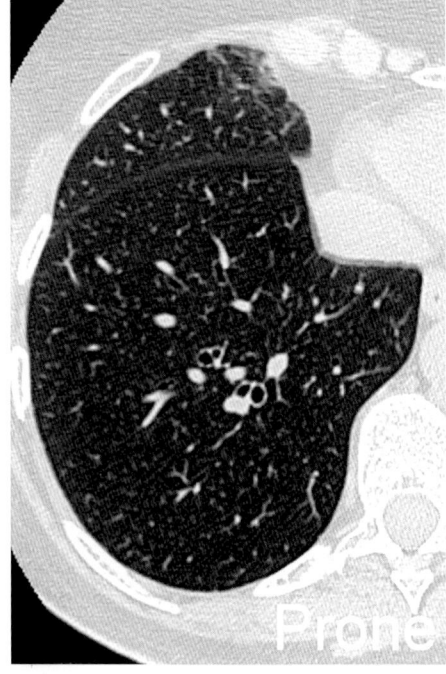

Figure 3-13. Supine (*top*) and prone (*bottom*) axial views of the right lung approximately at the same level. In the supine scan, there is an area of faint increased attenuation in the subpleural region (*arrow*). The opacity disappears in the prone position, so it should be functional and not due to lung pathology.

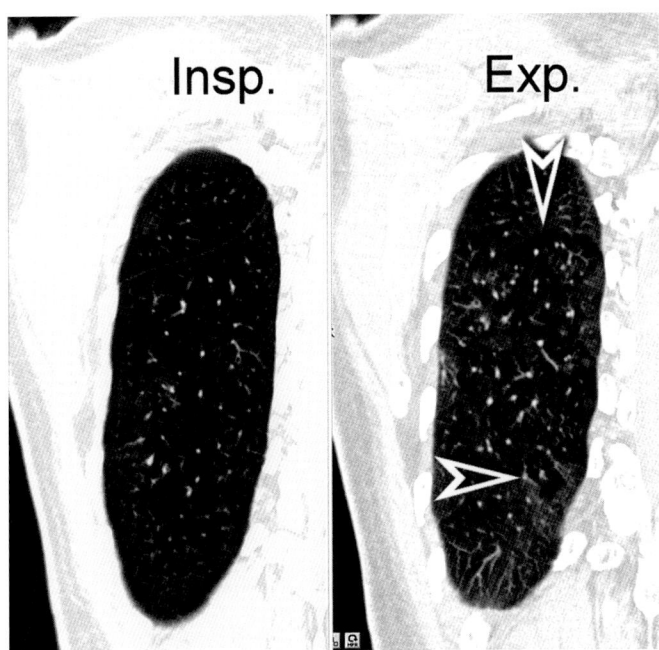

Figure 3-14. Frontal view of the right lung of a patient with constrictive bronchiolitis. The existence of patchy areas of different density due to air trapping is better demonstrated by the expiratory scan (*arrowheads*). Insp., inspiratory scan; Exp., expiratory scan.

In normal subjects, an expiratory scan shows a uniform reduction in size of the lungs together with a homogeneous increase of their density, due to the reduced amount of air within the alveoli. When an arterial obstructive or a bronchial stenotic disease is present, variable portions of lung become darker than normal because of the reduced blood supply caused directly by hampered vascular filling or indirectly caused by hypoxemic vasoconstriction. However, in the expiratory CT, the hyperlucent areas due to vascular obstruction physiologically increase their density, whereas in the case of bronchial stenosis they do not because the air does not exit from the alveoli (air trapping) (Fig. 3-14). When arterial obstructive or bronchial stenotic diseases are suspected, supplementary expiratory scans should then be added to complete the investigative process.

Diffuse Lung Diseases

Elementary Lesions

The radiologic appearance of each DLD depends on the elementary lesions and their distribution throughout the lung. The beginning of the radiologic process should involve verifying the existence of abnormalities, in particular of elements causing an increased absorption of the x-rays (opacities) or a reduced attenuation of them (hyperlucencies). If abnormalities exist, the next step should entail identifying their prevalent aspect, which in turn depends on the underlying pathology. Another step should involve localizing the abnormalities, both in relation to the lobular architecture (when possible) and their topographic distribution throughout the lung. The lobular approach presents valuable information about the modalities of arrival/onset of the lesions and their spreading routes, and the topographic approach helps discriminate among diseases with similar presentation.

The lobular approach should be quite obvious for the pathologist, who will find it extraordinarily easy to recognize many radiologic aspects of diseases with which he or she is acquainted from gross organ inspection (a radiologic image is essentially a black-and-white representation of gross lung examined with a magnifying glass). The possibility of confirming and specifying a disease using its distribution throughout the lung may be less intuitive but will become excitingly new and beneficial with practice. After all, the two modalities are not mutually exclusive; on the contrary, they strengthen each other through the concept of pattern.

Patterns

Patterns in practice of medicine are the ensemble of characteristic elements that give proof and name to a disease or to a family of diseases. In the DLD universe, basic radiologic patterns play an important role at the beginning of the diagnostic assessment. According to the literature and on the basis of the personal experience, the distinction of six main radiologic patterns is suggested:

- Septal pattern (linear pattern, preserved architecture)
- Fibrotic pattern (linear pattern, distorted architecture)
- Nodular pattern
- Alveolar pattern
- Cystic pattern (focal lucencies pattern)
- Dark lung pattern (diffuse lucencies pattern)

There are some limitations when thinking in terms of patterns. First, the same disease may present with different radiologic patterns. This may result from its variable pathologic expression in a given patient (e.g., pulmonary manifestations of progressive systemic sclerosis may show histologic usual interstitial pneumonia [UIP], nonspecific interstitial pneumonia [NSIP], organizing pneumonia [OP], and even diffuse alveolar damage patterns), from its temporal phase (e.g., a hypersensitivity pneumonitis may present in the acute, subacute, or chronic stage) or from its natural progression (e.g., an NSIP may proceed from a minimal changes pattern to end-stage lung disease). Second, the same pattern may be present in several diseases (a classical model being the systemic collagen vascular diseases [CVDs]), and also this is not unexpected because the lung has a limited number of reactions to different insults. These caveats are not an absolute limit to the diagnostic approach using patterns, but they underscore the necessity of a tight integration of imaging with clinical presentation and pathology in arriving at a meaningful diagnosis for the patient, as widely recognized in the literature.[5]

Septal Pattern

Definition

A septal pattern is present when a thickening of the perilobular interstitium is appreciable, making the lobular boundaries evident. The bronchovascular bundle is also usually thickened, producing changes both at the central parahilar level and in the centrilobular core (Fig. 3-15). The final effect is of that of a regular network of white lines with increased evidence of the perilobular interstitial architecture but without retraction or remodeling of pulmonary structures. For this reason, the septal pattern is also called *regular linear pattern* or *linear pattern with preserved architecture.*

High-Resolution Computed Tomography Signs

A network of white lines due to thickened septal, peribronchovascular, and subpleural interstitium is the trademark of this pattern. The thickened interlobular septa appear as white lines 1 to 2 cm in length outlining the polygonal boundaries of secondary lobules (interlobular or perilobular reticulation) (Fig. 3-16). Normally, these septa are not recognizable, so their presence points to an abnormality. A few lines inside the lobule may be also visible.[2,6]

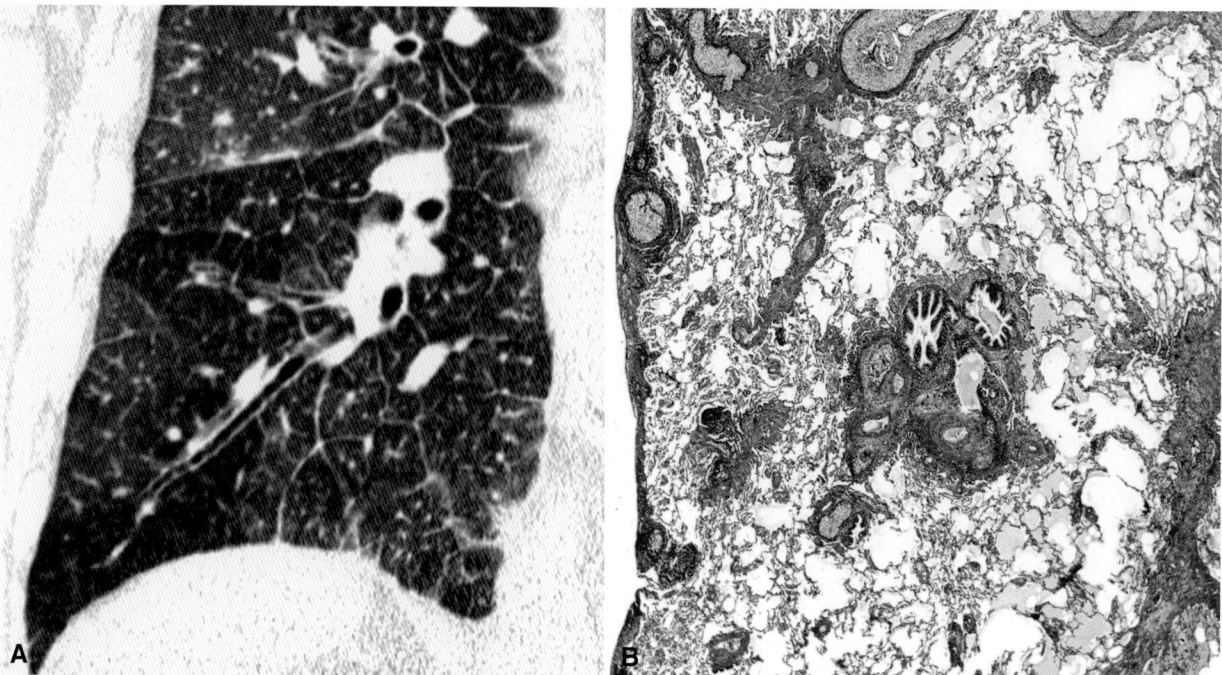

Figure 3-15. Radiology (**A**) and pathology (**B**) of septal diseases. Thickening of septal and fissural interstitium associated with peribronchovascular cuffing is the key element of this pattern.

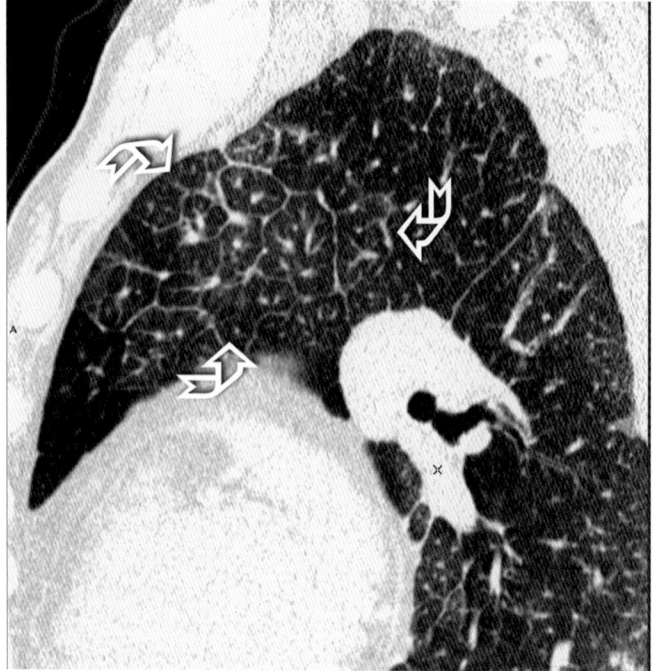

Figure 3-16. Septal thickening. This sagittal view shows thickened septa in the upper lobe (*curved arrows*). The thickening of the interlobular septa outlines secondary pulmonary lobules of various sizes.

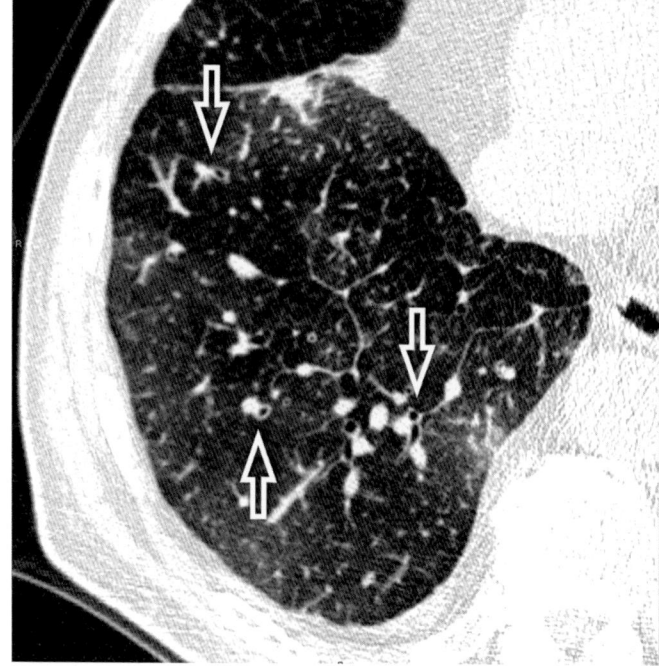

Figure 3-17. The centrilobular peribronchovascular thickening manifests itself as increased visibility of the centrilobular structures (*arrows*).

Centrilobular peribronchovascular thickening becomes manifest as a cuffing of the core structures of the lobule. The bronchiole, usually invisible under normal conditions, becomes evident as a white ring adjacent to a white dot of similar size (the centrilobular arteriole). It is enlarged compared with those identifiable in adjacent portions of pulmonary parenchyma (Fig. 3-17).

The thickened peribronchovascular bundle at a more central level is also perceived as arteries of increased size, compared with similar portions of pulmonary parenchyma, and as thickening of bronchial walls (Fig. 3-18). As a rule, vessel size and bronchial wall thickness in corresponding regions of one or both lungs should be similar, and a comparative evaluation of different lung regions is helpful and makes the recognition of the abnormalities easier.[2]

The subpleural interstitial thickening should be evaluated at the edges of the lung as a white enveloping line simulating thickened pleura. This sign is often easier to identify at the fissural level, where two layers of subpleural interstitium coexist[7] (Fig. 3-19).

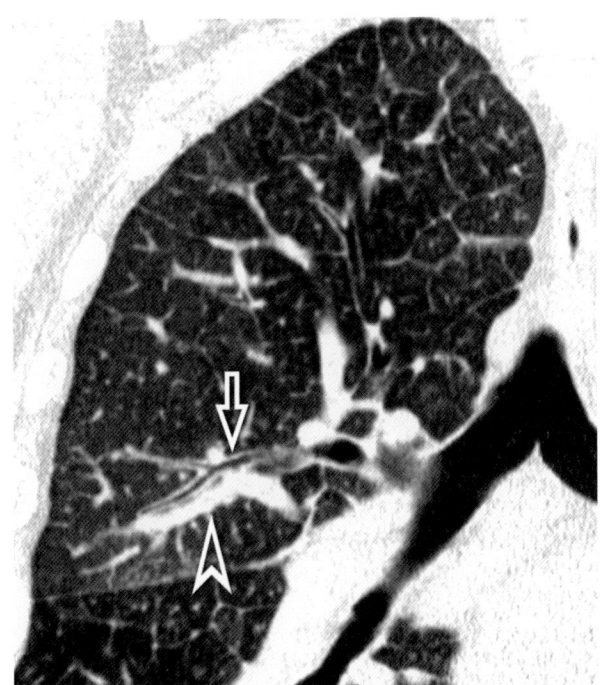

Figure 3-18. Central peribronchovascular thickening. In this coronal image, there is a thickening of the central peribronchovascular interstitium that manifests as peribronchial cuffing of segmental bronchi *(arrow)* and increased size of the companion arteries *(arrowhead)*.

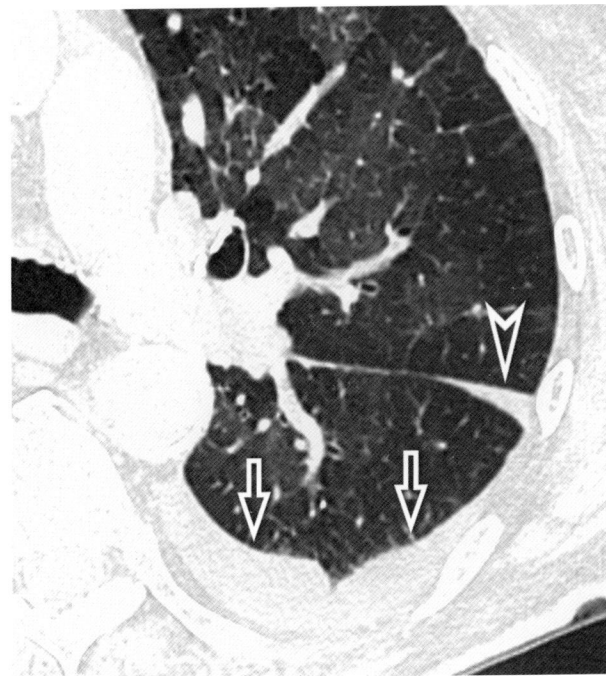

Figure 3-20. A pleural effusion is visible in this image along the costovertebral angle as a meniscus *(arrows)* and along the fissure *(arrowhead)*.

Subset Smooth

The anatomy of the three interstitial compartments (perilobular, peribronchovascular, and subpleural) is thickened more-or-less regularly with smooth profiles. The polygonal outlines of the lobules are visible without focal abnormalities. Their shape is variable, depending on the CT plane (Fig. 3-21).

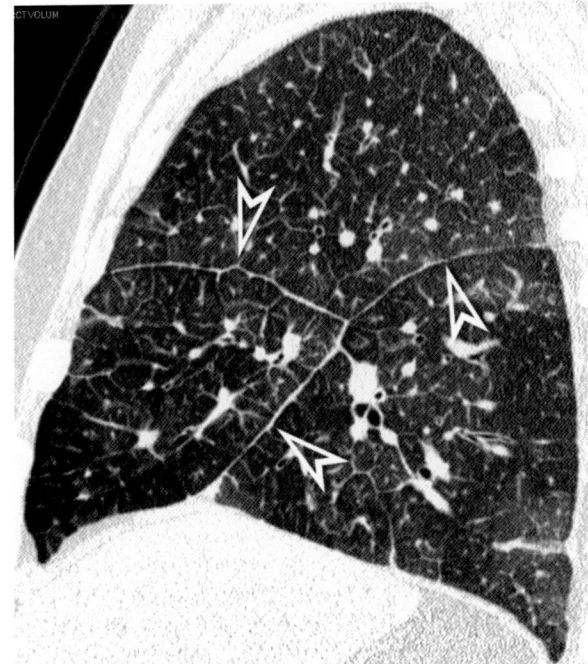

Figure 3-19. Subpleural interstitial thickening. The sagittal view shows thickening of subpleural interstitium, which is easily recognizable in relation to the fissures *(arrowheads)*.

Pleural effusion may be an additional finding in some septal disorders. It can be small and may be seen along the costovertebral angles or fissures (Fig. 3-20), where large, significant compressive effects on the adjacent parenchyma may be present.

Subsets

Morphologic characteristics of the septal thickening pattern allow the distinction of two possible subsets of the septal pattern: smooth and nodular.

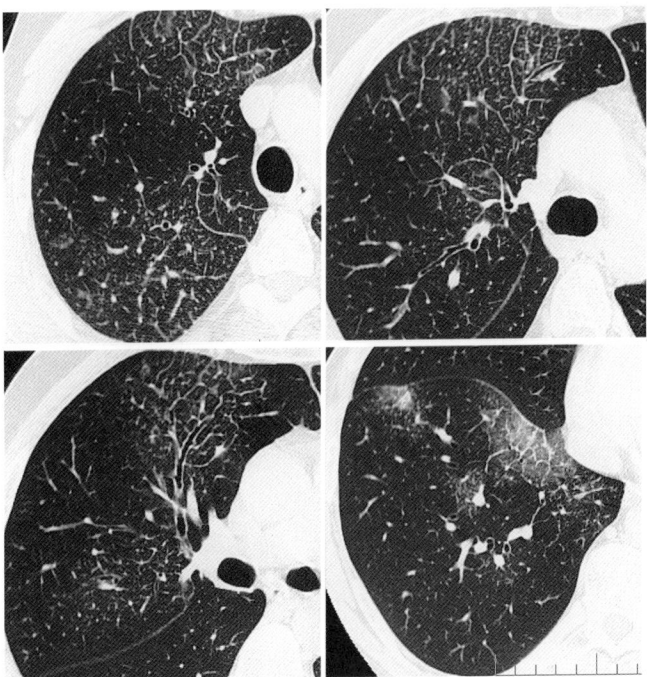

Figure 3-21. Four images of the right lung in a disease presenting with Septal Pattern, subset Smooth. A patchy distribution of thickened septa creates polygonal networks with smooth profiles.

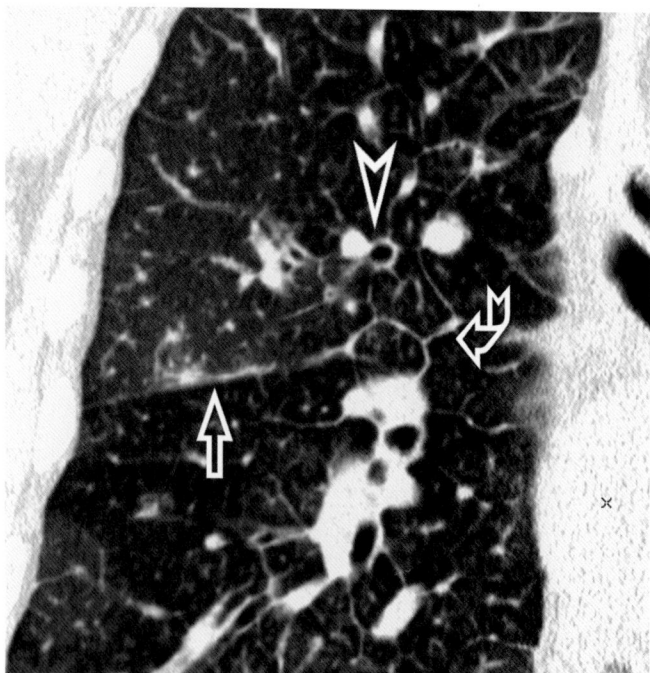

Figure 3-22. This coronal view shows smooth thickening of a fissure (*arrow*), of the perilobular interstitium (*curved arrow*), and of the peribronchovascular interstitium (*arrowhead*).

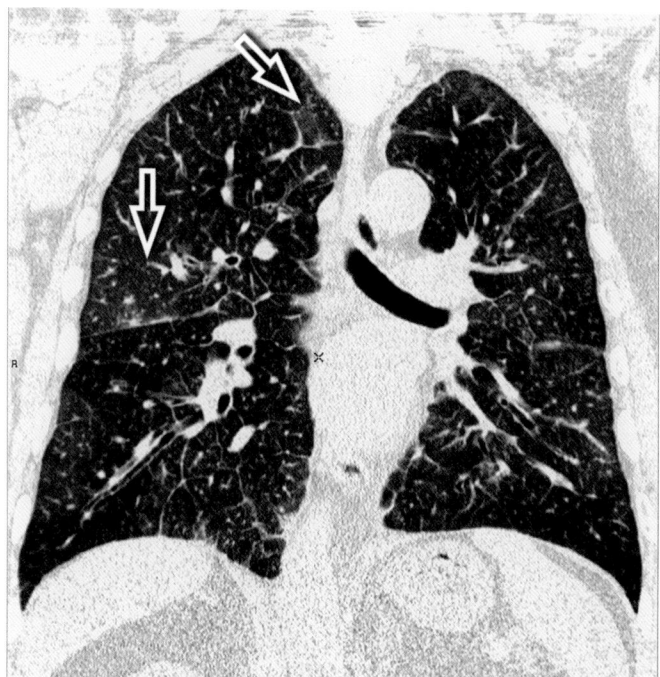

Figure 3-23. This coronal view shows bilateral smooth perilobular, peribronchovascular, and subpleural thickening in a patient with hydrostatic pulmonary edema (Fig. 3-22 is a close-up of this image). Areas of faint GGO are also present (*arrows*).

Inside the lobules, enlarged arteries and bronchioles with thickened walls are often visible. Smoothly thickened fissures are recognizable (Fig. 3-22), in particular with multiplanar reconstructions.[8] Coexisting patches of faint opacities are possible, due to partial alveolar filling (ground glass opacity [GGO]). However, these patches should not overshadow the septal aspects; otherwise, an alveolar pattern should be considered.

Diseases in the Septal Pattern, subset Smooth, are listed in Box 3-2.

Interstitial Hydrostatic Pulmonary Edema

The septal lines of pulmonary edema are usually associated with smooth subpleural and peribronchovascular interstitial thickening (peribronchial cuffing). Patchy lobular GGO often coexists, due to minimal alveolar edema[9] (Fig. 3-23). There is a tendency for the hydrostatic edema to show a symmetrical basal and posterior distribution (in supine patients) (Fig. 3-24), but patchy nongravitational distributions are not impossible.[10]

Heart enlargement and bilateral pleural effusion are common findings in cardiogenic pulmonary edema (see Fig. 3-24), and in a number of patients also a pericardial effusion may coexist. When the flow of the lymph to the systemic veins decreases, an enlargement of mediastinal lymph nodes due to fluid stagnation may occur[11] (Fig. 3-25).

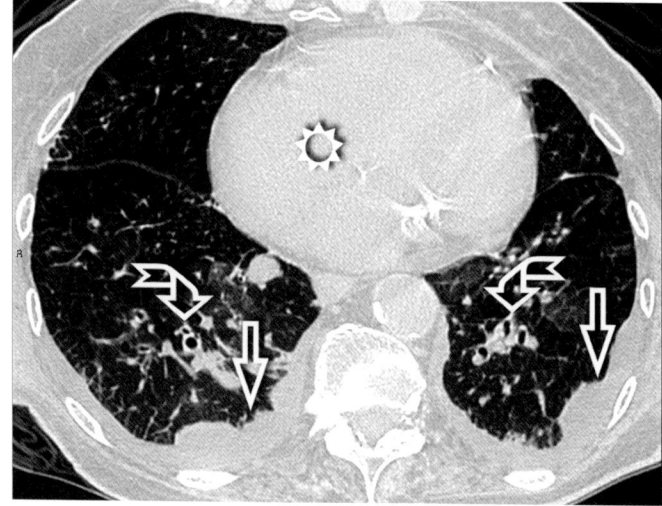

Figure 3-24. Supine patient, axial scan at the lung bases. The image reveals the posterior (gravitational) prevalence of bronchial cuffing (*curved arrows*) and bilateral pleural effusion (*arrows*) in a patient with congestive heart failure. Note also the enlarged heart (*sun*).

Lymphangitic Carcinomatosis

Lymphangitic carcinomatosis may present with a fully smooth subset[12] (Fig. 3-26), but not infrequently nodular irregularities (beaded appearance of septa and fissures) and random micronodules in areas of thickening occur. Nodules result from focal growth of cells within the lymphatics and local extensions into the parenchyma.[6,13] Subpleural thickening, when present, may also be smooth or nodular. Pleural effusion is unilateral in 50% of cases.

The lesions of lymphangitic carcinomatosis are typically patchy, often unilateral, and not gravity-dependent[12] (Fig. 3-27). Hilar

Box 3-2. Diseases Presenting with Septal Pattern, Subset Smooth

Frequent
Interstitial hydrostatic pulmonary edema
Lymphangitic carcinomatosis

Rare
Erdheim-Chester disease
Veno-occlusive disease

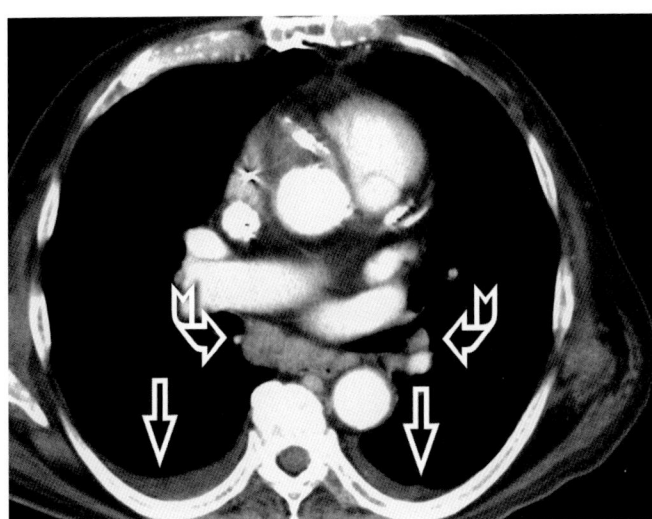

Figure 3-25. Axial scan (mediastinal window) in a patient with congestive heart failure. Subcarinal enlarged lymph nodes are visible in the mediastinum (*curved arrows*). A small bilateral pleural effusion coexists (*arrows*).

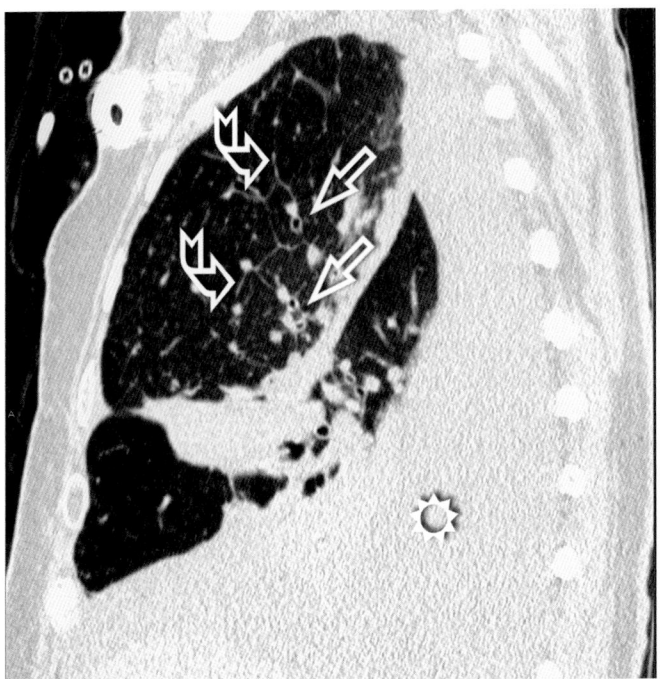

Figure 3-26. Sagittal view in a patient with lymphangitic carcinomatosis. The image shows smooth thickening of interlobular septa in the right upper lobe (*curved arrows*) and a thickening of the peribronchovascular interstitium, resulting in an increased thickness of bronchial walls and increased size of companion arteries (*arrows*). A pleural effusion is also present, with basal (*sun*) and intrafissural distribution.

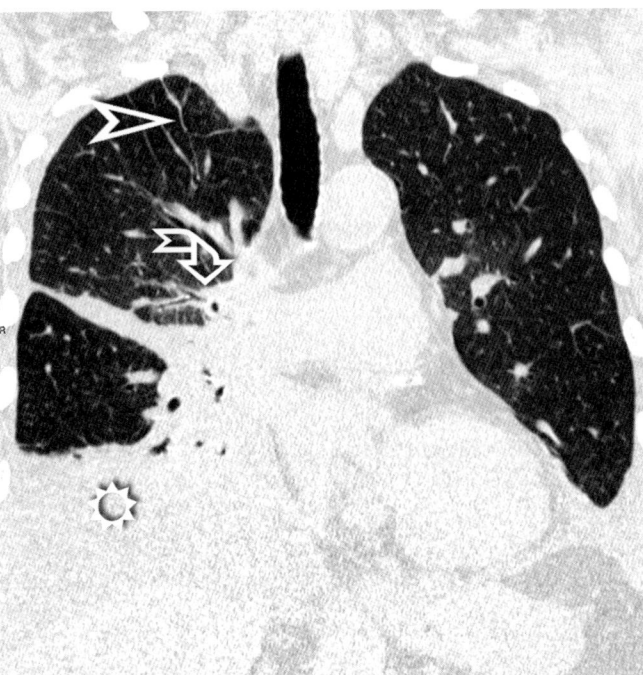

Figure 3-27. This coronal view shows a unilateral lymphangitic carcinomatosis. Note the non–gravity-dependent smooth septal thickening in the right upper lobe (*arrowhead*), the thickening of the peribronchovascular interstitium (*curved arrow*), and a pleural effusion (*sun*), together with lower lobe atelectasis.

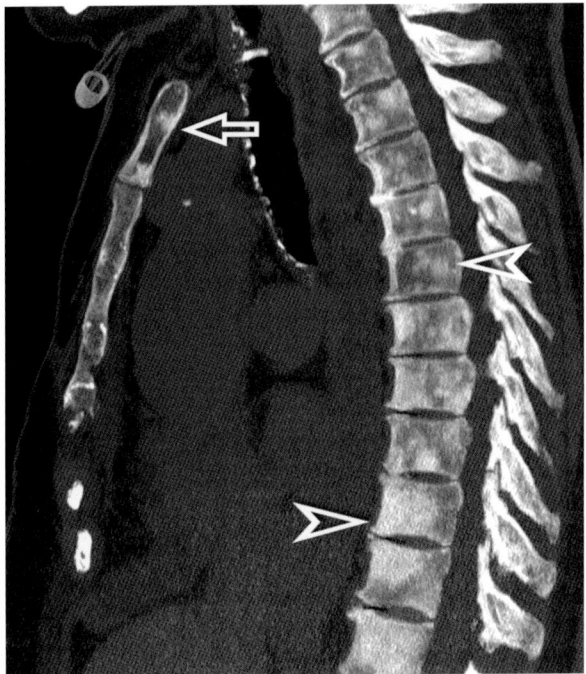

Figure 3-28. Sagittal view at the level of the midline in a patient with multiple skeletal metastases. The image has been documented with bone window settings and shows multifocal spotty white areas in the sternum (*arrow*) and thoracic vertebrae (*arrowheads*).

lymphadenopathy is visible in 50% of patients. Enlarged mediastinal lymph nodes can be also seen in a number of cases (25% to 50%).[13] Dedicated CT window settings may demonstrate metastatic lesions elsewhere (Fig. 3-28).

Veno-occlusive Disease

The presentation of veno-occlusive disease is similar to that of hydrostatic pulmonary edema. Smooth septal lines, bronchial cuffing, and patches of GGO related to alveolar wall thickening and pulmonary edema are apparent[14,15] (Fig. 3-29).

The lesions present a geographical appearance with variable localization. They are always bilateral and may have a gravitational preference[15] (Fig. 3-30).

A key radiologic sign is a coexisting enlargement of the central pulmonary arteries compatible with arterial pulmonary hypertension[16] (Fig. 3-31). The right side of the heart also may be dilated without

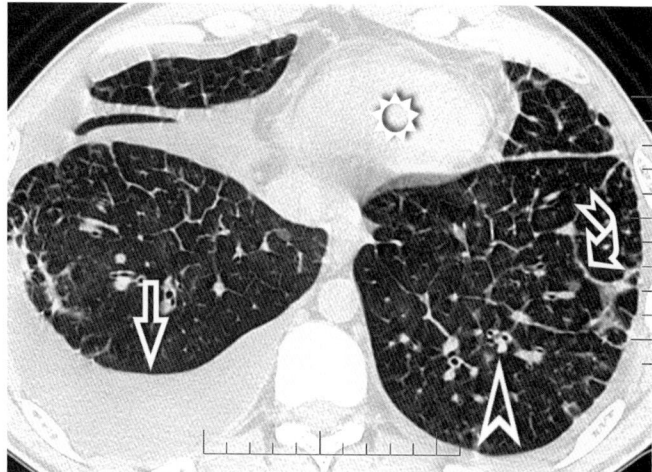

Figure 3-29. Pulmonary veno-occlusive disease in a 25-year-old man. The axial CT image shows widespread smoothly thickened interlobular septa (*curved arrow*), bronchial cuffing in the centrilobular area (*arrowhead*), and a right pleural effusion (*arrow*). The *sun* indicates the heart.

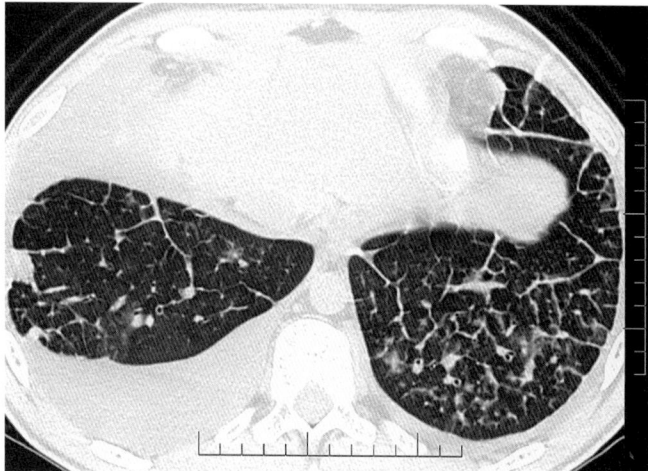

Figure 3-30. An axial scan of the same patient as in Figure 3-29 confirms the gravitational distribution of the lesions.

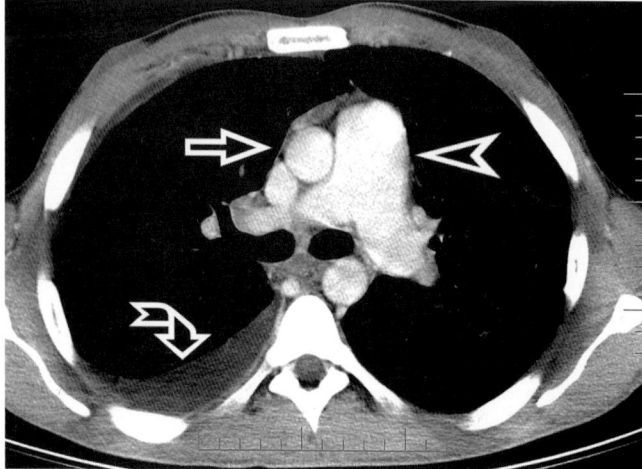

Figure 3-31. A contrast-enhanced axial scan (mediastinal window) of the same patient as in Figure 3-29 reveals a dilated central pulmonary artery (*arrowhead*) and a right pleural effusion (*curved arrow*). Compare the size of the main pulmonary artery with the diameter of the ascending aorta (*arrow*): they should be the same in a normal individual.

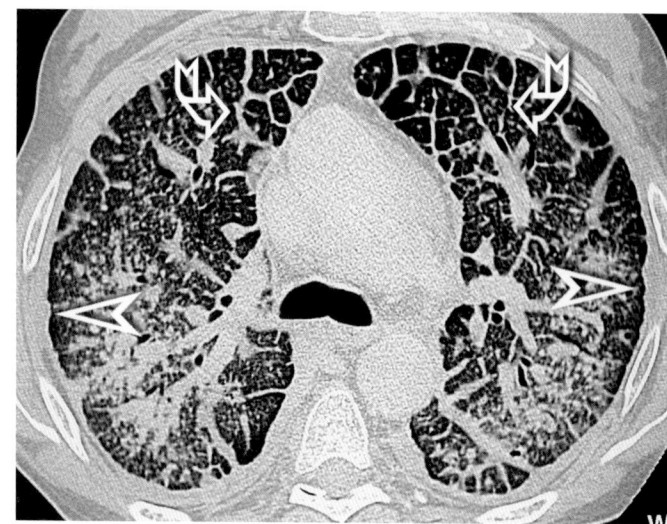

Figure 3-32. Computed tomography scan of a patient with Erdheim-Chester disease. The image shows a caricatural bilateral smooth thickening of interlobular septa (*curved arrow*) and subpleural interstitium along the costal margins (*arrowheads*) and the fissures.

evidence of left atrial or ventricular enlargement. In addition, pericardial or pleural effusion and enlargement of the mediastinal lymph nodes may be visible.[14]

Erdheim-Chester Disease

Erdheim-Chester disease is a non–Langerhans cell systemic histiocytosis that produces smooth septal and subpleural interstitial thickening, with more-or-less regular contours (Fig. 3-32). Multifocal areas of ground glass attenuation, small centrilobular nodular opacities, and pleural effusion may be also present.[17,18]

The septal lesions of Erdheim-Chester disease involve both lungs diffusely (Fig. 3-33), but in some cases they may predominate in the upper or lower lobes.[18] In addition, the pleura and the mediastinal structures may be involved (Fig. 3-34). The superior vena cava, along with the pulmonary trunk and main arteries, may be "coated" by anomalous tissue, and in case of severe involvement, a reduction of the vascu-

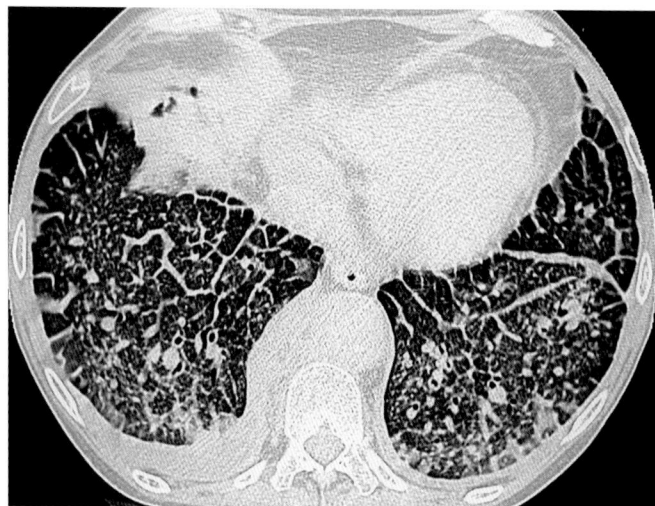

Figure 3-33. Widespread basal septal thickening in the same patient as in Figure 3-32.

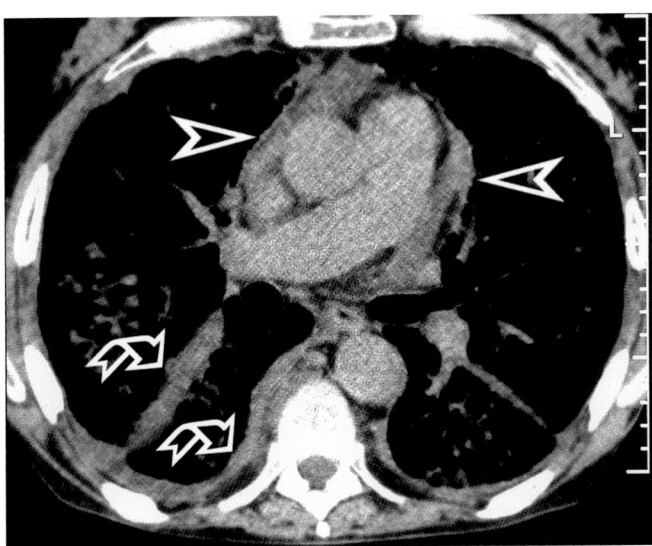

Figure 3-34. Axial scan (mediastinal window) of the same patient as in Figure 3-32. An abnormal dense tissue thickens the subpleural spaces (*curved arrows*) and infiltrates the mediastinal fat (*arrowheads*).

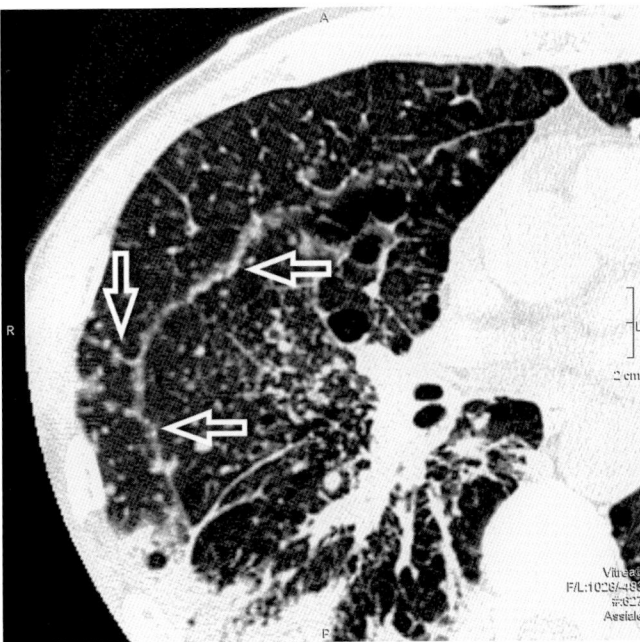

Figure 3-36. Septal Pattern, subset Nodular. The nodules inside the thickened septa and subpleural interstitium have high-density and well-defined margins (*arrows*).

lar lumen is also possible. The cardiac involvement may be endocardial or myocardial (not visible with HRCT) or pericardial, the latter being the most frequent and best visible on images, thanks to the contrast provided by the adjacent pericardial fat[19] (see Fig. 3-34).

Subset Nodular

The interstitial compartments are thickened in nodular form, testifying to the existence of locally growing cells or extracellular deposits within the interstitial boundaries[20] (Fig. 3-35). Being interstitial, these nodules are dense with well-defined margins[2] (Fig. 3-36), embedded as they are inside thickened interlobular septa and interstitial lines with an overall beaded appearance.[21]

The Septal Pattern, subset Nodular, differs from the Nodular Pattern, subset Lymphatic, where the nodules are more-or-less individually seen along appropriate routes that are not thickened. This important distinction helps the radiologist distinguish the two diseases (e.g., lymphangitic carcinomatosis [Septal Pattern, subset Nodular] from sarcoidosis [Nodular Pattern, subset Lymphatic]).

Lymphoid interstitial pneumonia is a multifaceted disease that may present with different patterns, including septal. However, it tends to show more often nodules along lymphatic routes, so it has been placed in the Nodular Pattern, subset Lymphatic. Diseases in the Septal Pattern, subset Nodular, are listed in Box 3-3.

Diffuse Interstitial Amyloidosis

The diffuse interstitial form of amyloidosis is characterized by smooth or nodular septal, peribronchovascular, and subpleural thickening, frequently (50%) associated with well-defined subpleural nodules that are often calcified (Fig. 3-37).[22,23] The lesions of diffuse pulmonary amyloidosis show a basal and peripheral prevalence[24] (Fig. 3-38).

The key to the diagnosis is the existence of subpleural, confluent, calcified consolidations (Fig. 3-39). Associated findings are lymph node enlargement and unilateral or bilateral pleural effusions.[25] Tracheobronchial involvement may be also present, with thickening of the tracheal and bronchial walls due to deposition of amyloid.

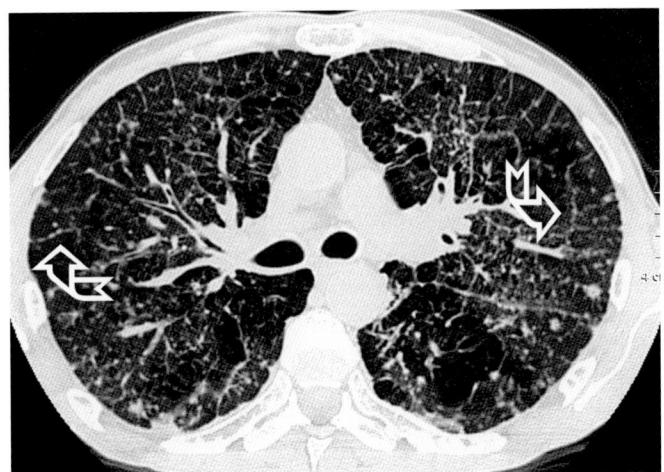

Figure 3-35. Septal Pattern, subset Nodular, showing both smooth and beaded septal thickening of the peripheral interstitium (interlobular septa) in which small nodules are visible (*curved arrows*).

Box 3-3. Diseases Presenting with Septal Pattern, Subset Nodular

Frequent
Lymphangitic carcinomatosis (see Septal Pattern, subset Smooth)

Rare
Diffuse interstitial amyloidosis
Lymphoid interstitial pneumonia (see Nodular Pattern, subset Lymphatic)

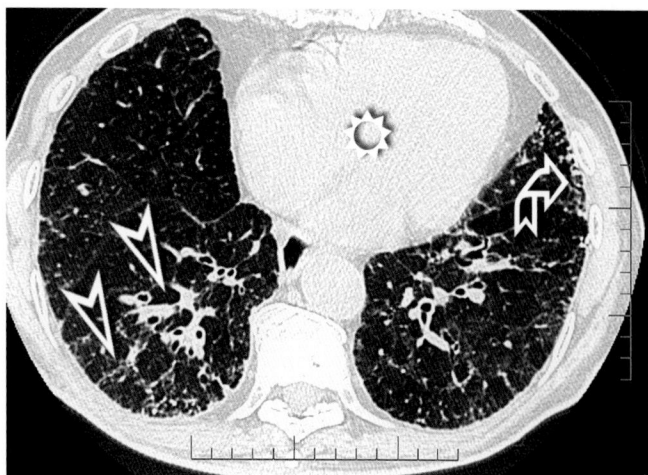

Figure 3-37. Diffuse interstitial amyloidosis. This axial scan at the level of the heart (*sun*) shows both smooth and nodular septal thickening (*arrowheads*) associated with well-defined subpleural nodules (*curved arrow*).

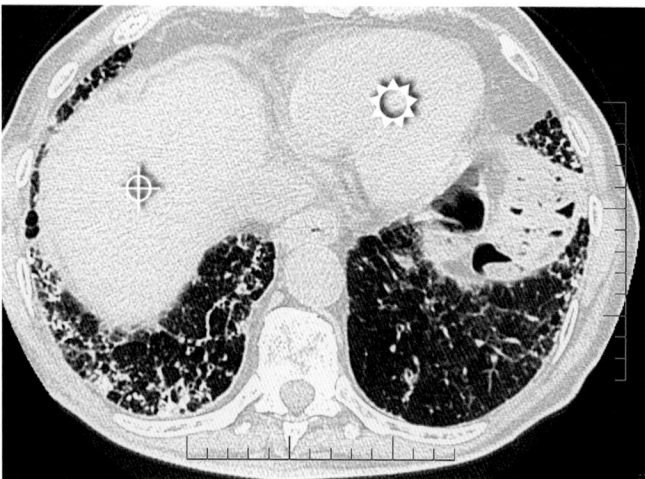

Figure 3-38. This is a more basal scan from the same patient as in Figure 3-37. *Bull's-eye*, liver; *sun*, heart.

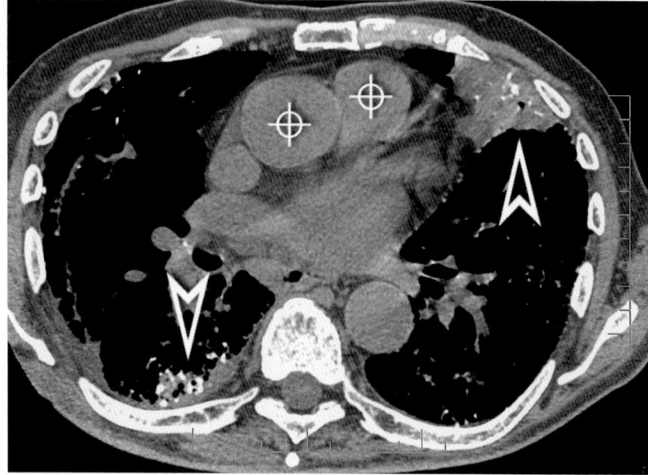

Figure 3-39. Mediastinal window at the level of the great vessels (*bull's-eyes*) in the same patient as Figure 3-37. The image shows patchy peripheral calcified consolidations in both lungs (*arrowheads*).

Fibrotic Pattern

Definition

A fibrotic pattern is present when signs of retraction and remodeling of thoracic structures are recognizable at the lobular level and/or in correspondence of larger portions of lung (Fig. 3-40).

High-Resolution Computed Tomography Signs

The signs of fibrotic disease are associated with the direct visualization of fibrotic elements or to the effects of retraction and remodeling on pulmonary structures. Direct signs of fibrosis are irregular linear opacities (irregular reticulation), vessel enlargement, traction bronchiectasis, and bronchiolectasis with bronchial wall thickening, parenchymal bands, and honeycombing. The effects of lung retraction and remodeling are identifiable as irregular displacement of fissures, crowding of vessels, and retraction of the pleural/mediastinal surfaces with interface signs. These features are all due to shrinking of the pulmonary parenchyma with volume loss.

Irregular linear opacities (irregular reticulation) are crisscrossing, not uniform, wavering, white lines that appear as though they were traced by an unsteady hand on the lung background (Fig. 3-41). Sporadically, one could imagine that one or more of these lines represent remnants of interlobular septa (interlobular reticulation), but the visibility of interlobular septa is not the rule. On the contrary, the distortion due to fibrosis tends to reduce the recognition of the lobular architecture.[2] Most of these lines criss-cross spaces of lobular size, so they are also called intralobular reticulation (see Fig. 3-41).

The vessels may appear enlarged with shaggy margins (interface sign), and the bronchi are irregularly ectatic with thickened walls and a winding or corkscrew appearance (Fig. 3-42). In the periphery of the lung, the bronchioles may be also ectatic (so visible) with the same appearance (traction bronchiectasis and bronchiolectasis) (see Fig. 3-41). Finally, parenchymal bands are long lines representing thickened connected septa marginating several lobules but also focal scarring or linear atelectasis.[2]

As a whole, the described lesions may vary in size and aspect, from a more-or-less coarse obvious pattern to a subtle hazy opacification of the lung referred to as fibrotic GGO that is only minimally inhomogeneous. In the latter case, ectatic bronchioles inside the GGO and superimposing irregular reticulation (indicating fibrosis) are the discriminant features[26] (see Fig. 3-42).

A peculiar feature of destructive fibrosis is honeycombing. In honeycombing, small hyperlucent areas of variable size (from 2 mm to 1 cm) and shape separated by well-defined thick walls are crowded in an area where the lung architecture is lost[27] (Fig. 3-43). They should be distinguished (not easy and not always possible, especially in the early cases) from also roundish or elongated, windingly linear, transparencies corresponding to ectatic bronchioles (called *microscopic honeycombing* by Nishimura[28]).

Signs of retraction and remodeling give further, at times striking, evidence of the existence of a fibrotic disorder. At the pulmonary interface, a pleural line with shaggy margins and connections with parenchymal irregular lines (interface signs) may be evident (Fig. 3-44). A thickening of the subpleural interstitium may also be obvious, as well as an increased thickness of extrapleural/mediastinal fat, the latter compensating for the shrinking lung (see Fig. 3-44). A shaggy thickening may be also observed at the interface of the visceral pleura, which becomes angulated and displaced.

When fibrosis advances, one or more lobes and even the entire lung may become reduced in size. The signs associated with this are

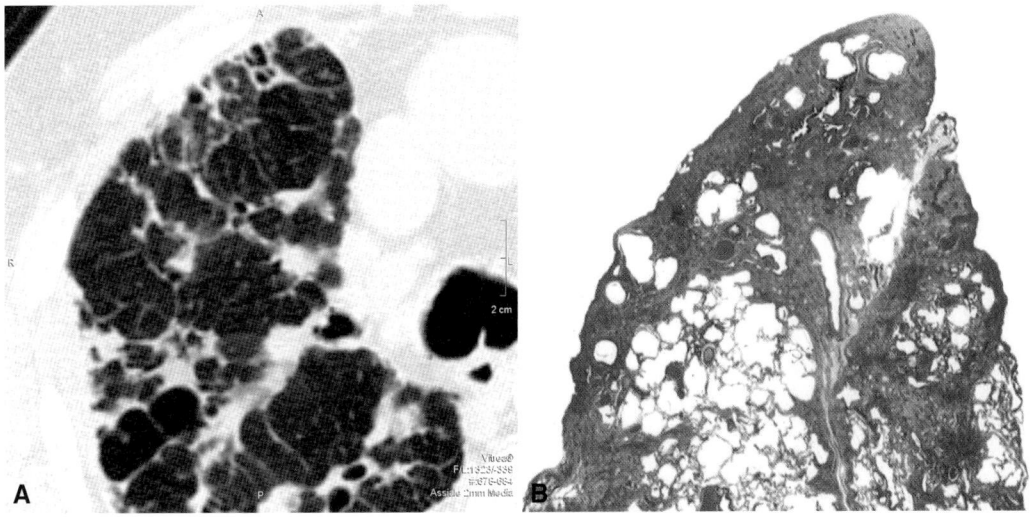

Figure 3-40. Radiology (**A**) and pathology (**B**) of fibrotic diseases. The signs of retraction and remodeling on the pulmonary structures are the key elements to identify this pattern.

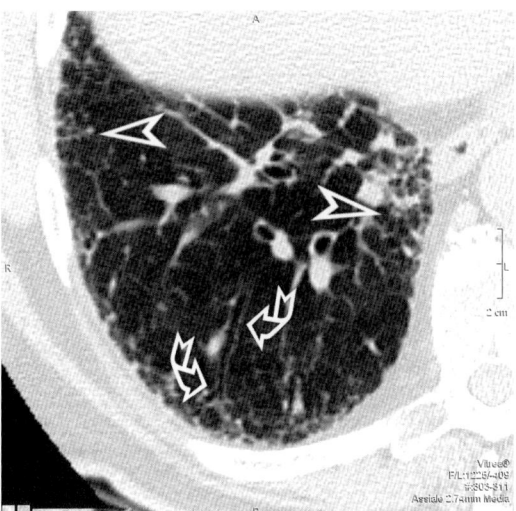

Figure 3-41. Irregular linear opacities (irregular reticulation) in the periphery of the lung (*arrowheads*) with remodeling of the lobular architecture, that indeed is no more recognizable. Signs of retraction are also evident on the bronchial structures with bronchiectasis and bronchiolectasis (*curved arrows*).

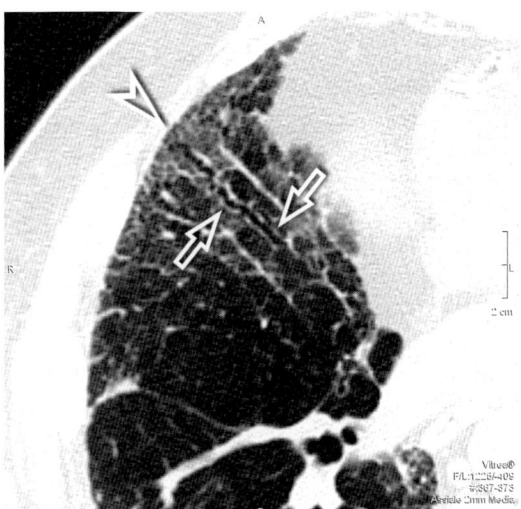

Figure 3-42. Tiny irregular lines in the anterior portion of the right lung. A long, ectatic winding bronchus with thickened walls is well appreciable (*arrows*). The ground glass component of the image is reasonably a fibrotic GGO, due to concomitant irregular reticulation and bronchiolectasis (*arrowhead*).

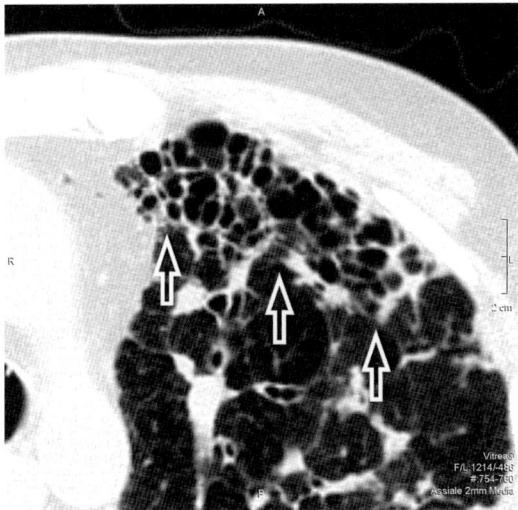

Figure 3-43. This is an example of what is called honeycombing radiologically (*arrows*)—multiple air-containing hyperlucent spaces (black holes) with well-defined thick walls grouped in several layers in an area of complete loss of the lobular architecture.

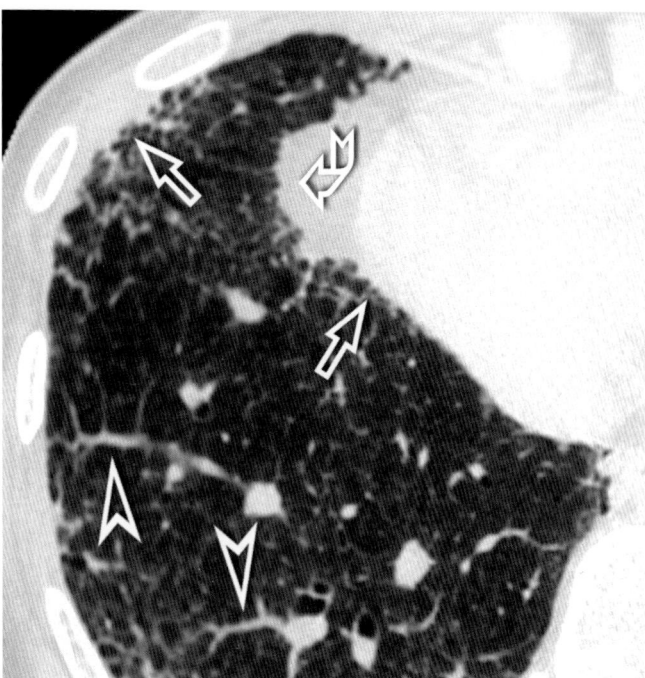

Figure 3-44. Shaggy margins of pleura (*arrows*) and vessels (*arrowheads*) (interface sign) and retraction of extrapulmonary structures toward the shrunk lung (*curved arrow*) are also indications of an underlying pulmonary fibrosing disorder.

angulation and displacement of fissures, crowding of vessels and bronchi, and mediastinal and diaphragmatic attraction toward the affected lung (Fig. 3-45).

Subsets

Depending on the underlying disease, the morphologic elements and their topographic distribution may be arranged in subsets that are helpful in focusing the observer on definite categories of fibrotic

disorders and at times even on specific diseases. The main subsets of the fibrotic pattern are UIP, NSIP, tug-of-war fibrosis, and bronchocentric fibrosis.

Subset Usual Interstitial Pneumonia

The UIP subset is defined by the presence of patchy areas of irregular reticulation and gross honeycombing with prominent signs of architectural distortion (Fig. 3-46). Traction bronchiectasis and microscopic honeycombing in connection with the pathologic areas are also characteristic.[28] Some GGO is possible but less extensive than the reticulation.[29] Signs of retraction and remodeling of vessels, fissures, lobes, and pulmonary boundaries are common, especially in advanced cases (Fig. 3-47).

The UIP subset may be seen both in idiopathic pulmonary fibrosis (IPF) and, with identical aspects, in several CVDs or, more rarely, chronic drug toxicity. Aspects of UIP are present also in individuals who develop an acute clinical course (acute exacerbation or acceleration of IPF), where the histologic findings show superimposed features of acute lung injury; in these cases, the radiologic presentation is usually dominated by the alveolar densities of acute lung injury and it is consequently discussed under the Alveolar Pattern, subset Acute. Diseases in the Fibrotic Pattern, subset UIP, are listed in Box 3-4.

Asbestosis

The early lesions of this disease are a combination of centrilobular dotlike and branching[30] opacities, which are often arranged in clusters or connected in form of subpleural curvilinear lines[31] (Fig. 3-48). These nodular opacities correspond to peribronchiolar nodular fibrosis responsible also for hyperlucent areas (mosaic perfusion) of lobular size from air trapping.[31] The subsequent evolution may lead to an

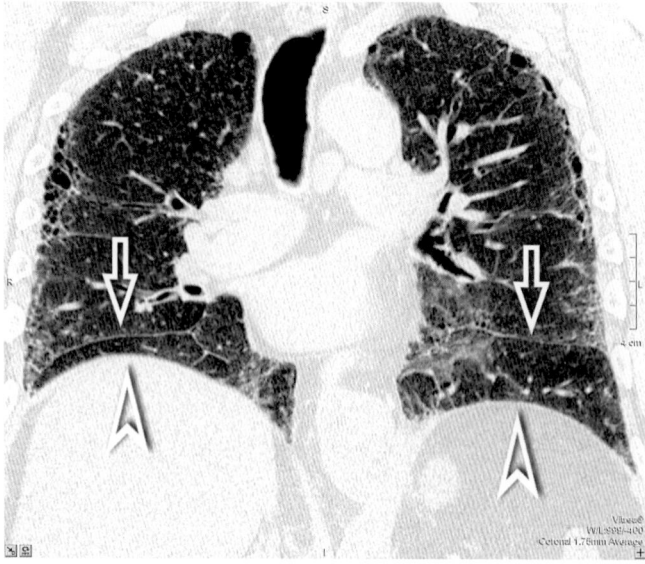

Figure 3-45. In this advanced fibrosing disease, the volume of the lower lung is markedly reduced, as shown by high diaphragmatic domes (*arrowheads*) approaching lowered fissures (*arrows*).

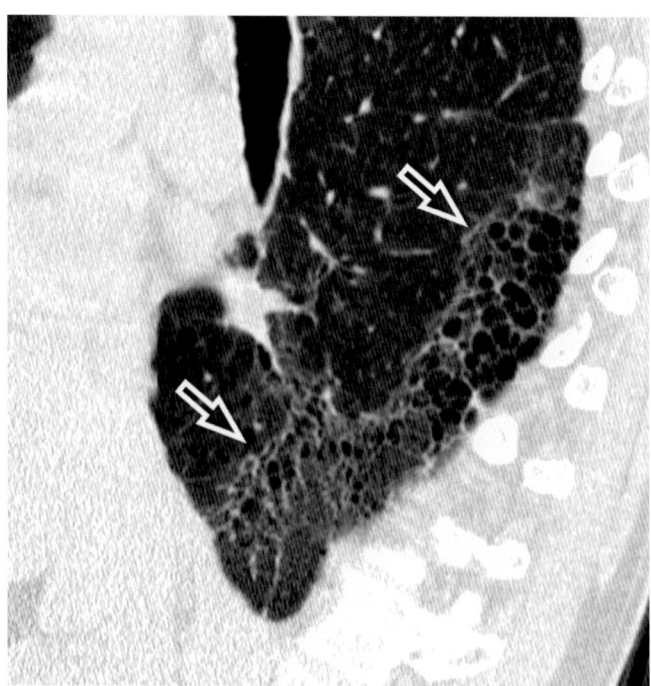

Figure 3-46. Honeycombing in the posterior costophrenic lung in a sagittal view. Note the sharp demarcation of the diseased lung with the normal pulmonary parenchyma (*arrows*).

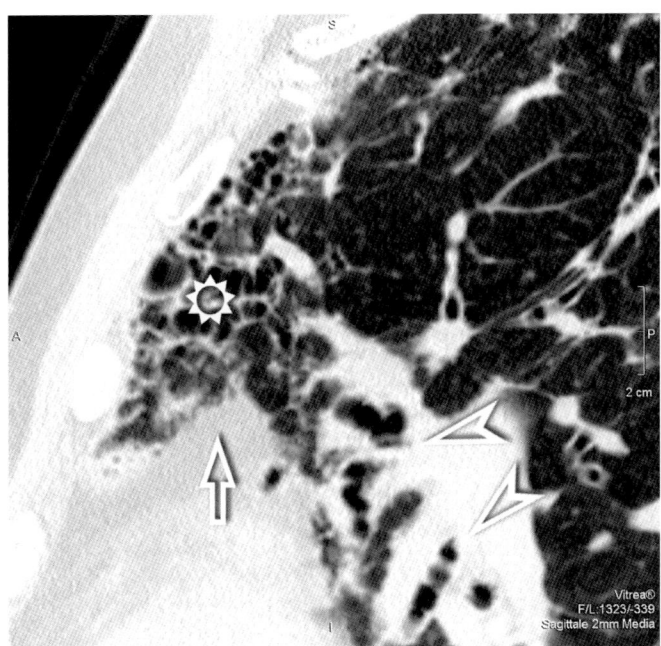

Figure 3-47. This sagittal view shows several signs of an important fibrosing pulmonary disorder: honeycombing in the anterior portions of the lung (*sun*), retraction of the mediastinal fat (*arrow*), and displacement of several ectatic bronchi (*arrowheads*).

Box 3-4. Diseases Presenting with Fibrotic Pattern, Subset Usual Interstitial Pneumonia

Frequent
Idiopathic usual interstitial pneumonia (UIP) (clinical idiopathic pulmonary fibrosis)
Collagen vascular diseases (see Idiopathic UIP)
Chronic hypersensitivity pneumonitis (HP)

Rare
Asbestosis
Chronic drug toxicity (see Idiopathic UIP)
Accelerated UIP and HP (see Alveolar Pattern, subset Acute)

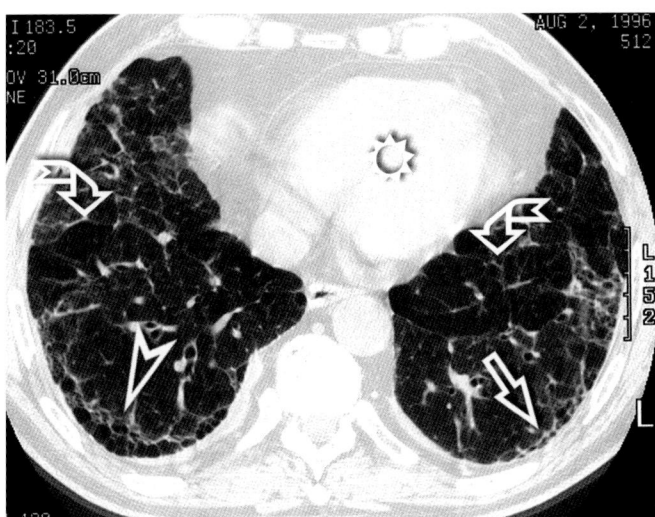

Figure 3-48. Axial scan at the level of the heart (*sun*) in a patient with asbestosis. Areas of advanced fibrosis with honeycombing (*arrowhead*), but also more initial subpleural lines with beaded appearance (*arrow*) are evident. The pattern is completed in this case by patchy areas of mosaic oligemia (*curved arrows*).

irregular interlobular and intralobular reticulation with bronchiectasis, architectural distortion, and honeycombing.[32]

The lesions are predominantly or exclusively located in the subpleural lobules of the posterior regions of the lower lobes in the early phases of disease,[30] but they may become more extensive as the disease progresses (Fig. 3-49).

Diffuse parietal pleural thickening and pleural plaques with or without calcifications (Fig.3-50; see also Figs. 3-48 and 3-49) are considered typical of the asbestos-related disease, but not all patients with

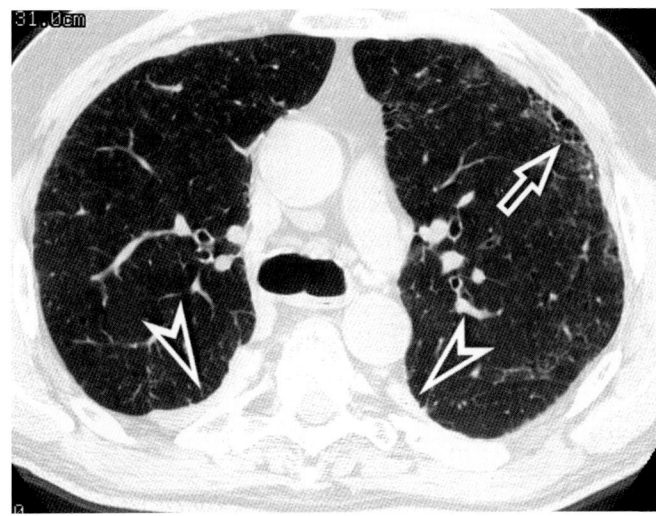

Figure 3-49. Axial scan at the carinal level in the same patient as in Figure 3-48. At this transversal level, the fibrotic involvement of the lung is only initial, and the honeycomb changes are confined in restricted areas (*arrow*). Bilaterally, there are pleural plaques of typical aspect (*arrowheads*).

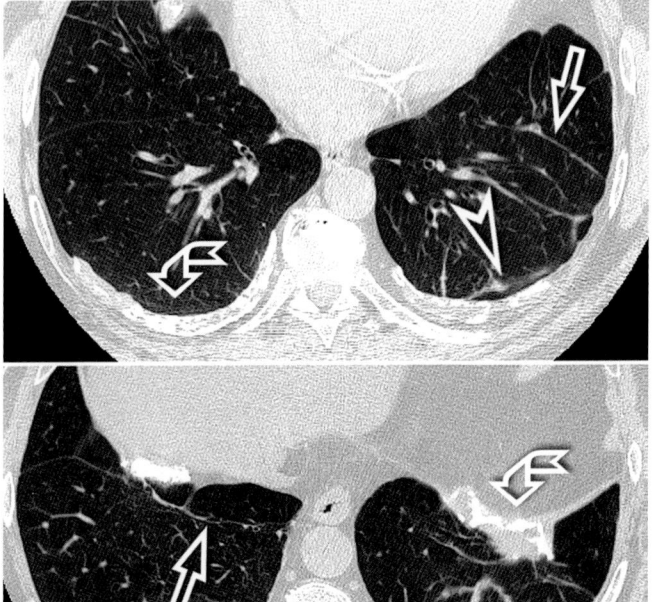

Figure 3-50. Calcified pleural plaques (*curved arrows*), subpleural lines (*arrowhead*), and parenchymal bands (*arrows*) are variably distributed in this patient with initial parenchymal asbestosis.

asbestosis show pleural abnormalities.[2] Parenchymal bands are also characteristic of this disease (see Fig. 3-50) and may reflect thickening of interlobular septa, fibrosis along bronchovascular sheaths, coarse scars, or areas of atelectasis adjacent to pleural plaques or visceral pleural thickening.[32,33]

Chronic Hypersensitivity Pneumonitis

Fibrotic GGO and irregular reticulation with traction bronchiectasis and bronchiolectasis are the most common features of hypersensitivity pneumonitis, but honeycombing is also a frequent finding. Characteristically, the fibrotic lesions may be associated to a mixture of lobular areas with decreased attenuation, centrilobular nodules, and cysts inside the GGO[34] (Fig. 3-51).

Both reticulation and honeycombing may prevail in the periphery of the lung and may show upper lung predominance (Fig. 3-52). However, a random distribution is also common. Lower lobe predominance is uncommon.[34]

Accompanying signs of retraction on the pleural surfaces and on the mediastinal profiles are generic consequences of the underlying fibrosis. Some volume loss may occur, particularly in the upper lungs[35] (Fig. 3-53).

Idiopathic Usual Interstitial Pneumonia (Clinical Idiopathic Pulmonary Fibrosis)

Patchy areas of dense irregular reticulation and macro,[31] as well as micro[28] honeycombing alternating with normal lung (morphologic heterogeneity), are the most specific feature. Some focal areas of only slightly increased attenuation (due to uneven fibrosis) interspersed with relatively normal alveoli may coexist.[28] Rugged pleural surfaces (due to the tendency for fibrosis to occur in the periphery of the secondary lobule) are very frequent.[28] Characteristically, the patches of fibrosis are intermingled and sharply marginated with areas of normal parenchyma[36] (Fig. 3-54).

The disease is typically subpleural,[29,37] with some extension to the inner lung in connection with thickened vessels and ectatic bronchi.[28] The longitudinal distribution of the lesions is interesting. Although the more complex lesions with traction bronchiectasis and honeycombing show middle and lower predominance,[34] a contemporary irregular reticulation is frequently seen in the upper peripheral lung[38] (Fig. 3-55). Especially in advanced fibrosis, the lung becomes smaller and the indirect signs of retraction and remodeling striking.

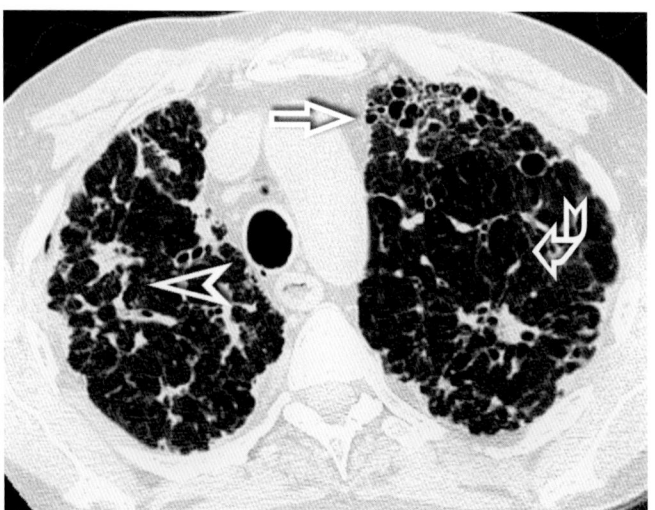

Figure 3-51. Mixed densities pattern in a patient with chronic hypersensitivity pneumonitis. Coarse irregular linear opacities (*arrowhead*) coexist with patchy honeycombing (*arrow*) and areas of hyperlucent lung with reduced vascularity (*curved arrow*).

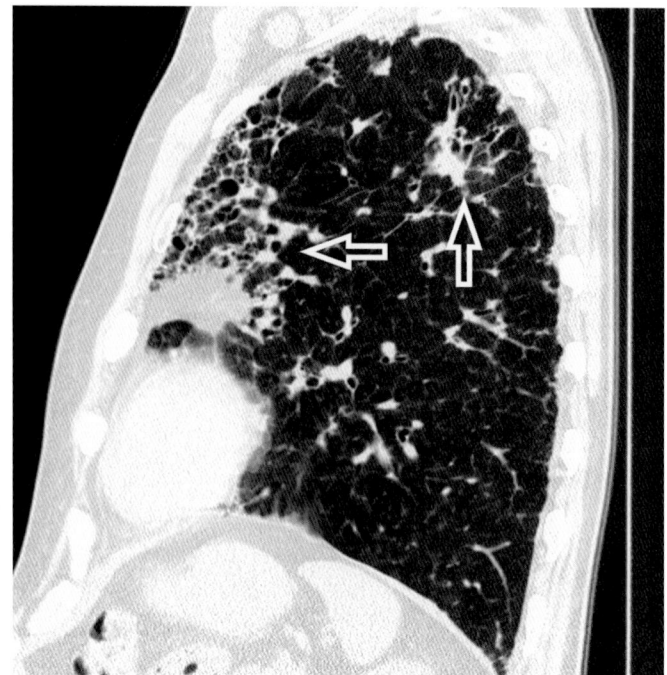

Figure 3-52. The lesions of chronic HP tend to prevail in the upper regions of the lung (*arrows*), and this is true also for honeycombing. In this sagittal view of the left lung, the base of the lung is relatively free of lesions, and this is an important element in the differential diagnosis with idiopathic UIP.

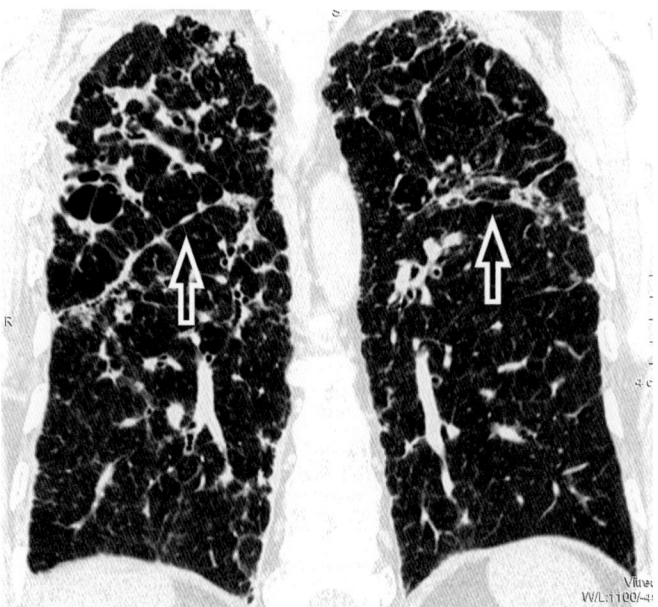

Figure 3-53. In chronic HP, interface signs, and evidence of architectural derangement are prevalently located in shrunken upper lobes, indicated here by the upward bowing of the major fissures (*arrows*).

Focal emphysematous hyperlucencies in the upper zones of the lung[28] but also inside the basal lesions are possible,[39] and these may create diagnostic problems of differential diagnosis with honeycombing.[40] A mild enlargement of mediastinal lymph nodes is present in approximately 70% of cases.[41] Occasionally, small nodular foci of calcification[25] or a disseminated dendriform pulmonary ossification[42] may be found. Associated solitary pulmonary opacities from lung cancer are possible,[43] as much as in all fibrotic disorders.

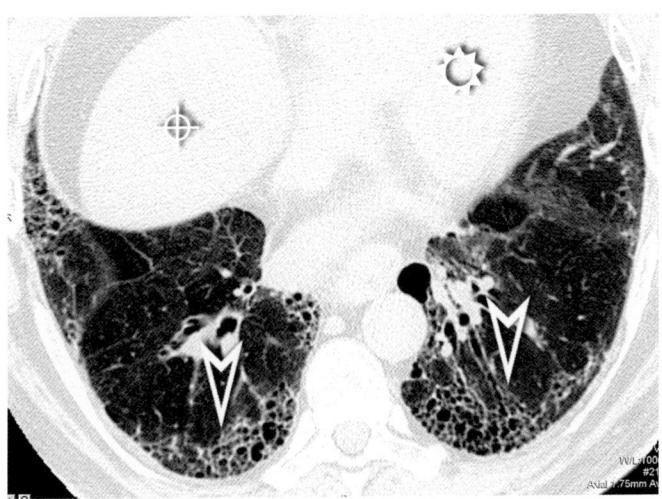

Figure 3-54. Axial scan at the level of the right liver dome (*bull's-eye*) and of the heart base (*sun*) in a patient with idiopathic UIP. Areas of patchy honeycombing alternating with normal lung are present (*arrowheads*) and are typical of this disease.

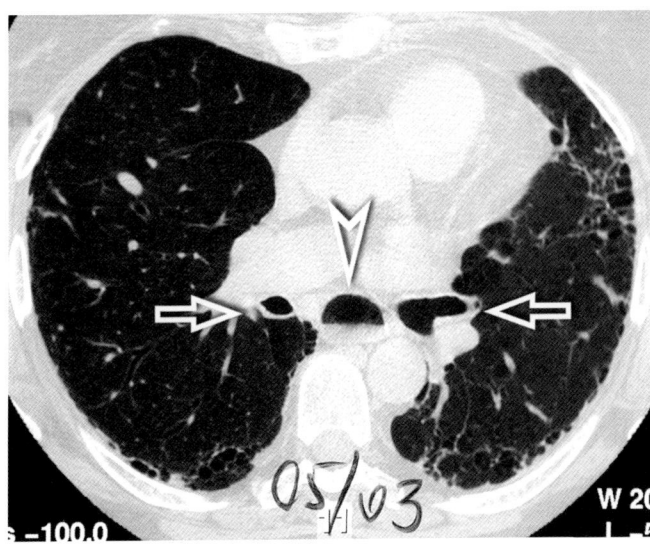

Figure 3-56. Patchy honeycombing alternating with normal lung (UIP subset) in a patient with systemic sclerosis. In this axial scan at the subcarinal level, an enlarged esophagus with air-fluid level is visible (*arrowhead*) between the intermediate bronchus to the right and the junction of the upper and lower lobe bronchus to the left (*arrows*).

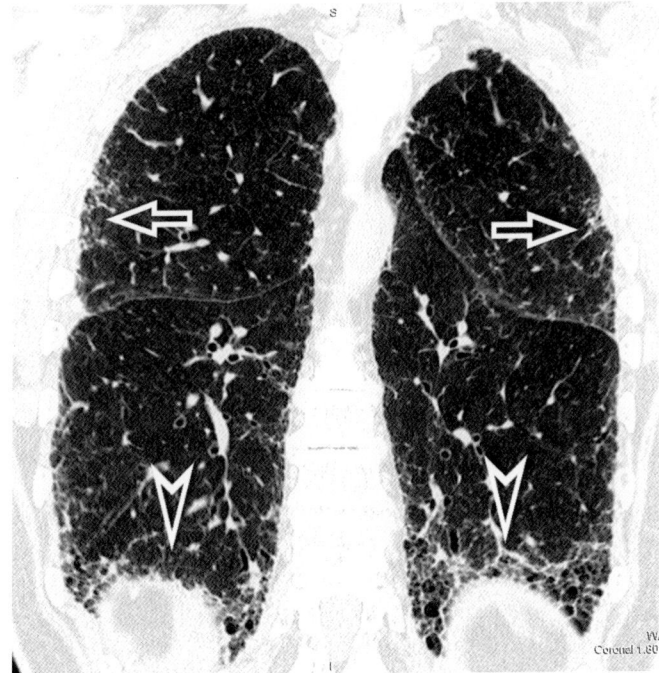

Figure 3-55. The peripheral regions of both lungs in this frontal view of a patient with idiopathic UIP show an irregular reticulation superiorly (*arrows*), and typical honeycombing is present at the basal level (*arrowheads*).

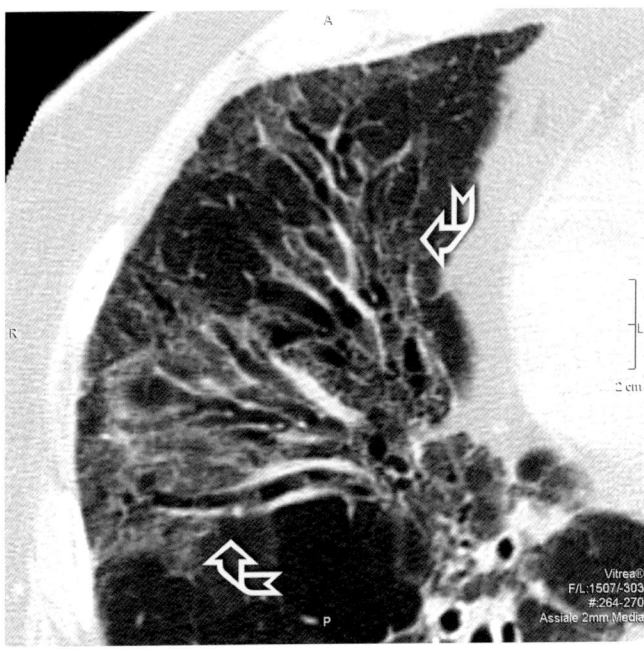

Figure 3-57. The typical fibrotic NSIP subset is characterized by areas of GGO and irregular reticulation associated with more-or-less evident bronchiectasis (*curved arrows*) but without significant honeycombing.

Some CVDs[44] and, more rarely, drug reactions[45] may present with aspects indistinguishable from the idiopathic UIP. Consequently, the suspicion of the underlying disorder may be formulated only on clinical grounds, but occasionally specific signs of the original disease are also seen radiologically[46–48] (Fig. 3-56).

Subset Fibrotic Nonspecific Interstitial Pneumonia

The NSIP pattern is defined by the presence of homogeneous areas of GGO associated with irregular reticulation[49] (Fig. 3-57). The percentage of each likely depends on the proportions of inflammation and fibrosis within the lung, and some authors have even attempted to identify definite subgroups based on the extent of reticulation and traction

bronchiectasis.[50] Traction bronchiectasis is characteristic (Fig. 3-58). Honeycombing, on the contrary, should be absent or minimal.[51]

The NSIP subset may be seen both in idiopathic NSIP and in several CVD and drug reactions, but NSIP aspects also may be present in patients with acute exacerbation of NSIP (accelerated NSIP) where the histologic findings show superimposed features of acute lung injury. In latter cases, the radiologic presentation is dominated by the alveolar densities of acute lung injury, and this is consequently discussed in the Alveolar Pattern, subset Acute. Diseases in the Fibrotic Pattern, subset Fibrotic NSIP, are listed in Box 3-5.

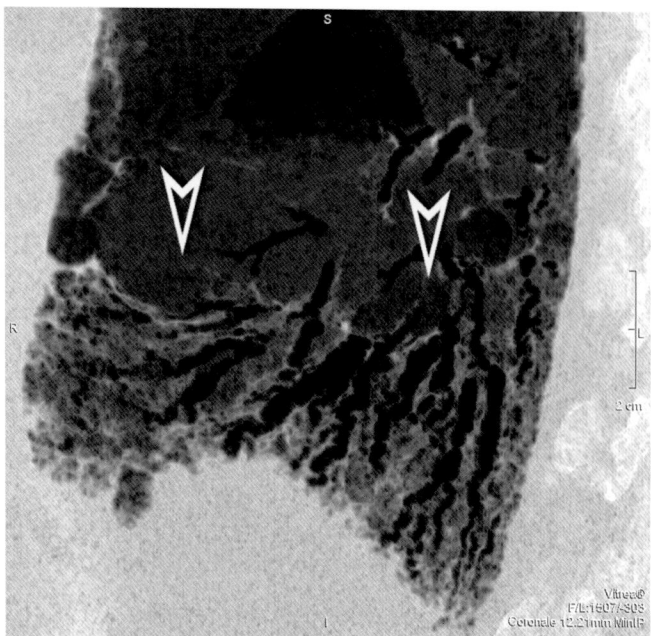

Figure 3-58. The minIP technique is valuable in showing size and extension of the bronchiectatic abnormalities inside the GGO (*arrowheads*). Note the absence of honeycomb cysts inside the pathologic area.

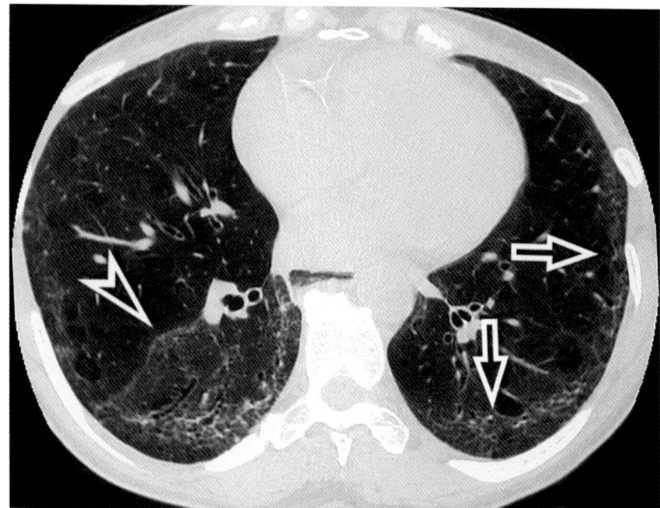

Figure 3-59. This is a patient with a typical fibrotic NSIP subset, possibly from systemic sclerosis because the esophagus is enlarged. Mainly the periphery of both lungs is involved by a subtle reticular GGO (*arrows*) without significant honeycombing. A shrunk right lower lobe (*arrowhead*) is more extensively involved, and it contains some bronchiectasis.

Box 3-5. Diseases Presenting with Fibrotic Pattern, Subset Fibrotic Nonspecific Interstitial Pneumonia

Frequent
Idiopathic fibrotic nonspecific interstitial pneumonia (NSIP)
Collagen vascular diseases (see Idiopathic Fibrotic NSIP)
Chronic drug toxicity (see Idiopathic Fibrotic NSIP)

Rare
Acute exacerbation of NSIP (see Alveolar Pattern, subset Acute)

Idiopathic Fibrotic Nonspecific Interstitial Pneumonia

Characteristic features of disease include reticular/GGO opacities with homogeneous aspect in affected areas. Inside the lesions, traction bronchiectasis and bronchiolectasis are common, and their extent has been shown to be a reliable indicator of fibrosis[50] (Fig. 3-59). Dense consolidations, on the contrary, are uncommon, and their presence should raise the suspicion of another disease (such as OP, chronic eosinophilic pneumonia, or bronchioloalveolar carcinoma) or, in the appropriate clinical setting, of an acute exacerbation (see Alveolar Pattern, subsets Acute and Chronic).[49] Honeycombing, if present, is mild and otherwise should raise the suspicion of UIP[51]; however, it has been reported that, over time, a number of NSIP originally presenting with NSIP pattern progress to UIP pattern.[52]

The disease is bilateral and symmetric,[49] involving mainly the lower lungs in more than 90% of the cases[51] (Fig. 3-60), otherwise equally distributed. On the contrary, primarily upper lobe lesions are very rare.[49] Axially, the pattern is diffuse in more than 50% of the cases or predominantly peripheral subpleural, but in a number of cases (20% to 43% according to some authors[27,51]) the immediate subpleural regions are relatively spared.

Volume loss, mostly of the lower lobes, is fairly common,[51] usually in conjunction with other indirect signs of fibrosis. Lymphadenopathy is possible at the mediastinal level,[49] usually mild and involving not more than two nodal stations.[41]

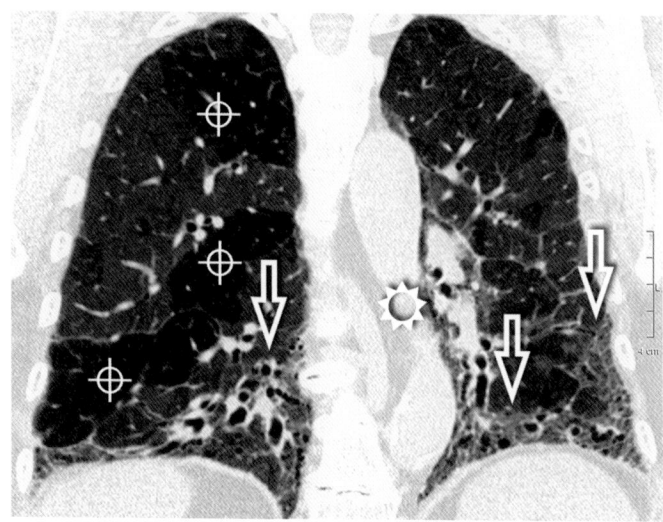

Figure 3-60. Frontal view of both lungs at the level of the descending aorta (*sun*). A basal fibrotic GGO with reticulation and bronchiectasis and bronchiolectasis is indicated by the *arrows*. In this patient, several areas of mosaic oligemia are also present (*bull's-eyes*).

Several CVDs[41] and adverse reactions to therapeutic drugs[53,54] may present with aspects indistinguishable from the idiopathic NSIP. Consequently, the suspicion of the underlying disorder should be formulated on clinical grounds. Occasionally, specific signs of the original disease are visible radiologically[46–49] (Fig. 3-61).

Subset Tug-of-War

Tug-of-war subset is defined by the presence of irregular linear opacities stretching between the mediastinum and the thoracic boundaries, bridging over variably involved bronchi, fissures, and more generally anatomical structures and even pathologic elements found on their way (Fig. 3-62). The mediastinal profiles are variably stretched outward and the thoracic pleural profiles inward, hence the proposal for the name of

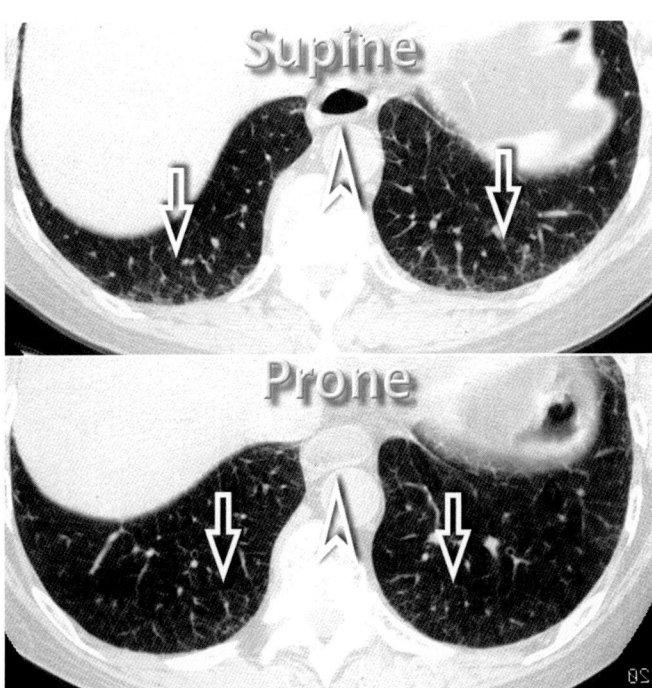

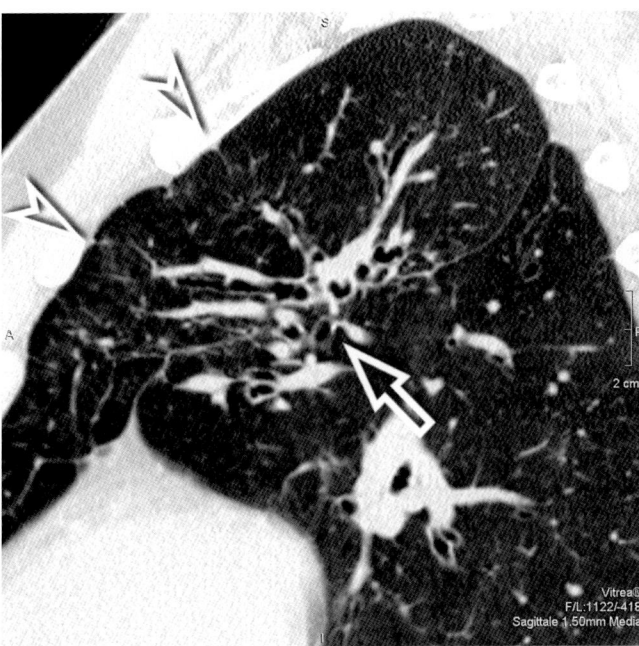

Figure 3-61. Supine and prone scans at a same axial level (costophrenic angles) in a patient with systemic sclerosis. In the supine image, there is some faint increased attenuation with irregular reticulation in the subpleural lung (*arrows*). In the prone scan, the GGO is gone (hence reversible) but the reticulation persists (*arrows*). In both images, the esophagus is enlarged (*arrowheads*).

Figure 3-63. Tug-of-war fibrosis, sagittal image. Straight interstitial connection lines bridge the bronchovascular bundle, entirely stretched anteriorly and superiorly (*arrow*), and several peripheral irregularities point inward (*arrowheads*).

Box 3-6. Diseases Presenting with Fibrotic Pattern, Subset Tug-of-War

Frequent
Sarcoidosis

Rare
Berylliosis (see Sarcoidosis)

nodules, distortion of fissures, bronchial irregularities, traction bronchiectasis, and more-or-less coarse linear opacities corresponding to the fibrotic component of the disease.[55] The elements of the bronchovascular bundle become crowded and show a zigzagging course with angulations[55,56] (Fig. 3-64). Progressive fibrosis leads to central conglomeration of parahilar bronchi embedded in a dense agglomerate of tissue

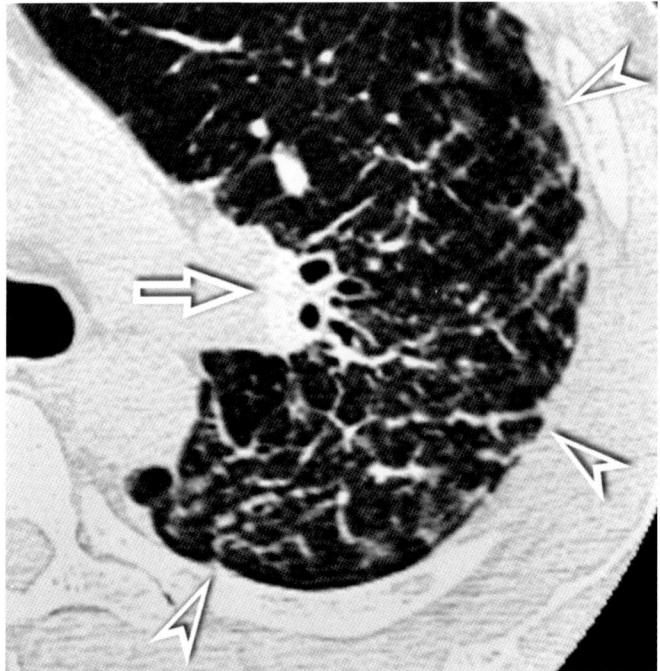

Figure 3-62. Tug-of-war fibrosis, axial scan. Several irregular white lines extend from the hilum, which is stretched outward (*arrow*) to the pulmonary periphery, which in turn is irregular for the presence of several spicules directed inward (*arrowheads*).

this fibrotic subset (Fig. 3-63). Diseases in the Fibrotic Pattern, subset Tug-of-War, are listed in Box 3-6.

Sarcoidosis

Fibrosis may present early in the history of the disease, when nodular elements are fairly well visible. Irregularities of the margin of the

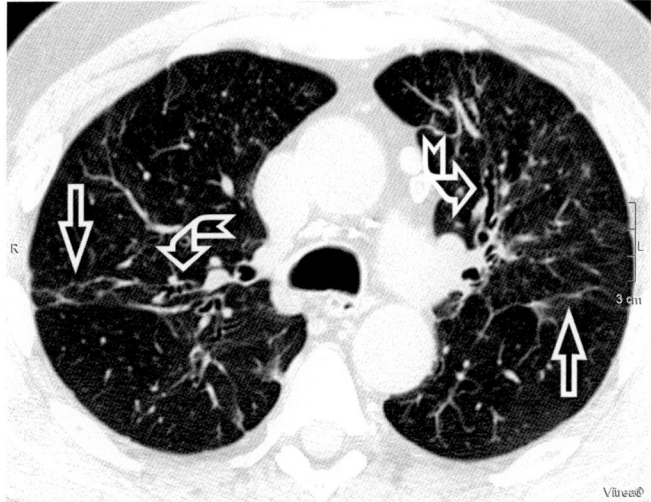

Figure 3-64. Axial scan of a patient with mild fibrosing sarcoidosis. There are some white irregular lines outstretched between the hilum and the periphery (*arrows*). Slightly ectatic bronchi with thickened wall (*curved arrows*) contribute to the feeling of a tug-of-war fibrosis. Calcified lymph nodes can be seen inside the mediastinum.

radiating from the center to the periphery.[56] Honeycombing and cystic abnormalities may be also seen, but rarely the honeycombing involves mainly the lower lung zones, mimicking UIP/IPF.[57]

The disease shows parahilar predominance between the central and the peripheral middle and upper lung, with patchy accentuation of parenchymal distortion and severity of the lesions[55,58] (Fig. 3-65).

Mediastinal lymphadenopathy frequently coexists, often calcified. CT findings suggestive of pulmonary hypertension are possible in the late disease.[2] Cavitation of conglomerated masses may be seen in patients with necrotizing sarcoid granulomatosis, the entity first described by Liebow characterized by sarcoid-like granulomas and vasculitis associated with variable degrees of necrosis[56] (Fig. 3-66).

Subset Bronchocentric Fibrosis

The bronchocentric subset is defined by the presence of a disease in which signs of traction and remodeling prevail at the level of the bronchial elements. The fibrosis may be focal or diffuse.

Focal fibrosis from constrictive bronchiolitis is concentrated on the bronchioli and too subtle to be appreciated radiologically. However, indirect signs of bronchial narrowing are visible, namely a patchy dark lung (Fig. 3-67). This condition is subsequently discussed in the Dark Lung Pattern.

Pulmonary Langerhans cell histiocytosis, also a prominently centrilobular fibrotic process, on the contrary is well visible in form of thick walls around enlarged airways (Fig. 3-68) that assume early a cystic aspect.[59] Consequently, its insertion in the cystic pattern has been considered more suitable. Diseases in the Fibrotic Pattern, subset Bronchocentric Fibrosis, are listed in Box 3-7.

Airway-Centered Interstitial Fibrosis

The main findings of airway-centered interstitial fibrosis are peribronchovascular interstitial thickening with traction bronchiectasis,

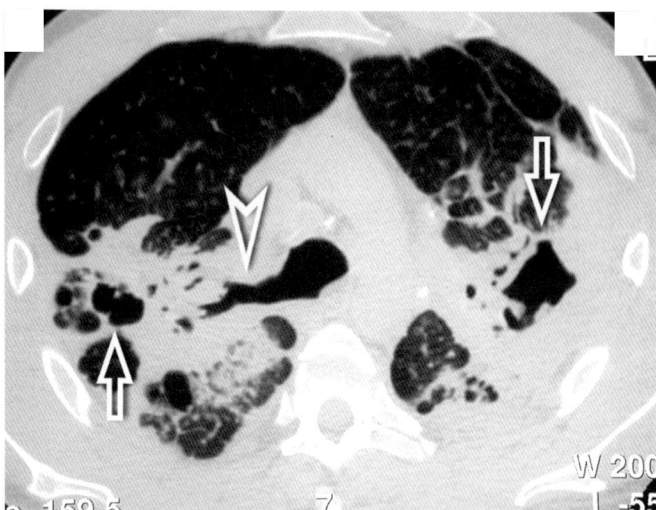

Figure 3-66. Necrotizing sarcoid granulomatosis. Here the lesions extending between the hila and the periphery are dense opacities containing air hyperlucencies from cavitation (*arrows*). Large bronchi stand out; they are embedded and irregularly stretched inside the opacities (*arrowhead*).

thickened airway walls, and surrounding dense tissue with irregular margins (Fig. 3-69). Bronchiolectasis and honeycombing may also occur in a limited number of cases. GGO, poorly defined centrilobular micronodules, and lobular air trapping with the mosaic attenuation of the dark lung pattern are lacking.[59]

The lesions show a central rather than a peripheral distribution. They consistently show scarring around the airways[60] (Fig. 3-70).

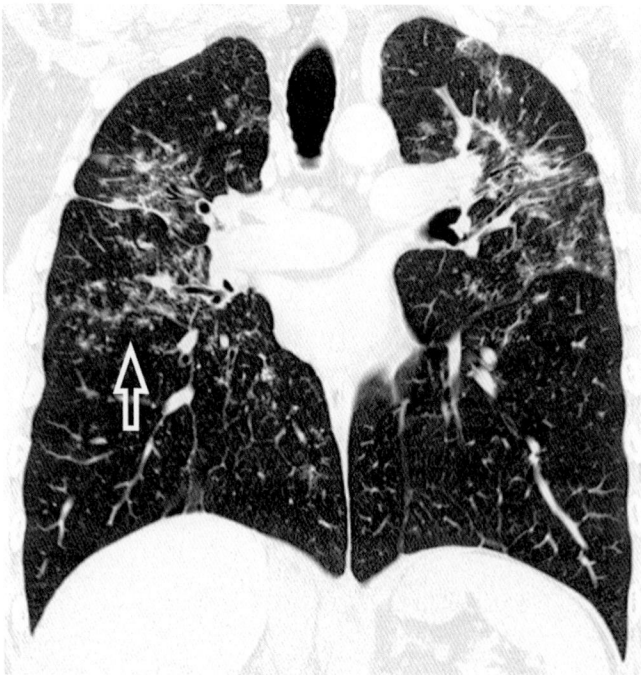

Figure 3-65. Frontal scan of a patient with sarcoidosis. The tug-of-war aspect of the fibrosing component of the disease is well appreciable in the upper lung fields. Several micronodules are also identifiable, in particular in the right middle lung field (*arrow*).

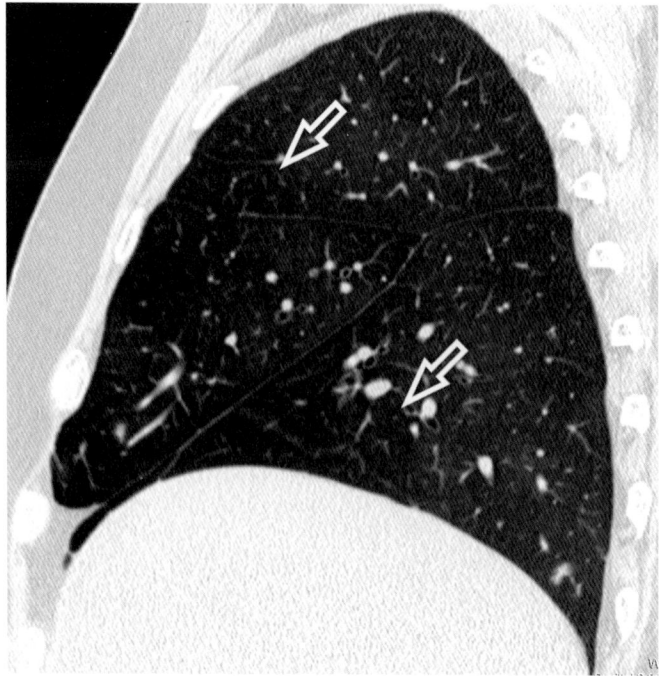

Figure 3-67. Patient with constrictive bronchiolitis post-transplantation. In this sagittal scan, there are vast areas of hyperlucent lung (dark lung) anteriorly (*arrows*), where vessel size and number is reduced.

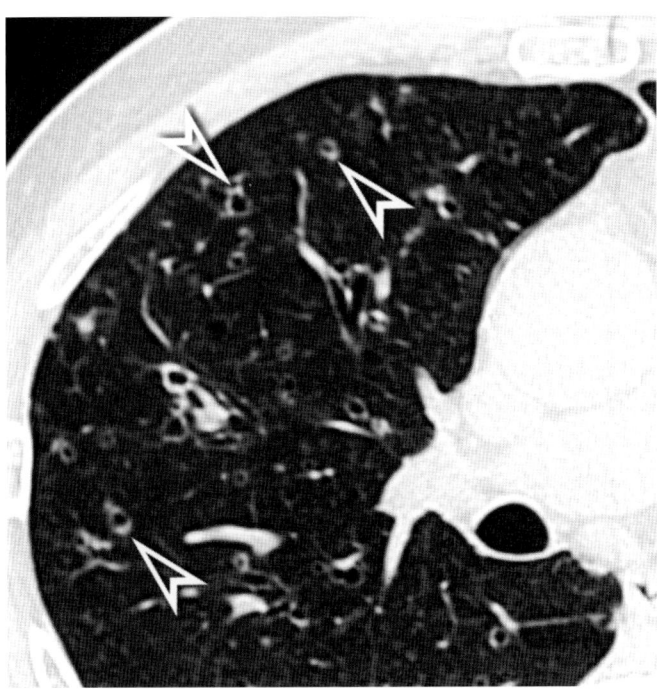

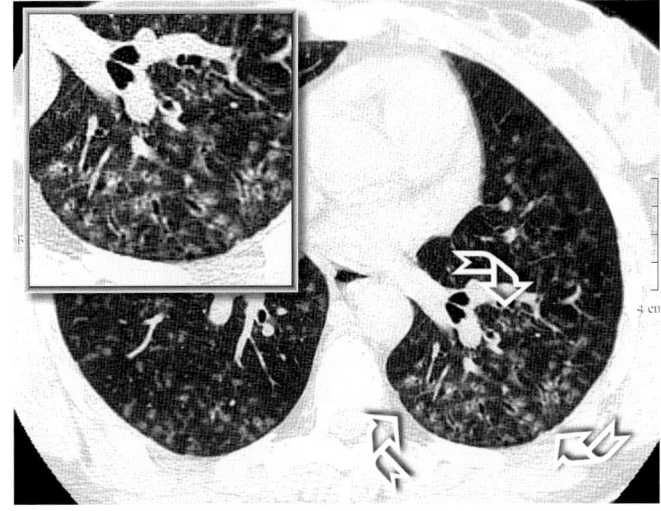

Figure 3-70. Another image of the same patient as in Figure 3-69. In the posterior left lung (*curved arrows*), the insistent thickening of the peripheral airways is well evident (*inset*). (Courtesy of Fabrizio Luppi, MD, Modena, Italy.)

Figure 3-68. Patient with early PLCH. Several ringlike opacities visible in this image represent enlarged bronchi with thickened walls, as indicated by the tiny white dot (the companion artery) nearby (*arrowheads*).

Box 3-7. Diseases Presenting with Fibrotic Pattern, Subset Bronchocentric Fibrosis

Frequent
Constrictive bronchiolitis (see Dark Lung Pattern)
Langerhans cell histiocytosis (see Cystic Pattern)

Rare
Airway-centered interstitial fibrosis

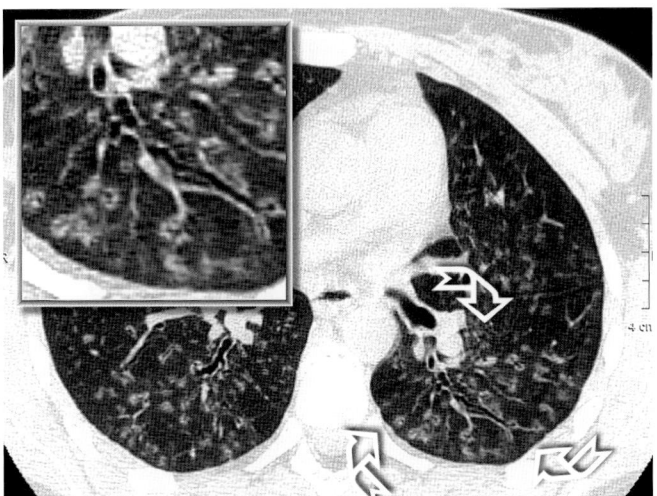

Figure 3-69. At a first glance, the lesions in this patient with ACIF mimic a nodular disease. Actually, the faint opacities scattered throughout the lungs are due to thickening of bronchial walls (better seen in the *inset,* where an enlarged view of the area between the *curved arrows* is shown). (Courtesy of Fabrizio Luppi, MD, Modena, Italy.)

Nodular Pattern

Definition

A nodular pattern is defined by the presence of multiple roundish opacities ranging in diameter from 2 to 10 mm (Fig. 3-71).

High-Resolution Computed Tomography Signs

On HRCT, lung nodules appear as white, roundish lesions with variable morphology and lobular distribution, depending on the route of arrival and on the modality of spread.[2,7,61]

Nodules that have low-density and ill-defined margins (nodular GGO) have a characteristic soft aspect, like snowflakes (Fig. 3-72). Sometimes they are very tiny and difficult to recognize.[20] They are commonly seen in patients with disease that primarily affects centrilobular bronchioles and the immediate area around them. The low-density CT aspect is due to minimal thickening of the peribronchiolar interstitium or partial filling of the peribronchiolar alveoli.[2] Both conditions are below the CT spatial resolution, and thus the common final effect is a focal low-density lesion. The ill-defined margins are due to progressive reduction of interstitial or alveolar involvement extending away from the centrilobular area to the periphery. These types of nodules may coalesce, resulting in the appearance of extensive GGO.

Nodules with high-density and well-defined margins are commonly seen in patients with diseases primarily affecting the interstitium and growing spherically in it surrounded by aerated parenchyma.[2,61] They present a solid aspect like opaque beads and obscure the edges of vessels or other structures that they touch (Fig. 3-73). They may have regular or lobulated contours, the latter aspect secondary to asymmetrical growth. The nodules may coalesce with development of larger opacities or pseudoplaques along the costal or fissural margins.[62]

On occasion, the nodules may have shaggy profiles, especially in diseases with a fibrotic component (Fig. 3-74). The existence of small black areas inside these high-density nodules may be due to necrosis (see Fig. 3-74) or traction bronchiolectasis. The presence of faint increased lung attenuation around the nodules (*halo sign*) is most often an expression of hemorrhage (see Fig. 3-74) or of inflammatory infiltrates from any origin.[62,65] Regarding the lobular distribution, this is the result of the route of arrival and of their modality of spread, both underlying their distinction in subsets.

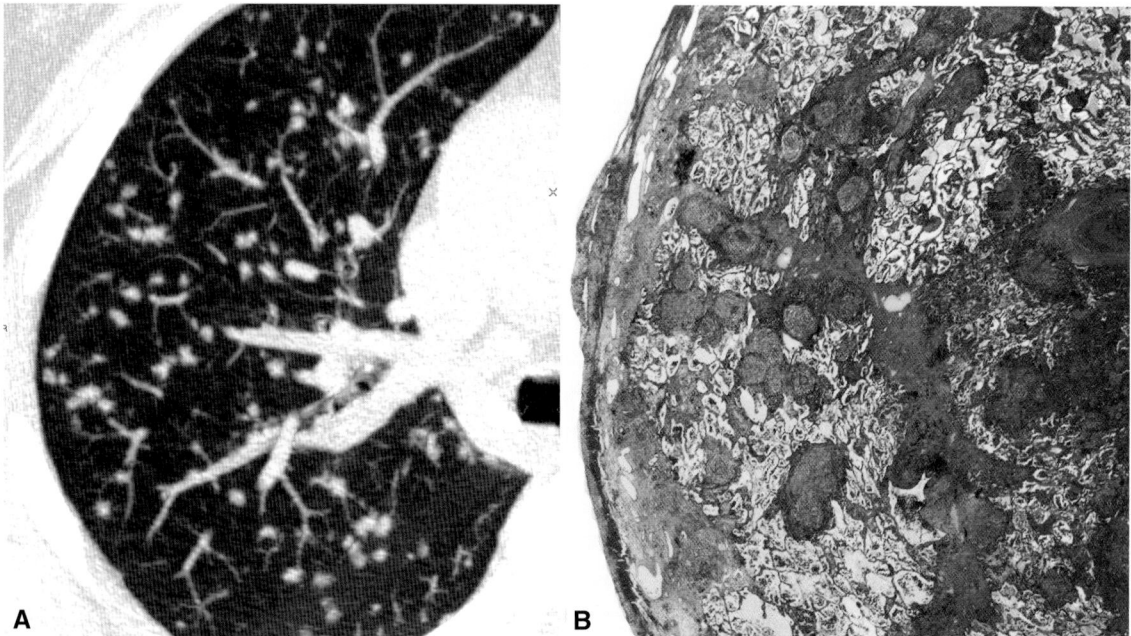

Figure 3-71. Radiology (**A**) and pathology (**B**) of a patient with nodular disease. The presence of multiple small roundish opacities scattered throughout the lung is the key element to identify this pattern.

Subsets

The inhaled diseases show nodules close to the bronchiole in the center of lobules (see subset Centrilobular). The diseases that grow along the lymphatics are more present in the periphery of the lobules and in particular along the fissures (see subset Lymphatic). The lesions that spread hematogenously are visible everywhere, so they may be seen in the core but also in the periphery (see subset Random), sometimes in connection with blood vessels.[61,64]

Subset Centrilobular

On CT images, one can assume a centrilobular distribution of nodules when they stop at a certain distance from the pleural surfaces ("avid of pleura").[7,64] This feature is well demonstrated on the sagittal MIP images with the visibility of thin black lines of normal lung along the fissures (Fig. 3-75).

In the early stage, Langerhans cell histiocytosis is characterized by the presence of centrilobular nodules that, however, become cysts early.[65] Consequently, the inclusion of this disease in the cystic pattern has been considered more suitable. Diseases in the Nodular Pattern, subset Centrilobular, are listed in Box 3-8.

Follicular Bronchiolitis

The basic features of follicular bronchiolitis consist of bilateral well-defined or ill-defined small centrilobular nodules (Fig. 3-76). In

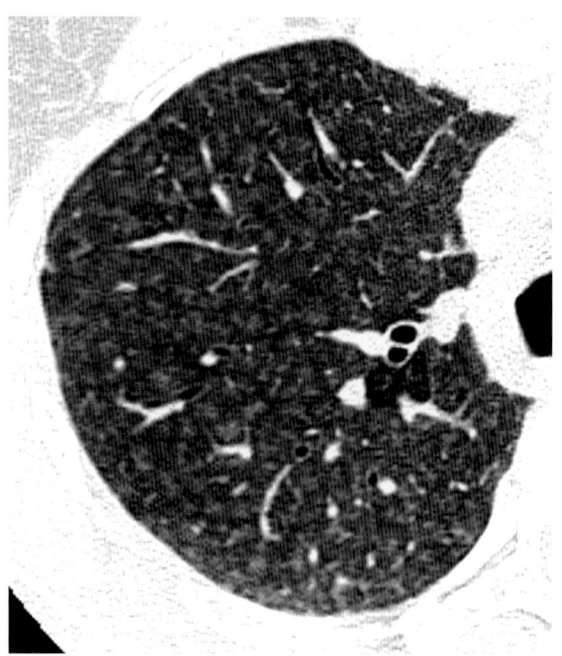

Figure 3-72. Nodules with low-density and ill-defined margins (nodular GGO). Innumerable white soft roundish lesions are visible, with an aspect similar to snowflakes.

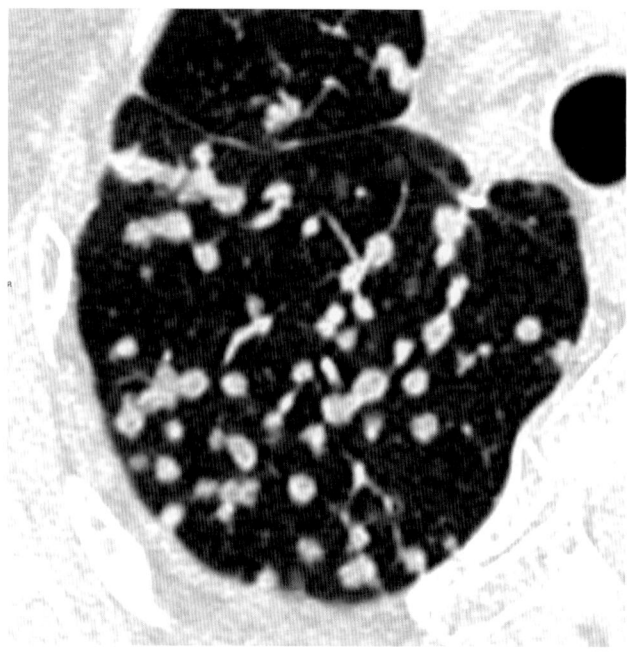

Figure 3-73. Nodules with high-density and well-defined margins. Several white dense roundish lesions are visible with an aspect similar to opaque beads.

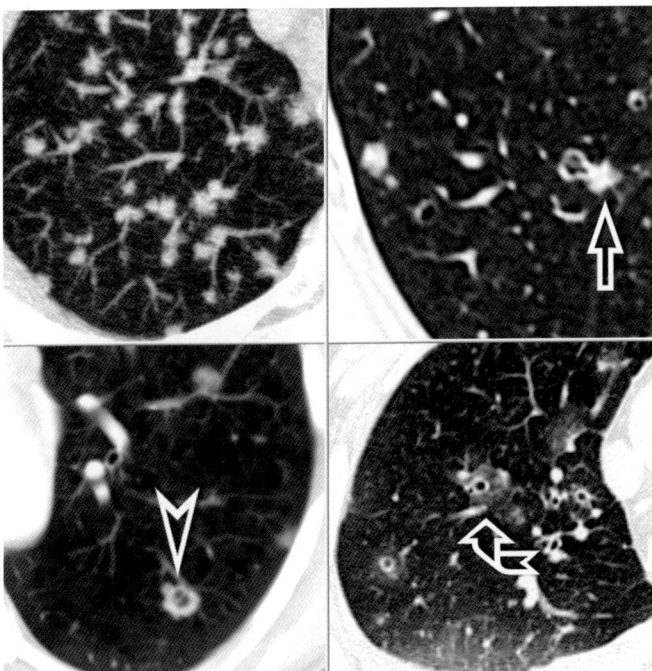

Frequent
Follicular bronchiolitis
Subacute hypersensitivity pneumonitis
Respiratory bronchiolitis–interstitial lung disease

Rare
Langerhans cell histiocytosis (see Cystic Pattern)
Lymphoid interstitial pneumonia (see Nodular Pattern, subset Lymphatic)

Figure 3-74. *Upper left,* In this patient with sarcoidosis, the nodules present shaggy profiles related to their fibrotic component. *Upper right,* Nodules with shaggy profiles (*arrow*) are quite typical also of patients with Langerhans cell histiocytosis. *Lower left,* Cavitated nodule (*arrowhead*) in a patient with pulmonary metastatic disease. *Lower right,* Cavitated nodules with *halo sign* (*curved arrow*) in a patient with metastatic angiosarcoma.

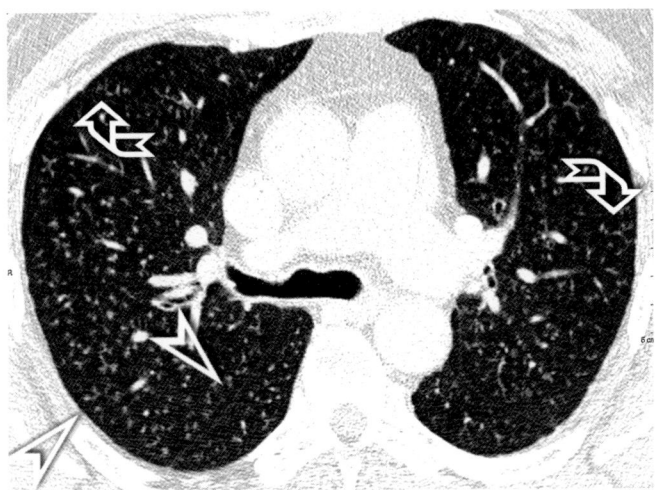

Figure 3-76. Axial view of a patient with follicular bronchiolitis. Innumerable small nodules are scattered throughout both lungs, but they spare the subpleural region (*arrowheads*), which indicates a centrilobular distribution. In the periphery of the lungs, there are also branching structures with *tree-in-bud* aspect (*curved arrows*).

some patients, the centrilobular opacities may present a branching appearance reflecting the morphology of the small airways involved, thereby with aspects mimicking an aspect called *tree-in-bud*[66-68] (see Fig. 3-76).

The lesions are bilateral and diffuse (Fig. 3-77), sometimes with a predominant involvement of the lower zones.[66]

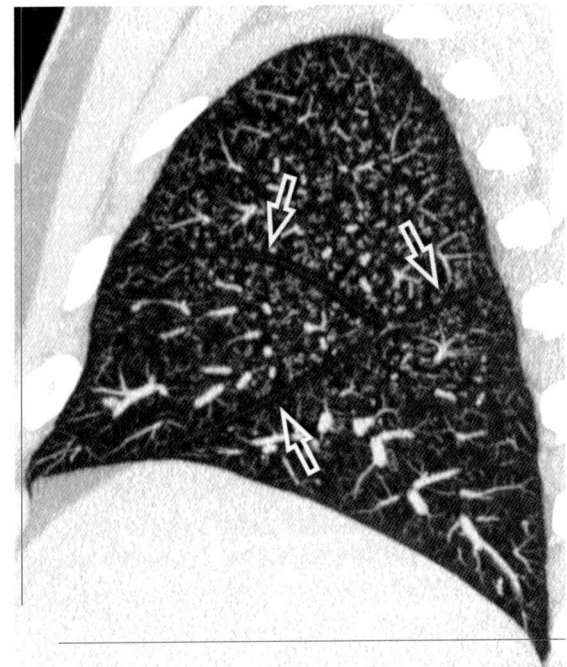

Figure 3-75. Nodular Pattern, subset Centrilobular. The sagittal MIP image highlights the centrilobular arrangement of the nodules that stop a certain distance from the pleural surface. As a result, they are separated from the fissures by a dark rim (*arrows*).

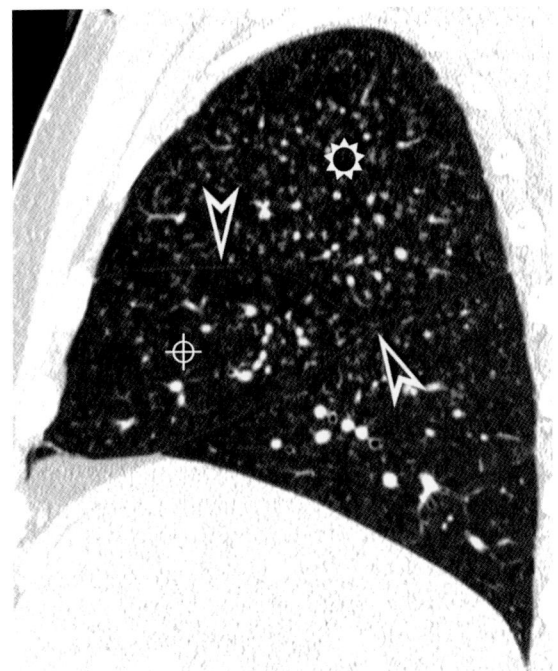

Figure 3-77. Sagittal view of the same patient as in Figure 3-76. This computed tomography plane highlights the visibility of the fissures (*arrowheads*) that are not involved by the nodules. This view also shows the craniocaudal distribution of the lesions that prevail in the right upper (*sun*) and middle (*bull's-eye*) lobes.

Patchy areas of GGO are present in 75% of patients, and mild bronchial wall thickening often exists[68] (Fig. 3-78). Rare subpleural nodules also may be present (20%), and thin-walled cysts may occur due to "check-valve" obstruction of small bronchioles by lymphoid tissue.[69,70]

Subacute Hypersensitivity Pneumonitis

The hypersensitivity pneumonitis pattern is defined by the presence of numerous centrilobular nodules with low-density and ill-defined margins (nodular GGO), usually less than 5 mm in diameter (Fig. 3-79).[35] The key to the diagnosis is the coexistence of sporadic lobular areas of air trapping appearing as patches of black lung (see Fig. 3-79). These regions of lobular air trapping are caused by concomitant bronchiolar inflammation and obstruction.[71]

The lesions are uniformly distributed, with possible middle-lower predominance[35,71] (Fig. 3-80).

Areas of GGO often coexist. These are usually bilateral and symmetric, but sometimes they can be patchy. Another significant diagnos-

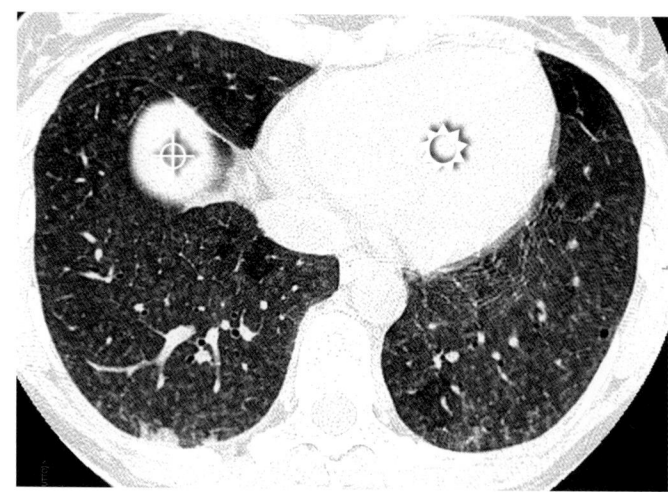

Figure 3-80. This axial scan of the same patient as in Figure 3-79, but at a lower level, confirms a high prevalence of lesions in the basal lung. The heart is indicated by the *sun*, the hepatic dome by the *bull's-eye*.

tic finding is the combination of patchy GGO, normal lung, and dark lung from air trapping. This mixture of densities gives the lung a distinctive appearance that has been nicknamed "head cheese" because of its resemblance to the variegated cross-sectional appearance of sausage made from parts of the head of a hog[72] (Fig. 3-81).

Bronchiolar wall thickening may also occur, and lung cysts have been found occasionally. The latter are probably caused by partial obstruction of bronchioles ("check-valve" mechanism).[71] Mediastinal lymph node enlargement has been described in approximately 30% of patients. In patients with an insidious onset of disease, focal areas of consolidation may be occasionally present, presumably representing OP or superimposed unrelated processes such as aspiration injury or infectious pneumonia.

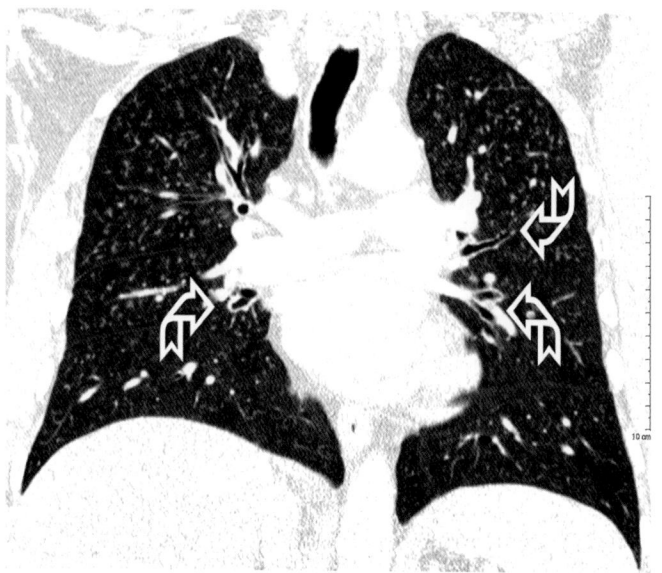

Figure 3-78. Coronal view of the same patient as in Figure 3-76. Bronchial wall thickening is visible in both parahilar zones (*curved arrows*).

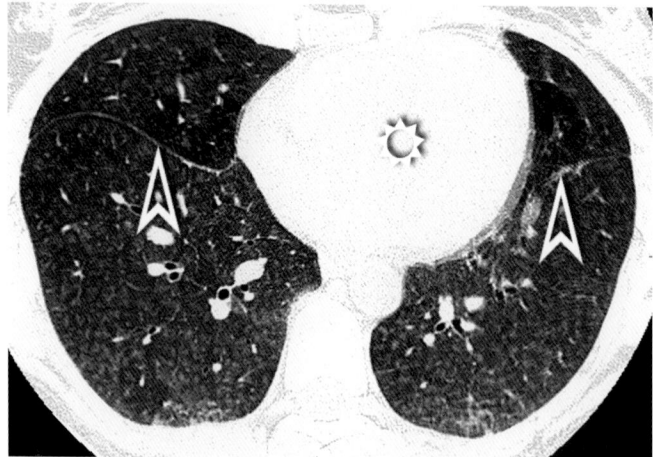

Figure 3-79. Subacute hypersensitivity pneumonitis. The axial scan at the level of the heart (*sun*) shows low-density, ill-defined, uniformly distributed nodules. In terms of their aspect, the nodules are similar to snowflakes. A few dark areas of lobular size due to air trapping are also visible in the middle lobe and in the lingula (*arrowheads*).

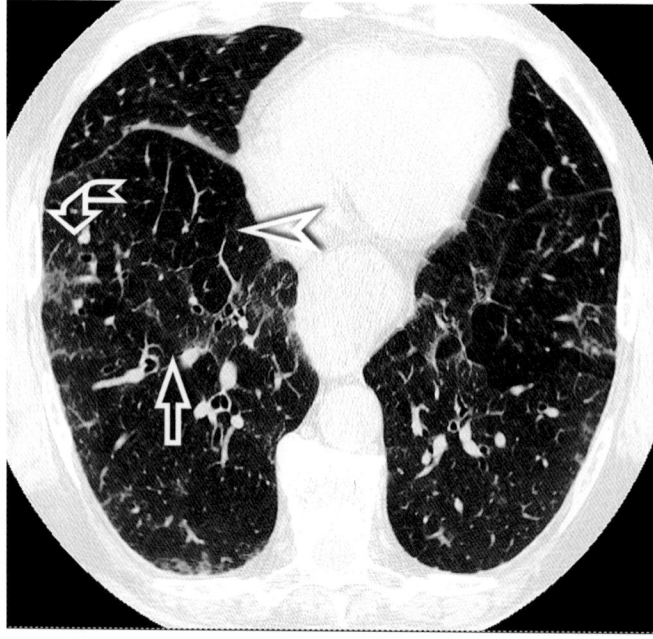

Figure 3-81. Another patient with hypersensitivity pneumonitis in the subacute phase. The image shows a patchy mixture of normal parenchyma (*arrow*), areas of GGO (*curved arrow*), and dark lobules (*arrowhead*), resulting in the so-called "head cheese" aspect.

Respiratory Bronchiolitis–Interstitial Lung Disease

The typical presentation of respiratory bronchiolitis–interstitial lung disease (RB-ILD) is that of centrilobular nodularity (Fig. 3-82), often in combination with areas of GGO and moderate centrilobular emphysema. The nodules present low-density and ill-defined margins (nodular GGO) and may be tiny and difficult to recognize[73,74] (see Fig. 3-82). Centrilobular nodules reflect accumulation of macrophages and inflammation in and around the respiratory bronchioles.

The nodules have an even uniform distribution in the axial plane, and they predominate in the upper lobes[76] (Fig. 3-83). The areas of GGO involve the lung zones diffusely with a patchy distribution; this

sign is thought to reflect the macrophage accumulation in the alveoli and alveolar ducts.[75]

Another common finding in RB-ILD is central and peripheral bronchial wall thickening caused by airway inflammation (90%) (Fig. 3-84). Areas of hypoattenuation are noted in 38% of patients and are most likely related to air trapping.[75,77] Sometimes signs of other smoking-related interstitial lung diseases may coexist (i.e., desquamative interstitial pneumonitis, pulmonary Langerhans cell histiocytosis, smoking-related pulmonary fibrosis), creating mixed patterns.[76]

Subset Lymphatic

Lymphatic nodules commonly occur along lymphatic routes. They tend to be concentrated and more visible along the costal margins and/or the fissures ("avid of pleura")[7] (Fig. 3-85). They are also visible in the perilobular interstitium, as much as along vessels and bronchi.[61,64]

In the lymphatic subset, however, the nodules are more-or-less individually seen along appropriate routes that are not intrinsically thickened. In contrast, in the Septal Pattern, subset Nodular, the nodules appear embedded within thickened interlobular septa and subpleural lines, with an overall beaded appearance. As previously stated, this important distinction helps the radiologist distinguish the two diseases (e.g., sarcoidosis [Nodular Pattern, subset Lymphatic] from lymphangitic carcinomatosis [Septal Pattern, subset Nodular]).

In the interstitial form of amyloidosis, the abnormalities may occur as distinct subpleural nodules, but nodular septal thickening and confluent subpleural consolidative opacities are more commonly observed (see Septal Pattern, subset Nodular). Diseases in the Nodular Pattern, subset Lymphatic, are listed in Box 3-9.

Sarcoidosis

The most characteristic abnormality in patients with sarcoidosis is the presence of small, high-density nodules with well-defined margins, sometimes with shaggy profiles (see Fig. 3-74). The nodules are distributed along the costal margins and the fissures, but they are also

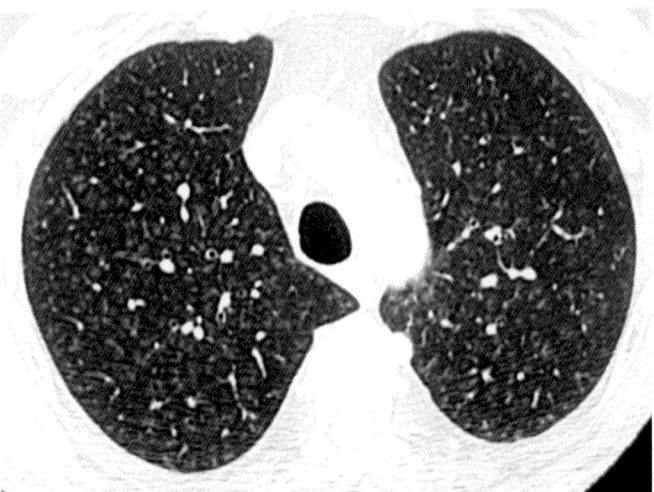

Figure 3-82. RB-ILD in a heavy smoker with cough. The axial image, obtained through the upper lungs, shows diffuse centrilobular nodules bilaterally. The tiny nodules have a very low density; hence, they are difficult to recognize unless a narrow radiologic window is set.

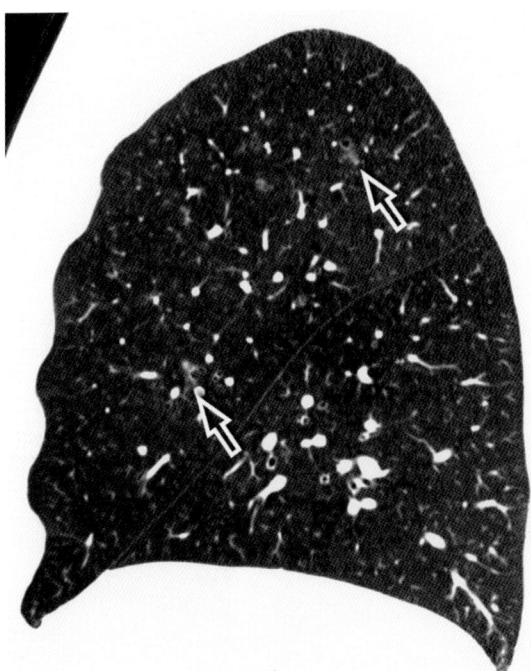

Figure 3-83. Sagittal view of another patient with RB-ILD. Scattered small opacities of faint density (*arrows*) are present, predominantly in the upper lobes.

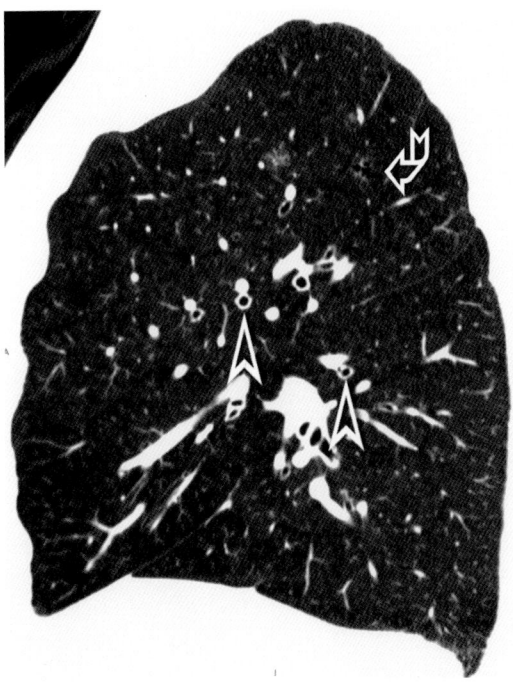

Figure 3-84. Sagittal view of the same patient as in Figure 3-83. The findings range from barely visible micronodular GGOs to a more convincing bronchial wall thickening (*arrowheads*) and some centrilobular emphysema (*curved arrow*).

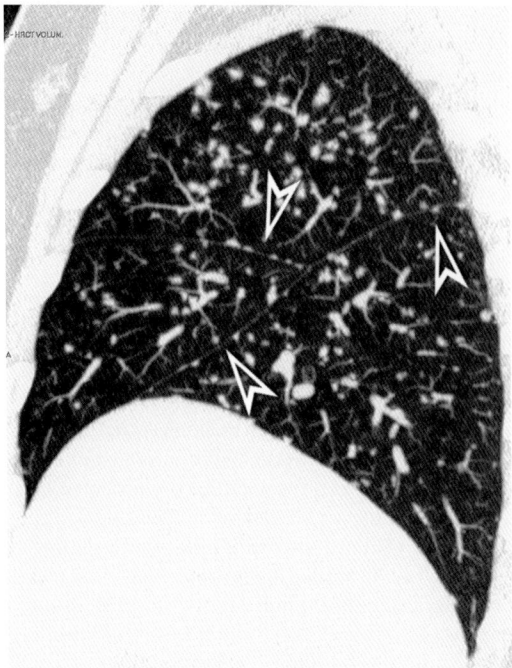

Figure 3-85. Nodular Pattern, subset Lymphatic. The sagittal view beautifully shows the affinity of the nodules for the subpleural spaces—in this case, especially for the fissures (*arrowheads*).

Box 3-9. Diseases Presenting with Nodular Pattern, Subset Lymphatic

Frequent
Sarcoidosis

Rare
Interstitial amyloidosis (see Septal Pattern, subset Nodular)
Lymphoid interstitial pneumonia
Silicosis and coal worker pneumoconiosis

concentrated along the bronchovascular sheath[56,78] (Fig. 3-86). They may coalesce to form large nodules or pseudoplaques along the pleural margins[62] (see Fig. 3-86).

The distribution of the lesions is patchy, with a parahilar predominance (see Fig. 3-86). A predilection for the upper-dorsal lung zones is often present[56,78] (Fig. 3-87).

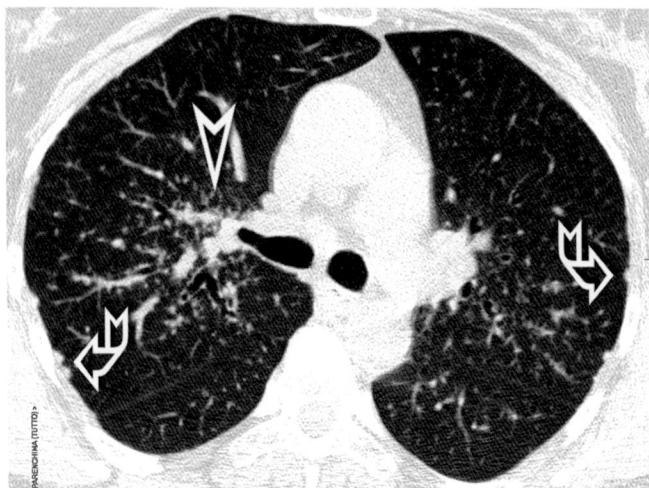

Figure 3-86. Sarcoidosis. Several small nodules with well-defined margins and high density are distributed along the costal margins (*curved arrows*) and the bronchovascular bundle (*arrowhead*).

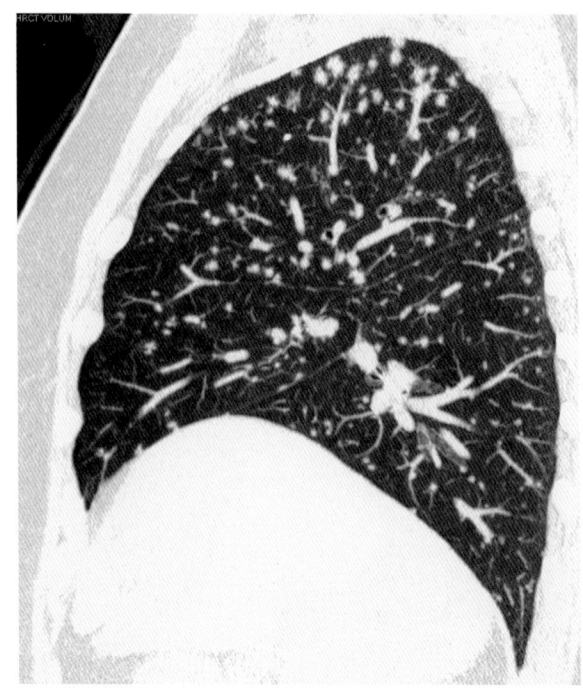

Figure 3-87. Sagittal view of a patient with sarcoidosis. A middle-upper predominance of the nodules is evident.

Lymphadenopathy is the most common finding in sarcoidosis, and typically it is hilar, bilateral, and symmetrical. In addition, mediastinal lymph node enlargement is often present, especially in the right paratracheal and subcarinal node groups (Fig. 3-88). Lymph node calcifications are visible in 25% to 50% of cases, and these may be amorphous, punctate, dense, or eggshell and suggest chronic disease.[78]

Occasionally, the confluence of several interstitial granulomas may result in large, irregular, masslike nodules without or with air bronchogram, resembling air-space consolidations. Small satellite nodules may be present at the periphery of these opacities, an

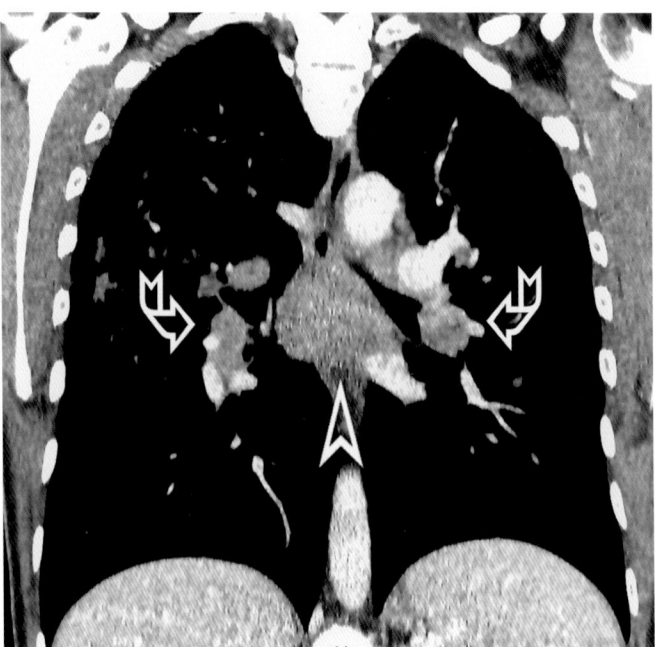

Figure 3-88. Contrast-enhanced frontal view through the middle of the mediastinum in a patient with sarcoidosis. Large subcarinal (*arrowhead*) and hilar (*curved arrows*) adenopathies are present. They are quite typical of this disease.

occurrence referred to as the "galaxy sign," given its resemblance to collections of stars.[79] In some cases, on the contrary, the nodules can be so small that they are not distinctly visible, but their attenuation produces patchy areas of finely granular increased opacity (granular GGO). Finally, granulomas situated in the small airways can cause lobular air trapping.[80]

Lymphoid Interstitial Pneumonia

Lymphoid interstitial pneumonia is a multifaceted disease that may present with different patterns depending at least in part on the underlying disease. In patients with acquired immunodeficiency syndrome (AIDS), HRCT most often shows nodular aspects along lymphatic routes. The well-defined nodules range from 1 to 3 mm (Fig. 3-89). This pattern may be associated with thickening of the bronchovascular bundles, mild interlobular septal thickening, and tiny ill-defined centrilobular nodules.[81]

The lesions involve mainly the lower lung zones[82] (Fig. 3-90).

In Sjögren syndrome, lymphoid interstitial pneumonia is typically associated with round or oval thin-walled cysts of variable size (Fig. 3-91). They may be seen in up to 80% of patients and are typically few in number, and they measure less than 3 cm in diameter. They presumably result from air trapping due to peribronchiolar lymphoid infiltration.[83,84]

Other possible findings include bilateral areas of ground glass attenuation and poorly defined centrilobular nodules, most often in congenital immunodeficiency syndromes. Lymphadenopathy is variably associated with lymphoid interstitial pneumonia, according to different series (0% to 68%).[81,83,85]

Silicosis and Coal Worker's Pneumoconiosis

The characteristic feature of silicosis and coal worker's pneumoconiosis (CWP) is the presence of multiple nodules with a lymphatic distribution. Usually the nodules predominate in the subpleural regions, but they are also observed in the centrilobular regions (Fig. 3-92). The high-density nodules often have well-defined margins, sometimes with calcification. Subpleural nodules have a rounded or triangular configuration, and if they are confluent, they may resemble pleural plaques (pseudoplaques)[86] (see Fig. 3-92).

The lesions of pneumoconiosis mainly involve the upper and posterior lung zones. Bilateral and symmetrical distributions may be observed, although a right-sided predominance is common[86,87] (Fig. 3-93).

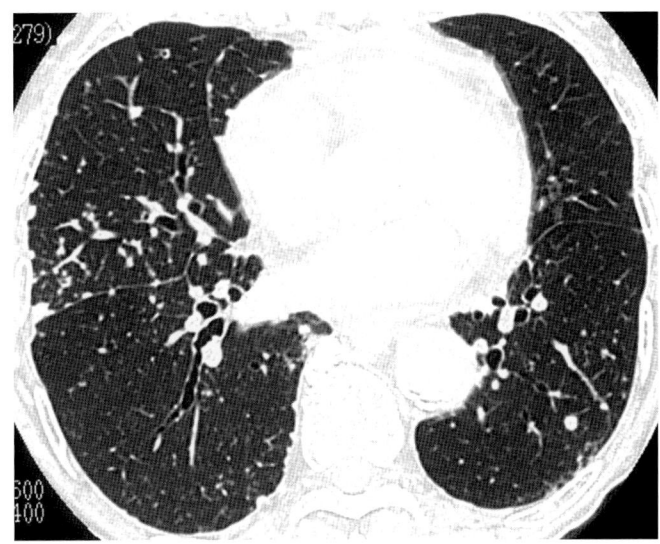

Figure 3-90. Same patient as in Figure 3-89. The axial scan at a lower level shows some prevalence of the nodules in the lower lung.

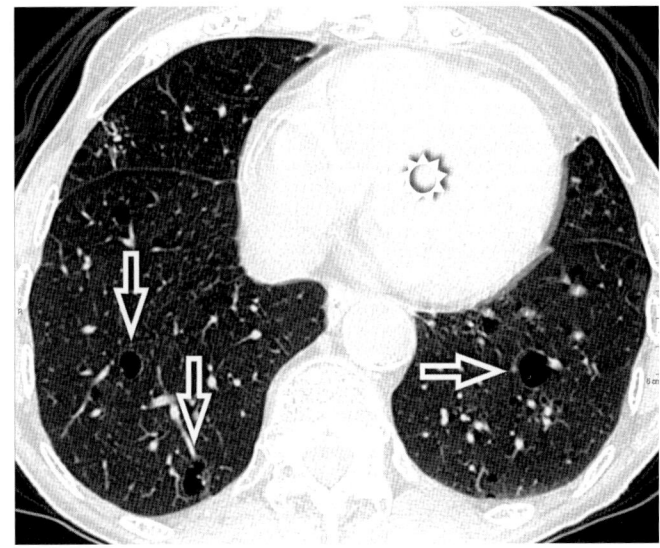

Figure 3-91. Axial scan at the level of the heart (*sun*) in a patient with Sjögren syndrome. The image shows several cysts in both lungs; they appear as small, black, rounded lesions with very thin walls (*arrows*).

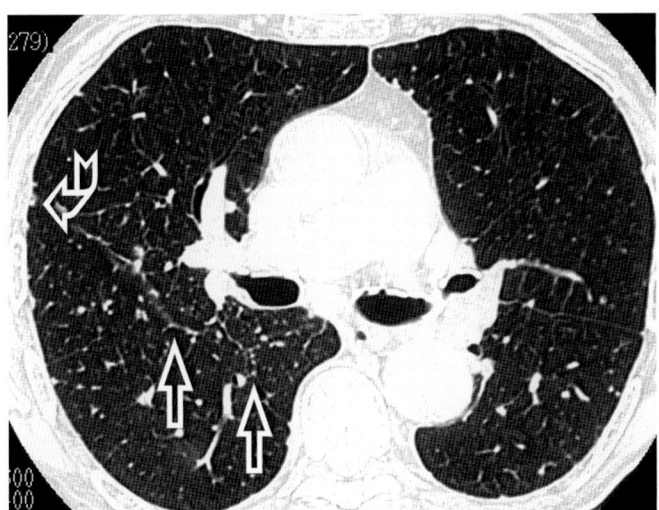

Figure 3-89. This axial image in a patient with LIP shows subpleural micronodules (*curved arrow*) and nodular thickening of interlobular septa (*arrows*). In this case, the lesions prevail to the right.

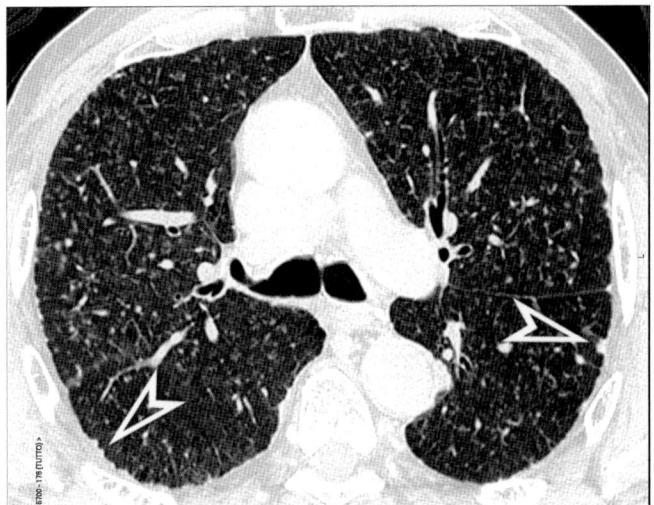

Figure 3-92. Axial thin-section computed tomogram in a patient with silicosis. The image shows numerous small nodules in both lungs. Note also the pseudoplaques that represent aggregates of several subpleural nodules (*arrowheads*).

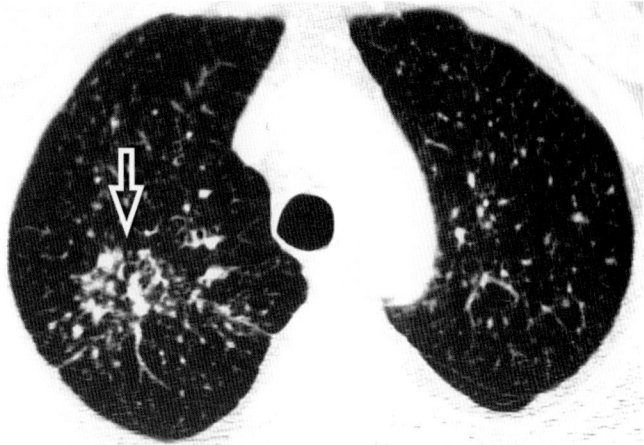

Figure 3-93. Axial scan of a patient with silicosis. The image shows a posterior predominance of the nodules and a higher profusion to the right (*arrow*).

Hilar and mediastinal lymph node enlargement may precede the appearance of parenchymal nodular lesions. Calcification of lymph nodes is common (Fig. 3-94) and may occur at the periphery of the node, producing an "eggshell" appearance. This so-called "eggshell calcification pattern" is highly suggestive of silicosis.[87]

The appearance of large parenchymal opacities or hyperdense areas greater than 1 cm in diameter indicates the presence of complicated silicosis/CWP (progressive massive fibrosis). These masses are often bilateral, symmetrical, and calcified, and they can demonstrate cavitations.[88]

Subset Random

Random nodules are visible everywhere and also touching the pleural surfaces but without a consistent relationship with them ("indifferent to the pleura") (Fig. 3-95). At times, they can be seen in contact with the extremities of the vascular structures from which they seem to originate ("feeding vessel" sign)[7,64] (see Fig. 3-95). Diseases in the Nodular Pattern, subset Random, are listed in Box 3-10.

Hematogenous Metastases
The nodules, usually dense and well defined, tend to appear evenly distributed. Individual nodules may have "feeding vessels" consistent with

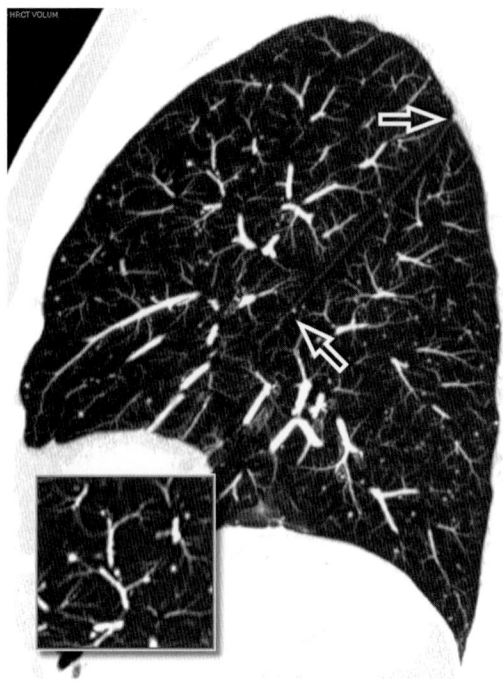

Figure 3-95. Nodular Pattern, subset Random. This sagittal MIP shows sharply defined nodules randomly distributed throughout both lungs. Some of these lie along the pleural surfaces (*arrows*) but without an elective affinity. Some nodules seem related to adjacent vessels (*inset*).

Box 3-10. Diseases Presenting with Nodular Pattern, Subset Random

Frequent
Hematogenous metastases
Miliary tuberculosis

Rare
Miliary fungal infection (see Miliary Tuberculosis)

their hematogenous origin (Fig. 3-96). Nodules with poorly defined margins can be identified in 16% to 30% of cases; these may reflect lepidic growth of tumor.[64,89] Nodules may also be cavitated and/or surrounded by a "halo" of ground glass attenuation, which is typical of hemorrhage.[89,90]

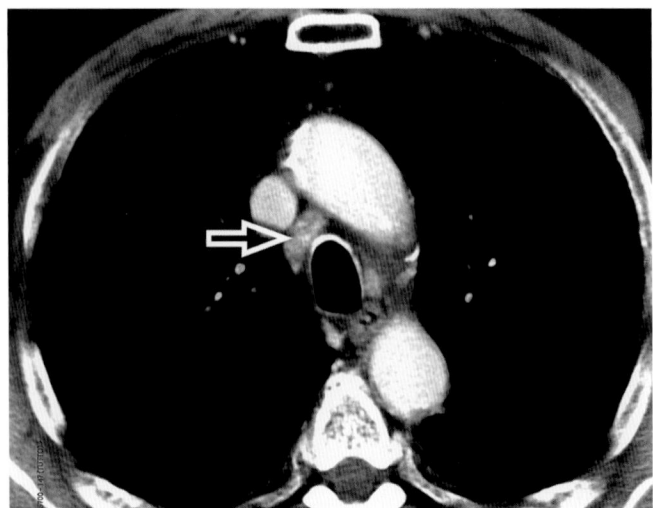

Figure 3-94. The computed tomography scan, documented with a mediastinal window, shows tiny calcifications in the pretracheal lymph nodes (*arrow*).

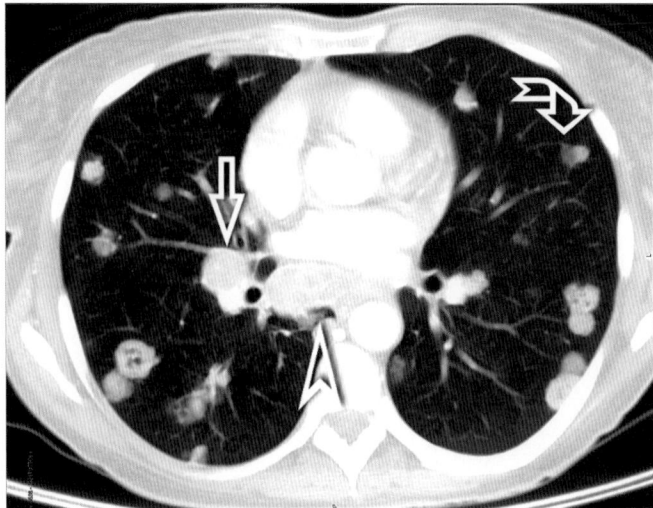

Figure 3-96. Metastatic nodules. The image shows random nodules of different size, and one of them seems to present a "feeding vessel" (*curved arrow*). Note also enlarged hilar (*arrow*) and subcarinal (*arrowhead*) lymph nodes.

A basilar predominance is typically noted due to preferential blood flow to the lung bases. When limited in number, metastatic nodules may be seen primarily in the lung periphery. In patients who have innumerable metastases, a uniform distribution throughout the lung is common[89] (Fig. 3-97).

Macronodules, carcinomatous lymphangitis, and enlarged lymph nodes also may be present (Fig 3-98; see also Fig. 3-96). Occasionally, intravascular tumor emboli may result in nodular or beaded enlargement of the peripheral pulmonary arteries with a *tree-in-bud* appearance[91] (see Fig. 3-98).

Miliary Tuberculosis

Numerous dense 1- to 3-mm nodules that are uniform in size, either sharply or poorly defined, are characteristic of this disease (Fig. 3-99).

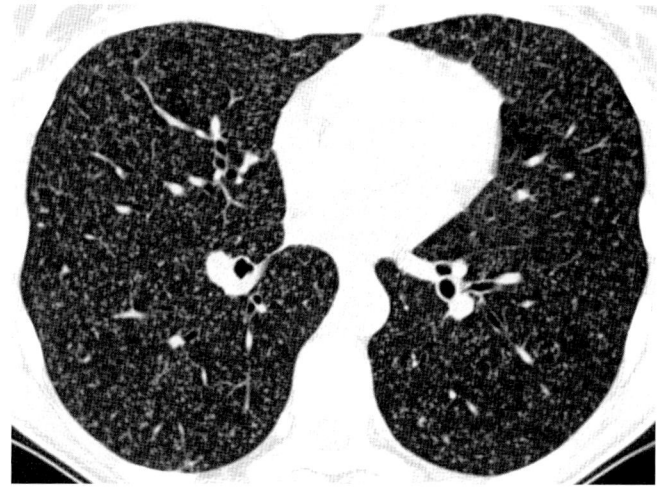

Figure 3-99. Miliary tuberculosis. The axial image shows innumerable noncalcified nodules of miliary size scattered throughout both lungs with random distribution. The nodules are dense and uniform in size.

The nodules may be observed in the subpleural regions or along the fissures, but the general impression is of a random distribution. At times, a relationship may be observed with the most peripheral vessels.[92,93] Macronodules resulting from the fusion of several granulomas are sometimes seen. GGOs are common in these patients and may represent areas of edema or multiple microgranulomas.[94,95] The nodules are distributed uniformly throughout the lungs without cephalocaudal or central-to-peripheral preference[92] (Fig. 3-100).

Associated findings that may suggest the diagnosis are present in up to 30% of affected persons and include consolidation, cavitation, and signs of bronchogenic spread of the disease with *tree-in-bud* pattern (see Fig. 3-100) and lymphadenopathy.[92] Necrotic lymph nodes may be observed in 70% of seropositive patients and in 20% of

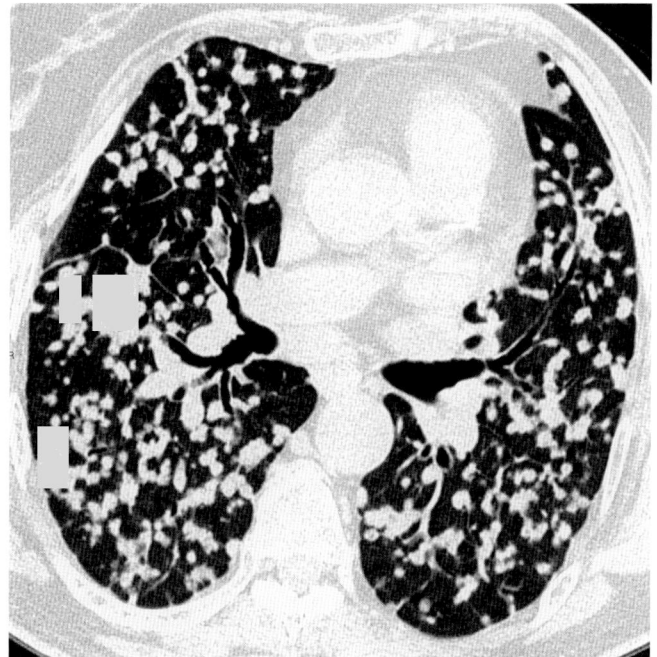

Figure 3-97. The axial image taken through the middle lung zone shows innumerable nodules with uniform random distribution in this patient with metastatic disease.

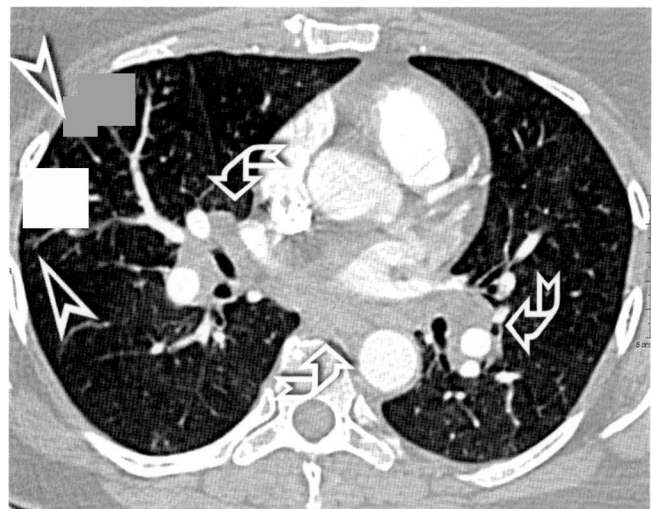

Figure 3-98. Axial image in a patient with metastatic breast carcinoma. A micronodularity is intuitable in the middle lobe, where some lesions assume a *tree-in-bud* appearance (*arrowheads*). Note also the mediastinal and hilar soft tissue density due to enlarged lymph nodes (*curved arrows*).

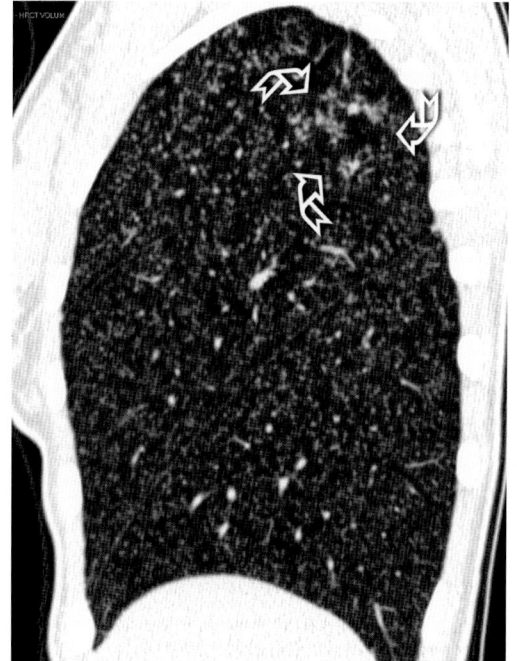

Figure 3-100. Sagittal view of the same patient as in Figure 3-99. The tiny nodules are scattered quite uniformly all through the lungs. In the upper lobe, there are also signs of bronchogenic spread of the disease with a *tree-in-bud* pattern (*curved arrows*).

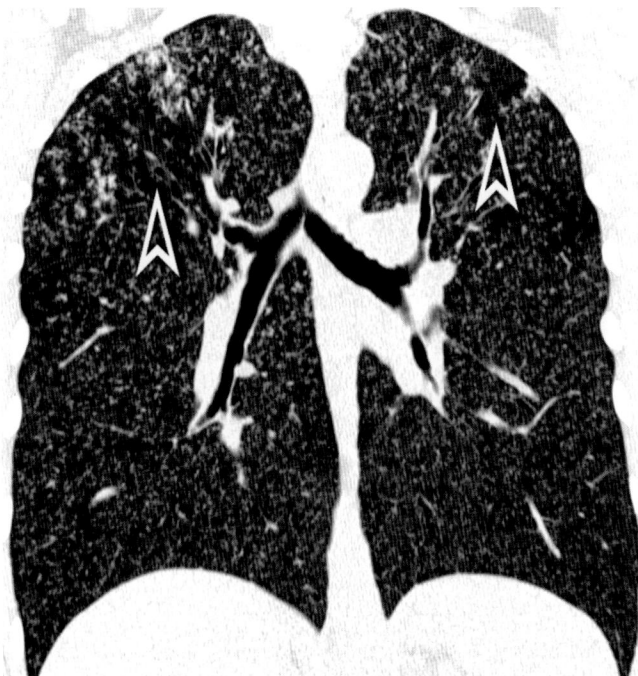

Figure 3-101. Coronal view of the same patient as in Figure 3-99. Patchy areas of oligemic dark lung (*arrowheads*) are present in the upper lung fields.

seronegative patients.[93] Diffuse or localized GGO is sometimes seen, and it may herald acute respiratory distress syndrome.[94,95] Changes from previous tuberculosis are seen in 50% of the patients and provide an aid in the differential diagnosis. Such changes often occur in the upper lobes as fibrotic bands with traction bronchiectasis, apical calcified nodules, and areas of oligemia due to previous bronchiolitis obliterans[95,96] (Fig. 3-101).

Fungal infection may produce diffuse interstitial lung disease characterized by small nodules with random distribution like miliary tuberculosis.[97] Also in this type of infection, signs of bronchiolar spreading with bronchioles filled with infected material are often present and result in a *tree-in-bud* appearance.[98] All these aspects are most commonly seen in immunocompromised patients.[99] The presence of cavitation inside the nodules and large nodules with a *halo sign* are both suggestive of fungal infection. The nodules may be associated with areas of air-space consolidation.[62,100]

Alveolar Pattern

Definition

An alveolar pattern is present when more-or-less broad portions of lung become more opaque than normal, due to a partial or complete filling of alveoli (Fig. 3-102). The pulmonary architecture is overall preserved, and if signs of interstitial involvement are present, they are not prevalent. Alveolar filling may be due to fluid, cells, or other material that in most cases, radiology is not able to discriminate. Nevertheless, size and aspect of the opacities, their distribution within the lung, and a number of ancillary signs provide useful diagnostic clues in several conditions.

Pure interstitial thickening from accumulation of cells, fluid, or other substances (including fibrosis) may simulate an alveolar pattern. However, when this occurs, associated evidence of spreading along interstitial routes (see Septal Pattern) or traction/remodeling of the pulmonary structures (see Fibrotic Pattern) should be evident.

High-Resolution Computed Tomography Signs

The main signs of an alveolar disorder are GGO and consolidation. GGO appears as hazy increase of lung attenuation with preservation of the bronchial and vascular margins[20,26] (Fig. 3-103). GGO may be caused by partial filling of air spaces, interstitial thickening, partial collapse of alveoli, increased capillary blood volume, or a combination of

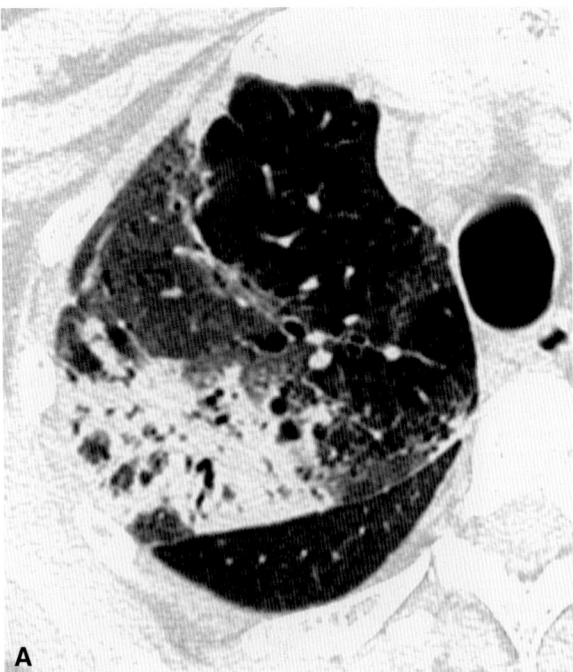

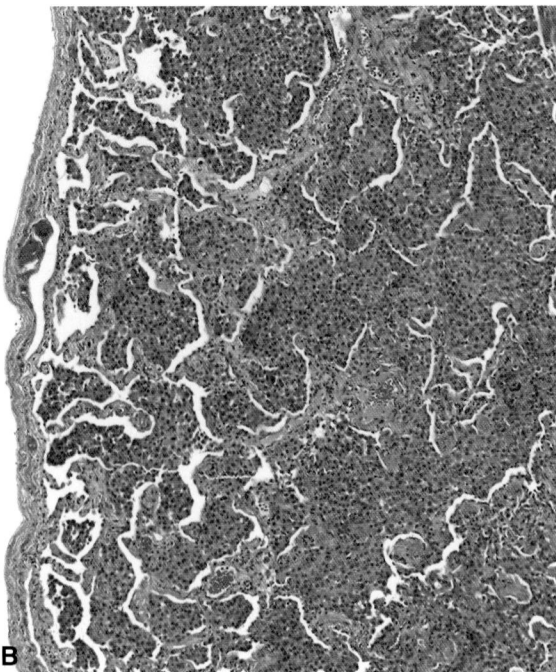

Figure 3-102. Radiology (**A**) and pathology (**B**) of alveolar opacities. Radiologically, a portion of lung becomes whiter than normal for the presence of material filling the alveoli. The different intensity of white depends on the percentage of alveolar filling in different areas.

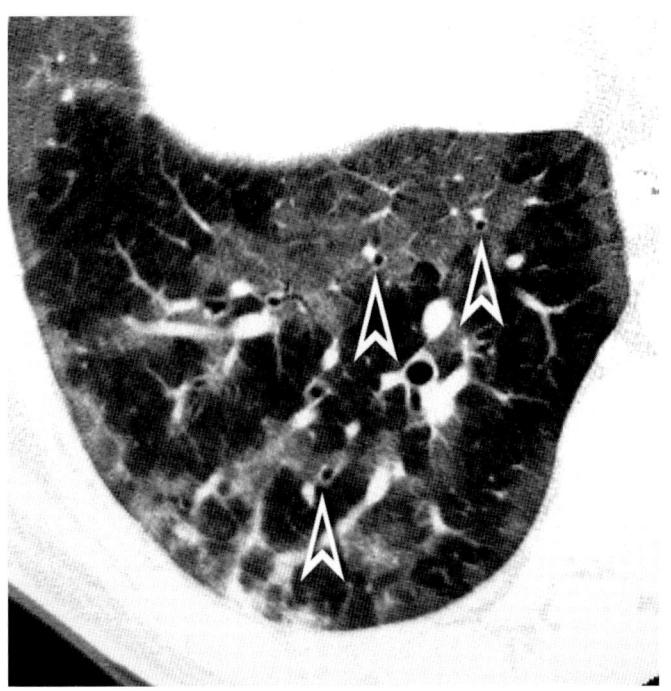

Figure 3-103. Ground glass opacity: hazy increase of lung attenuation with preservation of the bronchial and vascular margins (*arrowheads*).

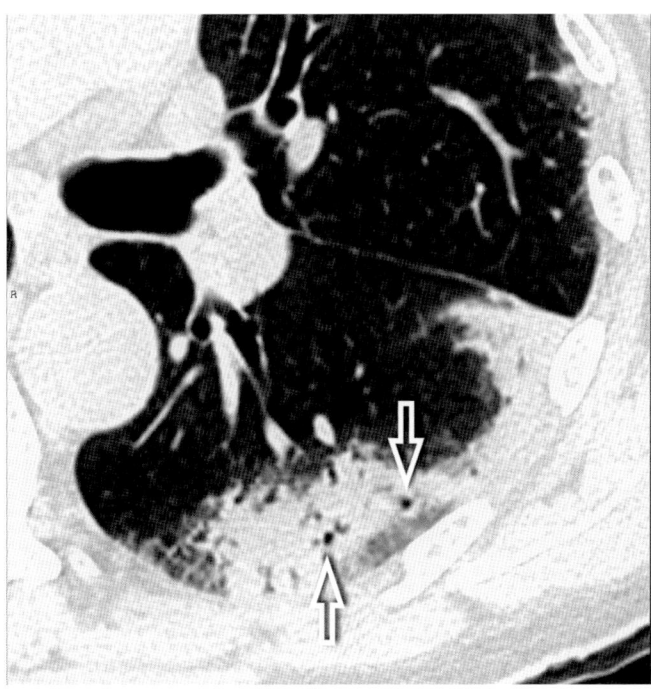

Figure 3-104. Consolidation is an increase in pulmonary attenuation that obscures the vessels and the airway walls. On the contrary, the bronchial lumen may remain visible (*arrows*) inside the consolidation (air bronchogram).

these, the common factor being the partial displacement of air.[20] The lobular elements and, more in general, the pulmonary architecture are not distorted (see Fig. 3-103). Consolidation appears as an intense increase in pulmonary attenuation that obscures the margins of vessels and airway walls.[8,20] Consolidation is due to a complete filling of alveoli by any material (exudate, cells or other product of disease cause a same radiologic aspect), the common factor being the full displacement of air from alveoli.[20] However, if air persists in the lumen of the bronchi, they remain visible inside the opacity (air bronchogram) (Fig. 3-104). An area of consolidation may contain hypodensities or hyperdensities, reflecting the presence of differently attenuating substances such as fat, metals, calcium, or air (Fig. 3-105). GGO and consolidation may coexist in the same patient, creating mixed densities aspects (see Fig. 3-102A).

Ancillary signs are *crazy paving*, *tree-in-bud*, *halo sign*, *reversed halo sign*, and *perilobular* pattern. These are imaginative but effective descriptive terms that help focus attention on subset disorders of the pulmonary parenchyma and airways.

Crazy paving is a smooth, fairly regular network of white lines superimposed on a background of GGO, resembling shaped paving stones[20,101] (see Fig. 3-105). These white lines may represent thickened intralobular/interlobular interstitium but also purely alveolar deposition of material within the air spaces at the borders of unit structures such as acini or secondary lobules.[102,103]

Tree-in-bud is the name given to centrilobular dense branching linear structures originating from a single stalk and often ending in a nodular form (thus, resembling a budding tree)[20,98] (Fig. 3-106). The "tree" reflects the existence of luminal dilatation, bronchiolar wall thickening, and impaction[104] for a spectrum of endobronchiolar and peribronchiolar diseases,[20] the most common being infectious disorders.[98,105] The "buds" are micronodular opacities due to concomitant nearby filling of airway lumina[106] or infiltration of the centrilobular interstitium. Rarely, a *tree-in-bud* aspect may represent an intravascular pulmonary tumor embolism[107,108] (see Hematogenous Metastases in Nodular Pattern, subset Random).

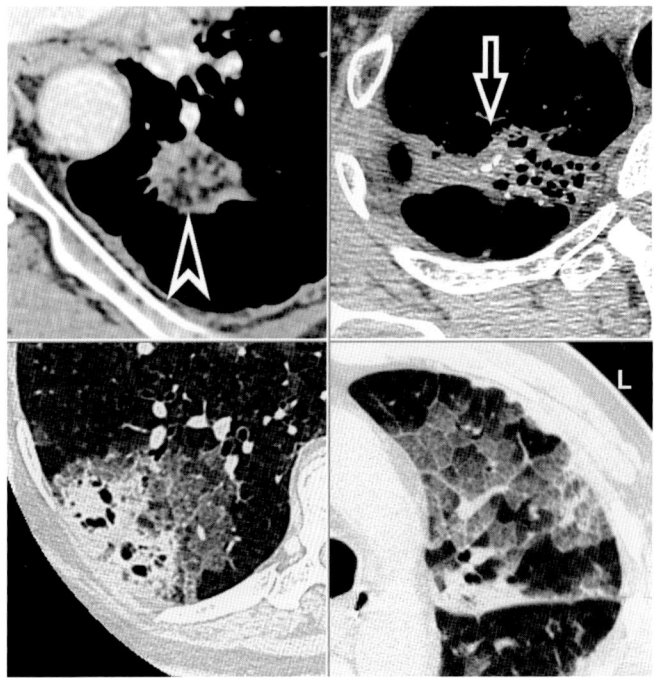

Figure 3-105. *Upper left,* The tiny dots with computed tomography attenuation inside this pulmonary lesion (*arrowhead*) have a fatty density. *Upper right,* The black dots inside this opacity (*arrow*) are bronchi, and the white dots are calcifications. *Lower left,* The black hyperlucencies inside this bronchioloalveolar carcinoma contain air (cystic BAC). *Lower right,* A fairly regular network of white lines is superimposed on a background of GGO. This appearance is called "crazy paving."

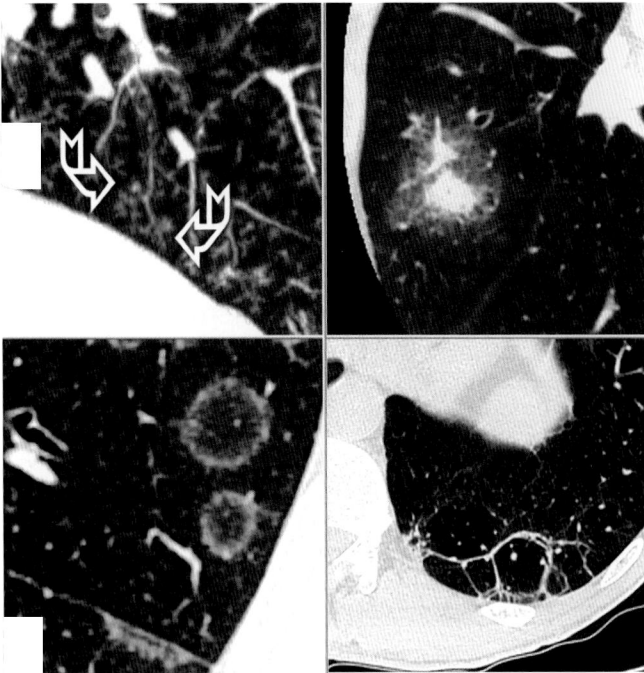

Figure 3-106. *Upper left,* Several branching linear structures in the lobular context (*curved arrows*) evoke the aspect of a *tree-in-bud* pattern. *Upper right,* The GGO surrounding central opacities is called *halo sign. Lower left,* A rim of denser opacity surrounding a central area of GGO is called *reversed halo sign* or *atoll sign. Lower right,* This aspect of polygonal bandlike opacities bordering elements of lobular size is known as *perilobular pattern.*

A *halo sign* occurs when a central area of consolidation is surrounded by a halo of GGO attenuation[63,109–111] (see Fig. 3-106). This sign suggests that a disease might be pathologically active with hemorrhage, inflammation, or tumor spread at its periphery.[109,112]

A *reversed halo sign* occurs when, on the contrary, a ring or crescent of dense consolidation surrounds a core of GGO (see Fig. 3-106). This often corresponds to patches of alveolar/septal inflammation and cellular debris surrounded by a rim of denser OP.[113,114]

A *perilobular pattern* occurs when poorly defined bandlike opacities with an arcade-like or polygonal appearance border the interlobular septa. They have greater thickness and are less sharply defined than true interlobular thickening encountered in the septal pattern (see Fig. 3-106). Indeed, these opacities are due to accumulation of organizing exudate in the perilobular alveoli even without septal thickening.[115,116]

Subsets

The clinical presentation of the patient represents the leading and most important discriminating element that allows dividing the alveolar pattern in two subsets: acute and chronic.

Subset Acute

An alveolar pattern is acute when the onset of respiratory symptoms dates back to days or a few weeks (1–14 days, according to Schwarz and King[117]).

The opacities are more often bilateral and diffuse, and they may change in appearance quite rapidly. With the exception of the presence of an underlying fibrotic disease, signs of distortion or remodeling of the pulmonary structures are not evident, at least in the early phases of disease (Fig. 3-107).

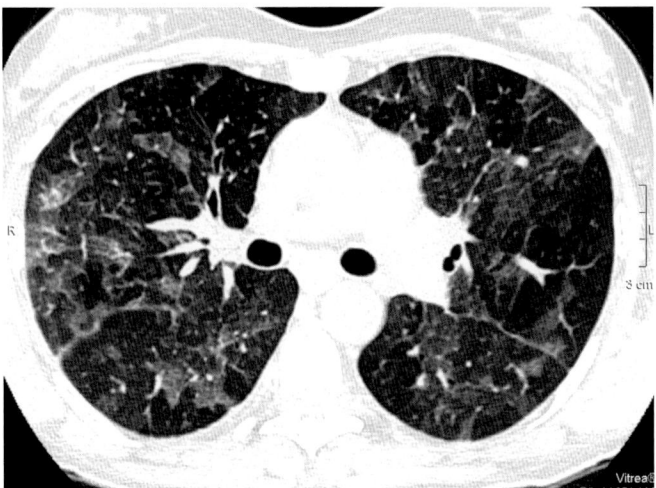

Figure 3-107. Diffuse, bilateral ground glass opacities are often the modality of presentation of the acute alveolar disorders.

Airborne diseases can be responsible for signs of bronchial wall involvement, peribronchial consolidations, poorly defined air-space nodules of acinar aspect (4–10 mm) (Fig. 3-108), and even lobular hyperinflation as a consequence of the reduction in caliper of the bronchiolar lumen. Diseases in the Alveolar Pattern, subset Acute, are listed in Box 3-11.

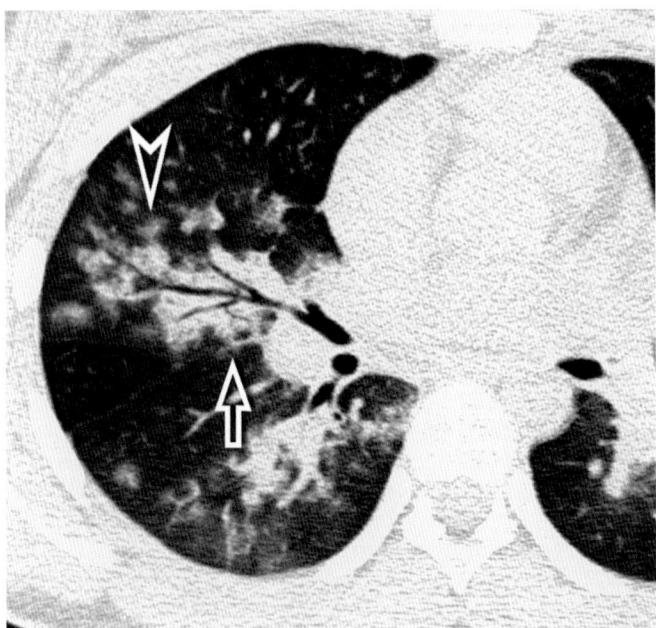

Figure 3-108. In an acute clinical context, peribronchial consolidations (*arrow*) and nodular opacities with ill-defined margins (*arrowhead*) may testify to the existence of an alveolar disease arriving through the airways.

Box 3-11. Diseases Presenting with Alveolar Pattern, Subset Acute

Frequent
Acute respiratory distress syndrome (ARDS)
Drug toxicity (see AIP/ARDS and DAH)
Hydrostatic pulmonary edema
Infectious diseases

Rare
Acceleration (acute exacerbation) of fibrosing diseases
Acute eosinophilic pneumonia (see AIP/ARDS)
Acute interstitial pneumonia (AIP)
Diffuse alveolar hemorrhage (DAH)

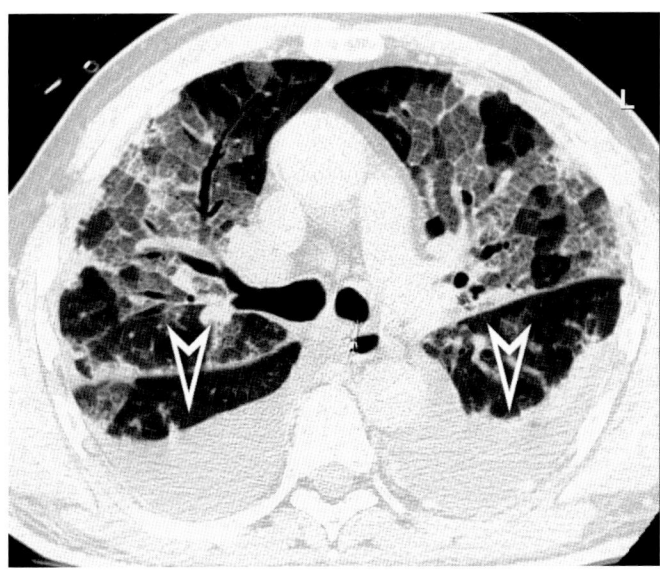

Figure 3-109. Acute respiratory distress syndrome. Bilateral patchy areas of GGO with *crazy paving* aspect and an air bronchogram are visible. A bilateral pleural effusion coexists in this patient (*arrowheads*).

Acute Interstitial Pneumonia/Acute Respiratory Distress Syndrome

Areas of GGO (100%) and patchy air-space consolidation (92%)[118] with air bronchogram[119] are the main findings in patients with both acute respiratory distress syndrome and acute interstitial pneumonia[120] (Fig. 3-109). Interlobular septal thickening (89%) and intralobular reticulation (78%)[118] with aspects of crazy paving,[102,103] thickening of the bronchovascular bundle (86%), and nodular (86%) opacities[118] are also very frequent. Similar findings with variants have been described in acute eosinophilic pneumonia[121–123] and acute reactions to therapeutic[45,53,54,124,125] and illicit[126] drugs.

The distribution of the lesions is variable, a specific predominance either in the craniocaudal or axial directions being possible in single cases.[118] During the progression of disease, the extent of GGO tends to increase, and more homogeneous, gravity-dependent consolidative opacities appear[118,120] (Fig. 3-110).

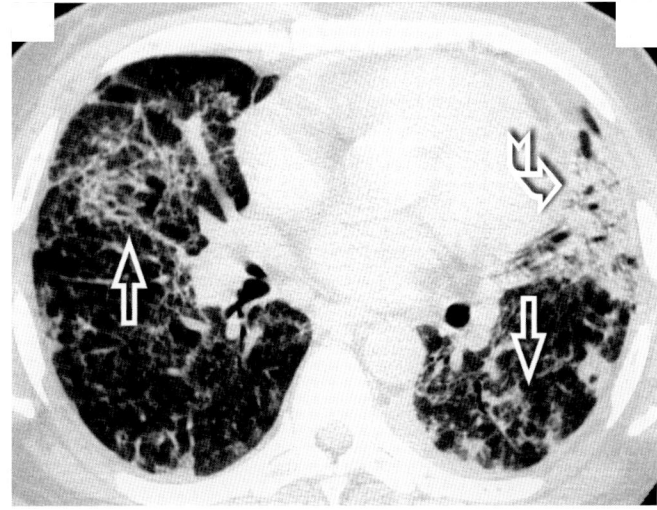

Figure 3-111. Late phase of ARDS. An alveolar opacity is still present in the left pericardial region (*curved arrow*); elsewhere (*arrows*), there is a network of irregular linear opacities due to residual fibrotic processes.

Moving from the acute and subacute to the chronic fibrotic phase, a distortion of the interstitial and bronchovascular markings is frequent (Fig. 3-111), and beyond the first week or two, a dramatic increase of subpleural cysts and bullae also occurs.[127] On the contrary, if signs of retraction and remodeling are evident in the early phases of disease, an acute exacerbation (acceleration) of a fibrosing disorder should be suspected (see Acceleration of Fibrosing Diseases). Late radiologic features of both acute interstitial pneumonia/acute respiratory distress syndrome are a piling up of findings from original disease, atelectasis, inflammation, and side effects of mechanical ventilation.

Acceleration (Acute Exacerbation) of Fibrosing Diseases

The radiologic presentation of accelerated fibrosing diseases (also called acute exacerbation) is a coexistence of more-or-less extensive GGO with or without consolidation and signs of the underlying disorder (Fig. 3-112). In patients with UIP, irregular reticulation with patchy areas of honeycombing[128,129] is visible. In contrast, in patients with

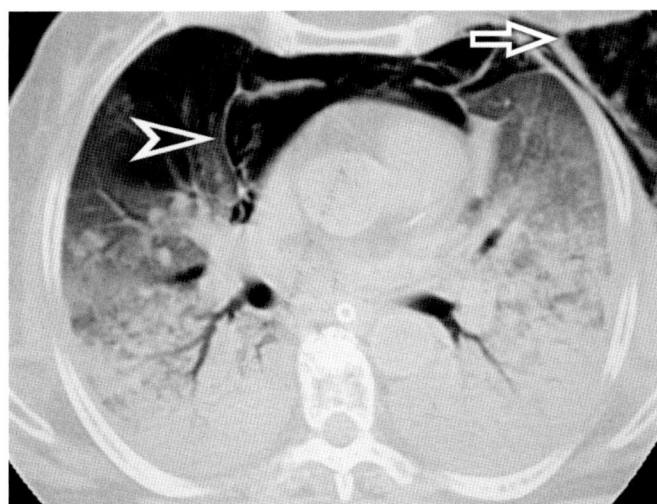

Figure 3-110. Extensive bilateral opacification of the lung in a patient with ARDS. The opacities are denser posteriorly, due to progressively atelectatic parenchyma. Note the air bronchogram inside the consolidations, which is typical of the injury edema. There are also abnormal collections of air at the mediastinal (*arrowhead*) and soft tissue (*arrow*) level, from barotrauma.

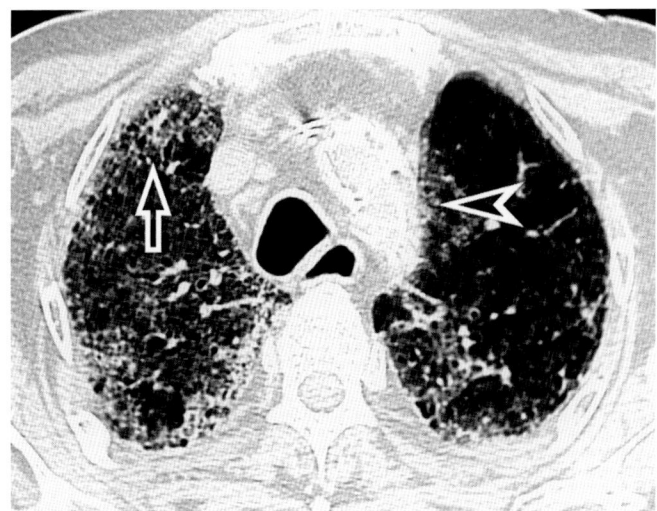

Figure 3-112. Accelerated UIP. Areas of opacity and GGO prevalent to the right are superimposed to a fine reticulation with subtle honeycombing (*arrow*). The mediastinum is enlarged, due to traction fibrosis testified by interface signs (*arrowhead*).

NSIP, irregular reticulation and bronchiectasis, as well as increasing of previous GGO, are present.[130]

The distribution of the alveolar densities may be multifocal, diffuse (Fig. 3-113) (and when multifocal it tends to evolve rapidly to the diffuse form), or peripheral. In a series of accelerated UIP, multifocal and diffuse disease corresponded to pathologic diffuse alveolar damage, whereas peripheral disease is mainly correlated with OP and numerous fibroblastic foci.[131]

The possibility of an acute exacerbation (Fig. 3-114) has been described for idiopathic UIP (clinical IPF), idiopathic NSIP, and both UIP and NSIP associated with connective tissue disorders.[131,132] The

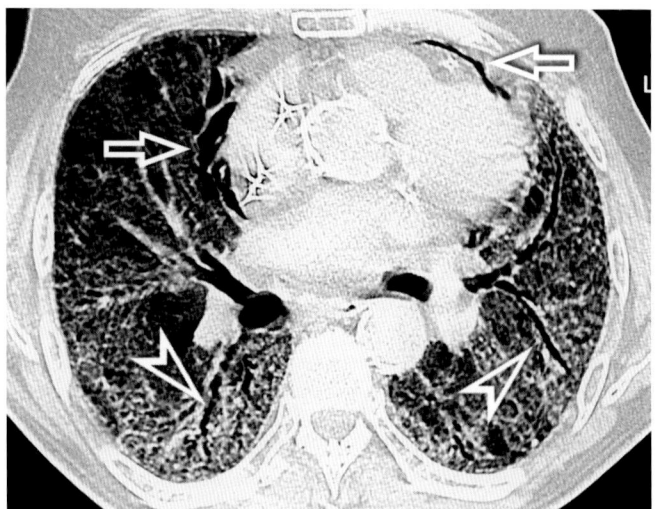

Figure 3-113. Accelerated fibrosing disease. There is an intense opacification of most lung parenchyma at this basal level, with a "scratched" aspect due to underlying fibrosing disease. Several ectatic bronchi coexist (*arrowheads*), and there is also a collection of mediastinal air from barotrauma due to mechanical ventilation (*arrows*).

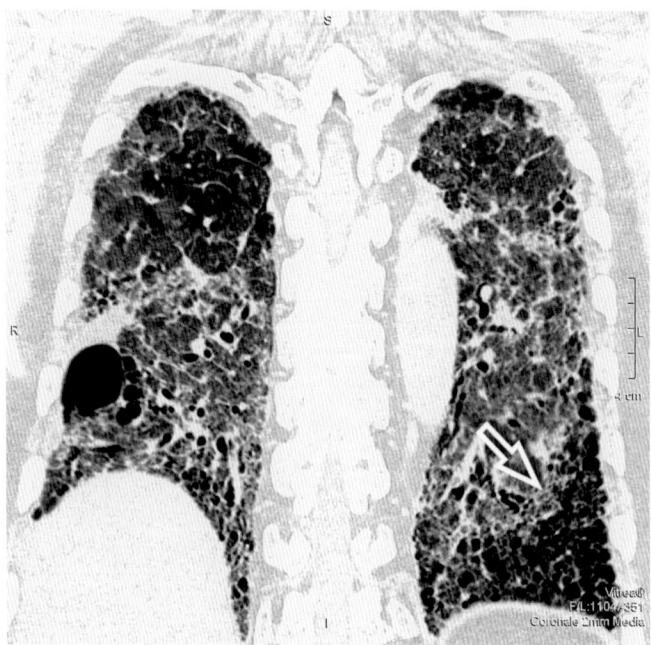

Figure 3-114. An extensive honeycombing (*arrow*) prevails at the basal level of this patient with accelerated usual interstitial pneumonia. The rest of the lung is extensively opacified, pointing to an acutely exacerbated fibrosing disorder.

specific aspect of the two leading subsets has been described in detail in Fibrotic Pattern.

Diffuse Alveolar Hemorrhage

Whatever the underlying cause (e.g., vasculitides, drug reactions, coagulopathies), limited free blood within the lobular boundaries gives origin to ill-defined centrilobular nodules. Larger amounts of fluid flooding the alveoli cause more-or-less extended opacities, ranging in intensity from vague GGO (Fig. 3-115) to intense consolidation.[133]

The distribution of the lesions is variable and depends on both the anatomical location and the mechanism by which the hemorrhage occurs. Extended areas of opacification may be patchy or uniform, tend to spare lung apices, and often show parahilar predominance[134] (Fig. 3-116).

Within days of an acute episode, the interlobular thickening due to hemosiderin-laden macrophages accumulating in the interstitium may give a *crazy paving* aspect to the opacities (Fig. 3-117). After

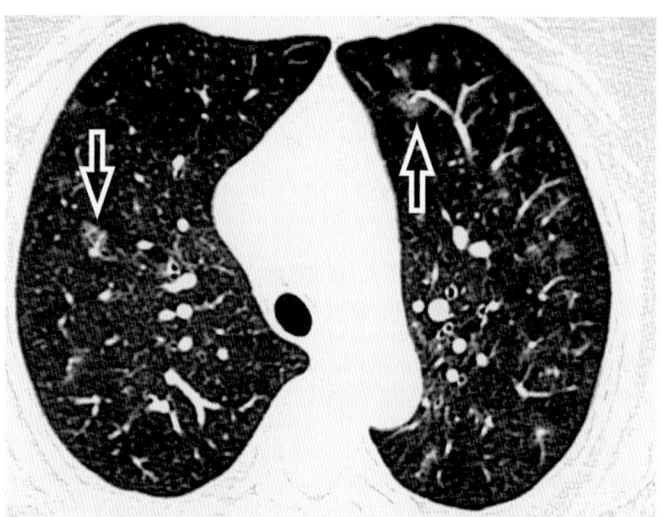

Figure 3-115. Patient with microscopic polyangiitis. There is a diffuse granular GGO with some discrete ill-defined nodules that seem connected to small vessels (*arrows*).

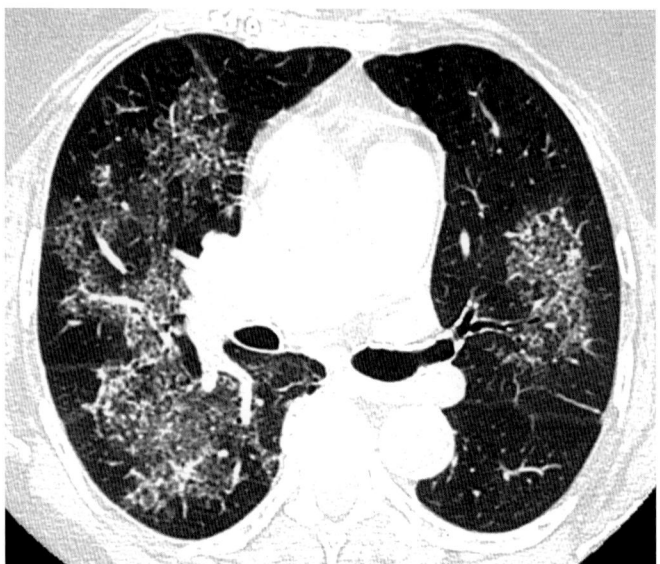

Figure 3-116. The alveolar opacities in this patient with alveolar hemorrhage show neat parahilar predominance.

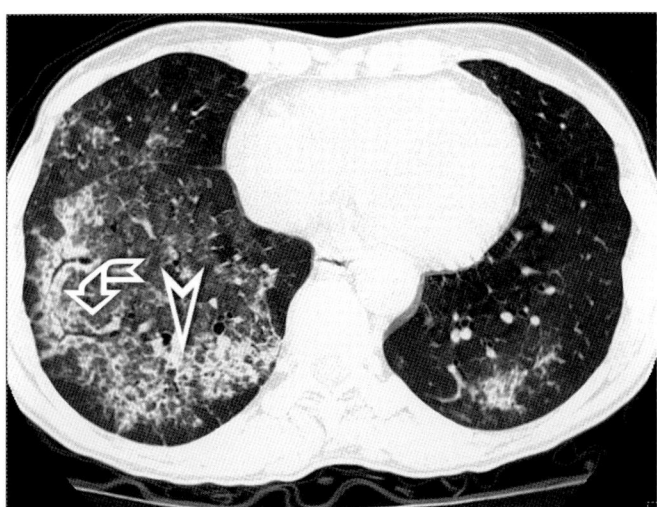

Figure 3-117. Long-standing alveolar hemorrhage. There is a fine reticular pattern intermingled with the alveolar opacities (*arrowhead*) and a modest distortion of bronchiolar elements (*curved arrow*).

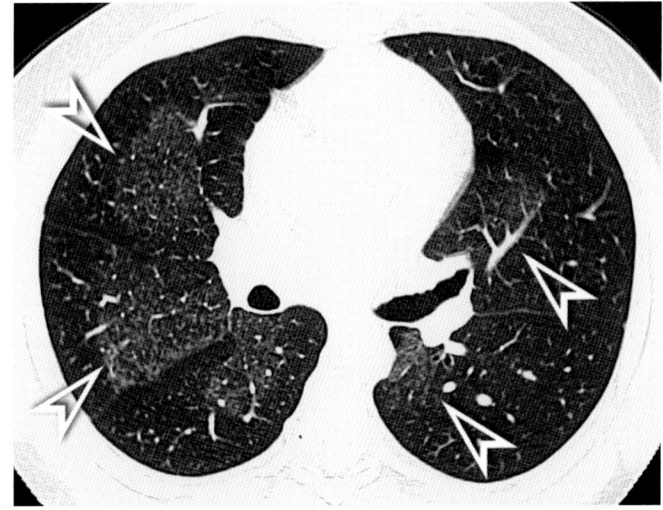

Figure 3-119. Pulmonary edema. In this patient, a hazy GGO from partial alveolar filling shows a noticeable central predominance (*arrowheads*) with sparing of the most peripheral lung.

repeated episodes, a persistent irregular reticular pattern with traction bronchiectasis, sometimes even with honeycombing, may be seen.[133]

Hydrostatic Pulmonary Edema

GGOs accompanied by visible interlobular septa and thickened peribronchovascular bundle are the most common findings[10,135] (Fig. 3-118). Frank parenchymal consolidations may coexist, but they are more typical of advanced cases. Usually, they are not investigated with CT (frank alveolar edema is simply diagnosed with radiography). The specific aspects of the interstitial involvement in pulmonary edema are described in detail in Septal Pattern, subset Smooth.

The opacities are diffuse or patchy and bilateral if no reasons for unilaterality exist (e.g., patient's lateral decubitus, fibrosing mediastinitis).[135] The lesions often show gravitational or parahilar predominance related to pressure dynamics[9] (Fig. 3-119). However, in these early phases of edema, the gravitational predominance may be subtle, and in selected cases even an upper lobe distribution of lesions may occur.[10] A characteristically asymmetrical involvement of right middle and upper

lobes is the rule in case of myocardial infarction, papillary muscle rupture, and mitral valve insufficiency.[10]

Unilateral or bilateral pleural effusion and thickening of the interlobar fissures are common in hydrostatic pulmonary edema[10] (Fig. 3-120). In addition, mediastinal lymphadenopathy is not rare at all in patients with left-sided heart failure.[11]

Infectious Diseases

A mixture of lobular or diffuse GGO/consolidation, centrilobular ill-defined nodules, and thickened interlobular septa may be seen, with a prevalence depending on the specific disease and its severity. The lesions reflect the variable extent of underlying histopathologic features: bronchial and bronchiolar participation, interstitial and alveolar inflammatory cell infiltration, intra-alveolar hemorrhage, and diffuse alveolar damage[134,136] (Fig. 3-121).

More than 60% of patients with *Mycoplasma pneumoniae* pneumonia have lower zone predominance, whereas 50% of patients with fungi have upper zone predominance of the lesions.[137] In influenza

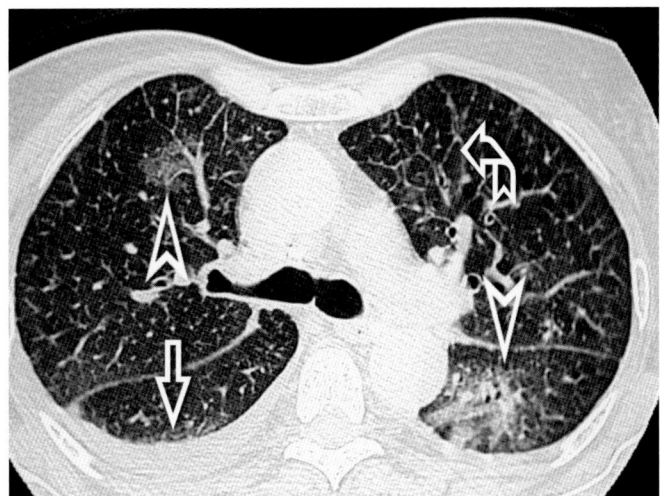

Figure 3-118. Patient with mild pulmonary edema. In this axial plane, there are patchy areas of GGO (*arrowheads*) and septal lines (*curved arrow*), highlighting the lobular boundaries. Some pleural effusion coexists to the right (*arrow*).

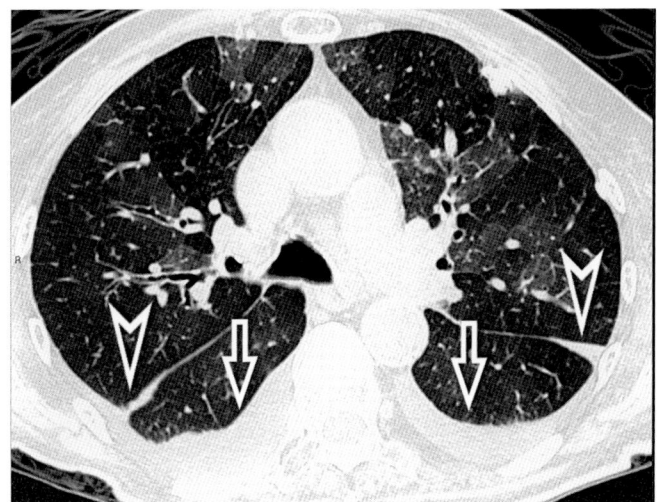

Figure 3-120. In this patient with patchy parahilar GGO from pulmonary edema, a pleural effusion is also visible on both sides posteriorly (*arrows)* and inside the fissures (*arrowheads*).

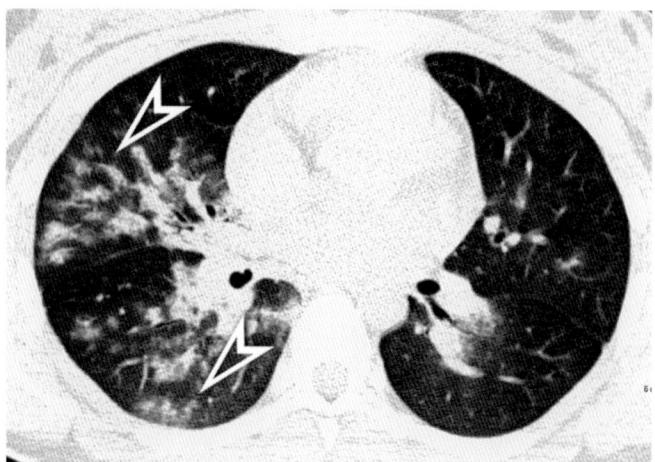

Figure 3-121. Patient with H1N1 influenza virus pneumonia. The pattern is dominated by dense homogeneous parahilar consolidations and peripheral nodules of hazy GGO (*arrowheads*) in centrilobular position.

pneumonia, the opacities may show a preference for perivascular (Fig. 3-122) and subpleural areas.[136] Pneumocystis presents a striking upper lobe predominance of GGO.[138]

Nodules are frequent in patients with fungal (65%), viral (77%), and *M. pneumoniae* pneumonia (89%), and they are much less common in patients with bacterial pneumonia (17%).[139] In varicella-zoster virus pneumonia, well-defined and ill-defined nodules of 1 to 10 mm diameter are diffusely scattered throughout the lungs (Fig. 3-123); coalescence of nodules and patches of GGO are also possible.[136] In immunocompromised subjects, especially HIV patients, the presence of extensive, diffuse, bilateral GGO is suggestive (although not specific) for *Pneumocystis jiroveci* pneumonia;[139,140] it becomes very typical if cystic lesions are contemporarily present.[137] On the contrary, nodules are absent.[139]

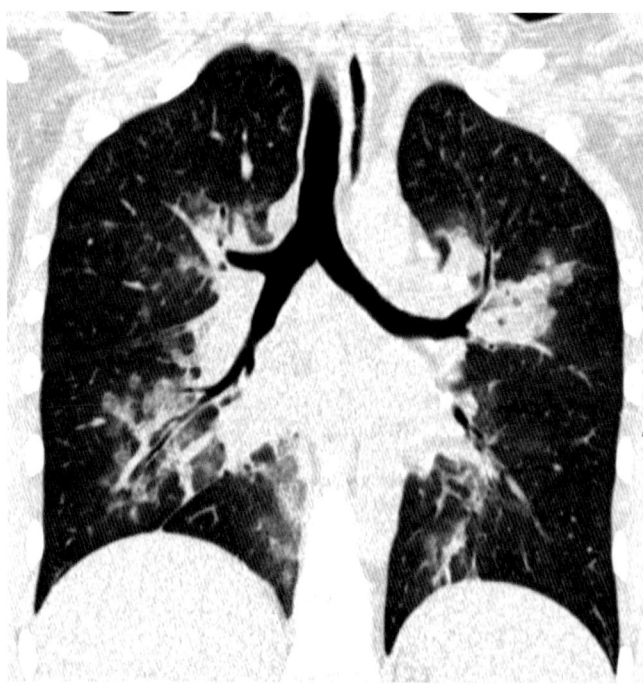

Figure 3-122. Patient with H1N1 influenza virus pneumonia. In this frontal view, the consolidations tend to aggregate in the parahilar areas along the bronchovascular bundles.

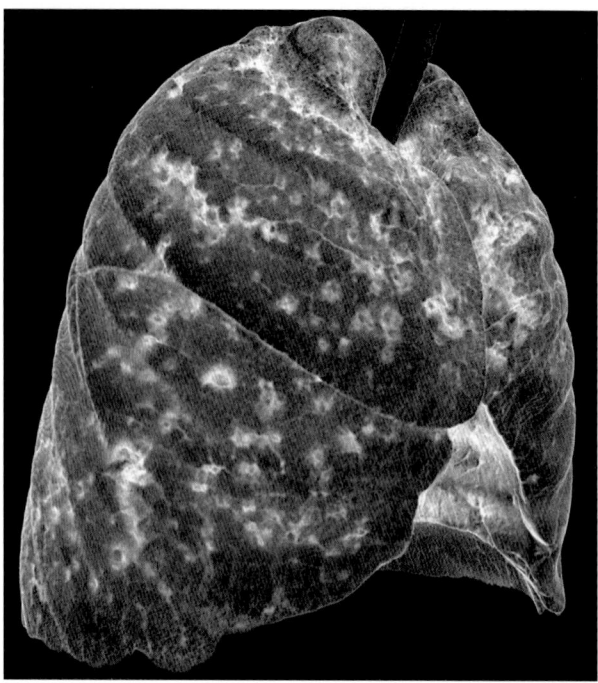

Figure 3-123. External view of the lungs in a subject with varicella-zoster virus pneumonia. The nodular lesions characteristic of this virus are well evident on the surface of the pulmonary parenchyma.

Subset Chronic

An alveolar pattern is chronic when the onset of respiratory symptoms dates back from months to years from the time of diagnosis.[117]

The lesions may be bilateral but also unilateral (Fig. 3-124), and with a few exceptions they tend to clear up slowly over time (unless they worsen and proceed to fibrosis). Often arranged in patches of conspicuous size, they entertain tight relationships with the large airways, but a participation of the small airways in the lobular area is also possible. The variety of chronic lung disorders may produce more multifaceted aspects than the acute forms (Fig. 3-125). However, within the range of the alveolar signs, it is often possible to identify prevalent

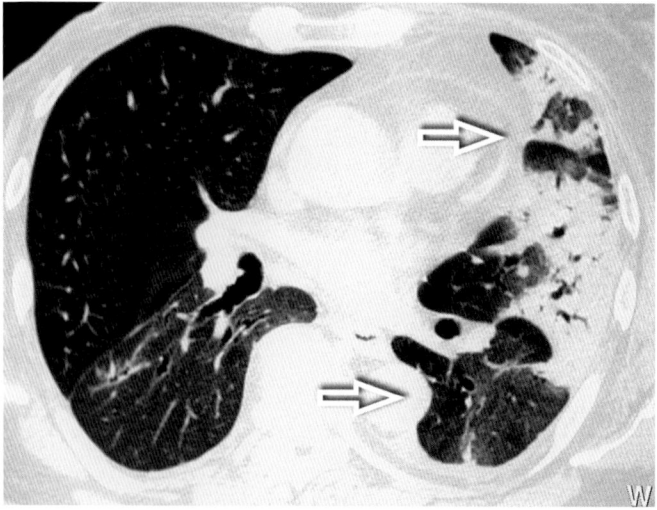

Figure 3-124. Typical presentation of an alveolar disease of chronic type (in this case, the recurrence of organizing pneumonia): unilateral, patchy, mixed densities (GGO and consolidation) with air bronchogram, and some remodeling of thoracic structures (the *arrows* point at the mediastinum shifted to the left).

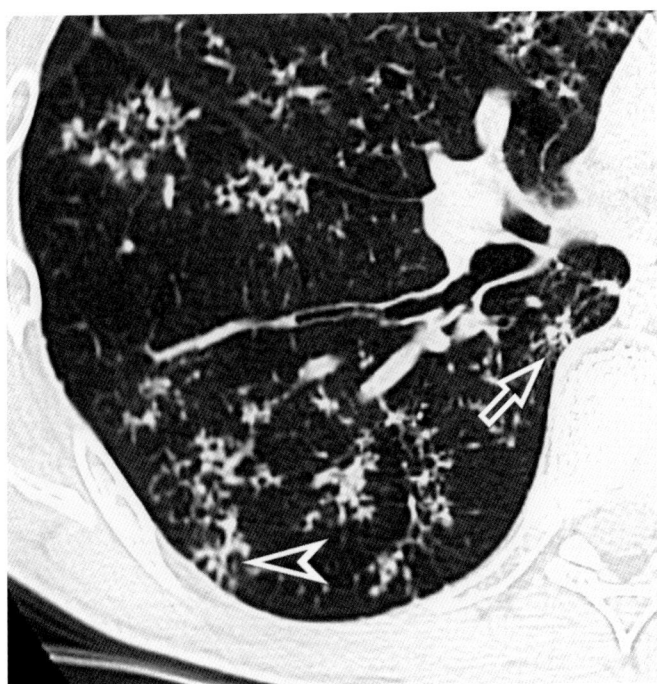

Figure 3-125. This is an exquisite example of a chronic airborne disease showing a *tree-in-bud* pattern (*arrowhead*) that testifies spreading through the airways. Here and there, the bronchioli are not filled with material, so their lumen is appreciable as much as their thickened walls (*arrow*).

aspects useful for narrowing the diagnostic possibilities: pure GGO, mixed densities, and *crazy paving* and *tree-in-bud* signs; these will be declared at the beginning of each disease presentation.

Some diseases tend to develop alveolar opacities but show prevalent aspects that make preferable their inclusion in another pattern. These are hypersensitivity pneumonitis and RB-ILD, described in the Nodular Pattern, subset Centrilobular, and the fibrosing disorders showing as GGO, discussed in the Fibrotic Pattern. Diseases in the Alveolar Pattern, subset Chronic, are listed in Box 3-12.

Bronchioloalveolar Carcinoma

The diffuse form of bronchioloalveolar carcinoma is a mixed densities disease. Patchy areas of GGO/consolidation and/or multifocal macronodular lesions with a *halo sign* are the most common

---

Box 3-12. Diseases Presenting with Alveolar Pattern, Subset Chronic

Frequent
Bronchioloalveolar carcinoma
Chronic eosinophilic pneumonia (CEP)
Drug toxicity (see CEP, Idiopathic Cellular NSIP, and OP)
Infectious and inflammatory diseases
Organizing pneumonia (OP)
Subacute hypersensitivity pneumonitis (see Nodular Pattern, subset Centrilobular)

Rare
Idiopathic cellular nonspecific interstitial pneumonia (NSIP)
Collagen vascular diseases (see Idiopathic Cellular NSIP and OP)
Desquamative interstitial pneumonia
Lipoid pneumonia (see Infectious and Inflammatory Diseases)
Mucosa-associated lymphoid tissue lymphoma
Pulmonary alveolar proteinosis
Respiratory bronchiolitis–interstitial lung disease (see Nodular Pattern, subset Centrilobular)

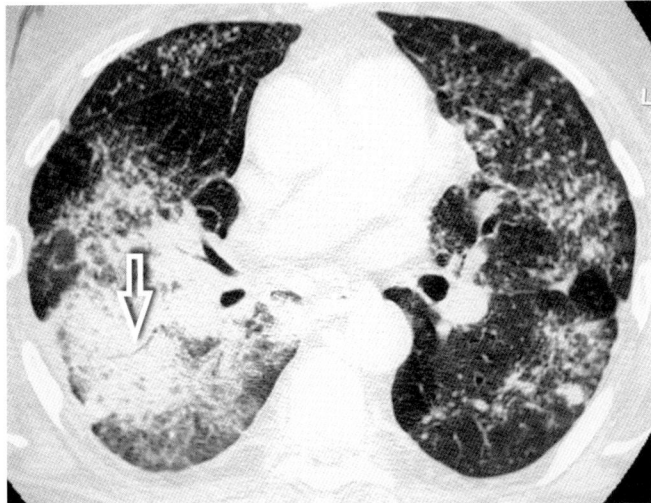

Figure 3-126. Bronchioloalveolar carcinoma. A large consolidation to the right possibly points at the origin of the disease, and elsewhere there are the signs of diffuse spreading. The *arrow* points to a narrowed and stretched bronchus inside the main opacity.

presentations.[141–143] A skeletal, stretched, air bronchogram is frequently seen inside the opacities[144] (Fig. 3-126). *Crazy paving* aspects and collections of air within consolidations (known as cystic bronchioloalveolar carcinoma) (see Fig. 3-105) are also possible.[143,145] When nodules are present at the lobular level, they assume the aspect of centrilobular ill-defined opacities or, rarely, a *tree-in-bud* appearance.[141]

Central or peripheral, a quite characteristic aspect is that of a more dense consolidation (possibly, the origin of the neoplasm), with GGO nearby. There are scattered patches of GGO and/or consolidation with a *halo sign* elsewhere, ipsilaterally and/or contralaterally[143] (Fig. 3-127). Bulging of fissures is possible in the presence of dense lobar consolidation[144] (Fig. 3-128), and pleural effusion and mediastinal lymph node enlargement are also possible.[143]

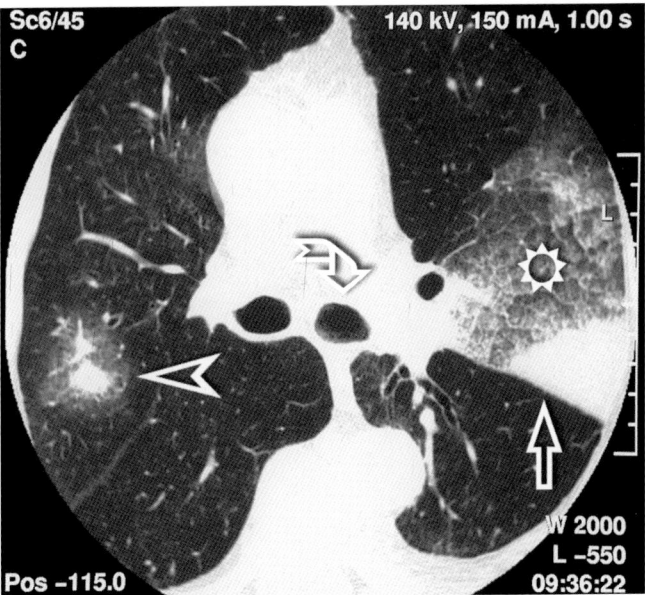

Figure 3-127. Axial scan in a patient with multifocal bronchioloalveolar carcinoma. To the left, there is a homogeneous alveolar opacity posteriorly (*arrow*) and a GGO with crazy paving anteriorly (*sun*). To the right, a focal lesion (*arrowhead*) has the typical aspect of a roundish consolidation surrounded by a rim of GGO (halo sign). Note the presence of low-density material (mucus) inside the left main bronchus (*curved arrow*).

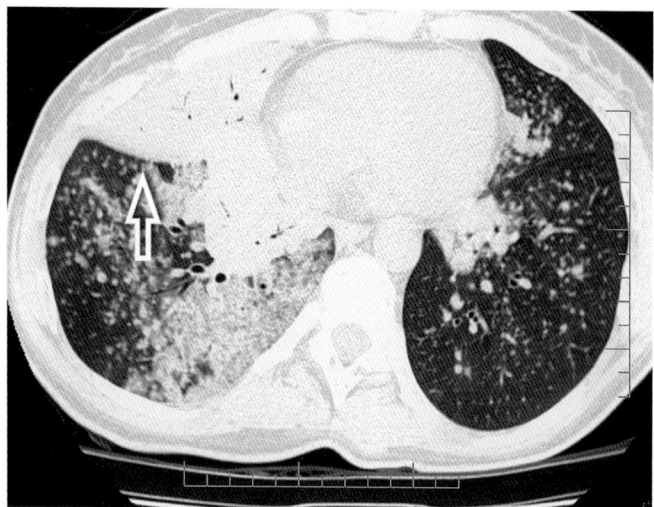

Figure 3-128. Bronchioloalveolar carcinoma. The dense, homogeneous opacity in the right cardiophrenic angle is an entire consolidated lobe. Note the bulging of the fissure posteriorly (*arrow*). Note also the black remnants of bronchi stretched inside the opacities.

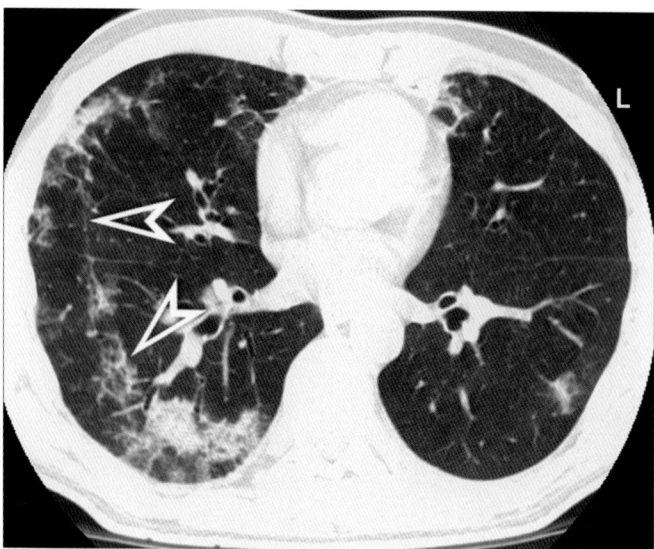

Figure 3-130. The opacities of this CEP are essentially peripheral, and to the right there is also a bizarre connecting trail (*arrowheads*) between two main foci of consolidation.

Chronic Eosinophilic Pneumonia

Chronic eosinophilic pneumonia is a mixed densities disease. In the early phases, bilateral homogenous air-space consolidations are the most frequent modality of presentation (65%). However, GGO may also be the predominant pattern (35%), and septal lines often coexist (72%)[146] (Fig. 3-129). In the later stages, GGO, nodules, some reticulation and, after weeks, linear bandlike opacities parallel to the pleural surface can be seen.[122] The opacities are quite characteristically arranged in the periphery of the upper lung zones in 50% of the cases,[122] with a less frequent "hinging on the bronchi" appearance compared with OP lesions (Fig. 3-130).

In drug-induced eosinophilic pneumonia, areas of ground glass attenuation, air-space consolidation, nodules, and interlobular septal thickening are common.[123,147] The clinical response to corticosteroids is usually excellent and, typically, accompanied by rapid clearing of the opacities[117] (Fig. 3-131). Pleural effusion is possible in 10% of cases.[122]

Desquamative Interstitial Pneumonia

Desquamative interstitial pneumonia is a GGO disease. Quite extensive areas of pure GGO are indeed the dominant finding[148,149] (Fig. 3-132). Centrilobular nodules are uncommon,[149] and consolidative and reticular opacities are also uncommon.[148]

The lesions start typically in the lower lungs and peripherally[149,150] (Fig. 3-133).

Emphysema (Fig. 3-134; see also Fig. 3-133) has been reported in about 50% of patients with desquamative interstitial pneumonia.[151] In late disease, signs of fibrosis may superimposed, with interstitial irregular lines, interface signs, and cystic hyperlucencies inside the GGO[149,152] (see Fig. 3-134).

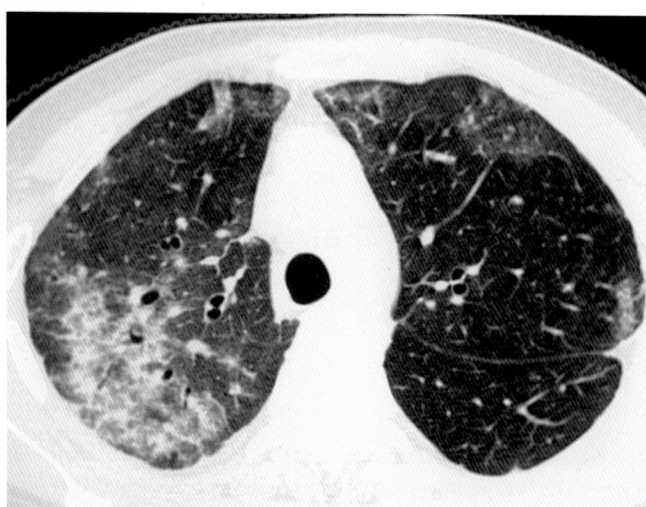

Figure 3-129. Chronic eosinophilic pneumonia. Inhomogeneous consolidation with septal lines to the right and spotty areas of GGO bilaterally are the modality of presentation of the disease in this axial scan.

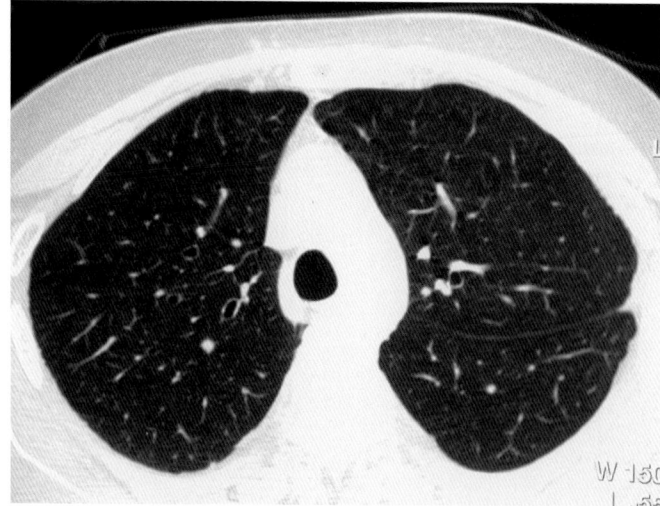

Figure 3-131. CEP in the same patient as in Figure 3-129. This is a comparable axial image of the patient after a brief period of steroid therapy: the parenchymal opacities have simply disappeared.

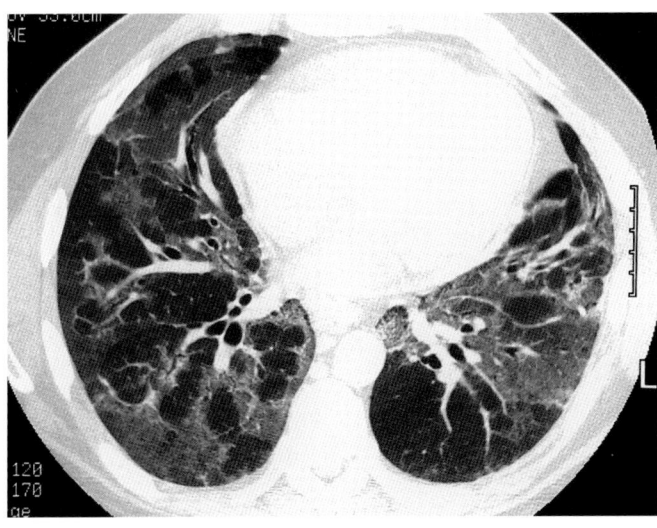

Figure 3-132. Desquamative interstitial pneumonia. Patches of GGO are visible at the level of the lower lungs in this axial CT scan. At this time, no opacities were visible at the upper levels.

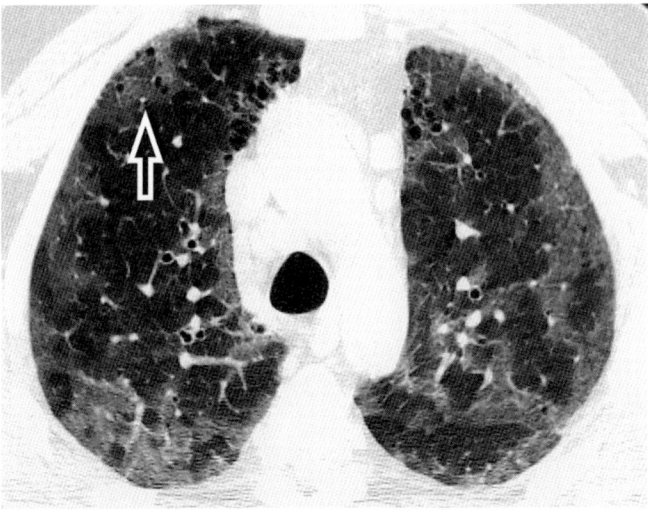

Figure 3-134. This is the same patient as in Figure 3-132, but after several years of a disease poorly managed. Now there are several patches of GGO in the upper lungs (this is an axial view at the level of the aortic arch). Some paraseptal emphysema is appreciable in the anterior paramediastinal area, but also tiny hyperlucencies inside the GGO are visible (*arrow*).

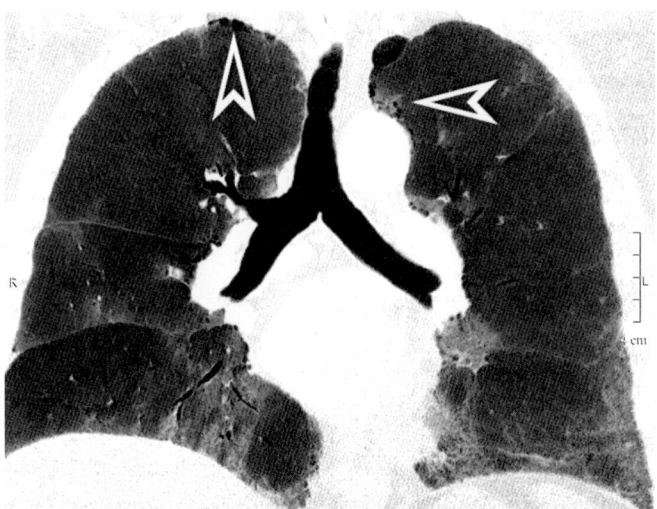

Figure 3-133. Coronal view of both lungs in a patient with DIP. This minIP image allows better recognition of patchy areas of GGO in the lower lung fields. The *arrowheads* point to small areas of paraseptal emphysema.

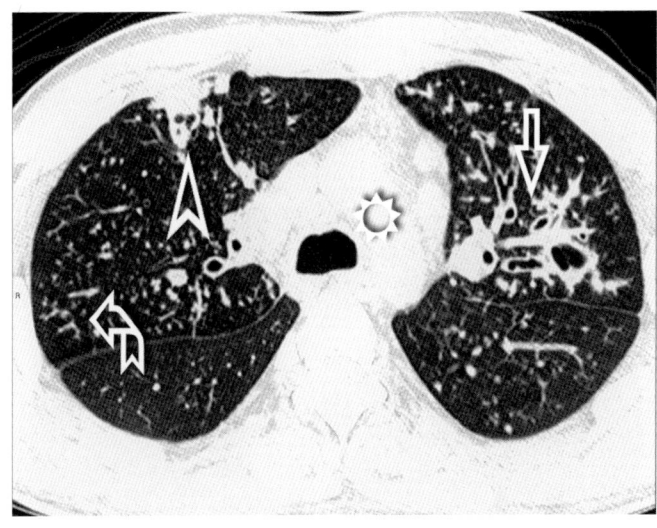

Figure 3-135. Disseminated tuberculosis. To the left, there is a cavitated process surrounded by bronchi with thickened walls (*arrow*). To the right, anteriorly, there is a triangular consolidation with air bronchogram (*arrowhead*) and in the posterior area of the same lobe there are *tree-in-bud* opacities (*curved arrow*), indicating a bronchial spread of the process. Enlarged lymph nodes are present in the mediastinum, to the left of the aortic arch (*sun*).

Infectious and Inflammatory Diseases

These are mixed densities and *tree-in-bud* entities. Single or multiple areas of consolidation/GGO alert to the existence of an alveolar disorder.[67] Signs of bronchial and bronchiolar involvement (bronchiectasis and bronchial wall thickening, bronchiolectasis with *tree-in-bud* or centrilobular nodules) often coexist and at times are the dominant pattern.[66,67,70] In areas of bronchiolar involvement, expiratory air trapping is frequently evident.[67,70] Cavitated opacities should raise the possibility of mycobacterial disease, and a surrounding (but also at a distance) *tree-in-bud* pattern should raise the suspicion of an aerogenous spread of disease (Fig. 3-135).

Bronchiolitis of infectious origin often has a patchy distribution, whereas noninfectious, inflammatory bronchiolitis tends to have a more uniform, bilaterally symmetrical involvement. Diffuse panbronchiolitis, in particular, presents with centrilobular nodules, *tree-in-bud* pattern, bronchiectasis, and bronchiolectasis with a dominant symmetrical lower lobe distribution.[67] If signs of bronchial involvement (including bronchiectasis) and/or alveolar opacities are found

predominantly in the right middle lobe and lingula, an infection from nontuberculous mycobacteria ("Lady Windermere" syndrome) should be suspected[153-155] (Fig. 3-136).

Unresolving consolidative opacities with low CT attenuation values (or frankly fatty densities) point to the possibility of an exogenous lipoid pneumonia[156,157] (see Fig. 3-105). In chronic mycobacterial infections, signs of retraction at the segmental or lobar level may be seen[155] (Fig. 3-137).

Mucosa-Associated Lymphoid Tissue Lymphoma

Mucosa-associated lymphoid tissue lymphoma (MALToma) is a mixed densities disease. Air-space consolidations with air bronchogram, from unifocal or multifocal lesions to pneumonic-like opacities of lobar size, are the most common findings[158-160] (Fig. 3-138). In the

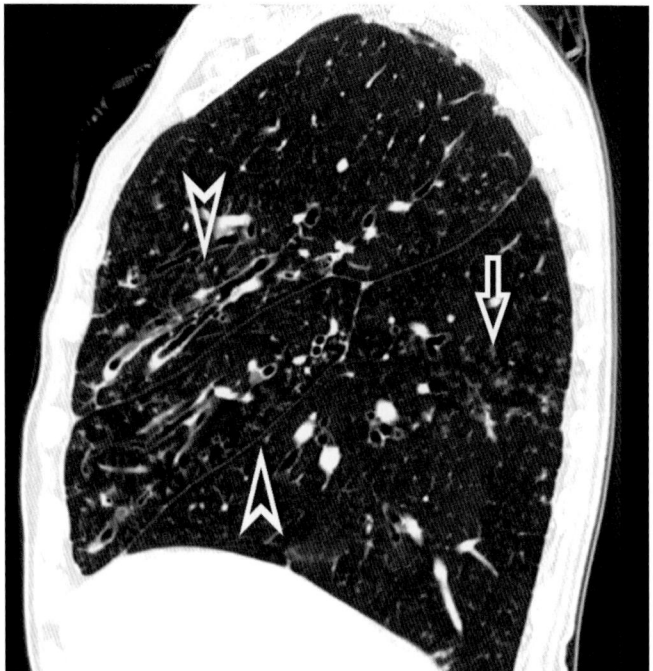

Figure 3-136. "Lady Windermere" syndrome. Several ectatic bronchi with thickened walls are visible in the anterior segment of the right upper lobe (upper *arrowhead*) and in the middle lobe (lower *arrowhead*). A patchy hyperlucent lung and some *tree-in-bud* opacities (*arrow*) are visible in the lower lobe in this sagittal scan.

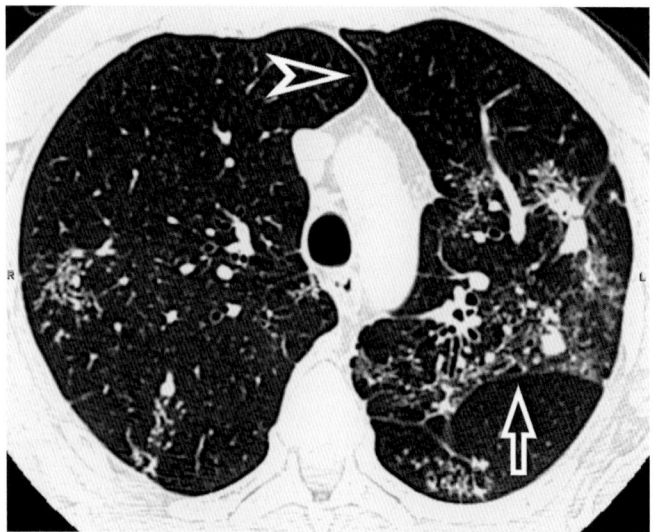

Figure 3-137. Some GGO and several ectatic bronchi with thickened walls are visible bilaterally in this axial scan, due to a tubercular process. Both the mediastinum (*arrowhead*) and the major fissure to the left (*arrow*) are retracted in connection with the parenchymal process.

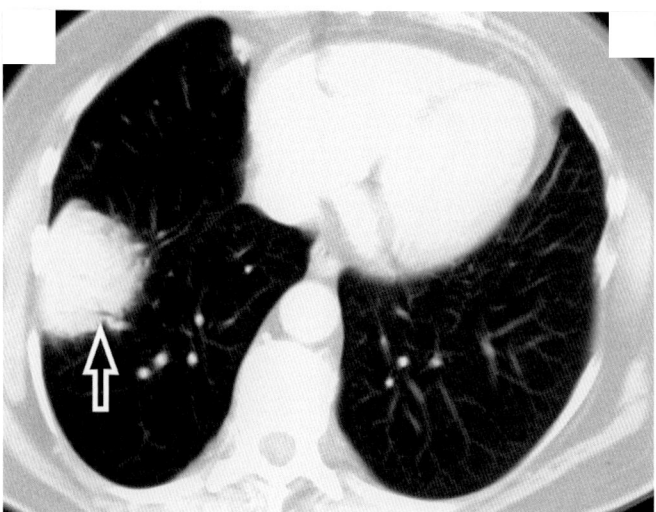

Figure 3-138. Pulmonary MALT lymphoma. In this case, the lesion is in form of a mass in the right lung, in contact with the pleural surface. Note a stretched bronchus entering the mass (*arrow*): this is uncommon in lung cancer so it might arouse the suspicion of a different lesion.

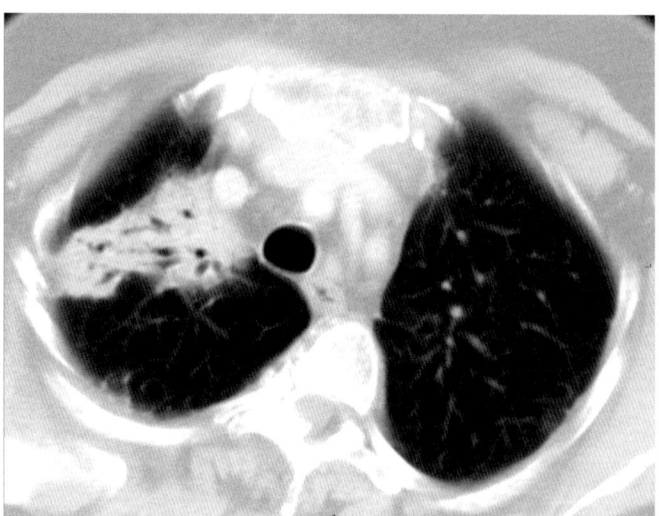

Figure 3-139. Pulmonary MALT lymphoma. This tumor assumes the aspect of a pulmonary consolidation that determines a modest attraction of the mediastinum to which it adheres. An air bronchogram is well recognizable inside the opacity.

surrounding area, spreading of disease along lymphatic routes may be responsible for a GGO with septal lines, some bronchial thickening, and micronodules with lymphatic distribution.[158,161,162] Centrilobular nodules are also possible.[159]

The disease may be unilateral or bilateral, seemingly with no vertical or horizontal zonal predominance.[158] The infiltration along bronchovascular bundles may result in focal lesions typically centered on the bronchi[159,162] (Fig. 3-139).

The lesions show a temporally indolent nature[160] and do not present a tendency to cavitation.[162] Significant hilar and mediastinal lymphadenopathies or pleural effusion are not a characteristic feature of the disease[159,162] (Fig. 3-140).

Cellular Nonspecific Interstitial Pneumonia

Cellular NSIP is a GGO disease. The opacities involve the lungs more-or-less extensively and are homogeneous. Significant reticulation, traction bronchiectasis, or other signs of architectural distortion should be minimal or absent[49,163] (Fig. 3-141), and honeycombing is typically absent.[164]

The disease is bilateral and symmetrical,[163] involving mainly the lower lung in more than 90% of cases[51] (else equally distributed). The opacities may show some tendency to distribute along the bronchovascular bundles.[50] Axially, the disease is diffuse in more than half of the cases or predominantly peripheral and subpleural. However, in a number of cases (20% to 43%), the extreme subpleural lung is relatively spared[27,51] (Fig. 3-142).

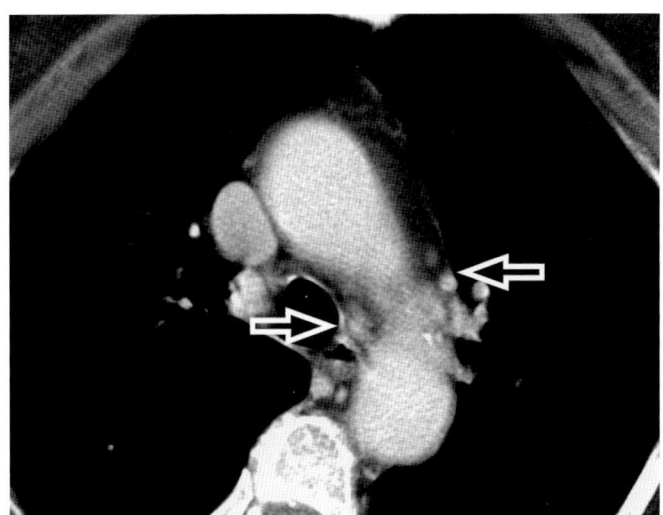

Figure 3-140. MALT lymphoma in the same patient as in Figure 3-139. Small lymph nodes are visible in the paratracheal area and at the level of the aortopulmonary window (*arrows*), but no definite adenopathic masses are present.

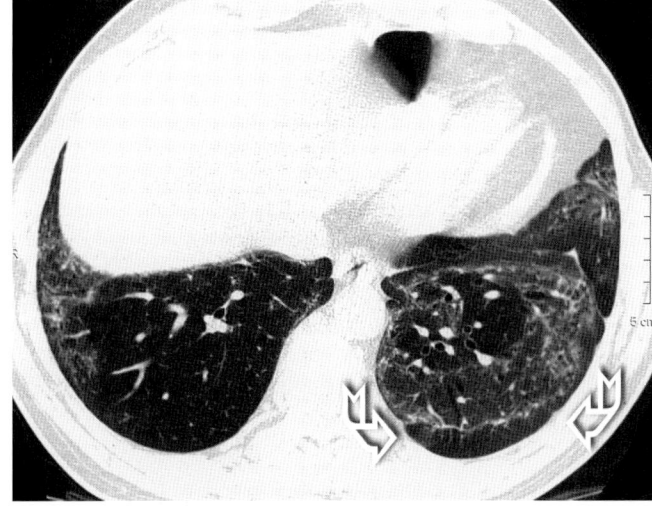

Figure 3-142. Axial scan at the level of the costophrenic angles in a subject with NSIP. There is quite homogeneous peripheral GGO; however, it spares the most subpleural lung (*curved arrows*). The opacities are more extensive to the left.

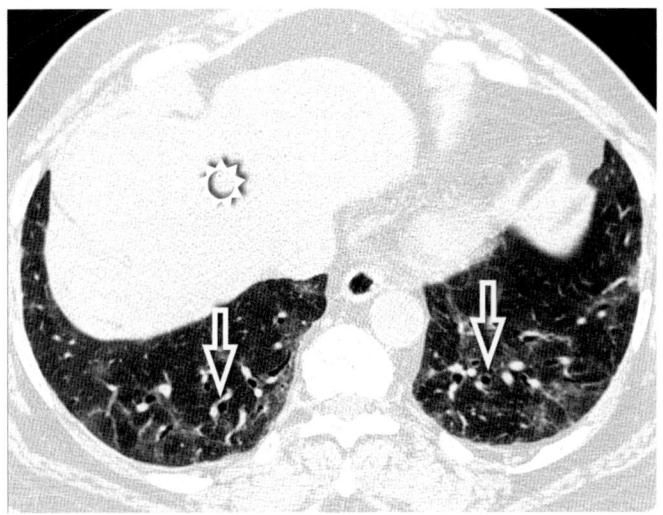

Figure 3-141. The scan is an axial view at the level of the costophrenic angles in a patient with NISP. The liver is evident (*sun*). The transparency of the basal lung is inhomogeneous because of the presence of patchy areas of pure GGO. Some slightly ectatic bronchi are recognizable (*arrows*).

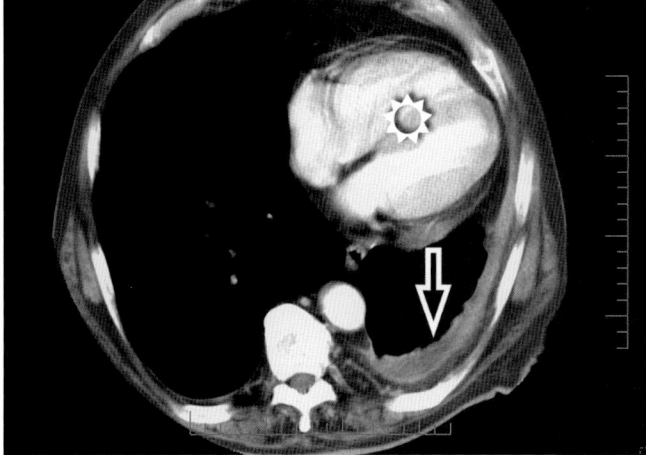

Figure 3-143. The pulmonary window shows NSIP-compatible lesions in this patient with rheumatoid arthritis, and this mediastinal window shows a chronic pleural effusion to the left (*arrow*). The heart (*sun*) is severely shifted ipsilaterally.

Several CVDs[44] and chronic drug reactions[165] may present with aspects indistinguishable from idiopathic NSIP. Consequently, a search for a nonidiopathic underlying disorder should be always undertaken clinically, although occasionally other signs of the original disease are visible radiologically[46,49] (Fig. 3-143).

Organizing Pneumonia

OP is a mixed densities disease. The classic presentation (60% to 80% of cases[27]) of the cryptogenic OP but also of other OP reactions (e.g., from pulmonary infection, connective tissue disease, drug toxicity) is characterized by unilateral or bilateral areas of patchy consolidation in which an air bronchogram is often recognizable[166] (see Fig. 3-124). Areas of GGO attenuation (60%) with septal lines (40%) may coexist.[27,146] Several variants of the classic presentation have been described for this protean disease, including multiple nodules (Fig. 3-144) that may cavitate; solitary focal lesions that may resemble a lung cancer; and

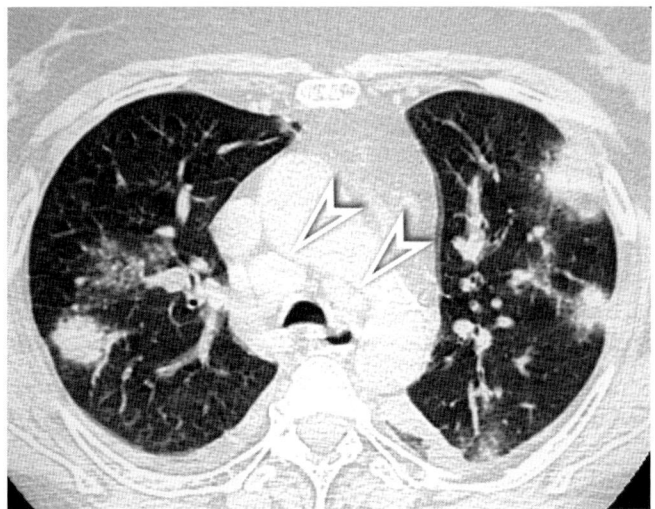

Figure 3-144. Organizing pneumonia presenting in nodular form. Note also the presence of mediastinal enlarged lymph nodes, especially in the paratracheal area (*arrowheads*). This is not the most typical aspect of this protean disease. The most frequent, mixed densities presentation is illustrated in Figure 3-124.

a peripheral distribution of disease in the context of the secondary lobule, thereby mimicking a linear septal pattern (see Fig. 3-106). All are detailed in the excellent review by Oikonomou.[166]

The consolidative lesions are often (60% to 80%) peripheral and/or centered on bronchial branches,[27] with the latter being a striking feature in a number of cases (17%)[167] (Fig. 3-145). Cryptogenic OP often involves the lower lung zones to a greater degree than the upper ones.[27] When focal, the lesions are often located in the upper lobes and they may be cavitary, thus creating problems of differential diagnosis with lung cancer.[168]

The opacities of OP vary in size from a few centimeters to an entire lobe.[168] Most patients respond to corticosteroid therapy (Fig. 3-146) or, in cases due to drug toxicity, to cessation of therapy. On occasion, the lesions may disappear spontaneously, only to reappear elsewhere (migrating disease).[169]

Pulmonary Alveolar Proteinosis

Pulmonary alveolar proteinosis is a GGO disease with *crazy paving*. The typical presentation of the disease (100% of cases) is dominated radiologically by *crazy paving*,[103] often in the form of sharply marginated areas with a geographical distribution[170] (Fig. 3-147). The extension of the pulmonary abnormalities is often impressive in comparison with the mild respiratory conditions of the patient. This clinicoradiologic discrepancy is considered quite typical of this disease.[171]

The areas of *crazy paving* are more often bilateral and symmetrical, sparing apices and costophrenic angles. Some central predominance has been suggested, but extensive or multifocal asymmetrical distributions without zonal preference are possible[171] (Fig. 3-148).

The natural course of disease is an evolution of the opacities over a period of months or years[171] (Fig. 3-149). Pleural effusion and cardiomegaly are absent.[171]

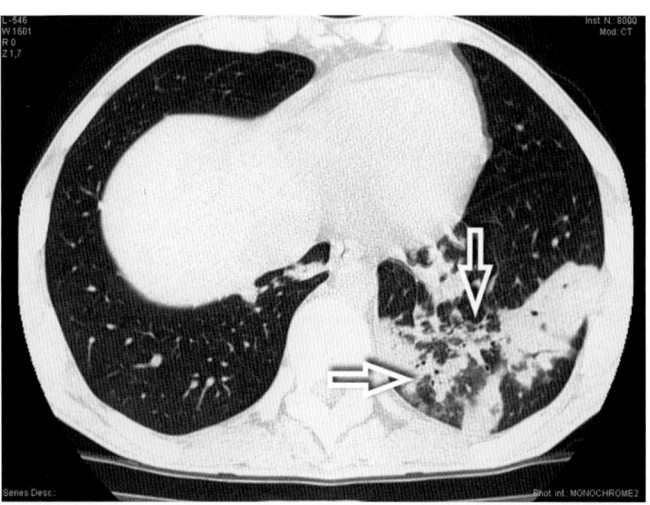

Figure 3-145. The consolidations of OP are often centered on the bronchial elements, as in the case shown (*arrows*).

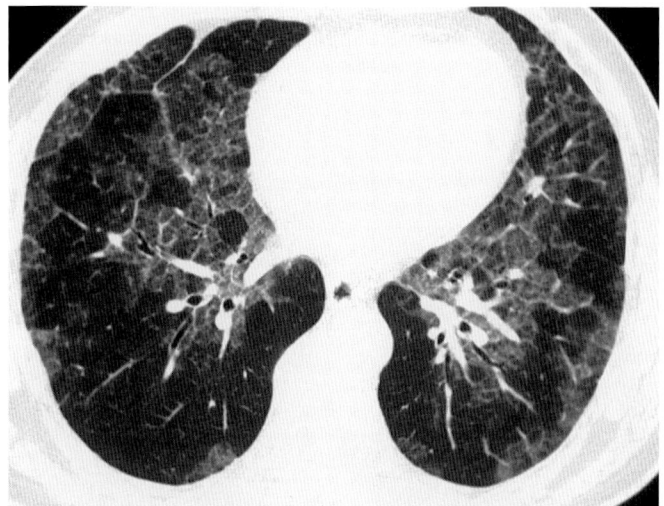

Figure 3-147. Pulmonary alveolar proteinosis. This patient presents very typical patchy areas of GGO with superimposed septal pattern (crazy paving).

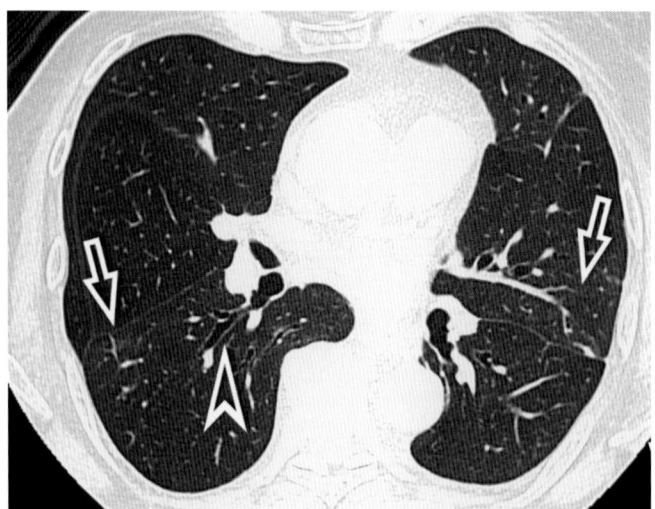

Figure 3-146. Healed OP after corticosteroid therapy. Only a minimal GGO (*arrows*) with some bronchial rigidity (*arrowhead*) persists. Usually, the response of the opacities to the therapy is striking; however, the possibility of a relapse is high.

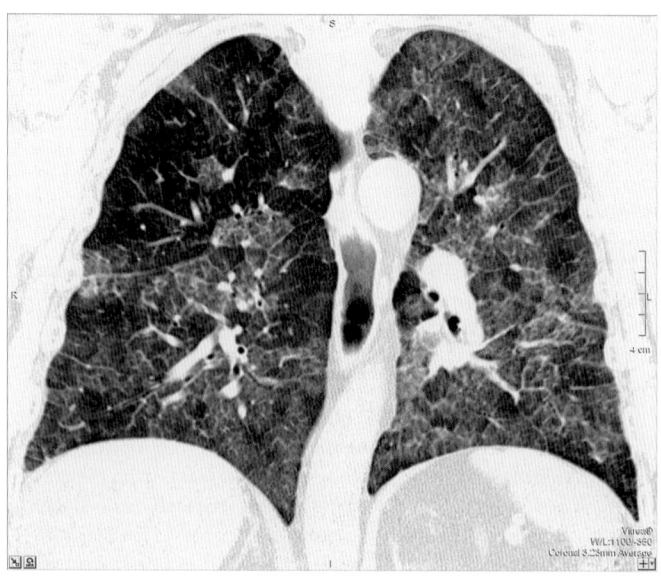

Figure 3-148. In this case, the areas of crazy paving are more-or-less extended throughout the lung without considerable geographical preferences.

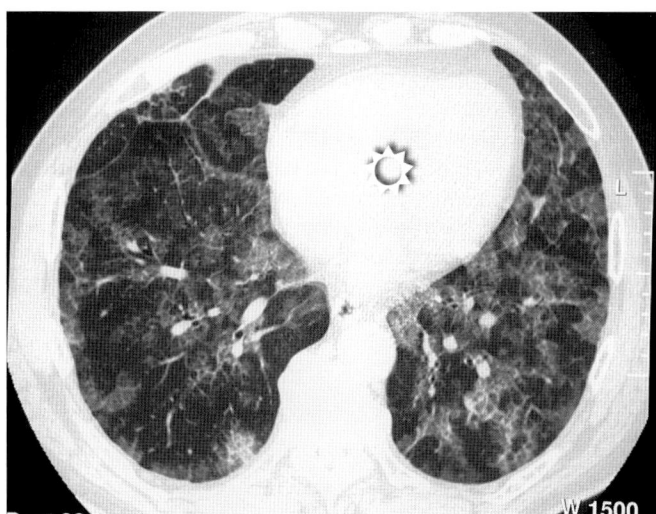

Figure 3-149. In this image, the lung involved by the crazy paving is intermingled with normal lung. There are no signs of pulmonary parenchymal distortion or of pleural effusion, and the heart (*sun*) is of normal size.

Cystic Pattern

Definition

A cystic pattern is present when multiple roundish, well-defined air-containing spaces (black holes) are variably scattered throughout the lung parenchyma (Fig. 3-150). These "holes in the lung" may be due to dilatation of the bronchial structures, abnormal distension of alveolar spaces, focal destruction of lung parenchyma, or even to cavitation of solid lesions.[172,173]

The cystic pattern should not be confused with the dark lung pattern. In both models, the elementary lesions are hyperlucent but in the cystic pattern, these lesions are focal and not diffuse and their density is that of pure air containing units, as black as the ambient air outside the chest.

High-Resolution Computed Tomography Signs

The cysts appear as multiple "black holes" that may differ by morphologic features (walls, shape, and contents) and distribution. When present, the walls of the cysts appear as white encircling lines (Fig. 3-151) of a thickness depending on the constituent elements (e.g., cells, fibrosis) and on

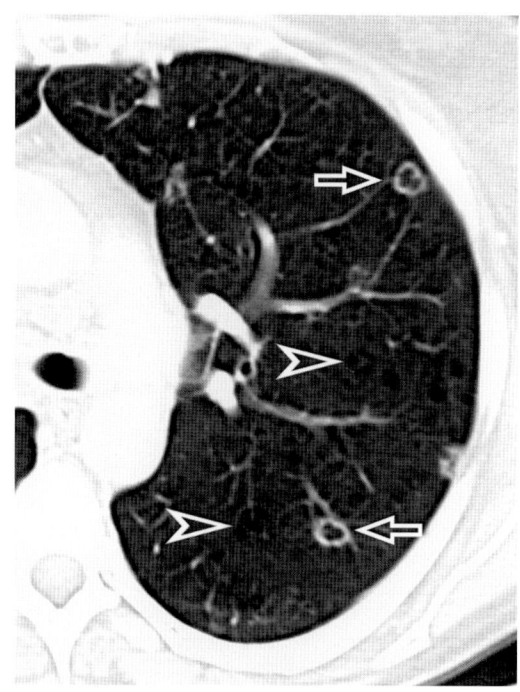

Figure 3-151. Cystic lesions. In this case, there are two associated diseases. The first is responsible for multiple focal hyperlucencies without walls (*arrowheads*). The second shows cysts with evident walls and also some material inside the central lucency (*arrows*).

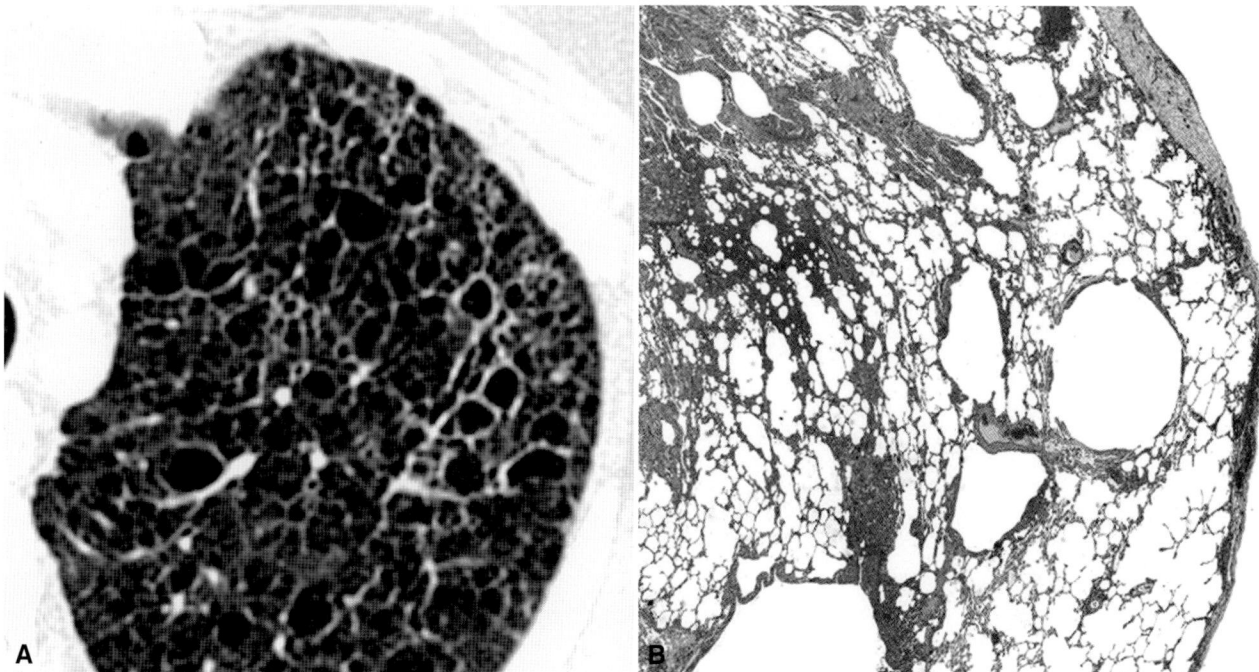

Figure 3-150. Radiology (**A**) and pathology (**B**) of patients with cystic diseases. Innumerable roundish lesions are scattered throughout the lung. The cysts appear hyperlucent (black) radiologically and white pathologically.

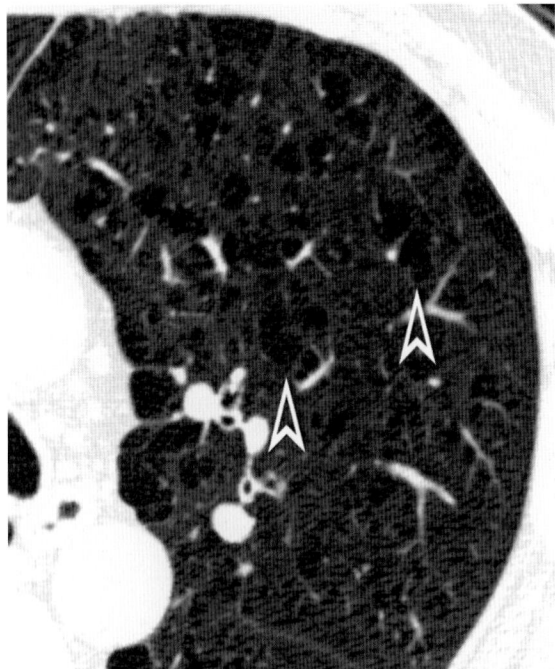

Figure 3-152. Typical "black holes" from destruction of lung parenchyma (patient with centrilobular emphysema). In the image, multiple black areas of different size and shape and with no recognizable walls are visible (*arrowheads*). Some lesions have a tiny white dot inside.

the phase of disease.[152] Cysts without walls are usually the result of local destruction of lung parenchyma[8] (Fig. 3-152; see also Fig. 3-151).

The shape of the cysts depends on the mechanism of their formation, on their relationships with each other, and on the concomitance of traction phenomena in the surrounding parenchyma.[2] Cysts with regular shape, for example, are usually secondary to "check-valve" mechanisms with localized hyperinflation occurring in the context of a normal parenchyma (Fig. 3-153). Cysts with bizarre shape, in contrast,

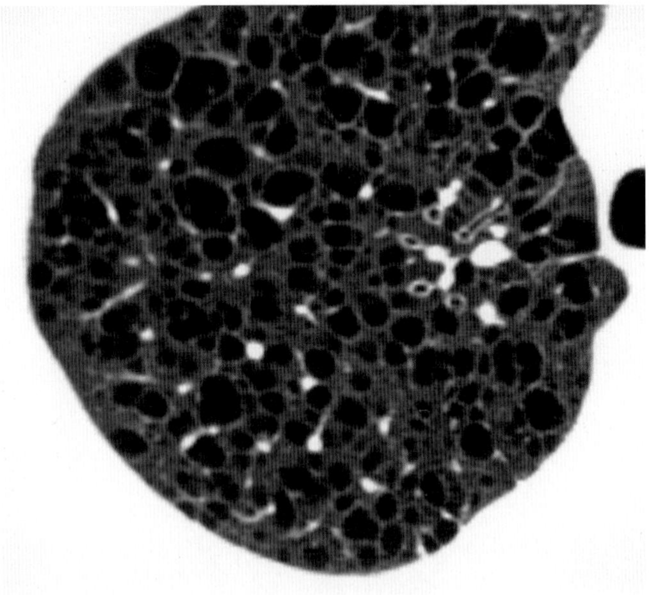

are often due to fusion of several single lesions and even incorporation of ectatic thick-walled bronchi for the presence of fibrotic phenomena with multifocal distortion[2,8] (Fig. 3-154).

The content of the cysts should be black because, by definition, it is pure air; however, when the cysts are due to destruction or necrosis of lung parenchyma, some remnants may persist within the blackness. For example, some cystic spaces may contain a small nodular opacity representing the centrilobular artery[174] (see Fig. 3-152), and others may contain solid material due to their neoplastic nature or to a fungus ball growing inside their lumen. When infected, the cysts may contain air-fluid levels (Fig. 3-155).

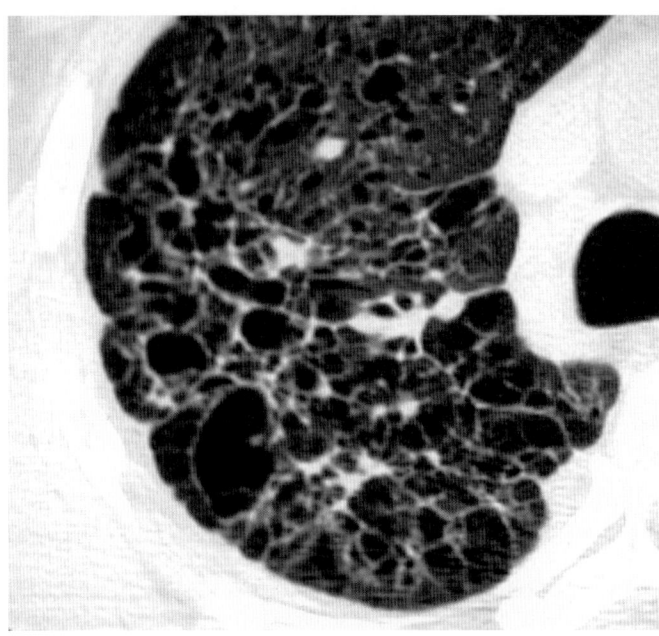

Figure 3-154. Cysts of a disease (PLCH) characterized by the phenomena of fibrosis with distortion and remodeling. The lesions are of variable size and shape, and their walls have an irregular thickness. It is difficult to recognize any normal lung parenchyma in between them. Compare with Figure 3-153.

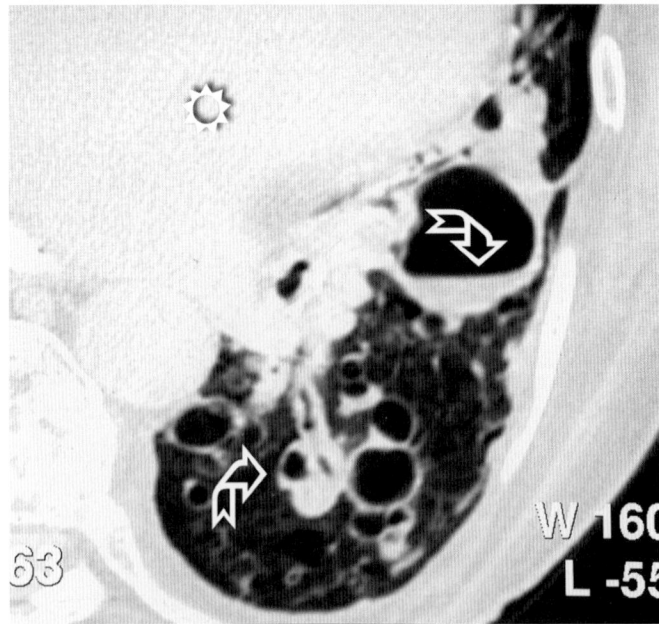

Figure 3-153. Cysts of a disease (LAM) surrounded by normal parenchyma. The lesions are roundish, homogeneously scattered throughout the lung, more or less regularly interspersed with vascular structures of adequate size, and their wall presents uniform thickness. Compare with Figure 3-154.

Figure 3-155. Axial view of multiple hyperlucent lesions (cystic bronchiectasis) in the lower left lung, behind the heart (*sun*). The fluid material inside some hyperlucencies forms what is called radiologically an air-fluid level (*curved arrows*).

Finally, the distribution of the cysts within the lungs varies with the underlying disease, and this element is often useful in the diagnosis. In this regard, the usage of multiplanar reconstructions is particularly useful because it supplies a panoramic comprehensive assessment of the regional distribution of the lesions along different axes, and the use of the minIP technique reveals itself to be helpful for quantifying them.[3]

Some diseases, partly belonging to this category, however, develop prevalent aspects that make preferable their inclusion in a different pattern. Consequently, lymphoid interstitial pneumonia is included in the Nodular Pattern, subset Lymphatic, and *Pneumocystis jiroveci* pneumonia is described in Infectious Diseases, Alveolar Pattern, subset Acute.

Honeycombing, the more distinguishing feature of some fibrosing diseases (IPF, CVD, chronic hypersensitivity pneumonitis, asbestosis, chronic drug toxicity), is also made of well-defined, pure air spaces separated by dense, thick, walls, but here the cysts are only an aspect of an entire fibrotic environment dominating the scene; consequently, honeycombing is discussed in the Fibrotic Pattern, subset Usual Interstitial Pneumonia. Disease in the Cystic Pattern are listed in Box 3-13.

Centrilobular Emphysema

In the early stage of disease, the cysts appear as tiny roundish black holes with invisible walls, and they are surrounded by normal lung parenchyma (Fig. 3-156). The lesions are homogeneously lucent. However, sometimes a central nodular or branching opacity representing the centrilobular artery is seen, and this finding may be helpful for distinguishing emphysema from other diffuse cystic diseases.[175] When emphysema enlarges and involves the entire secondary lobule, remnants of vessels and septa may simulate the appearance of thin walls, usually incomplete.[2]

Typically, in centrilobular emphysema, the lesions involve predominantly the upper lobes and the superior segment of both lower lobes[175] (Fig. 3-157). The distribution of the cysts in the affected regions is diffuse or patchy, and often the single lesions appear grouped in the centrilobular area and around the centrilobular artery (see Fig. 3-156). With more severe disease, the areas of destruction become confluent. CT documents a peripheral pruning of pulmonary vessels that are decreased in number, size, and arborization, closely mimicking the appearance of the panlobular emphysema[176] (see Fig. 3-157).

Paraseptal emphysema and bullae, bronchial and tracheal abnormalities, infections, pneumothorax, and pulmonary arterial hypertension are possible associated findings[175,177,178] (Fig. 3-158). The pulmonary volume is increased due to overinflation.

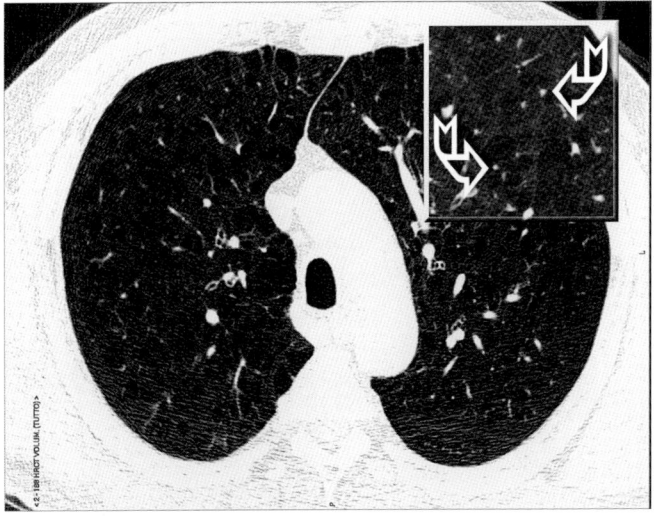

Figure 3-156. Centrilobular emphysema. Multiple focal hyperlucencies with no evident walls are scattered throughout both lungs in this axial scan. Note that some of these "black holes" have a central white tiny dot, the remnant of the centrilobular artery (*curved arrows* [*inset*]).

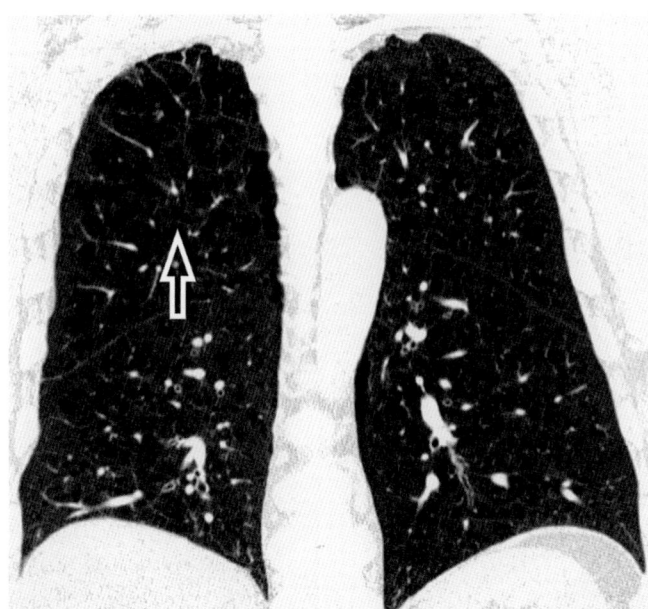

Figure 3-157. Frontal view of the lungs in a patient with emphysema from cigarette smoking. The areas of emphysema are more extended cranially, especially to the right where they involve the totality of the pulmonary lobules (*arrow*).

Box 3-13. Diseases Presenting with Cystic Pattern

Frequent
Centrilobular emphysema
Collagen vascular diseases (see Fibrotic Pattern, subset UIP)
Chronic hypersensitivity pneumonitis (see Fibrotic Pattern, subset UIP)
Idiopathic UIP (clinical IPF) (see Fibrotic Pattern, subset UIP)
Langerhans cell histiocytosis

Rare
Asbestosis (see Fibrotic Pattern, subset UIP)
Birt-Hogg-Dubé syndrome
Cystic metastases
Chronic drug toxicity (see Fibrotic Pattern, subset UIP)
Laryngotracheobronchial papillomatosis
Lymphangioleiomyomatosis
Lymphoid interstitial pneumonia (see Nodular Pattern, subset Lymphatic)
Pneumocystis jiroveci pneumonia (see Alveolar Pattern, subset Acute)

UIP, usual interstitial pneumonia.

Langerhans Cell Histiocytosis

Thin-walled and thick-walled cysts with bizarre shapes (e.g., bilobed, cloverleaf) are typically seen in the late phase of disease. The presence of a distinct wall allows their differentiation from areas of emphysema, which can be also seen in some patients.[76] The lesions, usually less than 10 mm in diameter, are due to coalescence of single cysts, ectatic bronchi, and surrounding paracicatricial emphysema[179,180] (Fig. 3-159). Signs of architectural distortion may be seen in the intervening lung parenchyma.[59]

The distribution of the cysts may be diffuse or patchy in the axial plane, whereas in the craniocaudal directions they present a mid and

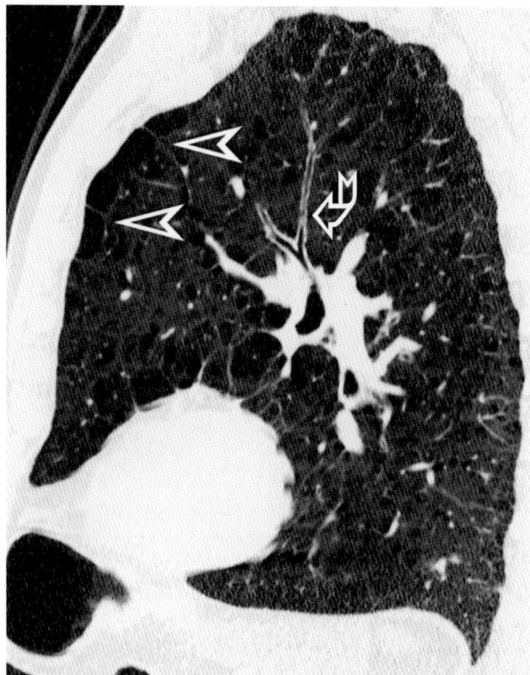

Figure 3-158. Sagittal view of a patient with emphysema from cigarette smoking. Several areas of centrilobular emphysema are scattered throughout the lung. Anteriorly, there also lesions from paraseptal emphysema (*arrowheads*) and, close to the hilum, bronchi with thickened walls are present (*curved arrow*).

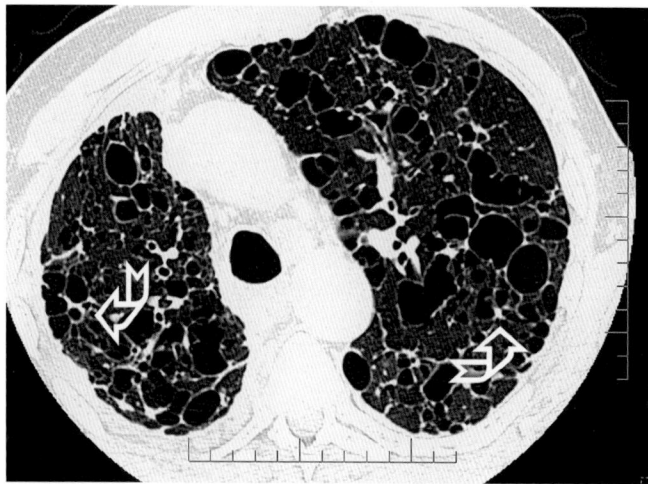

Figure 3-159. Axial view of a subject with advanced LCH. Innumerable cystic lesions with a distinct wall are variously scattered throughout both lungs. They assume various shapes and are not a uniform size. In some regions (*curved arrows*), there is evidence of centrilobular structures surrounded by areas of absolute hyperlucency. In this patient, the asymmetry of the chest with a noticeably smaller right hemithorax is due to a right pleural mesothelioma.

upper lung zone predominance with relative sparing of the lung bases[180] (Fig. 3-160).

In the advanced stages of disease, the cystic pattern is the only abnormality visible in CT but in the early and intermediate stages, more or less numerous centrilobular dense, often cavitated nodules with shaggy margins are present (Fig. 3-161). In some patients, a progression from cavitated nodules to cystic lesions has been observed.[180] Recurrent or bilateral pneumothorax occurs in up to 25% of patients over the course

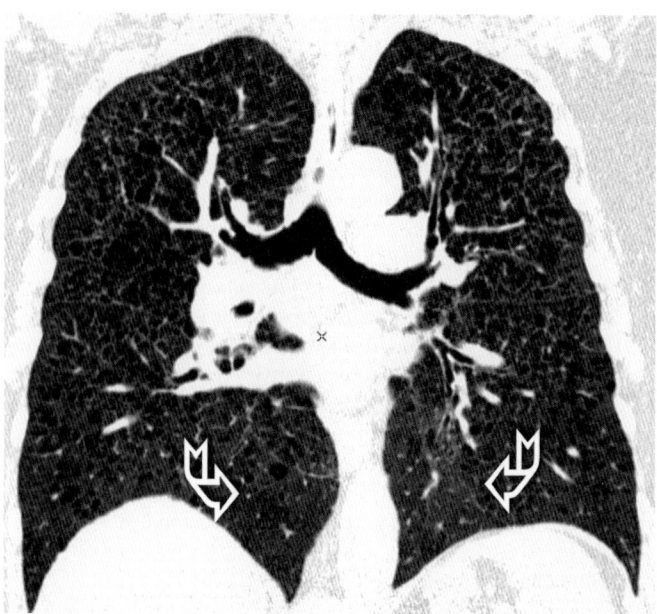

Figure 3-160. Coronal view of a subject with PLCH. The hyperlucent lesions extensively occupy the upper and middle zones of the lung, whereas at the lung bases there are still areas of relatively normal lung (*curved arrows*).

of their disease.[181] Signs of other smoking-related interstitial lung diseases (respiratory bronchiolitis, emphysema) may coexist, creating mixed patterns.[77]

Laryngotracheobronchial Papillomatosis
Laryngotracheobronchial papillomatosis is a viral infection that usually affects the upper airways but that may rarely spread along the airways disseminating to the lung parenchyma. The most common CT findings are intratracheal polypoid lesions, resulting in focal or diffuse narrowing of the trachea and pulmonary multilobulated nodules, many of which are cavitated[182] (Fig. 3-162). The cavitated lesions may have thin or thick walls with irregularly nodular inner walls. Air-fluid levels inside the cysts are not uncommon, and they are secondary to infection.

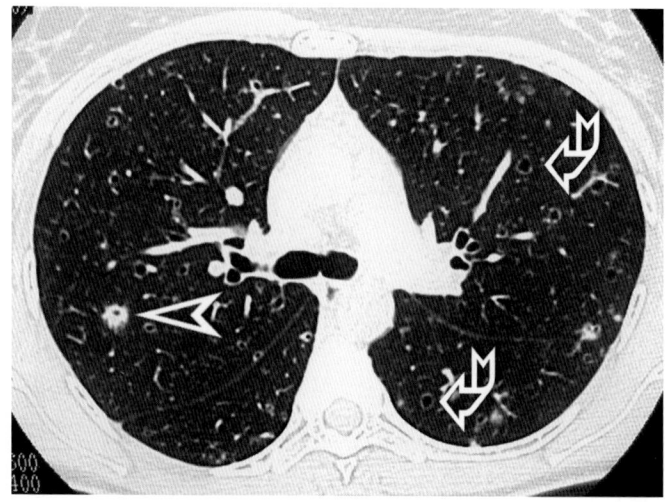

Figure 3-161. Early PLCH. The axial scan documents the coexistence of frankly cystic lesions (*curved arrows*) and nodules with shaggy margins (*arrowhead*). There is a hyperlucency inside the nodules, possibly centrilobular bronchioles.

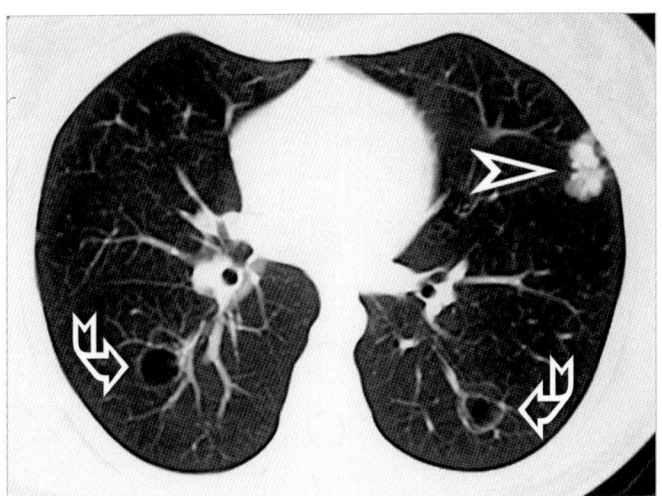

Figure 3-162. Axial scan of a patient with laryngotracheobronchial papillomatosis. In the image, a lobulated solid nodule (*arrowhead*) coexists with two fully cystic lesions (*curved arrows*).

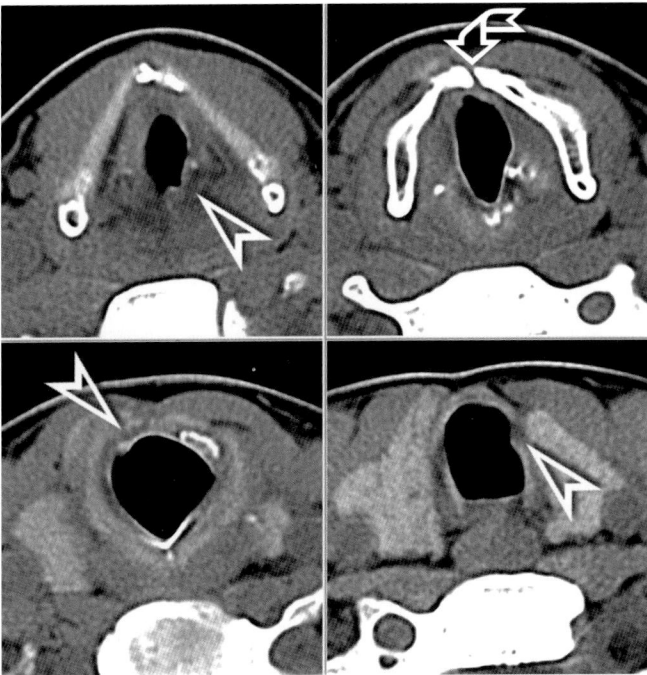

Figure 3-164. Four axial images from the laryngeal (*upper left*) to the upper tracheal level (*lower right*) of a patient with laryngotracheobronchial papillomatosis who has already undergone surgery (*curved arrow*). The lumen of the upper airways shows focal irregularities (*arrowheads*) at least partially related to previous surgery.

Some reports emphasize the possibility of a predominant lower lobe distribution, but the involvement of the upper lobes is not uncommon[183] (Fig. 3-163).

At the central airways level, CT shows multiple small nodules projecting into the airway lumen (Fig. 3-164) or a diffuse nodular thickening of the airway walls. Findings related to the airways obstruction are infections, atelectasis, air-trapping phenomena, and bronchiectasis.[182] There is also a risk of malignant transformation of the pulmonary lesions.[184]

Lymphangioleiomyomatosis

The cysts of lymphangioleiomyomatosis are multiple, round, and relatively uniform in size and shape, and they have homogenously thin walls[185] (Fig. 3-165). Typically, the size of the cysts ranges from 0.5 to 2 cm in diameter and tends to increase with the progression of the disease. In patients with mild disease, 25% to 80% of the lung parenchyma

are replaced by cysts, characteristically surrounded by normal lung[186] (see Fig. 3-165).

The cysts are uniformly and symmetrically distributed throughout the lungs, equally affecting the upper-lower and the central-peripheral lung parenchyma[185,187] (Fig. 3-166).

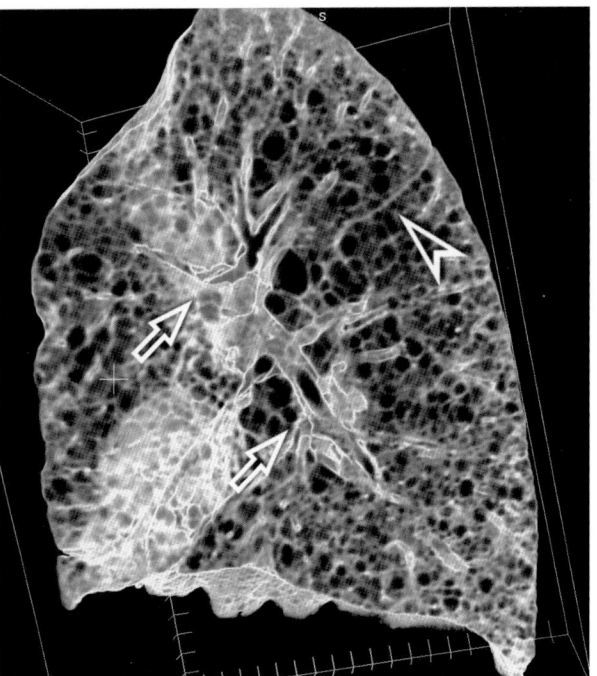

Figure 3-165. Anatomical volume rendering of a sagittal slab in a female with LAM. The image shows the cystic lesions well identified by thin regular walls. Note the regular arborization of the large vessels (*arrows*) and the normal position of the superior portion of the major fissure (*arrowhead*).

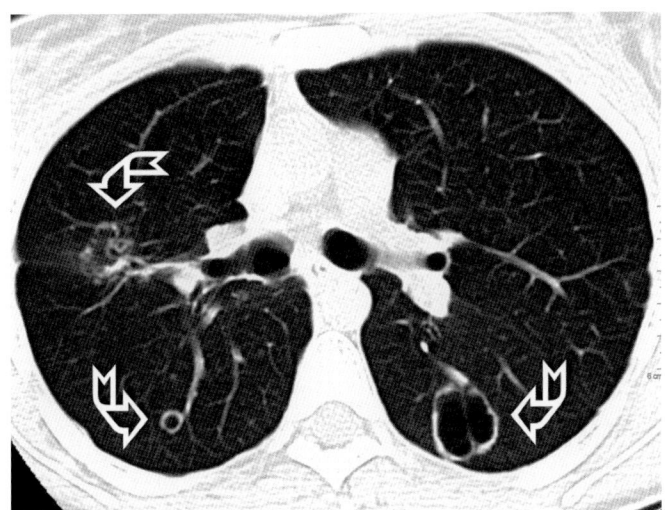

Figure 3-163. Axial scan of the same patient as in Figure 3-162, but at a higher level (carina). Multiple cystic lesions are documented also (*curved arrows*); the one to the left is bilobed.

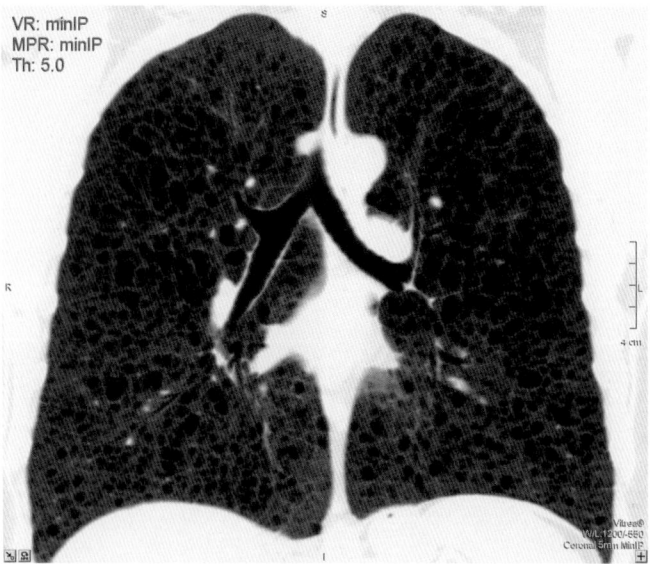

Figure 3-166. Minimum intensity projection (minIP) in a coronal view of the same patient as in Figure 3-165. The minIP technique enhances the visibility of the lesions that are scattered quite uniformly all through the lungs.

In patients with advanced disease, the parenchyma are completely replaced by cysts, and the pulmonary volume is increased (Fig. 3-167). Possible areas of GGO may result from edema or hemorrhage; pulmonary hemorrhage occurs in 8% to 14% of women with lymphangioleiomyomatosis.[187] The incidence of pneumothorax in lymphangioleiomyomatosis is high (40%) due to the thin wall of the cysts and their proximity with the pleural surface. Pleural effusion may also be seen, and other associated abnormalities, including mediastinal or retrocrural lymph node enlargement (40%) just as often.[185,186]

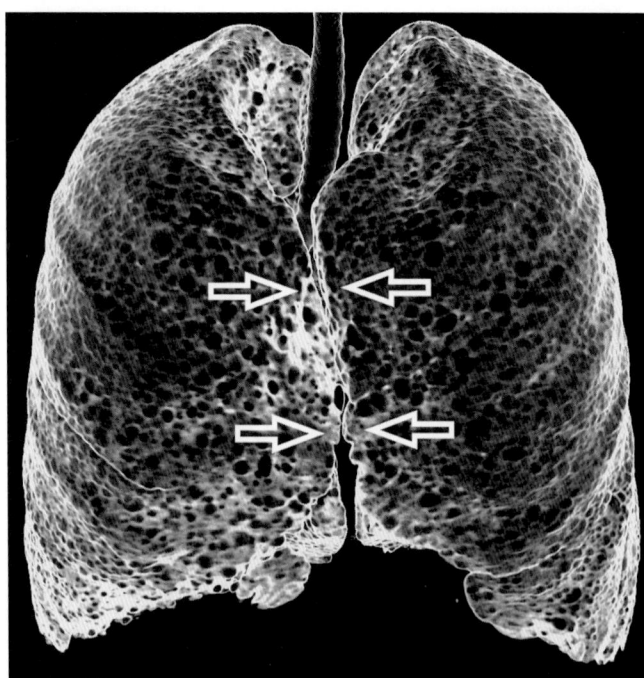

Figure 3-167. External volume rendering of the same patient as in Figure 3-165. This anterior rendering shows how the lungs are hyperinflated through the abnormal touching of their anterior borders (*arrows*).

Cystic Metastases

Although rare (4%), pulmonary metastases may present with a cystic pattern. Most of the lesions are roundish, of variable size, and often have irregularly thickened walls with septations (Fig. 3-168).[90] However, thin-walled cysts with smooth walls may be also observed, particularly after chemotherapy.[188] On the contrary, metastases from angiosarcoma may have an external halo of ground glass attenuation (30%) and an internal air-fluid level, both due to hemorrhage.[188,189]

The lesions occur in a random distribution, often showing a "feeding vessel" sign (Fig. 3-169). Most pulmonary metastases are located in the basal and peripheral zones.[90]

Hemothorax and pneumomediastinum are rare associated conditions.[189] An uncommon complication is the occurrence of a pneumothorax due to ruptured subpleural cavities into the pleural space. Enlarged hilar and mediastinal lymph nodes may be also present (Fig. 3-170).

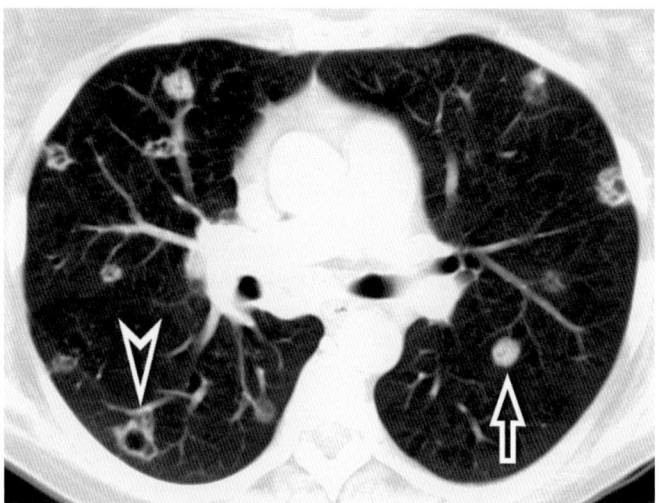

Figure 3-168. Axial view at the level of the carina in a patient with multiple metastases. There is a range of lesions, from solid nodules (*arrow*) to fully cavitated elements (*arrowhead*).

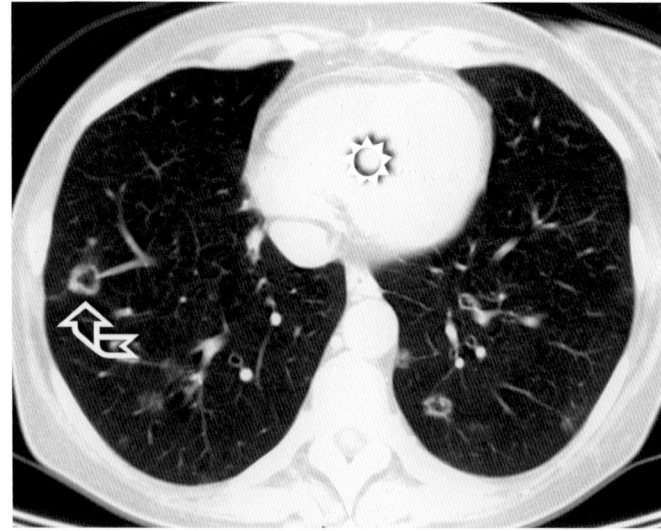

Figure 3-169. Axial scan of the same patient as in Figure 3-168, but at a lower level. The heart is indicated by the symbol of the sun (*sun*). One of the cystic metastases to the right (*curved arrow*) seems connected to an artery ("feeding vessel" sign).

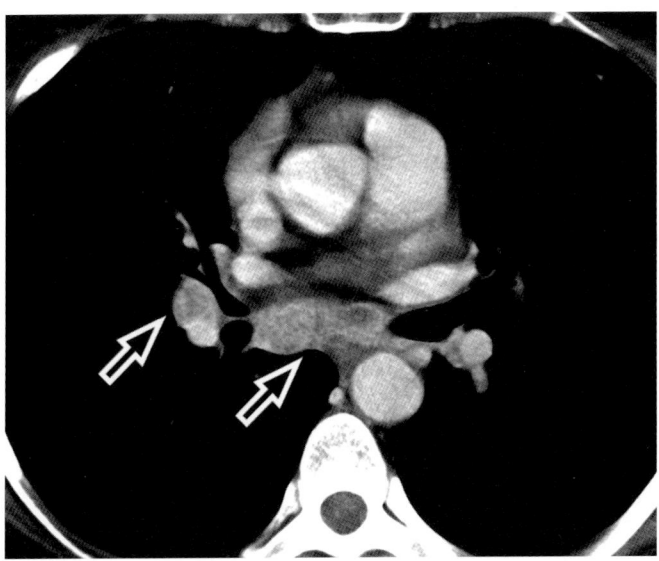

Figure 3-170. Same patient as in Figure 3-168. Note the enlarged and colliquated lymph nodes at the right hilar level and in the subcarinal area (*arrows*).

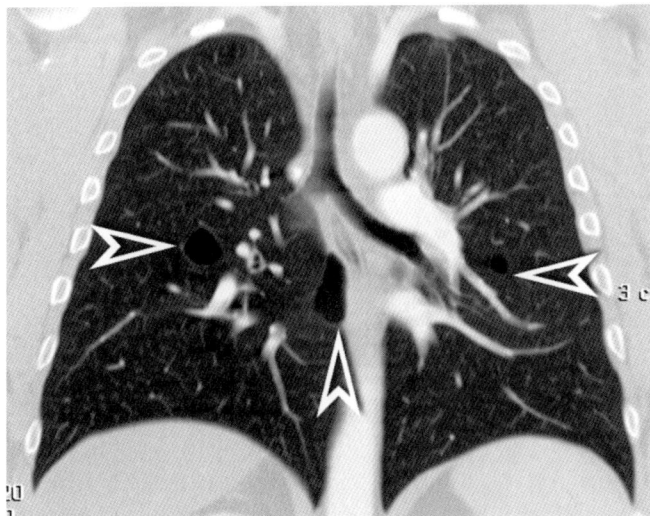

Figure 3-172. Frontal view of the same patient as in Figure 3-171. The scan nicely shows the relationship of the cysts with the pleural boundaries. The contact with them is indicated by the *arrowheads*. (Courtesy of Angelo Carloni, MD, Terni, Italy.)

Birt-Hogg-Dubé Syndrome

Birt-Hogg-Dubé syndrome[190] is a rare, inheritable, multisystem disorder (autosomal dominant) characterized by skin lesions, renal tumors, and multifocal pulmonary cysts. Radiologically, multiple thin-walled cysts round to oval in shape, ranging widely in size (a few millimeters to several centimeters) have been reported[191,192] (Fig. 3-171). The cysts are not numerous; in a paper on 12 patients, the mean extent score was 13% of the whole lung.[193]

The cysts are variably distributed but tend to predominate in the middle and lower lung[191]; characteristically, they are located along the pleural margins in 40% of patients[193] (Fig. 3-172). Cysts abutting or including the proximal portion of the lower pulmonary arteries and veins have been also described.[193]

The lung looks normal in between the cysts (Fig. 3-173). Birt-Hogg-Dubé syndrome can be associated with recurrent spontaneous pneumothoraces.[194]

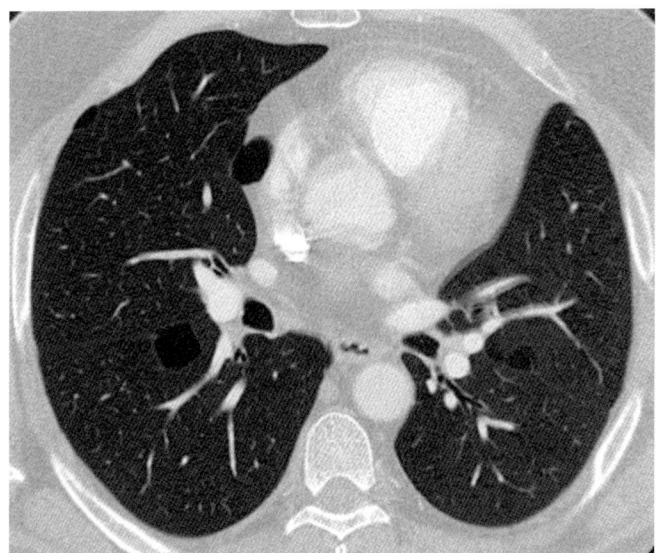

Figure 3-173. Another axial scan of the same patient as in Figure 3-171. The image shows the cysts and the intervening parenchyma that looks normal. (Courtesy of Angelo Carloni, MD, Terni, Italy.)

Dark Lung Pattern

Definition

A dark lung pattern is present when variable portions of lung parenchyma present a reduced attenuation to the x-rays, then are darker than normal (Fig. 3-174). In a lung image, the peak of gray of the background is determined by the relative amount of air and non-air components per volume unit: the more air (i.e., from obstructive emphysema) and/or the less "non-air" (i.e., from hampered vascular filling or from hypoxic vasoconstriction) components, the darker the background.[2]

Unlike the cystic pattern, the basic abnormality here is not pure black (like the ambient air outside the chest), but rather a dark gray due to lung tissue attenuating less than normal. In fact, bronchi and vessels are usually recognizable within the darkness.

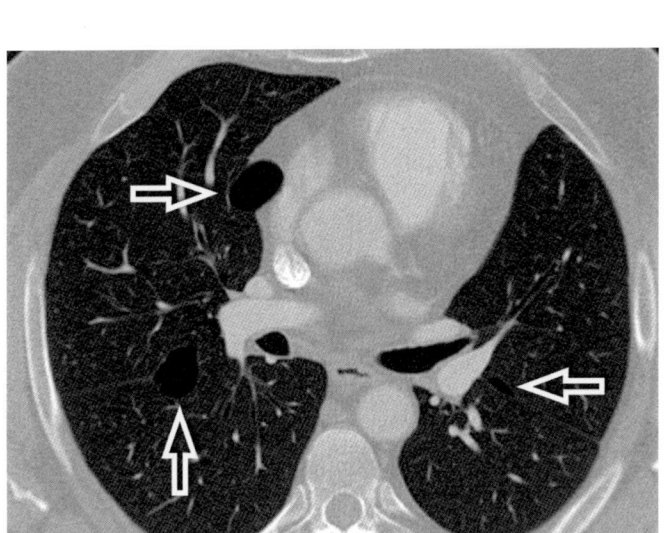

Figure 3-171. Axial scan of a patient with Birt-Hogg-Dubé syndrome. There are scattered small, thin-walled cysts of various size and shape (*arrows*). (Courtesy of Angelo Carloni, MD, Terni, Italy.)

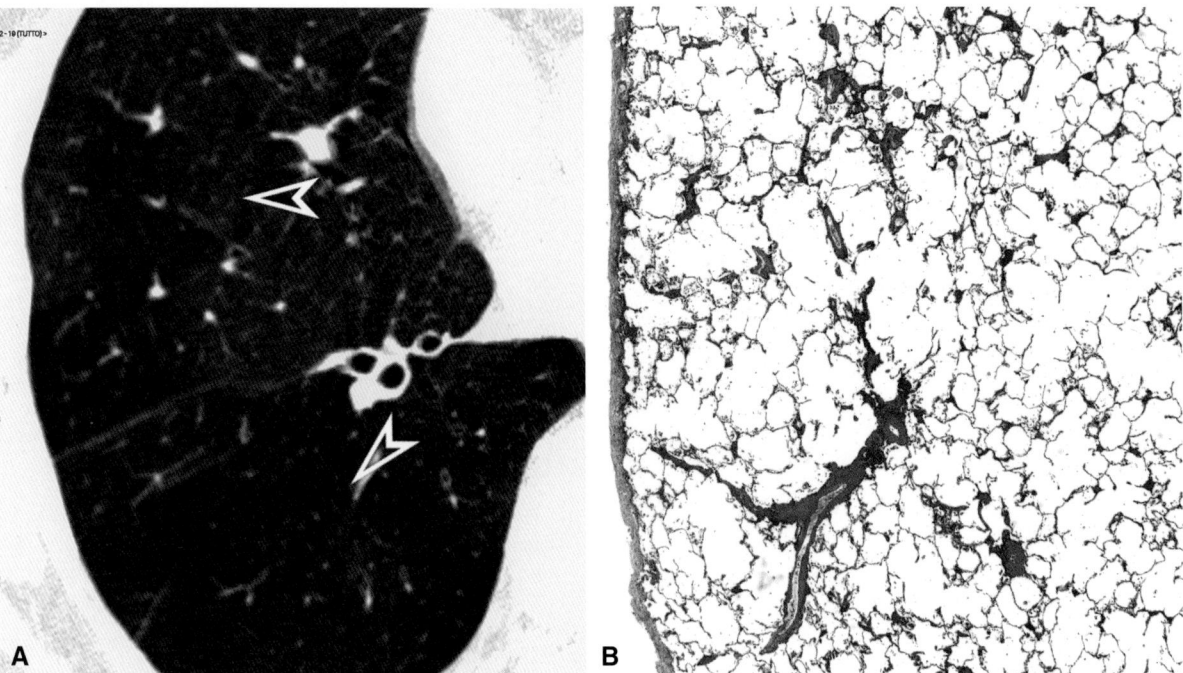

Figure 3-174. A, The high-resolution computed tomography image shows a "dark lung," with extensive areas of decreased attenuation (*arrowheads*) and reduced number and size of the pulmonary vessels. **B,** Pathologically, the low-magnification images may show nearly normal appearing lung (note the absence of visible bronchioles in the image).

High-Resolution Computed Tomography Signs

Patchy or diffuse, the dark lung appears more black than normal and is associated with a simplification of the vascular tree (see Fig. 3-174A); when patchy, the aspect is also called mosaic perfusion (Fig. 3-175).

In detail, the diagnostic elements to evaluate are the extent of the areas of decreased attenuation, the number and size of the vessels

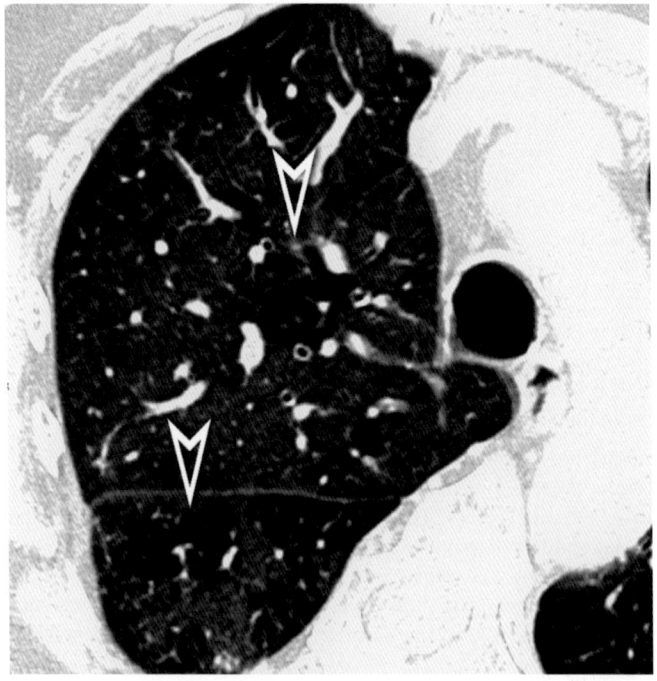

Figure 3-175. Patchwork of different attenuations secondary to small airways disease (mosaic oligemia). Some areas of dark lung are of lobular size and have well-defined contours (*arrowheads*). In the dark regions, the vessels are smaller than in the lighter region, where they are enlarged.

within them, and how the different attenuations vary in the expiratory scans. An involvement of airways may be contemporarily present.

The extent of the dark areas varies, from a lobular size to an entire lung, depending on the severity of the disease.[195] In patients with mosaic perfusion secondary to airway diseases, hyperlucent areas of lobular size are common, usually with well-defined margins (see Fig. 3-175). In patients with vascular diseases, on the contrary, the areas of low attenuation are often larger and poorly defined.[2]

The vessels inside the areas of decreased attenuation are smaller and less numerous than the companion vessels in the unaffected regions where, by contrast, they may be enlarged (see Fig. 3-175). The appearance of heterogeneous lung attenuation may be simulated by areas of GGO interspersed with patches of normal lung; however, in the latter case, the size of the vessels within different areas should be equal. Vessels and bronchi within the involved regions do not show distortion unless some pulmonary derangement exists.[7,196]

The differentiation between vascular or bronchial origin of a dark lung is achieved by repeating a number of CT expiratory scans. Normally, in an expiratory scan, the overall density of the lung increases homogenously. In the dark lung of vascular origin, a homogeneous increase in density occurs everywhere so that the contrast between areas of different attenuation is maintained. On the contrary, when the dark lung is due to airway stenosis, the contrast increases (air trapping)[197] (Fig. 3-176).

Some patients with dark lung pattern show smooth thickening of bronchial walls (Fig. 3-177) and occasionally central and peripheral cylindrical or cystic bronchiectasis. Rarely, centrilobular branching linear densities and centrilobular nodules may be also be apparent.[197] Diseases in the Dark Lung Pattern are listed in Box 3-14.

Chronic Pulmonary Thromboembolism

The most characteristic feature of chronic pulmonary thromboembolism is a mosaic perfusion that does not accentuate with expiratory scans (there is no air trapping). The low attenuation areas may be due both to hypoperfusion distal to occluded vessels and to peripheral

Figure 3-176. High-resolution computed tomography scans at the end of an inspiration *(left)* and expiration *(right)*, where several areas of dark lung are more visible. In the expiratory scan, the areas of normal lung show an increased attenuation (which is normal) *(arrows)* while the dark areas do not change (air trapping).

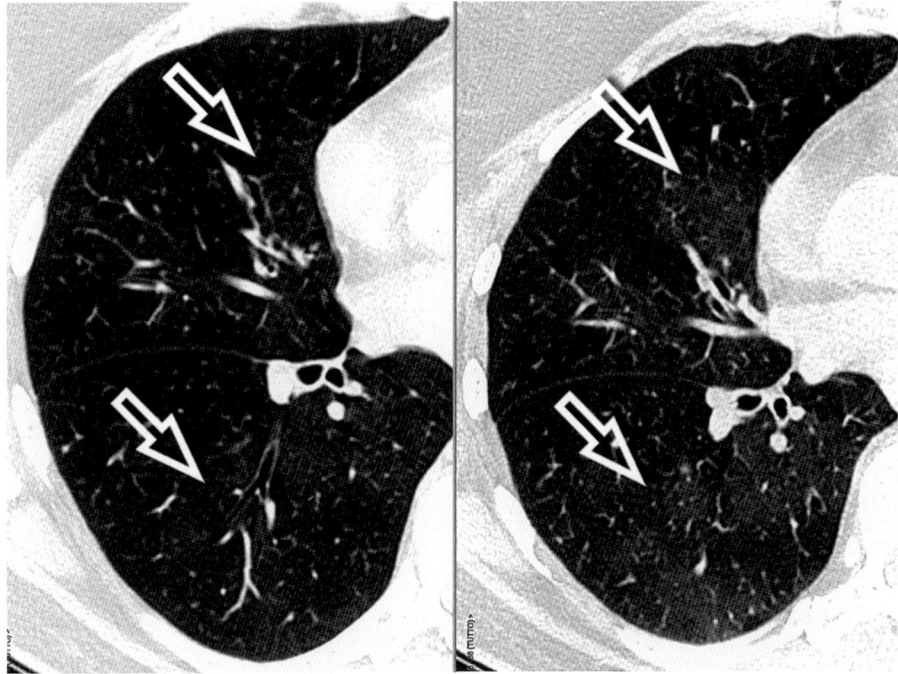

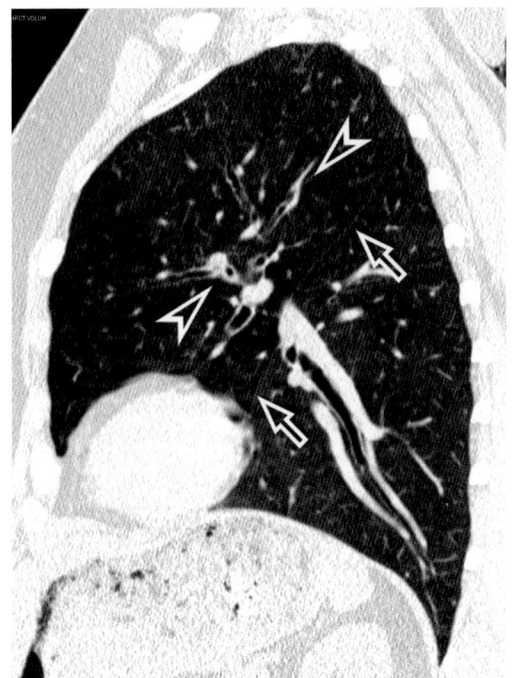

Figure 3-177. This is a sagittal image of the left lung of a patient with a dark lung pattern prevalent in the upper lobe *(arrows)*. The image shows also a thickening of the bronchial walls at the level of the central airways *(arrowheads)*.

Box 3-14. Diseases Presenting with Dark Lung Pattern

Frequent
Chronic pulmonary thromboembolism
Constrictive bronchiolitis (bronchiolitis obliterans)

Rare
Diffuse idiopathic pulmonary neuroendocrine cell hyperplasia
Panlobular emphysema
Swyer-James syndrome

vasculopathy. The areas of increased attenuation have been related to redistribution of blood flow toward the remaining patent vascular bed,[198] and indeed, in these areas, the vessels are larger and often tortuous (Fig. 3-178). Scars from prior pulmonary infarctions are often found in the lower lobes, and pleural thickening from previous pleural effusion is not uncommon.[199]

The areas of low attenuation are usually wide (larger than lobules) with ill-defined margins[198] (Fig. 3-179).

The direct signs of chronic thromboembolism are often visible at the level of the central vessels; these include partial arterial obstruction with mural thrombi (Fig. 3-180), intraluminal bands and webs, calcifications within chronic thrombi, and signs of pulmonary arterial hypertension (dilatation of the central pulmonary arteries secondary to the obstructed vascular lung bed, right ventricular enlargement and hypertrophy, tortuous arteries at the pulmonary level[198]) (see Fig. 3-178). In some cases, a collateral systemic blood supply may be evident with abnormal dilatation and tortuosity of the bronchial, phrenic,

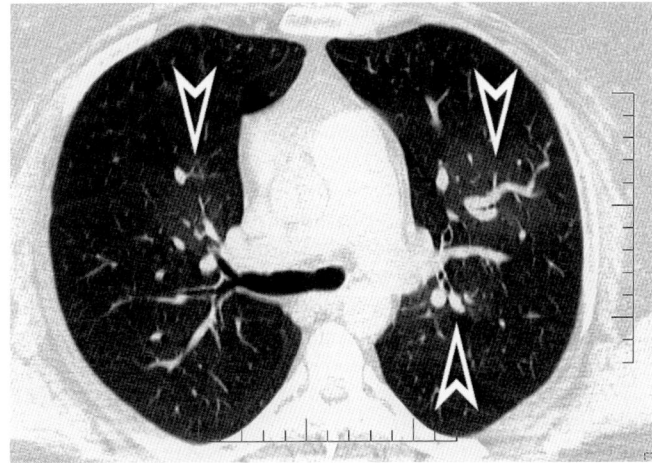

Figure 3-178. Chronic pulmonary thromboembolism. Mosaic perfusion with disparity in the size of the segmental vessels, larger, and also tortuous in the areas of higher attenuation *(arrowheads)*.

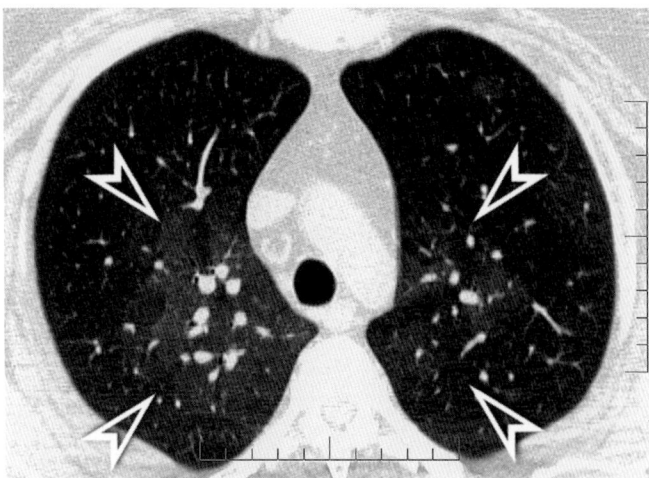

Figure 3-179. Chronic pulmonary thromboembolism. The dark, hypoperfused areas are extensive and prevalent in the lung periphery; their margins with the normal lung (*arrowheads*) are quite ill defined.

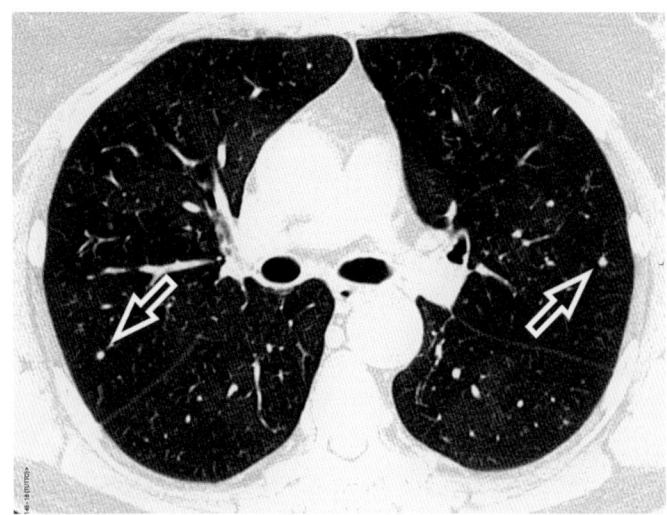

Figure 3-181. Axial scan of a patient with chronic cough and dyspnea. The combination of a mosaic perfusion pattern with air trapping and of sporadic bilateral micronodules (*arrows*) suggests the diagnosis of diffuse idiopathic pulmonary neuroendocrine cell hyperplasia.

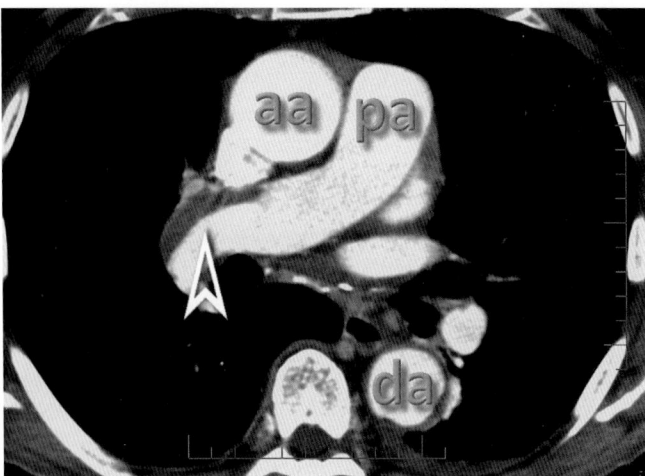

Figure 3-180. Axial contrast-enhanced computed tomography scan of a patient with chronic pulmonary thromboembolism. This axial image demonstrates an eccentric thrombus (*arrowhead*) showing as a thickening of the anterior wall of the right pulmonary artery. aa, ascending aorta; da, descending aorta; pa, main pulmonary artery.

intercostal and internal mammary arteries. Such systemic perfusion of the peripheral pulmonary arterial bed may account for the presence of focal areas of ground glass attenuation within the lung.[200] Patients with severe pulmonary hypertension may also show a mild pericardial thickening or a small pericardial effusion.

Diffuse Idiopathic Pulmonary Neuroendocrine Cell Hyperplasia

The narrowing of the bronchiolar lumen due to the neuroendocrine cellular hyperplasia and fibrosis[201] is not directly visible with HRCT, but it can show up indirectly as mosaic perfusion (Fig. 3-181) with air trapping.[202] Small, well-defined, randomly distributed nodules less than 5 mm in diameter may be also identified in the CT images, especially when obtained with multislice volumetric equipment. The nodules correspond to the neuroendocrine "tumorlets" present histologically (see Fig. 3-181).[203]

Usually, both hyperlucent dark lung and nodules are randomly distributed throughout both lungs. However, at times, the coronal MIP images may show a prevalence of the nodules in the lower zones[203,204] (Fig. 3-182).

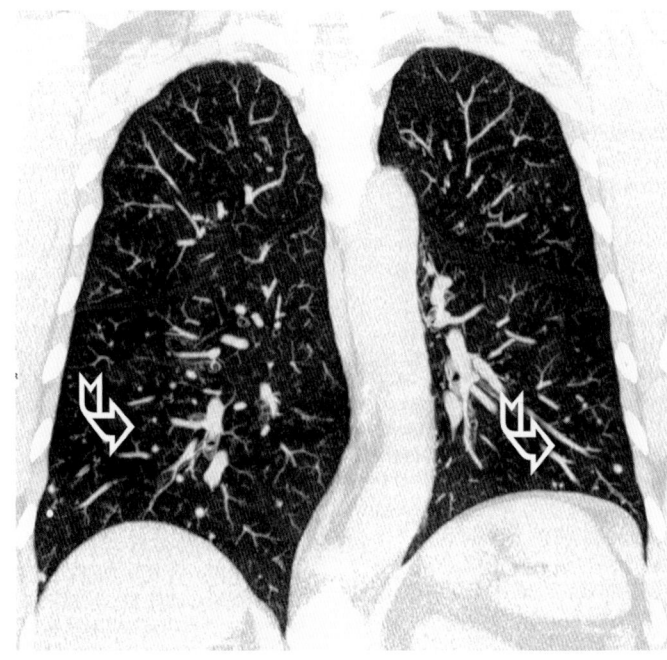

Figure 3-182. Maximum intensity projection (MIP) in a coronal view of the same patient as in Figure 3-181. The MIP technique highlights the visibility of the small nodules that are more numerous at the basal level, in the area indicated by the *curved arrows*.

Round lesions of more than 5 mm in diameter may suggest the existence of carcinoid tumors (grade 1 neuroendocrine carcinomas) (Fig. 3-183). Some patients may also show bronchial wall thickening and cylindrical bronchiectasis.[204]

Constrictive Bronchiolitis (Bronchiolitis Obliterans)

HRCT shows patchy areas of mosaic perfusion secondary to hypoxic vasoconstriction from bronchiolar obstruction (phlogosis/fibrosis). The reason for the narrowing is not directly visible with CT, but it shows up indirectly as dark lung.

The blood vessels in the low attenuation areas are smaller and less numerous than vessels in the areas of relatively high attenuation[67,69]

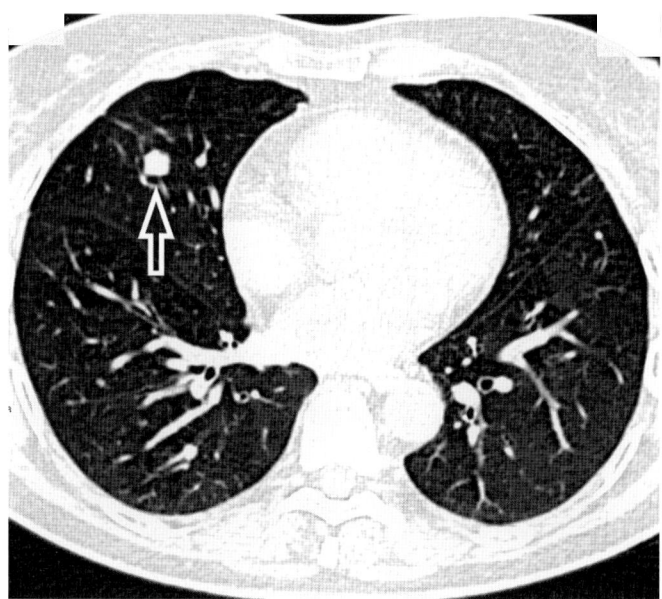

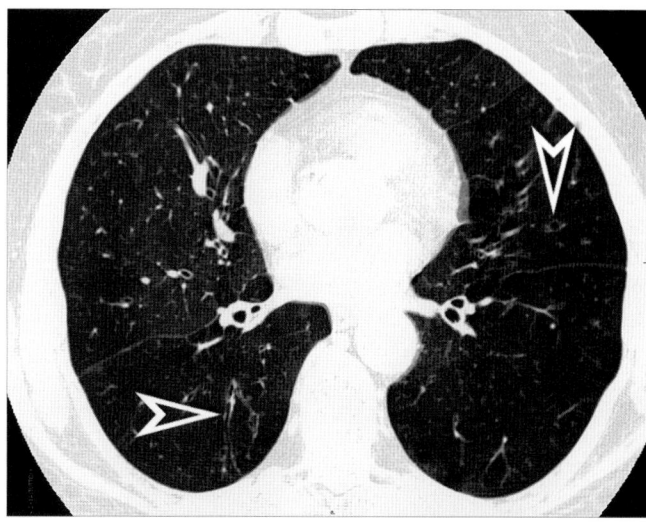

Figure 3-183. Axial view of a subject with diffuse idiopathic neuroendocrine cell hyperplasia. In the middle lobe, there is a nodule of a diameter > 5 mm (*arrow*) that could be a low-grade neuroendocrine carcinoma (carcinoid tumor).

Figure 3-185. Axial scan of the same patient as in Figure 3-184, but at a lower level. Extensive geographic areas of low attenuation are present (in particular to the left), interspersed with less frequent areas of relatively increased opacity. Evidence of mild bronchiectasis is present in the right lower lobe and in the lingula (*arrowheads*).

(Fig. 3-184). The dark lung often presents sharply defined margins and lobular or segmental extension. Air trapping on expiratory scans appears as an accentuated contrast between differently attenuating areas and may be helpful for the early detection and confirmation of the bronchial origin of the oligemia, particularly after lung transplantation.[197]

The disease is diffuse and bilateral, with more common and extensive involvement of the lower lobes[68] (Fig. 3-185). Some patients with constrictive bronchiolitis show also central and peripheral cylindrical bronchiectasis (Fig. 3-186). The cause of the bronchiectasis associated with bronchiolitis obliterans remains unclear, but it seems most likely due to concomitant injury of the large airways.[205,206] Rarely, centrilobular nodules or branching linear densities can also be observed.[205]

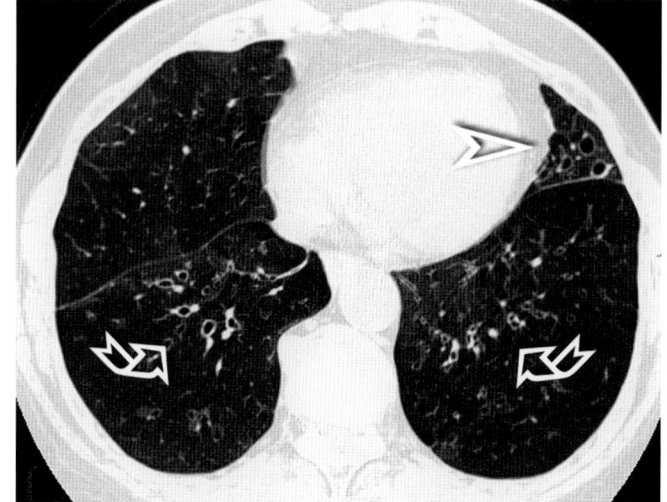

Figure 3-186. Axial scan of the same patient as in Figure 3-184, at the lung bases. Bronchiectasis is visible in the lower lobes (*curved arrows*) and in the basal portion of the lingula (*arrowhead*).

Panlobular Emphysema

Panlobular emphysema is characterized anatomically by a uniform destruction of the pulmonary lobule, and it appears radiologically as extensive areas of dark lung associated with a diffuse "simplification" of the pulmonary architecture (Fig. 3-187). The vessels appear reduced in number and size, at times as if they were stretched and rigid inside the darkness.[8] This is the pattern of emphysema seen in patients with alpha-1-antiprotease deficiency,[175] and it may be indistinguishable from the appearance of severe constrictive bronchiolitis.[20]

Panlobular emphysema is generalized within the lungs, but it can be more severe in the lower lobes[175] (Fig. 3-188).

In approximately 40% of patients with alpha-1-antiprotease deficiency, bronchiectasis is present due to destruction of the elastic

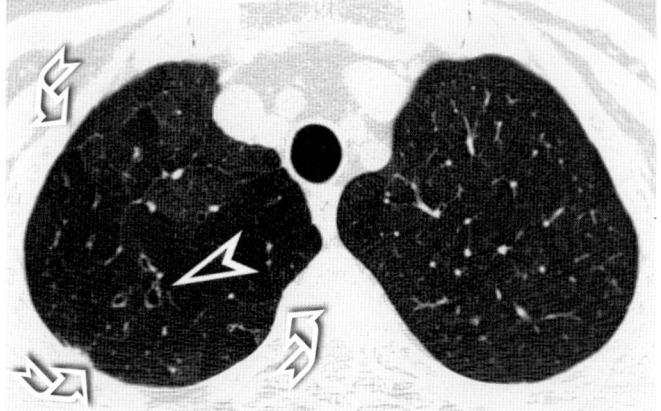

Figure 3-184. High-resolution computed tomography of a patient with constrictive bronchiolitis. The image shows multiple patchy dark areas, especially in the right lung, associated with decreased size of pulmonary vessels (*curved arrows*). Note the concomitant bronchiectasis with mild bronchial wall thickening (*arrowhead*).

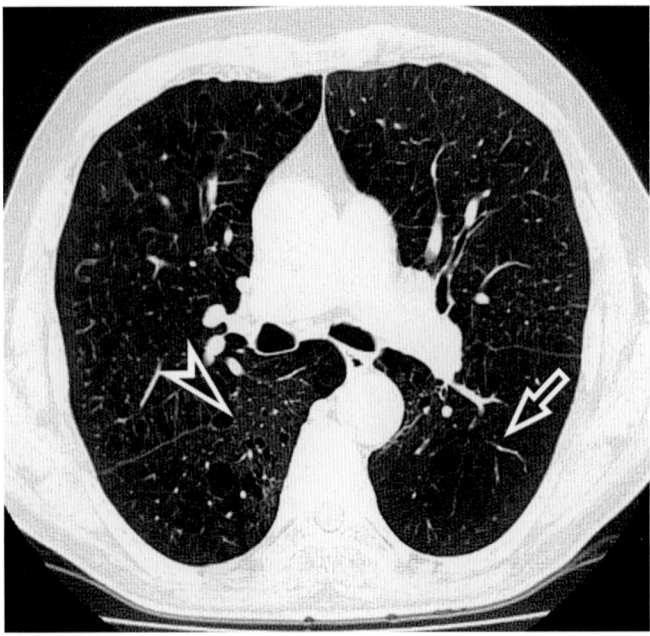

Figure 3-187. Extensive areas of low attenuation with stretched vessels typical of panlobular emphysema are visible everywhere, in particular in the left lower lobe (*arrow*). The right lower lobe is less extensively involved (*arrowhead*).

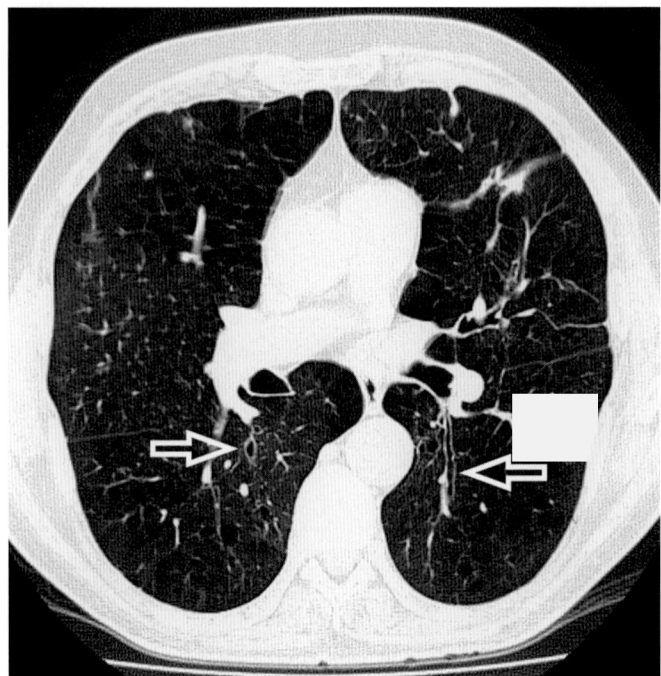

Figure 3-189. Patients with panlobular emphysema often have minimal bronchiectasis associated with bronchial wall thickening (*arrows*).

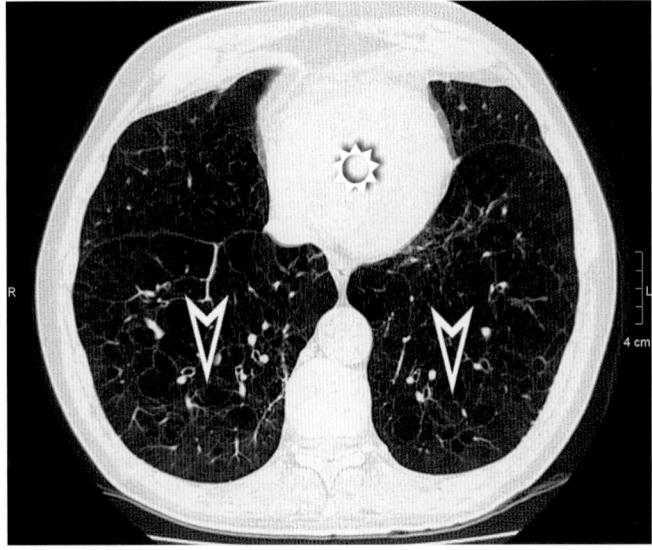

Figure 3-188. Axial scan of the same patient as in Figure 3-187 at the axial level of the heart (*sun*). The hyperlucent transformation of the lung is more extended and more severe at this basal level, where there is only little relatively normal surviving parenchyma posteriorly (*arrowheads*).

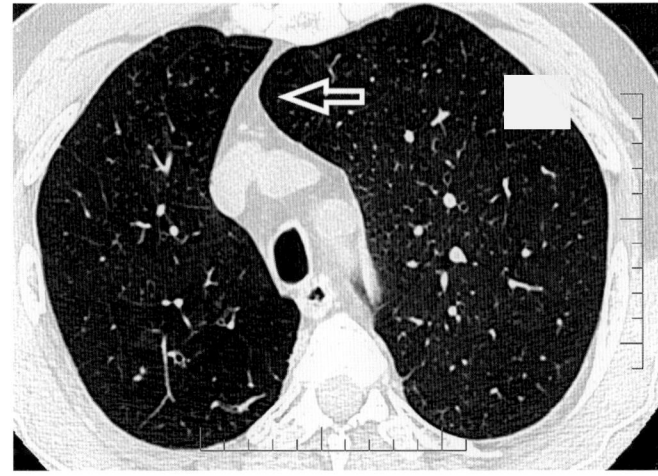

Figure 3-190. Patient with Swyer-James syndrome. The image shows unilaterally reduced right lung attenuation; in the dark lung, the vessels are smaller than contralaterally. The right lung is also smaller, and in fact the mediastinum is shifted ipsilaterally (*arrow*).

lamina[207] (Fig. 3-189). Associated paraseptal emphysema and bullae are relatively uncommon.

Swyer-James (MacLeod Syndrome)

Swyer-James syndrome is a peculiar postinfectious constrictive bronchiolitis that affects the lung asymmetrically[208] (Fig. 3-190). Consequently, the CT hallmark of this syndrome is a dark pattern that can be unilateral and even limited to one lobe. An associated decreased vascularity in the affected areas and air trapping during expiration are the rule.[68]

For decades, based on chest radiographs, authorities have believed that the damage had to be unilateral, but the advent of CT has made it increasingly clear that bilateral involvement is a rule rather than an exception.[208] However, a predominant involvement of one lung and even of one lobe is very frequent[209] (Fig. 3-191).

Ectatic bronchi with thickened walls are often present, sometimes severely[209] (Fig. 3-192).

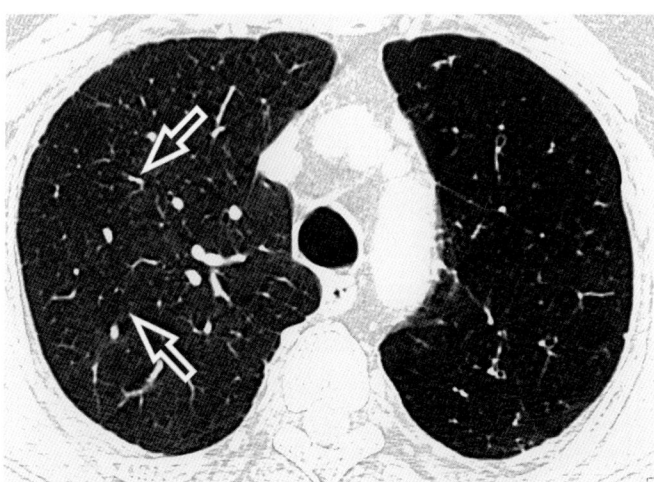

Figure 3-191. Another patient with Swyer-James syndrome. The left lobe is extensively involved, but also some portions of the right lung are relatively hyperlucent with simplified vascular tree (*arrows*).

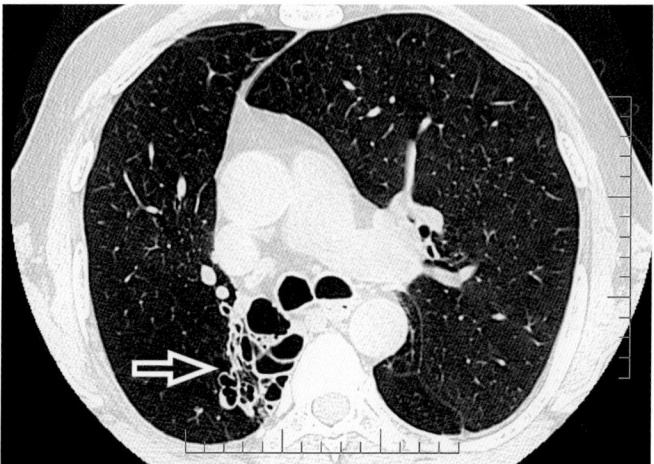

Figure 3-192. Axial scan of the same patient as in Figure 3-190, but at a lower level. Note the cluster of cystic bronchiectasis in the azygos-esophageal recess (*arrow*).

Imaging of the Solitary Pulmonary Nodule

Rationale for the Diagnostic Approach

The increasing availability of multidetector CT equipment continually contributes to the accidental discovery of solitary pulmonary nodules (SPNs). An SPN is a round opacity of the lung less than 3 cm in diameter (if <1 cm, the term *small nodule* is used). Eventually, at least in the United States, most of these SPNs turn out to be benign. However, to ensure that they are not malignant, a careful assessment should be done before establishing the optimal management: follow-up, biopsy, or surgery.

The diagnostic process for the SPNs develops through a decision analysis algorithm coupling the a priori probability of malignancy (risk factors) with the elements of the imaging, where CT is the standard basic imaging technique. CT has a higher sensitivity and specificity than chest radiography and gives extra information about the density of the nodule and its vascularization. Supplementary information about tumor metabolism can be further acquired by the means of

positron emission tomography (PET). PET uses 18F-labeled fluoro-2-deoxy-D-glucose (FDG) as a metabolic marker on the assumption that the metabolism of glucose is typically increased in malignancies. PET relies on a discriminating value of the maximum standardized uptake value (SUV_{max}) of FDG, expressing the highest nodular uptake, as an aid in predicting malignancy.

The PET technique proves reliable for solid nodules larger than 1 cm, for which it can predict a malignant tumor in 90% of cases. However, a number of malignancies, namely bronchioloalveolar carcinoma, well-differentiated adenocarcinomas, and carcinoid tumors, are often negative on PET and, conversely, infective and inflammatory nodules can present with high SUV_{max} uptakes. Said another way, PET (similarly to CT) should not be considered an absolute gold standard for the diagnosis of the SPN. Even when the PET scan is negative, when there is a mismatch of risk factors, clinical data, and elements of the imaging, further diagnostic procedures should be carried out.

Most of the elements summarized in the subsequent text and references have been derived from the excellent review of Truong and colleagues.[210] The interested reader is encouraged to refer to the original paper for further details.

Static Elements

Risk Factors

A given patient's likelihood of having a pulmonary malignancy increases with older age; current or past smoking habits; extrathoracic cancer more than 5 years before nodule detection[211]; exposure to asbestos, uranium, or radon; occurrence of symptoms[210] (in particular hemoptysis[212]); and a family history of lung cancer.[213] These risk factors do not enter in the radiologic evaluation of the nodule per se, but they represent key elements to match with the radiologic data in the final diagnostic algorithm. The differential diagnosis of SPNs is presented in Box 3-15.

Morphologic Aspects

The risk of malignancy is increased when the nodule has ill-defined margins and lobulated or spiculated contours. In particular, spiculation with the so-called sunburst aspect (corona radiata) has a 90% predictive value of malignancy[214] (Fig. 3-193). Unfortunately, this does

---

Box 3-15. Differential Diagnosis of Solitary Pulmonary Nodules

Frequent
Primary lung malignancies
Solitary metastasis
Granuloma
Intrapulmonary lymph node
Focal scarring

Rare
Hamartoma (or other benign tumor)
Arteriovenous malformation
Round pneumonia
Rounded atelectasis
Abscess
Septic embolus
Amyloidoma
Rheumatoid nodule
Pulmonary infarct
Bronchogenic cyst
Wegener granulomatosis
Pulmonary sequestration
Bronchial atresia with mucoid impact

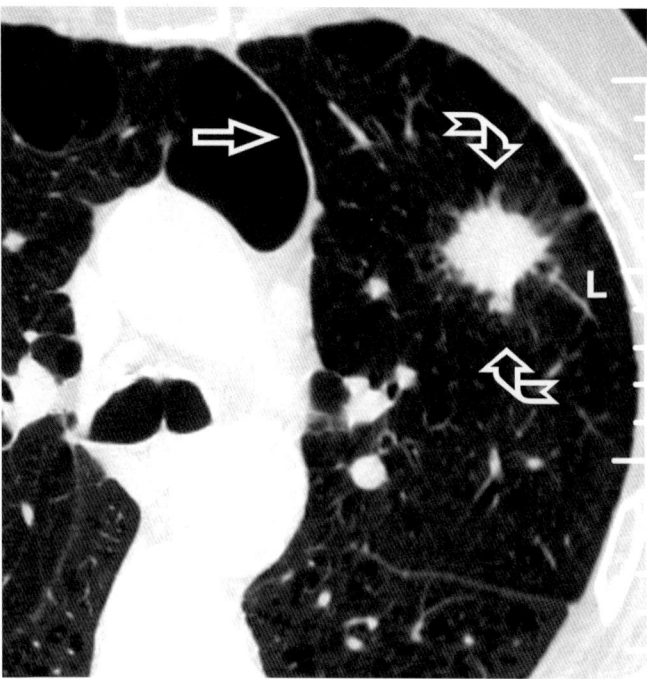

Figure 3-193. Solitary pulmonary nodule (*curved arrows*) in a heavy smoker with COPD. In this clinical context, the spicules that form the margins of the lesion (seen in the sunburst aspect) have a high probability of malignancy. A large bulla is responsible for the shifting of the anterior junction line to the left (*arrow*).

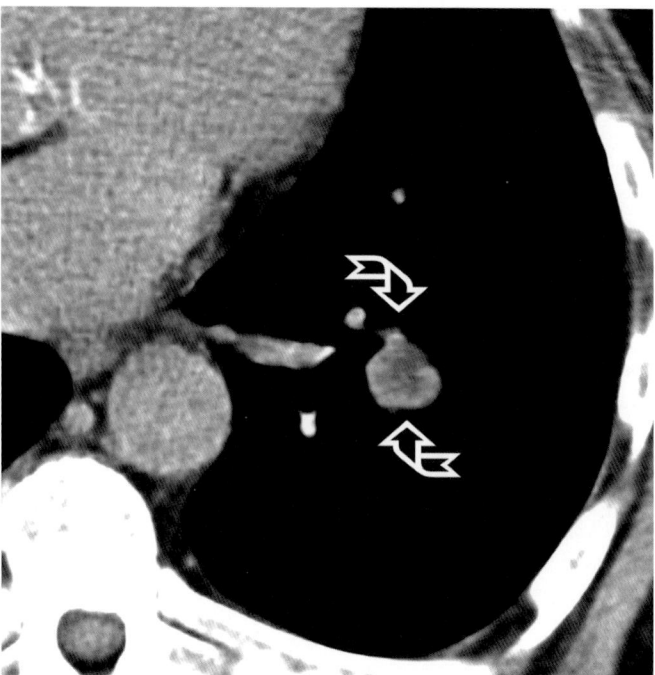

Figure 3-194. Solitary pulmonary nodule. The density of the nodule (*curved arrows*), solid in the periphery, is reduced in the center with attenuation values of −15 HU; this density might correspond to a fatty content.

not mean that a well-marginated SPN with regular contours cannot be malignant, and on the contrary one of five malignancies has these characteristics.[212] Also, size correlates with malignancy. An incidentally discovered SPN with a diameter less than 4 mm has a less than 1% chance of being a primary lung cancer, but if the diameter is in the 8-mm range, the probability is approximately 10% to 20%.[215-217]

Computed Tomography Densitometry

Fat densities inside the nodule (Fig. 3-194) are typical of hamartoma (50%),[218] but metastases from liposarcoma and renal carcinoma also may have fatty components.[219] Central, laminated, or popcorn calcifications inside the nodule are usually benign, but lung metastases from chondrosarcoma or osteosarcoma may present similar aspects.[90]

An SPN may be uniformly dense (solid) or contain ground glass components (subsolid). For solid nodules, the chance of malignancy is 7%, but for subsolid nodules, this percentage rises to 34%.[220] However, when the density is mixed (solid + GGO), this percentage rises to 63%, whereas for pure GGO lesions (Fig. 3-195) the rate of malignancy is "only" 18%. In a large series, 20% of the lesions detected during a CT screening program represented subsolid densities.[220] A halo of GGO around a nodule (*halo sign*) may be due to hemorrhage, inflammation, or tumoral infiltration. This sign is not specific, and it may be found also in benign conditions (e.g., nodular OP).[210]

Cavitation and Air Bronchogram

Cavitation may be benign or malignant; however, cavitation of malignant lesions tends to have more irregular and thicker walls than benign ones.[221] It has been reported that 95% of cavitary lesions with wall thickness greater than 15 mm are malignant.[222] Up to 15% of primary lung malignancies, in particular squamous cell carcinomas, cavitate.[210]

An air bronchogram is not present in the solid lesions, but it is possible inside the nodules of GGO (Fig. 3-196). It may also be seen in

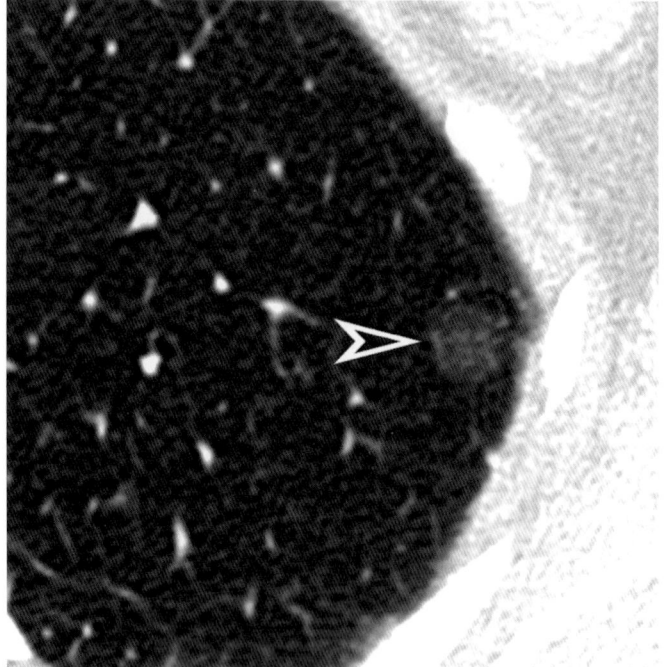

Figure 3-195. Barely visible solitary pulmonary nodule of faint density (nodular GGO) in the peripheral left upper lung (*arrowhead*). The surgical diagnosis was of a focal bronchioloalveolar carcinoma.

bronchioloalveolar carcinoma and pulmonary lymphoma, as well as in some benign lesions.

Dynamic Elements

Doubling Time

The doubling time is the time taken by a lesion to double its volume. The basic assumption is that, except for the infectious and

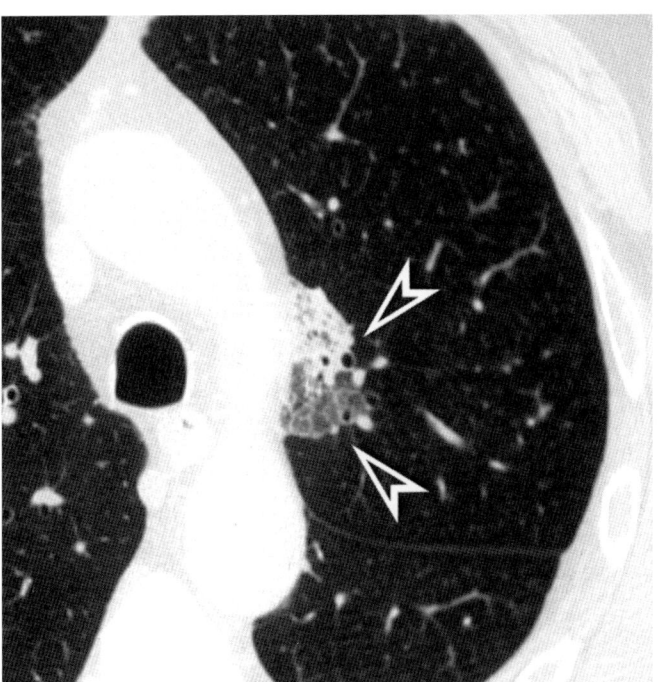

Figure 3-196. Initial presentation of a diffuse bronchioloalveolar carcinoma. In this phase, the lesion has a lobular size, and the appearance is of a mixed densities disease with consolidative and GGO aspects. A few small hyperlucent bronchi can be appreciated inside the opacity.

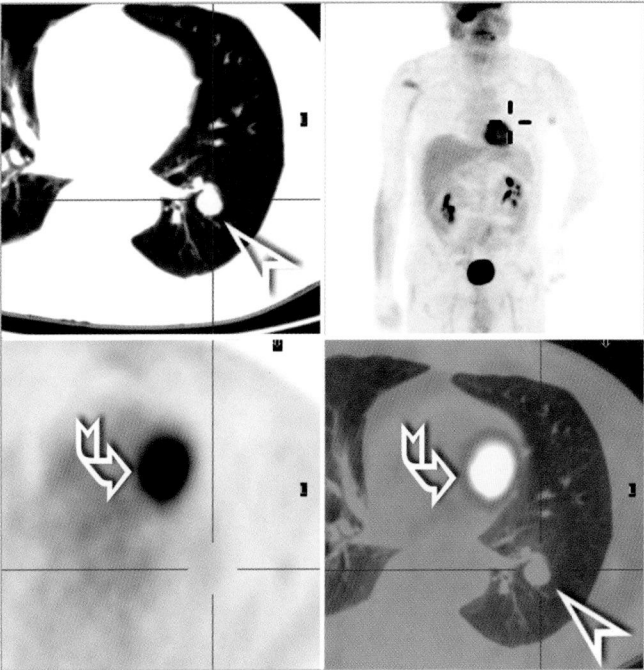

Figure 3-197. Same patient as in Figure 3-194. Here a computed tomography image is shown together with the results of a PET examination where the nodule (*arrowhead*) does not appear to concentrate the fluoro-2-deoxy-D-glucose. The cardiac uptake is indicated by a *curved arrow*.

inflammatory lesions, the faster the growth, the greater the chance a nodule is malignant. Indeed, the doubling time of a solid malignant nodule is in the range of 1 to 13 months, whereas that of a benign lesion tends to be shorter or longer.[210] The subsolid lesions, on the contrary, are another story. Approximately 20% of well-differentiated adenocarcinomas have a doubling time greater than 2 years,[223] and some bronchioloalveolar carcinomas may show a doubling time even greater than 3.5 years.[224]

In summary, the old adage that "a nodule should be considered benign if unvaried after two years" is still acceptable now,[210,225,226] but it is suitable only for solid lesions. Note that the recommendations of the literature refer to the volume of a nodule. However, more often in practice, the measures are done on two-dimensional images using diameter so the volume should be corrected accordingly (to double its volume, a nodule should increase its diameter by about 25%).[227]

The timing of the follow-up of a nodule incidentally discovered on CT depends on the priori probability of malignancy (risk factors), size, and density. The appropriate timing has been recently recommended in detail in a statement from the Fleischner Society.[228]

Computed Tomography Contrast Enhancement

The radiologic density of a nodule increases after administration of contrast medium; this is called contrast enhancement, and it depends on the lesion's vascularity. From the diagnostic point of view, the assumption is that the greater the contrast enhancement, the greater the probability of a nodule's being malignant. In fact, malignancies have contrast enhancements of 20 HU or more and benign lesions less than 15 HU. Again, these data are suitable only for relatively homogeneous solid nodules measuring between 5 mm and 3 cm in diameter, where the negative predictive value for malignancy of a contrast enhancement less than 15 HU is 96%.[229]

Positron Emission Tomography Metabolism

Typically, the metabolism of glucose is increased in malignancies, and this peculiarity is exploited with a technique of nuclear medicine known as PET (Fig. 3-197). For lung nodules, an SUV_{max} cutoff of FDG of 2.5 is used as the discriminating level between benign and malignant.[230] Unfortunately, PET is most efficient only for solid lesions with a diameter greater than 10 mm, where the sensitivity and specificity of the technique for detection of malignancy are about 90%.[231] On the contrary, a well-differentiated adenocarcinoma that shows a GGO appearance in CT is (falsely) negative in nine of ten cases, and a benign nodule that shows a GGO appearance in CT is (falsely) positive in four of five cases.[232]

The SUV has to be considered in connection with the pretest likelihood of malignancy. For example, a negative PET reduces the likelihood of malignancy to 1% in an individual with a pretest likelihood of 20% but only to 14% in one with a pretest likelihood of 80%.[210]

Self-assessment questions related to this chapter can be found online on the Expert Consult site for this title.

References

1. Naidich DP, Muller NL, Krinsky GA, et al. *Computed Tomography and Magnetic Resonance of the Thorax.* 4th ed Philadelphia: Lippincott Williams & Wilkins; 2007.
2. Webb WR, Müller NL, Naidich DP. *High-Resolution CT of the Lung.* 4th ed. Philadelphia: Wolters Kluwer Health/Lippincott Williams & Wilkins; 2009.
3. Beigelman-Aubry C, Hill C, Guibal A, et al. Multi-detector row CT and postprocessing techniques in the assessment of diffuse lung disease. *Radiographics.* 2005;25(6):1639–1652.
4. Aberle DR, Gamsu G, Ray CS, et al. Asbestos-related pleural and parenchymal fibrosis: detection with high-resolution CT. *Radiology.* 1988;166(3):729–734.
5. Flaherty KR, King Jr TE, Raghu G, et al. Idiopathic interstitial pneumonia: what is the effect of a multidisciplinary approach to diagnosis? *Am J Respir Crit Care Med.* 2004;170(8):904–910 [Epub July 15, 2004].
6. Webb WR. Thin-section CT of the secondary pulmonary lobule: anatomy and the image–the 2004 Fleischner lecture. *Radiology.* 2006;239(2):322–338.

7. Maffessanti M, Dalpiaz G. *Diffuse Lung Diseases: Clinical Features, Pathology, HRCT*. New York: Springer; 2006.

8. Gotway MB, Reddy GP, Webb WR, et al. High-resolution CT of the lung: patterns of disease and differential diagnoses. *Radiol Clin North Am*. 2005;43:513–542.

9. Gluecker T, Capasso P, Schnyder P, et al. Clinical and radiologic features of pulmonary edema. *Radiographics*. 1999;19(6):1507–1531.

10. Storto ML, Kee ST, Golden JA, et al. Hydrostatic pulmonary edema: high-resolution CT findings. *AJR Am J Roentgenol*. 1995;165(4):817–820.

11. Chabbert V, Canevet G, Baixas C, et al. Mediastinal lymphadenopathy in congestive heart failure: a sequential CT evaluation with clinical and echocardiographic correlations. *Eur Radiol*. 2004;14(5):881–889.

12. Munk PL, Müller NL, Miller RR, et al. Pulmonary lymphangitic carcinomatosis: CT and pathologic findings. *Radiology*. 1988;166(3):705–709.

13. Johkoh T, Ikezoe J, Tomiyama N, et al. CT findings in lymphangitic carcinomatosis of the lung: correlation with histologic findings and pulmonary function tests. *AJR Am J Roentgenol*. 1992;158(6):1217–1222.

14. Frazier AA, Franks TJ, Mohammed TL, et al. From the archives of the AFIP: pulmonary veno-occlusive disease and pulmonary capillary hemangiomatosis. *Radiographics*. 2007;27(3):867–882.

15. Mandel J, Mark EJ, Hales CA. Pulmonary veno-occlusive disease. *Am J Respir Crit Care Med*. 2000;162(5):1964–1973.

16. Montani D, Kemp K, Dorfmuller P, et al. Idiopathic pulmonary arterial hypertension and pulmonary veno-occlusive disease: similarities and differences. *Semin Respir Crit Care Med*. 2009;30(4):411–420.

17. Wittenberg KH, Swensen SJ, Myers JL. Pulmonary involvement with Erdheim-Chester disease: radiographic and CT findings. *AJR Am J Roentgenol*. 2000;174(5):1327–1331.

18. Chung JH, Park MS, Shin DH, et al. Pulmonary involvement in Erdheim-Chester disease. *Respirology*. 2005;10(3):389–392.

19. Dion E, Graef C, Haroche J, et al. Imaging of thoracoabdominal involvement in Erdheim-Chester disease. *AJR Am J Roentgenol*. 2004;183(5):1253–1260.

20. Hansell DM, Bankier AA, MacMahon H, et al. Fleischner Society: glossary of terms for thoracic imaging. *Radiology*. 2008;246(3):697–722.

21. Ren H, Hruban RH, Kuhlman JE, et al. Computed tomography of inflation-fixed lungs: the beaded septum sign of pulmonary metastases. *J Comput Assist Tomogr*. 1989;13:411–416.

22. Chung MJ, Lee KS, Franquet T, et al. Metabolic lung disease: imaging and histopathologic findings. *Eur J Radiol*. 2005;54(2):233–245.

23. Graham CM, Stern EJ, Finkbeiner WE, et al. High-resolution CT appearance of diffuse alveolar septal amyloidosis. *AJR Am J Roentgenol*. 1992;158(2):265–267.

24. Marchiori E, Franquet T, Gasparetto TD, et al. Consolidation with diffuse or focal high attenuation computed tomography findings. *J Thorac Imaging*. 2008;23:298–304.

25. Marchiori E, Souza Jr AS, Franquet T, et al. Diffuse high-attenuation pulmonary abnormalities: a pattern-oriented diagnostic approach on high-resolution CT. *AJR Am J Roentgenol*. 2005;184(1):273–282.

26. Remy-Jardin M, Giraud F, Remy J, et al. Importance of ground-glass attenuation in chronic diffuse infiltrative lung disease: pathologic-CT correlation. *Radiology*. 1993;189(3):693–698.

27. Silva CI, Müller NL. Idiopathic interstitial pneumonias. *J Thorac Imaging*. 2009;24(4):260–273.

28. Nishimura K, Kitaichi M, Izumi T, et al. Usual interstitial pneumonia: histologic correlation with high-resolution CT. *Radiology*. 1992;182(2):337–342.

29. American Thoracic Society, European Respiratory Society. American Thoracic Society/European Respiratory Society International Multidisciplinary Consensus Classification of the Idiopathic Interstitial Pneumonias. *Am J Respir Crit Care Med*. 2002;165(2):277–304.

30. Silva CI, Müller NL, Neder JA, et al. Asbestos-related disease: progression of parenchymal abnormalities on high-resolution CT. *J Thorac Imaging*. 2008;23(4):251–257.

31. Akira M, Yamamoto S, Inoue Y, et al. High-resolution CT of asbestosis and idiopathic pulmonary fibrosis. *AJR Am J Roentgenol*. 2003;181(1):163–169.

32. Akira M, Yamamoto S, Yokoyama K, et al. Asbestosis: high-resolution CT-pathologic correlation. *Radiology*. 1990;176(2):389–394.

33. Gevenois PA, de Maertelaer V, Madani A, et al. Asbestosis, pleural plaques and diffuse pleural thickening: three distinct benign responses to asbestos exposure. *Eur Respir J*. 1998;11(5):1021–1027.

34. Silva CI, Müller NL, Lynch DA, et al. Chronic hypersensitivity pneumonitis: differentiation from idiopathic pulmonary fibrosis and nonspecific interstitial pneumonia by using thin-section CT. *Radiology*. 2008;246(1):288–297.

35. Hirschmann JV, Pipavath SN, Godwin JD. Hypersensitivity pneumonitis: a historical, clinical, and radiologic review. *Radiographics*. 2009;29(7):1921–1938.

36. Sverzellati N, De Filippo M, Bartalena T, et al. High-resolution computed tomography in the diagnosis and follow-up of idiopathic pulmonary fibrosis. *Radiol Med*. January 15, 2010; [Epub ahead of print].

37. Elliot TL, Lynch DA, Newell Jr JD, et al. High-resolution computed tomography features of nonspecific interstitial pneumonia and usual interstitial pneumonia. *J Comput Assist Tomogr*. 2005;29(3):339–345.

38. Hunninghake GW, Lynch DA, Galvin JR, et al. Radiologic findings are strongly associated with a pathologic diagnosis of usual interstitial pneumonia. *Chest*. 2003;124(4):1215–1223.

39. Sverzellati N, Wells AU, Tomassetti S, et al. Biopsy-proved idiopathic pulmonary fibrosis: spectrum of nondiagnostic thin-section CT diagnoses. *Radiology*. 2010;254(3):957–964.

40. Akira M, Inoue Y, Kitaichi M, et al. Usual interstitial pneumonia and nonspecific interstitial pneumonia with and without concurrent emphysema: thin-section CT findings. *Radiology*. 2009;251(1):271–279 [Epub February 12, 2009].

41. Souza CA, Müller NL, Lee KS, et al. Idiopathic interstitial pneumonias: prevalence of mediastinal lymph node enlargement in 206 patients. *AJR Am J Roentgenol*. 2006;186(4):995–999.

42. Kim TS, Han J, Chung MP, et al. Disseminated dendriform pulmonary ossification associated with usual interstitial pneumonia: incidence and thin-section CT-pathologic correlation. *Eur Radiol*. 2005;15(8):1581–1585 [Epub April 23, 2005].

43. Kishi K, Homma S, Kurosaki A, et al. High-resolution computed tomography findings of lung cancer associated with idiopathic pulmonary fibrosis. *J Comput Assist Tomogr*. 2006;30(1):95–99.

44. Kim EA, Lee KS, Johkoh T, et al. Interstitial lung diseases associated with collagen vascular diseases: radiologic and histopathologic findings. *Radiographics*. 2002;22(spec no):S151–S165.

45. Mellot F, Scherrer A. Imaging features of drug-induced lung diseases. *J Radiol*. 2005;86(5 pt 2):550–557 [in French].

46. Mayberry JP, Primack SL, Müller NL. Thoracic manifestations of systemic autoimmune diseases: radiographic and high-resolution CT findings. *Radiographics*. 2000;20(6):1623–1635.

47. Desai SR, Veeraraghavan S, Hansell DM, et al. CT features of lung disease in patients with systemic sclerosis: comparison with idiopathic pulmonary fibrosis and nonspecific interstitial pneumonia. *Radiology*. 2004;232(2):560–567.

48. Tanaka N, Newell JD, Brown KK, et al. Collagen vascular disease-related lung disease: high-resolution computed tomography findings based on the pathologic classification. *J Comput Assist Tomogr*. 2004;28(3):351–360.

49. Kligerman SJ, Groshong S, Brown KK, et al. Nonspecific interstitial pneumonia: radiologic, clinical, and pathologic considerations. *Radiographics*. 2009;29(1):73–87.

50. Johkoh T, Müller NL, Colby TV, et al. Nonspecific interstitial pneumonia: correlation between thin-section CT findings and pathologic subgroups in 55 patients. *Radiology*. 2002;225(1):199–204.

51. Travis WD, Hunninghake G, King Jr TE, et al. Idiopathic nonspecific interstitial pneumonia: report of an American Thoracic Society project. *Am J Respir Crit Care Med*. 2008;177(12):1338–1347.

52. Silva CI, Müller NL, Hansell DM, et al. Nonspecific interstitial pneumonia and idiopathic pulmonary fibrosis: changes in pattern and distribution of disease over time. *Radiology*. 2008;247(1):251–259.

53. Erasmus JJ, McAdams HP, Rossi SE. High-resolution CT of drug-induced lung disease. *Radiol Clin North Am*. 2002;40(1):61–72.

54. Rossi SE, Erasmus JJ, McAdams HP, et al. Pulmonary drug toxicity: radiologic and pathologic manifestations. *Radiographics*. 2000;20(5):1245–1259.

55. Abehsera M, Valeyre D, Grenier P, et al. Sarcoidosis with pulmonary fibrosis: CT patterns and correlation with pulmonary function. *AJR Am J Roentgenol*. 2000;174(6):1751–1757.

56. Hoang DQ, Nguyen ET. Sarcoidosis. *Semin Roentgenol*. 2010;45(1):36–42.

57. Padley SP, Padhani AR, Nicholson A, et al. Pulmonary sarcoidosis mimicking cryptogenic fibrosing alveolitis on CT. *Clin Radiol*. 1996;51(11):807–810.

58. Nishino M, Lee KS, Itoh H, et al. The spectrum of pulmonary sarcoidosis: variations of high-resolution CT findings and clues for specific diagnosis. *Eur J Radiol*. 2010;73(1):66–73.

59. Abbott GF, Rosado-de-Christenson ML, Franks TJ, et al. From the archives of the AFIP: pulmonary Langerhans cell histiocytosis. *Radiographics*. 2004;24(3):821–841.

60. Churg A, Myers J, Suarez T. Airway-centered interstitial fibrosis: a distinct form of aggressive diffuse lung disease. *Am J Surg Pathol*. 2004;28(1):62–68.

61. Gruden JF, Webb WR, Naidich DP, et al. Multinodular disease: anatomic localization at thin-section CT—multireader evaluation of a simple algorithm. *Radiology*. 1999;210(3):711–720.

62. Remy-Jardin M, Beuscart R, Sault MC, et al. Subpleural micronodules in diffuse infiltrative lung diseases: evaluation with thin-section CT scans. *Radiology*. 1990;177(1):133–139.

63. Parrón M, Torres I, Pardo M, et al. The halo sign in computed tomography images: differential diagnosis and correlation with pathology findings. *Arch Bronconeumol*. 2008;44(7):386–392.

64. Raoof S, Amchentsev A, Vlahos I, et al. Pictorial essay: multinodular disease: a high-resolution CT scan diagnostic algorithm. *Chest*. 2006;129(3):805–815.

65. Abbott GF, Rosado-de-Christenson ML, Franks TJ, et al. From the archives of the AFIP: pulmonary Langerhans cell histiocytosis. *Radiographics*. 2004;24(3):821–841.

66. Howling SJ, Hansell DM, Wells AU, et al. Follicular bronchiolitis: thin-section CT and histologic findings. *Radiology*. 1999;212(3):637–642.

67. Pipavath SN, Stern EJ. Imaging of small airway disease (SAD). *Radiol Clin North Am*. 2009;47(2):307–316.

68. Kang EY, Woo OH, Shin BK, et al. Bronchiolitis: classification, computed tomographic and histopathologic features, and radiologic approach. *J Comput Assist Tomogr*. 2009;33(1):32–41.

69. Pipavath SJ, Lynch DA, Cool C, et al. Radiologic and pathologic features of bronchiolitis. *AJR Am J Roentgenol*. 2005;185(2):354–363.

70. Ryu JH, Myers JL, Swensen SJ. Bronchiolar disorders. *Am J Respir Crit Care Med*. 2003;168(11):1277–1292.

71. Silva CI, Churg A, Müller NL. Hypersensitivity pneumonitis: spectrum of high-resolution CT and pathologic findings. *AJR Am J Roentgenol*. 2007;188(2):334–344.

72. Chung MH, Edinburgh KJ, Webb EM, et al. Mixed infiltrative and obstructive disease on high-resolution CT: differential diagnosis and functional correlates in a consecutive series. *J Thorac Imaging*. 2001;16(2):69–75.

73. Mueller-Mang C, Grosse C, Schmid K, et al. What every radiologist should know about idiopathic interstitial pneumonias. *Radiographics*. 2007;27(3):595–615.

74. Hidalgo A, Franquet T, Giménez A, et al. Smoking-related interstitial lung diseases: radiologic-pathologic correlation. *Eur Radiol*. 2006;16(11):2463–2470.

75. Park JS, Brown KK, Tuder RM, et al. Respiratory bronchiolitis-associated interstitial lung disease: radiologic features with clinical and pathologic correlation. *J Comput Assist Tomogr*. 2002;26(1):13–20.

76. Attili AK, Kazerooni EA, Gross BH, et al. Smoking-related interstitial lung disease: radiologic-clinical-pathologic correlation. *Radiographics*. 2008;28(5):1383–1396 discussion 1396–1398.

77. Galvin JR, Franks TJ. Smoking-related lung disease. *J Thorac Imaging*. 2009;24(4):274–284.

78. Koyama T, Ueda H, Togashi K, et al. Radiologic manifestations of sarcoidosis in various organs. *Radiographics*. 2004;24(1):87–104.

79. Nakatsu M, Hatabu H, Morikawa K, et al. Large coalescent parenchymal nodules in pulmonary sarcoidosis: "sarcoid galaxy" sign. *AJR Am J Roentgenol*. 2002;178(6):1389–1393.

80. Davies CW, Tasker AD, Padley SP, et al. Air trapping in sarcoidosis on computed tomography: correlation with lung function. *Clin Radiol*. 2000;55(3):217–221.

81. Becciolini V, Gudinchet F, Cheseaux JJ, et al. Lymphocytic interstitial pneumonia in children with AIDS: high-resolution CT findings. *Eur Radiol*. 2001;11(6):1015–1020.

82. Johkoh T, Müller NL, Pickford HA, et al. Lymphocytic interstitial pneumonia: thin-section CT findings in 22 patients. *Radiology*. 1999;212(2):567–572.

83. Wittram C, Mark EJ, McLoud TC. CT-histologic correlation of the ATS/ERS 2002 classification of idiopathic interstitial pneumonias. *Radiographics*. 2003;23(5):1057–1071.

84. Swigris JJ, Berry GJ, Raffin TA, et al. Lymphoid interstitial pneumonia: a narrative review. *Chest*. 2002;122(6):2150–2164.

85. Honda O, Johkoh T, Ichikado K, et al. Differential diagnosis of lymphocytic interstitial pneumonia and malignant lymphoma on high-resolution CT. *AJR Am J Roentgenol*. 1999;173(1):71–74.

86. Chong S, Lee KS, Chung MJ, et al. Pneumoconiosis: comparison of imaging and pathologic findings. *Radiographics*. 2006;26(1):59–77.

87. Oikonomou A, Muller NL. Imaging of pneumoconiosis. *Imaging*. 2003;15:11–22.

88. Kim KI, Kim CW, Lee MK, et al. Imaging of occupational lung disease. *Radiographics*. 2001;21(6):1371–1391.

89. Hirakata K, Nakata H, Haratake J. Appearance of pulmonary metastases on high-resolution CT scans: comparison with histopathologic findings from autopsy specimens. *AJR Am J Roentgenol*. 1993;161(1):37–43.

90. Seo JB, Im JG, Goo JM, Chung MJ, et al. Atypical pulmonary metastases: spectrum of radiologic findings. *Radiographics*. 2001;21(2):403–417.

91. Franquet T, Giménez A, Prats R, et al. Thrombotic microangiopathy of pulmonary tumors: a vascular cause of tree-in-bud pattern on CT. *AJR Am J Roentgenol*. 2002;179(4):897–899.

92. Leung AN. Pulmonary tuberculosis: the essentials. *Radiology*. 1999;210(2):307–322.

93. Kim JY, Jeong YJ, Kim KI, et al. Miliary tuberculosis: a comparison of CT findings in HIV-seropositive and HIV-seronegative patients. *Br J Radiol*. 2010;83(987):206–211.

94. Van Dyck P, Vanhoenacker FM, Van den Brande P, et al. Imaging of pulmonary tuberculosis. *Eur Radiol*. 2003;13(8):1771–1785.

95. Jeong YJ, Lee KS. Pulmonary tuberculosis: up-to-date imaging and management. *AJR Am J Roentgenol*. 2008;191(3):834–844.

96. Burrill J, Williams CJ, Bain G, et al. Tuberculosis: a radiologic review. *Radiographics*. 2007;27(5):1255–1273.

97. Cheung OY, Muhm JR, Helmers RA, et al. Surgical pathology of granulomatous interstitial pneumonia. *Ann Diagn Pathol*. 2003;7(2):127–138.

98. Rossi SE, Franquet T, Volpacchio M, et al. Tree-in-bud pattern at thin-section CT of the lungs: radiologic-pathologic overview. *Radiographics*. 2005;25(3):789–801.

99. Escuissato DL, Gasparetto EL, Marchiori E, et al. Pulmonary infections after bone marrow transplantation: high-resolution CT findings in 111 patients. *AJR Am J Roentgenol*. 2005;185(3):608–615.

100. Kishi K, Homma S, Kurosaki A, et al. Clinical features and high-resolution CT findings of pulmonary cryptococcosis in non-AIDS patients. *Respir Med*. 2006;100(5):807–812.

101. Rossi SE, Erasmus JJ, Volpacchio M, et al. "Crazy-paving" pattern at thin-section CT of the lungs: radiologic-pathologic overview. *Radiographics*. 2003;23(6):1509–1519.

102. Johkoh T, Itoh H, Müller NL, et al. Crazy-paving appearance at thin-section CT: spectrum of disease and pathologic findings. *Radiology*. 1999;211(1):155–160.

103. Lee CH. The crazy-paving sign. *Radiology*. 2007;243(3):905–906.

104. Collins J, Blankenbaker D, Stern EJ. CT patterns of bronchiolar disease: what is "tree-in-bud"? *AJR Am J Roentgenol*. 1998;171(2):365–370.

105. Eisenhuber E. The tree-in-bud sign. *Radiology*. 2002;222(3):771–772.

106. Müller NL, Miller RR. Diseases of the bronchioles: CT and histopathologic findings. *Radiology*. 1995;196(1):3–12.

107. Franquet T, Giménez A, Prats R, et al. Thrombotic microangiopathy of pulmonary tumors: a vascular cause of tree-in-bud pattern on CT. *AJR Am J Roentgenol*. 2002;179(4):897–899.

108. Tack D, Nollevaux MC, Gevenois PA. Tree-in-bud pattern in neoplastic pulmonary emboli. *AJR Am J Roentgenol*. 2001;176(6):1421–1422.

109. Gaeta M, Blandino A, Scribano E, et al. Computed tomography halo sign in pulmonary nodules: frequency and diagnostic value. *J Thorac Imaging*. 1999;14(2):109–113.

110. Pinto PS. The CT halo sign. *Radiology*. 2004;230(1):109–110.

111. Primack SL, Hartman TE, Lee KS, et al. Pulmonary nodules and the CT halo sign. *Radiology*. 1994;190(2):513–515.

112. Lee YR, Choi YW, Lee KJ, et al. CT halo sign: the spectrum of pulmonary diseases. *Br J Radiol*. 2005;78(933):862–865.

113. Kim SJ, Lee KS, Ryu YH, et al. Reversed halo sign on high-resolution CT of cryptogenic organizing pneumonia: diagnostic implications. *AJR Am J Roentgenol*. 2003;180(5):1251–1254.

114. Voloudaki AE, Bouros DE, Froudarakis ME, et al. Crescentic and ring-shaped opacities. CT features in two cases of bronchiolitis obliterans organizing pneumonia (BOOP). *Acta Radiol*. 1996;37(6):889–892.

115. Johkoh T, Müller NL, Ichikado K. Perilobular pulmonary opacities: high-resolution CT findings and pathologic correlation. *J Thorac Imaging*. 1999;14(3):172–177.

116. Ujita M, Renzoni EA, Veeraraghavan S, et al. Organizing pneumonia: perilobular pattern at thin-section CT. *Radiology*. 2004;232(3):757–761.

117. Schwarz M, King T, eds. *Interstitial Lung Disease*. 3rd ed. Hamilton, Ontario, Canada: BC Decker; 1998.

118. Johkoh T, Müller NL, Taniguchi H, et al. Acute interstitial pneumonia: thin-section CT findings in 36 patients. *Radiology*. 1999;211(3):859–863.

119. Tomiyama N, Müller NL, Johkoh T, et al. Acute parenchymal lung disease in immuno-competent patients: diagnostic accuracy of high-resolution CT. *AJR Am J Roentgenol*. 2000;174(6):1745–1750.

120. Tomiyama N, Müller NL, Johkoh T, et al. Acute respiratory distress syndrome and acute interstitial pneumonia: comparison of thin-section CT findings. *J Comput Assist Tomogr*. 2001;25(1):28–33.

121. Daimon T, Johkoh T, Sumikawa H, et al. Acute eosinophilic pneumonia: thin-section CT findings in 29 patients. *Eur J Radiol*. 2008;65(3):462–467.

122. Jeong YJ, Kim KI, Seo IJ, et al. Eosinophilic lung diseases: a clinical, radiologic, and pathologic overview. *Radiographics*. 2007;27(3):617–637 discussion 637–639.

123. Johkoh T, Müller NL, Akira M, et al. Eosinophilic lung diseases: diagnostic accuracy of thin-section CT in 111 patients. *Radiology*. 2000;216(3):773–780.

124. Camus P, Kudoh S, Ebina M. Interstitial lung disease associated with drug therapy. *Br J Cancer*. 2004;91(suppl 2):S18–S23.

125. Cleverley JR, Screaton NJ, Hiorns MP, et al. Drug-induced lung disease: high-resolution CT and histological findings. *Clin Radiol*. 2002;57(4):292–299.

126. Nguyen ET, Silva CI, Souza CA, et al. Pulmonary complications of illicit drug use: differential diagnosis based on CT findings. *J Thorac Imaging*. 2007;22(2):199–206.

127. Gattinoni L, Caironi P, Pelosi P, et al. What has computed tomography taught us about the acute respiratory distress syndrome? *Am J Respir Crit Care Med*. 2001;164(9):1701–1711.

128. Churg A, Müller NL, Silva CI, et al. Acute exacerbation (acute lung injury of unknown cause) in UIP and other forms of fibrotic interstitial pneumonias. *Am J Surg Pathol*. 2007;31(2):277–284.

129. Collard HR, Moore BB, Flaherty KR, the Idiopathic Pulmonary Fibrosis Clinical Research Network Investigators. Acute exacerbations of idiopathic pulmonary fibrosis. *Am J Respir Crit Care Med*. 2007;176(7):636–643.

130. Park IN, Kim DS, Shim TS, et al. Acute exacerbation of interstitial pneumonia other than idiopathic pulmonary fibrosis. *Chest*. 2007;132(1):214–220.

131. Akira M, Kozuka T, Yamamoto S, et al. Computed tomography findings in acute exacerbation of idiopathic pulmonary fibrosis. *Am J Respir Crit Care Med*. 2008;178(4):372–378.

132. Silva CI, Müller NL, Fujimoto K, et al. Acute exacerbation of chronic interstitial pneumonia: high-resolution computed tomography and pathologic findings. *J Thorac Imaging*. 2007;22(3):221–229.

133. Castañer E, Alguersuari A, Gallardo X, et al. When to suspect pulmonary vasculitis: radiologic and clinical clues. *Radiographics*. 2010;30(1):33–53.

134. Primack SL, Miller RR, Müller NL. Diffuse pulmonary hemorrhage: clinical, pathologic, and imaging features. *AJR Am J Roentgenol*. 1995;164(2):295–300.

135. Ribeiro CM, Marchiori E, Rodrigues R, et al. Hydrostatic pulmonary edema: high-resolution computed tomography aspects. *J Bras Pneumol*. 2006;32(6):515–522.

136. Kim EA, Lee KS, Primack SL, et al. Viral pneumonias in adults: radiologic and pathologic findings. *Radiographics*. 2002;22(spec no):S137–S149.

137. Reittner P, Ward S, Heyneman L, et al. Pneumonia: high-resolution CT findings in 114 patients. *Eur Radiol*. 2003;13(3):515–521.

138. Gruden JF, Huang L, Turner J, et al. High-resolution CT in the evaluation of clinically suspected *Pneumocystis carinii* pneumonia in AIDS patients with normal, equivocal, or nonspecific radiographic findings. *AJR Am J Roentgenol*. 1997;169(4):967–975.

139. Reittner P, Müller NL, Heyneman L, et al. *Mycoplasma pneumoniae* pneumonia: radiographic and high-resolution CT features in 28 patients. *AJR Am J Roentgenol*. 2000;174(1):37–41.

140. Demirkazik FB, Akin A, Uzun O, et al. CT findings in immunocompromised patients with pulmonary infections. *Diagn Interv Radiol*. 2008;14(2):75–82.

141. Akira M, Atagi S, Kawahara M, et al. High-resolution CT findings of diffuse bronchioloalveolar carcinoma in 38 patients. *AJR Am J Roentgenol*. 1999;173(6):1623–1629.

142. Lee KS, Kim Y, Han J, et al. Bronchioloalveolar carcinoma: clinical, histopathologic, and radiologic findings. *Radiographics*. 1997;17(6):1345–1357.

143. Patsios D, Roberts HC, Paul NS, et al. Pictorial review of the many faces of bronchioloalveolar cell carcinoma. *Br J Radiol*. 2007;80(960):1015–1023.

144. Jung JI, Kim H, Park SH, et al. CT differentiation of pneumonic-type bronchioloalveolar cell carcinoma and infectious pneumonia. *Br J Radiol*. 2001;74(882):490–494.

145. Aquino SL, Chiles C, Halford P. Distinction of consolidative bronchioloalveolar carcinoma from pneumonia: do CT criteria work? *AJR Am J Roentgenol*. 1998;171(2):359–363.

146. Arakawa H, Kurihara Y, Niimi H, et al. Bronchiolitis obliterans with organizing pneumonia versus chronic eosinophilic pneumonia: high-resolution CT findings in 81 patients. *AJR Am J Roentgenol*. 2001;176(4):1053–1058.

147. Padley SP, Adler B, Hansell DM, et al. High-resolution computed tomography of drug-induced lung disease. *Clin Radiol*. 1992;46(4):232–236.

148. Ryu JH, Myers JL, Capizzi SA, et al. Desquamative interstitial pneumonia and respiratory bronchiolitis-associated interstitial lung disease. *Chest*. 2005;127(1):178–184.

149. Lynch DA, Travis WD, Müller NL, et al. Idiopathic interstitial pneumonias: CT features. *Radiology*. 2005;236(1):10–21.

150. Hartman TE, Primack SL, Swensen SJ, et al. Desquamative interstitial pneumonia: thin-section CT findings in 22 patients. *Radiology*. 1993;187:787–790.

151. Heyneman LE, Ward S, Lynch DA, et al. Respiratory bronchiolitis, respiratory bronchiolitis-associated interstitial lung disease, and desquamative interstitial pneumonia: different entities or part of the spectrum of the same disease process? *AJR Am J Roentgenol*. 1999;173(6):1617–1622.

152. Koyama M, Johkoh T, Honda O, et al. Chronic cystic lung disease: diagnostic accuracy of high-resolution CT in 92 patients. *AJR Am J Roentgenol*. 2003;180(3):827–835.

153. Levin DL. Radiology of pulmonary *Mycobacterium avium-intracellulare* complex. *Clin Chest Med*. 2002;23(3):603–612.

154. Jeong YJ, Lee KS, Koh WJ, et al. Nontuberculous mycobacterial pulmonary infection in immunocompetent patients: comparison of thin-section CT and histopathologic findings. *Radiology*. 2004;231(3):880–886.

155. Erasmus JJ, McAdams HP, Farrell MA, et al. Pulmonary nontuberculous mycobacterial infection: radiologic manifestations. *Radiographics*. 1999;19(6):1487–1505.

156. Laurent F, Philippe JC, Vergier B, et al. Exogenous lipoid pneumonia: HRCT, MR, and pathologic findings. *Eur Radiol*. 1999;9(6):1190–1196.

157. Lee JS, Im JG, Song KS. Exogenous lipoid pneumonia: high-resolution CT findings. *Eur Radiol*. 1999;9(2):287–291.

158. King LJ, Padley SP, Wotherspoon AC, et al. Pulmonary MALT lymphoma: imaging findings in 24 cases. *Eur Radiol*. 2000;10(12):1932–1938.

159. McCulloch GL, Sinnatamby R, Stewart S, et al. High-resolution computed tomographic appearance of MALToma of the lung. *Eur Radiol*. 1998;8(9):1669–1673.

160. Bae YA, Lee KS, Han J, et al. Marginal zone B-cell lymphoma of bronchus-associated lymphoid tissue: imaging findings in 21 patients. *Chest*. 2008;133(2):433–440.

161. Lee DK, Im JG, Lee KS, et al. B-cell lymphoma of bronchus-associated lymphoid tissue (BALT): CT features in 10 patients. *J Comput Assist Tomogr*. 2000;24(1):30–34.

162. Wislez M, Cadranel J, Antoine M, et al. Lymphoma of pulmonary mucosa-associated lymphoid tissue: CT scan findings and pathological correlations. *Eur Respir J*. 1999;14(2):423–429.

163. Churg A, Müller NL. Cellular vs fibrosing interstitial pneumonias and prognosis: a practical classification of the idiopathic interstitial pneumonias and pathologically/radiologically similar conditions. *Chest*. 2006;130(5):1566–1570.

164. Tsubamoto M, Müller NL, Johkoh T, et al. Pathologic subgroups of nonspecific interstitial pneumonia: differential diagnosis from other idiopathic interstitial pneumonias on high-resolution computed tomography. *J Comput Assist Tomogr*. 2005;29(6):793–800.

165. Erasmus JJ, McAdams HP, Rossi SE. Drug-induced lung injury. *Semin Roentgenol*. 2002;37(1):72–81.

166. Oikonomou A, Hansell DM. Organizing pneumonia: the many morphological faces. *Eur Radiol*. 2002;12(6):1486–1496.

167. Johkoh T, Müller NL, Cartier Y, et al. Idiopathic interstitial pneumonias: diagnostic accuracy of thin-section CT in 129 patients. *Radiology*. 1999;211(2):555–560.

168. Cordier JF. Cryptogenic organising pneumonia. *Eur Respir J*. 2006;28(2):422–446.

169. Epstein DM, Bennett MR. Bronchiolitis obliterans organizing pneumonia with migratory pulmonary infiltrates. *AJR Am J Roentgenol*. 1992;158(3):515–517.

170. Wang BM, Stern EJ, Schmidt RA, et al. Diagnosing pulmonary alveolar proteinosis. A review and an update. *Chest*. 1997;111(2):460–466.

171. Frazier AA, Franks TJ, Cooke EO, et al. From the archives of the AFIP: pulmonary alveolar proteinosis. *Radiographics*. 2008;28(3):883–899, quiz 915.

172. Lee KH, Lee JS, Lynch DA, et al. The radiologic differential diagnosis of diffuse lung diseases characterized by multiple cysts or cavities. *J Comput Assist Tomogr*. 2002;26(1):5–12.

173. Schoepf UJ, ed. *Multidetector-Row CT of the Thorax*. Berlin-Heidelberg: Springer-Verlag; 2006.

174. Collins J. CT signs and patterns of lung disease. *Radiol Clin North Am*. 2001;39(6):1115–1135.

175. Takahashi M, Fukuoka J, Nitta N, et al. Imaging of pulmonary emphysema: a pictorial review. *Int J Chron Obstruct Pulmon Dis*. 2008;3(2):193–204.

176. Pipavath SN, Schmidt RA, Takasugi JE, et al. Chronic obstructive pulmonary disease: radiology-pathology correlation. *J Thorac Imaging*. 2009;24(3):171–180.

177. Takasugi JE, Godwin JD. Radiology of chronic obstructive pulmonary disease. *Radiol Clin North Am*. 1998;36(1):29–55.

178. Webb EM, Elicker BM, Webb WR. Using CT to diagnose nonneoplastic tracheal abnormalities: appearance of the tracheal wall. *AJR Am J Roentgenol*. 2000;174(5):1315–1321.

179. Vassallo R, Ryu JH, Colby TV, et al. Pulmonary Langerhans'-cell histiocytosis. *N Engl J Med*. 2000;342(26):1969–1978.

180. Brauner MW, Grenier P, Mouelhi MM, et al. Pulmonary histiocytosis X: evaluation with high-resolution CT. *Radiology*. 1989;172(1):255–258.

181. Mendez JL, Nadrous HF, Vassallo R, et al. Pneumothorax in pulmonary Langerhans cell histiocytosis. *Chest*. 2004;125(3):1028–1032.

182. Marchiori E, Araujo Neto C, Meirelles GS, et al. Laryngotracheobronchial papillomatosis: findings on computed tomography scans of the chest. *J Bras Pneumol*. 2008;34(12):1084–1089.

183. Park CM, Goo JM, Lee HJ, et al. Tumors in the tracheobronchial tree: CT and FDG PET features. *Radiographics*. 2009;29(1):55–71.

184. Katz SL, Das P, Ngan BY, et al. Remote intrapulmonary spread of recurrent respiratory papillomatosis with malignant transformation. *Pediatr Pulmonol*. 2005;39(2):185–188.

185. Chu SC, Horiba K, Usuki J, et al. Comprehensive evaluation of 35 patients with lymphangioleiomyomatosis. *Chest*. 1999;115(4):1041–1052.

186. Abbott GF, Rosado-de-Christenson ML, Frazier AA. From the archives of the AFIP: lymphangioleiomyomatosis: radiologic-pathologic correlation. *Radiographics*. 2005;25(3):803–828.

187. Pallisa E, Sanz P, Roman A, et al. Lymphangioleiomyomatosis: pulmonary and abdominal findings with pathologic correlation. *Radiographics*. 2002;22(spec no):S185–S198.

188. Tateishi U, Hasegawa T, Kusumoto M, et al. Metastatic angiosarcoma of the lung: spectrum of CT findings. *AJR Am J Roentgenol*. 2003;180(6):1671–1674.

189. Park SI, Choi E, Lee HB, et al. Spontaneous pneumomediastinum and hemopneumothoraces secondary to cystic lung metastasis. *Respiration*. 2003;70(2):211–213.

190. Birt AR, Hogg GR, Dubé WJ. Hereditary multiple fibrofolliculomas with trichodiscomas and acrochordons. *Arch Dermatol*. 1977;113(12):1674–1677.

191. Ayo DS, Aughenbaugh GL, Yi ES, et al. Cystic lung disease in Birt-Hogg-Dube syndrome. *Chest*. 2007;132(2):679–684.

192. Souza CA, Finley R, Müller NL. Birt-Hogg-Dubé syndrome: a rare cause of pulmonary cysts. *AJR Am J Roentgenol*. 2005;185(5):1237–1239.

193. Tobino K, Gunji Y, Kurihara M, et al. Characteristics of pulmonary cysts in Birt-Hogg-Dubé syndrome: thin-section CT findings of the chest in 12 patients. *Eur J Radiol*. September 24, 2009 [Epub ahead of print].

194. Pittet O, Cristodoulou M, Staneczek O, et al. Diagnosis of Birt-Hogg-Dube syndrome in a patient with spontaneous pneumothorax. *Ann Thorac Surg*. 2006;82(3):1123–1125.

195. Stern EJ, Mülller NL, Swensen SJ, et al. CT mosaic pattern of lung attenuation: etiologies and terminology. *J Thorac Imaging*. 1995;10(4):294–297.

196. Schoepf UJ, ed. *Multidetector-Row CT of the Thorax*. Berlin-Heidelberg: Springer-Verlag; 2006.

197. Arakawa H. Expiratory high-resolution CT: diagnostic value in diffuse lung diseases. *AJR Am J Roentgenol*. 2000;175:1537–1543.

198. Castañer E, Gallardo X, Ballesteros E, et al. CT diagnosis of chronic pulmonary thromboembolism. *Radiographics*. 2009;29(1):31–50 discussion 50–53.

199. Frazier AA, Galvin JR, Franks TJ, et al. From the archives of the AFIP: pulmonary vasculature: hypertension and infarction. *Radiographics*. 2000;20(2):491–524.

200. Do KH, Goo JM, Im JG, et al. Systemic arterial supply to the lungs in adults: spiral CT findings. *Radiographics*. 2001;21(2):387–402.

201. Aguayo SM, Miller YE, Waldron Jr JA, et al. Brief report: idiopathic diffuse hyperplasia of pulmonary neuroendocrine cells and airways disease. *N Engl J Med*. 1992;327(18):1285–1288.

202. Brown MJ, English J, Müller NL. Bronchiolitis obliterans due to neuroendocrine hyperplasia: high-resolution CT—pathologic correlation. *AJR Am J Roentgenol*. 1997;168(6):1561–1562.

203. Lee JS, Brown KK, Cool C, et al. Diffuse pulmonary neuroendocrine cell hyperplasia: radiologic and clinical features. *J Comput Assist Tomogr*. 2002;26(2):180–184.

204. Davies SJ, Gosney JR, Hansell DM, et al. Diffuse idiopathic pulmonary neuroendocrine cell hyperplasia: an under-recognised spectrum of disease. *Thorax*. 2007;62(3):248–252.

205. Lynch DA. Imaging of small airways disease and chronic obstructive pulmonary disease. *Clin Chest Med*. 2008;29:165–179.

206. Rice A, Nicholson AG. The pathologist's approach to small airways disease. *Histopathology*. 2009;54(1):117–133.

207. King MA, Stone JA, Diaz PT, et al. Alpha 1-antitrypsin deficiency: evaluation of bronchiectasis with CT. *Radiology*. 1996;199(1):137–141.

208. Marti-Bonmati L, Ruiz Perales F, Catala F, et al. CT findings in Swyer-James syndrome. *Radiology*. 1989;172(2):477–480.

209. Moore AD, Godwin JD, Dietrich PA, et al. Swyer-James syndrome: CT findings in eight patients. *AJR Am J Roentgenol*. 1992;158(6):1211–1215.

210. Truong MT, Sabloff BS, Ko JP. Multidetector CT of solitary pulmonary nodules. *Radiol Clin North Am*. 2010;48(1):141–155.

211. Herder GJ, van Tinteren H, Golding RP, et al. Clinical prediction model to characterize pulmonary nodules: validation and added value of 18F-fluorodeoxyglucose positron emission tomography. *Chest*. 2005;128(4):2490–2496.

212. Gurney JW, Lyddon DM, McKay JA. Determining the likelihood of malignancy in solitary pulmonary nodules with Bayesian analysis. Part II. Application. *Radiology*. 1993;186(2):415–422.

213. Bailey-Wilson JE, Amos CI, Pinney SM, et al. A major lung cancer susceptibility locus maps to chromosome 6q23–25. *Am J Hum Genet*. 2004;75(3):460–474.

214. Winer-Muram HT. The solitary pulmonary nodule. *Radiology*. 2006;239(1):34–49 [review].

215. Swensen SJ, Jett JR, Hartman TE, et al. Lung cancer screening with CT: Mayo Clinic experience. *Radiology*. 2003;226(3):756–761.

216. Henschke CI, Naidich DP, Yankelevitz DF, et al. Early lung cancer action project: initial findings on repeat screenings. *Cancer*. 2001;92(1):153–159.

217. Pastorino U, Bellomi M, Landoni C, et al. Early lung-cancer detection with spiral CT and positron emission tomography in heavy smokers: 2-year results. *Lancet*. 2003;362(9384):593–597.

218. Siegelman SS, Khouri NF, Scott Jr WW, et al. Pulmonary hamartoma: CT findings. *Radiology*. 1986;160(2):313–317.

219. Muram TM, Aisen A. Fatty metastatic lesions in 2 patients with renal clear-cell carcinoma. *J Comput Assist Tomogr*. 2003;27(6):869–870.

220. Henschke CI, Yankelevitz DF, Mirtcheva R, et al, for the ELCAP Group. CT screening for lung cancer: frequency and significance of part-solid and nonsolid nodules. *AJR Am J Roentgenol*. 2002;178(5):1053–1057.

221. Zwirewich CV, Vedal S, Miller RR, et al. Solitary pulmonary nodule: high-resolution CT and radiologic-pathologic correlation. *Radiology*. 1991;179(2):469–476.

222. Woodring JH, Fried AM, Chuang VP. Solitary cavities of the lung: diagnostic implications of cavity wall thickness. *AJR Am J Roentgenol*. 1980;135(6):1269–1271.

223. Hasegawa M, Sone S, Takashima S, et al. Growth rate of small lung cancers detected on mass CT screening. *Br J Radiol*. 2000;73(876):1252–1259.

224. Aoki T, Nakata H, Watanabe H, et al. Evolution of peripheral lung adenocarcinomas: CT findings correlated with histology and tumor doubling time. *AJR Am J Roentgenol*. 2000;174(3):763–768.

225. Leef III JL, Klein JS. The solitary pulmonary nodule. *Radiol Clin North Am*. 2002;40(1):123–143, ix.

226. Hartman TE. Radiologic evaluation of the solitary pulmonary nodule. *Radiol Clin North Am*. 2005;43(3):459–465, vii [review].

227. Lillington GA, Caskey CI. Evaluation and management of solitary and multiple pulmonary nodules. *Clin Chest Med*. 1993;14(1):111–119.

228. MacMahon H, Austin JH, Gamsu G, et al, the Fleischner Society. Guidelines for management of small pulmonary nodules detected on CT scans: a statement from the Fleischner Society. *Radiology*. 2005;237(2):395–400.

229. Swensen SJ, Viggiano RW, Midthun DE, et al. Lung nodule enhancement at CT: multicenter study. *Radiology*. 2000;214(1):73–80.

230. Lowe VJ, Hoffman JM, DeLong DM, et al. Semiquantitative and visual analysis of FDG-PET images in pulmonary abnormalities. *J Nucl Med*. 1994;35(11):1771–1776.

231. Gould MK, Maclean CC, Kuschner WG, et al. Accuracy of positron emission tomography for diagnosis of pulmonary nodules and mass lesions: a meta-analysis. *JAMA*. 2001;285(7):914–924.

232. Nomori H, Watanabe K, Ohtsuka T, et al. Evaluation of F-18 fluorodeoxyglucose (FDG) PET scanning for pulmonary nodules less than 3 cm in diameter, with special reference to the CT images. *Lung Cancer*. 2004;45(1):19–27.

4

Developmental and Pediatric Lung Disease

Kirk D. Jones, MD, Megan K. Dishop, MD, and Thomas V. Colby, MD

The diagnostic approach to pediatric lung biopsy differs somewhat from that in the adult patient. Many of the usual questions that arise in adult pulmonary pathology are replaced by separate issues involving abnormal development, altered lung growth due to prematurity, genetic disease, and infections secondary to an immature immune system.[1] The spectrum of diseases observed in the pediatric lung biopsy differs from its adult counterpart and it is important to approach these biopsies with knowledge of lung development and anatomy. In addition, communication with the clinician, the radiologist, and the surgeon is essential, because a tentative list of diagnostic considerations usually can be built on the basis of clinical, radiologic, and intraoperative findings. This chapter covers a spectrum of common and rare entities that the surgical pathologist may encounter when examining biopsied and resected specimens from pediatric patients.

Processing of Pediatric Lung Biopsy Specimens

General processing of lung biopsy specimens is covered in Chapter 2. Recommendations have been published for processing of pediatric biopsy specimens for diffuse lung disease.[2] A point worthy of emphasis is that in both diffuse and localized disease of the pediatric lung, infection should always be considered, and a substantial portion (one third to one half) of the surgical lung biopsy specimen should be sent for cultures if the surgeon has not already sent culture samples directly from the operating room. Touch imprints of the biopsy cut surface can be made and rapidly stained with silver stains for fungi or acid-fast stains for mycobacteria, a technique that is particularly useful for processing of lung biopsy specimens from immunosuppressed or immunocompromised patients. A few small pieces should be retained in glutaraldehyde for electron microscopy, which may have utility in the diagnosis of genetic disorders of surfactant metabolism and viral infections. Additional tissue should be snap-frozen and retained for potential molecular diagnosis of genetic disorders or infectious processes. For patients with suspected autoimmune diseases or chronic hemorrhage syndromes, a piece of lung tissue should be frozen in cryomatrix for possible immunofluorescence study. The remaining lung tissue should be expanded with formalin using a tuberculin syringe or other fine needle by transpleural injection, fixed for approximately 10 minutes, and sectioned for histologic examination. Inflation of pediatric lung biopsy is essential to reproduce the in vivo lung architecture and enables microscopic assessment of alveolar growth and development. In addition to standard hematoxylin and eosin (H&E) stains, many cases of diffuse disease benefit from the addition of connective tissue stains, such as trichrome, Verhoeff-van Gieson, or Movat pentachrome stains, for further evaluation of vascular disease or small-airway scarring, both of which may be under-recognized with use of routine stains. Additional staining for microorganisms, iron, glycogen, and alveolar proteinosis should be performed when indicated.

Processing of Pediatric Cystic Lung Lesion Specimens

Gross examination is a critical component of the pathologic assessment of cystic malformations. In particular, the diagnosis of bronchial atresia and intralobar sequestration requires attention to gross characteristics that cannot be replicated microscopically. Lesions submitted with a working diagnosis of "congenital cystic adenomatoid malformation" may yield a wide array of pathologic diagnoses, including bronchial atresia, intralobar sequestration, large cyst congenital pulmonary airway malformation, and congenital lobar overinflation.

Accurate classification of these lesions is facilitated by use of a standard approach to identification of specific anatomic features. The pleura should be examined for accessory pseudofissures, which often mark the contour of underlying maldeveloped lung, typically corresponding to a segmental distribution in bronchial atresia or intralobar sequestration. Intralobar sequestration is often distinguishable by a segmental region of pulmonary congestion and hemorrhage. The pleural surface is examined for the presence or absence of ligated vessels correlating with entry of an aberrant systemic artery, typically at the medial basal aspect of a lower lobe lesion.

The hilum is examined for a bulging mucocele that may correspond with an atretic bronchial segment. The patent airways at the hilum are inflated with formalin by transbronchial injection, and the distribution of parenchymal expansion is observed, with uninflated segments potentially corresponding to a region of lung distal to a bronchial atresia or intralobar sequestration. The lobe is sectioned in a parasagittal plane from lateral to medial, preserving the hilum for the last section. Areas of abnormally congested, hyperinflated, or cystic lung parenchyma are documented. A region of microcystic lung parenchyma can be traced with each plane of section toward the hilum until a larger mucus-filled cyst (mucocele) or other dilated airway is recognized, at which point retrograde probing of the airway may assist in documenting the blind-ending point of an atretic bronchus in either isolated bronchial atresia or intralobar sequestration (bronchial atresia with systemic arterial supply). Microscopic sections should represent central and peripheral aspects of both normal lung and abnormal cystic regions, with interface sections providing a useful histologic contrast between normally developed alveoli and abnormally developed parenchyma. Hyperinflated lobes typical

of congenital lobar overinflation should prompt attention to the hilar bronchi for identification of stenotic lesions or bronchomalacia. Large unilocular or multilocular cysts need to be sampled extensively to distinguish congenital pulmonary airway malformation from the cystic form of pleuropulmonary blastoma.

Cysts and Masses

Many pediatric lung biopsies and resections are performed for localized abnormalities within the lungs, and these may be solid or cystic (Box 4-1). A number of clues can be obtained from the history and findings on diagnostic imaging and intraoperative inspection, and these can be helpful in making the correct diagnosis, even before slides have been reviewed. The location of the mass, the presence of cystic or solid areas, the vascular and bronchial supply, and the onset of symptoms can all be useful in narrowing the scope of the differential diagnosis.[3]

Bronchogenic Cysts

Bronchogenic cysts (or bronchial cysts) are developmental anomalies formed by abnormal budding of the tracheobronchial anlage of the primitive foregut in early development.[4,5] They commonly are found in the anterior mediastinum or along the tracheobronchial tree. Less often, they are found within the pulmonary parenchyma, within or below the diaphragm, or even within the pericardium.[6,7] Patients with bronchogenic cysts can present with infection or obstruction, although frequently these lesions are an incidental radiologic finding.[5] The cyst often is unilocular and lined by ciliated columnar epithelium. Many bronchogenic cysts communicate with the tracheobronchial tree. On occasion, they show squamous metaplasia or mild chronic inflammation.

Considerations in the differential diagnosis for bronchogenic cyst include esophageal duplication cyst for lesions occurring in the mediastinum and congenital pulmonary airway malformations (CPAMs) for lesions occurring within the substance of the lung. The bronchogenic cyst typically has cartilage plates and submucosal glands in the wall, similar to the normal microscopic anatomy of bronchi (Fig. 4-1).

Box 4-1. Intrathoracic Cystic Lesions in Neonates and Children

Mediastinal cysts
  Bronchogenic cyst
  Bronchopulmonary foregut malformation
  Esophageal duplication cyst
  Thymic cyst
  Pericardial cyst
Bronchial atresia
Pulmonary sequestrations
  Intralobar sequestration
  Extralobar sequestration
Congenital pulmonary airway malformation
Acquired cysts
  Abscess
  Pneumatocele
  Cystic bronchiectasis
  Post-infarction cyst
  Pulmonary interstitial emphysema, acute or persistent
  Peripheral cysts of pulmonary maldevelopment (Down syndrome) or chronic
    lung disease
Neoplasia
  Pleuropulmonary blastoma
  Cystic teratoma

Bronchial Atresia

Bronchial atresia is one of the most common forms of congenital pulmonary malformation. Atresia of a segmental or subsegmental bronchus classically results in a central mucus-filled cyst (mucocele) at the point of atresia, dilated distal airways with mucous plugs, and hyperinflated microcystic distal parenchyma (Fig. 4-2). Microscopically, the abnormally developed cystic parenchyma has a pattern identical to that described in type 2 CPAM, consisting of increased numbers of abnormal bronchiolar structures surrounded by variably abundant alveolar spaces which are typically distended and either round or elongated in shape.[8,9] Abundant mucus and muciphages typically are noted within proximal airway lumens and adjacent air spaces. Bronchial atresia often is detected prenatally or in infancy as an asymptomatic cystic lesion. Because of interconnection with the normal parenchyma through alveolar pores of Kohn, the abnormal lung distal to a bronchial atresia may potentially become secondarily infected, and presentation in later childhood, adolescence, or adulthood typically is due to symptoms of recurrent pneumonia. The primary considerations in the differential diagnosis are congenital lobar overinflation, which is characterized by normally developed (albeit markedly distended) air spaces, and intralobar sequestration, which is distinguished by the additional finding of aberrant systemic arterial supply.[3]

Pulmonary Sequestration

Pulmonary sequestration refers to the occurrence of lung tissue that does not communicate with the tracheobronchial tree and that typically has a systemic, rather than pulmonary, arterial supply.[10–13] Such lung tissue is therefore "sequestered" from the usual pulmonary airway and vascular connections. These lesions are further subdivided into an extralobar type, which occurs outside the visceral pleura of the adjacent lung, and an intralobar type, which resides within the visceral pleural investment of a lung lobe. Although there is general agreement that extralobar sequestrations represent congenital malformations, the origin of intralobar sequestrations has been more controversial. More

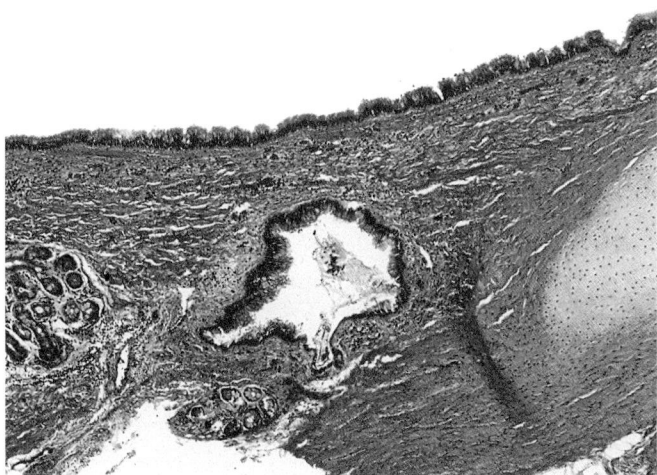

Figure 4-1. Bronchogenic cyst. The wall of a bronchogenic cyst shows features similar to those of a normal bronchus, including submucosal glands (*left* and *center*) and cartilage (*right*).

These structures may be sparse but can help differentiate this lesion from the esophageal duplication cyst, which lacks these structures and has a double muscular layer in its wall. Both of these entities can be lined by ciliated mucosa. The bronchogenic cyst lacks connection with alveolar tissue, a feature that aids in its distinction from CPAM. On occasion, with inflamed cysts within the lung, the nature of the specific lesion or underlying disorder may be impossible to ascertain. In such situations, a generic diagnosis of "inflamed intraparenchymal cyst," accompanied by a differential diagnosis summary that includes abscess, CPAM, bronchogenic cyst, esophageal cyst, and intralobar sequestration, is appropriate. Radiologic and clinical features may help in further differentiating among these entities.

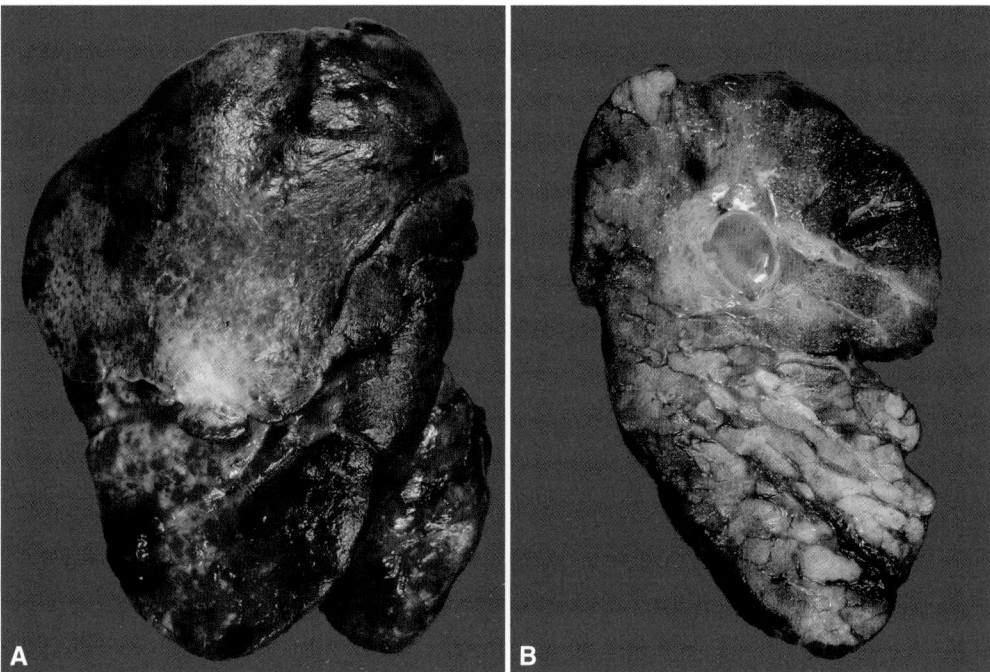

Figure 4-2. Bronchial atresia: resected specimens. **A,** The left upper lobe is enlarged with a region of hyperinflation marked by an irregular pleural pseudofissure. **B,** The site of bronchial atresia is indicated by a central mucus-filled cyst (mucocele) and surrounding microcystic parenchyma.

Table 4-1. Pulmonary Sequestration: Extralobar versus Intralobar

Clinical/Historical Feature	Extralobar Sequestration	Intralobar Sequestration
Location	Outside pleura of lung ("accessory lobe") Commonly, left lung base	Within pleura of lung lobe Lower lobe (98%)
Gross	Pyramidal structure	Congested, hemorrhagic segment(s) of lobe
Age at diagnosis	60% < 6 months	50% > 20 years
Arterial supply	Systemic	Systemic
Origin	Congenital anomaly	Congenital anomaly; possibly acquired in adults
Histologic appearance	CPAM type 2 pattern Hyperinflated air spaces	CPAM type 2 pattern with mucus stasis Hyperinflated, hemorrhagic segment(s) of lobe Inflamed, chronic pneumonia

CPAM, congenital pulmonary airway malformation.
Modified from Stocker JT. Sequestrations of the lung. *Semin Diagn Pathol.* 1986;3(2):106–121; and Langston C. New concepts in the pathology of congenital lung malformations. *Semin Pediatr Surg.* 2003;12(1):17–37.

frequent diagnosis in adults has led to the theory that they are post-inflammatory lesions with acquired loss of bronchial connection and development of collateral systemic circulation from hypertrophied pulmonary ligament arteries.[11] However, intralobar sequestrations diagnosed prenatally or in association with congenital malformations support the concept that the pathogenic mechanisms for extralobar and intralobar sequestrations are similar, and that adult lesions may represent occult malformation detected later in life. Specific features of extralobar and intralobar sequestrations, summarized in Table 4-1, are discussed next.[11]

Extralobar Sequestration

Extralobar sequestrations (ELSs) are thought to arise a a result of abnormal budding from the tracheobronchial anlage. Lying outside the normal lung, these structures appear as "accessory lobes," completely surrounded by their own visceral pleura.[10–15] ELSs usually are found in the lower thoracic cavity but may be found above, within, or below the diaphragm. On gross inspection, they appear as irregularly ovoid or pyramidal portions of lung tissue surrounded by pleura and with a vascular pole at one edge (see Fig. 4-3A). The radiographic or intraoperative finding of a systemic arterial supply confirms the diagnosis of ELS. The systemic artery can arise from a source above or below the diaphragm.[16,17] The microscopic appearance may vary but the histologic pattern typically is that of type 2 CPAM and less often resembles that of normal lung[11,14,15,18–21] (see Fig. 4-3B and C). Striated muscle occasionally is present within the interstitium of the lesion; this feature is called *rhabdomyomatous dysplasia*.

Intralobar Sequestration

Intralobar sequestrations (ILSs) lie within the parenchyma of the lung. Most ILSs occur in the medial area of a lower lobe, and the abnormal systemic elastic artery can usually be identified in the region of the inferior pulmonary ligament[22] (Fig. 4-4A). Radiologic studies can be

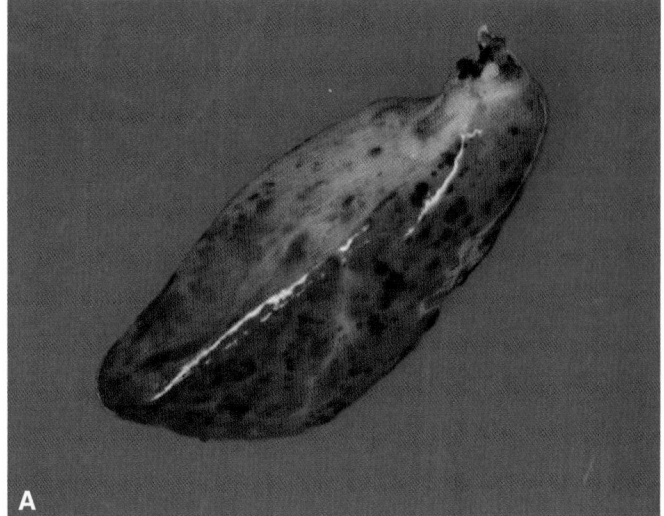

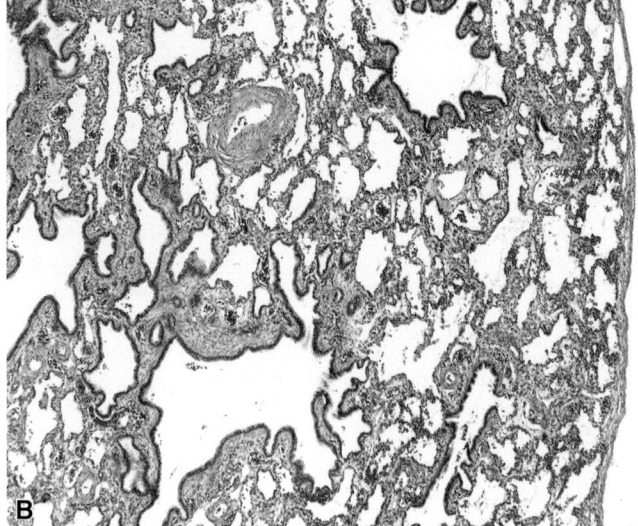

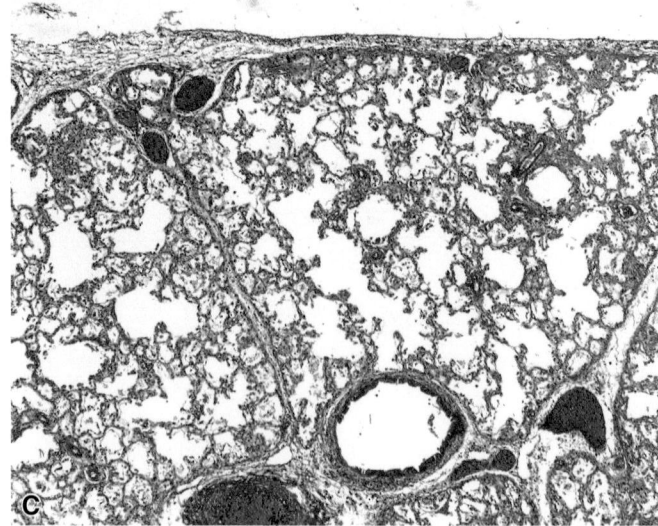

Figure 4-3. Extralobar sequestration. Extralobar sequestrations often are small pyramidal "accessory lobes" with a vascular pole on one side (**A**). They can have various histologic appearances, most often resembling the type 2 (small cyst) CPAM pattern (**B**), and occasionally showing near-normal lung parenchyma with only mildly enlarged air spaces (**C**).

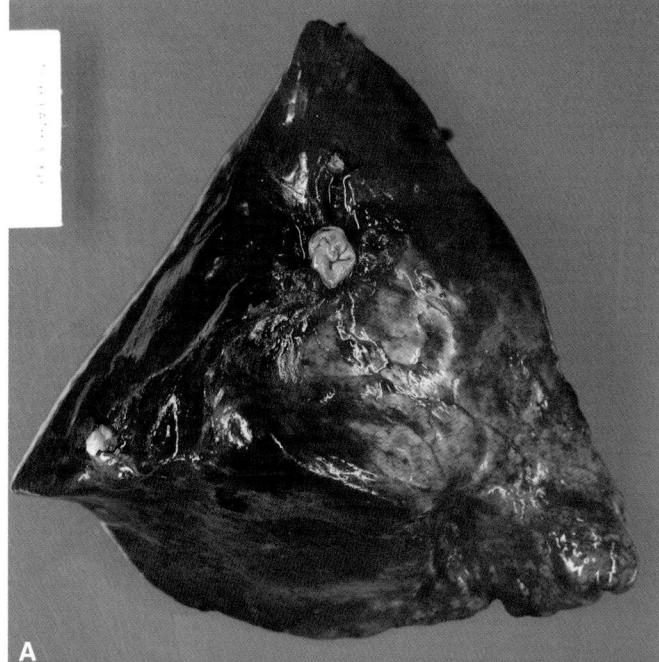

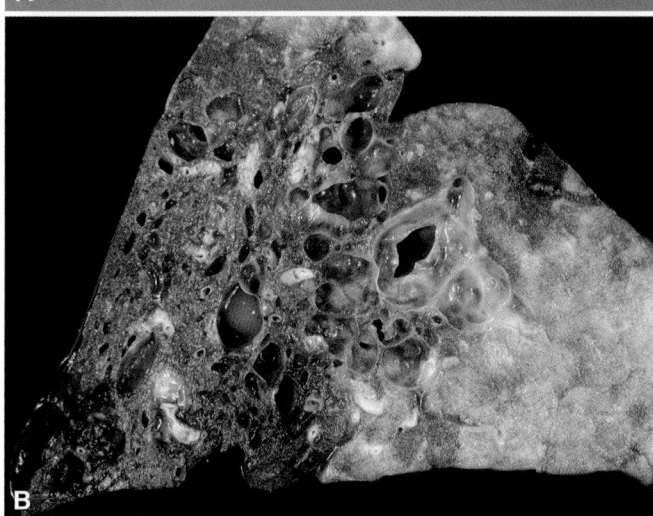

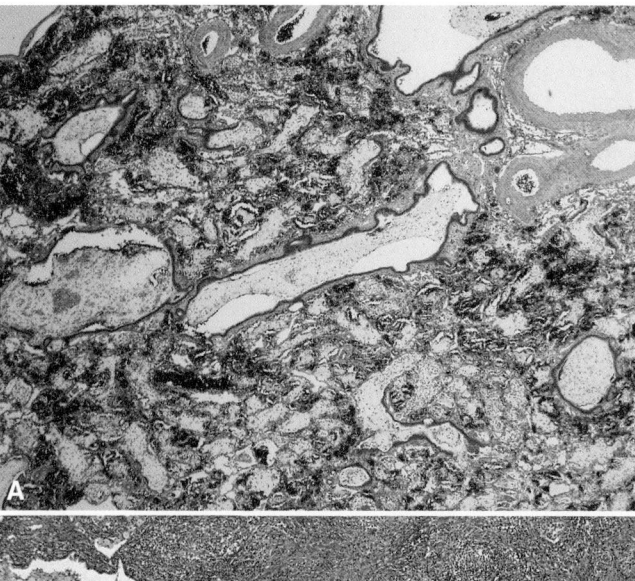

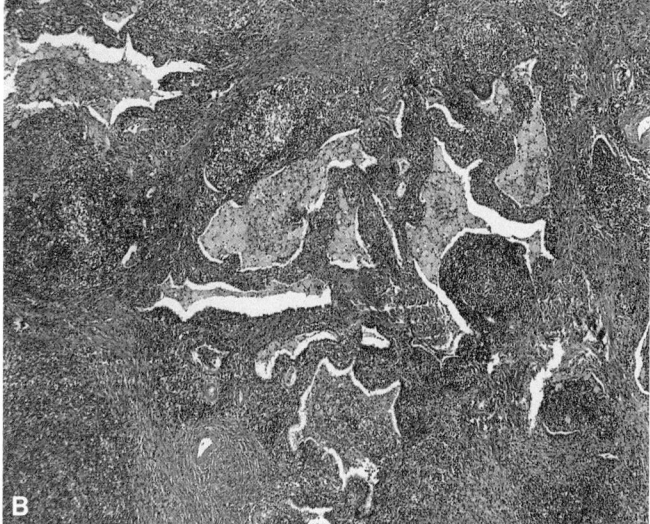

Figure 4-4. Intralobar sequestration. The sequestered lung is marked on the pleural surface by a region of congestion and hemorrhage. **A,** An elastic artery of systemic origin typically is present on the inferomedial aspect of the lower lobe. **B,** The cut surface similarly is congested and also demonstrates cystic change and mucus stasis, as seen in isolated segmental bronchial atresia.

Figure 4-5. Intralobar sequestration. **A,** Intralobar sequestrations typically show dilated central airways with mucous plugging and peripheral microcystic parenchyma, as well as alveolar hemorrhage due to the high-pressure systemic arterial circulation. **B,** In older children and adults, there may be evidence of chronic infection, including lymphoid hyperplasia, accumulation of foamy macrophages, and fibrosis.

extremely helpful in supporting the diagnosis.[23,24] Various modalities, including computed tomography (CT) and magnetic resonance imaging (MRI), will show a solid or cystic mass that lacks normal bronchovascular patterns. A systemic arterial supply may be confirmed radiologically or at the time of surgery. The gross and microscopic findings are markedly influenced by age at resection and presence or absence of any accrued chronic inflammatory insults (usually secondary infections) within the sequestered lung tissue. In infants with asymptomatic lesions, the lobe contains a segmental region of congestion and hemorrhage due to the high flow of the systemic circulation, accompanied by microcystic parenchyma (see Fig. 4-4B). The maldeveloped parenchyma shows mucus stasis, identical to that in segmental bronchial atresia (Fig. 4-5A). In older children and adults with recurrent pneumonia, the histologic findings are similar in appearance

to those in localized bronchiectasis with recurrent infection. Other features include marked acute and chronic inflammation with fibrosis and cyst formation (see Fig. 4-5B).

Congenital Pulmonary Airway Malformations

Congenital malformations of the pulmonary airways (i.e., CPAMs), also called congenital cystic adenomatoid malformations (CCAMs), are masses of maldeveloped lung tissue that are classified according to their gross and microscopic appearance.[12,25-34] These lesions are identified most commonly in stillborn infants or in newborns with respiratory distress, but they can be discovered in adolescents and rarely in adults.[35] Stocker and colleagues initially proposed a classification scheme for CCAM that divided these malformations into three subtypes.[36] This scheme was later expanded to five subtypes (types 0 to 4), with a subsequent change in terminology from CCAM to CPAM, acknowledging that not all of these malformations are cystic and not all are adenomatoid.[37] The overriding principle of this subclassification is that the dominant morphologic constituent of each type of CPAM reflects the morphology of the normal tracheobronchial tree from proximal to distal—that is, from malformed bronchi, to bronchioles, to distal lung (alveolar) tissue. This construct has provided useful morphologic distinctions and will continue to be revised as the pathogenesis of these lesions is better understood. CPAM classification may be difficult in immature or fetal lungs, and an alternate classification has been proposed for fetal lung resections.[33,34]

Type 0 CPAM, also called *acinar dysplasia*, is a rare lesion composed of cartilaginous airways and loose mesenchyme (see later discussion).[38–41] Types 1 to 3 have a common general overall appearance of cystic spaces (distorted airways) with intervening structures more or less resembling alveoli (Figs. 4-6 to 4-8). Type 1 CPAM shows larger cysts, having some bronchial differentiation in that they contain ciliated epithelial lining or mucinous-type epithelium or have cartilage in their walls. Type 2 CPAM shows smaller cystic spaces that resemble ectatic irregular bronchioles, evenly separated from each other by alveolar structures, and represents a histologic pattern that implies intrauterine bronchial obstruction, typically from bronchial atresia or pulmonary sequestration. Type 3 CPAM is a rare solid lesion typically encompassing an entire lobe or lung and resembles pulmonary hyperplasia or immature lung in the early canalicular stage of development. Type 4 CPAM has been described as a peripheral large cyst with thin walls and flattened alveolar-type epithelial lining. Existence of this type is controversial, because it may represent unrecognized, undersampled, or completely differentiated examples of cystic pleuropulmonary blastoma (PPB).[42–48] Large cysts resembling type 1 or type 4 CCAM should be extensively sampled to exclude the presence of small foci of either malignant primitive spindled cells beneath the alveolar epithelium ("cambium layer") or immature chondroid foci, diagnostic of cystic (type I) PPB. Immunohistochemical staining for myogenin, desmin, and MyoD1 may be helpful in differentiating the cells of PPB from reactive fibroblastic proliferation or cellular mesenchyme in CPAM. Cystic PPBs have potential for recurrence as high-grade tumors, particularly if incompletely resected.

Although the prognosis in most cases is favorable following resection, there are rare reported cases of patients developing carcinomas in association with CPAM.[49–55] Many of these lesions are mucinous bronchioloalveolar carcinomas, which has led to the proposal that the mucigenic epithelium in type 1 CPAM is preneoplastic (see Fig. 4-6C). Multifocal bilateral mucinous bronchioloalveolar carcinomas after

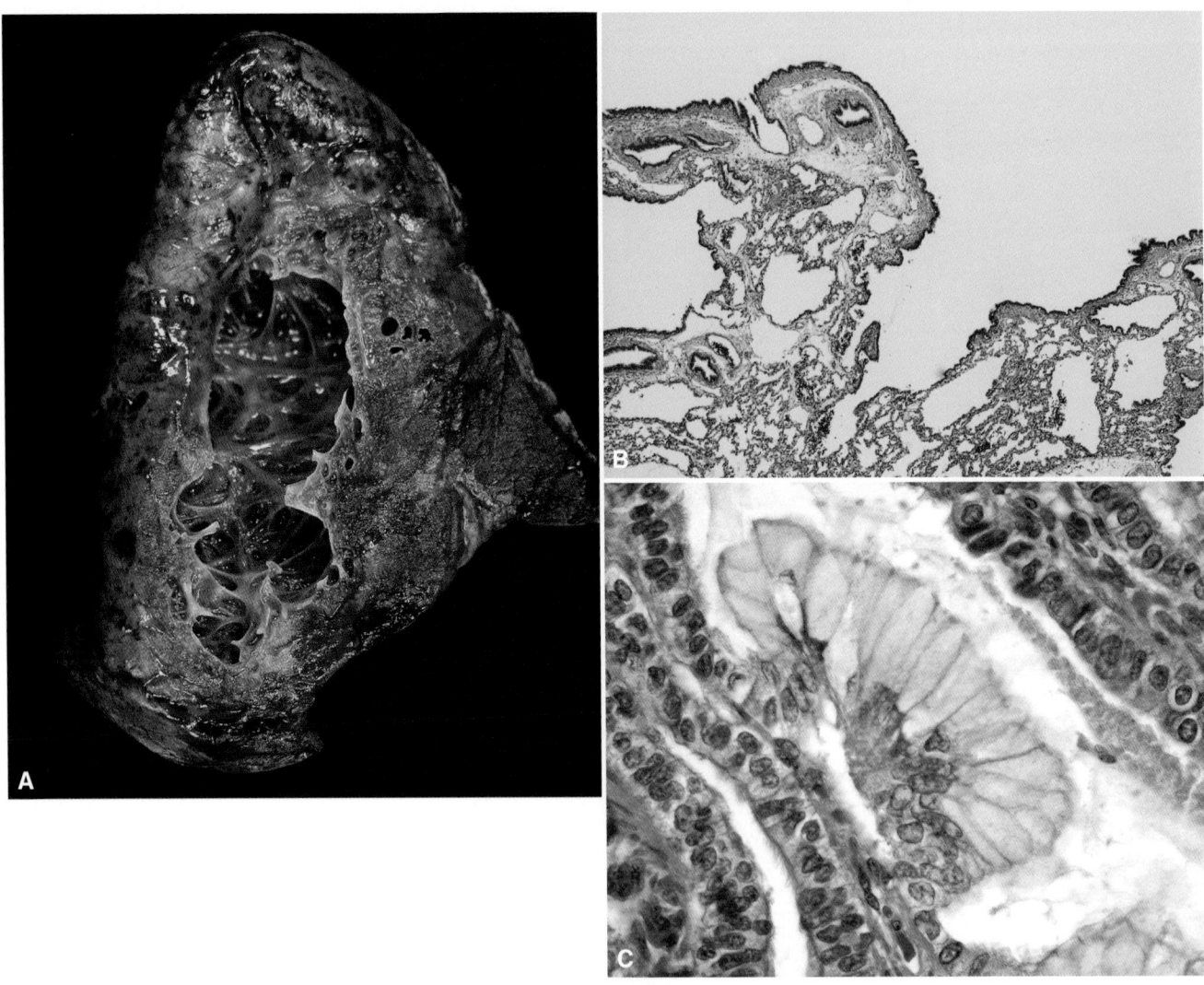

Figure 4-6. Congenital pulmonary airway malformation (CPAM). **A,** The type 1 lesion typically is composed of a single large trabeculated cyst or a large multilocular cyst, as in this gross specimen. **B,** Microscopically, the cyst wall is lined by ciliated columnar respiratory-type epithelium with underlying smooth muscle. The lining characteristically interdigitates with the surrounding alveolar parenchyma. **C,** Small foci of mucigenic epithelium are seen occasionally and are considered the precursor lesions for the rare complication of mucinous bronchioloalveolar carcinoma arising in a congenital cyst.

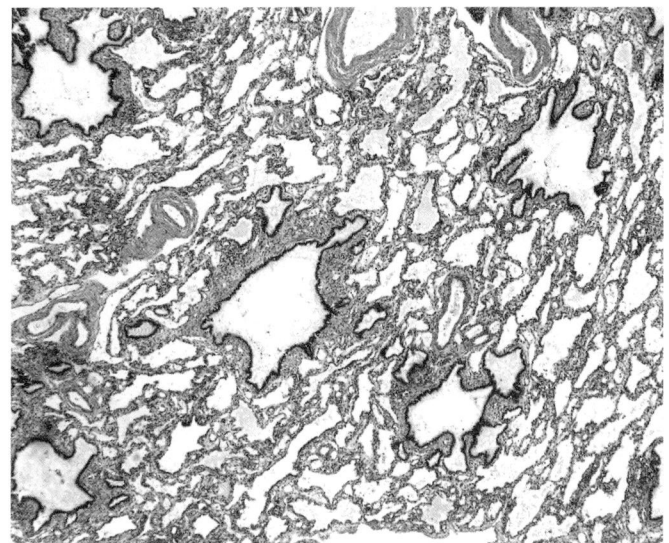

Figure 4-7. Congenital pulmonary airway malformation (CPAM). This type 2 CPAM shows numerous dilated bronchiolar structures within a background of enlarged irregular alveolar structures. This pattern is associated with intrauterine bronchial obstruction, for example bronchial atresia, intralobar sequestration, and extralobar sequestration.

incomplete resection of CPAM have been described in patients as young as 11 years of age.[51] In light of these rare cases, the presence of mucinous epithelium in CPAM and completeness of resection should be documented for follow-up purposes.

Pulmonary Interstitial Emphysema

Pulmonary interstitial emphysema (PIE) results from dissection of air into the interstitial connective tissue of the lung. Rupture of alveoli or disruption of airway walls often is responsible for this phenomenon.[12,56–59] Air accumulates in the interstitium along bronchovascular bundles and interlobular septa, creating cystic spaces that may at first resemble tissue architecturally torn during sectioning (Fig. 4-9A and B). The usual clinical scenario is that of a premature infant with neonatal respiratory distress syndrome receiving mechanical ventilation. Acute PIE usually resorbs over time, but the chronic form persists as cystic lesions lined by fibrous tissue or

multinucleate giant cells (see Fig. 4-9C). Grossly, the process can involve both lungs diffusely or may be localized to one or two lobes. Multiple small cysts can be seen to extend along interlobular septa.

Peripheral Cysts Secondary to Lung Maldevelopment

Hypoplastic lungs, and those damaged in the neonatal period, are susceptible to persistent alterations in alveolar growth. This maldevelopment frequently appears as alveolar enlargement or cysts, particularly in the subpleural areas and peripheral lobules. Microscopic examination reveals irregular air space enlargement with fibrovascular walls lined by alveolar cells (Fig. 4-10). Peripheral cysts have been described in the lungs of several patients with Down syndrome.[60–65]

Pulmonary Hyperlucency

Several conditions may lead to the radiologic appearance of hyperlucency (Box 4-2). Clinical history and knowledge of the indication for resection are helpful, because the pathologic findings can be extremely subtle histologically. The clinical presentation may include shortness of breath, tachypnea, wheezing, or cough, typically in infants. The chest radiograph shows marked lobar enlargement with displacement of the mediastinum. The two most commonly occurring histologic patterns are congenital lobar overinflation (so-called congenital lobar emphysema) (in 70% of the cases) and polyalveolar lobe (30%).

Congenital Lobar Overinflation

Congenital lobar overinflation (CLO), or congenital lobar emphysema, occurs when there is overdistention of the normal alveolar parenchyma[12,66,67] (Fig. 4-11). The etiology is variable, but the underlying cause frequently is a partial or intermittent high-grade obstruction of the bronchus supplying the affected lobe.[68] Bronchomalacia may result in collapse of the lobar bronchus with expiration, resulting in progressive air-trapping in the affected lobe. The obstruction can occur as a result of other intrinsic factors such as bronchial stenosis, abnormal "kinked" bronchial anatomy, mucosal webs, or mucous plugging. Alternatively, congenital lobar emphysema can be extrinsic as a result of various vascular or neoplastic etiologies.

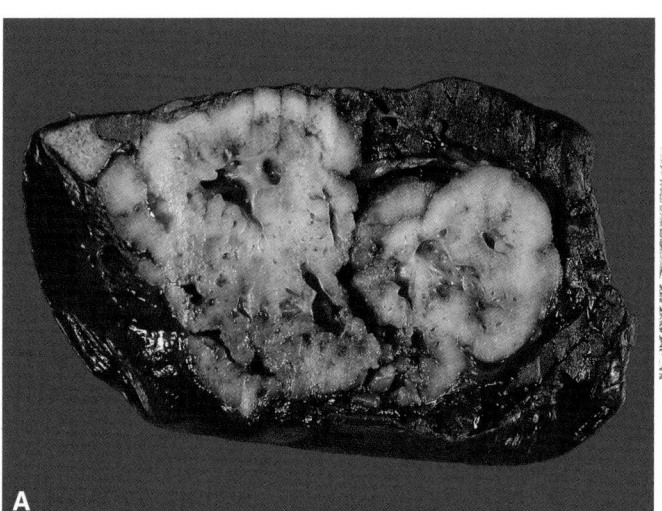

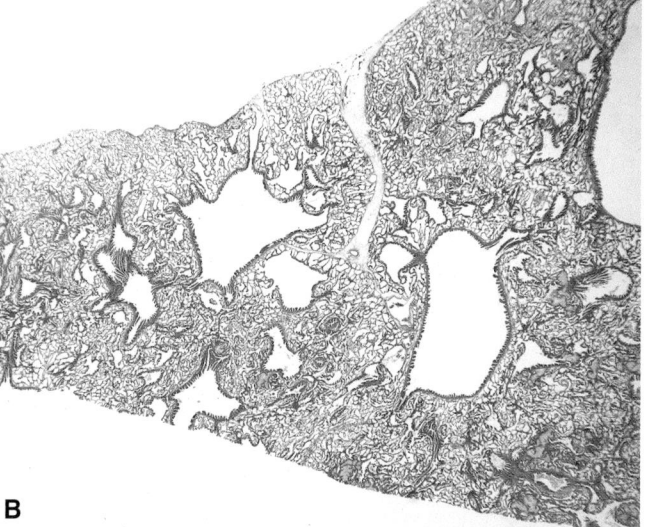

Figure 4-8. Congenital pulmonary airway malformation (CPAM). **A,** Grossly, this CPAM shows a spongy mass of abnormal tissue replacing the lobe. **B,** The abnormally developed parenchyma shows dilated bronchiolar structures surrounded by elongated hyperplastic air spaces.

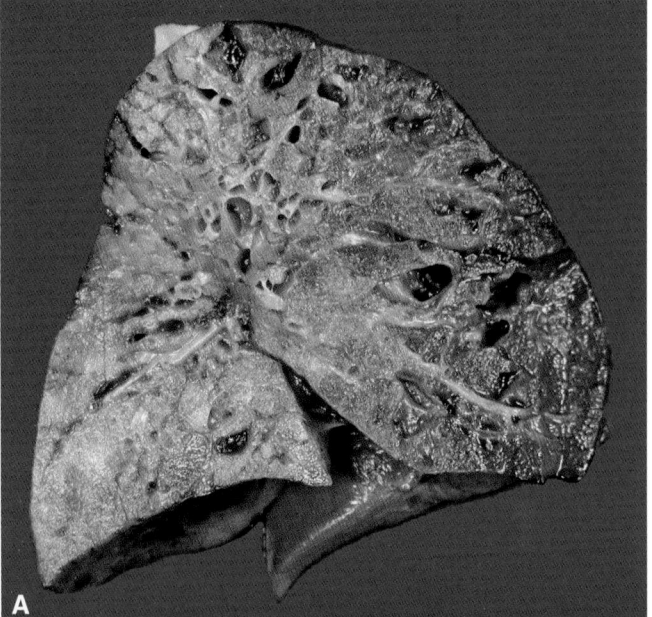

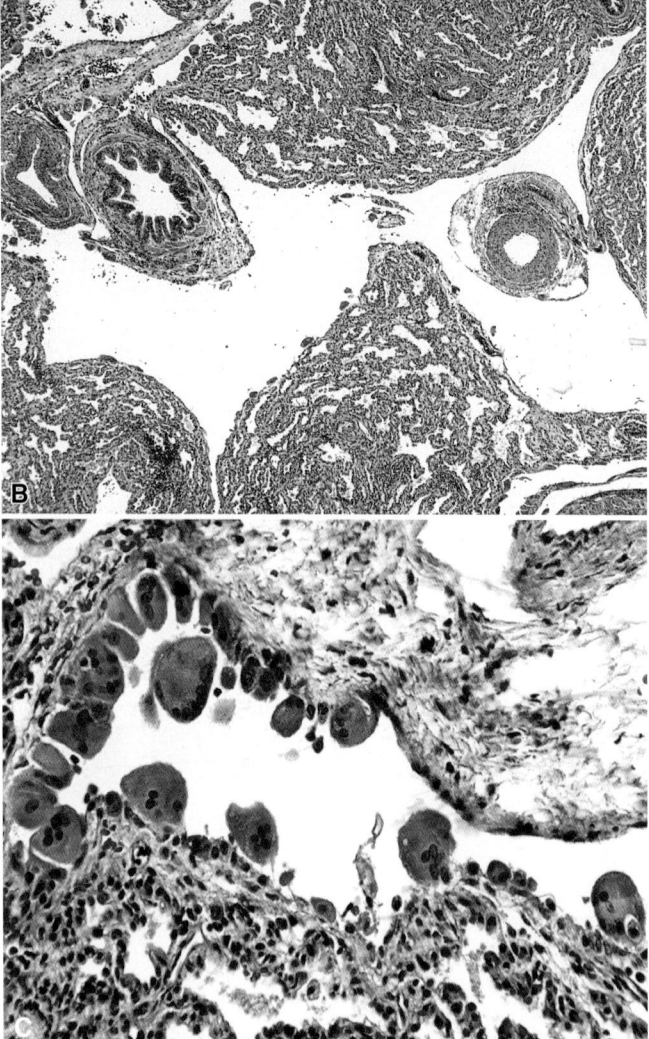

Figure 4-9. Pulmonary interstitial emphysema (PIE). PIE is caused by air leak from ruptured alveoli, with dissection of air into the interstitium along bronchovascular bundles and interlobular septa, producing angular elongated cysts, seen grossly (**A**) and microscopically (**B**). **C,** Multinucleate giant cells line the cysts in persistent PIE.

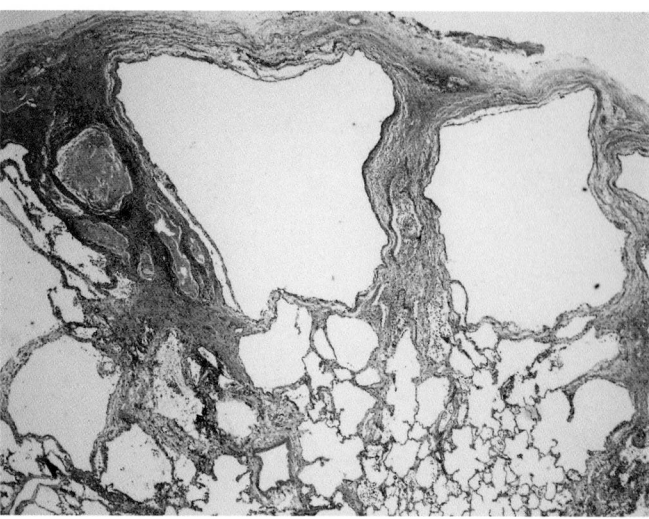

Figure 4-10. Down syndrome: pulmonary involvement. Peripheral cysts and alveolar simplification are prominent features in some children with Down syndrome.

Box 4-2. Disorders and Conditions Causing Radiologic Hyperlucency in the Lung

Congenital lobar overinflation
Idiopathic
Bronchial stenosis
Bronchial mucosal folds/webs
Extrinsic airway compression by mass or abnormal vasculature
Lobular hyperinflation due to small airway disease
    Obliterative bronchiolitis (postinfectious, bronchopulmonary dysplasia)
    Meconium aspiration
    Mucous plugging
    Polyalveolar lobe

Approximately one half of the cases are idiopathic. The upper lobe is involved in nearly all cases. Lower lobe involvement is highly unusual except in acquired cases in patients with previous hyaline membrane disease or bronchopulmonary dysplasia (BPD). Some cases may arise secondary to trauma from tracheal suctioning during respiratory support.[69]

On gross examination, CLO is characterized by a markedly enlarged lobe, which generally retains its basic shape. Alveoli, alveolar ducts, and respiratory bronchioles typically are dilated on histologic examination. Unlike bronchial atresia and CPAM, CLO shows otherwise normal alveolar development, with appropriate numbers of bronchiolar structures and appropriate alveolar septation. The source of obstruction is identified only occasionally by gross and microscopic examination[70–72] (Fig. 4-12).

Polyalveolar Lobe

Polyalveolar lobe occurs when there is an increase in the regional number of alveoli relative to the corresponding conducting airways and arteries.[73–75] Whereas the arteries and airways in these lungs are normal, the alveolar regions are enlarged by an increased number of nearly normal alveoli. The diagnosis can be made by radial alveolar counts, which are performed by counting the number of alveoli transected by a line drawn from the respiratory bronchiole to the nearest acinar edge (pleura or septum).[76] The normal count varies with age but should be between 5 and 10 for infants, and 10 and 12 for young children. Radial alveolar counts in polyalveolar lobe will be approximately two to three times that number (Fig. 4-13).

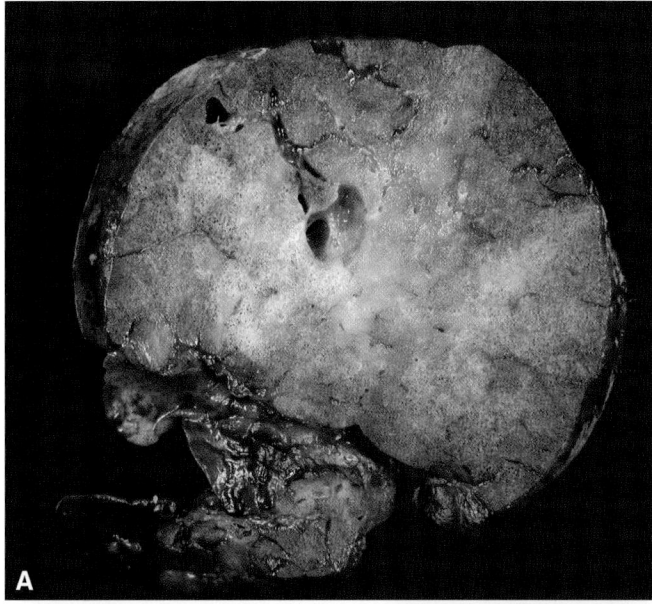

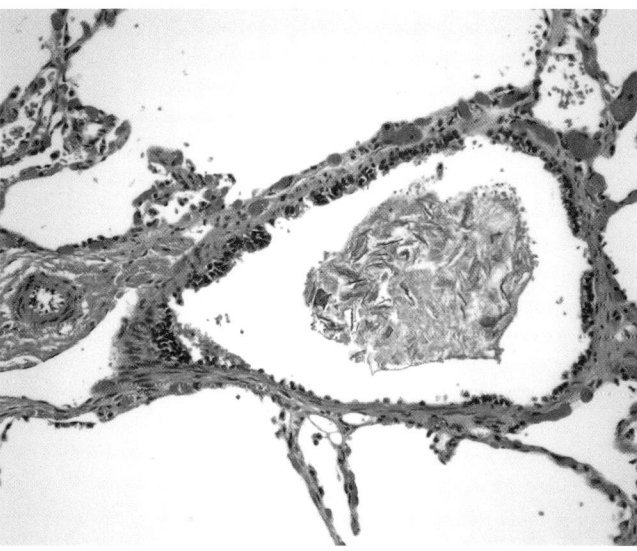

Figure 4-12. Meconium aspiration. Lung injury from meconium aspiration is one of many small-airway processes that can result in regional air-trapping and hyperlucency.

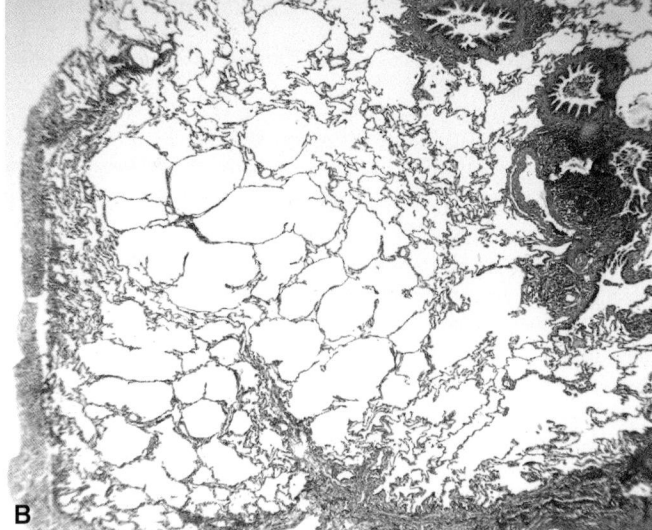

Figure 4-11. Congenital lobar overinflation. **A,** The major portion of a lobe in this specimen is massively overinflated, typically as a result of progressive air-trapping by bronchial stenosis or bronchomalacia, resulting in a region of pallor and accentuated air spaces. This specimen also shows focal pulmonary interstitial emphysema due to air leak. **B,** Microscopically, the overinflated alveoli are enlarged and distended but typically show normal development.

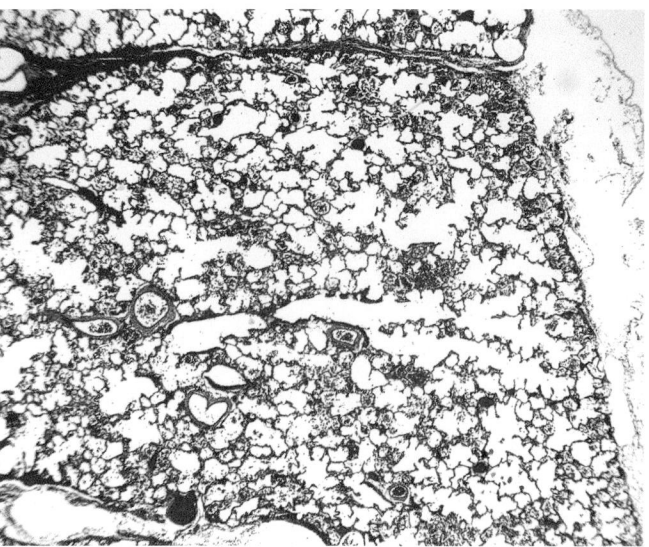

Figure 4-13. Polyalveolar lobe. An increased number of alveoli can be seen within the affected region. Radial alveolar counts can be performed to determine increased values.

Disorders of Lung Development

Acinar Dysplasia

Described in 1986, acinar dysplasia is a rare severe diffuse developmental lung disorder resulting in marked deficiency of acinar development, identical to the entity described as type 0 CPAM.[38-41] The lungs are small, with accentuation of small lobules by white interlobular septa (Fig. 4-14A). Microscopically, the lobular bronchi are surrounded by only few primitive air spaces, with virtually no alveolar development (see Fig. 4-14B). This disorder is uniformly fatal within the first few hours of life and typically is diagnosed at autopsy. Although acinar dysplasia is presumed to be of genetic origin, the etiology is unknown.

Congenital Alveolar Dysplasia

Congenital alveolar dysplasia also is a rare diffuse developmental lung disorder with incomplete air space development.[77] Relative to those in

acinar dysplasia, the air spaces are more numerous and exhibit greater complexity, but completely mature alveoli are lacking. The air spaces show primary septation but insufficient secondary septation, generally resembling the saccular stage of development (Fig. 4-15). This disorder can be difficult to distinguish from prematurity of lungs with superimposed injury and remodeling due to prolonged ventilation, and on a practical level, the diagnosis is reserved for term infants, in whom the disorder is more likely to be a developmental abnormality, rather than an acquired impairment of alveolar growth. The etiology is unknown.

Pulmonary Hypoplasia

Pulmonary hypoplasia refers to abnormally small size of the lungs due to limitation of intrauterine development. Although primary forms of hypoplasia exist, this term most commonly refers to the secondary forms of lung hypoplasia in which physical compression of the lungs, by extrathoracic or intrathoracic processes, limits intrauterine growth.

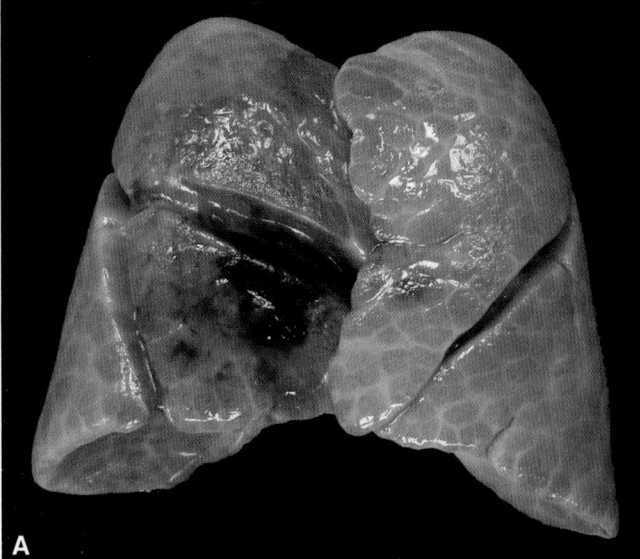

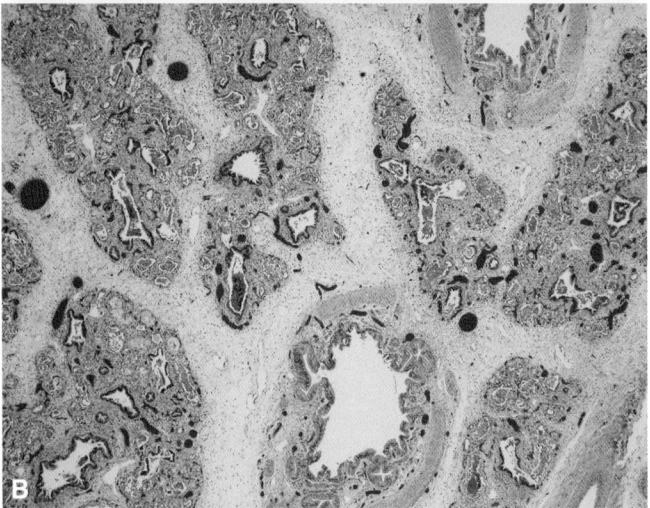

Figure 4-14. Acinar dysplasia. In this rare, uniformly fatal form of primary pulmonary hypoplasia, the acinar parenchyma fails to develop. **A,** The lobules in this specimen are accentuated by thickened interlobular septa. **B,** On microscopic examination, the parenchyma is seen to be composed of bronchi surrounded by primitive lobules, with lack of subdivision and alveolarization.

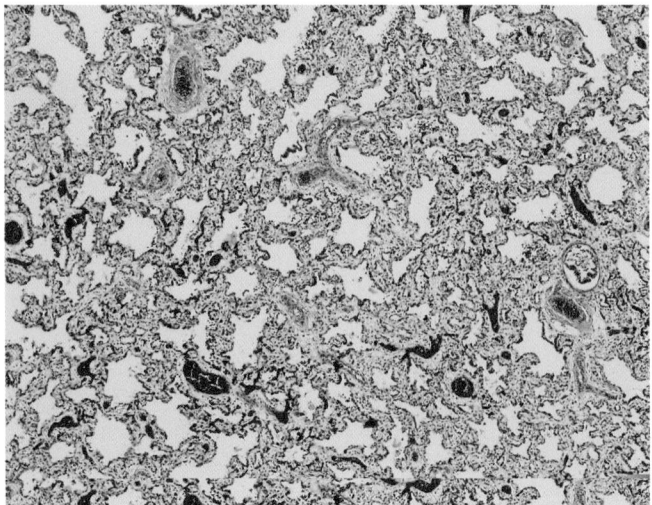

Figure 4-15. Congenital alveolar dysplasia. This rare diffuse developmental disorder microscopically resembles the saccular phase of development, despite term gestation.

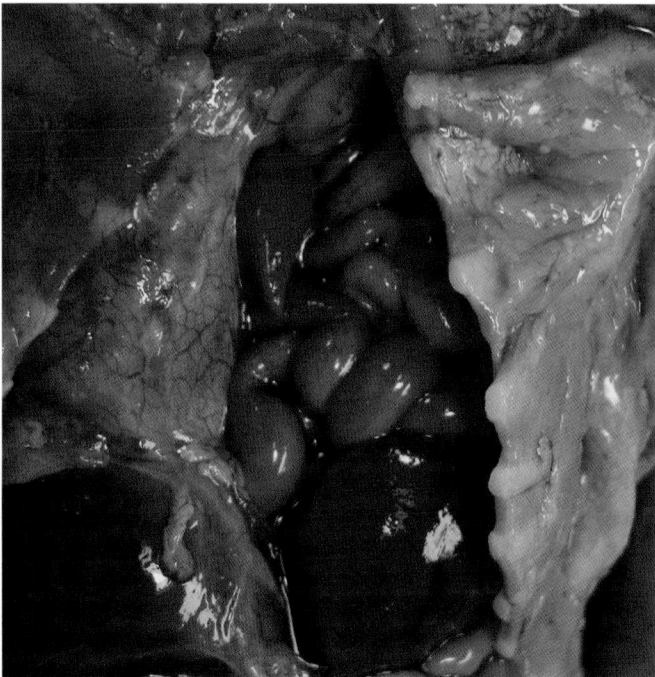

Figure 4-16. Pulmonary hypoplasia. In this case, the hypoplasia was secondary to a large left-sided congenital diaphragmatic hernia. The small left lung is compressed within the superomedial aspect of the thoracic cavity.

Common causes include congenital diaphragmatic hernia (Fig. 4-16), intrauterine chylothorax or pleural effusion, osteochondrodysplasia with small thorax, neuromuscular disorders with poor respiratory effort, and intrathoracic or intra-abdominal lesions with mass effect on thoracic contents.[78] Grossly, lung hypoplasia can be documented by low lung-to-body weight ratio or by low lung volumes.[79,80] Microscopically, the lobules are small, with a reduced radial alveolar count. Hypoplastic lungs are prone to development of hyaline membrane disease, even at term gestation. Beyond the postnatal period, the simplification of lobules manifests on biopsy as alveolar enlargement and simplification, identical in appearance to chronic neonatal lung disease due to prematurity (see the discussion in section "Alveolar Growth Abnormalities").

Pulmonary Hyperplasia

Pulmonary hyperplasia refers to enlargement of the lungs due to increased mass and volume, typically due to high-grade obstruction of the larynx (laryngeal atresia) or trachea (tracheal compression).[81,82] Morphologically, the air spaces are abnormally elongated and increased in number (Fig. 4-17).

Vascular Disorders

Alveolar Capillary Dysplasia with Misalignment of Pulmonary Veins

Alveolar capillary dysplasia is a disease characterized by a distinctive pattern of diffuse pulmonary vascular maldevelopment (Fig. 4-18). The disease typically manifests clinically soon after birth with profound respiratory distress, often after a brief asymptomatic period.[83–85] The clinical picture is one of severe persistent pulmonary hypertension, and survival beyond the neonatal period is rare.[86–88] Some cases are associated with other visceral malformations, and familial cases have been reported as well, supporting a genetic etiology.[89] Histopathologic examination reveals abnormal lobular architecture with a diminished number of capillaries within alveolar walls. These alveolar capillaries are abnormally located within the central portion of the septa, rather than adjacent to the alveolar epithelial cells. The pulmonary arteries show marked medial hypertrophy, and the smaller branches show increased muscle, including

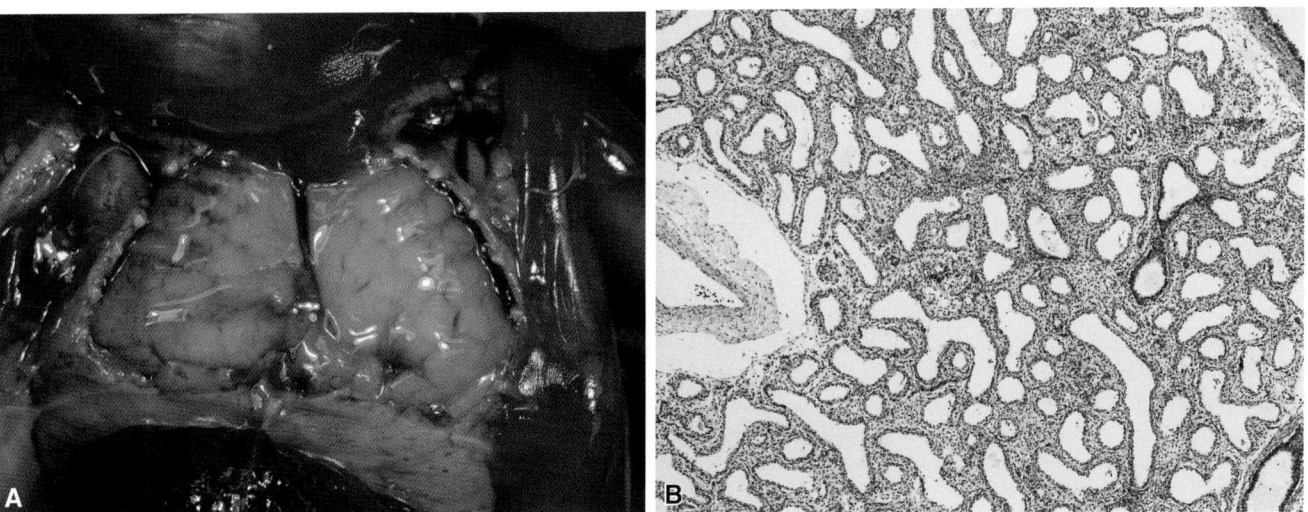

Figure 4-17. Pulmonary hyperplasia. **A,** In this case, pulmonary hyperplasia was due to laryngeal atresia. The lungs are markedly enlarged and cover the anterior mediastinum. Bilateral rib markings are due to overgrowth and compression within the thoracic cavity. **B,** Pulmonary hyperplasia is reflected microscopically by abnormally developed tubular and elongated air spaces. (**A,** Courtesy of Dr. Edwina Popek, Texas Children's Hospital, Houston, TX.)

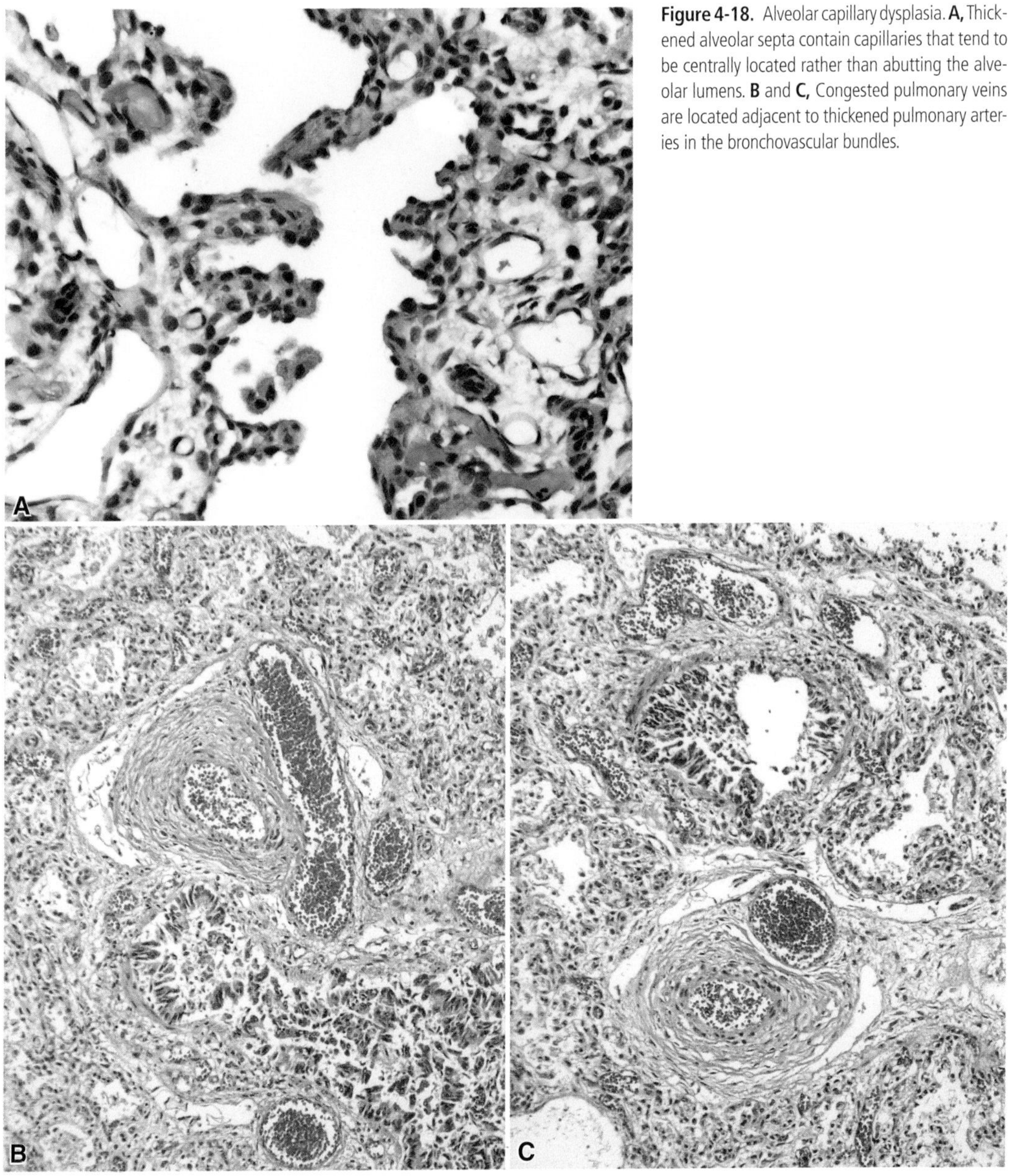

Figure 4-18. Alveolar capillary dysplasia. **A,** Thickened alveolar septa contain capillaries that tend to be centrally located rather than abutting the alveolar lumens. **B** and **C,** Congested pulmonary veins are located adjacent to thickened pulmonary arteries in the bronchovascular bundles.

the arterioles within the alveolar walls. Additional features include misalignment of the pulmonary veins, with congested pulmonary veins abnormally located adjacent to pulmonary arteries within bronchovascular sheaths and congested venules accompanying the hypertrophied arterioles within the lobular parenchyma. Of note, some pulmonary veins may lie in their normal location within interlobular septa, and misalignment of small pulmonary veins and venules within the lobules is more reliably identified. Lymphangiectasia is a variable feature.

Congenital Pulmonary Lymphangiectasis

Congenital pulmonary lymphangiectasis is a disease of newborns that manifests with dyspnea and cyanosis and often is lethal.[90–95] Panlobar diffuse ectasia of lymphatic channels along normal lymphatic routes (bronchovascular bundles, interlobular septa, and subpleural regions) is characteristic (Fig. 4-19). Localized lymphangiectasis occasionally is observed in adults and children and usually is found as an incidental radiographic abnormality.[96,97] Of note, chronic heart failure or pulmonary venous obstruction can lead to secondary lymphangiectasis, which has a similar histologic appearance, and clinical correlation is important in distinguishing between primary and secondary forms of lymphangiectasia.[98]

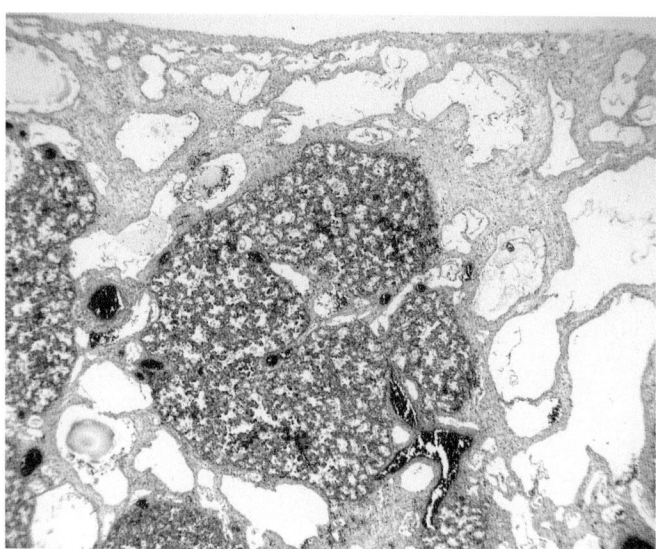

Figure 4-19. Lymphangiectasis. Characteristic dilated tortuous lymphatic vessels are present in the subpleural and septal regions.

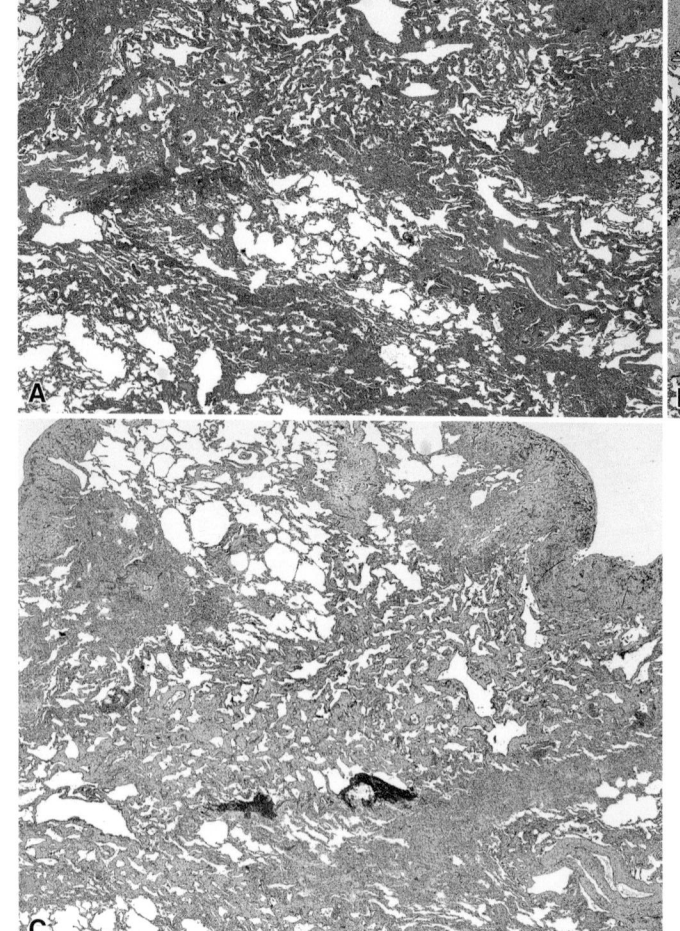

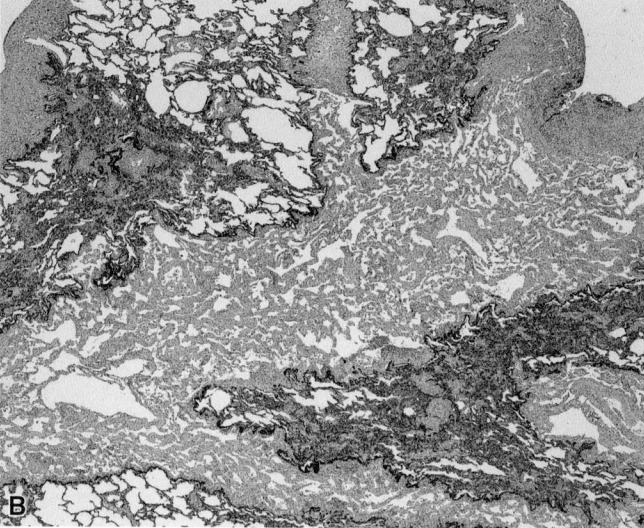

Figure 4-20. Diffuse lymphangiomatosis. **A,** The thin lymphatic channels of lymphangiomatosis can sometimes be difficult to distinguish from alveolar spaces. Use of immunohistochemical markers such as keratin (**B**), CD31 (**C**), or the lymphothelial marker D2-40 can be helpful in demonstrating the increased numbers of lymphatic vessels.

Diffuse Pulmonary Lymphangiomatosis

Diffuse pulmonary lymphangiomatosis is a rare disease, occurring in children or young adults, in which the normal lymphatic regions show an increased number of complex lymphatic channels.[93,95,99,100] The patients generally present with dyspnea and occasionally with hemoptysis. Microscopic examination reveals increased numbers of anastomosing lymphatic channels with interspersed fibroblasts, collagen, and small vessels distributed along the usual lymphatic routes of the lung. The lymphatics can be more easily observed with use of connective tissue stains and immunohistochemical stains for keratin (to demonstrate these structures in negative relief), or CD31 (which stains the lymphatic endothelium) (Fig. 4-20). Some cases have an associated hemorrhagic "kaposiform" spindle cell component.

Pulmonary Arteriovenous Malformations

Pulmonary arteriovenous malformations (PAVMs) are defined as direct connections between branches of the pulmonary artery and the pulmonary vein.[101] Common signs and symptoms are dyspnea, hemoptysis, palpitations, and chest pain. Initial clinical presentation of pulmonary arteriovenous malformations is fairly rare in young children and infants and tends to occur in older children and adults. The diagnosis can be made on clinical and radiologic grounds, followed by pathologic confirmation. Grossly, the malformations can be single or multiple and show ectatic vessels scattered amidst lung parenchyma (Fig. 4-21). Microscopic examination reveals dilated vessels and vascular tangles. The vessels are irregular and are not always in their usual position adjacent to bronchioles, in the case of pulmonary arteries, or in the interlobular septa, in the case of pulmonary veins. Otolaryngologic examination is suggested in patients with PAVM to rule out Osler-Weber-Rendu disease, because approximately one third of patients with single PAVM and one half of patients with multiple PAVMs will have this disease.[101,102] Rare cases of multiple small PAVMs and polysplenia have been described in young children.[103,104]

Complications of Prematurity

Hyaline Membrane Disease

Hyaline membrane disease is a form of acute lung injury seen in neonates and is the pathologic correlate of neonatal respiratory distress syndrome (RDS). Hyaline membrane disease arises as a result of surfactant deficiency due to prematurity.[105] Although surfactant granules can be observed in lung cells at a gestational age of 20 weeks, surfactant is not produced in sufficient amounts until 34 weeks. Lack of surfactant can result either from prematurity or, less commonly, from inadequate resorption of lung liquid at birth leading to a dilutional deficiency. Surfactant deficiency results in increased alveolar surface tension, with subsequent resistance to inflation and alveolar collapse at end-expiration. In this process, the alveoli become injured,[106] presumably as a result of shear stresses on the alveolar walls. Increases in either respiratory effort or mechanical ventilation pressures can increase the severity of the injury. This injury in turn leads to diffuse alveolar damage, which is similar in appearance to that observed in adult cases of acute respiratory distress syndrome (ARDS).[107]

Grossly, the lungs are firm, red, and consolidated, without significant aeration. Microscopic examination reveals the presence of homogeneous lightly eosinophilic linear material closely adherent to the alveolar surface (Fig. 4-22A). These hyaline membranes may look relatively uniform, but they are actually composed of a myriad of materials, including cytoplasm and nucleoplasm of dead cells, plasma transudate, and amniotic fluid. Hyaline membranes form within 3 to 4 hours of birth and are well developed by 12 to 24 hours.

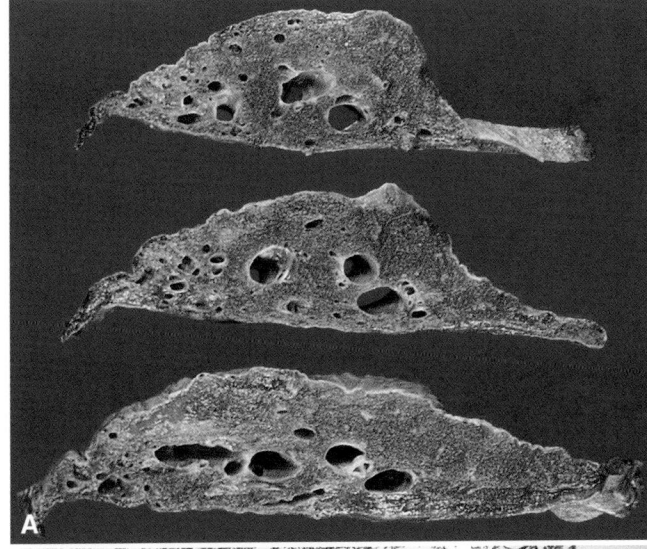

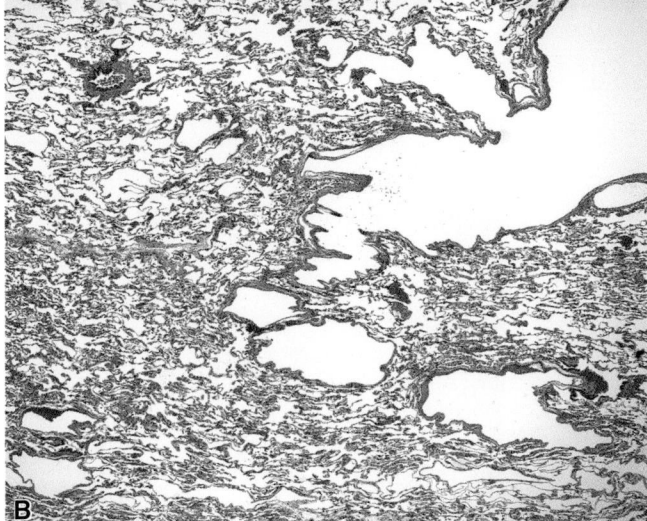

Figure 4-21. Arteriovenous malformation. **A,** Multiple ectatic vessels may be seen grossly in arteriovenous malformations. **B,** These enlarged dilated vessels are abnormally distributed within the lung parenchyma.

An interesting finding in jaundiced infants with acute lung injury is the presence of yellow hyaline membranes secondary to bilirubin staining[108] (see Fig. 4-22B). Complications of BPD have become relatively rare as a result of improvements in therapy, including surfactant replacement and advances in mechanical ventilation and oxygen therapy.[109] Of note, if numerous neutrophils accompany hyaline membranes, the possibility of acute infection should be considered, because these are not usual components of hyaline membrane disease.

Bronchopulmonary Dysplasia

BPD is a chronic lung disease that occurs in a proportion of children who require respiratory support in the neonatal period.[107,110-112] As the clinical treatment of prematurity has evolved, the pathologic appearance of this disease has changed.[109] The designation was first used for the chronic lung disease that developed subsequently in patients with previous hyaline membrane disease.[113] Examination of the lung in "classic" BPD showed a variegated pattern, with some lobules showing alveolar fibrosis and collapse, whereas adjacent lobules showed overdistention (Fig. 4-23A).[114-116] This appearance of the chronic disease

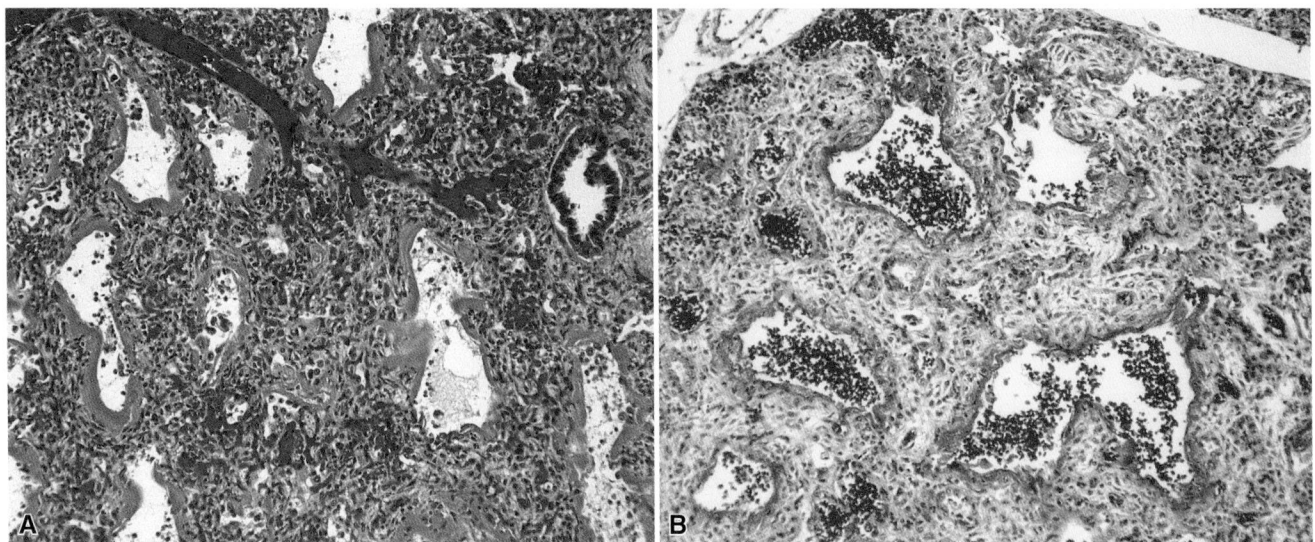

Figure 4-22. Hyaline membrane disease. **A,** Numerous hyaline membranes are seen lining the alveolar ducts and air spaces. Interstitial fibroblasts and congested alveolar capillaries thicken the alveolar septa. **B,** Yellow hyaline membranes may be observed in infants with respiratory distress syndrome and hyperbilirubinemia.

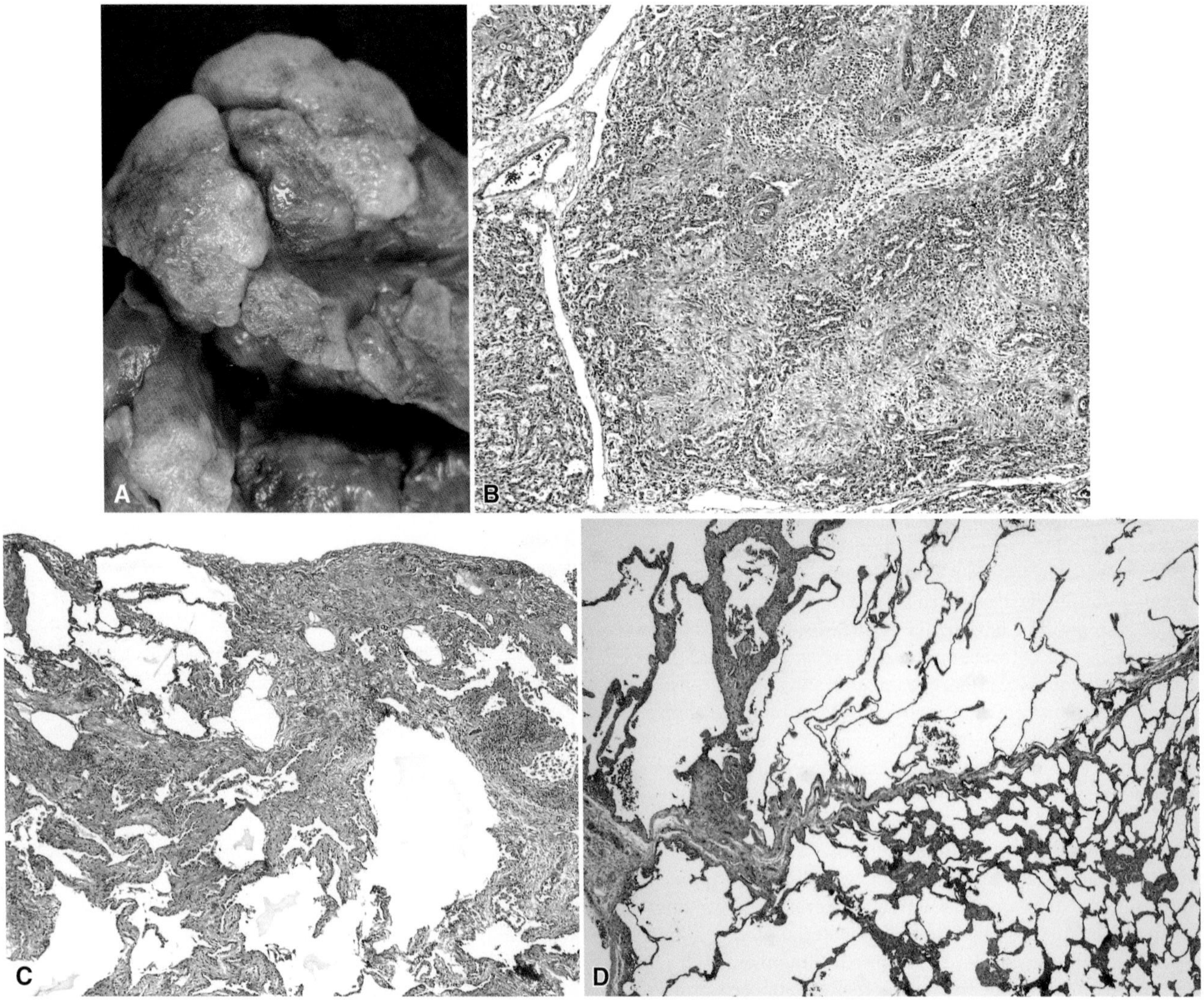

Figure 4-23. Bronchopulmonary dysplasia (BPD). **A,** Grossly, "classic" BPD shows pleural pseudofissures caused by septal fibrosis, pleural retraction, and regions of lobular hyperinflation. **B,** In the organizing phase, organization within alveolar ducts of a lobule is evident. The surrounding alveoli are atelectatic. **C,** In chronic BPD, patchy fibrosis and abnormally enlarged air spaces may be seen. **D,** Alternating zones of hyperinflation and parenchymal collapse are the result of proximal airway injury and stenosis of variable degree.

was explained by observations in the pre-existing hyaline membrane disease. Early cases of hyaline membrane disease showed areas of necrotizing bronchiolitis with poor aeration of distal alveolar parenchyma. These areas were subsequently spared from the continuous alveolar insult related to oxygen therapy and mechanical ventilation. As the bronchioles and hyaline membranes healed, airway and interstitial fibroblast proliferation occurred (see Fig. 4-23B). After fibrosis of the injured areas ensued, and healing of the bronchiole was complete, patchy fibrosis was evident in the affected regions, and nearly normal, overdistended alveoli were seen in the spared regions (see Fig. 4-23C and D).

In current practice, neonates at risk for hyaline membrane disease are treated with respiratory support and surfactant replacement therapy. This strategy obviates the need for intense oxygen therapy and the mechanical stress that occurred historically. Nevertheless, it is proposed that the lower levels of oxygen treatment in the current regimen result in a generalized uniform alveolar injury.[109] The injured alveoli continue to show maturation by thinning of their septa; however, there is a lack of additional subdivision and branching of the alveolar units of the lobule, thereby leading to an alveolar simplification, so-called "new" BPD.[109,112,117] This lack of normal maturation results in a decrease in the absolute numbers of alveoli. The alveolar walls may be of normal thickness or may be mildly fibrotic. As in polyalveolar lobe, radial alveolar counts can be used in BPD to assess the number of alveoli within lobules.[76,109]

Pediatric Interstitial Lung Disease

Attempts to classify pediatric interstitial lung disease with the same categories used in adults can result in difficulties in classification and even misclassification.[1] Several of the patterns of disease are similar in adults and in children, but the underlying etiology and prognosis may be different in pediatric cases.[118-123] So-called usual interstitial pneumonia (UIP) is virtually nonexistent in children.[124] Despite these differences, recognition of patterns of interstitial disease remains as important in the diagnosis of diffuse lung disease in children as it is in adults[125] (Box 4-3 and Table 4-2). The subtypes of interstitial lung disease are described separately in this section. Even if a precise diagnosis or underlying etiologic disorder cannot be established histologically, the pattern of injury should guide further diagnostic evaluation and in many cases will help to determine prognosis. Assessment of inflammation, and exclusion of infection, may be helpful in evaluating the potential role of steroid therapy also. Practically speaking, the most important diseases to recognize in the neonatal period are the abnormalities of alveolar development and growth, congenital disorders of surfactant metabolism, and alveolar capillary dysplasia. The most important diseases to consider in older children with chronic diffuse lung disease include obliterative bronchiolitis, collagen vascular disease, and hypersensitivity pneumonitis.

Alveolar Growth Abnormalities

Alveolar growth abnormalities are a group of disorders characterized morphologically by the presence of enlarged and simplified air spaces, indicating incomplete or altered alveolarization, either due to prenatal or postnatal factors. A common example of an alveolar growth abnormality, previously discussed, is chronic neonatal lung disease due to prematurity (see earlier section on BPD) (Fig. 4-24). However, sometimes a similar pattern is seen on lung biopsy from infants and young children, despite history of term gestation or lack of respiratory distress syndrome in the neonatal period. Considerations in the differential diagnosis in term infants include pulmonary hypoplasia; disordered lung growth due to underlying chromosomal syndromes

Box 4-3. Differential Diagnosis of Pediatric Diffuse Lung Disease

Alveolar growth abnormalities
    Chronic neonatal lung disease due to prematurity (bronchopulmonary dysplasia)
    Pulmonary hypoplasia
    Associated with Down syndrome, other chromosomal disorders, or congenital heart disease
Pulmonary interstitial glycogenosis (infantile cellular interstitial pneumonitis)
Infection—viral, mycoplasmal, fungal, mycobacterial, bacterial, parasitic
Hypersensitivity pneumonitis
Aspiration injury
Eosinophilic pneumonia
Drug reaction
Obliterative bronchiolitis (postviral, graft-versus-host disease, lung transplant rejection, Stevens-Johnson syndrome)
Neuroendocrine cell hyperplasia of infancy
Lymphoid hyperplasia due to primary or acquired immunodeficiency
    Lymphocytic interstitial pneumonitis
    Follicular bronchiolitis
Collagen vascular disease–related lung disease
Inflammatory bowel disease–related lung disease
Pulmonary hemosiderosis/capillaritis
Vasculopathy secondary to congenital heart disease or cardiomyopathy
    Pulmonary arteriopathy due to overcirculation (e.g., left to right cardiac shunt)
    Chronic congestive vasculopathy (e.g., pulmonary vein stenosis, chronic left ventricular failure)
Veno-occlusive disease
Alveolar capillary dysplasia with misalignment of pulmonary veins
Pulmonary lymphangiectasia or lymphangiomatosis
Genetic disorders of surfactant metabolism
    Pulmonary alveolar proteinosis
    Chronic pneumonitis of infancy
    Desquamative interstitial pneumonia
    Nonspecific interstitial pneumonia
    Pulmonary fibrosis
Other metabolic/storage diseases (e.g., Niemann-Pick disease, Gaucher disease)

Data from Swensen SJ, Hartman TE, Mayo JR, et al. Diffuse pulmonary lymphangiomatosis: CT findings. *J Comput Assist Tomogr.* 1995;19(3):348–352; Coren ME, Nicholson AG, Goldstraw P, et al. Open lung biopsy for diffuse interstitial lung disease in children. *Eur Respir J.* 1999;14(4):817–821; Fan LL, Mullen AL, Brugman SM, et al. Clinical spectrum of chronic interstitial lung disease in children. *J Pediatr.* 1992;121(6):867–872; Deutsch GH, Young LR, Deterding RR, et al: Diffuse lung disease in young children: application of a novel classification scheme. *Am J Respir Crit Care Med.* 2007;176:1120–1128; and Katzenstein AL, Myers JL. Idiopathic pulmonary fibrosis: clinical relevance of pathologic classification. *Am J Respir Crit Care Med.* 1998;157(4 Pt 1):1301–1315.

(e.g., Down syndrome, other trisomies), malformation syndromes, or congenital heart disease; and disordered lung growth due to poor postnatal alveolarization in the setting of severe neonatal illness. In some patients, impaired alveolarization is considered to be multifactorial—for example, a premature infant with Down syndrome and atrioventricular canal. This morphologic category, described as *alveolar growth abnormalities*, accounts for the largest subset of diffuse lung disease in infants,[123] and attention to alveolar architecture in a well-inflated lung biopsy specimen is essential for diagnosis. Generally speaking, this type of abnormality is likely to be underappreciated by pathologists who interpret predominantly adult lung biopsy specimens, because of the similarity of the enlarged infant air spaces to those in normal adult lung tissue or in emphysematous lung. Lack of interstitial fibrosis or inflammation in most cases also prevents recognition of impaired alveolar architecture as the primary abnormality. Other pathologic findings commonly associated with alveolar growth problems include pulmonary interstitial glycogenosis (discussed next) and secondary pulmonary arteriopathy. In infants with chronic lung disease due to prematurity, these findings may help to explain exacerbation of disease or clinical severity that is disproportionate to that expected for gestational age.

Table 4-2. Histologic Clues in Interstitial Lung Disease

Histologic Finding	Consider
Diffuse type II pneumocyte hyperplasia	Acute lung injury (proliferative diffuse alveolar damage, viral pneumonitis) Genetic disorders of surfactant metabolism
Alveolar macrophages	
Siderophages	Pulmonary capillaritis Collagen vascular disease Coagulopathy with recurrent hemorrhage Chronic congestive vasculopathy (PVS, VOD, left ventricular obstruction) Idiopathic pulmonary hemosiderosis
Foamy (vacuolated) macrophages	Aspiration pneumonia Metabolic storage disorders Genetic disorders of surfactant metabolism Airway obstruction, postobstructive pneumonia Endogenous lipoid pneumonia in peripheral lung cysts
With eosinophils and fibrin	Eosinophilic pneumonia
Lightly pigmented or nonpigmented	Desquamative interstitial pneumonia Drug reaction
Granular proteinaceous material	Genetic disorders of surfactant metabolism Pulmonary alveolar proteinosis *Pneumocystis* infection Infection (especially viral pneumonitis with epithelial necrosis)
Organizing pneumonia	Infection Collagen vascular disease Hypersensitivity pneumonitis Idiopathic
Alveolar septal thickening by lymphocytes	
Bronchiolocentric	Hypersensitivity pneumonitis Infection (e.g., viral bronchiolitis) Aspiration pneumonia Cystic fibrosis Collagen vascular disease Primary ciliary dyskinesia
Nonspecific interstitial pneumonia	Collagen vascular disease Hypersensitivity pneumonitis Genetic disorders of surfactant metabolism (older children)
Lymphocytic interstitial pneumonia	Primary immunodeficiency HIV infection Sjögren syndrome
Follicular bronchiolitis	Primary immunodeficiency (e.g., CVID) HIV infection Epstein-Barr virus infection Collagen vascular disease
Alveolar septal thickening	
By fibrosis	Bronchopulmonary dysplasia
By increased cellularity	Pulmonary interstitial glycogenosis (infantile cellular interstitial pneumonia)
By edema or muscular arterioles	Vascular/cardiogenic disease
With few central capillaries	Alveolar capillary dysplasia with misalignment of pulmonary veins

CVID, common variable immunodeficiency; PVS, pulmonary vein stenosis; VOD, veno-occlusive disease.

Pulmonary Interstitial Glycogenosis (Infantile Cellular Interstitial Pneumonitis)

Pulmonary interstitial glycogenosis (PIG), also called infantile cellular interstitial pneumonitis, is a disorder that occurs in infants younger than than 6 months of age, with the highest frequency in neonates. These infants develop tachypnea and respiratory distress, and chest radiographs may show bilateral interstitial infiltrates. Microscopic evaluation shows variable thickening of the alveolar septa due to a proliferation of round to oval bland mesenchymal cells (Fig. 4-25), with a paucity of inflammatory cells.[126] The spindle cells contain cytoplasmic glycogen granules demonstrable by their periodic acid/Schiff (PAS)–positive, diastase-digestible staining characteristics.[127,128] The process may be diffuse or patchy, with great variability in severity. It is vastly underreported in the medical literature and can be identified in the setting of a wide variety of associated conditions, including chronic neonatal lung disease due to prematurity, hypoplasia, congenital heart disease, and even congenital cystic malformations. Although initially proposed to be a genetic or developmental condition,[129] recognition of the many associated conditions has led to the concept that PIG is a reactive response to injury unique to the infant lung, perhaps reflecting differences in the proliferative capacity of the growing neonatal lung. Affected patients sometimes require ventilatory support, but they tend to show good recovery from their disease over the course of weeks, and steroid therapy has been used with symptomatic improvement in some cases. Prognosis generally is thought to relate to the severity of any underlying associated pathology, such as chronic neonatal lung disease.

Genetic Disorders of Surfactant Metabolism

The genetic disorders of surfactant metabolism have been associated with several different histologic patterns, including pulmonary alveolar proteinosis (PAP), chronic pneumonitis of infancy (CIP), desquamative interstitial pneumonia (DIP), nonspecific interstitial pneumonia (NSIP), and idiopathic pulmonary fibrosis.[130,131] The dominant histologic features probably depend on the genotype and the age at presentation. Generally speaking, neonates and infants have more abundant alveolar proteinosis material and more prominent alveolar epithelial hyperplasia, whereas older children and adolescents have less conspicuous globular proteinosis material, less epithelial hyperplasia, more abundant cholesterol clefts, and more abundant fibrosis. Presentation in the neonatal period is typical of surfactant protein B gene mutations and *ABCA3* mutations. Presentation in later infancy, childhood, or adolescence is more typical of *ABCA3* mutations or surfactant protein C gene mutations.

The histologic patterns associated with these genetic surfactant disorders are discussed next, including practical considerations for differential diagnosis.

Pulmonary Alveolar Proteinosis

PAP is characterized by the accumulation of granular-appearing proteinaceous material within the alveolar spaces[132] and is subdivided into congenital, acquired, and secondary forms.

Congenital forms of pulmonary alveolar proteinosis are progressive fatal diseases caused by defects in surfactant production and metabolism, and have been reported from mutations of the surfactant protein B gene and the *ABCA3* gene, the latter probably related to packaging and secretion of surfactant proteins[133–137] (Fig. 4-26A to C). This form of PAP typically is accompanied by prominent diffuse type 2 alveolar epithelial hyperplasia, increased alveolar macrophages, and occasional cholesterol clefts. Over a period of weeks, diffuse interstitial widening and chronic remodeling of air spaces can be recognized. Electron microscopy may be helpful in assessing lamellar body ultrastructure.[138,139] Presence of multivesicular bodies associated

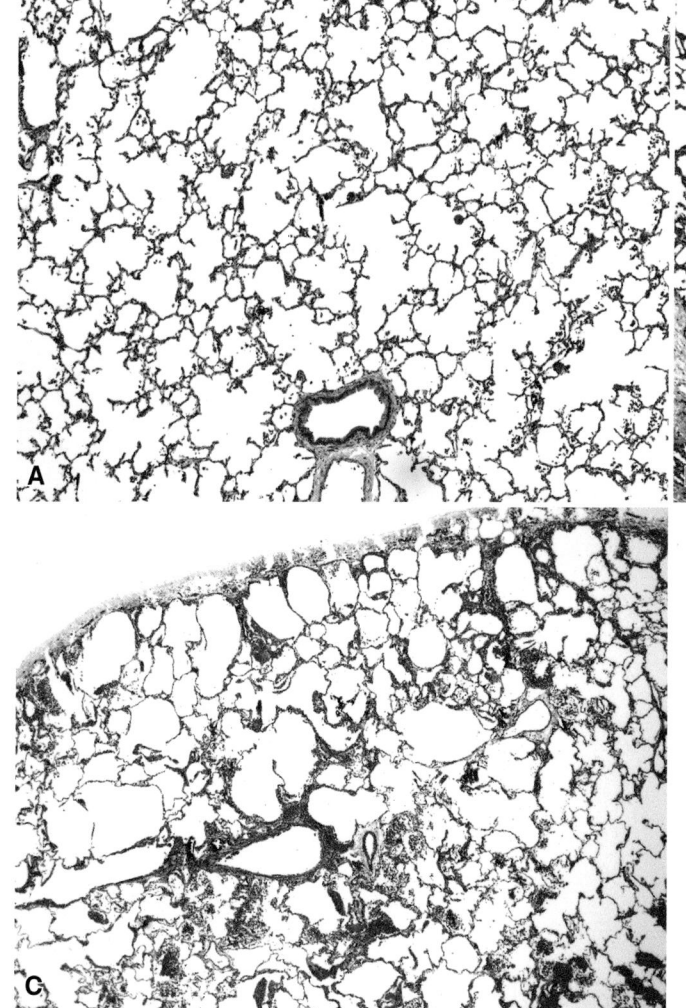

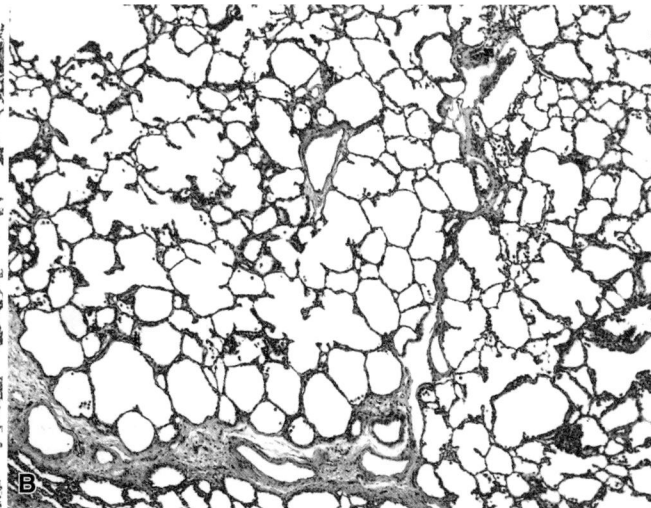

Figure 4-24. Alveolar growth abnormalities. In the post–surfactant era, chronic neonatal lung disease due to prematurity ("new" bronchopulmonary dysplasia) is characterized by impaired alveolarization. Compared with lung from a normal term infant (**A**), lung from a premature infant shows mildly enlarged and simplified air spaces with deficient septation (**B**). **C,** The deficient alveolarization often is accentuated in the subpleural region. A similar histologic pattern is seen in the setting of pulmonary hypoplasia and in some infants with chromosomal syndromes and/or cardiac malformations.

with *SFTPB* gene mutations or dense bodies associated with *ABCA3* mutations (see Fig. 4-26D) help to confirm the diagnostic impression based on histologic pattern, although normal lamellar bodies do not exclude a genetic disorder of surfactant metabolism. Definitive characterization of disease also requires correlation with mutation testing. Considerations in the differential diagnosis for congenital PAP include acquired PAP and secondary PAP.

Acquired PAP is unusual in infants and children but may be observed in adolescents. Acquired PAP is thought to arise as a result of autoantibodies to granulocyte-macrophage colony-stimulating factor (GM-CSF) and is more common in adults. Of interest, an identical pattern of disease has been described in children with genetic mutations in the GM-CSF receptor.[140,141] The same pattern is occasionally seen in children and adolescents with underlying systemic disorders such as leukemia, bone marrow transplantation, and collagen vascular diseases, despite absence of autoantibodies to GM-CSF. PAP in this setting generally is considered to be a problem of macrophage dysfunction and impaired surfactant recycling, although the mechanism of disease is not clear.

Finally, *secondary* PAP is observed in infants and children with infections causing extensive alveolar epithelial necrosis. The most common infections implicated are those caused by respiratory syncytial virus, cytomegalovirus, and parainfluenza virus. Occasionally, it is possible to recognize increased inflammation or viral cytopathic changes such as multinucleate giant cells in secondary PAP (Fig. 4-27). Affected patients frequently are immunosuppressed with severe

combined immunodeficiency syndrome, leukemia, or lysinuria.[142-145] *Pneumocystis* infection also should be excluded in this clinical setting.

Chronic Pneumonitis of Infancy

Initially recognized in 1992 and later named by Katzenstein and colleagues in 1995, CPI is a pattern of diffuse interstitial lung disease in infants and young children, which has now been recognized to be associated with the genetic disorders of surfactant metabolism, most commonly mutations in the surfactant protein C gene (*SFTPC*)[146–149] (Fig. 4-28). Microscopically, the lungs show alveolar septal thickening by fibroblastic spindle cells, and marked type II pneumocyte hyperplasia. Inflammation and fibrosis are sparse, although conspicuous remodeling of air spaces and interstitial extension of airway smooth muscle are commonly seen. Consolidation by air space macrophages, proteinaceous material, and cholesterol clefts is a frequent finding. Prognosis generally is poor, with development of chronic lung disease or death in a majority of affected infants. Surfactant protein C gene mutations are inherited in an autosomal dominant fashion, and pulmonary fibrosis has been recognized in some families of infants with CPI.

Desquamative Interstitial Pneumonia

In adults, DIP generally is a smoking-related illness resulting in filling of the alveoli with lightly pigmented macrophages. In children, a DIP pattern evokes an array of possible diagnoses including the genetic disorders of surfactant metabolism, particularly surfactant protein B and ABCA3 defects, various viral infections, aspiration, drug

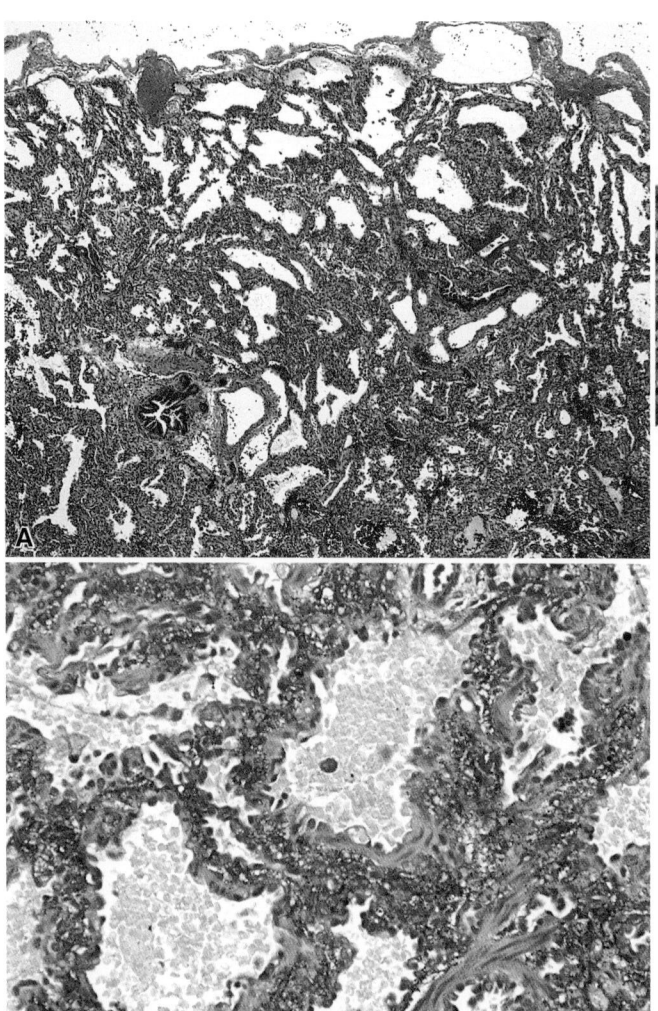

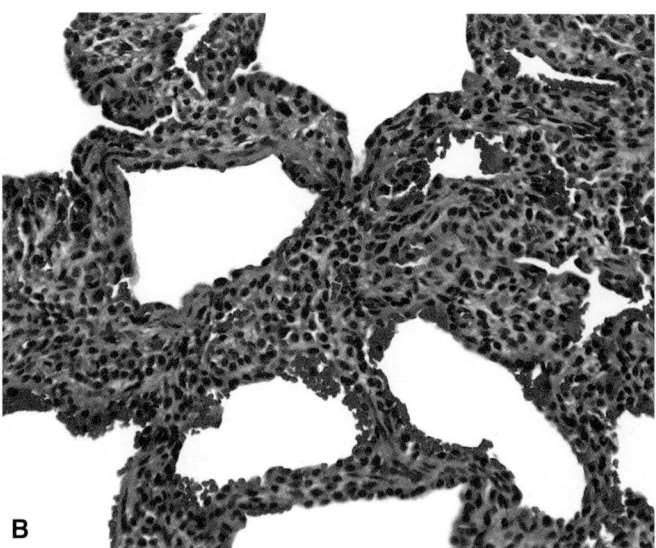

Figure 4-25. Pulmonary interstitial glycogenosis (infantile cellular interstitial pneumonia). Probably a reactive condition unique to the infant lung, pulmonary interstitial glycogenosis often is associated with abnormalities of alveolar growth or pulmonary arteriopathy. **A** and **B,** The alveolar septa are thickened by numerous round and spindle mesenchymal cells. **C,** Periodic acid–Schiff reagent (PAS) staining highlights cytoplasmic glycogen in these cells.

reactions, and inhalational injury. In some cases of DIP occurring in early childhood, stabilization has been achieved with systemic corticosteroid treatment.[118,125]

Nonspecific Interstitial Pneumonia

The term *nonspecific interstitial pneumonia* (NSIP) is used to describe idiopathic pulmonary diseases that show a uniform expansion of the alveolar septa by inflammation, fibrosis, or both.[150] NSIP is a relatively commonly observed interstitial disease pattern in children,[118] but further investigation often allows identification of a specific etiologic disorder. Presence of mild to moderate diffuse lymphocyte infiltrates (NSIP pattern) in the pediatric population raises various diagnostic possibilities including chronic disease due to the genetic disorders of surfactant metabolism (*ABCA3*, *SFTPC*), viral pneumonitis, hypersensitivity pneumonitis, and collagen vascular diseases.

Lymphocytic Interstitial Pneumonia and Follicular Bronchiolitis

Follicular bronchiolitis and lymphocytic interstitial pneumonia in children is histologically identical to that observed in adults. The presence of lymphocyte aggregates with germinal centers surrounding

bronchioles is characteristic of follicular bronchiolitis (Fig. 4-29), whereas a robust and diffuse lymphocytic interstitial infiltrate of the alveolar walls is the key finding in lymphocytic interstitial pneumonia (Fig. 4-30). Both patterns represent forms of pulmonary lymphoid hyperplasia, and may be observed in the same biopsy. Follicular bronchiolitis can be observed in patients with immune deficiencies such as common variable immune deficiency or hypogammaglobulinemia,[125,151] collagen vascular diseases such as juvenile rheumatoid arthritis or Sjögren syndrome,[125,152–154] or acquired immunodeficiency due to maternal-fetal transmission of human immunodeficiency virus (HIV).[155–160] Follicular bronchiolitis also should prompt consideration of Epstein-Barr virus infection.

Hypersensitivity Pneumonitis (Extrinsic Allergic Alveolitis)

Hypersensitivity pneumonitis in children is clinically and histologically similar to that seen in adults. The patient generally presents with exercise intolerance and cough. Although the list of antigens in the adult form of the disease is relatively broad as a result of a vast array of occupational exposures, a majority of the cases in children involve either bird antigens (70%) or molds (15%).[161,162] Histologically, hypersensitivity pneumonitis is characterized by a diffuse interstitial

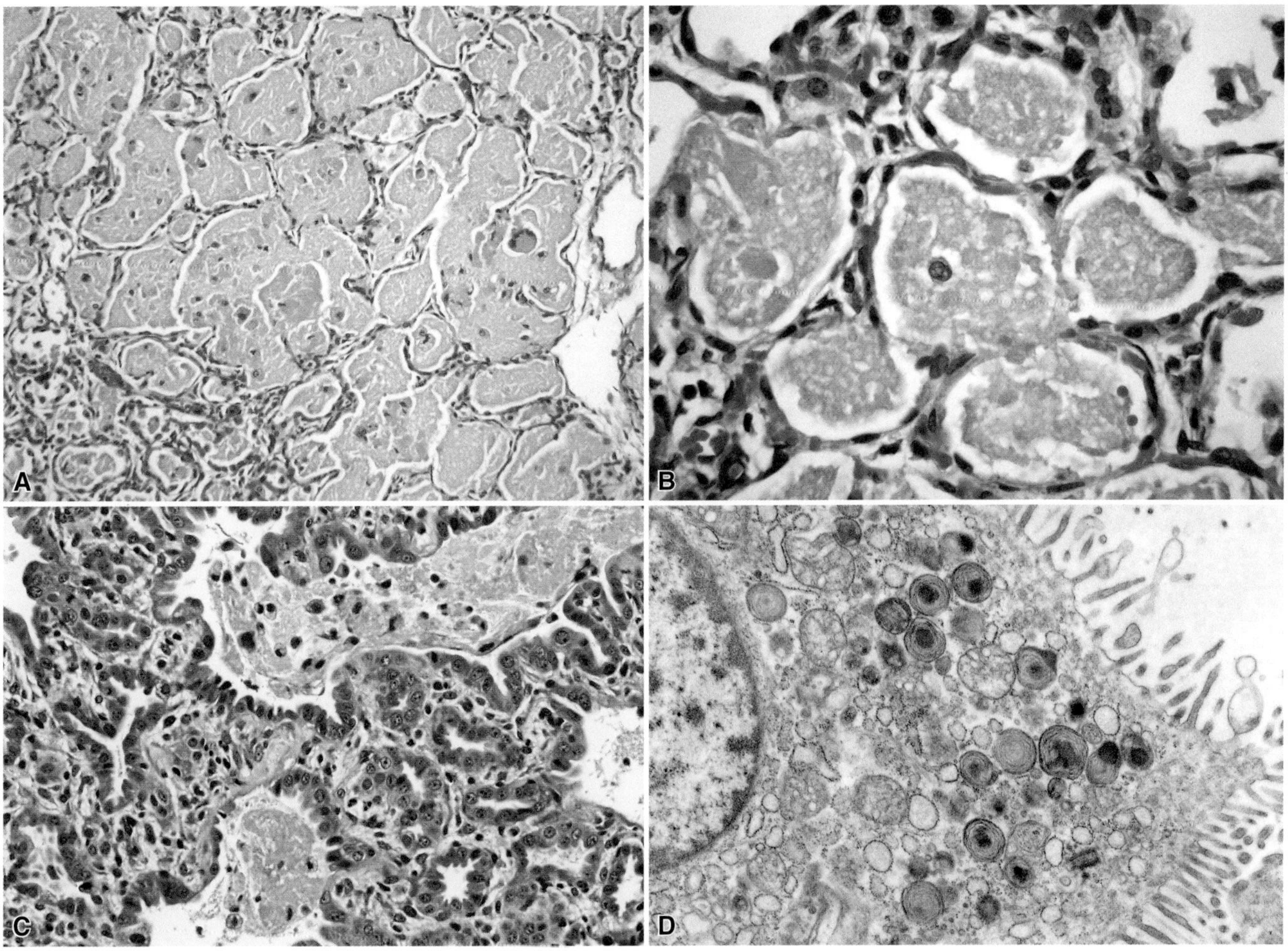

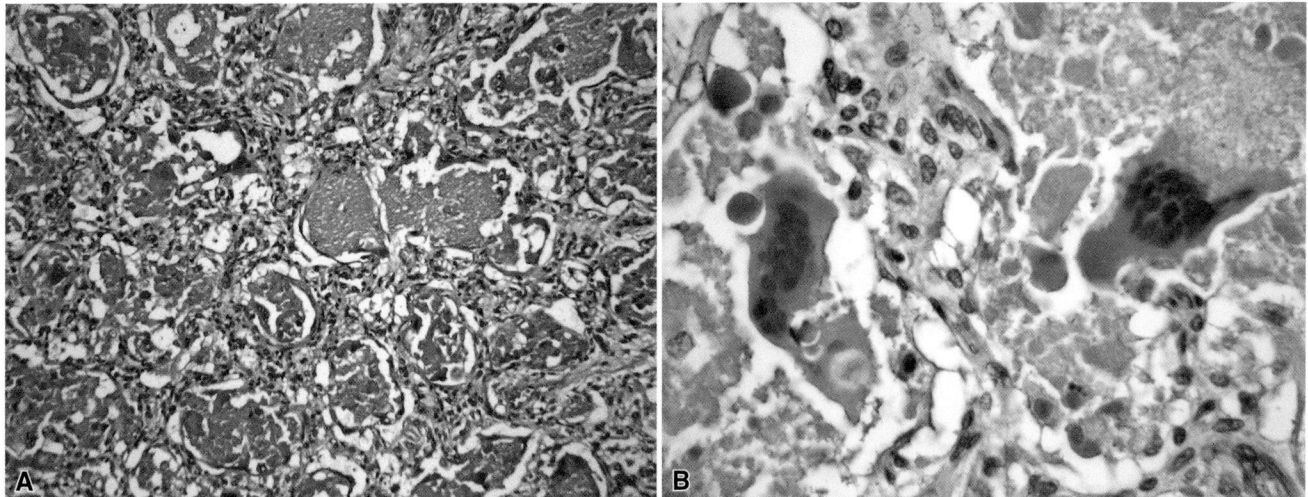

Figure 4-26. Genetic disorders of surfactant metabolism. Mutations in genes affecting surfactant metabolism result in various histologic patterns in infancy. **A** and **B,** Surfactant protein B gene (*SFTPB*) mutations cause accumulation of alveolar proteinaceous material and increased alveolar macrophages. **C,** Alveolar proteinosis typically is accompanied by diffuse alveolar epithelial hyperplasia, as in this patient with homozygous *ABCA3* gene mutations. **D,** Electron microscopy confirms the presence of abnormal small lamellar bodies with round dense bodies, characteristic of *ABCA3* mutations.

Figure 4-27. Pulmonary alveolar proteinosis. The differential diagnosis for pulmonary alveolar proteinosis includes the surfactant gene abnormalities, antibody-mediated dysfunction of the GM-CSF receptor, *Pneumocystis jiroveci* infection, and extensive alveolar epithelial necrosis. **A** and **B,** The alveolar epithelial necrosis evident in these photomicrographs was due to florid respiratory syncytial virus infection in an immunocompromised child.

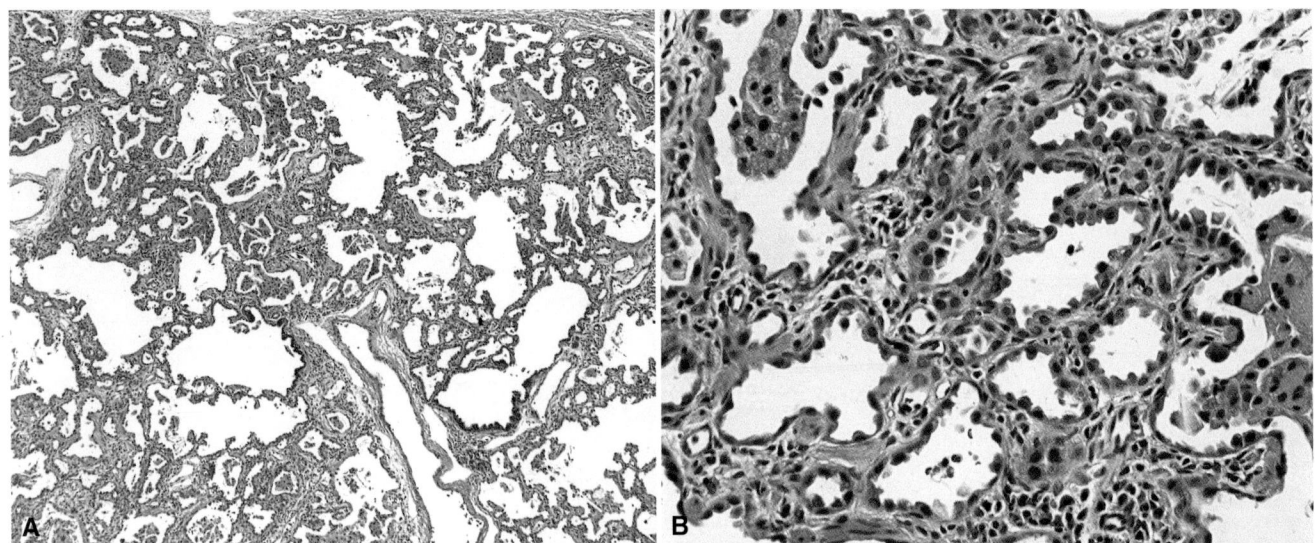

Figure 4-28. A and **B**, Genetic disorders of surfactant metabolism. Chronic pneumonitis of infancy is a histologic pattern often associated with mutations in the surfactant protein C (*SFTPC*) gene. This pattern is characterized by remodeled air spaces with thickened septa, sparse interstitial inflammation, prominent type II pneumocyte hyperplasia, clustered foamy alveolar macrophages, and occasional cholesterol clefts.

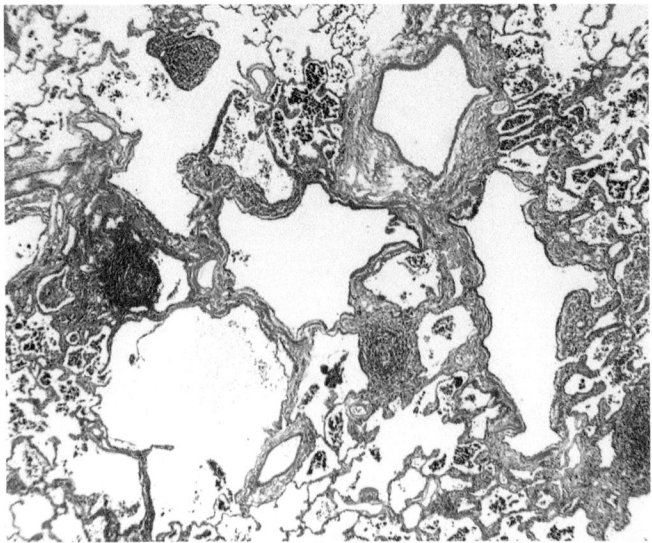

Figure 4-29. Lymphoid hyperplasia. In this example of lung involvement in juvenile rheumatoid arthritis, hemosiderin-filled macrophages are noted in air spaces, prominent lymphocyte follicles (follicular bronchiolitis) are present, and there is overinflation. Cystic changes were noted on computed tomography.

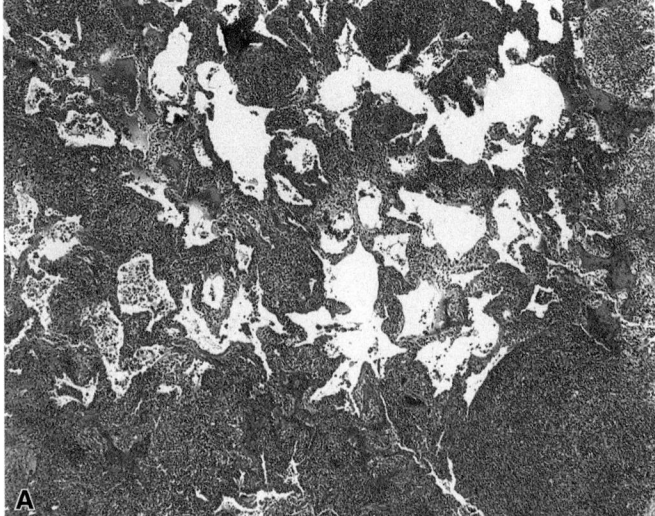

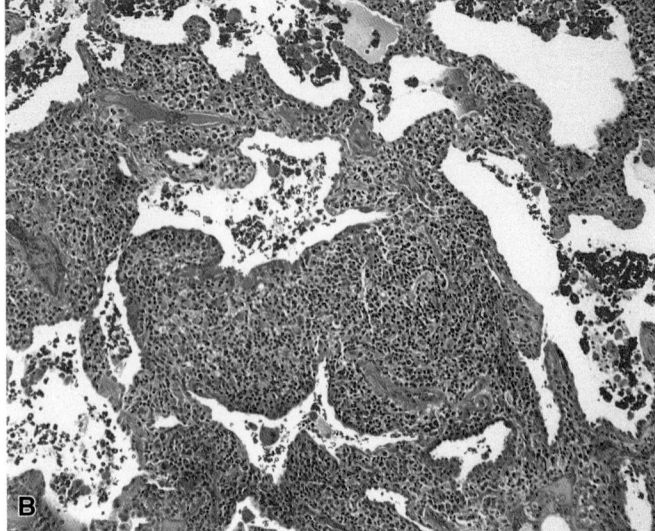

Figure 4-30. Congenital human immunodeficiency virus (HIV) infection. **A** and **B**, Numerous lymphocyte follicles are present, and the interstitium is broadly expanded by a lymphocytic infiltrate.

lymphocytic infiltrate with bronchiolocentric accentuation and scattered poorly formed granulomas. The air spaces may show consolidation, with macrophages or organizing pneumonia.

Eosinophilic Pneumonia

Eosinophilic pneumonia in children is similar in appearance to that in adults. The causes also are similar, with many cases being secondary to drug reactions, parasite infections, or systemic diseases.[163] Many cases are idiopathic. The histologic triad of eosinophils, macrophages, and fibrin filling the alveolar spaces usually is easily appreciated in acute eosinophilic pneumonia (Fig. 4-31).

Aspiration Injury

Children with abnormal swallowing function, or gastroesophageal reflux, may aspirate food or gastric fluids into the lung, resulting in aspiration injury. Diagnosis using oil red O stains for lipophages on bronchoalveolar lavage specimens has been suggested. Although this method is relatively sensitive, it is not very specific, since many other diseases including storage diseases, resolving hemorrhage, and resolving pneumonia can result in increased lipophages.[164] The histologic features associated with aspiration are variable and often nonspecific, making aspiration a difficult diagnosis to make with certainty. Accumulation of intra-alveolar foamy macrophages and cholesterol clefts occasionally is observed (Fig. 4-32A). Presence of aspirated food particles or interstitial lipid vacuoles, as in exogenous lipoid pneumonia due to mineral oil aspiration (see Fig. 4-32B), will point to a specific diagnosis. Chronic airway irritation can result in follicular bronchiolitis or organizing pneumonia with granulation tissue plugs occurring within airway lumina. In severe chronic cases, bronchiectasis can occur.[165] Aspirated food particles may elicit a surrounding granulomatous reaction.[166] An interesting but unusual interaction has been described in infants in whom aspiration of fat or oils occurs coincident with the development of infection by rapid-growing mycobacteria, resulting in a lipoid pneumonia with granulomas.[167] Acid-fast bacteria can be demonstrated within the lipid droplets in such cases (see Fig. 4-32C).

Obliterative Bronchiolitis

In children, airway obliteration may follow any form of chronic small- and large-airway injury, particularly that resulting in airway mucosal necrosis followed by fibrosis. Common etiologic conditions include

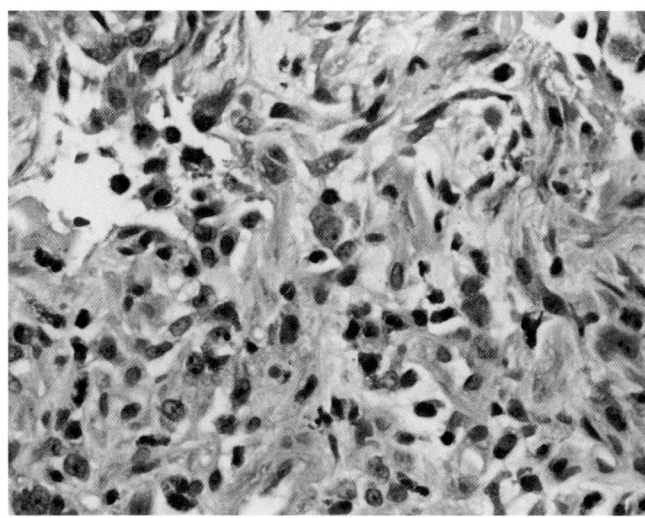

Figure 4-31. Eosinophilic pneumonia. Histopathologic features include interstitial eosinophils and alveolitis, often with organization of hyaline membranes and fibroblast proliferation.

preceding severe viral bronchiolitis (e.g., adenovirus or influenza infection), chronic aspiration injury, Stevens-Johnson syndrome, chronic graft-versus-host disease in bone marrow transplant recipients, and chronic airway rejection in lung transplant recipients[168] (Fig. 4-33).

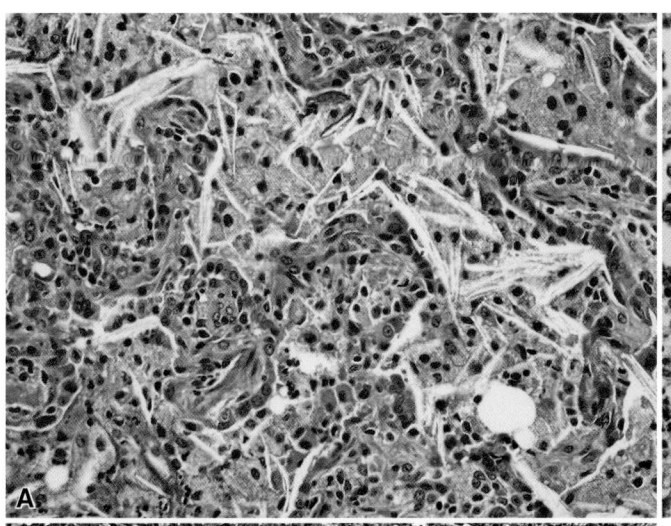

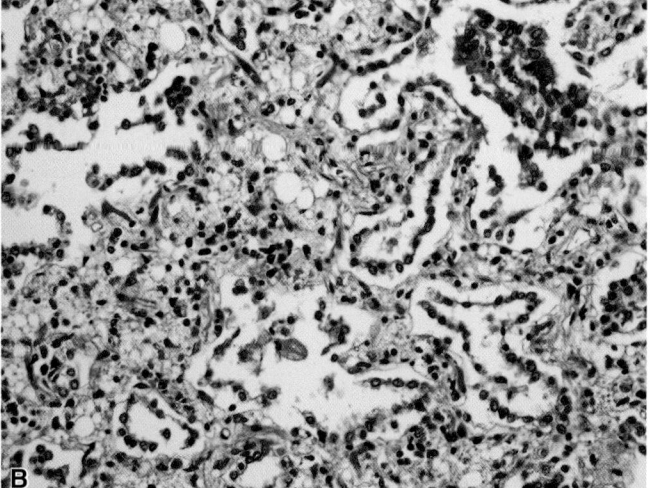

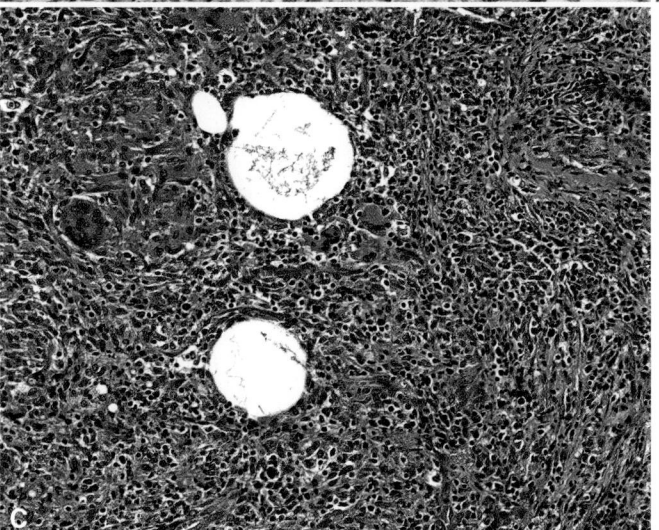

Figure 4-32. Aspiration injury. Aspiration injury may be difficult to diagnosis with certainty, but in florid examples as in part **A,** findings will include abundant foamy macrophages and cholesterol clefts. Food particles and granulomatous inflammation may be seen in older children and adolescents. **B,** Exogenous lipoid pneumonia due to mineral oil aspiration is characterized by interstitial vacuoles as well as foamy macrophages and areas of reactive alveolar epithelial hyperplasia. **C,** The interaction of aspirated lipid and rapid-growing mycobacteria creates an unusual lipoid granulomatous pneumonia with vacuoles surrounded by neutrophils and a histiocytic reaction with multinucleate giant cells. Stains for acid-fast bacilli revealed clusters of organisms within the vacuoles in this case.

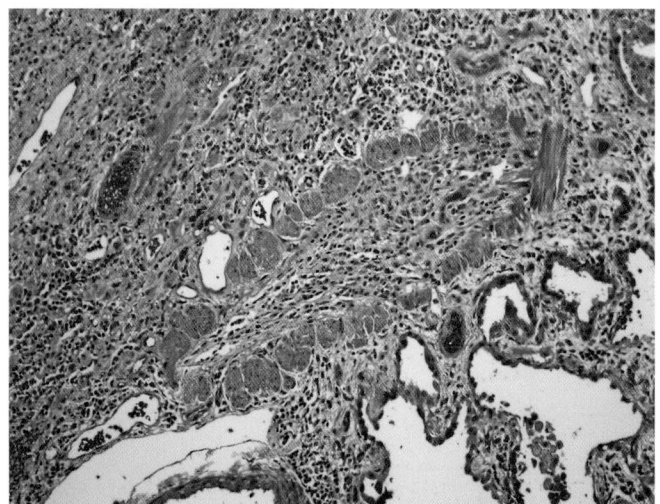

Figure 4-33. Obliterative bronchiolitis. Obliterated small airways may be a complication of preceding viral bronchiolitis, aspiration injury, graft-versus-host disease, and chronic airway rejection in transplant recipients.

Asthma and cystic fibrosis also may result in focal obliterative bronchiolitis.

Neuroendocrine Cell Hyperplasia of Infancy (Persistent Tachypnea of Infancy)

Neuroendocrine cell hyperplasia of infancy (NEHI) is a more recently described pathologic correlate to the clinical syndrome of persistent tachypnea of infancy.[169–171] Patients with NEHI are infants and young children with clinical signs and symptoms of chronic tachypnea and hypoxia, often with chronic oxygen requirement, and evidence of hyperinflated lungs on the chest radiograph and patchy perihilar ground-glass opacity on the chest CT scan.[172] Morphologically, the lung biopsy tissue appears almost normal, with only mild lymphoid hyperplasia and subtle alveolar duct expansion (Fig. 4-34). The virtually "normal" biopsy specimen and presence of appropriate alveolarization should prompt further evaluation for NEHI. The diagnosis is made by identifying increased numbers of airway neuroendocrine cells and large neuroepithelial bodies on special stains (e.g., bombesin

immunohistochemistry). It remains unknown whether this is a disorder with genetic predisposition or a reactive condition secondary to other forms of small- or large-airway injury. Some children have a history of preceding viral bronchiolitis, and familial cases have been recognized.

Storage Disorders

Lysosomal storage disorders, such as Niemann-Pick disease and mucolipidosis, may manifest with infiltrative lung disease. The histologic hallmark is the presence of confluent foamy, finely vacuolated macrophages, not only within air spaces but also within the interstitium or connective tissue of the bronchovascular bundles, interlobular septa, or pleura. Glycogen storage disease and Gaucher disease may also manifest with accumulation of macrophages within air spaces and within the septal connective tissues.

Vascular Disease as a Cause of Interstitial Lung Disease

Vascular diseases, especially those related to congenital heart defects, can mimic interstitial lung disease (ILD) clinically and radiologically.[119,120,173–175] Although many of these cases are identified before biopsy, it is important to consider a vascular cause in analysis of a wedge biopsy specimen from a patient being evaluated for ILD.

Hemorrhage Syndromes in Children

Chronic recurrent hemorrhage in children may result from recurrent episodes of pulmonary vasculitis, often small-vessel vasculitides such as capillaritis (Fig. 4-35A and B).[176,177] Other considerations in the differential diagnosis include chronic recurrent hemorrhage due to coagulopathy, chronic hemorrhage due to pulmonary arteriopathy, chronic congestive vasculopathy and pulmonary veno-occlusive disease (see Fig. 4-35C), and idiopathic pulmonary hemosiderosis. Chronic pulmonary hemorrhage has been described in milk aspiration (Heiner syndrome). Of note, idiopathic pulmonary hemosiderosis is a clinicopathologic diagnosis applied when abundant hemosiderin-laden macrophages are present on biopsy, without other associated pathologic changes, and the clinical etiology remains unknown.

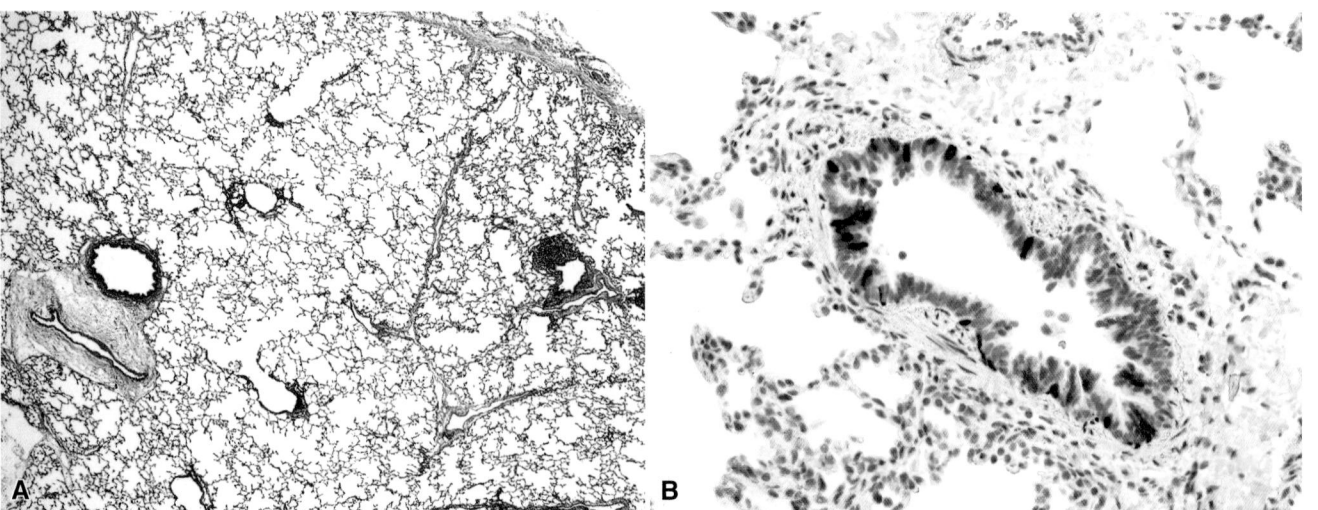

Figure 4-34. Neuroendocrine cell hyperplasia of infancy (NEHI). In some infants with persistent tachypnea and chronic oxygen requirement, the degree of clinical severity is disproportionate to pathologic findings on lung biopsy. **A,** A near-normal lung biopsy specimen with only mild lymphoid hyperplasia and alveolar duct distention raises consideration of NEHI. **B,** Immunohistochemical staining for bombesin confirms increased numbers of airway neuroendocrine cells. Obliterative bronchiolitis should be ruled out.

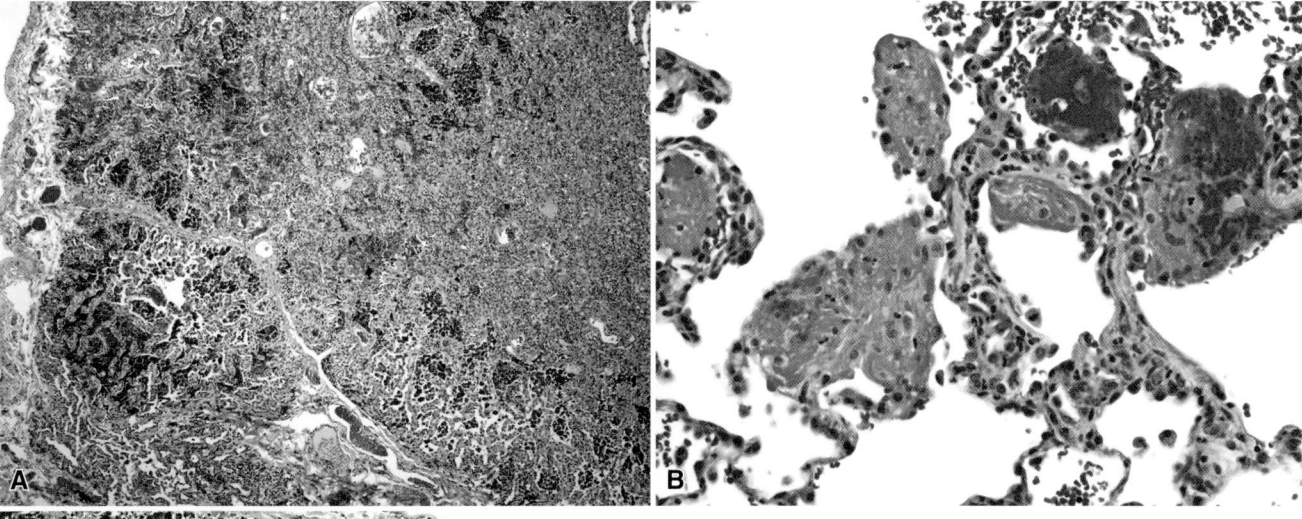

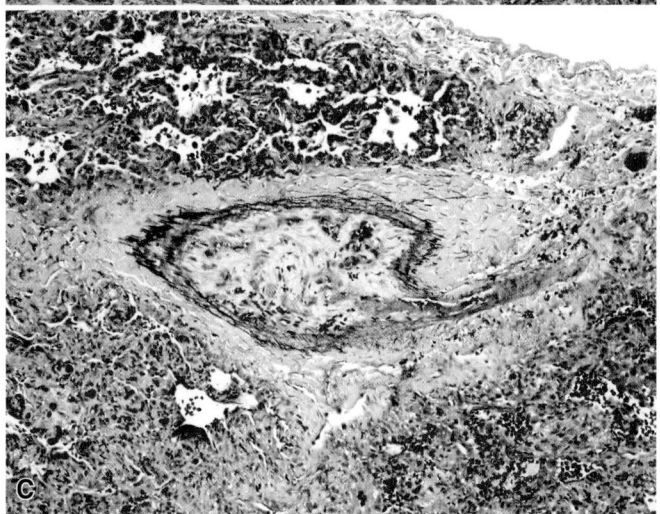

Figure 4-35. Pulmonary hemorrhage syndromes. **A,** Depending on timing of biopsy, chronic hemorrhage syndromes produce abundant hemosiderin-laden macrophages, with or without an admixture of acute alveolar hemorrhage. **B,** In acute capillaritis, common histopathologic features include subtle infiltrates of neutrophils in the alveolar walls and alveolar spaces, admixed with focal fibrin aggregates and acute hemorrhage. **C,** Abundant hemosiderin-laden macrophages also should prompt a search for chronic congestive vasculopathy and other causes of venous obstruction, as in this case of pulmonary veno-occlusive disease (Movat pentachrome stain).

Self-assessment questions related to this chapter can be found online on the Expert Consult site for this title.

References

1. Fan LL, Langston C. Pediatric interstitial lung disease: children are not small adults. *Am J Respir Crit Care Med.* 2002;165(11):1466–1467.
2. Langston C, Patterson K, Dishop MK, et al. A protocol for the handling of tissue obtained by operative lung biopsy: recommendations of the Child Pathology Co-operative Group. *Pediatr Dev Pathol.* 2006;9:173–180.
3. Langston C. New concepts in the pathology of congenital lung malformations. *Semin Pediatr Surg.* 2003;12(1):17–37.
4. Aktogu S, Yuncu G, Halilcolar H, et al. Bronchogenic cysts: clinicopathological presentation and treatment. *Eur Respir J.* 1996;9(10):2017–2021.
5. Cioffi U, Bonavina L, De Simone M, et al. Presentation and surgical management of bronchogenic and esophageal duplication cysts in adults. *Chest.* 1998;113(6):1492–1496.
6. Coselli MP, de Ipolyi P, Bloss RS, et al. Bronchogenic cysts above and below the diaphragm: report of eight cases. *Ann Thorac Surg.* 1987;44(5):491–494.
7. Kanemitsu Y, Nakayama H, Asamura H, et al. Clinical features and management of bronchogenic cysts: report of 17 cases. *Surg Today.* 1999;29(11):1201–1205.
8. Riedlinger WF, Vargas SO, Jenning RW, et al. Bronchial atresia is common to extralobar sequestration, intralobar sequestration, congenital cystic adenomatoid malformation, and lobar emphysema. *Pediatr Dev Pathol.* 2006;9:361–373.
9. Kunisaki SM, Fauza DO, Nemes LP, et al. Bronchial atresia: the hidden pathology within a spectrum of prenatally diagnosed lung masses. *J Pediatr Surg.* 2006;41(1):61–65.
10. Louie HW, Martin SM, Mulder DG. Pulmonary sequestration: 17-year experience at UCLA. *Am Surg.* 1993;59(12):801–805.
11. Stocker JT. Sequestrations of the lung. *Semin Diagn Pathol.* 1986;3(2):106–121.
12. Stocker JT, Drake RM, Madewell JE. Cystic and congenital lung disease in the newborn. *Perspect Pediatr Pathol.* 1978;4:93–154.
13. Stocker JT, Kagan-Hallet K. Extralobar pulmonary sequestration: analysis of 15 cases. *Am J Clin Pathol.* 1979;72(6):917–925.
14. Aulicino MR, Reis ED, Dolgin SE, et al. Intra-abdominal pulmonary sequestration exhibiting congenital cystic adenomatoid malformation. Report of a case and review of the literature. *Arch Pathol Lab Med.* 1994;118(10):1034–1037.
15. Morad NA, al-Malki T, e-Tahir M. Intra-abdominal pulmonary sequestration: diagnostic difficulties. *Pathology.* 1997;29(2):218–220.
16. Chan YF, Oldfield R, Vogel S, et al. Pulmonary sequestration presenting as a prenatally detected suprarenal lesion in a neonate. *J Pediatr Surg.* 2000;35(9):1367–1369.
17. Rosado-de-Christenson ML, Frazier AA, Stocker JT, et al. From the archives of the AFIP. Extralobar sequestration: radiologic-pathologic correlation. *Radiographics.* 1993;13(2):425–441.
18. Zangwill BC, Stocker JT. Congenital cystic adenomatoid malformation within an extralobar pulmonary sequestration. *Pediatr Pathol.* 1993;13(3):309–315.
19. Conran RM, Stocker JT. Extralobar sequestration with frequently associated congenital cystic adenomatoid malformation, type 2: report of 50 cases. *Pediatr Dev Pathol.* 1999;2(5):454–463.
20. Cass DL, Crombleholme TM, Howell LJ, et al. Cystic lung lesions with systemic arterial blood supply: a hybrid of congenital cystic adenomatoid malformation and bronchopulmonary sequestration. *J Pediatr Surg.* 1997;32(7):986–990.
21. Fraggetta F, Cacciaguerra S, Nash R, et al. Intra-abdominal pulmonary sequestration associated with congenital cystic adenomatoid malformation of the lung: just an unusual combination of rare pathologies? *Pathol Res Pract.* 1998;194(3):209–211.
22. Frazier AA, Rosado-De-Christenson ML, Stocker JT, et al. Intralobar sequestration: radiologic-pathologic correlation. *Radiographics.* 1997;17(3):725–745.
23. Zylak CJ, Eyler WR, Spizarny DL, et al. Developmental lung anomalies in the adult: radiologic-pathologic correlation. *Radiographics.* 2002;22(Spec No):S25–S43.
24. Au VW, Chan JK, Chan FL. Pulmonary sequestration diagnosed by contrast enhanced three-dimensional MR angiography. *Br J Radiol.* 1999;72(859):709–711.
25. Bale PM. Congenital cystic malformation of the lung. A form of congenital bronchiolar ("adenomatoid") malformation. *Am J Clin Pathol.* 1979;71(4):411–420.
26. Benning TL, Godwin JD, Roggli VL, et al. Cartilaginous variant of congenital adenomatoid malformation of the lung. *Chest.* 1987;92(3):514–516.
27. Cloutier MM, Schaeffer DA, Hight D. Congenital cystic adenomatoid malformation. *Chest.* 1993;103(3):761–764.

28. Luck SR, Reynolds M, Raffensperger JG. Congenital bronchopulmonary malformations. *Curr Probl Surg.* 1986;23(4):245–314.

29. Miller RK, Sieber WK, Yunis EJ. Congenital adenomatoid malformation of the lung. A report of 17 cases and review of the literature. *Pathol Annu.* 1980;15(Pt 1):387–402.

30. Moerman P, Fryns JP, Vandenberghe K, et al. Pathogenesis of congenital cystic adenomatoid malformation of the lung. *Histopathology.* 1992;21(4):315–321.

31. Nakamura Y. Pulmonary disorders in infants. *Acta Pathol Jpn.* 1993;43(7–8):347–359.

32. Rosado-de-Christenson ML, Stocker JT. Congenital cystic adenomatoid malformation. *Radiographics.* 1991;11(5):865–886.

33. Cha I, Adzick NS, Harrison MR, et al. Fetal congenital cystic adenomatoid malformations of the lung: a clinicopathologic study of eleven cases. *Am J Surg Pathol.* 1997;21(5):537–544.

34. Kreiger PA, Ruchelli ED, Mahboubi S, et al. Fetal pulmonary malformations: defining histopathology. *Am J Surg Pathol.* 2006;30(5):643–649.

35. Avitabile AM, Greco MA, Hulnick DH, et al. Congenital cystic adenomatoid malformation of the lung in adults. *Am J Surg Pathol.* 1984;8(3):193–202.

36. Stocker JT, Madewell JE, Drake RM. Congenital cystic adenomatoid malformation of the lung. Classification and morphologic spectrum. *Hum Pathol.* 1977;8(2):155–171.

37. Stocker JT. Congenital and developmental diseases. In: Hammar SP, ed. *Pulmonary Pathology.* New York: Springer-Verlag; 1994:155–190.

38. Rutledge JC, Jensen P. Acinar dysplasia: a new form of pulmonary maldevelopment. *Hum Pathol.* 1986;17(12):1290–1293.

39. Chambers HM. Congenital acinar aplasia: an extreme form of pulmonary maldevelopment. *Pathology.* 1991;23:69–71.

40. Davidson LA, Batman P, Fagan DG. Congenital acinar dysplasia: a rare cause of poulmonary hypoplasia. *Histopathology.* 1998;32(1):57–59.

41. Moerman P, Vanhole C, Devlieger H, Fryns JP. Severe primary pulmonary hypoplasia ("acinar dysplasia") in sibs: a genetically determined mesodermal defect? *J Med Genet.* 1998;35(11):964–965.

42. Federici S, Domenichelli V, Tani G, et al. Pleuropulmonary blastoma in congenital cystic adenomatoid malformation: report of a case. *Eur J Pediatr Surg.* 2001;11(3):196–199.

43. MacSweeney F, Papagiannopoulos K, Goldstraw P, et al. An assessment of the expanded classification of congenital cystic adenomatoid malformations and their relationship to malignant transformation. *Am J Surg Pathol.* 2003;27(8):1139–1146.

44. Dehner LP. Pleuropulmonary blastoma is THE pulmonary blastoma of childhood. *Semin Diagn Pathol.* 1994;11(2):144–151.

45. Manivel JC, Priest JR, Watterson J, et al. Pleuropulmonary blastoma. The so-called pulmonary blastoma of childhood. *Cancer.* 1988;62(8):1516–1526.

46. Merriman TE, Beasley SW, Chow CW, et al. A rare tumor masquerading as an empyema: pleuropulmonary blastoma. *Pediatr Pulmonol.* 1996;22(6):408–411.

47. Indolfi P, Casale F, Carli M, et al. Pleuropulmonary blastoma: management and prognosis of 11 cases. *Cancer.* 2000;89(6):1396–1401.

48. Priest JR, Williams GM, Hill DA, et al. Pulmonary cysts in early childhood and the risk of malignancy. *Pediatr Pulmonol.* 2009;44:14–30.

49. Sheffield EA, Addis BJ, Corrin B, et al. Epithelial hyperplasia and malignant change in congenital lung cysts. *J Clin Pathol.* 1987;40(6):612–614.

50. Benjamin DR, Cahill JL. Bronchioloalveolar carcinoma of the lung and congenital cystic adenomatoid malformation. *Am J Clin Pathol.* 1991;95(6):889–892.

51. Kaslovsky RA, Purdy S, Dangman BC, et al. Bronchioloalveolar carcinoma in a child with congenital cystic adenomatoid malformation. *Chest.* 1997;112(2):548–551.

52. Usui Y, Takabe K, Takayama S, et al. Minute squamous cell carcinoma arising in the wall of a congenital lung cyst. *Chest.* 1991;99(1):235–236.

53. Ribet ME, Copin MC, Soots JG, et al. Bronchioloalveolar carcinoma and congenital cystic adenomatoid malformation. *Ann Thorac Surg.* 1995;60(4):1126–1128.

54. Ota H, Langston C, Honda T, et al. Histochemical analysis of mucous cells of congenital adenomatoid malformation of the lung: insights into the carcinogenesis of pulmonary adenocarcinoma expressing gastric mucins. *Am J Clin Pathol.* 1998;110(4):450–455.

55. Granata C, Gambini C, Balducci T, et al. Bronchioloalveolar carcinoma arising in congenital cystic adenomatoid malformation in a child: a case report and review on malignancies originating in congenital cystic adenomatoid malformation. *Pediatr Pulmonol.* 1998;25(1):62–66.

56. Yao JL, Fasano M, Morotti R, et al. Demonstration of communication between alveolus and interstitium in persistent interstitial pulmonary emphysema: case report. *Pediatr Dev Pathol.* 1999;2(5):484–487.

57. Zimmermann H. Progressive interstitial pulmonary lobar emphysema. *Eur J Pediatr.* 1982;138(3):258–262.

58. Stocker JT, Madewell JE. Persistent interstitial pulmonary emphysema: another complication of the respiratory distress syndrome. *Pediatrics.* 1977;59(6):847–857.

59. Brewer LL, Moskowitz PS, Carrington CB, et al. Pneumatosis pulmonalis: a complication of the idiopathic respiratory distress syndrome. *Am J Pathol.* 1979;95(1):171–190.

60. Cooney TP, Thurlbeck WM. Pulmonary hypoplasia in Down's syndrome. *N Engl J Med.* 1982;307(19):1170–1173.

61. Cooney TP, Wentworth PJ, Thurlbeck WM. Diminished radial count is found only postnatally in Down's syndrome. *Pediatr Pulmonol.* 1988;5(4):204–209.

62. Gonzalez OR, Gomez IG, Recalde AL, et al. Postnatal development of the cystic lung lesion of Down syndrome: suggestion that the cause is reduced formation of peripheral air spaces. *Pediatr Pathol.* 1991;11(4):623–633.

63. Gyves-Ray K, Kirchner S, Stein S, et al. Cystic lung disease in Down syndrome. *Pediatr Radiol.* 1994;24(2):137–138.

64. Schloo BL, Vawter GF, Reid LM. Down syndrome: patterns of disturbed lung growth. *Hum Pathol.* 1991;22(9):919–923.

65. Tyrrell VJ, Asher MI, Chan Y. Subpleural lung cysts in Down's syndrome. *Pediatr Pulmonol.* 1999;28(2):145–148.

66. Hislop A, Reid L. New pathological findings in emphysema of childhood. 2. Overinflation of a normal lobe. *Thorax.* 1971;26(2):190–194.

67. Mani H, Suarez E, Stocker JT. The morphologic spectrum of infantile lobar emphysema: a study of 33 cases. *Paediatr Respir Rev.* 2004;5(suppl A):S313–S320.

68. Stanger P, Lucas Jr RV, Edwards JE. Anatomic factors causing respiratory distress in acyanotic congenital cardiac disease. Special reference to bronchial obstruction. *Pediatrics.* 1969;43(5):760–769.

69. Miller KE, Edwards DK, Hilton S, et al. Acquired lobar emphysema in premature infants with bronchopulmonary dysplasia: an iatrogenic disease? *Radiology.* 1981;138(3):589–592.

70. Newman B, Yunis E. Lobar emphysema associated with respiratory syncytial virus pneumonia. *Pediatr Radiol.* 1995;25(8):646–648.

71. Nathan L, Leveno KJ, Carmody 3rd TJ, et al. Meconium: a 1990s perspective on an old obstetric hazard. *Obstet Gynecol.* 1994;83(3):329–332.

72. Swaminathan S, Quinn J, Stabile MW, et al. Long-term pulmonary sequelae of meconium aspiration syndrome. *J Pediatr.* 1989;114(3):356–361.

73. Hislop A, Reid L. New pathological findings in emphysema of childhood. 1. Polyalveolar lobe with emphysema. *Thorax.* 1970;25(6):682–690.

74. Tapper D, Schuster S, McBride J, et al. Polyalveolar lobe: anatomic and physiologic parameters and their relationship to congenital lobar emphysema. *J Pediatr Surg.* 1980;15(6):931–937.

75. Munnell ER, Lambird PA, Austin RL. Polyalveolar lobe causing lobar emphysema of infancy. *Ann Thorac Surg.* 1973;16(6):624–628.

76. Emery JL, Mithal A. The number of alveoli in the terminal respiratory unit of man during late intrauterine life and childhood. *Arch Dis Child.* 1960;35:544–557.

77. MacMahon HE. Congenital alveolar dysplasia: a developmental anomaly involving pulmonary alveoli. *Pediatrics.* 1948;2:43–57.

78. Greenough A. Factors adversely affecting lung growth. *Paediatr Respir Rev.* 2000;1(4):314–320.

79. Langston C, Kida K, Reed M, Thurlbeck WM. Human lung growth in late gestation and in the neonate. *Am Rev Respir Dis.* 1984;129:607–613.

80. DePaepe ME, Friedman RM, Gundogan F, Pinar H. Postmortem lung weight/body weight standards for term and preterm infants. *Pediatr Pulmonol.* 2005;40:445–448.

81. Wigglesworth JS, Desai R, Hislop AA. Fetal lung growth in congenital laryngeal atresia. *Pediatr Pathol.* 1987;7:515–525.

82. Silver MM, Thurston WA, Patrick JE. Perinatal pulmonary hyperplasia due to laryngeal atresia. *Hum Pathol.* 1988;19:110–113.

83. Wagenvoort CA. Misalignment of lung vessels: a syndrome causing persistent neonatal pulmonary hypertension. *Hum Pathol.* 1986;17(7):727–730.

84. Janney CG, Askin FB, Kuhn 3rd C. Congenital alveolar capillary dysplasia—an unusual cause of respiratory distress in the newborn. *Am J Clin Pathol.* 1981;76(5):722–727.

85. Langston C. Misalignment of pulmonary veins and alveolar capillary dysplasia. *Pediatr Pathol.* 1991;11(1):163–170.

86. Tibballs J, Chow CW. Incidence of alveolar capillary dysplasia in severe idiopathic persistent pulmonary hypertension of the newborn. *J Paediatr Child Health.* 2002;38(4):397–400.

87. Alameh J, Bachiri A, Devisme L, et al. Alveolar capillary dysplasia: a cause of persistent pulmonary hypertension of the newborn. *Eur J Pediatr.* 2002;161(5):262–266.

88. Haraida S, Lochbuhler H, Heger A, et al. Congenital alveolar capillary dysplasia: rare cause of persistent pulmonary hypertension. *Pediatr Pathol Lab Med.* 1997;17(6):959–975.

89. Boggs S, Harris MC, Hoffman DJ, et al. Misalignment of pulmonary veins with alveolar capillary dysplasia: affected siblings and variable phenotypic expression. *J Pediatr.* 1994;124:125–128.

90. Case records of the Massachusetts General Hospital. Weekly clinicopathological exercises. Case 13-1992. A full-term newborn boy with chronic respiratory distress. *N Engl J Med.* 1992;326(13):875–884.

91. Noonan JA, Walters LR, Reeves JT. Congenital pulmonary lymphangiectasis. *Am J Dis Child.* 1970;120(4):314–319.

92. Hunter WS, Becroft DM. Congenital pulmonary lymphangiectasis associated with pleural effusions. *Arch Dis Child.* 1984;59(3):278–279.

93. Hilliard RI, McKendry JB, Phillips MJ. Congenital abnormalities of the lymphatic system: a new clinical classification. *Pediatrics.* 1990;86(6):988–994.

94. Brown M, Pysher T, Coffin CM. Lymphangioma and congenital pulmonary lymphangiectasis: a histologic, immunohistochemical, and clinicopathologic comparison. *Mod Pathol.* 1999;12(6):569–575.

95. Faul JL, Berry GJ, Colby TV, et al. Thoracic lymphangiomas, lymphangiectasis, lymphangiomatosis, and lymphatic dysplasia syndrome. *Am J Respir Crit Care Med.* 2000;161(3 Pt 1):1037–1046.

96. Wagenaar SS, Swierenga J, Wagenvoort CA. Late presentation of primary pulmonary lymphangiectasis. *Thorax.* 1978;33(6):791–795.

97. Verlaat CW, Peters HM, Semmekrot BA, et al. Congenital pulmonary lymphangiectasis presenting as a unilateral hyperlucent lung. *Eur J Pediatr.* 1994;153(3):202–205.

98. France NE, Brown RJ. Congenital pulmonary lymphangiectasis. Report of 11 examples with special reference to cardiovascular findings. *Arch Dis Child.* 1971;46(248):528–532.

99. Tazelaar HD, Kerr D, Yousem SA, et al. Diffuse pulmonary lymphangiomatosis. *Hum Pathol.* 1993;24(12):1313–1322.

100. Swensen SJ, Hartman TE, Mayo JR, et al. Diffuse pulmonary lymphangiomatosis: CT findings. *J Comput Assist Tomogr.* 1995;19(3):348–352.

101. Burke CM, Safai C, Nelson DP, et al. Pulmonary arteriovenous malformations: a critical update. *Am Rev Respir Dis.* 1986;134(2):334–339.

102. Sawyer SM, Menahem S, Chow CW, Robertson CF. Progressive cyanosis in a child with hereditary hemorrhagic telangiectasia (Osler–Weber–Rendu disease). *Pediatr Pulmonol.* 1992;13(2):124–127.

103. Kapur S, Rome J, Chandra RS. Diffuse pulmonary arteriovenous malformation in a child with polysplenia syndrome. *Pediatr Pathol Lab Med.* 1995;15(3):463–468.

104. Papagiannis J, Kanter RJ, Effman EL, et al. Polysplenia with pulmonary arteriovenous malformations. *Pediatr Cardiol.* 1993;14(2):127–129.

105. Farrell PM, Avery ME. Hyaline membrane disease. *Am Rev Respir Dis.* 1975;111(5):657–688.

106. Ikegami M, Jacobs H, Jobe A. Surfactant function in respiratory distress syndrome. *J Pediatr.* 1983;102(3):443–447.

107. O'Brodovich HM, Mellins RB. Bronchopulmonary dysplasia. Unresolved neonatal acute lung injury. *Am Rev Respir Dis.* 1985;132(3):694–709.

108. Morgenstern B, Klionsky B, Doshi N. Yellow hyaline membrane disease. Identification of the pigment and bilirubin binding. *Lab Invest.* 1981;44(6):514–518.

109. Husain AN, Siddiqui NH, Stocker JT. Pathology of arrested acinar development in postsurfactant bronchopulmonary dysplasia. *Hum Pathol.* 1998;29(7):710–717.

110. Bonikos DS, Bensch KG, Northway WH, et al. Bronchopulmonary dysplasia: the pulmonary pathologic sequel of necrotizing bronchiolitis and pulmonary fibrosis. *Hum Pathol.* 1976;7:643–666.

111. Nickerson BG. Bronchopulmonary dysplasia. Chronic pulmonary disease following neonatal respiratory failure. *Chest.* 1985;87(4):528–535.

112. Jobe AH, Bancalari E. Bronchopulmonary dysplasia. *Am J Respir Crit Care Med.* 2001;163(7):1723–1729.

113. Northway Jr WH, Rosan RC, Porter DY. Pulmonary disease following respirator therapy of hyaline-membrane disease. Bronchopulmonary dysplasia. *N Engl J Med.* 1967;276(7):357–368.

114. Northway Jr WH. Bronchopulmonary dysplasia: then and now. *Arch Dis Child.* 1990;65(10 Spec No):1076–1081.

115. Stocker JT. Pathologic features of long-standing "healed" bronchopulmonary dysplasia: a study of 28 3- to 40-month-old infants. *Hum Pathol.* 1986;17(9):943–961.

116. Northway Jr WH, Moss RB, Carlisle KB, et al. Late pulmonary sequelae of bronchopulmonary dysplasia. *N Engl J Med.* 1990;323(26):1793–1799.

117. Coalson JJ. Pathology of new bronchopulmonary dysplasia. *Semin Neonatol.* 2003;8(1):73–81.

118. Coren ME, Nicholson AG, Goldstraw P, et al. Open lung biopsy for diffuse interstitial lung disease in children. *Eur Respir J.* 1999;14(4):817–821.

119. Fan LL, Mullen AL, Brugman SM, et al. Clinical spectrum of chronic interstitial lung disease in children. *J Pediatr.* 1992;121(6):867–872.

120. Fan LL, Langston C. Chronic interstitial lung disease in children. *Pediatr Pulmonol.* 1993;16(3):184–196.

121. Fan LL, Deterding RR, Langston C. Pediatric interstitial lung disease revisited. *Pediatr Pulmonol.* 2004;38:369–378.

122. Clement A, ERS Task Force. Task force on chronic interstitial lung disease in immunocompetent children. *Eur Respir J.* 2004;24:686–697.

123. Deutsch GH, Young LR, Deterding RR, et al. Diffuse lung disease in young children: application of a novel classification scheme. *Am J Respir Crit Care Med.* 2007;176:1120–1128.

124. Katzenstein AL, Myers JL. Idiopathic pulmonary fibrosis: clinical relevance of pathologic classification. *Am J Respir Crit Care Med.* 1998;157(4 Pt 1):1301–1315.

125. Nicholson AG, Kim H, Corrin B, et al. The value of classifying interstitial pneumonitis in childhood according to defined histological patterns. *Histopathology.* 1998;33(3):203–211.

126. Schroeder SA, Shannon DC, Mark EJ. Cellular interstitial pneumonitis in infants. A clinicopathologic study. *Chest.* 1992;101(4):1065–1069.

127. Canakis AM, Cutz E, Manson D, et al. Pulmonary interstitial glycogenosis: a new variant of neonatal interstitial lung disease. *Am J Respir Crit Care Med.* 2002;65(11):1557–1565.

128. Smets K, Dhaene K, Schelstraete P, et al. Neonatal pulmonary interstitial glycogen accumulation disorder. *Eur J Pediatr.* 2004;163:408–409.

129. Onland W, Molenaar JJ, Leguit RJ, et al. Pulmonary interstitial glycogenosis in identical twins. *Pediatr Pulmonol.* 2005;40:362–366.

130. Cole FS, Hamvas A, Nogee LM. Genetic disorders of neonatal respiratory function. *Pediatr Res.* 2001;50:157–162.

131. Whitsett JA, Wert SE, Xu Y. Genetic disorders of surfactant homeostasis. *Biol Neonate.* 2005;87:283–287.

132. Rosen SH, Castleman B, Liebow AA. Pulmonary alveolar proteinosis. *N Engl J Med.* 1958;258(23):1123–1142.

133. Nogee LM, de Mello DE, Dehner LP, et al. Brief report: deficiency of pulmonary surfactant protein B in congenital alveolar proteinosis. *N Engl J Med.* 1993;328(6):406–410.

134. deMello DE, Heyman S, Phyelps DS, et al. Ultrastructure of lung in surfactant protein B deficiency. *Am J Respir Cell Mol Biol.* 1994;11:230–239.

135. Nogee LM, Garnier G, Dietz HC, et al. A mutation in the surfactant protein B gene responsible for fatal neonatal respiratory disease in multiple kindreds. *J Clin Invest.* 1994;93(4):1860–1863.

136. Shulenin S, Nogee LM, Annilo T, et al. ABCA3 gene mutations in newborns with fatal surfactant deficiency. *N Engl J Med.* 2004;350(13):1296–1303.

137. Bullard JE, Wert SE, Whitsett JA, et al. ABCA3 mutations associated with pediatric interstitial lung disease. *Am J Respir Crit Care Med.* 2005;172:1026–1031.

138. Tryka AF, Wert SE, Mazursky JE, et al. Absence of lamellar bodies with accumulation of dense bodies characterizes a novel form of congenital surfactant defect. *Pediatr Dev Pathol.* 2000;3(4):335–345.

139. Edwards V, Cutz E, Viero S, et al. Ultrastructure of lamellar bodies in congenital surfactant deficiency. *Ultrastruct Pathol.* 2005;29:503–509.

140. Martinez-Moczygemba M, Doan ML, Elidemir O, et al. Pulmonary alveolar proteinosis caused by deletion of the GM-CSFRα gene in the X chromosome pseudoautosomal region 1. *J Exp Med.* 2008;205(12):2711–2716. Epub 2008 Oct 27.

141. Suzuki T, Sakagami T, Rubin BK, et al. Familial pulmonary alveolar proteinosis caused by mutations in *CSF2RA. J Exp Med.* 2008;205(12):2703–2710. Epub 2008 Oct 27.

142. Bedrossian CW, Luna MA, Conklin RH, et al. Alveolar proteinosis as a consequence of immunosuppression. A hypothesis based on clinical and pathologic observations. *Hum Pathol.* 1980;11(5 suppl):527–535.

143. Nachajon RV, Rutstein RM, Rudy BJ, et al. Pulmonary alveolar proteinosis in an HIV-infected child. *Pediatr Pulmonol.* 1997;24(4):292–295.

144. Samuels MP, Warner JO. Pulmonary alveolar lipoproteinosis complicating juvenile dermatomyositis. *Thorax.* 1988;43(11):939–940.

145. Parto K, Svedstrom E, Majurin ML, et al. Pulmonary manifestations in lysinuric protein intolerance. *Chest.* 1993;104(4):1176–1182.

146. Fisher M, Roggli V, Merten D, et al. Coexisting endogenous lipoid pneumonia, cholesterol granulomas, and pulmonary alveolar proteinosis in a pediatric population. *Pediatr Pathol.* 1992;12:365–383.

147. Katzenstein AL, Gordon LP, Oliphant M, et al. Chronic pneumonitis of infancy. A unique form of interstitial lung disease occurring in early childhood. *Am J Surg Pathol.* 1995;19(4):439–447.

148. Nogee LM, Dunbar 3rd AE, Wert SE, et al. A mutation in the surfactant protein C gene associated with familial interstitial lung disease. *N Engl J Med.* 2001;344(8):573–579.

149. Tredano M, Griese M, Brasch F, et al. Mutation in SFTPC in infantile pulmonary alveolar proteinosis with or without fibrosing lung disease. *Am J Med Genet A.* 2004;126A:18–26.

150. Katzenstein AL, Fiorelli RF. Nonspecific interstitial pneumonia/fibrosis. Histologic features and clinical significance. *Am J Surg Pathol.* 1994;18(2):136–147.

151. Yousem SA, Colby TV, Carrington CB. Follicular bronchitis/bronchiolitis. *Hum Pathol.* 1985;16(7):700–706.

152. Athreya BH, Doughty RA, Bookspan M, et al. Pulmonary manifestations of juvenile rheumatoid arthritis. A report of eight cases and review. *Clin Chest Med.* 1980;1(3):361–374.

153. Uziel Y, Hen B, Cordoba M, et al. Lymphocytic interstitial pneumonitis preceding polyarticular juvenile rheumatoid arthritis. *Clin Exp Rheumatol.* 1998;16(5):617–619.

154. Lovell D, Lindsley C, Langston C. Lymphoid interstitial pneumonia in juvenile rheumatoid arthritis. *J Pediatr.* 1984;105(6):947–950.

155. Grieco MH, Chinoy-Acharya P. Lymphocytic interstitial pneumonia associated with the acquired immune deficiency syndrome. *Am Rev Respir Dis.* 1985;131(6):952–955.

156. Kornstein MJ, Pietra GG, Hoxie JA, et al. The pathology and treatment of interstitial pneumonitis in two infants with AIDS. *Am Rev Respir Dis.* 1986;133(6):1196–1198.

157. Teirstein AS, Rosen MJ. Lymphocytic interstitial pneumonia. *Clin Chest Med.* 1988;9(3):467–471.

158. Pitt J. Lymphocytic interstitial pneumonia. *Pediatr Clin North Am.* 1991;38(1):89–95.

159. Marchevsky A, Rosen MJ, Chrystal G, et al. Pulmonary complications of the acquired immunodeficiency syndrome: a clinicopathologic study of 70 cases. *Hum Pathol.* 1985;16(7):659–670.

160. Rubinstein A, Morecki R, Silverman B, et al. Pulmonary disease in children with acquired immune deficiency syndrome and AIDS-related complex. *J Pediatr.* 1986;108(4):498–503.

161. Fan LL. Hypersensitivity pneumonitis in children. *Curr Opin Pediatr.* 2002;14(3):323–326.

162. Yee WF, Castile RG, Cooper A, et al. Diagnosing bird fancier's disease in children. *Pediatrics.* 1990;85(5):848–852.

163. Oermann CM, Panesar KS, Langston C, et al. Pulmonary infiltrates with eosinophilia syndromes in children. *J Pediatr.* 2000;136(3):351–358.

164. Colombo JL, Hallberg TK. Recurrent aspiration in children: lipid-laden alveolar macrophage quantitation. *Pediatr Pulmonol.* 1987;3(2):86–89.

165. Annobil SH, Morad NA, Kameswaran M, et al. Bronchiectasis due to lipid aspiration in childhood: clinical and pathological correlates. *Ann Trop Paediatr.* 1996;16(1):19–25.

166. Gadol CL, Joshi VV, Lee EY. Bronchiolar obstruction associated with repeated aspiration of vegetable material in two children with cerebral palsy. *Pediatr Pulmonol.* 1987;3(6):437–439.

167. Annobil SH, Benjamin B, Kameswaran M, et al. Lipoid pneumonia in children following aspiration of animal fat (ghee). *Ann Trop Paediatr.* 1991;11(1):87–94.

168. Moonnumakal SP, Fan LL. Bronchiolitis obliterans in children. *Curr Opin Pediatr.* 2008;20(3):272–278.

169. Deterding RR, Fan LL, Morton R, et al. Persistent tachypnea of infancy (PTI)—a new entity. *Pediatr Pulmonol.* 2001;32(suppl 23):72–73.

170. Deterding RR, Pye C, Fan LL, Langston C. Persistent tachypnea of infancy is associated with neuroendocrine cell hyperplasia. *Pediatr Pulmonol.* 2005;40:157–165.

171. Cutz E, Yeger H, Pan J. Pulmonary neuroendocrine cell system in pediatric lung disease—recent advances. *Pediatr Dev Pathol.* 2007;10(6):419–435.

172. Brody AS, Crotty EJ. Neuroendocrine cell hyperplasia of infancy (NEHI). *Pediatr Radiol.* 2006;36:1328.

173. Sondheimer HM, Lung MC, Brugman SM, et al. Pulmonary vascular disorders masquerading as interstitial lung disease. *Pediatr Pulmonol.* 1995;20(5):284–288.

174. Rabinovitch M, Haworth SG, Castaneda AR, et al. Lung biopsy in congenital heart disease: a morphometric approach to pulmonary vascular disease. *Circulation.* 1978;58:1107–1122.

175. Haworth SG. Pulmonary vascular disease in different types of congenital heart disease: implications for interpretation of lung biopsy findings in early childhood. *Br Heart J.* 1984;52:557–571.

176. Susarla SC, Fan LL. Diffuse alveolar hemorrhage syndromes in children. *Curr Opin Pediatr.* 2007;19:314–320.

177. Fullmer J, Langston C, Dishop MK, Fan LL. Pulmonary capillaritis in children: a review of eight cases with comparison to other alveolar hemorrhage syndromes. *J Pediatr.* 2005;146:376–381.

Acute Lung Injury

Oi-Yee Cheung, MD, Paolo Graziano, MD, and Kevin O. Leslie, MD

A wide variety of insults can produce acute lung damage, inclusive of those that injure the lungs directly. Early terms for diffuse acute lung injury occurring indirectly in the setting of overwhelming nonthoracic trauma accompanied by hypovolemia were "shock lung," "postperfusion lung," "traumatic wet lung," and "congestive atelectasis."[1,2]

In 1967, Ashbaugh and coworkers formally described a syndrome characterized by acute onset of severe respiratory distress after an identifiable injury. Clinical signs included dyspnea, reduced lung compliance, diffuse chest radiographic infiltrates, and hypoxemia refractory to supplementary oxygen.[3] Today this sequence of clinical events is referred to as the *acute respiratory distress syndrome* (ARDS). The clinical course is rapid and the mortality rate is high, with more than one half of affected patients dying of respiratory failure within days to weeks.[2,4,5] A recent meta-regression analysis performed by Zambon and Vincent[6] of mortality rates from 72 published studies of ARDS identified a decrease of 1.1% per year for the period 1994 to 2006, with an overall pooled mortality rate for all studies of 43%.

The American-European Consensus Conference (AECC) formally defined ARDS in 1994 using the following criteria: acute onset; bilateral chest radiographic infiltrates; hypoxemia regardless of the positive end-expiratory pressure oxygen concentration, an arterial partial pressure of oxygen to inspired oxygen fraction ratio less than 200, and no evidence of left atrial hypertension.[7] The AECC also agreed that ARDS represents the most severe form on a spectrum of disease conditions encompassed under the general term *acute lung injury*.

The histopathologic counterpart of ARDS is distinctive and referred to as *diffuse alveolar damage* (DAD). DAD is the most extreme manifestation of lung injury and can occur as a result of a large number of direct injuries to the lungs (e.g., infection). In this chapter, the emphasis is on DAD and less severe manifestations of acute lung injury. Some authors have considered organizing pneumonia to be a form of acute lung injury, but we and others believe that organization is a subacute phenomenon with a more protracted clinical course (extending over several days to weeks). Subacute organizing pneumonia of unknown etiology (previously known as idiopathic bronchiolitis obliterans organizing pneumonia)[8] is discussed with the chronic diffuse diseases (see Chapter 7).

Diffuse Alveolar Damage: The Morphologic Prototype of Acute Lung Injury

The causes of acute lung injury are numerous (Box 5-1). The lung reacts to various types of insults in similar ways, regardless of etiology. The resultant endothelial and alveolar epithelial cell injury is attended by fluid and cellular exudation. Subsequent reparative fibroblastic proliferation is accompanied by type II pneumocyte hyperplasia.[4,9] The microscopic appearance depends on the time interval between insult and biopsy, and on the severity and extent of the injury.[2] DAD is the usual pathologic manifestation of ARDS and is the best-characterized prototype of acute lung injury. From studies of ARDS, the pathologic changes appear to proceed consistently through discrete but overlapping phases (Fig. 5-1)—an early exudative (acute) phase (Fig. 5-2A and B), a subacute proliferative (organizing) phase (see Fig. 5-2C), and a late fibrotic phase (Fig. 5-3).[2,4,5,8,10] The exudative phase is most prominent in the first week of injury. The earliest changes include interstitial and intra-alveolar edema with variable amounts of

Box 5-1. Etiology of Diffuse Alveolar Damage

Idiopathic
  Acute interstitial pneumonia (Hamman-Rich syndrome)
Infection
  Any infection in the immunosuppressed patient, especially *Pneumocystis jiroveci* infection
  Viral infection: adenovirus, influenzavirus, herpesvirus, CMV, and hantavirus infections; SARS; coronavirus and RSV infections, others
  Legionella infection
  Mycoplasma/Chlamydia infection
  Rickettsial infection
Drugs
  Chemotherapeutic drugs: busulfan, bleomycin, methotrexate, azathioprine, BCNU, cytoxan, melphalan, mitomycin-C
  Amiodarone
  Gold
  Nitrofurantoin
  Hexamethonium
  Placidyl
  Penicillamine
Collagen vascular disease
  Systemic lupus erythematosus
  Rheumatoid arthritis
  Polymyositis/dermatomyositis
  Scleroderma
  Mixed connective disease
Pulmonary hemorrhage syndrome and vasculitis
  Goodpasture syndrome
  Microscopic polyangiitis
  Polyarteritis nodosa
  Wegener granulomatosis
  Vasculitis associated with collagen vascular disease
Ingestants
  Paraquat
  Kerosene
  Denatured rapeseed oil
Inhalants
  Oxygen

Inhalants—cont'd
  Amitrole-containing herbicide
  Ammonia and bleach mixture
  Chlorine gas
  Hydrogen sulfide
  Mercury vapor
  Nitric acid fumes
  Nitrogen dioxide
  Paint remover
  Smoke
  Smoke bomb
  Sulfur dioxide
  War gases
Shock
  Traumatic
  Hemorrhage
  Neurogenic
  Cardiogenic
Sepsis
Radiation exposure
Other etiologic factors/conditions
  Acute massive aspiration
  Acute pancreatitis
  Burn
  Cardiopulmonary bypass
  Heat
  High altitude
  Intravenous administration of contrast material
  Leukemic cell lysis
  Molar pregnancy
  Near-drowning
  Peritoneal-venous shunt
  Post-lymphangiography
  Toxic shock syndrome
  Transfusion therapy
  Uremia
  Venous air embolism

BCNU, carmustine; CMV, cytomegalovirus; RSV, respiratory syncytial virus; SARS, severe acute respiratory syndrome.
Modified from Katzenstein A, Askin F, eds. *Katzenstein and Askin's Surgical Pathology of Non-Neoplastic Lung Disease,* 3rd ed. Philadelphia: Saunders; 1997:16.

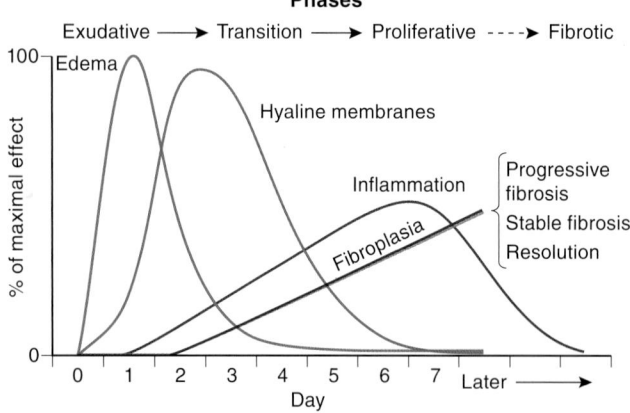

Figure 5-1. Acute respiratory distress syndrome (ARDS) timeline. The phases of ARDS are reproducible and reflect the global mechanisms of wound repair (exudation, proliferation, variable fibrogenesis). The indefinite relationship between proliferation and fibrogenesis is depicted as a *hashed line* in the sequence at the top of the figure. In experimental ARDS, the exact time of injury is known, and the entire lung proceeds through the phases at the same time. In a patient who develops diffuse alveolar damage from any cause, the acute lung injury may begin in different areas at different times, so a biopsy specimen may demonstrate injury at various phases in this sequence. (Modified from Katzenstein A: Acute lung injury patterns: diffuse alveolar damage and bronchiolitis obliterans–organizing pneumonia. In: Katzenstein A, Askin F, eds. *Katzenstein and Askin's Surgical Pathology of Non-Neoplastic Lung Disease,* 3rd ed. Philadelphia: Saunders; 1997.)

hemorrhage and fibrin deposition (Fig. 5-4). Hyaline membranes (Fig. 5-5), the histologic hallmark of the exudative phase of ARDS, are most prominent at 3 to 7 days after injury. Minimal interstitial mononuclear inflammatory infiltrates (Fig. 5-6) and fibrin thrombi in small pulmonary arteries (Fig. 5-7) also are seen. Type II pneumocyte hyperplasia (Fig. 5-8) begins by the end of this phase and persists through the proliferative phase. The reactive type II pneumocytes may demonstrate marked nuclear atypia, with numerous mitotic figures (Fig. 5-9). The proliferative phase begins at 1 week after the injury and is characterized by fibroblastic proliferation, seen mainly within the interstitium but also focally in the alveolar spaces (Fig. 5-10). The fibrosis consists of loose aggregates of fibroblasts admixed with scattered inflammatory cells (Fig. 5-11); collagen deposition is minimal. Reactive type II pneumocytes persist. Immature squamous metaplasia may occur (Fig. 5-12) in and around terminal bronchioles. The degree of cytologic atypia in this squamous epithelium can be so severe as to mimic malignancy (Fig. 5-13). The hyaline membranes are mostly resorbed by the late proliferative stage, but a few remnants may be observed along alveolar septa. Some cases of DAD resolve completely, with few residual morphologic effects, but in other cases, fibrosis may progress to extensive structural remodeling and honeycomb lung. As might be expected, a recent review of outcomes for 109 survivors of ARDS revealed persistent functional disability at 1 year after discharge from intensive care.[11]

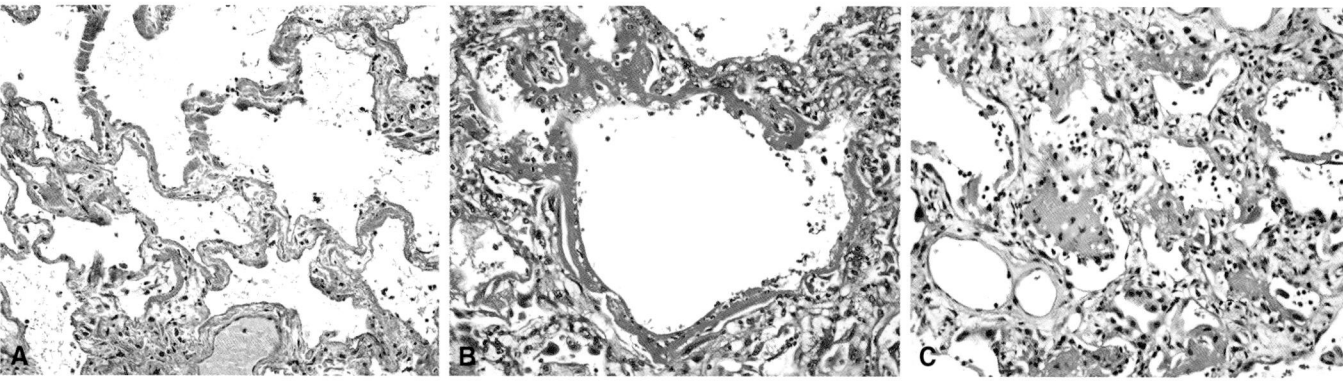

Figure 5-2. Acute respiratory distress syndrome (ARDS): exudative and proliferative phases. The early exudative phase of ARDS, characterized by some edema, cellular debris, and early hyaline membrane formation (**A**) evolves to include well-defined hyaline membranes (**B**). Note the increased cellularity in the interstitium, with some spindled fibroblast-like cells evident. **C,** Organization of hyaline membranes occurs in the early proliferative phase. Another feature specific to this stage is increased air space cellularity.

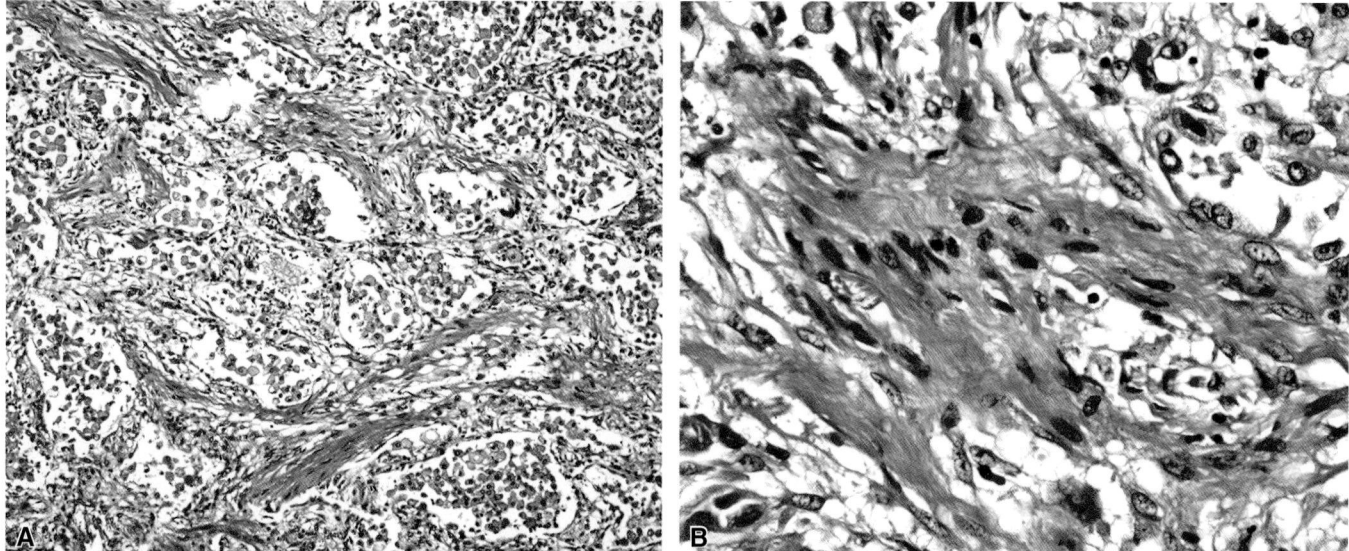

Figure 5-3. Acute respiratory distress syndrome (ARDS): late proliferative and fibrotic stages. The late proliferative phase of ARDS (**A**) may evolve to fibrosis (**B**), with cellular fibroblastic proliferation and collagen deposition.

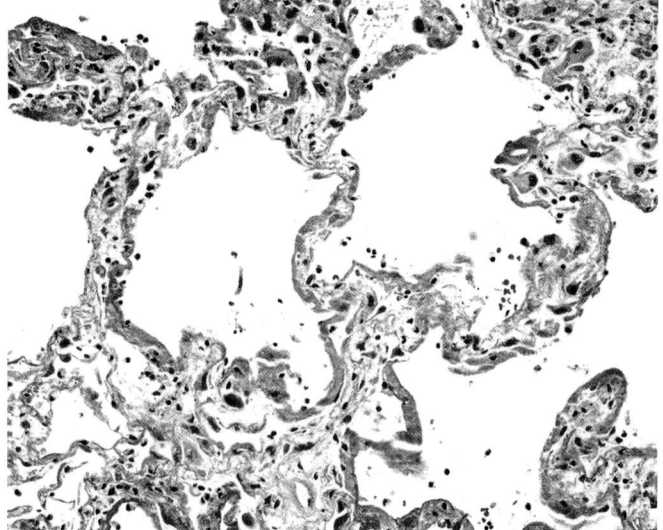

Figure 5-4. Acute respiratory distress syndrome: early exudative phase. Mild interstitial edema with hyaline membranes outlining alveolar spaces is characteristic.

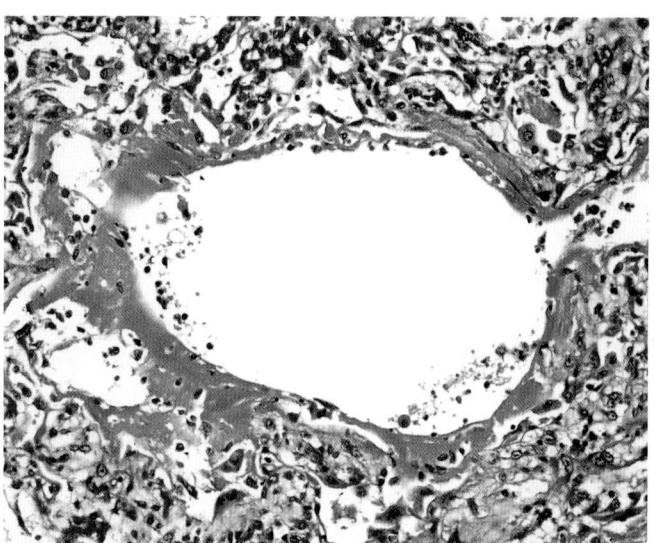

Figure 5-5. Acute respiratory distress syndrome: hyaline membranes. Proteinaceous alveolar exudates accumulate along the periphery of alveoli, closely adherent to alveolar wall–air space interface.

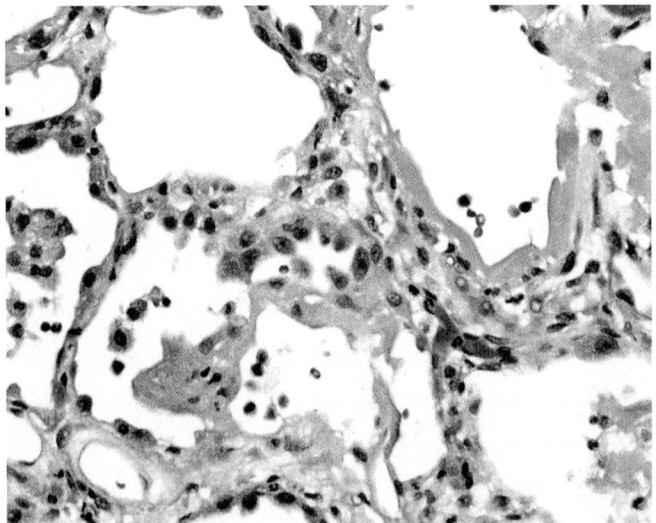

Figure 5-6. Acute respiratory distress syndrome (ARDS): mild interstitial inflammation. In ARDS, the inciting event is frequently extrathoracic, and lung injury is therefore superimposed on normal pre-existing structure.

By definition, ARDS has a known inciting event. The foregoing description is based on a model of ARDS due to oxygen toxicity, wherein the evolution of histopathologic abnormalities can be studied over a defined time period.[2,5] In practice, lung biopsy most often is performed in patients without a known cause or specific time of onset of injury. Moreover, with some causes of acute lung injury, the damage evolves over a protracted period of time, or the lung may be injured in repetitive fashion (e.g., with drug toxicity). In such circumstances, the pathologic changes do not necessarily progress sequentially through defined stages as in ARDS, so both acute and organizing phases may be encountered in the same biopsy specimen. The basic histopathologic elements of acute lung injury are presented in Box 5-2.

Acute fibrinous and organizing pneumonia (AFOP) is a recently recognized histologic pattern of acute lung injury with a clinical presentation similar to that of classic DAD, in terms of both potential etiologic disorders and outcome. It differs from DAD in that hyaline membranes are absent. The dominant feature is intra-alveolar fibrin "balls" or aggregates, typically in a patchy distribution. Organizing pneumonia in the form of luminal loose fibroblastic tissue is present surrounding the fibrin. The alveolar septa adjacent to areas of fibrin deposition show a variety of changes similar to those of DAD, such as septal edema, type II pneumocyte hyperplasia, and acute and chronic inflammatory infiltrates. The intervening lung shows minimal histologic changes. AFOP may represent a fibrinous variant of DAD. In some patients, both DAD and AFOP disease patterns may be present simultaneously.[12,13]

Specific Causes of Acute Lung Injury

Infection

Infection is one of the most common causes of acute lung injury. Among infectious organisms, viruses most consistently produce DAD.[2,5] Occasionally, fungi (e.g., *Pneumocystis*) and bacteria (e.g., *Legionella*) also can cause infections manifesting as DAD. Some of the organisms that are well known to cause acute lung injury with characteristic histopathologic changes are discussed next.

Viral Infection

Influenza is a common cause of viral pneumonia. The histopathology ranges from mild organizing acute lung injury (resembling organizing pneumonia) in nonfatal cases to severe DAD with necrotizing tracheobronchitis (Fig. 5-14) in fatal cases.[14,15] Specific viral cytopathic effects are not identifiable by light microscopy. On ultrastructural examination, intranuclear fibrillary inclusions may be seen in epithelial and endothelial cells.[16]

The *coronavirus* responsible for severe acute respiratory syndrome (SARS) produces the acute lung injury associated with this disorder.[17-20] Both DAD and AFOP patterns have been identified in affected patients. On ultrastructural examination, involved lung tissue revealed numerous to moderate numbers of cytoplasmic viral particles in pneumocytes, many within membrane-bound vesicles.[21-23] The virus particles were spherical and enveloped, with spike-like projections on the surface and coarse clumps of electron-dense material in the center. Most had sizes ranging from 60 to 95 nm in diameter, but some were as large as 180 nm.

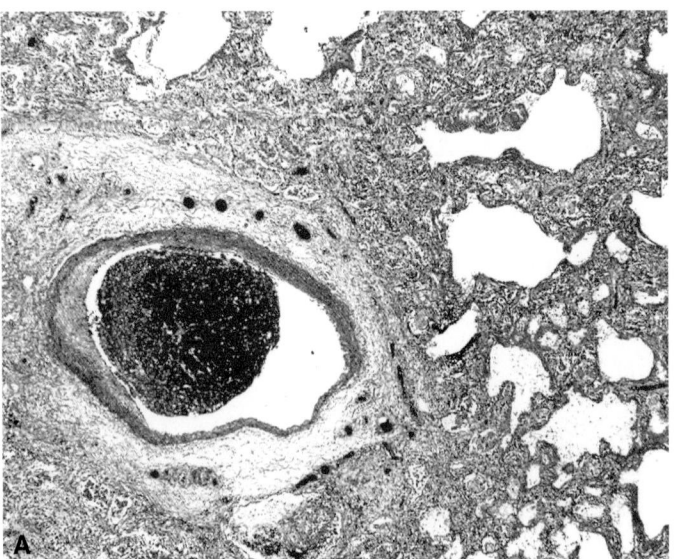
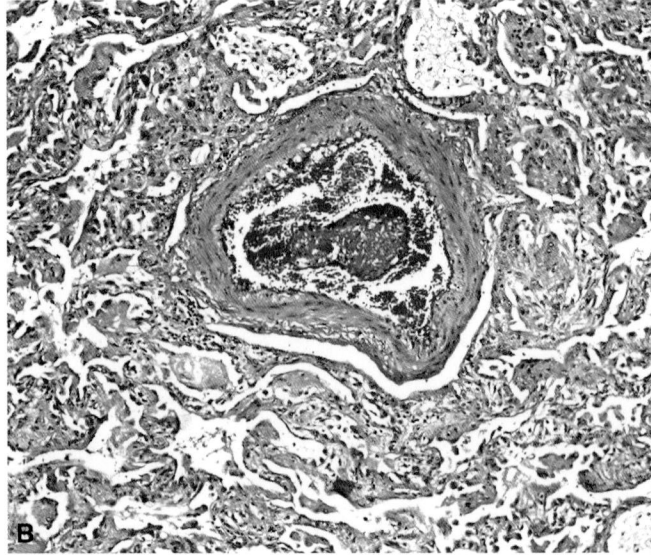

Figure 5-7. Acute respiratory distress syndrome: fibrin thrombi in arteries. Acute lung injury results in local conditions that lead to arterial thrombosis. Thrombi in various stages of organization may be seen (larger pulmonary artery in part **A**, smaller pulmonary artery in part **B**).

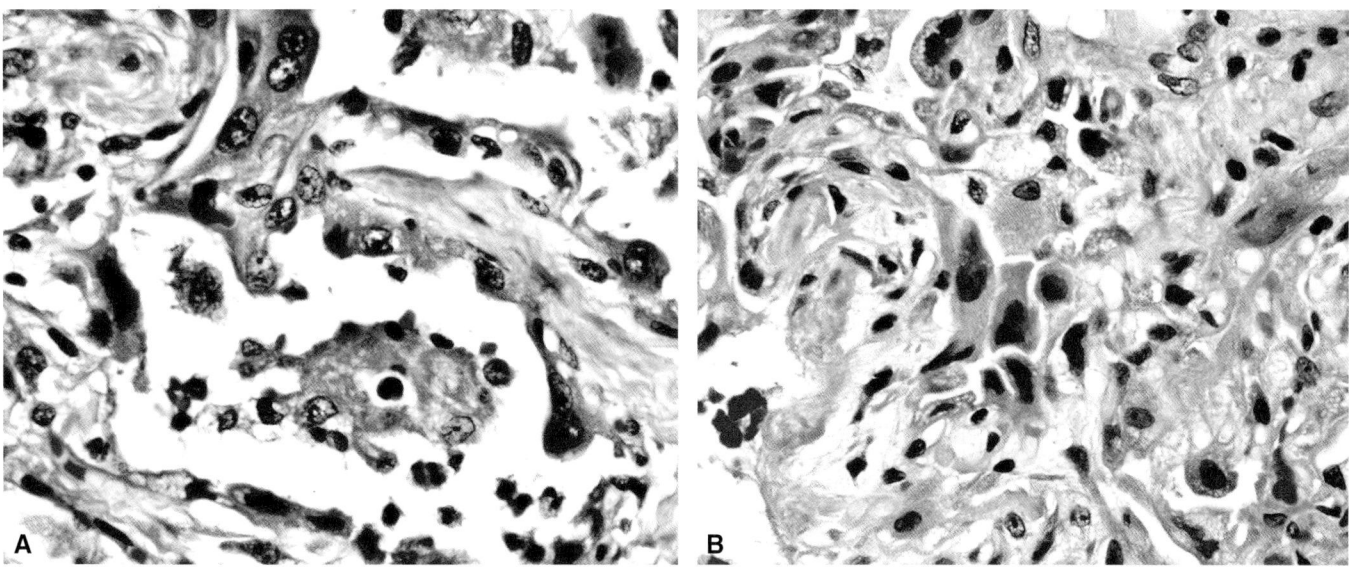

Figure 5-8. Acute respiratory distress syndrome (ARDS): type II cell hyperplasia. Cuboidal type II cells are nearly always prominent in the late exudative phase and throughout the proliferative phase of ARDS. These hyperchromatic and enlarged epithelial cells repopulate the damaged type I cell lining of the alveolar spaces. Depending on the mechanism of injury, atypia of regenerating type II cells may be mild, moderate, or severe. **A,** Prominent type II cells have a "hobnail" appearance simulating viropathic change. **B,** Brightly eosinophilic type II cells are aggregated at the center of a collapsed alveolus. Considerable structural remodeling may take place after ARDS as these atelectatic spaces fuse to form consolidated areas of lung parenchyma at the microscopic level.

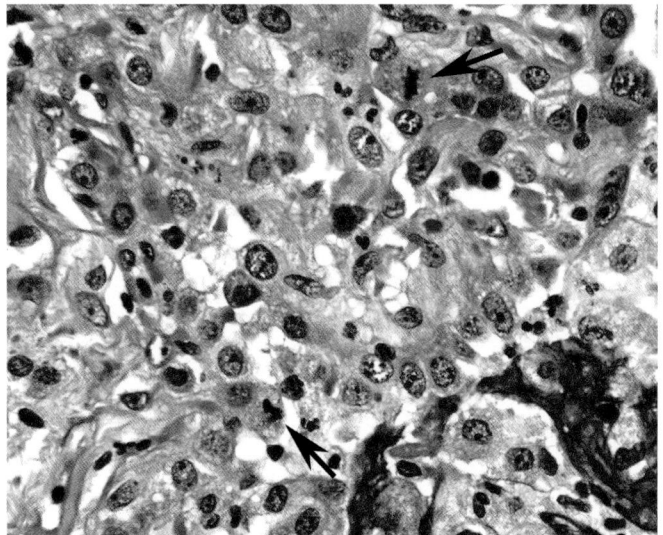

Figure 5-9. Acute respiratory distress syndrome: mitotic figures in type II cells. Mitotic activity can be quite brisk in all forms of acute lung injury (mitotic figures at *arrows*).

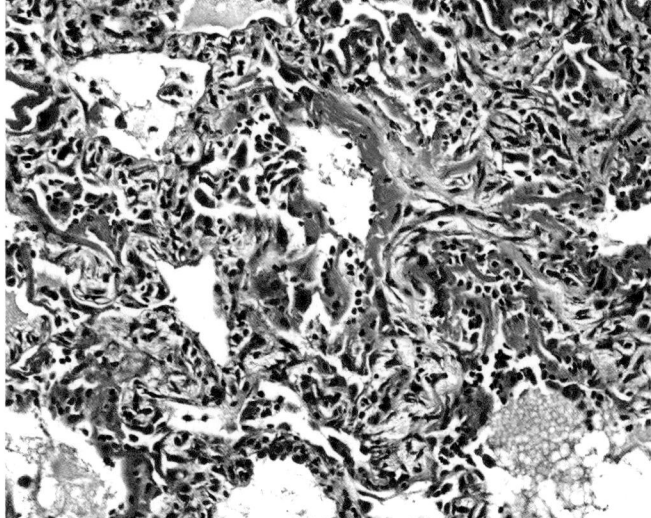

Figure 5-10. Acute respiratory distress syndrome (ARDS): fibroblastic proliferation. Fibroblastic proliferation occurs to a variable degree both in the interstitium and within air spaces in the proliferative and early fibrotic phases of ARDS.

Measles virus produces a mild pneumonia in the normal host but can cause serious pneumonia in immunocompromised children. Histopathologic features of such infection include interstitial pneumonia, bronchitis and bronchiolitis, and DAD.[24] The characteristic histologic feature is the presence of multinucleated giant cells (Fig. 5-15A) with characteristic eosinophilic intranuclear and intracytoplasmic inclusions.[24-28] These cells are found in the alveolar spaces and within alveolar septa (see Fig. 5-15B). Viral inclusions are seen on ultrastructural examination as tightly packed tubules.[28]

Adenovirus is an important cause of lower respiratory tract disease in children,[29,30] although adults (particularly those who are immunocompromised)[31] and military recruits also are occasionally affected.[32] The lung shows necrotizing bronchitis, or bronchiolitis, accompanied by DAD. The pathologic changes are more severe in bronchi,

bronchioles, and peribronchiolar regions (Fig. 5-16A). Two types of inclusions can be observed in lung epithelial cells: An eosinophilic intranuclear inclusion with a halo usually is less conspicuous than the more readily identifiable "smudge cells" (see Fig. 5-16B). These latter cells are larger than normal and entirely basophilic, with no defined inclusion or halo evident by light microscopy.[29] On ultrastructural examination, smudge cell inclusions are represented by arrays of hexagonal particles.[33]

Herpes simplex virus is mainly a cause of respiratory infection in the immunocompromised host. Two patterns of infection are recognized: airway spread resulting in necrotizing tracheobronchitis (Fig. 5-17) and blood-borne dissemination producing miliary necrotic parenchymal nodules. DAD and hemorrhage can occur in both forms.[34,35] Characteristic inclusions may be seen in bronchial and alveolar

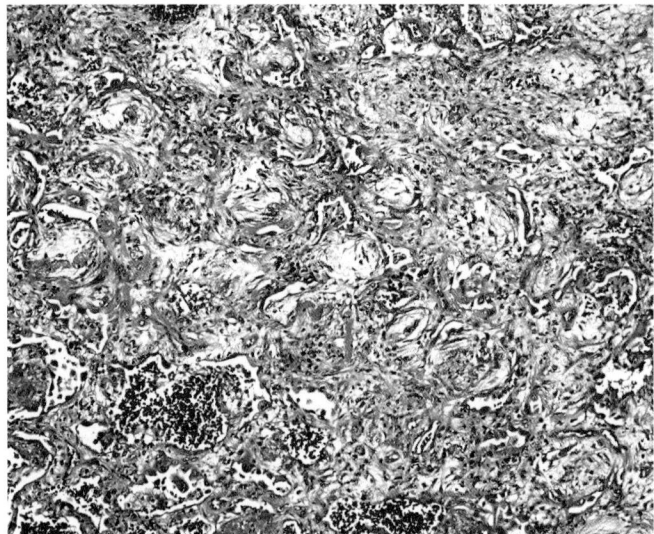

Figure 5-11. Acute respiratory distress syndrome (ARDS): air space organization. Organizing pneumonia–like air space organization can be quite prominent in the late proliferative phase of ARDS.

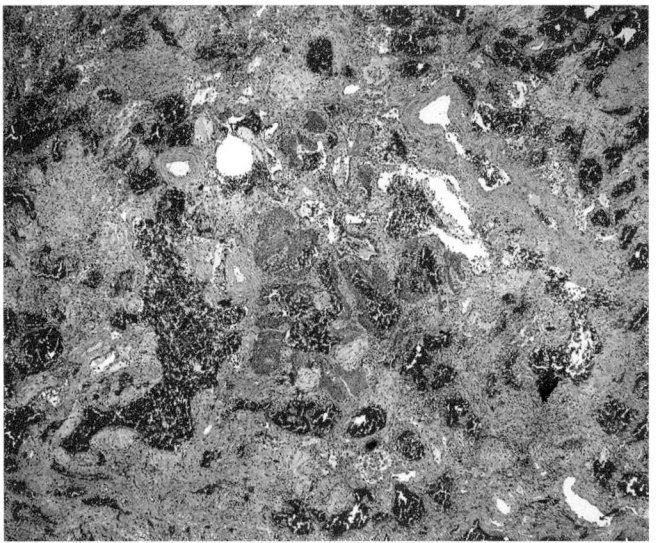

Figure 5-12. Acute respiratory distress syndrome (ARDS): squamous metaplasia. Squamous metaplasia of terminal airways may develop as a subacute proliferative event in ARDS and other forms of diffuse alveolar damage. The nested squamous epithelium often is nodular-appearing at scanning magnification by virtue of patchy terminal airway involvement.

epithelial cells (Fig. 5-18). The more obvious type is an intranuclear eosinophilic inclusion surrounded by clear halo (Cowdry A inclusion), and the other is represented by a basophilic to amphophilic ground-glass nucleus (Cowdry B inclusion). Rounded viral particles with double membranes are seen under the electron microscope.[34,35]

Varicella-zoster virus causes disease predominantly in children and is the agent of chickenpox.[36] Pulmonary complications of chickenpox are rare in children with normal immunity (accounting for less than 1% of the cases). By contrast, however, pneumonia develops in 15% of adults with chickenpox; immunocompetent and immunocompromised persons are equally affected.[32,36] The histopathologic picture in varicella pneumonia (Fig. 5-19) is similar to that in herpes simplex. Although identical intranuclear inclusions are reported to occur,[32,36] these can be considerably more difficult to identify in chickenpox pneumonia.

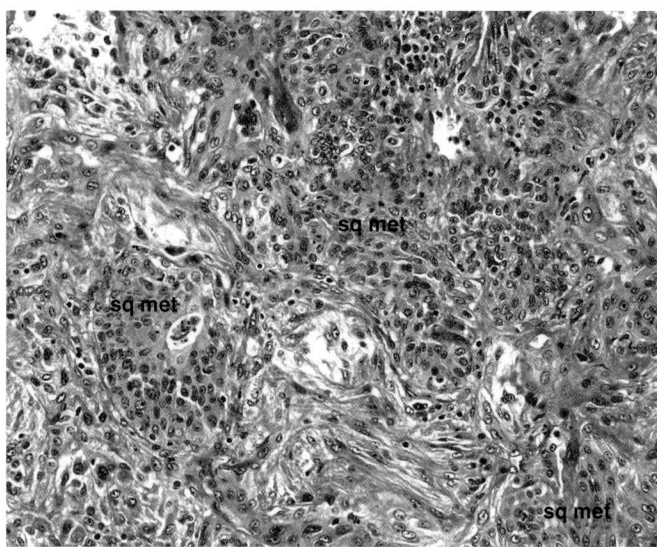

Figure 5-13. Acute respiratory distress syndrome: squamous metaplasia (sq met), high-magnification view. In some instances, squamous metaplasia may be so prominent as to suggest neoplasm.

Box 5-2. Defining Histopathologic Features of Acute Lung Injury

Interstitial (alveolar septal) edema
Fibroblastic proliferation in alveolar septa
Alveolar edema
Alveolar fibrin and cellular debris, with or without hyaline membranes
Reactive type II pneumocytes

Cytomegalovirus is an important cause of symptomatic pneumonia in immunocompromised persons, especially those who have received bone marrow or solid organ transplants, and in patients with human immunodeficiency virus (HIV) infection.[37–39] The histopathologic findings range from little or no inflammatory response to hemorrhagic nodules with necrosis (Fig. 5-20A) and DAD.[37] The diagnostic histopathologic pattern, seen in endothelial cells, macrophages, and epithelial cells, consists of cellular enlargement, a prominent intranuclear inclusion, and an intracytoplasmic basophilic inclusion[37] (see Fig. 5-20B).

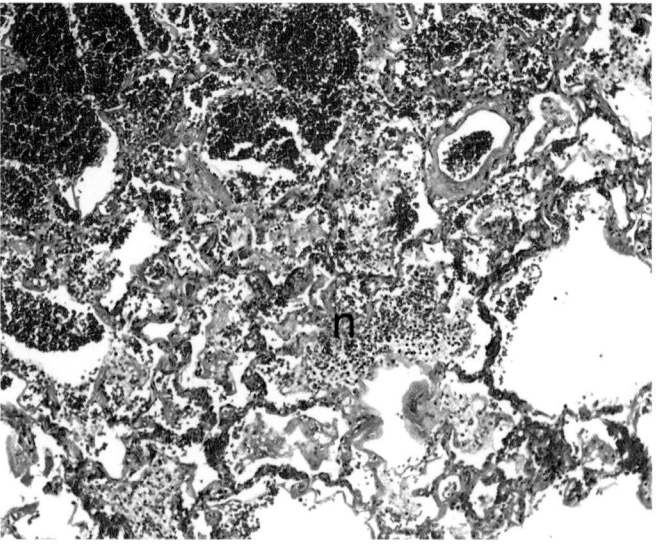

Figure 5-14. Diffuse alveolar damage in influenza pneumonia. Fibrinous and focally neutrophilic diffuse alveolar injury is characteristic. In this case, note the sparse neutrophils present in an air space (n) and abundant blood. No specific viral inclusions are produced by the influenzavirus.

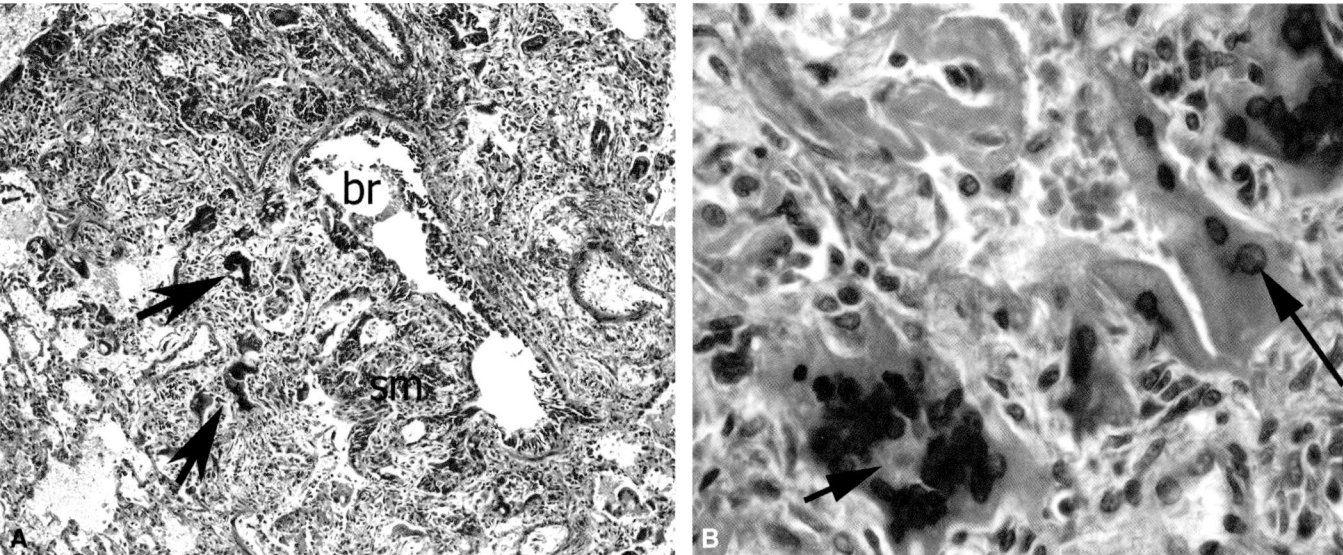

Figure 5-15. Diffuse alveolar damage (DAD) in measles pneumonia. **A,** A terminal airway (br) in a case of acute measles pneumonia with DAD. Squamous metaplasia of the airway also is present (sm). The *arrows* denote multinucleate giant cells, present here in a bronchiolocentric distribution. **B,** The characteristic multinucleate giant cells of measles pneumonia. Note the glassy intranuclear inclusions (*long arrow*) and occasional eosinophilic cytoplasmic inclusions (*short arrow*).

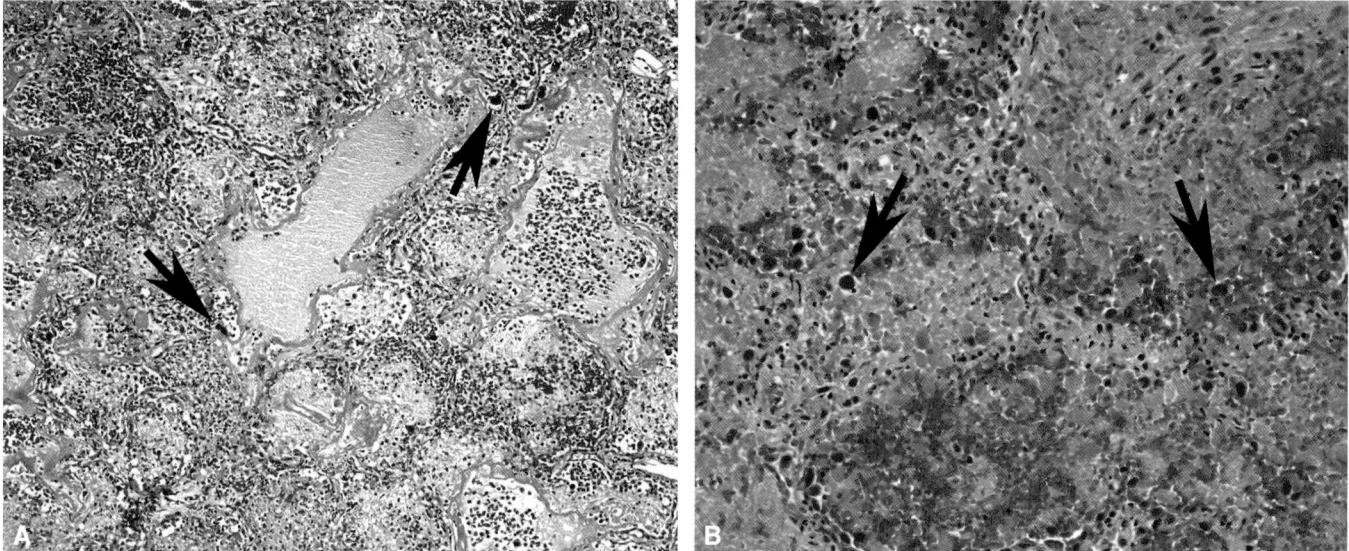

Figure 5-16. Diffuse alveolar damage (DAD) in adenovirus pneumonia. Adenovirus infection produces necrotizing bronchitis/bronchiolitis, and this is especially prominent in the setting of DAD caused by this infection. **A,** The "smudge cells" of adenovirus infection can be seen at scanning magnification (*arrows*). **B,** Smudge cells at higher magnification (*arrows*).

Hantavirus is a rare cause of acute lung injury.[40–42] The infection produces alveolar edema, hyaline membranes, and atypical interstitial mononuclear inflammatory infiltrates[40–42] (Fig. 5-21). Spherical membrane-bound viral particles have been found in the cytoplasm of endothelial cells by electron microscopy.

Fungal Infection

Pneumocystis jiroveci (previously known as *Pneumocystis carinii*) is the most common fungus to cause DAD.[43–45] The histopathology of *Pneumocystis* infection in the setting of profound immunodeficiency is one of frothy intra-alveolar exudates (Fig. 5-22A) (so-called "alveolar casts"), with many organisms[44,45] (see Fig. 5-22B). In the mildly immunocompromised patient, however, this feature is not observed, or the pathologic changes may be subtle. In such cases, several "atypical" manifestations have been described.[43,45,46] DAD is the most dramatic of these atypical presentations (Fig. 5-23A), with the organisms present within hyaline membranes (see Fig. 5-23B) and in isolated intra-alveolar fibrin deposits.[46] The Grocott methenamine silver method (GMS) is routinely used to stain the organisms, which typically are seen in small groups and clusters (see Figs. 5-22B and 5-23B).[43,45,46]

Bacterial Infection

Common bacterial pneumonias rarely cause DAD; however, this lung injury pattern has been described in legionnaires disease, *Mycoplasma* pneumonia, and rickettsial infection.[47–51]

Legionella is a fastidious gram-negative bacillus that causes acute respiratory infection in elderly and immunodeficient individuals.[47,48,51] The histopathologic pattern is that of a pyogenic necrotizing bronchopneumonia (Fig. 5-24A) affecting the respiratory bronchioles, alveolar ducts, and adjacent alveolar spaces. DAD is common.[47,48,51] The rod-shaped organisms (see Fig. 5-24B) can be identified by Dieterle silver stain.[51]

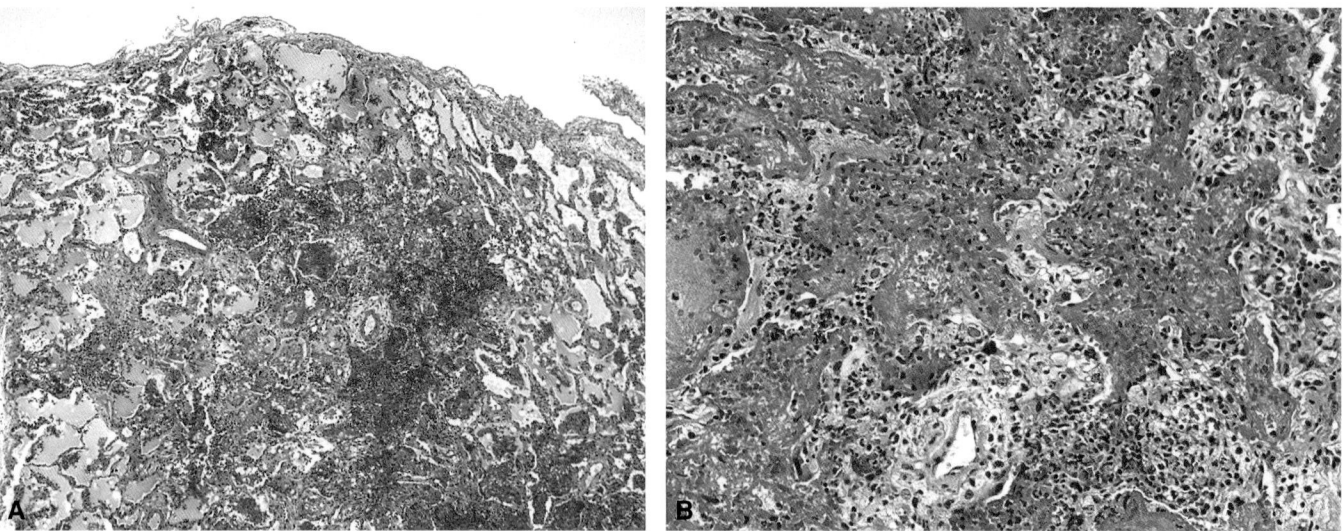

Figure 5-17. Diffuse alveolar damage in herpes simplex pneumonia. Herpesviridae viruses are capable of producing nodular necrotizing pneumonia (see Chapter 6). **A,** The nodular appearance of lung involved by herpes simplex pneumonia is evident, with zonal areas of hemorrhage and necrosis. **B,** A higher-magnification view of the hemorrhagic and necrotizing pneumonia.

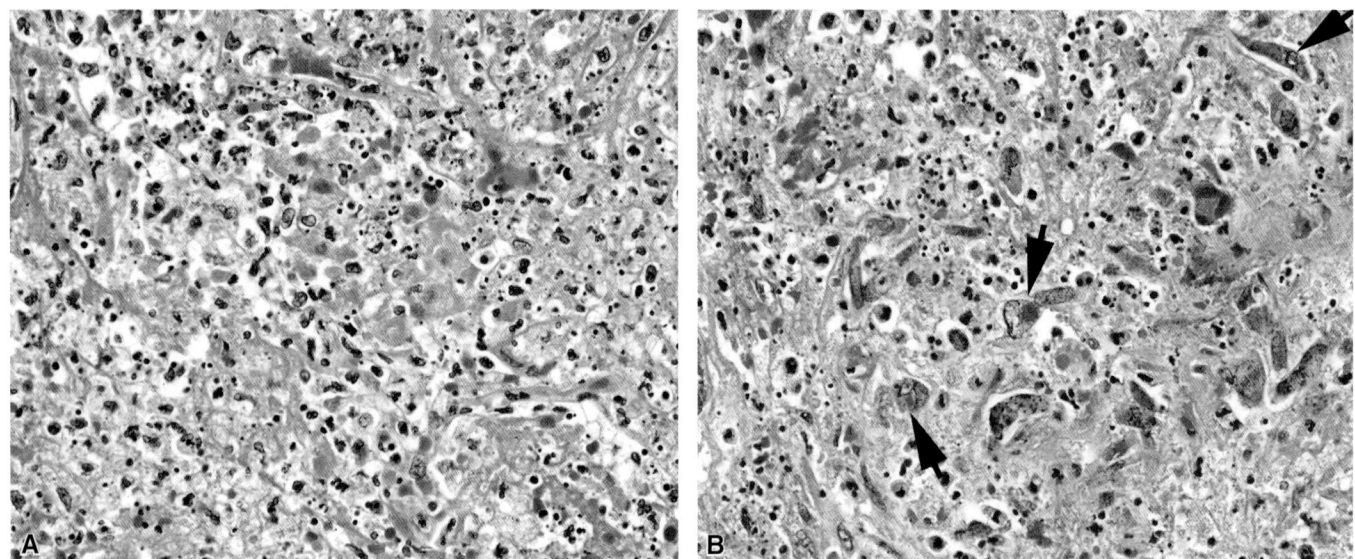

Figure 5-18. Herpes simplex pneumonia: inclusions. **A,** Diffuse alveolar damage associated with herpes simplex pneumonia. **B,** The viral cytopathic effects on bronchial and alveolar epithelium. The classic Cowdry A intranuclear inclusions (*arrows*) usually are easy to find, compared with the basophilic, smudged or ground-glass Cowdry B nuclear inclusions.

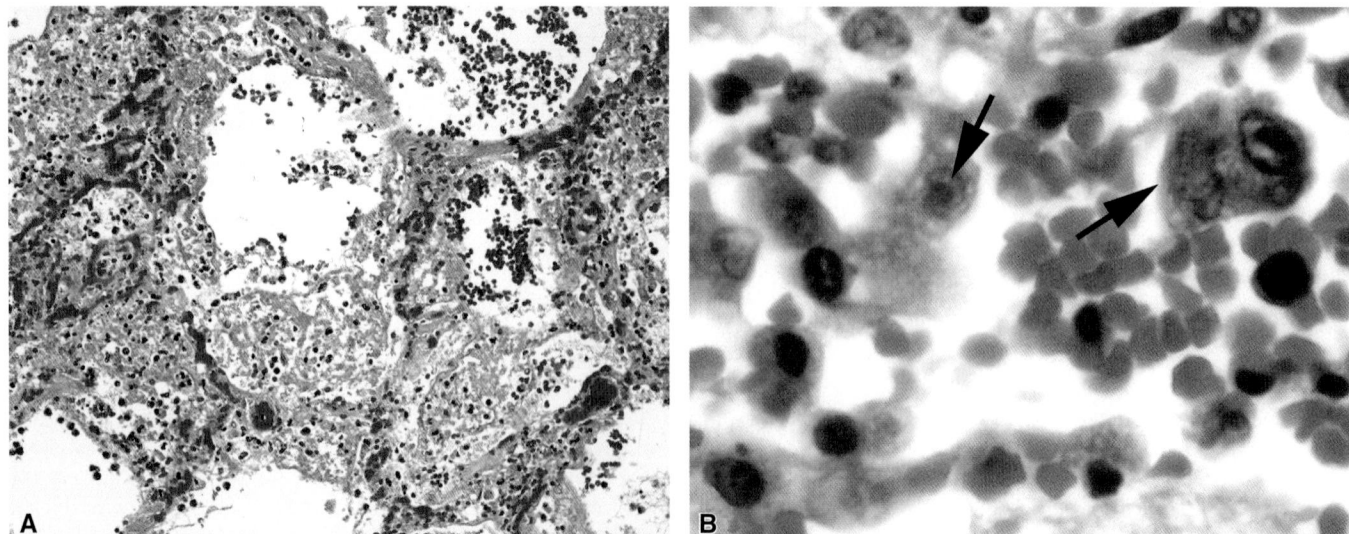

Figure 5-19. Diffuse alveolar damage (DAD) in varicella-zoster. The inclusions are similar to those produced by herpes simplex. **A,** Fibrinous DAD with neutrophils in air spaces in a case of chickenpox pneumonia. **B,** Rare intranuclear eosinophilic inclusions (*arrows*) are identifiable.

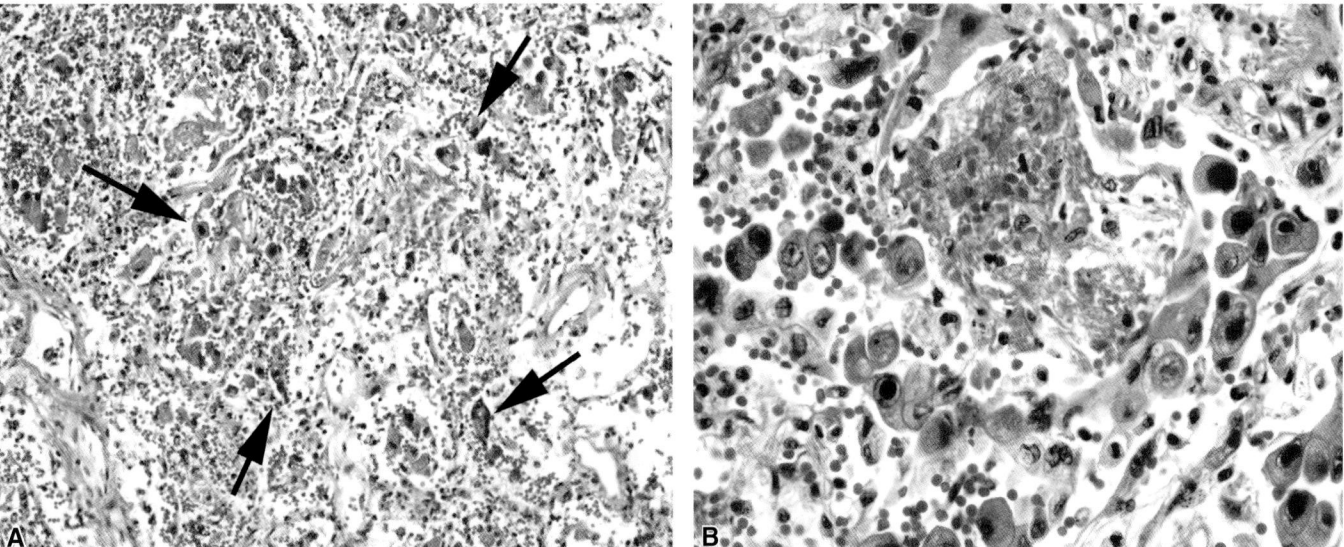

Figure 5-20. Diffuse alveolar damage (DAD) in cytomegalovirus (CMV) pneumonia. DAD from CMV infection can be quite dramatic in the immunocompromised host. **A,** DAD with numerous CMV cells evident at scanning magnification (*arrows*). **B,** CMV-infected cells at higher magnification. Prominent intranuclear inclusions are evident.

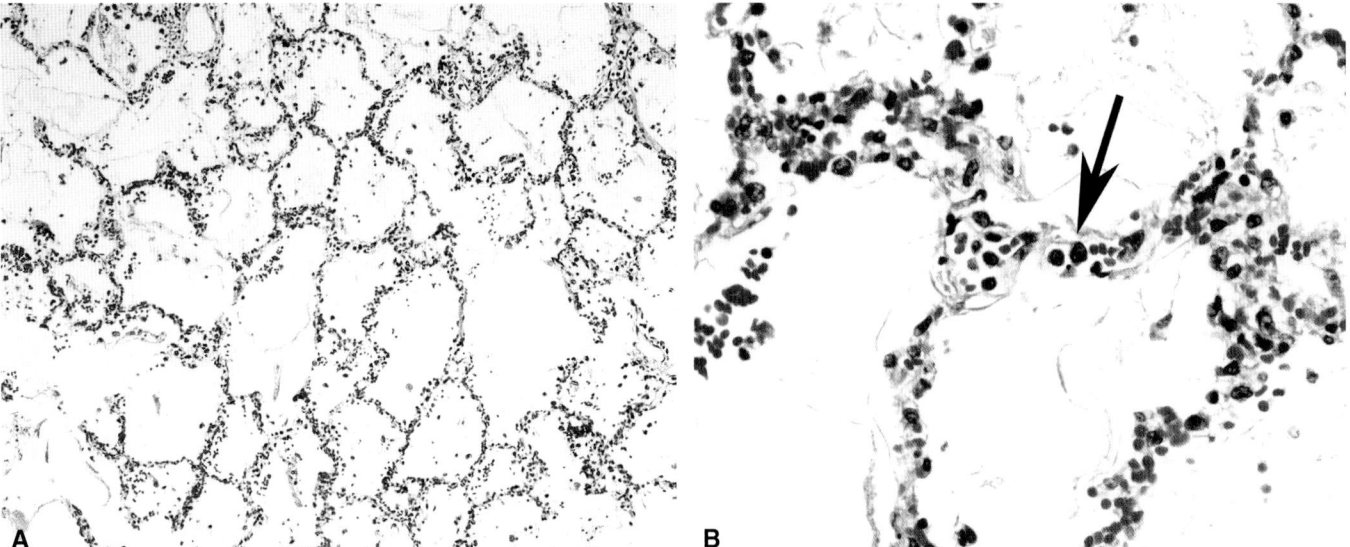

Figure 5-21. Diffuse alveolar damage in hantavirus pneumonia. Hantavirus pneumonia is characterized by alveolar edema, hyaline membranes (**A**), and scattered atypical interstitial mononuclear cells (**B,** *arrow*).

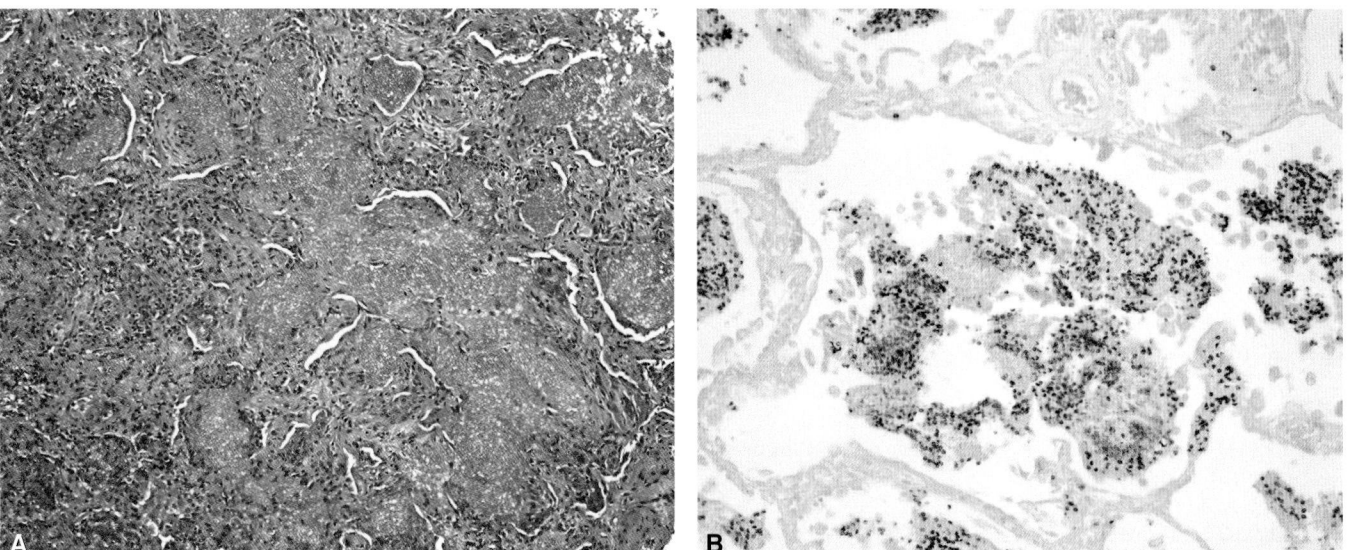

Figure 5-22. Diffuse alveolar damage in *Pneumocystis* pneumonia. **A,** The frothy "alveolar casts" characteristic of *Pneumocystis* pneumonia in the profoundly immunocompromised host (classically, the patient with AIDS or human immunodeficiency virus infection). **B,** Numerous silver-stained organisms are evident within these eosinophilic exudates (methenamine silver stain).

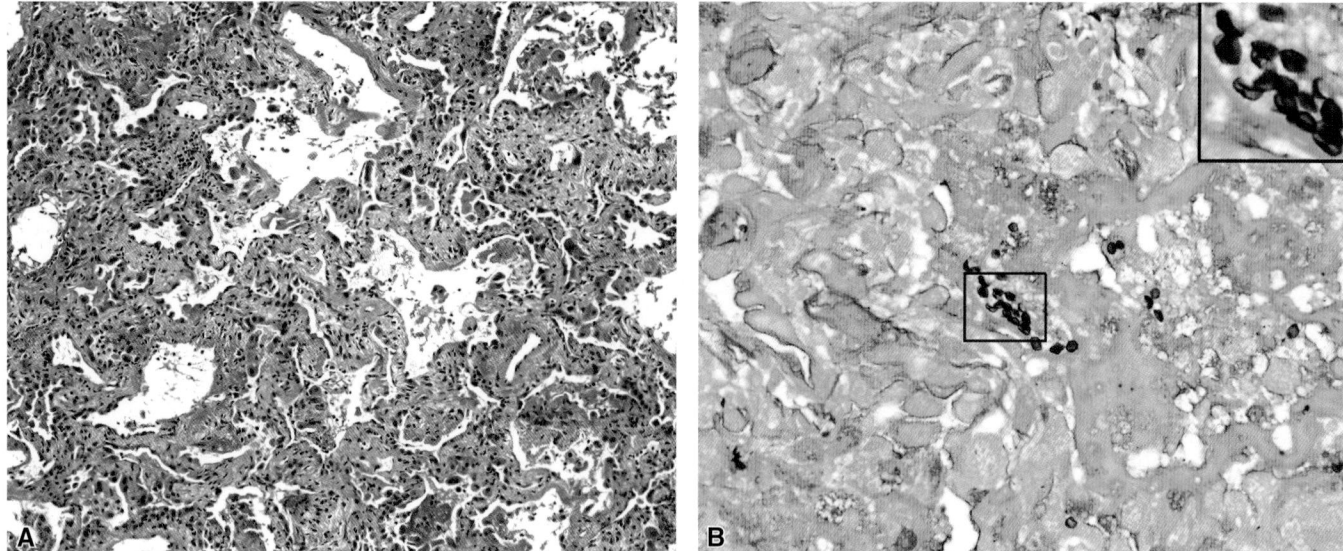

Figure 5-23. Diffuse alveolar damage in *Pneumocystis* pneumonia. **A,** Such diffuse damage also may occur in less severely immunocompromised patients. **B,** In such patients, few organisms may be identifiable by silver stains (methenamine silver stain). A colony of *Pneumocystis* organisms is shown in the *inset*.

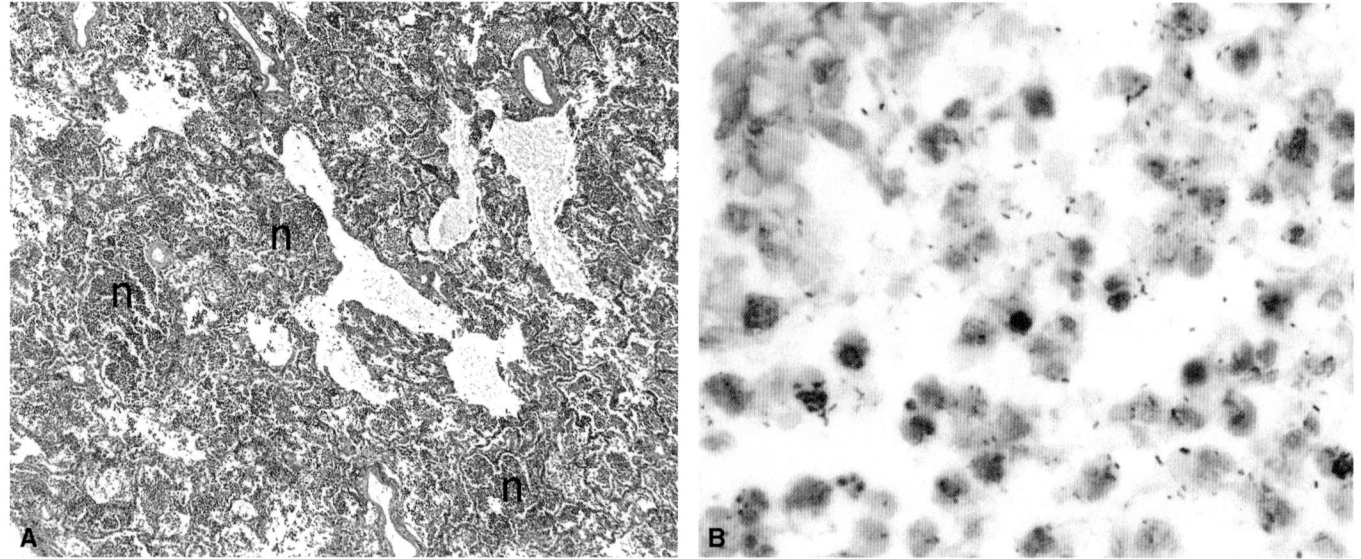

Figure 5-24. Diffuse alveolar damage in *Legionella* pneumonia. **A,** The diffuse alveolar injury caused by *Legionella* infection is prominently neutrophilic (n). **B,** Within these areas, a silver stain shows numerous rod-shaped stained organisms (Dieterle silver method).

Of note, in immunocompromised patients, any type of infection can cause DAD, with *Pneumocystis* pneumonia being the most common.[28] For this reason, it is essential to use special stains (acid-fast bacilli [AFB] stains or GMS or Warthin-Starry silver stain, and so on) on every lung biopsy specimen exhibiting DAD.

Collagen Vascular Diseases

Systemic collagen vascular disorders are a well-known cause of diffuse lung disease.[52–59] In some cases, lung involvement may be the first manifestation of the systemic disease, even without identifiable serologic evidence.[57] Acute lung injury has been reported to occur in the following collagen vascular diseases.

Systemic Lupus Erythematosus

Pulmonary involvement in SLE may manifest as pleural disease, acute or chronic diffuse inflammatory lung disease, airway disease, or vascular disease (vasculitis and thromboembolic lesions). Acute lupus pneumonitis (ALP) is a form of fulminant interstitial disease (Fig. 5-25A) with a high mortality rate.[52] Patients present with severe dyspnea, tachypnea, fever and arterial hypoxemia. ALP represents the first manifestation of SLE in approximately 50% of affected persons.[52,58] The most common histopathologic feature of this acute disease is DAD. Alveolar hemorrhage, with capillaritis and small-vessel vasculitis (see Fig. 5-25B), and pulmonary edema also may be observed.[52,57,60] Immunofluorescence studies demonstrate immune complexes in lung parenchyma, and both immune complexes and tubuloreticular inclusions may be seen on ultrastructural examination.[57,58,60]

Rheumatoid Arthritis

A significant percentage of patients with rheumatoid arthritis have lung disease.[53,54,61–64] Many different morphologic patterns of lung disease in rheumatoid arthritis have been described,[54,57,59] with the rheumatoid nodule being the most specific. Acute lung injury has been reported

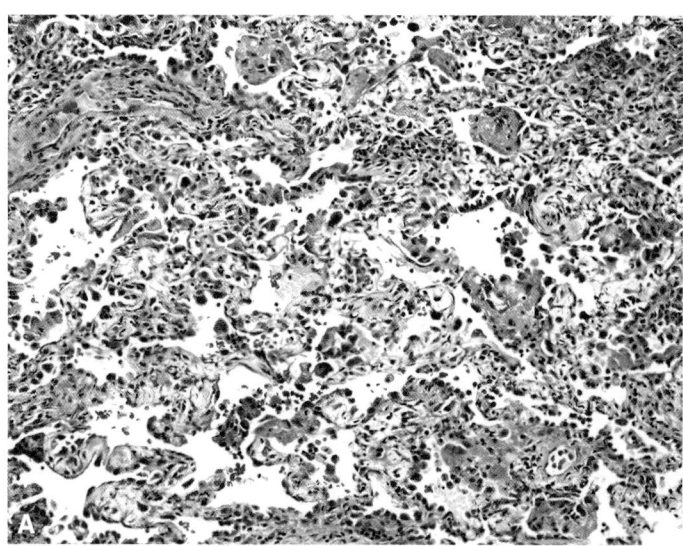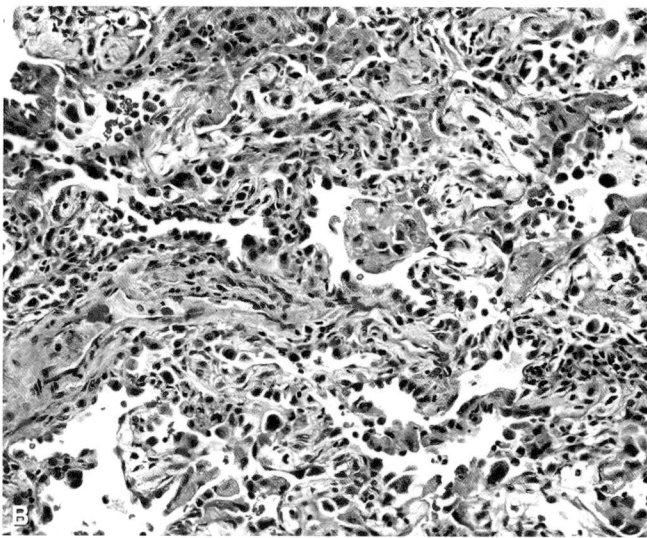

Figure 5-25. Diffuse alveolar damage (DAD) in systemic lupus erythematosus (SLE). The DAD associated with lupus may be quite hemorrhagic and associated with a "pneumonitis." Note the increased mononuclear cells within the alveolar interstitium in both parts **A** and **B**. Sometimes the alveolar hemorrhage of SLE may overlap with diffuse alveolar damage on morphologic grounds.

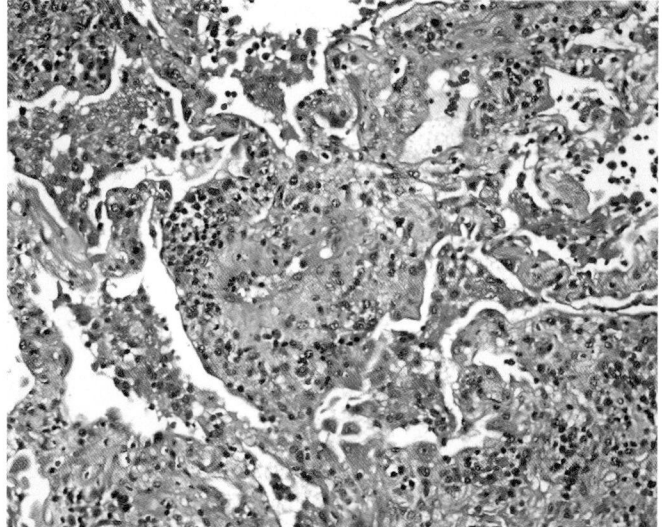

Figure 5-26. Diffuse alveolar damage (DAD) in rheumatoid arthritis. With DAD in rheumatoid arthritis, histopathologic hints of more chronic disease sometimes may be present, with lymphoplasmacellular infiltrates, chronic bronchiolitis, and chronic pleuritis. Here, a perivascular lymphoplasmacellular infiltrate is evident with surrounding air space fibrin and macrophages.

(Fig. 5-26), referred to as acute interstitial pneumonia in some publications[65] and as DAD in others.[54]

Polymyositis/Dermatomyositis

Polymyositis/dermatomyositis, a systemic connective tissue disorder, is well known to be associated with interstitial lung disease.[55,56] Three main clinical presentations are recognized: (1) acute fulminant respiratory distress resembling the so-called Hamman-Rich syndrome, (2) slowly progressive dyspnea, and (3) an asymptomatic form with abnormalities on radiologic and pulmonary function studies.[59] Three major histopathologic patterns have been observed: DAD (Fig. 5-27A), organizing pneumonia (see Fig. 5-27B), and chronic fibrosis (see Fig. 5-27C)—the so-called usual interstitial pneumonia (UIP) pattern.[66] The rapidly progressive clinical presentation is associated with a DAD histopathologic pattern on lung biopsy studies and carries the worst prognosis.[56]

DAD associated with *scleroderma* and *mixed connective disease* also has been described.[57,67]

Many patients with collagen vascular disease receive drug therapy during the course of their illness. A large number of drugs, including cytotoxic agents used for immunosuppression, are known to cause DAD. Also, as a desired result of therapy, patients may be immunosuppressed, making the exclusion of infection a high priority in the case of acute clinical lung disease.

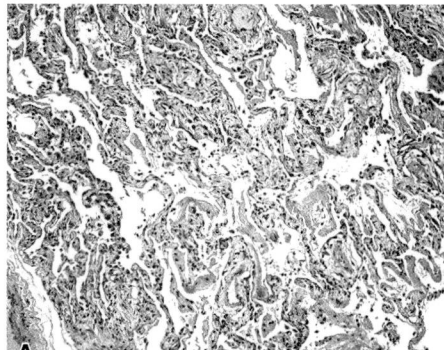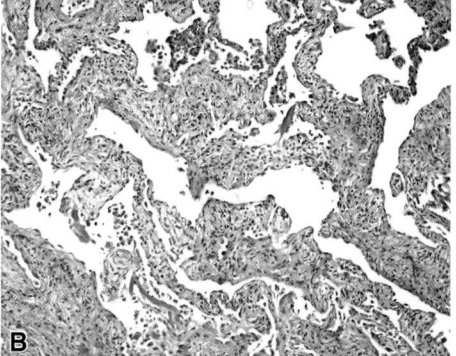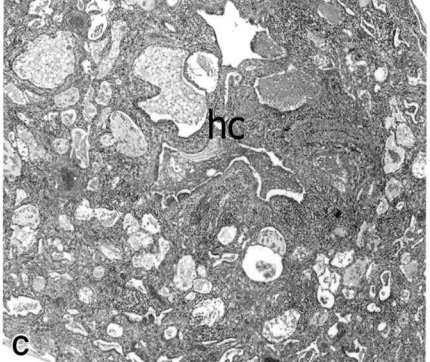

Figure 5-27. Diffuse alveolar damage (DAD) in polymyositis/dermatomyositis. All of the systemic connective tissue diseases can manifest with acute, subacute, and chronic lung disease. Three examples of diffuse lung disease accompanying polymyositis/dermatomyositis are presented: **A,** DAD; **B,** a subacute organizing pneumonia with an interstitial mononuclear infiltrate (nonspecific interstitial pneumonia [NSIP]-like; see Chapter 7); and **C,** a usual interstitial pneumonia (UIP)-like pattern of lung fibrosis with microscopic honeycomb remodeling (hc).

Drug Effect

Drugs can produce a wide range of pathologic effects with lung manifestations, and the causative agents are numerous.[68–81] The spectrum of drug-induced lung disease runs the entire gamut from DAD to fibrosis. Between these two extremes, subacute clinical manifestations may include organizing pneumonia, chronic interstitial pneumonia, eosinophilic pneumonia, obliterative bronchiolitis, pulmonary hemorrhage, pulmonary edema, pulmonary hypertension, veno-occlusive disease, and granulomatous interstitial pneumonia.[78,82,83]

DAD is a common and dramatic manifestation of pulmonary drug toxicity.[78] Many drugs are known to cause DAD.[82] A few of the more common ones are discussed next. (Drug-related lung disease is also discussed in Chapter 7.)

Chemotherapeutic Agents

DAD frequently is caused by cytotoxic drugs, and the commonly implicated ones include bleomycin (Fig. 5-28), busulfan (Fig. 5-29), and carmustine.[5,78,82] Patients usually present with dyspnea, cough, and diffuse pulmonary infiltrates.[84–88] The histologic pattern most commonly is one of nonspecific acute lung injury with hyaline membranes, but some changes may be present to at least suggest a causative agent. For example, the presence of acute lung injury with associated atypical type II pneumocytes with markedly enlarged pleomorphic nuclei[89] and prominent nucleoli (see Fig. 5-29) is characteristic for busulfan-induced pulmonary toxicity, and on ultrastructural examination, intranuclear tubular structures have been found in type II pneumocytes in association with administration of busulfan and bleomycin.[89–92] In most cases, the possibility that a drug is the cause of DAD can only be inferred from the clinical history. Considerations in the differential diagnosis typically include other treatment-related injury or complication of therapy (e.g., concomitant irradiation or infection). For example, oxygen therapy is a well-recognized cause of DAD (Fig. 5-30) and also may exacerbate bleomycin-induced lung injury.[93] Methotrexate (Fig. 5-31) is

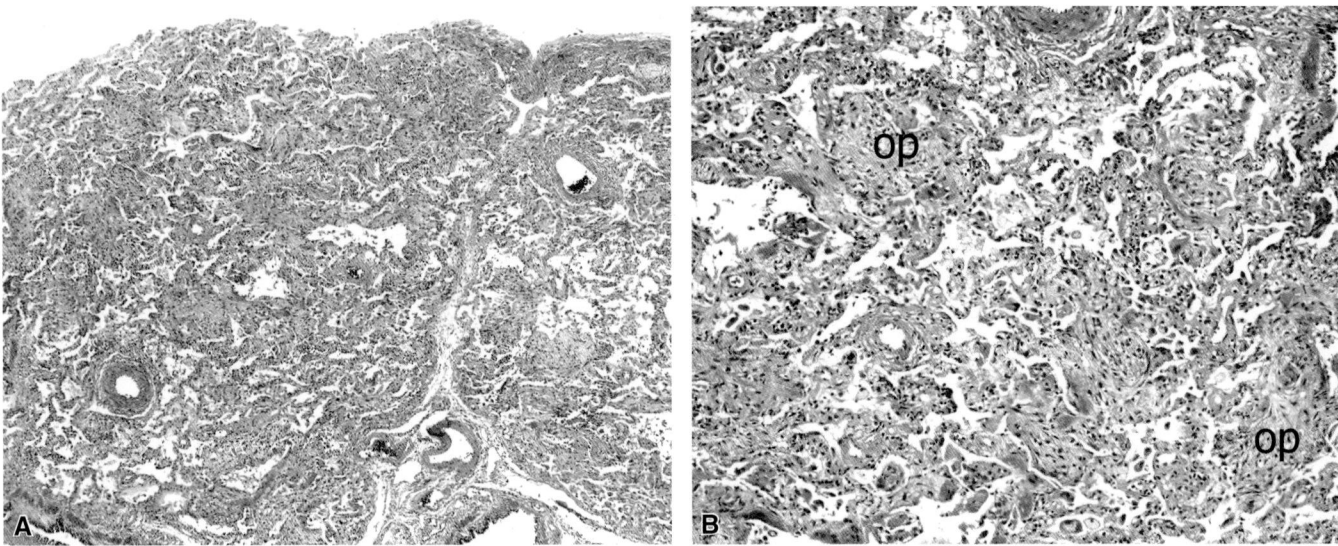

Figure 5-28. Diffuse alveolar damage from bleomycin toxicity. Bleomycin produces a characteristic lung injury in experimental animal models. Such damage has been observed to occur in humans as well (**A**), often typified by the presence of reactive type II cells and organizing pneumonia (op) (**B**).

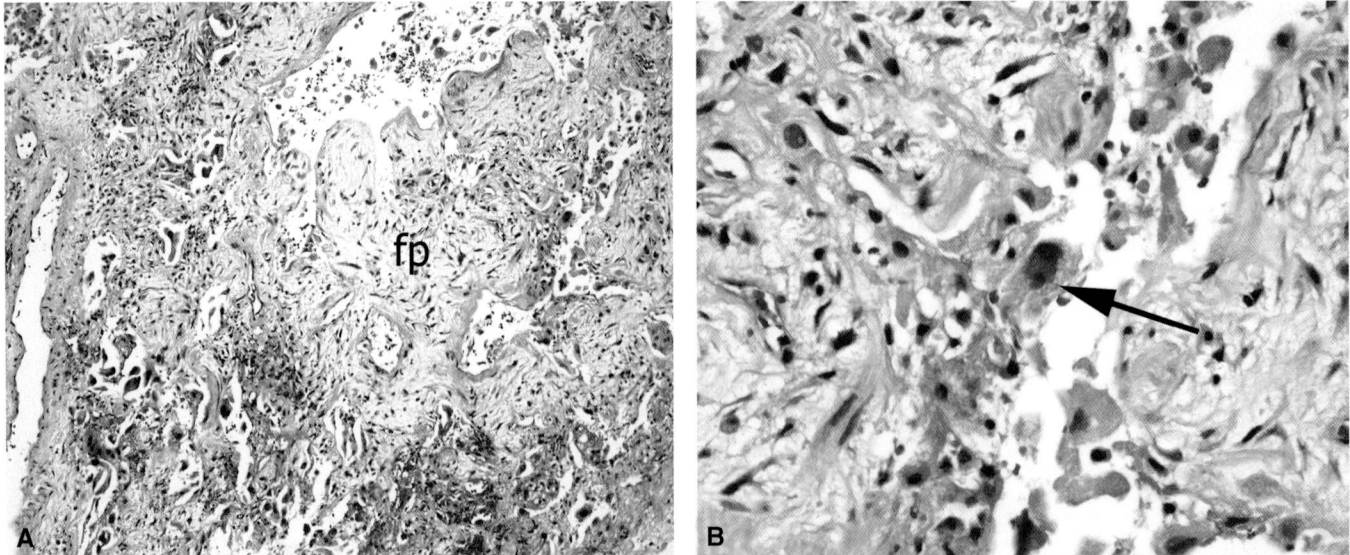

Figure 5-29. Diffuse alveolar damage from busulfan toxicity. Busulfan can produce diffuse injury characterized by the presence of prominently atypical type II cells. **A,** In this case, prominent interstitial organization with edematous fibroblastic proliferation is seen (fp), and hyaline membranes are evident. **B,** Reactive type II cells may appear alarmingly atypical (*arrow*).

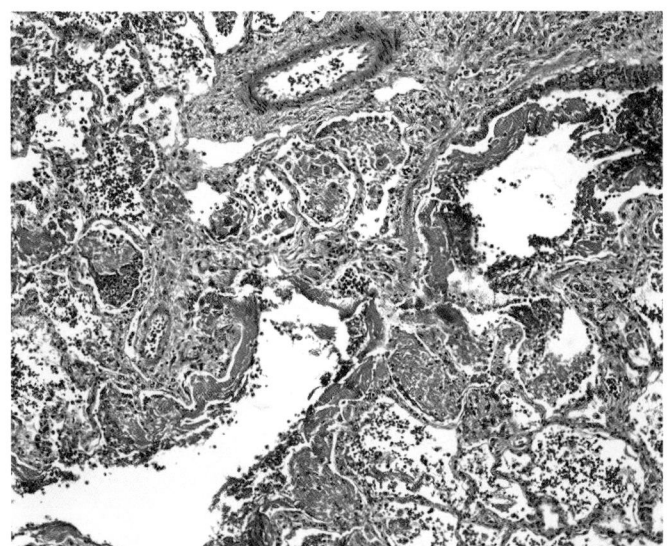

Figure 5-30. Diffuse alveolar damage from oxygen toxicity. Classic oxygen toxicity causes diffuse alveolar injury and necrosis of terminal airway epithelium, as illustrated in this photomicrograph.

another commonly used cytotoxic drug that can cause acute and organizing DAD.[94] Methotrexate also produces other distinctive patterns, such as granulomatous interstitial pneumonia (see Chapter 7) that is seldom seen in association with other commonly used chemotherapeutic agents. To complicate matters further, methotrexate also is used in the treatment of rheumatoid arthritis, a disease known to produce DAD independently as one of its pulmonary manifestations.[57,62]

Amiodarone

Amiodarone is a highly effective antiarrhythmic drug that is increasingly recognized as a cause of pulmonary toxicity.[77,95-99] Because patients taking amiodarone have known cardiac disease, the clinical presentation often is complicated, with several superimposed processes potentially affecting the lungs in various ways. Clinical and radiologic

considerations typically include congestive heart failure, pulmonary emboli, and acute lung injury from other causes.[77,99]

Distinctive features may be present on chest CT scans.[77] The lung biopsy commonly shows acute and organizing lung injury (Fig. 5-32A). Other patterns include chronic interstitial pneumonitis with fibrosis and organizing pneumonia.[97] Characteristically, type II pneumocytes and alveolar macrophages show finely vacuolated cytoplasm in response to amiodarone therapy (see Fig. 5-32B), but these changes alone are not evidence of toxicity because they also may be seen in patients taking amiodarone who do not have evidence of lung toxicity.[95-98]

Anti-inflammatory Drugs

Methotrexate and gold, common agents for treatment of rheumatoid arthritis, are frequently implicated in lung toxicity. Methotrexate is discussed earlier in this chapter. Organizing DAD (Fig. 5-33) and chronic interstitial pneumonia are commonly described pulmonary manifestations of so-called gold toxicity.[74,76,100]

Acute Eosinophilic Pneumonia

Acute eosinophilic pneumonia was first described in 1989[101] and is characterized by acute respiratory failure, fever of days' to weeks' duration, diffuse pulmonary infiltrates on radiologic studies, and eosinophilia in bronchoalveolar lavage (BAL) fluid or lung biopsy specimens in the absence of infection, atopy, and asthma.[102] Peripheral eosinophilia frequently is described but is not a consistent finding at initial presentation.[103,104] Acute eosinophilic pneumonia is easily confused with acute interstitial pneumonia because both manifest as acute respiratory distress without an obvious underlying cause.[102] Histologically, the disease is characterized by acute and organizing lung injury showing classic features (Fig. 5-34) of (1) alveolar septal edema, (2) eosinophilic air space macrophages, (3) tissue and air space eosinophils in variable numbers, and (4) marked reactive atypia of alveolar type II cells. Intra-alveolar fibroblastic proliferation (patchy organizing pneumonia) and inflammatory cells are present to a variable degree. Hyaline membranes and organizing intra-alveolar fibrin also may be present (Fig. 5-35). The most significant feature is the presence of interstitial and alveolar eosinophils. Infiltration of small blood vessels by eosinophils also may be seen. It is important to

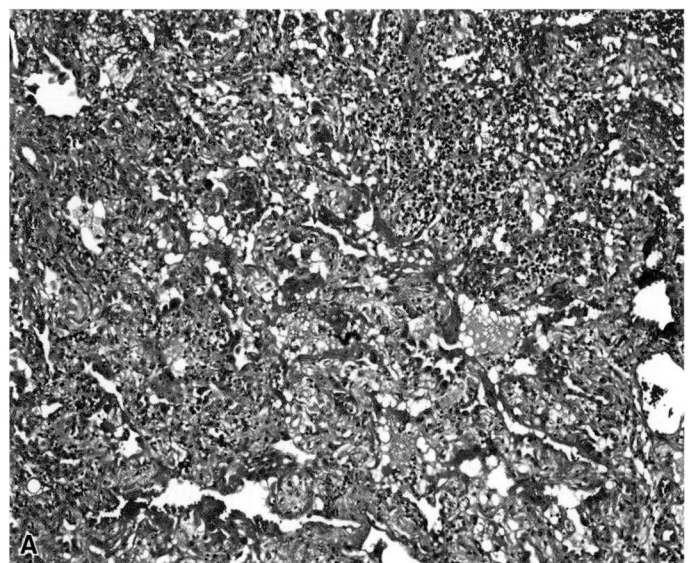

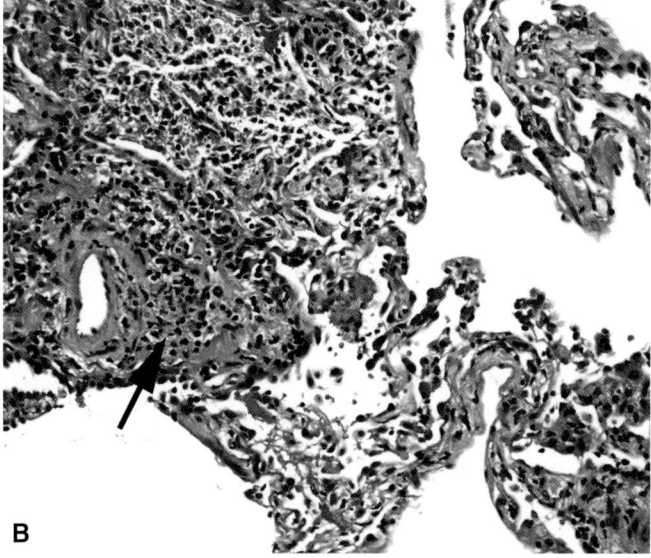

Figure 5-31. Diffuse alveolar damage (DAD) from methotrexate toxicity. **A** and **B,** Methotrexate produces small, poorly formed granulomas in subacute and chronic manifestations of lung toxicity. Early aggregations of macrophages may be seen resembling poorly formed granulomas in cases in which DAD is the manifestation of injury, but these are not required for the diagnosis (*arrow*).

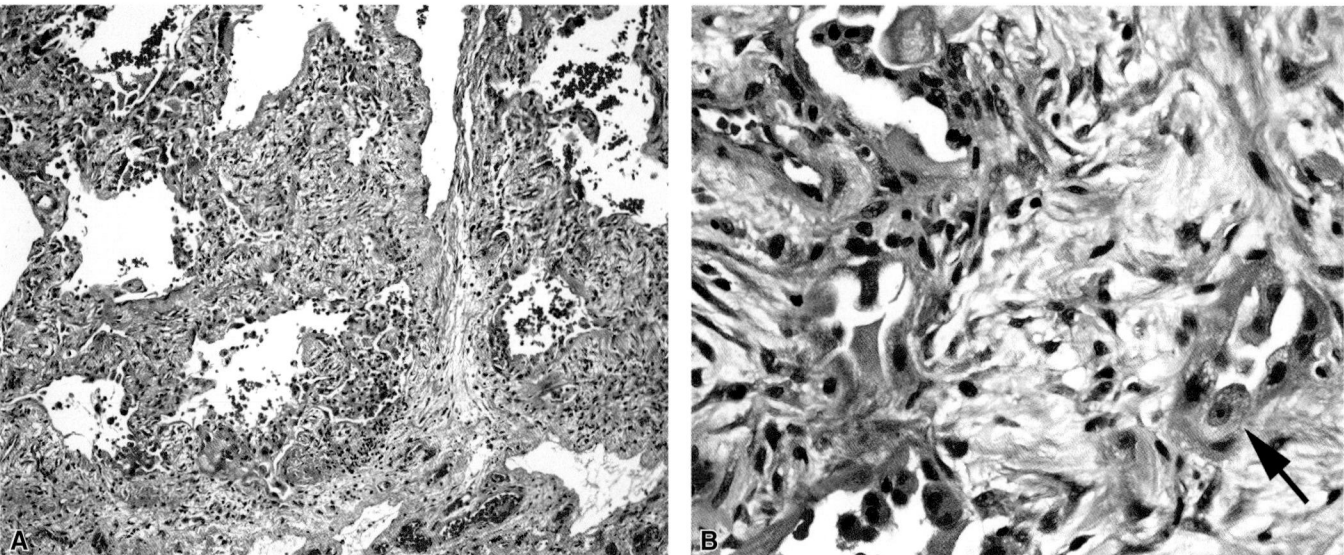

Figure 5-32. Diffuse alveolar damage from amiodarone toxicity. Amiodarone can produce acute, subacute, and chronic lung toxicity. **A,** Scanning magnification of amiodarone-induced diffuse alveolar injury. **B,** The finely vacuolated macrophages in type II cells are clearly evident (*arrow*).

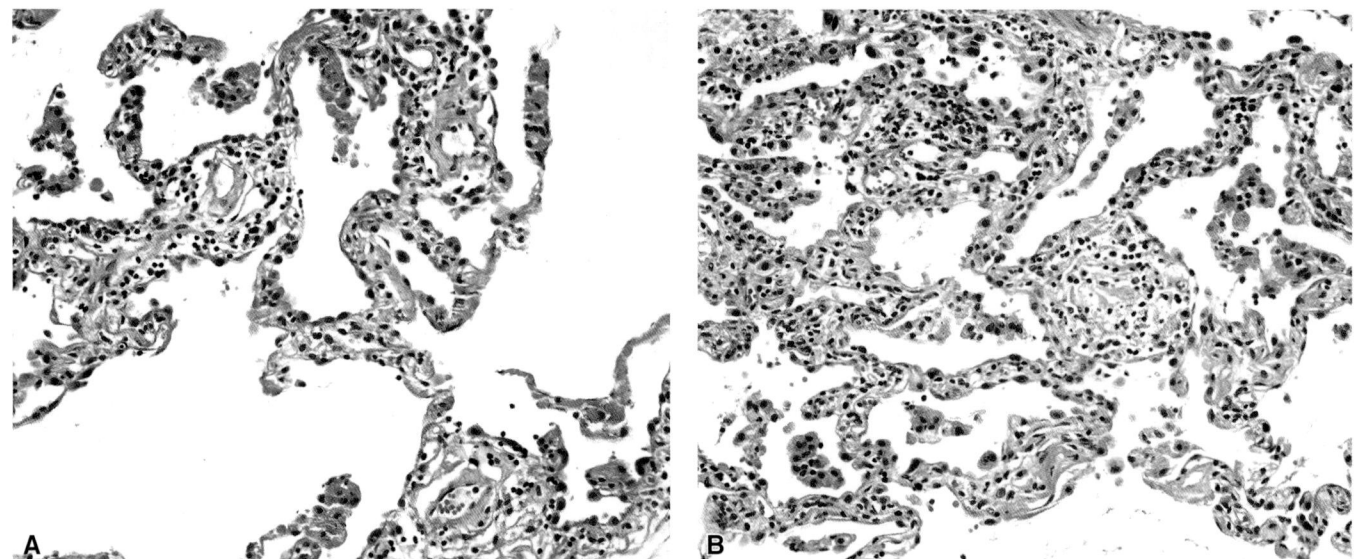

Figure 5-33. Diffuse alveolar damage from gold therapy toxicity. **A,** Gold therapy for rheumatoid arthritis may produce diffuse alveolar injury with hyaline membranes. **B,** A chronic or subacute cellular inflammatory process also has been described.

distinguish acute eosinophilic pneumonia from other causes of DAD, because patients typically benefit from systemic corticosteroid treatment, with prompt recovery. Before initiation of immunosuppressive therapy, however, infection should be rigorously excluded by culture and special stains, because parasitic and fungal infections also can manifest as tissue eosinophilia.

Acute Interstitial Pneumonia

Acute interstitial pneumonia, also commonly referred to as Hamman-Rich syndrome, is a fulminant lung disease of unknown etiology occurring in previously healthy patients.[105–107] Patients usually report a prodromal illness simulating viral infection of the upper respiratory tract, followed by rapidly progressive respiratory failure. The mortality rate is high, with death occurring weeks or months after the acute onset.[105,107] The classic histopathologic pattern is that of acute and organizing DAD,[105,107] with septal edema and hyaline membranes in the early phase and septal fibroblastic proliferation with reactive type II pneumocytes prominent in the organizing phase. In practice, a combination of acute and organizing changes (Fig. 5-36) often are seen in the lung at the time of biopsy.[108] A variable degree of air space organization, mononuclear inflammatory infiltrates, thrombi in small pulmonary arteries, and reparative peribronchiolar squamous metaplasia also are seen in most cases.

Because acute interstitial pneumonia is idiopathic, other specific causes of acute lung injury must be excluded before making this diagnosis. Considerations in the differential diagnosis include infection, collagen vascular disease, acute exacerbation of idiopathic pulmonary fibrosis (IPF), drug effect, and other causes of DAD.[108] Most cases of DAD are not acute interstitial pneumonia, and detailed clinical information, radiologic findings (localized versus diffuse disease), serologic data, and microbiologic results will often point to or rule out a specific etiologic condition. Use of special stains

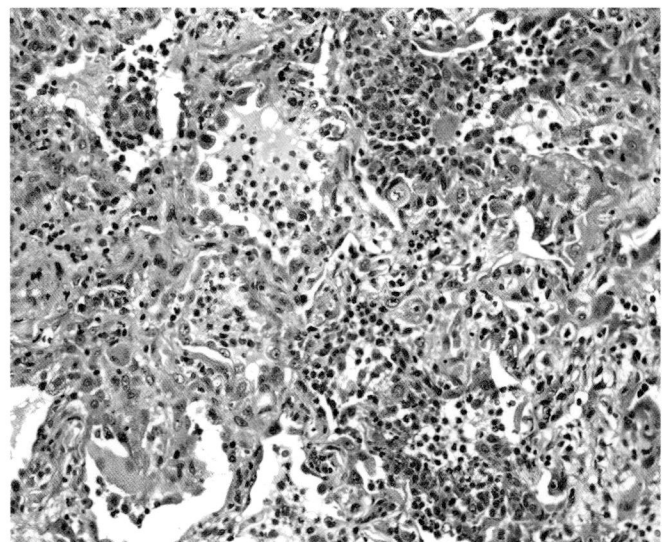

Figure 5-34. Acute eosinophilic pneumonia. The histopathologic changes seen in eosinophilic pneumonia are well known to most pathologists. Reactive type II cell hyperplasia in combination with the pesence of air space fibrin, eosinophilic air space macrophages, and scattered eosinophils yields a characteristic picture.

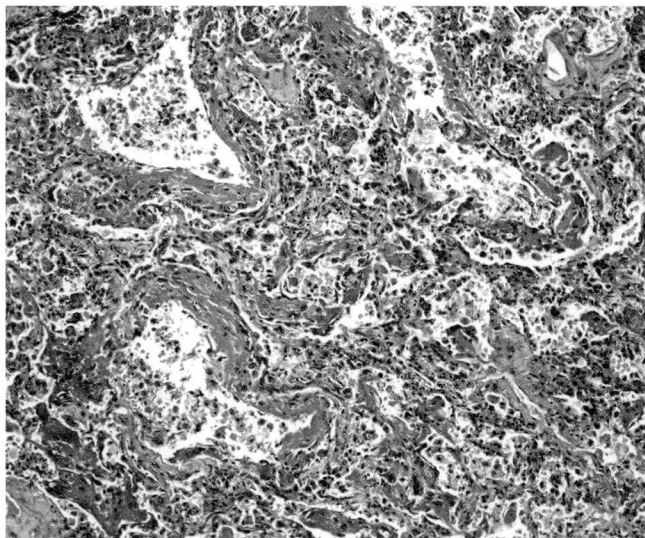

Figure 5-36. Acute interstitial pneumonia (AIP). Idiopathic AIP may take the form of every possible morphologic manifestation of acute respiratory distress syndrome, depending on the timing of biopsy relative to the onset of symptoms. Here, a classic pattern of diffuse alveolar damage (DAD) with hyaline membranes of variable cellularity is seen (midproliferative phase). Interstitial fibroblastic proliferation may be more or less prominent from case to case and should not serve as a qualifying morphologic finding for the diagnosis. AIP is nothing more than DAD of unknown causation.

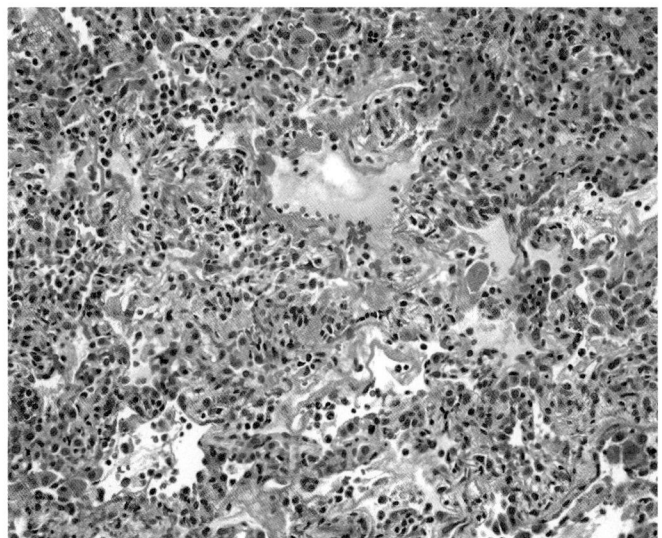

Figure 5-35. Diffuse alveolar damage (DAD) with acute eosinophilic pneumonia: hyaline membranes. Organization of hyaline membranes may occur in the acute lung injury of eosinophilic pneumonia. An awareness of this association is important, so that eosinophilic pneumonia is not overlooked as a potential cause of DAD with hyaline membranes.

applied to tissue sections or cytologic preparations (e.g., AFB, GMS or Warthin-Starry silver stain) also is essential to rule out infectious organisms in this setting.

Immunologically Mediated Pulmonary Hemorrhage and Vasculitis

So-called "pulmonary hemorrhage syndromes" may feature the histopathologic changes of acute lung injury,[109] in addition to the characteristic alveolar hemorrhage and hemosiderin-laden macrophages. In some patients, DAD may be the dominant histopathologic pattern.[110] In the study by Lombard and colleagues in patients with Goodpasture syndrome, all showed acute lung injury ranging in distribution from focal to diffuse lung involvement.[110] Histopathologic

examination demonstrated typical acute and organizing DAD, with widened and edematous alveolar septa, fibroblastic proliferation, reactive type II pneumocytes, and, rarely, even hyaline membranes (Fig. 5-37). Alveolar hemorrhage, either focal or diffuse, was present in all cases. Capillaritis, an important finding indicating true alveolar hemorrhage,[109] also was seen, as evidenced by marked septal neutrophilic infiltration. Capillaritis was absent in one case for which DAD was the dominant histopathologic pattern.

Microscopic polyangiitis can manifest as an acute interstitial pneumonia both clinically and histopathologically. Affected patients have vasculitis as the known cause of acute lung injury.[111] Alveolar hemorrhage with arteritis, capillaritis and venulitis may be seen in some cases.[111]

Polyarteritis nodosa and vasculitis associated with systemic connective tissue disease (notably systemic lupus erythematosus and rheumatoid arthritis) can also show acute lung injury with alveolar hemorrhage as the dominant histopathologic finding.[57,112]

Radiation Pneumonitis

Radiation can produce both acute and chronic damage to the lung, manifesting as acute radiation pneumonitis and chronic progressive fibrosis, respectively.[113] The effect is dependent on radiation dosage, total time of irradiation, and tissue volume irradiated. Concomitant chemotherapy and infections, which in themselves are causes of DAD, may potentiate the effect of radiation injury.[5,79,114,115] Acute radiation pneumonitis manifests 1 to 2 months after radiation therapy.[5,115] Clinical findings include dyspnea, cough, pleuritic pain, fever, and chest infiltrates. The lung biopsy specimen shows acute and organizing DAD.[113,115] Markedly atypical type II pneumocytes with enlarged hyperchromatic nuclei and vacuolated cytoplasm constitute a hallmark of the disease (Fig. 5-38A), and increased numbers of alveolar macrophages are seen. Foamy cells are present in the intima and media of pulmonary blood vessels in some cases, and thrombosis (see Fig. 5-38B), with or without transmural fibrinoid necrosis, is common.[79,116-118]

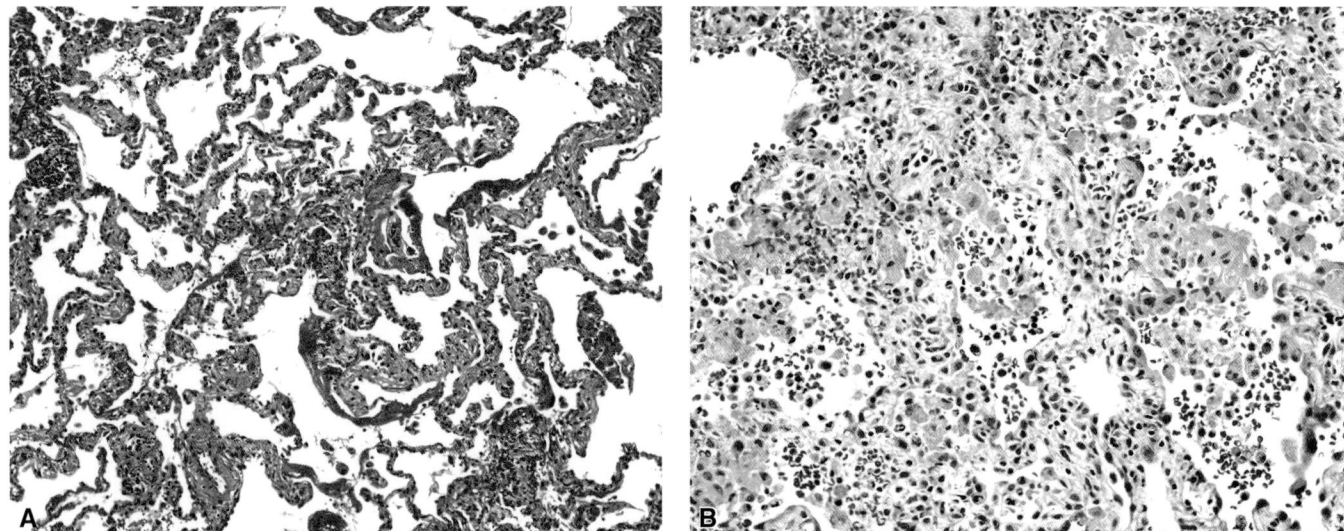

Figure 5-37. Diffuse alveolar damage (DAD) in Goodpasture syndrome. **A,** Goodpasture syndrome characteristically produces alveolar hemorrhage, but acute lung injury with hyaline membranes also can occur. **B,** In another example of DAD in Goodpasture syndrome, greater interstitial fibroblast proliferation is evident, along with more numerous air space macrophages.

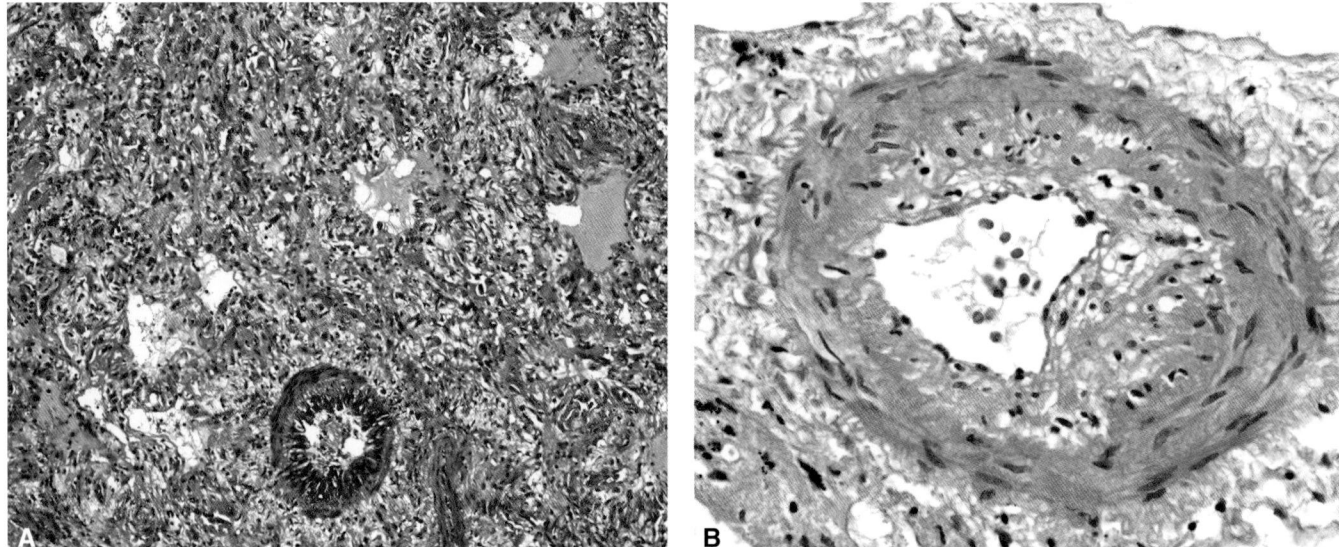

Figure 5-38. Diffuse alveolar damage (DAD) from radiation injury. **A,** Radiation injury to the lung can produce DAD with striking reactive type II cell hyperplasia. **B,** Foamy macrophages are present in the wall of a pulmonary artery involved in radiation pneumonitis.

Disease Presenting as Classic Acute Respiratory Distress Syndrome

By definition, ARDS must be associated with an identifiable inciting event. The histopathologic pattern is that of classic DAD. The histopathologic changes should be consistent with those expected for the time interval from the onset of clinical disease (see further on). In many cases, the ARDS may be caused by a combination of factors, each potentiating the other.[4] For the purposes of illustration, a few thoroughly studied causes are discussed next.

Oxygen Toxicity and Inhalants

Oxygen is a well-known cause of ARDS and a useful model for all types of DAD.[4,119,120] Oxygen toxicity also is important in that it is widely used in the care of patients, often in the setting of other injuries that can potentially cause ARDS, such as sepsis, shock, and trauma. Exposure to high concentrations of oxygen for prolonged periods can lead to characteristic pulmonary damage. In 1958, Pratt first noted pulmonary changes due to high concentrations

of inspired oxygen.[121] In 1967, Nash and colleagues described the sequential histopathologic changes of this injury,[119] later reemphasized by Pratt.[120] In neonates receiving oxygen for hyaline membrane disease, bronchopulmonary dysplasia was reported to occur. [122] As might be expected, the features of hyaline membrane disease in neonates and oxygen-induced DAD in adults are indistinguishable (see Fig. 5-30). Other inhalants such as chlorine gas, mercury vapor, carbon dioxide in high concentrations, and nitrogen mustard all have been reported to cause ARDS.[2,4,5]

Shock and Trauma

Massive extrapulmonary trauma and shock first became recognized as causes of unexplained respiratory failure during the wars of the second half of the 20th century. A variety of names were assigned to this wartime condition, including shock lung, congestive atelectasis, traumatic wet lung, Da Nang lung, respiratory insufficiency syndrome, post-traumatic pulmonary insufficiency, and progressive pulmonary consolidation.[2] It became clear that shock of any cause (e.g., hypovolemia due to hemorrhage, cardiogenic shock, sepsis), could cause ARDS, and that in most cases, a number of factors come into play. In the typical presentation, dyspnea of rapid onset is accompanied by development of diffuse chest infiltrates several hours to days after an episode of shock. Once ARDS begins, the mortality rate is high.[1,2,123]

Ingested Toxins

Paraquat is a potent herbicide that causes the release of hydrogen peroxide and superoxide free radicals, resulting in damage to cell membranes.[124–126] Oropharyngitis is the initial sign of poisoning, followed by impaired renal and liver function. Approximately 5 days later, ARDS develops. The histolopathologic pattern in most cases is one of organizing DAD (Fig. 5-39). The diagnosis is confirmed by tissue analysis for paraquat, which can be performed even on autopsy specimens. Other ingested toxins (e.g., kerosene, rapeseed oil) also have been reported to cause ARDS.[5]

Additional Features in the Differential Diagnosis of Acute Lung Injury

Acute lung injury is a pathologic pattern and by itself is a nonspecific finding. The following additional features often help narrow the list of possible causes (summarized in Table 5-1).

Presence of hyaline membranes. The most commonly encountered potential etiologic disorders include infection, collagen vascular disease, drug toxicity, and an idiopathic form (i.e., acute interstitial pneumonia).[2,5]

Presence of neutrophils. The presence of neutrophils in lung alveolar spaces should always raise the possibility of infection.[115,127] For example, legionnaires disease characteristically is associated with acute bronchopneumonia with DAD.[51]

Presence of frothy exudates. The presence of frothy exudates in alveolar spaces is a classic feature of *Pneumocystis* pneumonia. However, this feature is not always present. In some cases, especially in mildly immunocompromised patients, DAD may be the only finding.[46]

Presence of necrosis. Among the infectious causes of DAD, viral infection figures prominently. Influenzavirus, herpes simplex virus, varicella-zoster virus, and adenovirus infections are well known to produce DAD,[29,31,34–36] and all of these viral infections typically are accompanied by necrosis. *Legionella* and

Table 5-1. Key Histopathologic Findings in Acute Lung Injury, with Possible Causes

Finding	Possible Causes
Hyaline membranes	Infection, collagen vascular disease, drug toxicity, oxygen and inhalant toxicity, idiopathic (acute interstitial pneumonia); acute exacerbation of idiopathic pulmonary fibrosis (characteristic associated findings: background fibrosis and microscopic honeycombing)
Neutrophils and fibrinous exudates	Infection (viral, fungal, bacterial), alveolar hemorrhage
Diffuse alveolar hemorrhage (with or without capillaritis and small-vessel vasculitis)	Collagen vascular diseases (SLE, RA, MCTD, polymyositis/dermatomyositis, scleroderma), Goodpasture syndrome, microscopic polyangiitis, Wegener granulomatosis (organizing pneumonia— capillaritis variant)
Organizing pneumonia (alveolar organization)	Resolving infection, drug toxicity, collagen vascular diseases, idiopathic (cryptogenic organizing pneumonia); acute exacerbation of idiopathic pulmonary fibrosis
Fibrin and organization	Infection, drug toxicity, idiopathic (acute fibrinous and organizing pneumonitis), collagen vascular diseases; acute exacerbation of idiopathic pulmonary fibrosis
Alveolar eosinophils with fibrin	Infection, collagen vascular disease, drug toxicity; idiopathic acute eosinophilic pneumonia
Necrosis	Infection and infarction
Atypical cells	Infection (especially viral), radiation pneumonitis, chemotherapy-related changes (and effects of other drugs)
Foamy alveolar cells	Amiodarone and other drug toxicity, radiation pneumonitis

MCTD, mixed connective tissue disease; RA, rheumatoid arthritis; SLE, systemic lupus erythematosus.

Pneumocystis infections also can produce acute lung injury with necrosis.[46,51,128]

Presence of eosinophils. Acute and organizing DAD with prominent interstitial and alveolar eosinophils is characteristic of acute eosinophilic pneumonia.[102] However, if the patient has been treated with

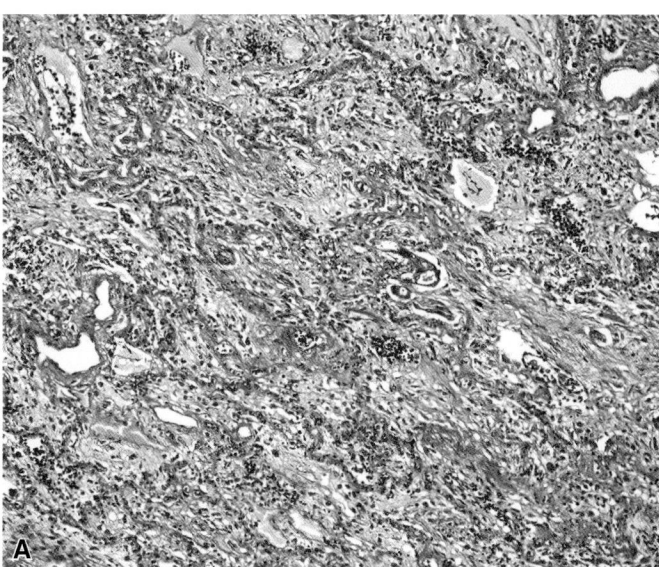

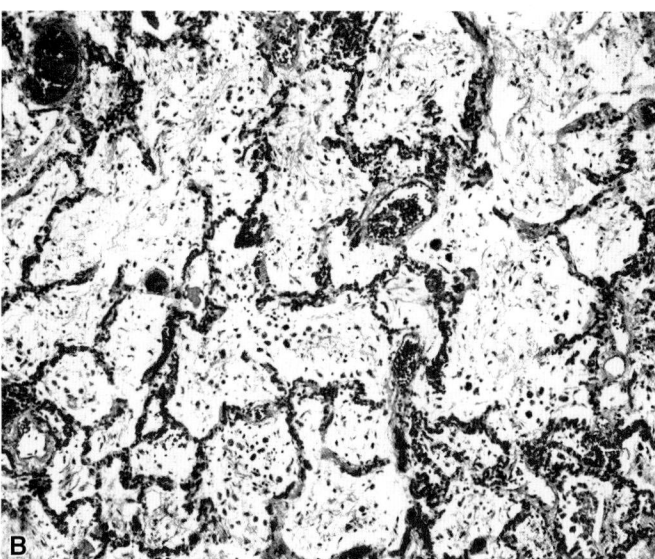

Figure 5-39. Diffuse alveolar damage from paraquat poisoning. Paraquat produces a dramatic and characteristic pattern of lung injury with prominent air space fibroplasia (**A**) and eventual fibrosis with collagen deposition in a loose pattern (**B**).

steroid before biopsy, very few eosinophils may remain, and the diagnosis may be difficult or impossible.

Presence of siderophages and capillaritis. Hemosiderin-laden macrophages with or without capillaritis in the setting of acute lung injury should raise consideration of immunologically mediated pulmonary hemorrhage.[109] Care must be taken not to interpret the pigmented macrophages seen in the lungs of cigarette smokers as evidence of hemorrhage.[129] The hemosiderin in macrophages related to true hemorrhage in the lung (from any cause) is globular, often slightly refractile, and golden-brown in color.[57,109-111]

Presence of atypical cells. Viral infections often produce cytopathic effects, including intracellular inclusions (see Chapter 6). Examples of intracellular inclusions are the Cowdry A and B inclusions seen in herpesvirus infection, cytomegaly with intranuclear and intracytoplasmic inclusions of cytomegalovirus, the multinucleated giant cells of measles virus and respiratory syncytial virus, and the smudged cells of adenovirus infection.[33,37,38,130,131] Chemotherapeutic drugs such as busulfan and bleomycin often are associated with markedly atypical type II pneumocytes, which may have enlarged pleomorphic nuclei and prominent nucleoli.[90,91] Markedly atypical type II pneumocytes that may be suggestive of a viropathic effect also are seen in radiation pneumonitis.[79,117,118]

Presence of foamy cells. Alveolar lining cells with vacuolated cytoplasm accompanied by intra-alveolar foamy macrophages are characteristic features seen in patients taking amiodarone, and amiodarone toxicity may lead to acute lung injury changes.[95-97,99] In some cases of radiation pneumonitis, foam cells are seen in the intima and media of blood vessels.[79,118]

Presence of advanced interstitial fibrosis. Clinical idiopathic pulmonary fibrosis is associated with the changes of UIP on pathologic examination (see Chapter 7), with advanced lung remodeling. Of interest, idiopathic pulmonary fibrosis undergoes episodic exacerbation, and on occasion such exacerbation may be overwhelming, with resultant DAD.[132] It is prudent to examine lung biopsy sections for the presence of dense fibrosis with structural remodeling (microscopic honeycombing) in cases of DAD, to identify the rare case of idiopathic pulmonary fibrosis that manifests for the first time as an acute episode of "exacerbation."

Clinicopathologic Correlation

Because the morphologic manifestations of acute diffuse lung disease may be relatively stereotypical, clinicopathologic correlation is often helpful in arriving at a specific diagnosis. A summary of the more important history and laboratory data pertinent to this correlation is presented in Box 5-3.

Box 5-3. Essential Information for Determining the Underlying Cause of Acute Lung Injury

Immune status
Acuity of onset
Radiologic distribution and character of abnormalities
History of inciting event (e.g., shock)
History of lung disease (e.g., "usual interstitial pneumonia" with current acute exacerbation)
History of systemic disease (e.g., connective tissue disease, heart disease)
History of medication use or drug abuse
History of other recent treatment (e.g., radiotherapy for malignancy)
Results of serologic studies: erythrocyte sedimentation rate determination, assays for autoimmune antibodies (e.g., ANA, RF, ANCA, Scl-70, Jo-1)
Results of microbiology studies

ANA, antinuclear antibody; ANCA, anti-neutrophil cytoplasmic antibody; RF, rheumatoid factor.

One of the first questions to be addressed is whether or not a known inciting event was identified clinically (i.e., Is this ARDS?). Next, the results of any sampling procedures to identify infection should be checked, along with application of special stains to the tissue sections, to exclude infection. Finally, data regarding related disease, such as infection, autoimmune disease, underlying lung disease, are needed. For example, if the patient is immunosuppressed, infection should always be the leading consideration in the differential diagnosis. Another point to keep in mind is that patients with certain diseases may be taking medications with the potential to cause DAD (e.g., amiodarone for cardiac arrhythmia). Moreover, laboratory studies may reveal antibodies related to connective tissue disease (e.g., antineutrophil antibody [ANA], rheumatoid factor [RF], Jo-1, Scl-70, anti-fibrillarin, anti-Mpp10, SS-A, SS-B).

Regarding the pathologist's role and responsibility in biopsy cases of acute lung injury, use of special stains for organisms (at a minimum, methenamine silver and acid-fast stains) is indicated. Additional stains (auramine-rhodamine, Dieterle or Warthin-Starry silver stain, immunohistochemical stains for specific organisms, or molecular probes) may be used, especially in patients known to be immunocompromised from any cause.

Self-assessment questions related to this chapter can be found online on the Expert Consult site for this title.

References

1. Petty T. 41st Aspen Lung Conference: Overview. *Chest.* 1999;116:1S–2S.
2. Tomashefski Jr J. Pulmonary pathology of acute respiratory distress syndrome. *Clin Chest Med.* 2000;21(3):435–466.
3. Ashbaugh D, Bigelow DB, Petty TL, Levine BE. Acute respiratory distress in adults. *Lancet.* 1967;2:319–323.
4. Katzenstein A, Bloor C, Liebow A. Diffuse alveolar damage—the role of oxygen, shock and related factors. *Am J Pathol.* 1976;85:209–228.
5. Katzenstein A. Acute lung injury patterns: diffuse alveolar damage and bronchiolitis obliterans–organizing pneumonia. In: Katzenstein A, Askin F, eds. *Katzenstein and Askin's Surgical Pathology of Non-Neoplastic Lung Disease.* Philadelphia: Saunders; 1997.
6. Zambon M, Vincent JL. Mortality rates for patients with acute lung injury/ARDS have decreased over time. *Chest.* 2008;133(5):1120–1127.
7. Bernard G, Artigas A, Brigham KL, et al. The American-European Consensus Conference on ARDS. Definitions, mechanisms, relevant outcomes, and clinical trial coordination. *Am J Respir Crit Care Med.* 1994;149:818–824.
8. Wright J. Adult respiratory distress syndrome. In: Thurlbeck W, Churg A, eds. *Pathology of the Lung.* New York: Thieme; 1995.
9. Bellingan G. The pulmonary physician in critical care 6: the pathogenesis of ALI/ARDS. *Thorax.* 2002;57:540–546.
10. Colby T, Lombard C, Yousem SA, Kitaichi M. *Atlas of Pulmonary Surgical Pathology.* Philadelphia: Saunders; 1991.
11. Herridge MS, Cheung AM, Tansey CM, et al. One-year outcomes in survivors of the acute respiratory distress syndrome. *N Engl J Med.* 2003;348(8):683–693.
12. Hwang DM, Chamberlain DW, Poutanen SM, et al. Pulmonary pathology of severe acute respiratory syndrome in Toronto. *Mod Pathol.* 2005;18(1):1–10.
13. Cincotta DR, Sebire NJ, Lim E, Peters MJ. Fatal acute fibrinous and organizing pneumonia in an infant: the histopathologic variability of acute respiratory distress syndrome. *Pediatr Crit Care Med.* 2007;8(4):378–382.
14. Oseasohn R, Adelson L, Kaji M. Clinicopathology study of 33 fatal cases of Asian influenza. *N Engl J Med.* 1959;260:509–518.
15. Yeldandi A, Colby T. Pathologic features of lung biopsy specimens from influenza pneumonia cases. *Hum Pathol.* 1994;25:47–53.
16. Tamura H, Aronson B. Intranuclear fibrillary inclusions in influenza pneumonia. *Pathol Lab Med.* 1978;102:252–257.
17. Cheung OY, Chan JW, Ng CK, Koo CK. The spectrum of pathological changes in severe acute respiratory syndrome (SARS). *Histopathology.* 2004;45(2):119–124.
18. Franks TJ, Chong PY, Chui P, et al. Lung pathology of severe acute respiratory syndrome (SARS): a study of 8 autopsy cases from Singapore. *Hum Pathol.* 2003;34(8):743–748.
19. Hwang D, Chamberlain DW, Poutanen SM, et al. Pulmonary pathology of severe acute respiratory syndrome in Toronto. *Mod Pathol.* 2005;18:1–10.
20. Nicholls JM, Poon LL, Lee KC, et al. Lung pathology of fatal severe acute respiratory syndrome. *Lancet.* 2003;361(9371):1773–1778.
21. Ksiazek TG, Erdman D, Goldsmith CS, et al. A novel coronavirus associated with severe acute respiratory syndrome. *N Engl J Med.* 2003;348(20):1953–1966.

22. Peiris JS, Lai ST, Poon LL, et al. Coronavirus as a possible cause of severe acute respiratory syndrome. *Lancet*. 2003;361(9366):1319–1325.

23. Lee N, Hui D, Wu A, et al. A major outbreak of severe acute respiratory syndrome in Hong Kong. *N Engl J Med*. 2003;348(20):1986–1994.

24. Sobonya RE, Hiller FC, Pingleton W, Watanabe I. Fatal measles (rubeola) pneumonia in adults. *Arch Pathol Lab Med*. 1978;102:366–371.

25. Enders JF, McCarthy K, Mitus A, Cheatham WJ. Isolation of measles virus at autopsy in cases of giant-cell pneumonia without rash. *N Engl J Med*. 1959;261:875–881.

26. Mitus A, Enders JF, Craig JM, Holloway A. Persistence of measles virus and depression of antibody formation in patients with giant-cell pneumonia after measles. *N Engl J Med*. 1959;261:882–889.

27. Haram K, Jacobsen J. Measles and its relationship to giant cell pneumonia (Hecht pneumonia). *Acta Pathol Microbiol Immunol Scand [A]*. 1973;81:761–769.

28. Katzenstein A. Infection. I. Unusual pneumonias. In: Katzenstein A, Askin F, eds. *Katzenstein and Askin's Surgical Pathology of Non-Neoplastic Lung Disease*. Philadelphia: Saunders; 1997.

29. Becroft D. Histopathology of fatal adenovirus infection of the respiratory tract in young children. *J Clin Pathol*. 1967;20:561–569.

30. Becroft D. Bronchiolitis obliterans, bronchiectasis and other sequelae of adenovirus type 21 infection in young children. *J Clin Pathol*. 1971;24:72–79.

31. Zahradnik J, Spencer M, Porter D. Adenovirus infection in the immunocompromised patient. *Am J Med*. 1980;68:725–732.

32. Miller R. Viral infections of the respiratory tract. In: Thurlbeck W, Churg A, eds. *Pathology of the Lung*. 2nd ed, New York: Thieme; 1995:195–222.

33. Abbondanzo S, English CK, Kagan E, McPherson RA. Fatal adenovirus pneumonia in a newborn identified by electron microscopy and in-situ hybridization. *Arch Pathol Lab Med*. 1989;113:1349–1353.

34. Ramsey P, Fife KH, Hackman RC, et al. Herpes simplex virus pneumonia: clinical, virologic, and pathologic features in 20 patients. *Ann Intern Med*. 1982;97:813–820.

35. Graham B, Snell JJ. Herpes simplex virus infection of the adult lower respiratory tract. *Medicine (Baltimore)*. 1983;62:384–393.

36. Pugh RN, Omar RI, Hossain MM. Varicella infection and pneumonia among adults. *Int J Infect Dis*. 1998;2(4):205–210.

37. Craighead J. Cytomegalovirus pulmonary disease. *Pathobiol Annu*. 1975;5:197–220.

38. Beschorner W, Hutchins GM, Burns WH, et al. Cytomegalovirus pneumonia in bone marrow transplant recipients: miliary and diffuse patterns. *Am Rev Respir Dis*. 1980;122:107–114.

39. Winston D, Ho W, Champlin R. Cytomegalovirus after allogeneic bone marrow transplantation. *Rev Infect Dis*. 1992;12(suppl):S776–S792.

40. Colby TV, Zaki SR, Feddersen RM, Nolte KB. Hantavirus pulmonary syndrome is distinguishable from acute interstitial pneumonia. *Arch Pathol Lab Med*. 2000;124(10):1463–1466.

41. Duchin J, Koster FT, Peters CJ, et al. Hantavirus pulmonary syndrome: a clinical description of 17 patients with a newly recognized disease. The Hantavirus Study Group. *N Engl J Med*. 1994;330:949–955.

42. Nolte K, Feddersen RM, Foucar K, et al. Hantavirus pulmonary syndrome in the United States. A new pathological description of a disease caused by a new agent. *Hum Pathol*. 1995;26:110–120.

43. Weber W, Askin F, Dehner L. Lung biopsy in *Pneumocystis carinii* pneumonia. A histopathologic study of typical and atypical features. *Am J Clin Pathol*. 1977;67:11–19.

44. Ognibene FP, Shelhamer J, Gill V, et al. The diagnosis of *Pneumocystis carinii* pneumonia in patients with the acquired immunodeficiency syndrome using subsegmental bronchoalveolar lavage. *Am Rev Respir Dis*. 1984;129:929–932.

45. Grimes M, LaPook JD, Bar MH, et al. Disseminated *Pneumocystis carinii* infection in a patient with acquired immunodeficiency syndrome. *Hum Pathol*. 1987;18:307–308.

46. Askin F, Katzenstein A. *Pneumocystis* infection masquerading as diffuse alveolar damage: a potential source of diagnostic error. *Chest*. 1979;4:420–422.

47. Blackmon J, Hicklin M, Chandler F. Legionnaires' disease. Pathological and historical aspects of a new disease. *Arch Pathol Lab Med*. 1978;102:337–343.

48. Lattimen G, Rachman R, Scarlato M. Legionnaires' disease pneumonia: histopathologic features and comparison with microbial and chemical pneumonias. *Ann Clin Lab Sci*. 1979;9:353–361.

49. Rollin S, Colby T, Clayton F. Open lung biopsy in *Mycoplasma pneumoniae* pneumonia. *Arch Pathol Lab Med*. 1986;110:34–41.

50. Torres A, de Celis MR, Roisin RR, et al. Adult respiratory distress syndrome in Q fever. *Eur J Respir Dis*. 1987;70:322–325.

51. Winn WJ, Myerowitz R. The pathology of the *Legionella* pneumonias. A review of 74 cases and the literature. *Hum Pathol*. 1981;12:401–422.

52. Matthay R, Schwarz MI, Petty TL, et al. Pulmonary manifestations of systemic lupus erythematosus: review of twelve cases of acute lupus pneumonitis. *Medicine*. 1974;54:397–409.

53. Hunninghake G, Fauci A. Pulmonary involvement in the collagen vascular diseases. *Am Rev Respir Dis*. 1979;119:471–503.

54. Yousem S, Colby T, Carrington C. Lung biopsy in rheumatoid arthritis. *Am Rev Respir Dis*. 1985;131:770–777.

55. Lakhanpal S, Lie JT, Conn DL, Martin 2nd WJ. Pulmonary disease in polymyositis/dermatomyositis: a clinicopathological analysis of 65 autopsy cases. *Ann Rheum Dis*. 1987;46:23–29.

56. Tazelaar H, Viggiano RW, Pickersgill J, Colby TV. Interstitial lung disease in polymyositis and dermatomyositis. Clinical features and prognosis as correlated with histologic findings. *Am Rev Respir Dis*. 1990;141:727–733.

57. Colby T. Pulmonary pathology in patients with systemic autoimmune disease. *Clin Chest Med*. 1998;19:587–612.

58. Quismorio Jr F, Cheema G. Interstitial lung disease in systemic lupus erythematosus. *Curr Opin Pulm Med*. 2000;6:424–429.

59. Lamblin C, Bergoin C, Saelens T, Wallaert B. Interstitial lung disease in collagen vascular disease. *Eur Respir J*. 2001;18(suppl 32):69s–80s.

60. Myers J, Katzenstein A. Microangiitis in lupus-induced pulmonary hemorrhage. *Am J Clin Pathol*. 1986;85:552–556.

61. Walker W, Wright V. Pulmonary lesions and rheumatoid arthritis. *Medicine (Baltimore)*. 1968;47:501–515.

62. Laitinen O, Nissilä M, Salorinne Y, Aalto P. Pulmonary involvement in patients with rheumatoid arthritis. *Scand J Respir Dis*. 1975;56:297–304.

63. Hakala M, Pääkkö P, Huhti E, et al. Open lung biopsy of patients with rheumatoid arthritis. *Clin Rheumatol*. 1990;9(4):452–460.

64. Gochuico BR. Potential pathogenesis and clinical aspects of pulmonary fibrosis associated with rheumatoid arthritis. *Am J Med Sci*. 2001;321(1):83–88.

65. Pratt D, Schwartz MI, May JJ, Dreisin RB. Rapidly fatal pulmonary fibrosis: the accelerated variation of interstitial pneumonitis. *Thorax*. 1979;34:587–593.

66. Douglas WW, Tazelaar HD, Hartman TE, et al. Polymyositis-dermatomyositis–associated interstitial lung disease. *Am J Respir Crit Care Med*. 2001;164(7):1182–1185.

67. Muir T, Tazelaar HD, Colby TV, Myers JL. Organizing diffuse alveolar damage associated with progressive systemic sclerosis. *Mayo Clin Proc*. 1997;72:639–642.

68. Clarysse A, Cathey WJ, Cartwright GE, Wintrobe MM. Pulmonary disease complicating intermittent therapy with methotrexate. *JAMA*. 1969;209:1861–1864.

69. Bone R, Wolfe J, Sobonya RE, et al. Desquamative interstitial pneumonia following chronic nitrofurantoin therapy. *Chest*. 1976;69(2):296–297.

70. Kruban Z. Pulmonary changes induced by amphophilic drugs. *Environ Health Perspect*. 1976;16:111–115.

71. Samuels ML, Johnson DE, Holoye PY, Lanzotti VJ. Large-dose bleomycin therapy and pulmonary toxicity. A possible role of prior radiotherapy. *JAMA*. 1976;235:1117–1120.

72. Kilburn K. Pulmonary disease induced by drugs. In: Fishman AP, ed. *Pulmonary Diseases and Disorders*. New York: McGraw-Hill; 1980:707–724.

73. Williams T, Eidus L, Thomas P. Fibrosing alveolitis, bronchiolitis obliterans and sulfalazine therapy. *Chest*. 1982;81:766–768.

74. Schapira C, Nahir M, Scharf Y. Pulmonary injury induced by gold salts treatment. *Med Interne*. 1985;23(4):259–263.

75. Yousem S, Lifson J, Colby T. Chemotherapy-induced eosinophilic pneumonia. Relation to bleomycin. *Chest*. 1985;88(1):103–106.

76. Slingerland R, Hoogsteden HC, Adriaansen HJ, et al. Gold-induced pneumonitis. *Respiration*. 1987;52(3):232–236.

77. Rosenow 3rd EC, Myers JL, Swensen SJ, Pisani RJ. Drug-induced pulmonary disease. An update. *Chest*. 1992;102:239–250.

78. Rossi SE, Erasmus JJ, McAdams HP, et al. Pulmonary drug toxicity: radiologic and pathologic manifestations. *Radiographics*. 2000;20(5):1245–1259.

79. Abid S, Malhotra V, Perry M. Radiation-induced and chemotherapy-induced pulmonary injury. *Curr Opin Oncol*. 2001;13(4):242–248.

80. Fassas A, Gojo I, Rapoport A, et al. Pulmonary toxicity syndrome following CDEP (cyclophosphamide, dexamethasone, etoposide, cisplatin) chemotherapy. *Bone Marrow Transplant*. 2001;28(4):399–403.

81. Erasmus J, McAdams H, Rossi S. Drug-induced lung injury. *Semin Roentgenol*. 2002;37(1):72–81.

82. Myers J. Pathology of drug-induced lung disease. In: Katzenstein A, Askin F, eds. *Katzenstein and Askin's Surgical Pathology of Non-Neoplastic Lung Disease*. Philadelphia: Saunders; 1997.

83. Cleverley JR, Screaton NJ, Hiorns MP, et al. Drug-induced lung disease: High-resolution CT and histological findings. *Clin Radiol*. 2002;57:292–299.

84. Cooper Jr J, White D, Mathay R. Drug-induced pulmonary disease (Parts 1 and 2). *Am Rev Respir Dis*. 1986;133:321–338, 488–502.

85. Limper AH, Rosenow 3rd EC. Drug-induced interstitial lung disease. *Curr Opin Pulm Med*. 1996;2(5):396–404.

86. Copper Jr JA. Drug-induced lung disease. *Adv Intern Med*. 1997;42:231–268.

87. Camus PH, Foucher P, Bonniaud PH, Ask K. Drug-induced infiltrative lung disease. *Eur Respir J*. 2001;32(suppl):93s–100s.

88. Ozkan M, Dweik RA, Ahmad M. Drug-induced lung disease. *Cleve Clin J Med*. 2001;68(9):782–785, 789–795.

89. Littler WA, Kay JM, Hasleton PS, Heath D. Busulphan lung. *Thorax*. 1969;24(6):639–655.

90. Koss L, Melamed M, Mayer K. The effect of bulsufan on human epithelia. *Am J Clin Pathol*. 1965;44:385–397.

91. Feingold M, Koss L. Effect of long-term administration of bulsufan. *Arch Intern Med*. 1969;124:66–71.

92. Gyorkey F, Gyorkey P, Sinkovies J. Origin and significance of intranuclear tubular inclusions in type II pulmonary alveolar epithelial cells of patients with bleomycin and bulsufan toxicity. *Ultrastruct Pathol*. 1980;1:211–221.

93. Ingrassia 3rd TS, Ryu JH, Trastek VF, Rosenow 3rd EC. Oxygen-exacerbated bleomycin pulmonary toxicity. *Mayo Clin Proc*. 1991;66:173–178.

94. Imokawa S, Colby TV, Leslie KO, Helmers RA. Methotrexate pneumonitis: review of the literature and histopathological findings in nine patients. *Eur Respir J*. 2000;15:373–381.

95. Dean PJ, Groshart KD, Porterfield JG, et al. Amiodarone-associated pulmonary toxicity: a clinical and pathologic study of eleven cases. *Am J Clin Pathol*. 1987;87:7–13.

96. Kennedy JI, Myers JL, Plumb VJ, Fulmer JD. Amiodarone pulmonary toxicity. Clinical, radiologic, and pathologic correlations. *Arch Intern Med*. 1987;147(1):50–55.

97. Myers JL, Kennedy JI, Plumb VJ. Amiodarone lung: pathologic findings in clinically toxic patients. *Hum Pathol*. 1987;18(4):349–354.

98. Martin 2nd W, Rosenow 3rd E. Amiodarone pulmonary toxicity. Recognition and pathogenesis (Part I). *Chest*. 1988;93:1067–1075.

99. Donaldson L, Grant IS, Naysmith MR, Thomas JS. Acute amiodarone-induced lung toxicity. *Intensive Care Med*. 1998;24(6):626–630.

100. Blancas R, Moreno JL, Martín F, et al. Alveolar-interstitial pneumopathy after gold-salts compounds administration, requiring mechanical ventilation. *Intensive Care Med*. 1998;24(10):1110–1112.

101. Allen JN, Pacht ER, Gadek JE, Davis WB. Acute eosinophilic pneumonia as a reversible cause of noninfectious respiratory failure. *N Engl J Med*. 1989;321:569–574.

102. Tazelaar HD, Linz LJ, Colby TV, et al. Acute eosinophilic pneumonia: histopathologic findings in nine patients. *Am J Respir Crit Care Med*. 1997;155:296–302.

103. Hayakawa H, Sato A, Toyoshima M. A clinical study of idiopathic eosinophilic pneumonia. *Chest*. 1994;105:1462–1466.

104. Pope-Harman AL, Davis WB, Allen ED, et al. Acute eosinophilic pneumonia: a review of 12 cases. *Chest*. 106:1994;156s.

105. Hamman L, Rich A. Acute diffuse interstitial fibrosis of the lungs. *Bull Johns Hopkins Hosp*. 1944;74:177–212.

106. Katzenstein A, Myers J, Mazur M. Acute interstitial pneumonia. A clinicopathologic, ultrastructural, and cell kinetic study. *Am J Surg Pathol*. 1986;10:256–267.

107. Olson J, Colby T, Elliott C. Hamman-Rich syndrome revisited. *Mayo Clin Proc*. 1990;65:1538–1548.

108. Bouros D, Nicholson AC, Polychronopoulos V, du Bois RM. Acute interstitial pneumonia. *Eur Respir J*. 2000;15:412–418.

109. Colby TV, Fukuoka J, Ewaskow SP, et al. Pathologic approach to pulmonary hemorrhage. *Ann Diagn Pathol*. 2001;5:309–319.

110. Lombard C, Colby T, Elliott C. Surgical pathology of the lung in anti-basement membrane antibody–associated Goodpasture syndrome. *Hum Pathol*. 1989;20:445–451.

111. Akikusa B, Kondo Y, Irabu N, et al. Six cases of microscopic polyarteritis exhibiting acute interstitial pneumonia. *Pathol Int*. 1995;45:580–588.

112. Matsumoto T, Homma S, Okada M, et al. The lung in polyarteritis nodosa: a pathologic study of 10 cases. *Hum Pathol*. 1993;24:717–724.

113. Fajardo L, Berthrong M. Radiation injury in surgical pathology. Part I. *Am J Surg Pathol*. 1978;2:159–199.

114. Einhorn L, Krause M, Hornback N, Furnas B. Enhanced pulmonary toxicity with bleomycin and radiotherapy in oat cell lung cancer. *Cancer*. 1976;37:2414–2416.

115. Flint A, Colby T. Diffuse alveolar damage. In: *Surgical Pathology of Diffuse Infiltrative Lung Disease*. Orlando: Grune and Stratton; 1987.

116. Gross N. Pulmonary effects of radiation therapy. *Ann Intern Med*. 1977;86:81–92.

117. Fajardo L. *Pathology of Radiation Injury*. Vol 1. New York: Masson Publishing; 1982.

118. Coggle J, Lambert B, Moores S. Radiation effects in the lung. *Environ Health Perspect*. 1986;70:261–291.

119. Nash G, Blennerhassett J, Pontoppidan H. Pulmonary lesions associated with oxygen therapy and artifical ventilation. *N Engl J Med*. 1967;276:368–374.

120. Pratt P. Pathology of pulmonary oxygen toxicity. *Am Rev Respir Dis*. 1974;110(suppl):51–57.

121. Pratt P. Pulmonary capillary proliferation induced by oxygen. *Am J Pathol*. 1958;34:1033–1050.

122. Northway Jr W, Rosan R, Porter D. Pulmonary disease following respirator therapy of hyaline-membrane disease: bronchopulmonary dysplasia. *N Engl J Med*. 1967;276:357–368.

123. Milberg JA, Davis DR, Steinberg KP, Hudson LD. Improved survival of patients with acute respiratory distress syndrome (ARDS): 1983–1993. *JAMA*. 1995;273(4):306–309.

124. Anderson C. Paraquat and the lung. *Australas Radiol*. 1970;14:409–412.

125. Dearden LC, Fairshter RD, McRae DM, et al. Pulmonary ultrastructure of the late aspects of human paraquat poisoning. *Am J Pathol*. 1978;93:667–680.

126. Fairshter R. Paraquat poisoning. An update. *West J Med*. 1978;128:56–58.

127. Chian CF, Chang FY. Acute respiratory distress syndrome in *Mycoplasma* pneumonia: a case report and review. *J Microbiol Immunol Infect*. 1999;32(1):52–56.

128. Weber W, Akin F, Dehner L. Lung biopsy in *Pneumocystis carinii* pneumonia: a histolopathologic study of typical and atypical features. *Am J Clin Pathol*. 1977;67:11–19.

129. Yousem S, Colby T, Gaensler E. Respiratory bronchiolitis–associated interstitial lung disease and its relationship to desquamative interstitial pneumonia. *Mayo Clin Proc*. 1989;64:1373–1380.

130. Everard M, Milner A. The respiratory syncytial virus and its role in acute bronchiolitis. *Eur J Pediatr*. 1992;151(9):638–651.

131. Ebsen M, Anhenn O, Roder C, Morgenroth K. Morphology of adenovirus type-3 infection of human respiratory epithelial cells in vitro. *Virchows Arch*. 2002;440(5):512–518.

132. Knodoh Y, Taniguchi H, Kawabata Y, et al. Acute exacerbation in idiopathic pulmonary fibrosis. Analysis of clinical and pathologic findings in three cases. *Chest*. 1993;103:1808–1812.

6

Lung Infections

Louis A. Rosati, MD, and Kevin O. Leslie, MD

Lower respiratory tract infections constitute a leading cause of morbidity and death worldwide.[1,2] Included in this category of infections are bronchitis and bronchiolitis, community-acquired and nosocomial pneumonias, and pneumonias in the immunocompromised patient. A relatively small percentage of these infections come to the attention of the surgical pathologist, because most are diagnosed in the microbiology laboratory. Nevertheless, as summarized in Box 6-1, the anatomic pathologist can play a pivotal role in the diagnosis of lung infections by identifying reaction patterns in tissue, and sometimes in the identification of an organism that microbiologic techniques fail to detect.[3] Despite significant advances in laboratory techniques, culture diagnosis is not always possible; the organism may not reproduce in culture, a culture study may not have been requested, or the culture technique may have failed for any of various technical reasons. Even when culture is successful, the time frame for diagnostic purposes may not be clinically useful, or the culture result, in the absence of an expected tissue response, may not permit distinction of pathogens from innocent bystanders, be they colonizers or contaminants. For all of these reasons, the pulmonary infection for which biopsy is performed often is one that has eluded standard microbiologic techniques, has not responded to empirical therapy, or requires morphologic analysis for clarification of a critical aspect of the differential diagnosis. In these situations, the diagnostic pathologist is indispensable,[4,5] if not for providing an immediate report intraoperatively (by frozen section or cytologic imprints or smears), then for dramatically improving diagnosis turnaround time with the use of newer rapid tissue-processing systems[6] (Table 6-1).

Box 6-1. Role of the Diagnostic Pathologist

Rapid diagnosis: frozen section; cytologic smears; rapid tissue process
Identify unculturable pathogens
Establish diagnosis when culture results are negative
Evaluate pathogenic significance of culture isolate
Define "new" infectious diseases
Exclude infection as etiologic disorder; detect comorbid process
Intraoperative triage of limited biopsy tissue
Clinicopathologic-microbiologic correlation

Modified from Watts J, Chandler F. The surgical pathologist's role in the diagnosis of infectious disease. *J Histotechnol.* 1995;18:191–193.

Table 6-1. Diagnostic Tools of the Pathologist

Activity	Objective
Pre-/intra-/postoperative consultation	Information exchange and strategies
Gross examination	Tissue handling and triage
Histopathologic examination	Organism morphology; cytopathic effect; host response
Histochemical stains	Detection and morphologic detail
Immunohistochemical stains	Detection of organisms; confirmation of genus/species
Electron microscopy	Selective use for virus, fungi, parasites, and bacteria
Molecular techniques: in situ hybridization, polymerase chain reaction	Sensitive and specific detection/identification of nonculturable organisms; stain-negative cases
Report	Clinicopathologic and microbiologic correlation

Table 6-2. Diagnostic Tools of the Microbiologist

Activity	Objective
Pre-/intra-/postoperative consultation	Information exchange and strategies
Direct visualization (smears and imprints)	Rapid detection
Culture	Identification of genus and species; susceptibility studies
Antigen detection	Rapid identification
Serologic testing	Specific antibody response
Molecular techniques	Sensitive and specific detection/identification
Report	Traditional versus interpretive format

Diagnostic Tools and Strategies

The history of the field of pathology is intertwined with the discovery of pathogenic bacteria and the development of the science of microbiology.[7] Today, pathologists and microbiologists approach the diagnosis of infection with techniques and methods that share some aspects but have important differences.[8] The surgical pathologist and the cytopathologist are in a position to apply the tools of both disciplines to achieve a clinically relevant diagnosis by correlating the histopathologic or cytopathologic examination findings with data obtained using microbiology techniques (Table 6-2). Unfortunately, the diagnostic workup and reporting of biopsy findings in surgical or cytopathology departments and those in the microbiology laboratory typically run along nonintersecting paths, often without one group knowing (or acknowledging) the findings of the other. An interdisciplinary approach that is based on mutual understanding and communication would seem to be a logical, if not ideal, scenario for optimal clinical management.[9] Our concept of an integrated morphologic and microbiologic approach is presented schematically in Figure 6-1, and with greater detail for specific situations in which bacterial (Fig. 6-2), mycobacterial (Fig. 6-3), fungal (Fig. 6-4), or viral (Fig. 6-5) pathogens are suspected.

In current medical practice, identification of the genus or species of an infectious organism can have important prognostic and therapeutic implications. Because histopathologic examination alone rarely provides this information, the findings should always be cor-

related with results of cultures. Accordingly, foresight is required on the part of the intraoperative pathologist in obtaining and properly handling tissues for culture.[10] The correlation of the morphologic and microbiologic data can be facilitated in the surgical pathology report by appending a comment that seeks to enhance the morphologic diagnosis by suggesting a specific etiologic disorder or agent, considerations for the differential diagnosis, or additional workup with culture, serology, or molecular studies. In certain situations, it is also appropriate to include the preliminary results of microbiology stains and cultures, and to correlate this information with the morphologic findings whenever possible.

Knowledge of the Clinical Setting

Identification of risk factors and determination of the immune status of the patient are of primary importance, because these parameters typically influence the spectrum of histopathologic changes and the type of etiologic agents and pathogen burden.[11–16] Also, because the degree of immunosuppression often influences the burden of organisms, different efforts may be required to identify the pathogen. For example, organisms are less often found in lung tissues from patients with normal or near-normal immunity. In this setting, cultures, serologic studies, and epidemiologic data must be relied on to provide the diagnosis.[17] By contrast, persons infected with the human immunodeficiency virus (HIV) in whom the acquired immunodeficiency syndrome (AIDS) or *Mycobacterium avium* infection develops typically manifest poorly formed granulomas, or simply histiocytic infiltrates, despite an overabundance of organisms identified by tissue acid-fast stains. *Pneumocystis* organisms may be easily identified in patients with AIDS, who manifest diffuse alveolar damage accompanied by abundant, foamy alveolar casts but when immunosuppression is less severe (such as that produced by corticosteroids therapy for arthritis), the morphologic features can be less typical, and the organisms sparse. The relationship among the level of immunity, burden of organisms, and patterns of disease is illustrated for cryptococcosis in Figure 6-6.

In the immunocompromised patient, one must also consider a broader differential diagnosis. In addition to infection, other disorders come into consideration such as pulmonary involvement by pre-existing disease, drug-induced and treatment-related injury, noninfectious interstitial pneumonias, malignancy, and new pulmonary diseases unrelated to the patient's immunocompromised state, such as aspiration, heart failure, and pulmonary embolism. When immunosuppression is intentional, as in transplant recipients, unique additional challenges

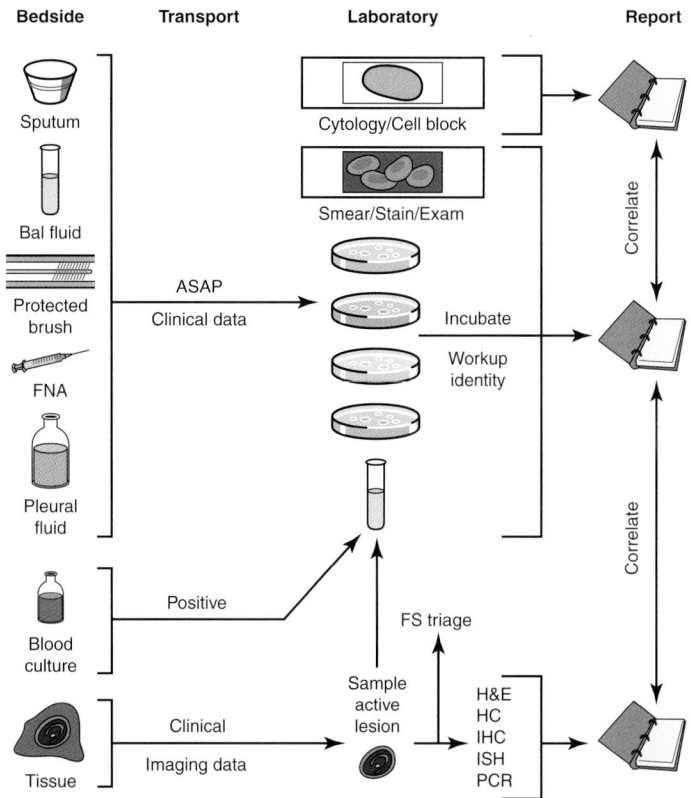

Figure 6-1. Schematic for workup of respiratory specimen for suspected infection. BAL, bronchoalveolar lavage; FNA, fine-needle aspiration; FS, frozen section; HC, histochemistry; H&E, hematoxylin-eosin [stain]; IHC, immmunohistochemistry studies; ISH, in situ hybridization; PCR, polymerase chain reaction [assay].

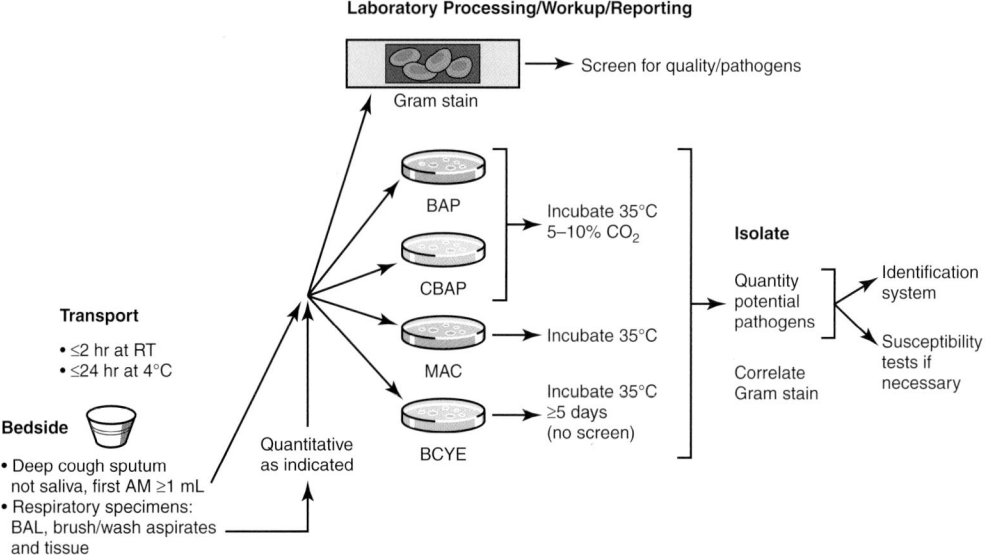

Figure 6-2. Integrated morphologic and microbiologic approach to laboratory diagnosis of bacterial infection. BAL, bronchoalveolar lavage; BAP, blood agar plate; BCYE, buffered charcoal yeast extract; CBAP, chocolate blood agar plate; MAC, MacConkey agar; RT, room temperature.

come into play, such as transplant rejection, graft-versus-host disease, and Epstein-Barr virus (EBV)-associated lymphoproliferative disorders. Immunosuppressed persons are at risk for multiple simultaneous infections, so when one organism is found, a careful search for others is always warranted (Fig. 6-7).

A number of well-characterized genetic disorders of immunity and cellular function are known to predispose affected persons to lung infection.[18–21] Cystic fibrosis bears special recognition in this context because it is associated with reproducible patterns of lung disease and susceptibility to a wide spectrum of infectious organisms. This genetic

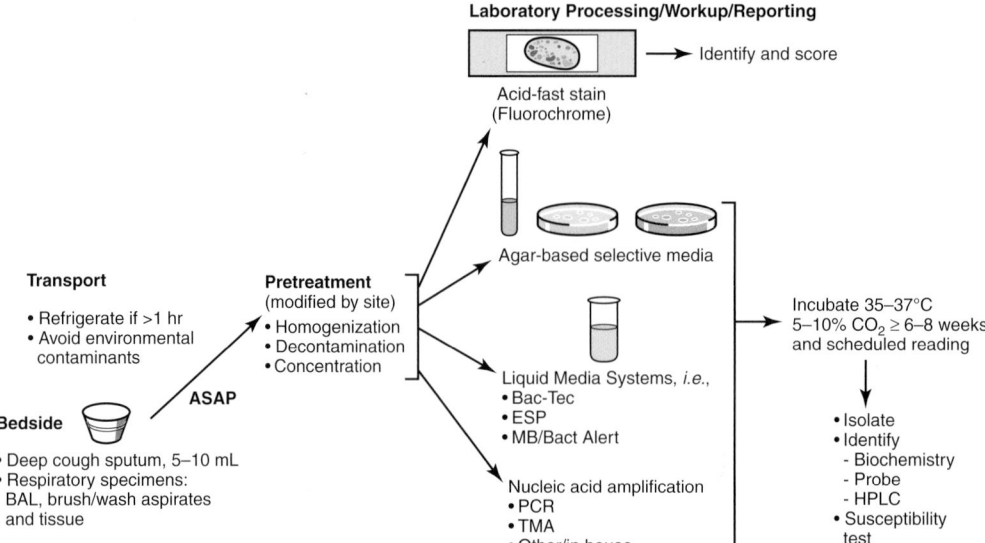

Figure 6-3. Integrated morphologic and microbiologic approach to laboratory diagnosis of mycobacterial infection. Bac-Tec, BD BACTEC Instrumented Mycobaterial Growth Systems; BAL, bronchoalveolar lavage; ESP, ESP Culture System; HPLC, high-performance liquid chromatography; MB/Bact Alert, Biomerieux Bact/alert 3D; PCR, polymerase chain reaction [assay]; TMA, transcription-mediated amplification.

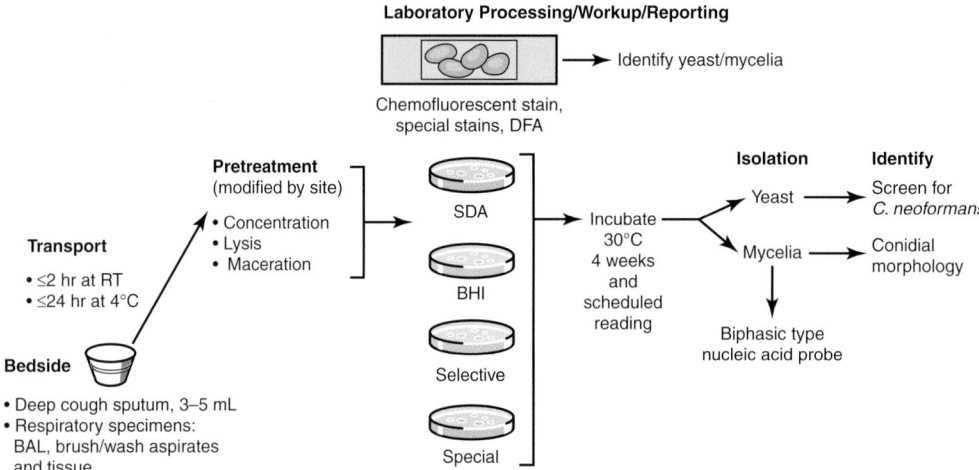

Figure 6-4. Integrated morphologic and microbiologic approach to laboratory diagnosis of fungal infection. BAL, bronchoalveolar lavage; BHI, brain-heart infusion; DFA, direct immunofluorescence assay; RT, room temperature; SDA, Sabouraud dextrose agar.

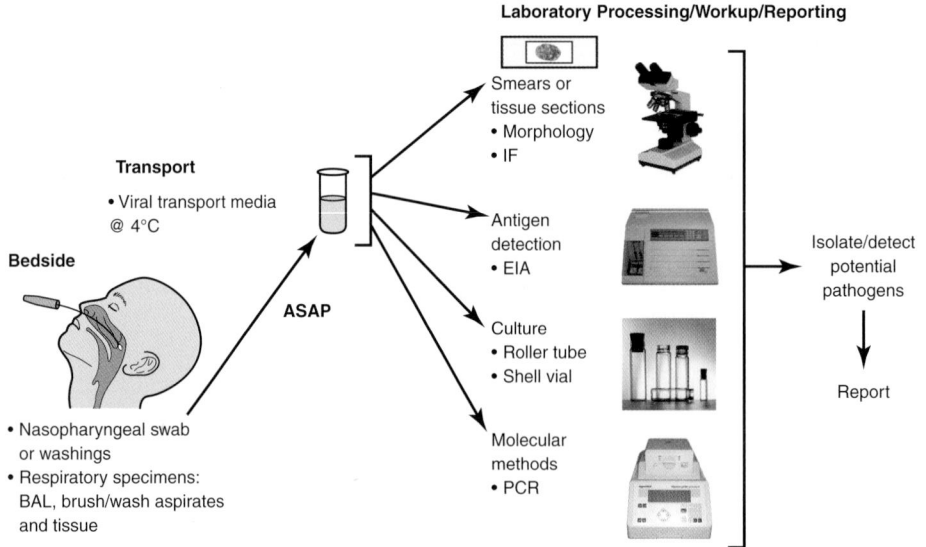

Figure 6-5. Integrated morphologic and microbiologic approach to laboratory diagnosis of viral infection. BAL, bronchoalveolar lavage; EIA, enzyme immunoassay; IF, immunofluorescence; PCR, polymerase chain reaction assay.

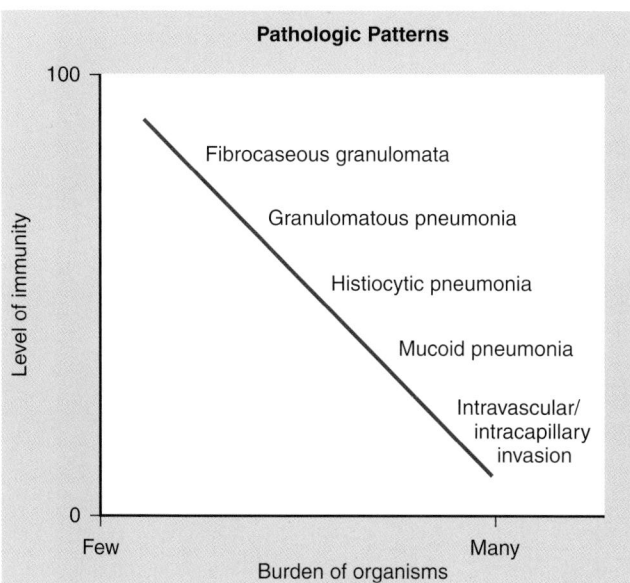

Pathologic Patterns

Fibrocaseous granulomata

Granulomatous pneumonia

Histiocytic pneumonia

Mucoid pneumonia

Intravascular/
intracapillary
invasion

Level of immunity — 0 to 100

Burden of organisms — Few to Many

Figure 6-6. Cryptococcosis: Correlation of pathologic patterns with immunity level and organism burden. With cryptococcal pneumonia in patients with normal or near-normal immunity, granuloma formation with few organisms is characteristic. In immunocompromised patients, typical findings include histiocytic infiltrates or mucoid pneumonia with little or no inflammatory reaction and many organisms. (Data from Mark EJ. Case records of the Massachusetts General Hospital. *N Engl J Med.* 2002;347:518–524.)

disease of autosomal recessive inheritance involves mutation of the *CFTR* gene that affects the ability of epithelial cells to effectively transport chloride and, secondarily, water across cell membranes. As a result, many organs, including the lungs, develop excessively viscous mucous secretions, which cannot be cleared effectively from the airways. In the lung, retention of such secretions leads to progressive and widespread bronchiectasis with airway obstruction that in turn paves the way for

recurrent infection (Fig. 6-8). Bacterial organisms commonly isolated include *Pseudomonas aeruginosa* (both mucoid and nonmucoid strains), *Haemophilus influenzae, Staphylococcus aureus, Escherichia coli, Klebsiella pneumoniae, Burkholderia cepacia* complex, *Stenotrophomonas maltophilia,* and *Achromobacter xylosoxidans.*[22] Polymicrobial infections are not uncommon, and some of these pathogens, especially certain subspecies within the *B. cepacia* complex, are linked to an adverse prognosis.[23] Cystic fibrosis also is a risk factor for non-tuberculous mycobacterial infection and allergic bronchopulmonary fungal disease, and the condition is potentially exacerbated by superimposed viral infections.[24–27]

Pattern Recognition

Knowledge of the radiologic pattern of infectious lung disease in a given patient often helps to narrow the scope of the differential diagnosis.[28,29] Patterns of lung infection seen on high-resolution computed tomography (HRCT) typically are dominated by increased attenuation (opacity). Such opacities may occur as one or more localized densities (nodule, mass, or localized infiltrate) or as more extensive infiltrates referred to as either *ground-glass opacities* (attenuation that allows underlying lung structures to be visible) or *consolidation* (attenuation that overshadows underlying structure).[30] Review of the chest imaging studies with the radiologist can be very helpful in arriving at a clinically relevant diagnosis. Correlating these data with the clinical history and pace of the disease under scrutiny (acute, subacute, chronic) allows a more accurate interpretation of the observed histopathologic pattern of disease in the tissue (Fig. 6-9). Fortunately, the recognized histopathologic patterns of lung infection are fairly limited (airway disease, acute lung injury, cellular infiltrates, alveolar filling, and nodules), and these typically correlate with a particular group of organisms (Table 6-3).

Useful Tissue Stains in Lung Infection

Many diagnostic pathologists have an aversion to the use of special stains for identifying organisms in tissue sections based on less than optimal specificity and sensitivity and the technical difficulty of performing some of these (especially silver impregnation methods, such

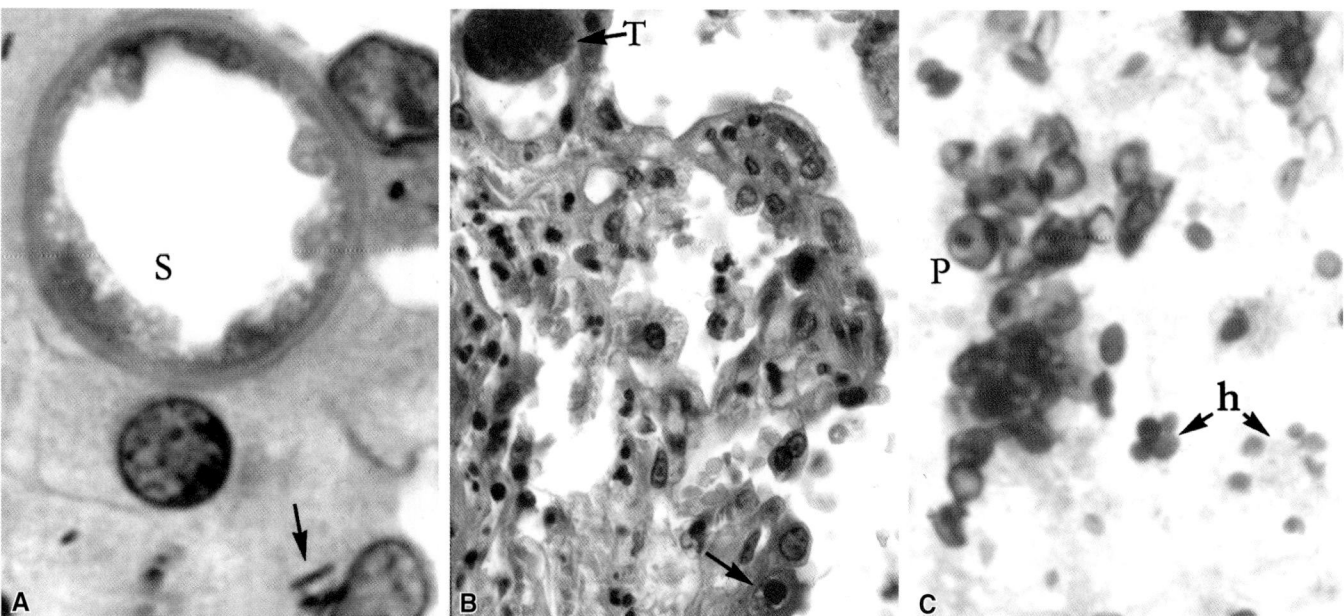

Figure 6-7. Co-infection with dual pulmonary pathogens. **A,** Spherule of *Coccidioides* (S) and *Mycobacterium avium* complex acid-fast bacilli (Ziehl-Neelsen/H&E stains). **B,** *Toxoplasma* pseudocysts (T) and cytomegalovirus-infected alveolar lining cell (*arrow*). **C,** Clusters of Pneumocystis cysts (P) in the midst of *H. capsulatum* yeast cells (h) (Grocott methenamine silver stain).

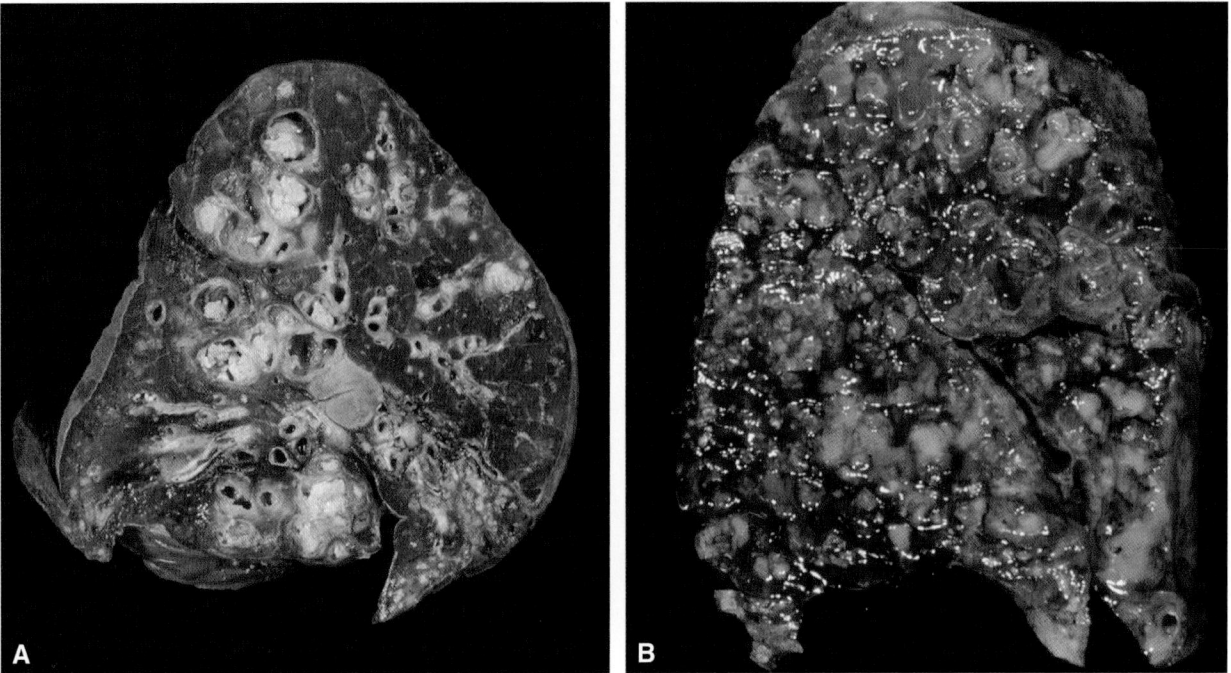

Figure 6-8. Changes of cystic fibrosis in the lung. **A,** Explant from a 13-year-old patient. **B,** Advanced disease at autopsy.

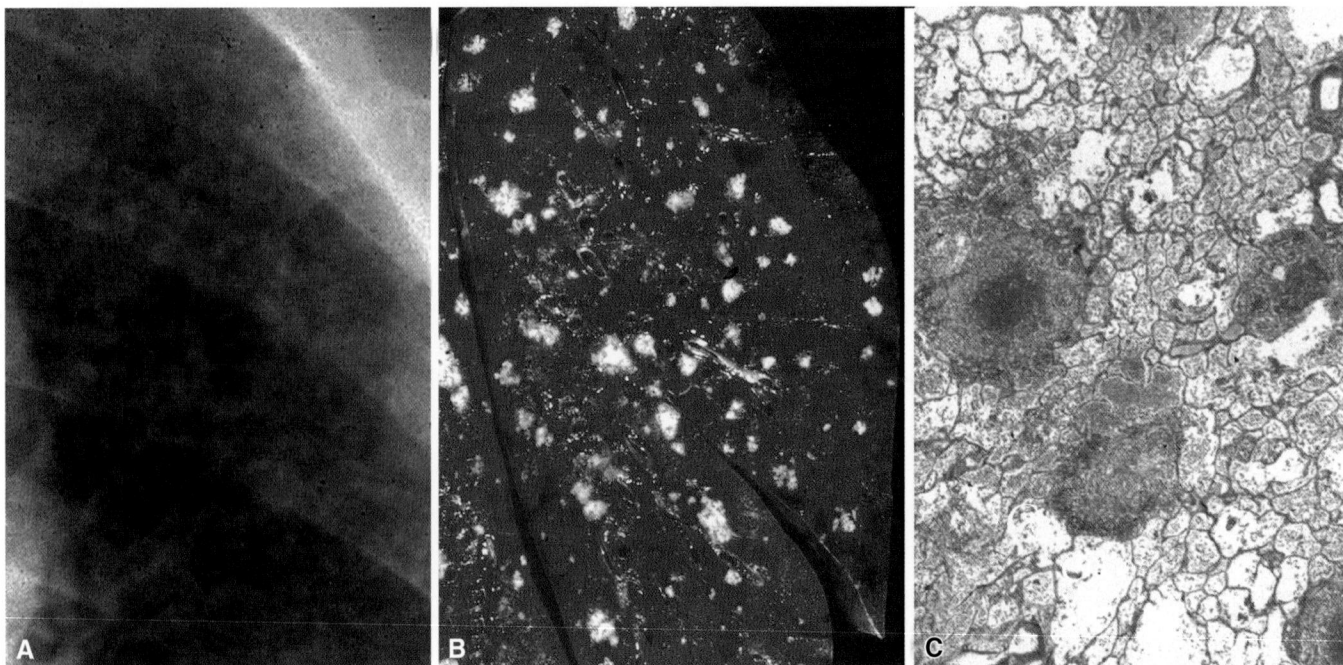

Figure 6-9. Miliary pattern of tuberculosis. **A,** Chest film, close-up view of miliary infiltrate. **B,** Gross cut surface of pulmonary parenchyma with miliary nodules. **C,** Histopathologic features of miliary necrotizing granulomas.

as the Dieterle, Steiner, and Warthin-Starry stains). Nevertheless, several tissue section staining techniques are quite useful in detecting bacteria, mycobacteria, and fungi in tissue sections. A list of these is presented in Box 6-2. These stains should always be applied as part of an algorithmic strategy for acute lung injury, but especially in the immunocompromised patient.[3] For example, when bacteria are being sought, some pathologists would prefer to begin with the tissue Gram stain (e.g., Brown and Hopps, Brown and Brenn)

(Fig. 6-10), but silver impregnation techniques (e.g., Warthin-Starry) are actually more sensitive and a good starting point for approaching a suspected bacterial infection. By coating the bacteria with metallic silver, the bacterial silhouettes are enhanced (Fig. 6-11) and become more visible.[3] Other stains (e.g., Giemsa) will sometimes detect bacteria that do not stain well with more conventional stains (Fig. 6-12). The Grocott methenamine silver (GMS) stain (Fig. 6-13) is the best stain for most fungi in tissue and also stains actinomycetes,

Table 6-3. Histopathologic Patterns and Most Agents of Pulmonary Infection

Pattern	Most Common Agent(s)
Airway disease	
Bronchitis/bronchiolitis	Virus; bacteria; *Mycoplasma*
Bronchiectasis	Bacteria; mycobacteria
Acute exudative pneumonia	
Purulent (neutrophilic)	Bacteria
Lobular (bronchopneumonia)	Bacteria
Confluent (lobar pneumonia)	Bacteria
With granules	Agents of botryomycosis (*Staphylococcus aureus*), actinomycosis (*Actinomyces israelii*)
Eosinophilic	Parasites
Foamy alveolar cast	*Pneumocystis*
Acute diffuse/localized alveolar damage	Virus; polymicrobial
Chronic pneumonia	
Fibroinflammatory	Bacteria
Organizing diffuse/localized alveolar damage	Virus
Eosinophilic	Parasite
Histiocytic	Mycobacteria
Interstitial pneumonia	
Perivascular lymphoid	Virus; atypical agents
Eosinophilic	Parasite
Granulomatous	Mycobacteria
Nodules	
Large	
Necrotizing	Fungi; mycobacteria
Granulomatous	Fungi; mycobacteria
Fibrocaseous	Fungi; mycobacteria
Calcified	Fungi; mycobacteria
Miliary	
Necrotizing	Viral; mycobacteria; fungi
Granulomatous	Fungi
Cavities and cysts	Fungi; mycobacteria
Intravascular/infarct	Fungi
Spindle cell pseudotumor	Mycobacteria
Minimal ("id") reaction	Polymicrobial

Box 6-2. Useful Tissue Stains in Lung Infection

Gram stain
  Brown and Brenn
  Brown and Hopps
Silver stains
  Warthin-Starry
  Steiner
  Dieterle
Fungal stains
  Grocott methenamine silver (GMS)
  Periodic acid/Schiff reagent (PAS)
Mycobacterial stains
  Ziehl-Neelsen (heat)
  Kinyon (cold)
  Auramine O (fluorochrome)
  Fite-Ferraco (peanut or mineral oil)
Other tissue stains
  Giemsa; Diff-Quik
  Mucicarmine
  Modified trichrome (Weber)
  Fontana-Masson
  Chemofluorescent (optical brighteners)
  Immunofluorescent antibodies
  Immunohistochemical

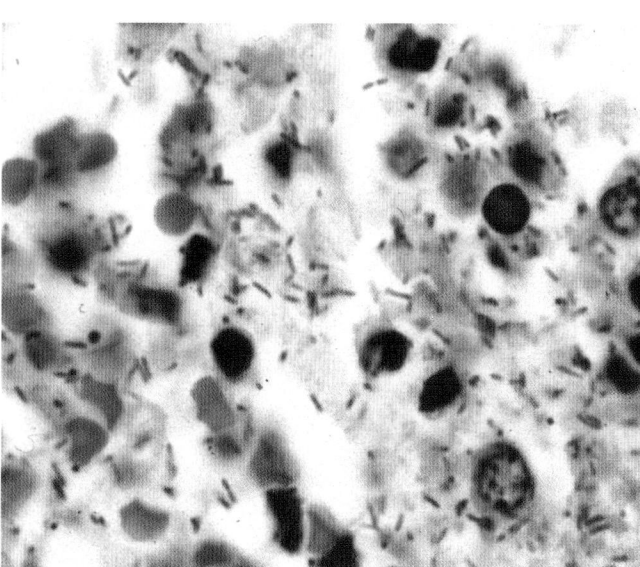

Figure 6-10. Gram-negative bacilli (*Escherichia coli*) in alveolar exudate (Brown and Hopps stain).

Nocardia, Pneumocystis (cysts), free-living soil amebae, algal cells, the spores of certain microsporidia, and the cytoplasmic inclusions of cytomegalovirus (CMV).[8]

Most mycobacteria stain well with the Ziehl-Neelsen procedure (Fig. 6-14), but the auramine-rhodamine fluorescent procedure is superior in terms of sensitivity (Fig. 6-15). *Nocardia* organisms, *Legionella micdadei*, and *Rhodococcus equi* are weakly or partially acid-fast, and use of modified acid-fast stains such as in the Fite-Faraco technique is more satisfactory for identification of these organisms. Some mycobacterial species, such as *M. avium* complex (MAC), also are periodic acid/Schiff reagent (PAS)-positive, GMS-positive, and weakly gram-positive.

Finally, for completeness, it can be said that for identification of most protozoa and helminths, as well as viral inclusions, a good-quality hematoxylin and eosin (H&E)-stained section suffices; in fact, a well-prepared H&E section alone is diagnostic for many infectious diseases. This stain often can detect and even distinguish between bacterial cocci and bacilli when the burden of organisms is high (Fig. 6-16).

Immunologic and Molecular Techniques

The application of ancillary studies, such as immunohistochemistry, in situ hybridization[31] (Fig. 6-17), or nucleic acid amplification technology, can provide a specific etiologic diagnosis in certain cases. These techniques have the best chance for diagnosing infections caused by fastidious species that are difficult or impossible to culture from fresh samples, and also for situations in which only formalin-fixed, paraffin-embedded tissues are available. Immunohistochemical reagents for microbiological detection are becoming increasingly available and provide added power to determining specific diagnoses on formalin-fixed paraffin-embedded tissue[32] (Fig. 6-18). Although these techniques provide the diagnostic equivalence of culture confirmation, they are

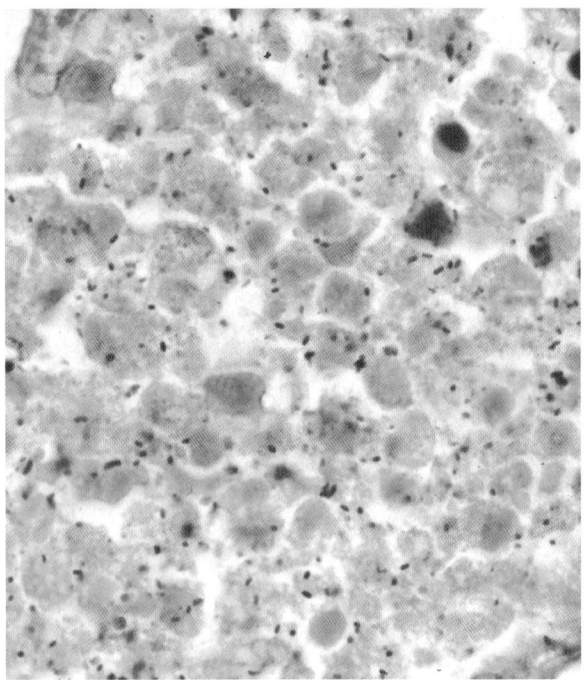

Figure 6-11. Black (silver-coated) bacilli (*Legionella pneumophila*) in alveolar exudate (Dieterle stain).

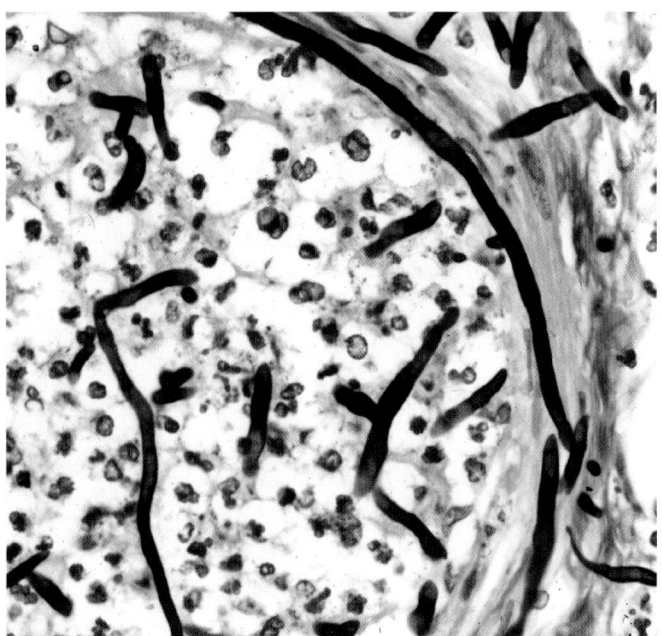

Figure 6-13. Angioinvasive *Aspergillus* species (Grocott methenamine silver stain). (Courtesy of Dr. Francis Chandler, Augusta, GA.)

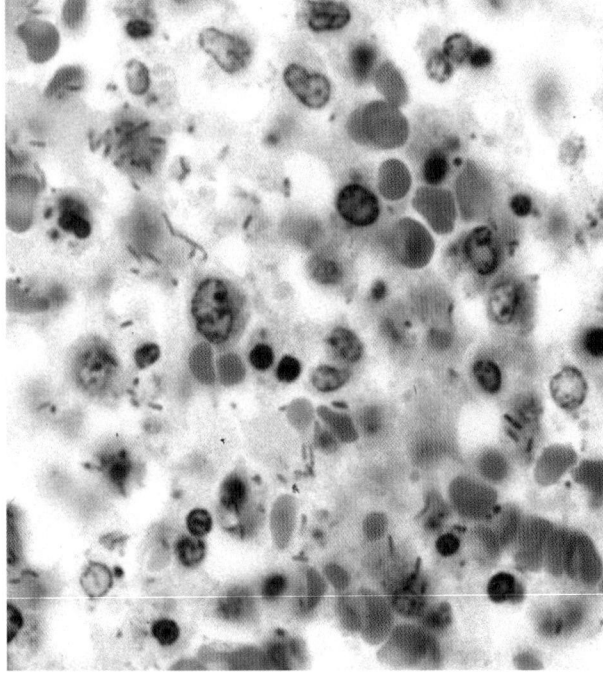

Figure 6-12. Bacillary organisms in alveolar exudates (Giemsa stain).

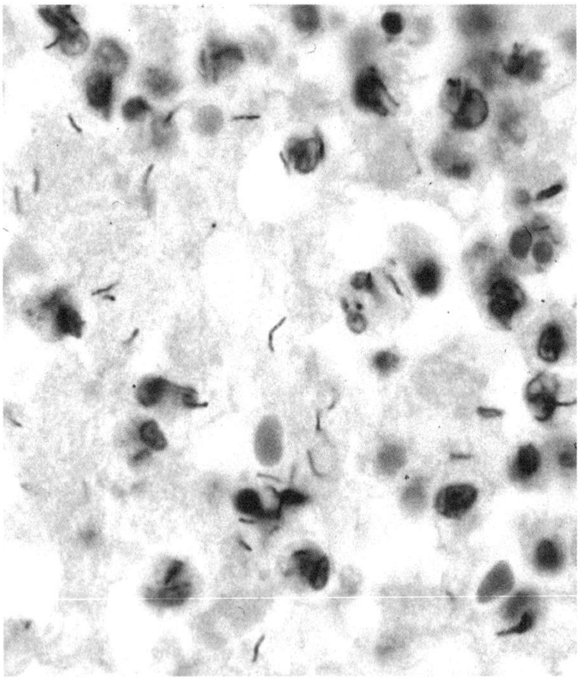

Figure 6-14. Acid-fast bacilli: *Mycobacterium tuberculosis* (Ziehl-Neelsen stain).

not without limitations and diagnostic pitfalls. The PCR method first introduced in the 1980s has undergone a number of modifications. Non-PCR DNA amplification methods and methods based not on the amplification of the DNA target per se, but on amplification of the signal or probe have also been introduced.[33] Among the more recently available technologies is the rapid-cycle "real-time" PCR assay, representing an especially powerful advance in that it is significantly more sensitive than culture. The adaptation of various amplification methods to real-time and multiplex formats enables laboratories to detect a wide range of respiratory pathogens. Furthermore, the transition from traditional and analyte-specific methods to more global technologies such as PCR arrays, liquid bead arrays, microarrays, and high-throughput DNA sequencing is under way. Over time, these methods will find a place in laboratories of all sizes, and dramatically impact the speed and accuracy of microbiologic testing practice for all types of microorganisms.[34–37]

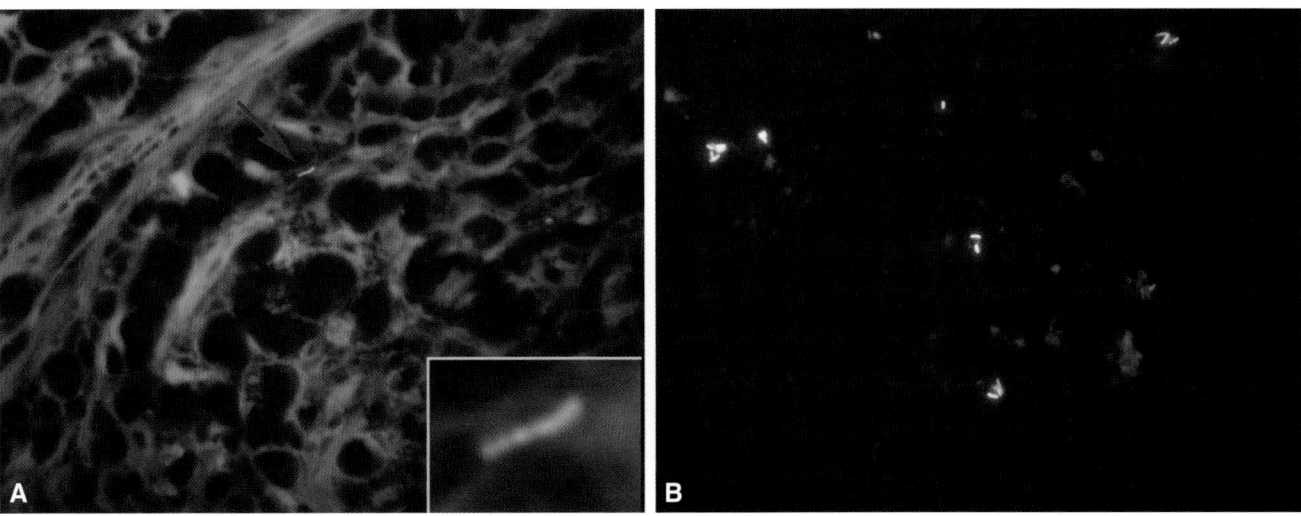

Figure 6-15. Fluorescent bacillary organisms: *Mycobacterium tuberculosis*. **A,** Tissue section with two bacilli. Note beaded character in closeup view (*inset*). (Auramine-rhodamine stain.) **B,** Low-power view.

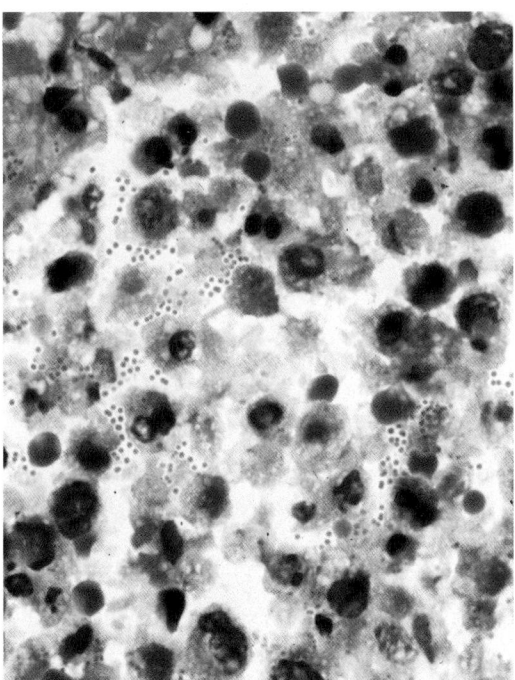

Figure 6-16. Streptococci in necrotizing pneumonia.

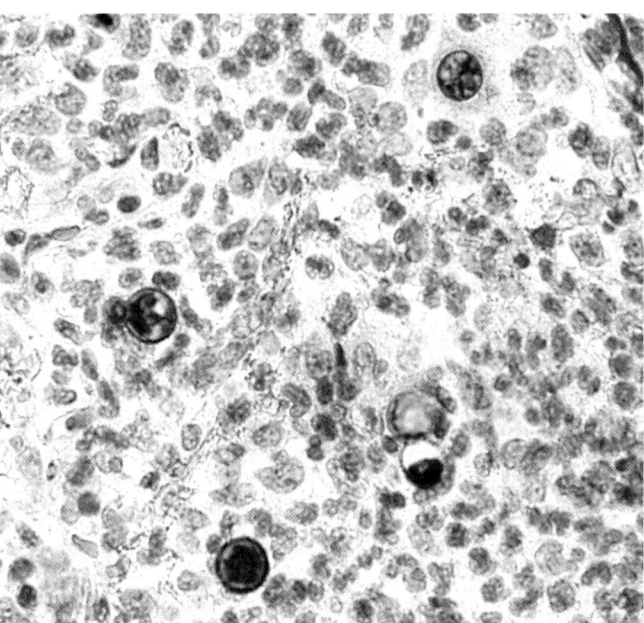

Figure 6-17. *Blastomyces dermatitidis*. In situ hybridization. (Courtesy of Ricardo Lloyd, MD, Rochester, MN.)

Limiting Factors in Diagnosis

Needless to say, the diagnostic tools employed by both pathologists and microbiologists have their limitations, in terms of sensitivity and specificity.[8] Some common tools are listed in Box 6-3. Culture alone cannot distinguish contamination from colonization, or in the case of viruses, asymptomatic shedding from true infection. Molecular tests also suffer from some of these problems; require specialized, often costly equipment; and are susceptible to false positive and false negative results.[36] If a surgical biopsy is available, correlation of the histopathologic features can help assign an etiologic role to an agent recovered in culture. The host inflammatory pattern and morphologic features of an organism can be characteristic for certain types of infections, but often the organism's morphology alone is not sufficient for a diagnosis at the genus or species level. Furthermore, the classic histopathologic findings for a given infection may be incomplete or lacking, making specific morphologic diagnosis possible for relatively few organisms. For example, the etiologic diagnosis is straightforward when large spherules with endospores characteristic of *Coccidioides* species are present, when small budding yeasts of *Histoplasma capsulatum* are seen, or yeasts with large mucoid capsules of *Cryptococcus neoformans* are identified. However, atypical forms of these organisms can be confusing.[38] Similarly, hyphal morphology is helpful when it is characteristic of a specific genus or group, but the many lookalikes (Fig. 6-19) require separation by searching for subtle differences under high magnification (or oil immersion), or reliance on special techniques and culture.[39]

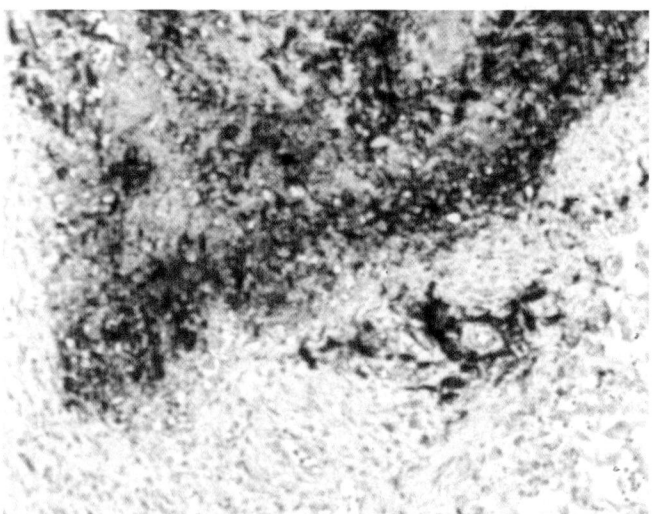

Figure 6-18. Herpes simplex virus necrotizing pneumonitis (immunohistochemical stain).

Box 6-3. Limitations of Diagnostic Tools

Morphology
- **Histopathologic examination:** Inflammatory changes nonspecific, atypical, or absent; organisms not visualized or nonspecific morphology (e.g., "*Aspergillus*-like"); unexpected or unfamiliar site
- **Special stains, immunohistochemical/molecular techniques:** Sensitivity and specificity issues; misinterpretation (e.g., aberrant forms, artifacts, nonmicrobial mimics); limited reagents, false-negative and false-positive results
- **Cytopathologic analysis:** Limitations similar to those with histopathologic examination

Microbiology
- **Direct visualization:** Sensitivity and specificity
- **Culture/identification:** Normal flora versus pathogens; colonization or asymptomatic shedding versus invasion; difficult, dangerous, or slow to grow; treated; fixed, contaminated tissue; too small or nonrepresentative sample
- **Serologic studies:** Single sample; no early response or lack of response; nondiagnostic for highly prevalent/persistent microbe; cross reaction; acute versus chronic; false-positive result on IgM tests

Certain viruses may have characteristic inclusions in tissue, but there are notable pitfalls. For example, eosinophilic intranuclear inclusions of adenovirus may resemble the early inclusions in herpes simplex virus or CMV, especially when the typical smudged cellular forms of adenovirus are absent. Also, simulators of viral cytopathic effect (CPE) can occur in a number of conditions and need to be recognized, such as macronucleoli, optically clear nuclei, and intranuclear cytoplasmic invaginations (Fig. 6-20).

Pseudo-microbe artifacts also have been recognized on routine and special stains for identification of bacteria and fungi. Such potential artifacts include fragmented reticulin fibers, pigments, calcium deposits, Hamazaki-Wesenberg (yellow-brown) yeast-like bodies (Fig. 6-21),

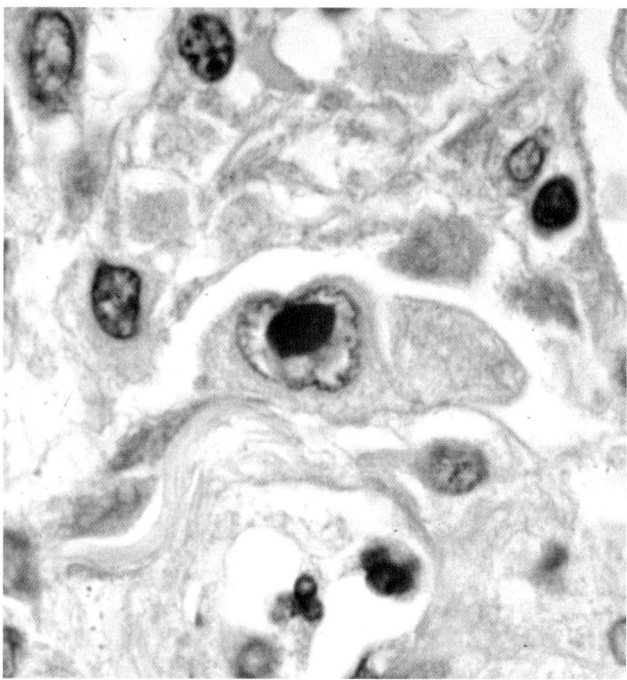

Figure 6-20. Macronucleolus mimicking a viral inclusion in an alveolar lining cell.

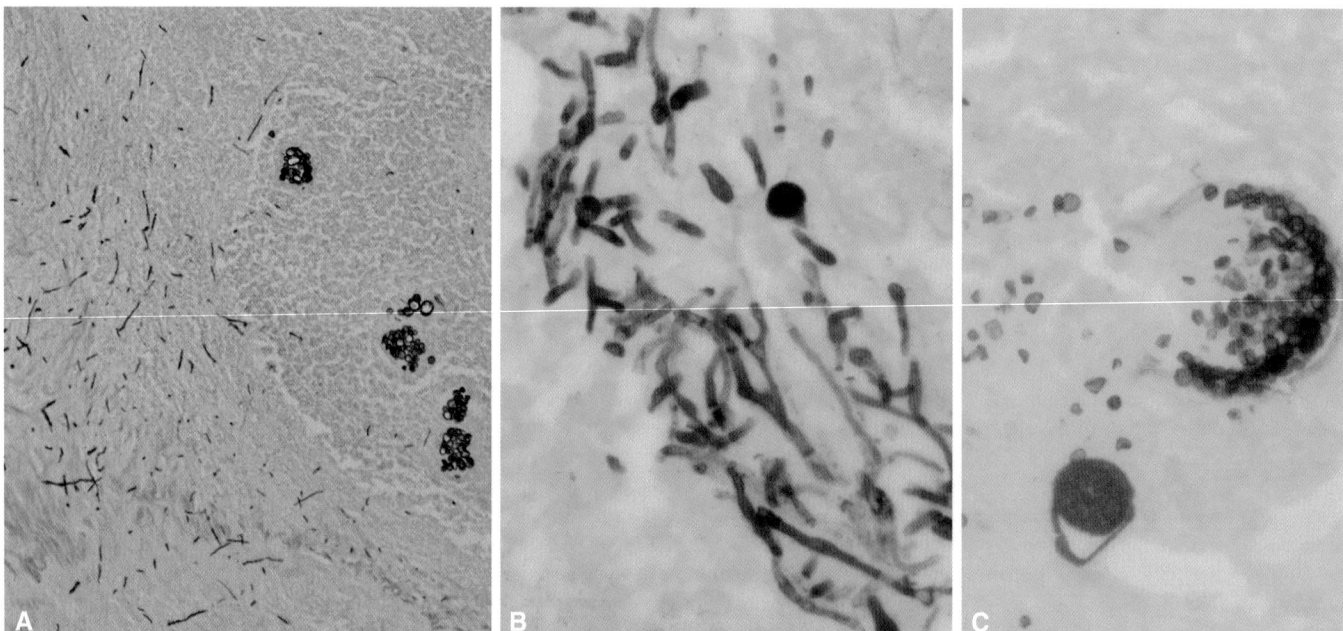

Figure 6-19. *Coccidioides immitis* demonstrating biphasic features versus those of other organisms. Culture grew *C. immitis* and *Fusarium* species. **A,** Spherules and mycelia; **B,** mycelia; **C,** ruptured spherules with endospores (Grocott methenamine silver stain).

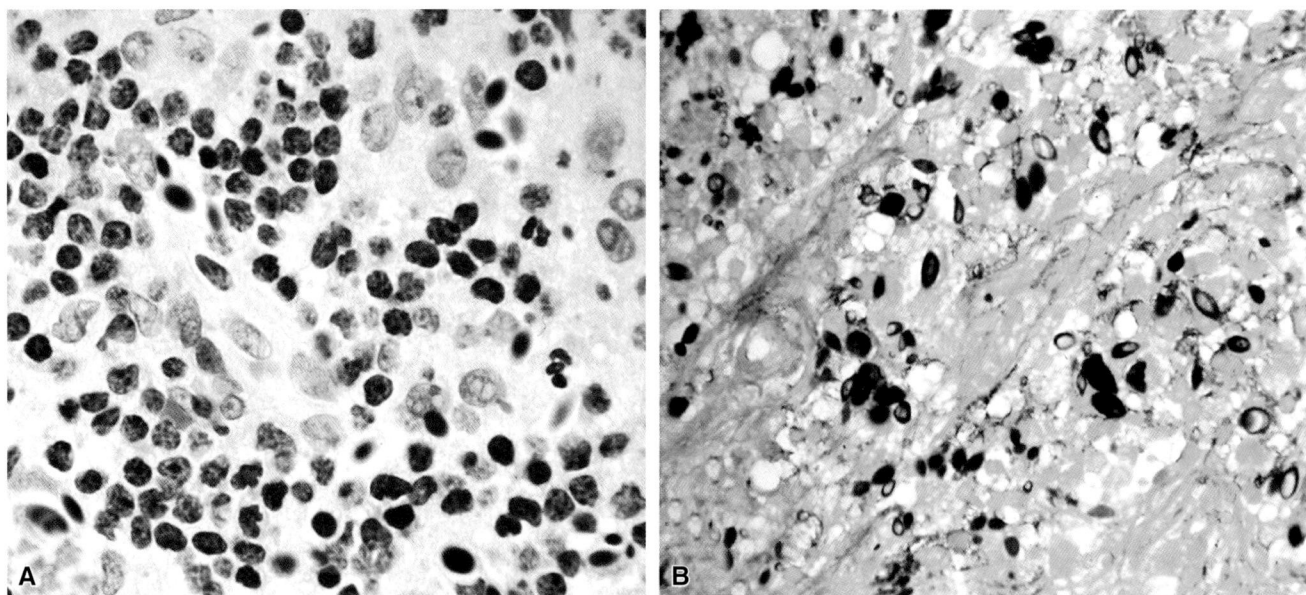

Figure 6-21. Yellow-brown Hamazaki-Wesenberg bodies (**A**, H&E; **B**, Grocott methenamine silver stain).

pollen grains, and even lymphoglandular bodies.[40] For all of these reasons, the pathologist must maintain a high threshold for diagnosing organisms on morphologic grounds. If any question remains, it is best to repeat special stains liberally on deeper levels or in different tissue blocks.

In some instances, presence of a specific infectious disease suggested by the clinical findings cannot be confirmed by the pathologist or the microbiologist, despite thorough microscopic evaluation and culture of the tissue. The histopathologic features indicative of infection may be lacking, and all stains and molecular techniques may yield negative results. Such information is nevertheless useful, however, because the clinical findings may actually reflect a noninfectious disease—for example, a pulmonary infiltrate in an immunocompromised patient may have a noninfectious etiology, such as a drug reaction, lymphangitic neoplasm, or graft-versus-host disease.

The Role of Cytopathologic Examination in Diagnosis of Lung Infection

A wide variety of infectious diseases of the lung, including bacterial, mycobacterial, fungal, viral, and parasitic, can be diagnosed through exfoliative or fine-needle aspiration cytologic techniques.[41–44] Fine-needle aspiration is an especially powerful tool, compared with exfoliative cytology study of respiratory secretions—sputum samples, bronchial washings, brushings, and bronchoalveolar lavage (BAL) fluid samples. The usefulness of exfoliative cytology examination often is limited owing to problems associated with distinguishing colonizing or oral contaminant organisms in the airways from true pathogens. Nonetheless, both diagnostic techniques are complementary and have been used in recent years to evaluate pneumonias and pulmonary nodules in both immunocompetent and immunocompromised patients.

Mass-like infiltrates are often the target of aspiration biopsy needles when suspicion or exclusion of an infectious process ranks high in the differential diagnosis. Besides the morphologic features of the microorganism, important cytologic clues to the diagnosis include the accompanying cellular response and the presence and character of any necrotic debris present, as outlined in Table 6-4. Although nonspecific, such features can suggest certain possibilities to the cytopathologist and assist the microbiology laboratory in triaging the specimen.[45] To this end, the presence of a cytopathologist, microscope, and staining setup during the aspiration process can be useful. The cytopathologist

Table 6-4. Fine-Needle Aspiration (FNA) Patterns of Pulmonary Infectious Diseases

Pattern	Possible Etiologic Agent(s)
Acute purulent inflammation/ abscess	Bacteria Fungi
Granuloma pattern (epithelioid cells with or without necrosis): Caseous/necrotizing Suppurative Epithelial Mixed	Mycobacteria Bacteria Parasite Fungi
Foamy alveolar cast pattern	*Pneumocystis jiroveci*
Histiocytic	Mycobacteria Bacteria Fungi
Chronic inflammation (lymphocyte and plasma cell)	Virus Other agent not otherwise specified
Null ("id") reaction	Virus Any other

can correlate the clinical setting, radiologic features, and clues from the gross character of the aspirate (color, consistency, odor, and so on), thereby assisting in narrowing the diagnostic possibilities and avoiding false-positive and false-negative diagnoses.[46] Also, immediate evaluation of smears by rapid stain procedures allows the cytopathologist to either make or suggest a specific diagnosis, as with preparation and evaluation of a frozen section during intraoperative consultation. Smears can be prepared for special stains, needle rinses can be performed for culture and other ancillary studies, and additional aspirations may be encouraged for these purposes.[47] Special stains for bacteria, mycobacteria, and fungi should be used whenever the character of the aspirate and the clinical setting (e.g., compromised immune status) indicate that such studies may be useful.

Some interventionists prefer to provide only a needle core biopsy in lieu of an aspirate for a variety of reasons. These two techniques can be viewed as complementary; while needle core biopsies work well for neoplasms and many granulomas, the aspirate is often superior for diagnosing many types of infections, especially bacterial abscesses. Sometimes a rapid and specific etiologic diagnosis is possible at the bedside, based on the microscopic features of the organism itself. However, when the organism is not readily apparent or its features are inconclusive, the microbiology laboratory can be invaluable for its role in isolation and identification.[47]

Summary

The successful treatment of pulmonary infections depends on accurate identification of the pathogen involved. In turn, this requires collecting the best specimens, transporting them to the anatomic and microbiology sections of the laboratory under optimal conditions, and processing them with techniques appropriate for the spectrum of possible etiologic disorders. An interdisiplinary approach enhances this process. It is in the best interest of all parties involved that pathologists, clinicians, and microbiologists communicate frequently and recognize the strengths and weaknesses of their respective disciplines. Joint strategies can be developed for the approach to certain types of suspected infections, helping to foster the development of laboratory "foresight" in surgical colleagues and medical consultants. As methods of diagnosis, treatment, and antimicrobial prophylaxis change, the pathologist must remain vigilant to a changing spectrum of etiologic agents and tissue injury patterns. The pathologist capable of integrating clinical and imaging data with morphologic and microbiologic findings can construct a comprehensive report useful for patient managment. The microbiology laboratory can be instrumental in delivery of more effective and efficient patient management if the microbiologist can capture this information, in view of its optimal position for choosing the appropriate combination of diagnostic methods (morphologic, culture, immunologic, molecular) for a particular type of sample. An example of such an operational protocol is presented in Box 6-4.

Box 6-4. Workup of Pulmonary Infections

Pre/Intraoperative Consultation
Inquiry regarding
- History
- Risk factors; immune status
- Radiographic pattern

Advise regarding
- How and what to collect
- What cultures and tests to order
- Devices, media, and containers for obtaining and transport of specimens
- Fixatives for morphologic study

Written Protocol
Handling tissue for cultures
Special stains and ancillary tests
Logistics
Requisition—designed to communicate

Morphologic Examination
Inflammatory pattern
Persistence and repeat studies
Oil immersion studies, if necessary
Strict criteria for positive
Consider multiple pathogens

Report
Presumptive versus definitive diagnosis; correlate with results of culture, other studies
Comment
- Clinicopathologic-microbiologic correlation
- Differential diagnosis
- Ancillary tests
- Suggestions for further workup

Bacterial Pneumonias

The surgical pathologist rarely receives biopsy specimens from patients with community-acquired or nosocomial pneumonias. Most of these infections are suspected clinically by symptoms and physical and radiologic findings; some are confirmed immediately by Gram stains (or later by culture) performed on respiratory secretions in the microbiology laboratory. Serologic studies sometimes prove to be diagnostic. Even when conventional microbiologic approaches are applied, however, approximately 50% of bacterial pneumonias remain undiagnosed.[48-50] Patients with mild disease often are not tested but simply treated empirically with antibiotic regimens following established guidelines. By contrast, patients with severe disease, whether immunocompromised or not, often become candidates for invasive procedures.

Etiologic Agents

Bacterial pneumonia may be classified according to various parameters including pathogenesis, epidemiology, anatomic pattern, clinical course, and organism type[51] (Box 6-5). Using bacterial type as a starting point allows the pathologist to correlate anatomic and histopathologic patterns of lung injury with categories of etiologic agents.

The **pyogenic bacteria** most commonly associated with community-acquired pneumonias include *S. pneumoniae*, *H. influenzae*, and *Moraxella catarrhalis*.[50] Other pathogens such as *Legionella* species, *Chlamydia pneumoniae*, and *Mycoplasma pneumoniae* (often referred to as the "atypical" group) are clinically important, but controversy exists with regard to the relative frequency of these organisms as etiologic agents. Although community-acquired pneumonia is considered to be fundamentally different in children and in adults, severe or complicated pneumonias in both of these age groups are of similar etiology.[52] The enteric gram-negative bacilli cause relatively few community-acquired pneumonias, whereas they account for most of the nosocomial pneumonias, along with *Pseudomonas* species, *Acinetobacter* species, *S. aureus*, and anaerobes.[53,54] Most nosocomial pneumonias result from aspiration of these bacterial species that colonize the oropharynx of hospitalized patients, and they are often polymicrobial. Any of the bacterial organisms listed (including mixtures with fungi and viruses) can cause pneumonia in immunocompromised patients.[15,55] Ventilator-associated pneumonia is a special subset of nosocomial pneumonia and an important cause of morbidity

---

Box 6-5. Classification of Bacterial Pneumonia

Pathogenesis
Primary
  Exogenous
  Endogenous
Secondary

Epidemiology
Community-acquired
Nosocomial

Anatomic Type
Lobular
Lobar

Clinical Course
Acute
Chronic

Bacterial Type
Pyogenic species
Atypical agents
Granule/filamentous group

---

and mortality in the intensive care unit.[56–58] The bacterial etiology in this setting is quite diverse and dependent on such factors as patient characteristics, underlying lung disease, and geographic location.[59] Most recently, an increase in skin and soft tissue staphylococcal infections due to methicillin-resistant strains has led to the recognition of these organisms as an important cause of both community-acquired and nosocomial pneumonia with attendant morbidity and mortality.[60] In rare nosocomial pneumonias, a number of unusual organisms, such as *Salmonella*, *Rhodococcus*, and *Leptospira* species, may be the etiologic agent.[61,62]

The **atypical pneumonia agents** are those that do not commonly produce lobar consolidation. Although this potentially implicates a wide variety of bacterial, viral, and protozoal pathogens, a selective list by convention includes *Mycoplasma pneumoniae*, *Legionella* species, and *C. pneumoniae* as the three dominant nonzoonotic pathogens, and *Coxiella burnetii* (the agent of Q fever), *Chlamydia psittaci* (causing psittacosis in people), and *F. tularensis* (causing tularemia) as the three more common zoonotic pathogens.[63,64]

The **filamentous/granule group** refers to those bacteria that form long, thin, branching filaments in tissues, such as *Actinomyces* (anaerobic actinomycetes) or *Nocardia* (aerobic actinomycetes).[65] Botryomycosis is caused by nonfilamentous bacteria, especially *Staphylococcus aureus*, or gram-negative bacilli, such as *P. aeruginosa* and *E. coli*, which form organized aggregates referred to as grains or granules.[66]

Histopathology

Bacterial lung injury patterns will vary in accordance with the virulence of the organism and the host response. These patterns are further modulated by therapeutic or immunologic factors. Although some of the patterns presented in Box 6-6 are characteristic, none are diagnostic. Overlap and mixed patterns occur.

Acute Exudative Pneumonia

Acute exudative pneumonia most often is caused by pyogenic bacteria, such as streptococci, which typically produce a neutrophil-rich intra-alveolar exudate (i.e., alveolar filling) with variable amounts of fibrin and red cells. Pathologists recognize this constellation of findings as acute lobular pneumonia (Fig. 6-22), which usually correlates with patchy segmental infiltrates on the chest film (consolidation pattern on HRCT).[29,67–69]

With increasing organism virulence and disease severity, lobular exudates may become confluent (i.e., lobar pneumonia). In milder cases, the disease may be limited to the airways (bronchitis/bronchiolitis) with a mixed cellular infiltrate of mononuclear cells and neutrophils (Fig. 6-23). One very common manifestation of such airway-limited infection has been designated as "acute exacerbation of chronic obstructive pulmonary disease" (COPD). A majority of these exacerbations are caused by particular bacteria, specifically *H. influenzae*, *S. pneumoniae*, and *M. catarrhalis*, with approximately one third

Box 6-6. Histopathologic Patterns in Bacterial Lung Injury

Bronchitis/bronchiolitis
Acute exudative pneumonia
    Lobular (bronchopneumonia)
    Confluent (lobar pneumonia)
    With granules
Fibroinflammatory and/or organizing pneumonia
Interstitial pneumonia
Nodular/necrotizing lesions
    Miliary lesions
    Abscess

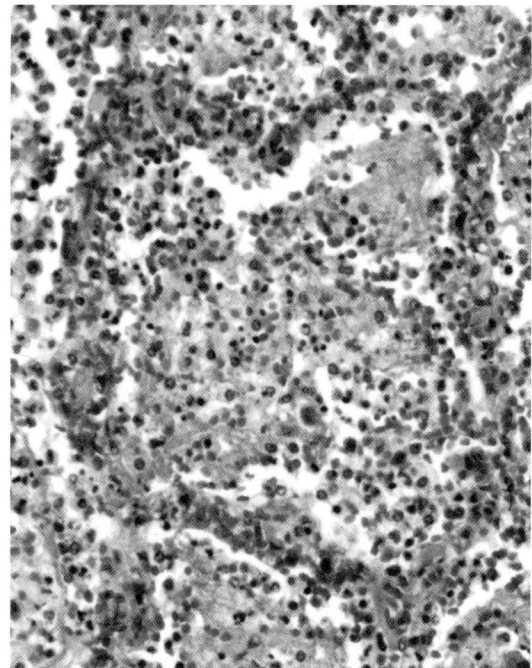

Figure 6-22. Alveoli filled with fibrinopurulent exudate with variable hemorrhage.

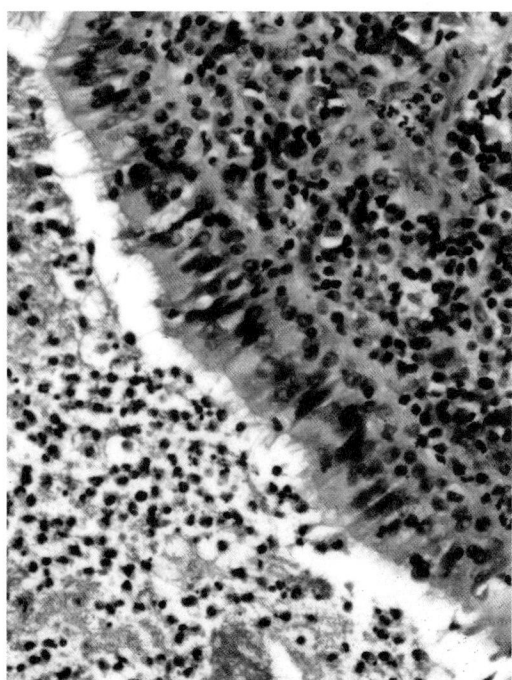

Figure 6-23. Bronchiolitis with intraluminal exudate.

resulting from viral airway infections, typically resulting from rhinovirus, respiratory syncytial virus (RSV), and human metapneumovirus.[70]

Nodular/Necrotizing Lesions

Nodular inflammatory infiltrates with or without necrotizing features (Fig. 6-24) are characteristic of infection by certain species, such as *Rhodococcus equi* (Fig. 6-25).[71] Necrotizing pneumonias also may be produced by pyogenic bacteria such as *Staphylococcus aureus*, *Streptococcus pyogenes*, and the gram-negative bacilli—*Klebsiella*, *Acinetobacter*, *Pseudomonas*, and *Burkholderia* species.

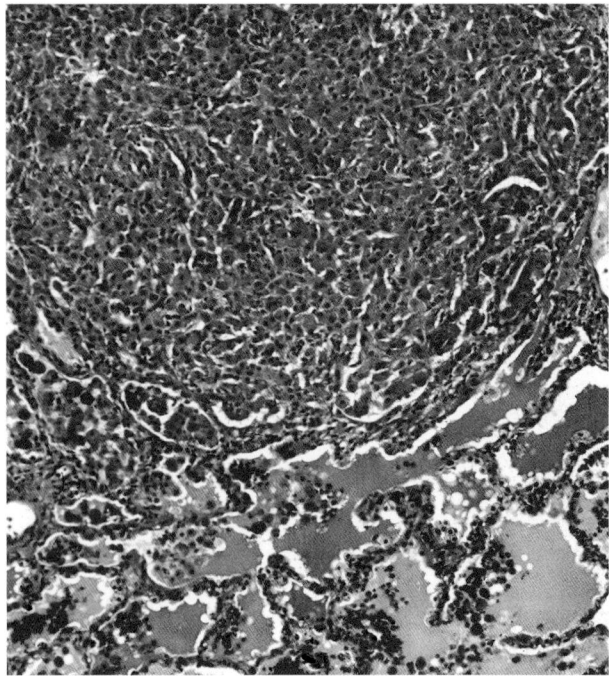

Figure 6-24. Nodular histiocytic infiltrate in rhodococcal pneumonia.

Miliary Lesions

A subset of the nodular histopathologic pattern, miliary infection (Fig. 6-26), strongly implies pneumonia secondary to hematogenous spread of bacteria (septicemia). This pattern of infection can be seen with other organisms, such as *Nocardia* and the anaerobic actionomycetes. In these settings, histopathologic examination may show a hybrid reaction with both nodular disease and alveolar filling.

Aspiration Pneumonia and Lung Abscess

Several pulmonary aspiration scenarios are recognized, including those caused by chemical pneumonitis (so-called Mendelsson syndrome), airway obstruction, exogenous lipoid pneumonia, chronic

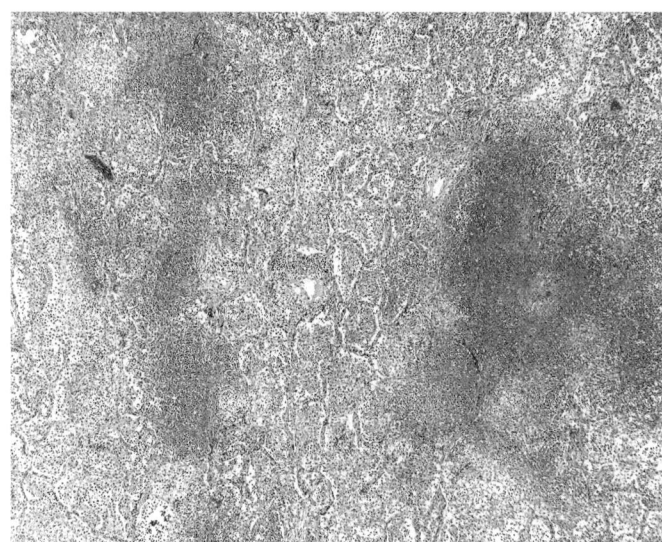

Figure 6-26. Necrotizing pneumonia, miliary pattern.

interstitial fibrosis, diffuse bronchiolar disease, bacterial pneumonia, and lung abscess.[72,73] *Aspiration pneumonia* refers specifically to aspiration of bacteria in oropharyngeal secretions and is classically a polymicrobial aerobic/anaerobic bacterial infection, with the bacterial species depending on whether the aspiration event occurs in the community or hospital setting. Recognition of food particles (so-called pulses) is key to the diagnosis. These may or may not be invested by giant cells but usually are found in purulent exudate or granulomatous foci. In the organizing phase of the pneumonia, food particles may be found within polyps of organizing pneumonia in the alveolar ducts and alveoli. Lobular pneumonia, lipoid pneumonia, organizing pneumonia, and bronchiolitis, alone or in combination, also may be seen.[69,74] The pathogens in lung abscess (Fig. 6-27) usually encompass a polymicrobic mixture of aerobic and anaerobic bacteria,[75] and formation of such abscesses most often is secondary to aspiration (Fig. 6-28). Infections due to *Actinomyces* species (Fig. 6-29) and *Nocardia* species also may manifest this pattern, as can those due to certain pyogenic bacteria, such as *Staphylococcus aureus* and the other organisms listed previously for necrotizing pneumonias. Granulomatous inflammation with foreign bodies may be present if aspiration is the cause (Fig. 6-30).

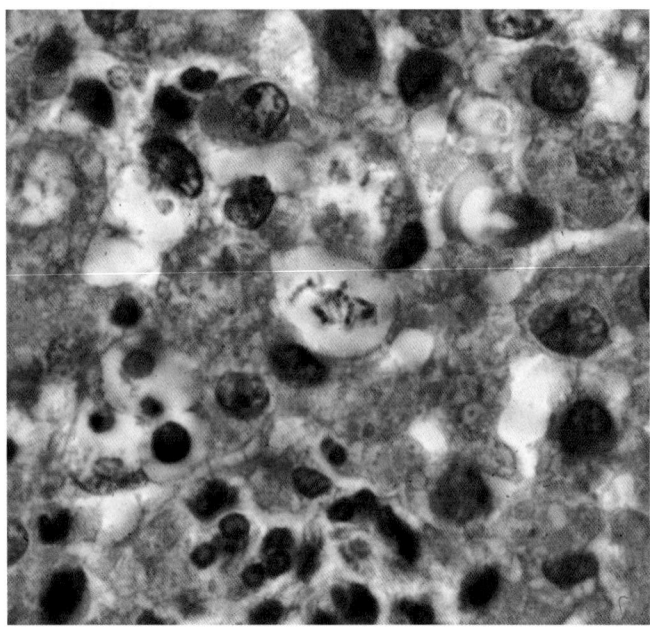

Figure 6-25. *Rhodococcus equi* bacilli in macrophage.

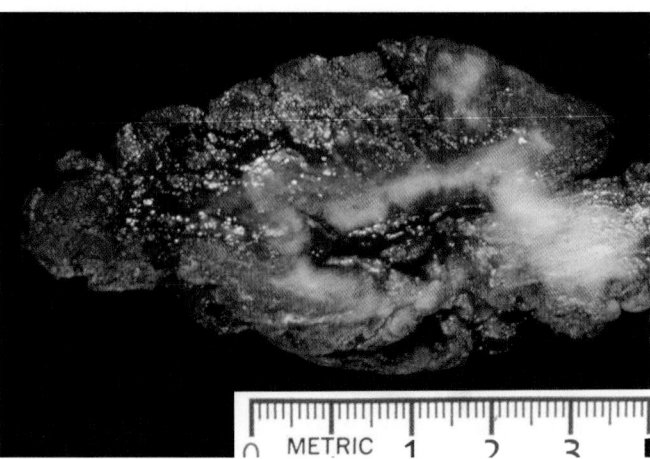

Figure 6-27. Lung abscess showing gross evidence of chronicity with fibrosis in surrounding parenchyma.

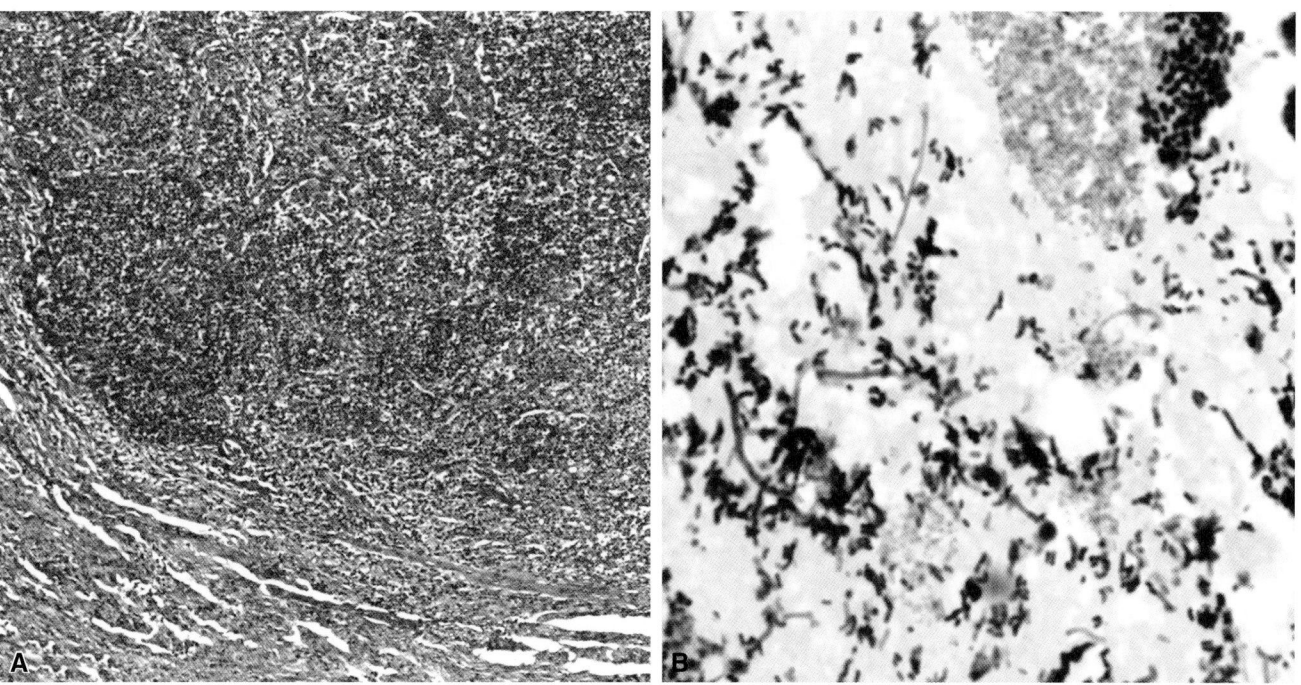

Figure 6-28. **A** and **B,** Lung abscess with polymicrobial bacterial population (Gram stain).

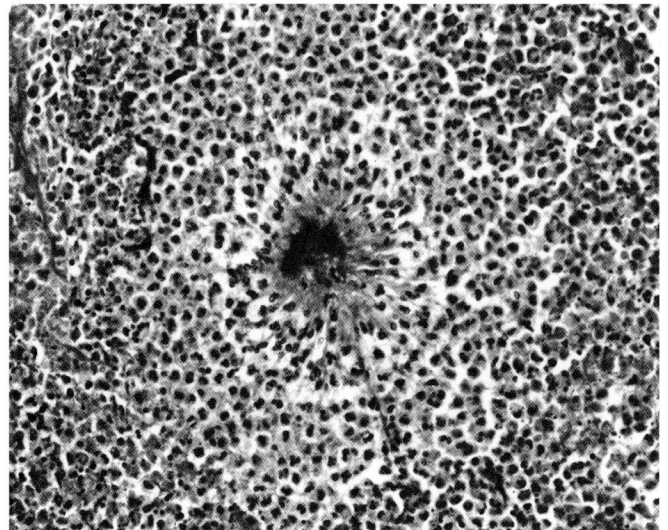

Figure 6-29. Lung abscess with sulfur granule of actinomycosis in purulent exudate.

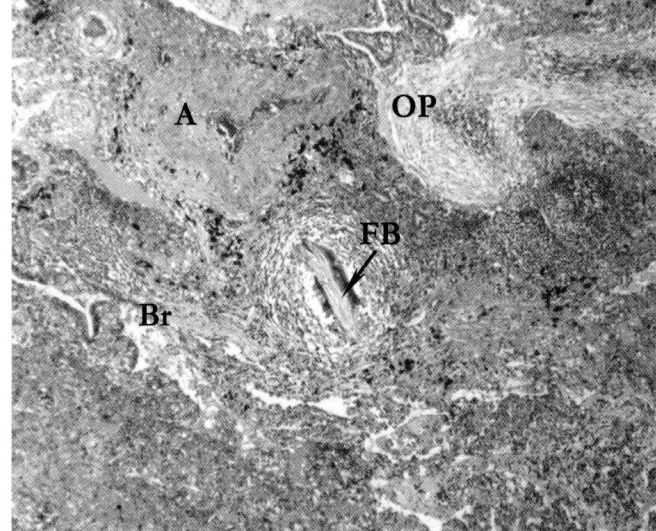

Figure 6-30. Aspiration pneumonia. Giant cells surround vegetable matter (FB) in purulent exudates, organizing pneumonia (OP), bronchiolitis (BR). A, artery.

Chronic Bacterial Pneumonias

Chronic bacterial infections (Fig. 6-31) that are slow to resolve as a result of inappropriate initial therapy, involvement with certain microbial species, a noninfectious comorbid process, or an inadequate host response can produce a nonspecific fibroinflammatory pattern, with lymphoplasmacytic infiltrates, macrophages, or organization with polyps of immature fibroblasts in alveolar ducts and alveolar spaces.[76-79] If not resorbed, polyps of air space organization may become polyps of intra-alveolar fibrosis, which sometimes ossify (dendriform ossification). Such scarring in chronic pneumonia often is associated with localized interlobular septal and pleural thickening (Fig. 6-32), producing a "jigsaw puzzle" pattern of scarring best seen at scanning magnification.

Diffuse alveolar damage is the histopathologic correlate of the acute repiratory distress syndrome (ARDS), and today, lung infection is the leading cause of diffuse alveolar damage and ARDS in the United States.[80] Diffuse alveolar damage may coexist with any of the necro-inflammatory patterns described earlier. The initial *exudative* phase of this process is accompanied by hyaline membranes (Fig. 6-33); the later *organizing* phase is attended by air space and interstitial fibroplasia. In clinical practice, diffuse alveolar damage accompanied by tissue necrosis is nearly always a manifestation of lung infection.

The **atypical pneumonias** include the well-described cases due to *Legionella* species and the less well-described cases caused by other organisims comprising the atypical group. *Legionella* infection typically results in an intensely neutrophilic acute fibrinopurulent lobular

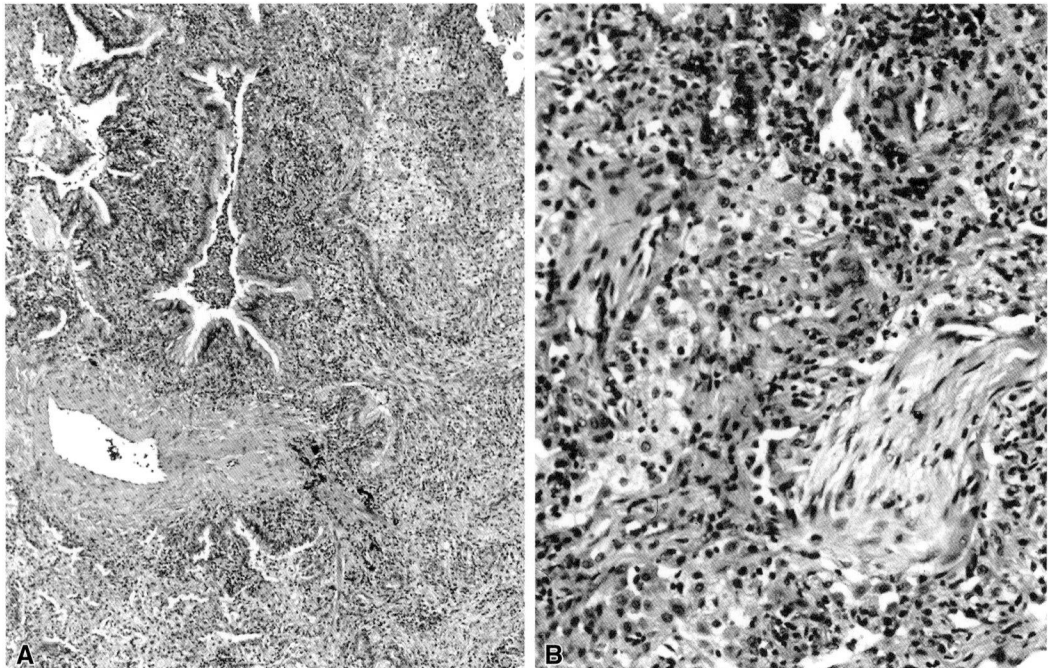

Figure 6-31. Chronic pneumonia. **A,** lymphoplasmacytic infiltrate. **B,** fascicles of fibroblasts in alveolar ducts and spaces.

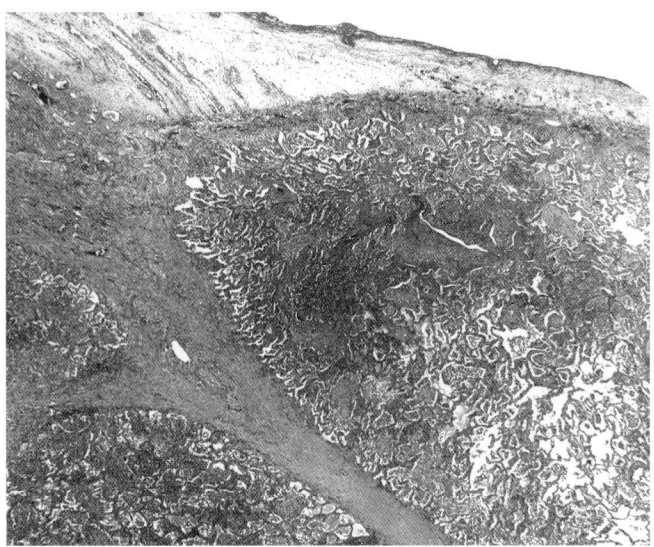

Figure 6-32. Chronic pneumonia with thickened interlobular septum.

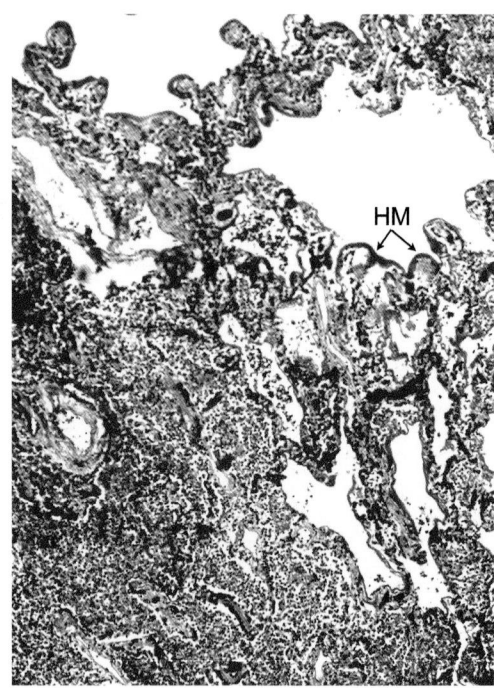

Figure 6-33. Bacterial pneumonia with hyaline membranes (HM) at periphery.

pneumonia[64,67] (Fig. 6-34A). *Legionella* bacilli often can be identified in silver impregnation-stained sections (see Fig. 6-34B) or recovered in culture, but newer diagnostic methods, such as real-time PCR and in situ hybridization (Fig. 6-35) also can be applied when standard approaches fail.[81] The histopathologic patterns associated with the other members of the atypical group (i.e., *Chlamydia, Mycoplasma*) are not well characterized, mainly because investigation of these pneumonias rarely includes biopsy. The few well-documented cases of *Mycoplasma, Chlamydia*, and *Coxiella* infections that have been described in the literature resemble viral bronchitis or bronchiolitis, with mixed inflammatory infiltrates in airway walls and in the adjacent interstitium[82,83] (Fig. 6-36). Relative sparing of the peribronchiolar alveolar spaces has been described, although patchy organized fibrinous exudates are seen in some cases, and complications may superimpose additional findings.

The **grains and granules** formed by the actinomycetes and bacteria of botryomycosis may have a uniform tinctorial hue on routine hematoxylin and eosin (H&E)–stained sections, but sometimes these bacterial aggregations display a distinctive body with a hematoxylinophilic core and an outer investment of eosinophilic material; formation of this array is referred to as the Splendore-Hoeppli phenomenon (Fig. 6-37). *Actinomyces* species tend to form similar-appearing granules, and both they and the bacteria of botryomycosis typically are found in the midst

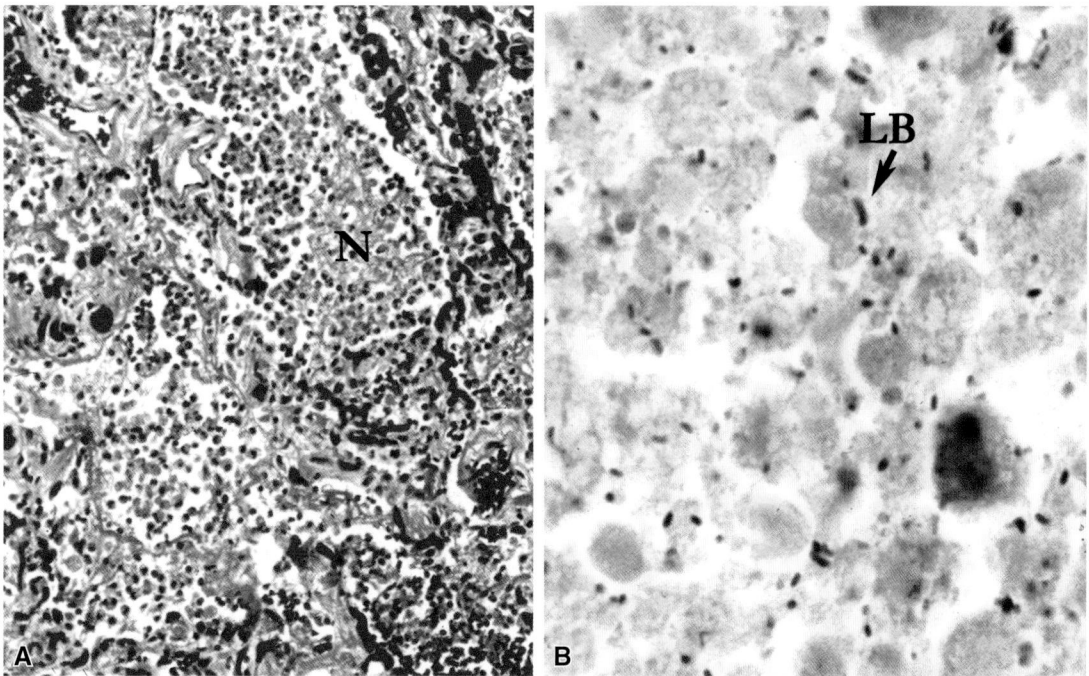

Figure 6-34. **A,** Legionnaires disease with intra-alveolar necroinflammatory exudates (N) and hemorrhage. **B,** Enhanced silhouette of *Legionella* bacilli (LB) in alveolar exudate with silver impregnation (Dieterle stain).

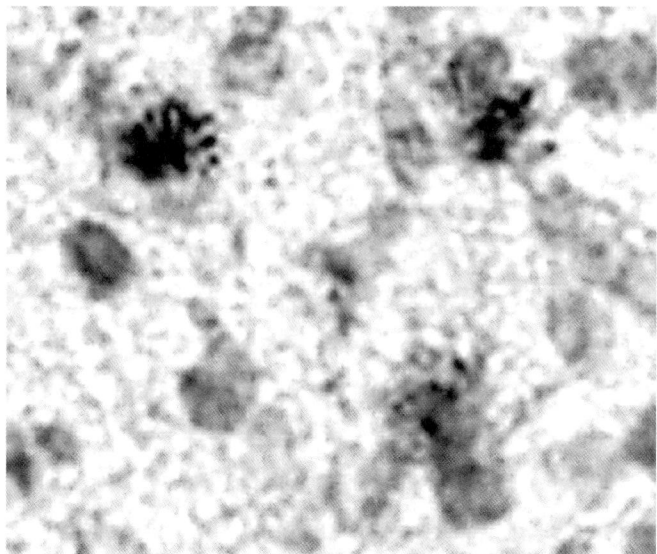

Figure 6-35. Legionnaire's disease. Detection of organisms by in situ DNA hybridization. (Courtesy of R. V. Lloyd, MD, Rochester, MN.)

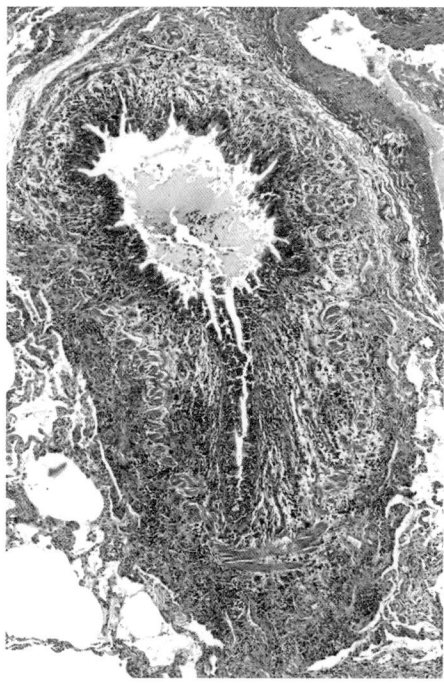

Figure 6-36. *Mycoplasma* pneumonia. Bronchiolitis with patchy infiltrates in peribronchial interstitium.

of purulent exudates.[65,84-86] The *Nocardia* species may aggregate in colonies simulating granules, but with a much looser texture (Fig. 6-38) and more monochromatic tinctorial properties.[87] Rarely, these colonies may be identical in appearance to the grains or granules of botryomycosis or actinomycosis in H&E sections.

Bacterial Agents of Bioterrorism

The potential for use of microbial pathogens as agents of bioterrorism requires that clinicians be alert to this possibility when community-acquired pneumonias are found to be caused by these agents. In turn, pathologists must become familiar with the histopathologic features these agents can produce.[88] Respiratory disease caused by the

inhalation of *Bacillus anthracis, Yersinia pestis*, and *Franciscella tularensis* is especially pertinent in this context and is discussed next.

Bacillus anthracis

In 1877, Robert Koch's conclusive demonstration that *B. anthracis* was the etiologic agent of anthrax revolutionized medicine by linking microbial cause and effect.[7] Set against its historical importance to medicine, the recent use of anthrax as a bioterrorism agent represents a sad contrast.

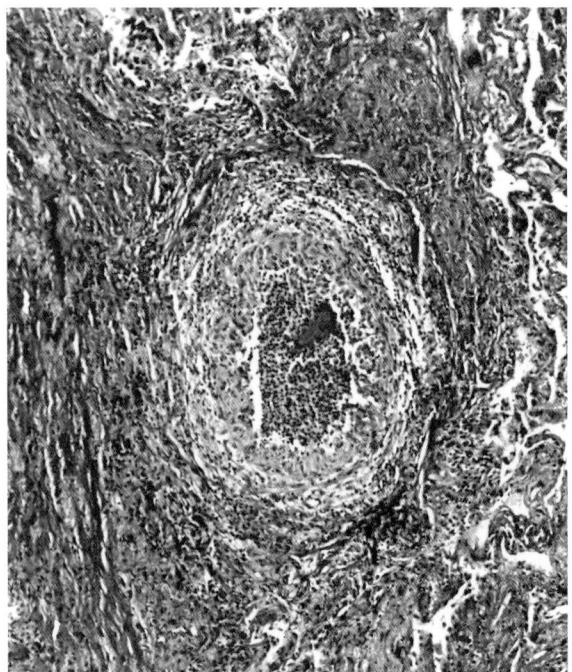

Figure 6-37. Botryomycosis granule with hematoxylinophilic core and eosinophilic investment known as Splendore-Hoeppli effect.

Inhalational anthrax causes a severe hemorrhagic mediastinitis.[89-93] This pathologic process, in combination with the toxemia (*B. anthracis* produces an exotoxin with three potent components—protective antigen, lethal factor, and edema factor) from the ensuing massive bacteremia, severely compromises pulmonary function, leading to death in 40% or more of the cases. Pleural effusion may be present, but pneumonia generally is minor and secondary. In those patients in whom pulmonary parenchymal changes are found, the alveolar spaces contain a serosanguineous fluid with minimal fibrin deposits and some mononuclear cells, but few if any neutrophils.[92] Large gram-positive bacilli (some may appear partially gram-negative) without spores, pervade the alveolar septal vessels, with a few in the alveolar spaces. This distribution suggests hematogenous rather than airway acquisition. Hemorrhagic mediastinitis in a previously healthy adult is essentially pathognomonic for

inhalational anthrax. The lymph node parenchyma generally is teeming with intact and fragmented gram-positive bacilli, which can be identified as *B. anthracis* by immunohistochemical studies.[91,92] Cultures of blood and pleural fluid, if available, are likely to yield the earliest positive diagnostic results.[93] Sputum studies are much less useful in this regard.

Yersinia pestis

Primary pneumonic plague follows inhalation of *Y. pestis* bacilli in a potential bioterrorism scenario.[94] The infection begins as bronchiolitis and alveolitis that progress to a lobular and eventual lobar consolidation.[95] The histopathologic features evolve over time, beginning with serosanguineous intra-alveolar fluid accumulation with variable fibrin deposits (Fig. 6-39), progressing through a fibrinopurulent phase, and culminating in a necrotizing lesion.[96] The presence of myriad bacilli in the intra-alveolar exudates, with significantly fewer organisms in the interstitium (a characteristic of primary pneumonia), is one of several pulmonary and extrapulmonary features used to distinguish primary from secondary pneumonic plague.[97] These bacilli may be obvious in H&E-stained sections (Fig. 6-40) but generally are better visualized

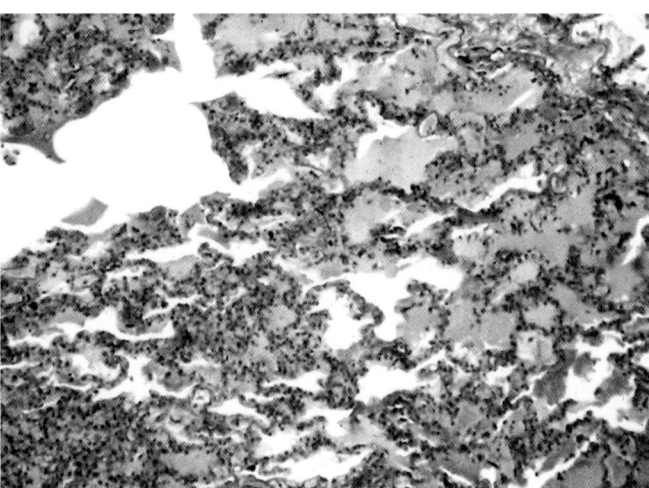

Figure 6-39. Plague pneumonia, early phase. Edema, fibrin, and sparse inflammatory cells are evident.

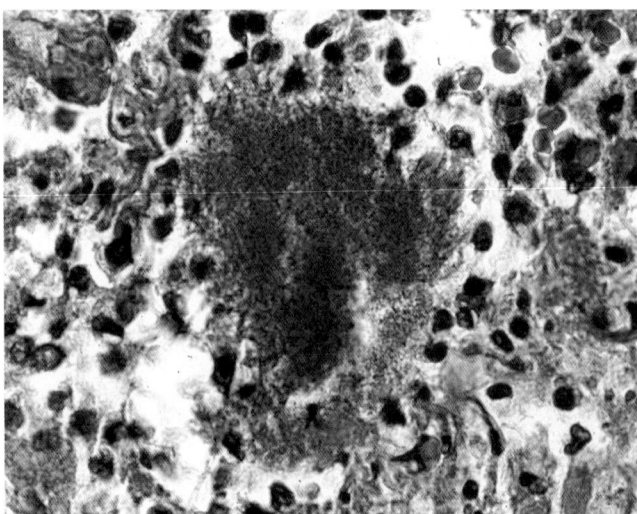

Figure 6-38. Loose-textured aggregate of *Nocardia* filamentous bacteria surrounded by neutrophils.

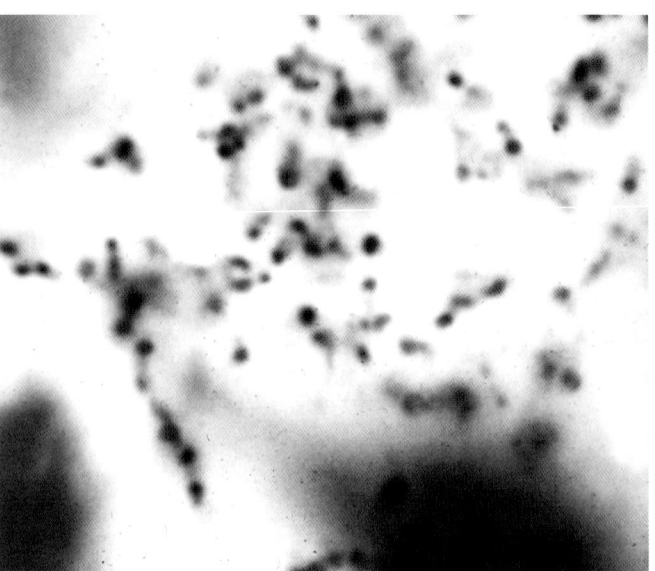

Figure 6-40. *Yersinia pestis* bacilli in alveolar space.

with Giemsa rather than Gram stain. Immunohistochemical staining provides a rapid and specific diagnosis.[95] Unlike with inhalational anthrax, sputum Gram stain and culture are useful tests that are likely to yield a positive result at clinical presentation. Also, because sepsis is an integral component of the pneumonia, it is important to collect blood culture specimens.

Francisella tularensis

Inhalation of *F. tularensis* bacilli, following a bioterrorism aerosol release, generally is expected to result in a slowly progressing pneumonia, with a lower case-fatality rate than with either inhalational anthrax or plague.[97] Initially, a hemorrhagic and ulcerative bronchiolitis is followed by a fibrinous lobular pneumonia with many macrophages but relatively few neutrophils (Fig. 6-41). Necrosis then supervenes and evolves into a granulomatous reaction. The small, gram-negative coccobacillary organisms are difficult to identify in a tissue Gram stain, and the use of silvering techniques (e.g., Steiner, Dieterle, Warthin-Starry)

is required to enhance their silhouette.[98] Specific fluorescent antibody testing for formalin-fixed tissue and immunohistochemical studies also are available through public health laboratories. In the microbiology laboratory, Gram stain and culture of respiratory secretions are useful for diagnosis, but blood culture results are not often positive. Antigen detection and molecular techniques, such as PCR amplification, can be used to identify *F. tularensis*. Serologic tests are available but probably would not provide timely information in an outbreak situation.[97]

Cytopathology

The stereotypic cellular response to pyogenic bacteria is acute inflammation, characterized by variable numbers of neutrophils. Bacteria may be visualized in various stained preparations made from respiratory tract secretions and washings using the Papanicolaou and Diff-Quik methods.[43] The clinical significance is rather limited in these specimens owing to the potential contamination by oral flora and the problem of distinguishing colonization from infection. However, when the upper respiratory tract can be bypassed, by means of either transtracheal or transthoracic needle aspiration, the presence of bacteria becomes much more significant, especially when sheets of neutrophils or necroinflammatory debris are present (Fig. 6-42A), as would be the case with a typical lobar or lobular consolidation, lung abscess, or other complex pneumonia.[49,86,99,100] In this context, transthoracic needle aspiration can establish the etiologic diagnosis of community-ascquired and nosocomial pneumonias in both children and adults when coupled with modern microbiologic methods.[47,54,101,102] Proponents consider it an underutilized technique whose potential benefits, in experienced hands, outweigh the modest associated risks.

Many types of bacilli and cocci can be seen within and around neutrophils on Diff-Quik–stained smears (see Fig. 6-42B). A smear also can be prepared for Gram stain and the aspirate needle rinsed in nonbacteriostatic sterile saline or nutrient broths for culture. The size (length and width) and shape of organisms and the Gram reaction allow rough categorization of organisms into groups such as enteric-type bacilli, pseudomonads, fusiform anaerobic-type bacilli, tiny coccobacillary types suggestive of the *Haemophilus-Bacteroides* group (Fig. 6-43), or gram-positive cocci.[103] Branching filamentous forms suggest actinomycetes or *Nocardia* organisms (Fig. 6-44), with the latter distinguished

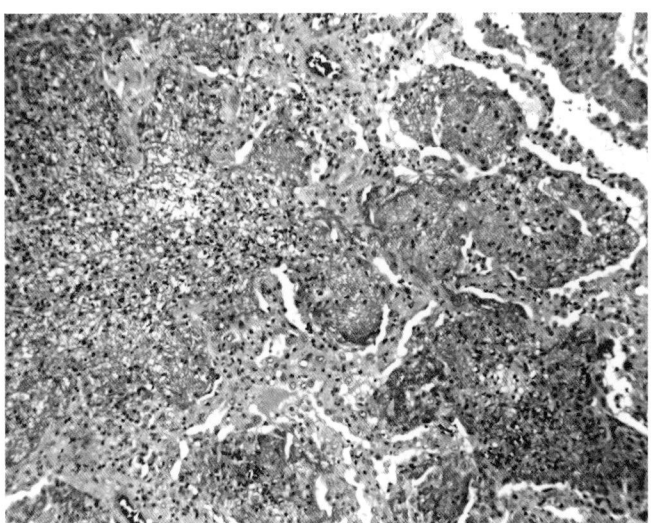

Figure 6-41. Tularemia. Fibrinous lobular pneumonia phase.

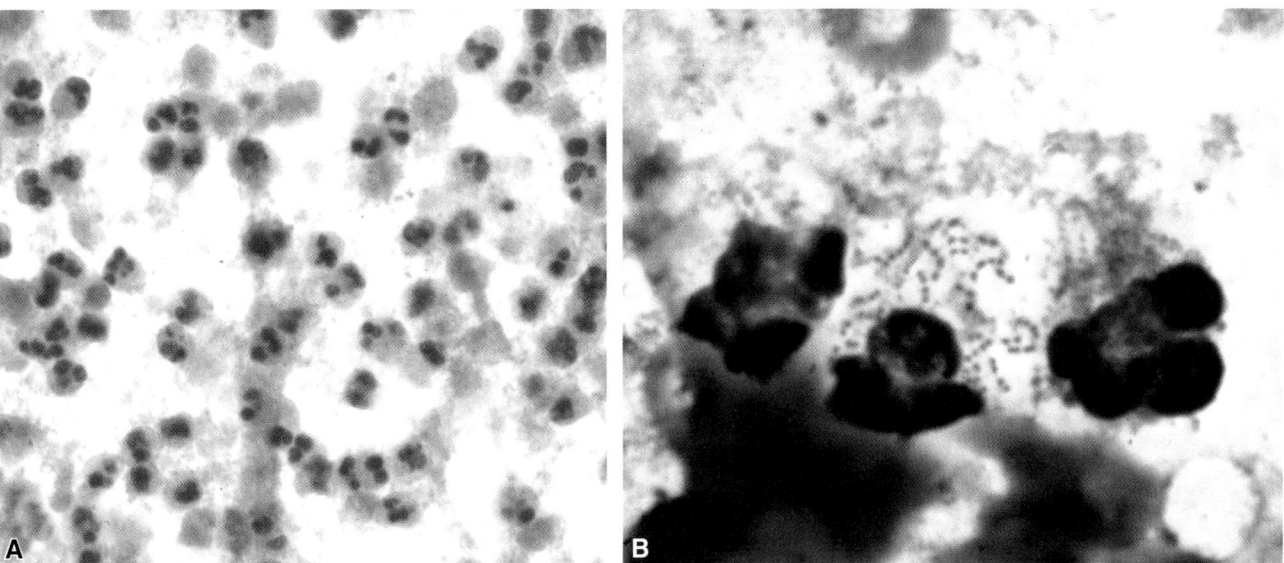

Figure 6-42. A, Purulent exudate of nodular pulmonary infiltrate in fine-needle aspirate (alcohol-fixed). **B,** Streptococci (viridans group) in cytoplasm of neutrophil seen in fine-needle aspirate (Diff-Quik preparation).

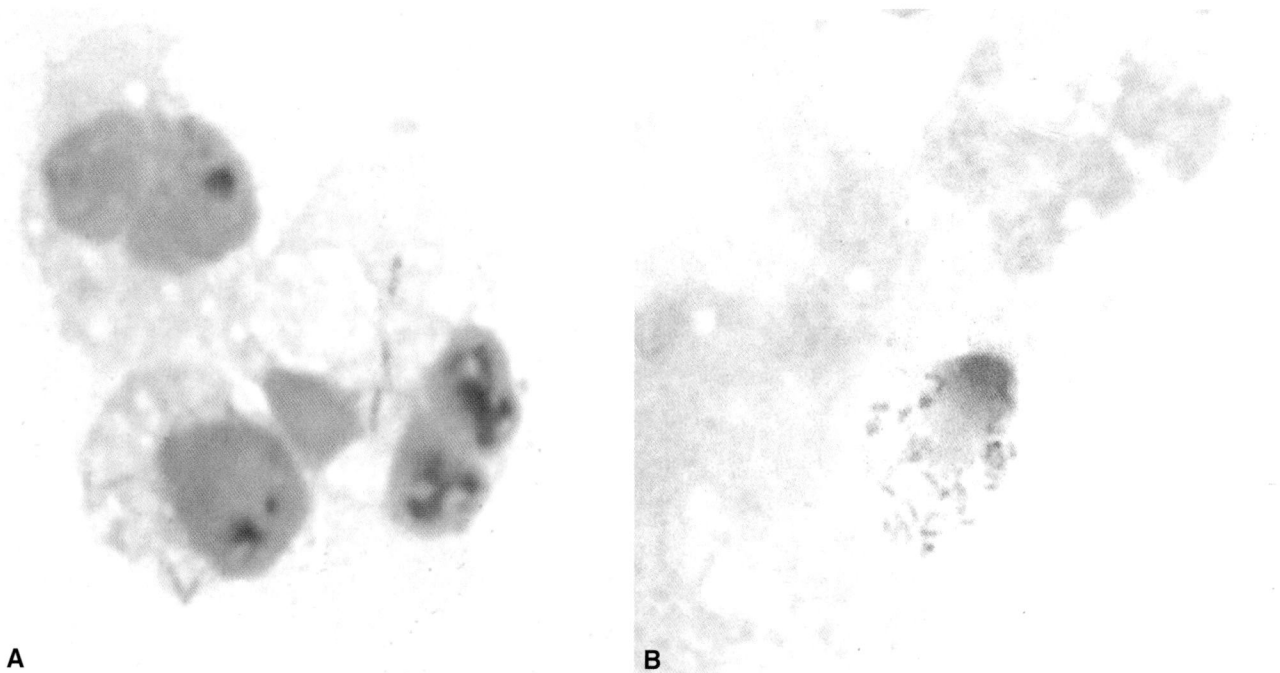

A

B

Figure 6-43. **A,** Fusiform bacteria (*Fusobacterium* organisms) in cytoplasm of neutrophil in fine-needle aspirate (Gram stain). **B,** Coccobacilli (*Haemophilus influenzae*) in cytoplasm of leukocyte in fine-needle aspirate (Gram stain).

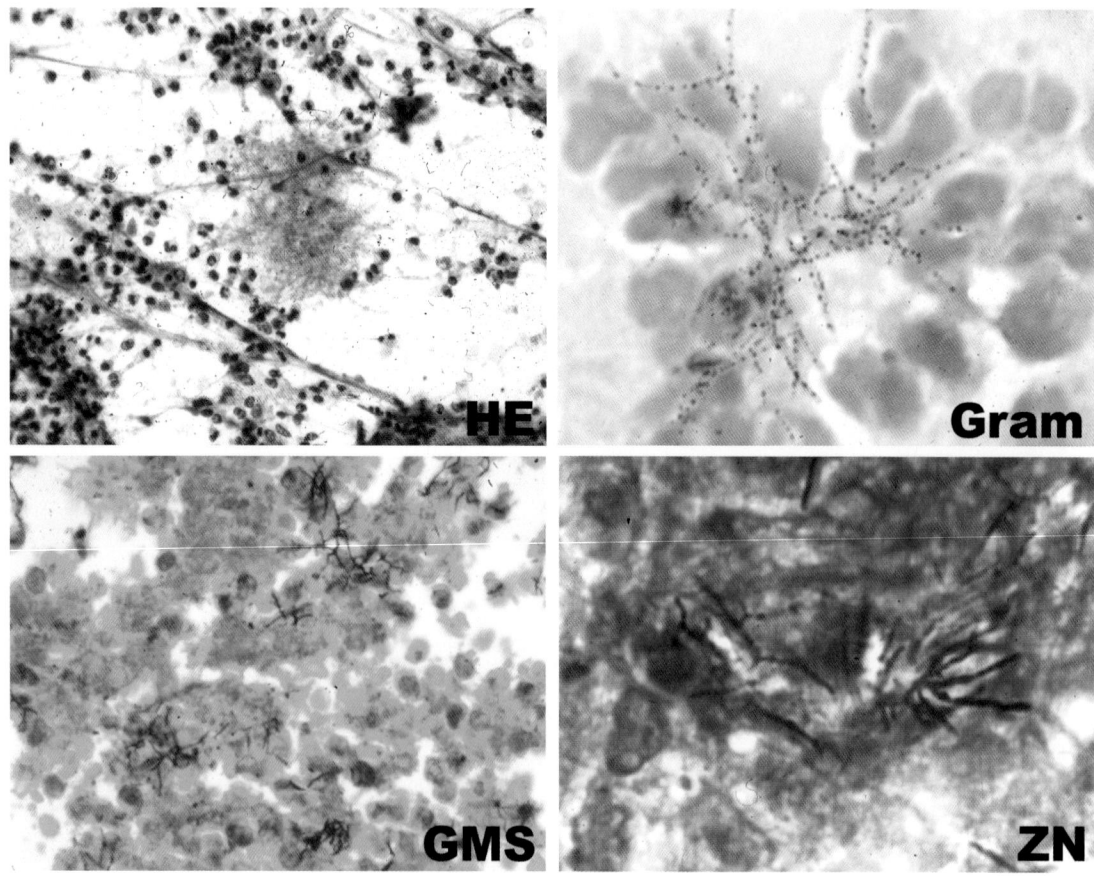

Figure 6-44. Nocardia. Loose, feathery cluster of bacilli in purulent exudate seen in a fine-needle aspirate: alcohol-fixed, H&E stain; Gram stain; Grocott methenamine silver stain; Ziehl-Neelsen stain.

by being partially acid-fast.[104,105] Extreme care must be exercised in the staining laboratory to prevent contamination of staining solutions, because this can be a cause of false-positive results.

Although most aspirated cavitary lung lesions with the abscess pattern are the result of bacterial infection, considerations in the differential diagnosis include necrotic neoplasm (particularly squamous cell carcinoma), Wegener granulomatosis, and nonbacterial infections associated with suppurative granulomas such as those due to fungi and mycobacteria.

Microbiology

Microbiology techniques in current use for the laboratory diagnosis of bacterial pneumonia are summarized in Box 6-7.[106-108] The traditional morphologic and functional approach to microbiologic diagnosis is gradually shifting to molecular methods, but their routine application continues to be a hope for the near future.

The workup of respiratory secretions, such as sputum, in the microbiology laboratory may or may not be indicated, based on the clinical and immunologic status of the patient. Certainly, the value of this workup for community-acquired pneumonias has been questioned for some time, and the guidelines from two specialty societies—the American Thoracic Society and the Infectious Disease Society of America—differ in this regard.[109-111] Nevertheless, when a carefully collected specimen reveals one or two predominant bacterial morphotypes on a well-prepared Gram stain (Fig. 6-45), especially in the presence of neutrophils and few or no squamous cells, a presumptive diagnosis can be offered and correlated with whatever grows on culture plates.[112,113] A mixed bacterial population usually is considered nondiagnostic, especially in the absence of inflammation or the presence of many benign oral squamous cells. By contrast, pneumonia in the hospitalized or immunocompromised patient requires an aggressive strategy to collect a good sputum sample for Gram stain and culture. If this attempt is unsatisfactory or the findings are nondiagnostic, then use of invasive techniques beginning with fiberoptic bronchocopy and BAL with protected catheters should be considered.[56,58,114] Anaerobic pulmonary infections, typically in the form of a lung abscess, also can be approached in this way or with transthoracic needle aspiration.[75]

Gram staining of tissue sections from bronchoscopic or surgical biopsy specimens is notoriously insensitive and nonspecific. As with sputum, the presence of a predominant bacterial morphotype in a distinctive necroinflammatory background carries diagnostic weight, especially when correlated with available clinical and laboratory data. Because histology laboratories do not generally observe the same level of caution in reagent preparation and storage as microbiology laboratoriess, it is worth remembering that tissue sections are prone to false-positive results from in vitro contamination.

In those cases in which bacteria are visible on H&E-stained sections, the Gram stain is especially helpful in confirming a presumptive etiology. For example, pairs and chains of gram-positive cocci in a necroinflammatory background suggest a streptococcal pneumonia, whereas numerous slender gram-negative bacilli investing and infiltrating blood vessels are characteristic of a *Pseudomonas* pneumonia (Fig. 6-46). Other types of gram-negative pneumonias (Fig. 6-47) also

Box 6-7. Laboratory Diagnosis of Bacterial Pneumonia

Direct detection of organisms
  Gram stain; other stains of respiratory secretions and fluids
  Direct fluorescent antibody stain
  Histopathologic/cytopathologic examination
  Immunohistochemistry
Antigen detection (with *Legionella pneumophila* [LP1] and *Streptococcus pneumoniae*)
Culture
  Conventional media for usual pyogenic bacteria
  Special media for fastidious or atypical agents
Serologic testing
Molecular methods
  In situ hybridization
  DNA amplification

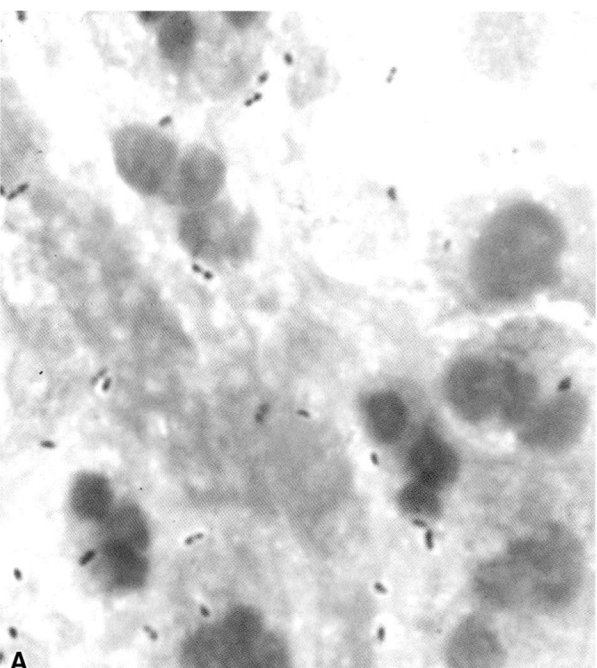 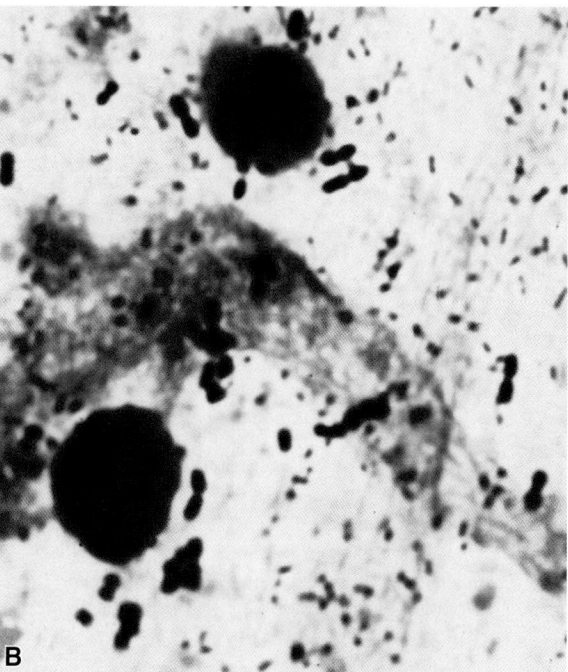

Figure 6-45. Sputum Gram stain. **A,** Gram-positive diplococci (*Streptococcus pneumoniae*) with neutrophils, but no squamous cells. **B,** Gram-positive diplococci (*S. pneumoniae*) and gram-negative coccobacilli (*Haemophilus influenzae*).

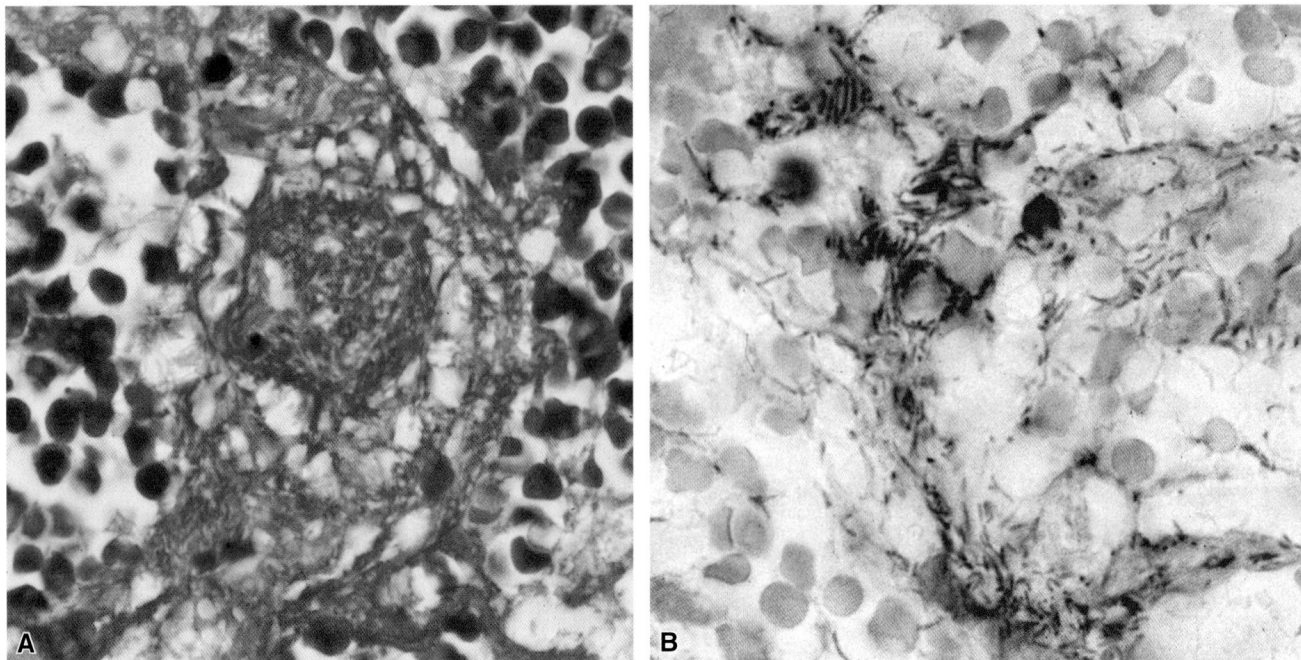

Figure 6-46. **A,** *Pseudomonas aeruginosa* bacilli investing interstitial vessels (Brown-Hopps stain). **B,** The slender gram-negative bacilli are nicely demonstrated on Gram stain.

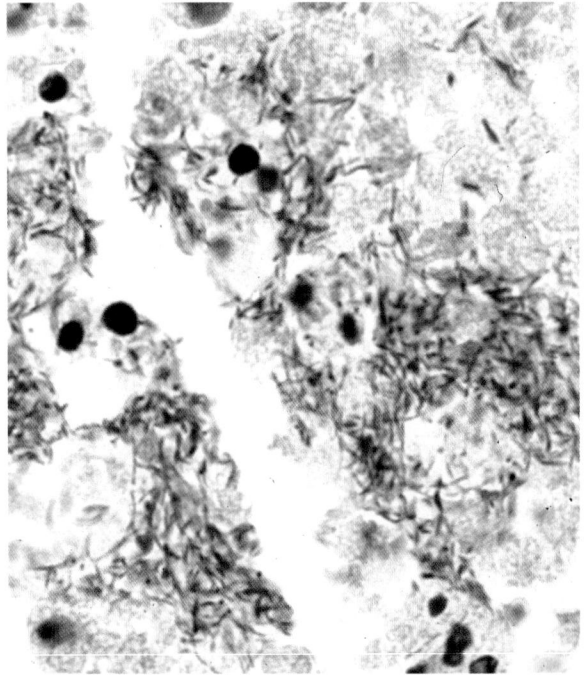

Figure 6-47. *Burkholderia cepacia* bacilli (Brown and Hopps stain).

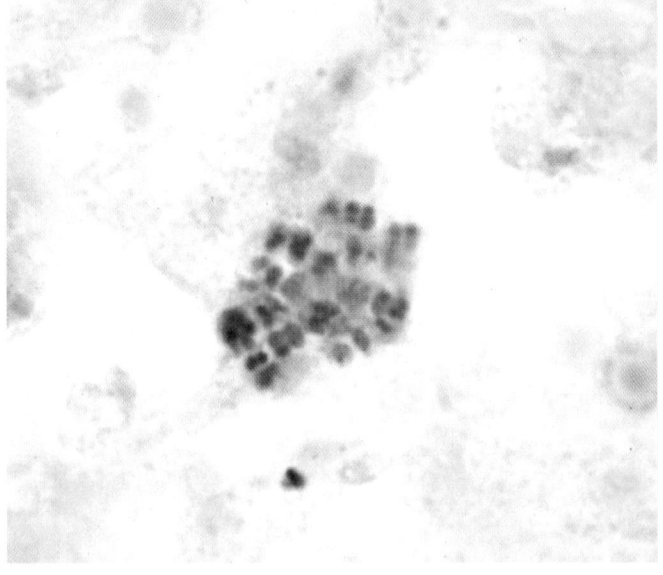

Figure 6-48. Bacterial tetrads in alveolar exudate (Giemsa stain).

can be confirmed with well-prepared Gram stains.[77] In the case of an abscess, a mixture of gram-positive cocci and gram-negative bacilli in tissue (illustrated earlier in Fig. 6-28) is a useful finding that is helpful in supporting a diagnosis of an anaerobic infection.

When organisms are sparse, other stains such as Giemsa or silver impregnation may highlight the organisms in the exudates (Fig. 6-48). The Gram stain also is useful for evaluating infections with granules and allows differentiation of the agents of botryomycosis (the gram-positive cocci or gram-negative bacilli) from the filamentous *Actinomyces* organisms (Fig. 6-49).

Staining with methenamine silver is the best procedure for detecting *Nocardia* organisms. The modified Ziehl-Neelsen stain allows for differentiation of *Nocardia* (positive) from the anaerobic *Actinomyces* (negative).[105]

Commercially available immunohistochemical reagents exist for relatively few bacterial species. Immunohistochemistry testing for the potential bioterrorist agents discussed in this chapter is available through the Centers for Disease Control and Prevention (CDC) in Atlanta, Georgia. It is expected that commercial reagents will become increasingly available for the common etiologic agents in the near future.[32]

Culture media that will allow recovery of common bacterial species causing pneumonia from various types of respiratory samples

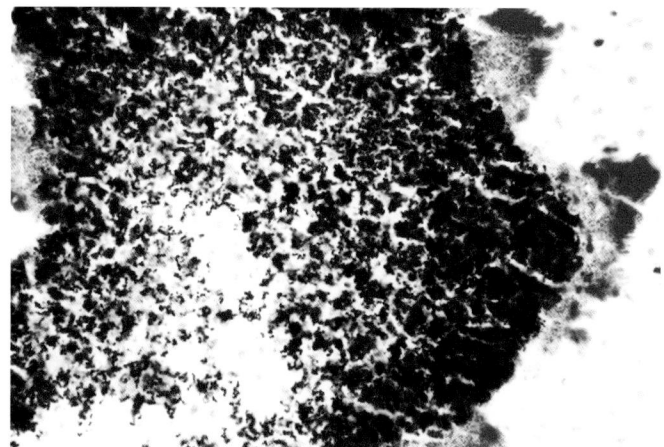

Figure 6-49. Botryomycosis. Cluster of gram-positive cocci (*Staphylococcus aureus*) invested by gram-negative–staining Splendore-Hoeppli material (Brown-Brenn stain). (Courtesy of Dr. Francis Chandler, Augusta, GA.)

(secretions, washings, brushings, aspirates, and tissues) include sheep blood agar, chocolate agar, and McConkey agar. These media also will support growth of *B. anthracis* and *Y. pestis*. Buffered charcoal yeast extract (BCYE) agar is the primary medium for *Legionella* species. Because *Legionella* organisms survive poorly in respiratory secretions, rapid transport and immediate plating is essential for recovery. BYE also is a good "all-purpose" medium for growing other fastidious species including *F. tularensis*. However, *F. tularensis* grows best in cysteine-enriched media.[115]

In addition to respiratory samples, blood can be otained for cultures in patients sick enough to suspect bacteremias and pleural fluid culture can be used when effusions are present. Positive cultures of these normally sterile fluids circumvent the interpretive problems associated with bacterial growth in sputum samples.

The actinomycetes are best isolated from invasive specimens such as needle aspirates and transbronchial and lung biopsy specimens. The laboratory should be alerted to search for these agents because special consideration must be given to culture setup and incubation conditions.[85] The actinomycetes responsible for actinomycosis require anaerobic media and atmosphere as well as prolonged incubation. *Nocardia*, an aerobic actinomycete, grows well on most nonselective media but requires extended incubation. Determination of colonial morphology, Gram and acid-fast stains, and a few biochemical tests generally suffice to identify these organisms at the genus level. However, genotype rather than phenotype characteristics are required to identify newly emergent species.[116]

In general, the laboratory diagnosis of pneumonia caused by most of the atypical agents is difficult because systems are not routinely available or are costly, cumbersome, or unsafe. For the atypical agents (*Mycoplasma*, *Chlamydia*, and *Coxiella* species), serologic testing has been the method of choice for diagnosis.[63,117] Classic cold agglutinin and complement fixation tests for these agents have largely been replaced by enzyme immunoassay and microimmunofluorescence testing.[83,118,119] Serologic methods also are useful for diagnosis of tularemia because of the difficulty in culturing the fastidious bacterium.

Legionella pneumonia is a common form of severe pneumonia not readily diagnosed for a number of reasons, including the organism's fastidiousness.[120] In the microbiology laboratory, the direct fluorescent antibody test and culture on buffered BCYE agar have been the mainstays of diagnosis. Culture is considered the diagnostic gold standard but is only 60% sensitive. Serologic testing is available for most of the *L. pneumophila* serotypes, which account for 90% of the pneumonia cases; however, the need to collect paired sera weeks apart limits

its usefulness in the acutely ill patient. Antigen detection in urine has become commercially available for both *L. pnemophila* and *S. pneumoniae*, and because the need to collect acute and convalesent sera is obviated, it has become a frequently used diagnostic test.[120,121] Its advantage lies in its potential to effect early treatment decisions through rapid diagnosis. Its disadvantage lies in the fact that it identifies only patients infected with *L. pneumophila* serogroup 1 (LP1), the most prevalent species and serotype, but none of the non-LP1 serotypes, or cases due to other *Legionella* species.[122–124]

The use of molecular diagnostic tools (in situ hybridization and nucleic acid amplification by PCR or other methods) to detect these agents has been reported.[81,124,125] Real-time PCR assay appears promising as a sensitive, specific, and rapid diagnostic technique that is likely to find routine clinical application. It provides a platform for the simultaneous amplification and detection of target DNA in a single tube through use of one of several types of fluorescence resonance transfer (FRET) fluorescent probe quencher techniques or melting curve analysis. Furthermore, it obviates the concern for amplicon contamination in the laboratory.[126] The development of a multiplex assay, to detect multiple agents in a single reaction, would seem to be an ideal pursuit for the laboratory diagnosis of the most common community-acquired pneumonias including those due to the atypical pneumonia agents.[35,127,128]

Differential Diagnosis

The key morphologic and microbiologic features of the bacterial pneumonias are summarized in Table 6-5. The presence of purulent exudates or significant numbers of neutrophils in biopsy or cytologic samples should always trigger a search for bacterial infection. Of note, however, because lung biopsies usually are performed late in the clinical course with respect to an evolving infiltrate, after many procedures have been performed and bacterial infections have been excluded or treated with antibiotics, neutrophilic exudates may not signify bacterial infection unless accompanied by necrosis, as in an abscess. Instead, consideration should be given to one of several noninfectious acute inflammatory diseases, with an immunologic basis, that can mimic bacterial infection. Some of these include Wegener granulomatosis, Goodpasture syndrome, systemic lupus erythematosus, and microscopic polyangiitis, all conditions that can produce acute inflammation predominantly involving alveolar septal blood vessels ("capillaritis"). On occasion, capillaritis can result in air space accumulation of neutrophils, further raising concern for bronchopneumonia. Centrally necrotic or cavitary neoplasms of various types may mimic abscesses grossly and microscopically, and exceptionally well-differentiated adenocarcinomas containing glands filled with detritus may mimic inflammatory and bacterial diseases. Suppurative granulomas can have a bacterial, mycobacterial, or fungal etiology. Even the miliary necroinflammatory lesion typical of bacterial infection can be produced by viruses, some fungi, and even protozoa (e.g., *Toxoplasma gondii*).

Mycobacterial Infections

The surgical pathologist tends to encounter mycobacterial infections in lung biopsies when standard clinical diagnostic approaches to pulmonary infiltrates are unsuccessful and the lesions persist or progress. Tuberculosis is but one of several different types of lung infection that can manifest clinically as community-acquired pneumonia, resulting in delay until an invasive procedure such as transbronchial biopsy, transthoracic needle biopsy, or surgical lung biopsy is performed, often a "last resort" effort.[129,130] In recent years, delays in diagnosis of mycobacterial infection have markedly decreased, thanks in part to recommendations from the CDC for improving laboratory turnaround time and to the response of the diagnostics industry with

Table 6-5. Bacterial Pneumonias: Summary of Pathologic Findings

Assessment Component	Findings
Pyogenic Bacteria	
Surgical pathology	Acute purulent inflammation with/without necrosis; organization; diffuse alveolar damage may be present
Cytopathology	Acute inflammation with/without visible bacteria on Diff-Quik–stained smear
Microbiology	Gram stain reactivity and morphology (visual detection requires heavy bacterial burden: 10^6 organisms/gram of tissue)
	Culture-sterile lung tissue on standard nonselective and selective media (blood, chocolate, MacConkey agars); anaerobic broth and agars for abscesses
	Urinary antigen for *Streptococcus pneumoniae*
Atypical Pneumonia Agents	
Surgical pathology	*Legionella* pneumonia: fibrinopurulent with bacilli visible in silver-stained (Dieterle; Warthin-Starry) sections
	DAD often present
	Chlamydia and *Mycoplasma* infection: polymorphous bronchiolar and interstitial infiltrate
Cytopathology	Acute inflammation with bacilli stained with silver or by immunofluorescence (*Legionella* pneumonia)
Microbiology	DFA for *L. pneumophila* serotypes
	Culture on selective (BCYE) agar for *Legionella*; urinary antigen for *Legionella*
	Serologic testing and/or PCR assay for *Mycoplasma* and *Chlamydia*
Filamentous-Granule Group	
Surgical pathology	Granules or loose filamentous aggregates in purulent exudate with abscess formation and poorly formed granuloma in some cases
Cytopathology	Filamentous tangles or aggregates or granules with neutrophils and/or necroinflammatory background
Microbiology	Gram-positive branching filaments: *Nocardia* (aerobic actinomycete) and *Actinomyces* (anaerobic actinomycete)
	Nocardia partially acid-fast and GMS-positive
	Gram-positive cocci or gram-negative bacilli (botryomycosis)
	Culture on standard nonselective media and selective (BCYE) media; anaerobic culture broths and media for *Actinomyces*

BCYE, buffered charcoal yeast extract; DAD, diffuse alveolar damage; DFA, direct fluorescence assay; GMS, Grocott methenamine silver.

better methods and technology. In fact, however, because direct acid-fast bacillary smears of respiratory specimens yield negative findings in at least one half of the cases,[131] and because many mycobacterial species are fastidious and slow-growing, the biopsy results may be the first suggestion of a mycobacterial infection. The biopsy findings also can define the organism's relationship to a histopathologic lesion, or host response. This is important in evaluating the significance of a culture result, because although an isolate of *M. tuberculosis* is always taken seriously, obtaining a single isolate of a nontuberculous mycobacterium from the respiratory tract does not necessarily implicate the organism as the cause of disease.[132]

Etiologic Agents

The mycobacterial species can be categorized in two clinically relevant groups: *Mycobacterium tuberculosis* complex (MTC) and the nontuberculous mycobacteria (NTM). MTC includes the subspecies *M. tuberculosis*, *Mycobacterium bovis*, *Mycobacterium africanum*, and *Mycobacterium microti*. The latter three species produce tuberculosis in some areas of the world, but in the United States the prevalence of such disease is very low.

Mycobacterium tuberculosis

M. tuberculosis is the most virulent mycobacterial species and an unequivocal pathogen that is responsible for more deaths worldwide than any single microbe. This organism is the etiologic agent of tuberculosis worldwide in its various forms, which are listed in Box 6-8.

Box 6-8. Classification of Tuberculosis

Primary tuberculosis
    Exogenous first infection
    Exogenous reinfection
Progressive primary tuberculosis
Post-primary tuberculosis
    Endogenous reactivation
    Exogenous infection in BCG-vaccinated persons
    Exogenous superinfection

BCG, bacille Calmette-Guérin.
Data from Allen E. Tuberculosis and other mycobacterial infections of the lung. In: Churg AM, Thurlbeck WM, eds. *Pathology of the Lung,* 2nd ed. New York: Thieme; 1995:233, Table 13-1.

Primary tuberculosis occurs in patients without previous exposure or loss of acquired immunity. Progressive primary tuberculosis occurs in patients with inadequate acquired immunity, that is, impaired cellular immunity. Post-primary tuberculosis, also referred to as secondary or reinfection-reactivation tuberculosis, occurs in patients with previous immunity to the organism and accounts for most clinical cases of tuberculosis.[133,134] Many clinical experts consider that most cases of active tuberculosis in adults with normal immunity arise from reactivation of latent infection (post-primary tuberculosis), whereas reinfection with a new strain derived from the environment (primary or post-primary tuberculosis) can occur in the immunocompromised patient. More recently, DNA fingerprinting methods (genotyping) have challenged this dogma, however, by showing that exogenous reinfection accounts for a significant percentage of cases in some areas of the world.[135] Miliary tuberculosis and extrapulmonary disease can occur with any of these forms.[133,136]

Primary tuberculosis usually is a mild illness that often is not clinically recognized. Of note, however, the bacillemia that occurs during its development can seed extrapulmonary organs and set the stage for subsequent reactivation. Approximately 5% of patients pass through latency to post-primary disease within 2 years of primary infection, and another 5% do so later in their lives.[137]

Non-Tuberculous Mycobacteria

Recognized NTM species number more than 125, many of which were identified during the past decade.[138,139] However, relatively few cause pulmonary disease.[132,140-142] These organisms are acquired from the environment, where they are ubiquitous. In contrast with *M. tuberculosis*, the NTM are not spread from person to person. In most instances, patients in whom NTM infection develops have chronic lung disease and other risk factors, such as AIDS, alcoholism, or diabetes. Reports of NTM infections in non-immunocompromised patients are increasing.[17,143] MAC and then *Mycobacterium kansasii* are the most frequent isolates in all settings. Among a growing number of species causing lung disease are *Mycobacterium abscessus*, *Mycobacterium fortuitum*, *Mycobacterium szulgai*, *Mycobacterium simiae*, *Mycobacterium xenopi*, *Mycobacterium malmoense*, *Mycobacterium celatum*, *Mycobacterium asiaticum*, and *Mycobacterium shimodii*. These latter species manifest marked geographic variability with respect to prevalence and severity. Of note, however, since 1985, more MAC isolates than *M. tuberculosis* have been reported in the United States.[132]

Histopathology

The histopathologic patterns produced by mycobacteria are listed in Box 6-9. The radiologic, gross, and microscopic patterns of mycobacterial disease reflect the virulence of the various mycobacterial species, as well as the patient's prior exposure and immune status.[144-146]

Primary Tuberculosis

Mycobacterium tuberculosis occurs typically in the best-aerated lung regions (anterior segments of the upper lobes, lingua and middle lobe, or basal segments of lower lobes.[145] The disease passes through progressive

Box 6-9. Histopathologic Patterns in Mycobacterial Lung Injury

Large nodules with or without cavities
   Well-formed granuloma
   Poorly formed granuloma
   Suppurative granuloma
   Histiocytic aggregates
Miliary nodules
Calcified nodules
Granulomatous interstitial pneumonitis
Bronchitis/bronchiectasis
Spindle cell pseudotumors

phases of exudation, recruitment of macrophages and T lymphocytes, and granuloma formation followed by repair with granulation tissue, fibrosis, and mineralization.[134,147] Macrophage-laden bacilli also travel to the hilar lymph nodes, where the phases are repeated. This combination of events produces the classic Ghon complex, consisting of a peripheral 1- to 2-cm lung nodule (Fig. 6-50) and an enlarged, sometimes calcified hilar lymph node. In both locations, the histopathologic hallmark is a necrotizing granuloma (Fig. 6-51) composed of epithelioid

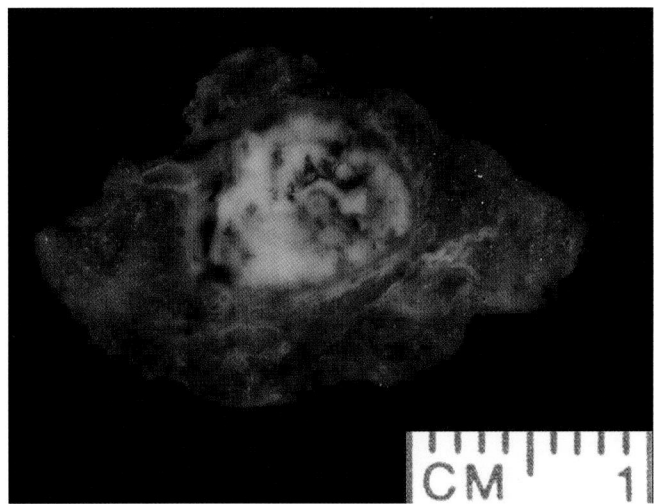

Figure 6-50. Tuberculoma removed from right upper lobe.

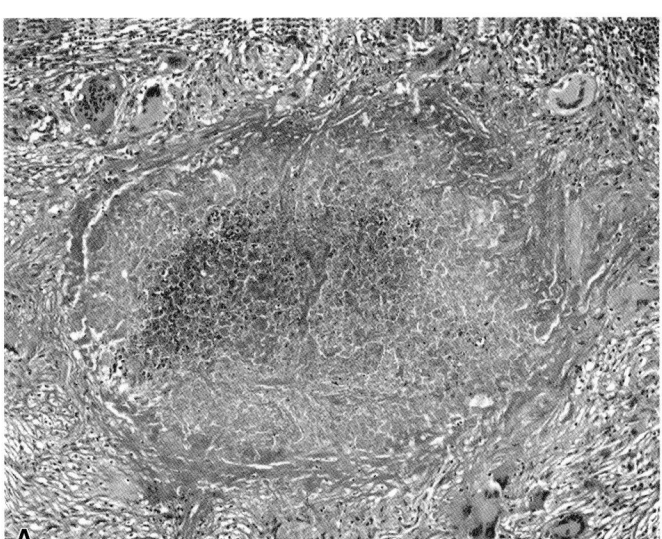

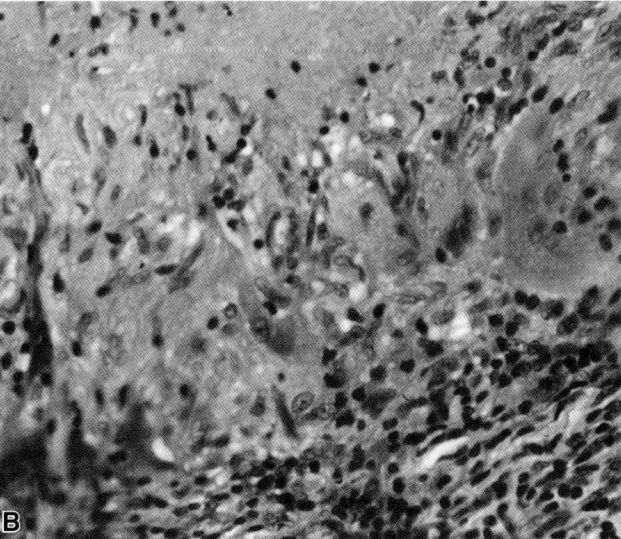

Figure 6-51. A, Tuberculoid granuloma with central zone of caseation necrosis surrounded by epithelioid cells, giant cells, and outer investment of lymphocytes. **B,** Palisade of epithelioid histiocytes in giant cells at edge of necrotic zone.

cells with variable numbers of Langhans giant cells, a peripheral invest-ment of lymphocytes, and a central zone of *caseation necrosis*, a form of necrosis attributed to apoptosis.[133,148] A spectrum of lesions may be seen, from the tuberculoid "hard" granuloma without necrosis and rare organisms, to the multibacillary necrotic lesion with scant epithelioid cells.[149] In a minority of patients the lesions enlarge and progress as a result of increased necrosis or liquifaction.

The complications of tuberculosis are listed in Box 6-10 and illus-trated in Figure 6-52. Other complications may include extension into blood vessels with miliary (Fig. 6-53) or systemic dissemination, lymphatic drainage into the pleura with granulomatous pleuritis and effusions, or to bronchi with bronchocentric granulomatous lesions (Fig. 6-54) or tuberculous bronchopneumonia. Granulomas also may encroach upon blood vessels, mimicking a "granulomatous" vasculitis. The hemophagocytic syndrome, which has been implicated in a vari-ety of bacterial, viral, and parasitic infections, also has been associated with tuberculosis.[150]

Post-primary Tuberculosis

Post-primary tuberculosis, the most common form in adults, typi-cally involves the apices of the upper lobes, producing granulomatous

Box 6-10. Complications of Tuberculosis

Miliary tuberculosis
Granulomatous pleuritis and effusions
Tuberculous bronchopneumonia
Extrapulmonary dissemination to:
    Meninges
    Kidney
    Bone
    Other

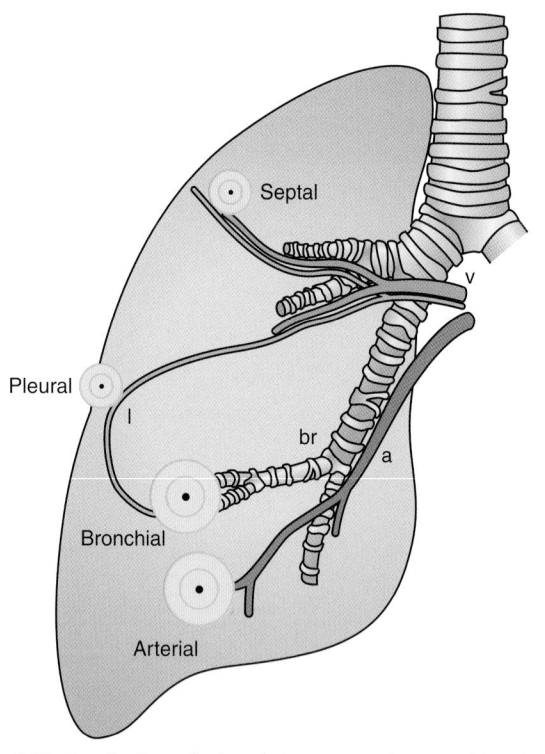

Figure 6-52. Complications of tuberculosis. Invasion of arteries (a) with miliary spread; bronchi (br) with tuberculous bronchopneumonia; lymphatics (l) with granu-lomatous pleuritis and effusions. Invasion of septal (s) veins (v) leads to extrapulmonary dissemination.

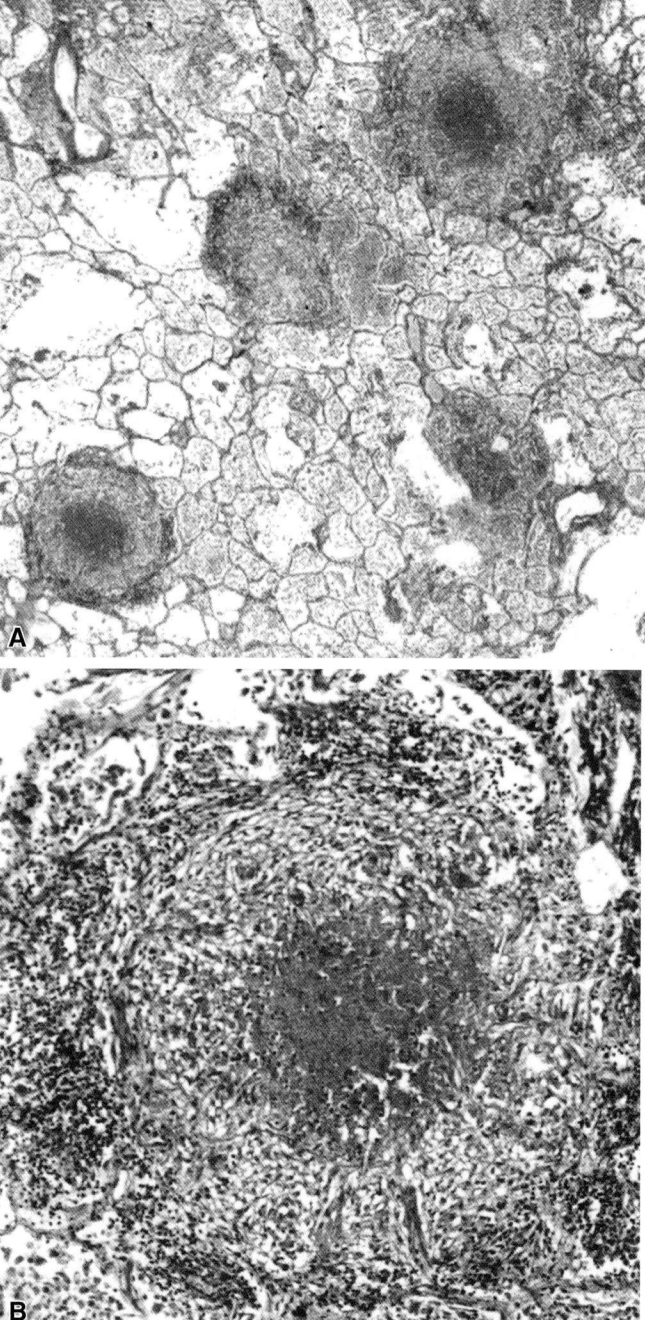

Figure 6-53. Miliary tuberculosis. **A,** Miliary pattern. **B,** Epithelioid granulomas with necrotic central zones.

lesions with greater caseation, often with cavities and variable degrees of fibrosis and retraction of the parenchyma.[136] Fibrosis and bron-chiectasis occurs with the healing of cavities and is the major cause of pulmonary disability in this disease.[151] Recent studies have proposed that post-primary disease begins as a form of lipoid pneumonia, with bacilli-laden foamy alvolar macrophages and bronchiolar obstruction progressing to cavitary disease, as a result of caseation, and micro-vascular occusion due to delayed-type hypersensitivity.[152] Extension to other lobes, hilar or mediastinal lymph nodes and miliary spread through the lungs and to extrapulmonary sites can complicate this form of disease. Other presentation patterns include acute and orga-nizing diffuse alveolar damage with advanced or miliary disease, acute

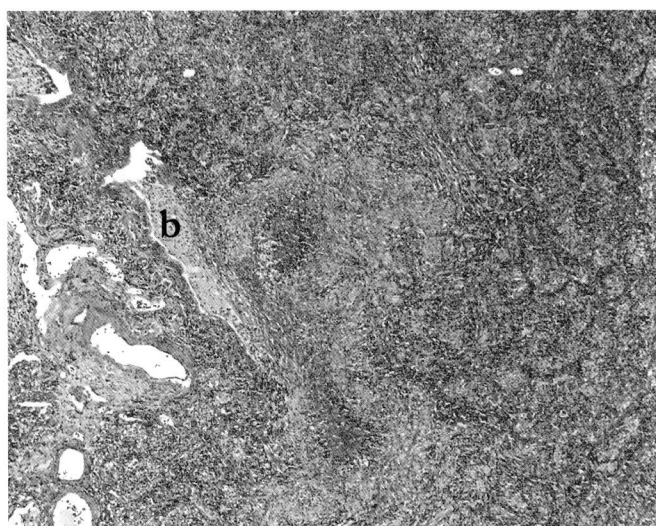

Figure 6-54. Bronchocentric granuloma in mycobacterial infection. Only a small focus of residual bronchial epithelium (b) remains.

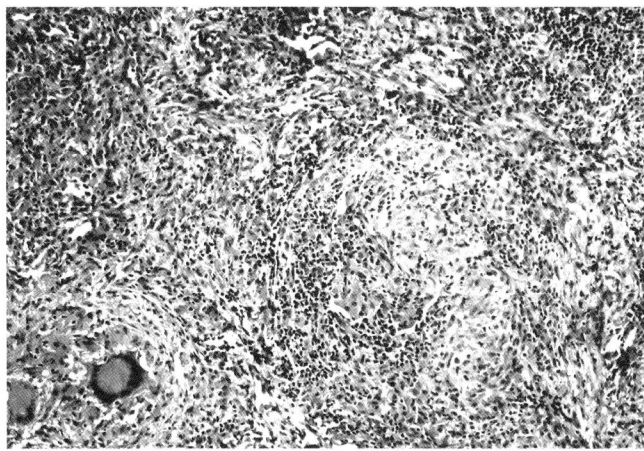

Figure 6-55. Non-necrotizing granuloma in infection due to *Mycobacterium avium* complex (MAC).

tuberculous bronchopneumonia, and the solitary pulmonary nodule (tuberculoma). A proximal endobronchial form may mimic a neoplasm and also is noteworthy for extensive necrosis and often large numbers of bacilli.[153] Because characteristic granulomatous morphology may not be visible around the necrotic material, stains for mycobacteria should be considered for all necrotic endobronchial samples.

Nontuberculous Mycobacterial Infections

NTM infections may be similar to those due to *M. tuberculosis*, but certain differences have been noted. For example, the NTM pathogens do not cause the same sequence of primary or post-primary disease, and systemic dissemination does not occur except in the immunocompromised patient. *M. kansasii* is more virulent than MAC, and the infection-associated histopathologic pattern is more like that produced by *M. tuberculosis*.[154]

Infections due to MAC and other common pulmonary NTM pathogens generally manifest as one of five clinicopathologic entities: solitary pulmonary nodule, chronic progressive pulmonary disease, disseminated disease, chronic bronchiolitis with bronchiectasis, and hypersensitivity-like pneumonitis.[134,155] Solitary pulmonary nodules generally exhibit granulomas resembling those caused by *M. tuberculosis*.

Chronic progressive disease also resembles tuberculosis, with upper lobe thin-walled cavities and granulomatous inflammation, with or without caseous necrosis (Fig. 6-55). Multiple confluent granulomas in fibrosis can mimic sarcoidosis. Organisms usually are sparse and more difficult to find in the immunocompetent patient. This presentation most often is seen in patients with underlying chronic lung disease such as COPD, bronchiectasis, cystic fibrosis, pneumoconiosis, reflux disease, or pre-existing cavitary lung disease of any cause (including old tuberculous cavities).

Disseminated disease typically is associated with the immunocompromise produced by HIV infection, in which the disease tends to target the gastrointestinal tract (the likely portal of entry), and pulmonary and reticuloendothelial disease signifies dissemination.[156] In this setting, NTM bacilli (predominantly MAC) proliferate characteristically to high levels in poorly formed granulomas, or in sheets and clusters of plump, finely vacuolated macrophages ("pseudo-Gaucher" cells) containing abundant phagocytosed intracytoplasmic bacilli (Fig. 6-56).

A distinctive form of NTM disease occurs as the "Lady Windermere syndrome." In the classic clinical scenario, an elderly, nonsmoking, immunocompetent woman of particular habits, demeanor, and body type presents with multiple pulmonary nodules, preferentially involving the middle lobe and lingula. The airway-centric granulomas and bronchiectasis can be subtle or pronounced (Fig. 6-57); this has

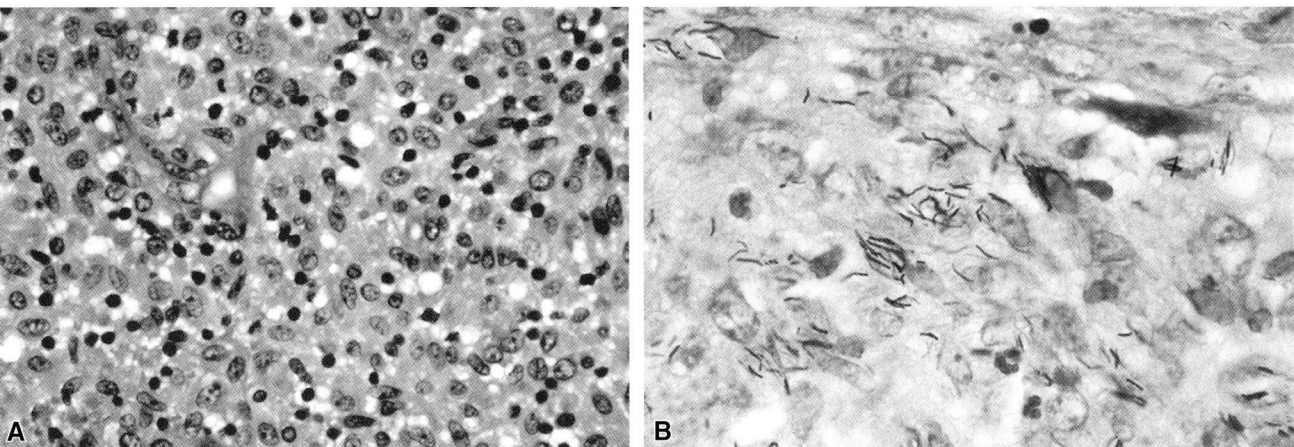

Figure 6-56. A, Clusters of macrophages in *Mycobacterium avium* complex (MAC) infection in a patient with AIDS. **B,** Myriad acid-fast bacilli (MAC) in histiocytic infiltrate (Ziehl-Neelsen stain).

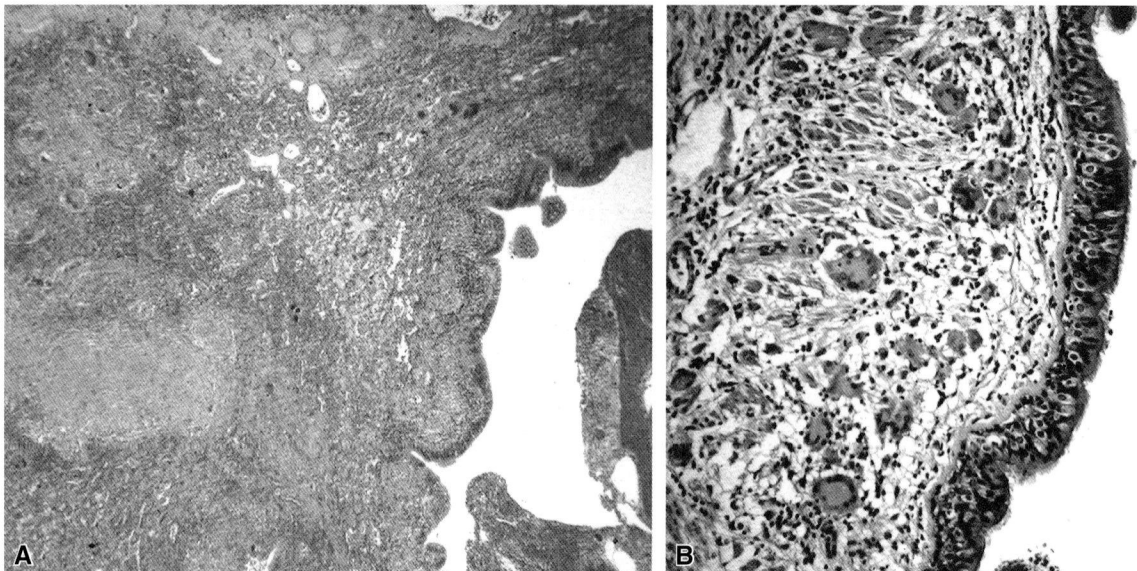

Figure 6-57. Middle lobe syndrome. **A,** Bronchiectasis with peribronchial granulomas containing *Mycobacterium avium* complex. **B,** Airway mucosa with granuloma.

been recognized as one of the patterns of middle lobe syndrome.[157] NTM bacilli also can colonize bronchiectatic lung from any cause, with resultant granulomatous inflammation predominantly affecting the airway walls—presumably a result of localized decreased mucociliary clearance.

Hypersensitivity-like pulmonary disease recently has been associated with contaminated water in hot tubs ("hot tub lung") and other environmental sources such as humidifiers and air conditioners.[17] Biopsy reveals a miliary bronchiolocentric and interstitial granulomatous pattern, similar to that produced by hypersensitivity pneumonitis (Fig. 6-58). A similar infection-colonization-hypersensitivity syndrome has been described in workers exposed to metal-working fluid aerosols.[158] The clinical, radiologic, and pathologic findings are similar to disease associated with hot tub use and other water sources except that a distinctive rapid-growing NTM species, *M. immunogenum*, has been recovered almost exclusively. Organisms are difficult to find in these cases but sometimes can be recovered in culture or with molecular techniques. Whether this entity represents an infection, a colonization, a hypersensitivity reaction, or a hybrid condition remains unresolved at this time.

A rare morphologic manifestation of mycobacterial infection is the so called "spindle cell inflammatory pseudotumor" (Fig. 6-59) which may occur in lung, skin, lymph nodes, and a number of other sites in immunocompromised patients.[159] The etiologic agents usually are NTM (MAC and *M. kansasii*), but *M. tuberculosis* has also been identified in some cases. Another uncommon variant is proximal endobronchial disease, discussed earlier in the spectrum of post-primary tuberculosis. Most cases are due to *M. avium* complex and manifest as polypoid lesions in immunocompromised HIV-infected patients, but this lesion also may be seen in immunocompetent persons.[160]

Certain species of rapidly growing mycobacteria (RGM) are capable of producing pulmonary disease, albeit infrequently.[132,161] Nevertheless, *M. abscessus* is the third most frequently recovered NTM respiratory pathogen in the United States, after *M. avium* complex and *M. kansasii*. It accounts for 80% of respiratory tract isolates, making it the leading rapidly growing mycobacterial species recovered from the lung. *M. abscessus* produces chronic lung infection that has a striking clinical and pathologic similarity to *M. avium* complex infection, including

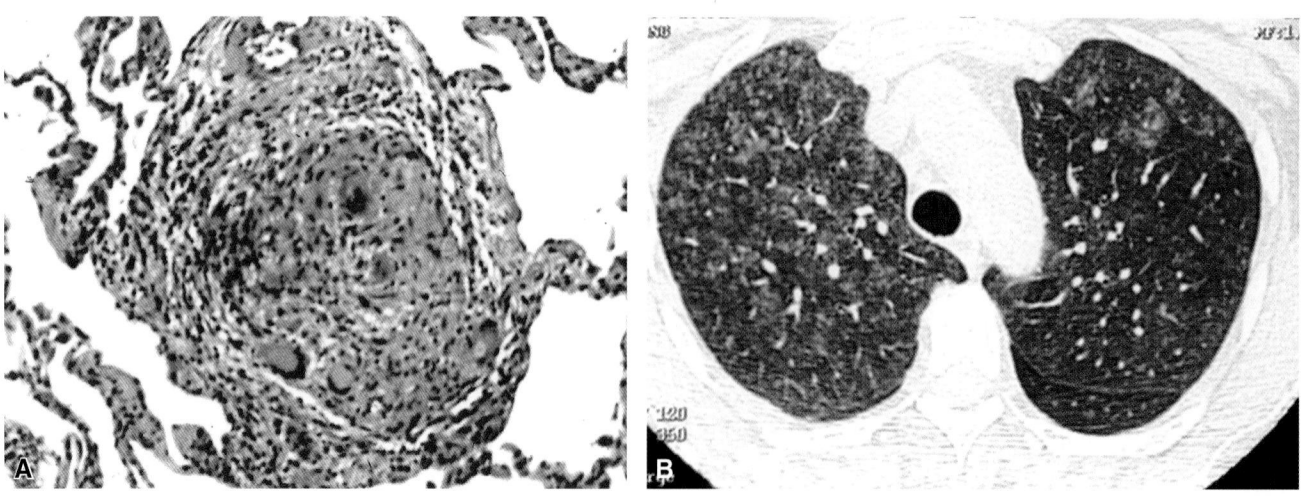

Figure 6-58. "Hot tub lung." **A,** Non-necrotizing granuloma. **B,** Computed tomographic image with features resembling those of hypersensitivity pneumonitis.

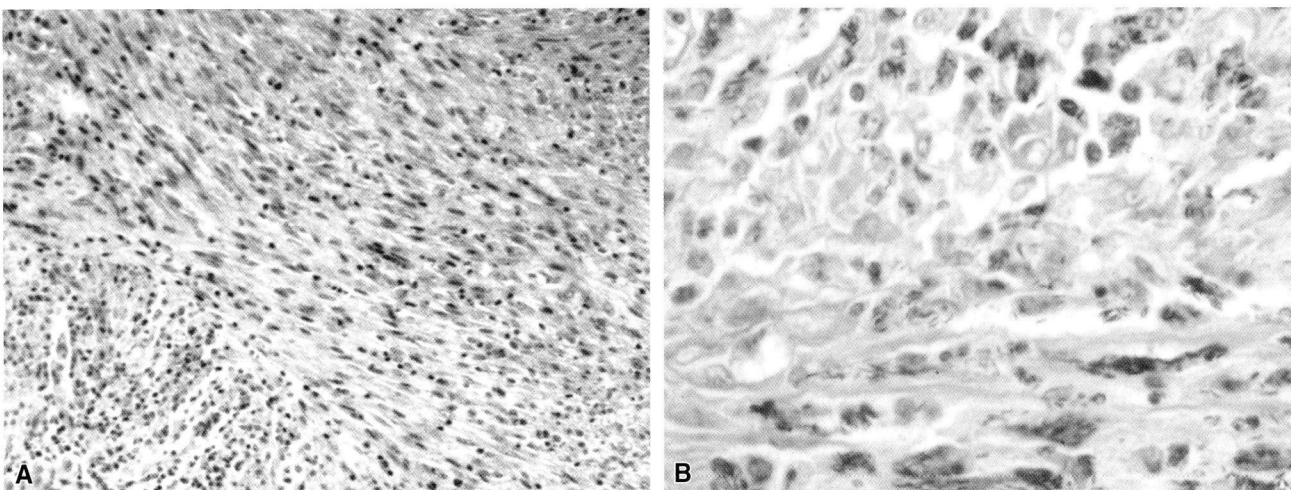

Figure 6-59. Spindle cell pseudotumor. **A,** The fascicles of fibroblasts with scattered lymphocytes. **B,** Myriad acid-fast bacilli (Ziehl-Neelsen stain).

the propensity to involve the lungs of patients with bronchiectasis. The RGM also have been thought to colonize lipoid pneumonia[162]; however, it is more likely that the pathogenesis of the lung injury pattern caused by the RGM is similar to that seen in skin and soft tissue cases, in which various combinations of suppurative foci, poorly formed or necrotizing granulomas, scattered multinucleated giant cells, and vacuoles are typical (termed "pseudocysts").[163] These combined features may mimic lipoid pneumonia and constitute an important clue to the presence of RGM infection.

Cytopathology

Fine-needle aspiration biopsy has been successfully used to diagnose both tuberculous pulmonary lesions and nontuberculous mycobacterial infections.[164] The finding of finely granular amorphous necrotic debris associated with aggregates of epithelioid histiocytes (with or without multinucleate giant cells) (Fig. 6-60) is suggestive of a mycobacterial or fungal infection.[165] In this setting, necrotic cancers must be excluded by a thorough search for atypical cells.

Special stains for acid-fast bacilli can be applied to aspirate smears, but culture of the aspirate is more likely to yield the etiologic agent when bacilli are sparse. Also, culture is still necessary for species identification and, if necessary, antimicrobial susceptibility testing. Epithelioid granulomas manifest a similar cellular pattern, but the granular necrotic debris is absent. Another pattern that may be seen, particularly in specimens from the immunocompromised patient, is a pure histiocytic or macrophage reaction with few or no epithelioid or multinucleate giant cells or necrotic debris. Numerous bacilli may be present in the distended cytoplasm of histiocytes and in the extracellular background. In air-dried (Diff-Quik) and alcohol-fixed (H&E- or Papanicolau-stained) smears, the bacilli may be recognized as negative images (Fig. 6-61).

Microbiology

The traditional as well as newer molecular approaches to the laboratory diagnosis of mycobacterial lung infection are outlined in Box 6-11. The mycobacterium is a slender but slightly curved bacillus, 4 μm in length, often with a beaded appearance; the length, curvature, and beadedness

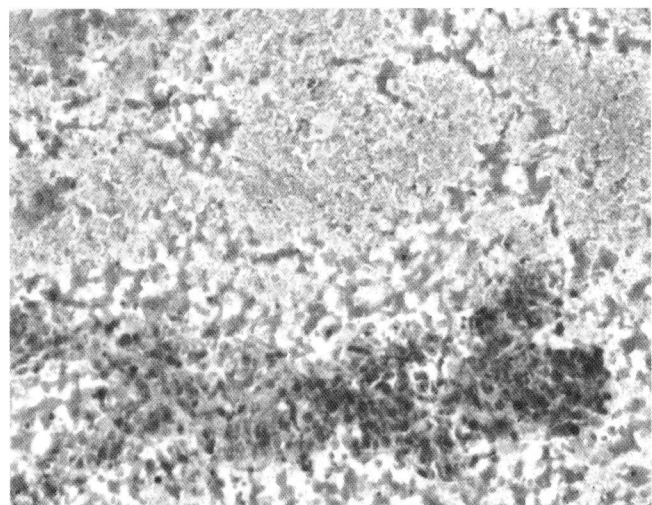

Figure 6-60. Necrotizing granuloma in *Mycobacterium kansasii* infection. Sheets of epithelioid cells in a background of granular necroinflammatory debris are evident in this fine-needle aspirate (Diff-Quik preparation).

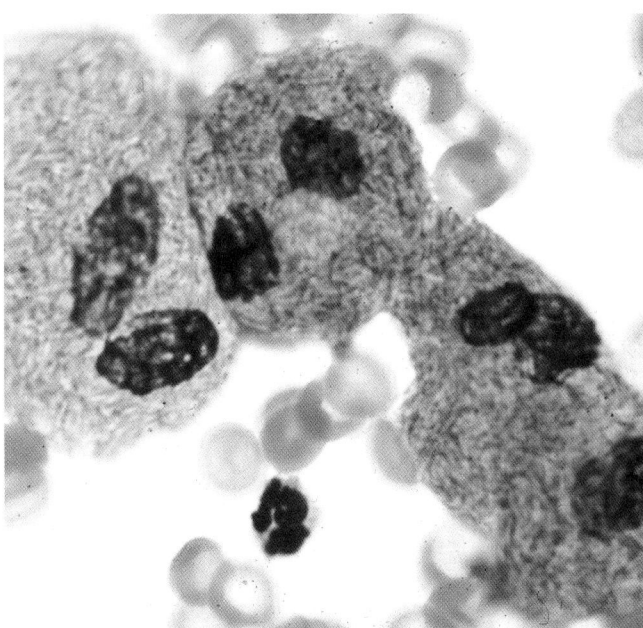

Figure 6-61. Pseudo-Gaucher histiocytes filled with myriad mycobacteria are seen as negative images in this fine-needle aspirate (Diff-Quik preparation).

Box 6-11. Laboratory Diagnosis of Mycobacterial Lung Infection

Direct detection of organisms
  Ziehl-Neelsen; Kinyon acid-fast stains
  Auramine O fluorescent stain
  Histopathologic/cytopathologic examination
  Immunohistochemical studies
Culture
  Conventional solid and broth media
  Radiometric liquid media system
  Nonradiometric (fluorescent; colorimetric) liquid media systems
Molecular methods
  In situ hybridization
  DNA amplification

sometimes are accentuated in *M. kansasii*.[166] In tissue sections or on smears, the Ziehl-Neelsen acid-fast stain or auramine-rhodamine fluorescent stains are most often recommended for best visualization. Organisms most often are found within the area of granulomatous reaction at the immediate periphery of the necrotic zone of the granulomas, or the cellular reactive process in the lining of cavities. Sections from several tissue blocks may be required to find organisms. Bacilli are rarely found in the absence of necrosis, except in smears from immunocompromised patients, in which they are visible and abundant within pseudo-Gaucher cells on H&E-stained sections, or as ghosted intracellular outlines with Giemsa-type stains. Dead bacilli lose their acid-fast character but sometimes may be identified with the GMS stain. The NTM, especially the RGM, may be more sensitive to acid alcohol decoloration and may not stain well or at all with the auramine-rhodamine method.[132] A commercial immunohistochemical reagent for mycobacteria is now available but is effective only in cases in which traditional acid-fast stains yield a positive result.[32] The differentiation of mycobacterial species in Ziehl-Neelsen–positive, formalin-fixed sections also has been achieved by in situ hybridization techniques with specific nucleic acid probes.[167–169] PCR amplification plus identification is likely to be the most sensitive technique in those cases in which the lesion is suspected to harbor mycobacteria but yields a negative result on acid-fast staining.[170] This technique may also be useful in cases in which the characteristic granulomatous pattern of inflammation is lacking, or mycobacteria have been identified in acid-fast–stained sections but culture results remain negative or cultures were not performed.[171,172]

Conventional wisdom states that culture is more sensitive than direct examination; however, the literature clearly documents cases in which acid-fast stains on tissue biopsies succeeded when cultures of tissue failed—an outcome that speaks to the virtue of perseverance in the face of compelling histopathologic findings.[173] Furthermore, tissue culture is prone to sampling error unless more than one site is sampled.[174] Specimens also may be smear positive and culture negative in patients whose disease has been treated. When only a rare bacillus is found, a strict criteria must be maintained and artifactual "pseudo" acid-fast bacilli excluded. As a general rule, a cutoff value of three organisms for a positive result seems prudent. False-positive smears also can result from contamination with local tap water, which may harbor mycobacteria.

Traditional solid media (Lowenstein-Jensen, Petragani, and Middlebrook agars) have given way to liquid media (radiometric and nonradiometric) as the first-line systems. Liquid media have demonstrated increased recovery of mycobacteria and decreased time to detection. They also facilitate rapid and accurate susceptibility testing.[131,175] Some of these liquid systems are manual with visual inspection, whereas others are fully automated and continuously monitored. Most laboratories back up liquid systems with conventional media, because no system, at this time, is capable of identifying all isolates. Commercially available DNA probes that hybridize to the mycobacterial RNA have largely replaced traditional biochemical testing, and these methods have significantly shortened the time to identification of *M. tuberculosis* and selected NTM.[176] For identification of the less frequently isolated species of NTM, for which probes are not available, it usually is necessary to send specimens to reference or state laboratories, where identification is accomplished by either biochemical testing, cell wall analysis using chromatographic techniques, or genotypic sequencing.[138]

The rapid differentiation of *M. tuberculosis* from NTM species is clinically very important, because the latter are much less infectious. In this context, molecular techniques have decreased the time to detection and identification of mycobacteria to less than three weeks in most instances. Direct nucleic acid amplification testing of clinical specimens using commercially available polymerase chain reaction (PCR) or transcription-mediated amplification (TMA) methods can reduce detection and identification times to less than 8 hours.[174] Immunochromatographic techniques based on the detection of secreted mycobacterial proteins have the potential to reduce these times even further.[177] Although NAA is faster, its overall accuracy is higher than that of smears but less than that of culture.[176] In fact, no single test at this time has sufficient sensitivity and specificity to stand alone, and use of a combination of available techniques, depending on the clinical and economic setting, may be the best overall strategy.[178,179]

Interpretation of a culture isolate can sometimes be difficult. The presence of *M. tuberculosis* is always significant. *M. kansasii* is an important pathogen, and its isolation usually is also significant, although it may represent colonization. The significance of other NTM isolates is variable, depending on whether there is clinical and radiologic evidence of disease. It is in this setting that histopathologic examination plays an important role. *M. avium* complex can be isolated from the respiratory tract of otherwise healthy adults, as well as HIV-infected patients with no clinical or radiologic evidence of disease. The American Thoracic Society has proposed diagnostic criteria requiring that certain clinical, radiologic, and laboratory parameters be met in order to prove pathogenicity.[132]

Differential Diagnosis

A synopsis of the key morphologic and microbiologic attributes of mycobacterial lung infections is presented in Table 6-6. Mycobacteria produce a wide spectrum of inflammatory patterns, both granulomatous and nongranulomatous. Although the potential differential diagnostic listing is long, in practical terms, major considerations are fungal infections, sarcoidosis, Wegener granulomatosis, and bacterial infections that produce suppurative granulomas, such as those due to *Nocardia*, *Actinomyces*, *Brucella*, and *Francisella* species. Generally, the use of special stains and cultures will resolve most diagnostic dilemmas. Wegener granulomatosis can usually be excluded based on the lack of the characteristic tinctorial properties of the necrosis in the granulomas, and absence of vasculitis or capillaritis. When necrosis is absent or sparse in a mycobacterial infection, sarcoidosis can be difficult to exclude. Radiologic evidence of bilateral hilar adenopathy and other systemic findings of sarcoidosis often resolve the issue.

Fungal Pneumonias

The pathologist examining tissue sections containing fungal forms is in a unique position to provide at least a provisional diagnosis at the group or genus level, and to make a judgment as to the significance of the organism in terms of its invasiveness or presence as a saprophobe or allergen. Indeed, often the most effective diagnostic strategy avail-

Table 6-6. Mycobacterial Pneumonias: Summary of Pathologic Findings

Assessment Component	Findings
Mycobacterium tuberculosis	
Surgical pathology	Necrotizing (tuberculoid) granulomas
Cytopathology	Epithelioid cells and necroinflammatory debris
	Acid-fast bacilli detected with Ziehl-Neelsen or auramine O stains of cell block sections, more sensitive than smears
Microbiology	Acid-fast bacilli detected with Ziehl-Neelsen; Kinyon stains or fluorescent bacilli with auramine O stain
	Culture on Lowenstein-Jensen and Middlebrook selective and nonselective agar and/or liquid media systems
	DNA probes or NAA for identification
Nontuberculous Mycobacteria (MOTT)	
Surgical pathology	Granulomas generally with less necrosis; often epithelioid only
	Unusual patterns, e.g., pseudo-Gaucher and spindle cell proliferation in immunocompromised patients
Cytopathology	Epithelioid cells; pseudo-Gaucher or spindle cells with little or no necrosis
	Negative images in Diff-Quik, confirmed as acid-fast bacilli with Ziehl-Neelsen
	Organisms sparse, except in immunocompromised patient
Microbiology	As for *Mycobacterium tuberculosis*

MOTT, mycobacteria other than *M. tuberculosis*; NAA, nucleic acid amplification.

Box 6-12. Common Fungal Pathogens in the Lung

Dimorphic fungi (mycelia at 25°C to 30°C; yeast at 37°C)
 Blastomyces dermatitidis
 Coccidioides immitis
 Histoplasma capsulatum
 Paracoccidioides braziliensis
 Sporothrix schenckii
 Penicillium marneffei
Yeasts
 Cryptococcus neoformans
 Candida spp.
Hyaline (non-pigmented) molds
 Aspergillus spp.
 Zygomycetes organisms
Phaeoid (pigmented; dematiaceous) molds
 Bipolaris spp., *Alternaria, Curvularia*
 Pseudoallescheria boydii/Scedosporium apiospermum
Miscellaneous pathogens
 Pneumocystis jiroveci

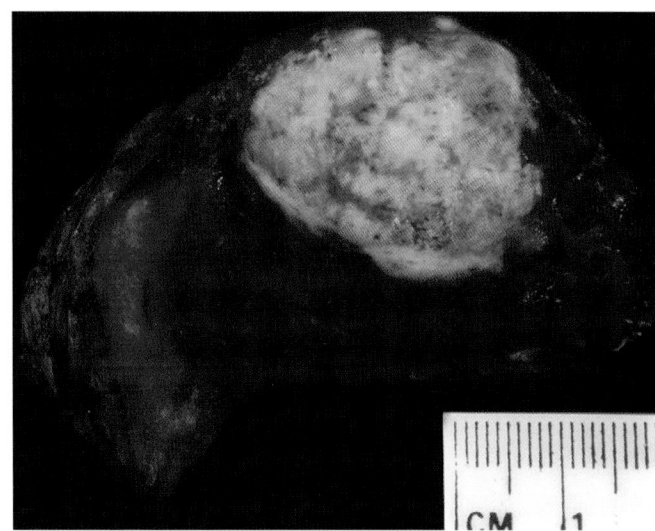

Figure 6-62. *Coccidioides* granuloma.

able is the rapid identification of fungi in tissue sections or cytologic samples.[43,180,181] This is especially important when opportunistic infection is being considered in the immunocompromised patient. However, optimal performance also requires knowing when the morphologic features of a fungal organism are insufficient to permit group or genus level diagnosis, and when integration of microbiologic data and histopathologic findings is required.

Etiologic Agents

Nearly 70,000 fungi are known, and approximately 100 have been recovered from respiratory infections.[182] Fortunately, only a small number are implicated as pathogenic on a consistent basis, and these are listed in Box 6-12.

Histopathology

Like mycobacterial species, fungal pathogens typically produce one or more nodular lesions in the normal host (Fig. 6-62) and these may become cavitary as the lesions evolve (Fig. 6-63). Inflammatory histopathologic patterns that suggest the presence of a fungal infection are summarized in Box 6-13. As is the case for other categories of etiologic agents, there are no absolutely characteristic or diagnostic patterns. Overlap is common and atypical reactions occur, ranging from overwhelming diffuse alveolar damage to little or no reaction in the immunocompromised patient. Proximal endobronchial disease mimicking neoplasm has also been described for various fungal species.[183] Detection of the etiologic agent in tissue by microscopic examination, ancillary tests, or culture confers specificity and significance to the listed patterns. Large spherules

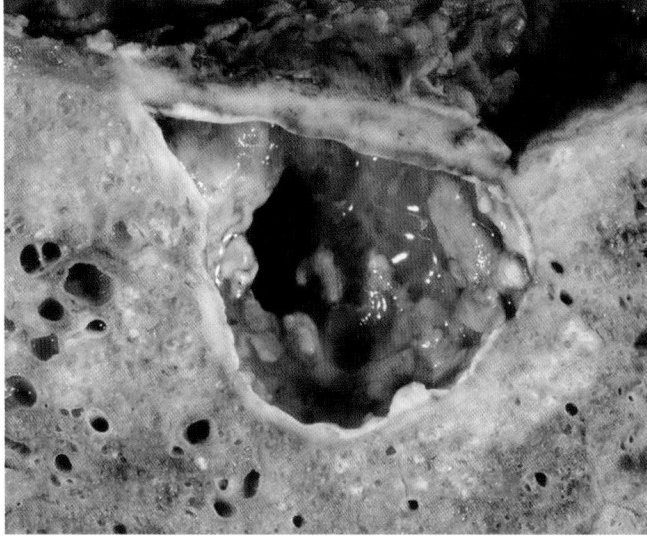

Figure 6-63. Cavitary aspergilloma.

Box 6-13. Histopathologic Patterns in Fungal Lung Injury

Large nodules
    Non-necrotizing granulomas
    Necrotizing granulomas
    Suppurative granulomas
    Poorly formed granulomas
Cavitary lesions
Miliary nodules
Acute bronchopneumonia
Airway disease
Intravascular changes/infarct
Diffuse alveolar damage, acute and organizing
Foamy alveolar casts

with endospores characteristic of *C. immitis* or yeast with large mucoid capsules of *C. neoformans* can be diagnostic. However, atypical forms of these organisms can be misleading and challenging. For example, in aerated cavities or in the setting of bronchopleural fistula, *Coccidioides* species may produce branching septate and moniliform hyphae or immature morula-like spherules mimicking other fungi (e.g., hyaline molds and *Blastomyces dermatitidis*).[38] Similarly, *C. neoformans*, *H. capsulatum*, and *S. schenckii* have been reported to produce hyphae or pseudohyphae in tissue, whereas acapsular *C. neoformans* may mimic other yeasts or *Pneumocystis* organisms.[184]

Mycelial morphology is helpful when it is characteristic of a specific genus or group. For example, broad, sparsely septate, nonparallel, twisted or irregular-diameter, thin-walled mycelia, with variable wide-angle branching, characterize zygomycetes, whereas progressively proliferating, regularly septate, 45-degree angle, dichotomously branching mycelia with parallel walls are typical of *Aspergillus* species (Fig. 6-64). In the case of *Aspergillus*, an important point is that *only the presence of a fruiting body* (conidiophore with sterigmata and conidia) permits diagnosis at the genus level, and there are many *Aspergillus* look-alikes in tissue, such as *Fusarium*, *Paecilomyces*, *Acremonium*, *Bipolaris*, *Pseudallescheria boydii*, and its asexual

anamorph, *Scedosporium apiospermum*.[184] Sometimes careful examination of tissue with special stains under high magnification or oil emersion will reveal clues, such as in situ sporulation, allowing a more definitive diagnosis.[39] However, these clues often are subtle, even for experienced microscopists, and it is important to defer to culture whenever possible.[185] Typical morphologic injury patterns and related etiologic agents are briefly highlighted below. The cited references should be consulted for further details.

Blastomycosis

Blastomycosis, the chronic granulomatous and suppurative infection produced by *B. dermatitidis*, is essentially a North American disease, concentrated in the Ohio and Mississippi river valleys. The prevalence of infection is particularly high in the state of Mississippi. Blastomycosis is the third most common endemic mycosis in North America, following histoplasmosis and coccidioidomycosis. It may occur in patients with normal immunity as well as those imunocompromised by diseases or medical therapy.[186] The isolated nodular manifestation can simulate lung cancer, radiologically.[187] The disease almost always begins in the lungs, although skin and bone are other common sites of involvement. In the lung, pathologic manifestations include focal or diffuse infiltrates; rare lobar consolidation; miliary nodules; solitary nodules; and acute or organizing diffuse alveolar damage[186-189] (Box 6-14). Necrotizing granulomas are characteristic and often of the suppurative type (Fig. 6-65A), but non-necrotizing granulomas may be found as well.

Box 6-14. Histopathologic Patterns in Pulmonary Blastomycosis

Acute pneumonia
    Lobular
    Lobar
Diffuse alveolar damage
Miliary nodule
Solitary nodule

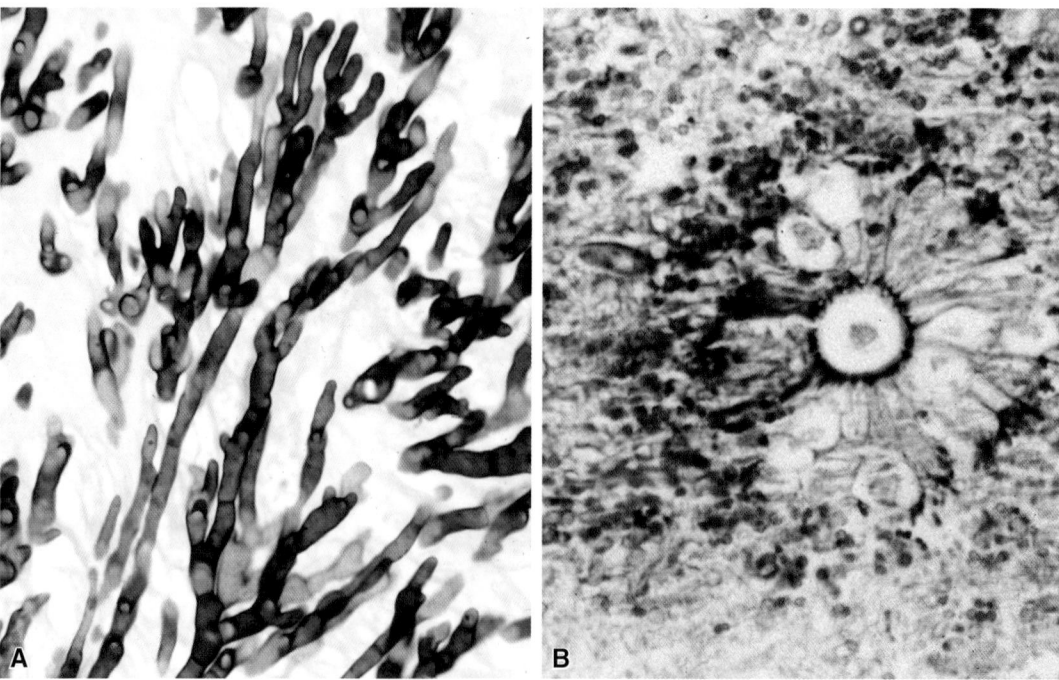

Figure 6-64. *Aspergillus* species. **A,** Septate mycelia with 45-degree angle branching (Grocott methenamine silver stain). **B,** Fruiting body (conidiophore with sterigmata and conidia) (Grocott methenamine silver stain).

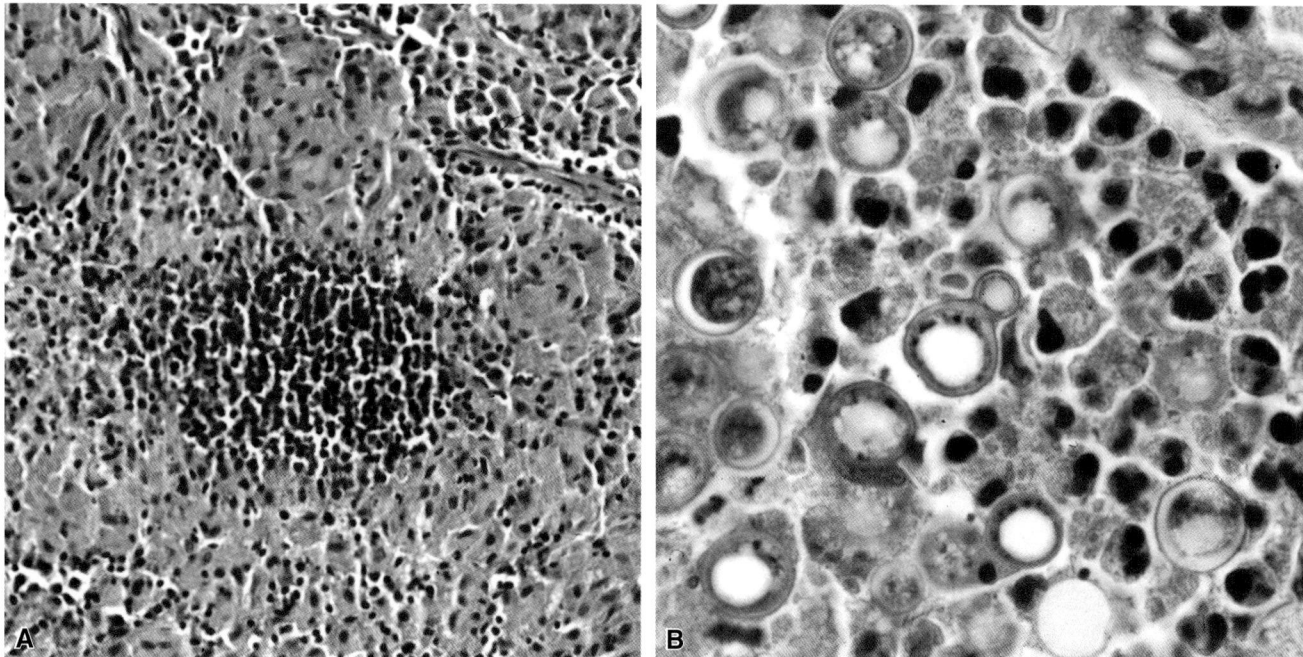

Figure 6-65. Blastomycosis. **A,** The suppurative granuloma is characteristic. **B,** Double-contour-wall yeast with broad-based budding.

The broad-based budding yeast forms of *Blastomyces* are refractile and have double-contoured walls. Multinucleate yeast cells typically are 8 to 15 μm in diameter, with some forms measuring up to 30 μm (see Fig. 6-65B). These large forms can mimic small *Coccidioides* spherules,[190] whereas smaller forms ("microforms") can mimic *C. neoformans*.[189]

Coccidioidomycosis

Endemic in the Lower Sonoran life zone of the southwestern United States, the soil fungus *Coccidioides immitis* and the more recently recognized, morphologically identical and genomically similar species *Coccidioides posadasii*[191] may be encountered outside the endemic area as a result of fomite transmission of arthroconidia (e.g., Asian textile workers handling imported Arizona cotton) or in travelers who have returned from an endemic area. Most primary pulmonary infections are asymptomatic. The exceptionally wide spectrum of pulmonary pathology in patients with clinically evident disease is outlined in Box 6-15. The true prevalence of the disease is significantly underestimated in endemic regions of the southwest, where it is thought to account for nearly 30% of community-acquired pneumonias in some metropolitan

Box 6-15. Histopathologic Patterns in Coccidioidal Respiratory Tract Disease

Airway disease
    Pharyngeal granuloma
    Laryngeal granuloma
    Tracheobronchial granuloma
Pulmonary parenchymal disease
    Acute pneumonia
    Eosinophilic pneumonia
    Chronic progressive infection
Fibrocavitary lesions
Bronchopleural fistula; empyema
Solitary pulmonary nodule
Disseminated disease
    Miliary
    Extrapulmonary

areas.[192-195] Granulomas are characteristic and may occur with or without necrosis. Intact spherules induce fibrocaseous granulomas (Fig. 6-66A) whereas ruptured spherules may incite suppurative and bronchocentric granulomatosis (BCG)-like reactions (see Fig. 6-66B).[192]

The large mature spherule (up to 40–60 μm in diameter) has a thick refractile wall lined by or filled with endospores and constitutes the key diagnostic finding (see Fig. 6-66C). This finding allows the distinction of coccidioidomycosis from other fungal infections such as blastomycosis and histoplasmosis, which are associated with similar histopathologic reaction patterns. In aerated cavities or the setting of bronchopleural fistula, mycelia resembling various hyaline molds may be seen with or without a variety of mature and immature spherules (see Figs. 6-19 and 6-66D). *Coccidioides* spherule look-alikes include large-variant *B. dermatitidis*, adiasporomycosis, pollen grains, and pulses (legume seeds).

Histoplasmosis

Histoplasmosis, the most common pulmonary fungal infection worldwide, is endemic in the Ohio and Mississippi river valleys of North America and is the most common endemic mycosis in AIDS.[196] The clinical forms of *H. capsulatum* infection[51,181,197] are presented in Box 6-16. The histopathologic correlates include a spectrum ranging from an exudative to a granulomatous process, influenced by such factors as the fungal burden and the immune status of the patient. In patients with normal defenses the characteristic histopathology is dominated by well-formed necrotizing and non-necrotizing granulomas occurring as solitary lesions indistinguishable from other granulomatous infections. Other presentations include miliary nodules (Fig. 6-67), cavitary lesions, and laminated fibrous solitary nodules (Fig. 6-68) that may be partially calcified (sometimes referred to as "residual granulomas"). In patients with impaired immunity, striking macrophage response with numerous intracellular yeasts is a characteristic pattern (Fig. 6-69A). The exudative lesion resembles acute lobular pneumonia with fibrinopurulent exudates.[198]

H. capsulatum organisms are yeasts (2–5 μm), with narrow-based unequal budding (see Fig. 6-69B). They may be seen on H&E-stained sections and, when numerous, appear as small refractile ovoid

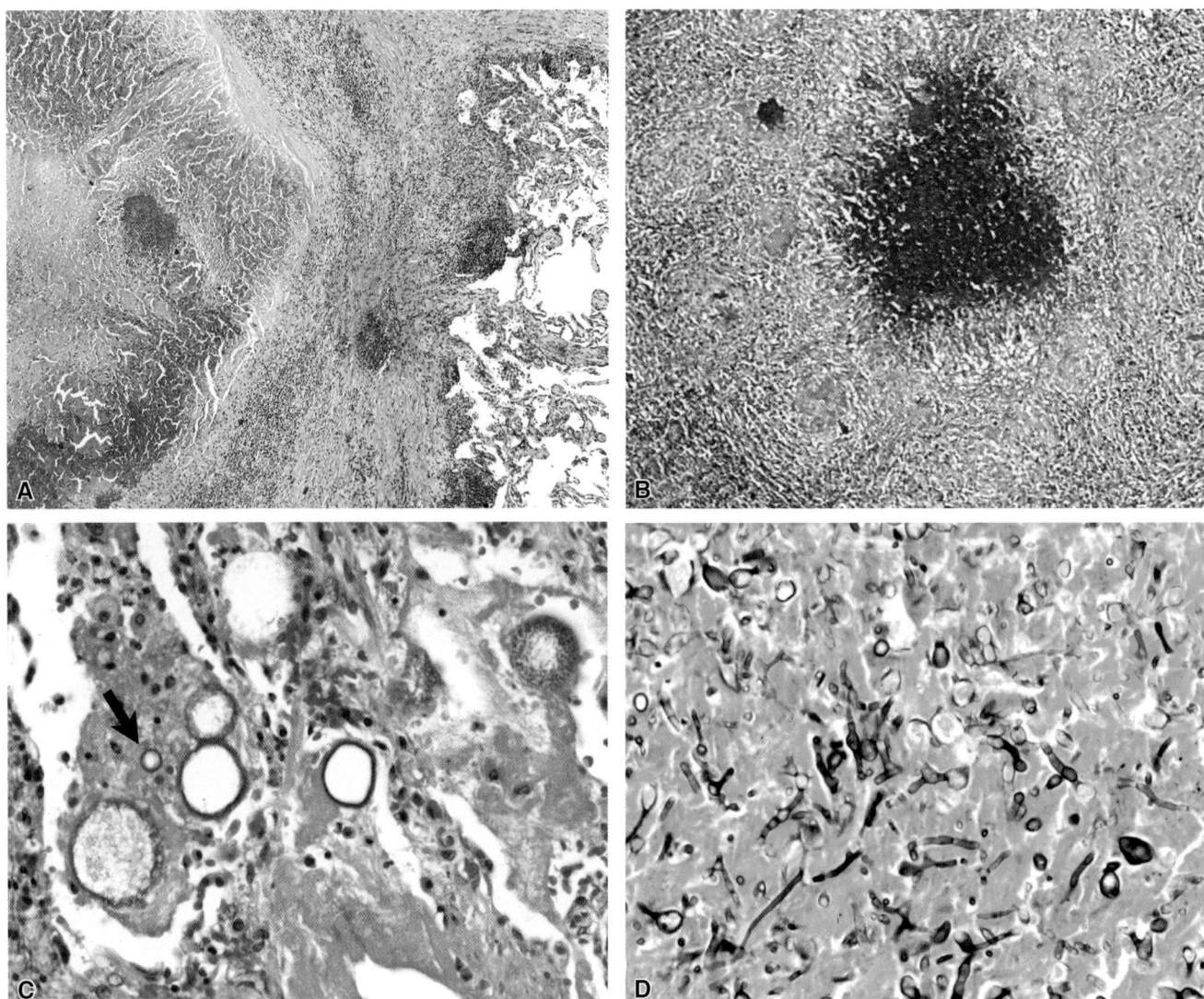

Figure 6-66. Coccidioidomycosis. **A,** Fibrocaseous granuloma. **B,** Bronchocentric granulomatosis–like granuloma. **C,** *Coccidioides immitis*. Both small (*arrow*) and large spherules with and without endospores can be seen. **D,** Biphasic pattern with mycelia and spore-like swellings (Grocott methenamine silver stain).

structures within macrophages. Yeasts typically occur in clusters but may be rare or very localized in old granulomas. A search for budding organisms in these situations may prove futile. Sometimes, yeasts may have dark-staining foci resembling pneumocystis organisms. Also,

Box 6-16. Clinical Forms of Pulmonary Histoplasmosis

Benign, self-limited
Acute
  Acute respiratory distress syndrome
  Acute self-limited, upper lobe (in smokers with emphysema)
Chronic
  Asymptomatic pulmonary nodule, with or without calcification
    ("histoplasmoma")
  Progressive (chronic cavitary) pulmonary
Progressive disseminated
Mediastinal
  Lymphadenopathy
  Middle lobe syndrome
  Fibrosis

Reprinted with permission from Travis WD, Colby TV, Koss MN, et al. Lung infections. In: King D, ed. *Atlas of Non-Tumor Pathology, Fascicle 2. Non-neoplastic Disorders of the Lower Respiratory Tract.* Washington, DC: American Registry of Pathology; 2002:539–728, Table 12-6.

some yeast cells may be surrounded by a clear space and may be mistaken for *Cryptococcus*.[51] Other look-alikes include *Candida* species, *P. marneffei*, capsule-deficient cryptococci, intracellular *B. dermatitidis*, and Hamazaki-Wesenberg bodies.

Paracoccidioidomycosis (South American Blastomycosis)

Seven clinical forms occur, but rarely cause lung infections in North America. The histopathology resembles other mycoses and can be exudative or granulomatous. *Paracoccidioides braziliensis* appears as a large spherical yeast (10–60 μm) with multiple buds attached by narrow necks ("steering wheel" or "ship's wheel").[199] When budding is sparse, look-alikes include *H. capsulatum* with small intracellular forms, *B. dermatitidis* and capsule-deficient cryptococci for medium-size forms, and *C. immitis* or *C. posadasii* for large forms.

Sporotrichosis

Infection by *Sporothrix schenckii* usually is confined to the skin, subcutis, and lymphatic pathways, but the organism can disseminate to the lungs. Rarely, *S. schenckii* is a primary pulmonary pathogen. The organism can produce cavitary disease in the form of a single lesion. Infection may be bilateral and apical, progressive and destructive, or may be identified clinically as a solitary pulmonary nodule. Microscopically, caseous

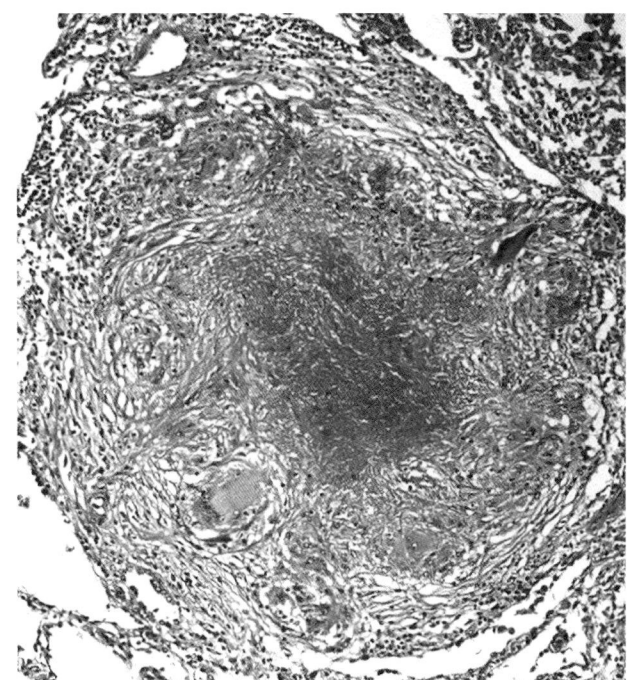

Figure 6-67. Histoplasmosis. Miliary nodule with central zone of necrosis invested by epithelioid histiocytes, multinucleate giant cells, and outer collarette of lymphocytes.

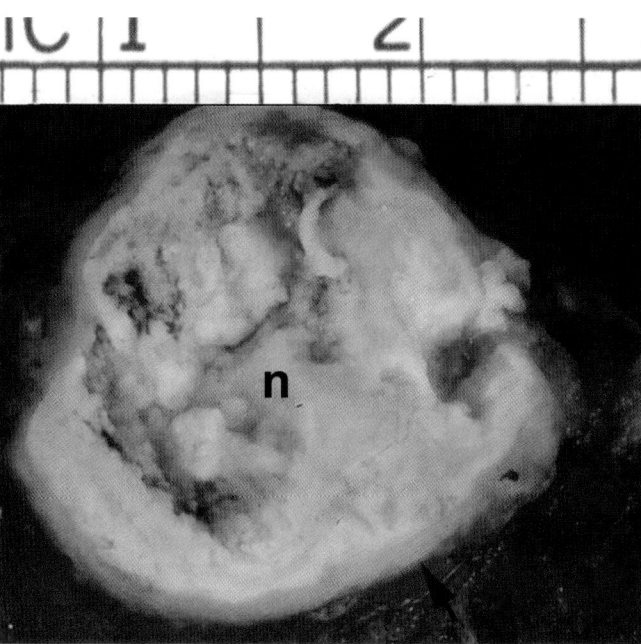

Figure 6-68. Histoplasmoma. Characteristic gross appearance of the persistent granulomatous nodule. Note the fibrous wall (*arrow*) surrounding caseous necrosis (n).

and suppurative type granulomas (Fig. 6-70A) occur with variable numbers of round to oval, small (2–3 µm) narrow budding yeast (see Fig. 6-70B) or cigar-shaped forms.[200] Non-necrotizing granulomas also occur. Asteroid bodies are an important clue, especially when organisms are sparse, as is often the case. Look-alikes include *H. capsulatum*, acapsular cryptococci, *Candida* organisms, and Hamazaki-Wesenberg bodies.

Penicilliosis

Southeast Asia is the endemic setting of the unique dimorphic fungus *Penicillium marneffei*. The disease it produces is not seen in North America except in travelers, especially immunocompromised persons.

It is one of the commonest opportunistic infections in AIDS patients in Southeast Asia and a significant clue to the presence of AIDS in that area. The respiratory tract is the portal of entry, with pulmonary infiltrates and disseminated disease, especially to skin. Microscopically, alveolar macrophages stuffed with spherical to oval yeast-like cells (2.5–5 µm) are seen, each with a single transverse septum; short hyphal forms and elongated, curved "sausage" forms may be formed in necrotic and cavitary lesions.[201,202] The septum distinguishes it from its look-alike, *H. capsulatum*.

Cryptococcosis

C. neoformans is a ubiquitous, facultative intracellular yeast. Pulmonary cryptococcosis occurs worldwide but has a particularly high

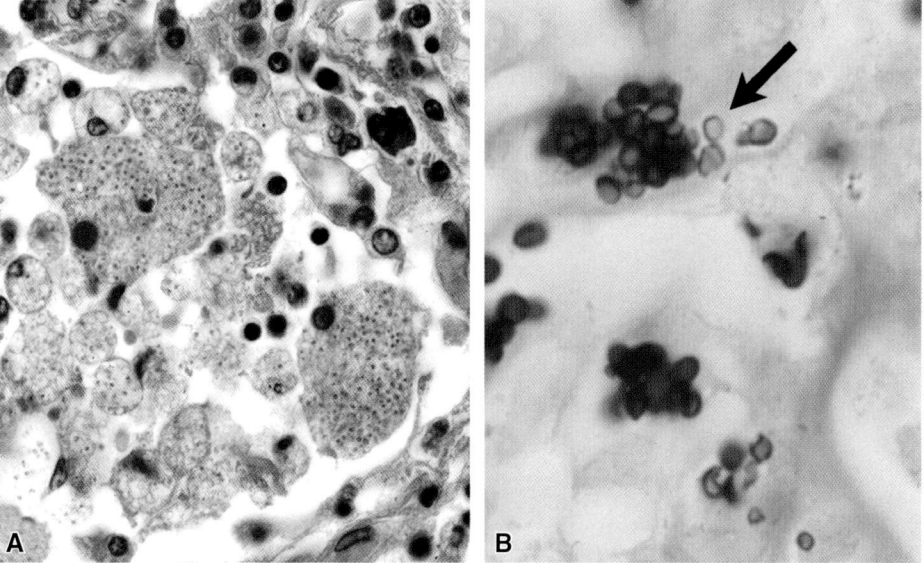

Figure 6-69. Histoplasmosis in an immunocompromised patient. **A,** Numerous *Histoplasma capsulatum* yeast cells in macrophages. **B,** Clusters of *H. capsulatum* yeast cells in macrophages. Note the narrow-based budding (*arrow*) (Grocott methenamine silver stain).

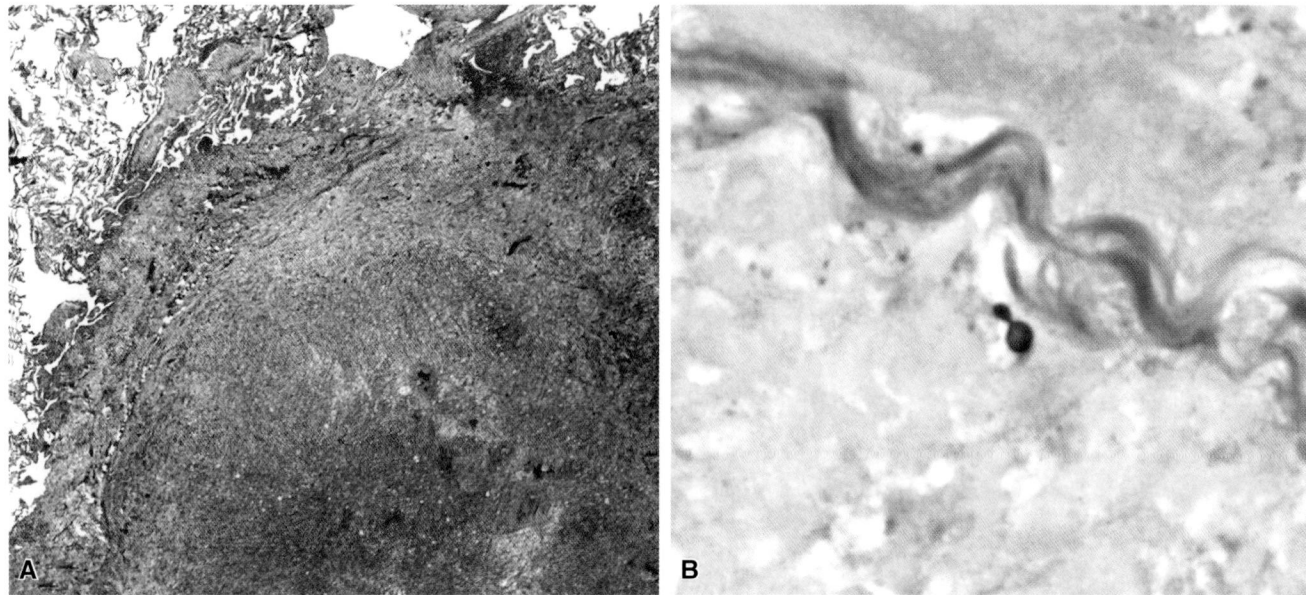

Figure 6-70. Sporotrichosis. **A,** Cavitary granuloma manifesting as a solitary pulmonary nodule. **B,** A rare, oval, narrow, budding yeast (Grocott methenamine silver stain).

incidence in the United States. The pathogenicity and histopathologic features of lung infection depends largely on the patient's immune status, as illustrated earlier in Figure 6-7 and summarized in Box 6-17. In the normal host, a substantial proportion of cryptococcal infections are asymptomatic while the remainders have respiratory symptoms associated with infiltrates or nodules. Immunocompromised patients are almost invariably symptomatic and often develop disseminated disease with a predilection for the brain and meninges. Pulmonary injury patterns include single or multiple large nodules, segmental or diffuse infiltrates, cavitary lesions, and miliary nodules. Normal hosts most often develop nodules comprised of fibrocaseous granulomas (Fig. 6-71A), or granulomatous pneumonia (see Fig. 6-71B). Immunocompromised patients are more likely to have histiocytic (see Fig. 6-71C) or mucoid infiltrates without inflammation (see Fig. 6-71D).

The cryptococcal organisms are round yeast forms ranging in diameter from 2 to 15 μm, with an average size of 4 to 7 μm. Cryptococcal yeasts are visible on H&E-stained sections as pale gray to light blue structures, frequently with attached smaller buds. They often occur in clusters and sometimes can be found within giant cells.[181] The mucicarmine stain highlights the capsule (Fig. 6-72A), but with capsule-deficient forms (see Fig. 6-72B), the pleomorphic appearance can be confused with that of other yeast forms (e.g., *H. capsulatum, B. dermatitidis, S. schenckii*) and sometimes *Pneumocystis.*

The lungs of patients with the most severe immunodeficiency may show myriad yeasts in alveolar septal capillaries (see Fig. 6-72A) with little if any intra-alveolar reaction[203] and this form of the disease also

may be associated with mucoid pneumonia.[204] The mucoid pneumonia (Fig. 6-73A) of cryptococcal infection can be confirmed with mucin stains such as Alcian blue (see Fig. 6-73B). Another microscopic pattern recently described in HIV-infected patients is the so-called "inflammatory spindle cell pseudotumor," a lesion much more commonly associated with mycobacterial infection.[205]

Candidiasis

Candida organisms are yeasts that can produce pseudohyphae and are the most common invasive fungal pathogens in humans. Secondary *Candida* pneumonia is relatively common, but primary *Candida* pneumonia is rare in other than immunocompromised patients in the intensive care unit.[51] In general, *C. albicans* is the most frequently isolated of the more than 100 known species which include a few rare and emerging human pathogens. *C. glabrata* and *C. tropicalis*, together with *C. albicans*, account for 95% of bloodstream infections, the principal route for acquisition of *Candida* pneumonia.[206] A non–blood-borne route to pneumonia results from aspiration of organisms from a heavily colonized or infected oropharynx. When blood-borne, miliary nodules with a necroinflammatory center and a hemorrhagic rim reflect an intravascular distribution of fungi. In the case of aspiration, the organisms may be found in the airways associated with an alveolar filling pattern of bronchopneumonia[207] (Fig. 6-74A) or, much less commonly, a bronchocentric granulomatosis pattern.

In tissue sections, oval budding yeast-like cells (blastoconidia) 2 to 6 μm in diameter may appear with pseudohyphae, which constrict at points of budding, creating the impression of bulging rather than parallel walls (see Fig. 6-74B). The pseudohyphae branch at acute angles and can overlap in width with the true hyphae of *Aspergillus*, from which they must be distinguished. Among the medically important species, *C. glabrata* (formerly *Torulopsis glabrata*) and *C. parapsilosis* produce only yeast cells in tissue, in contrast with most other *Candida* species, which produce both yeast and pseudohyphae.[181]

Other look-alikes include *H. capsulatum, Trichosporon beigeli*, and *Malassezia furfur*, depending on whether pseudohyphae or yeast forms alone are present. They can be distinguished from *Histoplasma* by their extracellular location and Gram stain positivity. *T. beigeli*

Box 6-17. Histopathologic Patterns in Cryptococcal Lung Disease

In order of associated decrease in immune function
- Fibrocaseous granuloma
- Granulomatous pneumonia
- Histiocytic pneumonia
- Mucoid pneumonia
- Intracapillary cryptococcosis

Reprinted with permission from Mark EJ. Case records of the Massachusetts General Hospital. *N Engl J Med.* 2002;347:518–524.

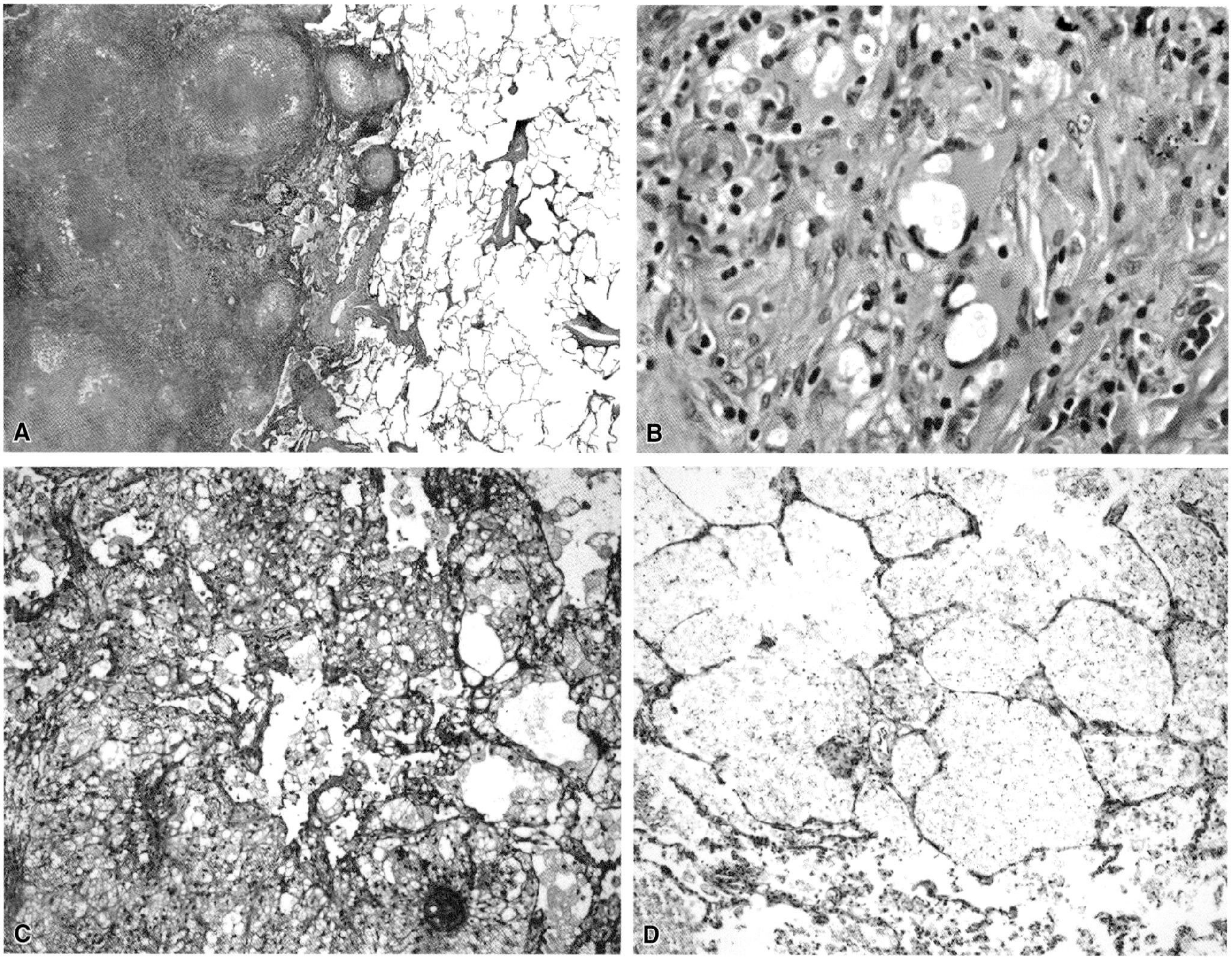

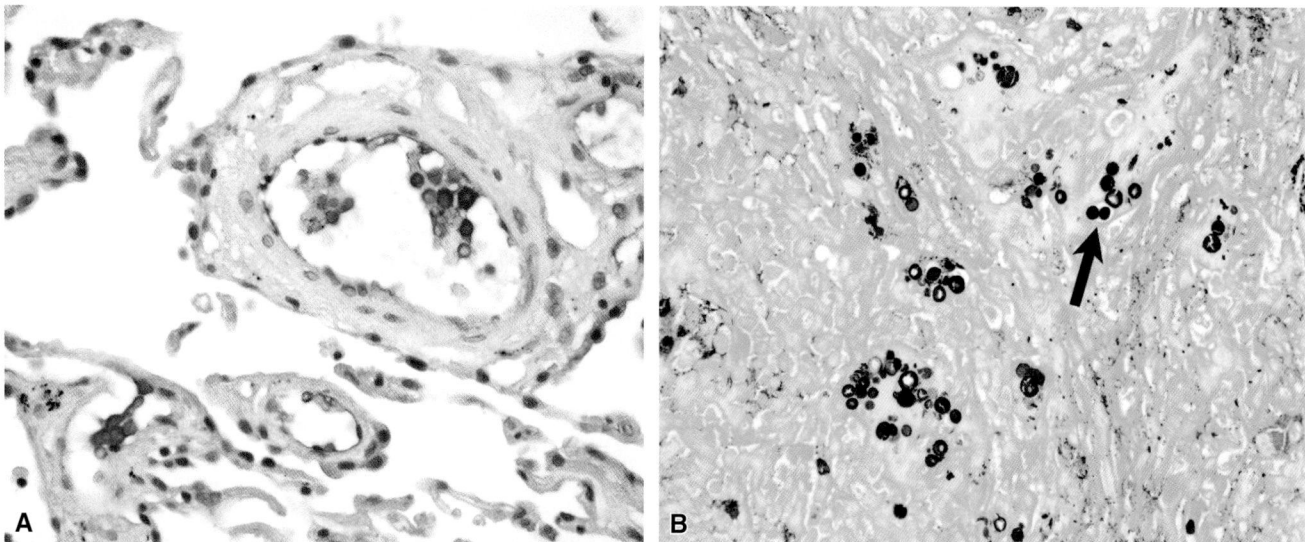

Figure 6-71. Cryptococcosis. **A,** Solitary pulmonary nodule with small satellite granulomas. **B,** Granulomatous pneumonia with clusters of pale staining yeast in clear spaces surrounded by histiocytes and multinucleated giant cells. **C,** Histiocytic pneumonia. **D,** Mucoid pneumonia with no inflammatory cell reaction.

Figure 6-72. **A,** Intravascular cryptococcus. Yeast cells with stained capsules (mucicarmine stain). **B,** Capsule-deficient cryptococcus (Grocott methenamine silver stain).

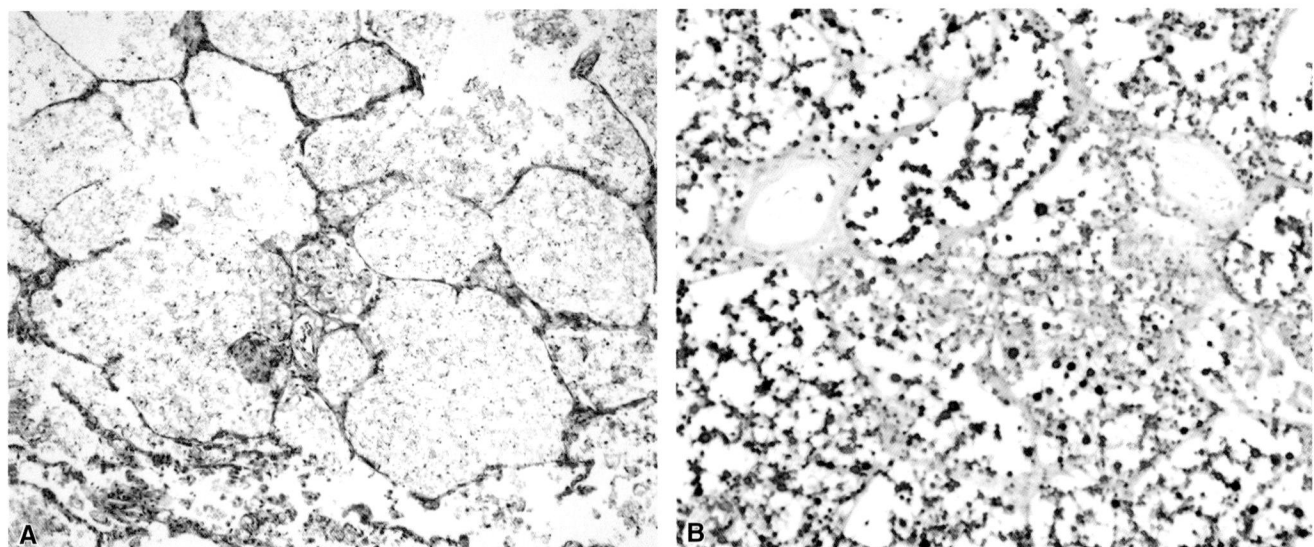

Figure 6-73. Cryptococcal mucoid pneumonia. **A,** Myriad blue-gray yeast in mucoid matrix. **B,** Alcian blue mucin stain accentuates the mucoid matrix.

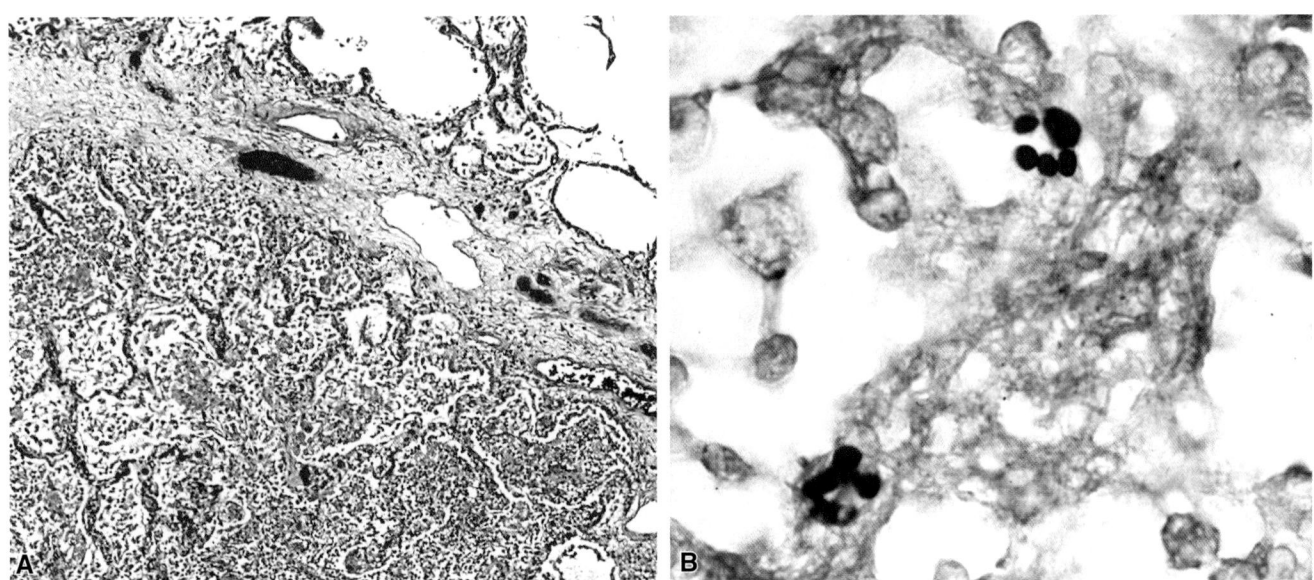

Figure 6-74. A, *Candida* bronchopneumonia. **B,** *Candida* yeast cells—blastoconidia (Grocott methenamine silver stain).

tends to be somewhat larger and more pleomorphic. Malasseziasis is clinically associated with parenteral nutrition, Intralipid, and indwelling catheters. Pulmonary lesions include pneumonia, mycotic thromboemboli, infarcts, and vasculitis. *M. furfur* may be found in small arteries, where the organisms appear as small, 2- to 5-μm yeast-like cells. They form distinctive unipolar broad-based buds but no pseudohyphae.[51]

Aspergillosis

Aspergillus species and other hyaline and dematiaceous molds have emerged as significant causes of morbidity and death in the immunocompromised host. Worldwide, species of *Aspergillus* are the most common invasive molds. They are the second most common fungal pathogens after *Candida* species but, in contrast with *Candida*, are more commonly isolated from the lung. Several species are recognized, but *A. fumigatus* is the one most often seen in the clinical laboratory and most often isolated from the lungs of immunocompromised patients.[208] Respiratory aspergillosis can be classified into a colonizing or saprophytic form (intrabronchial and pre-existing cavity fungus ball) (Fig. 6-75A); hypersensitivity forms (allergic bronchopulmonary aspergillosis, including mucoid impaction of bronchi and hypersensitivity pneumonitis) (see Fig. 6-75B); and invasive disease (minimally invasive–chronic necrotizing or angioinvasive–disseminated), as outlined in Box 6-18.[51,209-211] Invasive disease (Fig. 6-76) tends to occur in immunocompromised patients, including those with prolonged neutropenia, transplant recipients (especially hematopoietic stem cell and lung transplants), advanced AIDS, and and the inherited immune deficiency disorder referred to as "chronic granulomatous disease of childhood." The clinicopathologic features of invasive disease reflect these host-associated risk factors.[212] In patients with neutopenia, a charcteristic angioinvasive pattern occurs, with intravascular spread resulting in hemorrhagic infarcts (Fig. 6-77). In the non-neutropenic patient, the necroinflammatory pattern tends to lack this angioinvasive feature.[213] Some cases defy categorization; are unique, e.g. bronchocentric and miliary patterns (Fig. 6-78); or may be hybrids of infection and hypersensitivity.[214]

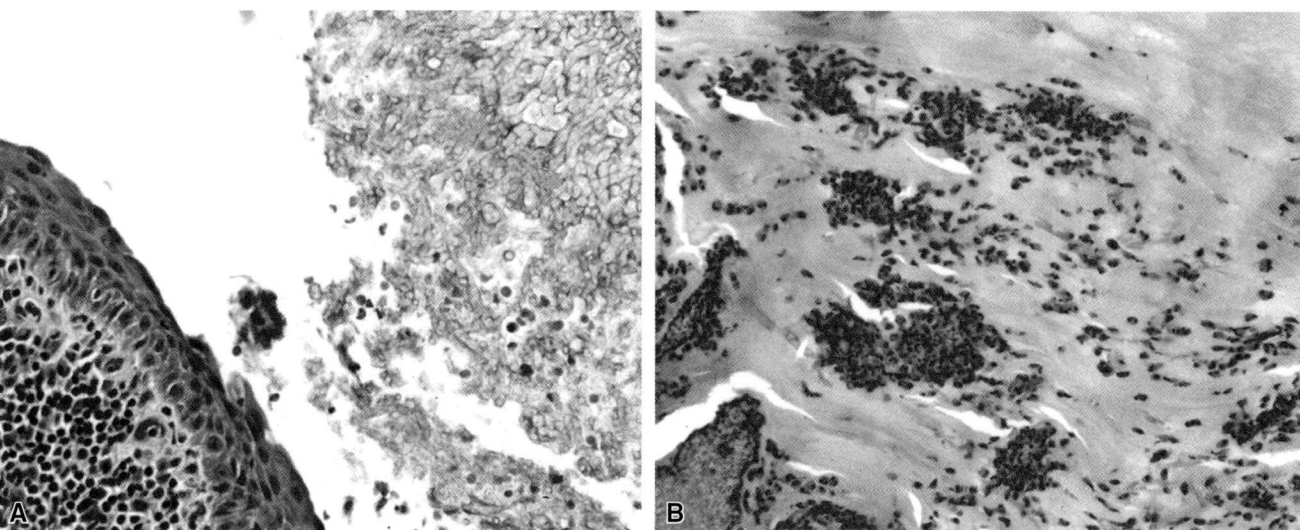

Figure 6-75. A, Aspergillosis fungus ball. **B,** Allergic bronchopulmonary aspergillosis. Intraluminal allergic mucin with laminated clusters of eosinophils can be seen in inspissated basophilic mucin with scattered Charcot-Leyden crystals.

Box 6-18. Histopathologic Patterns in Pulmonary Aspergillosis

Colonization
 Fungus ball
Hypersensitivity reaction
 Allergic bronchopulmonary aspergillosis
 Eosinophilic pneumonia
 Mucoid impaction
 Bronchocentric granulomatosis
 Hypersensitivity pneumonitis
Invasive
 Acute invasive aspergillosis
 Necrotizing pseudomembranous tracheobronchitis
 Chronic necrotizing pneumonia
 Bronchopleural fistula
 Empyema

Reprinted with permission from Travis WD, Colby TV, Koss MN, et al. Lung infections. In: King D, ed. *Atlas of Non-Tumor Pathology, Fascicle 2. Non-neoplastic Disorders of the Lower Respiratory Tract.* Washington, DC: American Registry of Pathology; 2002:539–728, Table 12-10.

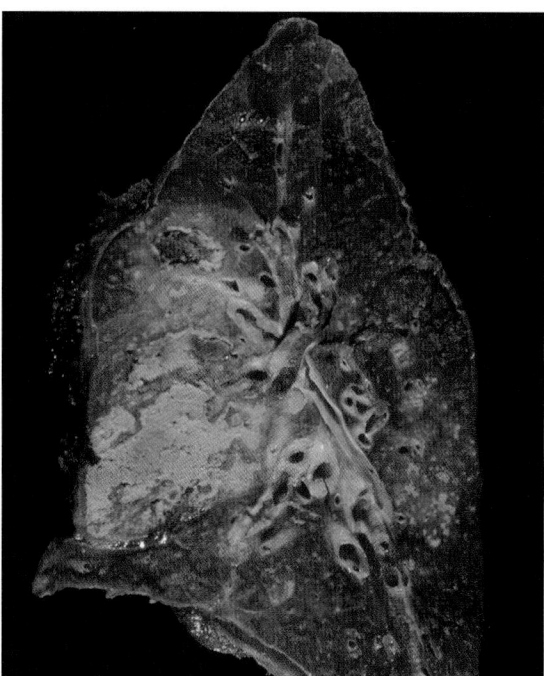

Figure 6-76. Resected lung specimen from an immunocompromised patient with necrotizing *Aspergillus* pneumonia.

Microscopically, septate hyphae, dichotomatously branched at 45-degree angle, have uniform, consistent width (3–6 µm) without constrictions at points of septation. When numerous, as in some angio-invasive lesions and fungus balls, these features can be readily appreciated in H&E-stained sections. Fruiting heads of *Aspergillus* (shown earlier in Fig. 6-64) are sometimes formed in cavities. Oxalate crystals, visible in plane-polarized light (Fig. 6-79), are an important clue to *Aspergillus* infection when hyphae cannot be identified.

Look-alikes include various hyaline molds such as zygomycetes and *Candida* species, as well as *P. boydii*.[215] Another look-alike is *Fusarium* species. Fusariosis is an emerging mycosis in the immunocompromised host, and *Fusarium* is the second most common opportunist after *Aspergillus* species in immunosuppressed patients with hematologic malignancies.[216] The clinical and pathological features in the lung and at sites of dissemination mimic those of aspergillosis, and the mycelia are essentially indistinguishable. Isolation in culture or by immunohistochemistry or molecular techniques, such as in situ hybridization or PCR amplification, is required for definitive diagnosis. Other previously uncommon but newly

emerging hyaline molds that may be difficult to distinguish from *Aspergillus* in tissue are *Paecilomyces, Acremonium, Scedosporium,* and *Basidiobolus*.[206,217,218]

Zygomycosis

The taxonomic organization of the fungal phylum Zygomycota includes the class Zygomycetes, which is subdivided into two orders: Mucorales and Entomophthorales. These orders contain the agents of human zygomycosis.[219] The order Mucorales includes the genera *Absidia, Apophysomyces, Rhizopus, Rhizomucor,* and *Mucor,* from which the often taxonomically incorrect term *mucormycosis* is derived. In fact, most infections are due to *Rhizopus* and *Absidia* species.[220] The zygomycete species share clinical and pathologic features with invasive

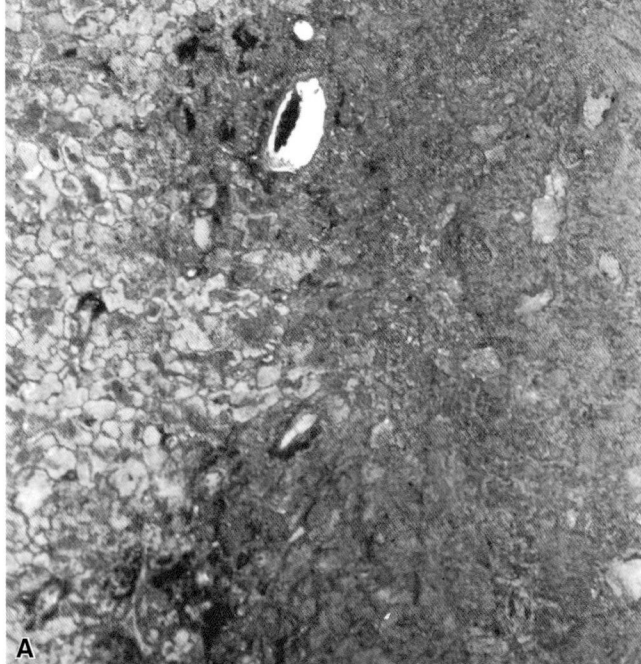

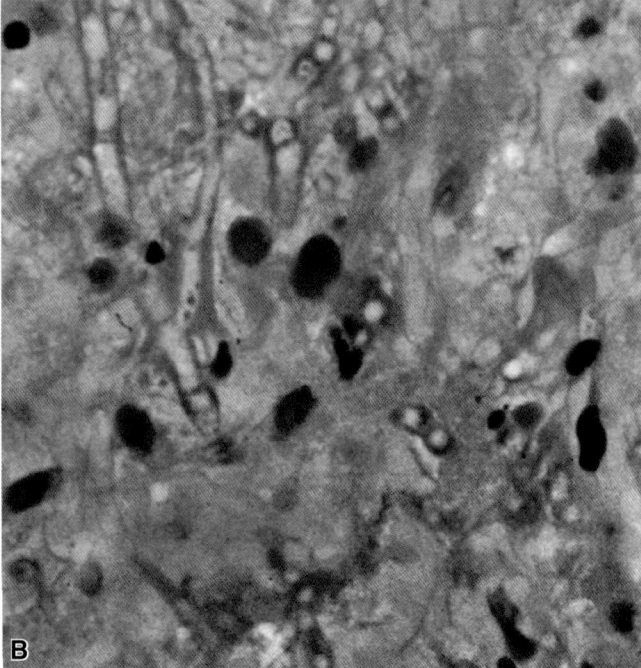

Figure 6-77. Invasive aspergillosis. **A,** Hemorrhagic infarct. **B,** 45-degree angle branching septate hyphae.

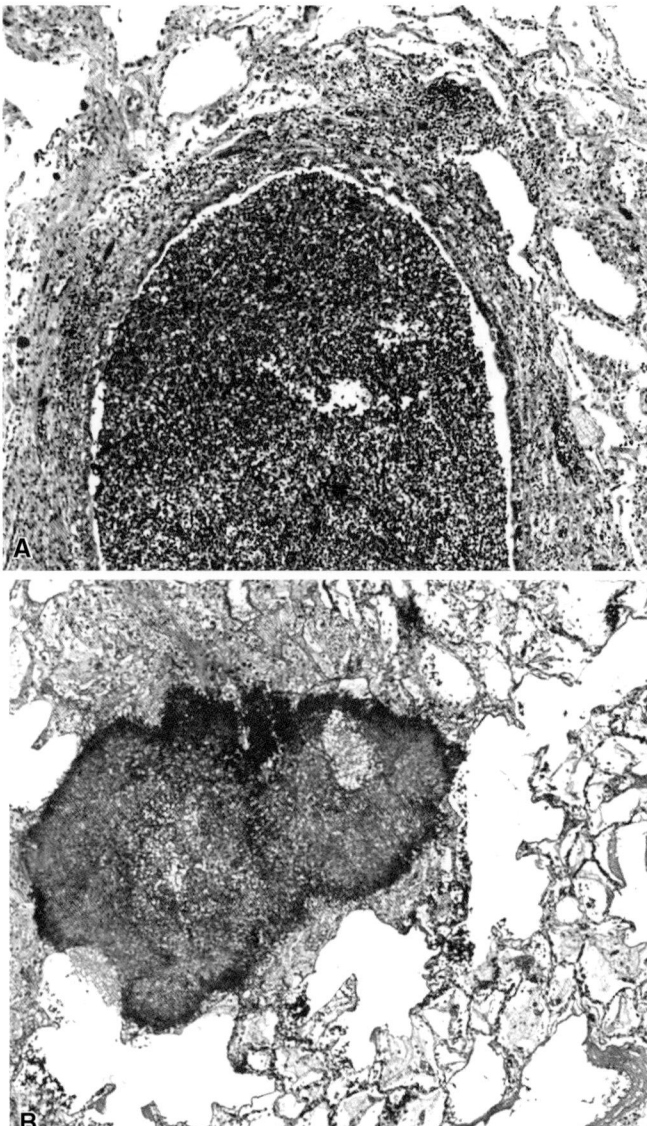

Figure 6-78. Bronchocentric aspergillosis. **A,** Bronchiole expanded and filled with purulent exudate. **B,** Miliary aspergillosis. Colony of organisms with hyaline membranes evident at periphery of the image (*lower right*).

Aspergillus species, being angiotropic and capable of inducing hemorrhagic infarcts with sparse inflammation.

Clinical syndromes produced by these fungi include rhinocerebral, pulmonary, cutaneous, and gastrointestinal infections, with a predilection for neonates. Hematopoietic malignancies and diabetes mellitus with acidosis underlie most cases of pulmonary infection in children and adults.[221] Box 6-19 lists a broad spectrum of pulmonary diseases that includes solitary or multiple and bilateral nodular lesions, segmental or lobar consolidation, cavitary lesions, fistulas, infarcts (Figs. 6-80 and 6-81); direct extension into mediastinal, thoracic soft tissue, chest wall and diaphragm; chronic tracheal and endobronchial infection; and fungus ball similar to aspergilloma.[222] An endobronchial syndrome with a propensity for blood vessel ersoion also has been described, sometimes resulting in fatal hemoptysis.[223]

Hyphae are broad (6–25 μm), thin-walled, and pauciseptate (Fig. 6-82A). They display considerable variation in width, with twisted, nonparallel contours and random wide-angle branching, nearing 90 degrees.[181] They also have a tendency to fragment more commonly than *Aspergillus* organisms, which tend to retain their elongate sweeping profiles. Additional features include variability in tinctorial staining in H&E sections, ranging from basophilia to eosinophilia. In frozen sections, hyphae may show weak staining, and they often have a bubbly or vacuolated appearance.[222] In addition to being angiotropic, they are neurotropic.[224] In lesions exposed to air, the hyphae may form ovoid or spherical thick-walled chlamydoconidia, within or at the terminal ends (see Fig. 6-82B).[225] Look-alikes at the lower-width range include *Aspergillus* and other *Aspergillus*-like hyaline molds. The pseudohyphae of *Candida* species sometimes can be closely simulated.

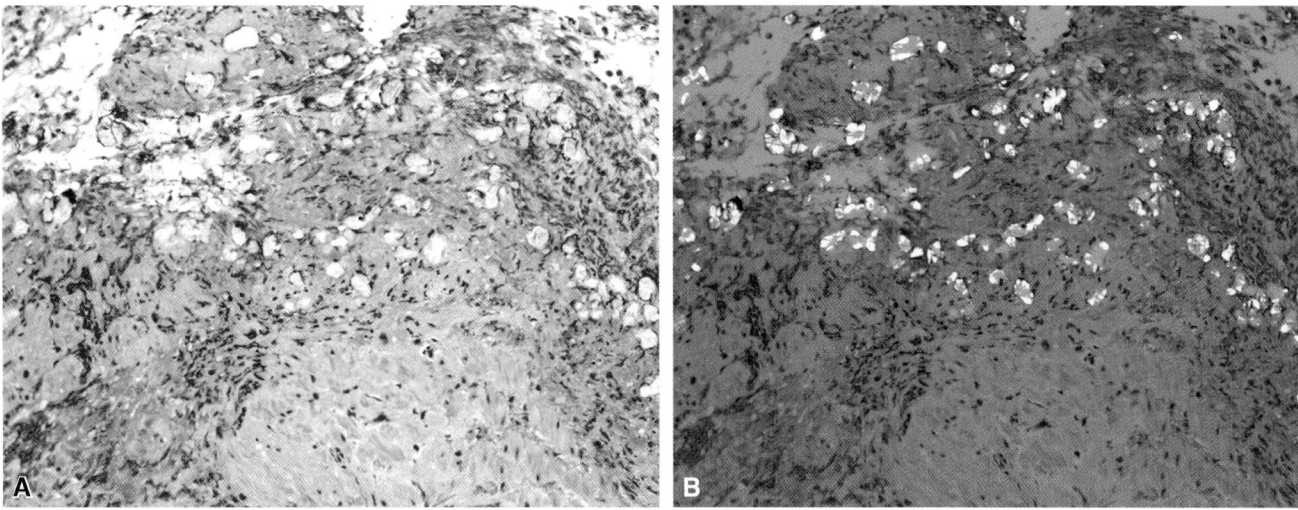

Figure 6-79. A, Pale yellow oxalate crystal sheaths in necroinflammatory debris. **B,** Birefringent oxalates seen under polarized light.

Box 6-19. Histopathologic Patterns in Pulmonary Zygomycosis

Acute lobular or lobar pneumonia
Nodules
Cavities
Endobronchial mass
Fistulas
Infarcts
Thoracic soft tissue/mediastinum
Fungus ball

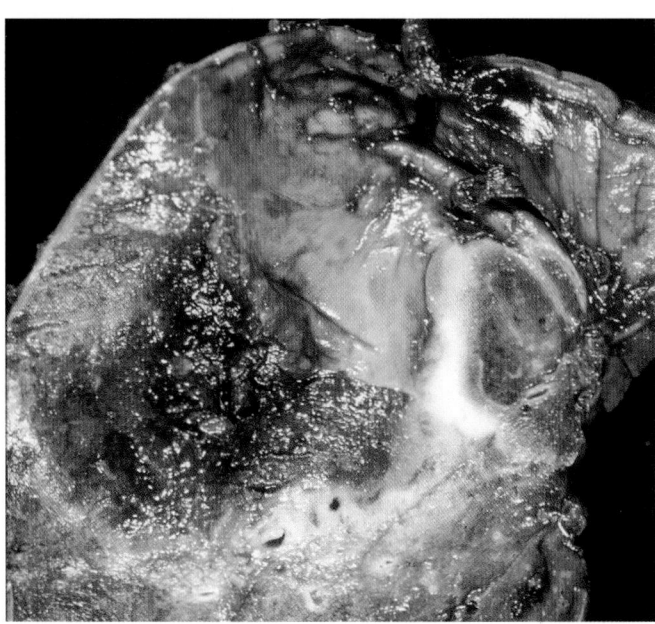

Figure 6-80. Resected lung specimen from patient with necrotizing pneumonia caused by zygomycosis.

Phaeohyphomycosis

A few genera of dematiaceous molds produce infections resembling those of *Aspergillus*, including allergic bronchopulmonary disease (Fig. 6-83A) and bronchocentric granulomatosis patterns.[226,227] The more than 80 genera and species of these saprophytes, which occur naturally in wood, soil, and decaying matter, include *Bipolaris, Exserohilum,*

Xylohypha, Alternaria, and *Curvularia,* among others.[181] The unique appearance of these fungi is due to their cell wall melanin content. In the allergic mucin or other deposits of necroinflammatory debris, the phaeoid (dark brown– to black-pigmented) hyphae (2–6 μm in diameter) generally are sparse but can resemble *Aspergillus* and other hyaline molds, especially when lightly pigmented or nonpigmented. Typically, only small mycelial fragments are seen, which may be mistaken for artifacts, sometimes with terminal swellings resembling chlamydoconidia (see Fig. 6-83B). The dematiaceous agents of subcutaneous forms of chromoblastomycosis appear as pigmented muriform cells in granulomas, and they do not form mycelia. Chromoblastomycosis is rarely encountered in the lung. Another *Aspergillus* look-alike is *P. boydii,* an organism that is sometimes grouped with the dematiaceous fungi. *P. boydii* usually exhibits a more ragged, disorganized, and densely clustered pattern of mycelia. Clinically, localized disease may be cured by excision alone; systemic disease often is refractory to treatment.[228]

Pneumocystosis

The face of *Pneumocystis* pneumonia continues to change. Once considered to be a protozoan, this organism is now classified as a fungus, and the species infecting humans has been renamed *Pneumocystis jiroveci* (formerly *Pneumocystis carinii*).[229] Once a disease primarily of malnourished children and occasionally occurring in the setting of treatment for childhood leukemia, today *Pneumocystis* infection is identified most commonly in patients with defective immunity, especially AIDS, or those on immunosuppressive therapies for hematopoietic malignancies, organ transplants, and collagen vascular diseases. With the success of contemporary therapy for AIDS, the pathologist is now more likely to encounter the disease in the latter group of patients in whom it is apt to be more subtle.[230] The classic pattern during the HIV epidemic was the foamy alveolar cast (Fig. 6-84) with moderate to numerous organisms, type II pneumocyte hyperplasia, and a scant to moderate interstitial lymphoplasmacytic infiltrate.[231,232]

In recent years a number of atypical and unusual patterns have been described that are worth recognizing.[51,233,234] These are listed in Box 6-20. *Pneumocystis jiroveci* infection can mimic any lung injury pattern, ranging from acute diffuse alveolar damage with hyaline membranes (Fig. 6-85) and minimal or no foamy exudates to an organizing phase with sparse organisms. There is also a spectrum of granulomatous infection, both non-necrotizing and necrotizing, that may overlap morphologically with mycobacterial or other fungal infections, particularly histoplasmosis (Fig. 6-86). Cavitary disease, solitary pulmonary

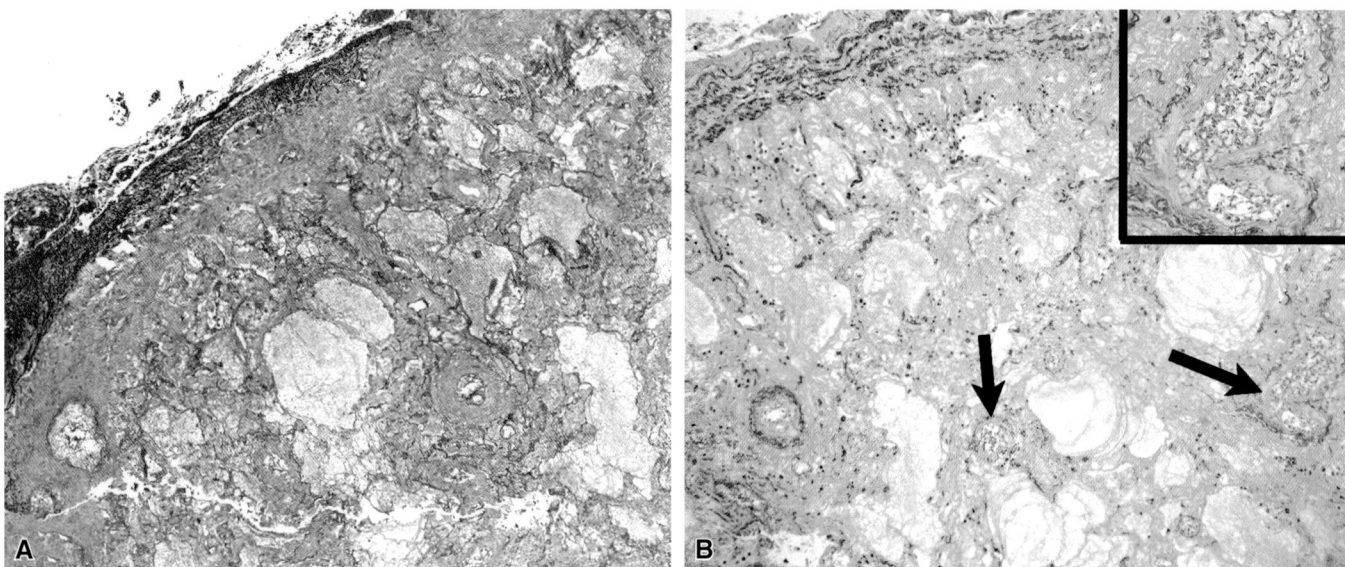

Figure 6-81. Zygomycosis. **A,** Nodular infarct. **B,** Intravascular organisms (*arrows*). Vessel at *right arrow* is shown at high magnification (*inset*) (Grocott methenamine silver stain).

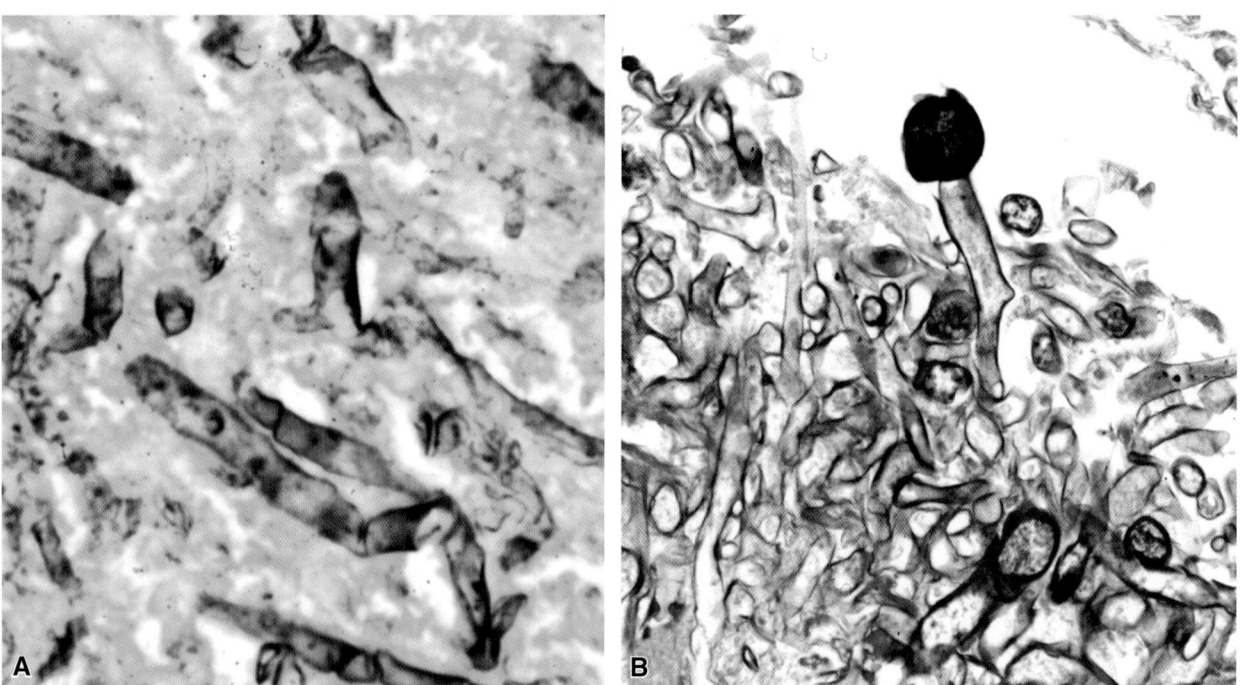

Figure 6-82. Zygomycosis. **A,** Twisted pauciseptate, broad mycelia characteristic of zygomycetes (Grocott methenamine silver stain). **B,** Endobronchial zygomycosis with chlamydospores.

nodules that may be relatively fibrotic, cysts, and dystrophic calcification also are described.[234-236]

Microscopically, the three life stages of the organism are still referred to by protozoan terminology as sporozoites, trophozoites, and cysts. The cyst is the most common form seen by pathologists. On silver stains the cyst is seen as an oval (4–7 μm) yeast-like cell that may be collapsed, helmet-shaped, or variably crescentic. The intracystic dot or paired-comma structures are important keys to distinguish *P. jiroveci* cysts from look-alikes such as *Histoplasma*, the capsule-deficient form of *Cryptococcus*, *Candida* species, and even overstained red blood cells. Sporozoites and trophozoites are

seen to best advantage in touch imprints and cytologic preparations of respiratory samples.

Cytopathology

Many of the fungal pathogens involving the respiratory tract can be detected by cytologic techniques in sputum samples, bronchial washings and brushings, BAL fluid samples, and needle aspirates.[44] The aspirates and other samples also can be submitted for culture and ancillary studies.[237] The four most common yeast forms—*C. neoformans*, *C. immitis* or *C. posadasii*, *H. capsulatum*, and *B. dermatitidis*—must be distinguished from each other, and *P. jiroveci* also can enter

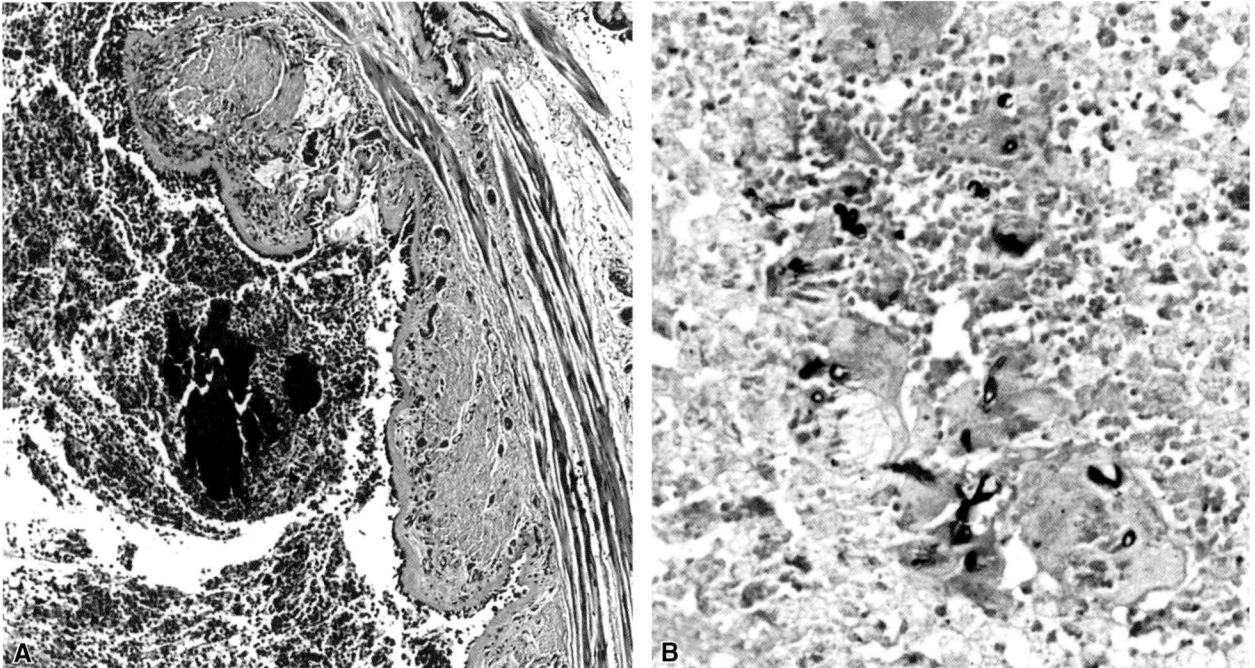

Figure 6-83. Allergic bronchopulmonary fungal disease. **A,** Ectatic bronchus with thick eosinophilic basement membrane and intraluminal necroinflammatory debris. **B,** Mycelial fragments of *Bipolaris* organisms (Grocott methenamine silver stain).

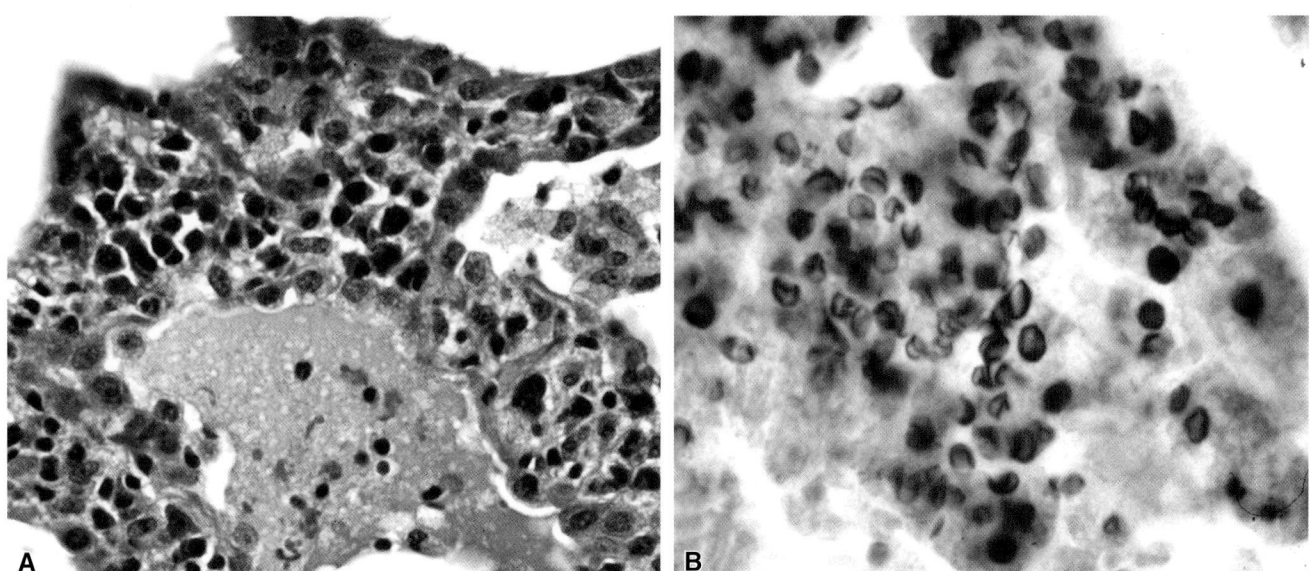

Figure 6-84. *Pneumocystis* pneumonia. **A,** Lymphoplasmacytic interstitial infiltrate and intra-alveolar foamy alveolar cast. **B,** Numerous yeast-like cells of *Pneumocystis jiroveci* of various shapes (Grocott methenamine silver stain).

Box 6-20. Histopathologic Patterns in Pulmonary *Pneumocystis* Infection

Foamy alveolar cast
Diffuse alveolar damage
"Id" reaction (minimal-change reaction)
Granulomas
Miliary disease
Vascular invasion/vasculitis/infarct
Lymphoid interstitial pneumonia
Cavities and cysts
Subpleural blebs and bullae
Microcalcification

the differential diagnosis.[43] Morphologic features of these organisms are often better visualized in cytologic preparations than in tissue sections, usually permitting a rapid and definitive diagnosis on smears prepared using routine stains (Papanicolaou, Diff-Quik, and H&E). More specific fungal stains (Grocott methenamine silver, Gridley, and Fontana-Masson) often can be held in reserve.

Amorphous granular debris and epithelioid cells characterize many necrotizing granulomas. Typically, a background of neutrophils is seen when suppurative granulomas are aspirated. *Histoplasma* infections may manifest an epithelioid or phagocytic cell population. Cryptococcal infections can be similar or may be

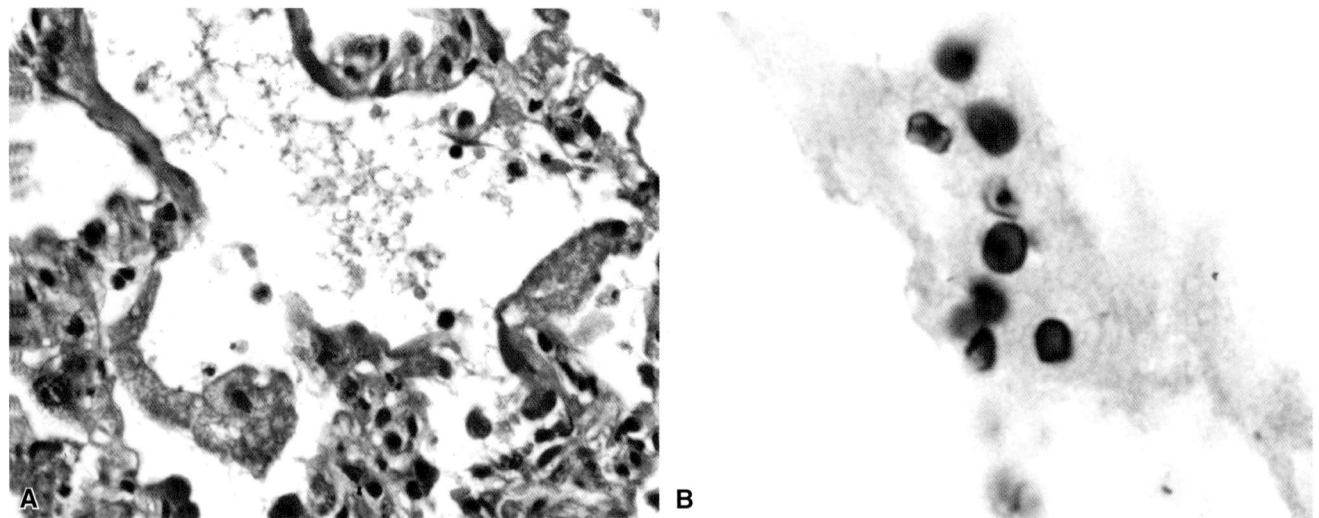

Figure 6-85. *Pneumocystis* pneumonia. **A,** Diffuse alveolar damage pattern with hyaline membranes. **B,** Cysts in hyaline membrane (Grocott methenamine silver stain).

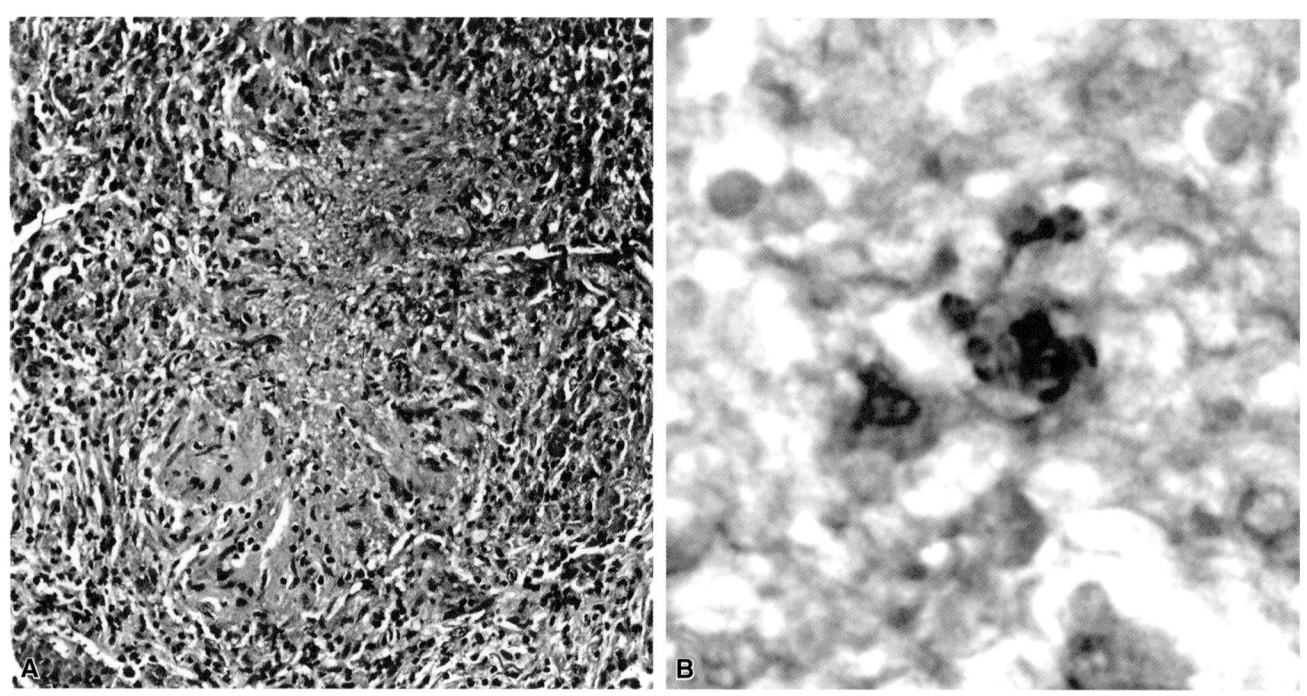

Figure 6-86. *Pneumocystis* pneumonia. **A,** Miliary granuloma with central necrosis. **B,** Sparse organisms in granuloma (Grocott methenamine silver stain).

associated with little or no accompanying inflammation in the immunocompromised patient.

Cytology of Common Yeast Forms

Morphologic features of some of the more common yeast forms that the pathologist may encounter in cytologic material are presented in Table 6-7.

C. neoformans organisms are seen as are single budding yeast forms with a narrow, pinched-off base, approximately 4 to 7 μm in diameter but ranging in size from 2 to 15 μm. In needle aspirates, the mucoid capsule investing the yeast imparts a "spare tire" appearance (Fig. 6-87).

B. dermatitidis organisms are refractile, double-contoured yeast forms and range in diameter from 8 to 15 μm with broad-based budding (Fig. 6-88). An internal amorphous mass can be appreciated in

some stained preparations. Smaller or larger yeast cells can be mistaken for *C. neoformans* or *C. immitis*, respectively.

C. immitis/C. posadasii spherules exhibit a variety of sizes and shapes, ranging from large spherules packed with endospores (Fig. 6-89A) to empty collapsed spheres and small immature spherules.[238] The latter may overlap with *Blastomyces* and other yeasts. Mycelial forms of *Coccidioides* species, with arthrospores, may be found in aspirates of cavitary nodules exposed to air (see Fig. 6-89B).

H. capsulatum yeast cells are small (2–5 μm) and stain poorly in routine smears, but presence of this pathogen can be suspected on the basis of the dot-like refractile appearance of these cells in the cytoplasm of macrophages. In Diff-Quik–stained smears, the characteristic purple, polarized yeast forms (Fig. 6-90) are discernible, and they are outlined entirely in GMS-stained smears.

Table 6-7. Morphologic Features of Selective Yeast Forms

	Small			Intermediate		Large
Feature	Candida	Pneumocystis	Histoplasma	Cryptococcus	Blastomyces	Coccidioides
Size (μm)	3–4	5–8	2–5	5–15	8–20	20–200
Shape	Oval	Pleomorphic	Oval	Pleomorphic	Round	Round
Budding	None	None	Narrow-based	Narrow-based	Broad-based	None
Wall thickness	Thin	Thin	Thin	Thin	Thick	Thick
Hyphae/ pseudohyphae	Common; characteristic	Absent	Rare	Rare	Rare	Occasional
Other features	Single and chains	Intracystic body Trophozoite forms	Intracellular Refractile	Mucicarmine + capsule Acapsular forms	Double-contour wall	Endospores, immature spherules

Modified from Chandler FW, Watts JC. *Pathologic Diagnosis of Fungal Infections.* ASCP Press: Chicago; 1987:87.

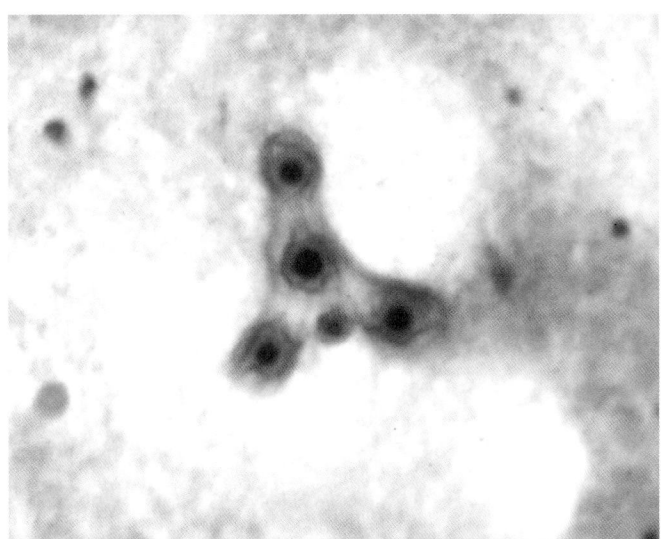

Figure 6-87. *Cryptococcus neoformans.* In this fine-needle aspirate, clusters of yeast cells resembling "spare tires" are invested by capsule in sparse inflammatory background (alcohol-fixed).

P. jiroveci most commonly is identified in exfoliative samples and aspirates by the presence of the foamy alveolar cast, which varies from eosinophilic to basophilic and is highly characteristic (Fig. 6-91A). These organisms rarely occur singly. The GMS stain outlines the characteristic cysts (see Fig. 6-91B).

Cytology of Common Mycelial Forms

The cytopathologist's most frequent challenge is the interpretation of mycelial forms in exfoliated material, especially the distinction between *Aspergillus* look-alikes—zygomycete and *Candida* hyphae. The morphologic features of some of the more common agents are compared in Table 6-8.

Candida species are readily seen and easily diagnosed when both yeasts and pseudohyphae are present. However, interpretation of their significance is difficult in all except transthoracic needle aspirates, where the presence of any mycelial structure, particularly in the setting of mass-like and cavitary infiltrates, provides strong morphologic evidence of infection.

Aspergillus species are characterized by septate mycelia that branch at angles approaching 45 degrees (Fig. 6-92). *Aspergillus* hyphae lack constrictions at points of septation. However, *Aspergillus* organisms cannot be differentiated from one of their mimics by morphology

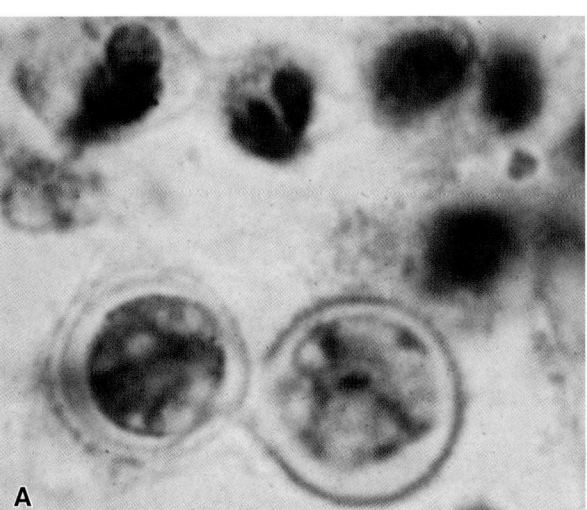
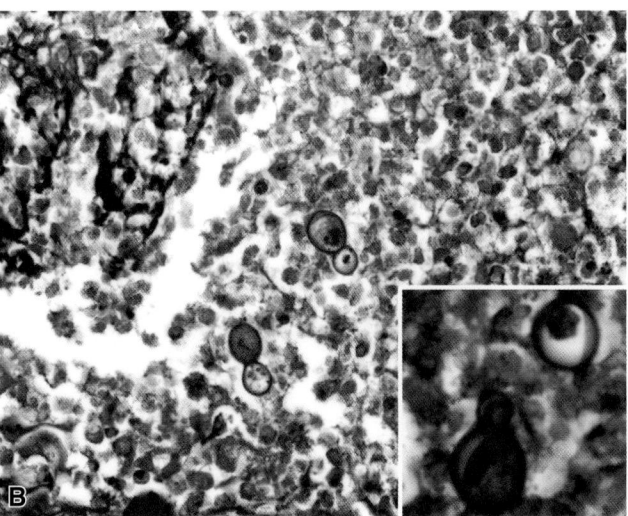

Figure 6-88. *Blastomyces dermatitidis.* **A,** Necroinflammatory infiltrate with refractile yeast forms. **B,** Periodic acid/Schiff staining highlights the double-contoured yeast with broad-based budding (see *inset* for greater detail).

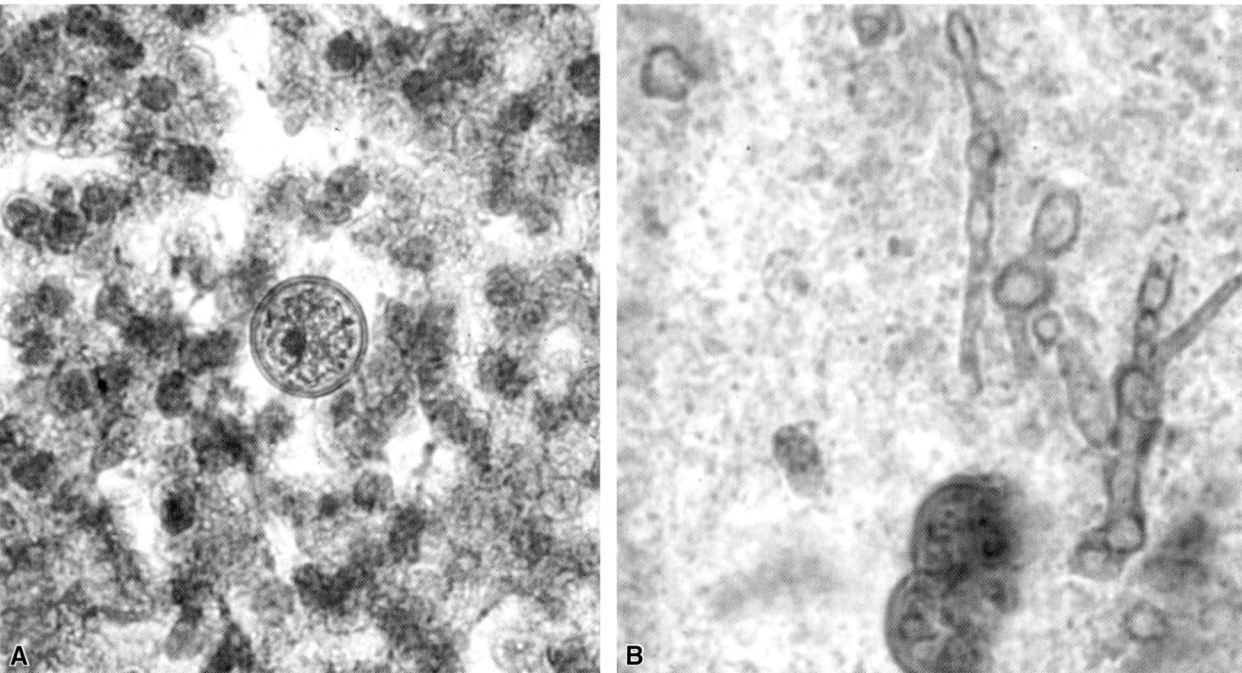

Figure 6-89. *Coccidioides* species. **A,** Negative-staining spherule in suppurative inflammatory background in a fine-needle aspirate (alcohol-fixed). **B,** Ruptured spherules and mycelia with arthrospores in granular necrotic background in another fine-needle aspirate (alcohol-fixed).

alone unless accompanied by a fruiting body. A rapid in situ hybridization technique specific for *Aspergillus* species can be performed on pulmonary cytocentrifuge preparations, as well as on tissue.[239] An additional advantage is that this technique may assist in this otherwise difficult differential diagnosis.

Zygomycete mycelia are distinguished from *Aspergillus* and *Candida* forms by their often broader width and their pleomorphic,

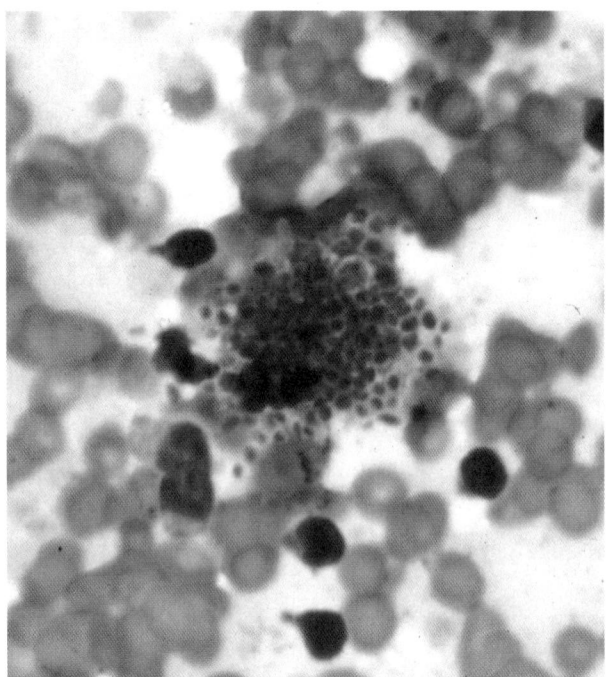

Figure 6-90. *Histoplasma capsulatum.* Clusters of purple polarized yeast cells are readily seen in this fine-needle aspirate (Diff-Quik preparation).

twisted ribbon-like, pauciseptate features. Of note, however, in aspirates of aspergilloma, the mycelia also may have a twisted appearance.

A potential pitfall in the evaluation of cytopathologic specimens in fungal infections (both exfoliative samples and needle aspirates) is the confounding presence of atypical reactive squamous cells and type II pneumocytes, which can mimic the cytologic atypia of malignant neoplasms.[46] Furthermore, the pathologist interpreting lung biopsy findings, especially with transbronchial specimens, should always attempt to correlate such findings with samples that may have been collected for cytologic or microbiologic study. This is especially advisable because etiologic agents that escape detection in tissue, such as *Pneumocystis, Aspergillus,* and CMV, may be found in washings or lavage fluid.[240]

Microbiology

Complementary laboratory methods are often required for diagnosis of fungal infection, and these are listed in Box 6-21.[182] Under the microscope, many fungi are readily apparent in H&E-stained sections, where they appear colorless (negative staining) or phaeoid (naturally pigmented). The GMS stain is the best histologic stain for demonstrating fungi when they are sparse or not visible on H&E sections. However, some fungi, notably the zygomycetes, may stain poorly with GMS. The GMS preparation can be counterstained with H&E, allowing co-evaluation of the host inflammatory response. The Fontana-Masson stain has been used to detect melanin in *C. neoformans* and phaeoid fungi, but many *Aspergillus* species and some zygomycetes also also will stain with this reagent.[225,241] The PAS stain can be useful in select circumstances, and histochemical stains for mucin (Alcian blue or mucicarmine) are useful for *C. neoformans* infections. The PAS and mucin preparations also can be counterstained with GMS or Fontana-Masson to simultaneously highlight cell walls and capsules of cryptococci. It is important to recognize that not everything that stains with the silver methods is a fungus, and care must be taken to distinguish organisms from pseudomicrobes, such as overstained red cells, white

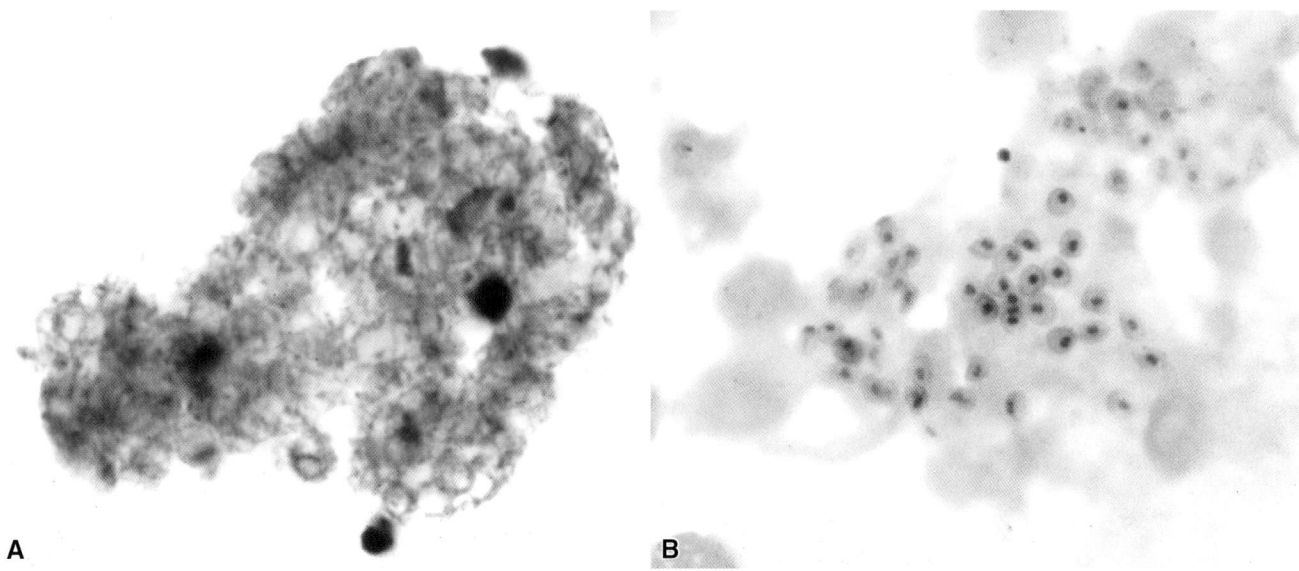

Figure 6-91. *Pneumocystis jiroveci.* **A,** Foamy alveolar cast in bronchial washing (ThinPrep Papanicolaou stain). **B,** Cysts with intracystic dot in bronchial washing (ThinPrep, Grocott methenamine silver stain).

Table 6-8. Morphologic Features of Selected Fungal Mycelia

Feature	*Aspergillus*	*Bipolaris*	Zygomycetes	*Pseudallescheria boydii*	*Fusarium*
Width (μm)	3–6	2–6	5–20	2–5	3–8
Contour	Parallel	Parallel	Irregular	Parallel	Parallel
Branching	Dichotomous	Haphazard	Wide angle	Haphazard	90-degree angle
Branch orientation	Parallel	Random	Random	Random	Random
Septation	Frequent	Frequent	Infrequent	Frequent	Frequent
Phaeoid (Brown)	No	Yes	No	Usually not	No
Angioinvasive	Yes	No	Yes	Yes	Yes
Other features	Fruiting body; oxalate crystals sometimes	Chlamydoconidia sometimes One of many dematiaceous genera	Rarely Chlamydoconidia	*Aspergillus* "look-alikes"	*Aspergillus* "look-alikes"

Modified from Chandler FW, Watts JC. *Pathologic Diagnosis of Fungal Infections.* ASCP Press: Chicago; 1987:204.

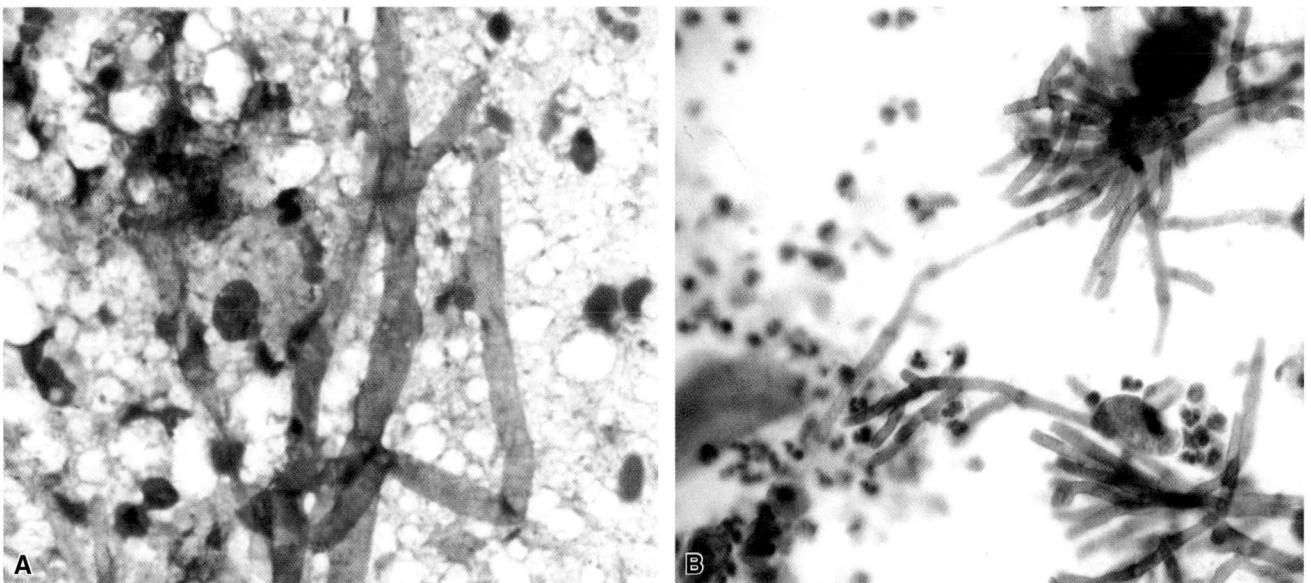

Figure 6-92. *Aspergillus* species. **A,** Twisted, sparsely septate mycelia are difficult to differentiate from mimics, including zygomycetes, in this fine-needle aspirate (Diff-Quik preparation). **B,** Characteristic mycelia in a bronchial washing (Papanicolaou stain).

Box 6-21. Laboratory Diagnosis of Fungal Pneumonia

Direct detection of organisms
    Chemofluorescence stains
    Direct fluorescent antibody stain
    Histopathologic/cytopathologic examination
    Immunohistochemical studies
Antigen detection (in suspected histoplasmosis and cryptococcosis)
Culture
    Emmons modified Sabouraud agar
    Brain-heart infusion agar
    Special and selective media
Serologic testing
Molecular methods
    In situ hybridization
    DNA amplification

blood cell nuclei, reticulin and elastic fibers, calcium deposits, and even Hamazaki-Wesenberg bodies.[40]

In the microbiology laboratory, the age-old technique of direct light microscopic visualization of fluids, exudates, and tissue homogenates treated with potassium hydroxide (KOH) is being replaced by chemofluorescent cotton-brightening agents (such as calcofluor white and fungiqual). Fluorescence microscopy with these reagents can detect a wide variety of fungi in wet mounts as well as frozen sections and paraffin-embedded tissue.[242,243]

The time-honored laboratory techniques for the identification of fungi (gross colonial and microscopic morphologic analysis after isolation on fungal media, followed by biochemical testing) may be the principal means to an etiologic diagnosis. For deep tissues, including the lung and other sterile sites, the Emmons modification of Saboraud glucose agar with chloramphenicol is recommended by many mycologists.[244] Additional use of enriched media such as brain-heart infusion agar can improve recovery of *C. neoformans, B. dermatitidis,* and *H. capsulatum*. Selective media containing cyclohexamide are not recommended for normally sterile sites, because they are potentially inhibitory for yeasts, such as *Cryptococcus* and *Candida* species, and molds, such as *Aspergillus* and zygomycetes.

The interpretation of a positive fungal culture must be made in the clinical context. In the absence of proof of tissue invasion, or compelling ancillary data, the interpretation of laboratory results requires considerable judgement. This is because many fungi are ubiquitous in the environment, and most fungal isolates from nonsterile respiratory samples do not represent disease unless there are also significant risk factors such as HIV infection, organ transplantation, or immunocompromising drug therapy.[245]

For most of the dimorphic fungi, in vitro hyphae-to-yeast conversion studies have given way to commercially available nucleic acid probes for rapid specific identification. Procurement of tissue for culture before formalin fixation is important whenever fungal infections are suspected. The tissue sample should be kept moist using sterile, nonbacteriostatic, saline or Ringers Solution. Specimens are minced, but not ground, before plating.

The value of bringing multiple, often complementary laboratory methods to bear on inconclusive morphologic findings cannot be overemphasized. In this context, while culture has been considered the most reliable method for definitive diagnosis, and histopathology often the fastest, the greatest yield results from combining histopathology with traditional culture and one or more of the newer molecular methods.[246,247] Culture may fail to yield an isolate even in the face of positive microscopic findings. In fact, the yield from tissue specimens, needle aspirates, BAL fluid samples, and bronchial washings is quite low for molds and other fungi, for reasons that are not entirely

clear.[47,248] Immunofluorescence testing using specific monoclonal antibodies can achieve rapid and specific diagnosis in selected infections, especially when tissue has not been submitted for culture. Antibodies directed against the antigens of *Aspergillus* species and selected other fungi have been described but most are not yet commercially available. For the problematic case, the mycology section of the CDC can provide assistance. Immunohistochemical identification of fungi can be accomplished fairly easily for those species for which reagents are commercially available.[32,249,250]

Molecular techniques, including in-situ hybridization and amplification technologies such as PCR, are other powerful tools that can provide rapid, accurate diagnosis for yeasts and molds which may be present in small numbers or manifest overlapping histologic features with one another.[243,251-253] A few laboratories (including the CDC) are performing such assays. Use of quantitative real-time PCR assays on blood, body fluids, and other samples holds promise for relatively rapid definitive diagnosis when routine methods of isolation and identification fail in critical situations.[254]

Serologic tests can support a morphologic diagnosis when positive titers are present, but effective serodiagnosis of systemic fungal infections is not available for most fungi.[255] Unfortunately, an antibody response does not necessarily correlate with invasive disease; and an antibody response may be lacking for various reasons. False-positive results due to cross reactions and false-negative results due to a variety of reasons plague many of these assays. Some of the most accurate serologic tests (with high sensitivity and specificity) for fungal infections are those for histoplasmosis and coccidioidomycosis, yet tests for both have limitations that must be recognized in interpreting results.[256,257]

The detection of macromolecular antigens shed into various body fluids requires a relatively large microbial burden which tends to limit sensitivity for most fungal infections except histoplasmosis and crytococcosis.[246] For these two fungi, useful antigen detection techniques are available using serum, urine, cerebrospinal and BAL fluids. They are especially sensitive in patients with defective immunity.[237,257] In patients with pneumonia and normal immunity, however, these tests may be positive in lavage fluid but negative in urine unless the disease has disseminated. Other assays designed to detect antigens or metabolites of invasive fungi include those for 1,3β-D-glucan, a cell wall component of several fungi such as *Aspergillus, Candida, Fusarium,* and others, and for galactomannin, a polysaccharide antigen in the cell wall of *Aspergillus,* have shown fair sensitivity and specificity.[181,258]

Differential Diagnosis

A synopsis of the key morphologic and mycologic features of the fungal pneumonias is presented in Table 6-9. When H&E and GMS stains fail to detect or clearly identify fungal elements in a suspected fungal infection, the use of ancillary procedures may provide the specific diagnosis. Sometimes, if tissue or other patient specimens have been submitted for culture, the answer may lie in the mycology section of the microbiology laboratory, as many species begin to grow in a matter of days. When fungi are not readily identified by any of these techniques or strategies, other granulomatous infections should be considered, especially mycobacterial, uncommon bacterial (e.g., tularemia, brucellosis), and parasitic infections. Noninfectious necrotizing and non-necrotizing granulomatous disorders also enter the differential diagnosis. These include Wegener granulomatosis, idiopathic bronchocentric granulomatosis, aspiration, sarcoidosis, rheumatoid nodules, pyoderma gangrenosum–like lung lesions in patients with inflammatory bowel disease, and Churg-Strauss syndrome.

Table 6-9. Fungal Pneumonias: Summary of Pathologic Findings

Assessment Component	Findings
Blastomycosis	
Surgical pathology	Suppurative granuloma most characteristic; also, tuberculoid (necrotizing) types Round, thick-walled (double-contour) yeast with broad-based budding
Cytopathology	Neutrophils and epithelioid cells with characteristic refractile yeast cell with double-contoured wall and broad-based budding
Microbiology	Characteristic yeast seen on wet mount, KOH- and calcofluor-stained smear Culture-sterile lung tissue on nonselective fungal media (e.g., Emmons modified Sabouraud) and enriched media (e.g., brain-heart infusion) Add selective media for bronchial/transbronchial samples Colonies produce oval conidia on terminal ends of conidiophore at right angle to mycelium Confirm with DNA probe Serologic studies not useful
Coccidioidomycosis	
Surgical pathology	Fibrocaseous granuloma Large intact and/or ruptured spherules, full or partially or completely empty of endospores Mycelial forms in aerated cavities and fistula
Cytopathology	Necroinflammatory debris with epithelioid histiocytes Intact, viable, colorless spherules with variable number of endospores and/or ruptured degenerating forms with stained wall; range in size from large mature to small immature types
Microbiology	Characteristic mature spherules in wet mount, KOH- and calcofluor-stained smear Culture of sterile lung tissue on nonselective fungal media yields mycelia with characteristic arthroconidia Confirm with DNA probe Serologic diagnosis with tests for IgG and IgM antibodies by immunodiffusion, EIA; complement fixation for titers
Histoplasmosis	
Surgical pathology	Macrophage reaction and/or granulomas, based on immunity, including miliary and solitary pulmonary, variably hyalinized nodule Small, thin-walled, oval yeasts with narrow-based buds, often refractile
Cytopathology	Macrophage and epithelioid cells with characteristic yeast cell, often intracellular, stained purple with Diff-Quik, black with GMS
Microbiology	Rarely detected by direct examination of most clinical specimens Culture sterile lung tissue on nonselective and enriched fungal media produces tuberculate macroconidia Confirm with DNA probe Antigen detection by EIA available for BAL fluid, CSF, serum, and urine
Paracoccidioidomycosis	
Surgical pathology	Exudative or granulomatous lesion with large, globose yeast cell with multiple buds
Cytopathology	Suppurative or granulomatous reaction with characteristic yeast cell
Microbiology	Direct detection in wet mount, KOH- and calcofluor-stained smear Culture-sterile lung tissue on standard nonselective fungal media Serologic testing by immunodiffusion, EIA; complement fixation for titer
Sporotrichosis	
Surgical pathology	Necrotizing granuloma, often cavitary with small, usually round, sometimes cigar-shape yeast with sparse, narrow buds
Cytopathology	Suppurative or necrotizing granuloma pattern Yeast cells generally sparse or absent
Microbiology	Rarely detected by direct examination of most clinical specimens Culture of sterile lung tissue on nonselective fungal media yield thin, hyphae-bearing conidia in a rosette pattern Converts to a yeast phase at 37°C on blood agar No serologic tests
Penicilliosis	
Surgical pathology	Alveolar macrophages stuffed with yeast cells resemble *Histoplasma* species, but with septum reflecting binary fission, not budding reproduction
Cytopathology	Macrophage with intracellular characteristic yeast forms

Continued

Table 6-9. Fungal Pneumonias: Summary of Pathologic Findings—cont'd

Assessment Component	Findings
Penicilliosis—cont'd	
Microbiology	Culture of sterile lung tissue on nonselective fungal media yields a mold with a red pigment evident as culture ages
	Erect conidiophores sometimes branched with metulae bearing one or several phialides with long, loose chains of oval conidia
	New urinary antigen test
Cryptococcosis	
Surgical pathology	Granulomas, histiocytic infiltrate or mucoid pneumonia, based on immunity with pale, round, budding pleomorphic yeast cells, often in clusters
	Mucoid capsules usually; acapsular types sometimes
Cytopathology	Yeast cell with mucoid capsular halo resembles "spare tire"
	Combination of mucicarmine and GMS or Fontana-Masson outlines capsule and cell wall
	Background of epithelioid cells or necroinflammatory debris may be sparse or absent
Microbiology	Oval to lemon-shaped calcofluor-positive yeast cell with capsule in India ink–stained touch imprint
	Culture on nonselective fungal media yields mucoid yeast-type colonies
	No pseudohyphae; germ tube–negative
	Dark brown pigment on birdseed (niger) agar
	Confirm with biochemical tests
	Antigen detection test (latex agglutination or EIA) on serum, BAL fluid, CSF, and needle aspirates
Candidiasis	
Surgical pathology	Miliary necroinflammatory lesions or bronchopneumonia with small, oval, budding yeasts with or without pseudohyphae
	C. glabrata yeast only
Cytopathology	Yeasts and/or pseudohyphae in a necroinflammatory background
Microbiology	Budding yeasts and pseudohyphae in wet mounts, KOH- and calcofluor-stained smears
	Cultures on selective and nonselective fungal media yield creamy tan to white yeast-type colonies
	Identification by germ tube production, carbohydrate assimilation, and cornmeal agar morphology
Aspergillosis	
Surgical pathology	Various forms include saprophytic (fungus ball), allergic (ABPA and mucoid impaction), hypersensitivity pneumonitis, and invasive disease, ranging in severity from minimal chronic necrotizing to extensive pneumonia
	Angiotrophic with necrotizing infarcts; also hybrid forms of disease
	Septate, dichotomous, 45-degree angle mycelia; oxalate crystals
	Presence of fruiting body is genus-specific
Cytopathology	Tangled clusters of septate mycelia in a necroinflammatory background
	May appear sparsely septate and twisted, mimicking zygomycetes
Microbiology	Positive staining of mycelia with calcofluor and GMS
	Culture of sterile lung tissue on nonselective fungal media produces mold-type colonies in a range of colors
	Species differentiation by conidial and conidiophore morphology
Zygomycosis	
Surgical pathology	Nodular lesions, lobar consolidations, cavitary lesions, fungus balls, and airway infections commonly necrotizing and ischemic secondary to angioinvasion
	Broad pauciseptate mycelia with 90-degree angle branching, often with twisted ribbon morphology
Cytopathology	Pauciseptate mycelia, often with twisted ribbon morphology in a necroinflammatory background
Microbiology	Positive staining of mycelia with calcofluor and GMS
	Rapidly growing cottony colonies are grown on most nonselective fungal media, but "controlled baiting" with bread sometimes necessary
	Identification based on presence and locations of rhizoids, shape of sporangia, presence of columellae, and shape of sporangiospores
Phaeohyphomycosis	
Surgical pathology	Allergic bronchopulmonary fungal disease similar to aspergillosis
Cytopathology	Similar to ABPA pattern—"allergic mucin" with eosinophils, Charcot-Leiden crystals in inspissated mucus
	Fungal mycelial fragments sparse or absent
Microbiology	Dematiaceous (phaeoid) dark brown to black colonies on nonselective fungal media
	Identified by shape and cross walls of multicell, pigmented conidia

Table 6-9. Fungal Pneumonias: Summary of Pathologic Findings—cont'd

Assessment Component	Findings
Pneumocystosis	
Surgical pathology	Pneumonia with foamy alveolar cast is classic; other patterns include diffuse alveolar damage, granulomatous lesions, and minimal changes Variable numbers of cysts noted in GMS-stained sections
Cytopathology	Foamy alveolar cast with characteristic cysts outlined by GMS
Microbiology	Causative organism: formerly *Pneumocystis carinii*, classified as a fungus and renamed *Pneumocystis jiroveci*; cannot be cultured Detection is with fluorescent monoclonal antibody assay or GMS-stained smears

ABPA, allergic bronchopulmonary aspergillosis; BAL, bronchoalveolar lavage; CSF, cerebrospinal fluid; EIA, enzyme immunoassay; GMS, Grocott methenamine silver; KOH, potassium hydroxide.

Viral Pneumonia

Viruses cause more infections than all other types of microorganisms combined, and involve the respiratory tract more commonly than other organ systems.[259] Fortunately, the lung diseases produced by viruses usually are mild and self-limited. Nevertheless, viruses cause major public health illnesses and account for many of the new and emerging diseases in today's headlines. At times, viruses also are capable of producing serious and life-threatening infections that come to the attention of pathologists in both immunocompromised patients and young, healthy persons.[260] The viruses that commonly infect the lung are listed in Table 6-10.

Etiologic Agents

The conventional respiratory viruses—influenza virus, parainfluenza virus, RSV, and adenovirus—cause outbreaks of respiratory illness in the general population each year. In infants, the elderly, and in those patients with chronic diseases, these pathogens can cause serious pneumonias. Pneumonia in immunocompromised persons usually is attributed to the herpesviruses (herpes simplex virus and CMV). Less appreciated is that the conventional respiratory viruses also are frequent causes of respiratory illness in these patients, and that such infections result in high rates of morbidity and mortality.[261]

Newly recognized respiratory viruses[262,263] include a highly pathogenic strain of influenza, H5N1. First detected in 1997 in Hong Kong, it has since spread to Europe, the Middle East and Africa. Another unique, triple-reassortment swine-origin influenza virus A, H1N1 (S-OIV), emerged in 2009 as the cause of outbreaks sustained by person-to-person transmission in multiple countries. It was characterized by respiratory illness of variable severity ranging from self-limited disease resembling seasonal flu to severe illness requiring hospitalization and occasionally eventuating in death from respiratory failure.[264] An acute cardiopulmonary syndrome in the southwest United States was etiologically linked to a new hantavirus referred to as *Sin Nombre* ("without a name"). The severe acute respiratory syndrome (SARS), which began in southern China and was carried by travelers to 33 other countries and 5 continents, was caused by a newly recognized coronavirus, SARS-CoV. Four other coronaviruses linked to respiratory illnesses (HCoV-229E; HCoV-NL63; HCoV-OC43;

HCoV-HKU1) have since been reported.[265] Human metapneumovirus, a paramyxovirus closely related to RSV, clinically and pathologically, has become recognized as one of the leading causes of respiratory illness in children and also can cause illness in adults and immunocompromised patients. Human bocavirus (h0bv) has been isolated in several countries from children with wheezing.[266] Qther viruses such as the picornavirus group (rhinovirus and enterovirus) can cause pneumonia, as can BK polyoma virus.[267] Other unusual viral lung infections have been attributed to henipah and hemorrhagic fever viruses.[268] Parvovirus B19, an erythrovirus, has long been known to cause disease, primarily in maternal-fetal and pediatric patients. Recently, an autoimmune-type pneumonitis associated with serologic evidence of parvovirus B19 also has been described.[269] The evolution of diagnostic laboratory methods and large-scale molecular screening suggests that more viruses will be linked to respiratory tract disease in the future.

Histopathology

The respiratory tract viruses have a tendency to target specific regions of the tracheobronchial tree and lungs, producing characteristic clinical syndromes. However, sufficient overlap clinically, radiologically, and pathologically often limits a strict interpretation of findings for a definitive diagnosis. Box 6-22 can sometimes be useful in narrowing the search for a specific etiologic agent. The microscopic findings in most pulmonary viral infections include the direct effect of the virus as well as the host's inflammatory response. The clinical outcome depends upon the virulence of the organism and the nature of the host response, be it diffuse alveolar damage, diffuse or patchy bronchiolitis and interstitial pneumonits, giant cell reactions, or even minimal change.[270]

The histopathologic diagnosis of viral infection is impossible without identification of the characteristic CPE. The term *cytopathic effect* traditionally has been used by virologists to describe cellular changes in unstained cell culture monolayers seen by light microscopy,[271,272] but it can be applied to all virus-associated nuclear and cytoplasmic alterations seen on H&E-stained slides or highlighted by immunohistochemical staining, molecular in situ–based methodology, or ultrastructural localization.[273,274] Diffuse alveolar damage, often with bronchiolitis, is the most typical pattern of viral lung injury. As noted earlier, however, diffuse alveolar damage also occurs in bacterial, mycobacterial, and fungal

Table 6-10. Viral Pathogens of the Lung

RNA Viruses	DNA Viruses
Influenza virus	Adenovirus
Parainfluenza virus	Herpes simplex virus
Respiratory syncytial virus	Varicella-zoster virus
Measles virus	Cytomegalovirus
Hantavirus	Epstein-Barr virus

Box 6-22. Histopathologic Patterns in Viral Lung Injury

Diffuse alveolar damage
Bronchitis and bronchiolitis
Diffuse interstitial pneumonia
Perivascular lymphoid infiltrates
Miliary small nodules
Air space organization—bronchiolitis obliterans–organizing pneumonia (BOOP) pattern
Calcified nodules

Table 6-11. Cytopathic Effects in Pulmonary Infections with Selected Viruses

Virus	Intranuclear	Intracytoplasmic	Inclusion Characteristics
	Presence of Inclusions		
Herpes simplex virus; varicella-zoster virus	+	−	Early ground-glass appearance; later eosinophilic (Cowdry A type) multinucleate cells
Adenovirus	+	−	Early eosinophilic (Cowdry A); later basophilic, smudged nucleus
Cytomegalovirus	+	+	Cytomegaly with large "owl eye" amphophilic (Cowdry A) nuclear and multiple smaller basophilic (GMS-positive), cytoplasmic type
Respiratory syncytial virus	−	+	Eosinophilic smooth, small, often indistinct Multinucleate syncytia in some cases
Measles virus	+	+	Eosinophilic nuclear (Cowdry A) in multinucleate cells Cytoplasmic type—eosinophilic, pleomorphic
Parainfluenza virus	−	+	Rarely observed, pleomorphic, eosinophilic Multinucleate syncytia rarely
Influenza virus	−	−	No inclusions or other distinctive cytopathic effects

pneumonias, so a careful search for specific viral CPE becomes important in this setting. For the surgical pathologist, CPE manifests mainly as the viral inclusion present in the nucleus or cytoplasm of an infected cell. Viral inclusions confer diagnostic specificity to the pathologic pattern of injury in which they are found, and for the common respiratory tract viruses, the features are presented in Table 6-11. Finally, it is worth mentioning that most clinically significant viral pneumonias that have CPE also show necrosis somewhere in the biopsy.

Influenza virus

Influenzaviruses are the most pathogenic of the respiratory viruses and predispose patients most commonly to secondary bacterial pneumonia. These viruses also account for the greatest public health burden. Annually, they cause epidemic outbreaks of respiratory disease that are often associated with considerable morbidity; periodically, they produce pandemics with high mortality rates. These viruses target the ciliated epithelium of the tracheobronchial tree, producing necrotizing bronchitis and bronchiolitis and a spectrum of changes that vary depending on the stage of the disease (early versus late), outcome (fatal versus nonfatal), and the presence or absence of secondary bacterial pneumonia. Uncomplicated influenza pneumonia is rarely biopsied today. Based on historical data from bronchoscopic biopsies performed in the 1950s and early 1960s, the histopathologic findings in nonfatal uncomplicated influenza are those of active tracheobronchitis.[275] Necrosis and desquamation of the epithelial cells to the basement membrane is associated with a relatively scant lymphocytic infiltrate; however, in more severe cases, the virus and its attendant inflammatory response spread more distally into the respiratory bronchioles and alveoli, with hemorrhage, edema, fibrinous exudate with hyline membranes, and patchy interstitial cellular infiltrates (Fig. 6-93). This constellation of findings comprises

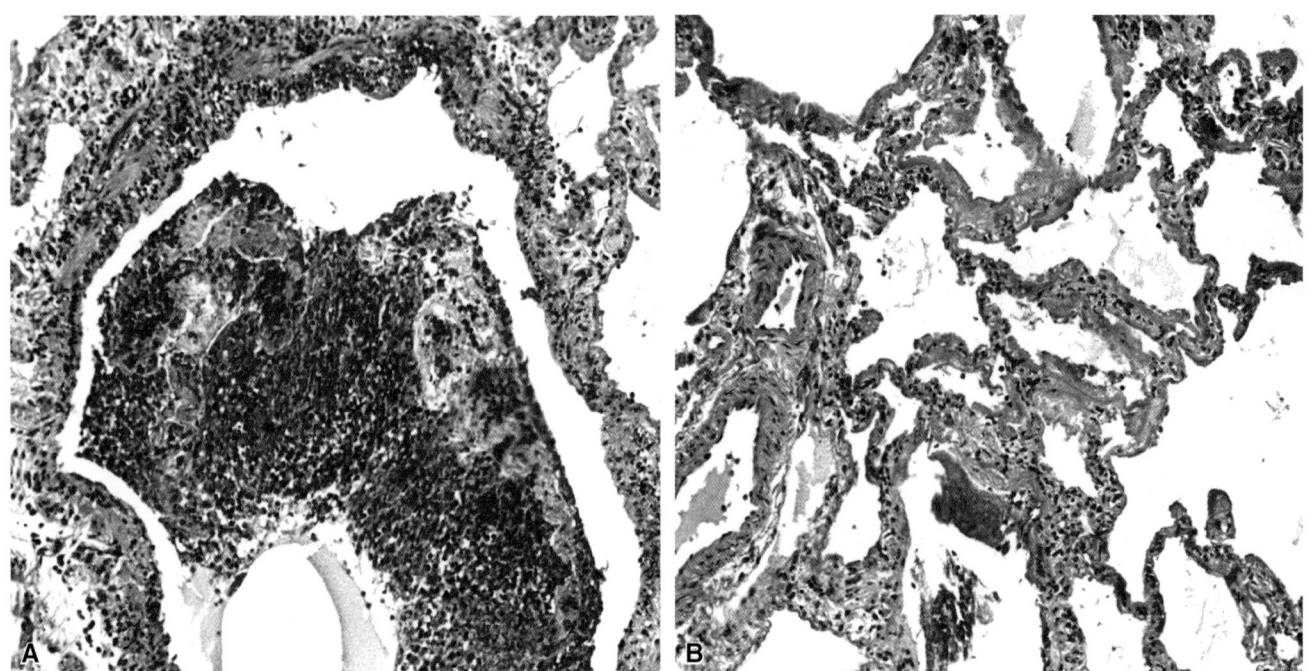

Figure 6-93. Influenza virus. **A,** Bronchiolitis with intraluminal necroinflammatory debris. **B,** Acute diffuse alveolar damage pattern with hyaline membranes.

the "lesion of characterization."[276] In contemporary pathologic terms this would correspond to diffuse alveolar damage, and clinically, a primary viral pneumonia. Depending on the clinical course and time of lung biopsy (or autopsy) within the first 2 weeks of illness, the process may be in the acute and/or organizing phase.[277,278] Later, the airway epithelial damage may pave the way for secondary bacterial pneumonia, which accounts for much of the morbidity and mortality of influenza and which may obscure the features of primary viral pneumonia.

From 2003 through 2008, 391 human cases of highly pathogenic avian influenza involving the H5N1 strain were recorded, with 247 deaths.[279] The histopathologic changes observed in the few autopsied cases fall within the spectrum of findings described during the pandemics of 1918, 1957, and 1968 and in fatal cases of interpandemic (seasonal) influenza.[278] A characteristic feature of the the H5N1 and 1918 cases is the high mortality rate, especially among previouly healthy older children and young adults. Excessively high levels of cytokine and chemokines are thought to play an important role in the pathogenesis of the acute lung injury pattern seen in these fatal cases of influenza.[280] Because these viruses produce no characteristic cellular inclusions, etiologic diagnosis is not possible by morphology alone, and requires antigen detection by immunofluorescence, immunohistochemistry, in situ hybridization, or culture.[281]

Parainfluenza Virus

Parainfluenza virus comprises four serotypes (I to IV) that typically target the upper respiratory tract, classically in the form of croup.[282] Some cases involve distal airways, as in infections due to RSV and influenza virus, but are milder, with less morbidity and requiring fewer hospitalizations. A few documented cases have been described with a diffuse alveolar damage pattern or an interstitial pneumonitis with giant cells, the latter resembling those of measles and respiratory syncytial virus infection. The giant cells of parainfluenza tend to be larger and have more intracytoplasmic inclusions.[51] Parainfluenza virus is a potential opportunist in immunocompromised patients, especially children with congenital immunodeficiency disorders[283] in whom fatal pneumonitis with disseminated disease may occur.[284]

Respiratory Syncytial Virus

RSV causes more significant respiratory infections in early childhood than those attributable to either influenza viruses or parainfluenza viruses.[285] The annual outbreaks of bronchiolitis and pneumonia in infants are especially severe during the first year of life, and in those of low birth weight or with cardiopulmonary disease.[282] Considered primarily a childhood virus, RSV has more recently been recognized as the etiologic agent of pneumonia in community-dwelling and high-risk adults with chronic lung disease requiring hospitalization.[283,286,287] Also, RSV is often an unsuspected opportunistic pathogen in immunocompromised patients.[261,288] RSV targets the epithelium of the distal airway, producing bronchiolitis with disorganization of the epithelium and epithelial cell sloughing[268] (Fig. 6-94A). In fatal cases, airway obstruction due to sloughed cell detritus, mucus, and fibrin is compounded by airway lymphoid hyperplasia.[289] Diffuse alveolar damage may be seen in immunocompromised patients. Giant cells (syncytia), similar to the cytopathic changes seen in cell culture, may be present in alveolar ducts and air spaces around areas of bronchiolitis (see Fig. 6-94B). Eosinophilic inclusions in cytoplasm may be seen in tissues and cytology specimens from immunosuppressed patients, but these are difficult to confirm as diagnostic of RSV without immunohistochemistry.

Human Metapneumovirus

Human metapneumovirus, a newly recognized paramyxovirus, is a leading cause of respiratory tract disease in infants, with annual epidemics occurring during the winter and early spring months.[290]

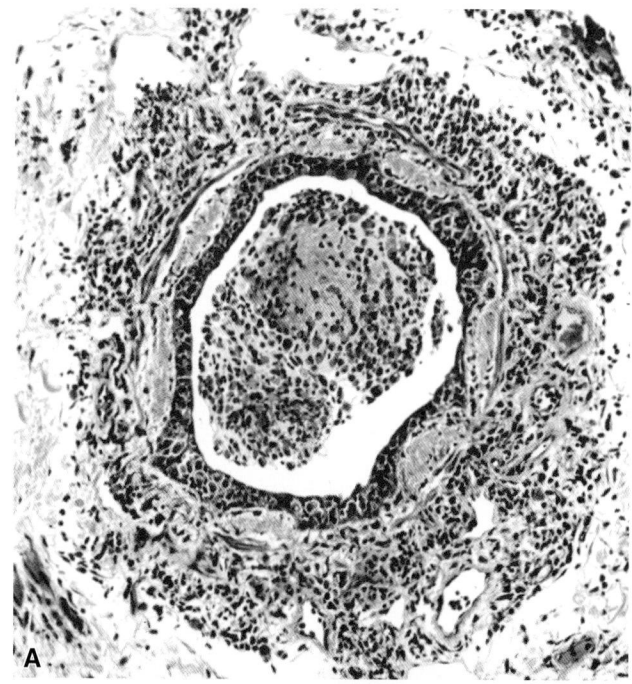

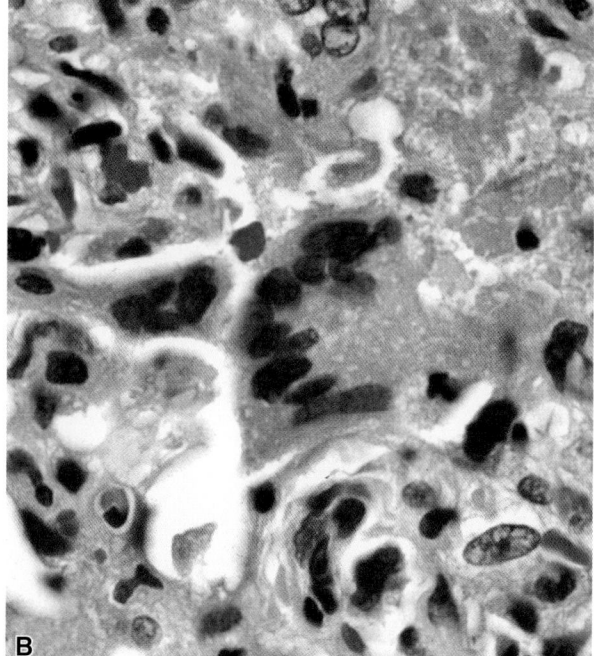

Figure 6-94. Respiratory syncytial virus. **A,** Bronchiolitis with intraluminal sloughing. **B,** Bronchiolitis with giant cell syncytia.

The virus also causes disease in immunocompromised patients and likely explains some lower respiratory tract infections in the elderly. The clinical spectrum of croup, bronchiolitis, and pneumonia is similar to that for infections due to other paramyxoviruses such as RSV and parainfluenza virus. The pathologic features are not well characterized, because few well-documented cases have included biopsy in the evaluation. However, histopathologic assessment of lung tissue in severe cases has revealed acute and organizing diffuse alveolar damage, as well as smudge cell formation.[291,292] The definitive identification of the virus can be established in tissue culture, but monoclonal antibody reagents and molecular techniques (real-time PCR assay) are the current diagnostic methods of choice.

Measles Virus

The measles virus causes a highly communicable childhood viral exanthema worldwide that, unlike varicella (chickenpox), leads to complications that are common and serious.[293] Measels pneumonia accounts for the vast majority of measles-related deaths and most of these are a consequence of secondary pneumonia (bacterial or viral), or attributable to an aberrant immune response. Primary viral pneumonia occurs, but is uncommon, even in immunocompromised hosts. Microscopically, bronchial and bronchiolar epithelial degeneration and reactive hyperplasia with squamous metaplasia is typically accompanied by peribronchial inflammation. Diffuse alveolar damage may occur and quantitative immmunohistochemical studies have revealed severe immune dysfunction with loss of key effector cells and their cytokines.[294] Characteristic giant cells show distintive intranuclear eosinophilic inclusions surrounded by halos (Fig. 6-95). This is the classic measles injury pattern[268] and is referred to as Hecht giant cell pneumonia. Minute intracytoplasmic eosinophilic inclusions precede the development of the intranuclear inclusions, and are often difficult to identify. Pneumonia with giant cells should always suggest measles, but similar changes can be seen in RSV and parainfluenza pneumonias, and not all cases of measles pneumonia have these giant cells.[268] Hard metal pneumoconiosis (giant cell interstitial pneumonia) is in the differential diagnosis, but the overall appearance of hard metal disease is one of a chronic disease with some fibrosis, and few if any acute changes. In the absence of giant cells, the cellular interstitial pneumonia must be differentiated from those caused by other viruses and atypical pneumonia agents, as well as from nonspecific interstitial pneumonia (NSIP).

Hantavirus

The recently identified hantavirus produces a rapidly evolving cardiopulmonary syndrome with a high mortality rate. This disorder first came to public attention as an emerging infection following an outbreak in the southwestern United States in 1993 that was causally linked to a previously unrecognized hantavirus. All members of this genus are zoonotic and are found in rodents around the world. The specific type responsible for the cardiopulmonary syndrome, designated *Sin Nombre* ("without a name"), is present in rodent feces and is acquired from the environment through inhalation. It produces florid pulmonary edema with pleural effusions, variable fibrin deposits, and focal wispy hyaline membranes[295] (Fig. 6-96A). Immunoblast-like cells are present in vascular spaces and in the peripheral blood (see Fig. 6-96B). Morphologic diagnosis is presumptive, because hantaviral antigen in endothelial cells, detected by immunohistochemistry, is required for definitive diagnosis.[296] In the appropriate clinical setting, clues to the diagnosis can sometimes be found in a constellation of morphologic findings on a peripheral blood smear, and confirmation can be achieved serologically by detection of hantavirus-specific immunoglobulin M (IgM) antibodies, or by detection of hantavirus RNA by PCR assay in peripheral blood leukocytes.[297,298]

Coronaviruses

Coronaviruses are ubiquitous RNA viruses known to cause disease in many animals. At least five different coronaviruses are known to infect humans and these cluster into two antigenic groups.[265] They are responsible for a majority of common colds, along with the rhinoviruses. Co-infections with other respiratory viruses occur in infants and children presenting with more severe respiratory disease. In certain

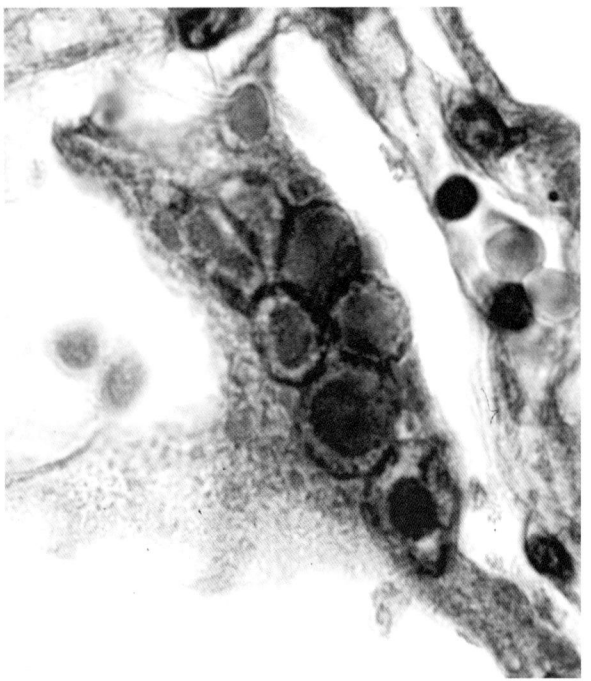

Figure 6-95. Measles virus pneumonia with characteristic eosinophilic intranuclear inclusions in giant cell.

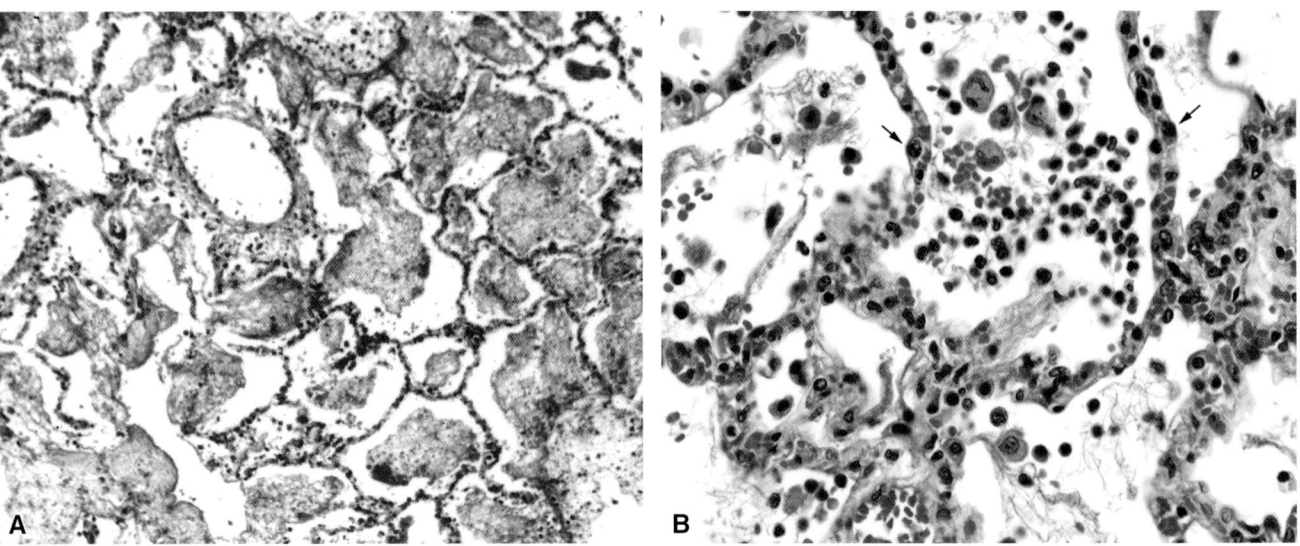

Figure 6-96. Hantavirus. **A,** Pulmonary edema with fibrin deposits. **B,** Immunoblast-like cells in alveolar capillaries at *arrows*.

epidemiologic situations, they can cause pneumonia in children, frail elderly individuals, and immunocompromised adults.[299,300]

In November 2002, the appearance of an atypical pneumonia in China, subsequently labeled *severe acute respiratory syndrome* (SARS), became an alarming global health problem in the period of a few months.[301] The disease was linked (Koch's postulates were fulfilled) by means of tissue culture isolation, electron microscopy, and molecular analysis to an emergent novel coronavirus, proposed as the Urbani strain of SARS-associated coronavirus.[302]

Clinically, the disease ranges from a nonhypoxemic febrile respiratory disease (with minimal symptoms in some patients) to one of severe pulmonary dysfunction, manifesting as acute respiratory distress syndrome and eventuating in death for approximately 5% of the patients affected.[303] In the reported cases, either the chest x-ray appearance on presentation was normal or the chest film showed unilateral, predominantly peripheral areas of consolidation that progressed to bilateral, patchy consolidation, the degree and extent of which correlated with the developmnent of respiratory failure. In patients who presented with normal x-ray appearance, CT scans often revealed bilateral ground-glass consolidation resembling that in bronchiolitis obliterans with organizing pneumonia (cryptogenic organizing pneumonia). Laboratory abnormalities in some but not all patients included leukopenia with lymphopenia and thrombocytopenia. The partial thromboplastin time and D-dimer levels were increased. Biochemical abnormalities included elevated lactate dehydrogenase (LDH), alanine aminotransferase, and creatinine levels. Lymphopenia and elevated LDH were helpful clues, but the clinical, radiologic, and laboratory features, although characteristic, were not distinguishable from those in patients with pneumonia caused by other viruses and bacteria and various atypical agents.

Histopathologic findings in lung biopsy and autopsy tissues included acute lung injury (diffuse alveolar damage) in various stages of organization.[304,305] Lung biopsy specimens in milder cases showed relatively scant intra-alveolar fibrin deposits with some congestion and edema (Fig. 6-97). However, the spectrum of findings included acute fibrinous pneumonia, hyaline membrane formation, interstitial lymphocytic infiltrates, desquamation of alveolar pneumocytes, and areas undergoing organization of the acute phase injury.[306] In some patients, multinucleate syncytial cells reminiscent of the CPE seen in influenza virus, RSV, and measles virus infections were noted. Viral inclusions were not identified, and initial immunohistochemical studies failed to reveal viral antigen. Subsequent investigations detected virus in epithelial cells

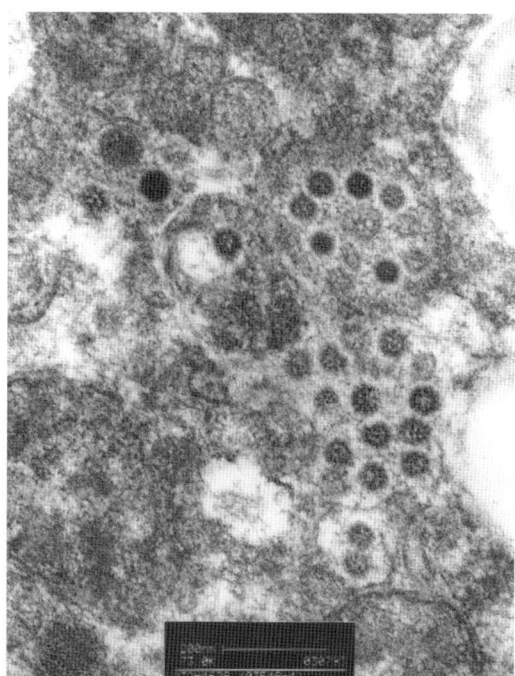

Figure 6-98. Coronavirus-infected cell can be seen in this electron photomicrograph. (Courtesy of Dr. Oi-Yee Cheung, Queen Elizabeth Hospital, Hong Kong, China.)

(predominantly type II pneumocytes) and alveolar macrophages using immunohistochemical staining, in situ hybridization, RT-PCR methods, and electron microscopy. A unique coronavirus (Fig. 6-98) was finally implicated as the etiologic agent.[306,307] Comparative histopathologic studies in fatal cases of SARS and H5N1 avian influenza reveal similarities and differences.[308] Both infections feature acute and organizing diffuse alveolar damage, but SARS appears to be more frequently associated with subacute injury with intra-alveolar organization, whereas H5N1 virus causes a more fulminant diffuse alveolar damage pattern with patchy intersitial inflammation and paucicellular fibrosis.

Adenovirus

Adenovirus comprises several genera, with multiple serotypes that cause infections of the upper and lower respiratory tract, conjunctiva,

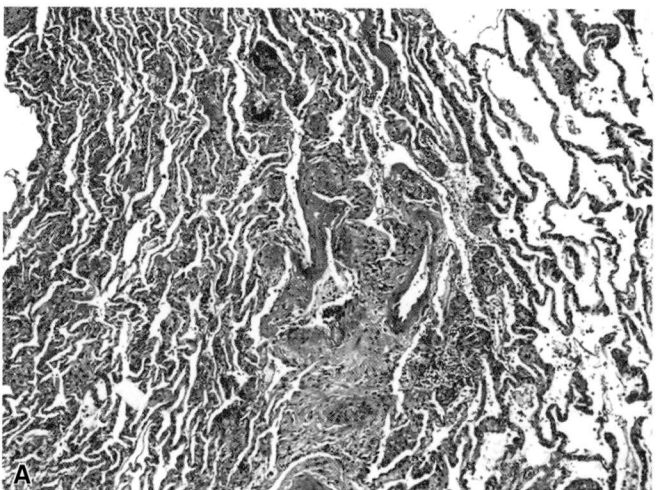
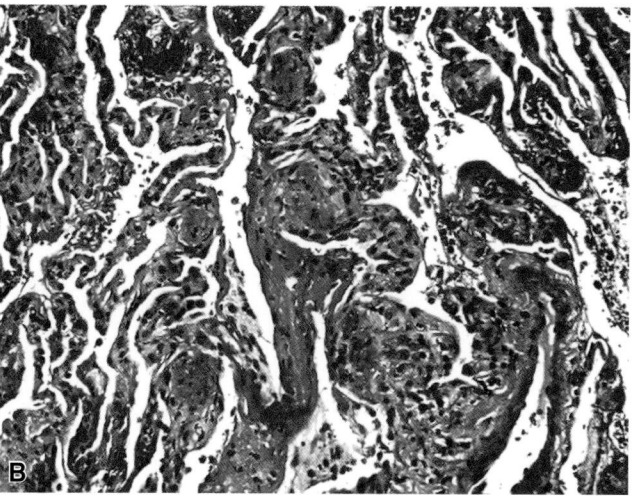

Figure 6-97. Coronavirus pneumonia: Severe acute respiratory syndrome (SARS). **A** and **B,** Acute fibrinous lung injury is evident. (Courtesy of Dr. Oi-Yee Cheung, Queen Elizabeth Hospital, Hong Kong, China.)

and gut. Respiratory tract infections are most common and account for approximately 5% to 10% of pediatric pneumonias. These can be especially severe in neonates and children and in immunocompomised persons.[268,309] In the lung, adenovirus infection produces two patterns of lung injury: diffuse alveolar damage, with or without necrotizing bronchiolitis, and pneumonitis with "dirty" or karyorrhectic necrosis[310] (Fig. 6-99). These patterns may coexist in some cases and the pneumonia may be accompanied by hemorrhage secondary to adenovirus-induced endothelial cell damage.[311] Two types of adenoviral CPE may be seen. Initially an eosinophilic (Cowdry A) intranuclear inclusion occurs surrounded by a halo with marginated chromatin, similar to herpes simplex virus (Fig. 6-100A). This later enlarges and becomes

amphophilic and then more basophilic, obliterating the nuclear membrane, producing the characteristic "smudge cell" (see Fig. 6-100B).[268]

Herpes Simplex Viruses

Herpes simplex virus (HSV) type I and type II have had traditional assigned roles as etiologic agents of mucocutaneous disease of the head and neck (type I) and genitalia (type II). Considerable crossover has been documented, however, with both types isolated from patients with disease at either site. Tracheobronchitis and pneumonia due to these viruses are rare in healthy adults with intact immune systems. They occur primarily in patients with underlying pulmonary disease and in association with inhalational and intubational trauma. They also occur

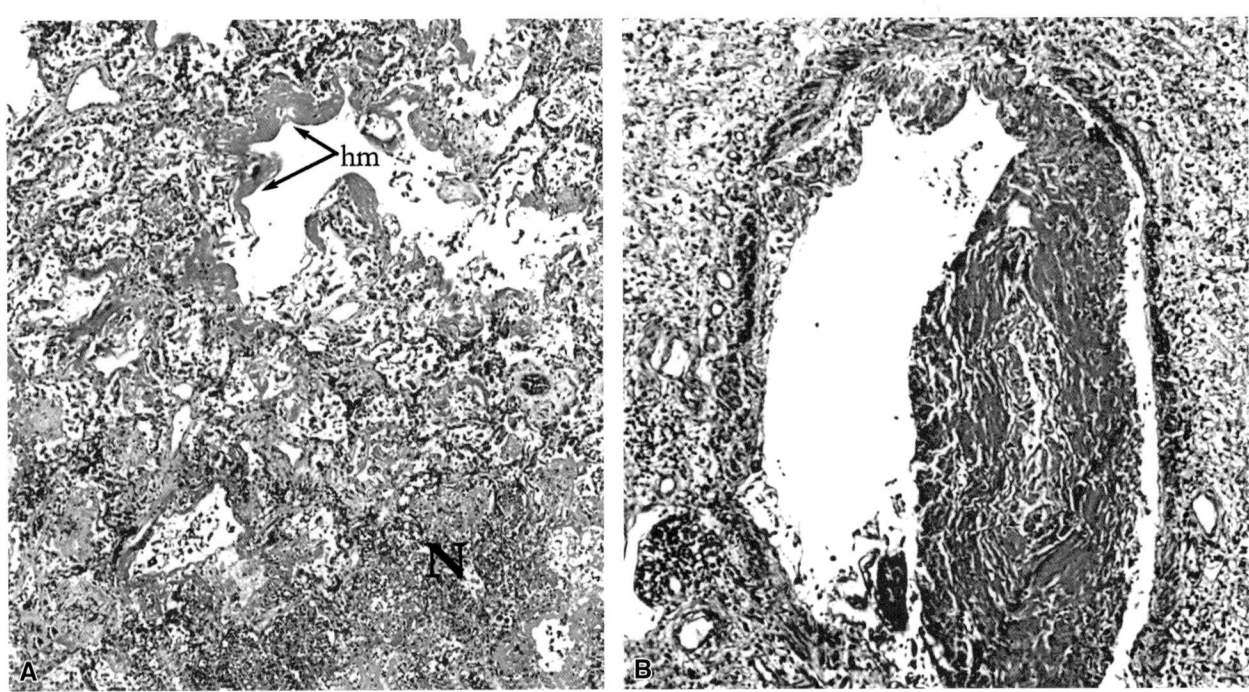

Figure 6-99. Adenoviral pneumonia. **A,** Necrosis (N) and diffuse alveolar damage (hm). **B,** Necrotizing bronchiolitis. hm, hyaline membrane.

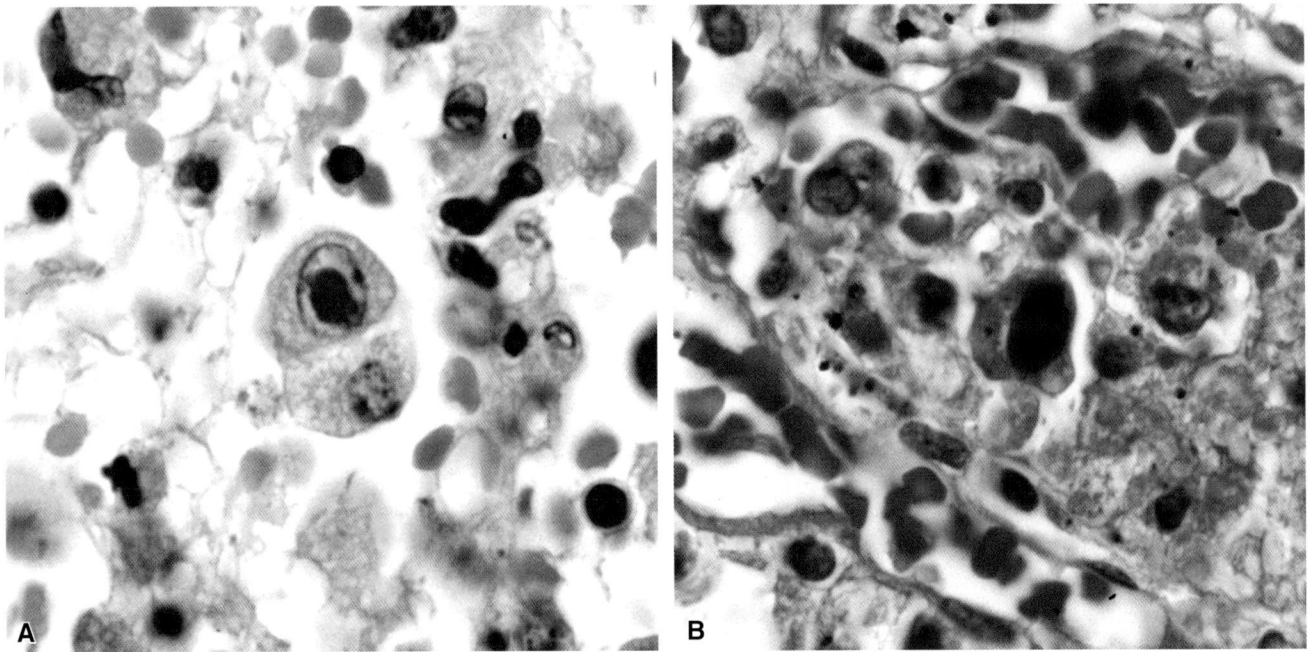

Figure 6-100. Adenovirus. **A,** Cowdry A intranuclear inclusions. **B,** Smudged cell.

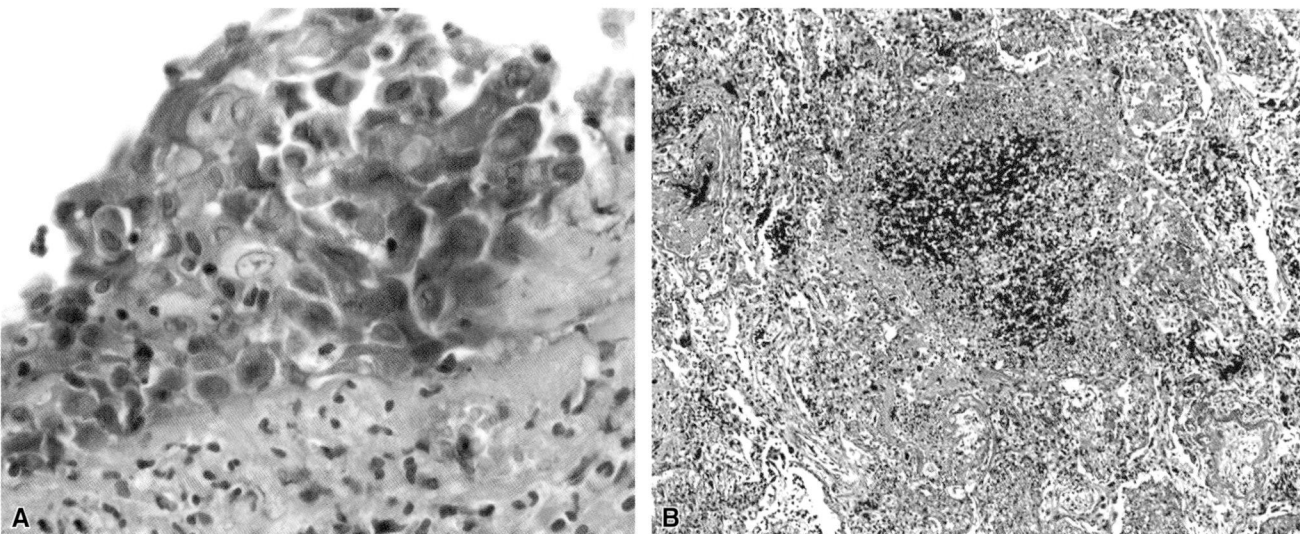

Figure 6-101. Herpes simplex virus pneumonia. **A,** Tracheobronchitis. Note cells with ground-glass inclusion. **B,** Miliary nodular pattern of hemorrhagic necrosis.

in neonates and in patients who are immunosuppressed or compromised by various chronic diseases. Characteristic lesions include tracheobronchitis (Fig. 6-101A) with ulcers and hemorrhagic diffuse alveolar damage. Necrosis in a miliary small, or rarely large, nodular pattern is a helpful clue and the best location to identify CPE[69] (see Fig. 6-101B). Like adenovirus, HSV also has two types of CPE: Initially a ground-glass amphophilic intranuclear inclusion, *Cowdry B*, appears with marginated chromatin. Later, a single eosinophilic, *Cowdry A* inclusion (Fig. 6-102) surrounded by a halo, similar to that seen with adenovirus, develops. The Cowdry A inclusion is considered noninfectious, as it is devoid of nucleic acid protein and is thought to represent the nuclear "scar" of HSV infection.[268] In the absence of smudge cells, HSV and adenoviral infections can look identical. Fortunately, immunohistochemistry or in situ hybridization can often resolve this differential diagnosis.

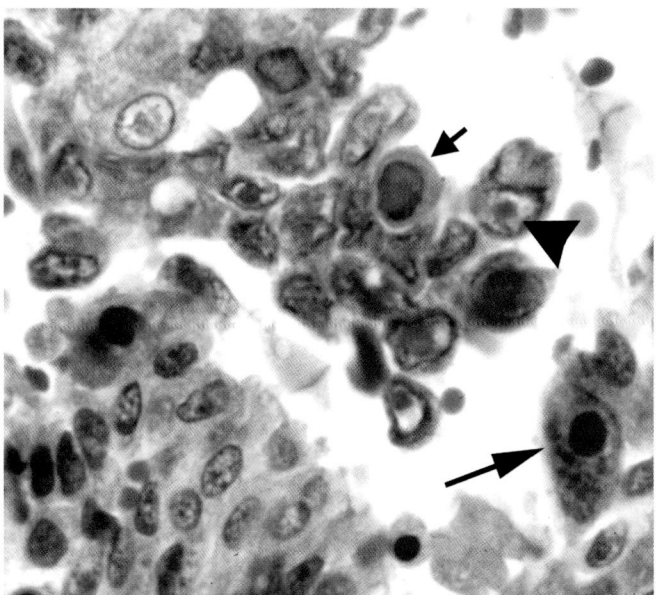

Figure 6-102. Herpes simplex virus pneumonia. Note two types of nuclear cytopathic effect: Cowdry A ground-glass type (*short arrow*) and Cowdry B eosinophilic inclusion (*arrowhead*). Compare with cytomegalovirus intranuclear and cytoplasmic inclusion at *long arrow*.

Varicella-Zoster Virus

Varicella-zoster virus (VZV) infection produces considerable morbidity in the newborn, the adult, and the immunocompromised host, both in its primary form (varicella) and in its reactivated form (zoster). Varicella pneumonia is rarely observed in otherwise healthy children but is a major complication of adult varicella, occurring in approximately 10% to 15% of adults with VZV. In affected adults without underlying diseases and normal immunity the course generally is mild and self-limited. Nevertheless, fatality rates of up to 10% have been reported.[268] By contrast, high mortality rates (25% to 45%) have been noted among some cohorts of immunosuppressed patients. Microscopically, small, miliary, nodules of necrosis are seen, associated with interstitial pneumonitis, edema, fibrin deposits, or patchy hyaline membranes (Fig. 6-103A). HSV-like intranuclear inclusions are present but may be sparse and difficult to identify. A miliary pattern of calcified nodules (see Fig. 6-103B) may be present in the healed phase.[312]

Cytomegalovirus

CMV infections are acquired throughout life. This virus can cause considerable morbidity and even death in the neonate, but infection generally is asymptomatic in older healthy children and adults. Like other herpesviruses, primary infection is followed by latency which persists until immune deficiency or immunosuppressive therapy causes it to reactivate and disseminate. CMV has therefore become one of the most common opportunists in patients with AIDS and those who receive organ transplants. In these settings, CMV can produce a variety of patterns, including one with minimal changes where only scattered alveolar lining cells with typical viropathic changes are seen. The CPE of CMV produces cytomegalic cells with large, round to oval, smooth "owl eye" eosinophilic to basophilic intranuclear inclusions surrounded by a clear halo (Fig. 6-104A).

Later, multiple eosinophilic cytoplasmic inclusions develop that may be positive on staining with PAS and GMS (see Fig. 6-104A, inset). The more numerous the cytomegalic cells, the greater the clinical significance. In some cases, atypical inclusions may be seen in cells that are not significantly enlarged and the nuclei may contain dark-staining homogeneous inclusions that may lack a clear halo. Despite their atypical appearance, these inclusions usually will be highlighted with immunohistochemical stains.[313] Another typical pattern that suggests viral infection is the presence of miliary small nodules with central

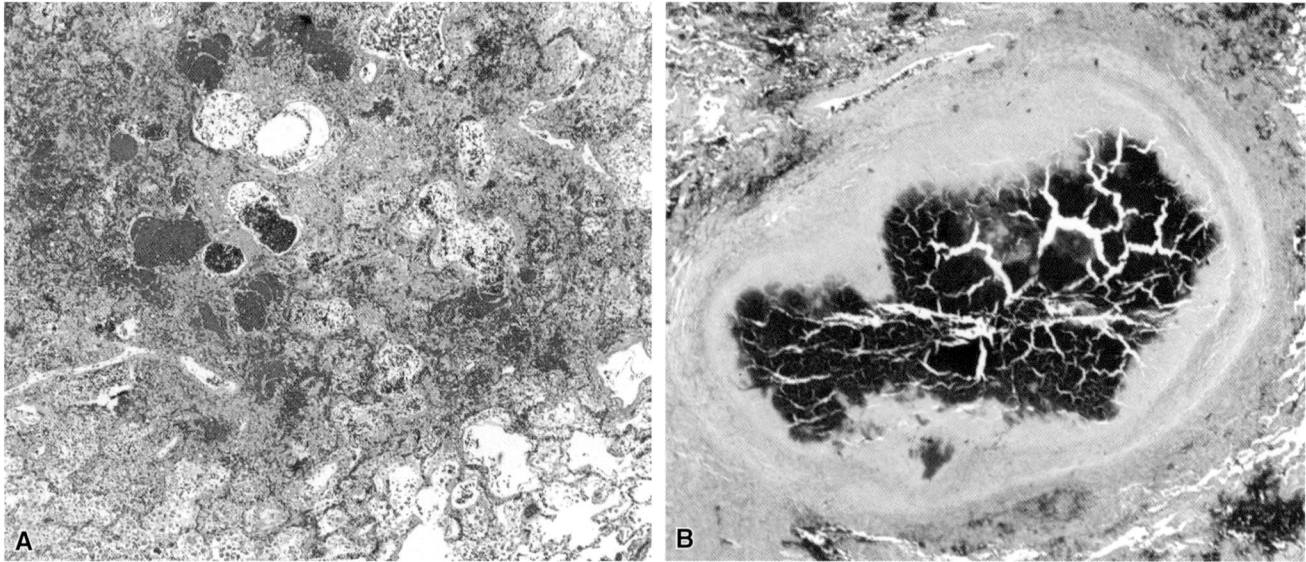

Figure 6-103. Varicella pneumonia. **A,** A hemorrhagic miliary nodule. **B,** Late phase with calcified nodules.

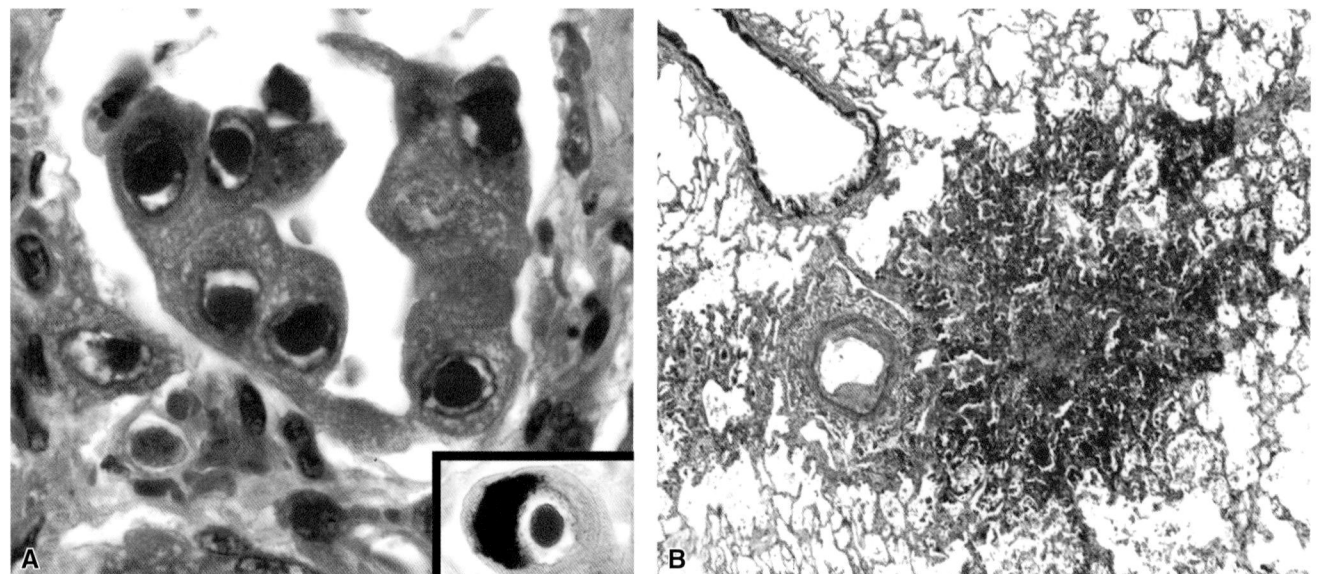

Figure 6-104. Cytomegalovirus (CMV) pneumonia. **A,** Multiple characteristic intranuclear and intracytoplasmic inclusions in alveolar lining cells. Note Grocott methenamine silver-positive staining of inclusions (*inset*). **B,** Miliary nodule pattern of CMV pneumonia. (**A,** Courtesy of Dr. Francis Chandler, Augusta, GA.)

hemorrhage surrounded by necrotic alveolar walls[69] (see Fig. 6-104B). Interstitial pneumonitis is the least common pattern of CMV infection. Ulcers may be seen in the trachea and bronchi, but occur less often than in herpetic infections. In CMV pneumonias, it is advisable to look for other pathogens, typically *P. jiroveci* (Fig. 6-105), but bacteria, fungi, protozoa, and other viruses all are possible co-infecting organisms.[314]

Epstein-Barr Virus

EBV infections usually are acquired in childhood and generally are asymptomatic. The pathologist most often encounters this virus in the lung in the context of pulmonary lymphomas or in other EBV-associated lymphoproliferative disorders that can occur in transplant recipients and other immunocompromised patients. However, the most common symptomatic primary EBV infection is infectious mononucleosis. Most of these patients recover uneventfully but a few develop one or more complications. Pneumonitis is one of them, albeit rare and not well

characterized. The few reports describing pathology indicate a nonspecific lymphocytic interstitial pneumonitis, which may be bronchiolo-centric[315,316] (Fig. 6-106). CPE is absent, and although serologic studies can be supportive of a clinicopathologic diagnosis, etiologic proof of EBV infection requires demonstration of the virus in lymphoid cells by in situ hybridization for EBV-encoded RNA-1 (EBER-1).

Cytopathology

The cytologic features of viral infections in the respiratory tract are most likely to be found in exfoliative specimens, such as bronchial washings and BAL fluid samples, rather than needle aspirates, although viral diagnosis has been achieved with this technique.[317,318] This is because viral infections are less likely to produce radiologic mass–like infiltrates, which are the most common targets of needle biopsy procedures. Herpes simplex virus, CMV (Fig. 6-107), and adenovirus are the most commonly identified viral pathogens in respiratory cytologic

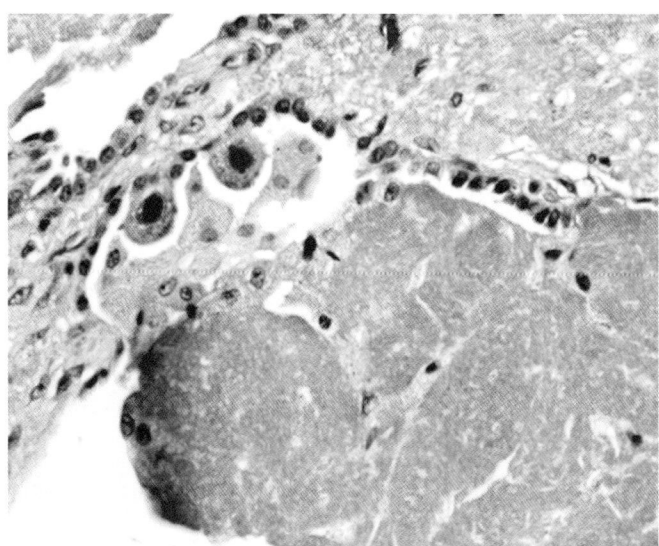

Figure 6-105. Cytomegalovirus-infected alveolar lining cells associated with the foamy alveolar casts of *Pneumocystis jiroveci*.

specimens, but varicella virus, parainfluenza virus, RSV, human metapneumovirus, and measles virus also have been detected.

Characteristic CPE produced by these viruses often is better appreciated in cytologic smears than in tissue sections, which may in fact yield a negative result. Therefore, review of any cytology sample taken at the time of biopsy can be valuable. Other, less specific changes may be found. These include ciliocytophoria (free cilia complexes with terminal bars) and cytologic atypia mimicking cancer.[44]

Microbiology

Diagnostic virology is the newest of the microbiology and infectious disease specialities to have benefited from the technologic revolution in laboratory medicine. Rapid and accurate diagnosis can often be achieved today using practical, convenient laboratory methods that employ reliable, commercially-available mammalian cells, media, and reagent systems.[260,319,320] This has allowed many rural and small urban hospital laboratories to provide timely viral diagnostic services not possible a short time ago. It is predicted that self-contained, rapid-cycle real-time PCR methods will one day account for a majority of viral assays in laboratories of all sizes. As a result, the pathologist who

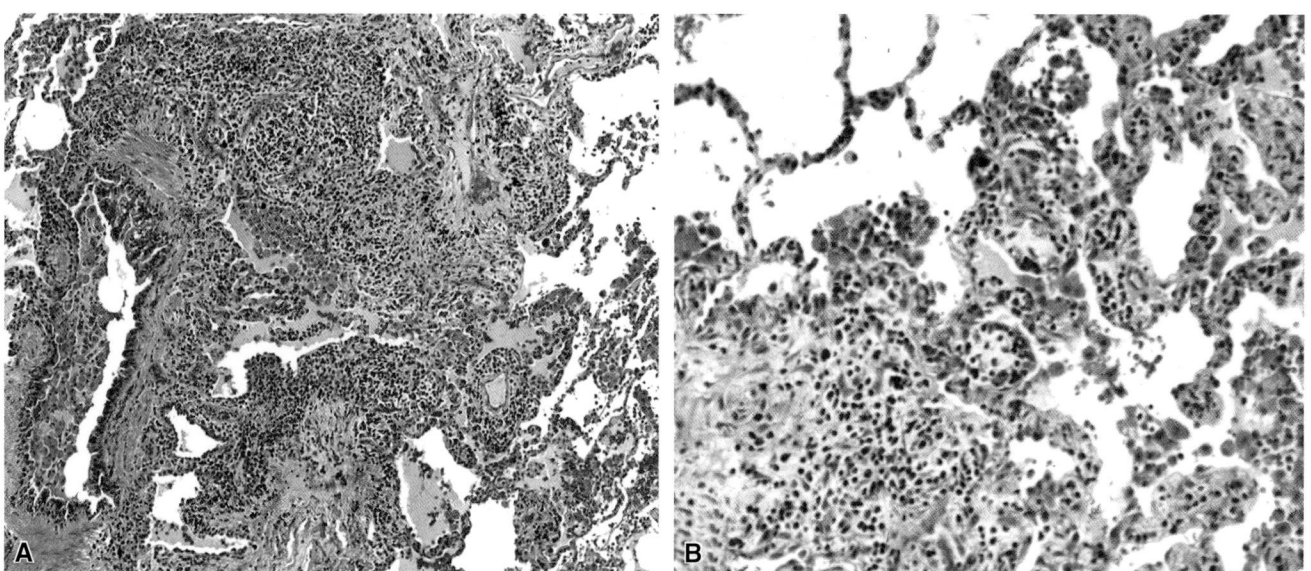

Figure 6-106. Epstein-Barr virus pneumonitis. **A,** Nonspecific cellular interstitial pneumonitis. **B,** Patchy interstitial infiltrate.

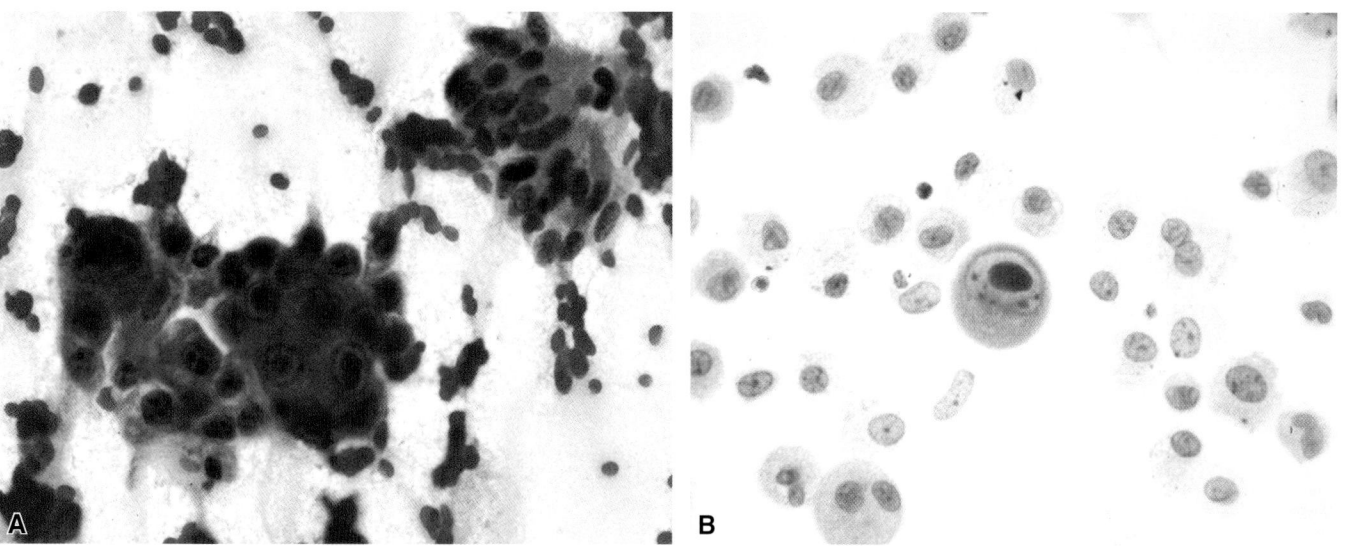

Figure 6-107. Cytomegalovirus pneumonitis with characteristic cytopathic effect. **A,** Fine-needle aspirate. **B,** Bronchoalveolar lavage specimen.

suspects a viral infection will increasingly have a variety of tools to obtain an etiologic diagnosis when morphologic manifestations are suggestive of viral infection.

The basic approaches to viral diagnosis in the laboratory are listed in Box 6-23. In questionable cases, confirmation by immunohistochemical studies (Fig. 6-108A), in situ hybridization (see Fig. 6-108B), or electron microscopy may be helpful.[31,321]

In the microbiology laboratory, the diagnosis of viral respiratory infections is based primarily on antigen detection and culture (Fig. 6-109). Direct antigen detection in clinical specimens collected by nasopharyngeal swabs, nasal washings, and aspirates or BAL fluid (but not sputum samples or, with rare exception, throat swabs) is performed using monoclonal antibodies by either immunofluorescence microscopy or enzyme immunoassay. By using a single reagent containing the monoclonal antibodies against several viruses and dual fluorochromes, the common respiratory viruses can be rapidly screened by direct immunofluoresence testing. Positive specimens can then be tested with individual reagents to determine the specific etiologic agent,

Box 6-23. Laboratory Diagnosis of Viral Pneumonia

Direct detection of organisms
    Histopathologic/cytopathologic examination for cytopathic effect (CPE)
    Immunohistochemical studies
    Electron microscopy
Antigen detection
    Direct fluorescent antibody test
    Enzyme immunoassay
Culture
    Conventional roller tube technique
    Shell vial technique
Serologic studies
Molecular methods
    In situ hybridization
    DNA amplification

while negative specimens can be submitted for culture.[322] Enzyme immunoassay includes methods that offer speed and convenience at the point of care. However, they are less sensitive than standard virologic methods, which still must be used to test negative specimens. Direct detection can also be accomplished in cellular samples, including tissue, by in situ hybridization or amplification techniques such as PCR. For RNA viruses, PCR amplification uses a reverse transcriptase (RT) step. Recently, PCR methodology has evolved into multiplex formats and novel systems have been introduced that combine multiplex PCR chemistry with electron microarray (DNA chip) technology or fluid microsphere-based systems, permitting the simultaneous detection of a wide array of respiratory viruses and other pathogens.[323-327] These systems have the potential to more rapidly and accurately diagnose acute infections and also may allow the study of complex coinfections and the active monitoring of outbreaks of influenza and other viral illnesses.[328] Current molecular diagnostic approaches are more technically demanding than culture, antigen detection by immunofluorescence, or enzyme immunoassay; and few are approved by the U.S. Food and Drug Administration (FDA). At present, isolation still remains useful for many respiratory viral infections, and antigen detection methods offer the speed and immediacy of reporting that many molecular methods lack.

Traditional viral cultures in tubes with various types of cell monolayers are currently performed with greater sensitivity and turnaround time using the shell vial technique. This technique uses centrifugation of clinical specimen suspensions onto coverslipped cell monolayers, followed by brief incubation (1–2 days) and antigen detection.[319] It is important therefore to preserve a portion of tissue from a bronchial or transbronchial biopsy or thoracotomy specimen in viral transport medium, especially in the immunocompromised patient, who may not have had BAL fluid submitted for culture.

Viral serologic testing commonly has been used for diagnosis but may be the least sensitive approach. A positive serodiagnosis typically is based on a fourfold rise in titer between acute and convalescent sera and therefore cannot be achieved by this means in the acutely ill

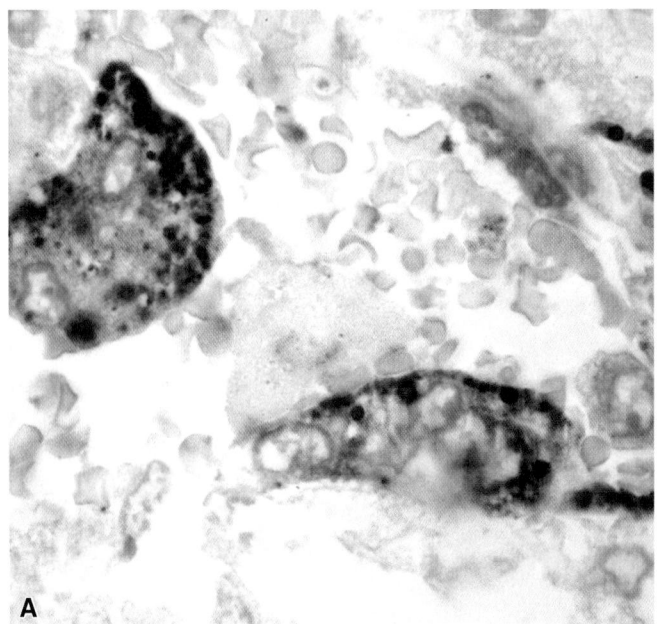

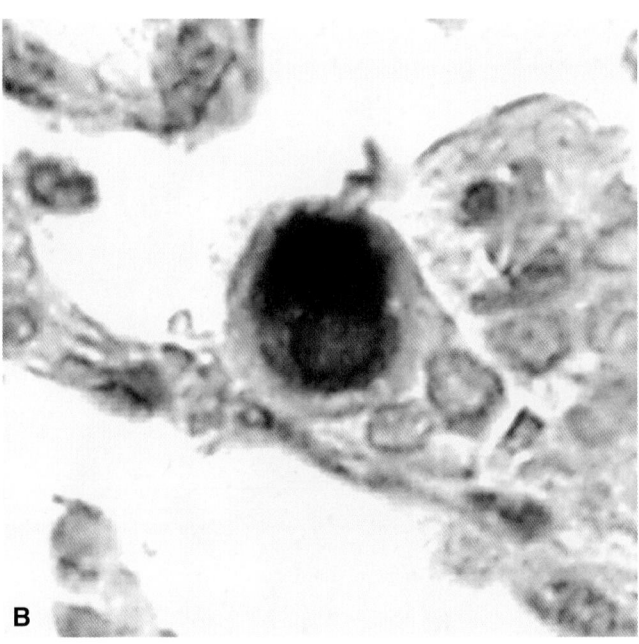

Figure 6-108. **A,** Respiratory syncytial virus cytoplasmic inclusions detected by immunohistochemical staining. **B,** Cytomegalovirus-infected cell with cytoplasmic inclusions detected by in situ hybridization. (Courtesy of R. V. Lloyd, MD, Rochester, MN.)

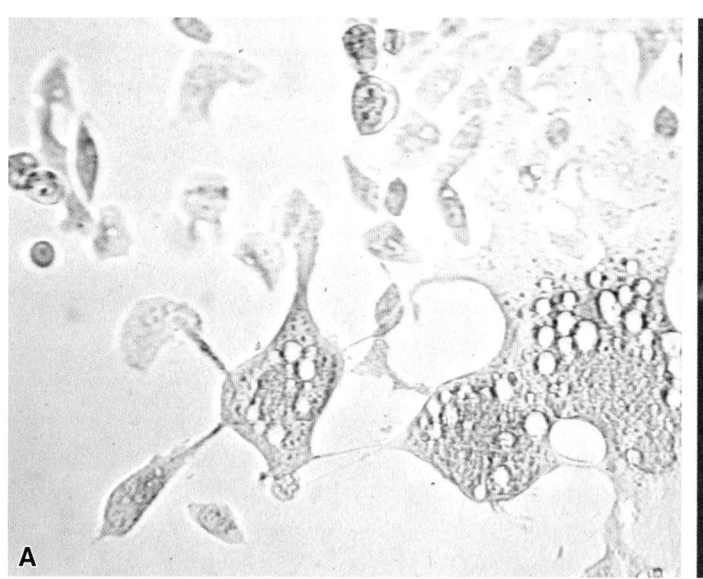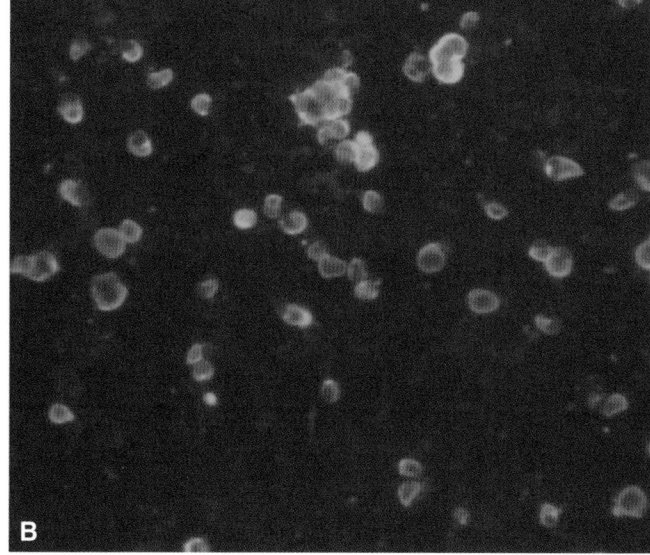

Figure 6-109. Respiratory syncytial virus (RSV) infection. **A,** RSV cytopathic effect in tissue culture. **B,** RSV antigen in nasopharyngeal swab specimen detected by direct immuno-fluorescence microscopy.

patient; antigen detection or culture of respiratory tract specimens is much preferred. However, a serologic strategy, utilizing a panel of antigens in an immunofluorescence or enzyme immunoassay format on a single specimen, is useful in suspected EBV infections.[329]

A case also can be made for the benefit of CMV serologic testing for assessment of the antibody status of organ donors and recipients for predicting risk of post-transplantation CMV disease. When tissue is not available or findings are inconclusive, tests for the detection of actual disease in these transplant recipients, include the p65 antigenemia assay on peripheral blood leukocytes and amplification or quantitation of CMV DNA in various peripheral blood compartments (plasma, whole blood, and leukocytes).[330] These assays may eventually replace culture of BAL fluid for surveillance of CMV infection in such patients.[331] The detection of virus in respiratory secretions (including BAL fluid), urine, or blood establishes the presence of virus but does not necessarily implicate it as the etiologic agent of a pneumonia. Quantitation of viral load by real-time PCR amplification, however, can be useful in this regard by linking high viral load with infection.[332]

Differential Diagnosis

A synopsis of the key morphologic and microbiologic features of the viral pneumonias is presented in Table 6-12. In the absence of CPE, diffuse alveolar damage and other patterns of lung injury are not diagnostic of viral infection. Diffuse alveolar damage is a nonspecific response to many types of infection, including bacterial, mycobacterial, fungal and protozoal, all of which must be considered in the differential diagnosis. In addition, other noninfectious causes include reactions to drugs, radiation, toxic inhalants, and shock of any type. Occasionally, CPE may not be diagnostic; for example, the early inclusions of adenovirus, herpes simplex virus, and CMV may be quite similar. In most cases, immunohistochemistry or molecular techniques can resolve the diagnostic dilemma. Mimics of CPE that must be ruled out include macronuclei in both reactive processes and occult neoplastic infiltrates, and intranuclear cytoplasmic invaginations which can occur in a variety of cells. Cytoplasmic viral inclusions also can be simulated by aggregated altered protein and particulate matter.

Table 6-12 Viral Pneumonias: Summary of Pathologic Findings

Assessment Component	Findings
Influenza Virus	
Surgical pathology	Diffuse alveolar damage, bronchitis and bronchiolitis Secondary acute purulent pneumonia Antigen detection by immunofluorescence, immunohistochemical, or in situ hybridization studies
Cytopathology	Nonspecific changes may include presence of reactive-type pneumocytes; ciliocytophoria
Microbiology	Antigen detection by DFA or EIA Culture on primary monkey kidney cells: noncytopathic Detection by hemadsorption
Respiratory Syncytial Virus	
Surgical pathology	Bronchiolitis with lumen detritus; may be associated with syncytial giant cells Diffuse alveolar damage in immunocompromised patients Confirm with immunohistochemistry
Cytopathology	Giant cell syncytia characteristic, but often not seen Eosinophilic inclusions may be seen in bronchial epithelial cells of immunocompromised patients; rarely in those of normal hosts Rarely diagnosed by cytology alone
Microbiology	Antigen detection by DFA and EIA usually more sensitive than culture Cultures on continuous epithelial cell lines (Hep-2) and primary monkey kidney yield characteristic syncytial CPEs
Measles Virus	
Surgical pathology	Bronchitis, bronchiolitis, diffuse alveolar damage with giant cells containing Cowdry A inclusions and small cytoplasmic inclusions
Cytopathology	Eosinophilic intranuclear and cytoplasmic inclusions Rarely diagnosed by cytology

Table 6-12   Viral Pneumonias: Summary of Pathologic Findings—cont'd

Assessment Component	Findings	Assessment Component	Findings
Measles Virus—cont'd		**Herpesvirus—cont'd**	
Microbiology	Antigen detection by DFA and EIA Culture on primary monkey kidney produces spindle cell or multinucleate CPE Serologic testing (for measles-specific IgM) available	Microbiology	Antigen detection by immunofluorescence Culture on diploid fibroblasts produces characteristic cytopathic effect, sometimes within 24 hours Serologic testing less useful
Hantavirus		**Varicella-Zoster Virus**	
Surgical pathology	Pulmonary edema pattern with variable fibrin deposits Immunoblast-like cells in vascular spaces Confirm by immunohistochemistry	Surgical pathology	Miliary necroinflammatory lesions; calcified nodules in healed phase
Cytopathology	Noncytopathic	Cytopathology	Intranuclear Cowdry A inclusions sparse and less well-defined than with herpes simplex
Microbiology	Serology: Hantavirus-specific IgM or detection of specific RNA by PCR assay in peripheral blood leukocytes	Microbiology	Antigen detection by immunofluorescence Culture on human embryonic lung or Vero cells produces CPE more slowly than for herpesviruses (3–7 days) Serologic testing available
Adenovirus		**Cytomegalovirus**	
Surgical pathology	Diffuse alveolar damage with or without necrotizing bronchiolitis and/or pneumonitis with necrosis and karyorrhexis	Surgical pathology	Minimal changes with scattered cytomegalic cells; miliary necroinflammatory lesions; interstitial pneumonitis
Cytopathology	Early Cowdry A intranuclear inclusions, later smudge cell Reactive and reparative-type atypia in background	Cytopathology	Large "owl eye" Cowdry A inclusions with halo; cytoplasmic inclusions stained with GMS
Microbiology	Antigen detection by EIA and DFA Culture on continuous epithelial cell lines produces characteristic grape-like clustered cytopathic effect	Microbiology	Culture on human diploid fibroblasts produces characteristic CPE slowly in traditional tube cultures but more rapidly with use of shell vial technique p65 antigenemia assay; PCR assay Selective application of serology useful
Herpesvirus		**Epstein-Barr Virus**	
Surgical pathology	Tracheobronchitis; diffuse alveolar damage; miliary necroinflammatory lesions	Surgical pathology	Polymorphous lymphoid interstitial pneumonitis Confirm by in situ hybridization
Cytopathology	Ground-glass (Cowdry B) intranuclear inclusions; later Cowdry A inclusions in multinucleated cells, often with a "seeds in a pomegranate" appearance on Pap-, H&E-, and Diff-Quik–stained smears Background reactive and reparative atypia	Cytopathology	Noncytopathic
		Microbiology	No routine culture; diagnosis by serologic testing using panel of antibodies (EA; IgG and IgM VCA; EBNA)

CPE, cytopathic effect; DFA, direct immunofluorescence antibody [test]; EA, early antigen; EBNA, Epstein-Barr virus–determined nuclear antigen; EIA, enzyme immunoassay; GMS, Grocott methenamine silver; H&E, hematoxylin-eosin; IgG, IgM, immunoglobulins G and M; Pap, Papanicolaou; PCR, polymerase chain reaction; VCA, viral capsid antigen.

Parasitic Infections

It is estimated that approximately 300 species of helminth worms and 70 species of protozoa have been acquired by humans during our short history on Earth.[333] Most of these are rare, but approximately 90 are relatively common, and some of them have been found in the lung.[334] A world made smaller by globalization and travel to endemic areas, in combination with the emergence (and re-emergence) of parasitic pathogens in immunocompromised patients, guarantees that pathologists will be increasingly challenged by diagnostic problems associated with these organisms.[335] Nevertheless, pulmonary parasitic infections are relatively rare and continue to be exotic diseases for surgical pathologists and cytopathologists in the United States.

Etiologic Agents

Several parasite species migrate through the lungs as part of their normal life cycle, but few preferentially infect the human lung.[336] Most are aberrant pulmonary localizations in the human host, where they become lost in transit or are part of a secondary disseminated infection from another organ system, often in the setting of compromised immunity. The etiologic listing in Box 6-24 is selective, based on the more common pathogens known to be associated with pulmonary involvement. The reader is encouraged to consult the References for a more comprehensive compilation.

Histopathology

When parasites, in the form of adult worms, larvae, or eggs, invade or become deposited in lung tissue, they usually provoke an intense inflammatory reaction with neutrophils, eosinophils, and various mononuclear cells. One or more of the patterns listed in Box 6-25 may be identified. When the predominant site of involvement is the bronchial mucosa, a bronchitis and bronchiolitis pattern is observed; when they become impacted in pulmonary arteries, a nodular angiocentric pattern is observed, although it may be overshadowed by thrombosis and infarction. Some parasites invade the alveolar parenchyma, resulting in a pattern of miliary small nodules or pneumonitis. Naturally, none of these patterns are consistently present and combinations of patterns may be seen. In some cases, an acute Loeffler-like eosinophilic pneumonia may reflect an allergic reaction to the transient passage of larvae through the pulmonary vasculature.

Box 6-24. Some Common Parasitic Lung Pathogens

Protozoa
Toxoplasma gondii
Entamoeba histolytica
Cryptosporidia
Microsporidia

Metazoa (Helminths)
Nematodes
    Dirofilaria immitis
    Strongyloides stercoralis
Cestodes
    Echinococcus spp.
Trematodes
    Paragonimus spp.
    Schistosoma spp.

Box 6-25. Histopathologic Patterns in Parasitic Lung Injury

Eosinophilic pneumonia
Large nodule(s)
Miliary small nodules
Bronchitis and bronchiolitis
Abscess, cavities, and cysts
Intravascular reaction

The various patterns, although nondiagnostic, can be suggestive of a parasitic infection, particularly when they incorporate a heavy eosinophilic infiltrate or granulomatous component. Eosinophilic lung disease, with or without blood eosinophilia, has a diverse etiology but is particularly characteristic of parasitic infection, especially in the tropics.[334] In the United States, other infections such as coccidioidomycosis must be considered, in addition to the many noninfectious causes of pulmonary eosinophilia. The challenge for the pathologist is the identification of a parasite, distinguishing it from artifact or foreign body, and classifying it as precisely as possible based on its size and unique morphologic features. Once the presence of suggestive morphologic features has been confirmed, the patient's travel history can help to further narrow the scope of the differential diagnosis. Of interest, a common "parasite" encountered in clinical practice is not a parasite at all but aspirated vegetable material simulating the complex structure of an organism.[337]

Toxoplasmosis

Toxoplasma gondii is an obligate, intracellular protozoan and a common opportunist in patients with AIDS, the disease underlying most cases of toxoplasmosis seen in recent years. The brain and retina are most commonly involved in these patients, but pulmonary lesions also may be present in cases of disseminated disease. These often take the form of miliary small nodules with fibrinous exudates, which may progress to a confluent fibrinopurulent pneumonia.[338] Free forms (crescent-shaped tachyzoites) and cysts may be identified (Fig. 6-110). Pseudocysts packed with tachyzoites can be distinguished from true cysts with bradyzoites by staining of the latter with PAS and GMS.[339]

Amebiasis

Amebic dysentery becomes invasive in a small percentage of patients. When the trophozoites leave the gut, they most commonly travel to the liver. From the liver, either by direct extension, or rarely by hematogenous spread, the lungs may become involved. In this scenario, abscesses composed of liquifactive debris—with few neutrophils, distinguishable

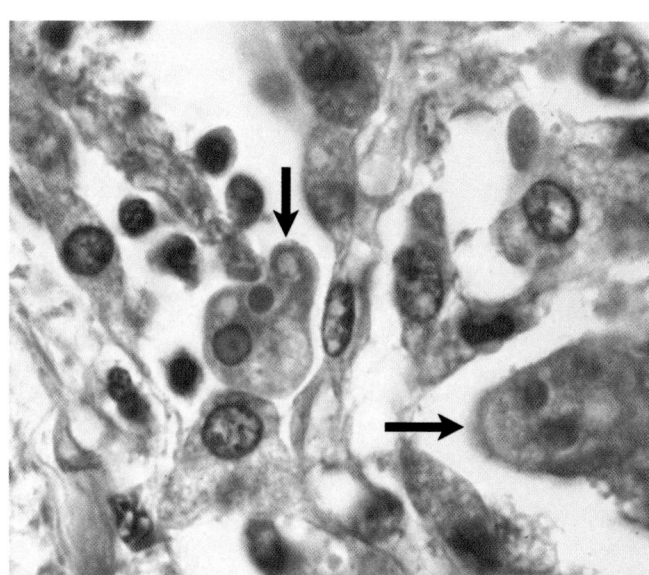

Figure 6-111. Amoebic trophozoite in lung tissue (*arrows*). Note delicate marginal nuclear chromatin with small central karyosome and small red blood cell in cytoplasm. (Courtesy of Ronald Neafi, Armed Forces Institute of Pathology, Washington, DC.)

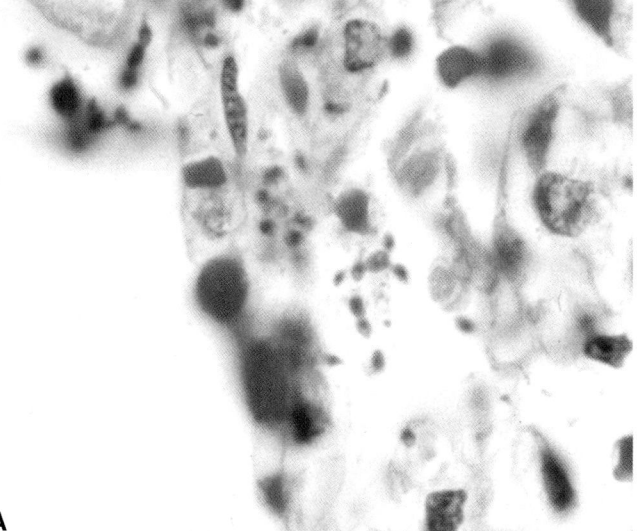

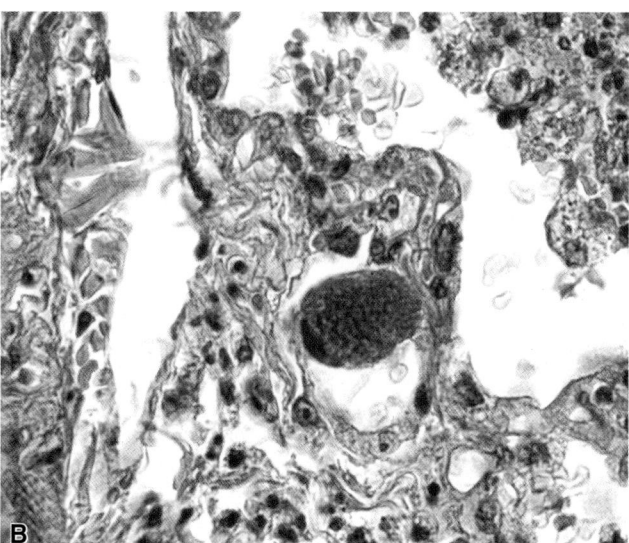

A

B

Figure 6-110. Toxoplasmosis. **A,** Tachyzoites. **B,** Pseudocysts packed with tachyzoites.

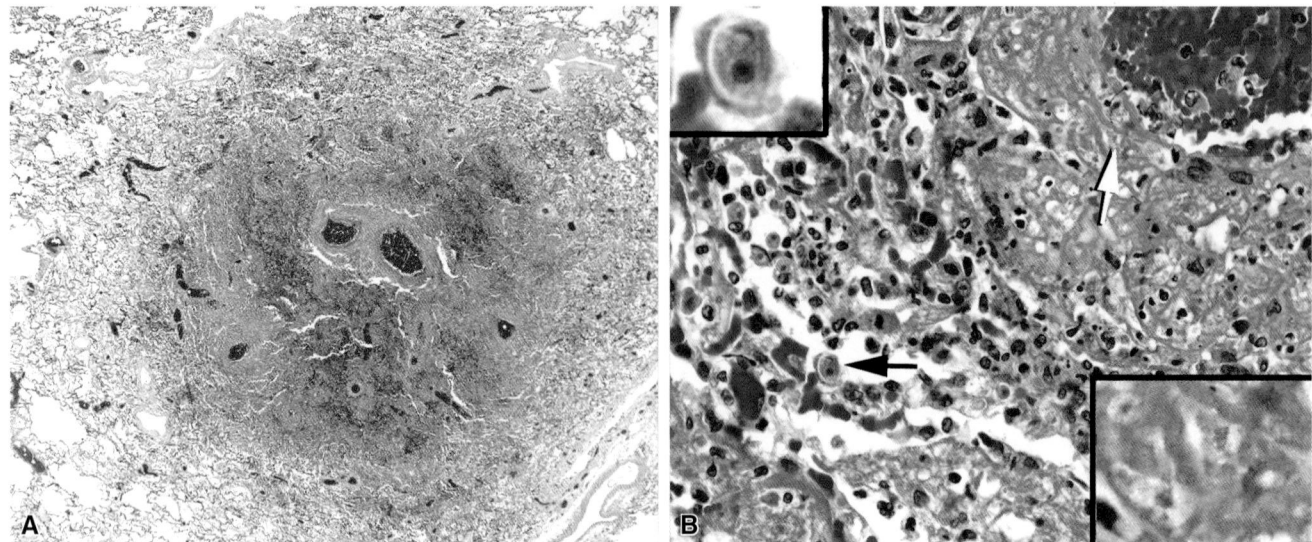

Figure 6-112. Free-living ameba in lung tissue from an immunocompromised patient. **A,** Necroinflammatory nodule. **B,** Encysted form, *black arrow* and *left upper inset*; trophozoite, *white arrow* and *right lower inset*.

from bacterial abscess where neutrophils are dominant—may be seen, most often in the right lower lobe adjacent to the liver.[340,341] Trophozoites can be best seen at the margin of viable tissue (Fig. 6-111). They resemble histiocytes but usually are larger, with a lower nucleocytoplasmic ratio. A tiny central karyosome within a round nucleus having vesicular chromatin is characteristic.[342,343] Bronchial fistula formation and empyema can occur as complications; amebae may be found in sputum and pleural fluid, respectively, in these situations. For free-living amebic species (those of the genera *Acanthamoeba, Balamuthia, Naegleria*), the central nervous system is the principal focus of infection. However, disseminated disease including lung infection (Fig. 6-112) may occur in certain epidemiologic situations, especially those involving compromised immune status.[344]

Cryptosporidiosis

Ten species of the intracellular coccidian protozoa are currently recognized, but one of them, *Cryptosporidium parvum*, causes most human infections.[345] Clinically, infection due to this organism may have three major manifestations: asymptomatic shedding, acute watery diarrhea that lasts for approximately 2 weeks, and persistent diarrhea that lasts several weeks. Patients with AIDS have a wider spectrum of disease severity and duration that includes a fulminant cholera-like illness.[345] These patients are most likely to manifest extraintestinal disease. In the lung, the organism targets the epithelium of the airways just as it does the surface epithelium of the gut and biliary tract.[346] In H&E sections, cryptosporidia appear as small (4–6 μm in diameter), round to oval protrusions from the cell surface. Electron microscopy reveals that they are intracellular but extracytoplasmic. In addition to H&E, they stain with Giemsa, PAS, GMS, and acid-fast stains. A mild to moderate chronic inflammatory cell infiltrate usually is present in the submucosa. Recognition of this disease in patients with AIDS can be challenging because the findings may be subtle and coexistent pneumonias caused by other pathogens can divert the pathologist's attention.

Microsporidiosis

The microsporidia are obligate intracellular, spore-forming protozoa. More than 140 genera and 1200 species are recognized, but only seven genera and a few species have been confirmed as human pathogens.[347] They are opportunists that have recently emerged in severely immunocompromised patients, especially people with AIDS and transplant recipients. They are found less often in persons with intact immunity. Clinically, they primarily cause chronic diarrhea and cholangitis. In the

lung, they cause bronchitis or bronchiolitis (or both), usually in patients who also have intestinal infection or disease in other sites, especially the biliary tract.[348] The predominant pathologic changes are in the airways, which show a mixed inflammatory cell infiltrate of mononuclear and polymorphonuclear leukocytes.[349] The organisms are found within vacuoles in the apical portion of epithelial cells lining the airways. They appear as very small (1–1.5 μm in diameter) basophilic dots, whose recognition depends on organism load. However, even when heavy, the findings can be subtle. Also, as with cryptosporidiosis, their presence often is overlooked or obscured by coexistent pneumonias. Special stains, such as modified trichrome, Warthin-Starry–type silver, and Gram stains, are more sensitive and specific, especially when used in combination.[350]

Leishmaniasis

Leishmaniasis (*Leishmania donovani* infection) is transmitted to humans by several species of the *Phlebotomus* sand fly.[351] Pulmonary leishmaniasis has been reported in HIV-infected patients and transplant recipients.[334] The organisms (*L. donovani* amastigotes) can be found in the alveoli and alveolar septa and may be recovered in BAL fluid from these patients.[352] They also can be found in bronchoscopic biopsies. (Fig. 6-113). Serologic testing for leishmaniasis has been suggested as part of the pre-transplantation workup in endemic areas.[353] A rapid PCR-amplified diagnostic method has been described.[354]

Dirofilariasis

The zoonosis caused by *Dirofilaria immitis*, a parasite of dogs and other mammals, is transmitted by mosquitos and black flies to humans. Larvae injected by these insect vectors migrate from the subcutis into veins and travel to the heart, where they die before maturing into adult worms. They are then washed into the lungs by the pulmonary arterial blood flow, where they form the nidus of a thrombus. Formation of an infarct follows, typically manifesting as an asymptomatic solitary pulmonary nodule ("coin lesion") in the lung periphery (Fig. 6-114) that may be visualized on a positron emission tomography (PET) scan.[355–357] Microscopically, the nodule resembles a typical infarct with a core of coagulation necrosis but also containing degenerated worm fragments in the remnant of an arteriole (Fig. 6-115). A peripheral investment of chronic granulation tissue forms an interface with the alveolated parenchyma. "Step" sections and trichrome stains may be needed when H&E sections do not show the parasite.[358]

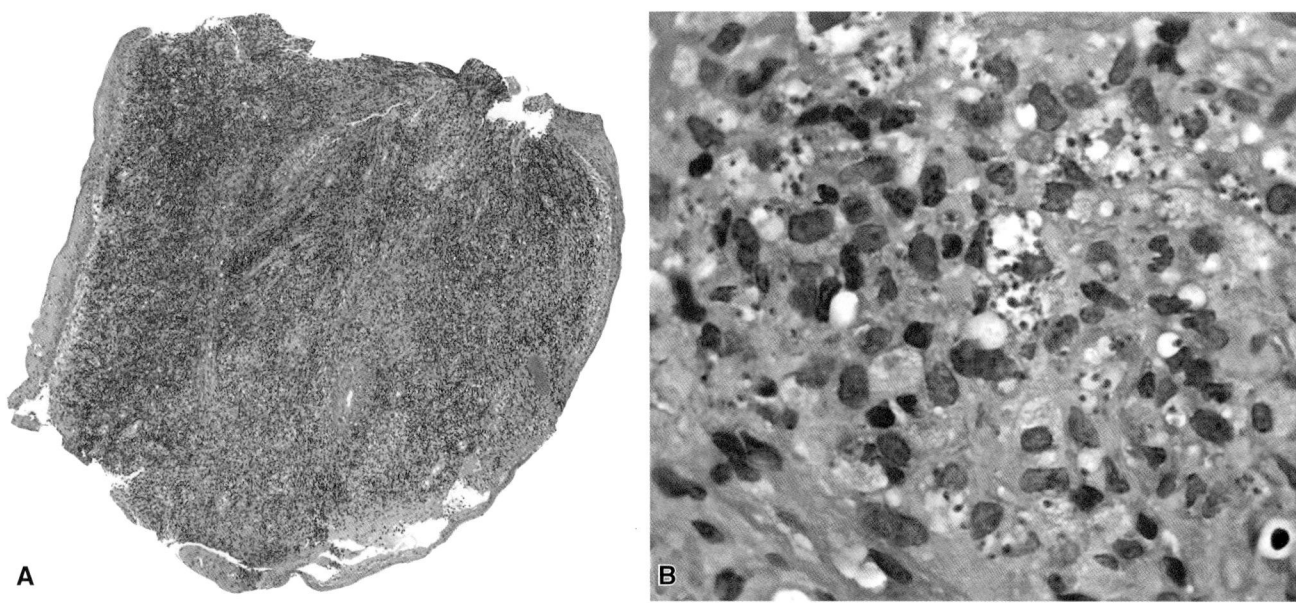

Figure 6-113. *Leishmania donovani* in bronchoscopic biopsy specimens obtained from a North African immigrant to Sicily. **A,** Lower-power view of cellular infiltrate. **B,** High-power view of dot-like organisms. (Courtesy of Dr. Francesca Guddo, Palermo, Italy.)

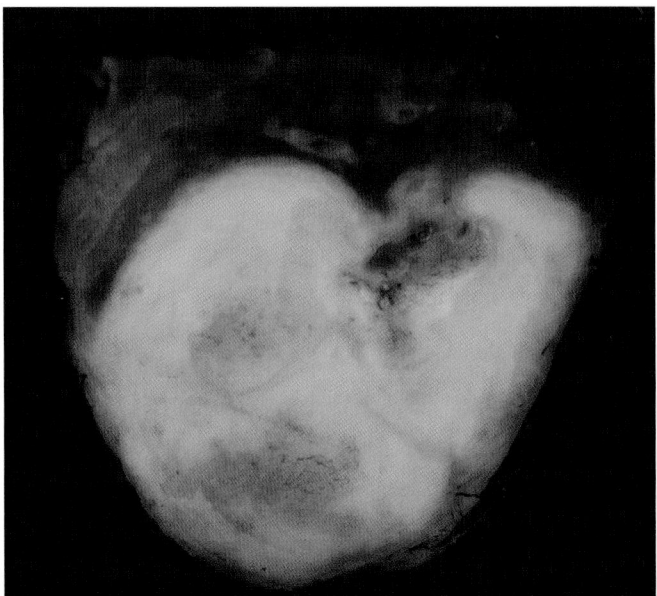

Figure 6-114. Dirofilarial nodule, gross specimen.

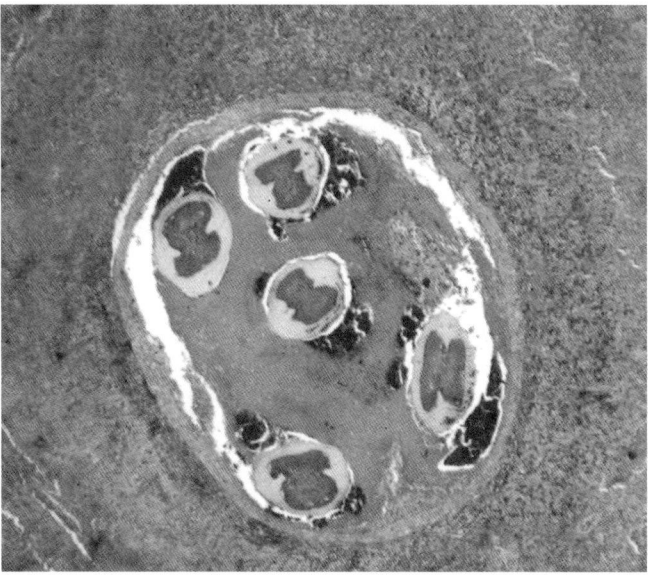

Figure 6-115. Dirofilarial nodule, with worm remnants in organizing thrombosed vessel.

Strongyloidiasis

Strongyloides is a parasite most often found in patients or travelers in the tropics, but endemic foci are present in the southeastern United States. Rabditiform larvae of the nematode *Strongyloides stercoralis*, after hatching from ingested eggs, invade the small intestinal mucosa. At this site occult infection may remain asymptomatic for years. Dissemination typically follows debilitation brought on by immuno-compromising diseases and therapies. When this occurs, filariform larvae leave the gut and travel through the pulmonary vasculature. When they penetrate alveoli (Fig. 6-116), they provoke hemorrhage and inflammation.[359] Loeffler syndrome, eosinophilic pneumonia, and abscesses may develop. When migration is interrupted, filariform larvae may metamorphose in situ to adult worms, which can produce eggs and rabidiform larvae. Larvae identified in the sputum indicate

hyperinfection.[360] Disseminated stronglyloidiasis is but one example of an infection that may become manifest, particularly in immunocompromised patients, years after emigration from or travel to an endemic area harboring pathogens considered unusual or exotic by pathologists in the United States.

Echinococcosis

Echinococcosis is a zoonosis that occurs wherever sheep, dogs or other canids, and humans live in close contact. Ingested eggs of the tapeworm *Echinococcus* hatch in the gut, releasing oncospheres, which then invade the mucosa, enter the circulation, and travel to various sites, where they develop into hydatid cysts. In the lung, unilocular slow-growing cysts are produced by *Echinococcus granulosus*.[361] *Echinococcus multilocularis* proliferates by budding, producing an alveolar pattern of *Paragonimus* species. Most cases worldwide are due to *P. westermani* but several other species exist in Asia, Africa, South and Latin America. In the United States, infections due to *P. kellicotti* have been reported.[336] The disease manifestations are related to the migratory route and the inflammatory response these hermaphroditic flukes stimulate as they enter lung parenchyma and travel to sites near larger bronchioles or bronchi. Typically, an area of eosinophil-rich inflammatory reaction surrounds them, and this reactive process may evolve to form a fibrous pseudocyst or capsule containing worms, exudate, and debris (Fig. 6-118A). Cysts rupturing into bronchioles may result in eggs, blood, and inflammatory cells being coughed up in the sputum. Alternatively, eggs may become embedded in parenchyma, producing nodular granulomatous lesions (see Fig. 6-118B) that progress to scars.[363] The eggs are yellowish, ovoid, and operculated, measuring 75 to 110 µm by 45 to 60 µm. The opercula unfortunately are not easily seen in tissue; however, the eggs are birefringent under polarized light, which helps to distinguish them from nonbirefringent schistosome eggs.[336]

Schistosomiasis

The public health burden of schistosomiasis is enormous: This parasitic infection affects 200 million people in 74 countries while continuing to expand its geographic range.[364,365] The life cycle and disease manifestations of the three major *Schistosoma* species—*Schistosoma mansoni*, *Schistosoma haematobium*, and *Schistosoma japonicum*—involve eggs, snail intermediate hosts, and free-swimming cercaria, which penetrate the skin of susceptible animals and people and develop into adult worms. The male and female worms eventually come to reside in various human venous plexuses, depending on the species, where egg deposition occurs. Pulmonary schistosomiasis comprises both acute and chronic forms. The acute disease, referred to as Katayama syndrome, manifests with fever, chills, weight loss, gastrointestinal symptoms, myalgia, and urticaria in patients with no previous exposure to the parasite. Acute larval pneumonitis and a Loeffler-like eosinophilic pneumonia may be seen in this setting.[364,366] Chronic pulmonary disease is almost always secondary to severe hepatic involvement with portal hypertension. In this setting, the eggs of *S. mansoni*, and rarely *S. japonicum* or *S. haematobium*, may

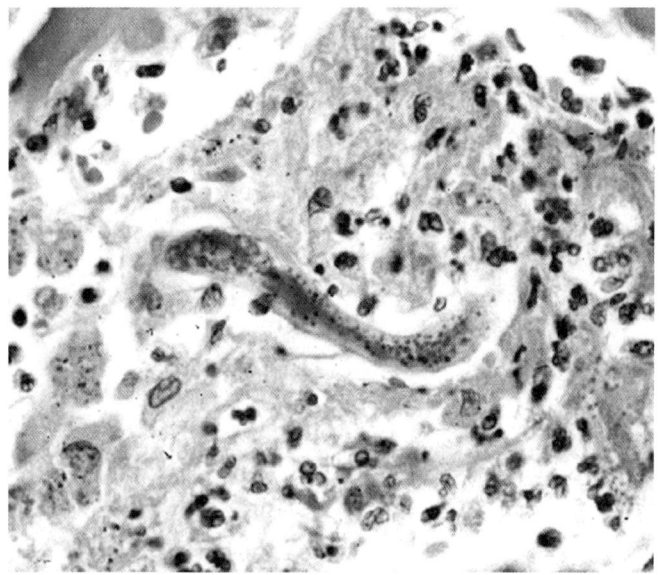

Figure 6-116. Filariform larva of *Strongyloides stercoralis* penetrating into alveolar space with associated inflammation.

of microvesicles.[343] The cyst of *E. granulosus* has a trilayered membrane (Fig. 6-117A) with an outer fibrous, middle-laminated hyaline, and inner germinal layer that gives rise to brood capsules containing infective protoscolices with hooklets and suckers (see Fig. 6-117B). The layers usually become separated in tissue, with the outer fibrous layer containing chronic inflammatory cells forming an interface with the alveolated parenchyma. Cysts that rupture into bronchi may be expectorated as debris with protoscolices or portions of the cyst wall. Abscesses and granulomas may also form in the lung, pleura, and chest wall.[362]

Paragonimoniasis

The parasite *Paragonimus* targets the lung and is acquired by the ingestion of freshwater crabs or crayfish infected with the metacercarial larvae

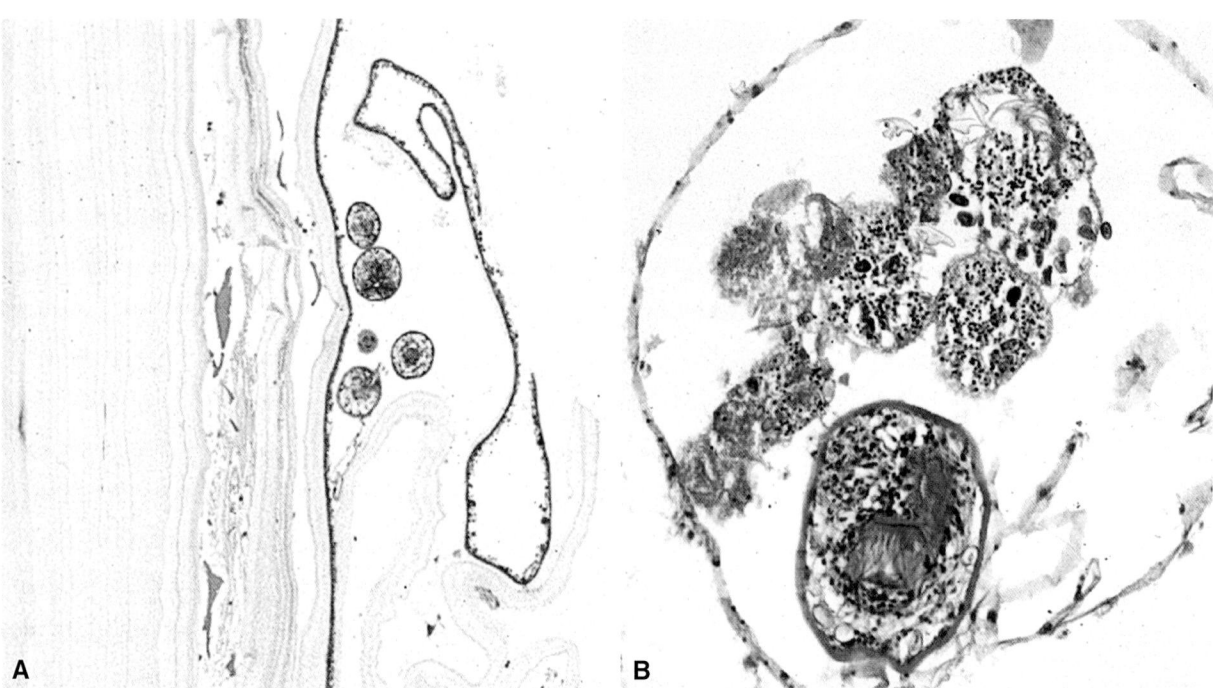

A   **B**

Figure 6-117. *Echinoccocus granulosus.* **A,** Cyst with trilayered membrane. **B,** Brood capsules.

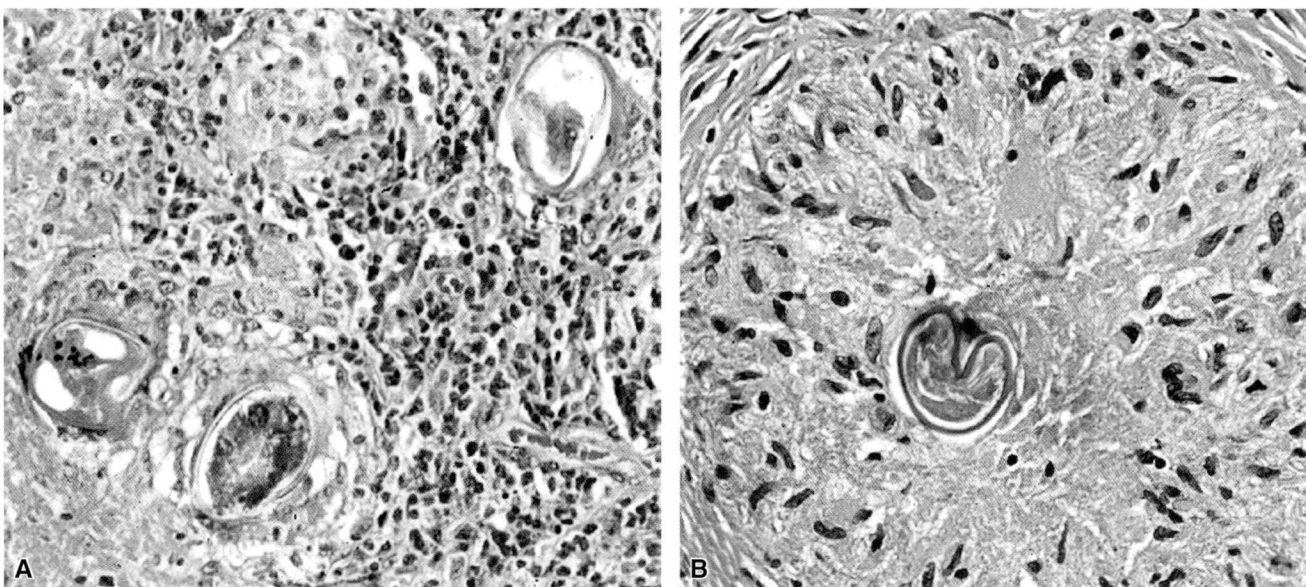

Figure 6-118. **A,** *Paragonimus westermani* with yellowish refractile eggs in eosinophil-rich exudates. **B,** Distorted egg of *Paragonimus kellicotti* in granuloma.

be shunted through portosystemic collateral veins to the lungs. The eggs lodge in arterioles, provoking a characteristic granulomatous endarteritis with pulmonary symptoms and radiologic infiltrates.[367,368] When the endarteritis is accompanied by angiomatoid changes, the lesion is considered pathognomonic for pulmonary schistosomiasis.[336]

Eggs typically are surrounded by epithelioid cells and collagen (Fig. 6-119). Most schistosome eggs do not exhibit birefringence and are larger than *Paragonimus* eggs, with which they share a superficial resemblance. Adult schistosomes may rarely be found in pulmonary blood vessels.

Visceral Larva Migrans

The common parasites that cause visceral larva migrans are the dog tapeworm, *Toxacara canis*, and the less common cat tapeworm,

Toxacara catis. When embryonated eggs are ingested by an intermediate host, typically a child with a history of pica, they hatch into infective larvae in the intestine. Subsequently, the larvae penetrate the intestinal wall, gain access to the circulation, and are carried to many organs, including the lungs. This is the end point, for their growth is arrested by a granulomatous reaction and they never mature into adult worms. The granulomatous reaction usually has a conspicuous eosinophilic component, and larvae may be seen.[369]

Cytopathology

The cytologic literature contains many reports of the successful identification of parasites in pulmonary specimens recovered by exfoliative (sputum, bronchial washing or brushing, BAL fluid, pleural fluid) and needle aspiration techniques. Some of these are listed in Box 6-26.[352,355–357,362,370–381]

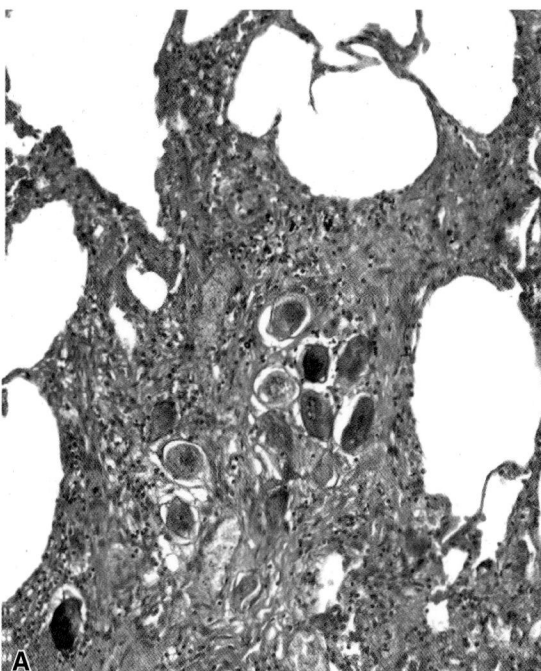
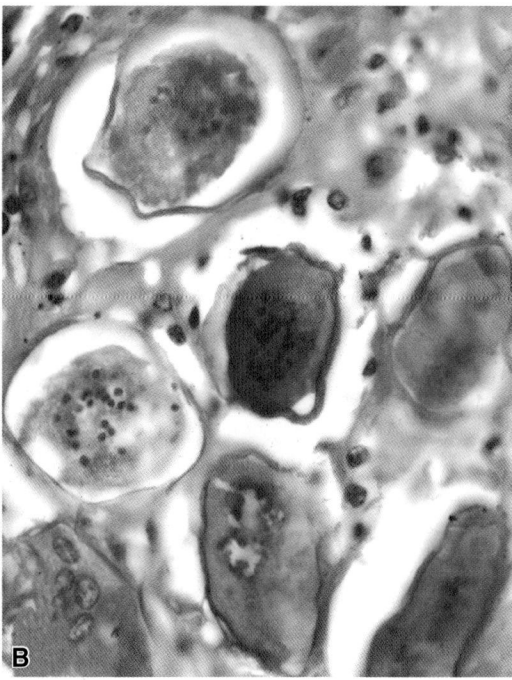

Figure 6-119. **A,** Schistosome eggs in lung parenchyma. **B,** Eggs of *Schistosoma japonicum.* (**A** and **B,** Courtesy of Ronald Neafi, Armed Forces Institute of Pathology, Washington, DC.)

Box 6-26. Parasites Reported in Respiratory Cytology Specimens

Toxoplasma
Amebae
Trichomonas
Cryptosporidia
Microsporidia
Leishmania
Paragonimus
Echinococcus
Strongyloides
Schistosoma
Dirofilaria
Microfilariae

Commonly cited in textbooks and reviews is the finding of *Strongyloides stercoralis* larvae in expectorated sputum or bronchial washings of patients with hyperinfections (Fig. 6-120). Also common are reports of *Echinococcus* protoscolices and hooklets in needle aspirates from patients with pleuropulmonary disease.[43,44] Use of large-bore and cutting needle biopsies traditionally has been contraindicated in the setting of suspected *Echinococcus* infections; reports of success with fine-needle aspiration, without untoward reactions, suggest that this latter technique is a relatively safe procedure in which the benefits outweigh the risks.[372]

Cytologic analysis is a sensitive and often preferred method to diagnose cryptosporidiosis, microsporidiosis, and other respiratory tract infections in the immunocompromised patient, because it has the advantage of being less invasive. Specimens such as bronchial washings and BAL fluids can be prepared by high-speed centrifugation followed by standard smear preparation, cytocentrifugation, or ThinPrep technology. A battery of special stains including Gram, modified trichrome, Giemsa, GMS, acid-fast, chemofluorescent, and immunofluorescent, depending on reagent availability, can then be applied to detect cryptosporidial oocysts, microsporidial spores, or other etiologic agents.

The morphologic features of many of the aforementioned organisms usually are better defined in cytologic preparations than in tissue biopsy specimens, provided that obscuring background debris is limited and that cytopreparation technique and staining have been well performed. Pseudoparasites such as vegtable matter, textile fibers, pollens, red cell "ghosts," and other extraneous material must be recognized and excluded. Thus, as for all of the various categories of microorganisms cited in this chapter, cytopathologic examination adds synergy to surgical pathologic and microbiologic methods.

Microbiology

The laboratory diagnosis of parasitic disease depends on the collection of appropriate specimens, which in turn requires appropriate clinical evaluation. For example, just as stool examination is the most efficient means of diagnosing most intestinal protozoa and helminths, respiratory specimens (e.g., sputum samples, bronchial washings, BAL fluid samples, touch imprints of lung biopsy tissue) can provide a specific etiologic diagnosis when pulmonary infections are suspected.[335] As in the case for cytologic samples, these specimens often reveal the characteristic micro-anatomic features of parasite larvae and eggs that usually cannot be readily seen when they are embedded in tissue. Moreover, the identification of organisms in respiratory specimens is diagnostic of pulmonary infection, whereas the presence of the organism in the feces of a patient suspected to have pulmonary disease provides only presumptive evidence.

Serodiagnosis with immunologic and molecular methods can be useful when parasites are located deep within tissue, such as the lung, and not easily accessible to biopsy or cytologic sampling.[341] The effectiveness of serodiagnosis of parasitic diseases has been hampered by tests with low sensitivity and specificity, mainly as a result of the complex composition of parasitic antigens and the occurrence of frequent cross reactions.[335] In recent years, however, significant refinements in antigenic preparations and improvements in technology have resulted in assays with greater predictive value. The newer tests are based on enzyme immunoassay and immunoblot methodology. Many test kits are commercially available, and diagnostic services are available from the CDC and other reference laboratories.[382]

With protozoal infections, serologic testing is especially useful for the diagnosis of toxoplasmosis. Several commercial kits are available for detection of immunoglobulin G (IgG) and IgM antibodies; however, false-negative results are possible in immunocompromised patients, and positive results must be interpreted with caution, especially when the index of clinical suspicion is low.[383] Real-time PCR analysis has been used for the diagnosis of toxoplasmosis in the immunocompromised patient.[384,385] Antibody determinations also have value in cases of pulmonary and other tissue-invasive forms of amebiasis, as compared with antigen detection methods, which are more useful for noninvasive amebic intestinal diseases. However, the best diagnostic approach

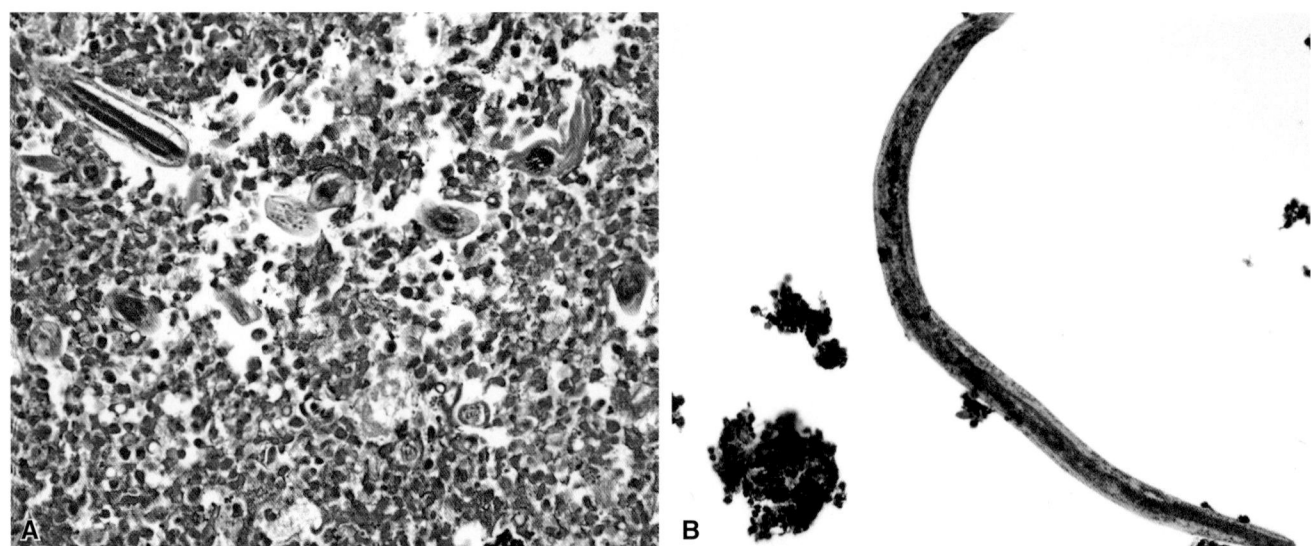

Figure 6-120. *Strongyloides stercoralis* larvae in bronchial washing. **A,** Larval fragments in cell block. **B,** ThinPrep smear.

to invasive disease may be the use of serologic testing, antigen detection, and PCR methods, in various combinations.[386] For identification of cryptosporidia, the new immunofluorescence tests and enzyme immunoassays that have been developed for intestinal infections may have application in respiratory infections. Similar tests are not available for the microsporidia, and diagnosis of infection with these organisms continues to rely on direct staining techniques at this time. For the helminths, serodiagnosis is possible for *Echinococcus, Paragonimus,*

Strongyloides, and *Schistosoma* species using enzyme immunoassay methods, which have fair sensitivity and specificity.[334,382] The available tests for *Dirofilaria* suffer from poor sensitivity and specificity and are not clinically useful at this time.

Differential Diagnosis

The key morphologic and microbiologic features of selected parasitic lung infections are summarized in Table 6-13. In the absence of eggs,

Table 6-13. Parasitic Pneumonias: Summary of Pathologic Findings

Assessment Component	Findings		Assessment Component	Findings
Toxoplasmosis			**Dirofilariasis**	
Surgical pathology	Miliary small necroinflammatory nodules with fibrin; fibrinous pneumonia		Surgical pathology	Solitary pulmonary nodule with infarct pattern and worm fragments
Cytopathology	Crescent-shaped tachyzoites, pseudocysts and true cysts		Cytopathology	Intact or fragmented worm in necroinflammatory debris
Microbiology	Serologic diagnosis by IFA or EIA Identification of tachyzoites or pseudocyst in tissue		Microbiology	Identification of characteristic roundworm in tissues Serologic studies not useful
Amebiasis			***Strongyloides* Infection**	
Surgical pathology	Lung abscess		Surgical pathology	Eosinophilic pneumonia, abscess, Loeffler syndrome with filariform larvae
Cytopathology	Trophozoite in necroinflammatory debris resembles histiocytes Confirm with immunohistochemistry		Cytopathology	Filariform larvae in sputum indicates hyperinfection
Microbiology	Identification of trophozoite characteristics Serologic methods positive in most cases of extraintestinal disease DNA probes		Microbiology	Primary diagnostic stage in stool is rhabitiform larvae; filariform larvae may be seen in sputum and lung tissue Eggs resemble hookworm eggs, but rarely seen
Cryptosporidiosis			***Echinococcus* Infection**	
Surgical pathology	Bronchitis and/or bronchiolitis with cryptosporidia seen on H&E sections as small, round protrusions along the epithelial surface of the mucosa		Surgical pathology	Trilayered cyst with brood capsules containing protoscolices Fibrous wall forms interface with lung parenchyma; sometimes abscess and granulomas
Cytopathology	Red oocysts in smears prepared from bronchial washes and BAL fluid stained with modified acid-fast stains		Cytopathology	Protoscolices with sucker and hooklets or detached hooklets in granular background debris
Microbiology	Findings on direct examination of specimens similar to those on cytologic examination Immunofluorescence and enzyme immunoassays developed for intestinal infection		Microbiology	Identification of hooklets and protoscolices in needle aspirates, pleural fluid, and sputum Serologic testing available
Microsporidiosis			**Paragonimiasis**	
Surgical pathology	Bronchitis and/or bronchiolitis Small basophilic dots in vacuoles may be visible in H&E-stained sections when burden of organism is heavy; highlighted with Gram and modified trichrome stains; toluidine blue stain on plastic sections; electron microscopy		Surgical pathology	Eosinophilic pneumonia Fibrous pseudocysts containing worms and necroinflammatory debris Egg granulomas
Cytopathology	Characteristic pink capsule-shaped spores with dark band in modified trichrome-stained preparations of BAL fluid Giemsa, Gram, and chemofluorescence stains also useful		Cytopathology	Yellow ovoid birefringent eggs with flattened operculum
			Microbiology	Identification of characteristic egg in sputum or tissue Serologic testing available
Microbiology	Findings on direct examination of fluids similar to those on cytologic examination Culture in research setting by special arrangement Molecular methods		**Schistosomiasis**	
			Surgical pathology	Granulomatous endarteritis; eggs in epithelioid granulomas
			Cytopathology	Characteristic nonbirefringent, nonoperculated eggs Presence and position of spine determines species
			Microbiology	Embryonated eggs may be present in feces or urine; not sputum Serologic testing available

BAL, bronchoalveolar fluid; EIA, enzyme immunoassay; H&E, hematoxylin-eosin; IFA, immmunofluoresence assay.

larvae, worms, or trophozoites, the various inflammatory patterns must be distinguished from those of other infections and various noninfectious processes due to toxins, drugs, and such entities as asthma, allergic bronchopulmonary aspergillosis, and pulmonary vasculitis syndromes including Churg-Strauss and hypereosinophilic syndromes.[387] Acute and chronic forms of eosinophilic pneumonia, as previously emphasized, have a varied etiology that includes parasitic infections.[388] False-positive morphologic diagnosis of a parasitic infection may be based on presence of objects resembling parasites[337,389] such as lentils in aspiration pneumonia, pollen grains, or Liesegang rings. These ring-like structures can simulate various types of nematodes.[390] Careful attention to the microanatomy of an apparent foreign body and comparison with parasites illustrated in atlases often can resolve such diagnostic dilemmas. Some cases, however, may require referral to pathologists with specialized training and experience in parasitic diseases.

Self-assessment questions related to this chapter can be found online on the Expert Consult site for this title.

References

1. Fauci AS. Infectious diseases: considerations for the 21st century. *Clin Infect Dis*. 2001;32(5):675–685.
2. Schmidt-Ioanas M. Treatment of pneumonia in elderly patient. *Exp Opin Pharmacol*. 2006;7:499–507.
3. Chandler F. Approaches to the pathologic diagnosis of infectious diseases. In: Chandler F, Connor D, Schwartz D, eds. *Pathology of Infectious Disease*. Stamford, CT: Appleton & Lange; 1997:3–7.
4. Watts J. The surgical pathologist's role in the diagnosis of infectious disease. *J Histotechnol*. 1995;18:191–193.
5. Watts JC. Surgical pathology and the diagnosis of infectious diseases. *Am J Clin Pathol*. 1994;102(6):711–712.
6. Morales AR, Essenfeld H, Essenfeld E, et al. Continuous-specimen-flow, high-throughput, 1-hour tissue processing. A system for rapid diagnostic tissue preparation. *Arch Pathol Lab Med*. 2002;126(5):583–590.
7. Rosati LA. The microbe, creator of the pathologist: an inter-related history of pathology, microbiology, and infectious disease. *Ann Diagn Pathol*. 2001;5(3):184–189.
8. Woods GL, Walker DH. Detection of infection or infectious agents by use of cytologic and histologic stains. *Clin Microbiol Rev*. 1996;9(3):382–404.
9. Procop GW, Wilson M. Infectious disease pathology. *Clin Infect Dis*. 2001;32(11):1589–1601.
10. Braunstein H. The value of microbiologic culture of tissue samples in surgical pathology. *Mod Pathol*. 1989;2(3):217–221.
11. Travis WD. Surgical pathology of pulmonary infections. *Semin Thorac Cardiovasc Surg*. 1995;7(2):62–69.
12. Colby TV, Weiss RL. Current concepts in the surgical pathology of pulmonary infections. *Am J Surg Pathol*. 1987;11(suppl 1):25–37.
13. Dunn DL. Diagnosis and treatment of opportunistic infections in immunocompromised surgical patients. *Am Surg*. 2000;66(2):117–125.
14. Levine SJ. An approach to the diagnosis of pulmonary infections in immunosuppressed patients. *Semin Respir Infect*. 1992;7(2):81–95.
15. Dichter JR, Levine SJ, Shelhamer JH. Approach to the immunocompromised host with pulmonary symptoms. *Hematol Oncol Clin North Am*. 1993;7(4):887–912.
16. Wilson WR, Cockerill 3rd FR, Rosenow 3rd EC. Pulmonary disease in the immunocompromised host (2). *Mayo Clin Proc*. 1985;60(9):610–631.
17. Khoor A, Leslie KO, Tazelaar HD, et al. Diffuse pulmonary disease caused by nontuberculous mycobacteria in immunocompetent people (hot tub lung). *Am J Clin Pathol*. 2001;115(5):755–762.
18. Gaspar HB, Goldblatt D. Immunodeficiency syndromes and recurrent infection. *Br J Hosp Med*. 1997;58(11):565–568.
19. Ming JE, Stiehm ER, Graham Jr JM. Immunodeficiency as a component of recognizable syndromes. *Am J Med Genet*. 1996;66(4):378–398.
20. Paller AS. Update on selected inherited immunodeficiency syndromes. *Semin Dermatol*. 1995;14(1):60–65.
21. Williams LW. Congenital immunodeficiency syndromes. *Chest Surg Clin N Am*. 1999;9(1):239–257.
22. Davies JC, Rudin BK. Emerging and unusual gram-negative infections in cystic fibrosis. *Semin Respir Crit Care Med*. 2007;28:312–321.
23. Sibley C, Rabin H, Surette M. Cystic fibrosis: a polymicrobial infection. *Future Microbiol*. 2006;1:53–61.
24. Hayes D. *Mycobacterium abscessus* and other nontuberculosus mycobacteria: Evolving respiratory pathogens in cystic fibrosis: a case report and review. *South Med J*. 2005;98:657–661.
25. Simmonds E, Littlewood J, Evans E. Cystic fibrosis and allergic bronchopulmonary aspergillosis. *Arch Dis Child*. 1990;65:507–511.
26. van Ewijk BE, van der Zalm MM, Wolfs TF, et al. Prevalence and impact of respiratory viral infections in young children with cystic fibrosis: prospective cohort study. *Pediatrics*. 2008;122:1171–1176.
27. Wat D, Gelder C, Hibbitts S, et al. The role of respiratory viruses in cystic fibrosis. *J Cystic Fibros*. 2008;7(4):320–328.
28. Colby TV, Swensen SJ. Anatomic distribution and histopathologic patterns in diffuse lung disease: correlation with HRCT. *J Thorac Imaging*. 1996;11(1):1–26.
29. Leslie KO. My approach to interstitial lung disease using clinical, radiological and histopathologic pattterns. *J Clin Pathol*. 2009;62(5):387–401.
30. Elicker B, Pereira CA, Webb R, Leslie KO. High-resolution computed tomography patterns of diffuse interstitial lung disease with clinical and pathological correlation. *J Bras Pneumol*. 2008;34(9):715–744.
31. Montone KT, Park C. In situ hybridization with oligonucleotide probes: applications to infectious agent detection. In: *Advances in Pathology*. London: Year Book–Mosby; 1996:329–357.
32. Cartun R. Use of immunohistochemistry in the surgical pathology laboratory for the diagnosis of infectious disease. *Pathol Case Rev*. 1999;4:260–265.
33. Wolk D, Mitchell S, Patel R. Principles of molecular microbiology testing methods. *Infect Dis Clin North Am*. 2001;15(4):1157–1204.
34. Versalovic J. Arrays and medical microbiology. *Arch Pathol Lab Med*. 2009;133:537–541.
35. Benson R, Tondella ML, Bhatnagar J, et al. Technology for molecular differential detection of bacterial respiratory disease pathogens. *J Clin Microbiol*. 2008;46:2074–2077.
36. Chan Y, Morris A. Molecular methods in pneumonia. *Curr Opin Infect Dis*. 2007;20:157–164.
37. Kumar S, Wang L, Fan J, et al. Detection of 11 common viral and bacterial pathogens causing community-acquired pneumonia or sepsis in assymptomatic patients by using a mutiplex reverse transcription–PCR assay with manual (enzyme hybridization) or automated (electronic microarray) detection. *J Clin Microbiol*. 2008;46:3063–3072.
38. Kaufman L, Valero G, Padhye AA. Misleading manifestations of Coccidioides immitis in vivo. *J Clin Microbiol*. 1998;36(12):3721–3723.
39. Liu K, Howell DN, Perfect JR, Schell WA. Morphologic criteria for the preliminary identification of *Fusarium*, *Paecilomyces*, and *Acremonium* species by histopathology. *Am J Clin Pathol*. 1998;109(1):45–54.
40. Gorelkin L, Chandler FW. Pseudomicrobes: some potential diagnostic pitfalls in the histopathologic assessment of inflammatory lesions. *Hum Pathol*. 1988;19(8):954–959.
41. Al-Za'abi AM, MacDonald S, Geddie W, Boerner SL. Cytologic examination of bronchoalveolar lavage fluid from immunosuppressed patients. *Diagn Cytopathol*. 2007;35:710–714.
42. DeMay RM. A micromiscellany. In: DeMay RM, ed. *The Art and Science of Cytopathology. Vol. 1, Exfoliative Cytology*. Chicago: ASCP Press; 1996:53–58.
43. Powers CN. Diagnosis of infectious disease: a cytopathologist's perspective. *Clin Microbiol Rev*. 1998;11:341–365.
44. Johnson W, Elson C. Respiratory tract. In: Bibbo M, ed. *Comprehensive Cytopathology*. Philadelphia: Saunders; 1991:340–352.
45. Silverman J, Gay J. Fine-needle aspiration and surgical pathology of infectious disease: morphologic features and role of the clinical microbiology laboratory for rapid diagnosis. *Clin Lab Med*. 1995;15:251–278.
46. Crapanzano JP, Zakowski MF. Diagnostic dilemmas in pulmonary cytology. *Cancer*. 2001;93(6):364–375.
47. Granville L, Laucirica R, Verstovek G. Cinical significance of cultures collected from fine-needle aspirates. *Diagn Cytopathol*. 2008;36:85–88.
48. Fang G, Fine M, Orloff J. New and emerging etiologies for community-acquired pneumonias with implications for therapy. *Medicine (Baltimore)*. 1990;69:307–316.
49. Ruiz-Gonzales A, Falquera M, Nogues A. Is *Streptococcus pneumoniae* the leading cause of pneumonia of unknown etiology? *Am J Med*. 1999;106:385–390.
50. Reimer L. Community-acquired bacterial pneumonia. *Semin Respir Infect*. 2000;15:95–100.
51. Travis WD, Colby TV, Koss MN, et al. Lung infections. In: King D, ed. *Atlas of Non-Tumor Pathology, Fascicle 2. Non-neoplastic Disorders of the Lower Respiratory Tract*. Washington, DC: American Registry of Pathology; 2002:539–728.
52. McIntosh K. Community-acquired pneumonia in children. *N Engl J Med*. 2002;346:429–436.
53. Pennington J. Hospital acquired pneumonia. In: Pennington J, ed. *Respiratory Infections. Diagnosis and Management*. New York: Raven Press; 1994:207–227.
54. Mayer J. Laboratory diagnosis of nosocomial pneumonia. *Semin Respir Infect*. 2000;15:119–131.
55. Baselski V, Mason K. Pneumonia in the immunocompromised host: the role of bronchoscopy and newer diagnostic methods. *Semin Respir Infect*. 2000;15:144–161.
56. Muscedere J, Dodek P, Keenan S, et al. Comprehensive evidence-based clinical practice guidelines for ventilator-associated pneumonia: diagnosis and treatment. *J Crit Care*. 2008;23:132–147.
57. Wall RJ, Ely EW, Talbot TR, et al. Evidence-based algorithms for diagnosing and treating ventilator-associated pneumonia. *J Hosp Med*. 2008;3:409–422.
58. Rea-Neto A, Youssef NC, Tuche F, et al. Diagnosis of ventilator-associated pneumonia: a systematic review of the literature. *Crit Care*. 2008;12:R56.
59. Park D. The microbiology of ventilator-associated pneumonia. *Respir Care*. 2005;50:742–763.
60. Rubinstein E, Kollef M, Nathwani D. Pneumonia caused by methicillin-resistant *Staphylococcus aureus*. *Clin Infect Dis*. 2008;46:S370–S385.
61. Genzen JR, Towle DM, Kravetz JD, Campbell SM. *Salmonella typhimurium* pulmonary infection in an immunocompetent patient. *Conn Med*. 2008;72:142–148.
62. Dolhnikoff M, Mauad T, Bethlem EP, Carvalho CR. Pathology and pathophysiology of pulmonary manifestations in leptospirosis. *Braz J Infect Dis*. 2007;11:142–148.

63. Hindizeh M, Carroll K. Laboratory diagnosis of atypical pneumonia. *Semin Respir Infect*. 2000;15:101–113.

64. Cunha B. The atypical pneumonias: clinical diagnosis and importance. *Clin Microbiol Infect Dis*. 2006;12:12–24.

65. Chandler F. Actinomycosis. In: Chandler F, Connor D, Schwartz D, eds. *Pathology of Infectious Disease*. Stamford, CT: Appleton & Lange; 1997:391–396.

66. de Montpreville V, Nashashibi N, Dulmet E. Actinomycosis and other bronchopulmonary infections with granules. *Ann Diagn Pathol*. 1999;3:67–74.

67. Winn W, LaSala P, Leslie KO. Bacterial infections. In: Tomashefski J, Farver C, Cagle P, Fraire A, eds. *Dail and Hammer's Pulmonary Pathology*. 3rd ed. New York: Springer; 2008:228–315.

68. Hazelton P. Pulmonary bacterial infections. In: Hazelton P, ed. *Spencer's Pathology of the Lung*. New York: McGraw-Hill; 1996:189–256.

69. Lombard C, Yousem S, Kitaichi M, Colby T, eds. *Atlas of Pulmonary Surgical Pathology*. Philadelphia: Saunders; 1991.

70. Sethi S, Murphy T. Infection in the pathogenesis and course of chronic obstructive pulmonary disease. *N Engl J Med*. 2008;359:2355–2365.

71. Kwon KY, Colby TV. *Rhodococcus equi* pneumonia and pulmonary malakoplakia in acquired immunodeficiency syndrome. Pathologic features. *Arch Pathol Lab Med*. 1994;118(7):744–748.

72. Manik P. Aspiration pneumonitis and aspiration pneumonia. *N Engl J Med*. 2001;344:665–671.

73. Barnes TW, Vassallo R, Tazelaar HD, et al. Diffuse bronchiolar disease due to chronic occult aspiration. *Mayo Clin Proc*. 2006;81:172–176.

74. Mukhopadhyay S, Katzenstein AL. Pulmonary disease due to aspiration of food and other particulate matter: a clinicopathologic study of 59 cases diagnosed on biopsy or resection specimens. *Am J Surg Pathol*. 2007;31(5):752–759.

75. Verma P. Laboratory diagnosis of anaerobic pleuropulmonary infections. *Semin Respir Infect*. 2000;15(2):114–118.

76. Corley DE, Winterbauer RH. Infectious diseases that result in slowly resolving and chronic pneumonia. *Semin Respir Infect*. 1993;8(1):3–13.

77. Belchis DA, Simpson E, Colby T. Histopathologic features of *Burkholderia cepacia* pneumonia in patients without cystic fibrosis. *Mod Pathol*. 2000;13(4):369–372.

78. Low D, Massulli T, Marrie T. Progressive and nonresolving pneumonia. *Curr Opin Pulm Med*. 2005;11:247–252.

79. Weyers C, Leeper K. Nonresolving pneumonia. *Clin Chest Med*. 2005;26:143–158.

80. Bauer T, Ewig S, Rodloff AC, Müller EE. Acute respiratory distress syndrome and pneumonia: a comprehensive review of clinical data. *Clin Infect Dis*. 2006;43:748–756.

81. Hayden RT, Uhl JR, Qian X, et al. Direct detection of *Legionella* species from bronchoalveolar lavage and open lung biopsy specimens: comparison of LightCycler PCR, in situ hybridization, direct fluorescence antigen detection, and culture. *J Clin Microbiol*. 2001;39(7):2618–2626.

82. Rollins S, Colby T, Clayton F. Open lung biopsy in *Mycoplasma pneumoniae* pneumonia. *Arch Pathol Lab Med*. 1986;110(1):34–41.

83. Waites K, Tarkington D. *Mycoplasma pneumoniae* and its role as a human pathogen. *Clin Microbiol Rev*. 2004;17:697–728.

84. Bartlett AH, Rivera AL, Krishnamurthy R, Baker CJ. Thoracic actinomycosis in children: case report and review of the literature. *Pediatr Infect Dis J*. 2008;27:165–169.

85. Yildz O, Doggoy M. Actinomycosis and nocardia pulmonary infections. *Curr Opin Pulm Med*. 2006;12:228–234.

86. Vera-Alvarez J, Marigil-Gómez M, García-Prats MD, et al. Primary pulmonary botryomycosis diagnosed by fine needle aspiration biopsy: a case report. *Acta Cytol*. 2006;50:331–334.

87. Oddo D, Gonzalez S. Actinomycosis and nocardiosis. A morphologic study of 17 cases. *Pathol Res Pract*. 1986;181(3):320–326.

88. Dattwyler R. Community-acquired pneumonia in the age of bioterrorism. *Allergy Asthma Proc*. 2005;26:191–194.

89. Bush LM, Abrams BH, Beall A, Johnson CC. Index case of fatal inhalational anthrax due to bioterrorism in the United States. *N Engl J Med*. 2001;345(22):1607–1610.

90. Borio L, Frank D, Mani V, et al. Death due to bioterrorism-related inhalational anthrax: report of 2 patients. *JAMA*. 2001;286(20):2554–2559.

91. Barakat LA, Quentzel HL, Jernigan JA, et al. Fatal inhalational anthrax in a 94-year-old Connecticut woman. *JAMA*. 2002;287(7):863–868.

92. Grinberg LM, et al. Quantitative pathology of inhalational anthrax I: quantitative microscopic findings. *Mod Pathol*. 2001;14(5):482–495.

93. Inglesby TV, Henderson DA, Bartlett JG, et al. Anthrax as a biological weapon: medical and public health management. Working Group on Civilian Biodefense. *JAMA*. 1999;281(18):1735–1745.

94. Inglesby TV, Dennis DT, Henderson DA, et al. Plague as a biological weapon: medical and public health management. Working Group on Civilian Biodefense. *JAMA*. 2000;283(17):2281–2290.

95. Guarner J, Shieh WJ, Greer PW, et al. Immunohistochemical detection of *Yersinia pestis* in formalin-fixed, paraffin-embedded tissue. *Am J Clin Pathol*. 2002;117(2):205–209.

96. Smith J, Reisner B. Plague. In: Chandler F, Connor D, Schwartz D, eds. *Pathology of Infectious Disease*. Stamford, CT: Appleton & Lange; 1997:729–738.

97. Dennis DT, Inglesby TV, Henderson DA, et al. Tularemia as a biological weapon: medical and public health management. *JAMA*. 2001;285(21):2763–2773.

98. Geyer S, Burkey A, Chandler F. Tularemia. In: Chandler F, Connor D, Schwartz D, eds. *Pathology of Infectious Disease*. Stamford, CT: Appleton & Lange; 1997:869–873.

99. Yang PC, Luh KT, Lee YC, et al. Lung abscesses: US examination and US-guided transthoracic aspiration. *Radiology*. 1991;180(1):171–175.

100. Grinan N, Lucerna F, Romero J. Yield of percutaneous aspiration in lung abscess. *Chest*. 1990;97:69–74.

101. Vuori-Holopainen E, Salo E, Saxén H, et al. Etiological diagnosis of childhood pneumonia by use of transthoracic needle aspiration and modern microbiological methods. *Clin Infect Dis*. 2002;34(5):583–590.

102. Garg S, Handa U, Mohan H, Janmeja AK. Comparative analysis of various cytohistological techniques in diagnosis of lung diseases. *Diagn Cytopathol*. 2007;35:26–31.

103. Bartlett R. Medical microbiology: How far to go—how fast to go in 1982. In: Lorian V, ed. *Significance of Medical Microbiology in the Care of Patients*. Baltimore/London: Williams & Wilkins; 1982:12–44.

104. Busmanis I, Harney M, Hellyar A. Nocardiosis diagnosed by lung FNA: a case report. *Diagn Cytopathol*. 1995;12(1):56–58.

105. Mathur S, Sood R, Aron M, et al. Cytologic diagnosis of pulmonary nocardiosis: a report of 3 cases. *Acta Cytol*. 2005;49:567–570.

106. Saubolle MA, McKellar PP. Laboratory diagnosis of community-acquired lower respiratory tract infection. *Infect Dis Clin North Am*. 2001;15(4):1025–1045.

107. Carroll KC. Laboratory diagnosis of lower respiratory tract infections: controversy and conundrums. *J Clin Microbiol*. 2002;40(9):3115–3120.

108. Stratton K. Usefulness of aetiological tests for guiding antibiotic therapy in community-acquired pneumonia. *Int J Antimicrob Agents*. 2008;31:3–11.

109. Barrett-Connor E. The nonvalue of sputum culture in the diagnosis of pneumococcal pneumonia. *Am Rev Respir Dis*. 1971;103(6):845–848.

110. American Thoracic Society. Diagnosis, treatment and prevention of non-tuberculous mycobacterial diseases. *Am J Respir Crit Care Med*. 2007;175:367–416.

111. Bartlett JG, Breiman RF, Mandell LA, File Jr TM. Community-acquired pneumonia in adults: guidelines for management. The Infectious Diseases Society of America. *Clin Infect Dis*. 1998;26(4):811–838.

112. Rosón B, Carratalà J, Verdaguer R, et al. Prospective study of the usefulness of sputum Gram stain in the initial approach to community-acquired pneumonia requiring hospitalization. *Clin Infect Dis*. 2000;31:869–874.

113. Musher D, Montoya R, Wanahita A. Diagnostic value of microscopic examination of gram-stained sputum and sputum cultures in patients with bacteremic pneumococcal pneumonia. *Clin Infect Dis*. 2004;39:165–169.

114. Danés C, González-Martín J, Pumarola T, et al. Pulmonary infiltrates in immunosuppressed patients: analysis of a diagnostic protocol. *J Clin Microbiol*. 2002;40(6):2134–2140.

115. Ellis J, Oyston PC, Green M, Titball RW. Tularemia. *Clin Microbiol Rev*. 2002;15(4):631–646.

116. Conville PS, Brown JM, Steigerwalt AG, et al. *Nocardia veterana* as a pathogen in North American patients. *J Clin Microbiol*. 2003;41(6):2560–2568.

117. Petitjean J, Vabret A, Gouarin S, Freymuth F. Evaluation of four commercial immunoglobulin G (IgG)- and IgM-specific enzyme immunoassays for diagnosis of *Mycoplasma pneumoniae* infections. *J Clin Microbiol*. 2002;40(1):165–171.

118. Blasi F, Tarsia P, Aliberti S, et al. *Chlamydia pneumoniae* and Mycoplasma pneumoniae. *Semin Respir Crit Care Med*. 2005;26:617–624.

119. Lee KY. Pediatric respiratory infection by *Mycoplasma pneumoniae*. *Exp Rev Anti Infect Ther*. 2008;6:509–521.

120. Fields BS, Benson RF, Besser RE. *Legionella* and legionnaires' disease: 25 years of investigation. *Clin Microbiol Rev*. 2002;15(3):506–526.

121. Boulware DR, Daley CL, Merrifield C, et al. Rapid diagnosis of pneumococcal pneumonia among HIV-infected adults with urine antigen detection. *J Infect*. 2007;55:300–309.

122. Muder RR, Yu VL. Infection due to *Legionella* species other than *L. pneumophila*. *Clin Infect Dis*. 2002;35(8):990–998.

123. Benin AL, Benson RF, Besser RE. Trends in legionnaires disease, 1980–1998: declining mortality and new patterns of diagnosis. *Clin Infect Dis*. 2002;35(9):1039–1046.

124. Waring AL, Halse TA, Csiza CK, et al. Development of a genomics-based PCR assay for detection of *Mycoplasma pneumoniae* in a large outbreak in New York State. *J Clin Microbiol*. 2001;39(4):1385–1390.

125. Reischl U, Linde HJ, Lehn N, et al. Direct detection and differentiation of *Legionella* spp. and *Legionella pneumophila* in clinical specimens by dual-color real-time PCR and melting curve analysis. *J Clin Microbiol*. 2002;40(10):3814–3817.

126. Krafft A, Kulesh D. Applying molecular biologic techniques in detection of biologic agents. *Clin Lab Med*. 2001;21:631–660.

127. Wittwer C, Hermann M, Gundry C. Real-time multiplex assays. *Methods*. 2001;25:132–143.

128. Loens K, Beck T, Ursi D, et al. Development of real-time multiplex nucleic acid sequence-based amplification for detection of *Mycoplasma pneumoniae*, *Chlymdia pneumoniae* and *Legionella* spp. in respiratory specimens. *J Clin Microbiol*. 2008;46:185–191.

129. Kunimoto D, Long R. Tuberculosis: still overlooked as a cause of community-acquired pneumonia—how not to miss it. *Respir Care Clin N Am*. 2005;11:25–34.

130. Storla D, Yimer S, Bjune GA. A systematic review of delay in the diagnosis and treatment of tuberculosis. *BMC Public Health*. 2008;8:15.

131. Gardiner DF, Beavis KG. Laboratory diagnosis of mycobacterial infections. *Semin Respir Infect*. 2000;15(2):132–143.

132. Griffith DE, Aksamit T, Brown-Elliott BA, et al. An official ATS/IDSA statement: diagnosis, treatment, and prevention of nontuberculous mycobacterial diseases. *Am J Respir Crit Care Med*. 2007;175(4):367–416.

133. Procop GW, Tazelaar HD. Tuberculosis and other mycobacterial infections of the lung. In: Churg AM, Myers JL, Tazelaar HD, Wright JL, eds. *Thurlbeck's Pathology of the Lung*. 3rd ed. New York/Stuttgart: Thieme Medical Publishers; 2005:219–248.

134. Tomashefski J, Farver C. Tuberculosis and nontuberculous mycobacterial infections. In: Tomashefski J, Farver C, Cagle P, Fraire A, eds. *Dail and Hammer's Pulmonary Pathology*. 3rd ed.New York: Springer; 2008:316–348.

135. Barnes P, Cave C. Molecular epidemiology of tuberculosis. *N Engl J Med*. 2003;12:1149–1156.

136. Lack E, Connor D. Tuberculosis. In: Chandler F, Connor D, Schwartz D, eds. *Pathology of Infectious Disease*. Stamford, CT: Appleton & Lange; 1997:857–868.

137. Small PM, Fujiwara PI. Management of tuberculosis in the United States. *N Engl J Med*. 2001;345(3):189–200.

138. Tortoli E. Impact of genotypic studies on mycobacterial taxonomy: the new mycobacteria of the 1990s. *Clin Microbiol Rev*. 2003;16(2):319–354.

139. Primm TP, Lucero CA, Falkinham 3rd JO. Health impacts of environmental mycobacteria. *Clin Microbiol Rev*. 2004;17(1):98–106.

140. Glassroth J. Pulmonary disease due to nontuberculous mycobacteria. *Chest*. 2008;133:243–251.

141. Field SK, Cowie RL. Lung disease due to more common mycobacteria. *Chest*. 2006;129:1653–1672.

142. Johnson MM, Waller EA, Leventhal JP. Nontuberculous mycobacterial pulmonary disease. *Curr Opin Pulm Med*. 2008;14:203–210.

143. Prince DS, Peterson DD, Steiner RM, et al. Infection with *Mycobacterium avium* complex in patients without predisposing conditions. *N Engl J Med*. 1989;321(13):863–868.

144. Marchevsky A, Damster B, Gribetz A. The spectrum of pathology of nontuberculous mycobacteria in open lung biopsy. *Am J Clin Pathol*. 1982;78:755.

145. Van Dyck P, Vanhoenacker FM, Van den Brande P, De Schepper AM. Imaging of pulmonary tuberculosis. *Eur Radiol*. 2003;13:1771–1785.

146. Martinez S, McAdams H, Batchu C. The many faces of nontuberculous mycobacterial infection. *Am J Roentgenol*. 2007;189:177–186.

147. Pieters J. Mycobacterium tuberculosis and the macrophage. *Cell Host Microbe*. 2008;3:399–407.

148. Leong AS, Wannakrairot P, Leong TY. Apotosis is a major cause of so-called "caseation necrosis" in mycobacterial granulomas in HIV-infected patients. *J Clin Pathol*. 2008;61:366–372.

149. Tang YW, Procop GW, Zheng H, et al. Histologic parameters predictive of mycobacterial infection. *Am J Clin Pathol*. 1998;109(3):331–334.

150. Brastianos PK, Swanson JW, Torbenson M, et al. Tuberculosis-associated haemophagocytic syndrome. *Lancet Infect Dis*. 2006;6:447–454.

151. Dehda K, Booth H, Huggett JF, et al. Lung remodeling in pulmonary tuberculosis. *J Infect Dis*. 2005;192:1201–1209.

152. Hunter R, Jagannath C, Actor J. Pathology of post primary tuberculosis in humans and mice: contradictions of long-held beliefs. *Tuberculosis*. 2007;87:267–278.

153. Hoheisel G, Chan BK, Chan CH, et al. Endobronchial tuberculosis: diagnostic features and therapeutic outcome. *Respir Med*. 1994;88(8):593–597.

154. Bloch KC, Zwerling L, Pletcher MJ, et al. Incidence and clinical implications of isolation of *Mycobacterium kansasii*: results of a 5-year, population-based study. *Ann Intern Med*. 1998;129(9):698–704.

155. Rotterdam H. *Mycobacterium avium* complex infection. In: Chandler F, Connor D, Schwartz D, eds. *Pathology of Infectious Disease*. Stamford, CT: Appleton & Lange; 1997:657–669.

156. Horsburgh Jr CR. *Mycobacterium avium* complex infection in the acquired immunodeficiency syndrome. *N Engl J Med*. 1991;324(19):1332–1338.

157. Kwon KY, Myers JL, Swensen SJ, Colby TV. Middle lobe syndrome: a clinicopathological study of 21 patients. *Hum Pathol*. 1995;26(3):302–307.

158. Wilson RW, Steingrube VA, Böttger EC, et al. *Mycobacterium immunogenum* sp. nov, a novel species related to *Mycobacterium abscessus* and associated with clinical disease, pseudo-outbreaks and contaminated metalworking fluids: an international cooperative study on mycobacterial taxonomy. *Int J Syst Evol Microbiol*. 2001;51:1751–1764.

159. Sekosan M, Cleto M, Senseng C, et al. Spindle cell pseudotumors in the lungs due to *Mycobacterium tuberculosis* in a transplant patient. *Am J Surg Pathol*. 1994;18(10):1065–1068.

160. Asano T, Itoh G, Itoh M. Disseminated *Mycobacterium intracellulare* infection in an HIV-negative, non-immunosuppressed patient with multiple endobronchial polyps. *Respiration*. 2002;69:175–177.

161. Brown-Elliott BA, Wallace Jr RJ. Clinical and taxonomic status of pathogenic nonpigmented or late-pigmenting rapidly growing mycobacteria. *Clin Microbiol Rev*. 2002;15(4):716–746.

162. Greenberger P, Katzenstein A. Lipoid pneumonia with atypical mycobacterial colonization. Association with allergic bronchopulmonary aspergillosis. *Arch Intern Med*. 1983;143:2003–2005.

163. Gable AD, Marsee DK, Milner DA, Granter SR. Suppurative inflammation with microabscess and pseudocyst formation is a characteristic histologic manifestation of cutaneous infections with rapid-growing *Mycobacterium* species. *Am J Clin Pathol*. 2008;130:514–517.

164. Das D. Fine needle aspiration cytology in the diagnosis of tuberculous lesions. *Lab Med*. 2000;31:625–632.

165. Dahlgren SE, Ekstrom P. Aspiration cytology in the diagnosis of pulmonary tuberculosis. *Scand J Respir Dis*. 1972;53(4):196–201.

166. Smith MB, Molina CP, Schnadig VJ, et al. Pathologic features of *Mycobacterium kansasii* infection in patients with acquired immunodeficiency syndrome. *Arch Pathol Lab Med*. 2003;127(5):554–560.

167. Zerbi P, Schønau A, Bonetto S, et al. Amplified in situ hybridization with peptide nucleic acid probes for differentiation of *Mycobacterium tuberculosis* complex and nontuberculous *Mycobacterium* species on formalin-fixed, paraffin-embedded archival biopsy and autopsy samples. *Am J Clin Pathol*. 2001;116(5):770–775.

168. Cho S, Brennan R. Tuberculosis diagnostics. *Tuberculosis*. 2007;87:s14–s17.

169. Tiwari RP, Hattikudur NS, Bharmal RN, et al. Modern approaches to a rapid diagnosis of tuberculosis: promises and challenges ahead. *Tuberculosis*. 2007;87:193–201.

170. Hardman WJ, Benian GM, Howard T, et al. Rapid detection of mycobacteria in inflammatory necrotizing granulomas from formalin-fixed, paraffin-embedded tissue by PCR in clinically high-risk patients with acid-fast stain and culture-negative tissue biopsies. *Am J Clin Pathol*. 1996;106(3):384–389.

171. Park DY, Kim JY, Choi KU, et al. Comparison of polymerase chain reaction with histopathologic features for diagnosis of tuberculosis in formalin-fixed, paraffin-embedded histologic specimens. *Arch Pathol Lab Med*. 2003;127(3):326–330.

172. Schulz S, Cabras AD, Kremer M, et al. Species identification of mycobacteria in paraffin-embedded tissues: frequent detection of non tuberculous mycobacteria. *Mod Pathol*. 2005;18:274–282.

173. Renshaw AA. The relative sensitivity of special stains and culture in open lung biopsies. *Am J Clin Pathol*. 1994;102(6):736–740.

174. O'Sullivan CE, Miller DR, Schneider PS, Roberts GD. Evaluation of Gen-Probe amplified *Mycobacterium tuberculosis* direct test by using respiratory and nonrespiratory specimens in a tertiary care center laboratory. *J Clin Microbiol*. 2002;40(5):1723–1727.

175. Bemer P, Palicova F, Rüsch-Gerdes S, et al. Multicenter evaluation of fully automated BacTec Mycobacteria Growth Indicator Tube 960 system for susceptibility testing of *Mycobacterium tuberculosis*. *J Clin Microbiol*. 2002;40(1):150–154.

176. Woods GL. Molecular techniques in mycobacterial detection. *Arch Pathol Lab Med*. 2001;125(1):122–126.

177. Hasegawa N, Miura T, Ishii K, et al. New simple and rapid test for culture confirmation of *Mycobacterium tuberculosis* complex: a multicenter study. *J Clin Microbiol*. 2002;40(3):908–912.

178. Al Zahrani K, Al Jahdali H, Poirier L, et al. Accuracy and utility of commercially available amplification and serologic tests for the diagnosis of minimal pulmonary tuberculosis. *Am J Respir Crit Care Med*. 2000;162(4 Pt 1):1323–1329.

179. Schluger NW. Changing approaches to the diagnosis of tuberculosis. *Am J Respir Crit Care Med*. 2001;164(11):2020–2024.

180. Sabonya R. Fungal disease, including *Pneumocystis*. In: Churg AM, Myers JL, Tazelaar HD, Wright JL, eds. *Thurlbeck's Pathology of the Lung*. 3rd ed.New York: Thieme Medical Publishers; 2005:283–314.

181. Haque A, McGinnis MR. Fungal infections. In: Tomashefski J, Farver C, Cagle P, Fraire A, eds. *Dail and Hammer's Pulmonary Pathology*. 3rd ed.New York: Springer; 2008:349–425.

182. Saubolle MA. Fungal pneumonias. *Semin Respir Infect*. 2000;15(2):162–177.

183. Karnak D, Avery RK, Gildea TR, et al. Endobronchial fungal disease: an under-recognized entity. *Respiration*. 2007;74:88–104.

184. Chandler F, Watts JC. *Pathologic Diagnosis of Fungal Infections*. Chicago: ASCP Press; 1987.

185. Watts JC, Chandler FW. Morphologic identification of mycelial pathogens in tissue sections. A caveat. *Am J Clin Pathol*. 1998;109(1):1–2.

186. Lemos LB, Baliga M, Guo M. Blastomycosis: The great pretender can also be an opportunist. Initial clinical diagnosis and underlying diseases in 123 patients. *Ann Diagn Pathol*. 2002;6(3):194–203.

187. Taxy J. Blastomycosis: contributions of morphology to diagnosis. A surgical pathology, cytopathology and autopsy study. *Am J Surg Pathol*. 2007;31:615–623.

188. Lemos LB, Guo M, Baliga M. Blastomycosis: organ involvement and etiologic diagnosis. A review of 123 patients from Mississippi. *Ann Diagn Pathol*. 2000;4(6):391–406.

189. Chandler F. Blastomycosis. In: Chandler F, Connor D, Schwartz D, eds. *Pathology of Infectious Disease*. Stamford, CT: Appleton & Lange; 1997:943–951.

190. Hussain Z, Martin A, Youngberg GA. *Blastomyces dermatitidis* with large yeast forms. *Arch Pathol Lab Med*. 2001;125(5):663–664.

191. Fisher MC, Koenig GL, White TJ, Taylor JW. Molecular and phenotypic description of *Coccidioides posadasii* sp. nov., previously recognized as the no-California population of *Coccidioides immitis*. *Mycologia*. 2002;94:73–84.

192. Pappagianis D, Chandler F. Coccidioidomycosis. In: Chandler F, Connor D, Schwartz D, eds. *Pathology of Infectious Disease*. Stamford, CT: Appleton & Lange; 1997:977–987.

193. DiTomasso JP, Ampel NM, Sobonya RE, Bloom JW. Bronchoscopic diagnosis of pulmonary coccidioidomycosis. Comparison of cytology, culture, and transbronchial biopsy. *Diagn Microbiol Infect Dis*. 1994;18(2):83–87.

194. Polesky A, Kirsch CM, Snyder LS, et al. Airway coccidioidomycosis—report of cases and review. *Clin Infect Dis*. 1999;28(6):1273–1280.

195. Valdivia L, Nix D, Wright M, et al. Coccidioidomycosis as a common cause of community-acquired pneumonia. *Emerg Infect Dis*. 2006;12:958–962.

196. Wheat J. Endemic mycoses in AIDS: A clinical review. *Clin Microbiol Rev*. 1995;8(1):146–159.

197. Goodwin Jr RA, Shapiro JL, Thurman GH, et al. Disseminated histoplasmosis: clinical and pathologic correlations. *Medicine (Baltimore)*. 1980;59(1):1–33.

198. Chandler F, Watts JC. *Histoplasmosis capsulati*. In: Chandler F, Connor D, Schwartz D, eds. *Pathology of Infectious Disease*. Stamford, CT: Appleton & Lange; 1997:1007–1015.

199. Londero A, Chandler F. Paracoccidioidomycosis. In: Chandler F, Connor D, Schwartz D, eds. *Pathology of Infectious Disease*. Stamford, CT: Appleton & Lange; 1997:1045–1053.

200. England DM, Hochholzer L. Primary pulmonary sporotrichosis. Report of eight cases with clinicopathologic review. *Am J Surg Pathol*. 1985;9(3):193–204.

201. Deng ZL, Connor DH. Progressive disseminated penicilliosis caused by *Penicillium marneffei*. Report of eight cases and differentiation of the causative organism from *Histoplasma capsulatum*. *Am J Clin Pathol*. 1985;84(3):323–327.

202. McGinnis MR, Chandler F. *Penicilliosis marneffei*. In: Chandler F, Connor D, Schwartz D, eds. *Pathology of Infectious Disease*. Stamford, CT: Appleton and Lange; 1997:1055–1058.

203. Mark EJ. Case records of the Massachusetts General Hospital. *N Engl J Med*. 2002;347:518–524.

204. Menefee J, Hutchins GM. Pulmonary cryptococcosis. *Hum Pathol*. 1985;16:121–128.

205. Singh Y, Pratistadevi K. Cryptococcal inflammatory pseudotumor. *Am J Surg Pathol*. 2007;31:1521–1527.

206. Pfaller M, Diekema D. Rare and emerging opportunistic fungal pathogens: concerns for resistance beyond *Candida albicans* and *Aspergillus fumigatus*. *J Clin Microbiol*. 2004;42:4419–4431.

207. Lun M. Candidiasis. In: Chandler F, Connor D, Schwartz D, eds. *Pathology of Infectious Disease*. Stamford, CT: Appleton & Lange; 1997:953–964.

208. Latge JP. *Aspergillus fumigatus* and aspergillosis. *Clin Microbiol Rev*. 1999;12(2):310–350.

209. Bosken CH, Myers JL, Greenberger PA, Katzenstein AL. Pathologic features of allergic bronchopulmonary aspergillosis. *Am J Surg Pathol*. 1988;12(3):216–222.

210. Yousem SA. The histological spectrum of chronic necrotizing forms of pulmonary aspergillosis. *Hum Pathol*. 1997;28(6):650–656.

211. Scully R, Mark E, McNeeley W. Case records of the Massachusetts General Hospital. *N Engl J Med*. 2001;345:443–449.

212. Segal B. Aspergillosis. *N Engl J Med*. 2009;360:1870–1884.

213. Stergiopoulou T, Meletiadis J, Roilides E, et al. Host-dependent patterns of tissue injury in invasive pulmonary aspergillosis. *Am J Clin Pathol*. 2007;127:349–355.

214. Kradin R, Mark EJ. The pathology of pulmonary disorders due to *Aspergillus* spp. *Arch Pathol Lab Med*. 2008;132:606–614.

215. Tadros TS, Workowski KA, Siegel RJ, et al. Pathology of hyalohyphomycosis caused by *Scedosporium apiospermum* (*Pseudallescheria boydii*): an emerging mycosis. *Hum Pathol*. 1998;29(11):1266–1272.

216. Boutati EI, Anaissie EJ. Fusarium, a significant emerging pathogen in patients with hematologic malignancy: ten years' experience at a cancer center and implications for management. *Blood*. 1997;90(3):999–1008.

217. Gutiérrez F, Masiá M, Ramos J, et al. Pulmonary mycetoma caused by an atypical isolate of *Paceilomyces* species in an immunocompetent individual: case report and literature review of *Paecilomyces* lung infections. *Eur J Clin Microbiol Infect Dis*. 2005;24:607–611.

218. Bigliazzi C, Poletti V, Dell'Amore D, et al. Disseminated basidiobolomycosis in an immunocompetent woman. *J Clin Microbiol*. 2004;42:1367–1369.

219. Guarro J, Gene J, Stchigel AM. Developments in fungal taxonomy. *Clin Microbiol Rev*. 1999;12(3):454–500.

220. Ribes JA, Vanover-Sams CL, Baker DJ. Zygomycetes in human disease. *Clin Microbiol Rev*. 2000;13(2):236–301.

221. Zaoutis T, Roilides E, Chiou C. Zygomycosis in children. *Pediatr Infect Dis J*. 2007;26:723–727.

222. Irwin R, Rinaldi M, Walsh T. Zygomycosis of the respiratory tract. In: Sarosi G, Davies S, eds. *Fungal Diseases of the Lung*. Philadelphia: Lippincott Williams & Wilkins; 2000:163–185.

223. Hansen LA, Prakash UB, Colby TV. Pulmonary complications in diabetes mellitus. *Mayo Clin Proc*. 1989;64(7):791–799.

224. Frater JL, Hall GS, Procop GW. Histologic features of zygomycosis: emphasis on perineural invasion and fungal morphology. *Arch Pathol Lab Med*. 2001;125(3):375–378.

225. Kimura M, Schnadig VJ, McGinnis MR. Chlamydoconidia formation in zygomycosis due to *Rhizopus* species. *Arch Pathol Lab Med*. 1998;122(12):1120–1122.

226. Lake FR, Froudist JH, McAleer R, et al. Allergic bronchopulmonary fungal disease caused by *Bipolaris* and *Curvularia*. *Aust N Z J Med*. 1991;21(6):871–874.

227. Travis WD, Kwon-Chung KJ, Kleiner DE, et al. Unusual aspects of allergic bronchopulmonary fungal disease: report of two cases due to *Curvularia* organisms associated with allergic fungal sinusitis. *Hum Pathol*. 1991;22(12):1240–1248.

228. Revankar S. Therapy of infections caused by dematiaceous fungi. *Exp Rev Anti Infect Ther*. 2005;3:601–612.

229. Stringer JR, Beard CB, Miller RF, Wakefield AE. A new name (*Pneumocystis jiroveci*) for Pneumocystis from humans. *Emerg Infect Dis*. 2002;8(9):891–896.

230. Zahar JR, Robin M, Azoulay E, et al. *Pneumocystis carinii* pneumonia in critically ill patients with malignancy: a descriptive study. *Clin Infect Dis*. 2002;35(8):929–934.

231. Schliep TC, Yarrish RL. *Pneumocystis carinii* pneumonia. *Semin Respir Infect*. 1999;14(4):333–343.

232. Wazir J, Ansari N. *Pneumocystis carinii* infection. Update and review. *Arch Pathol Lab Med*. 2004;128:1023–1027.

233. Travis WD, Pittaluga S, Lipschik GY, et al. Atypical pathologic manifestations of *Pneumocystis carinii* pneumonia in the acquired immune deficiency syndrome. Review of 123 lung biopsies from 76 patients with emphasis on cysts, vascular invasion, vasculitis, and granulomas. *Am J Surg Pathol*. 1990;14(7):615–625.

234. Haque A, Adegboyega P. *Pneumocystis jiroveci* pneumonia. In: Tomashefski J, Farver C, Cagle P, Fraire A, eds. *Dail and Hammar's Pulmonary Pathology*. 3rd ed.New York: Springer; 2008:426–475.

235. Hartz JW, Geisinger KR, Scharyj M, Muss HB. Granulomatous pneumocystosis presenting as a solitary pulmonary nodule. *Arch Pathol Lab Med*. 1985;109(5):466–469.

236. Couples JB, Blackie SP, Road JD. Granulomatous *Pneumocystis carinii* pneumonia mimicking tuberculosis. *Arch Pathol Lab Med*. 1989;113(11):1281–1284.

237. Liaw YS, Yang PC, Yu CJ, et al. Direct determination of cryptococcal antigen in transthoracic needle aspirate for diagnosis of pulmonary cryptococcosis. *J Clin Microbiol*. 1995;33(6):1588–1591.

238. Raab SS, Silverman JF, Zimmerman KG. Fine-needle aspiration biopsy of pulmonary coccidioidomycosis. Spectrum of cytologic findings in 73 patients. *Am J Clin Pathol*. 1993;99(5):582–587.

239. Zimmerman RL, Montone KT, Fogt F, Norris AH. Ultra fast identification of *Aspergillus* species in pulmonary cytology specimens by in situ hybridization. *Int J Mol Med*. 2000;5(4):427–429.

240. Aubry MC, Fraser R. The role of bronchial biopsy and washing in the diagnosis of allergic bronchopulmonary aspergillosis. *Mod Pathol*. 1998;11(7):607–611.

241. Kimura A, McGinnis MR. Fontana-Masson–stained tissue from culture-proven mycoses. *Arch Pathol Lab Med*. 1998;122(12):1107–1111.

242. Monheit JE, Cowan DF, Moore DG. Rapid detection of fungi in tissues using calcofluor white and fluorescence microscopy. *Arch Pathol Lab Med*. 1984;108(8):616–618.

243. Bialek R, Ernst F, Dietz K, et al. Comparison of staining methods and a nested PCR assay to detect *Histoplasma capsulatum* in tissue sections. *Am J Clin Pathol*. 2002;117(4):597–603.

244. Rosner ER, Reiss E, Warren NG, et al. Evaluation of the status of laboratory practices and the need for continuing education in medical mycology. *Am J Clin Pathol*. 2002;118(2):278–286.

245. Perfect JR, Cox GM, Lee JY, et al. The impact of culture isolation of *Aspergillus* species: a hospital-based survey of aspergillosis. *Clin Infect Dis*. 2001;33(11):1824–1833.

246. Yeo SF, Wong B. Current status of nonculture methods for diagnosis of invasive fungal infections. *Clin Microbiol Rev*. 2002;15(3):465–484.

247. Challier S, Boyer S, Abachin E, Berche P. Development of a serum based Taqman real-time PCR assay for diagnosis of invasive aspergillosis. *J Clin Microbiol*. 2004;42:844–846.

248. Tarrand JJ, Lichterfeld M, Warraich I, et al. Diagnosis of invasive septate mold infections. A correlation of microbiological culture and histologic or cytologic examination. *Am J Clin Pathol*. 2003;119(6):854–858.

249. Moskowitz LB, Ganjei P, Ziegels-Weissman J, et al. Immunohistologic identification of fungi in systemic and cutaneous mycoses. *Arch Pathol Lab Med*. 1986;110(5):433–436.

250. Choi J, Mauger J, McGowan K. Immunohistochemical detection of Aspergillus species in pediatric tissue samples. *Am J Clin Pathol*. 2004;121:18–25.

251. Hayden RT, Qian X, Roberts GD, Lloyd RV. In situ hybridization for the identification of yeastlike organisms in tissue section. *Diagn Mol Pathol*. 2001;10(1):15–23.

252. Sandhu GS, Kline BC, Stockman L, Roberts GD. Molecular probes for diagnosis of fungal infections. *J Clin Microbiol*. 1995;33(11):2913–2919.

253. Lindsley MD, Hurst SF, Iqbal NJ, Morrison CJ. Rapid identification of dimorphic and yeast-like fungal pathogens using specific DNA probes. *J Clin Microbiol*. 2001;39(10):3505–3511.

254. Pham AS, Tarrand JJ, May GS, et al. Diagnosis of invasive mold infection by real-time quantitative PCR. *Am J Clin Pathol*. 2003;119(1):38–44.

255. Wheat J. Serologic diagnosis of infectious disease. In: Sarosi G, Davies S, eds. *Fungal Disease of the Lung*. Philadelphia: Lippincott Williams & Wilkins; 2000:17–29.

256. Pappagianis D, Zimmer BL. Serology of coccidioidomycosis. *Clin Microbiol Rev*. 1990;3(3):247–268.

257. Wheat J. Laboratory diagnosis of histoplasmosis. *Semin Respir Infect*. 2001;16:141–148.

258. Kwak EJ, Husain S, Obman A, et al. Efficacy of galactomannan antigen in the Platelia Aspergillus antigen immunoassay for the diagnosis of invasive aspergillosis in liver transplants. *J Clin Microbiol*. 2004;42:435–438.

259. Treanor J. Respiratory infections. In: Richman R, Whitley R, eds. *Clinical Virology*. New York: Churchill Livingstone; 1997:5–34.

260. Storch GA. Diagnostic virology. *Clin Infect Dis*. 2000;31(3):739–751.

261. Rabella N, Rodriguez P, Labeaga R, et al. Conventional respiratory viruses recovered from immunocompromised patients: clinical considerations. *Clin Infect Dis*. 1999;28(5):1043–1048.

262. Gilliam-Ross L. Emerging respiratory viruses: challenges and vaccine strategies. *Clin Microbiol Rev*. 2006;19:614–636.

263. Kahn J. Newly identified respiratory viruses. *Pediatr Infect Dis J*. 2007;26:745–746.

264. WHO Writing Committee. Clinical aspects of pandemic 2009 influenza A (H1N1) virus infection. *N Engl J Med*. 2010;362.1708–1719.

265. Papa A, Papadimitriou E. Coronaviruses in children. Greece. *Emerg Infect Dis*. 2007;13:447–449.

266. Vicente D, Cilla G, Montes M, et al. Human bocavirus, a respiratory and enteric virus. *Emerg Infect Dis*. 2007;13:636–637.

267. Galan A, Rauch C, Otis C. Fatal BK polyoma viral pneumonia associated with immunosuppression. *Hum Pathol*. 2005;36:1031–1034.

268. Zaki SR, Paddock CD. Viral infections of the lung. In: Tomashefski J, Farver C, Cagle P, Fraire A, eds. *Dail and Hammar's Pulmonary Pathology*. 3rd ed.New York: Springer; 2008:426–475.

269. Magro CM, Wusirika R, Frambach GE, et al. Autoimmune-like pulmonary disease in association with parvovirus B19: a clinical, morphologic and molecular study of 12 cases. *Appl Immunohist Mol Morphol*. 2006;14:208–216.

270. Mizgard J. Acute lower respiratory tract infection. *N Engl J Med*. 2008;358:716–727.

271. Malherbe H, Strickland-Cholmley M. *Viral Cytopathology*. Boca Raton, FL: CRC Press; 1980.

272. Fields B, Knipe D. *Virology*. New York: Raven Press; 1990.

273. Shieh WJ, Hsiao CH, Paddock CD, et al. Immunohistochemical, in situ hybridization and ultrastructural localization of SARS-associated coronavirus in lung of a fatal case of severe acute respiratory syndrome in Taiwan. *Hum Pathol*. 2005;36:303–309.

274. Nuovo G. The utility of in situ-based methodologies including in situ polymerase chain reaction for the diagnosis and study of viral infections. *Hum Pathol*. 2007;38:1123–1136.

275. Walsh JJ, Dietlein LF, Low FN, et al. Broncheotracheal response in human influenza. Type A, Asian strain, as studied by light and electron microscopic esamination of bronchoscopic biopsies. *Arch Intern Med*. 1961;108:376–388.

276. Winternitz M, Wason I, McNamara F. *The Pathology of Influenza*. New Haven, CT: Yale University Press; 1920.

277. Anjuna V, Colby T. Pathologic features of lung biopsy specimens from influenza pneumonia cases. *Hum Pathol*. 1994;25:47–53.

278. Taubenberger J, Morens D. L The pathology of influenza virus infections. *Ann Rev Pathol*. 2008;3:499–522.

279. World Health Organization. Cumulative number of confirmed cases of avian influenza A/H5N1 reported to WHO. Available at: www.who.int/csr/disease/avian_influenza/country/cases_table_2008_06_19/en/index.html Accessed 25.12.09.

280. de Jong MD, Simmons CP, Thanh TT, et al. Fatal outcome of human influenza A (H5N1) is associated with viral load and hypercytokinemia. *Nat Med*. 2006;12:1203–1207.

281. Guarner J, Shieh WJ, Dawson J, et al. Immunohistochemical and in situ hybridization studies of influenza A virus infection in human lungs. *Am J Clin Pathol*. 2000;114(2):227–233.

282. Hall CB. Respiratory syncytial virus and parainfluenza virus. *N Engl J Med*. 2001;344(25):1917–1928.

283. Griffin MR, Coffey CS, Neuzil KM, et al. Winter viruses: influenza- and respiratory syncytial virus–related morbidity in chronic lung disease. *Arch Intern Med*. 2002;162(11):1229–1236.

284. Madden J, Burchette J, Hale L. Pathology of parainfluenza virus infection in patients with congenital immunodeficiency syndromes. *Hum Pathol*. 2004;35:594–603.

285. Hall CB, Weinberg G. The burden of respiratory syncytial virus infection in young children. *N Engl J Med*. 2009;360:588–598.

286. Falsey A, Walsh EE. Viral pneumonia in older adults. *Clin Infect Dis*. 2006;42:518–524.

287. Falsey AR, Formica MA, Walsh EE. Diagnosis of respiratory syncytial virus infection: Comparison of reverse transcription-PCR to viral culture and serology in adults with respiratory illness. *J Clin Microbiol*. 2002;40(3):817–820.

288. Krinzman S, Basgoz N, Kradin R, et al. Respiratory syncytial virus–associated infections in adult recipients of solid organ transplants. *J Heart Lung Transplant*. 1998;17(2):202–210.

289. Johnson J, Gonzales R, Olson S. The histopathology of fatal untreated human respiratory syncytial virus infection. *Mod Pathol*. 2007;20:108–119.

290. Williams JV, Harris PA, Tollefson SJ, et al. Human metapneumovirus and lower respiratory tract disease in otherwise healthy infants and children. *N Engl J Med*. 2004;350:443–450.

291. Sumino KC, Agapov E, Pierce RA, et al. Detection of severe human metapneumovirus infection by real-time polymerase chain reaction and histopathologic assessment. *J Infect Dis*. 2005;192:1052–1060.

292. Vargas SO, Kozakewich HP, Perez-Atayde AR, McAdam AJ. Pathology of human metapneumovirus infection: insights into pathogenesis of a newly identified respiratory virus. *Pediatr Dev Pathol*. 2004;7:478–486.

293. Duke T, Mgone C. Measles: not just another viral exanthem. *Lancet*. 2003;361:763–773.

294. Moussallem T, Guedes F, Fernandes E. Lung involvement in childhood measles: severe immune dysfunction revealed by quantitative immunohistochemistry. *Hum Pathol*. 2007;38:1239–1247.

295. Nolte KB, Feddersen RM, Foucar K, et al. Hantavirus pulmonary syndrome in the United States: a pathological description of a disease caused by a new agent. *Hum Pathol*. 1995;26(1):110–120.

296. Colby TV, Zaki SR, Feddersen RM, Nolte KB. Hantavirus pulmonary syndrome is distinguishable from acute interstitial pneumonia. *Arch Pathol Lab Med*. 2000;124(10):1463–1466.

297. Koster F, Foucar K, Hjelle B, et al. Rapid presumptive diagnosis of hantavirus cardiopulmonary syndrome by peripheral blood smear review. *Am J Clin Pathol*. 2001;116(5):665–672.

298. Peters CJ, Khan AS. Hantavirus pulmonary syndrome: the new American hemorrhagic fever. *Clin Infect Dis*. 2002;34(9):1224–1231.

299. MacIntosh K. Coronaviruses. In: Richman D, Whitley R, eds. *Clinical Virology*. New York: Churchill Livingstone; 1997:1123–1130.

300. Falsey AR, Walsh EE, Hayden FG. Rhinovirus and coronavirus infection–associated hospitalizations among older adults. *J Infect Dis*. 2002;185(9):1338–1341.

301. Wenzel RP, Edmond MB. Managing SARS amidst uncertainty. *N Engl J Med*. 2003;348(20):1947–1948.

302. Ksiazek TG, Erdman D, Goldsmith CS, et al. A novel coronavirus associated with severe acute respiratory syndrome. *N Engl J Med*. 2003;348(20):1953–1966.

303. Booth CM, Matukas LM, Tomlinson GA, et al. Clinical features and short-term outcomes of 144 patients with SARS in the greater Toronto area. *JAMA*. 2003;289(21):2801–2809.

304. Lee N, Hui D, Wu A, et al. A major outbreak of severe acute respiratory syndrome in Hong Kong. *N Engl J Med*. 2003;348(20):1986–1994.

305. Chow KC, Hsiao CH, Lin TY, et al. Detection of severe acute respiratory syndrome–associated coronavirus in pneumocytes of the lung. *Am J Clin Pathol*. 2004;121:574–580.

306. Hwang DM, Chamberlain DW, Poutanen SM, et al. Pulmonary pathology of severe acute respiratory syndrome in Toronto. *Mod Pathol*. 2005;18:1–10.

307. Ye J, Zhang B, Xu J, et al. Molecular pathology in the lungs of severe acute respiratory syndrome patients. *Am J Pathol*. 2007;170:538–545.

308. Ng WF, To KF, Lam WW, et al. The comparative pathology of severe acute respiratory syndrome and avian influenza A subtype H5N1—a review. *Hum Pathol*. 2006;37:381–390.

309. Peled N, Nakar C, Huberman H, et al. Adenovirus infection in hospitalized immunocompetent children. *Clin Pediatr (Phila)*. 2004;43:223–229.

310. Ohori NP, Michaels MG, Jaffe R, et al. Adenovirus pneumonia in lung transplant recipients. *Hum Pathol*. 1995;26(10):1073–1979.

311. Pham T, Burchette J, Hale L. Fatal disseminated adenovirus infection in immunocompromised patients. *Am J Clin Pathol*. 2003;120:575–583.

312. Floudas CS, Kanakis MA, Andreopoulos A, Vaiopoulos GA. Nodular lung calcifications following varicella-zoster pneumonia. *Q J Med*. 2008;101:159.

313. Andrade ZR, Garippo AL, Saldiva PH, Capelozzi VL. Immunohistochemical and in situ detection of cytomegalovirus in lung autopsies of children immunocompromised by secondary interstitial pneumonia. *Pathol Res Pract*. 2004;200(1):25–32.

314. Landry ML. Multiple viral infections in the immunocompromised host: recognition and interpretation. *Clin Diagn Virol*. 1994;2(6):313–321.

315. Schooley RT, Carey RW, Miller G, et al. Chronic Epstein-Barr virus infection associated with fever and interstitial pneumonitis. Clinical and serologic features and response to antiviral chemotherapy. *Ann Intern Med*. 1986;104(5):636–643.

316. Wick MJ, Woronzoff-Dashkoff KP, McGlennen RC. The molecular characterization of fatal infectious mononucleosis. *Am J Clin Pathol*. 2002;117(4):582–588.

317. Buchanan AJ, Gupta RK. Cytomegalovirus infection of the lung: cytomorphologic diagnosis by fine-needle aspiration cytology. *Diagn Cytopathol*. 1986;2(4):341–342.

318. Feldman P, Covell J. *Fine Needle Aspiration Cytology and Its Clinical Applications: Breast and Lung*. Chicago: ASCP Press; 1985.

319. Leland DS, Emanuel D. Laboratory diagnosis of viral infections of the lung. *Semin Respir Infect*. 1995;10(4):189–198.

320. Barenfanger J, Drake C, Leon N, et al. Clinical and financial benefits of rapid detection of respiratory viruses: an outcomes study. *J Clin Microbiol*. 2000;38(8):2824–2828.

321. Payne C. Electron microscopy in the diagnosis of infectious diseases. In: Chandler F, Connor D, Schwartz D, eds. *Pathology of Infectious Disease*. Stamford, CT: Appleton & Lange; 1997:9–34.

322. Murphy P, Roberts ZM, Waner JL. Differential diagnoses of influenza A virus, influenza B virus, and respiratory syncytial virus infections by direct immunofluorescence using mixtures of monoclonal antibodies of different isotypes. *J Clin Microbiol*. 1996;34(7):1798–1800.

323. Legoff J, Kara R, Moulin F, et al. Evaluation of the one-step multiplex real-time reverse transcription-PCR ProFlu-1 assay for the detection of influenza A and influenza B viruses in children. *J Clin Microbiol*. 2008;46:789–791.

324. Reijans M, Dingemans G, Klaassen CH, et al. RespiFinder: a new multiparameter test to differentially identify fifteen respiratory viruses. *J Clin Microbiol*. 2008;46:1232–1240.

325. Mahony J, Chong S, Merante F, et al. Development of a respiratory virus panel test for detection of twenty human respiratory viruses by use of multiplex PCR and fluid microbead–based assay. *J Clin Microbiol*. 2007;45:2965–2970.

326. Nolte FS, Marshall DJ, Rasberry C, et al. MultiCode-PLx system for multiplexed detection of seventeen respiratory viruses. *J Clin Microbiol*. 2007;45:2779–2786.

327. Takahashi H, Norman SA, Mather EL, Patterson BK. Evaluation of the Nanochip 400 system for detection of influenza A and B, respiratory syncytial virus and parainfluenza virus. *J Clin Microbiol*. 2008;46:1724–1727.

328. Wang W, Ren P, Mardi S, et al. Design of mutiplexed detection assays for identification of avian influenza A virus subtypes pathogenic to humans by SmartCycler real-time reverse transcription-PCR. *J Clin Microbiol*. 2009;47:86–92.

329. Rea TD, Ashley RL, Russo JE, Buchwald DS. A systematic study of Epstein-Barr virus serologic assays following acute infection. *Am J Clin Pathol*. 2002;117(1):156–161.

330. Razonable RR, Paya CV, Smith TF. Role of the laboratory in diagnosis and management of cytomegalovirus infection in hematopoietic stem cell and solid-organ transplant recipients. *J Clin Microbiol*. 2002;40(3):746–752.

331. Weinberg A, Schissel D, Giller R. Molecular methods for cytomegalovirus surveillance in bone marrow transplant recipients. *J Clin Microbiol*. 2002;40(11):4203–4206.

332. Chemaly R, Yen-Lieberman B, Castilla EA, et al. Correlation between viral loads of cytomegalovirus in blood and bronchoalveolar lavage specimens from lung transplant recipients determined by histology and immunohistochemistry. *J Clin Microbiol*. 2004;42:2168–2172.

333. Cox FE. History of human parasitology. *Clin Microbiol Rev*. 2002;15(4):595–612.

334. Vijuyan V. Tropical parasitic lung disease. *Indian J Chest Dis Allied Sci*. 2008;50:49–66.

335. Fritche TR, Selvarangan R. Medical parasitology. In: McPherson R, Pincus M, eds. *Henry's Clinical Diagnosis and Management by Laboratory Methods*. Philadelphia: Saunders/Elsevier; 2007:1119–1168.

336. Procop GW, Marty AM. Parasitic infections. In: Tomashefski J, Farver C, Cagle P, Fraire A, eds. *Dail and Hammer's Pulmonary Pathology*. 3rd ed. New York: Springer; 2008:515–560.

337. Ali A, Hoda S. Vegetable matter in histology sections may simulate pathogenic microorganisms [Abstract]. *Mod Pathol*. 2002;15:272A.

338. Nash G, Kerschmann RL, Herndier B, Dubey JP. The pathological manifestations of pulmonary toxoplasmosis in the acquired immunodeficiency syndrome. *Hum Pathol*. 1994;25(7):652–658.

339. Frenkel J. Toxoplasmosis. In: Chandler F, Connor D, Schwartz D, eds. *Pathology of Infectious Disease*. Stamford, CT: Appleton & Lange; 1997:1261–1278.

340. Lyche KD, Jensen WA. Pleuropulmonary amebiasis. *Semin Respir Infect*. 1997;12(2):106–112.

341. Wilson MR, Jorgensen JH, Yolken RH. Diagnosis of parasitic infection: Immunologic and molecular methods. In: Murray P, Baron E, Pfaller M, et al., eds. *Manual of Clinical Microbiology*. 6th ed. Washington, DC: ASM Press; 1995.

342. Ash L, Orihel T. *Atlas of Human Parasitology*. 4th ed. Chicago: ASCP Press; 1997.

343. Sun T. *Parasitic Disorders: Pathology, Diagnosis and Management*. 2nd ed. Baltimore: Williams & Wilkins; 1999.

344. Marciano-Cabral F, Cabral G. Acanthamoeba spp as agents of disease in humans. *Clin Micro Rev*. 2003;16:273–307.

345. Chen XM, Keithly JS, Paya CV, LaRusso NF. Cryptosporidiosis. *N Engl J Med*. 2002;346(22): 1723–1731.

346. Pearl M, Villanueva TG, Kauffman CA. Respiratory cryptosporidiosis in the acquired immune deficiency syndrome. *JAMA*. 1984;252:1290–1301.

347. Garcia LS. Laboratory identification of the microsporidia. *J Clin Microbiol*. 2002;40(6): 1892–1901.

348. Weber R, Bryan RT, Schwartz DA, Owen RL. Human microsporidial infections. *Clin Microbiol Rev*. 1994;7(4):426–461.

349. Schwartz DA, Visvesvara GS, Leitch GJ, et al. Pathology of symptomatic microsporidial (Encephalitozoon hellem) bronchiolitis in the acquired immunodeficiency syndrome: a new respiratory pathogen diagnosed from lung biopsy, bronchoalveolar lavage, sputum, and tissue culture. *Hum Pathol*. 1993;24(9):937–943.

350. Lamps LW, Bronner MP, Vnencak-Jones CL, et al. Optimal screening and diagnosis of microsporidia in tissue sections: a comparison of polarization, special stains, and molecular techniques. *Am J Clin Pathol*. 1998;109(4):404–410.

351. Piscopo T, Mallia A. Leishmaniasis. *Postgrad Med J*. 2006;82:649–657.

352. Jokipii L, Salmela K, Saha H, et al. Leishmaniasis diagnosed from bronchoalveolar lavage. *Scand J Infect Dis*. 1992;24(5):677–681.

353. Morales P, Torres JJ, Salavert M, et al. Visceral leishmaniasis in lung transplantation. *Transplant Proc*. 2003;35:2001–2003.

354. Deborggraeve S, Boelaert M, Rijal S, et al. Diagnostic accuracy of a new Leishmania PCR for clinical visceral leishmaniasis in Nepal and its role in diagnosis of disease. *Trop Med Int Health*. 2008;13:1378–1383.

355. Ro JY, Tsakalakis PJ, White VA, et al. Pulmonary dirofilariasis: the great imitator of primary or metastatic lung tumor. A clinicopathologic analysis of seven cases and a review of the literature. *Hum Pathol*. 1989;20(1):69–76.

356. Nicholson CP, Allen MS, Trastek VF, et al. Dirofilaria immitis: a rare, increasing cause of pulmonary nodules. *Mayo Clin Proc*. 1992;67(7):646–650.

357. Akaogi E, Ishibashi O, Mitsui K, et al. Pulmonary dirofilariasis cytologically mimicking lung cancer. A case report. *Acta Cytol*. 1993;37(4):531–534.

358. Flieder DB, Moran CA. Pulmonary dirofilariasis: a clinicopathologic study of 41 lesions in 39 patients. *Hum Pathol*. 1999;30(3):251–256.

359. Byard R, Bourne A, Matthews N. Pulmonary strongyloidiasis in a child diagnosed on open lung biopsy. *Surg Pathol*. 1993;109:55–61.

360. Upadhyay D, Corbridge T, Jain M, Shah R. Pulmonary hyperinfection syndrome with *Strongyloides stercoralis*. *Am J Med*. 2001;111(2):167–169.

361. Baden LR, Elliott DD. Case records of the Massachusetts General Hospital. Weekly clinicopathological exercises. Case 4–2003. A 42-year-old woman with cough, fever, and abnormalities on thoracoabdominal computed tomography. *N Engl J Med*. 2003;348(5):447–455.

362. Redington AE, Russell SG, Ladhani S, et al. Pulmonary echinococcosis with chest wall involvement in a patient with no apparent risk factors. *J Infect*. 2001;42(4):285–1258.

363. Sinniah B. Paragonimiasis. In: Chandler F, Connor D, Schwartz D, eds. *Pathology of Infectious Disease*. Stamford, CT: Appleton & Lange; 1997:1527–1530.

364. Ross AG, Bartley PB, Sleigh AC, et al. Schistosomiasis. *N Engl J Med*. 2002;346(16): 1212–1220.

365. King C. Toward the elimination of schistosomiasis. *N Engl J Med*. 2009;360:106–108.

366. Cooke GS, Lalvani A, Gleeson FV, Conlon CP. Acute pulmonary schistosomiasis in travelers returning from Lake Malawi, sub-Saharan Africa. *Clin Infect Dis*. 1999;29(4):836–839.

367. Bethlem EP, Schettino Gde P, Carvalho CR. Pulmonary schistosomiasis. *Curr Opin Pulm Med*. 1997;3(5):361–365.

368. Schwartz E, Rosenman J, Perlman M. Pulmonary manifestations of early schistosome infection among nonimmune travelers. *Am J Med*. 2000;9:718–722.

369. Despommier D. Toxacariasis: clinical aspects, epidemiology, medical ecology and molecular aspects. *Clin Microbiol Rev*. 2003;34:7–15.

370. Procop GW, Marty AM, Scheck DN, et al. North American paragonimiasis. A case report. *Acta Cytol*. 2000;44(1):75–80.

371. Singh A, Singh Y, Sharma VK, et al. Diagnosis of hydatid disease of abdomen and thorax by ultrasound guided fine needle aspiration cytology. *Indian J Pathol Microbiol*. 1999;42(2): 155–156.

372. Handa U, Mohan H, Ahal S, et al. Cytodiagnosis of hydatid disease presenting with Horner's syndrome: a case report. *Acta Cytol*. 2001;45(5):784–788.

373. Brown RW, Clarke RJ, Denham I, Trembath PW. Pulmonary paragonimiasis in an immigrant from Laos. *Med J Aust*. 1983;2(12):668–669.

374. Abdulla MA, Hombal SM, al-Juwaiser A. Detection of Schistosoma mansoni in bronchoalveolar lavage fluid. A case report. *Acta Cytol*. 1999;43(5):856–858.

375. Kramer MR, Gregg PA, Goldstein M, et al. Disseminated strongyloidiasis in AIDS and non-AIDS immunocompromised hosts: diagnosis by sputum and bronchoalveolar lavage. *South Med J*. 1990;83(10):1226–1229.

376. Kapila K, Verma K. Cytologic detection of parasitic disorders. *Acta Cytol*. 1982;26(3): 359–362.

377. Didier ES, Rogers LB, Orenstein JM, et al. Characterization of *Encephalitozoon (Septata) intestinalis* isolates cultured from nasal mucosa and bronchoalveolar lavage fluids of two AIDS patients. *J Eukaryot Microbiol*. 1996;43(1):34–43.

378. Weber R, Kuster H, Keller R, et al. Pulmonary and intestinal microsporidiosis in a patient with the acquired immunodeficiency syndrome. *Am Rev Respir Dis*. 1992;146(6):1603–1605.

379. Wheeler RR, Bardales RH, North PE, et al. Toxoplasma pneumonia: cytologic diagnosis by bronchoalveolar lavage. *Diagn Cytopathol*. 1994;11(1):52–55.

380. Radosavljevic-Asic G, Jovanovic D, Radovanovic D, Tucakovic M. Trichomonas in pleural effusion. *Eur Respir J*. 1994;7(10):1906–1908.

381. Newsome AL, Curtis FT, Culbertson CG, Allen SD. Identification of Acanthamoeba in bronchoalveolar lavage specimens. *Diagn Cytopathol*. 1992;8(3):231–234.

382. Maddison SE. Serodiagnosis of parasitic diseases. *Clin Microbiol Rev*. 1991;4(4):457–469.

383. Wilson M, Remington JS, Clavet C, et al. Evaluation of six commercial kits for detection of human immunoglobulin M antibodies to *Toxoplasma gondii*. The FDA Toxoplasmosis Ad Hoc Working Group. *J Clin Microbiol*. 1997;35(12):3112–3115.

384. Remington JS, Thulliez P, Montoya J. Recent developments for diagnosis of toxoplasmosis. *J Clin Microbiol*. 2004;42:941–945.

385. Petersen E, Edvinsson B, Lundgren B, et al. Diagnosis of pulmonary infection with *Toxoplasma gondii* in immunocompromised HIV-positive patients by real-time PCR. *Eur J Clin Microbiol Infec Dis*. 2006;25:401–404.

386. Tanyukjel M, Petri W. Laboratory diagnosis of amoebiasis. *Clin Microbiol Rev*. 2003;16:713–729.

387. Churg A. Recent advances in the diagnosis of Churg-Strauss syndrome. *Mod Pathol*. 2001;14(12):1284–1293.

388. Allen JN, Davis WB. Eosinophilic lung diseases. *Am J Respir Crit Care Med*. 1994;150(5 Pt 1):1423–1438.

389. Burgers JA, Sluiters JF, de Jong DW, et al. Pseudoparasitic pneumonia after bone marrow transplantation. *Neth J Med*. 2001;59(4):170–176.

390. Tuur SM, Nelson AM, Gibson DW, et al. Liesegang rings in tissue. How to distinguish Liesegang rings from the giant kidney worm, *Diotophyma renale*. *Am J Surg Pathol*. 1987;11:598–605.

7

Chronic Diffuse Lung Diseases

Junya Fukuoka, MD, PhD, and Kevin O. Leslie, MD

Diffuse or "interstitial" lung diseases (ILDs) include a spectrum of primarily non-neoplastic inflammatory conditions that share the common property of diffuse involvement of the lung parenchyma. The term "ILD" has become so thoroughly entrenched across multiple medical disciplines that it seems practical to continue its usage, although we would emphasize that many of the diseases discussed in this chapter also involve the alveolar spaces and terminal bronchioles to a variable extent and would therefore not be considered entirely "interstitial" by the anatomic purist.[1]

This chapter focuses on the subacute and chronic forms of ILD (acute ILDs are discussed in Chapter 5), which includes diseases that typically evolve over weeks, months, or years. Patients with ILD share a number of clinical and radiologic manifestations, including: (1) shortness of breath (dyspnea), (2) diffuse abnormalities in lung mechanics and gas transfer (pulmonary function), and (3) diffuse abnormalities on chest radiographs and computed tomography (CT) scans of the chest.[2]

An overview of ILD from the pathologist's perspective is presented in Box 7-1. In this chapter we will restrict our focus to a limited number of predominantly inflammatory diseases that come to biopsy relatively frequently (Box 7-2). Our emphasis is on the histopathologic patterns of these diseases as observed through the microscope. These patterns help narrow the differential diagnosis and often allow for a definitive diagnosis when coupled with clinical and radiologic data.

ILDs have in common the accumulation of inflammatory and immune effector cells in the lung interstitium as their main histopathologic finding. The interstitium of the lung is the compartment that exists between the basement membrane of lung epithelial cells (the lining cells of the airways and alveoli in direct contact with inspired air) and that of adjacent blood vessels. There is a general misconception that the lung interstitium is confined to the "space" that exists within the alveolar walls. In fact, this compartment extends as a continuum from the alveolar septa to the pleura.

Unlike neoplasms, which may have distinctive or even unique morphologic features, ILDs are distinguished from one another by (1) location involved (anatomic compartment or structure), (2) distribution (focal or diffuse), and (3) cellular composition (e.g., acute, chronic, histiocytic) of the inflammatory reaction. Additional identification criteria include the mechanism by which repair is taking place (organizing or not) and the stage of the reparative process (acute: fibroblastic proliferation; subacute: fibroblasts accompanied by matrix and epithelial regeneration; chronic: dense fibrosis and structural remodeling).[2]

Transbronchial and surgical wedge biopsy interpretation in the ILD patient is complicated by several factors.[3] First, these diseases involve the interstitium, but they are frequently attended by reactive changes in the surrounding alveolar spaces and associated terminal airways. Such reactive changes can be quite impressive and commonly distract the observer from recognizing the interstitial nature of the process. Second, the inherent variability and natural history of inflammatory diseases pose problems, wherein early phases of a disease may differ in appearance from later phases, and the intensity of a reaction may vary from individual to individual. Third, more than one inflammatory disease can involve the lung simultaneously, adding further complexity to the morphologic picture. Finally, and perhaps of greatest importance, these predominantly medical diseases cannot be diagnosed accurately without some clinical and radiologic correlation.[4]

Despite extensive clinical and experimental research efforts over the past several decades, the etiology and pathogenesis of most ILDs remain unknown. In certain ILDs, a specific exposure can be identified (e.g., in hypersensitivity pneumonitis or with toxic reaction to a drug), whereas in others, a systemic autoimmune disease may be present (e.g., rheumatoid arthritis manifesting in the lung). When no associated exposure or underlying condition is identified after rigorous evaluation, an ILD is considered to be "idiopathic."

Like most human organs, the lung has a limited repertoire of responses to injury of any type, and most of these responses are nonspecific. Without guidelines for interpretation and appropriate nomenclature, the surgical pathologist may experience difficulty coming to a clinically meaningful diagnosis for the patient with ILD. Additionally, because the lung biopsy for ILD is always a limited sampling, the pathologist and clinician must work cooperatively in establishing a differential diagnosis based on the clinical presentation, laboratory data, and radiologic findings. A purely descriptive pathologic diagnosis (e.g., "chronic lung fibrosis"), without clinical or radiologic correlation, or a focused differential diagnosis, is of marginal use in the contemporary practice of pulmonary medicine. In this chapter, we will present the essential clinical, radiologic, and histopathologic elements of chronic ILDs and will provide the reader with specific terminology for use in diagnosing these diseases, wherever possible.

One of the most important chronic lung diseases in pulmonary medicine today is known clinically as *idiopathic pulmonary fibrosis* (IPF). This most devastating of chronic ILDs is often the diagnosis of exclusion from a clinical perspective and one against which all other chronic lung diseases are judged. The reason for this is that IPF is a disease that progresses despite therapy and rivals many cancers in mortality rate, with death often occurring within 3 years of the diagnosis.[5] As emphasized in the 2002 joint consensus statement of the American Thoracic Society (ATS) and the European Respiratory Society (ERS), the pathologic manifestation of IPF in the lung is *usual interstitial pneumonia* (UIP).[6] UIP was a term introduced by Liebow in reference to one of five forms of *idiopathic interstitial pneumonia* (IIP).[7] In Liebow's words, UIP represents "chronic lung fibrosis of the common or usual type,"—a seemingly broad category of chronic lung disease.

As we explore chronic ILDs, it seems most appropriate to begin with UIP, with recognizing that our current concept of this disease is more restrictive than perhaps was initially intended. The pathologist who is able to recognize the subtle but distinctive features of UIP and confidently distinguish it from other ILDs is well on the way to mastering the art of pulmonary pathology.

Idiopathic Interstitial Pneumonias

Liebow's initial classification of IIPs is presented for historical purposes in Box 7-3. In the years following the introduction of this classification scheme, new information led to the modification or elimination of certain of these IIPs and the addition of others not previously included[8,9] (Box 7-4). Since Liebow's time, it has been established that *desquamative interstitial pneumonia* (DIP), initially thought to be an early manifestation of UIP,[10] is in fact a smoking-related disease in a majority of cases, most often affecting adults.[11,12] Subsequent investigation also showed that giant cell interstitial pneumonia (GIP) was actually a manifestation of cobalt exposure, as a pneumoconiosis in "hard metal disease" (see Chapter 8).[13] Finally, it became apparent that many early cases of lymphoid interstitial pneumonia (LIP) evolved into lymphoproliferative disease and probably did not constitute "inflammatory" disease in the true sense of the word.[14]

Box 7-4. Initial Revised Classification of Idiopathic Interstitial Pneumonias

Usual interstitial pneumonia (UIP)
Desquamative interstitial pneumonia (DIP)
Respiratory bronchiolitis interstitial lung disease (RBILD)
Acute interstitial pneumonia (AIP)
Nonspecific interstitial pneumonia (NSIP)

Reprinted with permission from Katzenstein A, Askin F, eds. *Surgical Pathology of Non-Neoplastic Lung Disease,* 2nd ed. Philadelphia: WB Saunders; 1990:49, Table 3-1.

Based on this evolution in our understanding, a modification to Liebow's original classification of the IIPs was proposed by Katzenstein.[8,9] This new schema included the major categories of UIP and DIP but coupled DIP with "respiratory bronchiolitis–associated interstitial lung disease" (RBILD) and acknowledged the strong relationship of these diseases to cigarette smoking. Katzenstein also proposed a new category of *acute interstitial pneumonia* (AIP)[15] as an entity separate from UIP, a distinction that Liebow did not make in his initial classification. Finally, Katzenstein created a new category to encompass a group of inflammatory diseases that differed in appearance from UIP, DIP, or AIP. The term *nonspecific interstitial pneumonia* (NSIP) was proposed for this "new" pattern.[16] In our experience, a majority of IIPs can be classified using this scheme. We would add *idiopathic (cryptogenic) organizing pneumonia,* previously known as "idiopathic bronchiolitis obliterans organizing pneumonia,"[17] to this classification, as has been recommended by the 2002 International Workshop on the classification of IIPs.[6] That workshop retained LIP in the classification (Table 7-1), acknowledging the presence of some morphologic overlap with NSIP once a lymphoproliferative disease has been excluded by all available means. Importantly, the consensus panel determined that NSIP should be included in the IIPs as a provisional category until additional data accrue.[6]

IIPs are classically defined as diffuse pulmonary diseases that involve two or more lobes of the lung; in most patients, such diseases are bilateral in distribution.[18] Some localized lesions (such as infection, atelectasis, or tumor) may mimic IIP in a biopsy specimen. It is safe to say that if a disease process is confined to the biopsy area sampled, it is unlikely to be an IIP. AIP is an acute form of IIP (discussed in detail in Chapter 5). A comparison of the histopathologic findings in each of the

Table 7-1. International Consensus Classification of Idiopathic Interstitial Pneumonias (2002)

Histopathologic Pattern	Clinical-Radiologic-Pathologic Diagnosis
Usual interstitial pneumonia	Idiopathic pulmonary fibrosis/cryptogenic fibrosing alveolitis
Nonspecific interstitial pneumonia	Nonspecific interstitial pneumonia ("provisional")
Respiratory bronchiolitis	Respiratory bronchiolitis interstitial lung disease
Desquamative interstitial pneumonia	Desquamative interstitial pneumonia
Organizing pneumonia	Cryptogenic organizing pneumonia
Diffuse alveolar damage	Acute interstitial pneumonia
Lymphoid interstitial pneumonia	Lymphoid interstitial pneumonia

Reprinted with permission from American Thoracic Society/European Respiratory Society international multidisciplinary consensus classification of the idiopathic interstitial pneumonias. *Am J Respir Crit Care Med.* 2002;165(2):277–304, Table 2.

IIPs is presented in Table 7-2. The importance of accurately diagnosing these IIPs lies mainly with differences in prognosis. UIP is a uniformly fatal disease for which the median survival period historically is less than 3 years in its classic presentation (CT with honeycombing), competing with many cancers in this respect.

Usual Interstitial Pneumonia

Pulmonary pathologists have debated for years what is, and what is not, UIP. To some, UIP is a relatively nonspecific pattern of chronic lung injury with fibrosis and "honeycomb" remodeling (see further on). Today it is recognized that not all lung diseases with fibrosis behave similarly and, in particular, do not run the aggressive course expected for clinical IPF. The most honest answer may be that clinical and radiologic IPF has UIP-type pathologic changes, but that a UIP pattern of parenchymal fibrosis with remodeling may be seen in biopsy specimens and may not necessarily correlate with clinical and radiologic

Table 7-2. Histopathologic Features of the Idiopathic Interstitial Pneumonias

Feature	NSIP	UIP	DIP	AIP	LIP	COP
Temporal appearance	Uniform	Variegated	Uniform	Uniform	Uniform	Uniform
Interstitial inflammation	Prominent	Scant	Scant	Scant	Prominent	Scant
Interstitial fibrosis: collagen	Variable, diffuse	Patchy	Variable, diffuse	No	Some cases	No
Interstitial fibrosis: fibroblasts	Occasional, diffuse	No	No	Yes, diffuse	No	No
OP pattern	Occasional, focal	Occasional, focal	No	Occasional, focal	No	Prominent
Fibroblast foci	Occasional, focal	Typical	No	No	No	No
Honeycomb areas	Rare	Typical	No	No	Sometimes	No
Intra-alveolar macrophages	Occasional, patchy	Occasional, focal	Yes, diffuse	No	Occasional, patchy	No
Hyaline membranes	No	No	No	Yes, focal	No	No
Granulomas	No	No	No	No	Focal, poorly formed	No

AIP, acute interstitial pneumonia; COP, cryptogenic organizing pneumonia; DIP, desquamative interstitial pneumonia; LIP, lymphocytic interstitial pneumonia; NSIP, nonspecific interstitial pneumonia; OP, organizing pneumonia; UIP, usual interstitial pneumonia.
Data from Katzenstein AL, Myers JL: Nonspecific interstitial pneumonia and the other idiopathic interstitial pneumonias: classification and diagnostic criteria. *Am J Surg Pathol.* 2000;24(1):1–3; and American Thoracic Society/European Respiratory Society international multidisciplinary consensus classification of the idiopathic interstitial pneumonias. *Am J Respir Crit Care Med.* 2002;165(2):277–304, Table 2.

IPF. Fortunately, not all lung diseases that produce scarring fit the pattern now defined as UIP. Asbestosis,[19-21] chronic hypersensitivity pneumonitis,[22-24] systemic collagen vascular diseases (CVDs),[25-28] and even some chronic toxic drug reactions[29] can all produce lung fibrosis. Unfortunately, in the 30 years following Liebow's introduction of UIP as an "idiopathic" interstitial disease, pathologists often used the designation of UIP in a variety of nonidiopathic settings (e.g., "UIP from asbestosis" or "UIP from rheumatoid arthritis"). If UIP is defined as simply any form of lung fibrosis, then applying UIP as a synonym for fibrosis is perfectly reasonable. On the other hand, if UIP is a distinctive pathologic entity that corresponds to an idiopathic clinical disease (IPF), then UIP should have identifiable features that afford it status as a unique disease process. That there is a continued misconception of UIP among pathologists is underscored by feedback from our clinical colleagues, who note that many diagnoses of UIP provided by the pathology laboratory do not correspond to clinical IPF in their patients' presentation, response to therapy, or observed outcome.

An examination of the subset of ILDs that correspond to clinical and radiologic IPF reveals a disease that is not overtly inflammatory but nevertheless has a clear tendency to produce fibrosis. Moreover, the fibrosis seen in the lungs of patients with IPF has a relatively reproducible pattern and distribution. Such a focused analysis can reveal the subtle differences between the UIP of IPF and the fibrosis that may occur in other lung diseases, most of which have an identifiable cause, etiologic agent, or associated systemic disease process.

Clinical Presentation

The incidence of UIP varies by gender, with males predominating. The disease may have a prevalence in the United States as high as 43 per 100,000, using broad criteria[30]; roughly two thirds of patients are older than 60 years of age at diagnosis.[5,31] For this reason, caution should be exercised when considering a diagnosis of UIP in patients who are younger than 50 years of age, and preferably expert consultation should be sought in this setting. Symptoms typically progress insidiously for months to years before diagnosis. The onset of a nonproductive cough and slowly progressive dyspnea are characteristic. Dry inspiratory crackles (so-called Velcro crackles) are detected at the lung bases on chest auscultation in more than 80% of patients at presentation.[5] Clubbing of the digits is seen in 25% to 50% of patients at presentation. Fever is rare, and its presence should suggest an alternate diagnosis, as should a significantly elevated erythrocyte sedimentation

rate (greater than 100 mm/hour). Serologic studies such as antinuclear antibody (ANA) or rheumatoid factor (RF) assays may reveal mildly elevated titers, but when significant elevation is present, a systemic connective tissue disease should be strongly considered. Also, in patients presenting with clinical features of UIP or IPF in whom a defined CVD develops later, reclassification of their disease may be necessary.

Radiologic Findings

On chest radiographs, peripheral reticular opacities involving the lung bases are a characteristic finding.[32] When present, these usually are bilateral and often asymmetrical. Lung volumes are typically decreased at presentation except in cases with severe upper lobe (centriacinar) emphysema.[33] Unfortunately, a normal chest radiograph does not exclude the diagnosis.[34] Confluent alveolar opacities are rare and, if present, suggest an alternate diagnosis or a comorbid process. CT scans, preferably of the high-resolution type (i.e., with scan sections ≤ 1 mm), commonly show patchy, predominantly peripheral (subpleural) reticular abnormalities involving the lung bases bilaterally.[35] Some asymmetry is expected between right and left lungs, and characteristic "skip" areas are present, with coarse pleural-based reticulation alternating with adjacent better-preserved lung (so-called "radiologic heterogeneity"). The earliest findings may be quite subtle, consisting of delicate, peripherally accentuated pleural-based reticular opacities in the lower lung zones (Fig. 7-1). Ground-glass opacities are not typical and, if present, should be limited in extent.[36-38] Subpleural cysts—ranging from a few millimeters to a centimeter or more in diameter ("radiologic honeycombing")—increase in prominence as the disease advances (Fig. 7-2). In areas of more severe involvement, traction bronchiectasis often is evident. Diagnostic accuracy for IPF on high-resolution CT scan by trained observers is in the range of 90% when typical findings are present (high specificity); however, approximately one third of cases of UIP will be missed when relying on high-resolution CT diagnosis alone (low sensitivity).[24,39]

Histopathologic Findings

UIP cannot be diagnosed with the bronchoscopic or transbronchial biopsy specimen. Surgically derived wedge lung biopsies (3–5 cm in length by 2–3 cm in breadth), obtained from video-assisted thoracoscopic surgery (VATS) or open thoracotomy, are the appropriate samples for diagnosis (see Chapter 2 for additional details on the lung biopsy). Occasionally, UIP will be evident in lobectomy and pneumonectomy specimens obtained for other diseases. UIP is a process that

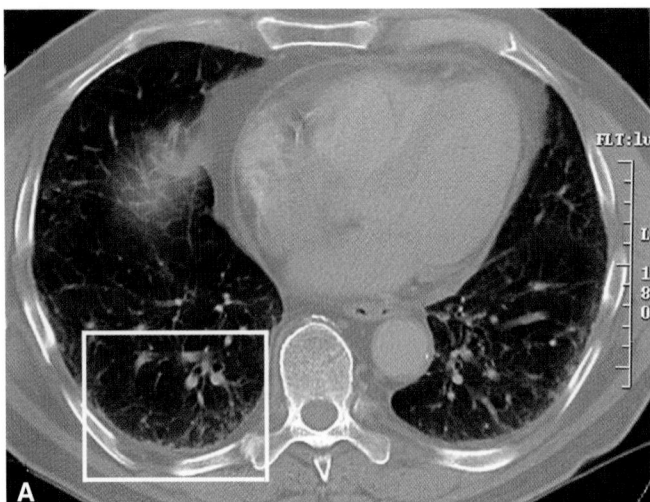
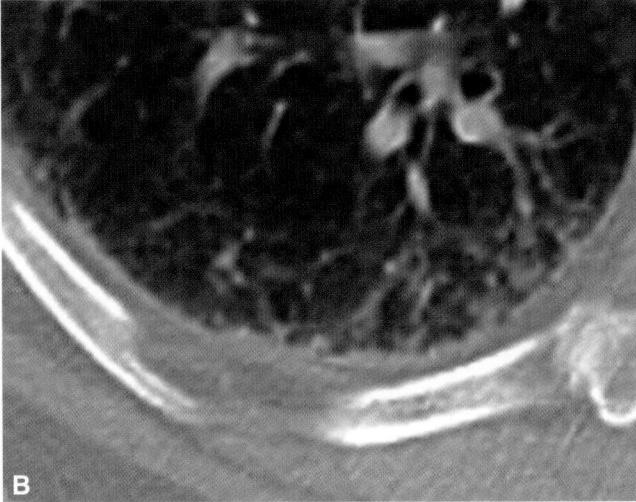

Figure 7-1. Usual interstitial pneumonia (UIP). **A,** This computed tomography scan shows the early subtle findings in UIP, with delicate pleura-based reticular opacities in the lower lung zones and a few small honeycomb cysts. **B,** Higher magnification of the boxed area from part **A.**

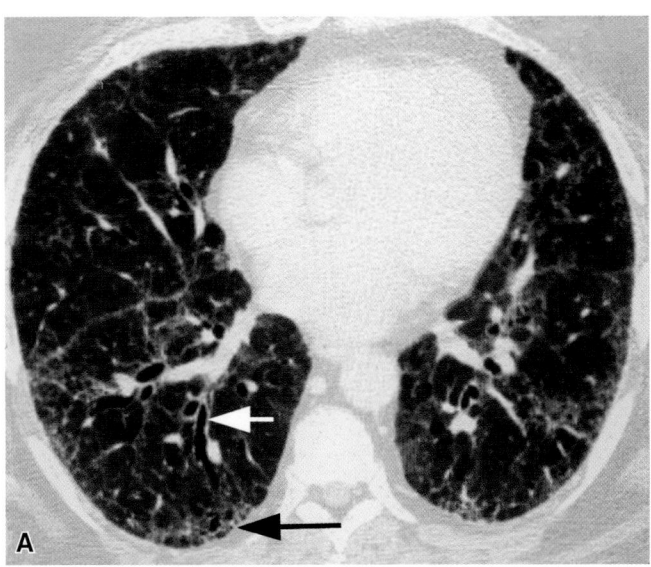
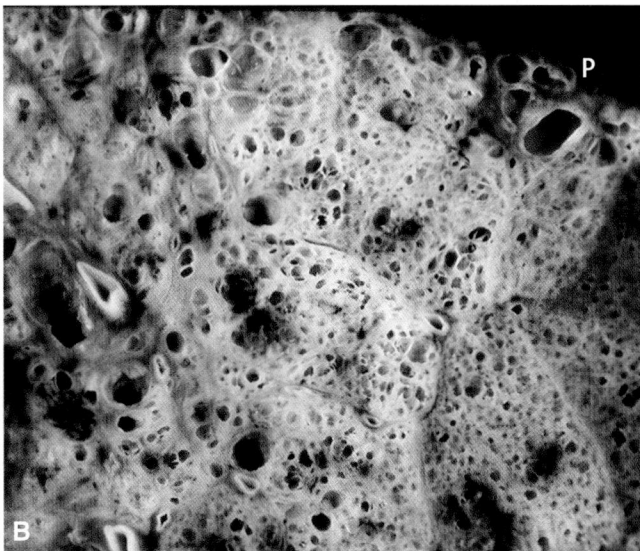

Figure 7-2. Usual interstitial pneumonia (UIP). **A,** Computed tomography scan showing characteristic changes of UIP, with subpleural cysts (*black arrow*) and traction bronchiectasis (*white arrow*). **B,** Gross lung specimen shows subpleural (P) cysts, ranging from a few millimeters to a centimeter or more in diameter (i.e., radiologic honeycombing), that increase in prominence as the disease advances.

involves the periphery of the lung lobule; these areas are not sampled adequately in even the most ambitious transbronchial biopsy scenario (where many large fragments of alveolar parenchyma may be present, but are mainly derived from the central portion of the lung lobules). More than one biopsy site should be sampled, and preferably a biopsy sample should be obtained from all lobes in the hemithorax chosen for surgical intervention. If only two areas can be sampled, mid-lung and lower lung are preferable to upper and mid-lung, and samples from the lower lobe should be taken above the most advanced areas of fibrosis.

The characteristic histopathologic findings of UIP have been referred to as being "temporally heterogeneous" or having a "patchwork quilt" appearance,[32,40–43] concepts and terms that are often misunderstood by surgical pathologists and pulmonologists. An expanded description of "temporal heterogeneity" is that of transitions in the biopsy from dense scar (the "past") to normal lung (the "future"—lung tissue yet to be involved). At the juncture of these, transitions occur through patches of active lung injury referred to as "fibroblast" or "fibroblastic" foci (Fig. 7-3). The remodeled lung is present mainly beneath the pleura and at the periphery of the secondary lobule, adjacent to interlobular septa (Fig. 7-4). When UIP is recognizable as a distinct pathologic entity, the pleural fibrosis contains smooth muscle proliferation in disorganized fascicles (Fig. 7-5) and foci of microscopic honeycombing are evident, even when the overall process appears to be mild or early in its evolution (Fig. 7-6). Microscopic honeycombing probably represents one of the early manifestations of the gross honeycomb cysts seen in the end-stage of UIP. As used by radiologists, the term *honeycombing* refers to an array of much larger cysts (in the range of 0.5–3 cm or larger) as a localized manifestation of advanced lung remodeling (Fig. 7-7). Microscopic honeycomb cysts are considerably smaller (in the range of 1–3 mm) and typically are present subpleurally (Fig. 7-8). The cysts are lined by columnar ciliated epithelium and typically are filled with mucus, with variable amounts of acute inflammation and inflammatory debris (Fig. 7-9). When dense chronic inflammation is present in UIP, it is seen around these localized inflammatory lesions.

Exactly how honeycomb cysts (gross or microscopic) form is unclear, but we believe they represent centrilobular airways, trapped in the fibrous remodeling, that are then pulled to the periphery of the lobule. In support

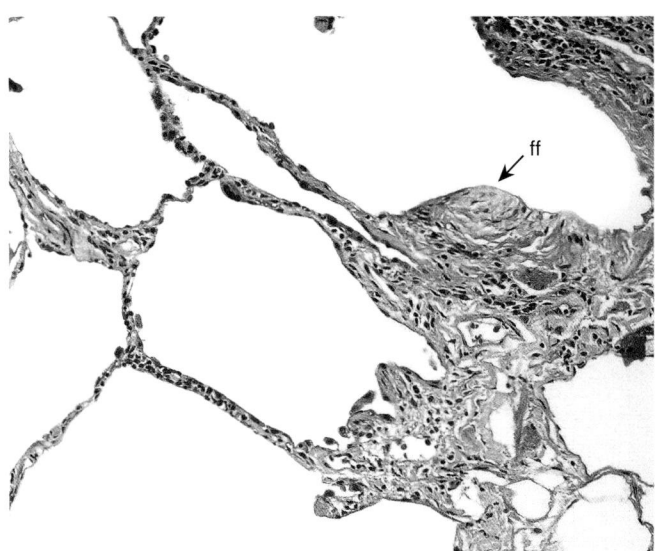

Figure 7-3. Usual interstitial pneumonia (UIP). The histopathologic temporal heterogeneity of UIP is characterized by abrupt transitions in the biopsy tissue, from dense remodeled lung parenchyma ("old" injury, evident at *right* in this image) to normal alveolar walls ("new" or not-yet-involved lung, *center* and *left* in this image) at the center of the lobule. This transition occurs through patchy areas of lung injury evidenced by the "fibroblast" or "fibroblastic" focus (ff).

of this concept, lobules with foci of microscopic honeycombing often lack a visible central airway, and tractional emphysema is nearly always present. This hypothesis also would explain the presence of smooth muscle fascicles in subpleural fibrosis and may thus be more tenable than the hypothesis that such muscle forms by fibroblast metaplasia.

Between the two temporal extremes of "old" peripheral fibrosis and uninvolved lung present centrally in the lobule is the presumed active zone of injury in UIP, evidenced by a crescent-shaped bulge of immature fibroblasts (technically, *myofibroblasts*) and ground substance (see Fig. 7-3). This lesion is known as the *fibroblastic focus* and typically is not extensive in the biopsy. Fibroblast foci have been shown to be continuous linear structures in three-dimensional reconstruction.[44]

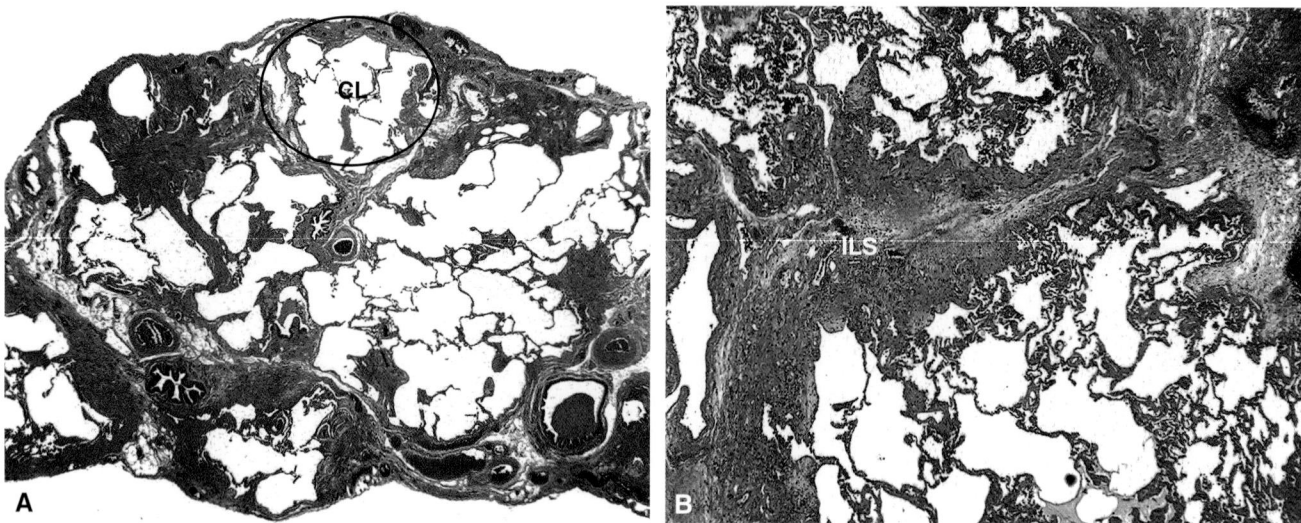

Figure 7-4. Usual interstitial pneumonia. **A,** The remodeled lung is present mainly beneath the pleura and at the periphery of the secondary lobule, adjacent to interlobular septa. A slightly shrunken lobule is *circled* at *upper center*. CL, center of lobule. **B,** An interlobular septum (ILS) widened by fibrosis is seen at *center*, with less involved lung lobules above and below.

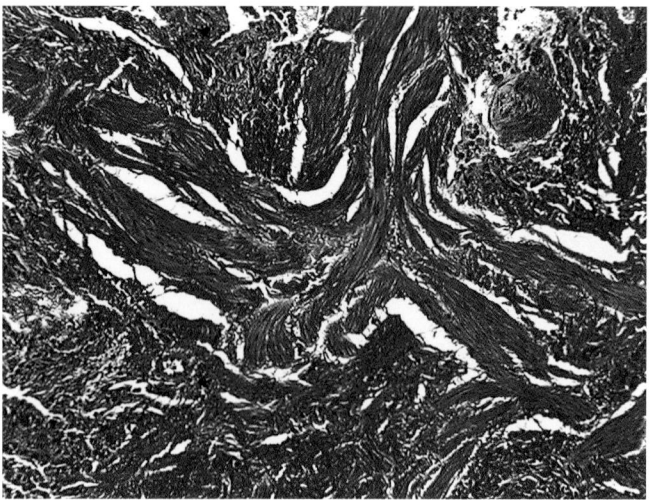

Figure 7-5. Usual interstitial pneumonia (UIP). When UIP is recognizable as a distinct pathologic entity, the subpleural fibrous tissue contains areas of smooth muscle proliferation, seen here as large disorganized fascicles.

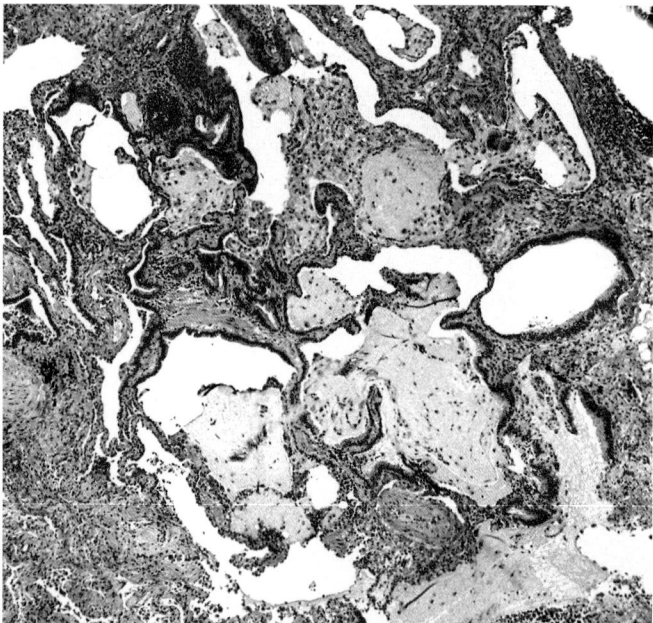

Figure 7-6. Usual interstitial pneumonia. Even in patients with "early" disease as determined radiologically, foci of microscopic honeycombing typically are present. To distinguish bronchiolar metaplasia from microscopic honeycombing, noting the location of the lesion often is helpful, because microscopic honeycombing is present more peripherally in lobules and associated with dense scar, whereas bronchiolar metaplasia develops at the center of lobules, in association with respiratory bronchioles.

Some investigators have postulated that the increased number of these foci in a given UIP patient's biopsy is associated with a worse prognosis, and that a relative lack of fibroblastic foci may be an explanation for the better prognosis observed for patients with UIP-like lung fibrosis related to systemic CVDs.[45]

UIP is not an overtly inflammatory condition, in the absence of so-called acute exacerbation (see further on). This is not to imply that fibrosis occurs "mysteriously" in the disease. Some form of injury is occurring in UIP, but it seems to be subtle and probably is directed at the alveolar epithelium and its underlying basement membrane (epithelial-mesenchymal transitions). The fibroblastic foci of UIP appear immediately beneath reactive-appearing alveolar lining epithelium, where they obscure the epithelial basement membrane and bulge into the adjacent air space (Fig. 7-10), as though they were aborted "Masson polyps" of the type seen in organizing pneumonia (see later under "Cryptogenic Organizing Pneumonia"). Further evidence of an injury repair phenotype for UIP/IPF is the consistent presence of reactive type

II cell proliferation overlying fibroblastic foci. Conceptually, the subtle inflammatory disease of UIP burns like a smoldering fire through the lung, leaving fibrosis, smooth muscle proliferation, microscopic honeycombing, and fibrosis in its path.

Acute Exacerbation
In his writings, Liebow conceived of UIP as a chronic lung disease resulting from repeated subclinical episodes of "diffuse alveolar damage" (DAD).[7] In support of this hypothesis, episodic deterioration is typical in patients with IPF.[5] In some patients with IPF, however,

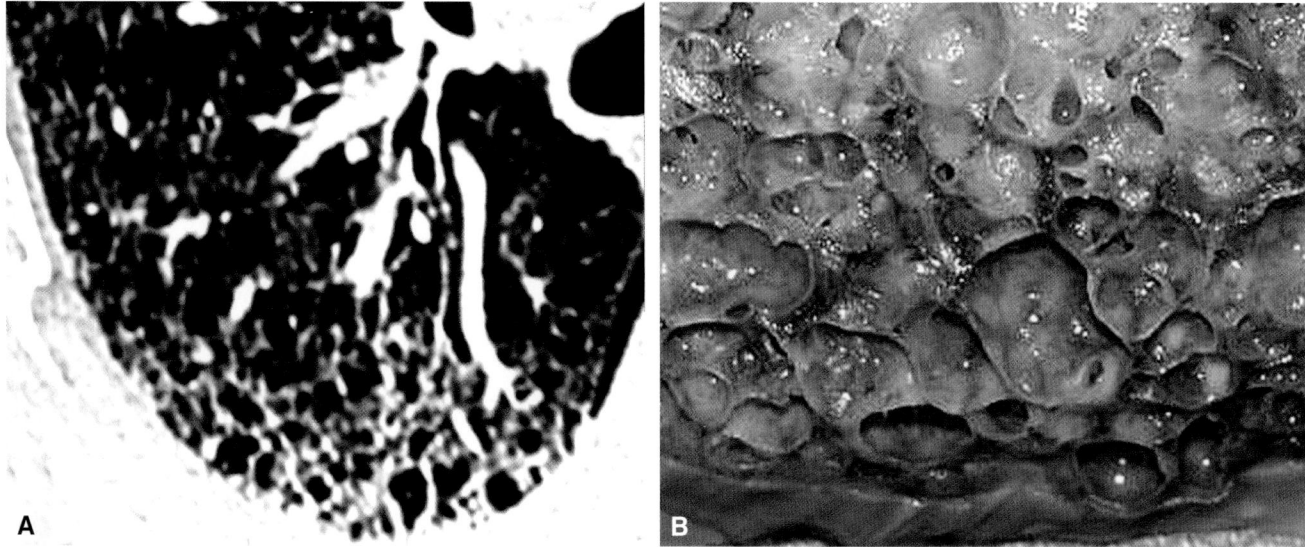

Figure 7-7. Usual interstitial pneumonia (UIP). As used by radiologists, the term *honeycombing* refers to an array of much larger cysts (in the range of 0.5 to 3 cm or more in diameter) as a localized manifestation of advanced lung remodeling. **A,** A patient with advanced UIP has many peripheral honeycomb cysts and traction bronchiectasis. **B,** The gross lung shows dramatic confluent cyst formation.

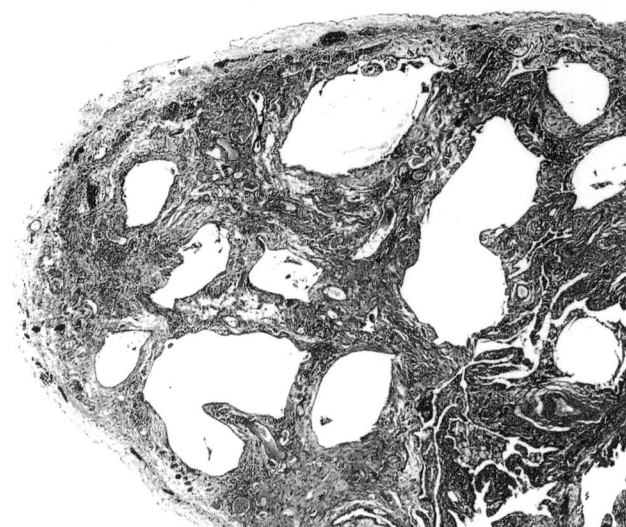

Figure 7-8. Usual interstitial pneumonia. Microscopic honeycomb cysts are considerably smaller (in the range of 1–3 mm in diameter) than those identified radiologically.

clinical deterioration is abrupt and overwhelming. Many of these acute deteriorations are of unidentifiable cause and have been referred to as "acute exacerbations of IPF." Acute exacerbations have been the subject of considerable laboratory investigation, but the mechanism of their occurrence remains unknown. We do know that when such episodes are biopsied, the most consistent pathologic finding is that of DAD.[46] Acute exacerbations of IPF can manifest as other patterns of acute lung injury, such as organizing pneumonia, and despite the implication of the term, the "acute" exacerbation tends to evolve over several weeks, rather than a few days.[47] The mixed histopathologic changes can be confusing to the surgical pathologist examining the lung biopsy (and to the radiologist) because the background older fibrosis with microscopic honeycombing of UIP is often overshadowed by diffuse acute lung injury (Fig. 7-11).

The three patients described by Kondoh and coworkers all showed some degree of improvement in the short term after high-dose corticosteroid therapy, but no consistently effective therapy has

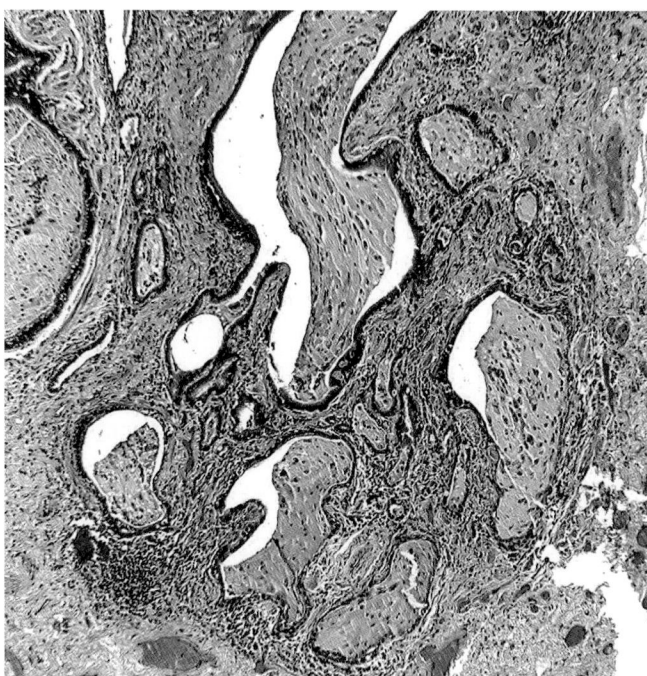

Figure 7-9. Usual interstitial pneumonia (UIP). Microscopic honeycomb cysts are lined by columnar ciliated epithelium and typically are filled with mucus, with variable amounts of acute inflammation and inflammatory debris. When dense chronic inflammation is present in UIP, it is most often seen around microscopic honeycombing.

emerged.[46] Several investigators have proposed that acute exacerbations may be the common terminal episode in many patients with IPF, even though respiratory failure has always been presumed to be of slower evolution.[48] Based on all available data, including data from the placebo arms of several large randomized, double-blind, placebo-controlled trials in patients with IPF, an estimated 10% to 15% of patients with UIP experience overwhelming acute exacerbation during the course of their disease, and this is often the fatal event for those affected.[47,49]

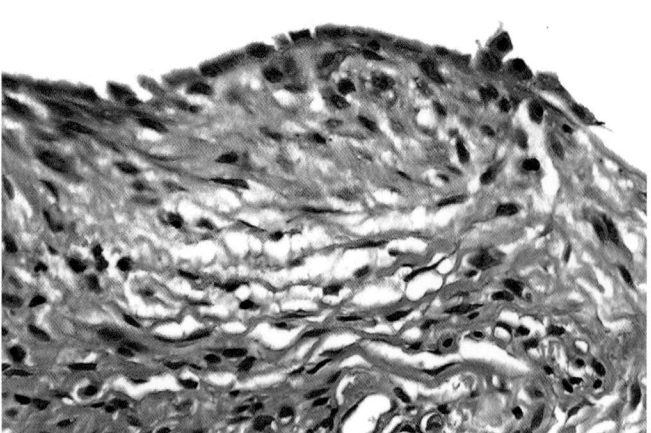

Figure 7-10. Usual interstitial pneumonia (UIP). The fibroblastic foci of UIP are patchy and present immediately beneath reactive-appearing cuboidal alveolar lining epithelium (type II cell hyperplasia). The fibroblastic proliferation bulges toward the air space but does not appear to make a polypoid structure.

Differential Diagnosis

The differential diagnosis for the UIP pattern includes a number of diseases that produce lung fibrosis. When this is a diffuse bilateral process, the main entities in the differential diagnosis are listed in Box 7-5. There are cases showing coexistence of histopathologic patterns of NSIP and UIP in the same patient in multiple lobe biopsies.[50] Such cases can be considered "discordant" UIP.[51] The clinical course of discordant UIP is still more like that of "non-discordant" UIP, however, with possibly longer survival.[52]

Clinical Course

The most common causes of death among patients with IPF are listed in Box 7-6. As defined clinically, IPF patients have a median survival time of less than 3 years.[53] At present, no effective therapy has been established for IPF, but newer therapies are on the horizon using human recombinant cytokines as agents antagonistic to the effects of potentially "responsible" molecules.

Box 7-5. Potential Causes of Lung Fibrosis, with or without Honeycomb Remodeling

Usual interstitial pneumonia (UIP)
Desquamative interstitial pneumonia (DIP)
Lymphoid interstitial pneumonia (LIP)
Systemic collagen vascular disease
Certain chronic drug reactions
Pneumoconioses
Sarcoidosis
Pulmonary Langerhans cell histiocytosis (pulmonary histiocytosis X)
Chronic granulomatous infections
Chronic aspiration
Chronic hypersensitivity pneumonitis
Organized chronic eosinophilic pneumonia
Healed diffuse alveolar damage
Chronic interstitial pulmonary edema/passive congestion
Radiation exposure (chronic)
Healed infectious pneumonias and other inflammatory processes
Nonspecific interstitial pneumonia (NSIP)
Hermansky-Pudlak syndrome (oculocutaneous albinism with platelet dysfunction)
Idiopathic pulmonary fibroelastosis
Idiopathic airway-centered fibrosis
Erdheim-Chester disease (non–Langerhans cell histiocytosis)

Modified from Leslie K, Colby T, Swensen S: Anatomic distribution and histopathologic patterns in interstitial lung disease. In: Schwarz M, King TJ, eds. *Interstitial Lung Disease.* Hamilton, ON: BC Decker; 2002:31–50.

Box 7-6. Cause of Death in 543 Patients with Idiopathic Pulmonary Fibrosis*

Respiratory failure, 38.7%
Infection, 6.5%
Lung cancer, 10.4%
Pulmonary embolism, 3.4%
Heart failure, 14.4%
Ischemic heart disease, 9.5%
Other, 17.1%†

*Of the 543 patients in the study, 60% died in the follow-up period, which ranged from 1 to 7 years.
†Including pneumothorax, corticosteroid-induced metabolic side effects and myopathy, and therapy-related immunosuppression.
Data from Panos RJ, Mortenson RL, Niccoli SA, King TE Jr: Clinical deterioration in patients with idiopathic pulmonary fibrosis: causes and assessment. *Am J Med.* 1990;88(4):396–404.

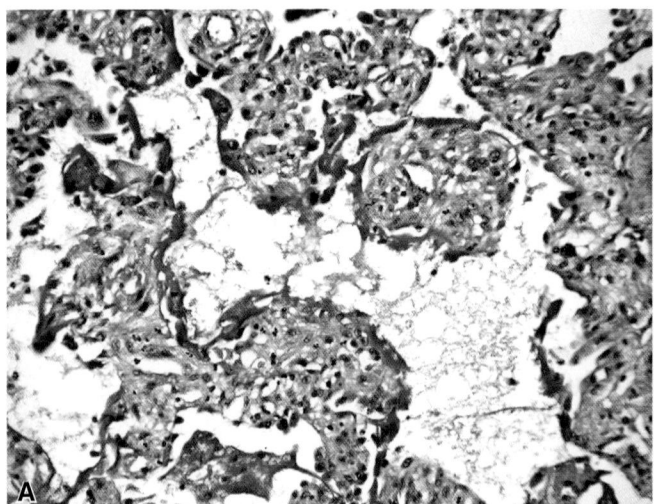
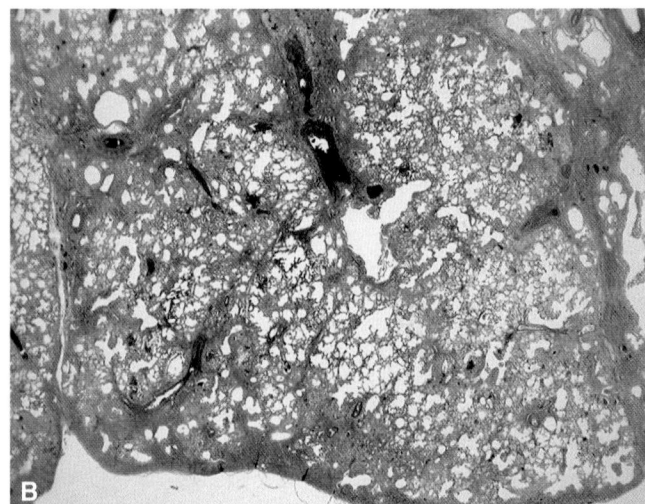

Figure 7-11. Usual interstitial pneumonia (UIP). Acute exacerbation of idiopathic pulmonary fibrosis is associated with mixed histopathologic changes, typically with diffuse alveolar damage (**A**) superimposed on a background of older fibrosis and microscopic honeycombing of UIP. The background disease may be highlighted with the trichrome stain (**B**), which shows peripherally accentuated perilobular fibrosis. These two images are of the same biopsy section.

A number of therapeutic approaches have been attempted in clinical trials. These include use of human recombinant interferon γ-1β, the antifibrotic compound pirfenidone, the antioxidant *N*-acetylcysteine, and several endothelin receptor antagonists (e.g., bosentan, ambrisentan). To date, no trial has revealed a successful cure for the disease. However, perfenidone has emerged as a candidate for slowing functional loss in IPF patients and is approved for the treatment of IPF in Japan.[54,55]

Essential Requirements for Accurate Diagnosis

For pulmonary physicians, a pathologic diagnosis of UIP implies clinical IPF; accordingly, UIP should never be diagnosed in the absence of clinical and radiologic correlation. The gravity of the prognosis and the lack of current available therapy strongly support this notion.[5] If the pathologic findings are compelling for a UIP pattern, it is reasonable to use a descriptive diagnosis such as that presented in Box 7-7. This approach provides an opportunity for further correlation by clinical colleagues and radiologists in solidifying the diagnosis.

Familial Idiopathic Pulmonary Fibrosis

There is a small subset of patients with IPF who have a history of unexplained lung disease in first-degree relatives. This form of pulmonary fibrosis has been referred to as *familial IPF* or *familial interstitial pneumonia* (although in most studies of familial interstitial pneumonia, fibrosis seems to be the dominant pattern of disease). A compelling body of evidence suggests that IPF is a genetic disorder,[56,57] and its familial occurrence is not surprising. Steele and colleagues examined the population of persons with familial interstitial pneumonia from 111 candidate families and found that more than 80% of these individuals had clinical IPF, followed by NSIP.[58] Genetic analysis was performed in search of the mechanism underlying familial IPF, and telomerase germ line mutations were identified in 8%.[59] The role of telomerase mutations was hypothesized to be a function of excess telomere shortening over time, resulting in cellular dysfunction and premature cell death.

Box 7-7. Sample Diagnosis for a Case with Histopathologic Pattern of Usual Interstitial Pneumonia at Surgical Lung Biopsy

Diagnosis
Fibrosing interstitial pneumonia with microscopic honeycombing and peripheral fibrosis with smooth muscle prominence. Fibroblast focus activity is [high / intermediate / low].

Comment
The histopathologic changes identified are characteristic of those seen in patients with clinical idiopathic pulmonary fibrosis. Radiologic and clinical correlation is required for a definitive diagnosis.

Criteria for the Usual Interstitial Pneumonia Pattern
Chronic fibrosing interstitial pneumonia with
    Patchy involvement
    Architectural loss with fibrous remodeling
    Mainly peripheral zones of chronic scarring with honeycomb change
    Marked smooth muscle metaplasia/hyperplasia
    Peripheral lobular and paraseptal accentuation
    Centrilobular sparing
    Fibroblastic foci are present at the junction of fibrosis with normal lung.

Data from Leslie K, Colby T, Swensen S: Anatomic distribution and histopathologic patterns in interstitial lung disease. In: Schwarz M, King TJ, eds. *Interstitial Lung Disease.* Hamilton, ON: BC Decker; 2002:31–50; and American Thoracic Society/European Respiratory Society international multidisciplinary consensus classification of the idiopathic interstitial pneumonias. *Am J Respir Crit Care Med.* 2002;165(2):277–304.

Nonspecific Interstitial Pneumonia

For many years after Liebow's classification of IIPs was widely adopted, a number of diffuse inflammatory lung diseases were identified that did not fit well within this classification scheme. Various terms were applied to such diffuse lung diseases, including "chronic cellular" and "unclassifiable" interstitial pneumonia.[60] In 1994 the term *nonspecific interstitial pneumonia* was proposed by Katzenstein and Fiorelli, based on data from 64 patients who presented with diffuse lung disease and a chief complaint of dyspnea, usually present for several months before evaluation.[16] Radiologic studies showed bilateral interstitial infiltrates with variable consolidation. Importantly, the 64 patients in this study had a significantly better prognosis than that observed for patients with UIP.

Katzenstein and Fiorelli recognized that the constellation of histopathologic patterns seen in NSIP did not represent one disease and, in follow-up investigations, found that these patients often had hypersensitivity, resolving infection, or systemic CVD, among other occurrences. Nagai and coworkers studied a group of patients with cellular interstitial pneumonia and rigorously excluded possible etiologies. The reported survival rate in this "idiopathic NSIP" was 90% at 5 years.[61] Thus, when used in the true idiopathic context, the designation "NSIP" may actually be useful if it consistently implies an interstitial chronic inflammatory disease of unknown etiology, with an expected good response to therapy and excellent survival rate. If, on the other hand, the term is applied indiscriminately as a substitute for any histopathologically unrecognized ILD, clinical behavior will be impossible to predict, thereby significantly reducing the benefit of lung biopsy.

Clinical Presentation

Some general statements can be made regarding the clinical presentation in NSIP, recognizing that most of the available data have been derived from studies in which a heterogeneous group of disorders were represented. Patients with NSIP histopathology in lung biopsies (that is, an NSIP pattern) tend to be younger than patients with UIP[61-63]; the NSIP pattern might also appear in children.[16] As with many of the chronic diffuse lung diseases, symptoms develop gradually. Shortness of breath, cough, fatigue, and weight loss are the most common complaints. Fever and digital clubbing have been reported but are uncommon.[16,62]

Radiologic Findings

As in UIP, most of the chest x-ray abnormalities in NSIP are confined to the lower lung zones and tend to be bilateral and symmetrical.[64] Less than 40% of the lung volume is typically involved. Patchy parenchymal (alveolar) opacification is a commonly reported abnormality,[64] but reticular (interstitial) changes have also been identified.[16] High-resolution CT findings are variable and nonspecific.[65] The most common findings are a reticular pattern and traction bronchiectasis, followed by lobar volume loss and ground-glass attenuation. As uncommon features, subpleural sparing, irregular linear opacities, patchy honeycombing, and nodular opacities can be seen.[61,62] As might be anticipated, some of the findings described for NSIP overlap with those in other ILDs, such as hypersensitivity pneumonitis and COP. In the stage before honeycomb cysts are visible, even UIP can be indistinguishable from NSIP.

Histopathologic Findings

Katzenstein and Fiorelli emphasized that the histopathologic pattern in NSIP was temporally uniform (Fig. 7-12), in contrast with the UIP pattern, in which variable zones of established (dense) fibrosis, more active fibroplasia, and normal lung all coexist in the same biopsy specimen (i.e., temporal heterogeneity). As initially defined, the inflammatory process

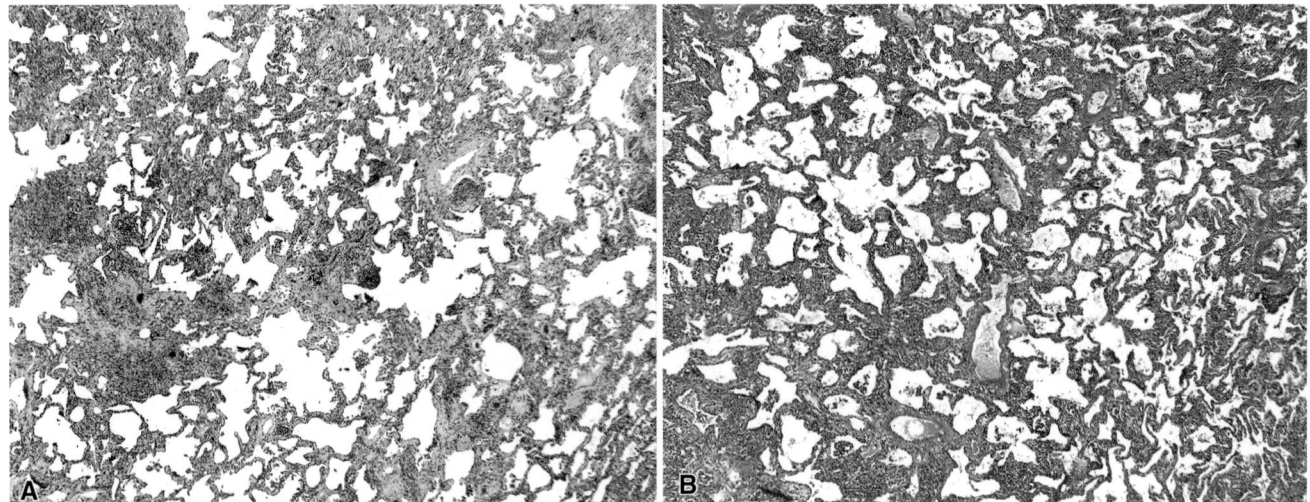

Figure 7-12. Nonspecific interstitial pneumonia (NSIP). The histopathology of NSIP is temporally uniform, in contrast with the temporal heterogeneity of the usual interstitial pneumonia pattern. Two examples are shown here: **A,** Small lymphoid aggregates can be appreciated at scanning magnification; **B,** the process is uniform and may be associated with interstitial widening and some interstitial fibrosis.

in NSIP is diffuse and uniform, mainly involving the alveolar walls (Fig. 7-13) and variably affecting the bronchovascular sheaths (Fig. 7-14) and pleura[16] (Fig. 7-15). In some patients, infiltrates are predominantly peribronchial, whereas in others, germinal centers may be seen along with chronic pleuritis. When air space organization (the organizing pneumonia pattern) is present, it is not uniformly distributed (Fig. 7-16) as might occur in organizing infectious pneumonia.[16] When fibrosis occurs in NSIP, it is usually mild and preserves lung structure (Fig. 7-17). Peribronchiolar metaplasia of variable extent may be seen, but microscopic honeycombing is characteristically absent.[16,66]

There has been debate as to whether NSIP is a new "interstitial lung disease" or simply a wastebasket category of diseases with some overlapping features. An American Thoracic Society project concluded that idiopathic NSIP is likely a distinct clinical entity with characteristic radiologic and pathologic features.[66] Caution is advised in using this term for any lung disease with interstitial inflammation, just as it is imprudent to diagnose all fibrosing lung diseases as UIP.

Differential Diagnosis

The main entities in the differential diagnosis of the NSIP pattern include hypersensitivity pneumonitis, systemic CVDs manifesting in the lung, resolving infection, and low-grade lymphoproliferative disease masquerading as LIP (see later on). Cellular NSIP and LIP may be difficult to distinguish from one another on histopathologic grounds, so they might be considered synonymous from the pathologist's perspective, once lymphoproliferative disease has been rigorously excluded. Kinder and associates hypothesized that a majority of NSIP cases fall into the category of undifferentiated connective tissue disease manifesting in the lung. Because of significant overlap between NSIP and ILD in CVD, careful follow-up with serologic testing is recommended.[67] In clinical practice, in view of the limited arsenal of available therapies for ILD, managing NSIP as a systemic autoimmune disorder with immunosuppressive strategies (even though it may not be initially diagnosable by a rheumatologist) often proves to be the best course of action for the patient.

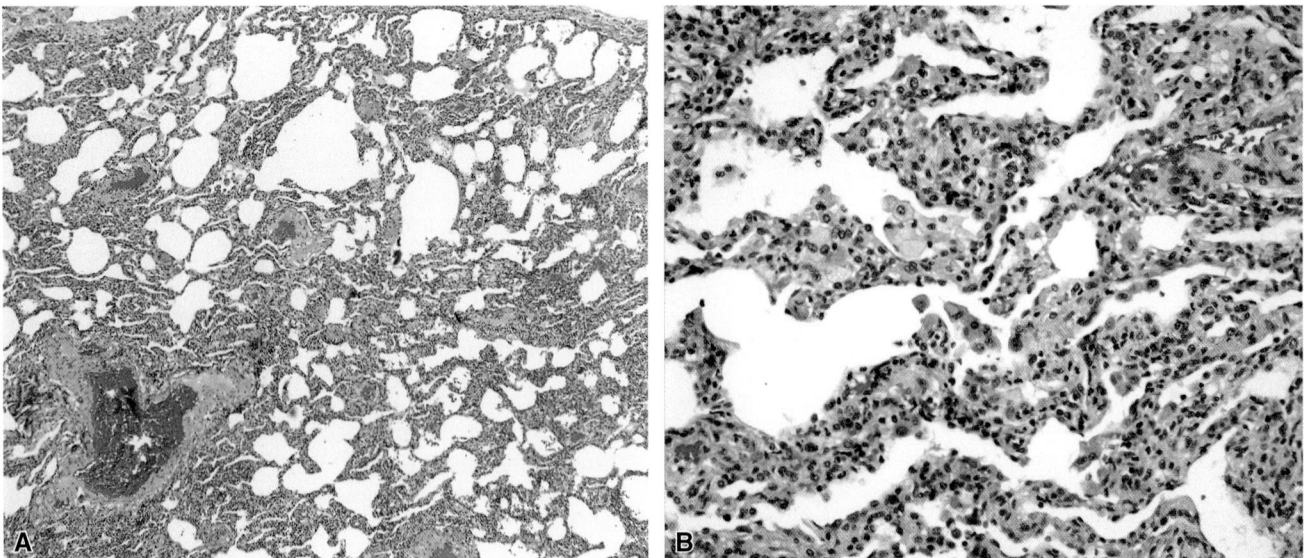

Figure 7-13. Nonspecific interstitial pneumonia (NSIP). **A,** The chronic inflammatory infiltration in NSIP is diffuse and relatively uniform, mainly involving the alveolar walls. **B,** Lymphocytes and plasma cells are the dominant cells.

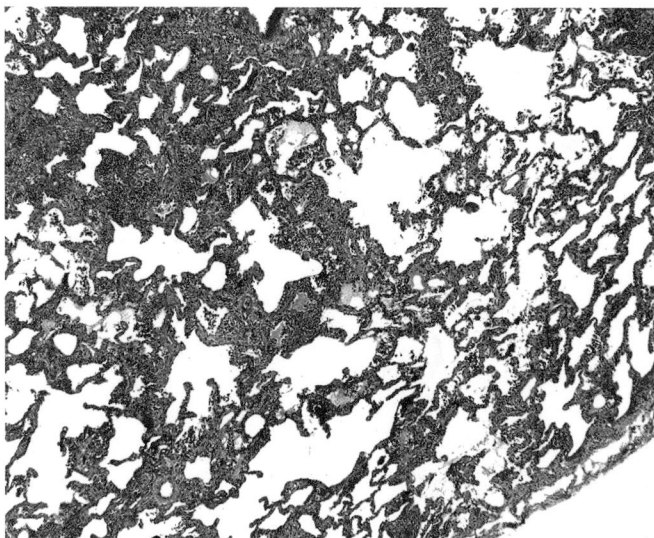

Figure 7-14. Nonspecific interstitial pneumonia. Variable widening of alveolar walls by chronic inflammation can be seen, with little if any spared alveolar parenchyma in the biopsy. Bronchovascular sheaths also typically are involved by the inflammatory process, to a variable degree.

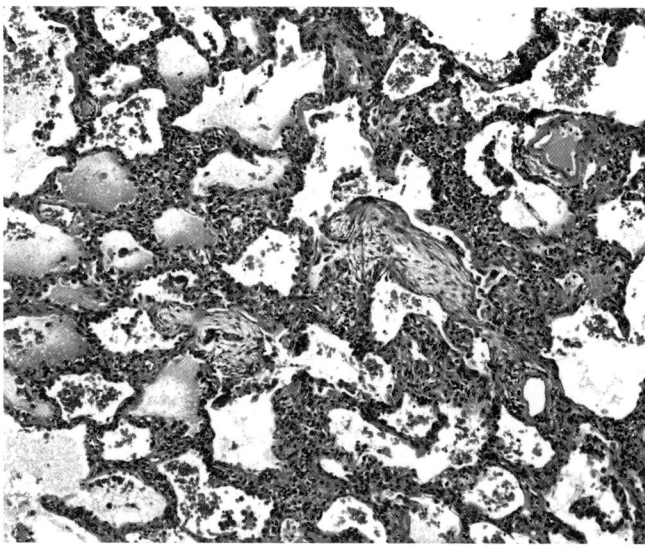

Figure 7-16. Nonspecific interstitial pneumonia. When air space organization (organizing pneumonia pattern) is seen (*center*), it is not diffusely or uniformly distributed, as might occur in organizing infectious pneumonia.

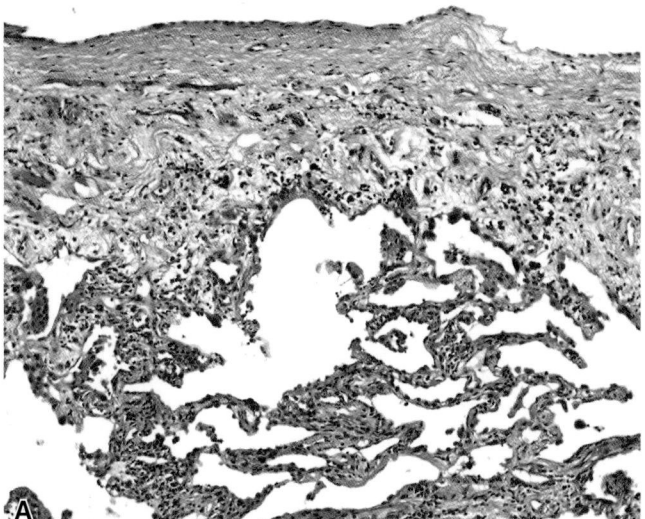

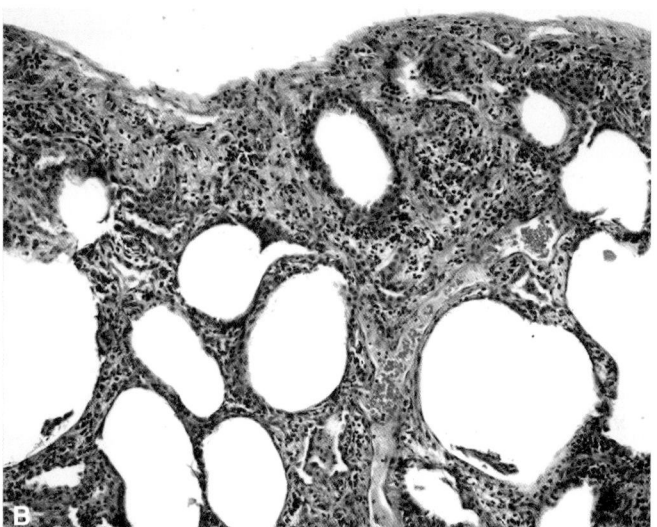

Figure 7-15. Nonspecific interstitial pneumonia (NSIP). **A** and **B,** Pleuritis is very common in NSIP, emphasizing the strong association between the NSIP pattern in biopsy tissue and the presence of known, or evolving, systemic collagen vascular disease.

Clinical Course

The overall survival rate for patients with NSIP is estimated to be in the range of 82.3% at 5 years and 73.2% at 10 years.[66] The purely "cellular" form of NSIP seems to be a disease with a good prognosis, compared with UIP and AIP.

When significant fibrous remodeling with microscopic honeycombing is permitted in the diagnosis of NSIP, 5- and 10-year survival rates change significantly for the worse.[61,68] This observation suggests that fibrotic forms of NSIP may be within the spectrum of other fibrosing lung diseases, such as UIP of IPF, and certain systemic connective tissue diseases that manifest in the lung with fibrosis.

Cryptogenic Organizing Pneumonia

Air space organization is an extremely common manifestation of lung injury and can be seen after a wide variety of insults, from organizing lung infarction to bacterial pneumonia (Box 7-8). For this reason, the organizing pneumonia pattern in the lung biopsy is the least specific and perhaps the most misunderstood.

It is well known that lung repair following a wide spectrum of injuries frequently evolves through a phase of air space organization. When organization is diffuse, involving the entire surgical biopsy, organizing pneumonia (or "diffuse air space organization") is an appropriate designation. When no etiology can be identified for an organizing pneumonia pattern, the clinical diagnosis of *cryptogenic organizing pneumonia* (COP) has been proposed (referred to previously as "idiopathic bronchiolitis obliterans organizing pneumonia").[6,17,69]

The term *bronchiolitis obliterans organizing pneumonia* (BOOP), as an idiopathic disease, was first proposed by Davison and coworkers,[69] and later used by Epler and associates,[17] to define a specific clinical disease course in a group of patients in whom lung biopsies showed variable amounts of air space organization (organizing pneumonia pattern) of unexplained etiology. The importance of recognizing the pattern of organizing pneumonia in the clinical context defined relates

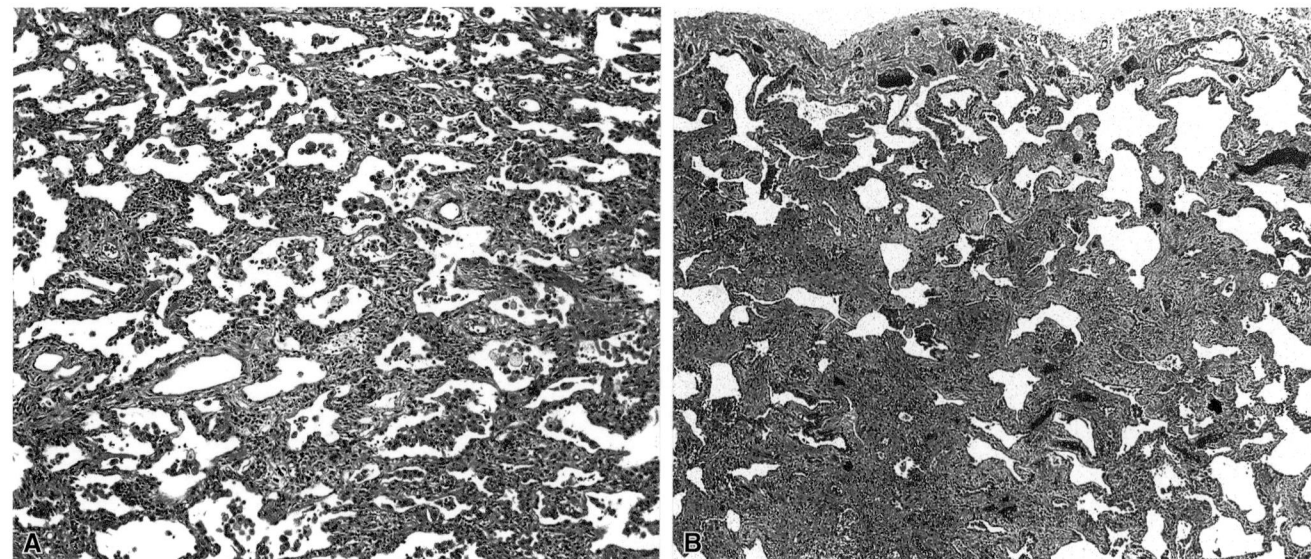

Figure 7-17. Nonspecific interstitial pneumonia (NSIP). When fibrosis occurs in NSIP (so-called "fibrotic NSIP"), it is usually mild to moderate in degree, with preservation of lung structure, and generally without microscopic honeycombing or heterogeneity (i.e., normal lung adjacent to advanced fibrosis). **A,** Changes of NSIP seen at low magnification. **B,** Different specimen showing more prominent fibrosis.

Box 7-8. Causes of the Organizing Pneumonia Pattern

Organizing infections
Organizing diffuse alveolar damage
Drug or toxic reactions
Collagen vascular diseases
Hypersensitivity pneumonitis
Chronic eosinophilic pneumonia
Airway diseases complicated by infection (bronchitis and emphysema, bronchiectasis, cystic fibrosis, aspiration pneumonia, and chronic bronchiolitis)
Airway obstruction
Peripheral reactive process surrounding pulmonary abscesses, infarcts, lesions of Wegener granulomatosis, others
Cryptogenic organizing pneumonia

Modified from Leslie K, Colby T, Swensen S: Anatomic distribution and histopathologic patterns in interstitial lung disease. In: Schwarz M, King TJ, eds. *Interstitial Lung Disease.* Hamilton, ON: BC Decker; 2002:31–50.

to therapy and prognosis. Patients with clinical COP respond well to systemic corticosteroid administration, and pulmonologists expect a good prognosis when this diagnosis is implied histopathologically. When "BOOP" is used in a pathology report as a descriptive term for the occurrence of organizing pneumonia in a biopsy, the clinician may misinterpret this to mean "idiopathic BOOP" is the correct diagnosis. For example, the "BOOP" pattern may be seen in a disease with abundant background lung fibrosis. In this setting, the prognosis is best considered to be guarded.[70]

Clinical Presentation

As described by Epler and coworkers for the original "idiopathic BOOP," the patient typically presents several weeks after an episode of clinical symptoms suggesting upper respiratory tract infection.[17] The mean age at onset is 55 years, and a majority of patients are nonsmokers.[71,72] Slowly worsening symptoms of cough (sometimes productive) and dyspnea are typically present, often leading to surgical lung biopsy within 3 months of disease onset. Weight loss, night sweats, chills, intermittent fever, and myalgias are common. Mild to moderate restrictive pulmonary function studies are identified in a majority of patients.[72–74]

Hemoptysis and wheezing typically are absent. Often there is a marked increase in the erythrocyte sedimentation rate (ESR). Digital clubbing is not a feature of the disease.

Radiologic Findings

Chest radiography and CT show a number of abnormalities, none of which are specific for one disease. Patchy air space consolidation (loss of visible structure underlying opacification) is the most consistent finding and is present in 90% of cases.[75,76] Air bronchograms can be seen in areas of consolidation. Ground-glass attenuation accompanies consolidation in more than one half of the patients. The disease involves the lower lung zones more often than the upper lung zones.[77] Small nodular opacities can be seen in 10% to 50% of patients.[78]

In a small percentage of patients, large nodules may be seen[78]; rarely, reticulonodular infiltrates occur.[74] It is speculated that this latter finding identifies a subset of COP that may not respond to therapy. Opacities may be recurrent and/or migratory.[79,80] Lung volumes are normal in most patients, and pleural effusions rarely occur.[75,76,81]

Histopathologic Findings

The organizing pneumonia pattern is characterized by variably dense air space aggregates of fibroblasts in ground substance (immature collagen matrix) (Fig. 7-18). This alveolar filling process can be seen to extend into or from terminal bronchioles (Fig. 7-19). Typically, the lung architecture is preserved in COP, and lymphocytes, plasma cells, and histiocytes are present in variable numbers within the interstitium[17,82,83] (Fig. 7-20). Fibrin may be seen focally in association with air space organization (Fig. 7-21). Alveolar macrophage accumulation may be present, attesting to some degree of airway obstruction.[17,82,83] When air space organization is confluent and diffuse in the biopsy, COP is less likely to be the accurate diagnosis. Interstitial fibrosis and honeycomb lung remodeling are not components of the cryptogenic (idiopathic) form of organizing pneumonia.[17,82,83]

Treatment and Prognosis

The expected response to systemic corticosteroid administration therapy is excellent.[17,79,84] Because relapses may occur if therapy is stopped abruptly, patients with COP generally require extended corticosteroid tapering, sometimes over a year or more.[17,79,84]

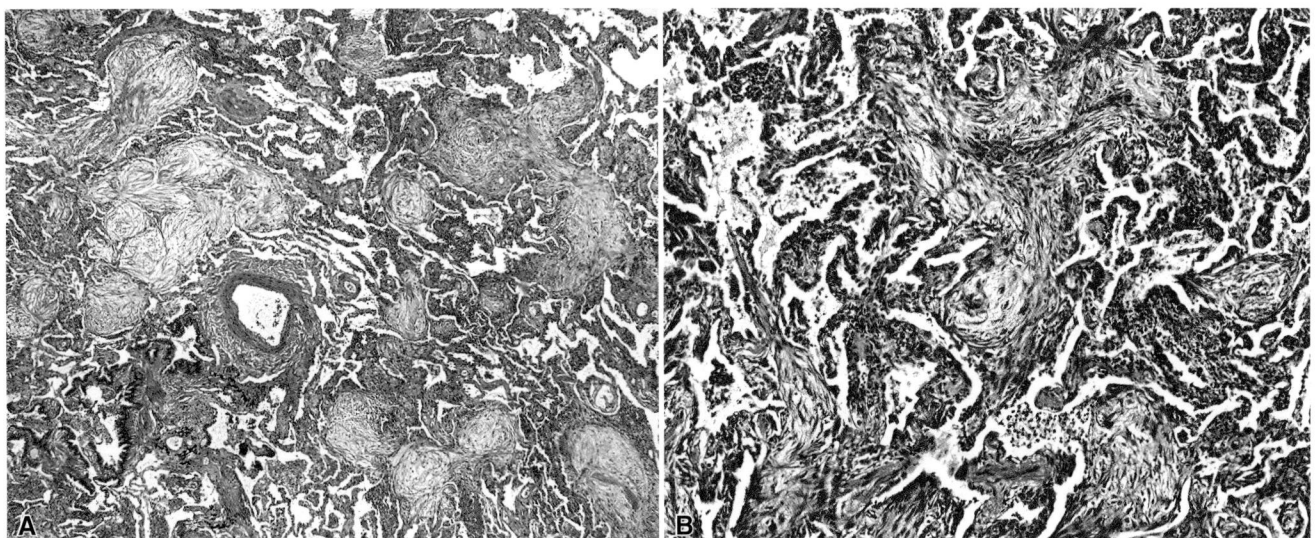

Figure 7-18. Organizing pneumonia pattern. This histopathologic pattern is characterized by variably dense air space aggregates of loose fibroblasts within ground substance (immature collagen associated with an acellular pale or basophilic matrix). **A,** At scanning magnification, slight nodularity of the process is evident. **B,** At higher magnification, growth of loose granulation tissue can be seen within terminal airways and adjacent alveolar spaces.

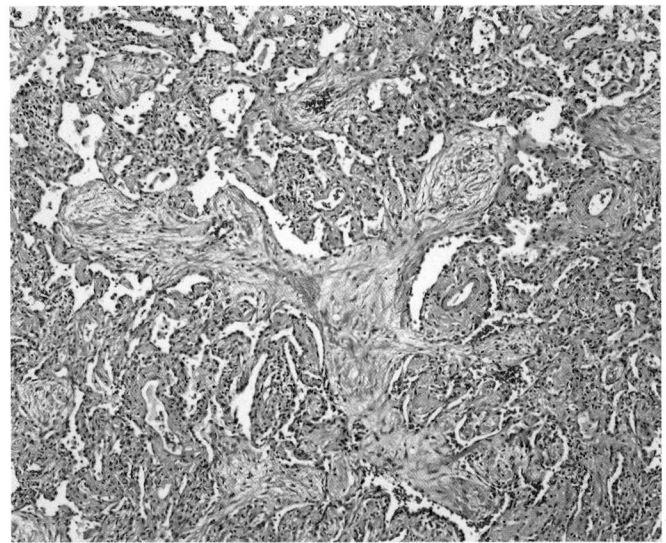

Figure 7-19. Organizing pneumonia pattern. A branching tongue of fibroblastic proliferation can be seen to extend into, or from, an alveolar duct. Note the mild inflammatory interstitial infiltrate in surrounding alveolar walls.

Differential Diagnosis

As mentioned previously, the differential diagnosis for the organizing pneumonia histopathologic pattern is too broad in scope to be of clinical use. In general, it is fair to say that the presence of the organizing pneumonia pattern is much more commonly associated with slowly organizing infection, systemic connective tissue diseases, hypersensitivity pneumonitis, and idiosyncratic reaction to drug or medication, rather than a "cryptogenic" disease. Rarely, air space organization may ossify and produced so-called "racemose" or "dendriform" ossification (Fig. 7-22).

Respiratory Bronchiolitis–Associated Interstitial Lung Disease

Respiratory bronchiolitis (RB) is a histopathologic lesion of the small airways that is common in cigarette smokers.[85] In some smokers, an exuberant form of RB occurs as a clinical and radiologic manifestation of diffuse "interstitial" lung disease. This ILD manifestation of RB has been referred to as *respiratory bronchiolitis–associated interstitial lung disease* (RBILD).[86] RB, RBILD, and DIP have been proposed as existing along a continuum in smokers,[87] with RB on the asymptomatic end of a spectrum that culminates in DIP on the other. Whether RB, RBILD, and DIP are truly manifestations of a single disease process remains to be proved. Certainly, all three have some histopathologic elements in common, but the two main clinical manifestations in the spectrum (RBILD and DIP) also differ in a number of ways clinically and radiologically.

Clinical Presentation

Patients with RBILD are typically a decade younger than those with DIP and present in early midlife, with a mean age of 36 years in two studies.[86,88] A relationship between smoking pack-years and onset of disease suggests a dose-related effect, with a threshold in the vicinity of 30 pack-years. There tends to be a gender predilection toward men,[87,89] but men and women were equally affected in one study.[88] Mild breathlessness and cough are the most common initial complaints.[86,88] Clubbing of the digits is unusual in RBILD.[88,90,91] Pulmonary function abnormalities parallel the mild clinical symptoms and may show evidence of both obstruction and restriction, with mild reduction in the diffusing capacity.[89]

Radiologic Findings

The chest x-ray appearance of RBILD reflects the presence of disease centered on the airways, mainly with thickening of airway walls.[87] Ground-glass opacity is seen in more than 50% of chest radiographs in RBILD. On CT scans, ground-glass opacities and centrilobular nodules are typical findings, often best seen at the periphery of the upper lung zones.[87]

Histopathologic Findings

RB is a common reactive process in the lungs of cigarette smokers; its presence alone does not imply the diffuse lung disease manifestation.[91] Moreover, even when the histopathologic changes are diffuse and distinctive in the biopsy specimen, clinical correlation is required for accurate diagnosis. For example, a patient with a lung mass, resected and found to be a bronchogenic carcinoma, may have extensive RB in surrounding lung parenchyma. In the absence of a clinically and radiologically defined ILD, a diagnosis of RBILD would be inappropriate.

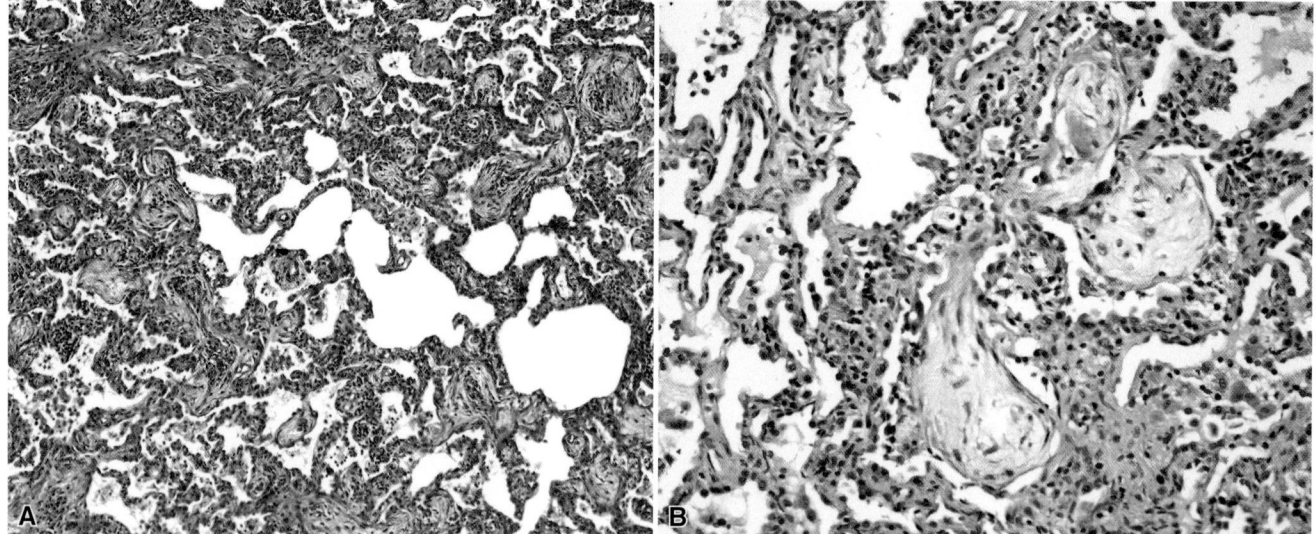

Figure 7-20. Organizing pneumonia pattern. In cryptogenic organizing pneumonia (COP), the lung architecture typically is preserved. Lymphocytes, plasma cells, and histiocytes are present to variable degree within the interstitium. **A,** Note the very patchy organization. **B,** The prototypical appearance of COP, with patchy organization and mild interstitial pneumonia.

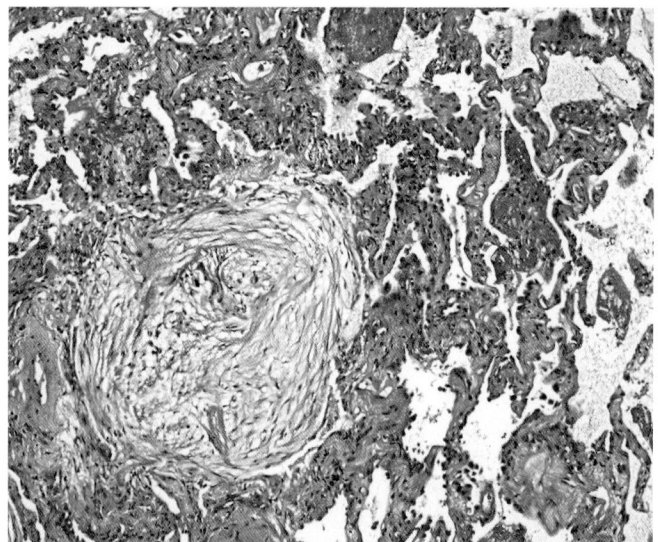

Figure 7-21. Organizing pneumonia pattern. Fibrin (*center right*) may be seen focally in association with air space organization (*center left*) in cryptogenic organizing pneumonia.

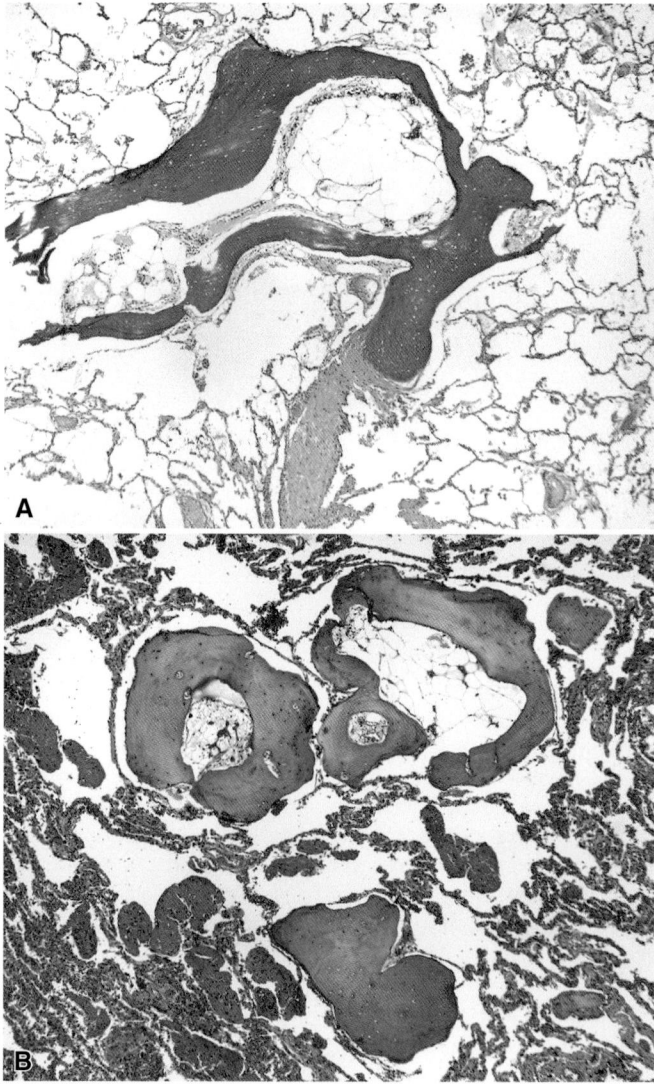

Figure 7-22. Racemose (dendriform) alveolar calcification. **A** and **B,** Rarely, air space organization may ossify, producing so-called "racemose" or "dendriform" ossification.

The essential morphologic constituents of RB are (1) scant inflammation around the terminal airways (Fig. 7-23), (2) metaplastic bronchiolar epithelium extending out from terminal airways to involve alveolar ducts (Fig. 7-24), and (3) variable numbers of lightly pigmented, dusty brown air space macrophages within bronchiolar lumens and in immediate surrounding alveoli (Fig. 7-25). Scant peribronchiolar fibrosis may be present and may extend to involve contiguous alveolar walls (Fig. 7-26). When bronchiolocentric scarring is prominent, an alternative diagnosis, such as chronic hypersensitivity pneumonitis, should be considered. Dense collagenous thickening of the alveolar septa without inflammation can be seen in RBILD. Such fibrosis does not appear to progress to honeycomb fibrosis.[92] Presence of fibroblastic foci or destruction of the lung architecture should always raise the possibility of an alternative diagnosis, especially undersampled UIP.

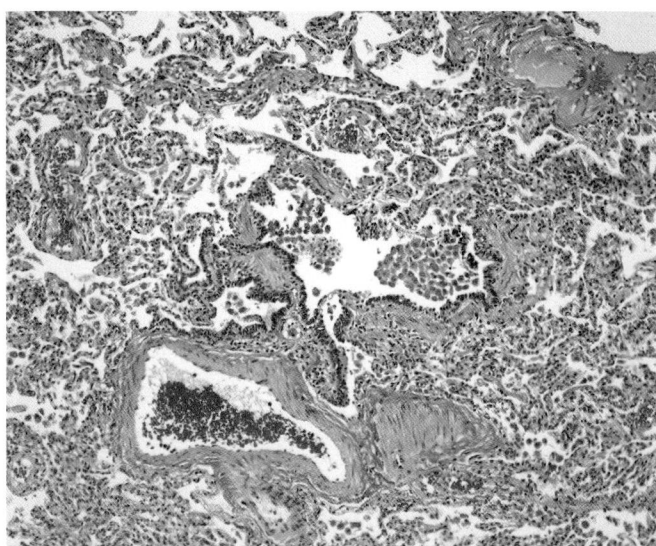

Figure 7-23. Respiratory bronchiolitis. This pathologic process is characterized by the presence of scant inflammation around the terminal airways.

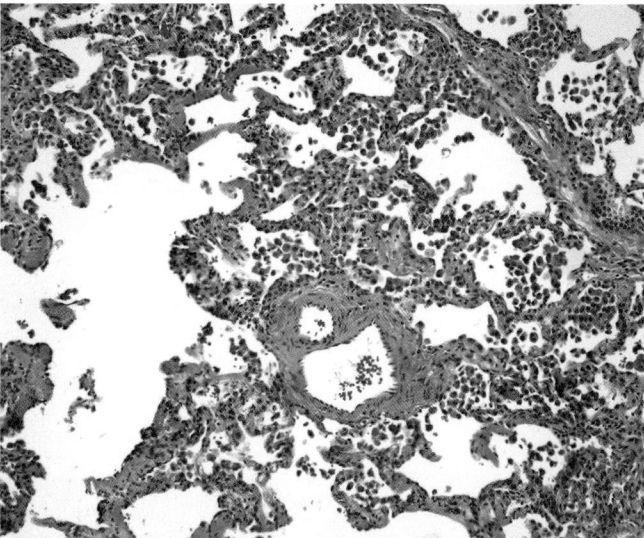

Figure 7-25. Respiratory bronchiolitis. Variable numbers of lightly pigmented (dusty brown) air space macrophages are seen within bronchiolar lumens and in immediate surrounding alveoli.

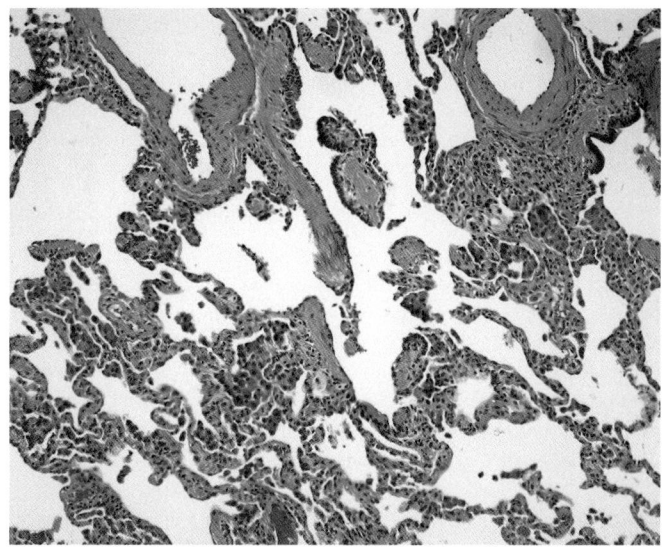

Figure 7-24. Respiratory bronchiolitis. Metaplastic bronchiolar epithelium extends out from terminal airways to involve alveolar ducts.

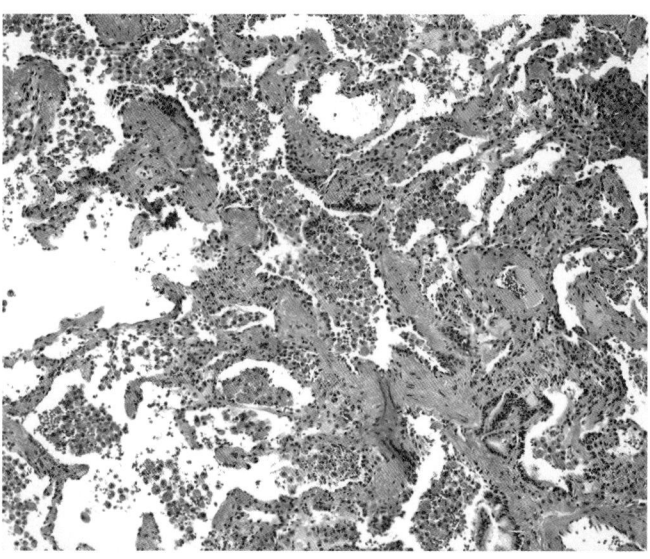

Figure 7-26. Respiratory bronchiolitis. Scant peribronchiolar fibrosis may be present; this may extend to involve contiguous alveolar walls, with or without prominent smooth muscle bundles.

Differential Diagnosis

RB may be confused with bronchiolitis of some other etiology. When bronchiolar metaplasia is a prominent component, distinction from other small-airway disease, such as idiopathic constrictive bronchiolitis, may be difficult. Patients with idiopathic constrictive bronchiolitis in surgical biopsies tend to have more severe pulmonary function abnormalities than patients with RB or RBILD (see Chapter 8 for a discussion of small airways disease).

Clinical Course

RBILD generally carries an excellent prognosis. However, symptomatic or physiologic improvement occurs in a limited number of patients. Smoking cessation, with or without immunosuppressive therapy, has been recommended, but a recent report demonstrated benefit in only a small subset of patients.[93]

Desquamative Interstitial Pneumonia

Leibow[7] proposed the term *desquamative interstitial pneumonia* for a diffuse lung disease that occurred in patients who were typically 10 years or more younger than patients who developed UIP. The disease often presented in mid-adulthood, and most patients were cigarette smokers.[94] Liebow also believed that the "desquamated" cells that filled the air spaces in DIP were epithelial cells. It has now been established that the air space cells of Liebow's DIP are actually macrophages, and that DIP is not a credible precursor lesion for UIP, as was proposed by a number of authorities.

Our current concept of DIP overlaps with that of RBILD, with both being considered components of the smoking-related diffuse lung diseases (see the section "Pulmonary Langerhans Cell Histiocytosis" in this chapter). Whether DIP occurs as a separate disease in nonsmoking adolescents remains debatable, but it is unlikely. Another debate is centered on whether a form of UIP coexists with DIP as a "hybrid" entity. Those who still believe DIP is a precursor lesion to UIP embrace this as proof of concept for instances in which this association is suggested in surgical lung biopsies. The counterargument is that smokers accumulate alveolar macrophages in areas of lung fibrosis, and because a majority of patients with UIP are current or former smokers, some of these patients will have prominent smoker-type macrophages coexistent with UIP.

Clinical Presentation

As currently defined, DIP is a very rare smoking-related lung disease. Patients with DIP are typically older than those with RBILD[87] and roughly a decade younger than those with UIP.[91,94] Most patients with DIP are cigarette smokers; men are more frequently affected than women. Like UIP, the clinical presentation is dominated by insidious onset of dyspnea and dry cough over several weeks or months.[91,95] Digital clubbing is present in 50% of patients with DIP, a finding in sharp contrast with RBILD. The symptoms of DIP are usually more pronounced and more severe than those of RBILD,[87] supported by pulmonary function testing showing mild restriction and moderate reduction in diffusing capacity.[95]

Radiologic Findings

The chest radiograph may be normal in 3% to 22% of patients. When abnormalities are present, patchy areas of ground-glass opacification predominate. The lung bases and periphery are most commonly affected.[87,96,97] On CT scans, ground-glass opacification is universally present, mostly in a bibasilar distribution.[96] Linear and reticular opacities may accompany ground-glass opacities at the bases but tend to be quite limited in extent. Focal areas of peripheral honeycombing may be identified in as many as one third of patients,[96] but when prominent and associated with more pronounced reticular abnormalities, an alternate diagnosis should be considered (probably UIP).

Histopathologic Findings

On scanning magnification, the surgical lung biopsy in DIP has an eosinophilic appearance due to the presence of eosinophilic macrophages uniformly filling air spaces[11,88] (Fig. 7-27). Mild interstitial thickening by fibrous tissue is the rule and is uniform in appearance

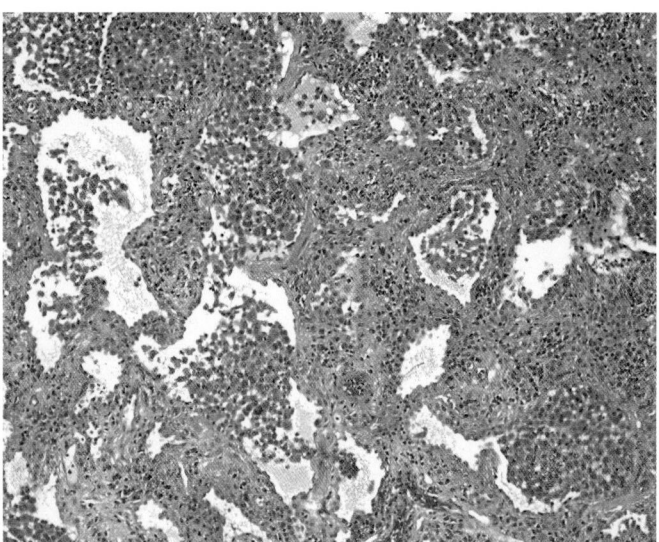

Figure 7-28. Desquamative interstitial pneumonia (DIP). Variable thickening of alveolar walls by fibrous tissue is the rule in DIP and typically is uniform in appearance. The expected presence of some alveolar wall fibrosis often makes the distinction of DIP from fibrotic forms of nonspecific interstitial pneumonia in heavy smokers the main issue, especially because the prognosis may be quite different for the two diseases.

(Fig. 7-28). When chronic inflammation is evident at scanning magnification, it is centrilobular and associated with respiratory bronchioles (Fig. 7-29). Scant numbers of plasma cells and rare eosinophils may be seen within slightly thickened alveolar walls at high magnification (Fig. 7-30).

Differential Diagnosis

Distinguishing DIP from RBILD is probably a useless exercise for pathologists; inclusion of these two smoking-related diseases together as a diagnostic entity seems reasonable in the absence of clinical and radiologic data. Eosinophilic lung disease can simulate the low-magnification appearance of DIP, as can chronic passive congestion, pulmonary hemorrhage syndromes, giant cell interstitial pneumonia in hard metal disease, and pulmonary Langerhans cell histiocytosis

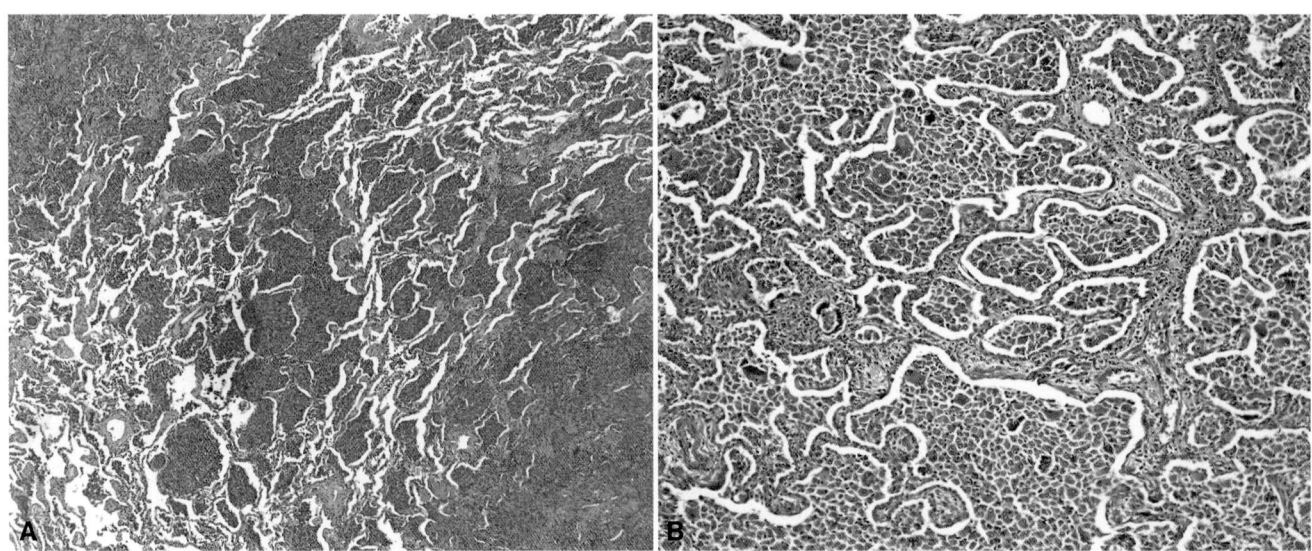

Figure 7-27. Desquamative interstitial pneumonia (DIP). **A,** DIP is often a scanning magnification diagnosis. **B,** The surgical lung biopsy has an eosinophilic appearance owing to the presence of eosinophilic macrophages uniformly filling air spaces.

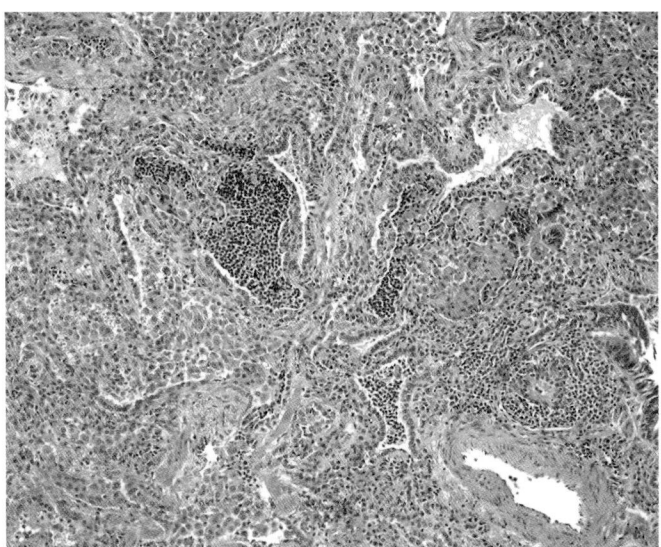

Figure 7-29. Desquamative interstitial pneumonia (DIP). When chronic inflammation is evident in DIP at scanning magnification, it is centrilobular and associated with respiratory bronchioles.

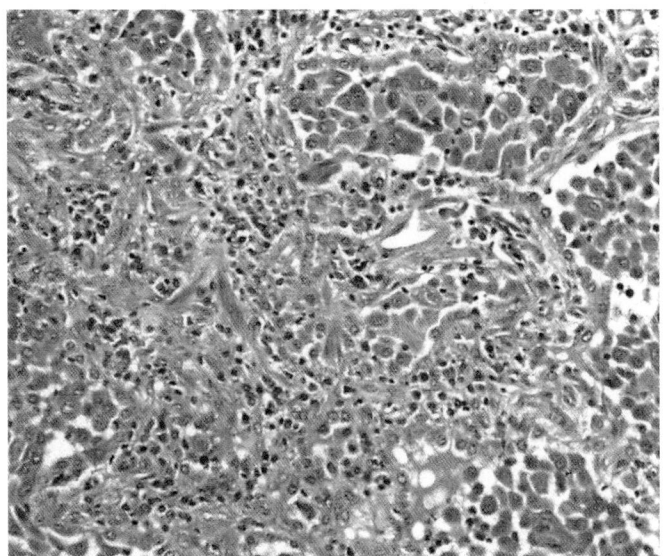

Figure 7-30. Desquamative interstitial pneumonia. Scant numbers of plasma cells and rare eosinophils may be seen within slightly thickened alveolar walls at high magnification.

(pulmonary histiocytosis X) when a prominent "DIP reaction" is identified. Progression to end-stage fibrotic lung disease is atypical and should raise consideration of alternative diagnoses including comorbid disease.

Clinical Course

As with RBILD, the prognosis for patients with DIP tends to be good, with an estimated 10-year survival rate of 70%.[95] Smoking cessation and corticosteroid therapy have proved effective in older studies.[94]

Lymphoid Interstitial Pneumonia

LIP was originally conceived as a chronic cellular interstitial pneumonia with distinctive histopathologic features, quite different in cellular composition and form from Liebow's other IIPs (e.g., UIP, BIP, DIP, GIP).[7] LIP became controversial because many of the cases originally

classified as LIP by Liebow (and his contemporaries) evolved into (or were actually indolent forms of) low-grade lymphoproliferative disease involving the lung.[98-100] It is now generally acknowledged that the accrual of dense lymphoid tissue in the lung carries strong implications for lymphoproliferative disease, especially small B cell lymphomas of extranodal marginal zone type (so-called lymphomas of the mucosa-associated lymphoid tissue [MALT]) and polymorphous lymphoproliferative disorders associated with viral infection, including EBV or HTLV-1.[98-103] "Lymphoid interstitial pneumonia," as currently defined, is included as an entity in this chapter because a recent international consensus panel chose to keep LIP as a form of IIP, partly for historical reasons. The panel participants acknowledged that many pulmonary pathologists might classify the described histopathologic findings of "idiopathic LIP" as a cellular form of NSIP.

More recently, Cha and colleagues[104] described a series of non-lymphoma LIP cases in which 9 of 15 patients were found to have a CVD, mainly Sjögren syndrome. In that series, three patients with idiopathic LIP were identified. All three survived longer than 10 years, and their disease did not progress to lymphoma or leukemia, despite the fact that one of them had a monoclonal gammopathy.[104]

Clinical Presentation

The clinical manifestations of the idiopathic form of the LIP pattern are not well studied but seem to be similar to those associated with definable systemic conditions, such as CVD. Women are more commonly affected than men; patients are typically between 40 and 50 years of age.[105] Interestingly, all of the "idiopathic LIP" patients described by Cha and colleagues were men, whereas most of secondary LIP patients were women.[104] Slowly progressive breathlessness is a common feature, with or without nonproductive cough; the disease may evolve over months or years.

In the classic description of LIP, systemic signs and symptoms such as weight loss, pleuritic pain, arthralgias, adenopathy, and fever were reported, depending on whether an associated systemic condition was present.[105-107] Findings may include bibasilar crackles, cyanosis, and clubbing. Immunoglobulin abnormalities in serum are present in some patients.[108] More commonly, the LIP pattern is associated with a systemic condition that dominates the clinical presentation and clinical course (e.g., Sjögren syndrome, pernicious anemia, hypogammaglobulinemia).

Radiologic Findings

The published radiologic features of idiopathic LIP seem to describe more than one pattern of disease.[109] Bibasilar reticular opacities along with ground-glass attenuation and thickening of interlobular septa are frequently observed abnormalities.[104,109-111] There may be mixed alveolar and interstitial infiltrates and thin-walled cysts, honeycombing, and changes suggesting pulmonary hypertension late in the disease.[112,113] Nodular patterns can also occur.[114] Pleural effusion is rare and, if present, should increase concern for low-grade malignant lymphoma.

A distinctive cystic disease has also been referred to by radiologists as "lymphocytic interstitial pneumonia" (or simply, LIP); on biopsy, however, the process has no significant interstitial inflammatory infiltrates or fibrosis, exhibiting only thin-walled, dilated airways with scant associated bronchiolitis.[115] An association with Sjögren syndrome has been documented.[116]

Histopathologic Findings

The histopathologic pattern in LIP is characterized by the presence of a *dense and diffuse* alveolar septal infiltrate made up of lymphocytes, plasma cells, and histiocytes (Fig. 7-31). This definition helps exclude diseases with less intense cellular interstitial infiltrates, such

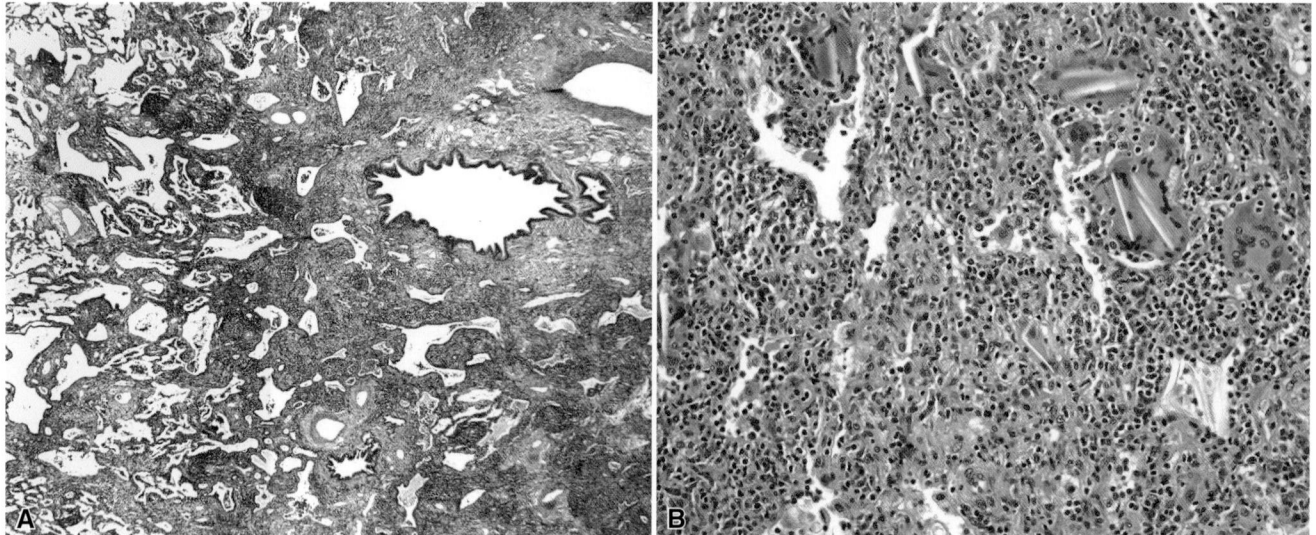

Figure 7-31. Lymphoid interstitial pneumonia. **A,** This histopathologic pattern is characterized by the presence of a dense and diffuse alveolar septal infiltrate made up of lymphocytes, plasma cells, plasmacytoid cells, and histiocytes. **B,** Multinucleate giant cells and small non-necrotizing granulomas are commonly present.

as certain hypersensitivity reactions and systemic connective tissue diseases. Multinucleated giant cells or small, ill-defined granulomas in the interstitium have been described in the idiopathic form of LIP, but microscopic honeycomb remodeling, with some interstitial fibrosis (Fig. 7-32), can also be a part of idiopathic LIP. To a variable extent, germinal centers may be present along airways and lymphatic routes (Fig. 7-33). When these are prominent and interstitial lymphocytic infiltration is less remarkable, *diffuse lymphoid hyperplasia* has been used as a preferable term. In this situation, lymphoproliferative disorders, such as multicentric Castleman disease, idiopathic plasmacytic lymphadenopathy with hyperimmunoglobulinemia, or even MALT lymphoma, are the main considerations.[117] When the idiopathic form of the LIP pattern is identified, immunophenotyping and gene rearrangement studies typically show an absence of clonality.[118] When nodular lymphoid hyperplasia is prominent around bronchioles, typically accompanied by an interstitial infiltrate, Sjögren syndrome should be rigorously investigated as a potential etiology.

Differential Diagnosis

The LIP pattern is most consistently seen when systemic CVDs manifest in the lung.[105,119] The LIP pattern may also be seen in the setting of bone marrow transplantation[120] and has frequently been observed in both children and adults who have congenital or acquired immunodeficiency syndromes[121] and in the setting of adult HIV infection including vertical transmission from mother to child.[122–124]

Much of what has been written about the histopathology of LIP is similar to that written about the histopathologic patterns of NSIP. If LIP and cellular NSIP can be distinguished from each other microscopically, it is usually on the basis of the sheer density of the lymphoid infiltrate in LIP, accompanied by fibrosis and some degree of remodeling (the latter would be unexpected for the cellular form of NSIP). Naturally, in this setting, gene rearrangement studies are important in distinguishing idiopathic LIP from low-grade lymphoproliferative disease (see Chapter 15 for further discussion). Once the pattern is established, it is useful to suggest the potential systemic conditions that may be associated with this pattern (Box 7-9) in a "comment" section of the surgical pathology report.

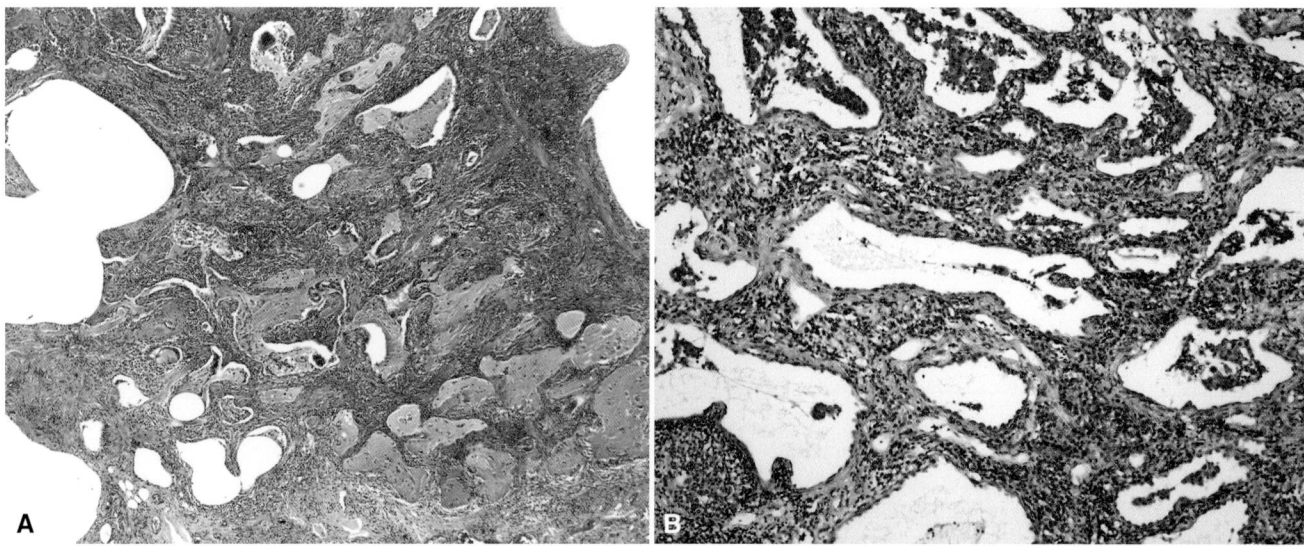

Figure 7-32. Lymphoid interstitial pneumonia (LIP). Microscopic honeycomb cystic remodeling (**A**), with some interstitial fibrosis (**B**), can also be components of idiopathic LIP.

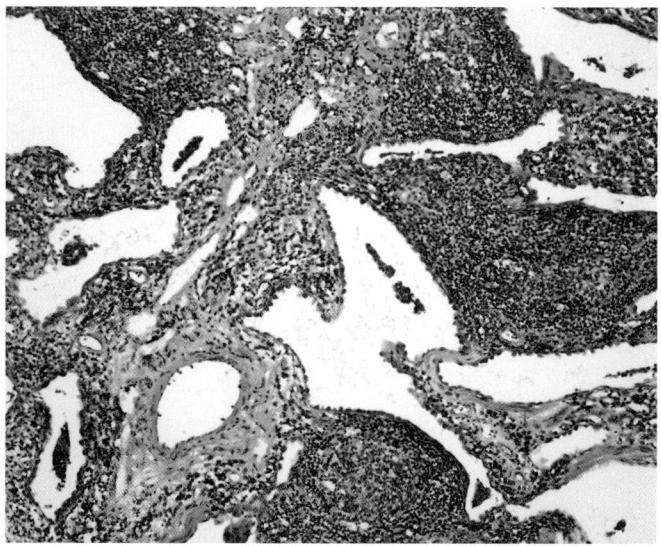

Figure 7-33. Lymphoid interstitial pneumonia. Germinal centers may be present to a variable extent along airways and lymphatic routes. When these are prominent, "diffuse lymphoid hyperplasia" has been used as a preferable alternative term for this clinical entity.

Box 7-9. Systemic Conditions Associated with the Lymphoid Interstitial Pneumonia Histopathologic Pattern

Certain infections (e.g., *Pneumocystis jiroveci* pneumonia, Epstein-Barr virus infection, HIV infection)
Connective tissue diseases (Sjögren syndrome, rheumatoid arthritis, systemic lupus erythematosus)
Immune deficiency diseases (HIV infection, heritable immunodeficiency syndromes)
Autoimmune diseases (Hashimoto thyroiditis, myasthenia gravis, pernicious anemia)
Drug- or toxin-related lung injury
Lymphoproliferative disorders (multicentric Castleman disease, idiopathic plasmacytic lymphoadenopathy with hypergammaglobulinemia, IgG4-related disease)

Modified from Leslie K, Colby T, Swensen S: Anatomic distribution and histopathologic patterns in interstitial lung disease. In: Schwarz M, King TJ, eds. *Interstitial Lung Disease*. Hamilton, ON: BC Decker; 2002:31–50.

Clinical Course

The clinical outcome and response to therapy for patients with the LIP pattern is largely dependant on whether systemic disease is present. In the idiopathic form, an accurate prognosis has not been forthcoming, although in the series reported by Cha and coworkers, three patients survived more than 10 years.[104] In symptomatic patients, corticosteroid administration may result in significant benefit,[105] lending further support to LIP's being an immunologic disease, rather than a neoplastic one, in most instances. When honeycomb cysts, clubbing, or cor pulmonale are present, the prognosis is less favorable, with as many as one third of patients succumbing to the disease.[105,114] Infection is a common complication, especially when LIP is associated with dysproteinemia.[105,106,125]

Chronic Manifestations of Systemic Collagen Vascular Disease

Systemic CVDs play an extremely important role in the etiology of ILDs. Knowledge of rheumatic ILD is derived mainly from retrospective studies, typically including small numbers of patients. Because of differences in patient populations reported and in the rheumatic disease severity (and duration) at the time of study, many important questions remain concerning the frequency, pathogenesis, natural history, clinical relevance, and prognosis of ILD occurring in the rheumatic diseases. It is estimated that ILD in CVD is responsible for 1600 deaths annually in the United States, accounting for roughly 25% of all ILD deaths and 2% of all deaths from respiratory causes.[126] Not suprisingly, most interstitial pneumonia patterns raise CVD as a consideration in the differential diagnosis. On the other hand, certain CVDs are associated with reasonably reproducible findings in the lung.[2] Table 7-3 summarizes the different patterns of inflammatory lung disease that have been described as lung manifestations of the known connective tissue diseases. The five rheumatic diseases that are more commonly associated with ILD are (1) rheumatoid arthritis (RA), (2) progressive systemic sclerosis (PSS), (3) systemic lupus erythematosus (SLE), (4) polymyositis-dermatomyositis (PM-DM), and (5) Sjögren syndrome. The estimated frequency of lung involvement and the patterns produced are presented in Table 7-4. This section is restricted to the more chronic manifestations of these diseases. Acute lung manifestations of the rheumatic diseases are described in Chapter 5.

Rheumatoid Arthritis

RA is a chronic systemic disease that produces symmetrical arthritis and occurs more commonly in women than in men. ILD was not recognized as a manifestation of RA until 1948,[138] possibly because lung manifestations of the disease are difficult to recognize on purely clinical grounds. Today, with the use of pulmonary function testing, bronchoalveolar lavage, and CT imaging, significant lung disease is identified in 14% of patients who meet the American College of Rheumatology (formerly the American Rheumatism Association) criteria for RA; subclinical disease is seen in as many as 44%.[139] Interestingly, men are three times more likely to develop ILD with RA than are women.[25] Clinically significant ILD in RA is associated with increased morbidity and mortality.[25]

Clinical Presentation

Diffuse lung disease in RA typically is noted in patients with diagnosed RA, but rarely, ILD may precede articular manifestations.[140,141] The clinical presentation is dominated by shortness of breath and cough. Adults are more commonly affected than children,[142] and despite a higher incidence of RA in women, men with long-standing rheumatoid disease and subcutaneous nodules seem to develop lung manifestations more often.[140] Physical examination may reveal bibasilar inspiratory crackles, digital clubbing, and evidence of cor pulmonale, the last due to pulmonary hypertension arising as a result of hypoxic vasoconstriction.[25,140] When fibrosis and honeycomb remodeling accompany diffuse lung disease in RA, UIP enters into the differential diagnosis. Affected patients often are younger than those with idiopathic UIP. Cigarette smoking has been reported to be an independent predictor of lung disease in persons with RA.[143]

Radiologic Findings

Several radiologic manifestations are described in RA, including reticular opacities with or without honeycombing, airway-associated abnormalities (bronchiectasis, nodules, centrilobular branching lines), and parenchymal opacities.[144] When ground-glass infiltrates and reticular opacities are present, there is a predilection for involving the bases and lung periphery. High-resolution CT findings include ground-glass attenuation with mixed alveolar and interstitial infiltrates. As lung disease advances, dense reticular and nodular opacities appear, and honeycomb lung may be seen in late stages of the disease.[144,145]

Histopathologic Findings

Despite the seemingly nonspecific nature of the histopathologic manifestations of RA, a few key elements emerge on review of many well-documented cases of RA-associated ILD. Chronic inflammation, in

Table 7-3. Lung Manifestations of the Collagen Vascular Diseases

Manifestation	RA	SLE	PSS	PM-DM	MCTD	SS	AS
Pleural inflammation, fibrosis, effusions	X	X	X	X	X	X	X
Airway disease							
Inflammation (bronchiolitis)	X	X		X	X	X	
Constrictive bronchiolitis	X				X		
Bronchiectasis	X				X		
Follicular bronchiolitis	X	X			X	X	
Interstitial disease							
Acute (DAD), with or without hemorrhage	X	X	X	X	X		
Subacute/organizing (OP pattern)	X	X	X	X	X	X	
Subacute cellular	X	X	X	X	X		
Chronic cellular and fibrotic	X	X	X	X	X	X	
Eosinophilic infiltrates	X				X		
Granulomatous interstitial pneumonia	X	X			X		
Vascular diseases; hypertension/vasculitis	X	X	X	X	X	X	
Parenchymal nodules	X						
Apical fibrobullous disease	X		X		X		
Lymphoid proliferation (reactive, neoplastic)	X		X		X		

AS, ankylosing spondylitis; DAD, diffuse alveolar damage; MCTD, mixed connective tissue disease; OP, organizing pneumonia; PM-DM, polymyositis-dermatomyositis; PSS, progressive systemic sclerosis; RA, rheumatoid arthritis; SLE, systemic lupus erythematosus; SS, Sjögren syndrome.
Modified from Colby TV, Lombard C, Yousem SA, et al: Atlas of pulmonary surgical pathology. In: Bordin G, ed. *Atlases in Diagnostic Surgical Pathology.* Philadelphia: WB Saunders; 1991:380; and Travis WD, Colby T, Koss M, et al: Non-neoplastic disorders of the lower respiratory tract. In: King DW, ed: *Atlases of Nontumor Pathology.* Washington, DC: Armed Forces Institute of Pathology: 2002.

Table 7-4. Pulmonary Manifestations of the Rheumatic Diseases

Disease	Estimated Frequency	Type of ILD	Anatomic Involvement/Dominant Finding
Rheumatoid arthritis (RA)[127]	20%	UIP/NSIP >> OP	Pleuritis > bronchiolitis > ILD > RA nodule
Progressive systemic sclerosis[128,129]	40%	NSIP >> OP > UIP > DAD	ILD > aspiration > PHT
Systemic lupus erythematosus[130,131]	<10%	DAD > DAH > OP > UIP/NSIP	Pleuritis > infection > ILD > PHT
Polymyositis-dermatomyositis[132]	10–35%*	NSIP > DAD > OP > UIP	Aspiration > ILD
Sjögren syndrome[133–135]	25%	NSIP > OP > UIP > LIP	Bronchiolitis > ILD
Mixed connective tissue disease[136]	40%	UIP/NSIP > OP > DAD > DAH	ILD > pleuritis > PHT > aspiration

*75% when patient is seropositive for Jo-1.[137]
DAD, diffuse alveolar damage; DAH, diffuse alveolar hemorrhage; DIP, desquamative interstitial pneumonia; ILD, interstitial lung disease; LIP, lymphocytic interstitial pneumonia; NSIP, nonspecific interstitial pneumonia; OP, organizing pneumonia; PHT, pulmonary hypertension; UIP, usual interstitial pneumonia.

the form of lymphocyte aggregates and germinal centers, is typical, although not unique (Fig. 7-34) Most of the lymphoid aggregations are present around the terminal airways ("follicular bronchiolitis" when lymphoid germinal centers are prominent) (Fig. 7-35), but lymphoid follicles may also present in the pleura. In fact, the presence of chronic pleuritis should always raise RA as a consideration in the differential diagnosis. Areas of subacute lung injury, attended by reactive type II cells and air space organization (Fig. 7-36), can be seen with cellular interstitial pneumonia (Fig. 7-37) and variable interstitial fibrosis (Fig. 7-38). This combination of subacute and chronic inflammatory reactions haphazardly involving the same lung biopsy, including the pleura, should raise the possibility of RA lung disease. When fibrosis is prominent, it is often difficult to classify as UIP or NSIP. That may be one of the reasons for the variable reported incidence of these two patterns of fibrosis in the disease. Fibroblastic foci are usually less prominent, and normal lung may be absent. Vasculitis (including capillaritis) and even

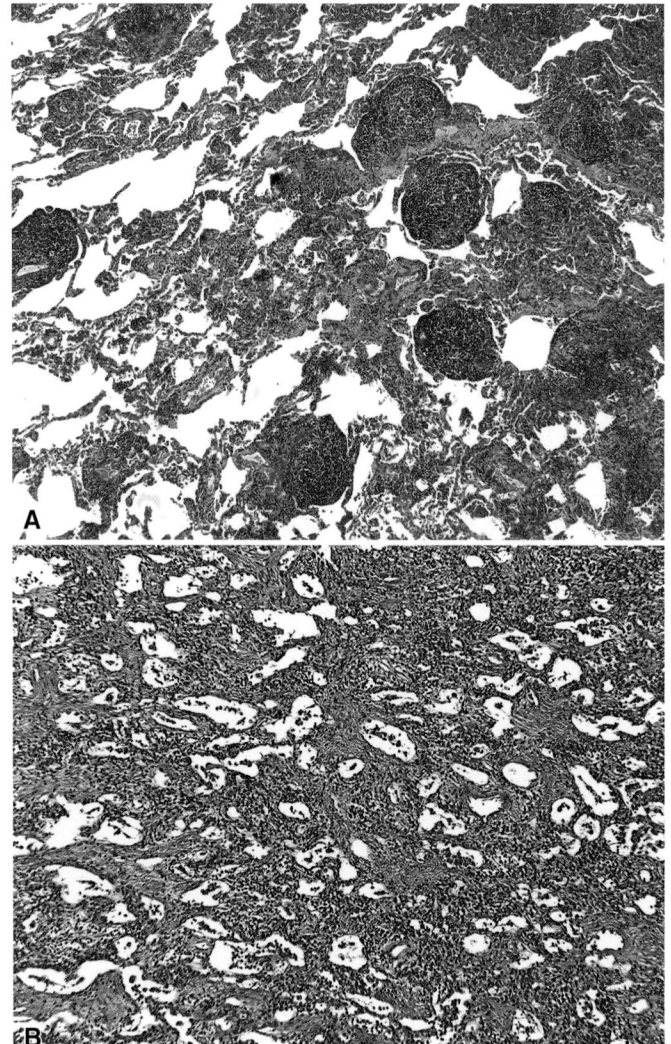

Figure 7-34. Rheumatoid arthritis (RA) lung disease. **A,** Chronic inflammation typically manifests in RA lung as lymphoid aggregates and follicular lymphoid germinal centers. **B,** A variably cellular chronic interstitial infiltrate rich in plasma cells and lymphocytes is typical.

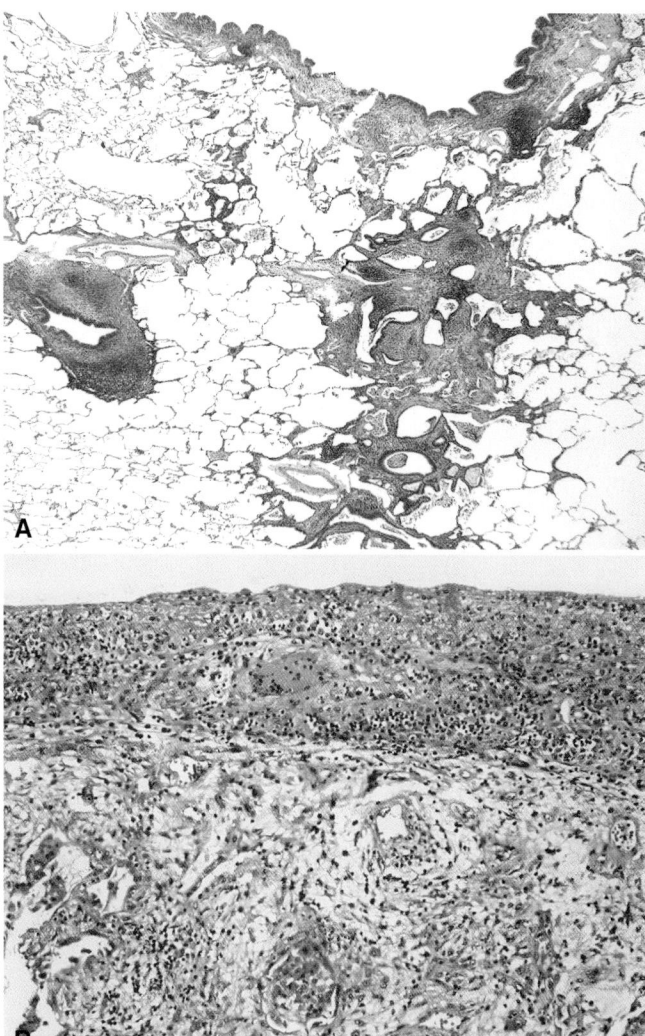

Figure 7-35. Rheumatoid arthritis (RA) lung disease. Most of the lymphoid aggregations in RA (**A**) are present around the terminal airways ("follicular bronchiolitis" when lymphoid germinal centers are prominent), but lymphoid follicles may also be present in the pleura. In fact, the presence of chronic pleuritis (**B**) should always raise the possibility of RA in the differential diagnosis.

pulmonary hemorrhage have been described as manifestations of RA lung. When silicosis occurs with RA, the resulting disease is referred to as *Caplan syndrome.* Rheumatoid nodules can occur in the lung and pleura and must be distinguished from granulomatous infection or Wegener granulomatosis. Intrapulmonary lymph nodes may become prominent in RA and typically show reactive lymphoid hyperplasia when subjected to biopsy.

Differential Diagnosis
RA lung manifestations are frequently confused with the idiopathic interstitial pneumonias (COP, NSIP, or even UIP), especially when the lung disease precedes the systemic disease. When patients with RA develop pulmonary symptoms, biopsies are usually performed only when superimposed lung infections or drug reactions are suspected clinically. Surgical lung biopsy in this context can be extremely difficult to interpret, given significant overlap in the morphologic patterns of drug reactions, low-grade infection, and the systemic CVD itself.

Clinical Course
As with other connective tissue diseases, therapeutic strategies in RA have focused on immunosuppression.[146] Although the reported survival significance of RA-ILD varies, a majority of published papers indicate

better survival rates for patients with RA-ILD than for those with UIP/IPF.[147] Needless to say, the development of pulmonary fibrosis with a UIP pattern has a significant negative impact on survival.[141,143,148,149]

Progressive Systemic Sclerosis

PSS is a relatively rare systemic autoimmune disease, with cutaneous manifestations (dermal sclerosis) frequently accompanied by Raynaud phenomenon. Pulmonary involvement (mainly ILD) occurs more commonly in patients with PSS than in those with any other connective tissue disease,[128,150] with lung disease ranking fourth in frequency (after skin, peripheral vascular, and esophageal manifestations) in the disease, but is the primary cause of death in PSS.[151] As in RA, lung involvement in PSS is associated with increased morbidity and mortality.[151]

Clinical Presentation
Chronic exertional dyspnea is the most common presentation, followed in frequency by chronic cough. Bibasilar inspiratory crackles are present in two thirds of patients.[128,152] Digital clubbing may be present but is

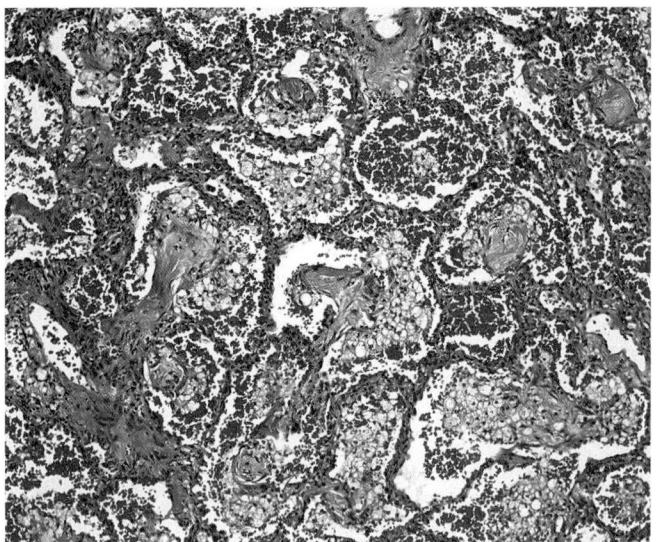

Figure 7-36. Rheumatoid arthritis (RA) lung disease. Areas of subacute lung injury, attended by reactive type II cells and air space organization, can be seen. Fresh hemorrhage, probably related to the biopsy procedure, also is evident.

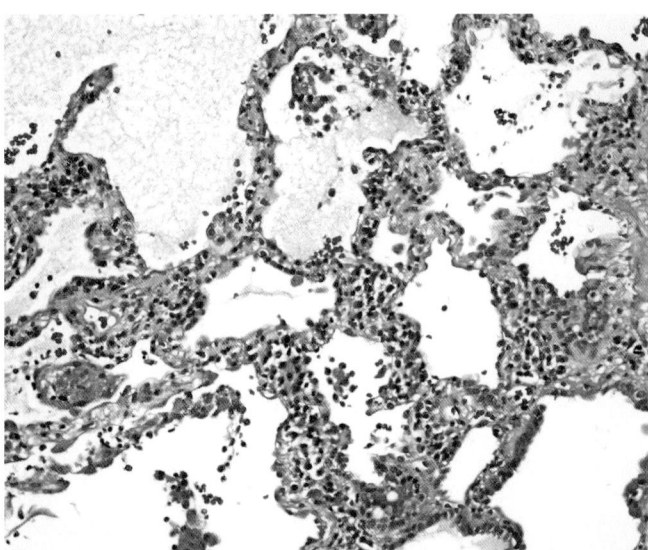

Figure 7-37. Rheumatoid arthritis (RA) lung disease. The cellular interstitial pneumonia of RA may be attended by diffuse reactive type II cell hyperplasia, but this finding is not particularly diagnostic absent other features more characteristic of RA (lymphoid germinal centers, follicular bronchiolitis, pleuritis, rheumatoid nodules).

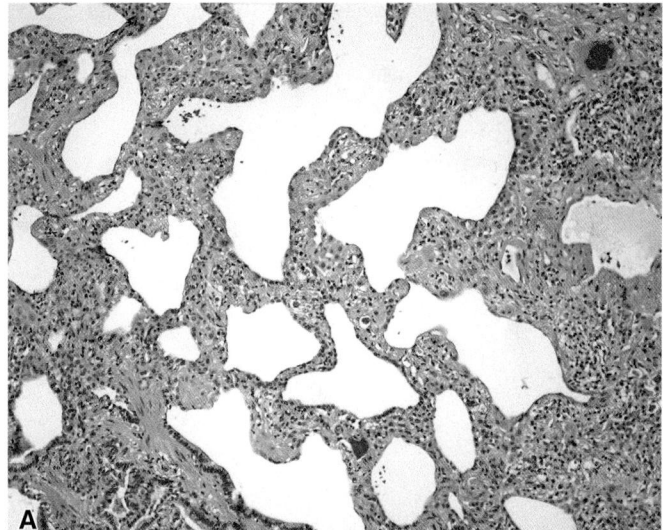

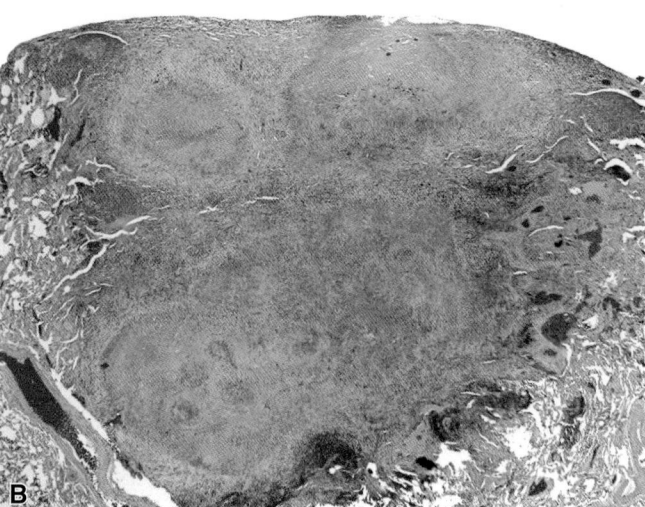

Figure 7-38. Rheumatoid arthritis (RA) lung disease. **A,** Variable interstitial fibrosis is typical and often resembles the fibrotic form of nonspecific interstitial pneumonia. **B,** Typical rheumatoid nodules may occur in RA lung and must be distinguished from lesions seen with infection and in Wegener granulomatosis.

uncommon. Pulmonary fibrosis and cor pulmonale may develop eventually.[153] As in other CVDs, lung involvement can precede the development of diagnostic systemic manifestations.[128,154]

Radiologic Findings

Bibasilar interstitial infiltrates with relative sparing of the upper lung zones are typical radiologic features.[155,156] Loss of lung volume, honeycomb cysts, and findings consistent with pulmonary hypertension may also be seen. Mixed reticular and nodular infiltrates are common.[155,156] Pleural effusion and pleural thickening may occur as minor findings.

Histopathologic Findings

The pulmonary manifestations of PSS can be quite characteristic. The interstitial fibrosis of PSS is paucicellular and diffuse, with preservation of underlying lung architecture (Fig. 7-39). This distinctive

"collagenization" of the lung interstitium has been confused with the pattern of lung fibrosis seen in idiopathic UIP.[153] The lack of so-called "temporal heterogeneity" (see the earlier section, "Usual Interstitial Pneumonia") is a useful finding and helps exclude UIP (of IPF) from the differential diagnosis. Pulmonary hypertensive changes (Fig. 7-40) may be present and merit careful attention because this is a major cause of death in patients with scleroderma and lung disease.[157] Because patients with PSS can also develop esophageal motility problems, subclinical chronic aspiration should be carefully excluded as a comorbid disease process.[158,159]

Clinical Course

The mean survival time for patients with scleroderma is 12 years from the time of diagnosis; pulmonary disease has emerged as the major cause of death.[160] Pulmonary function status at presentation is a reasonable predictor of survival; high-dose immunosuppressive therapy, typically in combination with a cytotoxic agent, seems to benefit those patients with severe manifestations.[161]

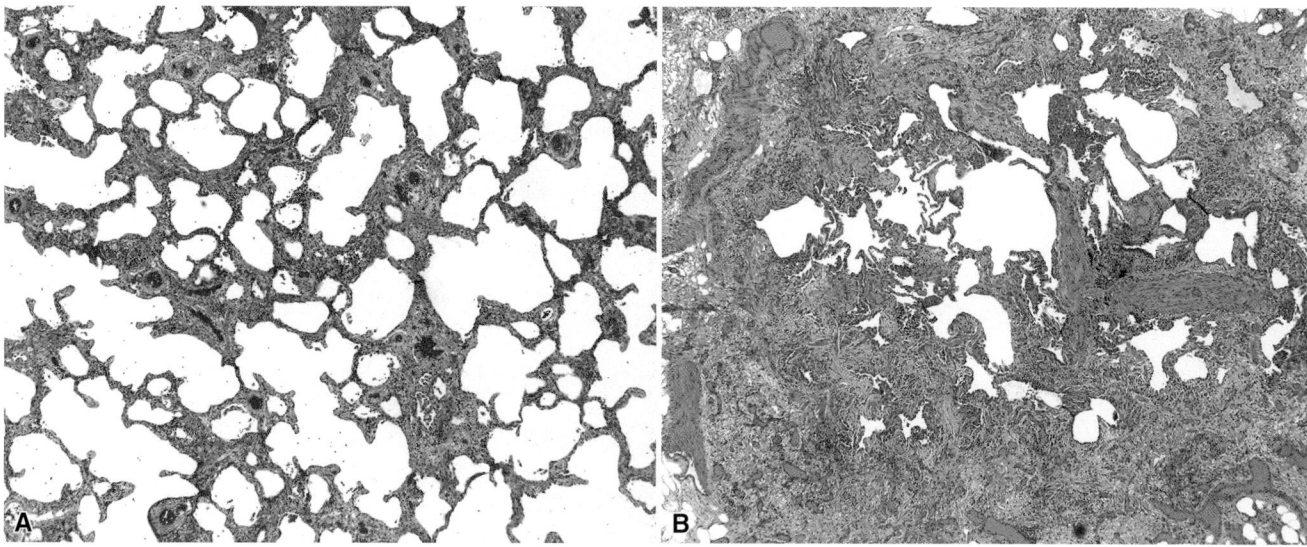

Figure 7-39. Progressive systemic sclerosis (PSS). **A,** The interstitial fibrosis of PSS is typically paucicellular and diffuse, with preservation of underlying lung architecture. **B,** When fibrosis is more advanced, distinction from usual interstitial pneumonia (of idiopathic pulmonary fibrosis) may be difficult on morphologic grounds.

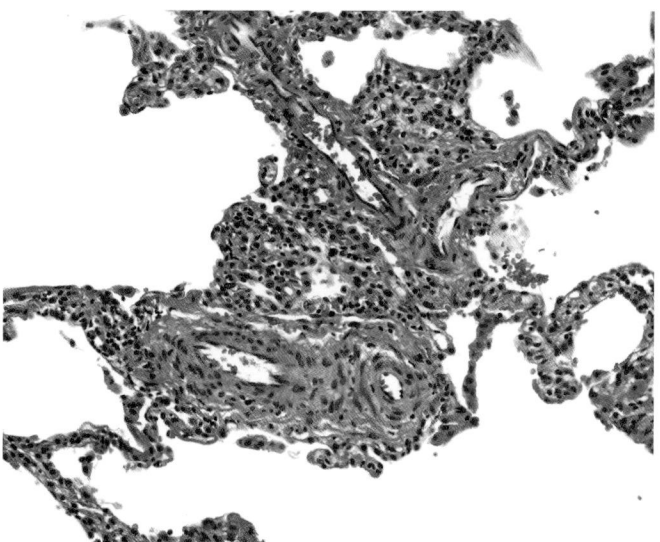

Figure 7-40. Progressive systemic sclerosis. Pulmonary hypertensive changes may be present and deserve careful attention, since this is a major cause of mortality in scleroderma patients with lung disease.

Systemic Lupus Erythematosus

SLE is a chronic systemic autoimmune disorder characterized by arthropathy, mucocutaneous manifestations, renal disease, and serositis.[162] The lung may be the major site of involvement in SLE, ranging from acute lupus pneumonitis on one end of the spectrum to fibrotic forms of NSIP on the other.[130,163,164] Acute lung injury and pulmonary hemorrhage are more commonly associated with SLE than with other systemic connective tissue diseases,[130,165] but hemoptysis occurs only in little more than one half of the affected patients.[166,167]

Clinical Presentation

SLE rivals PSS as the leader in pleuropulmonary manifestations in CVD.[131,163,168,169] The spectrum of lung disease in SLE is quite broad[130,164,165,170] and includes pleuritis (Fig. 7-41), acute lupus pneumonitis (Fig. 7-42), NSIP with fibrosis (Fig. 7-43), and diffuse alveolar hemorrhage (Fig. 7-44).

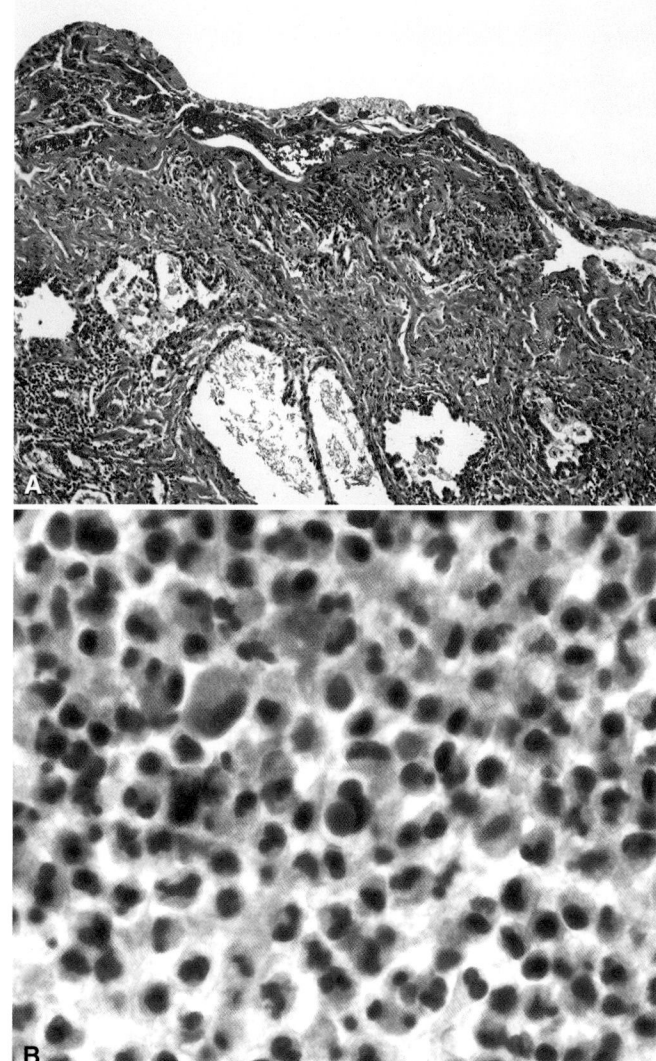

Figure 7-41. Systemic lupus erythematosus (SLE). The spectrum of lung disease in SLE is quite broad and includes pleuritis (**A**), sometimes accompanied by so-called "lupus erythematosis bodies" or simply, "LE bodies" (**B**, *center*).

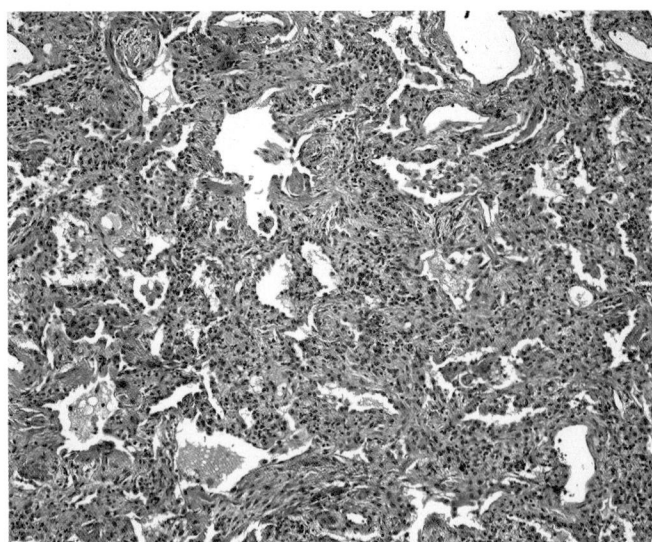

Figure 7-42. Systemic lupus erythematosus (SLE). Acute lupus pneumonitis is the most dramatic manifestation of SLE lung disease and is a form of acute lung injury.

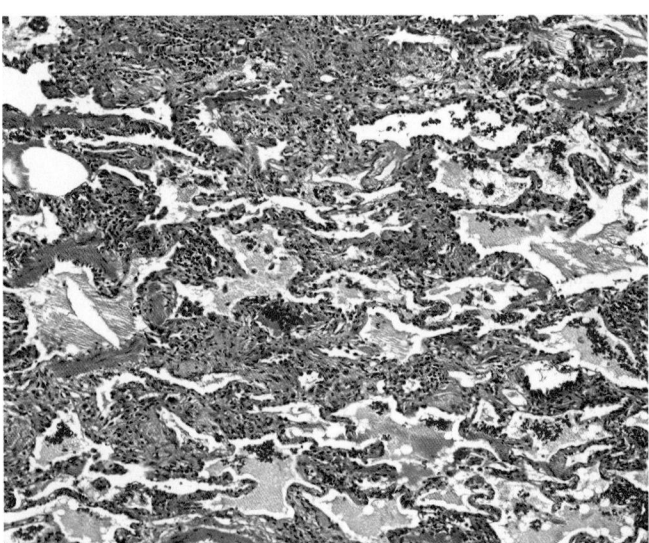

Figure 7-43. Systemic lupus erythematosus (SLE). The second most common manifestation of SLE lung disease is nonspecific interstitial pneumonia pattern cellular interstitial pneumonia with variable interstitial fibrosis.

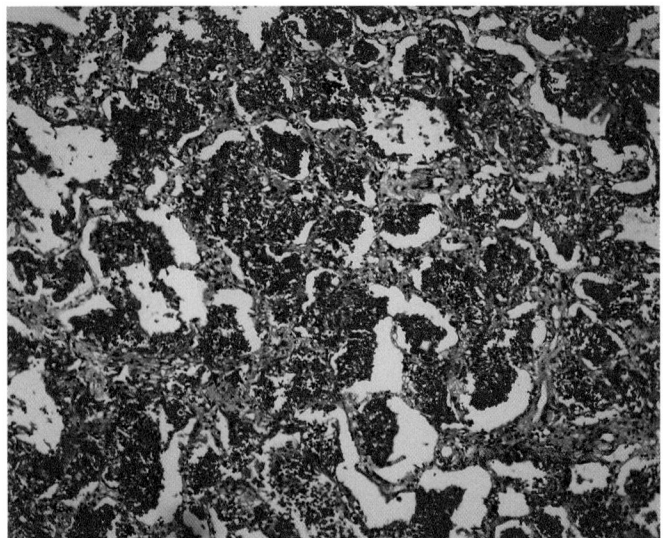

Figure 7-44. Systemic lupus erythematosus (SLE). Diffuse alveolar hemorrhage may occur in SLE, often without hemoptysis. In this specimen, prominent air space fibrin and blood are accompanied by siderophages and marked reactive type II cell hyperplasia. An interstitial pneumonia is also evident in the widened alveolar walls.

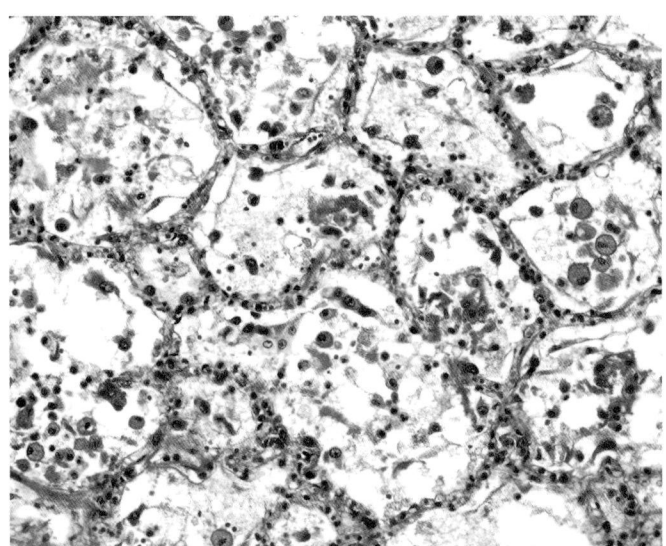

Figure 7-45. Systemic lupus erythematosus. At high magnification the acute lung injury of acute lupus pneumonitis is characterized by alveolitis with variable interstitial inflammation and edema.

Constrictive small-airway disease, pulmonary arterial hypertension, and pulmonary embolism can also occur as rare manifestations. Patients with lung disease often have high serum ANA or RF titers.

Radiologic Findings

The radiologic findings are similar to those in other connective tissue diseases: variable ground-glass attenuation, pleural thickening, pleural and pericardial effusions, and linear parenchymal opacities.[130,171–174] Acute pneumonitis can produce more extensive changes, but, rarely, chest radiography and high-resolution CT may show normal findings.[175]

Histopathologic Findings

Two general categories of pulmonary disease are described in SLE. The first is acute lupus pneumonitis (ALP). ALP is characterized by alveolitis with variable interstitial inflammation and edema (Fig. 7-45). Siderophages and capillaritis occur to a variable degree (Fig.

7-46). Pleuritis is commonly present. The second category of disease includes cellular interstitial pneumonia (lymphocytes and plasma cells) with variable interstitial fibrosis (Fig. 7-47). This latter NSIP pattern is associated with a better prognosis than that for ALP. When pulmonary hemorrhage occurs, the prognosis may be adversely affected. One dramatic but fortunately rare complication of SLE is the occurrence of lung infarction related to the lupus anticoagulant.[176–178] Whenever lung infarction is encountered in a young, otherwise healthy patient, this possibility should be considered (even if the patient does not have evident SLE).

Clinical Course

Systemic corticosteroid therapy may be effective in SLE-associated lung disease, although sometimes the addition of a cytotoxic agent (e.g., cyclophosphamide, azathioprine) may be required.[179] Acute lupus

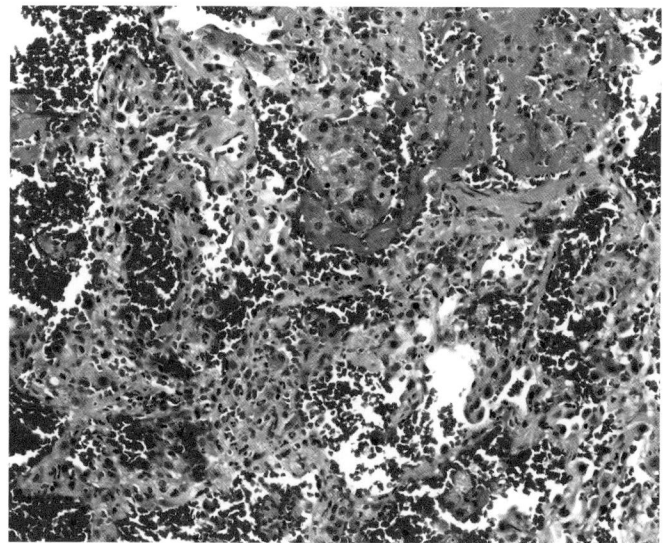

Figure 7-46. Systemic lupus erythematosus (SLE). Siderophages and capillaritis may be present in the diffuse alveolar hemorrhage of SLE.

pneumonitis carries a reported high mortality rate in some series.[168] More chronic forms of diffuse lung disease in SLE have a relatively good prognosis and response to therapy.[180]

Polymyositis-Dermatomyositis

Polymyositis and dermatomyositis (PM-DM) are inflammatory disorders of the skeletal muscle and dermis. Five groups of primary or secondary disease are recognized, including childhood forms and overlap syndromes.[181,182] Pulmonary complications in PM-DM occur less commonly than in other systemic connective tissue diseases, but in a percentage of patients, the pulmonary manifestations can be quite dramatic.[183]

Clinical Presentation

Although most patients with PM-DM develop lung manifestations after the clinical diagnosis has been established, occasionally lung disease can precede the clinical and serologic diagnosis by months or even years.[184] Onset of pulmonary symptoms may occur at any age, with a mean occurrence in the sixth decade.[150,184,185] Women are more commonly affected than men. Digital clubbing is rare. In contrast with most other systemic connective tissue diseases (with the exception of SLE), patients with PM-DM can present with acute lung disease, typically manifesting as rapidly progressive DAD.[183,185] Importantly, both acute aspiration pneumonitis secondary to underlying respiratory muscle weakness and bronchopneumonia occurring in the setting of immunosuppressive therapy are more common in PM-DM than is chronic diffuse lung disease.[186,187]

Radiologic Findings

As with other CVDs manifesting in the lung, radiologic abnormalities in PM-DM predominantly affect the lung bases.[185] Ikezoe and colleagues reviewed the high-resolution CT findings in 23 of 25 patients with PM-DM who had high-resolution CT abnormalities.[188] These researchers identified ground-glass opacities in 92%, linear opacities in 92%, irregular interfaces in 88%, air space consolidation in 52%, parenchymal micronodules in 28%, and honeycombing in 16% of the cases. The most dramatic radiologic finding associated with PM-DM is the rapid onset of air space consolidation associated with the development of DAD.[184,185]

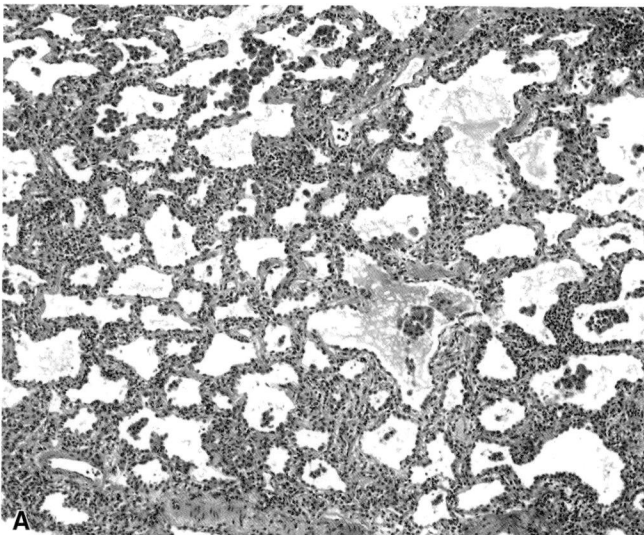

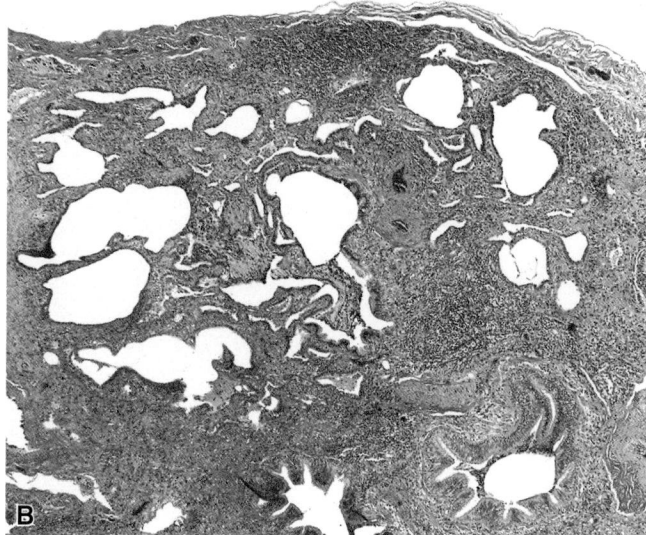

Figure 7-47. Systemic lupus erythematosus (SLE). The cellular interstitial pneumonia of SLE lung is often accompanied by subacute lung injury with reactive type II cells and variable amounts of air space fibrin (**A**). Some diffuse fibrosis typically is present in the nonspecific interstitial pneumonia manifestation of lupus, but advanced pulmonary fibrosis may occur in SLE, with chronic pleuritis (**B**).

Histopathologic Findings

The most frequent lung manifestation of PM-DM is a cellular interstitial pneumonia (Fig. 7-48) with some fibrosis,[184,185] indistinguishable from nonspecific interstitial pneumonia (see the later section, "Idiopathic Interstitial Pneumonias"). The next most common pattern is DAD (Fig. 7-49). The fibrosis associated with PM-DM is distinguishable from that of idiopathic UIP based on a relative lack of peripheral accentuation (Fig. 7-50) and absence of the typical transitions from older lung fibrosis to normal lung through fibroblastic foci. Pleuritis, inflammatory small-airway disease, and pulmonary hypertension are unusual findings; their occurrence should suggest a manifestation of a different connective tissue disease.

Sjögren Syndrome

Sjögren syndrome is an immune-mediated exocrinopathy characterized by lymphocytic infiltration of the salivary glands, with resulting dry mouth and dry eyes.[189] Lung involvement is common and is

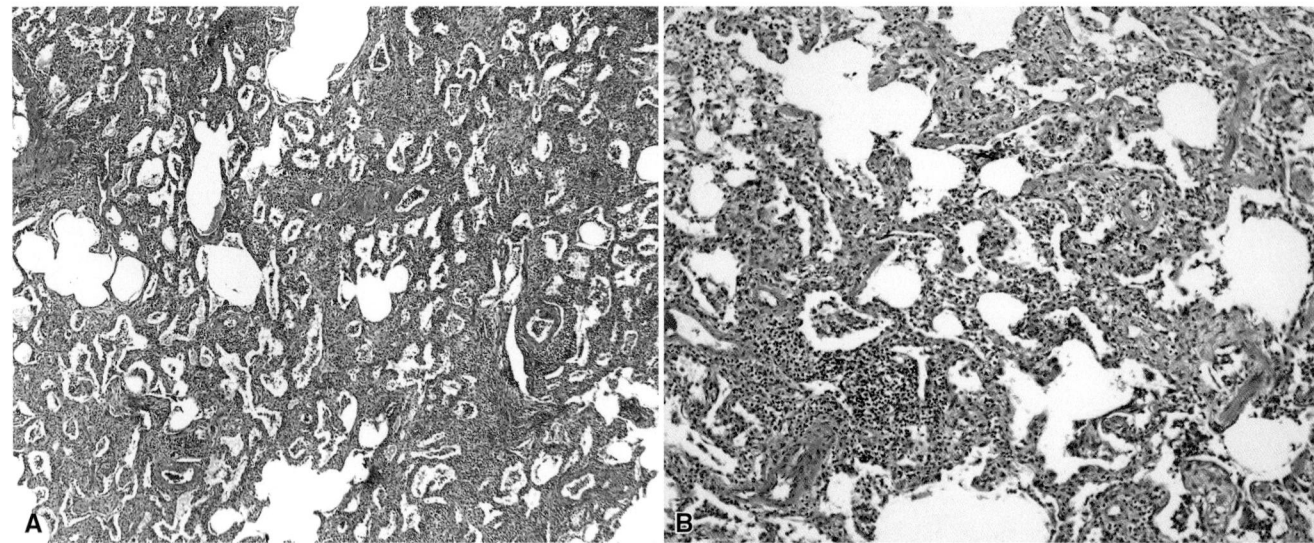

Figure 7-48. Polymyositis-dermatomyositis (PD-DM). **A** and **B,** The most frequent lung manifestation of PM-DM is a cellular interstitial pneumonia with some fibrosis, indistinguishable from cellular or fibrotic forms of nonspecific interstitial pneumonia.

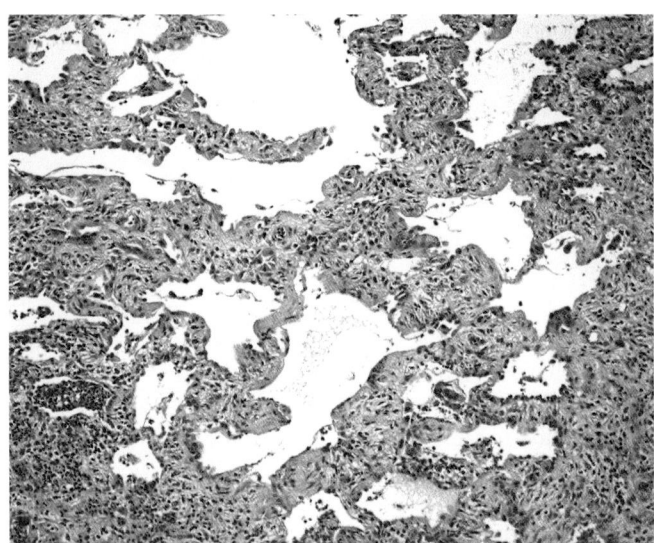

Figure 7-49. Polymyositis-dermatomyositis (PD-DM). PM-DM–associated diffuse alveolar damage may precede the systemic and serologic manifestations of the disease by a year or more. Note the prominent hyaline membranes. Without an explanation for this acute lung disease, idiopathic "acute interstitial pneumonia" may be the clinical diagnosis until the systemic disease manifests itself.

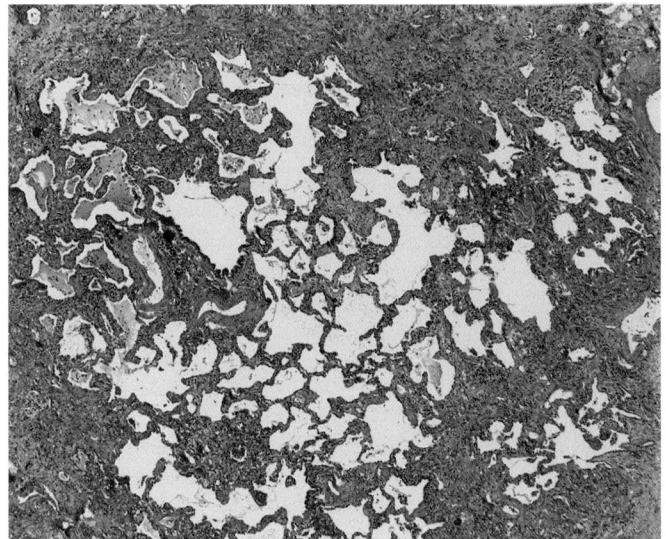

Figure 7-50. Polymyositis-dermatomyositis (PD-DM). The fibrosis associated with PM-DM may be indistinguishable from that of idiopathic usual interstitial pneumonia in limited samples. In general, there is a relative lack of peripheral accentuation and absence of the typical transitions from older lung fibrosis to normal lung through fibroblastic foci.

similar to that in other CVDs manifesting in the lung.[107,190,191] Sjögren syndrome can occur as a primary connective tissue disease or as a complication associated with other connective tissue diseases (occurrence rates for the two forms are approximately equal).[189] In both primary and secondary forms, the consistent pathologic manifestation is that of lymphoid accumulation in a bronchiolocentric distribution and the NSIP/LIP pattern of cellular interstitial pneumonia.

Clinical Presentation

Women are more commonly affected with lung disease in Sjögren syndrome than men; the most frequent presenting complaint is cough and dyspnea.[107,190] Positive results on rheumatoid factor and ANA assays are expected findings, as well as positive reactions to extractable nuclear antigens (anti-SSA, anti-SSB).[192] These latter serologic tests are specific for the primary form of the disease.[193]

Radiologic Findings

Mixed alveolar and interstitial infiltrates are characteristic in Sjögren syndrome; they usually have a finely reticular or nodular pattern.[191,194] The occurrence of pleural effusion or hilar/mediastinal adenopathy in patients with Sjögren syndrome should raise concern for lymphoma.[195]

Histopathologic Findings

The histopathologic spectrum of pulmonary Sjögren syndrome includes bronchiolitis (Fig. 7-51) with or without air space organization, follicular lymphoid hyperplasia along airways (Fig. 7-52), diffuse NSIP or LIP pattern interstitial inflammation (Fig. 7-53), and rarely, interstitial fibrosis (Fig. 7-54), the last raising concern for an inflammatory version of UIP. Small, non-necrotizing granulomas, resembling those of hypersensitivity pneumonitis, are frequently identified in the

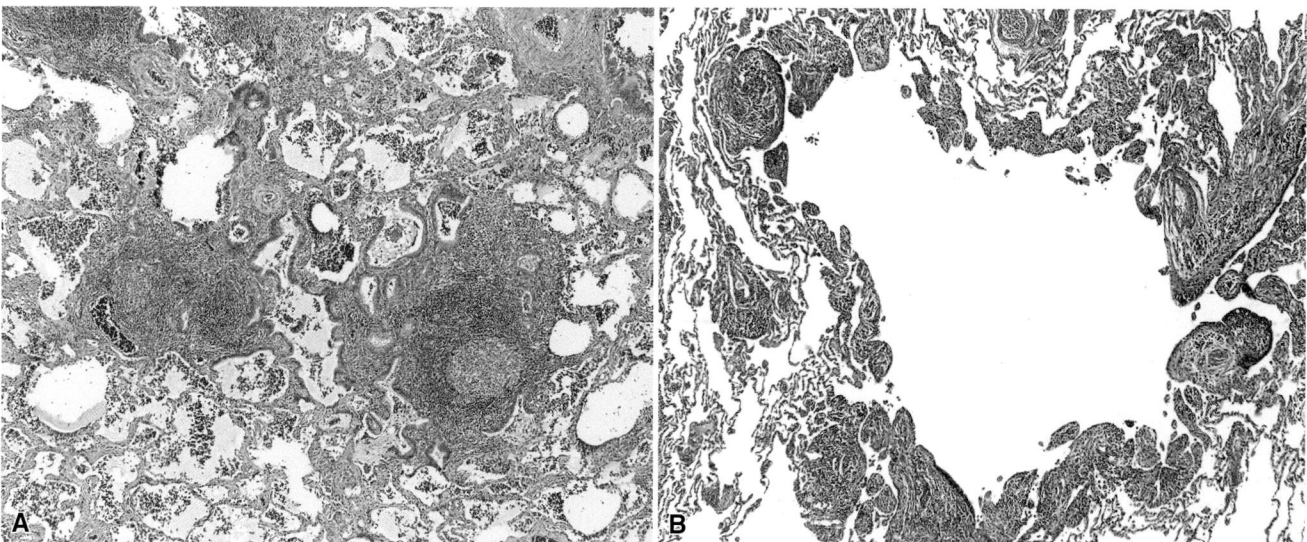

Figure 7-51. Sjögren syndrome (SS). **A,** The histopathologic spectrum of pulmonary SS includes bronchiolitis as the dominant and consistent feature. **B,** Cysts may occur in SS and may be seen both radiologically and in surgical biopsy specimens.

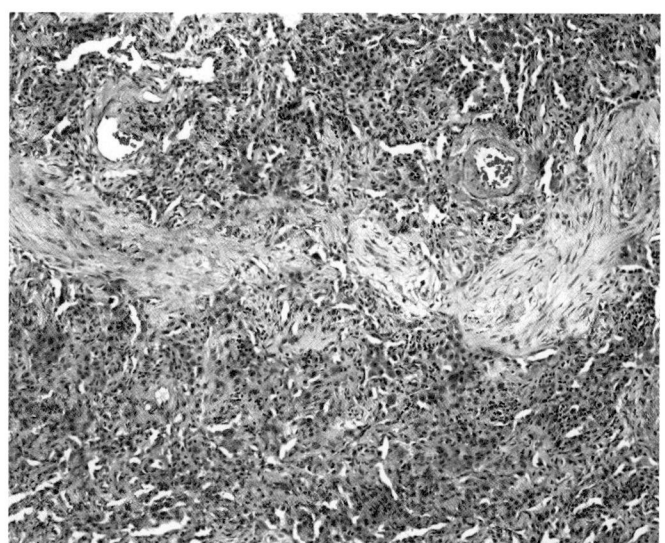

Figure 7-52. Sjögren syndrome (SS). Terminal airway and alveolar space organization commonly accompany the bronchiolitis and cellular interstitial pneumonia of SS.

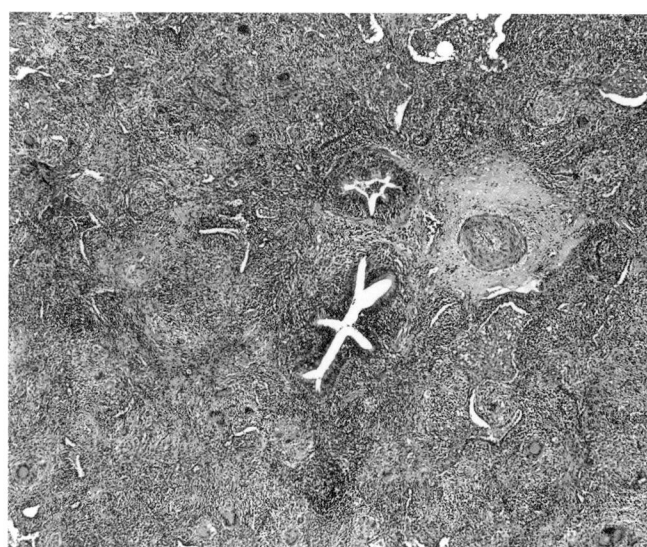

Figure 7-53. Sjögren syndrome (SS). Nonspecific interstitial pneumonia or lymphoid interstitial pneumonia pattern of interstitial inflammation in SS lung must be distinguished from low-grade lymphoproliferative disease when lymphocytes are dense and dominant. Note the numerous multinucleate giant cells and poorly formed granulomas in this specimen. Prominent arteriopathic changes with marked adventitial fibrosis can be seen in the pulmonary artery at *center right*.

interstitium (Fig. 7-55).[196] In some cases, more prominent granulomatous inflammation can be seen, especially in association with the LIP pattern of cellular infiltration. Patients with Sjögren syndrome are at risk of developing lymphoid hyperplasia and lymphoproliferative diseases; this predilection should be kept in mind in evaluating the lung biopsy in this setting.

Diffuse Eosinophilic Lung Disease (Pulmonary Eosinophilia)

Several conditions have been described in which the lungs become infiltrated by eosinophils.[197,198] An etiologic and clinical classification of the "eosinophil-rich lung diseases" is presented in Box 7-10. Asthma and hypersensitivity play important roles in a number of these. Eosinophilic lung diseases are discussed together here, but in practice, only acute onset of diffuse lung injury accompanied by extravascular eosinophils is relatively predictable in terms of clinical behavior and responsiveness to therapy (i.e., corticosteroids). When

pulmonary eosinophilia presents as a chronic condition, the behavior seems to be less predictable. The term *chronic eosinophilic pneumonia* has been applied in such cases, even though the histopathologic findings in biopsy specimens may not reflect this longer evolution with observable fibrosis or structural remodeling.

Clinical Features

Patients with the "chronic" form of eosinophilic pneumonia often exhibit a typical clinical syndrome and radiographic appearance.[199] The condition frequently affects middle-aged women, and asthma is present in approximately one fourth of the cases. Nasal symptoms occur in roughly one third of affected individuals. The disease typically presents with severe systemic symptoms, including fever, sweats, weight loss, cough, and dyspnea. Peripheral blood eosinophilia can often be identified, but this may be transient or absent altogether.

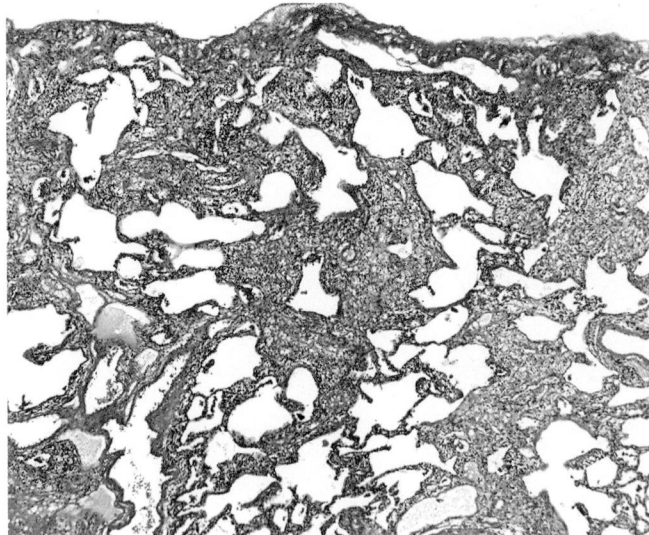

Figure 7-54. Sjögren syndrome (SS). Advanced interstitial fibrosis occurs rarely in SS lung disease and may raise concern for an inflammatory version of usual interstitial pneumonia. Note the absence of transitions to normal lung and absence of peripheral accentuation here.

Radiologic Findings

Chronic eosinophilic pneumonia presents the most consistent radiologic pattern, with bilateral, poorly defined, subpleural air space consolidation on chest radiographs, most commonly distributed at the lung apices and in the axillary region. One unifying concept for the diffuse forms of eosinophilic lung disease is the "migratory" infiltrate. These infiltrates may disappear spontaneously and recur in the same position or elsewhere. In the most extreme cases, the infiltrates are densest in the periphery of the lung and spare the central region. This phenomenon has been referred to as the *photographic negative of pulmonary edema*.[199] CT scans detect the peripheral location of infiltrates even when this distribution is not apparent on the chest radiograph.[200] Once the characteristic presentation is recognized, corticosteroid administration can lead to dramatic improvement in patients with some forms

Box 7-10. Etiologic and Clinical Classification of Eosinophilic Pneumonia

Idiopathic (Unknown Cause) Eosinophilic Pneumonia
Chronic eosinophilic pneumonia
Acute eosinophilic pneumonia
Simple eosinophilic pneumonia (Loeffler syndrome)
Incidental eosinophilic pneumonia

Secondary Eosinophilic Pneumonia
Infection
  Parasitic
    Tropical eosinophilic pneumonia
    Ascaris lumbricoides, Toxicara canis, filariae
    Dirofilaria
  Fungal
    Aspergillus
Drug-induced
  Antibiotics
  Cytotoxic drugs
  Anti-inflammatory agents
  L-Tryptophan
Immunologic or systemic diseases
  Allergic bronchopulmonary fungal disease
  Asthma
  Collagen vascular disease
  Churg-Strauss syndrome
  HIV infection
  Malignancy
  Hypereosinophilic syndrome
Smoking-induced

Modified from Travis WD, Colby T, Koss M, et al: Non-neoplastic disorders of the lower respiratory tract. In: King DW, ed: *Atlases of Nontumor Pathology.* Washington, DC: Armed Forces Institute of Pathology: 2002:161, Table 3-31.

of the disease and may even be used as a diagnostic test. Atypical presentations occur, so surgical wedge biopsy may be required to establish the diagnosis.

Histopathologic Findings

The histopathologic features of chronic pulmonary eosinophilia are similar to those of the acute form; it has been said that the distinction must rely on the clinical course rather than on the constellation

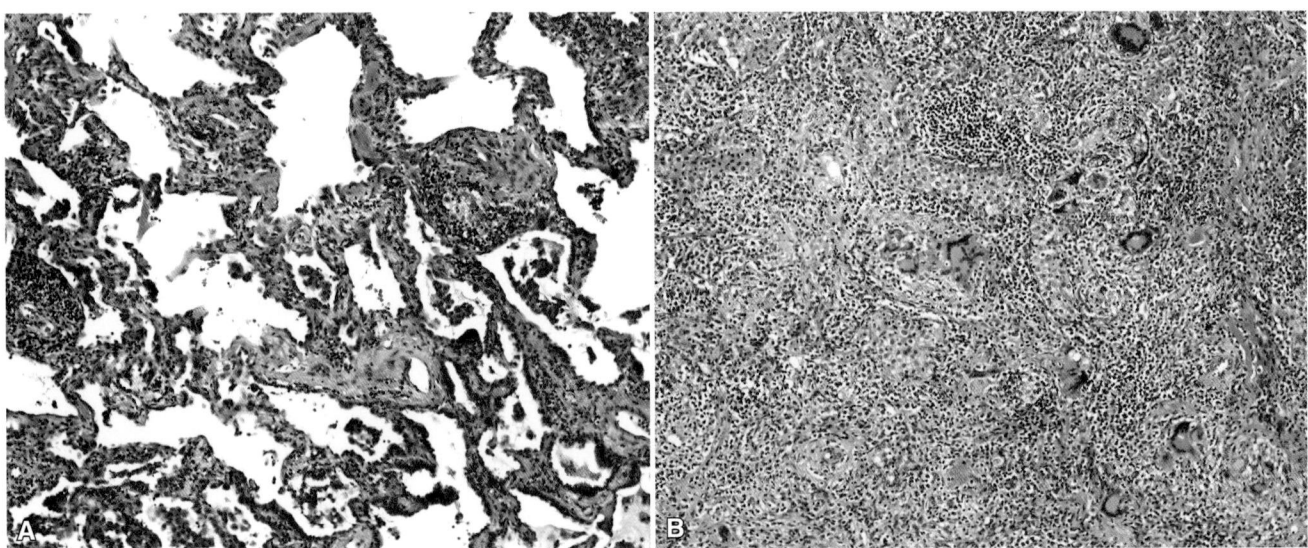

Figure 7-55. Sjögren syndrome (SS). **A,** Small, non-necrotizing granulomas, resembling those of hypersensitivity pneumonitis, are frequently identified in the interstitium in the lymphoid interstitial pneumonia pattern of SS. **B,** Sometimes the granulomas are more diffusely distributed; in such instances, infection and aspiration pneumonia will be important considerations in the differential diagnosis.

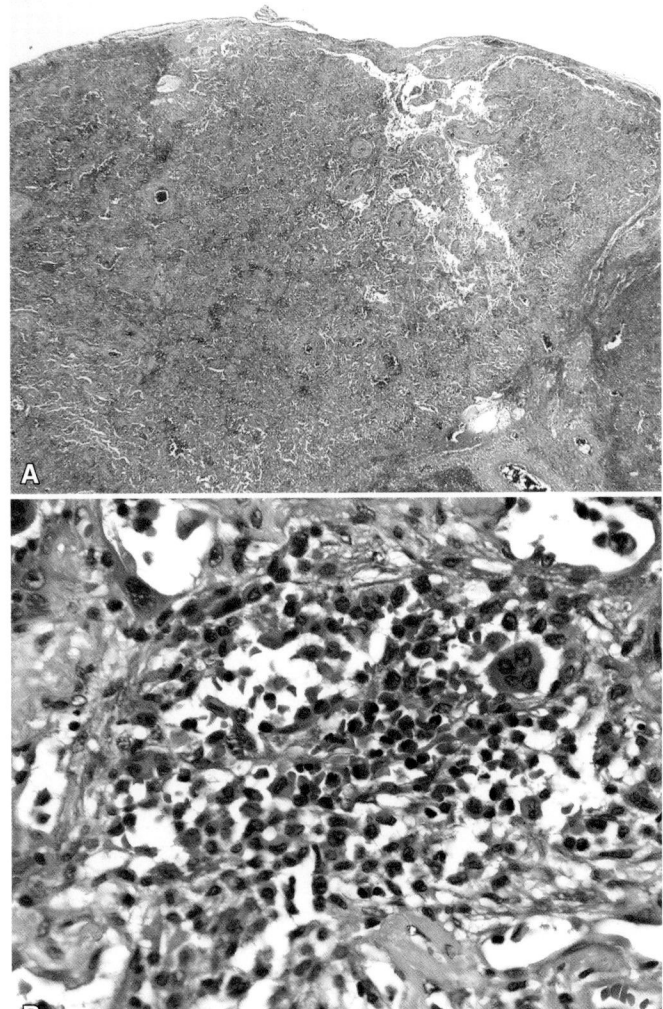

Figure 7-56. Eosinophilic pneumonia. **A,** In acute eosinophilic pneumonia, the alveolar spaces are diffusely filled with eosinophils and plump eosinophilic macrophages, sometimes with an associated mild interstitial pneumonia. **B,** Eosinophilic microabscesses may be present.

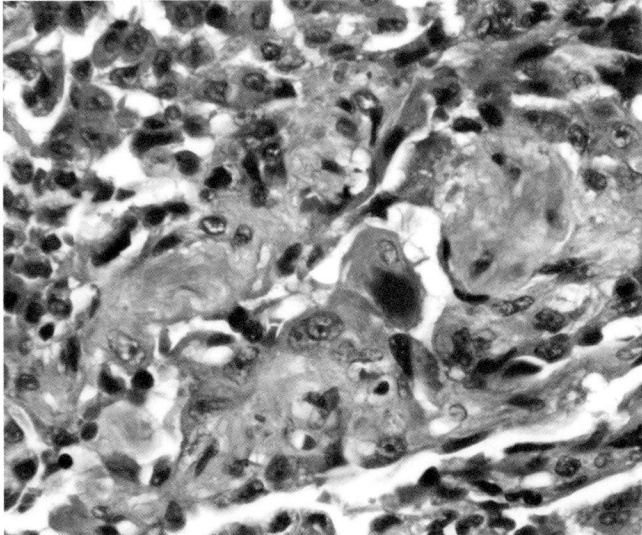

Figure 7-57. Eosinophilic pneumonia. Highly atypical type II hyperplasia is characteristic in acute eosinophilic pneumonia, often raising concern for viral cytopathic changes.

of morphologic findings.[1] Alveolar spaces are filled with eosinophils and plump eosinophilic macrophages (Fig. 7-56), and there is an associated mild interstitial pneumonia. Type II hyperplasia is characteristic (Fig. 7-57), and fibrin often is present in the air spaces (Fig. 7-58). Angiitis of small vessels may be seen, and patchy air space and alveolar duct organization may be present. A vaguely granulomatous accumulation of dense macrophages may be seen within the alveolar spaces (Fig. 7-59), sometimes accompanied by multinucleate giant cells whose nuclei and cytoplasm closely resemble those of adjacent macrophages (Fig. 7-60). Chronicity may be suggested by the presence of variable interstitial fibrosis on histopathologic examination, but as mentioned earlier, this is not a prerequisite for the diagnosis.

Differential Diagnosis

When air space organization is prominent, disorders with the organizing pneumonia pattern must be considered in the differential diagnosis (see Box 7-8). Some investigators have proposed an overlap syndrome between COP and eosinophilic pneumonia with subacute clinical course; it is interesting that both conditions are expected to have favorable responses to systemic corticosteroid administration. When corticosteroids have been administered before biopsy (which is quite

common), eosinophils may be absent or inconspicuous in lung sections. In such cases, the differential diagnosis may include granulomatous disease if the dense histiocytic response and multinucleate giant cells dominate the picture. When fibrin is prominent in the setting of pretreatment with corticosteroids, generic acute lung injury (including DAD and acute fibrinous and organizing pneumonia, because both patterns can be seen in acute eosinophilic pneumonia [AEP]; see Chapter 5) may enter the histopathologic differential diagnosis. Some patients with long-standing symptoms may have fibrosis on biopsy; in such cases, a fibrosing lung disease, such as UIP or NSIP, may enter the differential diagnosis, with eosinophilic pneumonia possibly manifesting as a comorbid process (e.g., drug reaction superimposed on NSIP).

Clinical Course

The clinical course is somewhat dependent on the underlying cause of the eosinophilic pneumonia, but in general, most affected individuals will benefit from high-dose corticosteroid therapy (although the speed of recovery may not be as rapid as that seen in acute onset eosinophilic pneumonia). As in all cases of eosinophilic pneumonia, it is always worthwhile to suggest the possibility of Churg-Strauss syndrome (see Chapter 10) because the pulmonary manifestations of that systemic vasculitic disease in the lung are most commonly those of eosinophilic pneumonia.

Drug-Associated Diffuse Lung Disease

An increasing number of medications have been implicated in chronic diffuse lung disease.[201,202] Three distinct forms are recognized: (1) drug-mediated chronic diffuse lung disease, (2) acute lung injury associated with drug administration, and (3) vascular diseases produced by medications.[203,204] The latter two conditions are dealt with in Chapters 5 and 10, respectively.

The recognition of drug-induced diffuse lung disease is a major challenge in lung pathology because most of the histopathologic changes identified are nonspecific (Table 7-5) and simulate those seen with other causes of diffuse lung disease.[262] Moreover, many affected patients have underlying diseases for which a drug has been administered, and some of these diseases also have pulmonary manifestations. The diagnosis of a drug-mediated diffuse lung disease requires careful exclusion of other causes.[262] Unfortunately, a clear onset of pulmonary

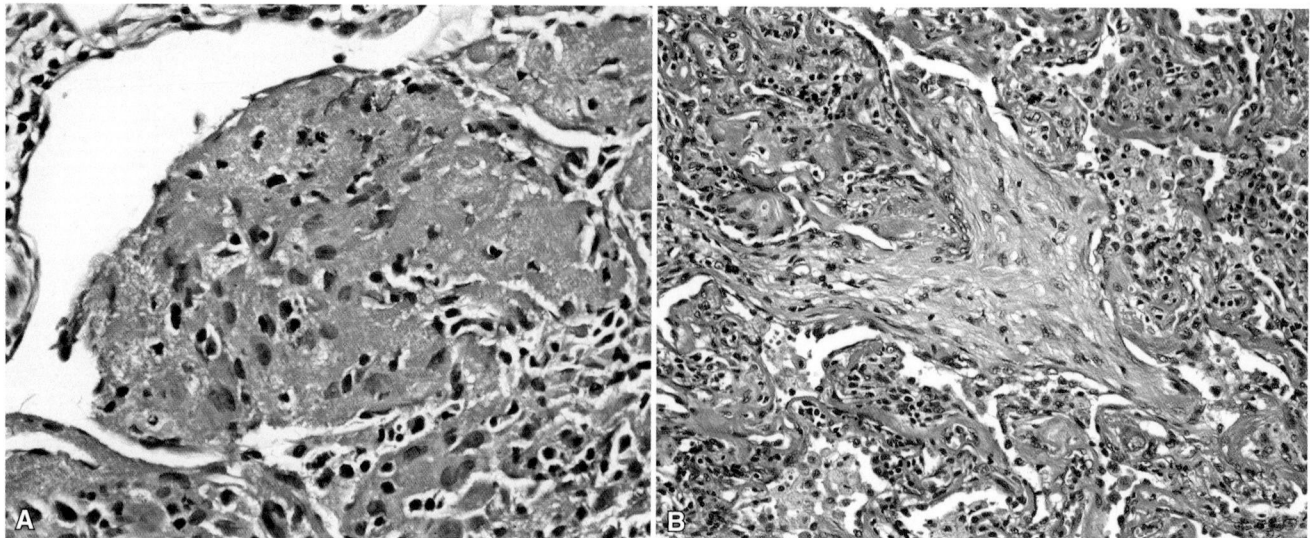

Figure 7-58. Eosinophilic pneumonia. **A,** Fibrinous air space exudates are commonly present, typically with admixed eosinophils, as seen in this specimen. **B,** Organizing pneumonia pattern repair may also occur.

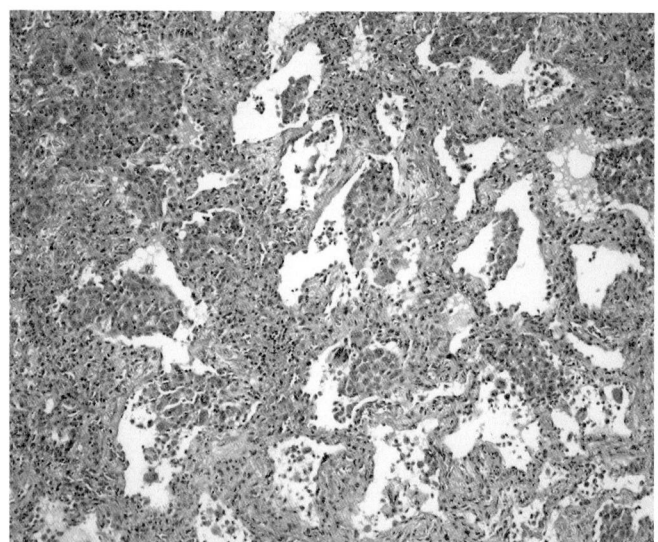

Figure 7-59. Eosinophilic pneumonia. A vaguely granulomatous accumulation of dense macrophages may be seen within the alveolar spaces, sometimes accompanied by plump multinucleate macrophages.

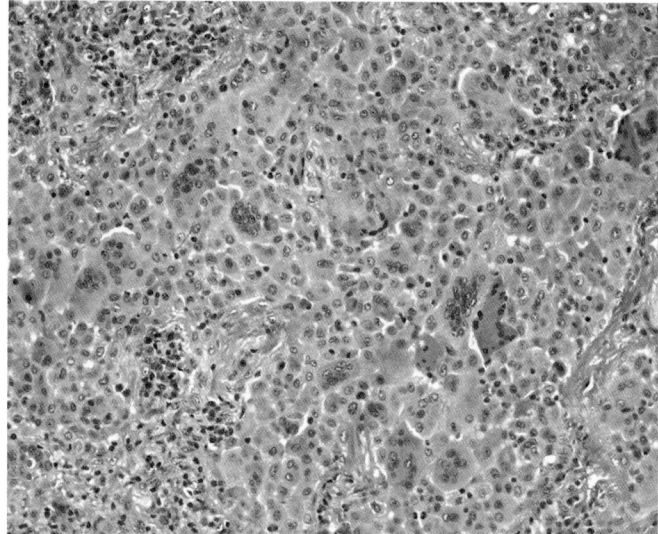

Figure 7-60. Eosinophilic pneumonia. The multinucleate giant cells of eosinophilic pneumonia have nuclei and cytoplasm that closely resemble those of adjacent alveolar macrophages, but occasionally they may be more brightly eosinophilic.

symptoms with drug administration and abatement of symptoms on cessation of the drug may not be easily discernable. Clinical information regarding specific drug type, dose, and timing of administration relative to onset of symptoms is essential to an accurate diagnosis.

General Histopathologic Findings

Most of the inflammatory changes in the lung related to drug toxicity are nonspecific. More often than not, a mixture of both acute and chronic disease is apparent and can be a clue to the diagnosis of drug-mediated injury.[238] In chronic drug toxicity, lung fibrosis may occur, sometimes with honeycomb remodeling. In such cases, UIP may be simulated. Type II cell hyperplasia with or without atypia, cytoplasmic vacuolation in type II cells and macrophages, and tissue eosinophilia can occur in drug reactions. Also, some drugs are associated with the production in the lung of small, poorly formed granulomas, simulating infection, hypersensitivity, or even Sjögren syndrome.[201]

General Treatment and Prognosis

Most patients with drug-mediated diffuse lung disease have a favorable prognosis when the implicated drug is withdrawn. Certain newer targeted molecular therapies have been associated with a higher mortality rate when diffuse acute injury occurs.[224,263] Once fibrosis has occurred, changes are likely to be stable, with little improvement. Systemic corticosteroid therapy may be added when symptoms are severe.

Specific Drugs Associated with Interstitial Lung Disease

Methotrexate

Methotrexate (MTX) lung toxicity is uncommon; when it occurs, it is predominantly a manifestation in women taking the drug.[264,265] Because MTX is used in the treatment of a variety of disorders (e.g., RA, some leukemias, some visceral cancers), these tend to be the associated underlying diseases that must be considered in the differential diagnosis for the lung manifestations identified. Interstitial inflammation and fibrosis

Table 7-5. Pulmonary Reactions and Associated Drugs

Drug	FIP	CIP	OP	Edema	DAD	Eos	AH	BO	PVOD	Gran
Amiodarone[205–207]	+	++	+	++	+	+	++			+
β-Blockers[208]	+	++	+			+				
Bevacizumab[209]							+			
Bleomycin[210,211]	++	++	+	++	+	+			+	
Busulfan[212,213]	+				+			+	+	
Carmustine (BCNU)[214,215]	+	++		++	+				+	
Cocaine[216,217]					+	+	+			+
Cyclophosphamide[218–221]	+		+	++	+		+			
Docetaxel[222]		+		+	+					
Ergolines[223]	+	++	+							
Erlotinib[224]					+					
Etoposide[225]		++			+					
Gefitinib[226]		+	+		++	+				
Gemcitabine[227]	+	+		+	+		+			
G(M)-CSF		++		++	+	+				
Gold[228]	+	++	+		++	+				
Heroin[229,230]		++		++			+			
Hexamethonium[231,232]	+		+		+					
Hydrochlorothiazide[233–235]		++		++	+	+				
Imatinib		+			+					
Infliximab[236]	+	+			+	+				
Leflunomide		+			++	+				+
Lomustine (CCNU)[237]	+				+					
Methotrexate[238,239]	++	++	+	+	+	+		+		+
Minocycline[240,241]		+		++		+				
Mitomycin C[242,243]	+	++		++	+		++		+	
Nitrofurantoin[244–246]	+	++	+	++	+	+	++			+
Paclitaxel[247]		+				+				
Penicillamine[248–250]		+	+		+	+	++	+		
Phenytoin[251,252]		+	+			+	++			
Procarbazine[253–255]		+			+	+				+
Prozac (fluoxetine)[256]		+								
Rituximab[257]	+	+			+		+			
Sulfasalazine[258]	+	++		++	+	+				
L-Tryptophan[259,260]		+				+				
Zinostatin[261]					+				+	

AH, alveolar hemorrhage; BO, bronchiolitis obliterans; CCNU, chloroethyl-cyclohexyl-nitrosourea; CIP, cellular interstitial pneumonia including cellular NSIP and LIP patterns; DAD, diffuse alveolar damage; Eos, tissue eosinophilia; FIP, fibrosing interstitial pneumonia including UIP and fibrosing NSIP pattern; G(M)-CSF, granulocyte (macrophage) colony-stimulating factor; Gran, granulomatous inflammation; LIP, lymphocytic interstitial pneumonia; OP, organizing pneumonia; NSIP, nonspecific interstitial pneumonia; PVOD, pulmonary veno-occlusive disease; UIP, usual interstitial pneumonia.

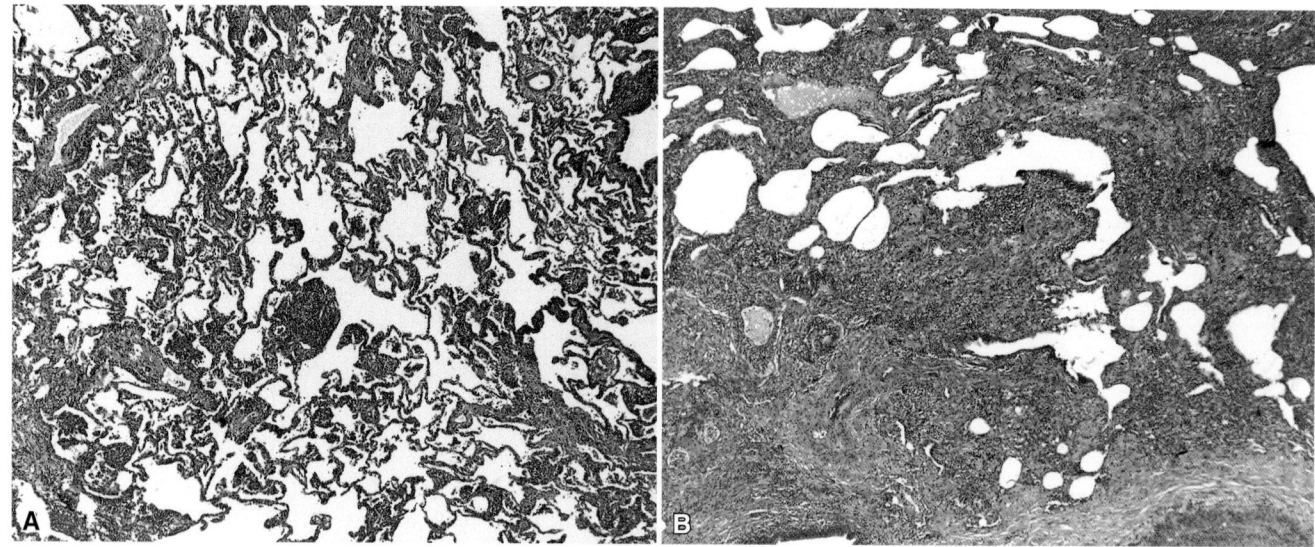

Figure 7-61. Methotrexate toxicity. Nonspecific interstitial inflammation (**A**) and fibrosis (**B**) are common findings, and scattered lymphoid aggregates may be seen. When the latter are prominent and accompanied by bronchiolitis, the possibility of exacerbation of an underlying connective tissue disease comes into the differential diagnosis (e.g., rheumatoid arthritis).

(Fig. 7-61) are common findings in the surgical lung biopsy.[239,266,267] Giant cells and small non-necrotizing granulomas (Fig. 7-62) are the only relatively specific markers for MTX, in comparison with other drugs.[239] Type II pneumocyte hyperplasia and tissue eosinophilia may be seen (Fig. 7-63). Hyaline membranes are rarely identified.[239]

Amiodarone

Amiodarone is the drug of choice for the treatment of certain refractory cardiac arrhythmias. Pulmonary toxicity has been reported in 5% to 10% of patients taking this medication. Older patients are more likely to develop lung disease. The clinical onset is characterized by slowly progressive dyspnea and dry cough, occurring within months of initiating therapy. Approximately one third of patients experience an acute febrile illness mimicking infectious pneumonia.[268–271] High-resolution CT scans show diffuse infiltrates combined with basal or peripheral high-attenuation opacities and nonspecific infiltrates.[272,273] The most common pathologic manifestation is a cellular interstitial pneumonia (Fig. 7-64) associated

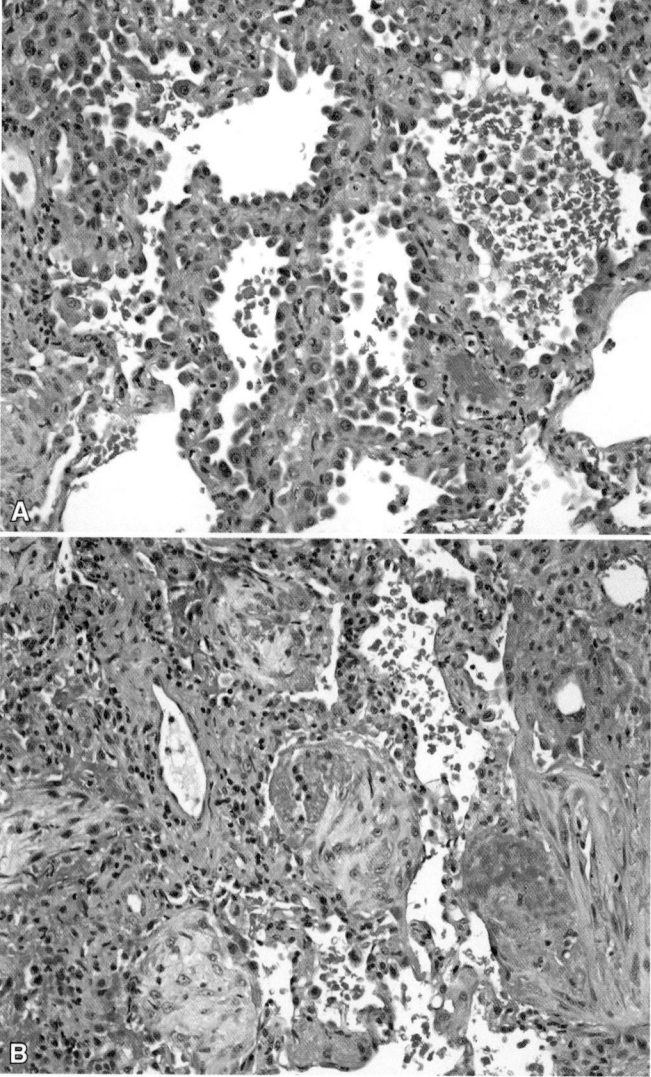

Figure 7-63. Methotrexate toxicity. Type II pneumocyte hyperplasia (**A**) and variable acute lung injury with air space organization (**B**), with or without tissue eosinophilia, can be seen.

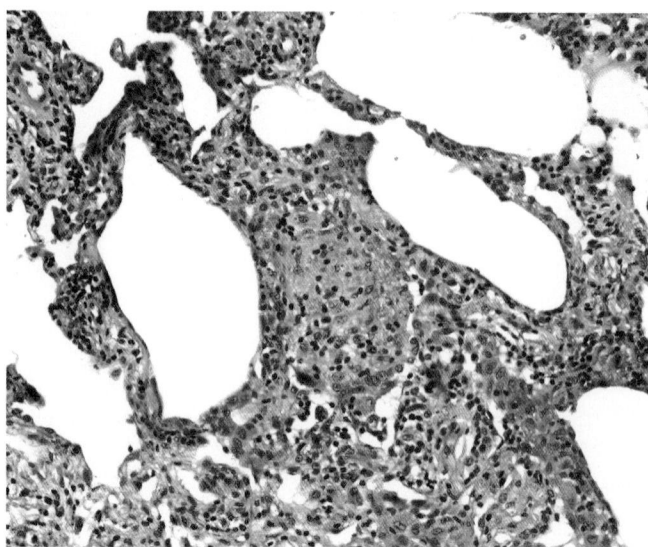

Figure 7-62. Methotrexate toxicity. Giant cells and scattered small non-necrotizing granulomas (*center*) are the only relatively specific markers for lung injury due to methotrexate.

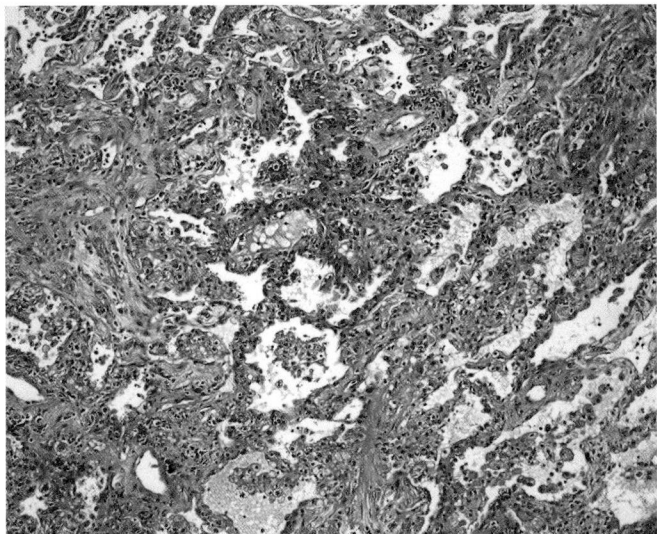

Figure 7-64. Amiodarone toxicity. The most common pathologic change seen in amiodarone toxicity is a cellular interstitial pneumonia associated with prominent intra-alveolar macrophages whose cytoplasm shows fine vacuolation.

with prominent intra-alveolar macrophages whose cytoplasm shows fine vacuolation.[268,274–276] This vacuolation can also be seen in reactive type II pneumocytes (Fig. 7-65); published reports have described the presence of characteristic lamellar cytoplasmic inclusions ultrastructurally.[200] Unfortunately, these cytoplasmic changes are an expected manifestation of the drug, so the mere presence of such changes is not sufficient to warrant a diagnosis of amiodarone toxicity.[274] Pleural inflammation and pleural effusion have also been reported.[277] Some patients with amiodarone toxicity may develop an organizing pneumonia (OP) pattern (Fig. 7-66), a nodular pattern,[278] or even DAD.[274,279,280] A majority of patients with amiodarone-related pulmonary toxicity will recover once the drug is discontinued.[268,269,274–276]

BCNU

BCNU (carmustine) is the treatment of choice for patients with certain brain tumors and is used in some combination chemotherapy regimens. Acute and organizing DAD is the most common manifestation

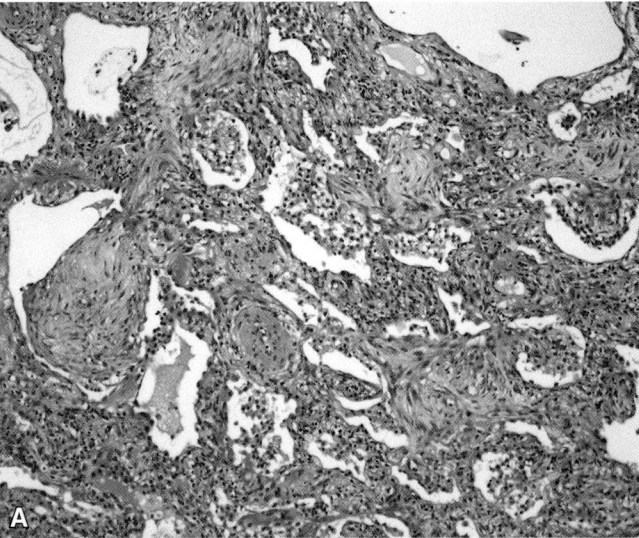

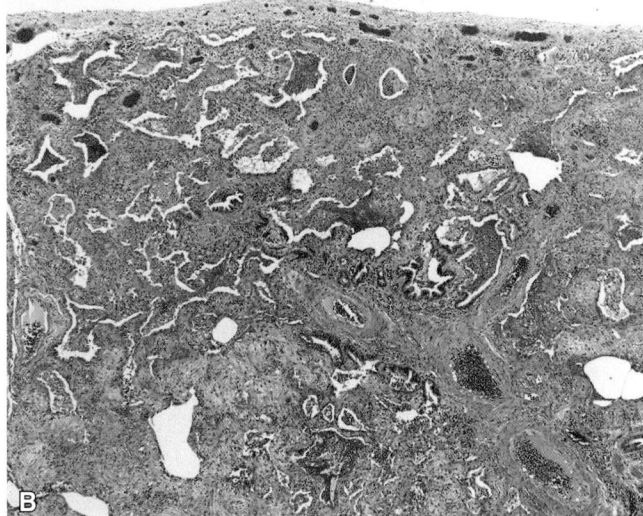

Figure 7-66. Amiodarone toxicity. **A,** In some patients with amiodarone toxicity, an organizing pneumonia pattern develops, resulting in a mass effect on thoracic imaging studies. **B,** Rarely, chronic toxicity may result in advanced lung fibrosis.

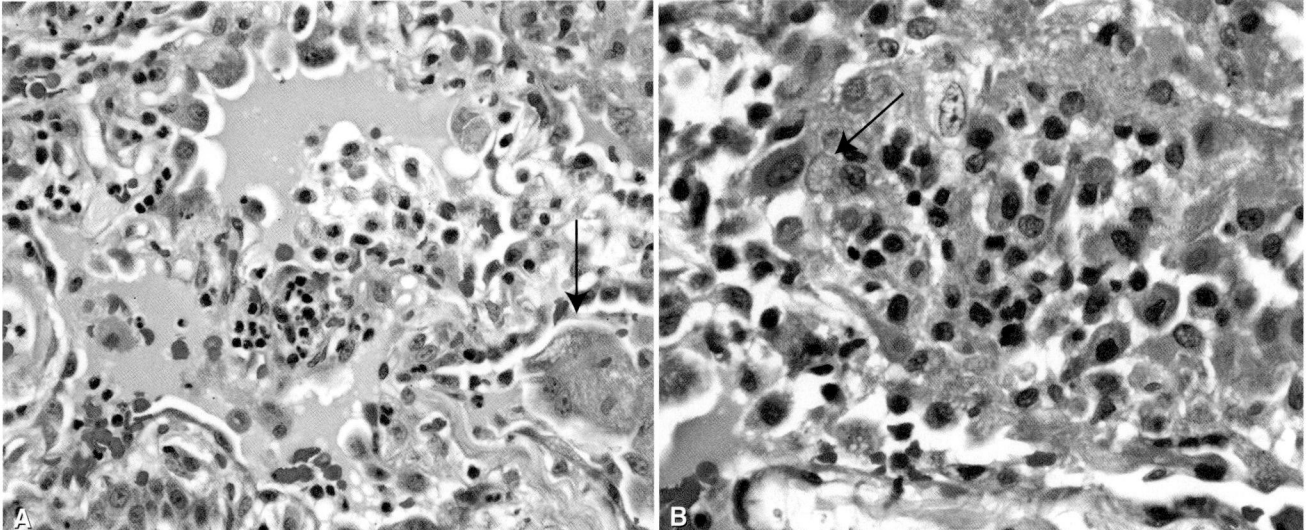

Figure 7-65. Amiodarone toxicity. **A** and **B,** Amiodarone effect (fine cytoplasmic vacuolation; *arrows*) can be seen and in reactive type II pneumocytes. Published reports have described the presence of characteristic lamellar cytoplasmic inclusions ultrastructurally. Unfortunately, these cytoplasmic and ultrastructural changes are expected with treatment with this drug, so that the mere presence of such changes is not sufficient to warrant a diagnosis of amiodarone toxicity.

of acute BCNU pulmonary toxicity.[281–284] Delayed lung toxicity has been described in survivors of childhood brain tumors who received BCNU, with lung changes appearing 8 to 20 years after cessation of treatment.[281,285,286] The histopathologic features of BCNU toxicity can be generally grouped within the NSIP pattern (Fig. 7-67). In children, fibrosis develops in the upper lung zones, with peripheral accentuation.[286] In adults, this upper lobe distribution is uncommon.[287] Pleural disease can accompany pulmonary abnormalities in some patients.

Busulfan

Busulfan is an alkylating agent that has been used in the treatment of chronic myelogenous leukemia. Pulmonary toxicity has been reported to occur in 4% of patients,[288–290] most commonly as acute lung injury. Unfortunately, the prognosis for patients with busulfan-induced acute lung disease is poor. Rarely, patients with busulfan toxicity develop chronic diffuse lung disease[212] (Fig. 7-68).

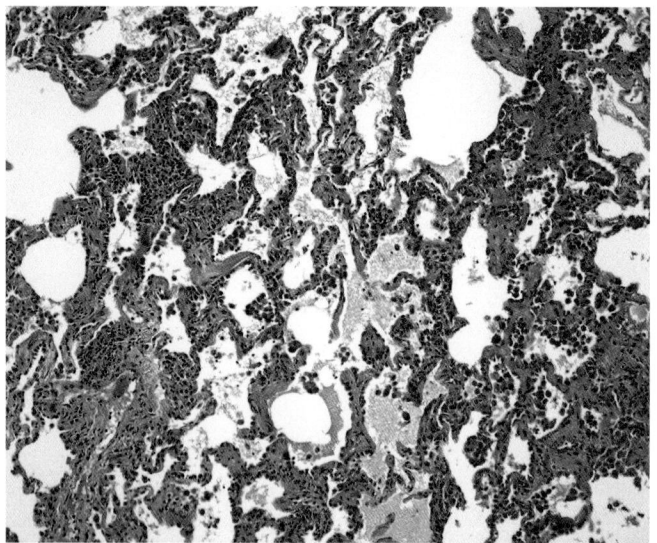

Figure 7-67. BCNU (carmustine) toxicity. The histopathologic features of BCNU toxicity are those of a nonspecific cellular interstitial pneumonia with variable interstitial fibrosis.

Bleomycin

Bleomycin is a chemotherapeutic agent used in the treatment of lymphomas, epidermoid carcinomas, and malignant testicular tumors. Lung toxicity appears to be dose-related, but irradiation or oxygen therapy may predispose the lung to injury.[210,291–293] The typical clinical presentation begins with dry cough and progresses to breathlessness. Chest imaging reveals areas of nodular consolidation or diffuse reticulation.[294] In experimental models, the initial site of injury seems to be the venous endothelial cell, followed by necrosis of type I cells with consequent fibroplasia.[295–298] In humans, toxicity results in acute lung injury with air space organization in the early phase and fibrosis as a late consequence (Fig. 7-69).

Targeted Molecular Therapies

Progress in the application of newer anti-cancer therapies using antibodies and small molecules directed at molecular signaling pathways has lead to increasing reports of pulmonary toxicity. For example, the epidermal growth factor receptor tyrosine kinase inhibitor (EGFR-TKI) gefitinib is said to produce ILD in 1% of patients treated with this agent (2% to 4% in Japanese patients and 0.3% in U.S. patients).[299,300] The most common histopathologic pattern associated with gefitinib use is DAD. The other main EGFR-TKI, erlotinib, is also reported to produce a DAD reaction pattern.[224] The common risk factors for toxicity with these agents are smoking history, age, and the presence of pre-existing ILD.[263] Similar trends are seen with conventional cytotoxic chemotherapies, such as paclitaxel, docetaxel, and gemcitabine.

Newer additions to the anti-inflammatory drug arsenal, such as the anti-TNF-α inhibitor infliximab, are also associated with adverse reactions, including an apparent risk for certain pulmonary infections, such as tuberculosis and aspergillosis, followed by DAD and pulmonary fibrosis.[301]

Illicit Drug Abuse

Many of the described pulmonary manifestations of illicit drug use (Box 7-11) are related to infections derived from the use of contaminated needles for intravenous injection or comorbidity related to the use of inhaled substances.[302] For a minority of substance abusers, intravenously injected solubilized analgesic tablets is the drug of

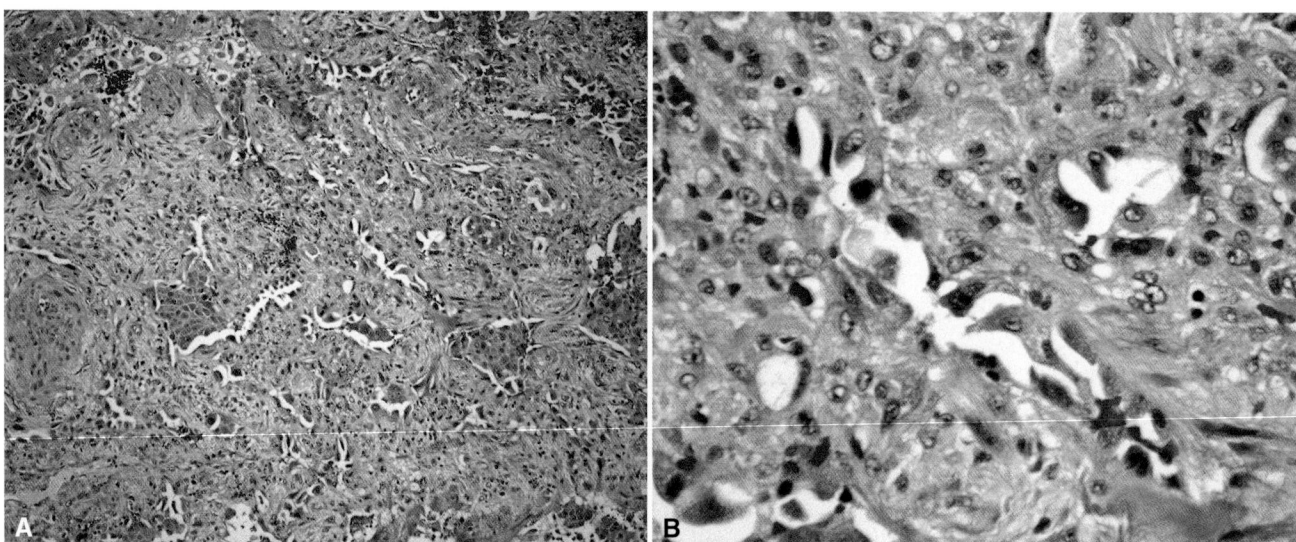

Figure 7-68. Busulfan toxicity. **A** and **B,** The prognosis for patients with busulfan-induced acute lung disease is poor. In the subacute form of injury, air space organization is often accompanied by marked atypia of reactive type II cells.

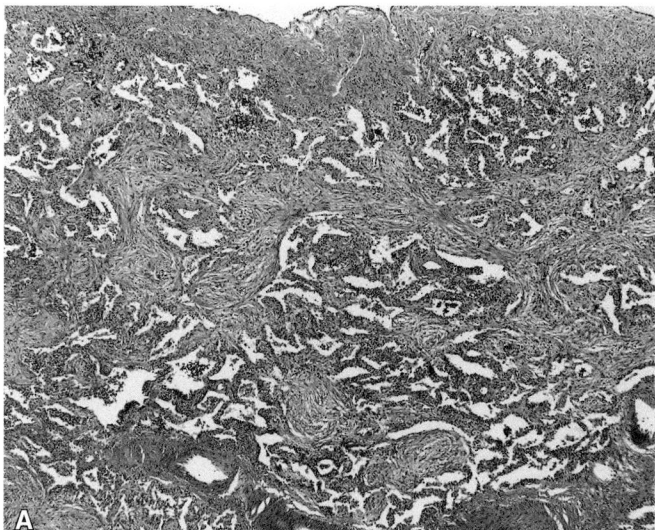

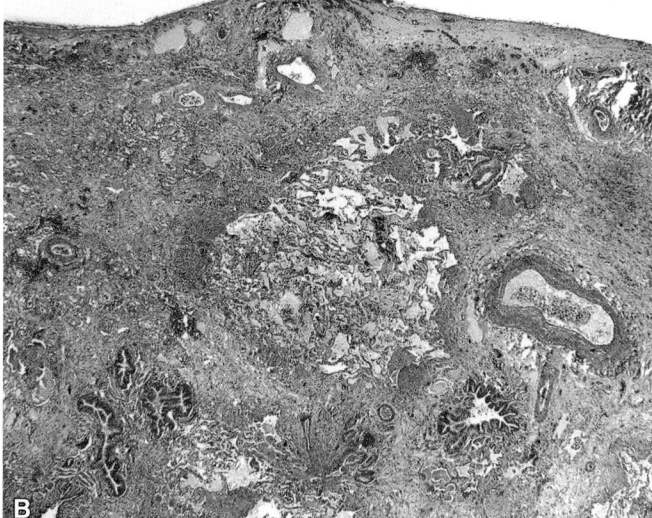

Figure 7-69. Bleomycin toxicity. Pulmonary changes may include acute lung injury with air space organization in the early phase (**A**) and fibrosis resembling that of usual interstitial pneumonia as a late consequence (**B**).

Box 7-11. Pulmonary Complications of Intravenous Drug Abuse

Infections (including HIV) and infection-related diseases
Pneumonia
Abscesses
Mycotic aneurysms
Septic emboli
Acute respiratory distress syndrome
Pulmonary hypertension
Interstitial fibrosis with interstitial lung disease
Massive fibrosis
Emphysema

choice. In current practice, the presence of perivascular talc particles in giant cells usually indicates a residual injury from earlier in the patient's life, because tablet manufacturers today most often use microcrystalline cellulose compounds as binding and filling agents, rather than talc, as was the practice several decades ago. When intravenous drug use entails injection of crushed analgesic tablets nowadays, microcrystalline cellulose is the commonly identified injurious particle in the lung parenchyma. The physical characteristics and histochemical staining reactions of this material are different than those of talc; these may be useful distinguishing features, on occasion.[303]

Injected particles generally average 10 to 15 μm in diameter,[303–305] in contrast with inhaled substances, for which particle sizes tend to be smaller, usually less than 5 μm (with red blood cells used for size comparison). Cornstarch is another filler agent; it appears as a spherical structure with a "Maltese cross" pattern under plane-polarized light. Talc appears as irregular, plate-like, crystals that are strongly birefringent (Fig. 7-70) and may be slightly yellow on routine hematoxylin and eosin staining when a single polarizing filter is in place. Microcrystalline cellulose particles appear as elongated crystalline structures (Fig. 7-71) that may stain positively using digested PAS, methenamine silver, and Congo red stains. The reaction in the lung is generally interstitial and perivascular (Fig. 7-72), rather than intraalveolar. Intravenous foreign material may rarely become encrusted with iron (ferruginated), and sometimes colored tablet coatings (such as blue crospovidone) may be present and quite striking in histopathologic appearance.

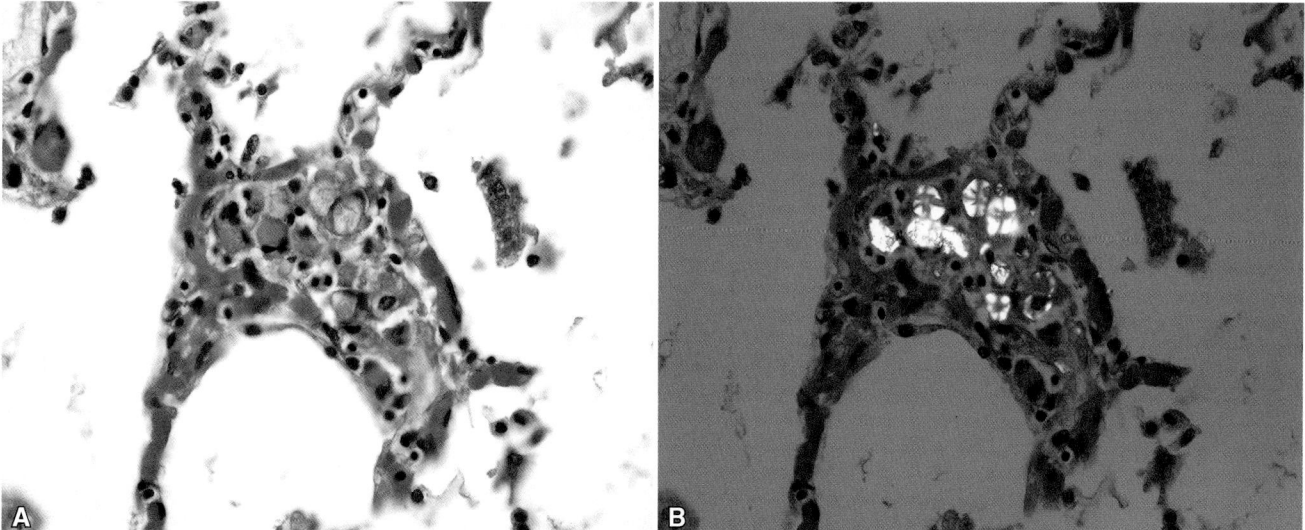

Figure 7-70. Intravenous drug: talc. **A,** The patient had intravenous talcosis, manifested on histopathologic examination as small clusters of multinucleate histiocytes containing irregular plate-like crystals that are strongly birefringent under full polarization. **B,** Birefringent talc particles may be seen in routine hematoxylin and eosin staining using plane-polarized light.

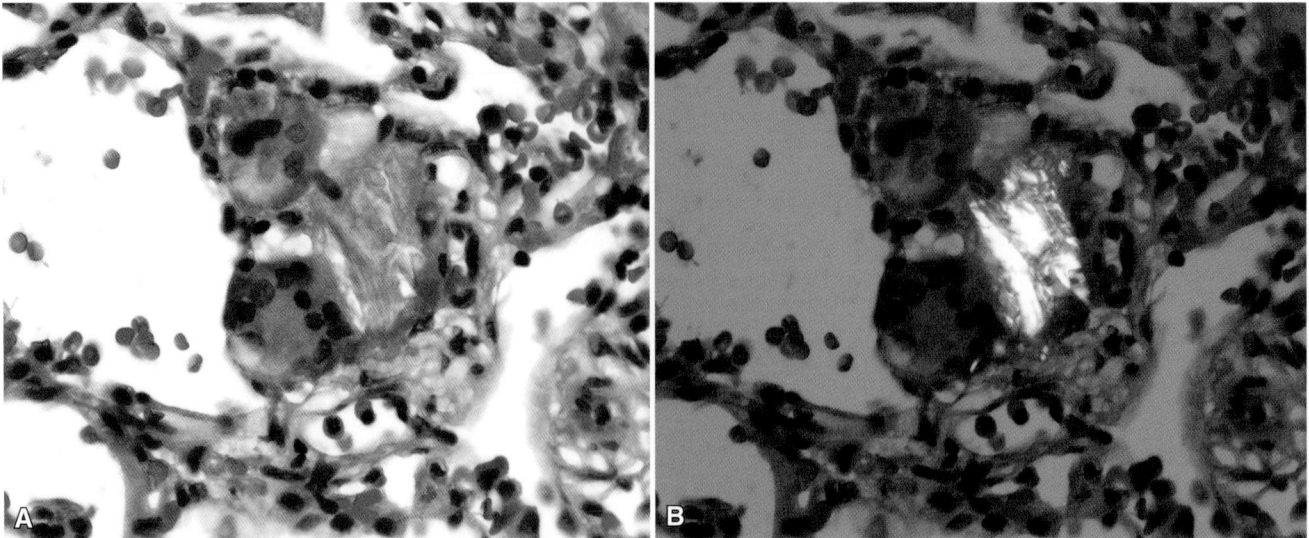

Figure 7-71. Intravenous drug: microcrystalline cellulose. **A,** Microcrystalline cellulose particles appear as elongated crystalline structures in the cytoplasm of foreign body giant cells in the perivascular interstitium. **B,** These particles are strongly birefringent in polarized light.

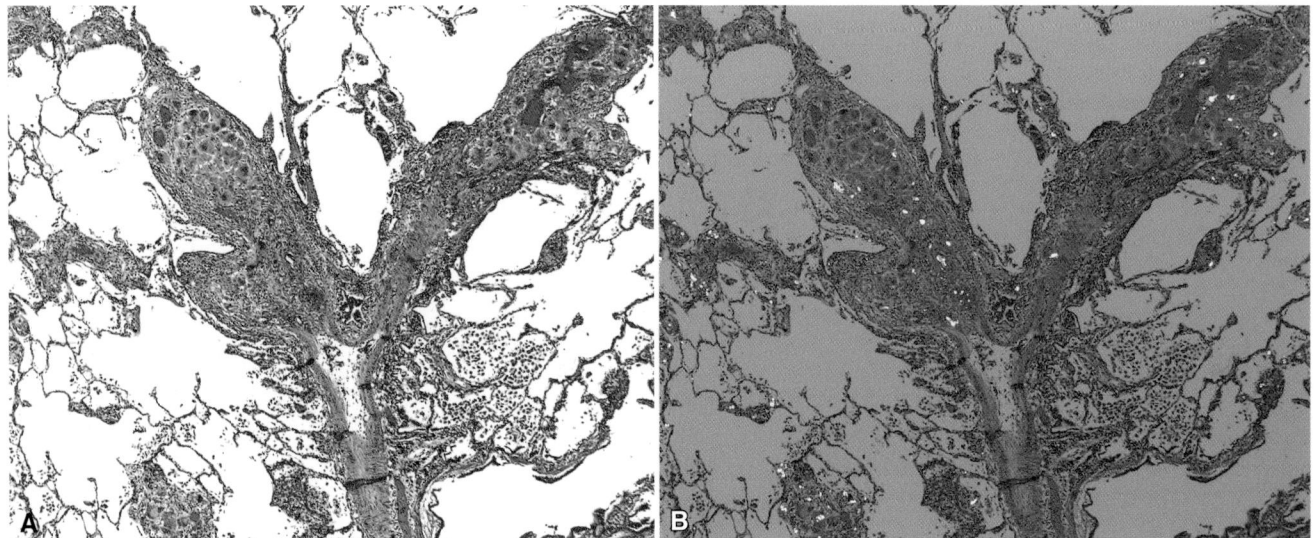

Figure 7-72. Intravenous drug: microcrystalline cellulose. **A,** The reaction in the lung is generally interstitial and perivascular, rather than intra-alveolar. **B,** The extent of intravenous foreign material may be better appreciated using polarizing filters.

Histopathologic Findings

As the intravenous material becomes lodged in the pulmonary microvasculature, a perivascular interstitial foreign body–type granulomatous reaction is produced (Fig. 7-73) that may be associated with prominent vascular changes (including pulmonary hypertension and thrombotic lesions and others),[306] as well as interstitial fibrosis (Fig. 7-74) that may be focal or diffuse and sometimes massive.[307] Among the pathologic manifestations presented in Table 7-6, pulmonary hypertension is the most common, whereas emphysema is quite uncommon. Emphysema associated with intravenous drug abuse is typically of the panacinar type (similar to that in α_1-antitrypsin deficiency) and has been most frequently associated with methylphenidate (Ritalin) abuse.[308] In contrast with smoking-associated emphysema, the radiologic changes seen in so-called "Ritalin lung" are more severe in the lower lobes. Bullae may be present. In one report it was suggested that the presence of basilar pulmonary emphysema should always alert the radiologist to the possibility of intravenous drug abuse.[308] The pathogenesis of panlobular emphysema associated with intravenous drug abuse is unknown.

Some of the postulated mechanisms include synergism with cigarette smoke, direct toxic effects of the drug, and induced intravascular leukocyte sequestration causing proteolytic pulmonary injury.

Because the foreign material remains in the lung, progression of the clinical and pathologic lesions may occur after discontinuation of intravenous drug use. Recurrence of the changes of intravenous drug abuse have been described rarely in transplanted lung tissue, although such recurrence appears to be a consequence of resumed intravenous drug abuse.[309]

Diffuse Lung Diseases with Granulomas

Granulomas occur in the lung in a variety of infectious and noninfectious diseases[310] (Box 7-12). Infectious diseases with granulomas are discussed in Chapter 6. Although non-infectious granulomas can occur diffusely in the lungs in certain drug reactions and in Sjögren syndrome, the relatively specific disease entities of sarcoidosis, berylliosis, and hypersensitivity pneumonitis are discussed here separately because of their distinctive clinical, radiologic, and histopathologic presentations.

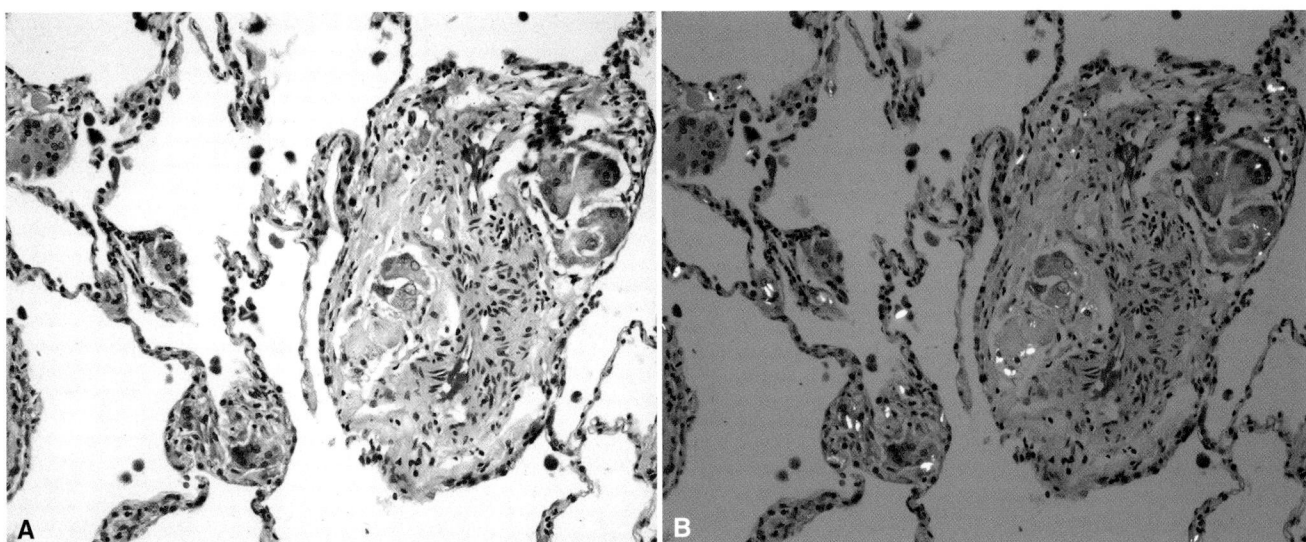

Figure 7-73. Intravenous drug. **A,** Normal light. **B,** Polarized light. A perivascular interstitial foreign body–type granulomatous reaction is associated with prominent vascular changes, as seen here.

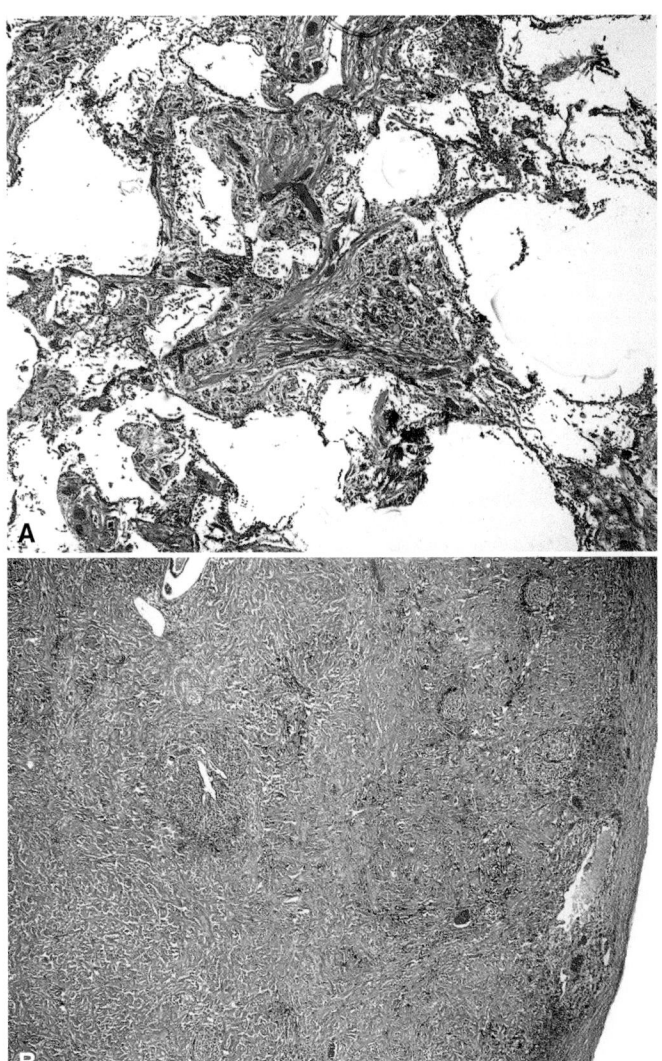

Figure 7-74. Intravenous drug. One complication of intravenous drug abuse is lung fibrosis (**A**); sometimes this can be massive (**B**).

Table 7-6. Pathologic Lesions and Clinical Syndromes Related to Intravenous Drug Use

Pathologic Lesion	Clinical Syndrome
Vascular, perivascular, and interstitial foreign body granulomas with:	
Pulmonary arterial hypertension (with or without thrombotic lesions)	Pulmonary hypertension (may cause sudden death)
Interstitial fibrosis	Interstitial lung disease
Massive fibrosis	Complicated "pneumoconiosis" (tends to be bilateral and involves mid- and upper lung zones)
Panacinar emphysema	Emphysema/chronic airflow obstruction

Box 7-12. Granulomatous Interstitial Pneumonias

Commonly Encountered Granulomas
Sarcoidosis/berylliosis
Infections (e.g., mycobacteria, fungi, pneumocystis, actinomyces, nocardia)
Hypersensitivity pneumonitis

Infrequently Encountered or Inconsistent Granulomas
Bronchiectasis/bronchiolitis with secondary granulomatous infection
Berylliosis and other pneumoconioses
Drug reactions
Collagen vascular diseases (e.g., Sjögren syndrome)
Intravenous talcosis
Vasculitis (Wegener granulomatosis, Churg-Strauss syndrome)*
Bronchocentric granulomatosis
Eosinophilic pneumonia
Foreign body granulomas (aspiration pneumonia)
Immunoglobulin deficiency
Lymphoid interstitial pneumonia/diffuse lymphoid hyperplasia
Giant cell interstitial pneumonia/hard metal lung disease
Diffuse neoplastic involvement of the lungs (e.g., lymphoma, leukemia)
Inflammatory bowel disease (Crohn disease)
Incidental granulomas
Unclassifiable

*Vasculitis syndromes rarely present as diffuse granulomatous lung disease.
Adapted from Cheung OY, Muhm JR, Helmers RA, et al: Surgical pathology of granulomatous interstitial pneumonia. *Ann Diagn Pathol.* 2003;7(2):127–138.

Sarcoidosis

Clinical Presentation

Sarcoidosis is a systemic disease of uncertain etiology, with frequent lung manifestations.[311] Lung disease is usually mild, accompanied by variable degrees of shortness of breath, chest pain, and cough.[311] As many as two thirds of patients are asymptomatic.[270,312] Sarcoidosis is predominantly a disease of young adults but has been described in patients of all ages.[313–315] Sarcoidosis can have an acute, subacute, or chronic presentation in the lung. In symptomatic patients, restrictive defects and decreased diffusing capacity are commonly described. Serum angiotensin-converting enzyme (ACE) is elevated in 30% to 80% of patients. ACE has also been detected within granulomas, bronchial alveolar lavage fluid, tears, and even cerebrospinal fluid in these patients. Unfortunately, ACE levels can be elevated in a variety of disorders, including infectious granulomatous diseases, lymphoma, hepatitis, and diabetes.[270] The Kveim test[270] is relatively specific for sarcoidosis, employing an injected antigenic extract derived from human sarcoid granulomas, but the test is not widely used today,[311] given the widespread adoption of bronchoscopic biopsy for confirming the diagnosis in patients suspected of having the disease on clinical and radiologic grounds.

Radiologic Findings

The clinical staging of sarcoidosis is based on chest radiographic findings. Five stages of pulmonary sarcoidosis are described, corresponding to the extent of disease. Stage I and stage II disease are most common, with only 15% of patients presenting with parenchymal infiltrates alone.[270,311] When sarcoidosis involves the lung parenchyma, the disease is upper lobe predominant.[311] CT scans are not usually necessary for the diagnosis but will show reticulonodular opacities along lymphatic routes, with or without alveolar infiltrates.[270,316–318] Bullae with honeycombing may be seen in advanced disease, sometimes associated with progressive lung fibrosis.[319,320] A peculiar form of sarcoidosis with rapid onset of symptoms and a diffuse alveolar filling pattern on CT scans has been referred to as "alveolar sarcoidosis."[321] The pathologic manifestations of this form of the disease are distinctive only for the large number of small interstitial granulomas present throughout the lung parenchyma.

Histopathologic Findings

The characteristic histopathologic lesion of pulmonary sarcoidosis is the non-necrotizing (immune) granuloma, typically occurring within areas of sclerotic fibrosis (Fig. 7-75). In sarcoidosis, small granulomas have a tendency to coalesce to form larger nodular lesions, all embedded in refractile eosinophilic collagen (Fig. 7-76). A narrow rim of lymphocytic inflammation is typically seen at the periphery of these confluent nodules (Fig. 7-77). Granulomas are distributed along lymphatic routes in the pleura, within the intralobular septa, and along the bronchovascular bundles (Fig. 7-78). Multinucleate giant cells are characteristically present in the disease, often accompanied by a variety of distinctive cytoplasmic inclusions (e.g., Schaumann bodies, asteroid bodies) (Fig. 7-79). A mild inflammatory interstitial infiltrate is said to occur occasionally in pulmonary sarcoidosis, but in practice this is rarely seen. In bronchoscopic or transbronchial biopsies, granulomas are typically seen immediately beneath the airway mucosa (Fig. 7-80).

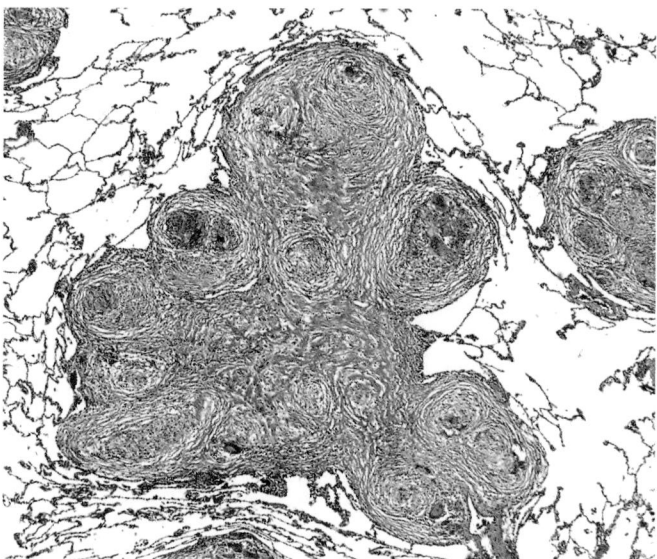

Figure 7-76. Sarcoidosis. In sarcoidosis, small granulomas have a tendency to coalesce to form larger nodular lesions, all embedded in refractile eosinophilic collagen.

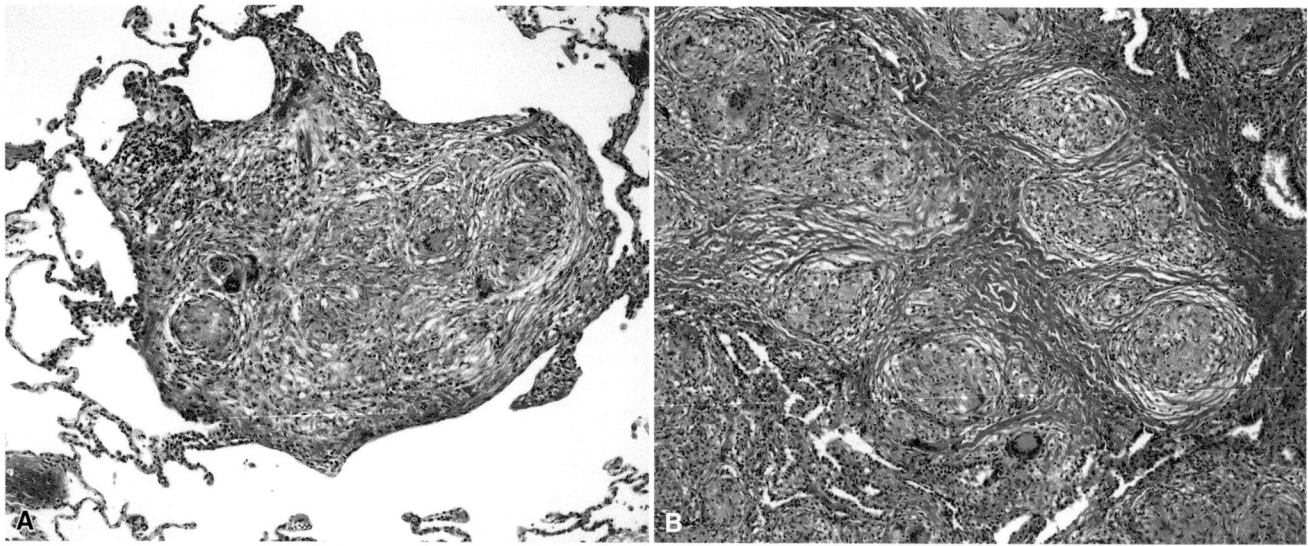

Figure 7-75. Sarcoidosis. The characteristic pathologic lesion of pulmonary sarcoidosis is the non-necrotizing (immune) granuloma (**A**), typically occurring within sclerotic fibrosis (**B**).

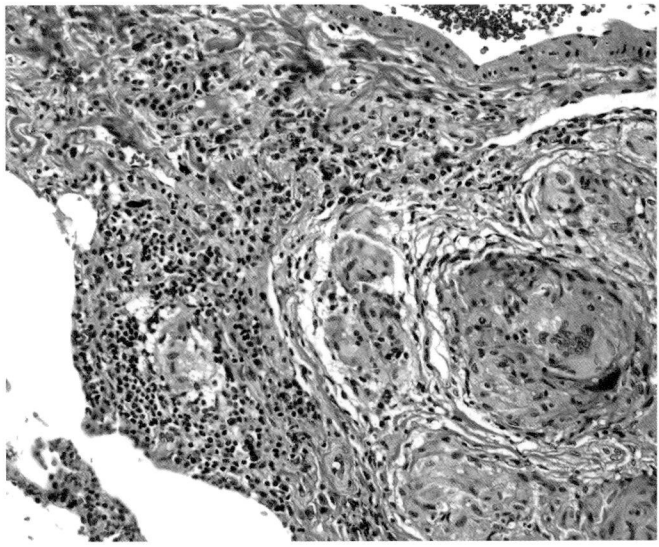

Figure 7-77. Sarcoidosis. A variable (but rarely intense) rim of lymphocytic inflammation is typically seen at the periphery of confluent granulomas.

Gilman and coworkers showed that the chance of obtaining a positive result in patients with sarcoidosis increased to 90% when four biopsy specimens were obtained.[322] When five to six samples were obtained, the probability rose to 100% for patients with stage II and stage III disease.

Special stains for organisms (acid-fast stains and silver stains) should be routinely used when granulomas are identified in lung biopsies to exclude infection, even in the absence of necrosis. In a retrospective study performed by Hsu and colleagues, positive microbiological cultures were identified in 11% of biopsies in which granulomas were present despite negative special stains of tissue sections.[323] In the culture-positive cases, clinical and radiographic findings were judged to be of low or intermediate suspicion for sarcoidosis. As might be expected, necrosis in granulomas was more frequently associated with culture-positive cases.

Differential Diagnosis

Granulomatous infection leads the differential diagnosis for sarcoidosis and is the diagnosis of exclusion. The granulomas of hypersensitivity pneumonitis are vague and poorly formed. Aspiration pneumonia can

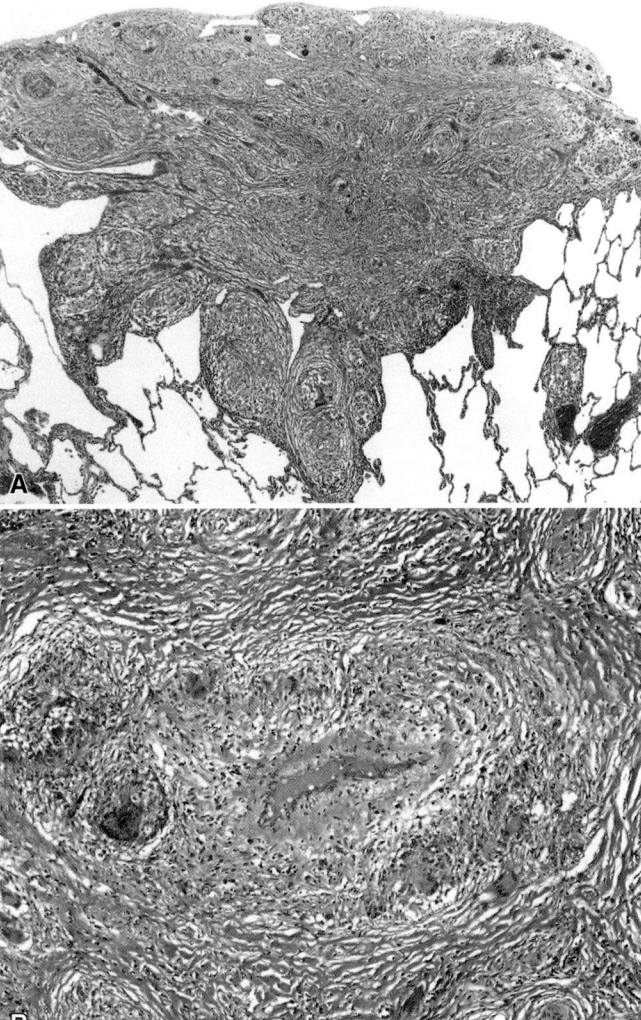

Figure 7-78. Sarcoidosis. **A,** Granulomas are distributed along lymphatic routes in the pleura, within the intralobular septa, and along the bronchovascular bundles. This image is diagnostic of sarcoidosis, but berylliosis should always be included as a diagnostic possibility. **B,** Perivascular granulomas embedded in sclerosis are commonly seen. Despite this potential for vasocentric growth, pulmonary hypertension is an uncommon complication of sarcoidosis.

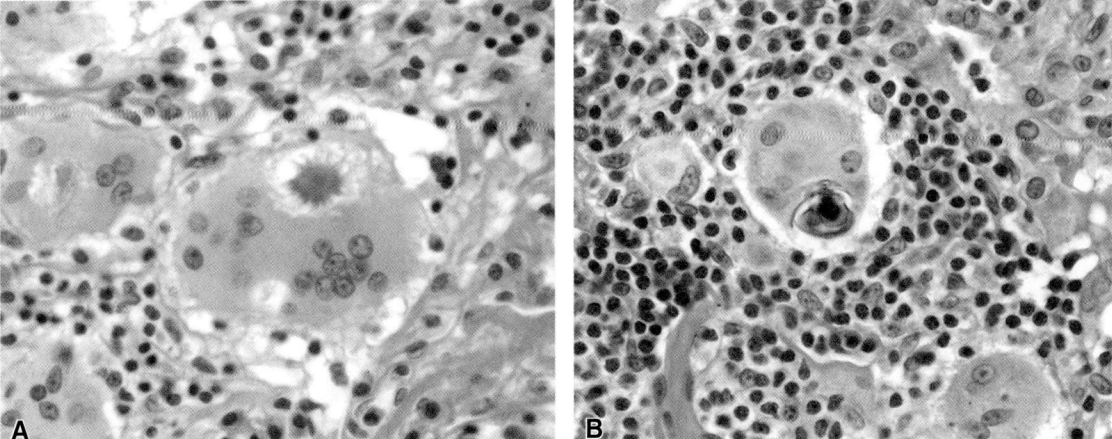

Figure 7-79. Sarcoidosis. Multinucleate giant cells characteristically are present, often accompanied by a variety of distinctive (but not specific) cytoplasmic inclusions: **A,** asteroid body; **B,** Schaumann body.

Continued

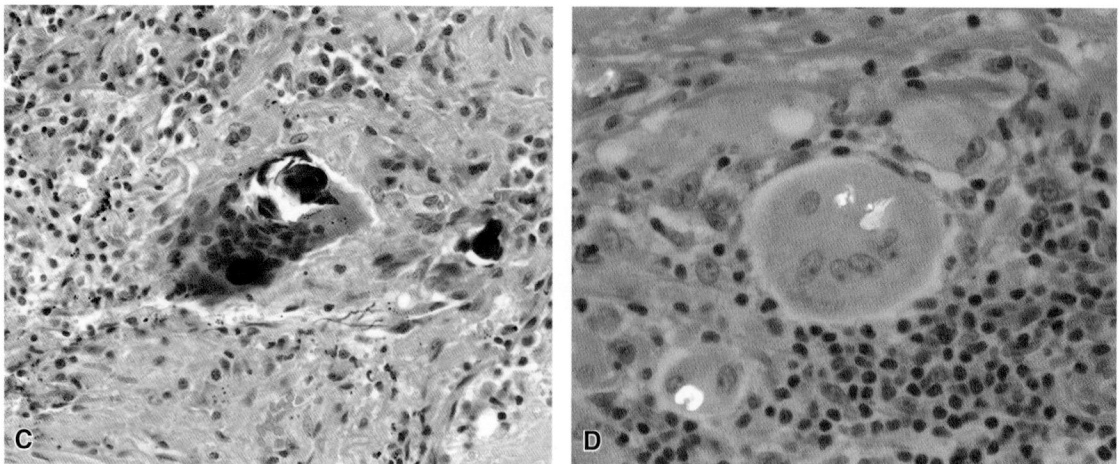

Figure 7-79—cont'd. C, Schaumann (conchoidal) bodies; **D,** Schaumann body in polarized light.

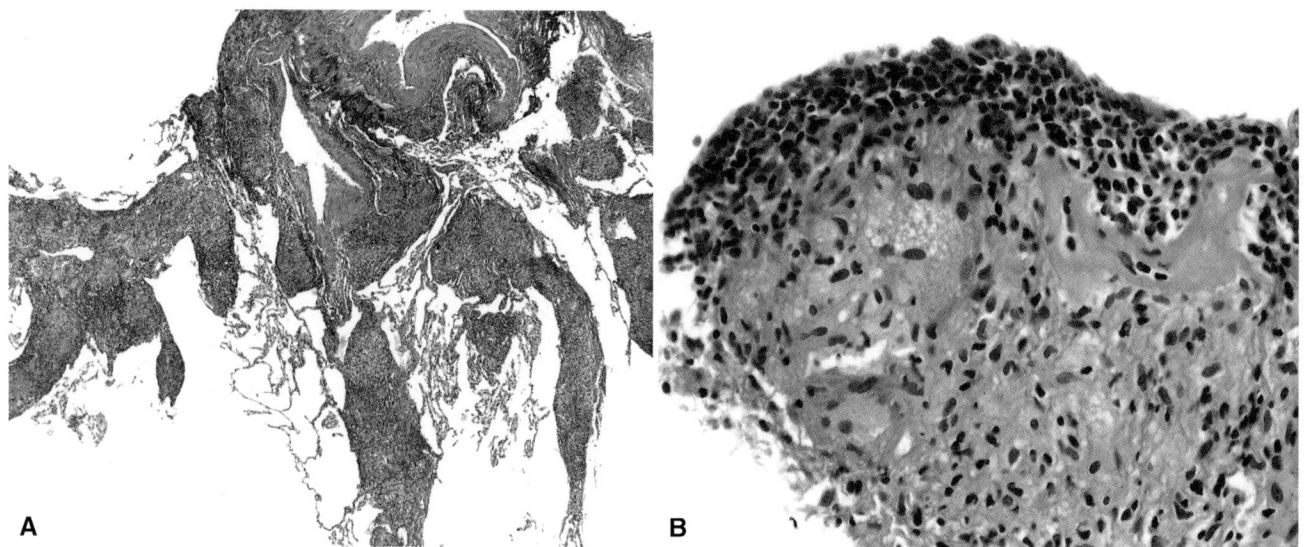

Figure 7-80. Sarcoidosis. In bronchoscopic or transbronchial biopsies, granulomas may be quite dramatic in appearance (**A**), but sometimes the histopathologic pattern is more subtle. **B,** In bronchial mucosal biopsies, lesions typically are present in the immediate subepithelial region of the airway.

be associated with granuloma formation, but these tend to resemble foreign body–type granulomas with characteristic multinucleate giant cells, often containing foreign material (partially digested food, primarily).

Chronic Berylliosis

Beryllium, derived from the mineral beryl, is the etiologic agent for berylliosis.[324–326] The disease occurs after inhalation of this metal or its salts.[327] Exposure to beryllium occurs today mainly as an occupational lung disease, particularly in the computer manufacturing and aerospace engineering fields. However, recent reports indicate that individuals with low-level exposure, such as residents living near facilities that use beryllium, can also develop berylliosis[328–330] (for additional discussion, see Chapter 8).

Acute berylliosis occurs after heavy exposure; fortunately, it is rare today as a consequence of strict industrial exposure regulations and aggressive surveillance in this setting. When acute berylliosis occurs, the histopathologic findings are similar to those of DAD. The chronic form of berylliosis is indistinguishable from sarcoidosis on histopathologic

grounds.[324–326] Like sarcoidosis, chronic berylliosis produces fibrosis of variable severity and has distinct granulomas with giant cells (Fig. 7-81). Chronic berylliosis may produce large, centrally hyalinized nodules (Fig. 7-82), which can mimick resolved lesions of histoplasmosis. When granulomas are less prominent, chronic berylliosis may also simulate hypersensitivity pneumonitis histopathologically (Fig. 7-83).

Hypersensitivity Pneumonitis (Extrinsic Allergic Alveolitis)

Environmental antigens (typically, "organic" protein antigens) are known to produce characteristic inflammatory reactions in the lung in certain predisposed individuals.[331–334] The classic descriptions of *farmer's lung*, resulting from exposure to thermophilic actinomycetes in hay, and *bird fancier's lung*, resulting from inhalation from avian antigens, are examples of hypersensitivity pneumonitis. Similar reactions to ingested antigens associated with some medications can also occur, but in general usage, hypersensitivity pneumonitis refers to disease occurring as a result of inhalation exposure. The more common antigens implicated in hypersensitivity pneumonitis are presented in Table 7-7.

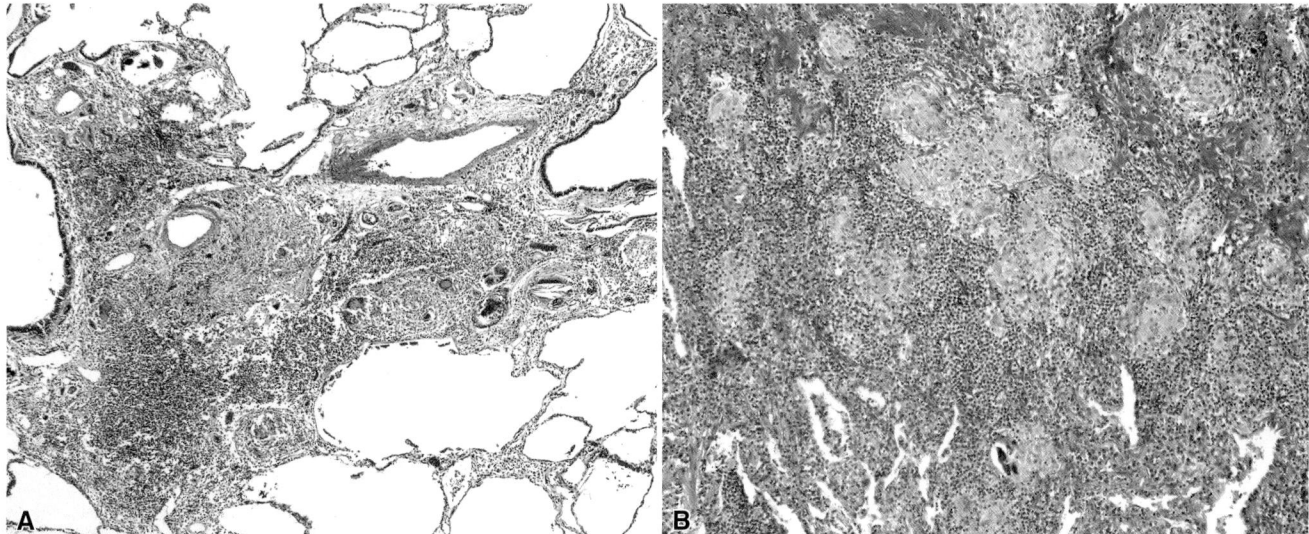

Figure 7-81. Berylliosis. Like sarcoidosis, chronic berylliosis produces variable fibrosis (**A**) and distinct granulomas with giant cells (**B**). There may be a suggestion of more lymphocytic inflammation, but this finding is not sufficiently reliable to be useful diagnostically.

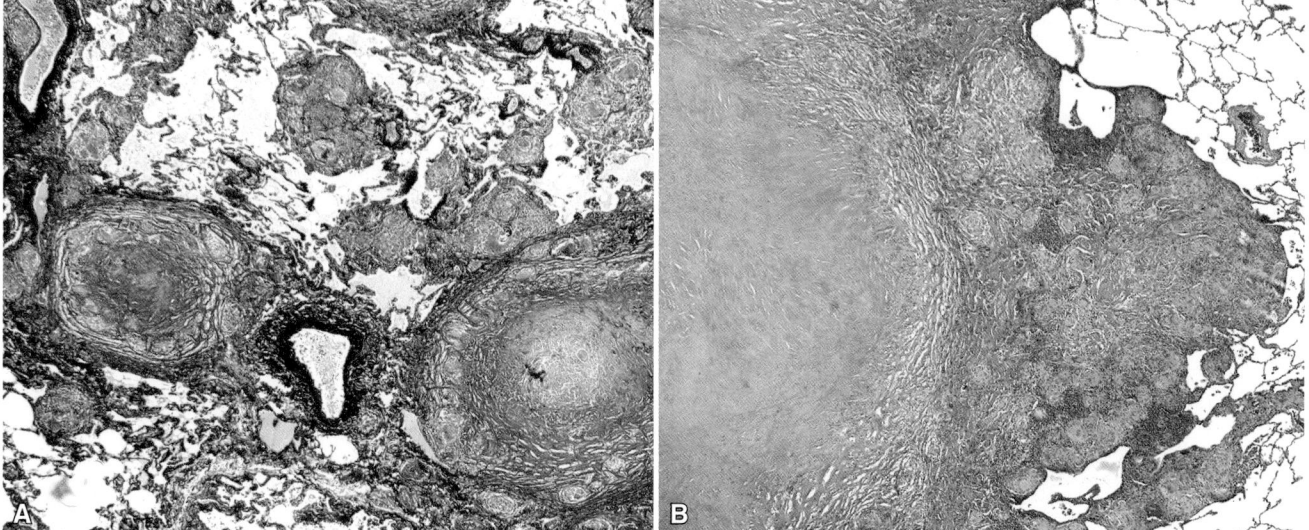

Figure 7-82. Berylliosis. **A** and **B**, Chronic berylliosis may produce large, centrally hyalinized nodules, which can mimick resolved lesions of histoplasmosis.

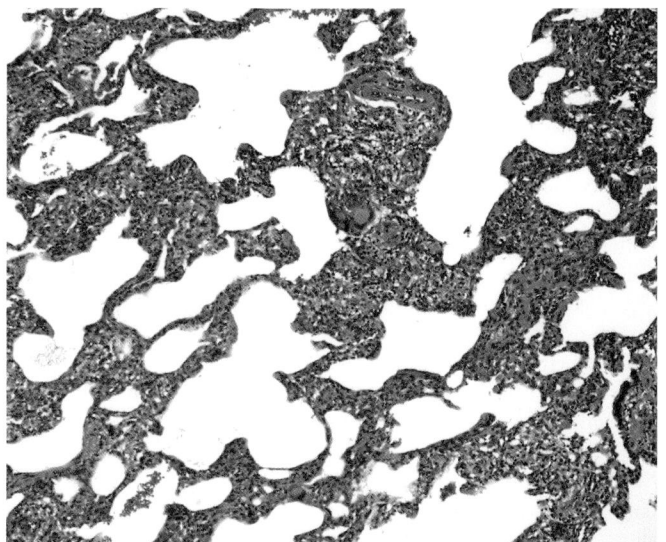

Figure 7-83. Berylliosis. When granulomas are less prominent, as in this specimen, hypersensitivity pneumonitis may enter the differential diagnosis.

Clinical Presentation

Hypersensitivity pneumonitis can occur as acute or subacute and chronic forms. The acute form occurs within hours of inhalational exposure to antigen. Affected individuals experience malaise, dyspnea, dry cough, and, occasionally, fever and chills. With this symptom complex, the differential diagnosis will include viral infection. Recurrence of symptoms and signs follows subsequent exposure episodes.[335] Women are more commonly affected than men. Cigarette smoking seems to reduce the risk of developing hypersensitivity, although the mechanism for this protective effect is unknown.[336]

The chronic form of hypersensitivity pneumonitis probably results from lower levels of antigen exposure over time, presumably accompanied by more subtle symptoms, so that the affected person may not associate the symptom with a specific exposure.[335,337] The frequency of disease occurrence in smokers and men is higher in the chronic form than in the acute and subacute forms of the disease. Unfortunately, the chronic form of hypersensitivity pneumonitis may be progressive, eventuating in death from end-stage lung fibrosis.[335,337] As in the acute phase, patients experience chronic malaise and varying degrees of breathlessness on exertion, sometimes accompanied by weight loss. Several excellent reviews of hypersensitivity pneumonitis are available.[333–335,337,338]

Table 7-7. Agents of Hypersensitivity Pneumonitis (Extrinsic Allergic Alveolitis)

Antigen	Source	Disease
Thermophilic bacteria		
Micropolyspora faeni	Moldy hay	Farmer's lung
Thermoactinomyces vulgaris	Moldy compost	Mushroom worker's disease
Thermoactinomyces saccharii	Moldy sugar cane	Bagassosis
Thermoactinomyces vulgaris	Air conditioners, humidifiers	Air conditioner lung/humidifier lung
Thermoactinomyces candidus	Air conditioners, humidifiers	Air conditioner lung/humidifier lung
Molds		
Cryptostroma corticale	Moldy maple bark	Maple bark stripper's disease
Aspergillus clavatus	Moldy barley	Malt worker's lung
Graphium spp.	Moldy wood dust	Sequoiosis
Pullularia spp.	Moldy wood dust	Sequoiosis
Trichosporon cutaneum	Home environment	Summer-type hypersensitivity pneumonitis (Japan)
Other bacteria		
Bacillus subtilis	Water	Detergent worker's lung
Bacillus cereus	Water	Humidifier lung
Bacterial products	Cotton	Byssinosis
Amebae	Water	Humidifier lung
Insect products	Grain	Wheat weevil disease
Chemicals		
Trimellitic anhydride (TMA)	Plastics, rubber manufacturing	Chemical worker's lung
Methylene diisocyanate (MDI)	Plastics, rubber manufacturing	Chemical worker's lung
Toluene diisocyanate (TDI)	Plastics, rubber manufacturing	Chemical worker's lung
Pyromellitic dianhydride (PMDA)	Epoxy resin	Chemical worker's lung

Reprinted with permission from Katzenstein A, Askin F, eds. *Surgical Pathology of Non-Neoplastic Lung Disease,* 2nd ed. Philadelphia: WB Saunders; 1990:139.

Radiologic Findings

In acute hypersensitivity pneumonitis, a diffuse ground-glass appearance is seen on CT scans of the chest, sometimes accompanied by fine nodules.[339] In subacute disease, abnormalities tend to be confined to the upper one half or two thirds of the lung and are characterized radiologically as *ill-defined centrilobular nodules.* In more chronic forms, small nodules, variable ground-glass change, and irregular linear opacities may be seen, most often in the middle lung zones (with relative sparing of the apices and bases) or without a specific zonal predilection.[23] The presence of irregular linear opacities correlates with the presence of lung fibrosis.[335,338] In very-late-stage chronic hypersensitivity pneumonitis, honeycomb remodeling may be identified radiologically, mimicking UIP.[23,24] Interestingly, the CT appearance of subacute hypersensitivity pneumonitis may be indistinguishable from that in low-grade atypical mycobacterial infection occurring in the immunocompetent host as a result of bioaerosol exposure to non-tuberculous mycobacteria[340,341] (so-called "hot tub lung"; see Chapter 6).

Histopathologic Findings

The histopathologic features of hypersensitivity pneumonitis are typically those of a chronic inflammatory interstitial pneumonia associated with bronchiolitis, and small, indistinct, non-necrotizing *interstitial* granulomas[331,342,343] (Fig. 7-84). In early reports of farmer's lung, acute inflammation and vasculitis were also observed.[344] The histopathology of hypersensitivity pneumonitis raises a differential diagnosis that includes other cellular interstitial pneumonias, such as NSIP. At low magnification, the surgical lung biopsy shows a moderately dense interstitial infiltrate, composed of plasma cells and small lymphocytes, causing slight widening of the alveolar walls (Fig. 7-85). A bronchiolocentric distribution may be evident, either by the presence of a terminal bronchiole or by some degree of nodularity in the infiltrates at low magnification (Fig. 7-86). The interstitial "granulomas" of hypersensitivity pneumonitis are inconspicuous (Fig. 7-87) and may easily escape notice in many cases. Multinucleate giant cells (Fig. 7-88) may be seen in the interstitium at scanning magnification and constitute a helpful feature in prompting closer examination of the interstitium for epithelioid histiocytes in small aggregates. Necrosis is not a component of the granulomatous reaction in hypersensitivity pneumonitis. Air space organization (Fig. 7-89) with immature fibroblast and matrix (organizing pneumonia pattern) can be seen in as many as 60% of patients with hypersensitivity pneumonitis.[342] In general, this is not confluent organization, as seen in organizing pneumonia of infectious etiology. Rather, small, tufted patches of organization can be seen scattered throughout the lung biopsy. Some degree of bronchiolitis is expected in hypersensitivity pneumonitis; this is characterized by aggregates of lymphocytes and plasma cells surrounding terminal airways (Fig. 7-90). A mild perivascular lymphoid accumulation typically is present in hypersensitivity pneumonitis, but prominent germinal centers or dense lymphoplasmacellular infiltration along vascular sheaths (especially veins in the interlobular septa) are not typical and should raise concern for lymphoproliferative disease (which on occasion can simulate the cellular phase of chronic hypersensitivity pneumonitis). In the chronic form, dense fibrosis with microscopic honeycombing can be seen (Fig. 7-91). Peribronchiolar metaplasia along with peribronchiolar fibrosis is frequent. There may be bridging formations between peribronchiolar areas and subpleural scar, analogous to "bridging fibrosis" in liver disease.[345] Refractile oxalate crystals in giant cells may be sufficiently prominent to suggest aspiration pneumonia or even pneumoconiosis (Fig. 7-92).

Clinical Course

The clinical course in hypersensitivity pneumonitis varies with the intensity and chronicity of exposure.[335,344,346] If an offending antigen cannot be identified in the patient's environment, the prognosis is guarded since patients may not respond to corticosteroid therapy in the continued presence of the initiating antigen.[347–351] Once lung fibrosis ensues, immunosuppressive therapy is of little benefit, especially if continued antigen exposure occurs.[351]

Differential Diagnosis

Cellular interstitial pneumonias with or without small non-necrotizing granulomas can be a component of drug reactions and low-grade infections (especially those produced by atypical mycobacterial species). Whether true hypersensitivity pneumonitis can occur due to ingestion of drugs is controversial. Early sarcoidosis is included in the differential diagnosis, but the presence of more characteristic, well-formed granulomas of sarcoidosis and the presence of sclerotic fibrous tissue matrix surrounding granulomas is helpful in differentiating sarcoidosis from hypersensitivity pneumonitis. Also, interstitial inflammation can be seen in sarcoidosis, but it is exceedingly mild, if present at all. As mentioned earlier, when lymphoplasmacellular infiltrates are dense or confluent, LIP or low-grade malignant

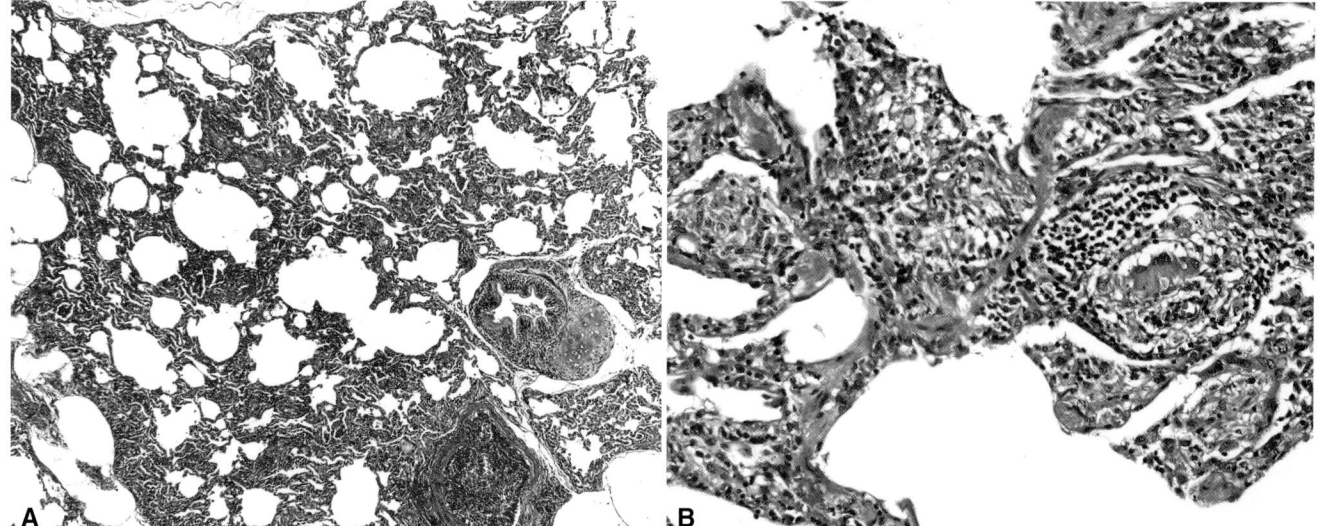

Figure 7-84. Hypersensitivity pneumonitis. This pathologic process manifests as a chronic inflammatory interstitial pneumonia associated with bronchiolitis (**A**) and small, indistinct, non-necrotizing interstitial granulomas (**B**).

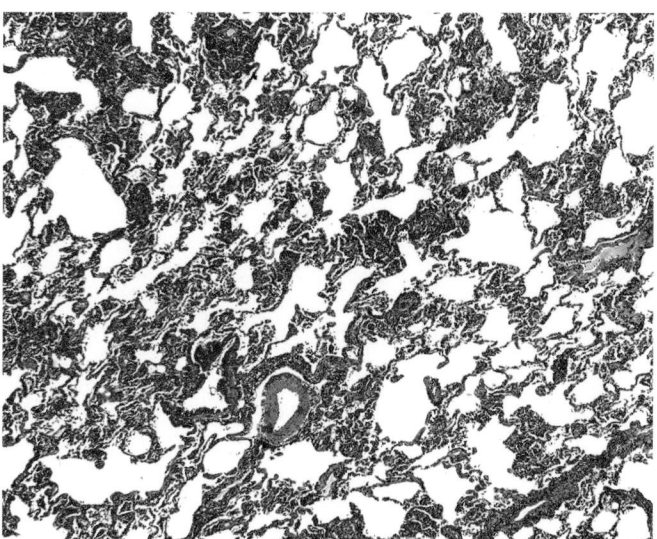

Figure 7-85. Hypersensitivity pneumonitis. At low magnification, the surgical lung biopsy shows a moderately dense interstitial infiltrate, causing slight widening of the alveolar walls.

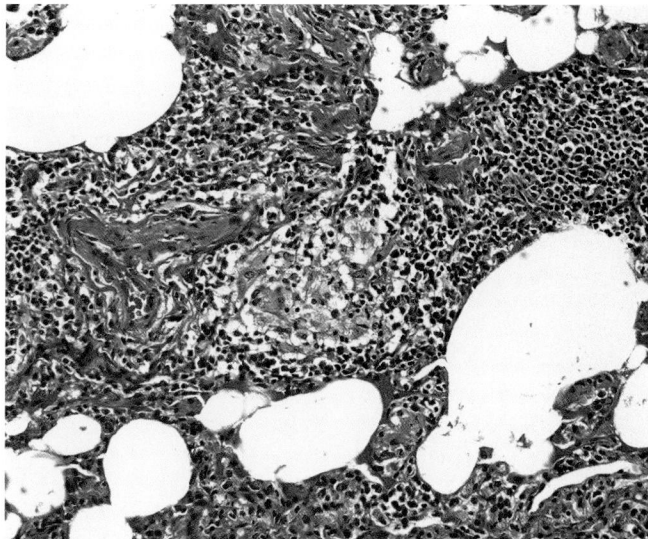

Figure 7-87. Hypersensitivity pneumonitis. The characteristic interstitial "granulomas" are sufficiently vague in appearance as to escape notice in many cases. Prominent, well-formed granulomas are not a typical manifestation of the disease.

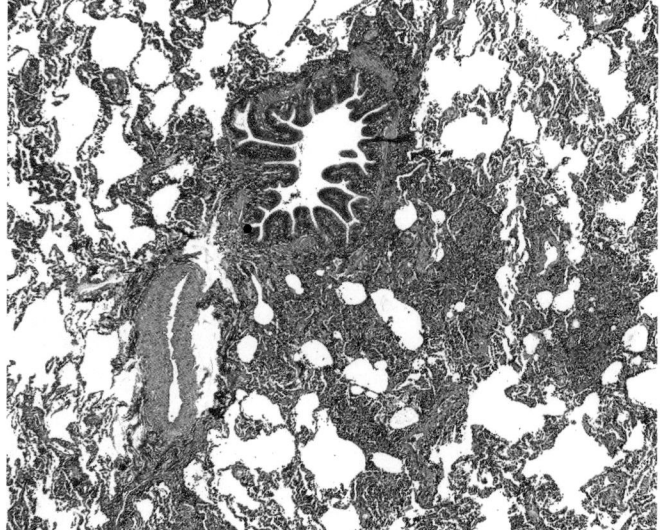

Figure 7-86. Hypersensitivity pneumonitis. A bronchiolocentric distribution may be evident, as indicated either by the presence of a terminal bronchiole or by some degree of nodularity to the infiltrates at low magnification.

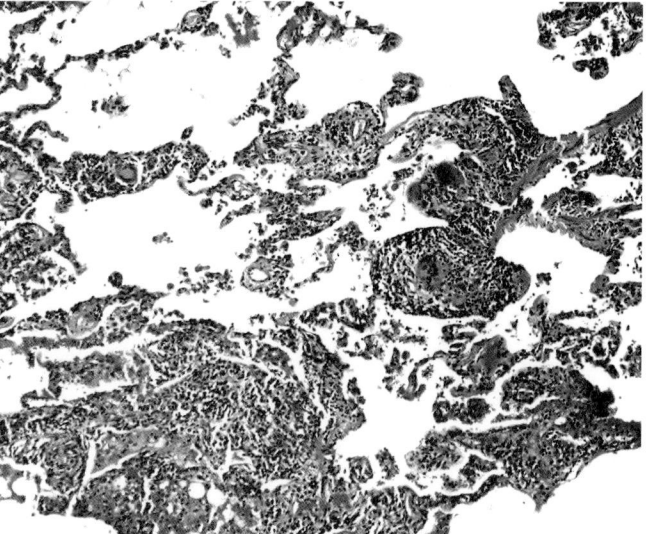

Figure 7-88. Hypersensitivity pneumonitis. Multinucleate giant cells may also be seen in the interstitium and constitute a helpful feature at low magnification in drawing the eye to features meriting closer examination.

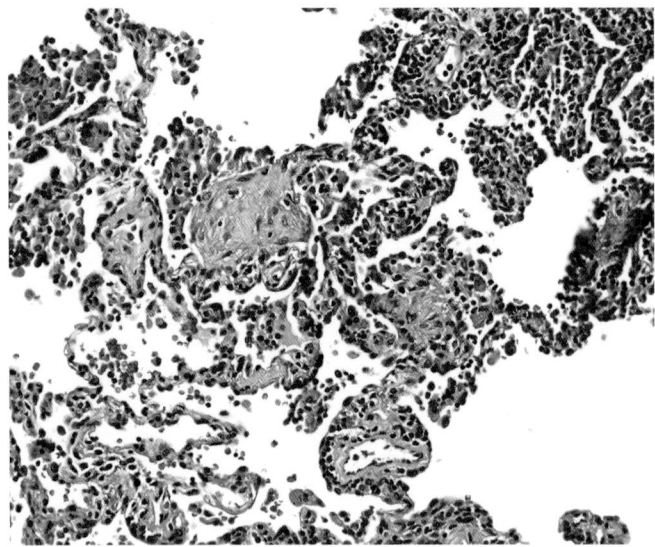

Figure 7-89. Hypersensitivity pneumonitis. Patchy air space organization can be seen in as many as 60% of affected patients.

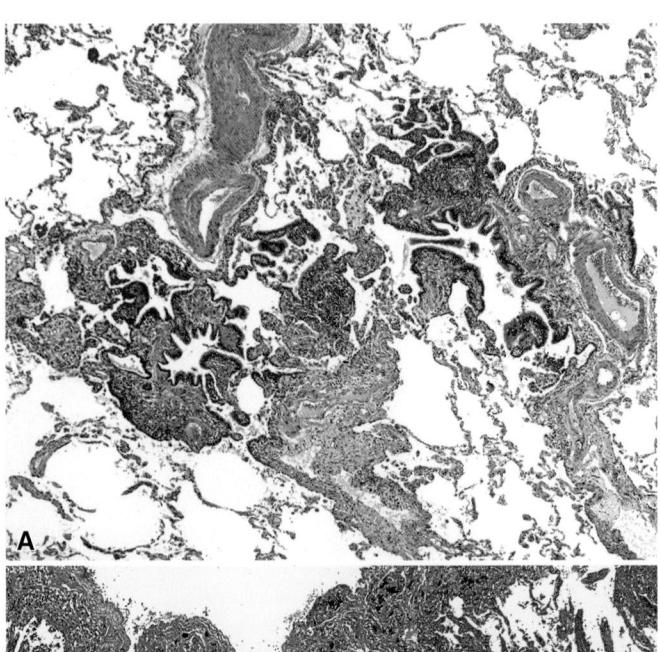

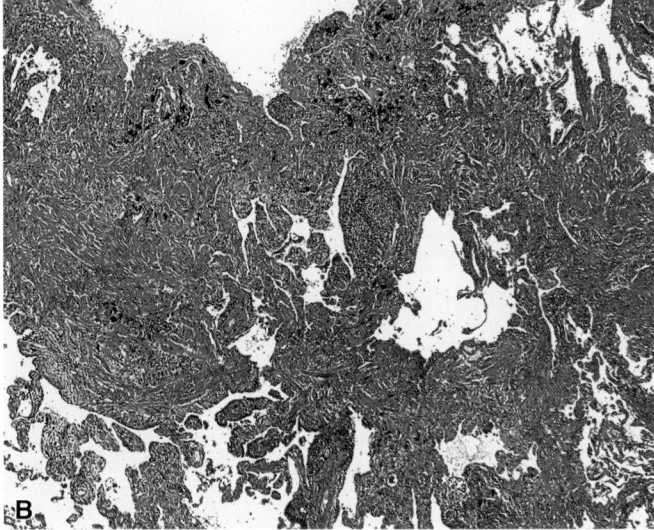

Figure 7-91. Hypersensitivity pneumonitis. **A,** In chronic hypersensitivity pneumonitis, prominent bronchiolization ("Lambertosis") attests to chronic airway injury from inhaled antigen. **B,** Dense fibrosis with microscopic honeycombing resembling that in usual interstitial pneumonia may also be seen.

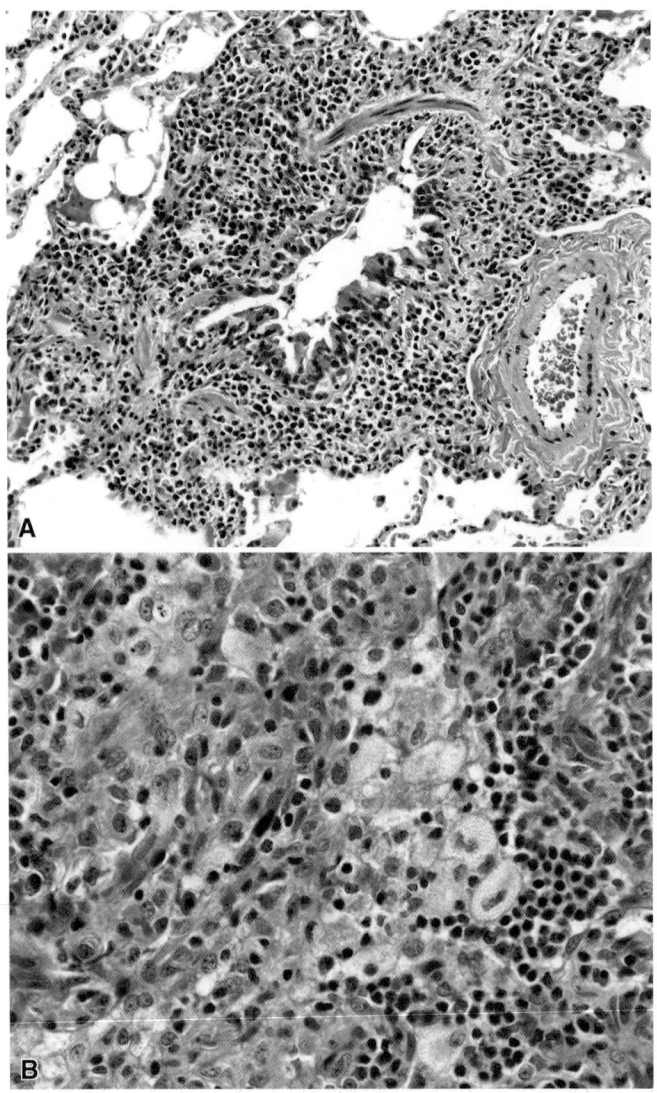

Figure 7-90. Hypersensitivity pneumonitis. **A,** Bronchiolitis, an expected feature in this disorder, is manifested here as aggregates of lymphocytes and plasma cells surrounding a terminal airway. **B,** Presumably, as a consequence of bronchiolitis and some degree of obstruction, prominently vacuolated macrophages may be present in a bronchiolocentric distribution.

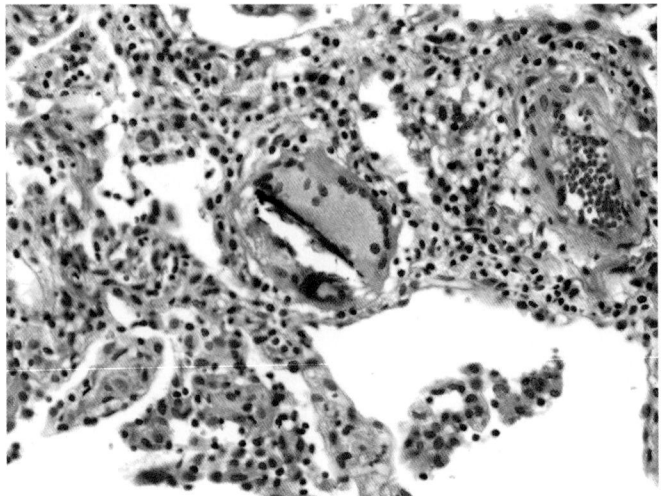

Figure 7-92. Hypersensitivity pneumonitis. Refractile oxalate crystals in giant cells may be sufficiently prominent to suggest aspiration pneumonia or even pneumoconiosis.

lymphoma of MALT enters the differential diagnosis. In the latter situation, immunohistochemical stains (CD20, CD3, kappa and lambda immunoglobulin light chains) may be helpful in demonstrating a predominance of CD20-positive B lymphocytes, or a lambda light chain predominance; such findings should raise serious consideration of malignant lymphoma.

Miscellaneous Diffuse Lung Diseases

Pulmonary Langerhans Cell Histiocytosis

In addition to smoking-related ILD (i.e., RBILD, as described earlier in the chapter), another important consequence of smoking is *pulmonary Langerhans cells histiocytosis* (PLCH), a lung disease previously referred to as "pulmonary eosinophilic granuloma" or "pulmonary histiocytosis X." PLCH is considered to be a reactive proliferative disease of Langerhans cells,[352,353] in contrast to extrapulmonary forms of Langerhans cell histiocytosis, which are thought to be neoplasms.[354] A compelling association with cigarette smoking has led to the general acceptance of this lung disorder as a smoking-related disease.[355,356] The pathobiology of PLCH has been comprehensively reviewed by Vassalo and associates.[353] Although PLCH is unrelated to the systemic diseases of Langerhans cells (eosinophilic granuloma, Letterer-Siwi disease, Hand-Schüller-Christian disease), systemic eosinophilic granuloma involving the lung, when it occurs, is said to be indistinguishable from the cellular phase of PLCH on histopathologic grounds.[357]

Two distinctive histopathologic manifestations of PLCH occur—a cellular form and a fibrotic form. The natural history of PLCH suggests that the early lesions of PLCH are cellular, with many Langerhans cells and tissue eosinophils, whereas older lesions are predominantly fibrotic. Such a natural progression may occur continuously in the same patient, with "younger" cellular lesions admixed with "older" ones, but in most surgical biopsy specimens, one form of the disease seems to predominate.[353] Often the fibrotic lesions of the disease are not recognized because of the paucity or absence of Langerhans cells, and the proliferative lesions are typically mistaken for neoplasm.

Clinical Presentation

The true incidence and prevalence of PLCH are unknown. Most patients are between 20 and 50 years of age at the onset of symptoms; women may be more commonly affected than men.[353,355,358] Chronic cough and dyspnea are typical presenting complaints. However, a significant percentage of patients are asymptomatic. Rarely, hemoptysis or pneumothorax can occur.

Radiologic Findings

PLCH is a disease of the upper lung zones. Small nodules and cysts are present to a variable degree as seen on plain films of the chest.[358–361] The nodules range in size from 0.2 to 1 cm. When fibrosis occurs, it is best seen on high-resolution CT scans and appears as reticular opacities.[360,362] When significant fibrosis occurs in PLCH, the disease may simulate IPF.[359,360,362]

Histopathologic Findings

Proliferative (Cellular) Phase

At scanning magnification, the nodules of PLCH have a stellate appearance and are centered on the small airways (Fig. 7-93). Cysts are formed at the periphery of nodules by traction on surrounding alveolar walls or the central terminal airway, resulting in variably sized spaces, typically lacking distinctive lining cells (Fig. 7-94). Stellate cellular nodules may be as large as 1.5 cm,[357] and confluence of nodules affecting adjacent

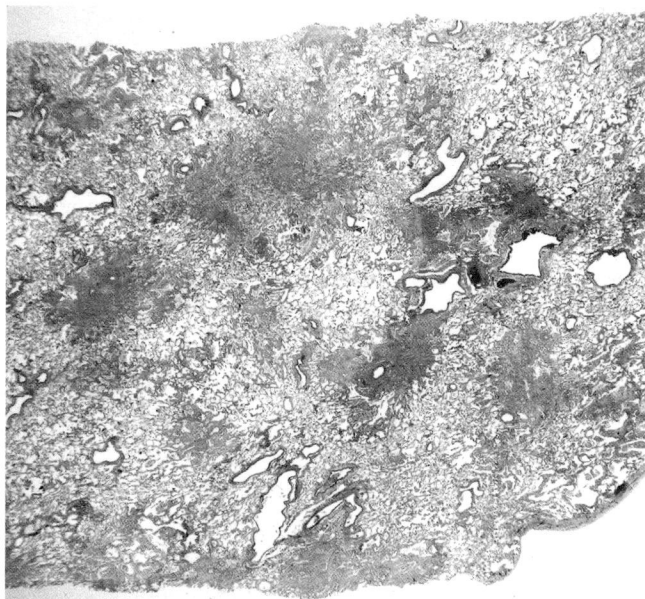

Figure 7-93. Pulmonary Langerhans cell histiocytosis. At scanning magnification, the characteristic nodules have a stellate appearance and are centered on the small airways.

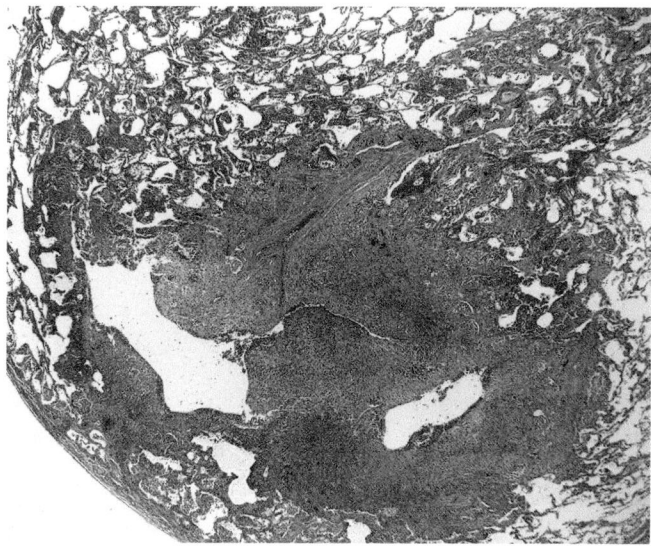

Figure 7-94. Pulmonary Langerhans cell histiocytosis. The characteristic cysts are formed by traction on surrounding alveolar walls or the central terminal airway, resulting in variably sized spaces, typically lacking distinctive lining cells.

airways may impart a serpentine outline to the lesions (Fig. 7-95). As suggested by a three-dimensional reconstruction study, the lesions of PLCH seem to form a sheath around the small airways exclusively and extend proximally and distally in a continuous fashion.[363] In many cases, lightly pigmented brown macrophages ("smoker's macrophages") are present in and around the nodules (Fig. 7-96). Eosinophils in variable numbers occupy the next innermost layer of the nodules (Fig. 7-97); this is the location in which aggregated Langerhans cells are most easily found in the thickened interstitium (Fig. 7-98). The Langerhans cells have a pale basophilic nucleus with characteristic sharp nuclear infoldings, imparting a "crumpled tissue paper" nuclear contour (Fig. 7-99). The cytoplasm of the Langerhans cell is granular and mildly eosinophilic, with indistinct margins. In these cellular lesions of PLCH, immunohistochemical stains for S100 protein and CD1a can be used to highlight the presence of Langerhans cells (Fig. 7-100), but in most instances, the morphology

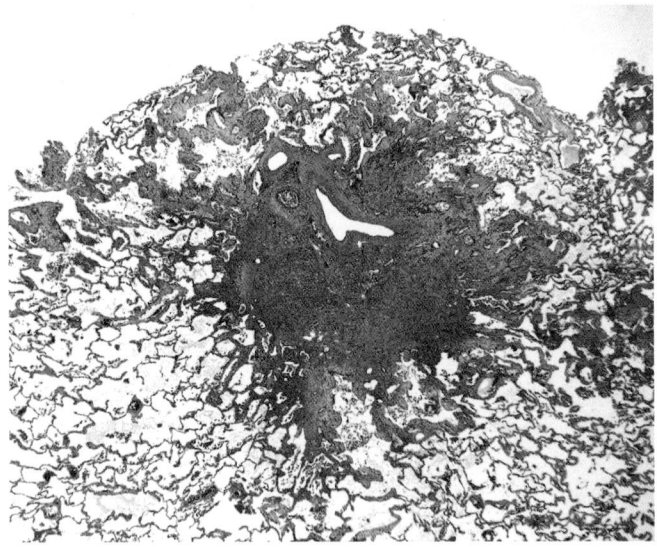

Figure 7-95. Pulmonary Langerhans cell histiocytosis. The characteristic stellate cellular nodules may be as large as 1.5 cm in diameter.

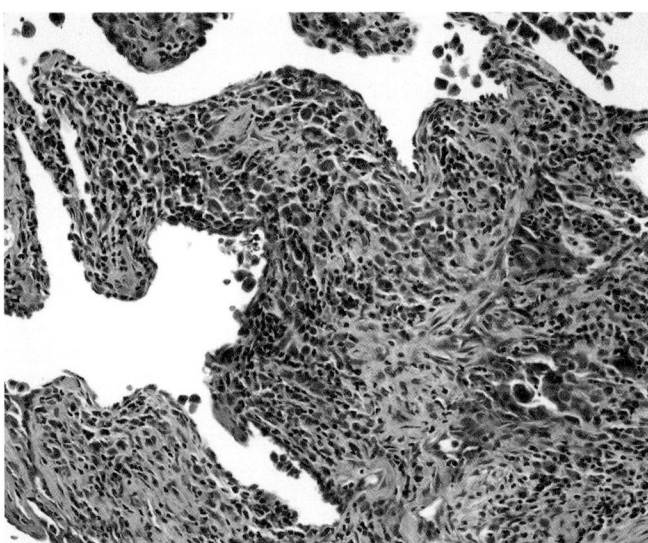

Figure 7-97. Pulmonary Langerhans cell histiocytosis. Eosinophils in variable numbers occupy the next innermost layer of the nodules.

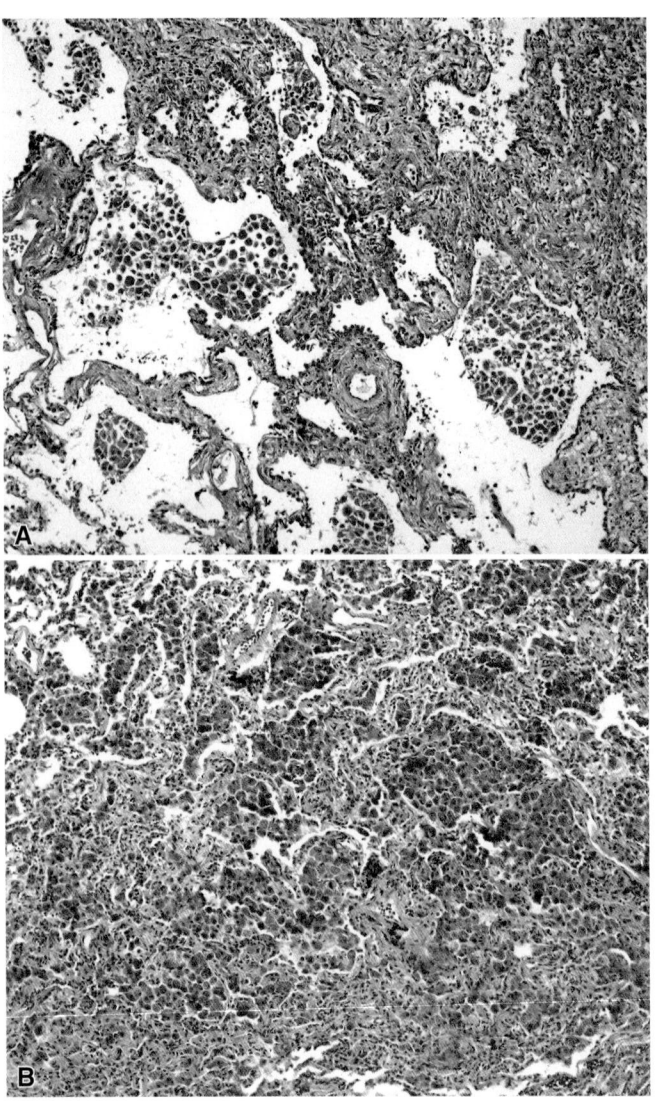

Figure 7-96. Pulmonary Langerhans cell histiocytosis. **A** and **B,** In many cases, a rim of lightly pigmented, brown macrophages ("smoker's macrophages") is present within and around the nodules.

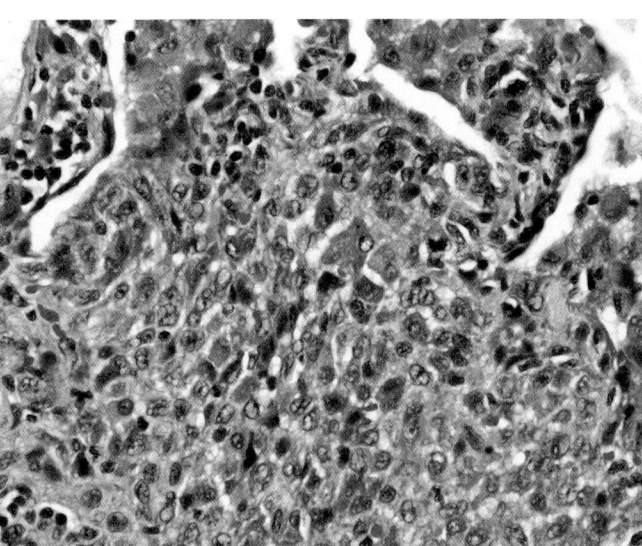

Figure 7-98. Pulmonary Langerhans cell histiocytosis. Aggregates of Langerhans cells are most readily found in the thickened interstitium of the stellate ramifications of the lesions.

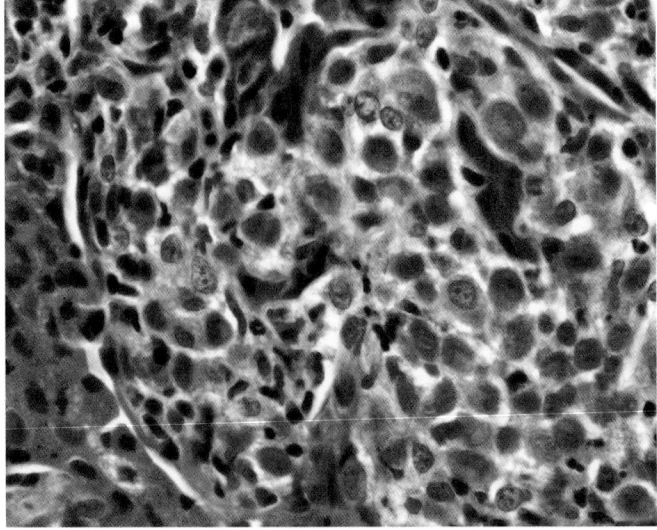

Figure 7-99. Pulmonary Langerhans cell histiocytosis. The Langerhans cells have a pale nucleus with characteristic sharp nuclear infoldings, imparting a "crumpled tissue paper" outline. The cytoplasm is variably eosinophilic and indistinct.

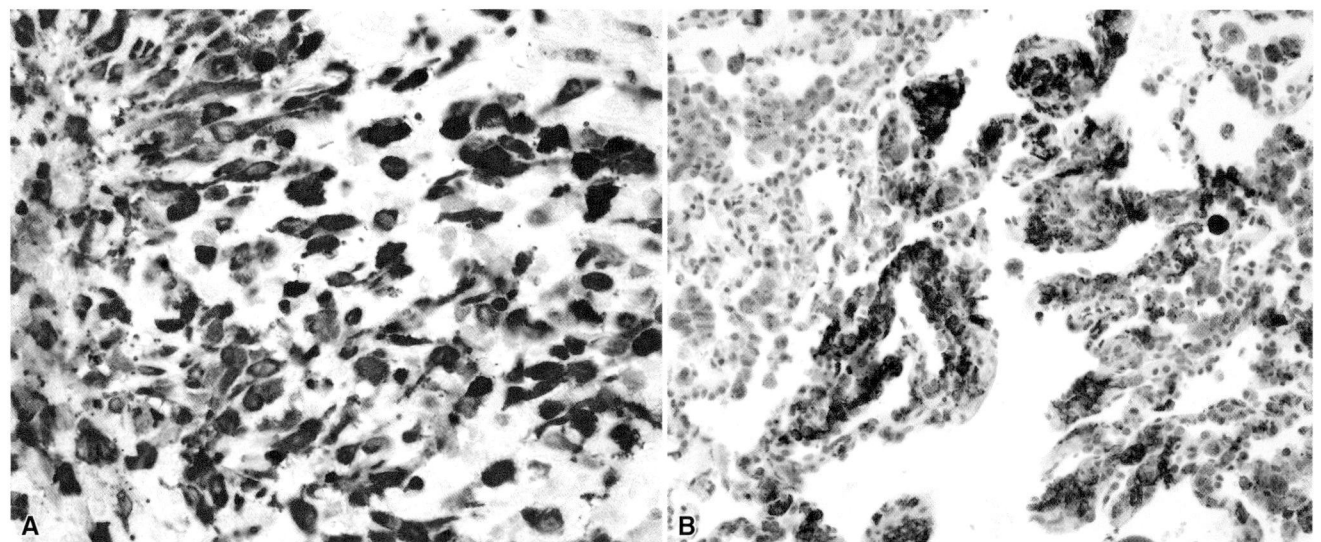

Figure 7-100. Pulmonary Langerhans cell histiocytosis (PLCH). In the cellular lesions of PLCH, immunohistochemical stains for S100 protein (**A**) and CD1a (**B**) can be used to highlight the presence of Langerhans cells (immunohistochemical stains; red chromogen). In most cases, however, the morphology of the lesions is sufficiently compelling that a definitive diagnosis can be established without the aid of special stains.

of the lesions is sufficiently compelling enough for a definitive diagnosis to be established without the aid of special stains. In some cases, patchy interstitial and air space organization (Fig. 7-101) may be seen, and RB is typically present. Other smoking-related lung changes may be present, adding further complexity to the morphologic picture (e.g., DIP/RBILD, small-airway disease with mucostasis, areas of bronchiolization).

Fibrotic Lesions

With "aging" of the lesions of PLCH, Langerhans cells become progressively depleted and overshadowed by fibrosis (Fig. 7-102). The mechanism for this transformation is unknown. In some patients, only residual stellate parenchymal scars are found, and in these patients, pulmonary function may be significantly compromised (by a process analogous to constrictive bronchiolitis). Lung function and radiologic studies may suggest a diffuse lung disease, but biopsy tissue may exhibit only stellate fibrotic lesions centered on the terminal airways, without an identifiable interstitial inflammatory disease (Fig. 7-103). Another scenario in

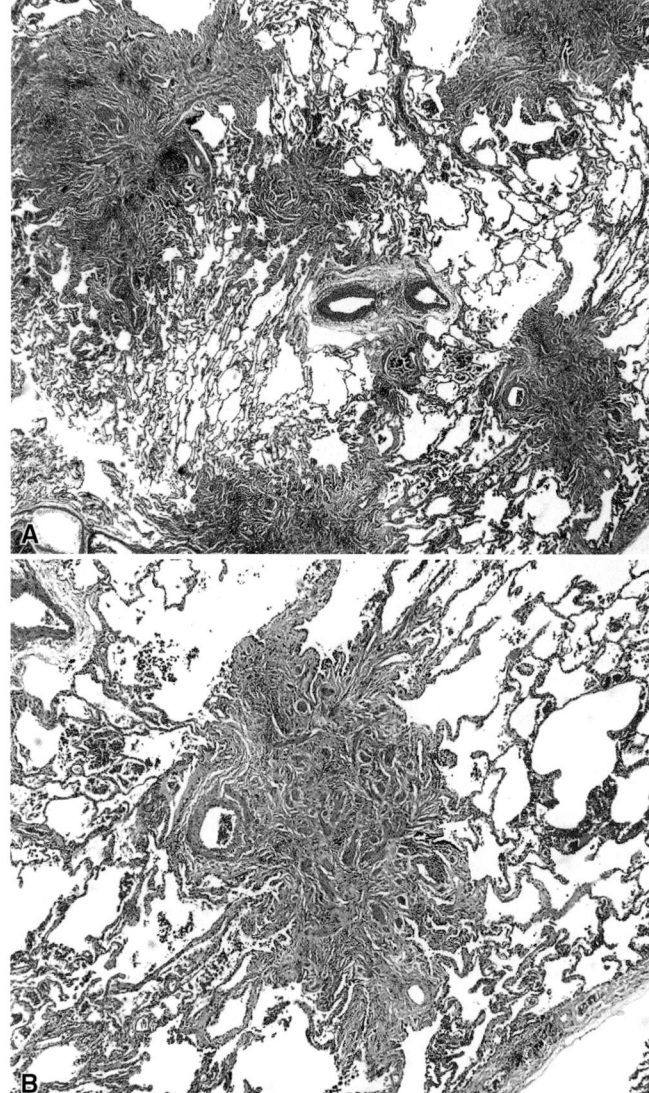

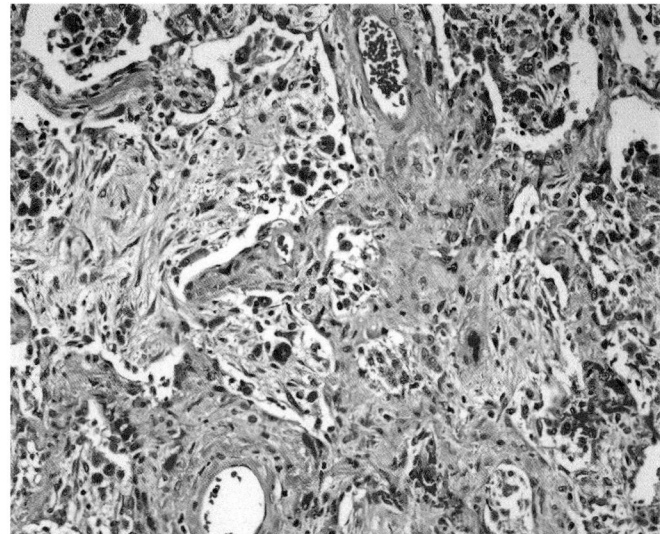

Figure 7-101. Pulmonary Langerhans cell histiocytosis. In some cases, patchy air space organization may be present, but it is not a particularly characteristic feature of the disease.

Figure 7-102. Pulmonary Langerhans cell histiocytosis (PLCH). As the lesions of PLCH "age," they become progressively fibrotic (**A**), and Langerhans cells become depleted and replaced by fibrosis (**B**).

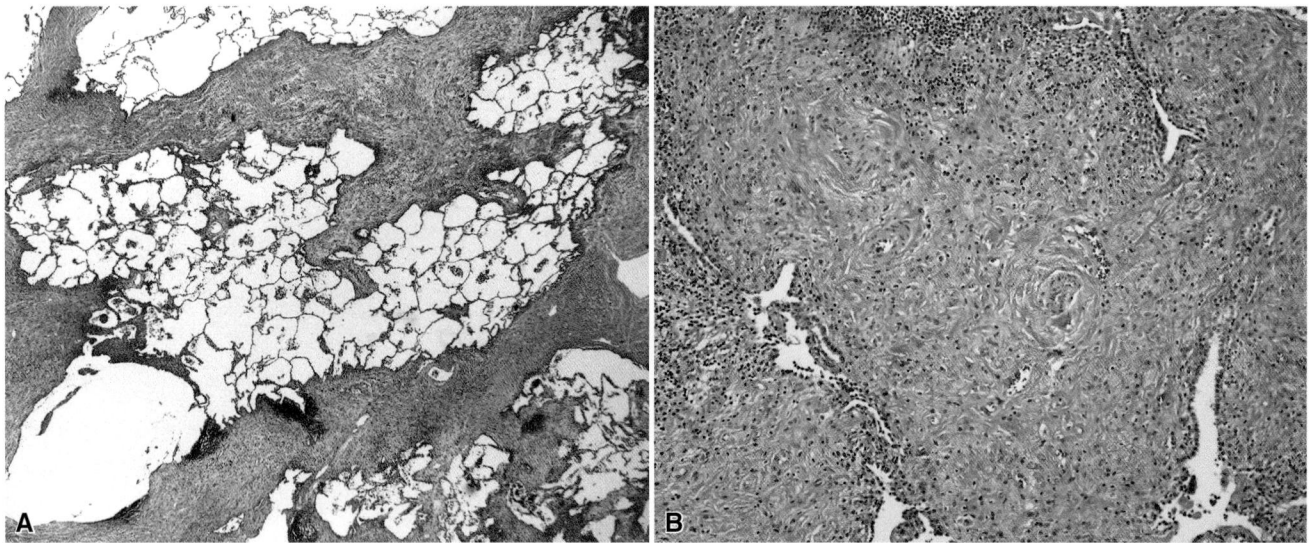

Figure 7-103. Erdheim-Chester disease. **A,** In surgical wedge lung biopsies or resected lung lobes, a distinctive pattern of pleural and septal fibrosis is evident, with a distinctive lymphatic distribution. **B,** Admixed lymphoid aggregates are typical. The interface with surrounding lung is generally abrupt.

which such scars can be seen is in portions of lung removed for other reasons (e.g., bronchogenic carcinoma). Presumably these "footprints" of previous PLCH are incidental findings and do not necessarily imply active disease elsewhere in the lung.

Differential Diagnosis
Nodular infections and neoplasm are common in the differential diagnosis radiologically, the latter especially in the setting of known breast carcinoma in a young woman undergoing screening for metastatic disease to the lungs. Pathologically, the proliferative lesions may be mistaken for neoplasm as well, but careful attention to the layered or zonal composition of the nodules and the distinctive morphology of the Langerhans cells will typically bring the diagnosis of PLCH to the forefront. When cysts are prominent, lymphangioleiomyomatosis (LAM) enters the differential diagnosis (see further on). In this setting, immunohistochemical stains may be useful in establishing the correct diagnosis (S100 protein immunoreactivity in Langerhans cells versus HMB45 and actin in LAM cells). Other nodular lung diseases are occasionally confused with PLCH, including Wegener granulomatosis, Hodgkin disease, and certain metastatic low-grade sarcomas. When fibrotic lesions are dominant, UIP (clinical IPF) and other fibrosing lung disorders may be suggested. Helpful distinguishing features include the stellate appearance of the PLCH lesion, the tendency for lesions to spare the pleura and immediate subpleural lung, and the association of scars with the airways. Rarely, pneumothorax (from any cause) can produce subpleural fibrosis with sheets of tissue eosinophils (so-called "reactive eosinophilic pleuritis").[364,365] Such lesions are not usually confused with PLCH but on occasion may be the only pathologic change identified on biopsy following pneumothorax (sometimes during surgical intervention for the pneumothorax), raising concern of undersampled or "upstream" PLCH. Radiologic correlation may be very helpful in this setting.

Clinical Course
Smoking cessation is the most effective management approach and is the "treatment" of choice.[353] Immunosuppression with corticosteroids, with or without the addition of a cytotoxic agent, has met with variable success. In larger reviews, the median survival time is 12 years,[353,366] with 5- and 10-year survival rates of 70% and 60%, respectively. The most frequent cause of death is the respiratory complications asso-

ciated with neoplasms of hematologic, pulmonary, or other organs. Survival rates are worse for patients with poorer respiratory function at diagnosis.[353]

Erdheim-Chester Disease

Erdheim-Chester disease (ECD) is a rare, nonfamilial, "non–Langerhans cell," systemic histiocytosis affecting middle-aged adults; it has no gender predilection.[367-369] The disease is characterized by xanthogranulomatous infiltration of the long tubular bones, resulting in symmetrical osteosclerosis.[367,370-373] Extraskeletal involvement is relatively common, occurring in approximately one half of patients. Of the reported extraskeletal sites, the pituitary area, skin, orbit, pericardium, and retroperitoneum are most often involved.

Clinical Presentation
Pulmonary involvement occurs in approximately one third of patients with ECD and is associated with significant morbidity and mortality.[367,374-378] Progressive breathlessness is the typical presentation.

Radiologic Findings
CT scans reveal thickening of the visceral pleura and interlobular septa, fine reticular and centrilobular opacities, and ground-glass attenuation.[377]

Histopathologic Findings
In surgical wedge lung biopsies, a distinctive interstitial infiltrate is observed consisting of xanthomatous histiocytes, lymphocytes, and scattered Touton-type giant cells[376] (Fig. 7-104). Prominent fibrosis is present in a characteristic subpleural and lymphatic distribution (Fig. 7-105). In immunohistochemical studies, the cells of ECD express histiocytic markers (CD68 and factor XIIIa) but typically lack CD1a immunoreactivity. S100 protein immunoreactivity occurs in a subset of patients.

Differential Diagnosis
The differential diagnosis includes advanced lung fibrosis associated with pulmonary Langerhans cell histiocytosis, and the exceedingly rare occurrence of lung manifestations of Rosai-Dorfman disease (sinus histiocytosis with massive lymphadenopathy—see Chapter 18 for discussion). In advanced PLCH, the fibrosis tends to be more confluent

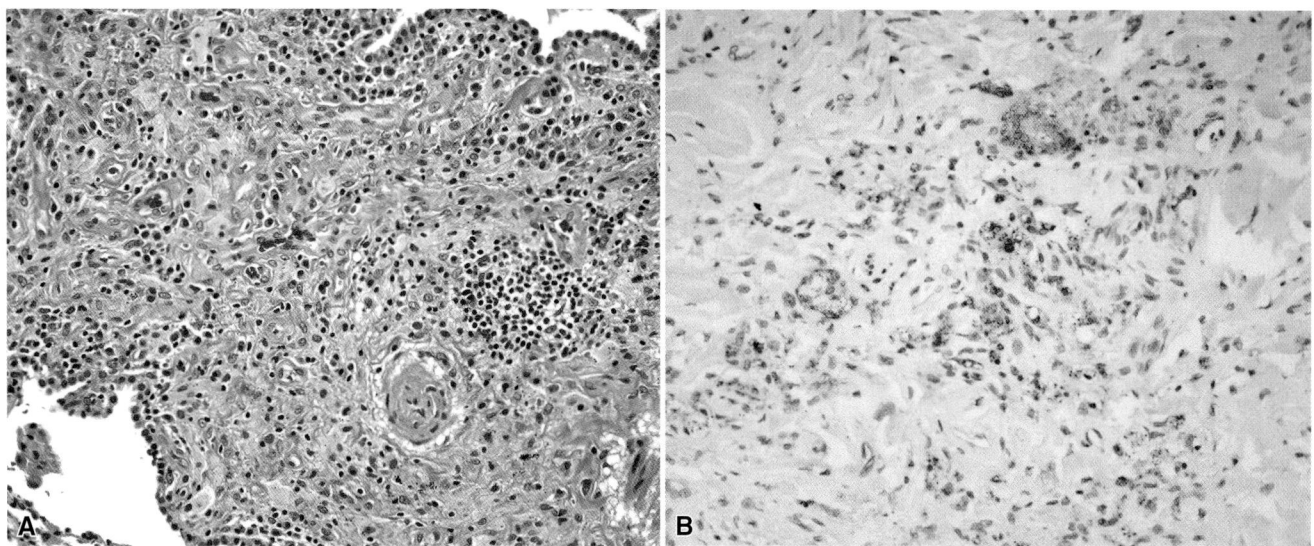

Figure 7-104. Erdheim-Chester disease. **A,** On closer inspection, the characteristic fibrotic process is seen to contain xanthomatous histiocytes, lymphocytes, and scattered Touton-type giant cells. **B,** These giant cells, along with other histiocytes in the infiltrate, can be highlighted with immunohistochemical stains for CD68 and factor XIIIa.

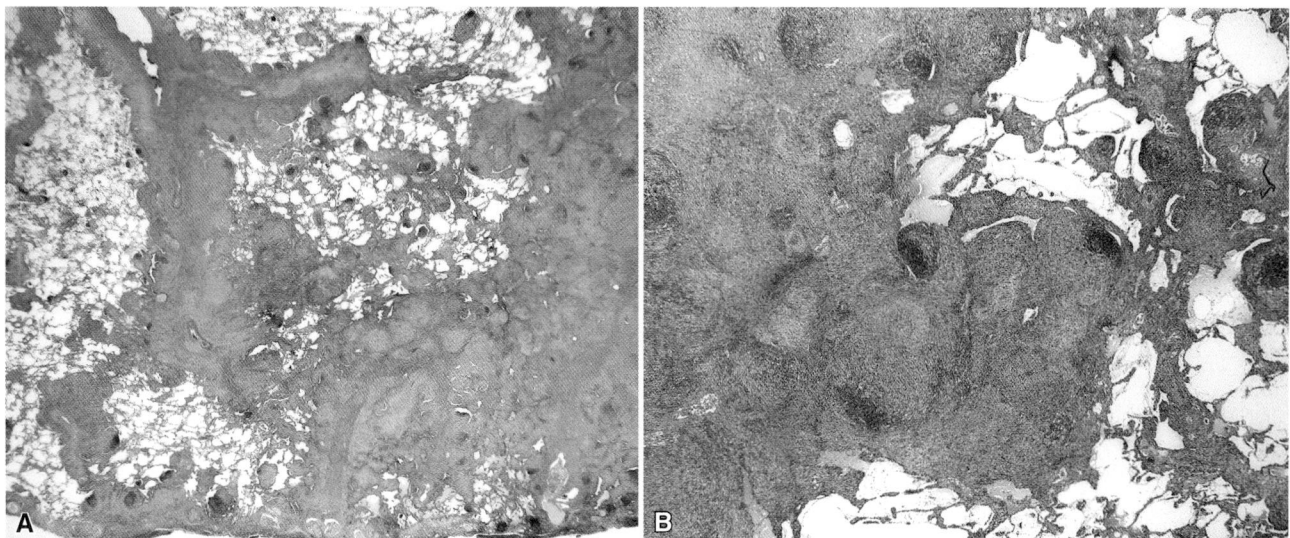

Figure 7-105. Rosai-Dorfman disease. **A,** Nodular expansion of interlobular septa, pleura, and bronchovascular sheaths is apparent at low magnification. **B,** The mixed inflammatory composition of the process becomes more evident at higher magnification.

and particularly bronchiolocentric, with blunt, stellate-shaped scars. In Rosai-Dorfman disease, the histiocytic nature of the process is often overshadowed by the inflammatory component (Fig. 7-106).

Clinical Course

Patients with pulmonary involvement by ECD typically follow a progressive downhill course with respiratory compromise and death. The disease is unresponsive to therapy.

Lymphangioleiomyomatosis

Lymphangioleiomyomatosis (LAM) is a rare chronic lung disease characterized by the presence of cysts accompanied by bundles of distinctive smooth muscle cells.[379-384] LAM is a disease that affects women; it has a distinctive relationship to the genetic disorder known as the tuberous sclerosis complex (TSC).[385] Recent experimental data have demonstrated loss of heterozygosity on 9p and and 16p and mutation in the tuberous

sclerosis complex gene (*TSC2*), suggesting that LAM is a neoplastic disease.[386-388] Nevertheless, debate continues as to whether LAM is a true neoplasm or represents hyperplasia of genetically aberrant cells. Although LAM was considered to be a disease unique to women, rare cases of LAM in males have been reported.[389] Likewise, we have seen an additional case in consultation (unpublished data) in a phenotypic male with TSC. LAM is included in this chapter because the disease typically presents as a chronic diffuse lung process clinically and radiologically.

Clinical Presentation

LAM occurs most frequently in women of childbearing age, with a peak incidence in the fourth decade of life.[379,383] Two forms of the disease occur, one sporadically and the other in association with the genetic marker for TSC. In both forms of the disease, extrathoracic (especially renal) angiomyolipomas are common.[390-395] Of note, the rare male patients reported to have LAM also had TSC.[389] LAM is

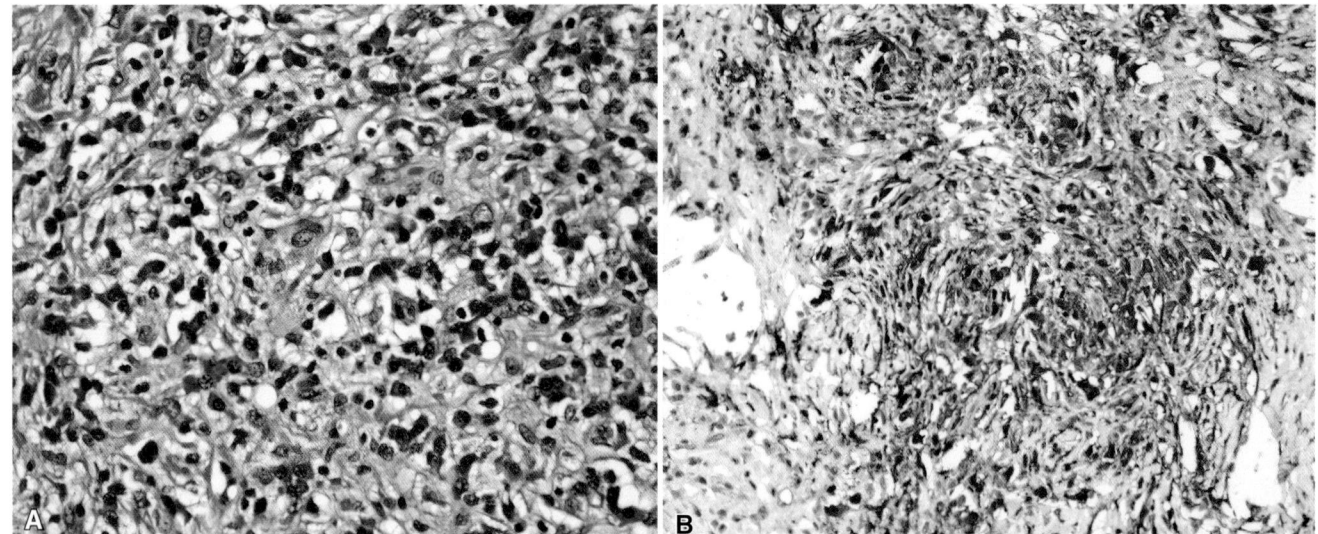

Figure 7-106. Rosai-Dorfman disease. **A,** The histiocytic nature of the disease process is often overshadowed by the inflammatory component. **B,** An S100 protein stain may be very useful in establishing the diagnosis. Emperipolesis, the typical finding in the more common lymph node manifestation of the disease, may be difficult to appreciate on routine hematoxylin and eosin–stained sections of lung tissue.

often asymptomatic in its early stage, and many affected individuals are diagnosed by chest radiographs performed for other reasons. The most common clinical complaint is shortness of breath.[379,383,384] Pneumothorax occurs, and pleurocentesis may reveal a chylous effusion.

Radiologic Features

Plain films of the chest may be interpreted as normal,[396] but with pneumothorax, air or fluid may be present in the pleural space. Small nodules and cysts may be detected and typically are present diffusely in the lungs, in contrast with the upper lobe distribution of lesions in PLCH. CT scans show diagnostic changes, with small nodules and thin-walled cysts seen throughout both lungs.[396–401]

Histopathologic Features

LAM lesions may be difficult to appreciate at scanning magnification, particularly in cases where smooth muscle lesions are sparse or of small size (Fig. 7-107). In most cases, thin walled cysts are easily visible (Fig. 7-108) and useful for identifying diagnostic smooth muscle bundles at higher magnification (Fig. 7-109). The smooth muscle of LAM is distinctive (Fig. 7-110). The LAM cell is fusiform and plump. The nucleus is larger than that of other smooth muscle cells in the lung (Fig. 7-111) and the nuclear-cytoplasmic ratio is typically higher. Smooth muscle bundles may be small or attenuated at the periphery of cysts (Fig. 7-112) or quite cellular and prominent (Fig. 7-113). In the lung lymphatics or pleural space, unattached aggregations of cells enveloped by lymphatic endothelium may be seen; these have been referred to as *LAM cell clusters*.[402] These unattached cell clusters have been proposed as the mechanism for dissemination of the disease.[402]

Differential Diagnosis

The differential diagnosis for LAM includes Birt-Hogg-Dubé syndrome,[403] alveolar duct smooth muscle hyperplasia, pulmonary Langerhans cell histiocytosis, metastatic low-grade sarcomas in the lung, thin-walled cysts seen in so-called "radiologic LIP" or in Sjögren syndrome, and cystic terminal airways in small-airway disease, especially when these diseases occur in the setting of recurrent pneumothorax in a woman.

Clinical Course

No effective therapy has emerged for LAM. Nevertheless, antihormonal therapy[404–407] has been the mainstay of treatment, based on the presence of estrogen and progesterone receptors in the abnormal smooth muscle cells in this disease.[270,384,406,408] There is no evidence of improvement with the use of estrogen antagonists.[409] Currently several multicenter clinical trials are under way using agents such as the mTOR inhibitor, sirolimus, Rheb inhibitors, selective estrogen antagonists, tyrosine kinase inhibitors, angiogenesis inhibitors, and lymphangiogenesis inhibitors (anti–vascular endothelial growth factor D antibody).[409] Lung transplantation may also be considered an effective option.[410] Recurrence of LAM in transplanted lung has been reported.[411] The median survival period is in the range of 10 years, with an early subset of deaths occurring within the first 5 years of diagnosis.[309,412]

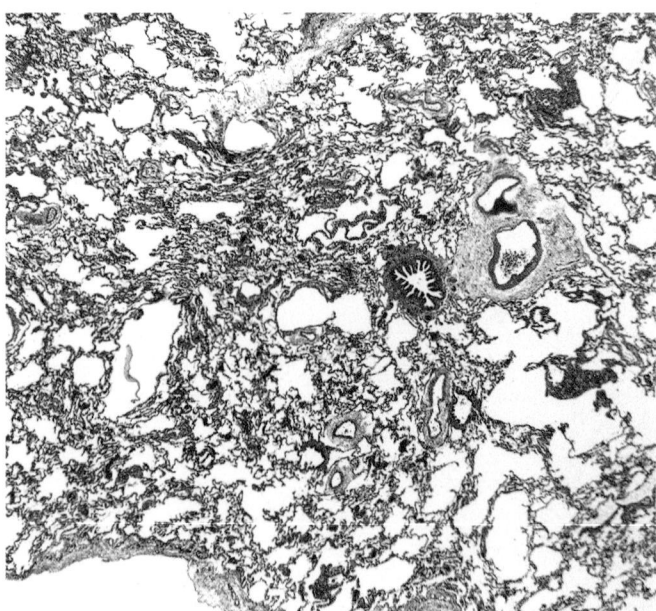

Figure 7-107. Lymphangioleiomyomatosis (LAM). LAM lesions may be difficult to appreciate at scanning magnification, particularly in cases in which smooth muscle lesions are sparse or of small size.

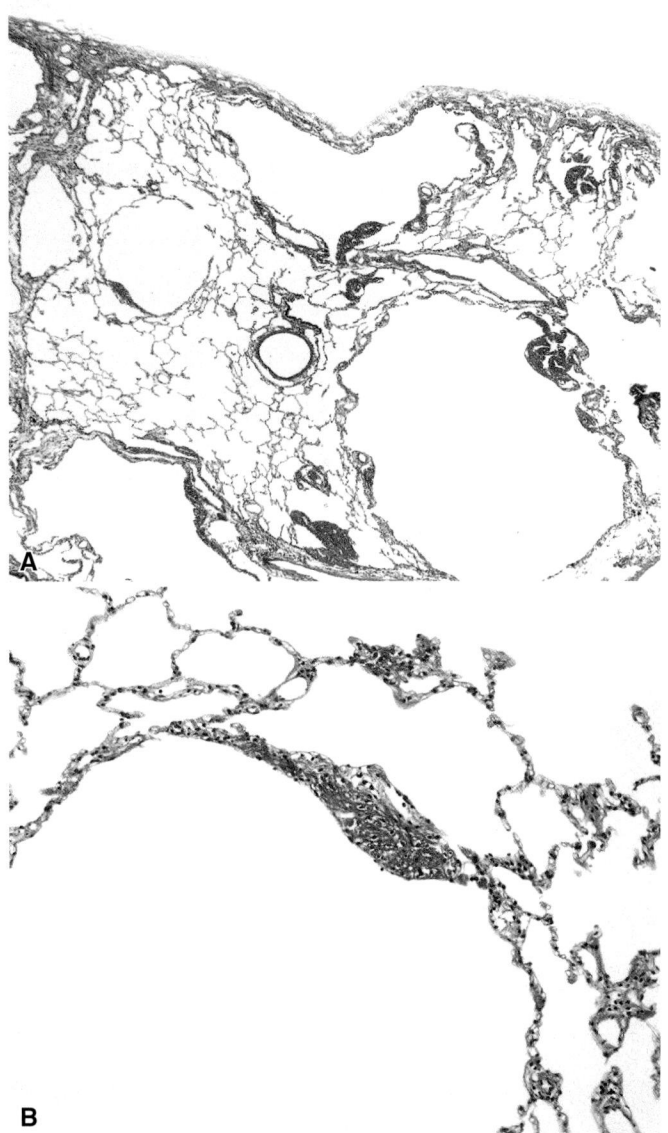

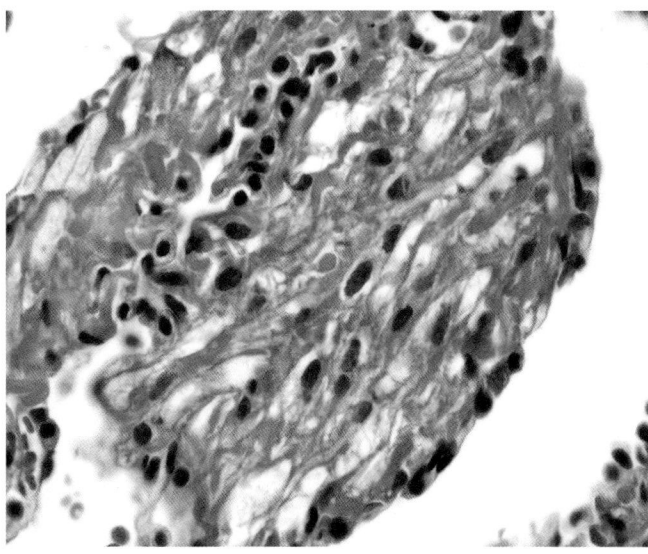

Figure 7-110. Lymphangioleiomyomatosis (LAM). The smooth muscle cells of LAM are distinctive in appearance. The LAM cell is fusiform and plump, with irregular pale vacuoles in its cytoplasm.

Hermansky-Pudlak Syndrome

The Hermansky-Pudlak syndrome (HPS) encompasses a group of genetic disorders of autosomal recessive inheritance that share features of oculocutaneous albinism, platelet storage pool deficiency, and variable tissue lipofuchsinosis.[413–415] The most common form of HPS arises from a 16–base pair duplication in the *HPS1* gene at exon 15 on the long arm of chromosome 10 (10q23).[416] This form is referred to as *HPS type 1* (HPS-1) and is associated with progressive, lethal pulmonary fibrosis.[417] HPS-1 affects between 400 and 500 individuals in northwest Puerto Rico.[418,419] Pulmonary fibrosis typically begins in the fourth decade and results in death from respiratory failure within 1 to 6 years of onset.[420] A granulomatous colitis may also occur in HPS patients.

Radiologic Findings

Avila and coworkers[421] reviewed chest radiographs and CT scans from 67 patients with HPS-1. CT scans with minimal abnormalities had normal corresponding chest radiographs. When abnormalities were present on the radiographs, these consisted of diffuse reticulonodular

Figure 7-108. Lymphangioleiomyomatosis (LAM). In most cases, thin-walled cysts are readily visible (**A**) and useful for searching out the characteristic smooth muscle of LAM (**B**).

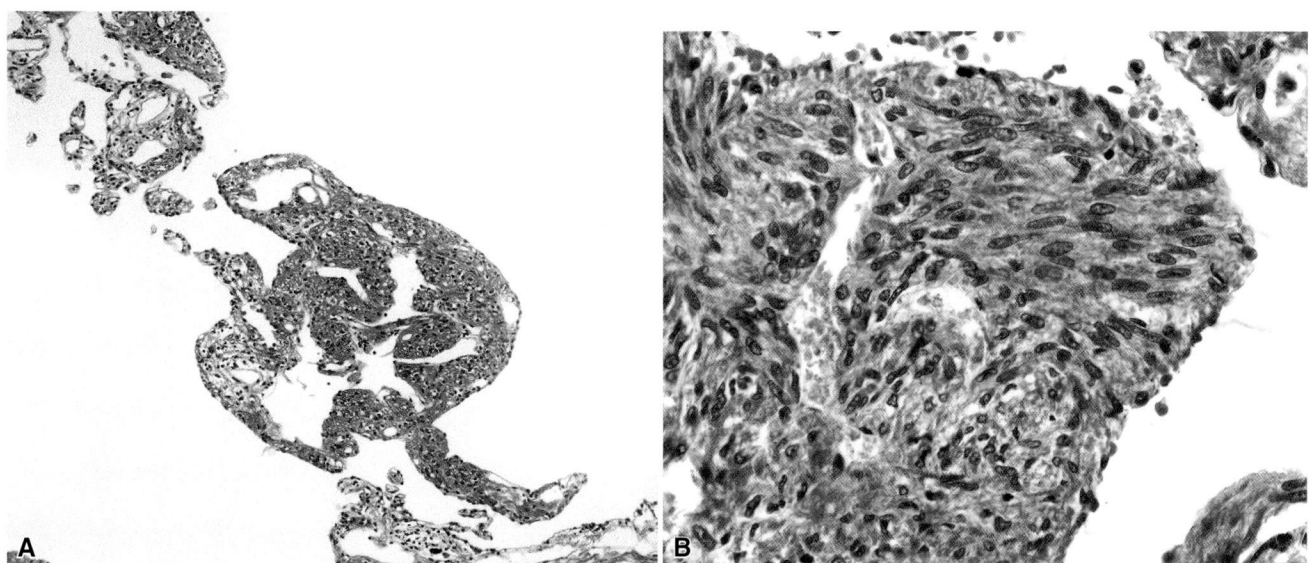

Figure 7-109. Lymphangioleiomyomatosis (LAM). **A** and **B,** The smooth muscle of LAM more closely resembles a low-grade neoplasm than any normally occurring smooth muscle.

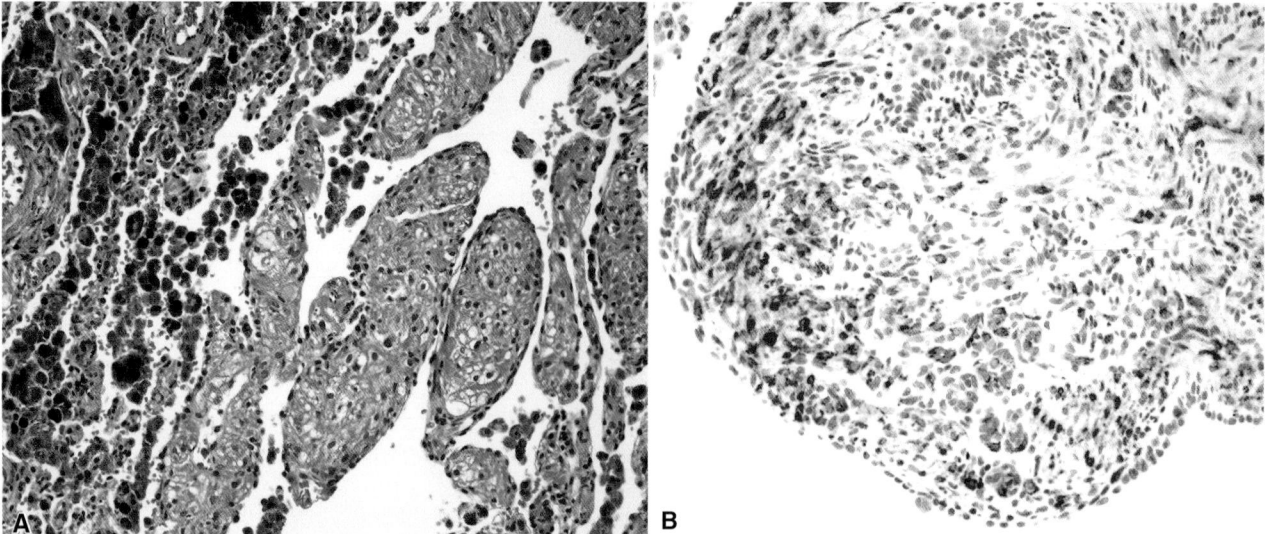

Figure 7-111. Lymphangioleiomyomatosis (LAM). **A,** The nucleus of the LAM smooth muscle cell is larger than that of other smooth muscle cells in the lung, and the nuclear-cytoplasmic ratio is typically higher. In this example, hemosiderosis is present in adjacent alveolar spaces. **B,** Immunohistochemical stains for HMB45 are very helpful in establishing the correct diagnosis.

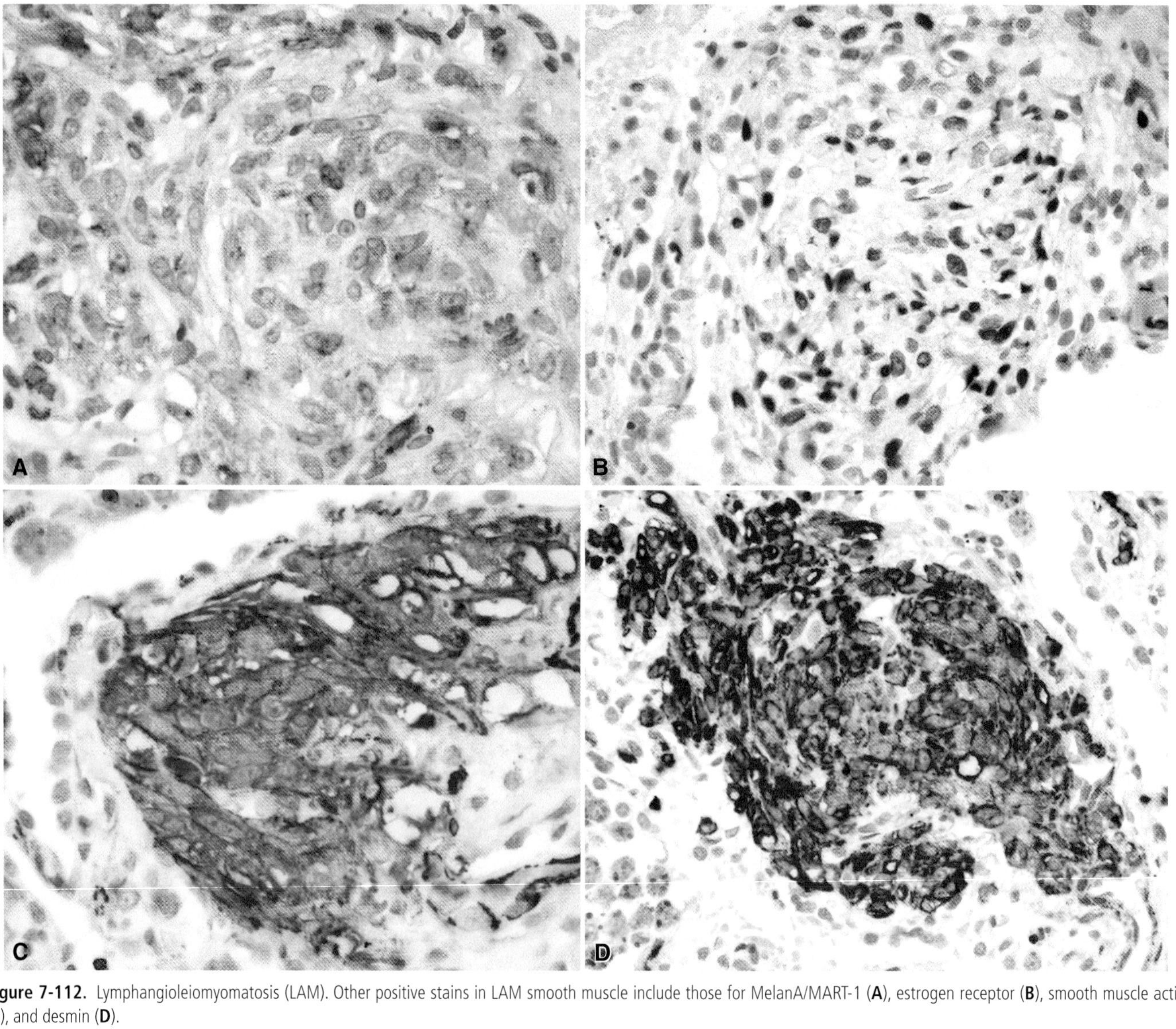

Figure 7-112. Lymphangioleiomyomatosis (LAM). Other positive stains in LAM smooth muscle include those for MelanA/MART-1 (**A**), estrogen receptor (**B**), smooth muscle actin (**C**), and desmin (**D**).

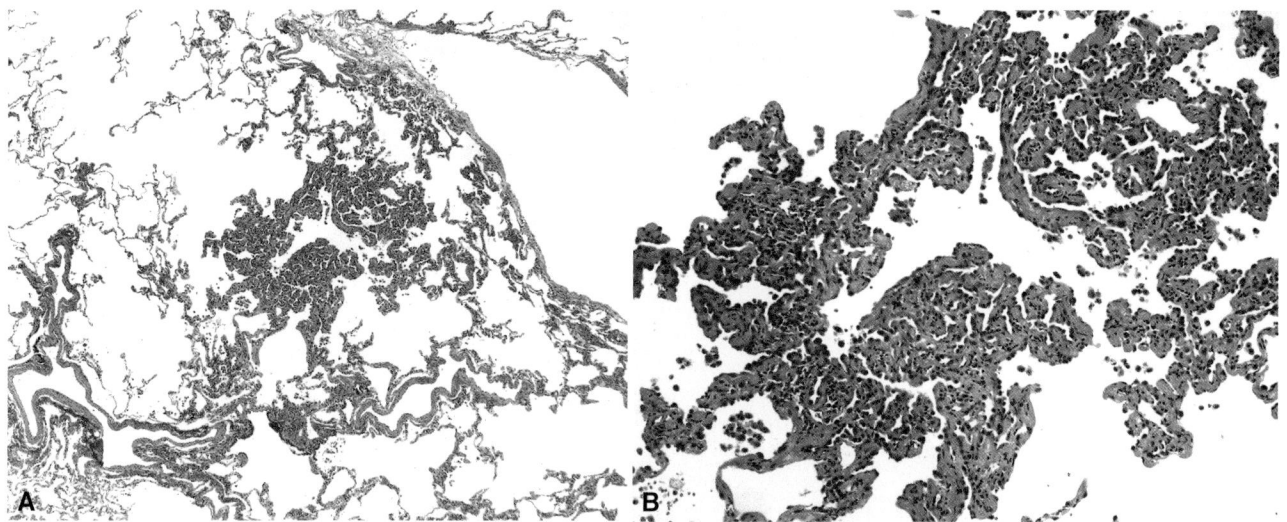

Figure 7-113. Lymphangioleiomyomatosis (LAM). **A,** Another distinctive lesion that may be seen in association with LAM, especially in those patients who also have tuberous sclerosis complex, is micronodular pneumocyte hyperplasia (MNPH). **B,** MNPH lesions are epithelial and probably represent a hamartomatous proliferation. The cells of MNPH do not stain with antibodies directed against HMB45 or MelanA/MART-1 but, rather, stain with cytokeratin and surfactant apoprotein antibodies.

interstitial infiltrates, perihilar fibrosis, and pleural thickening. High-resolution CT findings included peribronchovascular thickening, ground-glass opacification, and septal thickening. Increasing severity of these changes, as assessed using a fibrosis scoring system, was inversely correlated with forced vital capacity.

Histopathologic Findings

Surgical biopsies and autopsy lungs from five patients with HPS were studied by Nakatani and colleagues.[422] These researchers described alveolar septal thickening (Fig. 7-114) associated with prominent clear vacuolated type II pneumocytes (Fig. 7-115), patchy zones of fibrosis with an apparent bronchiolocentric distribution, some evidence of constrictive bronchiolitis, and haphazard microscopic honeycombing without a consistent peripheral lobular or subpleural distribution. Many giant lamellar bodies were present in the macrophages and type II cells on ultrastructural examination, and the phospholipid material in the vacuoles was weakly positive with antibodies directed against surfactant apoprotein by immunohistochemistry.

Clinical Course

No effective therapy has been identified for HPS patients with lung fibrosis, but newer antifibrotic therapies are being explored.[423]

Pulmonary Alveolar Microlithiasis

Pulmonary alveolar microlithiasis (PAM) is a rare but distinctive lung disease of autosomal recessive inheritance, with approximately 300 cases reported in the literature.[424–428] A significant number of cases identified are familial (affecting siblings); however, PAM occurring in both a parent and a child is uncommon. The exact incidence of the disease is unknown, but in a 46-year period, the Mayo Clinic identified only eight cases.[426] Patients are typically diagnosed in the fourth decade of life, but diagnosis can occur from childhood to 80 years of age.[426] There appears to be an increased incidence in individuals of Turkish descent; a Turkish family with six affected members has been described.[429] The responsible gene mutation has been found in the *SLC34A2* gene, which encodes the sodiumphosphate cotransporter in patients with PAM.[430]

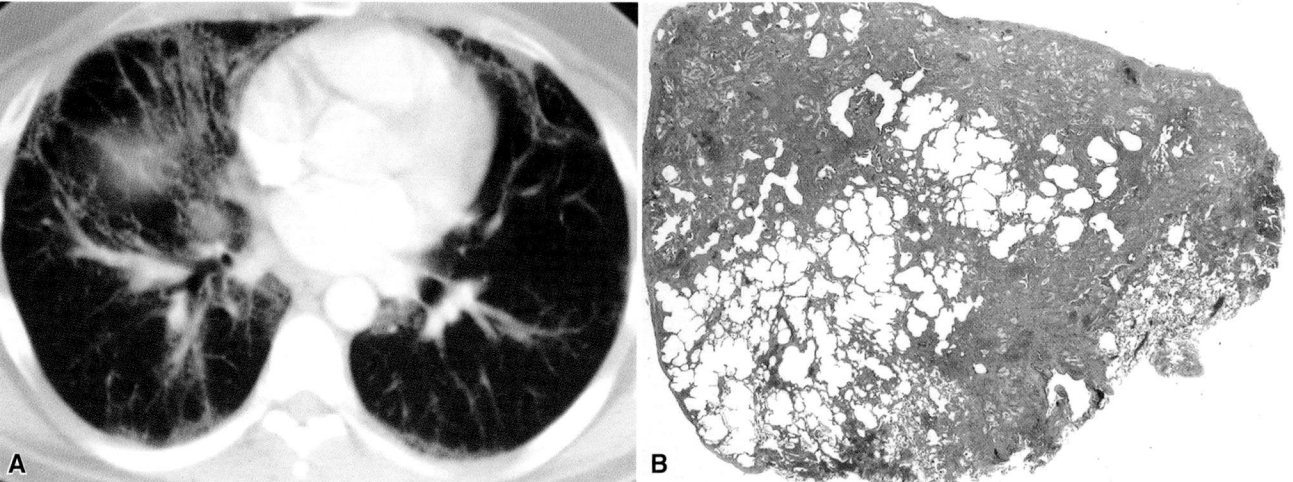

Figure 7-114. Hermansky-Pudlak syndrome. This genetic disease produces lethal lung fibrosis in affected persons. **A,** The computed tomography findings are dramatic and characterized by diffuse reticular opacities. **B,** Tissue sections show advanced lung remodeling with fibrosis, typically without an easily characterized distribution, but somewhat patchy and "UIP-like" at scanning magnification.

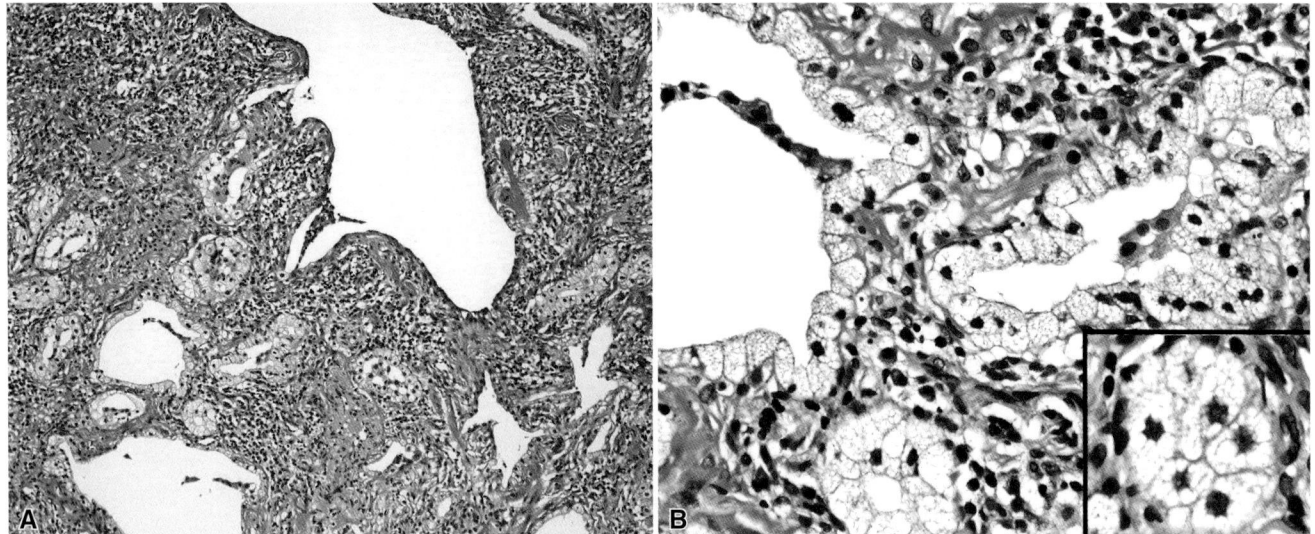

Figure 7-115. Hermansky-Pudlak syndrome. **A** and **B,** At higher magnifications, prominent clear vacuolated type II pneumocytes can be seen embedded in chronic inflammation within, patchy zones of fibrosis. *Inset* in part **B** shows the peculiar vacuolated cells of this disease, sometimes even confused for "clear cell carcinoma."

Clinical Presentation

Most cases are diagnosed in adult life, but the disease can manifest at any age.[425–427] It is hypothesized that the condition results from a congenital metabolic disorder, resulting in slowly progressive disease during life. The most common presentation is that of an asymptomatic patient. Some patients may experience various degrees of dyspnea, and death has been reported to occur after accelerated respiratory failure. Affected patients typically exhibit a restrictive pulmonary function defect,[425] but this is generally mild when compared with the dramatic appearance of the chest radiograph, especially in young patients. Associated nephrolithiasis and pleural calcification have been reported.[431]

Radiologic Findings

The chest radiograph is almost immediately diagnostic, with sand-like micronodular opacities present throughout both lungs diffusely. The lower lung zones tend to be more opacified than the upper lobes. Chest radiographs may remain static for many years.[425–427] High-resolution CT scans reveal intra-alveolar microcalcifications bilaterally, with increased concentration of microliths along bronchovascular bundles and interlobular fissures and in the subpleural lung parenchyma.[432]

Histopathologic Findings

On gross examination, the lungs are firm and gritty and rigidly maintain their shape before fixation. On microscopic examination, the air spaces contain innumerable tiny calcified bodies that are concentrically laminated and have radial striations (Fig. 7-116). These microliths are composed of calcium and phosphorus, in concentrations similar to those in bone.[427] Magnesium and iron are typically present in small amounts. Microliths may be as large as 1 mm or more in diameter, but usually they are of uniform size, with diameters in the range of 250 μm. Rarely, microlithiasis may involve the alveolar walls, often accompanied by some degree of interstitial thickening and chronic inflammation (Fig. 7-117).

Differential Diagnosis

The differential diagnosis includes corpora amylacea and alveolar calcification from any cause. The microliths of PAM can be distinguished from incidental corpora amylacea by the larger size of the former and the lack of calcification in the latter. Also, corpora amylacea typically have a small black pigment core while the microliths of PAM lack this

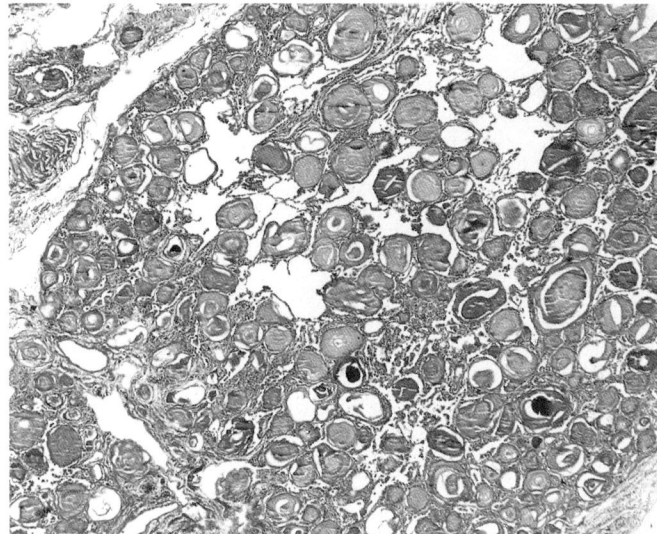

Figure 7-116. Pulmonary alveolar microlithiasis. The air spaces contain innumerable tiny calcified bodies that are concentrically laminated and have radial striations.

feature. The shear number of alveolar microliths in PAM distinguish this condition from other forms of lung calcification.

Clinical Course

A majority of patients with PAM survive for many years with little disease progression. No effective therapy is currently available for symptomatic patients.

Pulmonary Alveolar Proteinosis

Pulmonary alveolar proteinosis (PAP) is a diffuse lung process characterized by the presence of alveolar spaces filled with amorphous eosinophilic material. Recent data suggest that most patients with primary PAP develop this disorder as part of an autoimmune disease.[433,434] In a recent series of PAP patients, 223 of 248 were seropositive for anti–granulocyte-monocyte colony-stimulating factor (anti–GM-CSF) autoantibody.[435] PAP is often multilobar, bilateral, and of subacute or chronic onset. Other subacute or chronic ILDs that include an alveolar component are considerations in the differential diagnosis for PAP (e.g., COP, RBILD/DIP, LIP, NSIP).

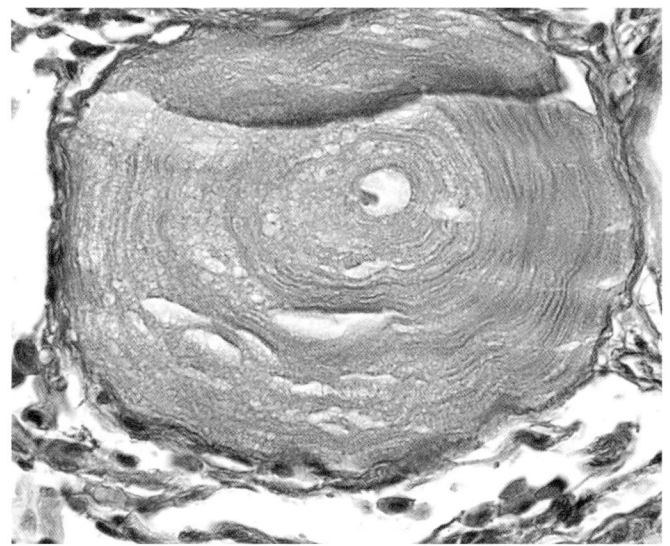

Figure 7-117. Pulmonary alveolar microlithiasis. Rarely, the calcifications may be present within the alveolar walls, often accompanied by some degree of interstitial thickening and chronic inflammation.

Clinical Presentation

The disease occurs commonly as a primary idiopathic form, whether congenital or adult onset. However, PAP may also be seen as a secondary phenomenon in the settings of occupational disease (especially dust-related), drug-induced injury, hematologic diseases, and in many settings of immunodeficiency.[436–440] The disease is commonly associated with exposure to crystalline material and silica, although other substances have also been implicated.[437,441] The idiopathic form is the most common presentation. Most PAP patients are male and range in age from 30 to 50 years. The usual presenting symptom is dyspnea on exertion, followed in frequency by insidious breathlessness, sometimes with cough.[435,440–442]

Radiologic Findings

Chest radiographs show extensive bilateral air space consolidation, involving mainly the perihilar regions; often the symptoms belie the severity of the radiologic abnormalities. CT demonstrates smooth thickening of lobular septa that is not seen on the chest radiograph.

Thickened lobular septa sharply demarcate areas of ground-glass attenuation. These characteristics of alveolar proteinosis on CT are referred to as "crazy paving pattern."[443]

Histopathologic Findings

PAP (i.e., alveolar lipoproteinosis) is characterized by an intra-alveolar accumulation of lipid-rich eosinophilic material.[436] In primary PAP, it occurs as a result of impaired clearance of surfactant by alveolar macrophages due to the effects of an autoantibody directed against GM-CSF. The gross lung shows firm yellow-white nodules, some as large as 2 cm in diameter. Microscopically, the scanning magnification appearance is distinctive, if not diagnostic. Pink granular material fills the air spaces, sometimes with a rim of retraction that separates the alveolar wall slightly from the exudates (Fig. 7-118). Closer inspection of this material shows embedded clumps of dense globular material and cholesterol clefts (Fig. 7-119). Amorphous solid eosinophilic globules are seen frequently inside the pools of proteinaceous material. The

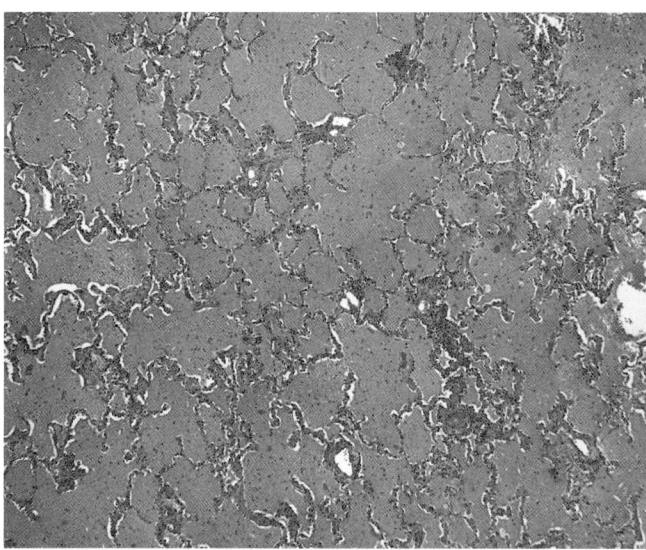

Figure 7-118. Pulmonary alveolar proteinosis (PAP). The nearly diagnostic appearance of PAP at scanning magnification demonstrates pink granular material filling the air spaces, sometimes with a rim of retraction that separates the alveolar wall slightly from the exudate.

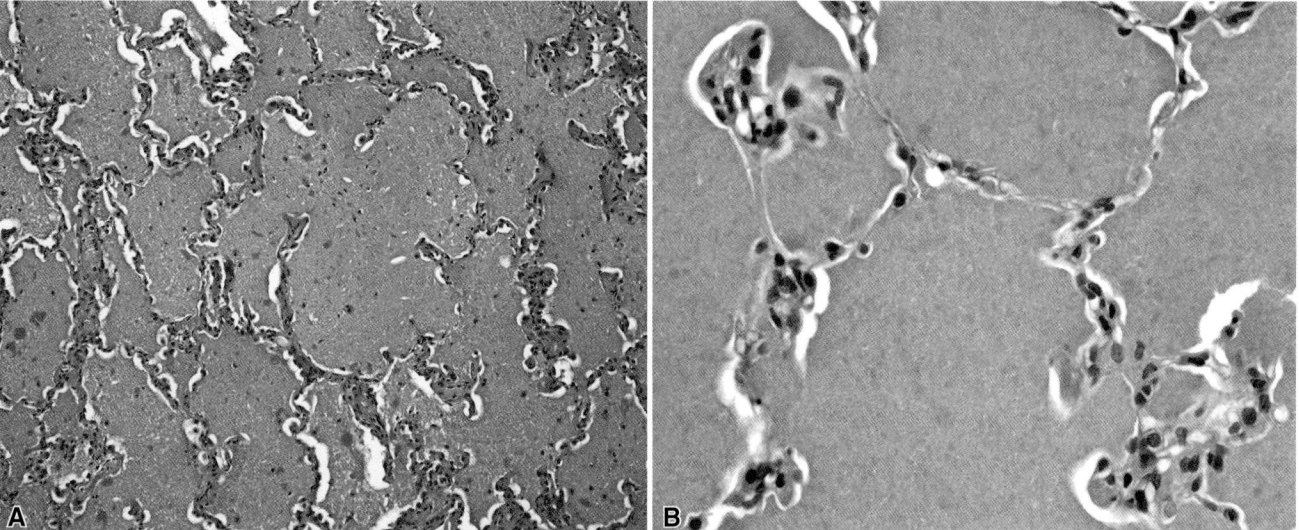

Figure 7-119. Pulmonary alveolar proteinosis (PAP). **A,** Closer inspection of the material seen in Figure 7-118 shows embedded clumps of dense globular material and cholesterol clefts. **B,** The clumps may be variably prominent; in this example, they are less distinct.

periodic acid/Schiff reagent (PAS) stain may be useful in demonstrating a diastase-resistant, positive reaction in the globular inclusions of PAP. By immunohistochemistry this material is immunoreactive with antibodies directed against surfactant. There may be few other associated changes in the lung biopsy, although patients with long-standing disease may develop some interstitial fibrosis and chronic inflammation. More dramatic inflammatory changes should suggest comorbid disease, such as infection. For example, *Nocardia*, *Aspergillus*, or mycobacterial infection can be associated with PAP.[435] PAP can be patchy in the lungs and even in biopsy specimens, so a high index of suspicion is required, coupled with good clinical and radiologic data.

Differential Diagnosis

The differential diagnosis includes pulmonary edema and *Pneumocystis* pneumonia. Pulmonary edema does not feature the globular material and cellular debris seen in PAP. *Pneumocystis* pneumonia can be distinguished from PAP by a more dramatic clinical presentation, exudates that appear finely vacuolated or foamy, and significantly more inflammatory changes in background lung. When fibrotic change is prominent, it may be difficult to distinguish from UIP because focal PAP reaction can occur in and around areas of microscopic honeycombing in UIP.

Clinical Course

Despite significant radiologic abnormalities, the disease may be unusually silent, producing few if any clinical manifestations in the absence of superimposed infection. When patients have severe dyspnea and hypoxemia, treatment can be accomplished using one or more sessions of whole-lung lavage, which usually induces remission and excellent long-term survival.[444] Based on the recent evidence of a high incidence of anti–GM-CSF antibody in primary PAP patients, clinical trials using aerosolized GM-CSF have been initiated with good results.[445,446]

Lymphangitic Carcinomatosis

Metastatic carcinoma involving the lung, primarily within lymphatics, is known as *pulmonary lymphangitic carcinomatosis* (lymphangitis carcinomatosa). The tumor type is most often adenocarcinoma; it accounts for as much as 8% of all cases of metastasis to the lung. The most common sites of origin are breast, lung, and stomach, although primary disease in pancreas, ovary, kidney, and uterine cervix can also spread to the lungs in this manner.[447,448] Published reports on this subject are found predominantly in the radiology literature.[447–450]

Clinical Presentation

Patients often present with insidious onset of dyspnea, frequently accompanied by an irritating/nonproductive cough.

Radiologic Findings

On plain chest films, the changes are often subtle and nonspecific. In one study, the correct diagnosis was made in only 20 of 87 cases (23%), and 50% of the films were interpreted as normal.[451] Abnormalities include linear opacities, horizontal linear lines abutting on the pleura, mostly the lower lobes (Kerley B lines), subpleural edema, and commonly, hilar and mediastinal lymph node enlargement.[449] By contrast, the high-resolution CT findings are highly characteristic and accurately reflect the macroscopic abnormalities in this disease. Because the major lymphatic vessels in the lung are located in the pleura, interlobular septa, and bronchovascular bundles, the abnormalities are found primarily in this distribution, thickening and accentuating these structures. High-resolution CT scanning shows irregular thickening of the bronchovascular bundles and lobular septa, giving them a beaded appearance.[448,450] Distinction from sarcoidosis (another "lym-

phatic" disease) can be made by examining distribution (sarcoidosis is an upper lung zone disease).

Histopathologic Findings

Small aggregates of tumor cells are present within lymphatic channels of the bronchovascular sheath and pleura (Fig. 7-120). Because the lymphatics of the bronchi are involved in this process, lymphangitic carcinoma is one of the few diffuse lung diseases that can be diagnosed definitively by bronchial or transbronchial biopsy[452] (Fig. 7-121). Variable amounts of tumor may be present throughout the lung, involving the interstitium of the alveolar walls, the air spaces themselves, and the lumens of small muscular pulmonary arteries. This latter finding (microangiopathic obliterative endarteritis) may be the origin of the edema, inflammation, and interstitial fibrosis that frequently accompany the disease and probably accounts for the clinical and radiologic impression of non-neoplastic diffuse lung disease.[447,449]

The pathogenesis of lymphangitic carcinoma is unknown. Seeding of the lung lymphatics from retrograde spread of microvascular tumor emboli has been postulated and supported by observations of intravascular tumor present in other organs at autopsy from patients so affected.[447,449]

Differential Diagnosis

Lesions that may mimic lymphangitic carcinoma include intravascular lymphoma, thromboembolic disease, and foreign material from intravenous injection.

Clinical Course

The prognosis is grim, with most patients dying within 6 months of diagnosis. Rarely, long-term survivors are reported.[447]

Idiopathic Pleuroparenchymal Fibroelastosis

In 2004, Frankel and coworkers described five distinctive cases of an ILD referred to as *idiopathic pleuroparenchymal fibroelastosis* (IPFE).[453] This upper lobe–predominant fibrotic disease slowly progresses to involve the lower lung. On histopathologic examination, elastotic fibrosis, similar to that seen in so-called apical cap, is the dominant feature. The major differences between apical cap and IPFE are that the patients with IPFE are symptomatic and the disease is progressive, even-

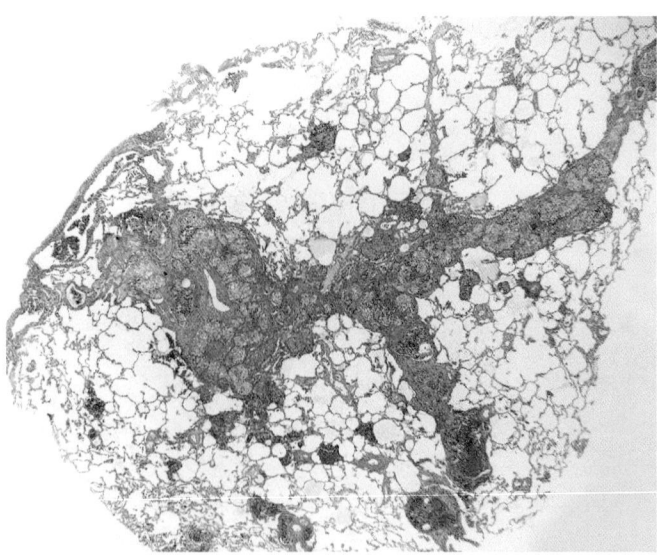

Figure 7-120. Lymphangitic carcinomatosis. Few lung diseases are as dramatic (or as devastating to those affected) than lymphangitic carcinomatosis. The characteristic distribution of the disease is demonstrated here at scanning magnification, with peribronchial and septal lymphatics filled by metastatic tumor.

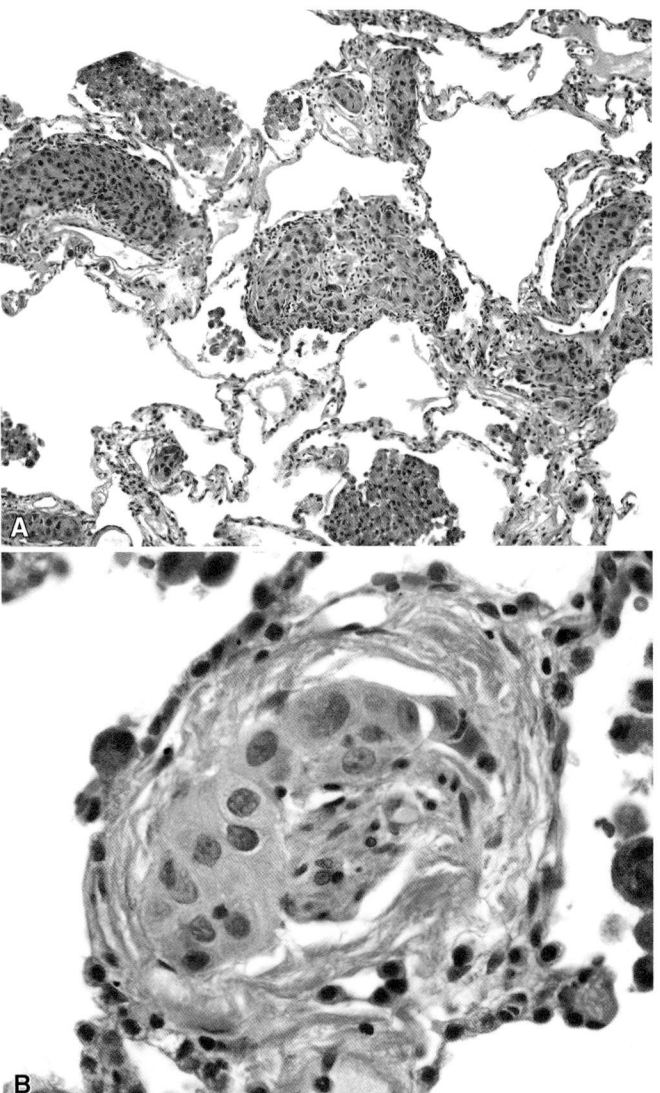

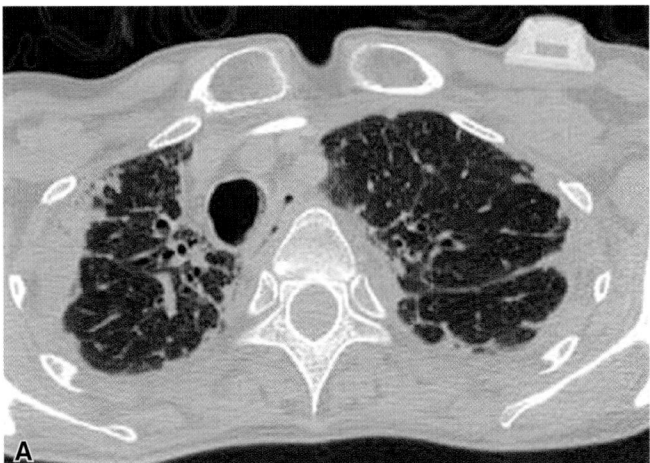

Figure 7-121. Lymphangitic carcinomatosis. **A,** At times the disease may be more subtle and manifest as an interstitial infiltrate in lung biopsies. **B,** Lymphangitic carcinoma is one of the few diffuse lung diseases that can be diagnosed definitively by bronchial or transbronchial biopsy.

tuating in death within several years. In addition to the original series described by Frankel's group, only two reports of IPFE have appeared in the English literature to date; however, several case reports from Japan and the United States seem to describe a similar disease.[454–457]

Clinical Presentation
IPFE patients range in age from 32 to 65 years. Most of the reported cases have been in women who present with dyspnea on exertion and cough. Pneumothorax has been reported in some patients. In a subset of reported cases of IPFE, the patients had a history of malignancy; however, many of them began to experience lung symptoms before their malignant neoplasm was diagnosed. There appears to be a familial association.

Radiologic Findings
Bilateral upper lung volume loss with marked apical pleural thickening is the most common finding on plain films. CT images show marked visceral pleural thickening extending into the lung parenchyma with subpleural reticular abnormalities. Traction bronchiectasis is a common finding in areas of fibrosis. Lower lung zones may be hyperinflated (Fig. 7-122A).

Histopathologic Findings
The histopathology of IPFE overlaps with that of apical cap. Fibrotic areas show dense elastotic scarring without inflammation. Scattered lymphoid aggregations are common, but there is no associated cellular interstitial pneumonia. Margins between normal lung and affected fibrotic areas are sharply defined. Uninvolved lung shows minimal abnormalities, mainly involving the airways (bronchiolar fibrosis or ectasia). Broad pleural adhesions, probably due to the common history of pneumothorax, may be present (see Fig. 7-122B).

Differential Diagnosis
Apical cap should be excluded from the differential diagnosis. IPFE is a progressive scarring disorder that can affect survival through eventual loss of lung compliance. The presence of dense collagenous fibrosis should raise an alternative diagnosis, such as UIP/NSIP. Honeycomb fibrosis in the lower lung is not an expected finding in patients with IPFE.

Clinical Course
The expected clinical course varies considerably from case to case; however, three of the seven patients were dead within the follow-up period.[453,454]

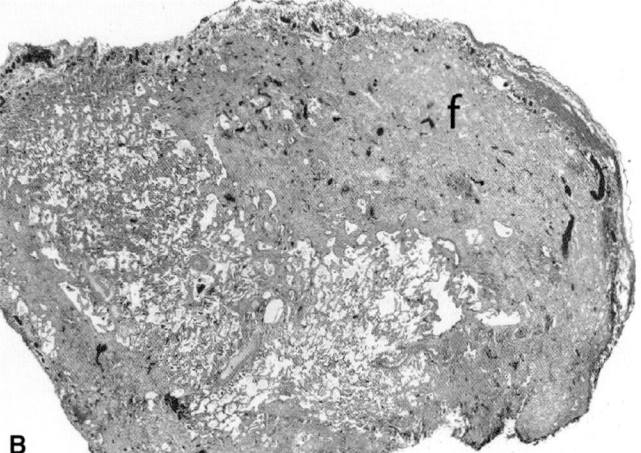

Figure 7-122. Idiopathic pleuroparenchymal fibroelastosis (IPFE). **A,** Biapical pleural fibrotic changes, more prominent on the right (CT image). Subcutaneous Port-A-Cath reservoir is present on the left anterior chest wall. **B,** An upper lobe biopsy from a patient with IPFE, seen at scanning magnification. Note the elastotic fibrosis (f) in a subpleural location, extending into the parenchyma. (**A,** Reprinted with permission from Becker CD, Gil J, Padilla ML: Idiopathic pleuroparenchymal fibroelastosis: an unrecognized or misdiagnosed entity? *Mod Pathol.* 2008;21(6):784–787, Case 2, Figure 4.)

Self-assessment questions related to this chapter can be found online on the Expert Consult site for this title.

References

1. Leslie K, Colby T. Classification and pathology of diffuse interstitial lung disease. *Semin Clin Immunol*. 1999;1:7–15.
2. Leslie KO. My approach to interstitial lung disease using clinical, radiological and histopathologic patterns. *J Clin Pathol*. 2009;62(5):387–401.
3. Leslie KO, Gruden JF, Parish JM, Scholand MB. Transbronchial biopsy interpretation in the patient with diffuse parenchymal lung disease. *Arch Pathol Lab Med*. 2007;131(3):407–423.
4. Elicker B, Pereira CA, Webb R, Leslie KO. High-resolution computed tomography patterns of diffuse interstitial lung disease with clinical and pathological correlation. *J Bras Pneumol*. 2008;34(9):715–744.
5. American Thoracic Society. Idiopathic pulmonary fibrosis: diagnosis and treatment. International consensus statement. American Thoracic Society (ATS), and the European Respiratory Society (ERS). *Am J Respir Crit Care Med*. 2000;161(2 Pt 1):646–664.
6. American Thoracic Society/European Respiratory Society. International Multidisciplinary Consensus Classification of the Idiopathic Interstitial Pneumonias. *Am Rev Respir Crit Care Med*. 2002;165(2):227–304.
7. Liebow AL, Carrington CB. The interstitial pneumonias. In: Simon M, Potchen EJ, LeMay M, eds. *Frontiers of Pulmonary Radiology: Pathophysiologic, Roentgenographic and Radioisotopic Considerations*. New York: Grune & Stratton; 1969:102–141.
8. Katzenstein AL. Idiopathic interstitial pneumonia: classification and diagnosis. *Monogr Pathol*. 1993;(36):1–31.
9. Katzenstein AL, Myers JL. Nonspecific interstitial pneumonia and the other idiopathic interstitial pneumonias. classification and diagnostic criteria. *Am J Surg Pathol*. 2000;24(1):1–3.
10. Crystal R, Fulmer JD, Roberts WC, et al. Idiopathic pulmonary fibrosis: clinical histologic, radiographic, physiologic, scintigraphic, cytologic and biochemical aspects. *Ann Intern Med*. 1976;85:769–788.
11. Carrington CB, Gaensler EA, Coutu RE, et al. Usual and desquamative interstitial pneumonia. *Chest*. 1976;69(suppl 2):261–263.
12. Aubry MC, Wright JL, Myers JL. The pathology of smoking-related lung diseases. *Clin Chest Med*. 2000;21(1):11–35, vii.
13. Ohori N, Sciurba FC, Owens GR, et al. Giant-cell interstitial pneumonia and hard-metal pneumoconiosis. A clinicopathologic study of four cases and review of the literature. *Am J Surg Pathol*. 1989;13(7):581–587.
14. Lewis CC, Yang JY, Huang X, et al. Disease-specific gene expression profiling in multiple models of lung disease. *Am J Respir Crit Care Med*. 2008;177(4):376–387.
15. Katzenstein A, Myers J, Mazur M. Acute interstitial pneumonia: a clinicopathologic, ultrastructural, and cell kinetic study. *Am J Surg Pathol*. 1986;10:256–267.
16. Katzenstein AL, Fiorelli RF. Nonspecific interstitial pneumonia/fibrosis. Histologic features and clinical significance. *Am J Surg Pathol*. 1994;18(2):136–147.
17. Epler GR, Colby TV, McLoud TC, et al. Bronchiolitis obliterans organizing pneumonia. *N Engl J Med*. 1985;312(3):152–158.
18. Leslie KO. Pathology of the idiopathic interstitial pneumonias. *Exp Lung Res*. 2005;31(suppl 1):23–40.
19. Gough J. Differential diagnosis in the pathology of asbestosis. *Ann N Y Acad Sci*. 1965;132:368–372.
20. Gadek J, Hunninghake G, Schoenberger C, et al. Pulmonary asbestosis and idiopathic pulmonary fibrosis: pathogenetic parallels. *Chest*. 1981;80(suppl 1):63–64.
21. Yamamoto S. Histopathological features of pulmonary asbestosis with particular emphasis on the comparison with those of usual interstitial pneumonia. *Osaka City Med J*. 1997;43(2):225–242.
22. Leslie K, King Jr TE, Low R. Smooth muscle actin is expressed by air space fibroblast-like cells in idiopathic pulmonary fibrosis and hypersensitivity pneumonitis. *Chest*. 1991;99(suppl 3):47S–48S.
23. Adler BD, Padley SP, Müller NL, et al. Chronic hypersensitivity pneumonitis: high resolution CT and radiographic features in 16 patients. *Radiology*. 1992;185:91–95.
24. Lynch DA, Newell JD, Logan PM, et al. Can CT distinguish hypersensitivity pneumonitis from idiopathic pulmonary fibrosis? *AJR Am J Roentgenol*. 1995;165(4):807–811.
25. Hunninghake G, Fauci A. Pulmonary involvement in the collagen vascular diseases. *Am Rev Respir Dis*. 1979;119:471–503.
26. Colby TV. Pathology of the lung in collagen vascular diseases. In: Cannon G and Zimmerman G, eds. *The Lung Rheumatic Diseases*. New York: Marcel Dekker; 1990:145–178.
27. Leslie KO, Trahan S, Gruden J. Pulmonary pathology of the rheumatic diseases. *Semin Respir Crit Care Med*. 2007;28(4):369–378.
28. Lamblin C, Bergoin C, Saelens T, Wallaert B. Interstitial lung diseases in collagen vascular diseases. *Eur Respir J Suppl*. 2001;32:69s–80s.
29. Rossi SE, Erasmus JJ, McAdams HP, et al. Pulmonary drug toxicity: radiologic and pathologic manifestations. *Radiographics*. 2000;20(5):1245–1259.
30. Raghu G, Weycker D, Edelsberg J, et al. Incidence and prevalence of idiopathic pulmonary fibrosis. *Am J Respir Crit Care Med*. 2006;174(7):810–816.
31. Coultas DB. Epidemiology of idiopathic pulmonary fibrosis. *Semin Respir Med*. 1993;14:181–196.
32. Guerry-Force M, Müller NL, Wright JL, et al. A comparison of bronchiolitis obliterans with organizing pneumonia, usual interstitial pneumonia and small airways disease. *Am Rev Respir Dis*. 1987;135:705–712.
33. Staples C, Müller NL, Vedal S, et al. Usual interstitial pneumonia: correlations of CT with clinical, functional and radiologic findings. *Radiology*. 1987;162:377–381.
34. Epler G, McLoud TC, Gaensler EA, et al. Normal chest roentgenograms in chronic diffuse infiltrative lung disease. *N Engl J Med*. 1978;298:934–939.
35. Akira M, Sakatani M, Ueda E. Idiopathic pulmonary fibrosis: progression of honeycombing at thin-section CT. *Radiology*. 1993;189(3):687–691.
36. Nishimura K, Itoh H. High-resolution computed tomographic features of bronchiolitis obliterans organizing pneumonia. *Chest*. 1992;102:26S–31S.
37. Lynch DA. Ground glass attenuation on CT in patients with idiopathic pulmonary fibrosis. *Chest*. 1996;110(2):312–313.
38. Kazerooni EA, Martinez FJ, Flint A, et al. Thin-section CT obtained at 10-mm increments versus limited three-level thin-section CT for idiopathic pulmonary fibrosis: correlation with pathologic scoring. *AJR Am J Roentgenol*. 1997;169(4):977–983.
39. Hunninghake GW, Zimmerman MB, Schwartz DA, et al. Utility of a lung biopsy for the diagnosis of idiopathic pulmonary fibrosis. *Am J Respir Crit Care Med*. 2001;164(2):193–196.
40. Katzenstein A, Myers JL, Prophet WD, et al. Bronchiolitis obliterans and usual interstitial pneumonia. A comparative clinicopathologic study. *Am J Surg Pathol*. 1986;10:373–376.
41. Lee JS, Gong G, Song KS, et al. Usual interstitial pneumonia: relationship between disease activity and the progression of honeycombing at thin-section computed tomography. *J Thorac Imaging*. 1998;13(3):199–203.
42. Myers JL. NSIP, UIP, and the ABCs of idiopathic interstitial pneumonias. *Eur Respir J*. 1998;12(5):1003–1004.
43. Nagao T, Nagai S, Kitaichi M, et al. Usual interstitial pneumonia: idiopathic pulmonary fibrosis versus collagen vascular diseases. *Respiration*. 2001;68(2):151–159.
44. Cool CD, Groshong SD, Rai PR, et al. Fibroblast foci are not discrete sites of lung injury or repair: the fibroblast reticulum. *Am J Respir Crit Care Med*. 2006;174(6):654–658.
45. Flaherty KR, Colby TV, Travis WD, et al. Fibroblastic foci in usual interstitial pneumonia: idiopathic versus collagen vascular disease. *Am J Respir Crit Care Med*. 2003;167(10):1410–1415.
46. Kondoh Y, Taniguchi H, Kawabata Y, et al. Acute exacerbation in idiopathic pulmonary fibrosis. Analysis of clinical and pathologic findings in three cases. *Chest*. 1993;103(6):1808–1812.
47. Collard HR, Moore BB, Flaherty KR, et al. Acute exacerbations of idiopathic pulmonary fibrosis. *Am J Respir Crit Care Med*. 2007;176(7):636–643.
48. Panos RJ, Mortenson RL, Niccoli SA, King Jr TE. Clinical deterioration in patients with idiopathic pulmonary fibrosis: causes and assessment. *Am J Med*. 1990;88(4):396–404.
49. Kim DS, Park JH, Park BK, et al. Acute exacerbation of idiopathic pulmonary fibrosis: frequency and clinical features. *Eur Respir J*. 2006;27(1):143–150.
50. Katzenstein AL, Zisman DA, Litzky LA, et al. Usual interstitial pneumonia: histologic study of biopsy and explant specimens. *Am J Surg Pathol*. 2002;26(12):1567–1577.
51. Flaherty KR, Travis WD, Colby TV, et al. Histopathologic variability in usual and nonspecific interstitial pneumonias. *Am J Respir Crit Care Med*. 2001;164(9):1722–1727.
52. Noth I, Martinez FJ. Recent advances in idiopathic pulmonary fibrosis. *Chest*. 2007;132(2):637–650.
53. Bjoraker JA, Ryu JH, Edwin MK, et al. Prognostic significance of histopathologic subsets in idiopathic pulmonary fibrosis. *Am J Respir Crit Care Med*. 1998;157(1):199–203.
54. Raghu G, Brown KK, Costabel U, et al. Treatment of idiopathic pulmonary fibrosis with etanercept: an exploratory, placebo-controlled trial. *Am J Respir Crit Care Med*. 2008;178(9):948–955.
55. Ask K, Martin GE, Kolb M, Gauldie J. Targeting genes for treatment in idiopathic pulmonary fibrosis: challenges and opportunities, promises and pitfalls. *Proc Am Thorac Soc*. 2006;3(4):389–393.
56. Grutters JC, du Bois RM. Genetics of fibrosing lung diseases. *Eur Respir J*. 2005;25(5):915–927.
57. Wang Y, Kuan PJ, Xing C, et al. Genetic defects in surfactant protein A2 are associated with pulmonary fibrosis and lung cancer. *Am J Hum Genet*. 2009;84(1):52–59.
58. Steele MP, Speer MC, Loyd JE, et al. Clinical and pathologic features of familial interstitial pneumonia. *Am J Respir Crit Care Med*. 2005;172(9):1146–1152.
59. Armanios MY, Chen JJ, Cogan JD, et al. Telomerase mutations in families with idiopathic pulmonary fibrosis. *N Engl J Med*. 2007;356(13):1317–1326.
60. Kitaichi M. Pathologic features and the classification of interstitial pneumonia of unknown etiology. *Bull Chest Dis Res Inst Kyoto Univ*. 1990;23(1–2):1–18.
61. Nagai S, Kitaichi M, Itoh H, et al. Idiopathic nonspecific interstitial pneumonia/fibrosis: Comparison with idiopathic pulmonary fibrosis and BOOP. *Eur Respir J*. 1998;12(5):1010–1019.
62. Cottin V, Donsbeck AV, Revel D, et al. Nonspecific interstitial pneumonia. Individualization of a clinicopathologic entity in a series of 12 patients. *Am J Respir Crit Care Med*. 1998;158(4):1286–1293.
63. Daniil ZD, Gilchrist FC, Nicholson AG, et al. A histologic pattern of nonspecific interstitial pneumonia is associated with a better prognosis than usual interstitial pneumonia in patients with cryptogenic fibrosing alveolitis. *Am J Respir Crit Care Med*. 1999;160(3):899–905.
64. Park JS, Lee KS, Kim JS, et al. Nonspecific interstitial pneumonia with fibrosis: radiographic and CT findings in seven patients. *Radiology*. 1995;195(3):645–648.

65. Hartman TE, Swensen SJ, Hansell DM, et al. Nonspecific interstitial pneumonia: variable appearance at high-resolution chest CT. *Radiology*. 2000;217(3):701–705.

66. Travis WD, Hunninghake G, King Jr TE, et al. Idiopathic nonspecific interstitial pneumonia: report of an American Thoracic Society project. *Am J Respir Crit Care Med*. 2008;177(12):1338–1347.

67. Kinder BW, Collard HR, Koth L, et al. Idiopathic nonspecific interstitial pneumonia: lung manifestation of undifferentiated connective tissue disease? *Am J Respir Crit Care Med*. 2007;176(7):691–697.

68. Travis WD, Matsui K, Moss J, Ferrans VJ. Idiopathic nonspecific interstitial pneumonia: prognostic significance of cellular and fibrosing patterns: survival comparison with usual interstitial pneumonia and desquamative interstitial pneumonia. *Am J Surg Pathol*. 2000;24(1):19–33.

69. Davison AG, Heard BE, McAllister WA, Turner-Warwick ME. Cryptogenic organizing pneumonitis. *Q J Med*. 1983;52:382–394.

70. Yousem SA, Lohr RH, Colby TV. Idiopathic bronchiolitis obliterans organizing pneumonia/cryptogenic organizing pneumonia with unfavorable outcome: pathologic predictors. *Mod Pathol*. 1997;10(9):864–871.

71. Izumi T, Nagai S, Nishimura K, et al. BALF cell findings in patients with BOOP, particularly in comparison with UIP. *Nihon Kyobu Shikkan Gakkai Zasshi*. 1989;27(4):474–480.

72. King TJ, Mortensen R. Cryptogenic organizing pneumonitis. *Chest*. 1992;102:8S–13S.

73. Müller NL, Guerry-Force ML, Staples CA, et al. Differential diagnosis of bronchiolitis obliterans with organizing pneumonia and usual interstitial pneumonia: clinical, functional, and radiologic findings. *Radiology*. 1987;162(1 Pt 1):151–156.

74. Cordier JF, Loire R, Brune J. Idiopathic bronchiolitis obliterans organizing pneumonia: definition of clinical profiles in a series of 16 patients. *Chest*. 1989;96:999–1004.

75. Müller NL, Staples CA, Miller RR. Bronchiolitis obliterans organizing pneumonia: CT features in 14 patients. *AJR Am J Roentgenol*. 1990;154(5):983–987.

76. Lee KS, Kullnig P, Hartman TE, Müller NL. Cryptogenic organizing pneumonia. CT findings in 43 patients. *AJR Am J Roentgenol*. 1994;62:543–546.

77. Preidler KW, Szolar DM, Moelleken S, et al. Distribution pattern of computed tomography findings in patients with bronchiolitis obliterans organizing pneumonia. *Invest Radiol*. 1996;31(5):251–255.

78. Akira M, Yamamoto S, Sakatani S. Bronchiolitis obliterans organizing pneumonia manifesting as multiple large nodules or masses. *AJR Am J Roentgenol*. 1998;170(2):291–295.

79. Izumi T, Kitaichi M, Nishimura K, Nagai S. Bronchiolitis obliterans organizing pneumonia. Clinical features and differential diagnosis. *Chest*. 1992;102(3):715–719.

80. King Jr TE. BOOP: An important cause of migratory pulmonary infiltrates? *Eur Respir J*. 1995;8(2):193–195.

81. Bouchardy LM, Kuhlman JE, Ball Jr WC, et al. CT findings in bronchiolitis obliterans organizing pneumonia (BOOP) with radiographic, clinical, and histologic correlation. *J Comput Assist Tomogr*. 1993;17:352–357.

82. Colby TV. Pathologic aspects of bronchiolitis obliterans organizing pneumonia. *Chest*. 1992;102(suppl 1):38S–43S.

83. Kitaichi M. Bronchiolitis obliterans organizing pneumonia (BOOP). In: Takishima T, ed. *Basic and Clinical Aspects of Pulmonary Fibrosis*. Boca Raton, FL: CRC Press; 1994:463–488.

84. Cordier JF. Cryptogenic organizing pneumonitis. Bronchiolitis obliterans organizing pneumonia. *Clin Chest Med*. 1993;14(4):677–692.

85. Niewoehner D, Kleinerman J, Rice D. Pathologic changes in the the peripheral airways in young cigarette smokers. *N Engl J Med*. 1974;291:755–758.

86. Myers J, Veal Jr CF, Shin MS, Katzenstein AL. Respiratory bronchiolitis causing interstitial lung disease. A clinicopathologic study of six cases. *Am Rev Respir Dis*. 1987;135:880–884.

87. Heyneman LE, Ward S, Lynch DA, et al. Respiratory bronchiolitis, respiratory bronchiolitis–associated interstitial lung disease, and desquamative interstitial pneumonia: different entities or part of the spectrum of the same disease process? *AJR Am J Roentgenol*. 1999;173(6):1617–1622.

88. Yousem SA, Colby TV, Gaensler EA. Respiratory bronchiolitis–associated interstitial lung disease and its relationship to desquamative interstitial pneumonia. *Mayo Clin Proc*. 1989;64(11):1373–1380.

89. Myers JL, Veal Jr CF, Shin MS, Katzenstein AL. Respiratory bronchiolitis causing interstitial lung disease. A clinicopathologic study of six cases. *Am Rev Respir Dis*. 1987;135(4):880–884.

90. King Jr TE. Respiratory bronchiolitis–associated interstitial lung disease. *Clin Chest Med*. 1993;14(4):693–698.

91. Moon J, du Bois RM, Colby TV, et al. Clinical significance of respiratory bronchiolitis on open lung biopsy and its relationship to smoking related interstitial lung disease. *Thorax*. 1999;54(11):1009–1014.

92. Yousem SA. Respiratory bronchiolitis–associated interstitial lung disease with fibrosis is a lesion distinct from fibrotic nonspecific interstitial pneumonia: A proposal. *Mod Pathol*. 2006;19(11):1474–1479.

93. Portnoy J, Veraldi KL, Schwarz MI, et al. Respiratory bronchiolitis–interstitial lung disease: long-term outcome. *Chest*. 2007;131(3):664–671.

94. Carrington CB, Gaensler EA, Coutu RE, et al. Natural history and treated course of usual and desquamative interstitial pneumonia. *N Engl J Med*. 1978;298(15):801–809.

95. Katzenstein AL, Myers JL. Idiopathic pulmonary fibrosis: clinical relevance of pathologic classification. *Am J Respir Crit Care Med*. 1998;157(4 Pt 1):1301–1315.

96. Hartman TE, Primack SL, Swensen SJ, et al. Desquamative interstitial pneumonia: thin-section CT findings in 22 patients. *Radiology*. 1993;187(3):787–790.

97. Gruden JF, Webb WR. CT findings in a proved case of respiratory bronchiolitis. *AJR Am J Roentgenol*. 1993;161(1):44–46.

98. Nicholson AG, Wotherspoon AC, Diss TC, et al. Pulmonary B-cell non-Hodgkin's lymphomas. The value of immunohistochemistry and gene analysis in diagnosis. *Histopathology*. 1995;26(5):395–403.

99. Nicholson AG, Wotherspoon AC, Diss TC, et al. Reactive pulmonary lymphoid disorders. *Histopathology*. 1995;26(5):405–412.

100. Nicholson AG, Wotherspoon AC, Jones AL, et al. Pulmonary B-cell non-Hodgkin's lymphoma associated with autoimmune disorders: a clinicopathological review of six cases. *Eur Respir J*. 1996;9(10):2022–2025.

101. Koss MN. Pulmonary lymphoproliferative disorders. *Monogr Pathol*. 1993;18(36):145–194.

102. Herbert A, Walters MT, Cawley MI, Godfrey RC. Lymphocytic interstitial pneumonia identified as lymphoma of mucosa-associated lymphoid tissue. *J Pathol*. 1985;146(2):129–138.

103. Schuurman HJ, Gooszen HC, Tan IW, et al. Low-grade lymphoma of immature T-cell phenotype in a case of lymphocytic interstitial pneumonia and Sjögren's syndrome. *Histopathology*. 1987;11(11):1193–1204.

104. Cha SI, Fessler MB, Cool CD, et al. Lymphoid interstitial pneumonia: clinical features, associations and prognosis. *Eur Respir J*. 2006;28(2):364–369.

105. Strimlan C, Rosenow 3rd EC, Weiland LH, Brown LR. Lymphocytic interstitial pneumonitis. Review of 13 cases. *Ann Intern Med*. 1978;88:616–621.

106. Liebow AA, Carrington CB. Diffuse pulmonary lymphoreticular infiltrations associated with dysproteinemia. *Med Clin North Am*. 1973;57:809–843.

107. Strimlan CV, Rosenow 3rd EC, Divertie MB, Harrison Jr EG. Pulmonary manifestations of Sjögren's syndrome. *Chest*. 1976;70(03):354–361.

108. DeCoteau WE, Tourville D, Ambrus JL, et al. Lymphoid interstitial pneumonia and autoerythrocyte sensitization syndrome. A case with deposition of immunoglobulins on the alveolar basement membrane. *Arch Intern Med*. 1974;134(3):519–522.

109. Julsrud PR, Brown LR, Li CY, et al. Pulmonary processes of mature-appearing lymphocytes: pseudolymphoma, well-differentiated lymphocytic lymphoma, and lymphocytic interstitial pneumonitis. *Radiology*. 1978;127(2):289–296.

110. Schwarz MI. A man with dyspnea, productive cough, and chest radiograph showing hyperinflation and a diffuse nodular pattern. *Chest*. 1998;113(4):1123–1124.

111. Johkoh T, Ichikado K, Akira M, et al. Lymphocytic interstitial pneumonia: follow-up CT findings in 14 patients. *J Thorac Imaging*. 2000;15(3):162–167.

112. Macfarlane A, Davies D. Diffuse lymphoid interstitial pneumonia. *Thorax*. 1973;28(6):768–776.

113. Strimlan C, Rosenow 3rd EC, Weiland LH, Brown LR. Lymphocytic interstitial pneumonitis. Review of 13 cases. *Ann Intern Med*. 1978;88:616–621.

114. Johkoh T, Müller NL, Pickford HA, et al. Lymphocytic interstitial pneumonia: thin-section CT findings in 22 patients. *Radiology*. 1999;212(2):567–572.

115. Silva CI, Flint JD, Levy RD, Müller NL. Diffuse lung cysts in lymphoid interstitial pneumonia: high-resolution CT and pathologic findings. *J Thorac Imaging*. 2006;21(3):241–244.

116. Lohrmann C, Uhl M, Warnatz K, et al. High-resolution CT imaging of the lung for patients with primary Sjögren's syndrome. *Eur J Radiol*. 2004;52(1):137–143.

117. Torii K, Ogawa K, Kawabata Y, et al. Lymphoid interstitial pneumonia as a pulmonary lesion of idiopathic plasmacytic lymphadenopathy with hyperimmunoglobulinemia. *Intern Med*. 1994;33(4):237–241.

118. Julsrud PR, Brown LR, Li CY, et al. Pulmonary processes of mature-appearing lymphocytes: pseudolymphoma, well-differentiated lymphocytic lymphoma, and lymphocytic interstitial pneumonitis. *Radiology*. 1978;127:289–296.

119. Strimlan CV. Pulmonary function in patients with primary Sjögren's syndrome. *Ann Rheum Dis*. 2001;60(4):429.

120. Palmas A, Tefferi A, Myers JL, et al. Late-onset noninfectious pulmonary complications after allogeneic bone marrow transplantation. *Br J Haematol*. 1998;100(4):680–687.

121. Grieco M, Chinoy-Acharya P. Lymphoid interstitial pneumonia associated with the acquired immune deficiency syndrome. *Am Rev Respir Dis*. 1985;131:952–955.

122. Berdon WE, Mellins RB, Abramson SJ, Ruzal-Shapiro C. Pediatric HIV infection in its second decade—the changing pattern of lung involvement. Clinical, plain film, and computed tomographic findings. *Radiol Clin North Am*. 1993;31(3):453–463.

123. Ikeogu MO, Wolf B, Mathe S. Pulmonary manifestations in HIV seropositivity and malnutrition in Zimbabwe. *Arch Dis Child*. 1997;76(2):124–128.

124. Khare MD, Sharland M. Pulmonary manifestations of pediatric HIV infection. *Indian J Pediatr*. 1999;66(6):895–904.

125. Church JA. Lymphoid interstitial pneumonia and rheumatoid arthritis. *J Pediatr*. 1985;107(3):485.

126. Black L, Katz S. *Respiratory Disease: Task Force Report on Problems, Research Approaches, Needs*. Washington, DC: Department of Health, Education, and Welfare, National Heart and Lung Institute; 1977.

127. Banks J, Banks C, Cheong B, et al. An epidemiological and clinical investigation of pulmonary function and respiratory symptoms in patients with rheumatoid arthritis. *Q J Med*. 1992;85:795–806.

128. Cheema GS, Quismorio Jr FP. Interstitial lung disease in systemic sclerosis. *Curr Opin Pulm Med*. 2001;7(5):283–290.

129. Minai OA, Dweik RA, Arroliga AC. Manifestations of scleroderma pulmonary disease. *Clin Chest Med*. 1998;19(4):713–731, viii–ix.

130. Cheema GS, Quismorio Jr FP. Interstitial lung disease in systemic lupus erythematosus. *Curr Opin Pulm Med*. 2000;6(5):424–429.

131. Murin S, Wiedemann HP, Matthay RA. Pulmonary manifestations of systemic lupus erythematosus. *Clin Chest Med*. 1998;19(4):641–665, viii.

132. Dickey BF, Myers AR. Pulmonary disease in polymyositis/dermatomyositis. *Semin Arthritis Rheum*. 1984;14(1):60–76.

133. Ito I, Nagai S, Kitaichi M, et al. Pulmonary manifestations of primary Sjogren's syndrome: a clinical, radiologic, and pathologic study. *Am J Respir Crit Care Med*. 2005;171(6):632–638.

134. Koyama M, Johkoh T, Honda O, et al. Pulmonary involvement in primary Sjögren's syndrome: spectrum of pulmonary abnormalities and computed tomography findings in 60 patients. *J Thorac Imaging*. 2001;16(4):290–296.

135. Sarkar PK, Patel N, Furie RA, Talwar A. Pulmonary manifestations of primary Sjögren's syndrome. *Indian J Chest Dis Allied Sci*. 2009;51(2):93–101.

136. Prakash UB. Respiratory complications in mixed connective tissue disease. *Clin Chest Med*. 1998;19(4):733–746, ix.

137. Tillie-Leblond I, Wislez M, Valeyre D, et al. Interstitial lung disease and anti-Jo-1 antibodies: difference between acute and gradual onset. *Thorax*. 2008;63(1):53–59.

138. Ellman P, Ball RE. "Rheumatoid disease" with joint and pulmonary manifestations. *BMJ*. 1948;2:816–820.

139. Gabbay E, Tarala R, Will R, et al. Interstitial lung disease in recent onset rheumatoid arthritis. *Am J Respir Crit Care Med*. 1997;156(2 Pt 1):528–535.

140. Anaya JM, Diethelm L, Ortiz LA, et al. Pulmonary involvement in rheumatoid arthritis. *Semin Arthritis Rheum*. 1995;24(4):242–254.

141. Hakala M. Poor prognosis in patients with rheumatoid arthritis hospitalized for interstitial lung fibrosis. *Chest*. 1988;93(1):114–118.

142. Athreya BH, Doughty RA, Bookspan M, et al. Pulmonary manifestations of juvenile rheumatoid arthritis. A report of eight cases and review. *Clin Chest Med*. 1980;1(3):361–374.

143. Saag KG, Kolluri S, Koehnke RK, et al. Rheumatoid arthritis lung disease. Determinants of radiographic and physiologic abnormalities. *Arthritis Rheum*. 1996;39(10):1711–1719.

144. Akira M, Sakatani M, Hara H. Thin-section CT findings in rheumatoid arthritis–associated lung disease: CT patterns and their courses. *J Comput Assist Tomogr*. 1999;23(6):941–948.

145. Remy-Jardin M, Remy J, Cortet B, et al. Lung changes in rheumatoid arthritis: CT findings. *Radiology*. 1994;193(2):375–382.

146. Hunninghake GW, Fauci AS. Pulmonary involvement in the collagen vascular diseases. *Am Rev Respir Dis*. 1979;119(3):471–503.

147. Hubbard R, Venn A. The impact of coexisting connective tissue disease on survival in patients with fibrosing alveolitis. *Rheumatology (Oxford)*. 2002;41(6):676–679.

148. Laitinen O, Nissilä M, Salorinne Y, Aalto P. Pulmonary involvement in patients with rheumatoid arthritis. *Scand J Respir Dis*. 1975;56:297–304.

149. Lee HK, Kim DS, Yoo B, et al. Histopathologic pattern and clinical features of rheumatoid arthritis–associated interstitial lung disease. *Chest*. 2005;127(6):2019–2027.

150. Schwarz MI, Matthay RA, Sahn SA, et al. Interstitial lung disease in polymyositis and dermatomyositis: analysis of six cases and review of the literature. *Medicine (Baltimore)*. 1976;55(1):89–104.

151. Khanna D, Brown KK, Clements PJ, et al. Systemic sclerosis-associated interstitial lung disease-proposed recommendations for future randomized clinical trials. *Clin Exp Rheumatol*. 2010;28(2 Suppl 58):S55–S62.

152. Hunninghake GW, Gadek JE, Kawanami O, et al. Inflammatory and immune processes in the human lung in health and disease: evaluation by bronchoalveolar lavage. *Am J Pathol*. 1979;97:149–206.

153. Bouros D, Wells AU, Nicholson AG, et al. Histopathologic subsets of fibrosing alveolitis in patients with systemic sclerosis and their relationship to outcome. *Am J Respir Crit Care Med*. 2002;165(12):1581–1586.

154. Kim DS, Yoo B, Lee JS, et al. The major histopathologic pattern of pulmonary fibrosis in scleroderma is nonspecific interstitial pneumonia. *Sarcoidosis Vasc Diffuse Lung Dis*. 2002;19(2):121–127.

155. Kim EA, Johkoh T, Lee KS, et al. Interstitial pneumonia in progressive systemic sclerosis: serial high-resolution CT findings with functional correlation. *J Comput Assist Tomogr*. 2001;25(5):757–763.

156. Cozzi F, Chiesura Corona M, Rizzi M, et al. Lung fibrosis quantified by HRCT in scleroderma patients with different disease forms and ANA specificities. *Reumatismo*. 2001;53(1):55–62.

157. Yamane K, Ihn H, Asano Y, et al. Clinical and laboratory features of scleroderma patients with pulmonary hypertension. *Rheumatology (Oxford)*. 2000;39(11):1269–1271.

158. Johnson DA, Drane WE, Curran J, et al. Pulmonary disease in progressive systemic sclerosis. A complication of gastroesophageal reflux and occult aspiration? *Arch Intern Med*. 1989;149(3):589–593.

159. Montesi A, Pesaresi A, Cavalli ML, et al. Oropharyngeal and esophageal function in scleroderma. *Dysphagia*. 1991;6(4):219–223.

160. Tashkin DP, Elashoff R, Clements PJ, et al. Effects of 1-year treatment with cyclophosphamide on outcomes at 2 years in scleroderma lung disease. *Am J Respir Crit Care Med*. 2007;176(10):1026–1034.

161. McSweeney PA, Nash RA, Sullivan KM, et al. High-dose immunosuppressive therapy for severe systemic sclerosis: initial outcomes. *Blood*. 2002;100(5):1602–1610.

162. Dubois E, Tufanelli DL. Clinical manifestations of systemic lupus erythematosus. *JAMA*. 1964;190:104–111.

163. Eisenberg H, Dubois EL, Sherwin RP, Balchum OJ. Diffuse interstitial lung disease in systemic lupus erythematosus. *Ann Intern Med*. 1973;79:37–45.

164. Gammon RB, Bridges TA, al-Nezir H, et al. Bronchiolitis obliterans organizing pneumonia associated with systemic lupus erythematosus. *Chest*. 1992;102:1171–1174.

165. Myers JL, Katzenstein AA. Microangiitis in lupus-induced pulmonary hemorrhage. *Am J Clin Pathol*. 1986;85(5):552–556.

166. Chang MY, Fang JT, Chen YC, Huang CC. Diffuse alveolar hemorrhage in systemic lupus erythematosus: a single center retrospective study in Taiwan. *Ren Fail*. 2002;24(6):791–802.

167. Santos-Ocampo AS, Mandell BF, Fessler BJ. Alveolar hemorrhage in systemic lupus erythematosus: presentation and management. *Chest*. 2000;118(4):1083–1090.

168. Matthay RA, Schwarz MI, Petty TL, et al. Pulmonary manifestations of systemic lupus erythematosus: review of twelve cases with acute lupus pneumonitis. *Medicine*. 1974;54:397–409.

169. Kim JS, Lee KS, Koh EM, et al. Thoracic involvement of systemic lupus erythematosus: clinical, pathologic, and radiologic findings. *J Comput Assist Tomogr*. 2000;24(1):9–18.

170. Hughson MD, He Z, Henegar J, McMurray R. Alveolar hemorrhage and renal microangiopathy in systemic lupus erythematosus. *Arch Pathol Lab Med*. 2001;125(4):475–483.

171. Bankier AA, Kiener HP, Wiesmayr MN, et al. Discrete lung involvement in systemic lupus erythematosus: CT assessment. *Radiology*. 1995;196(3):835–840.

172. Fenlon HM, Doran M, Sant SM, Breatnach E. High-resolution chest CT in systemic lupus erythematosus. *AJR Am J Roentgenol*. 1996;166(2):301–307.

173. Sant SM, Doran M, Fenelon HM, Breatnach ES. Pleuropulmonary abnormalities in patients with systemic lupus erythematosus: assessment with high resolution computed tomography, chest radiography and pulmonary function tests. *Clin Exp Rheumatol*. 1997;15(5):507–513.

174. Ooi GC, Ngan H, Peh WC, et al. Systemic lupus erythematosus patients with respiratory symptoms: the value of HRCT. *Clin Radiol*. 1997;52(10):775–781.

175. Susanto I, Peters JI. Acute lupus pneumonitis with normal chest radiograph. *Chest*. 1997;111(6):1781–1783.

176. Anderson NE, Ali MR. The lupus anticoagulant, pulmonary thromboembolism, and fatal pulmonary hypertension. *Ann Rheum Dis*. 1984;43(5):760–763.

177. Howe HS, Boey ML, Fong KY, Feng PH. Pulmonary haemorrhage, pulmonary infarction, and the lupus anticoagulant. *Ann Rheum Dis*. 1988;47(10):869–872.

178. Auger WR, Permpikul P, Moser KM. Lupus anticoagulant, heparin use, and thrombocytopenia in patients with chronic thromboembolic pulmonary hypertension: a preliminary report. *Am J Med*. 1995;99(4):392–396.

179. Urman JD, Rothfield NF. Corticosteroid treatment in systemic lupus erythematosus. Survival studies. *JAMA*. 1977;238(21):2272–1176.

180. Rosner S, Ginzler EM, Diamond HS, et al. A multicenter study of outcome in systemic lupus erythematosus. II. Causes of death. *Arthritis Rheum*. 1982;25(6):612–617.

181. Bohan A, Peter JB, Bowman RL, Pearson CM. Computer-assisted analysis of 153 patients with polymyositis and dermatomyositis. *Medicine (Baltimore)*. 1977;56(4):255–286.

182. Bohan A. History and classification of polymyositis and dermatomyositis. *Clin Dermatol*. 1988;6(2):3–8.

183. Nobutoh T, Kohda M, Doi Y, Ueki H. An autopsy case of dermatomyositis with rapidly progressive diffuse alveolar damage. *J Dermatol*. 1998;25(1):32–36.

184. Tazelaar HD, Viggiano RW, Pickersgill J, Colby TV. Interstitial lung disease in polymyositis and dermatomyositis. Clinical features and prognosis as correlated with histologic findings. *Am Rev Respir Dis*. 1990;141(3):727–733.

185. Douglas WW, Tazelaar HD, Hartman TE, et al. Polymyositis-dermatomyositis–associated interstitial lung disease. *Am J Respir Crit Care Med*. 2001;164(7):1182–1185.

186. Hepper N, Ferguson RH, Howard FM. Three types of pulmonary involvement in polymyositis. *Med Clin North Am*. 1964;48:1031–1042.

187. Benbassat J, Gefel D, Larholt K, et al. Prognostic factors in polymyositis/dermatomyositis. A computer-assisted analysis of ninety-two cases. *Arthritis Rheum*. 1985;28(3):249–255.

188. Ikezoe J, Johkoh T, Kohno N, et al. High-resolution CT findings of lung disease in patients with polymyositis and dermatomyositis. *J Thorac Imaging*. 1996;11(4):250–259.

189. Whaley K, Alspaugh MA. Sjögren's syndrome. In Kelley H, Harris Jr ED, Ruddy S, Sledge CB, eds. *Textbook of Rheumatology*. 2nd ed Philadelphia: WB Saunders; 1985:956.

190. Baruch HH, Firooznia H, Sackler JP, et al. Pulmonary disorders associated with Sjögren's syndrome. *Rev Interam Radiol*. 1977;2(2):77–81.

191. Franquet T, Giménez A, Monill JM, et al. Primary Sjögren's syndrome and associated lung disease: CT findings in 50 patients. *AJR Am J Roentgenol*. 1997;169(3):655–658.

192. Deheinzelin D, Capelozzi VL, Kairalla RA, et al. Interstitial lung disease in primary Sjögren's syndrome. Clinical-pathological evaluation and response to treatment. *Am J Respir Crit Care Med*. 1996;154(3 Pt 1):794–799.

193. Reveille JD, Wilson RW, Provost TT, et al. Primary Sjögren's syndrome and other autoimmune diseases in families. Prevalence and immunogenetic studies in six kindreds. *Ann Intern Med*. 1984;101(6):748–756.

194. Meyer CA, Pina JS, Taillon D, Godwin JD. Inspiratory and expiratory high-resolution CT findings in a patient with Sjögren's syndrome and cystic lung disease. *AJR Am J Roentgenol*. 1997;168(1):101–103.

195. Hansen LA, Prakash UB, Colby TV. Pulmonary lymphoma in Sjögren's syndrome. *Mayo Clin Proc*. 1989;64(8):920–931.

196. Kokosi M, Riemer EC, Highland KB. Pulmonary involvement in Sjögren syndrome. *Clin Chest Med*. 2010;31(3):489–500.

197. Carrington CB, et al. Chronic eosinophilic pneumonia. *N Engl J Med*. 1969;280:787–798.

198. Liebow A, Carrington C. The eosinophilic pneumonias. *Medicine (Baltimore)*. 1969;48: 251–285.

199. Gaensler E, Carrington C. Peripheral opacities in chronic eosinophilic pneumonia: the photographic negative of pulmonary edema. *AJR Am J Roentgenol*. 1977;128:1–13.

200. Mayo J, Müller NL, Road J, et al. Chronic eosinophilic pneumonia: CT findings in six cases. *AJR Am J Roentgenol*. 1989;153:727–730.

201. Copper Jr JA. Drug-induced lung disease. *Adv Intern Med*. 1997;42:231–268.

202. Camus PH, Foucher P, Bonniaud PH, Ask K. Drug-induced infiltrative lung disease. *Eur Respir J Suppl*. 2001;32:93s–100s.

203. Ozkan M, Dweik RA, Ahmad M. Drug-induced lung disease. *Cleve Clin J Med*. 2001;68(9): 782–785, 789–795.

204. Cuellar ML. Drug-induced vasculitis. *Curr Rheumatol Rep*. 2002;4(1):55–59.

205. Ruangchira-Urai R, Colby TV, Klein J, et al. Nodular amiodarone lung disease. *Am J Surg Pathol*. 2008;32(11):1654–1660.

206. Camus P, Lombard JN, Perrichon M, et al. Bronchiolitis obliterans organising pneumonia in patients taking acebutolol or amiodarone. *Thorax*. 1989;44(9):711–715.

207. Kennedy JI, Myers JL, Plumb VJ, Fulmer JD. Amiodarone pulmonary toxicity. Clinical, radiologic, and pathologic correlations. *Arch Intern Med*. 1987;147(1):50–55.

208. Musk AW, Pollard JA. Pindolol and pulmonary fibrosis. *BMJ*. 1979;2(6190):581–582.

209. Sandler A, Gray R, Perry MC, et al. Paclitaxel-carboplatin alone or with bevacizumab for non-small-cell lung cancer. *N Engl J Med*. 2006;355(24):2542–2550.

210. Iacovino JR, Leitner J, Abbas AK, et al. Fatal pulmonary reaction from low doses of bleomycin. An idiosyncratic tissue response. *JAMA*. 1976;235(12):1253–1255.

211. Luna MA, Bedrossian CW, Lichtiger B, Salem PA. Interstitial pneumonitis associated with bleomycin therapy. *Am J Clin Pathol*. 1972;58(5):501–510.

212. Feingold ML, Koss LG. Effects of long-term administration of busulfan. Report of a patient with generalized nuclear abnormalities, carcinoma of vulva, and pulmonary fibrosis. *Arch Intern Med*. 1969;124(1):66–71.

213. Littler WA, Kay JM, Hasleton PS, Heath D. Busulphan lung. *Thorax*. 1969;24(6):639–655.

214. Lombard CM, Churg A, Winokur S. Pulmonary veno-occlusive disease following therapy for malignant neoplasms. *Chest*. 1987;92(5):871–876.

215. Mitsudo SM, Greenwald ES, Banerji B, Koss LG. BCNU (1,3-*bis*-(2-chloroethyl)-1-nitrosurea) lung. Drug-induced pulmonary changes. *Cancer*. 1984;54(4):751–755.

216. Forrester JM, Steele AW, Waldron JA, Parsons PE. Crack lung: an acute pulmonary syndrome with a spectrum of clinical and histopathologic findings. *Am Rev Respir Dis*. 1990;142(2): 462–467.

217. Murray RJ, Albin RJ, Mergner W, Criner GJ. Diffuse alveolar hemorrhage temporally related to cocaine smoking. *Chest*. 1988;93(2):427–429.

218. Abdel Karim FW, Ayash RE, Allam C, Salem PA. Pulmonary fibrosis after prolonged treatment with low-dose cyclophosphamide. A case report. *Oncology*. 1983;40(3):174–176.

219. Patel AR, Shah PC, Rhee HL, et al. Cyclophosphamide therapy and interstitial pulmonary fibrosis. *Cancer*. 1976;38(4):1542–1549.

220. Spector JI, Zimbler H, Ross JS. Early-onset cyclophosphamide-induced interstitial pneumonitis. *JAMA*. 1979;242(26):2852–2854.

221. Slavin RE, Millan JC, Mullins GM. Pathology of high dose intermittent cyclophosphamide therapy. *Hum Pathol*. 1975;6(6):693–709.

222. Read WL, Mortimer JE, Picus J. Severe interstitial pneumonitis associated with docetaxel administration. *Cancer*. 2002;94(3):847–853.

223. Pfitzenmeyer P, Foucher P, Dennewald G, et al. Pleuropulmonary changes induced by ergoline drugs. *Eur Respir J*. 1996;9(5):1013–1019.

224. Liu V, White DA, Zakowski MF, et al. Pulmonary toxicity associated with erlotinib. *Chest*. 2007;132(3):1042–1044.

225. Gurjal A, An T, Valdivieso M, Kalemkerian GP. Etoposide-induced pulmonary toxicity. *Lung Cancer*. 1999;26(2):109–112.

226. Inoue A, Saijo Y, Maemondo M, et al. Severe acute interstitial pneumonia and gefitinib. *Lancet*. 2003;361(9352):137–139.

227. Briasoulis E, Froudarakis M, Milionis HJ, et al. Chemotherapy-induced noncardiogenic pulmonary edema related to gemcitabine plus docetaxel combination with granulocyte colony-stimulating factor support. *Respiration*. 2000;67(6):680–683.

228. Tomioka R, King Jr TE. Gold-induced pulmonary disease: clinical features, outcome, and differentiation from rheumatoid lung disease. *Am J Respir Crit Care Med*. 1997;155(3):1011–1020.

229. Warnock ML, Ghahremani GG, Rattenborg C, et al. Pulmonary complication of heroin intoxication. Aspiration pneumonia and diffuse bronchiectasis. *JAMA*. 1972;219(8):1051–1053.

230. Karne S, D'Ambrosio C, Einarsson O, O'Connor PG. Hypersensitivity pneumonitis induced by intranasal heroin use. *Am J Med*. 1999;107(4):392–395.

231. Petersen AG, Dodge M, Helwig FC. Pulmonary changes associated with hexamethonium therapy. *Arch Intern Med*. 1959;103:285–288.

232. Perry Jr HM, O'Neal RM, Thomas WA. Pulmonary disease following chronic chemical ganglionic blockade. *Am J Med*. 1957;22:37–50.

233. Beaudry C, Laplante L. Severe allergic pneumonitis from hydrochlorothiazide. *Ann Intern Med*. 1973;78(2):251–253.

234. Kaufman A, Montilla E, Helfgott M, et al. Pneumonitis and hydrochlorothiazide. *Ann Intern Med*. 1973;79(2):282–283.

235. Dorn MR, Walker BK. Noncardiogenic pulmonary edema associated with hydrochlorothiazide therapy. *Chest*. 1981;79(4):482–483.

236. Tengstrand B, Ernestam S, Engvall IL, et al. TNF blockade in rheumatoid arthritis can cause severe fibrosing alveolitis. Six case reports. *Lakartidningen*. 2005;102(49):3788–3790, 3793.

237. Cordonnier C, Vernant JP, Mital P, et al. Pulmonary fibrosis subsequent to high doses of CCNU for chronic myeloid leukemia. *Cancer*. 1983;51(10):1814–1818.

238. Myers JL. Pathology of drug-induced lung disease. In: Katzenstein AL, ed. *Katzenstein and Askin's Surgical Pathology of Non-Neoplastic Lung Disease*. Philadelphia: WB Saunders; 1997:81–111.

239. Imokawa S, Colby TV, Leslie KO, Helmers RA. Methotrexate pneumonitis: review of the literature and histopathological findings in nine patients. *Eur Respir J*. 2000;15(2):373–381.

240. Bentur L, Bar-Kana Y, Livni E, et al. Severe minocycline-induced eosinophilic pneumonia: extrapulmonary manifestations and the use of in vitro immunoassays. *Ann Pharmacother*. 1997;31(6):733–735.

241. Piperno D, Donné C, Loire R, Cordier JF. Bronchiolitis obliterans organizing pneumonia associated with minocycline therapy: a possible cause. *Eur Respir J*. 1995;8(6):1018–1020.

242. Waldhorn RE, Tsou E, Smith FP, Kerwin DM. Pulmonary veno-occlusive disease associated with microangiopathic hemolytic anemia and chemotherapy of gastric adenocarcinoma. *Med Pediatr Oncol*. 1984;12(6):394–396.

243. Fielding JW, Crocker J, Stockley RA, Brookes VS. Interstitial fibrosis in a patient treated with 5-fluorouracil and mitomycin C. *BMJ*. 1979;2(6189):551–552.

244. Israel KS, Brashear RE, Sharma HM, et al. Pulmonary fibrosis and nitrofurantoin. *Am Rev Respir Dis*. 1973;108(2):353–356.

245. Geller M, Dickie HA, Kass DA, et al. The histopathology of acute nitrofurantoin-associated pneumonitis. *Ann Allergy*. 1976;37(4):275–279.

246. Magee F, Wright JL, Chan N, et al. Two unusual pathological reactions to nitrofurantoin: case reports. *Histopathology*. 1986;10(7):701–706.

247. Ayoub JP, North L, Greer J, et al. Pulmonary changes in patients with lymphoma who receive paclitaxel. *J Clin Oncol*. 1997;15(6):2476.

248. Epler GR, Snider GL, Gaensler EA, et al. Bronchiolitis and bronchitis in connective tissue disease. A possible relationship to the use of penicillamine. *JAMA*. 1979;242(6):528–532.

249. Sternlieb I, Bennett B, Scheinberg IH. D-Penicillamine induced Goodpasture's syndrome in Wilson's disease. *Ann Intern Med*. 1975;82(5):673–676.

250. Davies D, Jones JK. Pulmonary eosinophilia caused by penicillamine. *Thorax*. 1980;35(12): 957–958.

251. Chamberlain DW, Hyland RH, Ross DJ. Diphenylhydantoin-induced lymphocytic interstitial pneumonia. *Chest*. 1986;90(3):458–460.

252. Michael JR, Rudin ML. Acute pulmonary disease caused by phenytoin. *Ann Intern Med*. 1981;95(4):452–454.

253. Dohner VA, Ward HP, Standord RE. Alveolitis during procarbazine, vincristine and cyclophosphamide therapy. *Chest*. 1972;62(5):636–639.

254. Farney RJ, Morris AH, Armstrong JD, Hammer S. Diffuse pulmonary disease after therapy with nitrogen mustard, vincristine, procarbazine, and prednisone. *Am Rev Respir Dis*. 1977;115(1):135–145.

255. Horton LW, Chappell AG, Powell DE. Diffuse interstitial pulmonary fibrosis complicating Hodgkin's disease. *Br J Dis Chest*. 1977;71(1):44–48.

256. Gonzalez-Rothi RJ, Zander DS, Ros PR. Fluoxetine hydrochloride (Prozac)-induced pulmonary disease. *Chest*. 1995;107(6):1763–1765.

257. Burton C, Kaczmarski R, Jan-Mohamed R. Interstitial pneumonitis related to rituximab therapy. *N Engl J Med*. 2003;348(26):2690–2691, discussion 2690–2691.

258. Parry SD, et al. Sulphasalazine and lung toxicity. *Eur Respir J*. 2002;19(4):756–764.

259. Travis WD, Kalafer ME, Robin HS, Luibel FJ. Hypersensitivity pneumonitis and pulmonary vasculitis with eosinophilia in a patient taking an L-tryptophan preparation. *Ann Intern Med*. 1990;112(4):301–303.

260. Catton CK, Elmer JC, Whitehouse AC, et al. Pulmonary involvement in the eosinophilia-myalgia syndrome. *Chest*. 1991;99(2):327–329.

261. Calvo 3rd DB, Legha SS, McKelvey EM, et al. Zinostatin-related pulmonary toxicity. *Cancer Treat Rep*. 1981;65(1–2):165–167.

262. Zitnik RJ, Matthay RA. Drug-induced lung disease. In: Schwartz MI, King TE, eds. *Interstitial Lung Disease*. London: BC Decker; 1998.423–449.

263. Kudoh S, Kato H, Nishiwaki Y, et al. Interstitial lung disease in Japanese patients with lung cancer: a cohort and nested case-control study. *Am J Respir Crit Care Med*. 2008;177(12):1348–1357.

264. Sostman HD, Matthay RA, Putman CE, Smith GJ. Methotrexate-induced pneumonitis. *Medicine (Baltimore)*. 1976;55(5):371–388.

265. Goodman TA, Polisson RP. Methotrexate: adverse reactions and major toxicities. *Rheum Dis Clin North Am*. 1994;20(2):513–528.

266. Bedrossian CW, Miller WC, Luna MA. Methotrexate-induced diffuse interstitial pulmonary fibrosis. *South Med J*. 1979;72(3):313–318.

267. Zisman DA, McCune WJ, Tino G, Lynch 3rd JP. Drug-induced pneumonitis: the role of methotrexate. *Sarcoidosis Vasc Diffuse Lung Dis*. 2001;18(3):243–252.

268. Kennedy JI, Myers JL, Plumb VJ, Fulmer JD. Amiodarone pulmonary toxicity. Clinical, radiologic, and pathologic correlations. *Arch Intern Med*. 1987;147(1):50–55.

269. Dusman RE, Stanton MS, Miles WM, et al. Clinical features of amiodarone-induced pulmonary toxicity. *Circulation*. 1990;82(1):51–59.

270. Newman LS, Rose CS, Bresnitz EA, et al. A case control etiologic study of sarcoidosis: environmental and occupational risk factors. *Am J Respir Crit Care Med*. 2004;170(12):1324–1330.

271. Fraire AE, Guntupalli KK, Greenberg SD, et al. Amiodarone pulmonary toxicity: a multidisciplinary review of current status. *South Med J*. 1993;86(1):67–77.

272. Nicholson AA, Hayward C. The value of computed tomography in the diagnosis of amiodarone-induced pulmonary toxicity. *Clin Radiol*. 1989;40(6):564–567.

273. Kuhlman JE, Teigen C, Ren H, et al. Amiodarone pulmonary toxicity: CT findings in symptomatic patients. *Radiology*. 1990;177(1):121–125.

274. Myers JL, Kennedy JI, Plumb VJ. Amiodarone lung: Pathologic findings in clinically toxic patients. *Hum Pathol*. 1987;18(4):349–354.

275. Martin 2nd WJ, Rosenow 3rd EC. Amiodarone pulmonary toxicity. Recognition and pathogenesis (Part I). *Chest*. 1988;93(5):1067–1075.

276. Martin 2nd WJ, Rosenow 3rd EC. Amiodarone pulmonary toxicity. Recognition and pathogenesis (Part 2). *Chest*. 1988;93(6):1242–1248.

277. Gonzalez-Rothi RJ, Hannan SE, Hood CI, Franzini DA. Amiodarone pulmonary toxicity presenting as bilateral exudative pleural effusions. *Chest*. 1987;92(1):179–182.

278. Ruangchira-Urai R, Colby TV, Klein J, et al. Nodular amiodarone lung disease. *Am J Surg Pathol*. 2008;32(11):1654–1660.

279. Wood DL, Osborn MJ, Rooke J, Holmes Jr DR. Amiodarone pulmonary toxicity: report of two cases associated with rapidly progressive fatal adult respiratory distress syndrome after pulmonary angiography. *Mayo Clin Proc*. 1985;60(9):601–603.

280. Van Mieghem W, Coolen L, Malysse I, et al. Amiodarone and the development of ARDS after lung surgery. *Chest*. 1994;105(6):1642–1645.

281. Durant JR, Norgard MJ, Murad TM, et al. Pulmonary toxicity associated with bischloroethylnitrosourea (BCNU). *Ann Intern Med*. 1979;90(2):191–194.

282. Lieberman A, Ruoff M, Estey E, et al. Irreversible pulmonary toxicity after single course of BCNU. *Am J Med Sci*. 1980;279(1):53–56.

283. Litam JP, Dail DH, Spitzer G, et al. Early pulmonary toxicity after administration of high-dose BCNU. *Cancer Treat Rep*. 1981;65(1–2):39–44.

284. Cao TM, Negrin RS, Stockerl-Goldstein KE, et al. Pulmonary toxicity syndrome in breast cancer patients undergoing BCNU-containing high-dose chemotherapy and autologous hematopoietic cell transplantation. *Biol Blood Marrow Transplant*. 2000;6(4):387–394.

285. Holoye PY, Jenkins DE, Greenberg SD. Pulmonary toxicity in long-term administration of BCNU. *Cancer Treat Rep*. 1976;60(11):1691–1694.

286. O'Driscoll BR, Hasleton PS, Taylor PM, et al. Active lung fibrosis up to 17 years after chemotherapy with carmustine (BCNU) in childhood. *N Engl J Med*. 1990;323(6):378–382.

287. Parish JM, Muhm JR, Leslie KO. Upper lobe pulmonary fibrosis associated with high-dose chemotherapy containing BCNU for bone marrow transplantation. *Mayo Clin Proc*. 2003;78(5):630–634.

288. Littler W, Kay JM, Hasleton PS, Heath D. Busulphan lung. *Thorax*. 1969;24(6):639–655.

289. Cooper Jr JA, White DA, Matthay RA. Drug-induced pulmonary disease. Part 1: Cytotoxic drugs. *Am Rev Respir Dis*. 1986;133(2):321–340.

290. Kreisman H, Wolkove N. Pulmonary toxicity of antineoplastic therapy. *Semin Oncol*. 1992;19(5):508–520.

291. Holoye PY, Luna MA, MacKay B, Bedrossian CW. Bleomycin hypersensitivity pneumonitis. *Ann Intern Med*. 1978;8:47–49.

292. Hay JG, Haslam PL, Dewar A, et al. Development of acute lung injury after the combination of intravenous bleomycin and exposure to hyperoxia in rats. *Thorax*. 1987;42(5):374–382.

293. Borzone G, Moreno R, Urrea R, et al. Bleomycin-induced chronic lung damage does not resemble human idiopathic pulmonary fibrosis. *Am J Respir Crit Care Med*. 2001;163(7):1648–1653.

294. Lien HH, Brodahl U, Telhaug R, et al. Pulmonary changes at computed tomography in patients with testicular carcinoma treated with cis-platinum, vinblastine and bleomycin. *Acta Radiol Diagn (Stockh)*. 1985;26(5):507–510.

295. Adler KB, Callahan LM, Evans JN. Cellular alterations in the alveolar wall in bleomycin-induced pulmonary fibrosis in rats. An ultrastructural morphometric study. *Am Rev Respir Dis*. 1986;133(6):1043–1048.

296. Lazo JS. Bleomycin. *Cancer Chemother Biol Response Modif*. 1999;18:39–45.

297. Bowler RP, Nicks M, Warnick K, Crapo JD. Role of extracellular superoxide dismutase in bleomycin-induced pulmonary fibrosis. *Am J Physiol Lung Cell Mol Physiol*. 2002;282(4):L719–L726.

298. Taatjes DJ, Leslie KO, von Turkovich M, et al. Alveolocapillary remodeling in bleomycin-induced rat lung injury: interpretation from lectin-binding studies. *Prog Histochem Cytochem*. 1991;23(1–4):194–199.

299. Cohen MH, Williams GA, Sridhara R, et al. FDA drug approval summary: gefitinib (ZD1839) (Iressa) tablets. *Oncologist*. 2003;8(4):303–306.

300. Ando M, Okamoto I, Yamamoto N, et al. Predictive factors for interstitial lung disease, antitumor response, and survival in non-small-cell lung cancer patients treated with gefitinib. *J Clin Oncol*. 2006;24(16):2549–2556.

301. Ostör AJ, Chilvers ER, Somerville MF, et al. Pulmonary complications of infliximab therapy in patients with rheumatoid arthritis. *J Rheumatol*. 2006;33(3):622–628.

302. Stern W, Subbarao K. Pulmonary complications of drug addiction. *Semin Roentgenol*. 1983;28:183–197.

303. Abraham J, Brambilla C. Particle size for differentiation between inhalation and injection pulmonary talcosis. *Environ Res*. 1980;21(1):94–96.

304. Abraham JL. Identification and quantitative analysis of tissue particulate burden. *Ann N Y Acad Sci*. 1984;428:60–67.

305. Abraham JL, Burnett BR, Hunt A. Development and use of a pneumoconiosis database of human pulmonary inorganic particulate burden in over 400 lungs. *Scanning Microsc*. 1991;5(1):95–104; discussion 105–108.

306. Tomashefski J, Hirsch C. The pulmonary vascular lesions of intravenous drug abuse. *Hum Pathol*. 1980;11:133–145.

307. Crouch E, Churg A. Progressive massive fibrosis of the lung secondary to intravenous injection of talc. A pathologic and mineralogical analysis. *Am J Clin Pathol*. 1983;80:520–526.

308. Stern EJ, Frank MS, Schmutz JF, et al. Panlobular pulmonary emphysema caused by i.v. injection of methylphenidate (Ritalin): findings on chest radiographs and CT scans. *AJR Am J Roentgenol*. 1994;162:555–560.

309. Schiavina M, Di Scioscio V, Contini P, et al. Pulmonary lymphangioleiomyomatosis in a karyotypically normal man without tuberous sclerosis complex. *Am J Respir Crit Care Med*. 2007;176(1):96–98.

310. Cheung OY, Muhm JR, Helmers RA, et al. Surgical pathology of granulomatous interstitial pneumonia. *Ann Diagn Pathol*. 2003;7(2):127–138.

311. Hunninghake GW, Costabel U, Ando M, et al. ATS/ERS/WASOG statement on sarcoidosis. American Thoracic Society/European Respiratory Society/World Association of Sarcoidosis and other Granulomatous Disorders. *Sarcoidosis Vasc Diffuse Lung Dis*. 1999;16(2):149–173.

312. Stirling RG, Cullinan P, Du Bois RMP. Sarcoidosis. In: Schwartz MI, King TE, eds. *Interstitial Lung Disease*. London: BC Decker; 1998:279–322.

313. Milman N, Selroos O. Pulmonary sarcoidosis in the Nordic countries 1950–1982. Epidemiology and clinical picture. *Sarcoidosis*. 1990;7(1):50–57.

314. Milman N, Selroos O. Pulmonary sarcoidosis in the Nordic countries 1950–1982. II. Course and prognosis. *Sarcoidosis*. 1990;7(2):113–118.

315. Sartwell PE, Edwards LB. Epidemiology of sarcoidosis in the U.S. Navy. *Am J Epidemiol*. 1974;99(4):250–257.

316. Lynch DA, Webb WR, Gamsu G, et al. Computed tomography in pulmonary sarcoidosis. *J Comput Assist Tomogr*. 1989;13:405–410.

317. Kuhlman JE, Fishman EK, Hamper UM, et al. The computed tomographic spectrum of thoracic sarcoidosis. *Radiographics*. 1989;9(3):449–466.

318. Müller NL, Kullnig P, Miller RR. The CT findings of pulmonary sarcoidosis: analysis of 25 patients. *AJR Am J Roentgenol*. 1989;152(6):1179–1182.

319. Padley SP, Padhani AR, Nicholson A, Hansell DM. Pulmonary sarcoidosis mimicking cryptogenic fibrosing alveolitis on CT. *Clin Radiol*. 1996;51(11):807–810.

320. Abehsera M, Valeyre D, Grenier P, et al. Sarcoidosis with pulmonary fibrosis: CT patterns and correlation with pulmonary function. *AJR Am J Roentgenol*. 2000;174(6):1751–1757.

321. Battesti JP, Saumon G, Valeyre D, et al. Pulmonary sarcoidosis with an alveolar radiographic pattern. *Thorax*. 1982;37:448–452.

322. Gilman MJ, Wang KP. Transbronchial lung biopsy in sarcoidosis. An approach to determine the optimal number of biopsies. *Am Rev Respir Dis*. 1980;122(5):721–724.

323. Hsu RM, Connors Jr AF, Tomashefski Jr JF. Histologic, microbiologic, and clinical correlates of the diagnosis of sarcoidosis by transbronchial biopsy. *Arch Pathol Lab Med*. 1996;120(4):364–368.

324. Freiman D, Hardy H. Beryllium disease: the relation of pulmonary pathology to clinical course and prognosis based on a study of 130 cases from the U.S. Beryllium Case Registry. *Hum Pathol*. 1970;1:25–44.

325. Matilla A, Galera H, Pascual E, Carapeto R. Chronic berylliosis. *Br J Dis Chest*. 1973;67:308–314.

326. Aronchik JM, Rossman MD, Miller WT. Chronic beryllium disease: diagnosis, radiographic findings, and correlation with pulmonary function tests. *Radiology*. 1987;163:677–678.

327. Kriebel D, Brain JD, Sprince NL, Kazemi H. The pulmonary toxicity of beryllium. *Am Rev Respir Dis*. 1988;137(2):464–473.

328. Kriebel D, Sprince NL, Eisen EA, Greaves IA. Pulmonary function in beryllium workers: assessment of exposure. *Br J Ind Med*. 1988;45(2):83–92.

329. Kriebel D, Sprince NL, Eisen EA, et al. Beryllium exposure and pulmonary function: a cross sectional study of beryllium workers. *Br J Ind Med*. 1988;45(3):167–173.

330. Maier LA, Martyny JW, Liang J, Rossman MD. Recent chronic beryllium disease in residents surrounding a beryllium facility. *Am J Respir Crit Care Med*. 2008;177(9):1012–1017.

331. Kawanami O, Basset F, Barrios R, et al. Hypersensitivity pneumonitis in man: light- and electron-microscopic studies of 18 lung biopsies. *Am J Pathol*. 1983;110:275–289.

332. Salvaggio J, Karr R. Hypersensitivity pneumonitis: state of the art. *Chest*. 1979;75(suppl 2):270–274.

333. Wild LG, Lopez M. Hypersensitivity pneumonitis: a comprehensive review. *J Investig Allergol Clin Immunol*. 2001;11(1):3–15.

334. Bourke SJ, Dalphin JC, Boyd G, et al. Hypersensitivity pneumonitis: current concepts. *Eur Respir J Suppl*. 2001;32:81s–92s.

335. Selman M. Hypersensitivity pneumonitis. In: Schwartz MI, King TE, eds. *Interstitial Lung Disease*. London: BC Decker; 1998:393–422.

336. McSharry C, Banham SW, Boyd G. Effect of cigarette smoking on the antibody response to inhaled antigens and the prevalence of extrinsic allergic alveolitis among pigeon breeders. *Clin Allergy*. 1985;15:487.

337. Patel AM, Ryu JH, Reed CE. Hypersensitivity pneumonitis: current concepts and future questions. *J Allergy Clin Immunol*. 2001;108(5):661–670.

338. Glazer C, Rose C, Lynch D. Clinical and radiologic manifestations of hypersensitivity pneumonitis. *J Thorac Imaging*. 2002;17(4):261–272.

339. Cook PG, Wells IP, McGavin CR. The distribution of pulmonary shadowing in farmer's lung. *Clin Radiol*. 1988;39(1):21–27.

340. Khoor A, Leslie KO, Tazelaar HD, et al. Diffuse pulmonary disease caused by nontuberculous mycobacteria in immunocompetent people (hot tub lung). *Am J Clin Pathol*. 2001;115(5):755–762.

341. Pham R, Vydareny K, Gal A. High-resolution computed tomography appearance of pulmonary *Mycobacterium avium* complex infection after exposure to hot tub: case of hot-tub lung. *J Thorac Imaging*. 2003;18(1):48–52.

342. Coleman A, Colby TV. Histologic diagnosis of extrinsic allergic alveolitis. *Am J Surg Pathol*. 1988;12(7):514–518.

343. Colby TV, Coleman A. Histologic differential diagnosis of extrinsic allergic alveolitis. *Prog Surg Pathol*. 1989;10:11–26.

344. Seal RM, Hapke EJ, Thomas GO, et al. The pathology of the acute and chronic stages of farmer's lung. *Thorax*. 1968;23(5):469–489.

345. Takemura T, Akashi T, Ohtani Y, et al. Pathology of hypersensitivity pneumonitis. *Curr Opin Pulm Med*. 2008;14(5):440–454.

346. Barbee RA, Callies Q, Dickie HA, Rankin J. The long-term prognosis in farmer's lung. *Am Rev Respir Dis*. 1968;97(2):223–231.

347. Kokkarinen J, Tukiainen H, Seppä A, Terho EO. Hypersensitivity pneumonitis due to native birds in a bird ringer. *Chest*. 1994;106(4):1269–1271.

348. Kokkarinen J, Tukiainen H, Terho EO. Mortality due to farmer's lung in Finland. *Chest*. 1994;106(2):509–512.

349. Kokkarinen JI, Tukiainen HO, Terho EO. Effect of corticosteroid treatment on the recovery of pulmonary function in farmer's lung. *Am Rev Respir Dis*. 1992;145(1):3–5.

350. Sansores R, Salas J, Chapela R, et al. Clubbing in hypersensitivity pneumonitis. Its prevalence and possible prognostic role. *Arch Intern Med*. 1990;150(9):1849–1851.

351. Pérez-Padilla R, Gaxiola M, Salas J, et al. Bronchiolitis in chronic pigeon breeder's disease. Morphologic evidence of a spectrum of small airway lesions in hypersensitivity pneumonitis induced by avian antigens. *Chest*. 1996;110(2):371–377.

352. Brabencova E, Tazi A, Lorenzato M, et al. Langerhans cells in Langerhans cell granulomatosis are not actively proliferating cells. *Am J Pathol*. 1998;152(5):1143–1149.

353. Vassallo R, Ryu JH, Colby TV, et al. Pulmonary Langerhans'-cell histiocytosis. *N Engl J Med*. 2000;342(26):1969–1978.

354. Willman CL, Busque L, Griffith BB, et al. Langerhans'-cell histiocytosis (histiocytosis X)—a clonal proliferative disease. *N Engl J Med*. 1994;331(3):154–160.

355. Travis WD, Borok Z, Roum JH, et al. Pulmonary Langerhans cell granulomatosis (histiocytosis X). A clinicopathologic study of 48 cases. *Am J Surg Pathol*. 1993;17(10):971–986.

356. Parambil JG, Myers JL, Aubry MC, Ryu JH. Causes and prognosis of diffuse alveolar damage diagnosed on surgical lung biopsy. *Chest*. 2007;132(1):50–57.

357. Colby TV, Lombard C. Histiocytosis X in the lung. *Hum Pathol*. 1983;14(10):847–856.

358. Niku S, Stark P, Levin DL, Friedman PJ. Lymphangioleiomyomatosis: clinical, pathologic, and radiologic manifestations. *J Thorac Imaging*. 2005;20(2):98–102.

359. Lacronique J, Roth C, Battesti JP, et al. Chest radiological features of pulmonary histiocytosis X: a report based on 50 adult cases. *Thorax*. 1982;37(2):104–109.

360. Moore AD, Godwin JD, Müller NL, et al. Pulmonary histiocytosis X: comparison of radiographic and CT findings. *Radiology*. 1989;172(1):249–254.

361. Kulwiec EL, Lynch DA, Aguayo SM, et al. Imaging of pulmonary histiocytosis X. *Radiographics*. 1992;12(3):515–526.

362. Brauner MW, Grenier P, Tijani K, et al. Pulmonary Langerhans cell histiocytosis: evolution of lesions on CT scans. *Radiology*. 1997;204(2):497–502.

363. Kambouchner M, Basset F, Marchal J, et al. Three-dimensional characterization of pathologic lesions in pulmonary Langerhans cell histiocytosis. *Am J Respir Crit Care Med*. 2002;166(11):1419–1421.

364. McDonnell TJ, Crouch EC, Gonzalez JG. Reactive eosinophilic pleuritis. A sequela of pneumothorax in pulmonary eosinophilic granuloma. *Am J Clin Pathol*. 1989;91(1):107–111.

365. Askin FB, McCann BG, Kuhn C. Reactive eosinophilic pleuritis: a lesion to be distinguished from pulmonary eosinophilic granuloma. *Arch Pathol Lab Med*. 1977;101:187–192.

366. Delobbe A, Durieu J, Duhamel A, Wallaert B. Determinants of survival in pulmonary Langerhans' cell granulomatosis (histiocytosis X). Groupe d'Etude en Pathologie Interstitielle de la Societe de Pathologie Thoracique du Nord. *Eur Respir J*. 1996;9(10):2002–2006.

367. Veyssier-Belot C, Cacoub P, Caparros-Lefebvre D, et al. Erdheim-Chester disease. Clinical and radiologic characteristics of 59 cases. *Medicine (Baltimore)*. 1996;75(3):157–169.

368. Cottin V, Nunes H, Brillet PY, et al. Combined pulmonary fibrosis and emphysema: a distinct underrecognised entity. *Eur Respir J*. 2005;26(4):586–593.

369. Bisceglia M, Cammisa M, Suster S, Colby TV. Erdheim-Chester disease: clinical and pathologic spectrum of four cases from the Arkadi M. Rywlin slide seminars. *Adv Anat Pathol*. 2003;10(3):160–171.

370. Bancroft LW, Berquist TH. Erdheim-Chester disease: radiographic findings in five patients. *Skeletal Radiol*. 1998;27(3):127–132.

371. Breuil V, Brocq O, Pellegrino C, et al. Erdheim-Chester disease: typical radiological bone features for a rare xanthogranulomatosis. *Ann Rheum Dis*. 2002;61(3):199–200.

372. Gottlieb R, Chen A. MR findings of Erdheim-Chester disease. *J Comput Assist Tomogr*. 2002;26(2):257–261.

373. Olmos JM, Canga A, Velero C, González-Macías J. Imaging of Erdheim-Chester disease. *J Bone Miner Res*. 2002;17(3):381–383.

374. Kambouchner M, Colby TV, Domenge C, et al. Erdheim-Chester disease with prominent pulmonary involvement associated with eosinophilic granuloma of mandibular bone. *Histopathology*. 1997;30(4):353–358.

375. Egan AJ, Boardman LA, Tazelaar HD, et al. Erdheim-Chester disease: clinical, radiologic, and histopathologic findings in five patients with interstitial lung disease. *Am J Surg Pathol*. 1999;23(1):17–26.

376. Rush WL, Andriko JA, Galateau-Salle F, et al. Pulmonary pathology of Erdheim-Chester disease. *Mod Pathol*. 2000;13(7):747–754.

377. Wittenberg KH, Swensen SJ, Myers JL. Pulmonary involvement with Erdheim-Chester disease: radiographic and CT findings. *AJR Am J Roentgenol*. 2000;174(5):1327–1331.

378. Shamburek RD, Brewer Jr HB, Gochuico BR. Erdheim-Chester disease: a rare multisystem histiocytic disorder associated with interstitial lung disease. *Am J Med Sci*. 2001;321(1):66–75.

379. Taylor JR, Ryu J, Colby TV, Raffin TA. Lymphangioleiomyomatosis. Clinical course in 32 patients. *N Engl J Med*. 1990;323(18):1254–1260.

380. Kitaichi M, Nishimura K, Itoh H, Izumi T. Pulmonary lymphangioleiomyomatosis: a report of 46 patients including a clinicopathologic study of prognostic factors. *Am J Respir Crit Care Med*. 1995;151(2 Pt 1):527–533.

381. Kalassian KG, Doyle R, Kao P, et al. Lymphangioleiomyomatosis: new insights. *Am J Respir Crit Care Med*. 1997;155(4):1183–1186.

382. Athavale A, Chhajed P, Singhal P, et al. Pulmonary lymphangioleiomyomatosis. *J Assoc Physicians India*. 1999;47(6):649–650.

383. Urban T, Lazor R, Lacronique J, et al. Pulmonary lymphangioleiomyomatosis. A study of 69 patients. Groupe d'Etudes et de Recherche sur les Maladies "Orphelines" Pulmonaires (GERM"O"P). *Medicine (Baltimore)*. 1999;78(5):321–337.

384. Chu SC, Horiba K, Usuki J, et al. Comprehensive evaluation of 35 patients with lymphangioleiomyomatosis. *Chest*. 1999;115(4):1041–1052.

385. Costello LC, Hartman TE, Ryu JH. High frequency of pulmonary lymphangioleiomyomatosis in women with tuberous sclerosis complex. *Mayo Clin Proc*. 2000;75(6):591–594.

386. Sato T, Seyama K, Fujii H, et al. Mutation analysis of the *TSC1* and *TSC2* genes in Japanese patients with pulmonary lymphangioleiomyomatosis. *J Hum Genet*. 2002;47(1):20–28.

387. Yu J, Astrinidis A, Henske EP. Chromosome 16 loss of heterozygosity in tuberous sclerosis and sporadic lymphangiomyomatosis. *Am J Respir Crit Care Med*. 2001;164(8 Pt 1):1537–1540.

388. Carsillo T, Astrinidis A, Henske EP. Mutations in the tuberous sclerosis complex gene *TSC2* are a cause of sporadic pulmonary lymphangioleiomyomatosis. *Proc Natl Acad Sci U S A*. 2000;97(11):6085–6090.

389. Aubry MC, Myers JL, Ryu JH, et al. Pulmonary lymphangioleiomyomatosis in a man. *Am J Respir Crit Care Med*. 2000;162(2 Pt 1):749–752.

390. Lack EE, Dolan MF, Finisio J, et al. Pulmonary and extrapulmonary lymphangioleiomyomatosis. Report of a case with bilateral renal angiomyolipomas, multifocal lymphangioleiomyomatosis, and a glial polyp of the endocervix. *Am J Surg Pathol*. 1986;10(9):650–657.

391. Uzzo RG, Libby DM, Vaughan Jr ED, Levey SH. Coexisting lymphangioleiomyomatosis and bilateral angiomyolipomas in a patient with tuberous sclerosis. *J Urol*. 1994;151(6):1612–1615.

392. Bernstein SM, Newell Jr JD, Adamczyk D, et al. How common are renal angiomyolipomas in patients with pulmonary lymphangiomyomatosis? *Am J Respir Crit Care Med*. 1995;152(6 Pt 1):2138–2143.

393. Maziak DE, Kesten S, Rappaport DC, Maurer J. Extrathoracic angiomyolipomas in lymphangioleiomyomatosis. *Eur Respir J*. 1996;9(3):402–405.

394. Neumann HP, Schwarzkopf G, Henske EP. Renal angiomyolipomas, cysts, and cancer in tuberous sclerosis complex. *Semin Pediatr Neurol*. 1998;5(4):269–275.

395. Tüzel E, Kirkali Z, Mungan U, et al. Giant angiomyolipoma associated with marked pulmonary lesions suggesting lymphangioleiomyomatosis in a patient with tuberous sclerosis. *Int Urol Nephrol*. 2000;32(2):219–222.

396. Müller NL, Chiles C, Kullnig P. Pulmonary lymphangiomyomatosis: correlation of CT with radiographic and functional findings. *Radiology*. 1990;175(2):335–339.

397. Rappaport DC, Weisbrod GL, Herman SJ, Chamberlain DW. Pulmonary lymphangioleiomyomatosis: high-resolution CT findings in four cases. *AJR Am J Roentgenol*. 1989;152(5):961–964.

398. Templeton PA, McLoud TC, Müller NL, et al. Pulmonary lymphangioleiomyomatosis: CT and pathologic findings. *J Comput Assist Tomogr*. 1989;13(1):54–57.

399. Sherrier RH, Chiles C, Roggli V. Pulmonary lymphangioleiomyomatosis: CT findings. *AJR Am J Roentgenol*. 1989;153(5):937–940.

400. Templeton PA, McLoud TC, Müller NL, et al. Pulmonary lymphangioleiomyomatosis: CT and pathologic findings. *J Comput Assist Tomogr*. 1989;13:54–57.

401. Kirchner J, Stein A, Viel K, et al. Pulmonary lymphangioleiomyomatosis: high-resolution CT findings. *Eur Radiol*. 1999;9(1):49–54.

402. Kumasaka T, Seyama K, Mitani K, et al. Lymphangiogenesis-mediated shedding of LAM cell clusters as a mechanism for dissemination in lymphangioleiomyomatosis. *Am J Surg Pathol*. 2005;29(10):1356–1366.

403. Toro JR, Wei MH, Glenn GM, et al. BHD mutations, clinical and molecular genetic investigations of Birt-Hogg-Dubé syndrome: a new series of 50 families and a review of published reports. *J Med Genet*. 2008;45(6):321–331.

404. Shen A, Iseman MD, Waldron JA, King TE. Exacerbation of pulmonary lymphangioleiomyomatosis by exogenous estrogens. *Chest*. 1987;91(5):782–785.

405. Eliasson AH, Phillips YY, Tenholder MF. Treatment of lymphangioleiomyomatosis. A meta-analysis. *Chest*. 1989;96(6):1352–1355.

406. Ohori NP, Yousem SA, Sonmez-Alpan E, Colby TV. Estrogen and progesterone receptors in lymphangioleiomyomatosis, epithelioid hemangioendothelioma, and sclerosing hemangioma of the lung. *Am J Clin Pathol*. 1991;96(4):529–535.

407. Rajjoub S, Blatt MW, Ritterspach J. Response to treatment with progesterone in a patient with pulmonary lymphangioleiomyomatosis. *W V Med J*. 1995;91(7):322–323.

408. Colley MH, Geppert E, Franklin WA. Immunohistochemical detection of steroid receptors in a case of pulmonary lymphangioleiomyomatosis. *Am J Surg Pathol*. 1989;13(9):803–807.

409. McCormack FX. Lymphangioleiomyomatosis: a clinical update. *Chest*. 2008;133(2):507–516.

410. Boehler A, Speich R, Russi EW, Weder W. Lung transplantation for lymphangioleiomyomatosis. *N Engl J Med*. 1996;335(17):1275–1280.

411. Bittmann I, Dose TB, Müller C, et al. Lymphangioleiomyomatosis: recurrence after single lung transplantation. *Hum Pathol*. 1997;28(12):1420–1423.

412. Gunji Y, Akiyoshi T, Sato T, et al. Mutations of the Birt Hogg Dube gene in patients with multiple lung cysts and recurrent pneumothorax. *J Med Genet*. 2007;44(9):588–593.

413. Davies BH, Tuddenham EG. Familial pulmonary fibrosis associated with oculocutaneous albinism and platelet function defect. A new syndrome. *Q J Med*. 1976;45(178):219–232.

414. DePinho RA, Kaplan KL. The Hermansky-Pudlak syndrome. Report of three cases and review of pathophysiology and management considerations. *Medicine (Baltimore)*. 1985;64(3):192–202.

415. Dimson O, Drolet BA, Esterly NB. Hermansky-Pudlak syndrome. *Pediatr Dermatol*. 1999;16(6):475–477.

416. Huizing M, Gahl WA. Disorders of vesicles of lysosomal lineage: the Hermansky-Pudlak syndromes. *Curr Mol Med*. 2002;2(5):451–467.

417. Pierson DM, Ionescu D, Qing G, et al. Pulmonary fibrosis in Hermansky-Pudlak syndrome. A case report and review. *Respiration*. 2006;73(3):382–395.

418. Anikster Y, Huizing M, White J, et al. Mutation of a new gene causes a unique form of Hermansky-Pudlak syndrome in a genetic isolate of central Puerto Rico. *Nat Genet*. 2001;28(4):376–380.

419. Hermos CR, Huizing M, Kaiser-Kupfer MI, Gahl WA. Hermansky-Pudlak syndrome type 1: gene organization, novel mutations, and clinical-molecular review of non–Puerto Rican cases. *Hum Mutat*. 2002;20(6):482.

420. Okano A, Sato A, Chida K, et al. Pulmonary interstitial pneumonia in association with Hermansky-Pudlak syndrome. *Nihon Kyobu Shikkan Gakkai Zasshi*. 1991;29(12):1596–1602.

421. Avila NA, Brantly M, Premkumar A, et al. Hermansky-Pudlak syndrome: radiography and CT of the chest compared with pulmonary function tests and genetic studies. *AJR Am J Roentgenol*. 2002;179(4):887–892.

422. Nakatani Y, Nakamura N, Sano J, et al. Interstitial pneumonia in Hermansky-Pudlak syndrome: significance of florid foamy swelling/degeneration (giant lamellar body degeneration) of type-2 pneumocytes. *Virchows Arch*. 2000;437(3):304–313.

423. Gahl WA, Brantly M, Troendle J, et al. Effect of pirfenidone on the pulmonary fibrosis of Hermansky-Pudlak syndrome. *Mol Genet Metab*. 2002;76(3):234–242.

424. Sosman MC, Dodd GD, Jones WD, Pillmore GU. The familial occurrence of pulmonary alveolar microlithiasis. *Am J Roentgenol Radium Ther Nucl Med*. 1957;77:947–952.

425. Fuleihan FJ, Abboud RT, Balikian JP, Nucho CK. Pulmonary alveolar microlithiasis: lung function in five cases. *Thorax*. 1969;24:84–90.

426. Prakash UB, Barham SS, Rosenow 3rd EC, et al. Pulmonary alveolar microlithiasis. A review including ultrastructural and pulmonary function studies. *Mayo Clin Proc*. 1983;58(5):290–300.

427. Edelweiss M, Medeiros LJ, Suster S, Moran CA. Lymph node involvement by Langerhans cell histiocytosis: a clinicopathologic and immunohistochemical study of 20 cases. *Hum Pathol*. 2007;38(10):1463–1469.

428. Castellana G, Gentile M, Castellana R, et al. Pulmonary alveolar microlithiasis: clinical features, evolution of the phenotype, and review of the literature. *Am J Med Genet*. 2002;111(2):220–224.

429. Senyiğit A, Yarami A, Gürkan F, et al. Pulmonary alveolar microlithiasis: a rare familial inheritance with report of six cases in a family. Contribution of six new cases to the number of case reports in Turkey. *Respiration*. 2001;68(2):204–209.

430. Huqun IS, Miyazawa H, Ishii K, et al. Mutations in the *SLC34A2* gene are associated with pulmonary alveolar microlithiasis. *Am J Respir Crit Care Med*. 2007;175(3):263–268.

431. Pant K, Shah A, Mathur RK, et al. Pulmonary alveolar microlithiasis with pleural calcification and nephrolithiasis. *Chest*. 1990;98:245–246.

432. Chang Y, Yang PC, Luh KT, et al. High-resolution computed tomography of pulmonary alveolar microlithiasis. *J Formos Med Assoc*. 1999;98(6):440–443.

433. Trapnell BC, Whitsett JA, Nakata K. Pulmonary alveolar proteinosis. *N Engl J Med*. 2003;349(26):2527–2539.

434. Kitamura T, Tanaka N, Watanabe J, et al. Idiopathic pulmonary alveolar proteinosis as an autoimmune disease with neutralizing antibody against granulocyte/macrophage colony-stimulating factor. *J Exp Med*. 1999;190(6):875–880.

435. Inoue Y, Trapnell BC, Tazawa R, et al. Characteristics of a large cohort of patients with autoimmune pulmonary alveolar proteinosis in Japan. *Am J Respir Crit Care Med*. 2008;177(7):752–762.

436. Singh G, Katyal SL, Bedrossian CW, Rogers RM. Pulmonary alveolar proteinosis. Staining for surfactant apoprotein in alveolar proteinosis and in conditions simulating it. *Chest*. 1983;83:82–86.

437. Miller RR, Churg AM, Hutcheon M, Lom S. Pulmonary alveolar proteinosis and aluminum dust exposure. *Am Rev Respir Dis*. 1984;130:312–315.

438. Bedrossian CW, Luna MA, Conklin RH, Miller WC. Alveolar proteinosis as a consequence of immunosuppression. A hypothesis based on clinical and pathologic observations. *Hum Pathol*. 1980;11(suppl 5):527–535.

439. Wang Y, Xia J, Wang QW. Clinical report on 62 cases of acute dimethyl sulfate intoxication. *Am J Ind Med*. 1988;13(4):455–462.

440. Seymour J, Presneill J. Pulmonary alveolar proteinosis: progress in the first 44 years. *Am J Respir Crit Care Med*. 2002;166(2):215–235.

441. Shah P, Hansell D, Lawson PR, et al. Pulmonary alveolar proteinosis: clinical aspects and current concepts in pathogenesis. *Thorax*. 2000;55:67–77.

442. Davidson J, MacLeod W. Pulmonary alveolar proteinosis. *Br J Dis Chest*. 1969;63:13–16.

443. Lynch DA, Godwin JD, Safrin S, et al. High-resolution computed tomography in idiopathic pulmonary fibrosis: diagnosis and prognosis. *Am J Respir Crit Care Med*. 2005;172(4):488–493.

444. Claypool W, Roger R, Matuschak G. Update on the clinical diagnosis, management, and pathogenesis of pulmonary alveolar proteinosis (phospholipidosis). *Chest*. 1984;85:550–558.

445. Wylam ME, Ten R, Prakash UB, et al. Aerosol granulocyte-macrophage colony-stimulating factor for pulmonary alveolar proteinosis. *Eur Respir J*. 2006;27(3):585–593.

446. Tazawa R, Hamano E, Arai T, et al. Granulocyte-macrophage colony-stimulating factor and lung immunity in pulmonary alveolar proteinosis. *Am J Respir Crit Care Med*. 2005;171(10):1142–1149.

447. Heitzman E. *The Lung: Radiologic-Pathologic Correlations*, 2nd ed. St. Louis: Mosby; 1984.

448. Munk PL, Müller NL, Miller RR, Ostrow DN. Pulmonary lymphangitic carcinomatosis: CT and pathologic findings. *Radiology*. 1988;166:705–709.

449. Janower M, Blennerhassett J. Lymphangitic spread of metastatic cancer to the lung: a radiologic-pathologic classification. *Radiology*. 1971;101:267–273.

450. Stein MG, Mayo J, Müller N, et al. Pulmonary lymphangitic spread of carcinoma: appearance on CT scans. *Radiology*. 1987;162:371–375.

451. Goldsmith HS, Bailey HD, Callahan EL, Beattie Jr EJ. Pulmonary lymphangitic metastases from breast carcinoma. *Arch Surg*. 1967;94:483–488.

452. Wall CP, Gaensler EA, Carrington CB, Hayes JA. Comparison of transbronchial and open biopsies in chronic infiltrative lung disease. *Am Rev Respir Dis*. 1981;123:280–285.

453. Frankel SK, Cool CD, Lynch DA, Brown KK. Idiopathic pleuroparenchymal fibroelastosis: description of a novel clinicopathologic entity. *Chest*. 2004;126(6):2007–2013.

454. Becker CD, Gil J, Padilla ML. Idiopathic pleuroparenchymal fibroelastosis: an unrecognized or misdiagnosed entity? *Mod Pathol*. 2008;21(6):784–787.

455. Shiota S, Shimizu K, Suzuki M, et al. Seven cases of marked pulmonary fibrosis in the upper lobe. *Nihon Kokyuki Gakkai Zasshi*. 1999;37(2):87–96.

456. Kamoi H, Okamoto T, Yoshimura N, et al. A case of interstitial pneumonia in the upper lung field histologically diagnosed as nonspecific interstitial pneumonia complicated by bilateral pneumothorax. *Nihon Kokyuki Gakkai Zasshi*. 2002;40(12):936–940.

457. Krakówka P, Meleniewska-Maciszewska A, Lesiak B, et al. Pulmonary fibrosis of the upper lobe resembling tuberculosis in patients without ankylosing spondylitis. *Pneumonol Pol*. 1985;53(1):39–47.

Non-Neoplastic Pathology of the Large and Small Airways

Mattia Barbareschi, MD, PhD, Alberto Cavazza, MD, and Kevin O. Leslie, MD

In this chapter, as elsewhere in this book, the focus is on those diseases and conditions that are likely to come to the attention of the surgical pathologist. Descriptions of individual lesions of the trachea and conducting airways, and of the different diseases in which these lesions may be encountered, are presented first. A few of the more specific clinicopathologic entities classically associated with disease of the airways, such as asthma, chronic obstructive pulmonary disease (COPD), and emphysema, are considered in a separate section.

The Conducting Airways

The trachea and conducting airways play a vital role in lung function. The diseases that affect these structures are commonly related to inhalation exposure but also may arise from developmental anomalies and systemic diseases (Box 8-1). In this section, topics are presented in anatomic order, beginning with the trachea and proceeding distally to the bronchi and bronchioles.

The Trachea

Non-neoplastic pathology of the trachea can be divided broadly into extrinsic and intrinsic diseases. Among extrinsic diseases are certain infections, such as rhinoscleroma (caused by *Klebsiella rhinoscleromatis*[1,2]) (Fig. 8-1), and systemic autoimmune diseases that affect cartilage (e.g., Wegener granulomatosis[3,4]). These diseases may cause tracheal obstruction or collapse and may also involve the larynx or the conducting airways, or both. Diseases intrinsic and unique to the trachea are few and mainly of congenital and/or metabolic origin. In the following section, we will describe three of these entities: tracheal amyloidosis, tracheobronchomalacia, and tracheobronchopathia osteochondroplastica. The latter may be rare but deserves mention as it can be encountered incidentally during bronchoscopy.

Tracheal Amyloidosis

Tracheobronchial amyloidosis is an idiopathic disease characterized by amyloid deposition, often throughout the tracheobronchial tree[5,6] but sometimes restricted to the larynx and trachea.[7] Approximately 150 cases have been reported in the literature. Tracheobronchial amyloidosis most frequently produces dyspnea, wheezing (sometimes misdiagnosed as asthma), recurrent pneumonia, and atelectasis, which are believed to be sequelae of the narrowed airways. Pulmonary function tests usually show fixed obstruction. On histopathologic examination, amyloid deposits usually are seen in the submucosa and may involve the entire tracheal or bronchial wall, occurring in irregular masses or sheets (Fig. 8-2). Amyloid may be accompanied by multinucleate giant cells; calcification and ossification are frequent[5,6,8,9] (Fig. 8-3). When amyloid is identified in bronchoscopic biopsy specimens, this typically is an organ-limited manifestation, similar to nodular lung parenchymal amyloid.[10] Of the three major types of amyloid, AL, AA, and transthyretin, the AL type is the most common in tracheobronchial amyloid deposits. The prognosis is poor: Nearly one third of patients die within 7 to 12 years of diagnosis.[6] Therapy is limited to debulking procedures and stent placement for localized lesions, although some evidence suggests that radiation therapy may provide more definitive treatment.[11–14]

Tracheobronchomalacia

Tracheobronchomalacia (TBM) is a term used to encompass a number of conditions characterized by a decrease in the structural rigidity of the trachea and conducting airways. Such changes are manifested clinically by excessive expiratory collapse of the central airways owing to increased flaccidity or redundancy of the posterior membranous airway wall, or to weakness of the supporting cartilage (a recent in-depth

Box 8-1. Non-Neoplastic Diseases of the Trachea and Bronchi

Asthma
Bronchitis related to:
    Infection
    Inhalational injury (including smoking)
    Collagen vascular disease
    Aspiration
    Miscellaneous inflammatory diseases (e.g., inflammatory bowel disease)
Bronchiectasis
Bronchocentric granulomatosis
Mucoid impaction of the bronchi
Allergic bronchopulmonary fungal disease
Plastic bronchitis
Tracheobronchomegaly
Congenital bronchial cartilage deficiency
Relapsing polychondritis
Broncholithiasis, bronchostenosis
Miscellaneous conditions (tracheobronchial amyloid, tracheomalacia, tracheobronchopathia osteochrondroplastica)

review of the disease is available[15]). Although typically a disease process of the central airways, TBM has been shown to frequently have associated air trapping on computed tomography (CT) scan, an indicator of small-airway disease.[16,17]

Both children and adults may be affected.[18] In children, the disease most often is related to prematurity and the requirement for prolonged mechanical ventilation. In these patients, TBM appears to be self-limited.[19,20] In adults, TBM is seen in the middle-aged and the elderly and is a progressive condition, commonly seen in association with COPD.[16] Other reported associations in adults include prolonged intubation, vascular anomalies, and exposure to mustard gas.[21] TBM may complicate amyloidosis and rheumatoid arthritis when these diseases affect the airways[22] and may be related to relapsing polychondritis, a systemic disease affecting the cartilaginous tissue in several organs, including the airways.[18,23–25] Pathologically, the tracheal wall is soft, as a result of inflammatory destruction of the cartilage (Fig. 8-4). Over time, the cartilage is replaced by fibrous tissue, accompanied by inflammatory infitration and reparative vascular proliferation.

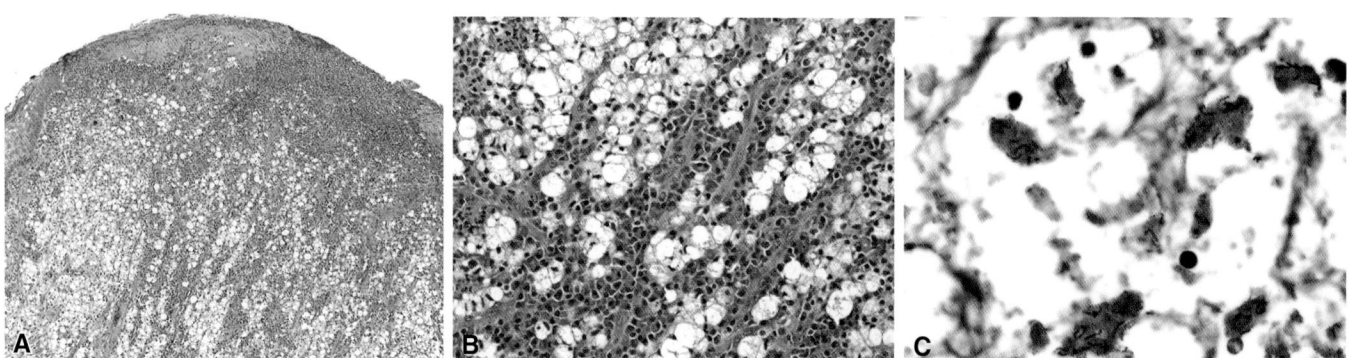

Figure 8-1. Tracheal rhinoscleroma. **A,** Low-power view showing the tracheal wall and mucosa infiltrated and expanded by inflammatory cells and histiocytes with clear cytoplasm, seen more clearly at higher magnification, as shown in part **B**. **C,** Warthin-Starry silver impregnation highlights (in *black*) the bacterial pathogen *Klebsiella rhinoscleromatis* in the cytoplasm of the histiocytes.

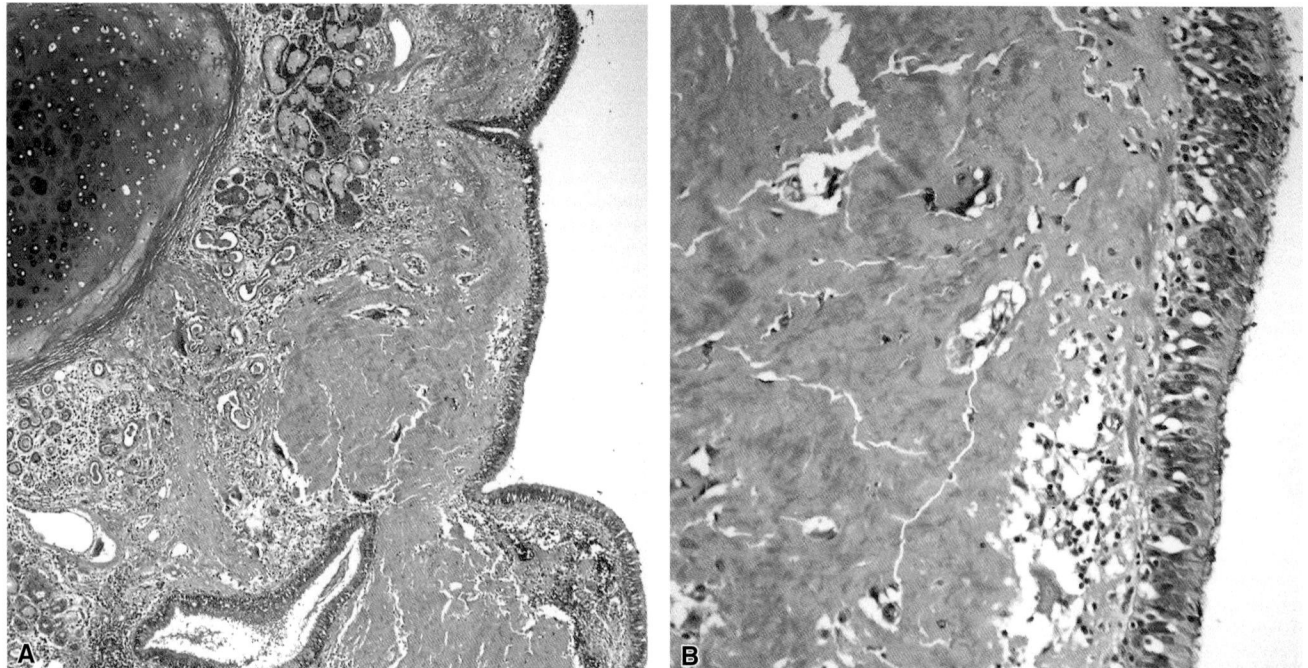

Figure 8-2. Tracheal amyloid. **A,** Low-power view showing the tracheal wall with diffuse amyloid deposition. **B,** At higher magnification, the amyloid is seen to be present just below the respiratory epithelium.

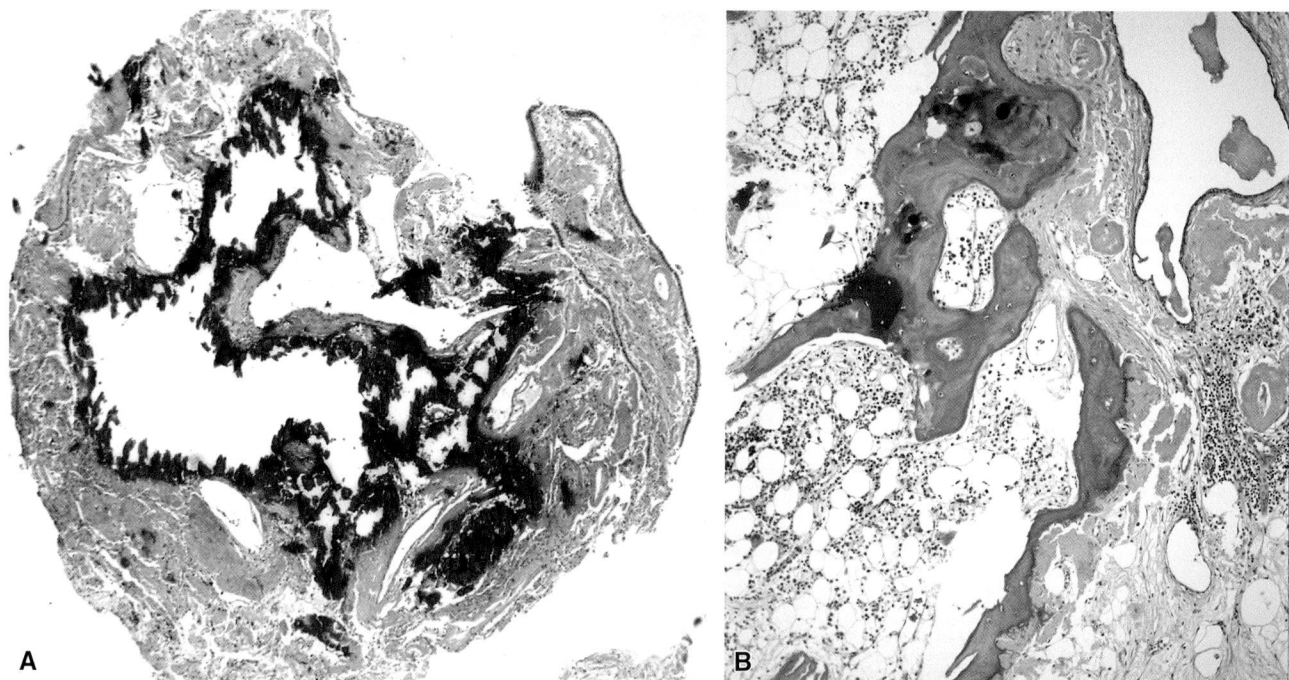

Figure 8-3. Tracheal amyloid. **A,** In this tracheal biopsy specimen, the amyloid is diffusely calcified. **B,** Osseous metaplasia can occur in tracheal amyloid.

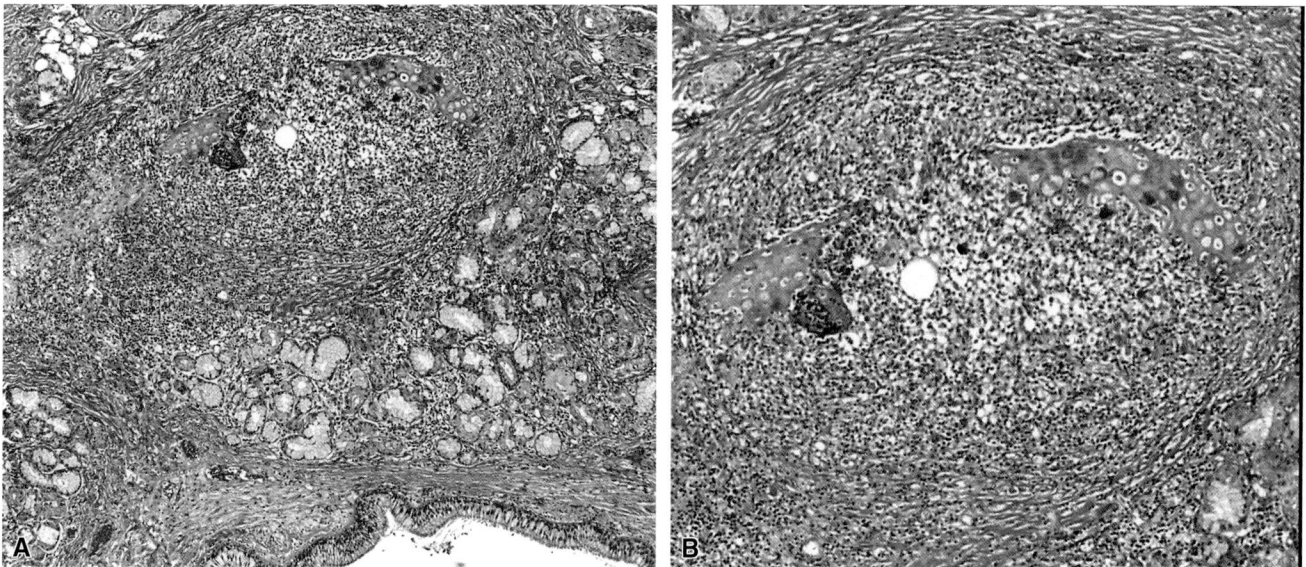

Figure 8-4. Tracheal chondritis. **A,** The cartilage of the tracheal wall is surrounded and replaced by inflammatory, vascular, and fibrous tissue. **B,** At higher magnification (*upper center* of part **A**), cartilage is seen to be disrupted and replaced by inflammatory cells.

Treatment is variable and depends on symptom severity, with conservative therapy appropriate for mildly symptomatic cases and more invasive therapy indicated for severely symptomatic cases, including tracheoplasty (for reduction of expiratory tracheal collapse and symptomatic improvement).[26] In the absence of treatment, severely symptomatic TBM can lead to significant respiratory morbidity and rarely may be fatal.

Tracheobronchopathia Osteochondroplastica

Tracheobronchopathia osteochondroplastica is a rare lung disease characterized by the presence of cartilaginous or osseous submucosal nodules that bulge into the lumen of the trachea and bronchi (Fig. 8-5), with sparing of the posterior membranous portion.[27–30] The etiology and pathogenesis are unknown. The disease affects adults more commonly than children, with a predilection for males. Most cases are asymptomatic, and are most often diagnosed incidentally during intubation or bronchoscopy. A minority of patients may experience cough, dyspnea, and hemoptysis.

The bronchoscopic appearance alone is usually diagnostic, and biopsy is seldom if ever required.[31] In the rare bronchoscopic biopsy showing the cartilaginous or ossified lesions of tracheobronchopathia osteochondroplastica (Fig. 8-6), the differential diagnosis includes ossified amyloid deposits. Other conditions associated with endoluminal nodular lesions include endobronchial sarcoidosis, endobronchial granulomatous infections, papillomatosis, and tracheobronchial calcinosis.

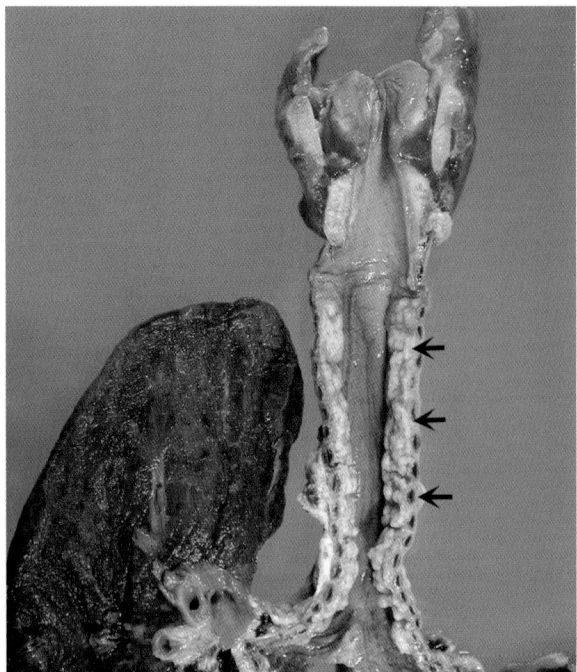

Figure 8-5. Tracheobronchopathia osteochondroplastica. Gross specimen of trachea showing prominent nodularity (*arrows*). This condition presents a striking bronchoscopic image (not shown).

The Bronchi

The conducting airways begin at the carina and extend distally in the lung to the level of the noncartilaginous bronchioles. Although many diffuse lung diseases may involve the large airways secondarily, some primary diseases also may affect the bronchi and are presented here. Asthma-associated diseases, typically observed in the large airways, are discussed later in the final section of this chapter. Cystic fibrosis and ciliary disorders are not discussed here, because detailed expositions can be found in other sources.[32,33]

Bronchitis

Infectious and inflammatory conditions of the large airways are particularly relevant to the surgical pathologist and the cytopathologist, given the prominence of inflammatory manifestations seen in biopsies obtained through the bronchoscope (endobronchial and transbronchial specimens). In practice, the presence of acute or chronic inflammation in endobronchial biopsies, in which bronchial mucosa and muscle or cartilage are evident, demands a descriptive diagnosis (Fig. 8-7). It is best to avoid the use of the term "chronic bronchitis" in reference to such inflammatory changes involving respiratory mucosa, because it carries a clinical implication regarding the diffuse nature of the disease and specific clinical manifestations. When bronchitis occurs as a direct result of respiratory infection, necrosis of the mucosa may be present (acute necrotizing bronchitis). In the postinfection period, residual chronic

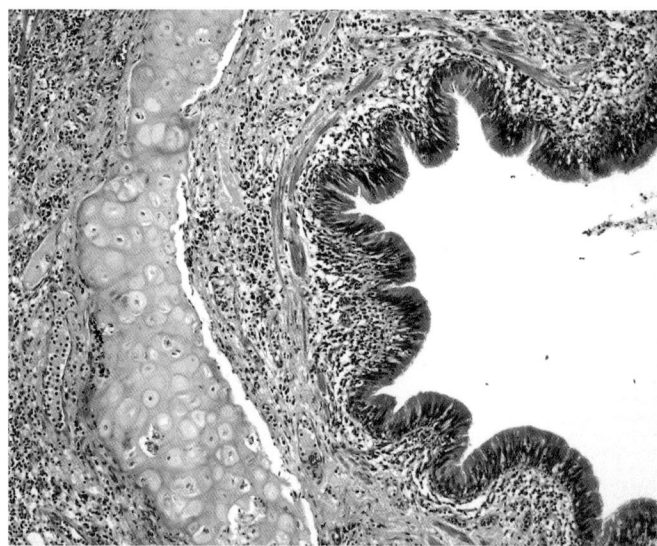

Figure 8-7. Bronchitis. The bronchial wall shows a chronic inflammatory infiltrate in the subepithelial connective tissue and surrounding cartilage.

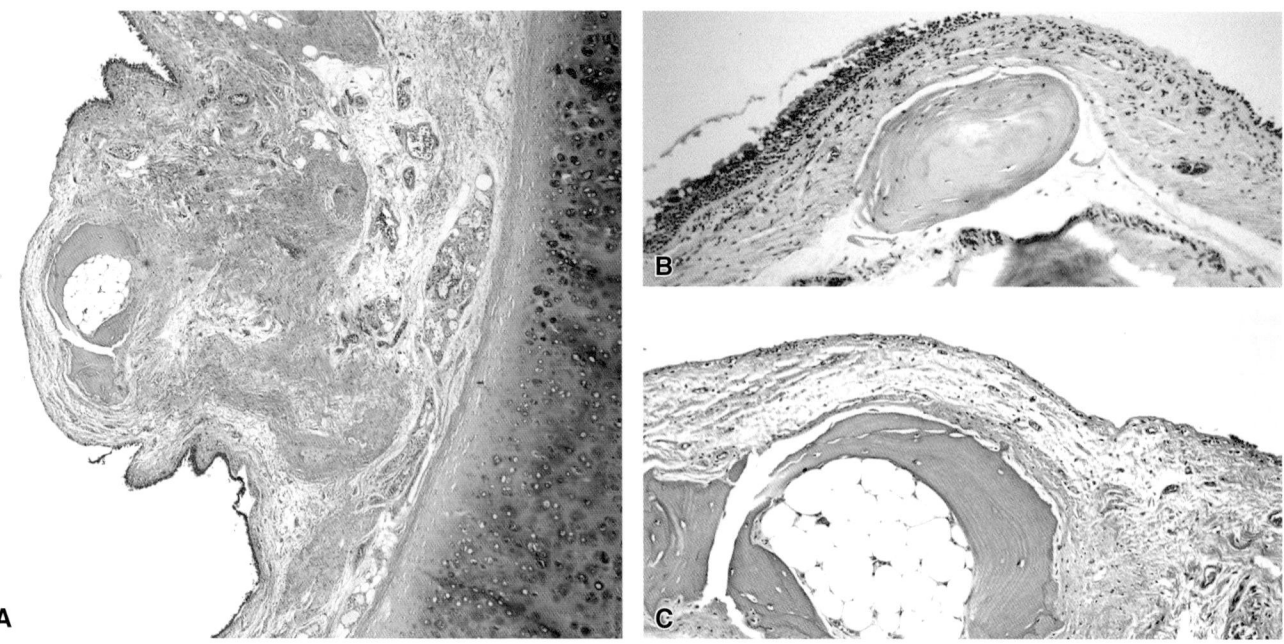

Figure 8-6. Tracheobronchopathia osteochondroplastica. **A,** The panoramic view shows a nodular protrusion into the tracheal lumen, composed of fibrous tissue and mature bone. **B,** A preparation from a different patient showing osseous metaplasia. **C,** An area from the same nodule as in part **A,** seen at higher magnification.

Box 8-2. Possible Causes of Dense Chronic Inflammation in Bronchoscopic Biopsies

Clinical chronic bronchitis
Postinfectious
Hypersensitivity reactions
Allergic bronchopulmonary fungal disease
Bronchiectasis
Reaction at the periphery of a tumor, abscess, or infection
Marginal zone lymphoma (of MALT)
Follicular bronchiolitis
Drug reactions
Toxic inhalation

MALT, mucosa-associated lymphoid tissue.

inflammatory changes may be the dominant findings. Unfortunately, the list of possible etiologic disorders associated with chronic inflammation in bronchial mucosa is quite long (Box 8-2) and sufficiently diverse as to not be useful in narrowing the scope of the clinical differential diagnosis. For this reason, a careful search for other, more specific findings is always in order, and these are worth mentioning as a list of pertinent negative findings (e.g., vasculitis, granulomas, necrosis, tumor).

Bronchiectasis

Bronchiectasis is defined as a permanent dilatation of the cartilaginous airways (bronchi), often attended by acute and chronic inflammation. Conceptually, bronchiectasis can be considered the end result of any number of conditions that damage the airway wall and result in weakening over time and dilatation.[34] Primary causes are most commonly related to inherited abnormalities (ciliary dysfunction, abnormal mucus production), whereas secondary causes are numerous. In a review of multiple published series of bronchiectasis between 1935 and 1981, Barker and Bardana[35] found a significant proportion of idiopathic cases (as much as 30% according to Nicotra and associates[36]). Among recognizable causes of bronchiectasis are infections, primary ciliary dyskinesia, immunodeficiency, cystic fibrosis, rheumatoid arthritis, inflammatory bowel disease,[37] and graft-versus-host disease.[38] An intriguing implication of *Helicobacter pylori* in the pathogenesis of bronchiectasis has been raised in some studies.[39–41] In specific conditions such as cystic fibrosis, bronchiectasis may dominate the pulmonary pathology. Bronchiectasis, outside the setting of cystic fibrosis, often is perceived to be rare in Western societies but remains an important cause of chronic suppurative lung disease in the developing world. The decline in hospital admission rates for pediatric bronchiectasis in the Western countries has been noted since the 1950s and has been attributed to improvements in sanitation and nutrition, introduction of childhood immunization (particularly against pertussis and measles), and the early and frequent use of antibiotics.

Bronchiectasis is a radiologic diagnosis in the living patient but has distinctive features in resected lungs (Fig. 8-8) and lobes and sometimes in surgical biopsies. The proposed historical classification of bronchiectasis divided the process into three types:

- Saccular, characterized by progressive dilatation of the bronchi from central to peripheral
- Varicose, in which combined dilatation and constriction dominate the picture without a consistent pattern
- Cylindrical, characterized by uniform dilatation, primarily a manifestation of loss of normal tapering

Such a classification has come under intense scrutiny with the advent of high-resolution CT (HRCT) scanning, whereby the airways can be better defined in three-dimensional space through computer-enhanced reconstruction.

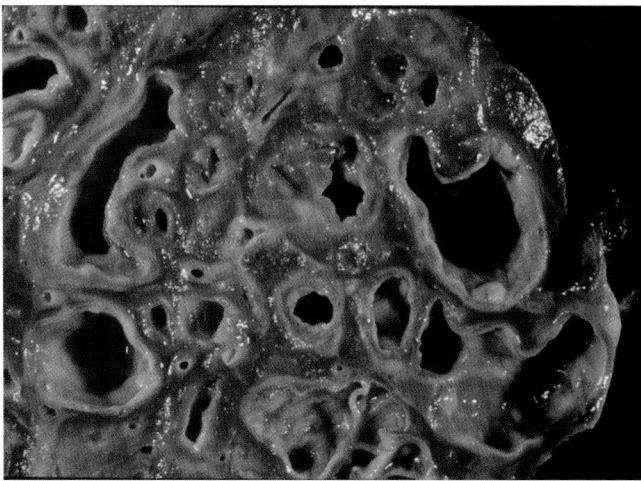

Figure 8-8. Bronchiectasis. Gross specimen showing classic saccular enlargement of the bronchi.

Presenting signs and symptoms include cough with production of purulent sputum, fever, shortness of breath, and, occasionally, hemoptysis. No age or sex predilection has been noted, and the disease tends to run a course of recurrent exacerbation, sometimes with superimposed infection. Inflammatory changes in biopsies obtained with the bronchoscope correlate poorly with the presence or absence of bronchiectasis. Nevertheless, such specimens may be useful for ancillary laboratory studies (such as ultrastructural studies in search of ciliary abnormalities). On plain films of the chest, classic parallel linear opacities (referred to as "tram tracks") correspond to thickened bronchial walls, whereas tubular opacities reflect mucus-filled bronchi. Today, most cases of bronchiectasis are diagnosed by HRCT.[42,43] Overall, the sensitivity of HRCT in detecting bronchiectasis is quite high.[44,45] The HRCT findings in bronchiectasis are summarized in Box 8-3.

The gross findings in bronchiectasis have been well described in autopsy series.[46] For the histopathologist, acute and chronic inflammatory changes dominate the bronchoscopic biopsy picture (Fig. 8-9). The presence of necrotic debris and mucus in airways may be a sign of coexistent bronchiectasis, but in most instances, even surgical lung biopsy findings only reflect "downstream" secondary manifestations of obstruction or infection occurring more proximally. Lymphoid hyperplasia surrounding the large airways may occur in bronchiectasis and bronchoscopically derived biopsies may sample such hyperplastic lymphoid tissue, raising concern for tumor on occasion (especially when a portion of a germinal center dominates the small biopsy specimen). Caution is always advisable in these settings to avoid the overdiagnosis of lymphoproliferative disease. Also, the necrotic granular debris that may accompany bronchiectasis may be sampled by bronchoscopic biopsy, thereby raising concern for necrotic neoplasm or abscess. Providing a broad differential diagnosis is the best approach here, to avoid confusion and possible misdirection of clinical management.

Box 8-3. High-Resolution Computed Tomography Findings in Bronchiectasis

Lack of bronchial tapering
Presence of visible bronchi within 1 cm of the costal pleura
Visible bronchial lumens abutting mediastinal pleura, bronchi seen as horizontal parallel lines ("tram tracks")
Bronchial diameter exceeding adjacent pulmonary diameter ("signet ring sign")
Irregular bronchial dilatation
Clustered thin-walled cystic spaces with or without air-fluid levels

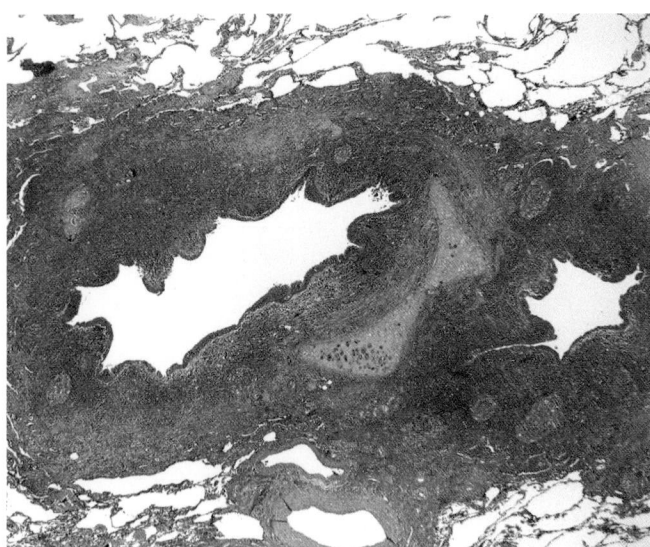

Figure 8-9. Bronchiectasis. The lumen of the bronchus is dilated, and there is prominent chronic inflammation in the bronchial wall.

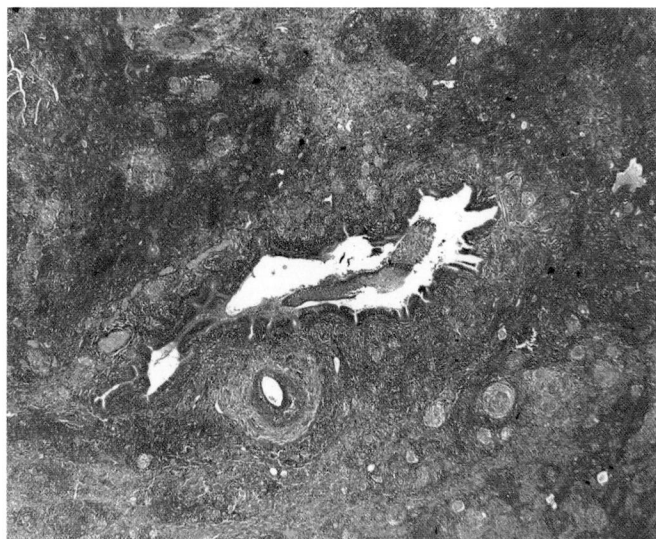

Figure 8-10. Middle lobe syndrome. The bronchial wall shows prominent lymphoid infiltration, with many germinal centers.

Middle Lobe Syndrome

Middle lobe syndrome is included in this disease category because the disorder is fundamentally one of chronic large airway obstruction with secondary bronchiectasis, bronchitis, and bronchiolitis-associated parenchymal changes that arise as additional "downstream" effects of these airway abnormalities.

The concept of "right middle lobe syndrome" was highlighted in studies of children with chronic failure to thrive and right middle lobe abnormalities on chest radiographs. The proposed hypothesis was based on the notion that lymphoid hyperplasia occurring around the right middle lobe bronchus produced compression and narrowing of the bronchial lumen. Also, the position of the middle lobe (and the lingula of the left lung) relative to the remainder of the tracheobronchial tree makes it susceptible to obstruction and secondary chronic inflammatory changes in the lobe (long narrow bronchus). In clinical practice, the disease occurs more frequently in adults and often without an identifiable obstructing lesion.[47] This population consists predominantly of middle-aged or elderly women, and the condition has been referred to as "Lady Windermere syndrome."[48-50] A role for *Mycobacterium avium* complex infection has been postulated in the pathogenesis of middle lobe syndrome, although it remains unclear whether this is an epiphenomenon related to the common occurrence of bronchiectasis in this condition. Consolidation of the right middle lobe, or lingula, attended by bronchiectasis, is typical.[34,47]

In surgical lung biopsies of the right middle lobe or lingula, advanced remodeling, granulomatous inflammation, extensive inflammatory infiltrates, and mucostasis, when present together, should always suggest the possibility of middle lobe syndrome (Fig. 8-10). The presence of granulomas in the context of middle lobe syndrome should raise suspicion for colonization by atypical mycobacterial species, and acid-fast organisms may be identified in granulomas.[48] A number of inflammatory changes are observed in middle lobe syndrome, and these are listed in Box 8-4.[47,51] Removal of any obstructing lesions, whether neoplasm or other, in early stages of the disease process may avoid the need for lobectomy.[52]

Box 8-4. Histopathologic Findings in Middle Lobe Syndrome

Bronchiectasis
Follicular bronchiolitis
Organizing pneumonia
Bronchial lithiasis
Atelectasis
Granulomas (mainly due to *Mycobacterium avium* complex)
Abscesses
Hemosiderosis
Interstitial fibrosis and honeycomb changes
Pleural fibrosis

Modified from Kwon KY, Myers JL, Swensen SJ, Colby TV. Middle lobe syndrome: a clinicopathological study of 21 patients. *Hum Pathol*. 1995;26(3):302–307.

The Small Airways (Bronchioles and Alveolar Ducts)

The small airways of the lung include the small bronchi, with a diameter less than 2 to 3 mm, and the membranous bronchioles (terminal and respiratory bronchioles). Terminal bronchioles have a diameter of less than 1 mm and are just proximal to the respiratory bronchioles, the first airways that have alveoli budding from their walls. The terminal bronchioles are located in the center of the pulmonary lobule and, like all conducting airways, are always accompanied by a pulmonary artery branch (Fig. 8-11). In cross-sectional views, their respective diameters are approximately equal (Fig. 8-12A). The lumen of the terminal bronchiole is uniform in longitudinal histologic sections, but minor variations in size can be seen (see Fig. 8-12B).

It is said that the small airways constitute the "Achilles heel" of the lung, because they play an important role in air distribution and flow but lack the rigid structure of the bronchi to protect them from collapse during exhalation, especially when affected by disease. The small airways can be affected secondarily by inflammatory diseases that involve primarily the bronchi or the alveoli, or both, or by primary diseases that selectively involve these delicate anatomic structures. No single classification of bronchiolar disorders has been widely accepted, although any number of classification schemes have been proposed based on cause

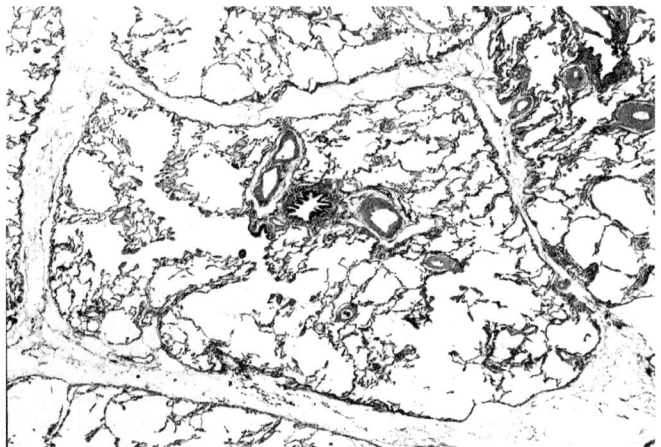

Figure 8-11. Normal lobule. A near-normal pulmonary lobule, whose outlines are enhanced in this preparation by a slight degree of septal edema. In the *middle* of the lobule is the bronchiole along with the adjacent pulmonary artery. Note that the diameter of the terminal bronchiole, seen here in cross section, is very similar to that of the nearby arteries.

Box 8-5. Classification of Bronchiolar Disorders

Primary bronchiolar disorders
    Respiratory bronchiolitis
    Acute bronchiolitis
    Constrictive/obliterative bronchiolitis
    Follicular bronchiolitis
    Mineral dust airway disease
Bronchiolar involvement in interstitial lung diseases
    RBILD/DIP
    Organizing pneumonia patterns
    Hypersensitivity pneumonitis
    Langherhans cell histiocytosis
    Sarcoidosis
Bronchiolar involvement in large-airway disease
    Chronic bronchitis
    Bronchiectasis
    Asthma

RBILD/DIP, respiratory bronchiolitis–associated interstitial lung disease/desquamative interstitial pneumonia.
Adapted from Ryu JH. Classification and approach to bronchiolar diseases. *Curr Opin Pulm Med.* 2006;12(2):145–151; and Ryu JH, Myers JL, Swensen SJ. Bronchiolar disorders. *Am J Respir Crit Care Med.* 2003;168(11):1277–1292.

and underlying diseases, radiologic features, histopathologic findings, or some combination of these parameters.[53–56] As recently proposed by Ryu and colleagues, bronchiolar disorders can be divided into three groups: primary bronchiolar disorders, bronchiolar involvement in interstitial lung diseases, and bronchiolar involvement in large airway disease[57,58] (Box 8-5). From a histopathologic point of view it should be pointed out that patients rarely come to lung biopsy with a preoperative diagnosis of "small airway disease." The reasons for this are legion but

mainly reflect the fact that disorders of the small airways are relatively "silent" clinically and radiologically. In addition, some of the small-airway lesions are quite subtle histologically and, at first glance, may be overlooked.[59,60]

It is the rare lung biopsy that does not show some degree of histopathologic alteration in the small airways. Critical to the evaluation of such changes is knowledge of the clinical manifestations, the radiologic distribution of disease (whether localized or

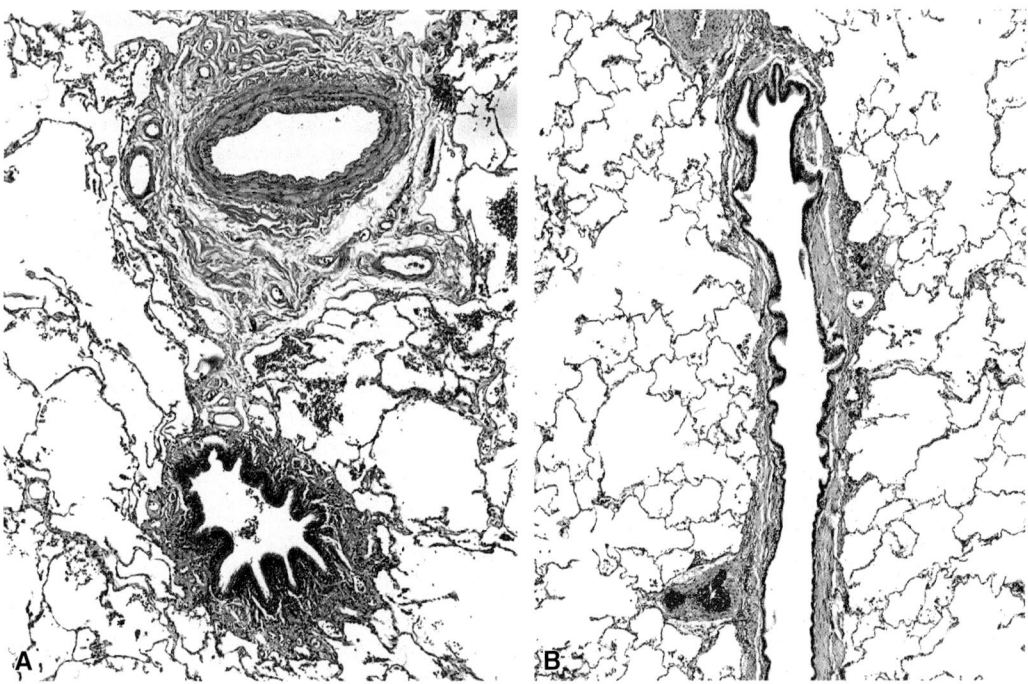

Figure 8-12. Terminal bronchiole. **A,** A cross section of a terminal bronchiole and adjacent artery. The normal terminal bronchiole has a thin wall and an open lumen. The wall is composed of a variably enfolded mucosa, showing a columnar to cuboidal epithelium with ciliated columnar cells and Clara cells. In longitudinal sections, the lumen of the normal bronchiole is regular, and little tortuosity is evident. **B,** This bronchiole is cut lengthwise, its major axis is relatively straight, and the lumen has a relatively constant diameter.

bilateral and diffuse), and the patient's cigarette smoking history. Attempts to predict clinical disease based on isolated abnormalities of the small airways, as viewed through the microscope, often are unrewarding. The HRCT scan may provide valuable information regarding the possible pathologic pattern of disease, as shown in Table 8-1.

What follows is a compilation of the specific elementary pathologic changes in the small airways that can be identified on histopathologic examination, along with the lists of conditions that should be considered when each such change is encountered. It is important to recognize that the elementary lesions rarely occur in isolation, and that they are frequently combined together. Also presented is a brief review of some general histopathologic patterns of lesions (or specific diseases) that may involve the small airways.

Conceptually, the elementary histopathologic lesions of the small airways can be subdivided into inflammatory (acute, chronic, granulomatous, with or without necrosis) and proliferative (epithelial or mesenchymal, concentric within the lumen or eccentric in peribronchiolar tissue) types. The foregoing reactions may lead to a number of distortions of the normal bronchiolar architecture, including occlusion, constriction, dilatation (with or without mucostasis), tortuosity, and nodularity. The lesion may be exquisitely bronchiolar or may extend to involve the surrounding parenchyma, and in the latter case it is important to distinguish between lesions that extend from the bronchiole to the parenchyma and those with the reverse orientation (as with organizing pneumonia patterns, in which the main lesion is in the parenchyma). All of these features must be considered in analyzing the histology of the small airways. An important point is that most of the described lesions (except perhaps scarring) typically are part of a dynamic process, whereby one single causative agent may produce distinct pathologic features at different times in the natural history of the disease. In addition, the same clinical disease manifestations may result in a variety of pathologic lesions. In practice, it is best not to assume an unequivocal relationship between the *histopathologic* lesions observed on biopsy and a specific *clinical* disease. The diagnosis of small-airway diseases is rarely possible in transbronchial biopsies but may be appreciated in surgical lung sections, often as a "minimal changes" pattern (see introductory section "Pattern-Based Approach to Diagnosis").

Table 8-1. High-Resolution Computed Tomography Abnormalities of the Small Airways

Radiologic Finding	Pathologic Pattern
Centrilobular nodularity	Cellular bronchiolitis Follicular bronchiolitis Respiratory bronchiolitis
Peribronchial nodules	Follicular bronchiolitis
"Tree in bud" pattern	Cellular bronchiolitis Panbronchiolitis
Diffuse or "geographic" air-trapping	
Mosaic pattern	Constrictive bronchiolitis
Bronchioloectasis, bronchiectasis	Panbronchiolitis
Patchy ground-glass attenuation	Respiratory bronchiolitis
Ground-glass opacity	Follicular bronchiolitis

Modified from Lynch DA. Imaging of small airways diseases. *Clin Chest Med.* 1993;14(4): 623–634.

Inflammatory Bronchiolitis

Inflammatory bronchiolitis, also known as cellular bronchiolitis, is a generic term that includes acute bronchiolitis, chronic bronchiolitis, and combined forms with variable amounts of both types of processes. All forms may be associated with bronchiolar fibrosis.[60] An important point is that both acute and chronic forms of bronchiolitis may have significant overlap, with one form typically being dominant. Diseases of the airways rarely have histopathologic features sufficiently specific to point to a single etiologic disorder or a specific disease in the absence of some characteristic finding (e.g., viral inclusions, aspirated foreign material). When the surgical pathologist is confronted with isolated inflammatory changes in the small airways, it is important to invoke a differential diagnosis to stimulate clinicopathologic correlation, and thereby help to narrow considerations in the clinical differential diagnosis.

Acute Bronchiolitis

Florid acute bronchiolitis is characterized by predominantly acute inflammation of the small airways, with variable epithelial sloughing. Extension of acute inflammation into surrounding peribronchiolar parenchyma is typical (Fig. 8-13). Very often, acute bronchiolitis is associated with some degree of chronic inflammatory infiltration, as described below. Conditions associated with relatively pure acute bronchiolitis include the early phase of certain infections (most of which also produce epithelial necrosis).[61,62] A careful search for viral inclusions is especially relevant in this scenario. Acute fume or toxic gas inhalation can also produce acute small-airway injury, with few if any chronic changes. Loose connective tissue polyps may develop as a consequence of basement membrane disruption with fibroblastic migration into the airway lumens from subepithelial regions (so-called Masson polyps). Acute aspiration can manifest occasionally as acute bronchiolitis (most commonly seen at autopsy, in cases in which aspiration may have been part of the terminal event). Acute bronchiolitis can be an uncommon manifestation of Wegener granulomatosis.[63]

Acute and Chronic Bronchiolitis

Acute and chronic inflammation of the small airways (Fig. 8-14) is one of the most common manifestations of so-called cellular bronchiolitis.[64] This inflammatory process frequently is associated with other bronchiolocentric manifestations, including intraluminal polyp formation, constriction and obliteration, and presence of lymphoid follicles within the peribronchiolar sheath (follicular bronchiolitis).

When acute and chronic bronchiolitis are the primary manifestation in the lung biopsy, clinical manifestations may be accompanied by completely obstructive, completely restrictive, or a mixture of obstructive and restrictive pulmonary physiology. HRCT scans may show a predominantly nodular pattern, although reticulonodular infiltrates are more commonly observed. Box 8-6 lists the most frequent diseases associated with acute and chronic bronchiolitis.

Chronic Bronchiolitis

Chronic inflammation within and surrounding the walls of small airways (Figs. 8-15 and 8-16) can be seen in several conditions (Box 8-7). Chronic bronchiolitis can occur with or without lymphoid follicles or some degree of fibrosis. *Follicular bronchiolitis* is a specific subtype of chronic bronchiolitis, characterized by the presence of lymphoid follicles with well-formed germinal centers surrounding the bronchiolar walls, sometimes with lymphocytes migrating

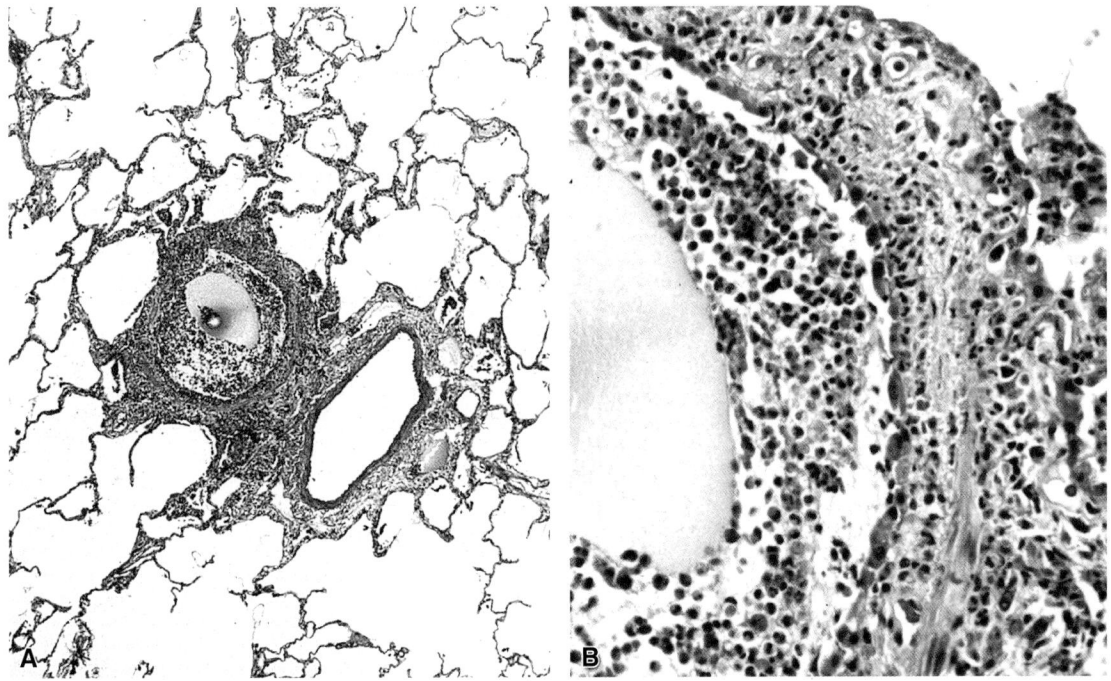

Figure 8-13. Acute bronchiolitis. **A,** A bronchovascular bundle with the small artery and the respiratory bronchiole. Increased cellularity of the bronchiolar wall is evident, and many neutrophils are present within its lumen, accompanied by some acellular exudate. The surrounding lung parenchyma is uninvolved by the disease. **B,** At higher magnification, the bronchiolar wall shows a cellular infiltrate composed of neutrophils, which expand the adventitial connective tissue and the subepithelial tissue.

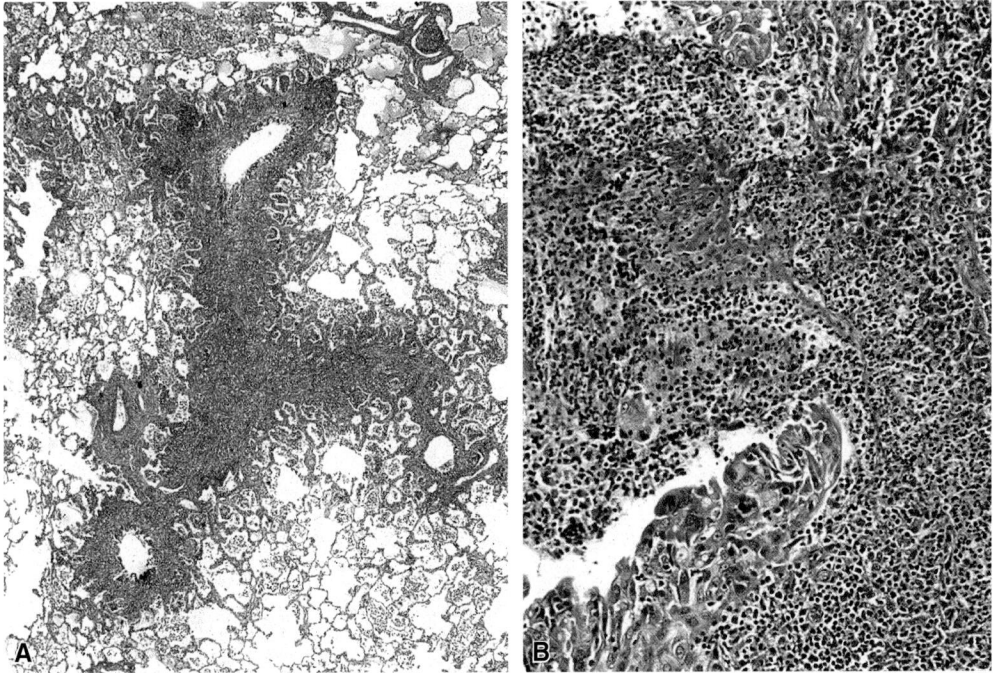

Figure 8-14. Acute and chronic bronchitis/bronchiolitis. **A,** At low magnification, a definite peribronchiolar lesion is seen that also involves the adjacent lung parenchyma. **B,** The cellular infiltrate is composed of neutrophils and lymphocytes. This preparation is from a patient with bronchiolocentric Wegener granulomatosis.

in the respiratory epithelium, either singly or in small clusters (Figs. 8-17 to 8-19). Follicular bronchiolitis may be seen in several connective tissue diseases.[65–69] In cases with dense and extensive lymphoid infiltrates, especially if lymphoepithelial lesions are prominent, one should always consider the possibility of a lung lymphoma, most of which are low-grade B cell lymphomas of extranodal marginal zone type, arising from the mucosa-associated lymphoid tissue (MALT)[70–72] (Fig. 8-20). Follicular bronchiolitis may also be seen in some occupational exposure settings, such as nylon flocking workers,[73–77] and in immunodeficiency syndromes including the acquired immunodeficiency syndrome (AIDS) related to human immunodeficiency virus (HIV) infection.[78]

Box 8-6. Diseases and Conditions Associated with Acute and Chronic Bronchiolitis

Infections
Allergic reactions
Collagen vascular diseases
Bronchocentric granulomatosis
Allergic bronchopulmonary fungal disease
Bronchiectasis
Inflammatory bowel disease
Aspiration pneumonia
Graft-versus-host disease
Wegener granulomatosis
Idiopathic forms

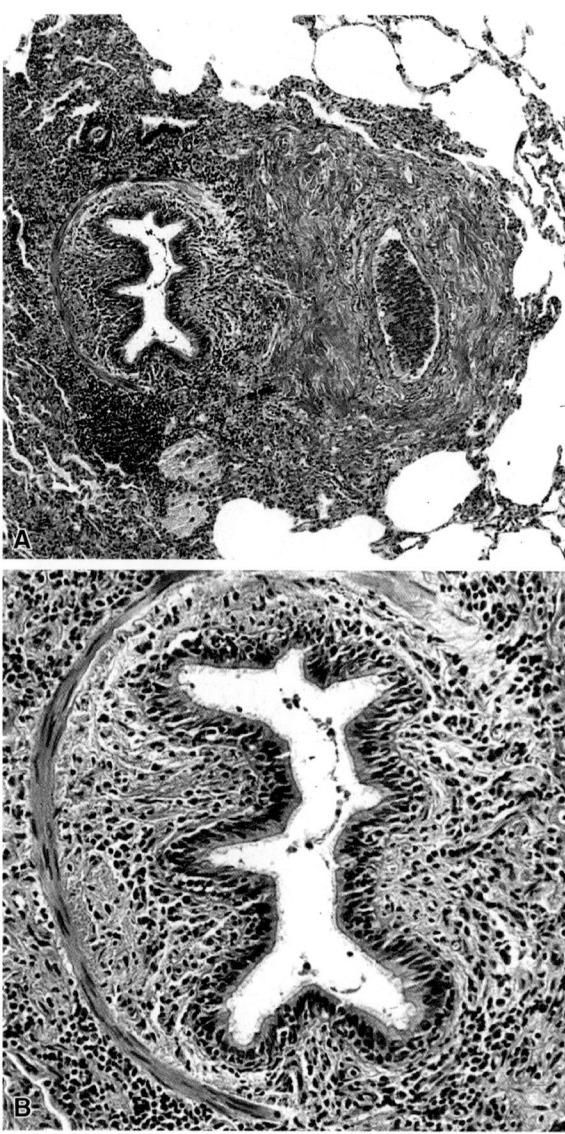

Figure 8-15. Chronic bronchiolitis. **A,** The bronchiole shows an inflammatory reaction that expands the subepithelial connective tissue, whereas the actual diameter of the airway is similar to that of the adjacent artery. **B,** At higher magnification, the chronic inflamatory infiltrate can be seen to fill the subepithelial area and also extends across the muscular wall to involve the bronchovascular sheath. The patient had a severe restrictive ventilatory defect.

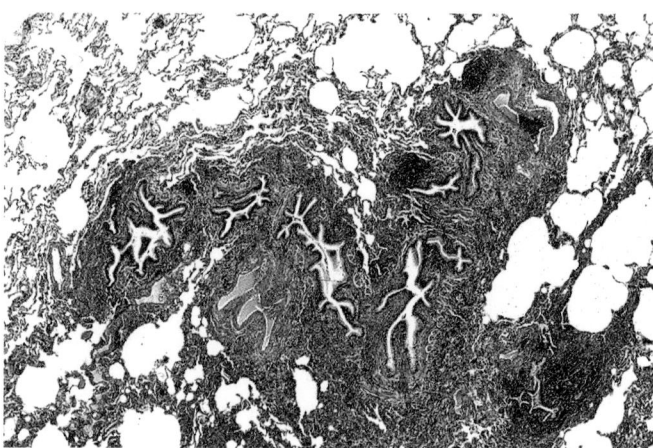

Figure 8-16. Chronic bronchiolitis: Effects on the structure of the terminal bronchioles. A longitudinal section of a terminal bronchiole along with the adjacent artery in a preparation from a patient with a severe restrictive ventilatory defect. The airway is surrounded by a prominent lymphocytic infiltrate and shows distortion of the lumen, with variable stricture and dilatation.

Box 8-7. Conditions Associated with Chronic Inflammation of the Small Airways

Bronchiectasis (especially in airways distal to markedly dilated airways)
Collagen vascular diseases
Asthma
Hypersensitivity pneumonitis
Graft-versus-host disease
Lymphoproliferative diseases (especially-low grade MALT lymphomas)
Respiratory bronchiolitis
Chronic aspiration pneumonia
Associated with inflammatory bowel disease
Nylon flocking–associated interstitial lung disease
As a minor component of a localized inflammatory reaction (e.g., in right middle lobe syndrome)
Idiopathic forms

MALT, mucosa-associated lymphoid tissue.

Granulomatous Bronchiolitis

Isolated granulomatous bronchiolitis is unusual. Sarcoidosis is the leading consideration in the differential diagnosis in the absence of necrosis (Fig. 8-21). Granulomas of sarcoidosis are usually distributed along the lymphatic routes in the lung and therefore are frequently bronchiolocentric, allowing bronchoscopic biopsy to provide excellent diagnostic material. On the other hand, when necrosis is present, granulomas are usually present in the surrounding lung parenchyma as well, and herald the strong possibility of infection (especially infection caused by mycobacteria and fungi)[79] (Fig. 8-22). Necrotizing granulomatous bronchiolitis also may be seen in the setting of middle lobe syndrome[47] and chronic necrotizing forms of pulmonary aspergillosis.[80] Even in the absence of necrosis, however, infection should still remain high in the differential diagnosis. Non-necrotizing granulomatous bronchiolitis can be seen in association with inflammatory bowel disease, such as Crohn disease, sometimes accompanied by microabscesses.[81] Non-necrotizing peribronchiolar granulomas are also seen in a majority of patients with hypersensitivity pneumonitis

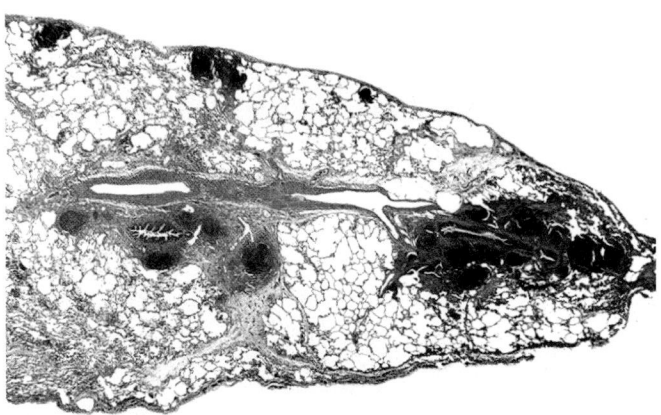

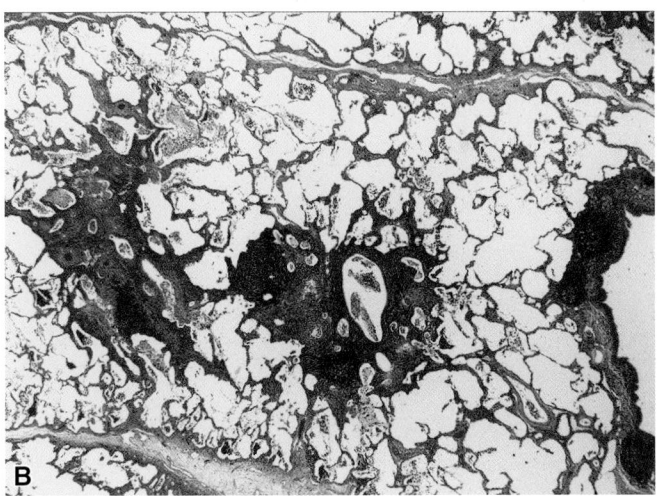

Figure 8-17. Follicular bronchiolitis. Biopsy specimen from a patient with Sjögren syndrome. **A,** At low magnification, the characteristic bronchiolocentric lymphoid infiltrate of follicular bronchiolitis can be seen. **B,** Lymphoid follicles with germinal centers are readily apparent and associated with bronchiolar injury (*center*). Follicular bronchiolitis may have a number of causes, including collagen vascular disease (as in this case), cystic fibrosis, ciliary defects, or immunodeficiency syndromes, or may be secondary to bronchiectasis, previous infection, or aspiration.

(Fig. 8-23). Generally, granulomas in hypersensitivity are less well delimited and well formed than in infectious diseases and may take the form of loose aggregations of histiocytic epithelioid cells, with or without giant cells.

Another frequent cause of granulomatous bronchiolitis is aspiration pneumonia,[64] which may be clinically occult and manifest as diffuse bronchiolar disease with bronchiolecentric granulomatous inflammation.[82,83] It is worth noting that aspirated food particles are not usually birefringent under polarized light. The exceptions are talc and microcrystalline cellulose, both used as inert components of oral pharmaceutical tablets and susceptible to accidental aspiration. Talc aspiration also has been rarely reported in children related to the liberal use of baby powder on the skin.[83] When isolated peribronchiolar multinucleated giant cells are the major finding, one should consider Wegener granulomatosis (Fig. 8-24), aspiration pneumonia (Figs. 8-25 and 8-26), and hard metal (cobalt) pneumoconiosis (so-called giant cell interstitial pneumonia of Liebow).

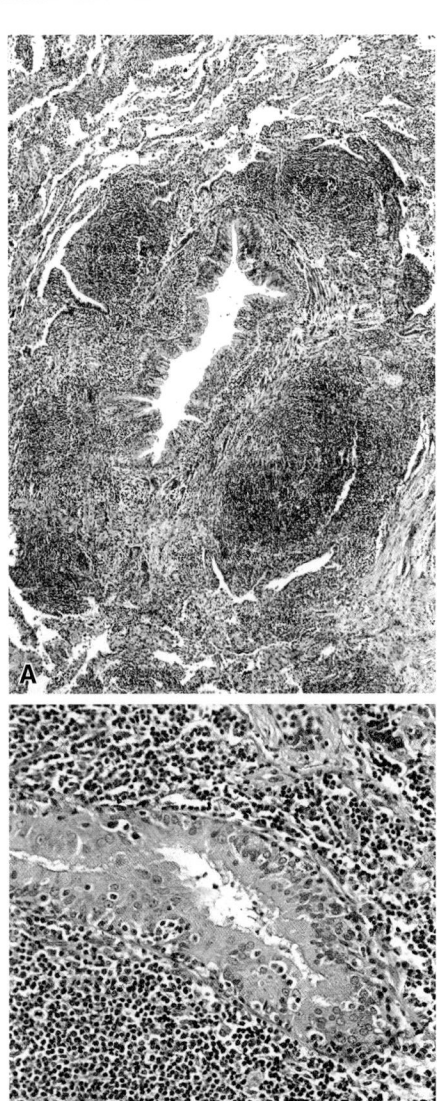

Figure 8-18. Follicular bronchiolitis. The patient presented with bronchiectasis in the setting of a middle lobe syndrome. **A,** The terminal bronchiole is surrounded by a prominent inflammatory infiltrate, with lymphoid follicles having well-formed germinal centers. The inflammatory process involves both the subepithelial layer and the adventitial tissue. **B,** The subepithelial layer has a diffuse lymphoid infiltrate composed of mature small lymphocytes, which may show a tendency toward intraepithelial migration, simulating the lymphoepithelial lesions seen in low-grade lymphomas of the MALT/BALT tissue.

Bronchiolar Necrosis

Complete mucosal necrosis with epithelial sloughing and variable acute inflammation is typical of a limited number of lung diseases, mainly those of infectious origin (Box 8-8). In the presence of bronchiolar necrosis, a careful search for viropathic changes or microorganisms

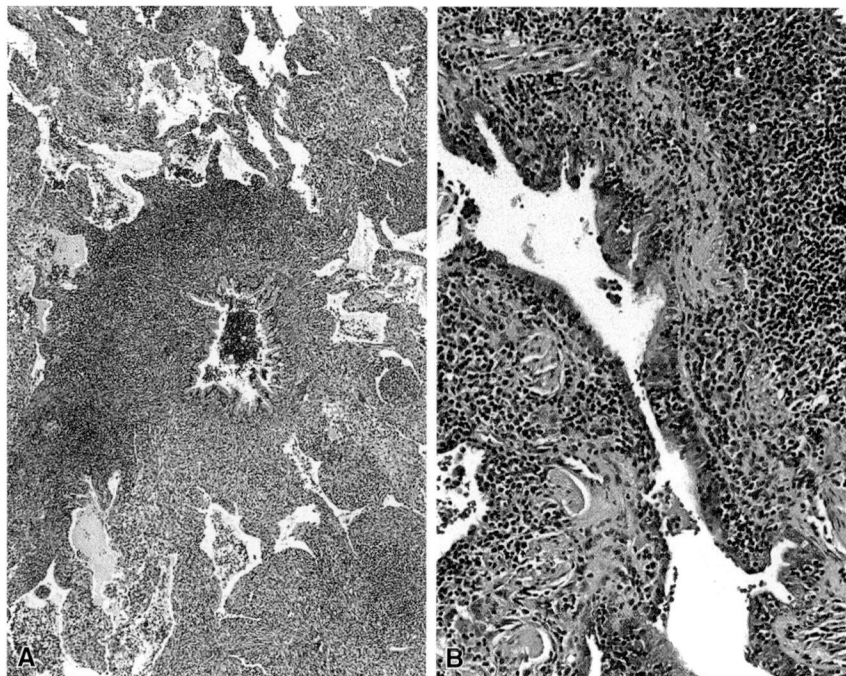

Figure 8-19. Follicular bronchiolitis. The patient had IgA deficiency. **A,** Respiratory bronchiole surrounded by several lymphoid follicles. **B,** The lymphoid tissue expands the bronchiolar wall, and many mononuclear cells are seen between the epithelial cell layer and the muscularis propria.

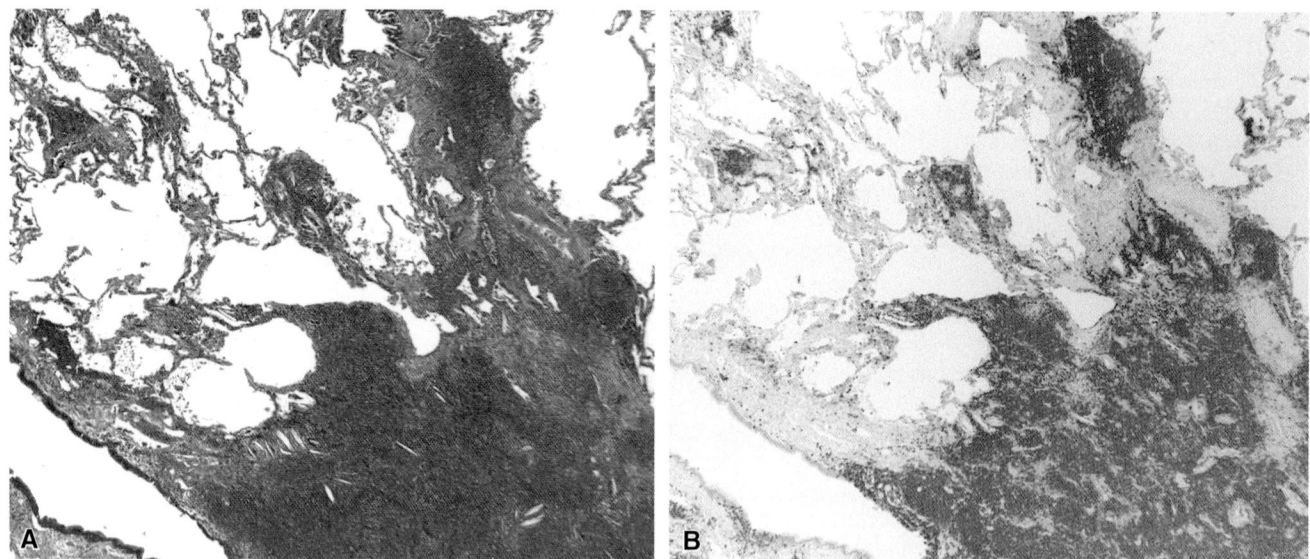

Figure 8-20. Low-grade lymphoma of the bronchus-associated lymphoid tissue (BALT). This lymphoma, the bronchial counterpart of gastric MALToma, is a marginal zone lymphoma that originated from the BALT lymphoid tissue. **A,** The present case shows a dense and homogeneous cellular infiltrate composed predominantly of small lymphocytes, which extends along the bronchiolar wall. **B,** A CD20 immunostain highlights the diffuse and monomorphous spread of small B lymphocytes.

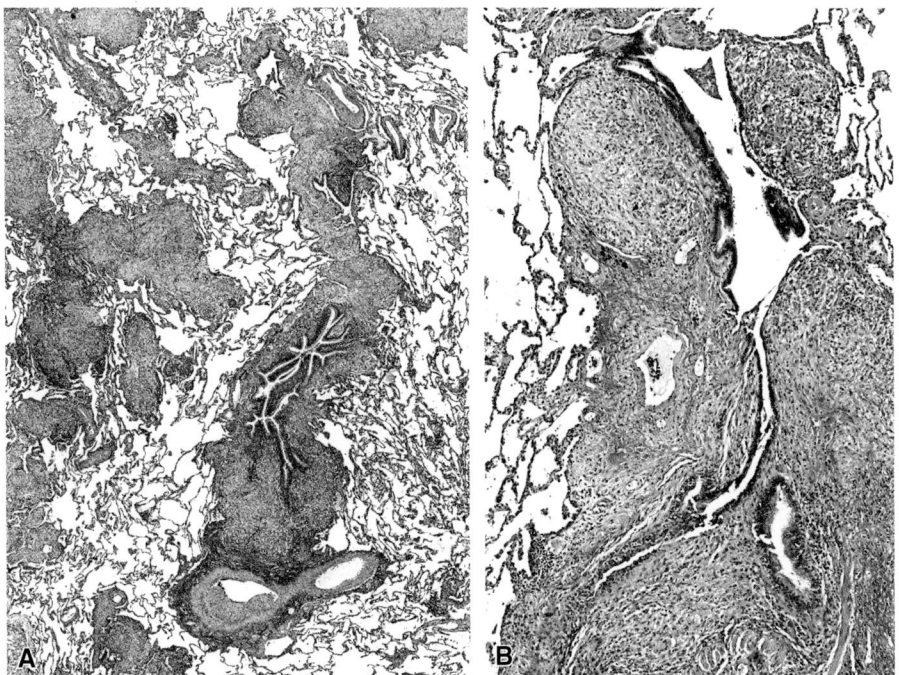

Figure 8-21. Sarcoidosis. **A,** At scanning magnification, the serpiginous outline of the bronchovascular bundle is accentuated by pale pink granulomas, collagen, and scant chronic inflammation. **B,** The bronchiole shows the typical granulomas and sclerotic background matrix of sarcoidosis, which involves the airway wall and impinges on the adjacent arterial wall. The granulomas are well formed, with a definite fibrous demarcation, and show a tendency toward coalescence. Inflammatory cells are scant, and the whole process has an eosinophilic appearance, which is clearly different from that of the lesions seen in granulomatous bronchiolitis due to infection (compare Fig. 8-22).

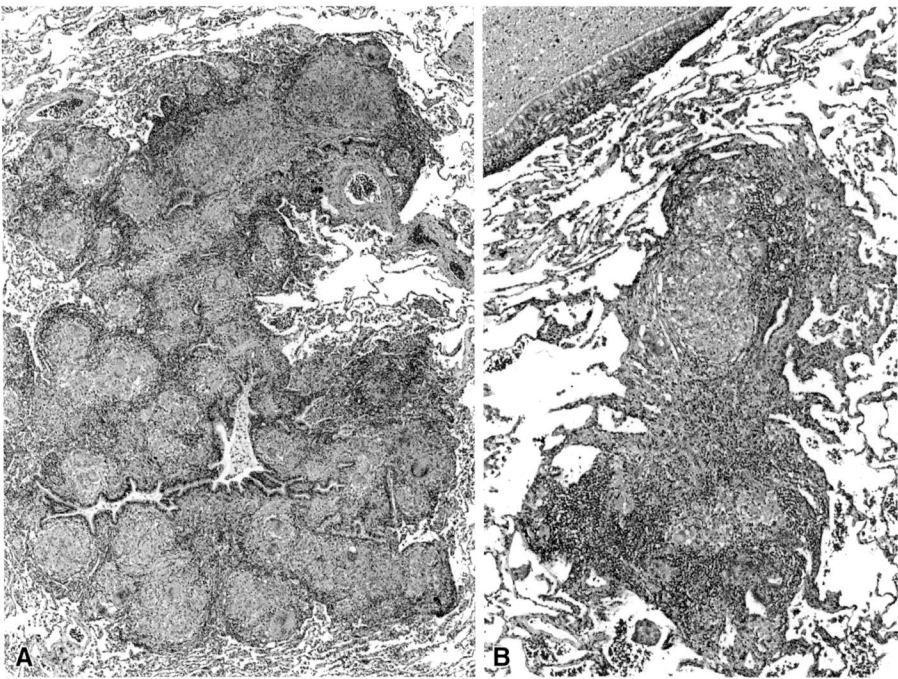

Figure 8-22. Granulomatous bronchiolitis due to infection. **A,** A granulomatous bronchiolitis in *Mycobacterium tuberculosis* infection: granulomas are abundant and have distinct giant cells. **B,** A case of *Mycobacterium avium* complex (MAC) infection, with non-necrotizing granulomas centered on the bronchioles (note the dilated bronchiole in the *left upper corner*). The small granulomas usually are solitary, with a cuff of lymphocytes, and involve respiratory and terminal bronchioles. These lesions frequently are seen in association with a predisposing factor (e.g., bronchiectasis) or in healthy patients exposed to a contaminated environment (such as associated with hot tub use). The inflammatory process surrounding the granulomas is more pronounced than that associated with sarcoidosis. On the other hand, MAC granulomas are much better organized than those seen in hypersensitivity pneumonitis, where "granulomas" tend to be nothing more than loose clusters of interstitial epithelioid histiocytes and giant cells.

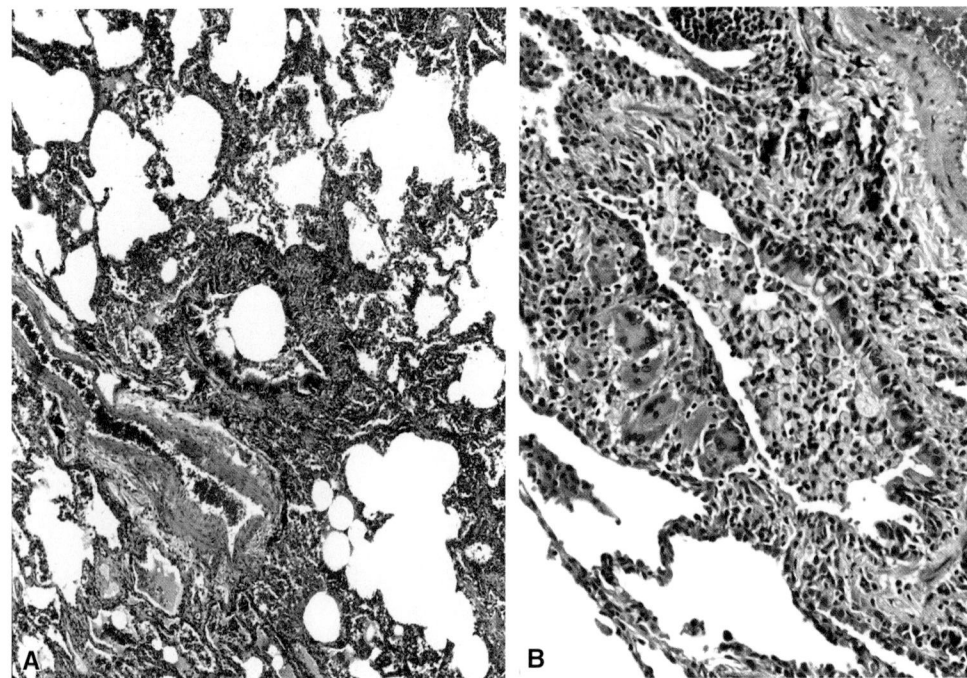

Figure 8-23. Hypersensitivity pneumonitis. **A,** A bronchiolocentric cellular infiltrate is typically present, accompanied by an ill-defined granulomatous reaction in the interstitium focally (**B**), and sometimes adjacent to the bronchioles. In this case, the patient had a hypersensitivity reaction after using a polyurethane spray indoors.

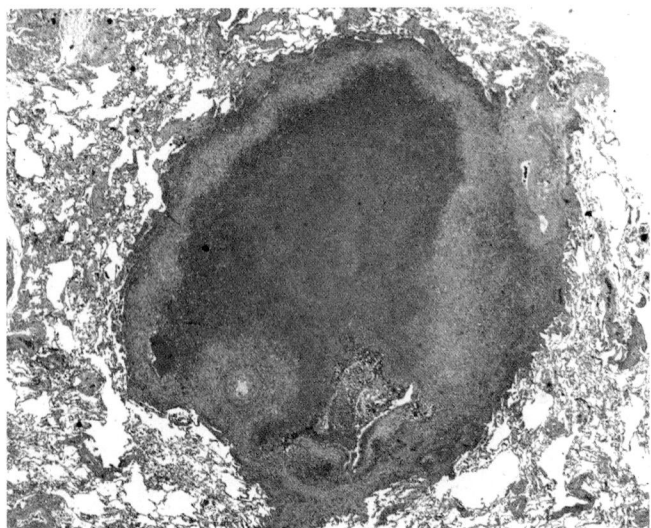

Figure 8-24. Bronchiolocentric granulomas in Wegener granulomatosis. This lung biopsy specimen shows a granulomatous reaction, with central necrosis, involving a small airway. Note the typical basophilic appearance of the necrosis.

(bacterial and fungal) should be undertaken (Fig. 8-27 to 8-29). When the process is intensely suppurative with large nodular foci of necrosis, consideration should be given to the possibility of pyoderma gangrenosum lesions in the lung associated with inflammatory bowel disease (e.g., ulcerative colitis)[84,85] or occurring de novo without inflammatory bowel disease.[86–91]

Respiratory (Smoker's) Bronchiolitis

Respiratory bronchiolitis is a very special marker for smoking-related lung injury and is extremely common in lung biopsy and surgical specimens (cigarette smoking being a cause of, or associated with, many lung diseases).[92–98] The histopathologic lesion of respiratory bronchiolitis is characterized by accumulation of lightly pigmented macrophages (smoker's macrophages) within the lumens of the respiratory bronchioles as well as in the surrounding peribronchiolar alveoli. This macrophage accumulation is associated with mild distortions of the overall architecture of the bronchiole, slight inflammation, fibrosis, and smooth muscle hyperplasia of the bronchiole wall. Minimal inflammation and interstitial fibrosis variably extends to the surrounding alveolar walls (Figs. 8-30 and 8-31). Sometimes respiratory bronchiolitis can be sufficiently extensive to produce clinical and radiologic manifestations of diffuse interstitial lung disease, so-called respiratory bronchiolitis–associated interstitial lung disease (RBILD) (see Chapter 7).[96,99,100] Desquamative interstitial pneumonia is also a consideration when this occurs. Histologically, RBILD is indistinguishable from respiratory bronchiolitis. A diagnosis of RBILD, as opposed to respiratory bronchiolitis, should be rendered only in the presence of clinically significant diffuse lung disease (shortness of breath, cough, mixed restrictive and obstructive physiology), if HRCT findings are compatible with the diagnosis (centrilobular micronodules, ground-glass opacities, and peribronchiolar thickening) and other causes of lung disease can be excluded with reasonable confidence.[96] In rare instances, RBILD can also be associated with significant panlobular and subpleural alveolar septa fibrosis, which may simulate fibrotic nonspecific interstitial pneumonia (NSIP).[101] Respiratory bronchiolitis is very commonly seen with Langerhans cell histiocytosis (pulmonary eosinophilic granuloma), because both have the same relationship to cigarette smoking.[92,102,103]

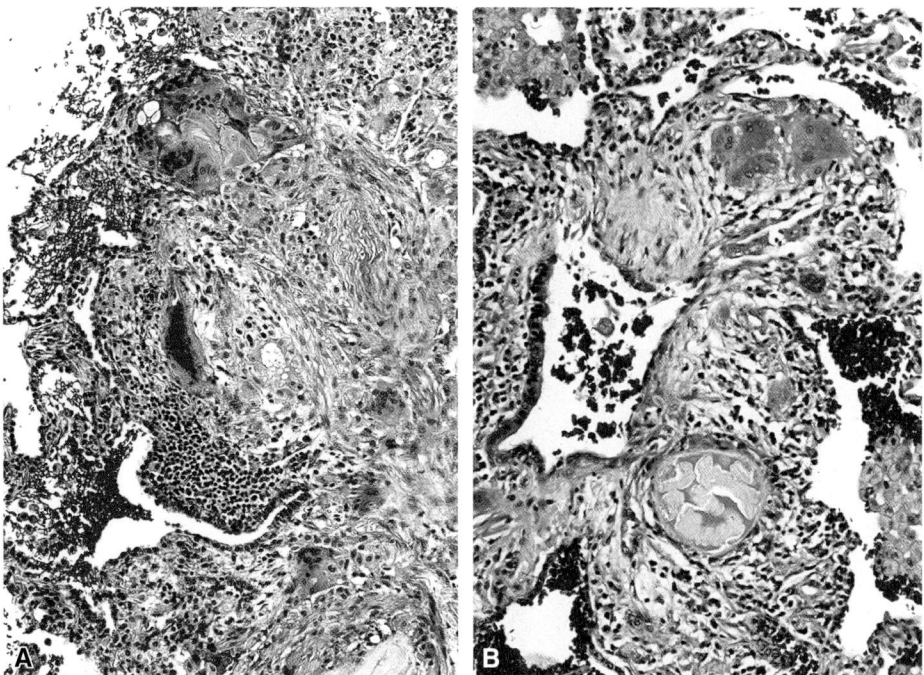

Figure 8-25. Aspiration bronchiolitis. This biopsy is from a patient who suffered from gastroesophageal reflux disease (GERD). He underwent lung biopsy 4 weeks after the sudden onset of pneumonia that failed to resolve. **A,** The pattern is one of non-necrotizing granulomatous bronchiolitis with many giant cells, some of which can be seen surrounding typical aspirated starch grains (**B**).

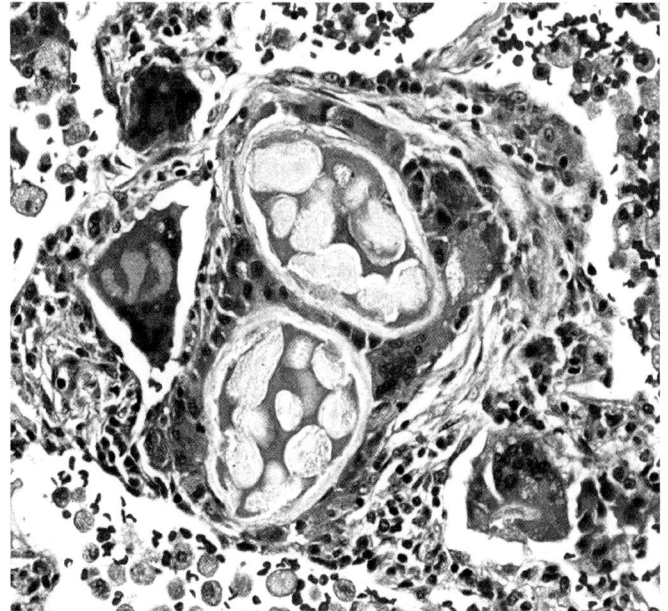

Figure 8-26. Aspiration bronchiolitis. Typical starch grains surrounded by foreign body–type giant cells.

When respiratory bronchiolitis is the sole pathologic finding in a smoker, a careful search for another disease process is in order, because mild respiratory bronchiolitis alone is probably an innocent bystander, unlikely to produce sufficient clinical and radiographic findings to warrant lung biopsy. Conversely, in a lifelong nonsmoker, changes

Box 8-8. Causes of Bronchiolar Necrosis (Mucosal Necrosis, Epithelial Sloughing, and Variable Acute Inflammation)

Infections (especially viral infections and certain bronchocentric fungal infections)
Aspiration
Toxic fume exposure
Bronchocentric granulomatosis
Wegener granulomatosis

resembling respiratory bronchiolitis usually indicate significant small-airway pathology, and some of these patients may have profound clinical symptoms with significant hypoxia and manifestations on CT scan suggesting interstitial lung disease (particularily mosaic perfusion). Trichrome and elastic tissue stains may be useful in this setting to highlight the occasionally subtle small airways pathology in the biopsy, such as excessive peribronchiolar fibrosis and obliterative scars. In this situation, high-resolution inspiratory and expiratory CT scans may provide additional radiologic evidence to support the small airways as the primary focus of the lung disease (see discussion of constrictive bronchiolitis later in this chapter).

Bronchiolar Metaplasia (Lambertosis)
Bronchiolar metaplasia is a pathologic process in which bronchiolar epithelial cells extend beyond the respiratory bronchioles along alveolar septa, replacing the normal alveolar lining cells, and is usually accompanied by some degree of stromal fibrosis (Fig. 8-32). This lesion is often referred to as "Lambertosis," because it is hypothesized that the metaplastic epithelium derives from the canals of Lambert that connect nonrespiratory bronchioles directly to adjacent alveoli. Lambertosis can be seen in a number of pathologic conditions, including COPD

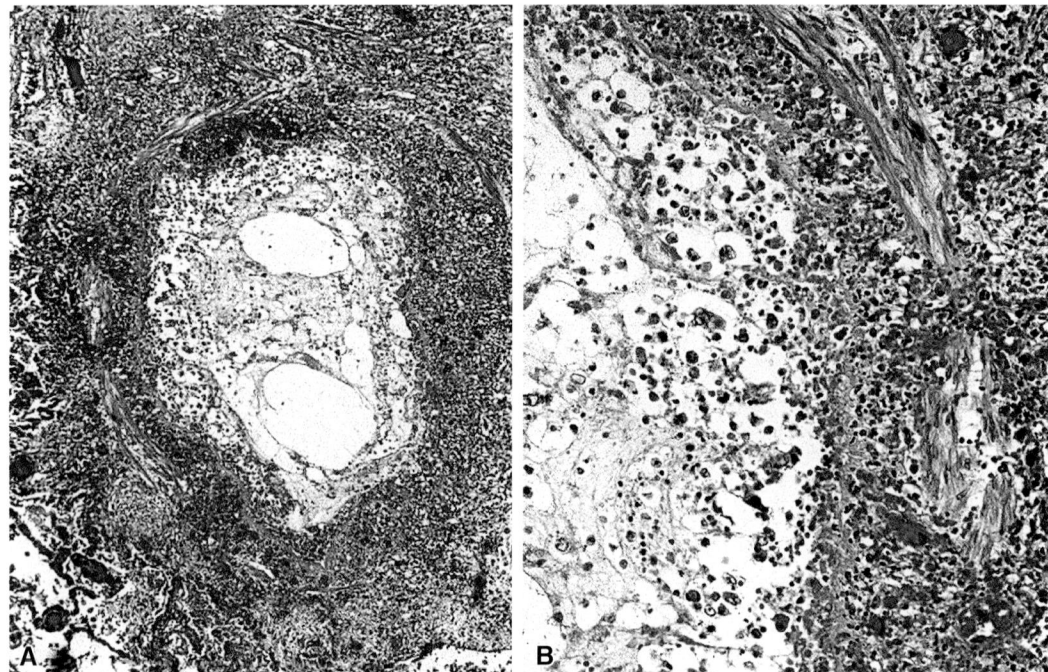

Figure 8-27. Herpetic necrotizing bronchiolitis. **A,** An acute necrotizing inflammatory process involves the entire bronchiolar wall, as well as surrounding alveolar septa. **B,** The lumen of the bronchiole contains exudate, red blood cells, and single epithelial cells.

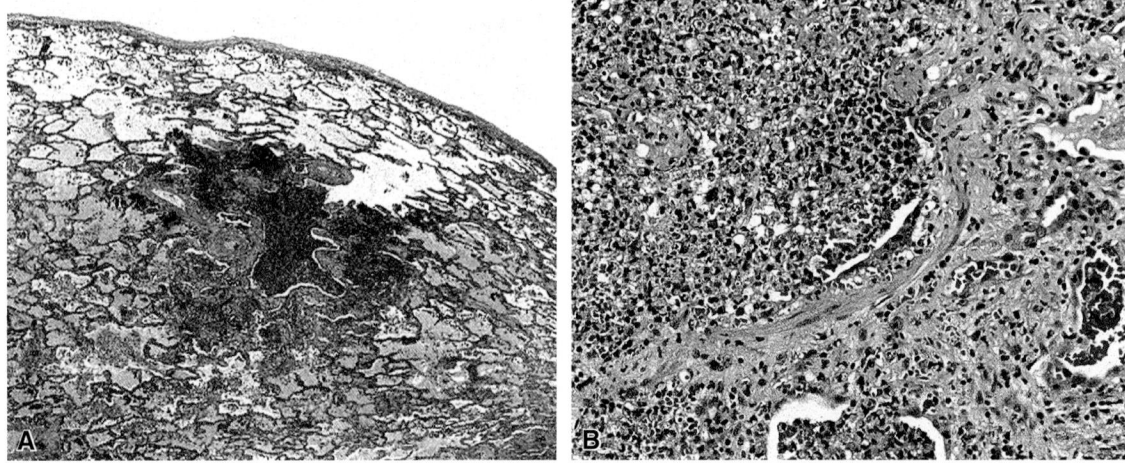

Figure 8-28. Adenovirus necrotizing acute bronchiolitis. This biopsy is from a renal transplant recipient undergoing immunosuppressive therapy. The lung tissue shows a bronchiolocentric acute inflammatory process characterized by prominent epithelial necrosis. **A,** The lumen of the bronchiole has been obliterated. **B,** At higher magnification, the presence of the muscular layer can be appreciated, whereas the epithelial layer is almost completely destroyed. Adenovirus was cultured from the biopsy specimen.

and constrictive bronchiolitis among others. In most cases the lesion is felt to be postinflammatory in origin and therefore could potentially be seen as a consequence of any number of inflammatory diseases involving the small airways. No specific cause is identified in some patients and the disease may be an idiopathic manifestation of an unidentified remote injury to the small airways. When this is the case, the disease may manifest clinically as an interstitial lung disease with restrictive physiology. The histopathology of bronchiolar metaplasia is one of variable extension of columnar, sometimes ciliated epithelium, beyond the alveolar ducts to involve alveolar walls. When the lesions are exuberant, they may appear as nodules 2 to 5 mm in diameter. These lesions must be distinguished from microscopic honeycombing, atypical adenomatous hyperplasia,[104–108] and the micronodular pneumocyte hyperplasia of tuberous sclerosis complex.[109–111]

When prominent bronchiolar metaplasia is identified, along with some other significant pathology (e.g., in association with a lobectomy for carcinoma), the exact significance of this process relative to the patient's clinical manifestations is unclear. In our

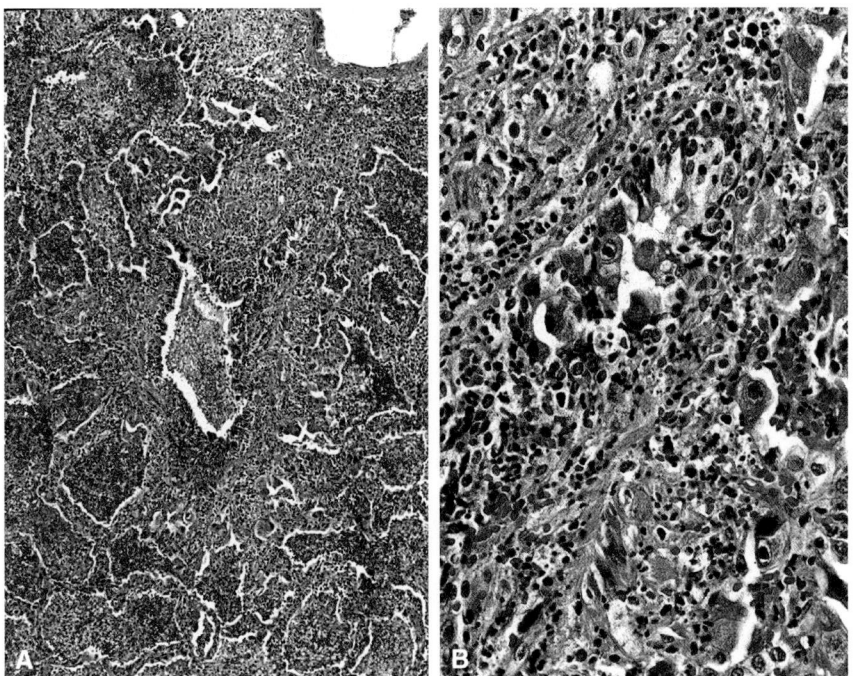

Figure 8-29. Cytomegalovirus bronchiolitis. **A,** The bronchiole shows an acute inflammatory necrotizing process. **B,** Viral inclusions are seen at higher magnification.

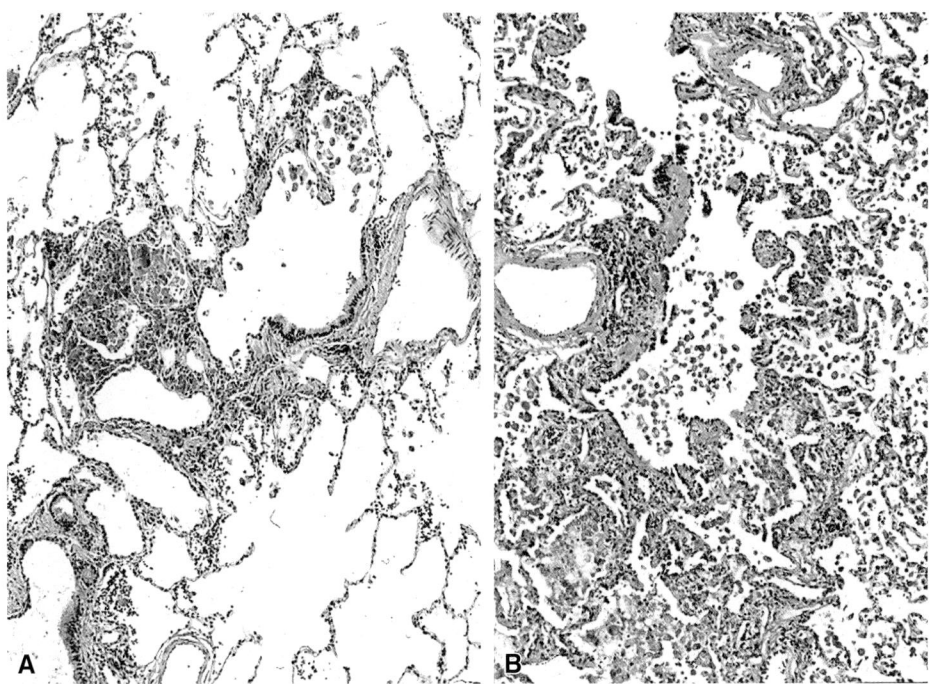

Figure 8-30. Respiratory bronchiolitis. Two different histopathologic patterns of distortion and inflammation in so-called smoker's bronchiolitis. **A,** The bronchiole is dilated and mildly distorted, and there is prominent filling of the alveolar spaces by finely granular and pigmented macrophages. **B,** The bronchiolar wall shows mild thickening with chronic inflammation, along with "smoker's macrophages" in the lumen.

experience, bronchiolar metaplasia in the setting of smoking-related lung disease may or may not have a clinical or radiologic correlation. Conversely, such changes in a nonsmoker are always significant. Diseases associated with prominent bronchiolar metaplasia are listed in Box 8-9.

Mucostasis

Mucostasis (also referred to as mucus stasis) is defined as visible amphophilic mucin within dilated terminal airways or in surrounding alveolar ducts and alveolar spaces[64,112] (Fig. 8-33). Mucostasis is a common finding in cigarette smokers and can occur in a number of other

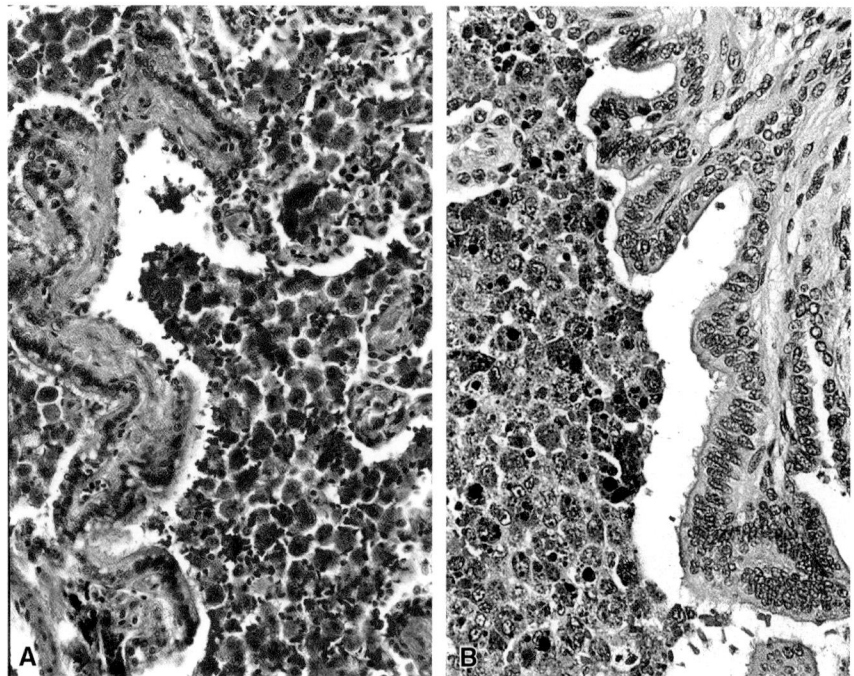

Figure 8-31. Respiratory bronchiolitis. **A,** Alveolar macrophages with finely granular, golden brown cytoplasmic pigment accumulate in the respiratory bronchiole, alveolar ducts, and peribronchiolar alveoli. **B,** On the *right*, by comparison, the heavily pigmented macrophages seen in hemorrhage syndromes. In pulmonary hemorrhage, the hemosiderin pigment granules are more abundant and more coarse.

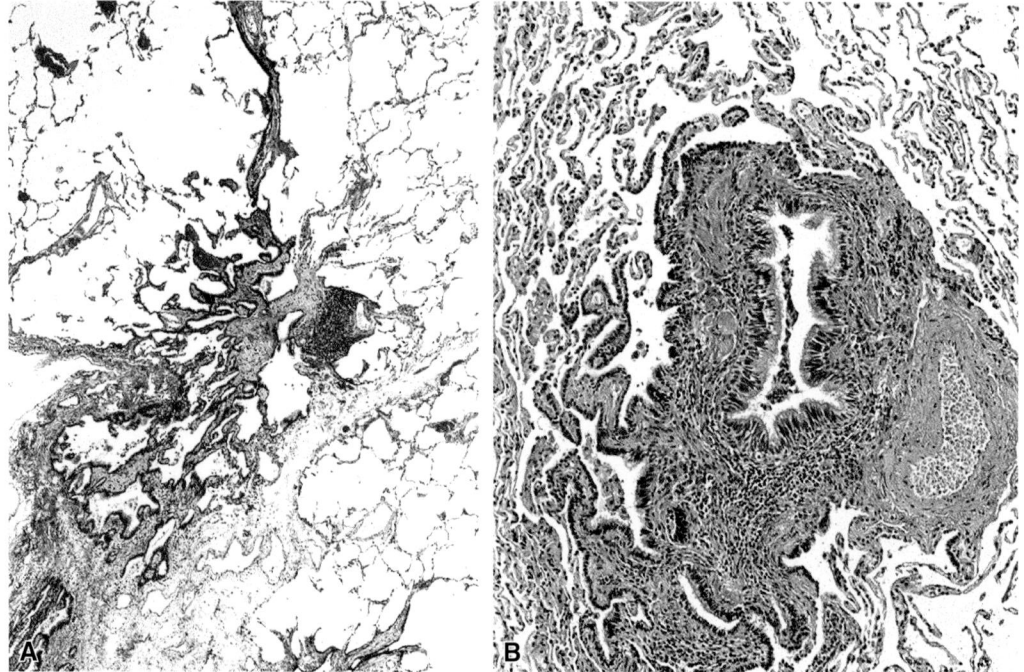

Figure 8-32. Bronchiolar metaplasia (so-called Lambertosis). **A,** Proliferation of cuboidal epithelial cells, extending from alveolar ducts into proximal lobular acini along the alveolar septa is a common finding in smokers and may be considered to represent a reactive or reparative process involving chronic injury to the terminal and respiratory bronchioles. **B,** At higher magnification, the bronchiolocentric nature is readily appreciated. This image is of a preparation from a patient who was a heavy smoker.

Box 8-9. Diseases Associated with Bronchiolar Metaplasia (Lambertosis)

Healed bronchiolitis (from any cause)
Chronic hypersensitivity pneumonitis (extrinsic allergic alveolitis)
Distal to bronchiectasis (from any cause)
As a component of constrictive bronchiolitis

settings, as detailed in Box 8-10. When mucus extrusion into alveolar spaces is extensive, a careful search for bronchioloalveolar carcinoma (BAC) is in order, especially in the absence of another specific pathologic entity in the biopsy. Correlation with imaging studies may be helpful in excluding BAC.

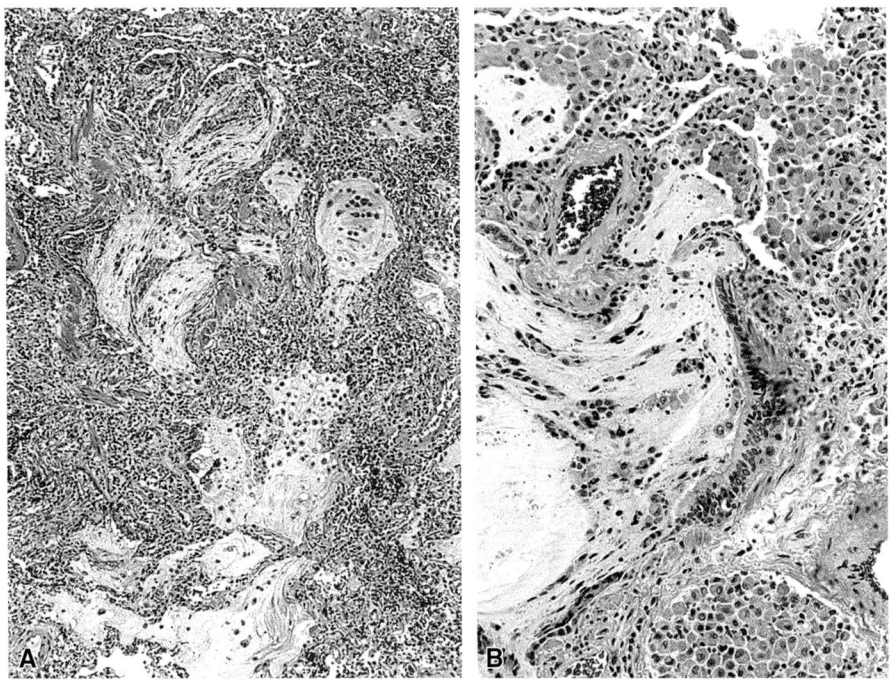

Figure 8-33. Mucostasis in respiratory bronchiolitis. **A,** The respiratory bronchioles and alveolar ducts are filled with mucinous material. **B,** Extension of free mucus into peribronchiolar alveoli is seen and many smoker's-type macrophages with dusty brown pigment are visible (*center right*).

Box 8-10. Diseases Associated with Mucostasis

Chronic obstructive pulmonary disease
Respiratory bronchiolitis
Asthma
Mucoid impaction/allergic pulmonary fungal disease
Constrictive bronchiolitis
Upstream bronchiectasis
Upstream bronchial obstruction, of any cause
As part of a localized inflammatory reaction (e.g., middle lobe syndrome)
Bronchioloalveolar carcinoma

Bronchiolar Smooth Muscle Hyperplasia

Generalized thickening of the smooth muscle around conducting airways and alveolar ducts can be seen in a number of inflammatory lung diseases (Fig. 8-34A). Sometimes smooth muscle nodules formed of haphazard fascicles can be seen in smokers and are of unknown clinical relevance (see Fig. 8-34B). Smooth muscle hyperplasia associated with subpleural fibrosis is common in usual interstitial pneumonia (UIP) as well. The diseases associated with smooth muscle hyperplasia are listed in Box 8-11.

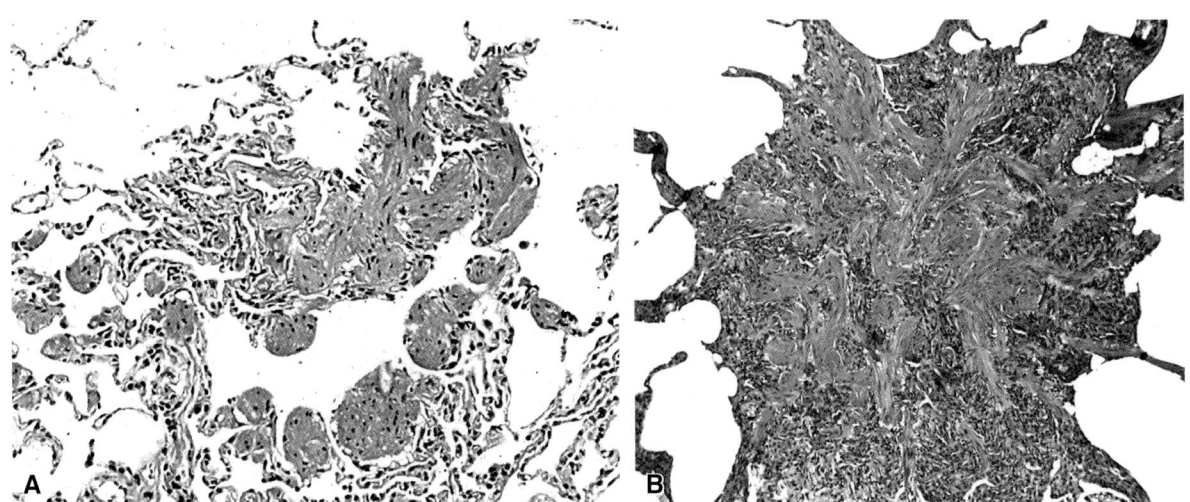

Figure 8-34. Smooth muscle hyperplasia. **A,** This terminal bronchiole is from a patient with previous history of radiation therapy and exhibits an irregular lumen with an excessively thick smooth muscle layer. **B,** A typical "smoker's nodule," characterized by radial fascicles of smooth muscle present in a centrilobular distribution.

Box 8-11. Diseases Associated with Airway Smooth Muscle Hyperplasia

Asthma
As a component of constrictive bronchiolitis
Associated with fibrosing lung diseases
As part of a localized inflammatory process
As a focal incidental finding
As a component of generalized bronchiolar scarring and peribronchiolar metaplasia
Aguayo-Miller disease (neuroendocrine cell hyperplasia with occlusive bronchiolar fibrosis)

Fibrous Proliferations in and around Bronchioles

Increase of fibrous tissue in the lumen or wall of bronchioles and in immediately surrounding tissue may be seen in several clinicopathologic conditions, particularly those associated with acute inhalational injury (Figs. 8-35 and 8-36). The fibrous proliferation seen at the microscopic level may be of recent development, characterized by a loose fibroblastic intraluminar proliferation having a fibromyxoid stroma. Alternatively, fibrosis may be more advanced, with fewer fibrocytes, more abundant extracellular collagen, and usually more prominent distortion of bronchiolar morphology. More advanced fibrotic processes

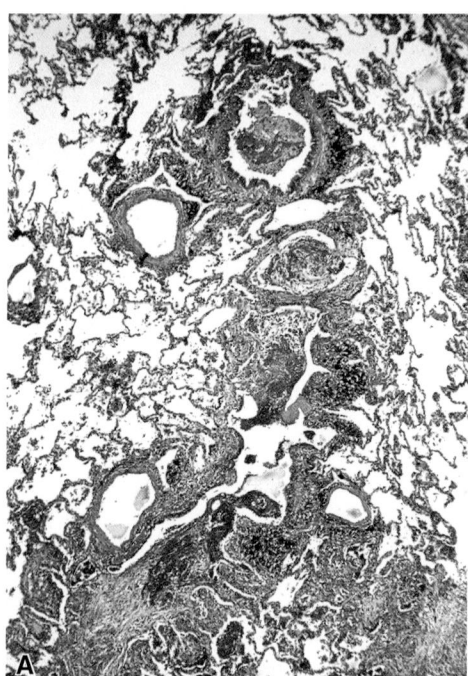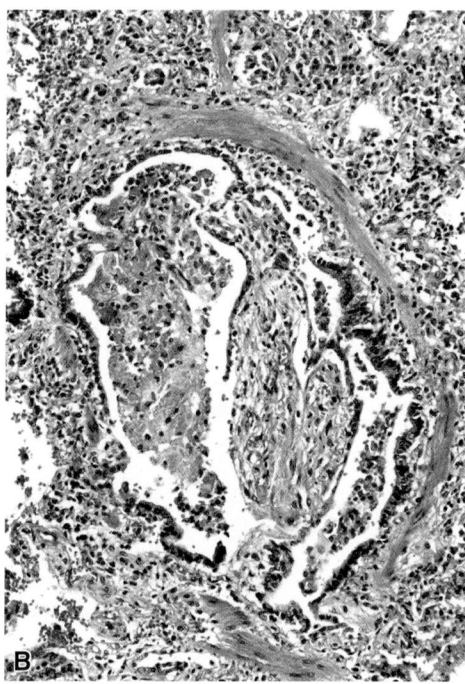

Figure 8-35. Organizing pneumonia with Masson polyps and fibrin (bronchiolitis obliterans). These images are from a silo filler's lung biopsy. The patient developed an acute illness and died 3 days after biopsy, despite steroid therapy. **A,** The bronchioles are filled with polypoid formations. **B,** Some of these formations are partially fibroblastic and partially fibrinous, whereas others are purely fibroblastic and show an investing epithelial layer.

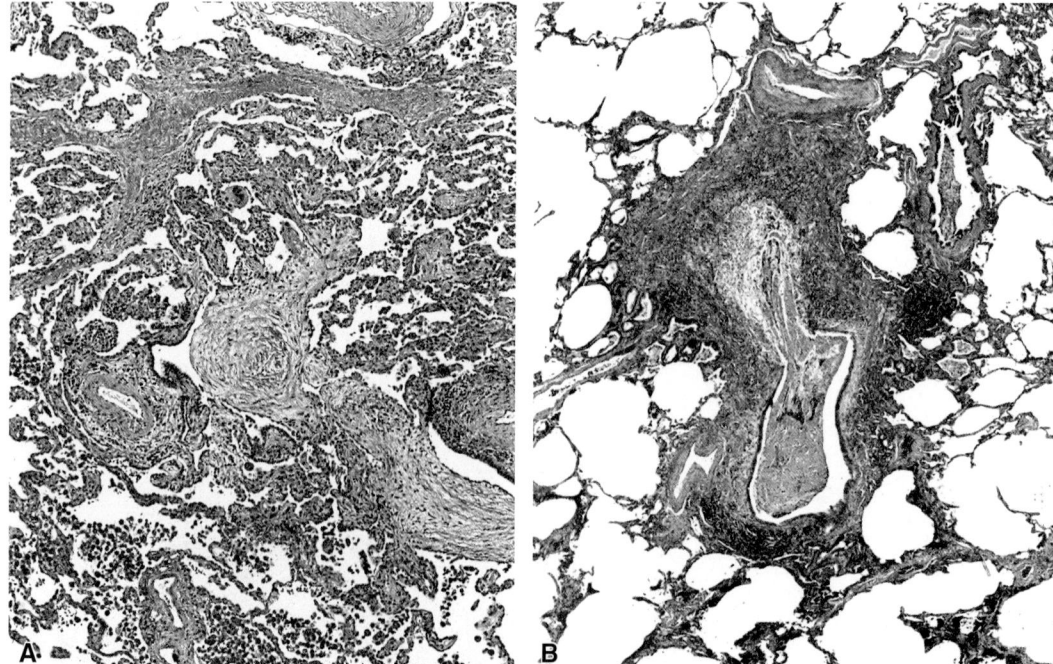

Figure 8-36. Organizing pneumonia with Masson polyps and fibrin (bronchiolitis obliterans). **A,** A polyp extending along the terminal airway in a patient with Wegener granulomatosis. **B,** A bronchiole in a patient with rheumatoid arthritis shows luminal polypoid myofibroblastic proliferation, accompanied by a peribronchiolar lymphoid infiltrate.

may have a predominant concentric growth pattern in and around the airway, resulting in narrowing or obliteration of the lumen. In other cases, fibrosis may have a predominant peribronchiolar-radiating pattern, involving the adventitia of the airway with variable extension into the adjacent lung parenchyma.

Affected bronchioles may show lesions of different ages, and the injury-related changes may not be uniform throughout the biopsy (or presumably the lung as a whole). Moreover, significant reduction of bronchiolar lumen may be seen in conjunction with aspects of bronchioloectasia and mucostasis, which can be consequences of the same pathogenetic event, with dilatation and mucostasis the possible effect of air trapping and defects in mucus clearance. Indeed, the bronchioles, seen in longitudinal sections, may exhibit an irregular distribution of constricted and dilated tracts, with a somehow "varicose" aspect. The fibrotic process may also be accompanied by variable amounts of bronchiolar and peribronchiolar inflammation, which may extend to involve the alveolar walls of the adjacent lung parenchyma. Increased fibrous tissue beneath the epithelium of the small airways, or around the airways, may be seen with or without smooth muscle hyperplasia and proliferation of respiratory epithelium, leading to peribronchiolar metaplasia of adjacent alveolar walls (Lambertosis).

Among fibrous proliferations mainly involving the luminal portion of the airway are those processes characterized by *loose fibroblastic polyps* (Fig. 8-36A)—so-called Masson bodies.[113] Rarely, bronchiolar intraluminal fibroblastic polyps may be the predominant finding in lung biopsies, such as in very acute fume inhalation. More frequently the polyps are located in the lumen of the bronchioles and, more conspicuously, in the surrounding distal air spaces representing a generalized parenchymal repair reaction. In these cases they are almost always associated with significant inflammatory changes in the airway wall and surrounding lung parenchyma, a feature now referred to as *organizing pneumonia pattern* (OP), or simply "air space organization."[114] When this type of fibroblastic proliferation has no apparent etiology, the condition is referred to clinically as *cryptogenic organizing pneumonia* (COP),[115] formerly known as "idiopathic bronchiolitis obliterans organizing pneumonia" (BOOP).[116] Intraluminal fibroblastic polyps can be seen in many lung disorders, as detailed in Box 8-12.

Bronchiolitis Obliterans Syndrome

Fibrous proliferation at the bronchiolar level may result in luminal constriction and ultimately complete obliteration of the the small airways. This process is best illustrated by chronic transplant rejection (see Chapter 12). In this setting the fibrotic process is referred to as *obliterative bronchiolitis* (OB)[117,118] and corresponds to the clinical entity referred to as "bronchiolitis obliterans syndrome" (BOS).[119–121] OB/BOS is not simply graft rejection but a complex multifactorial process involving immune-mediated and alloimmune dependent tissue injuries and aberrant reparative responses or remodeling.[122] Histopathologically, the earliest stage is characterized by eccentric subepithelial fibrosis with scattered admixed chronic inflammatory cells. Concentric fibrosis then progresses over time until the lumen becomes markedly narrowed, or entirely obliterated. In other instances, the lumen may be initially occluded by loose fibrous tissue, presumably as a manifestation of active repair following an injury to the airway epithelium and basal lamina. Some investigators have distinguished these latter lesions as more typical of bronchiolitis obliterans—asserting that the outer dimensions of the bronchiole remain stable (i.e., not necessarily constricted).

In the non-lung transplant patient, the term *constrictive bronchiolitis* is less prone to misunderstanding than the term *obliterative bronchiolitis*, and refers to a small-airway disease characterized by

Box 8-12. Conditions Associated with the Organizing Pneumonia Pattern

Organizing phase of diffuse alveolar damage
Result of infection
Distal to bronchial obstruction
With aspiration pneumonia
After certain drug reactions and toxic exposures
In association with systemic connective tissue disease
In hypersensitivity pneumonitis
In eosinophilic pneumonia
As a consequence of chronic bronchiolitis or diffuse panbronchiolitis
As an idiopathic process, usually associated with mild interstitial pneumonia
As a nonspecific reaction in other inflammatory lung diseases as in, for example, Wegener granulomatosis, abscesses, and necrosis and with tumors and infarcts
In lung transplants with graft-versus-host disease

Modified from Travis WD, et al. Non-neoplastic disorders of the lower respiratory tract. In: Kind DW, ed. *Atlases of Nontumor Pathology*. Washington: Armed Forces Institute of Pathology; 2002.

variable narrowing or obliteration of the small airways. Constrictive bronchiolitis not associated with lung transplantation may be a consequence of injuries resulting from infection, toxic fume inhalation, drug reaction, chemical toxins, hematopoietic stem cell transplantation, or connective tissue disease (Table 8-2). In some cases no etiology is identified.[60,64,68,123–133] It is worth noting that the pathologic findings in constrictive bronchiolitis may be quite subtle (see the introductory section "Pattern-Based Approach to Diagnosis," Pattern 6, Minimal changes). When no explanation for a patient's significant hypoxia is identifiable in lung biopsy sections, trichrome and elastic tissue stains may be helpful in highlighting the changes in small airways. Nevertheless, it is important to remember that some degree of subepithelial fibrosis in the small airways is almost a universal finding

Table 8-2. Known Causes of Constrictive Bronchiolitis

Category	Specific Agents
Infections	*Mycoplasma*, viruses (cytomegalovirus, adenovirus, influenzavirus, parainfluenza virus, varicella virus)
Fumes	Nitrogen dioxide, sulfur dioxide, ammonia, phosgene, chlorine, fly ash, styrene, fire fumes, possibly volatile chemicals used as flavoring ingredients in food industry
Toxins	Ingested toxins from juice of the plant *Sauropus androgynus*[132]
Massive dust exposure[127]	World Trade Center Disaster "Ground Zero" dust exposure
Drugs	Penicillamine, cocaine, gold, chemotherapeutic agents (lomustine, 5-fluorouracil)[177]
Paraneoplastic syndromes[126,178]	Paraneoplastic pemphigus in cases of malignant lymphomas and Castleman disease
Stevens-Johnson syndrome[130]	
Systemic connective tissue disease	Rheumatoid arthritis, mixed connective tissue disease
Idiopathic	

Data from Colby TV, Leslie KO. Small airway lesions. In: Cagle PT, ed. *Diagnostic Pulmonary Pathology*. New York: Marcel Dekker; 2000:231–249; King TE Jr. Bronchiolitis. In: Schwartz MI, King TE, eds. *Interstitial Lung Disease*. London: BC Decker; 1998:654–684; and Ryu JH. Classification and approach to bronchiolar diseases. *Curr Opin Pulm Med*. 2006;12(2):145–151.

in heavy cigarette smokers. Without clinical manifestations of lung disease, such findings are most often irrelevant. Examples of the spectrum of constrictive airway injury are presented in Figures 8-37 to 8-39.

Given the limited repertoire of airway repair after injury, it is probably best to think of constrictive and obliterative forms of bronchiolitis simply as a representation of a later evolution of the repair process, whereas organizing intraluminal polyps are a more subacute manifestation of injury.[121] Why some injuries resolve with little permanent structural abnormalities, whereas others result in persistent damage, is unknown.

Fibrosis centered on the small airway, involving the wall of the bronchiole and surrounding lung parenchyma with or without any degree of inflammation, may be descriptively termed *bronchiolocentric fibrosis* (Fig. 8-40). This may be seen as a late manifestation of several conditions, most notoriously hypersensitivity pneumonitis. In some cases the process appears to be idiopathic.[134-138]

Terminal Airway Fibrosis with Dust Deposition (Pneumoconiosis-Associated Small Airway Disease)

Variable dust deposition around airways, accompanied by fibrosis, can be seen commonly in smokers. Under polarized light, small refractile silicate particles (typically aluminum and magnesium silicates) may be identified within areas of pigment deposition, either as a consequence of lifelong dust exposure in the older patient or as a common finding in cigarette smokers. In addition to occupational exposure to dust, a slight degree of airway remodeling with increased amounts of muscle and fibrous tissue can be seen in people exposed to high concentrations of ambient particulate matter, as can occur in some highly polluted urban areas.[139]

When peribronchiolar dust deposition around airways is prominent and associated with numerous and large (typically larger than 1 cm in diameter) "dust nodules," a pneumoconiosis enters into the differential diagnosis. Fibrosis often accompanies such nodules.

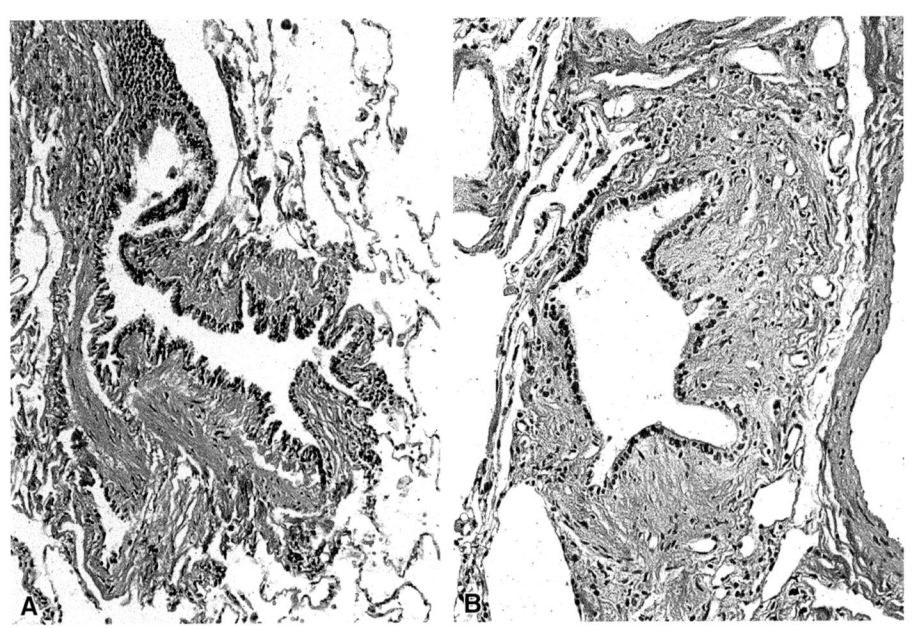

Figure 8-37. Idiopathic constrictive bronchiolitis. **A,** The wall of this bronchiole is thick and fibrotic without much associated inflammatory changes. **B,** The luminal profiles may be highly variable; here they appear slightly dilated and tortuous, despite abundant mural fibrosis.

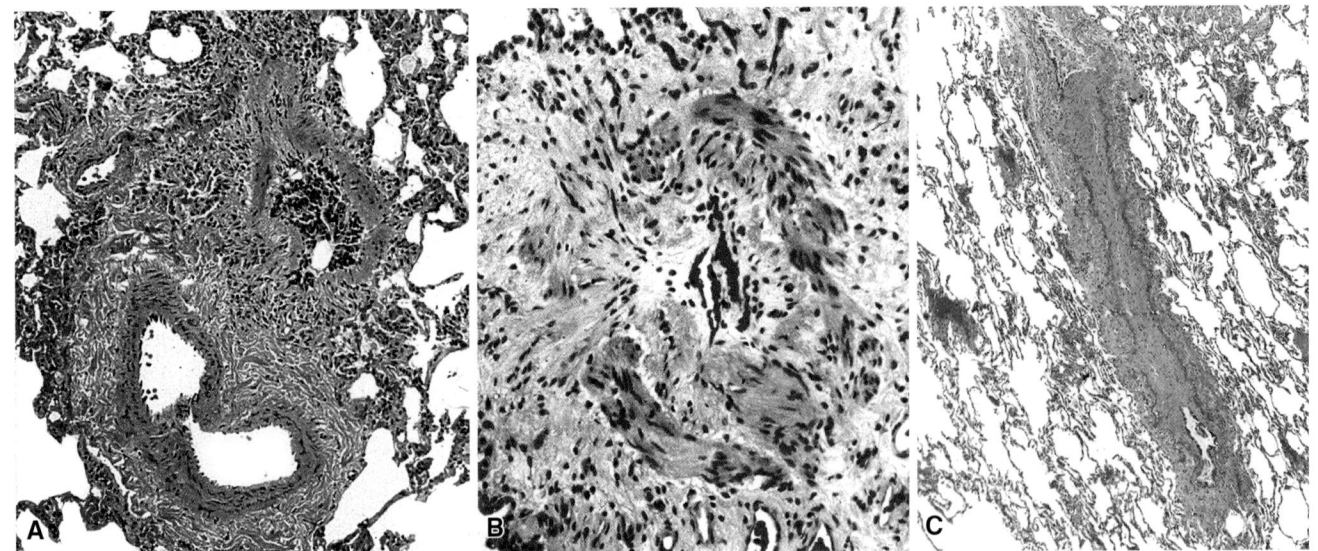

Figure 8-38. Constrictive bronchiolitis. **A,** Lung tissue from a child after a viral infection: The lumen of the bronchiole is small, the walls are fibrotic, and the epithelial cells are sloughed into the lumen. **B,** Lung preparation from a patient who developed obstructive lung disease after an acute pneumonia due to *Mycoplasma* infection. The bronchiole is almost completely obliterated by fibrous tissue. The epithelial cells are lost, although the muscularis propria is still preserved. **C,** Lung preparation from a bone marrow transplant recipient. Note the entire segmental obliteration by fibrous tissue.

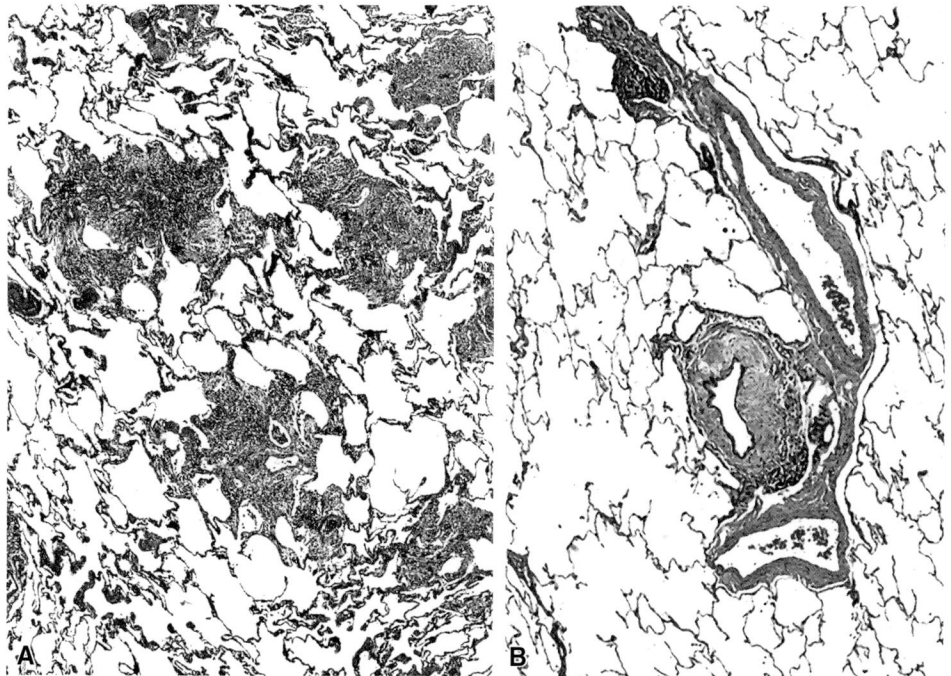

Figure 8-39. Constrictive bronchiolitis associated with inflammatory bowel disease. **A,** Low-magnification image showing bronchiolocentric lesions, characterized by fibrosis and a chronic inflammatory infiltrate with almost complete destruction of the terminal bronchioles. **B,** A higher-magnification image from another patient shows changes that are quite subtle. There is no inflammation in the bronchiolar wall, but the diameter of the airway is smaller than that of the artery, and the subepithelial connective tissue is dense and fibrotic.

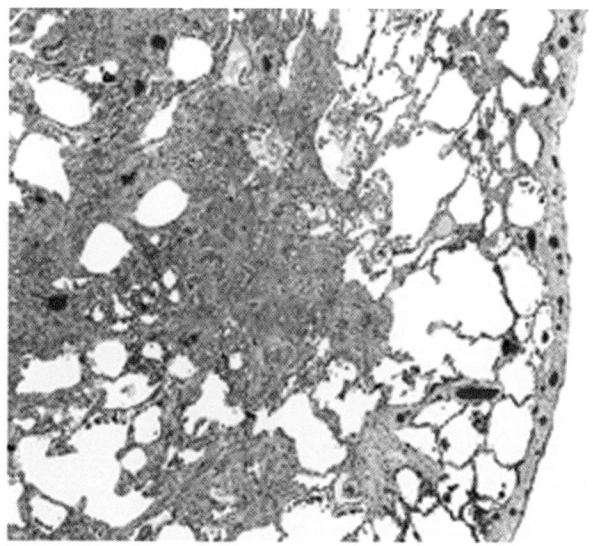

Figure 8-40. Airwway-centered fibrosis. An example of distinctive airway-centered fibrosis in a patient with chronic hypersensitivity pneumonitis.

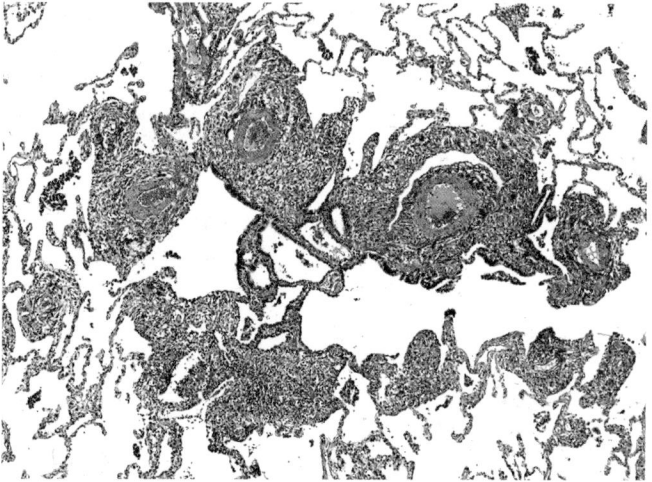

Figure 8-41. Silicatosis. A biopsy from a pottery factory worker showing the wall of a thickened and distorted respiratory bronchiole. A majority of cells in the wall are histiocytes. Under polarized light, many needle-shaped, birefringent silicate crystals are evident.

Small airway disease associated with exposure to a specific mineral dust, such as that from asbestos, aluminum oxide, iron oxide, silicates, or coal, is referred to as *pneumoconiosis-associated small-airway disease.*[118] Pneumoconiosis-associated small-airway injury frequently demonstrates only minimally inflammatory changes (Figs. 8-41 and 8-42). The alveolar duct walls are thickened by fibrous tissue, and dust deposition occurs along the small airways. Clinical and radiographic correlation is essential before a pathologic diagnosis of clinically significant pneumoconiosis is made (see Chapter 9). When hemosiderin is present along with alveolar duct fibrosis and other pigment deposition, a careful search for asbestos bodies is in order. In this setting, iron stains (Prussian blue) may be helpful

for identifying foci of iron deposition, thereby attracting the pathologist's attention to areas in which asbestos bodies (ferruginous bodies) are more likely to be identified (see Fig. 8-42B). Not all ferruginous bodies are asbestos-related, so it is important to establish the presence of a delicate translucent core fiber—the characteristic feature of asbestos bodies.

Dilated and Irregular Bronchiolar Shapes

Variation in the shape and other distortions of the terminal airways can be seen as a secondary phenomenon in many inflammatory airway diseases and is a common finding in smokers. A useful method for assessing such changes is to search for terminal airways that are

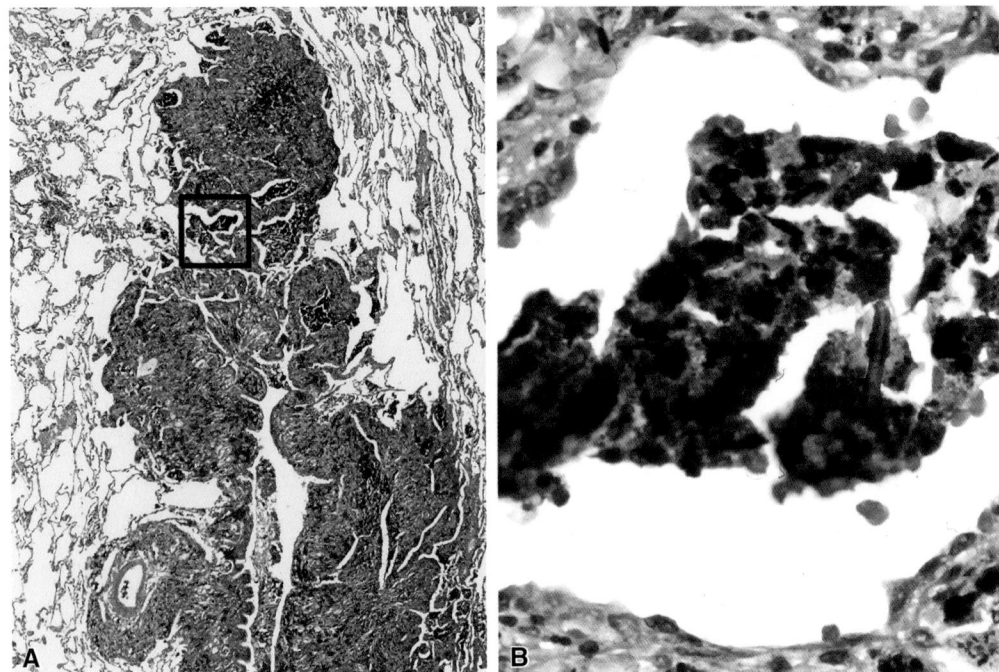

Figure 8-42. Mixed dust pneumoconiosis. **A,** At low magnification, the bronchiole and accompanying artery are surrounded by densely pigmented fibrous tissue, which distorts the normal architecture of the bundle. **B,** At higher magnification, the histiocytic cells within the fibrous tissue contain abundant black pigment, and the lumen of the bronchiole contains densely pigmented cells, most of which contain hemosiderin and, occasionally, ferruginous bodies.

visible in cross section, so that the diameter of the airway and of the adjacent artery can be compared. In this setting, the diameters should be equal. When considerable bronchiolar distortion is present, thin-walled dilated airways may greatly exceed the pulmonary artery in diameter or, alternatively, may be significantly smaller. Such variable saccular, or varicose, dilatation and constriction is common in chronic small-airway diseases that result in fibrosis.

Bronchiolocentric Nodules

A number of diseases may produce nodular lesions centered on the small airways (bronchiolocentric nodules).[60] The diseases that can produce bronchocentric nodules include primarily inflammatory lesions (e.g., panbronchiolitis—discussed further on), inflammatory and fibrotic lesions (e.g., pulmonary Langerhans cell histiocytosis) (Figs. 8-43 and 8-44), and miscellaneous disease processes (e.g., multiple

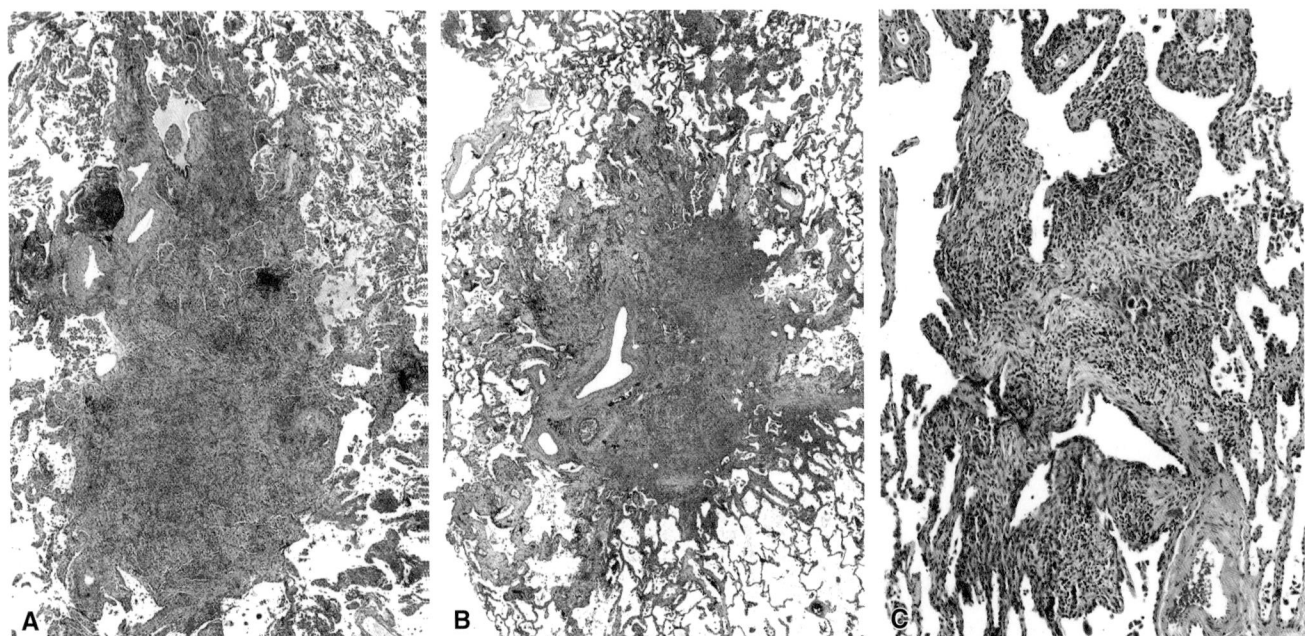

Figure 8-43. Pulmonary Langerhans cell histiocytosis (PLCH). Three different phases of the disease, with nodular cellular lesions (**A** and **B**) undergoing transition to characteristic stellate morphology (**C**). The diagnosis of PLCH can frequently be made at scanning magnification, at which one can easily appreciate the typical discrete, roughly symmetrical nodules, which have a stellate shape, a dense fibrotic core, and, frequently, a more cellular peripheral zone. The nodules involve the bronchiole and contain variable numbers of eosinophils and Langerhans cells.

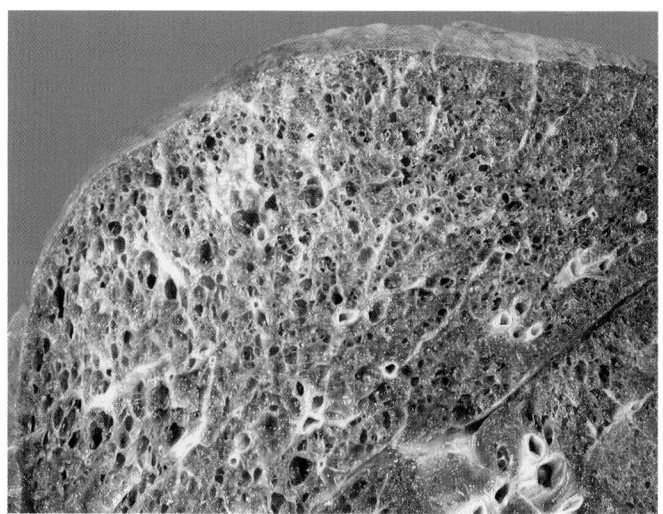

Figure 8-44. Pulmonary Langerhans cell histiocytosis (PLCH). Explanted lung from a patient with advanced airway-centered fibrosis from PLCH.

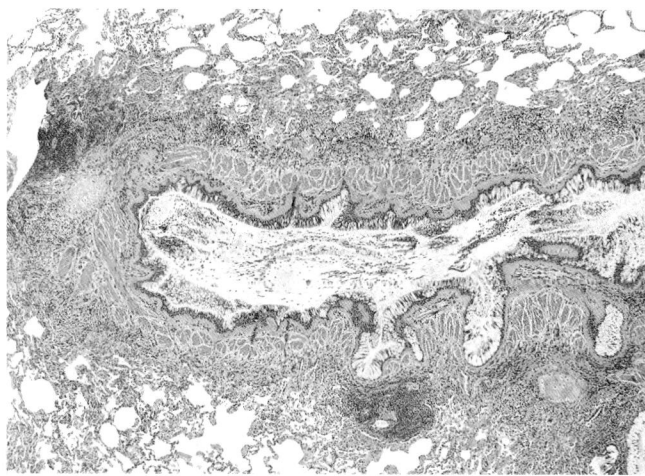

Figure 8-45. Asthmatic changes in a bronchus. The lumen is filled with mucus, the epithelium shows prominent goblet cell hyperplasia, the basal membrane is thick, smooth muscle is prominent, and there is a chronic inflammatory infiltrate extending through the bronchial wall.

carcinoid tumorlets, with or without constrictive bronchiolitis, or lymphangitic tumor, including malignant lymphoma).

Clinicopathologic Entities with Prominent Airway Manifestations

Defined clinical diseases with distinctive inflammatory reaction patterns in the airways are few. In this section, we examine two frequent diseases, asthma and COPD, and two additional rare but well-defined diseases, panbronchiolitis and neuroendocrine cell hyperplasia with occlusive bronchiolar fibrosis (Aguayo-Miller disease). Emphysema is also covered in this section, because it features a structural remodeling of the lung parenchyma that involves the small airways.

Asthma-Associated Airway Diseases

Asthma is a chronic inflammatory disease of the airways accompanied by bronchial hyperresponsiveness (the primary clinical manifestation). Affected individuals develop a number of well-characterized inflammatory changes in the large airways, including epithelial fragility, intraepithelial goblet cell hyperplasia, mural infiltration by eosinophils, smooth muscle hyperplasia, and enlargement of subepithelial mucous glands[140] (Fig. 8-45 and Box 8-13). In a subset of asthmatic individuals also will develop chronic disease of the small airways.[60,140–145] The large-airway pathology is seen mainly in lobectomy specimens removed for other causes and autopsy lungs from patients who die in status asthmaticus. The small-airway changes are more often observed in surgical biopsy specimens because these are taken from peripheral lung. These changes include chronic bronchiolitis, eosinophilic bronchiolitis, varicosity of bronchiolar lumens, bronchiolar metaplasia, constrictive bronchiolitis, and even features of bronchocentric granulomatosis (Figs. 8-46 to 8-49). These changes may also be appreciated in bronchoscopic biopsies. In addition to these bronchial and bronchiolar alterations, four distinctive, albeit partially overlapping, asthma-associated lung diseases are recognized: eosinophilic pneumonia, allergic bronchial pulmonary fungal disease, mucoid impaction of bronchi, and bronchocentric granulomatosis. Eosinophilic pneumonia is discussed in Chapter 5 (Acute Lung Injury) and Chapter 7 (Chronic Diffuse Lung Diseases); the other three asthma-associated diseases are described next.

Box 8-13. Pathologic Findings in Asthma

Mucous plugs
Mucosal eosinophils
Mucosal basement membrane thickening due to submembranous collagen deposition
Distinctive inclusions in airway mucus
    Charcot-Leyden crystals
    Creola bodies
    Curschmann spirals
Epithelial shedding (desquamation)
Goblet cell metaplasia/hyperplasia
Squamous metaplasia
Airway wall edema
Bronchial mucous gland hyperplasia
Airway wall smooth muscle hyperplasia

Data from Dunnill MS, Massarella GR, Anderson JA. A comparison of the quantitative anatomy of the bronchi in normal subjects, in status asthmaticus, in chronic bronchitis, and in emphysema. *Thorax.* 1969;24(2):176–179; Aikawa T, Shimura S, Sasaki H, et al. Marked goblet cell hyperplasia with mucus accumulation in the airways of patients who died of severe acute asthma attack. *Chest.* 1992;101(4):916–921; and Messer JW, Peters GA, Bennett WA. Causes of death and pathologic findings in 304 cases of bronchial asthma. *Dis Chest.* 1960;38:616–624.

Allergic Bronchopulmonary Fungal Disease

In certain predisposed individuals, *Aspergillus* and other fungi may colonize the mucus of the respiratory tract, resulting in a form of chronic inflammatory disease termed *allergic bronchopulmonary fungal disease* (ABFD).[146–148] Other fungi implicated in the pathogenesis of this disorder include *Pseudallescheria boydii*, *Bipolaris* species, *Torulopsis glabrata*, *Curvularia*, and *Lunata*. The hallmark of ABFD is the presence of so-called allergic mucin.[149] Allergic mucin is characterized by the presence of eosinophils and eosinophil cytoplasmic granular debris (Fig. 8-50). One or more additional manifestations are typical, such as mucoid impaction, bronchocentric granulomatosis, and eosinophilic pneumonia. Calcium oxalate crystals may be present in the granular debris of allergic mucin, similar to that seen with sinus hypersensitivity to *Aspergillus* and other fungi in asthmatic patients. When allergic mucin is present, silver stains for fungal organisms often are helpful in confirming the diagnostic impression of ABFD; however, the fungi often are focal and fragmented and can be easily overlooked. Because ABFD is considered an allergic manifestation, rather than a true infection, a course of oral corticosteroids is often the treatment of choice.

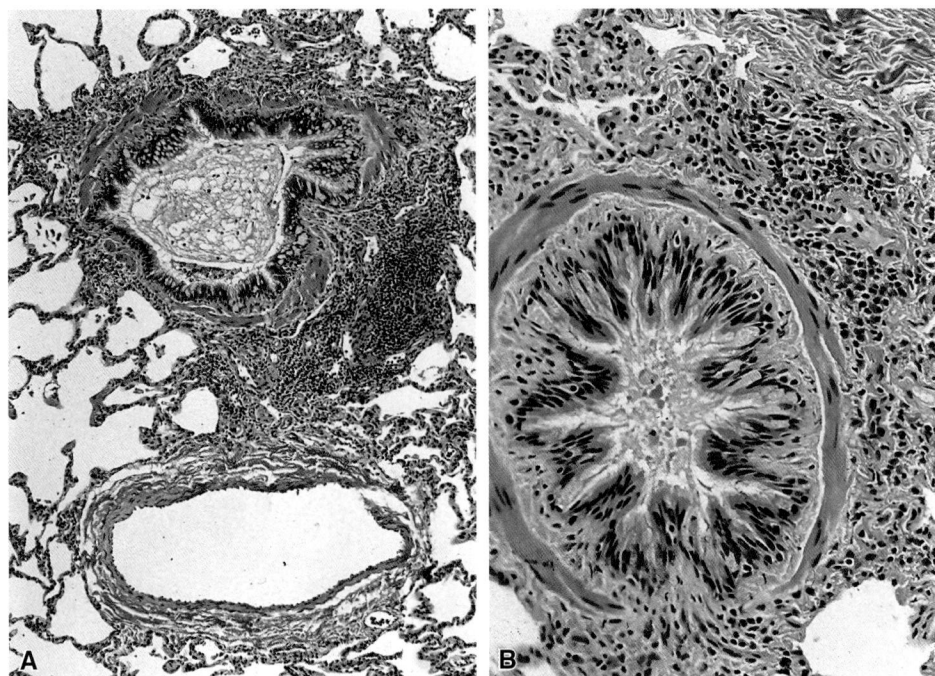

Figure 8-46. Constrictive bronchiolitis in asthma. A lung biopsy specimen showing some of the usual features of asthma, as well as some scarring of the small airways. The patient suffered from severe obstructive disease with a concurrent restrictive component. **A,** The bronchiole on the *left* is somewhat dilated and demonstrates mucostasis. **B,** The bronchiole on the *right* is smaller, with subepithelial and adventitial fibrosis and inflammation with a prominent eosinophilic component.

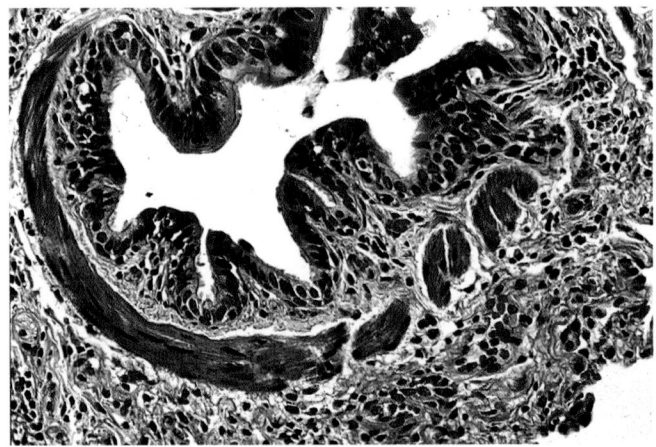

Figure 8-47. Constrictive bronchiolitis in asthma. This bronchiole shows a very corrugated mucosa, with collagen fibers in the subepithelial connective tissue and also between the muscle fibers (trichrome stain).

Figure 8-48. Bronchiolitis in asthma. This bronchiole shows prominent goblet cell metaplasia and basement membrane thickening: the mucus in the lumen shows eosinophils and there is also an increased number of eosinophils in the epithelium and in the subepithelial connective tissue.

Mucoid Impaction of Bronchi

A distinctive clinicopathologic syndrome is characterized by the presence of extensive mucous plugging of the airways accompanied by airway dilatation.[150–153] In this entity, termed *mucoid impaction of bronchi* (MIB), the mucus has the appearance of allergic mucin. MIB is considered to be one of the major manifestations of ABFD. Patients may be asymptomatic or may have obstructive pneumonia distal to the impaction. Radiologically, band-like or branching densities involving the upper lobes are characteristic findings ("gloved finger sign").[150] On occasion a solitary nodule may be seen. Branching strands of inspissated mucus may be coughed up by the patient (so-called plastic

bronchitis) (Fig. 8-51), and bronchoscopy may identify clues to the disease with the presence of impacted airways containing mucus.

Microscopically, the affected bronchi are dilated and contain brownish to green mucus of tenacious consistency. The mucus has a laminated appearance (Fig. 8-52) with eosinophilic debris and Charcot-Leyden crystals (hexagonal brightly eosinophilic crystals); this appearance defines allergic mucin. Asthma-type changes may be present in bronchoscopic biopsies from more central airways. Fungal stains may demonstrate hyphae, so use of such stains is recommended whenever

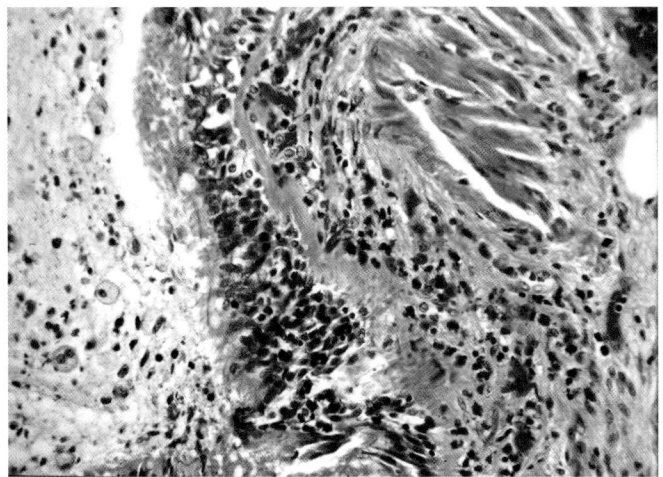

Figure 8-49. Small airway changes in a case of fatal asthma. In a small bronchiole, a very prominent goblet cell metaplasia with mucostasis is evident, and the basement membrane is thick and intensely eosinophilic. The smooth muscle layer is prominent.

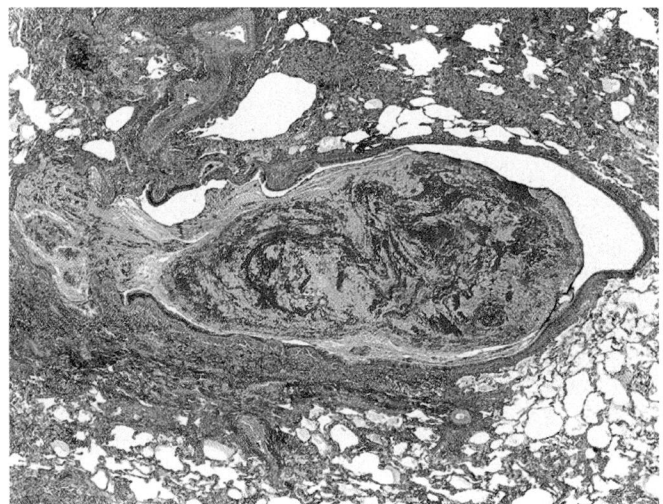

Figure 8-50. Allergic bronchopulmonary fungal disease. Allergic mucin (mucus, eosinophils, and eosinophilic necrosis) is filling a distended bronchiole.

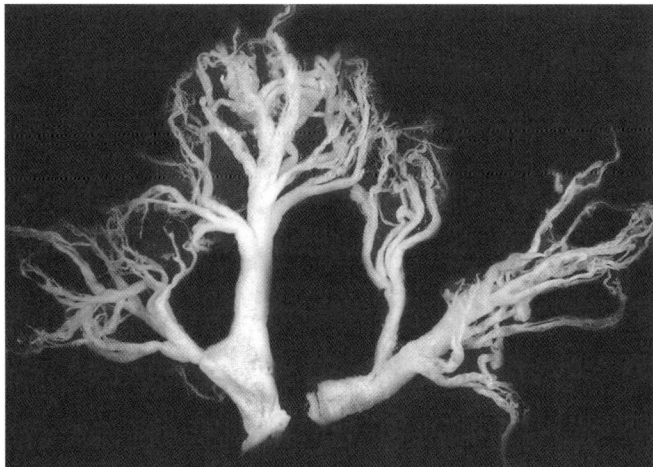

Figure 8-51. Plastic bronchitis. Solid mucous casts of the airways are expectorated or extracted.

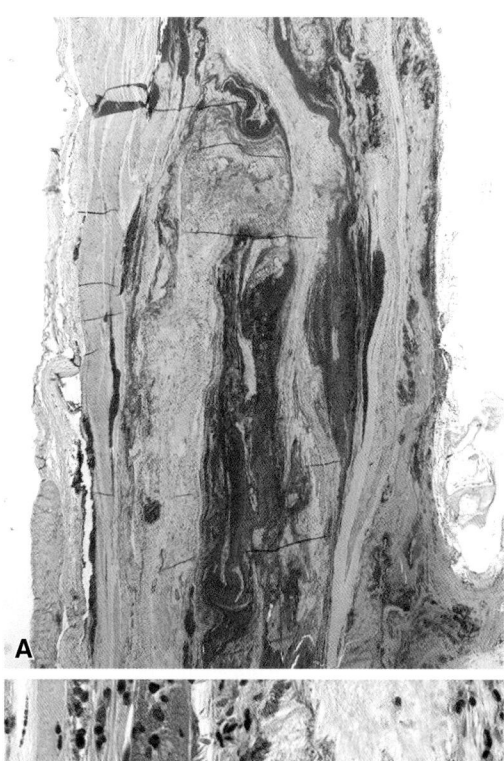

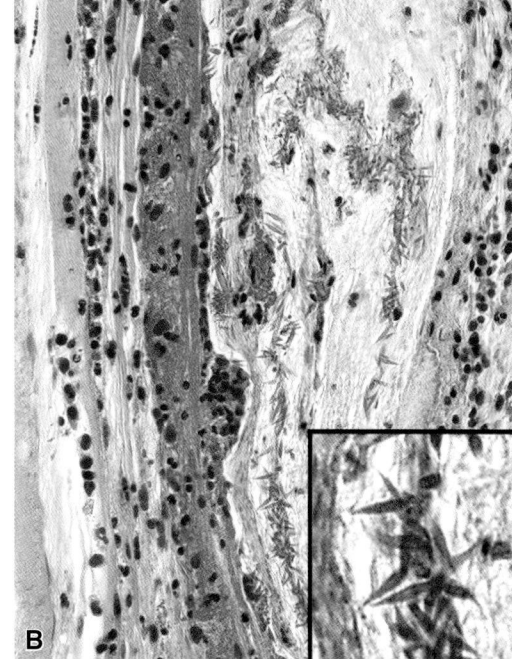

Figure 8-52. Mucoid impaction of bronchi. **A,** The characteristic laminated mucin. **B,** At higher magnification, eosinophils and Charcot-Leyden crystals (*inset*) can be seen.

allergic mucin is found. Polarizable calcium oxalate crystals may also be present. Because mucous plugging can occur in a number of airway diseases, a distinctive laminated appearance should be present before the diagnosis is invoked.

Bronchocentric Granulomatosis

Bronchocentric granulomatosis is a distinctive form of granulomatous inflammation that surrounds the larger airways, replacing bronchial walls and mucosa.[148,154–156] In bronchocentric granulomatosis, the lumen of the airway contains necrotic debris and palisaded histiocytes surround the lumen. Bronchocentric granulomatosis is not

Box 8-14. Common Causes of Bronchocentric Granulomatosis

Allergic bronchopulmonary fungal disease
Bacterial infection, fungal infection, parasitic infestation
Rheumatoid arthritis
Wegener granulomatosis
Necrotizing sarcoidosis

only confined to the larger bronchi but may also involve more distal bronchioles. Both infectious and noninfectious causes are described, and these are presented in Box 8-14. A useful distinguishing clinical feature for separating infectious and noninfectious bronchocentric granulomatosis is the presence or absence of asthma in the affected individual. In asthmatic patients, the disease may manifest as an exacerbation of the underlying airway disease, accompanied by wheezing, cough, and fever, or can be related to hypersensitivity and may be associated with mucoid impaction and ABFD. In nonasthmatic patients, infection should be the main consideration in the differential diagnosis, even when special stains are negative in tissue sections.

In the asthmatic patient, the radiographic findings are often accompanied by the changes of mucoid impaction (branching opacities in a bronchial distribution). In the nonasthmatic patient, given the propensity for infection as the etiology, the radiologic manifestations may be quite variable, ranging from localized consolidation to nodular parenchymal lesions on chest radiographs. Also, in the nonasthmatic patient, cavitation may be present in the nodules, attesting to the likelihood of an infectious etiology.[157]

The most prominent histologic manifestation of bronchocentric granulomatosis is the destruction of the airway wall (Fig. 8-53). This feature is helpful in distinguishing peribronchial granulomas that occur in a number of infectious and noninfectious conditions (e.g., sarcoidosis). As in all cases of necrotizing granulomatosis inflammation, special stains for organisms should always be performed, even in the asthmatic patient in whom a hypersensitivity disease process is suspected. Rarely, Wegener granulomatosis may be present in an exclusively airway-centered distribution, so clinical correlation and serologic studies may be useful. A feature helpful in excluding

Wegener granulomatosis is the presence of well-formed granulomas without necrosis in the surrounding parenchyma (see Chapter 10, on vasculitis). When well-formed granulomas without necrosis are present, Wegener granulomatosis is an unlikely etiology. If the biopsy is obtained from the middle lobe or lingula, middle lobe syndrome should be considered as an alternative diagnosis. Aspiration pneumonia is also in the differential diagnosis, and a careful search for foreign material or foreign body giant cells is always advisable. Vegetable material with thick cellular walls or meat (skeletal muscle fragments) implicates aspiration when present.[83] The presence of conchoidal calcifications, or calcium oxalate crystals in isolation, is not a sign of aspiration, but such bodies can occur in any granulomatous inflammatory reaction.

Chronic Obstructive Pulmonary Disease

COPD is a relatively common disease characterized by chronic airflow obstruction and small-airway abnormalities.[158-160] The disease usually is related to cigarette smoking. The small airways in COPD are often subtly abnormal, and this is the most common situation in which minor abnormalities of the bronchioles are seen, reflecting the high prevalence of smoking in affected patients. Histologically, there is a minor degree of inflammation in the walls of bronchioles, including respiratory bronchioles, with variable occurrence of fibrosis, mucus stasis, loss of radial attachments, and bronchiolectasia (with dilatation and distortion). Emphysema and chronic bronchiolitis both occur in COPD but vary in proportion and severity from patient to patient.

Emphysema

Emphysema may be classified according to the part of the lung acinus that is primarily affected.[161] *Proximal* (centrilobular, centriacinar) emphysema (Fig. 8-54A) involves the proximal part of the lung acinus. This form of emphysema is strongly associated with smoking. The respiratory bronchioles are enlarged and destroyed, and the enlarged air spaces are seen at the center of the secondary acinus; respiratory bronchiolitis of variable degree may be present. *Panacinar* emphysema (see Fig. 8-54B) affects the whole acinus and is characteristic of α_1-antitrypsin deficiency; the air spaces of the whole acinus

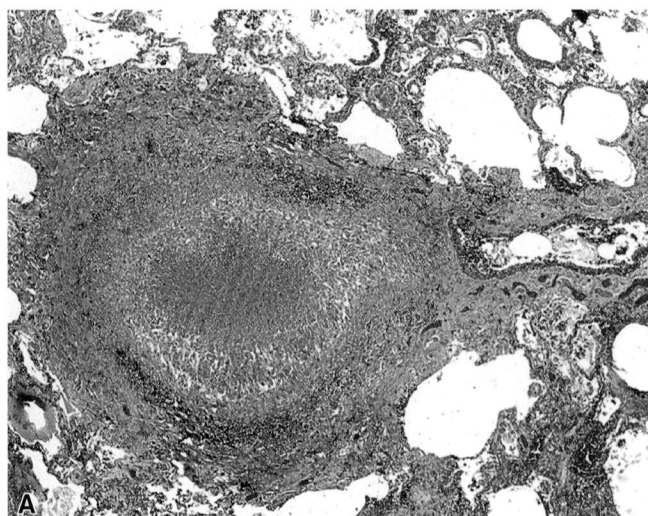
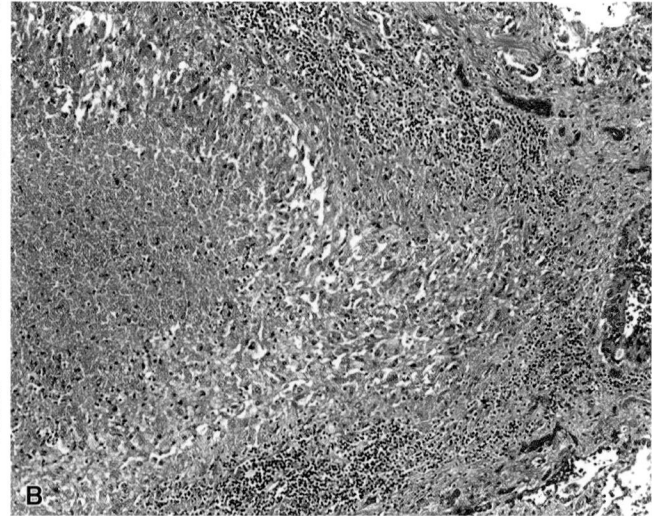

Figure 8-53. Bronchocentric granulomatosis. **A,** The disease is characterized by obliteration of the airway lumen by granulomatous inflammation and complete effacement of the airway epithelium. **B,** Note the prominent hystiocytic reaction at higher magnification.

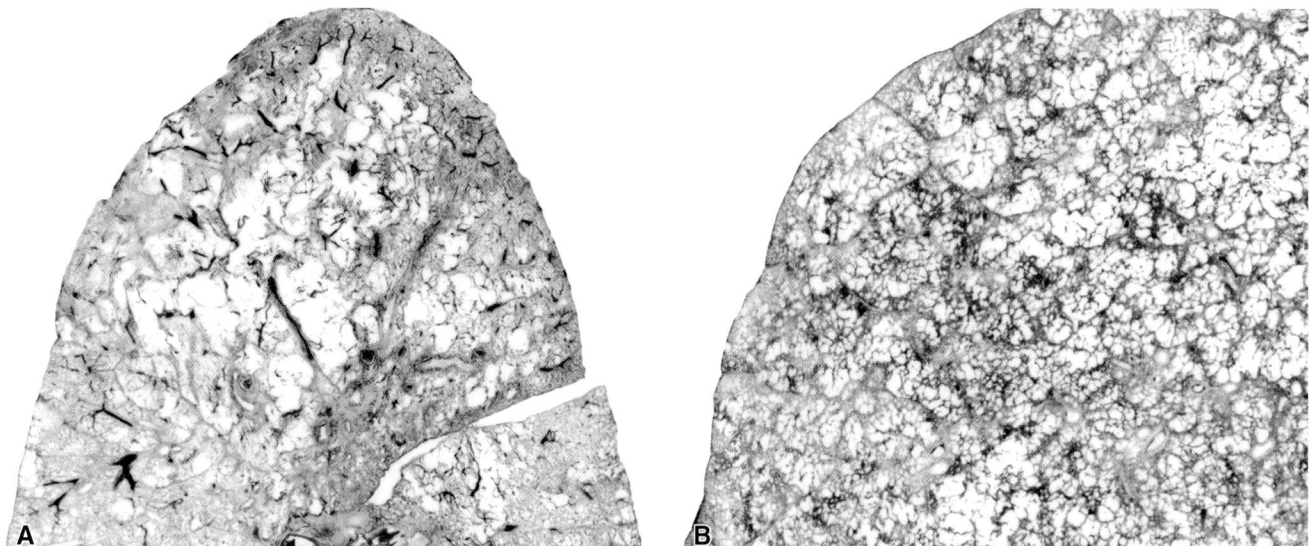

Figure 8-54. Emphysema. Paper-thin Gough-Wentworth sections prepared from whole lungs. **A,** Centriacinar emphysema in a smoker. **B,** Panacinar emphysema in α_1-antitrypsin deficiency. (Original Gough sections courtesy of T.V. Colby and the Charles B. Carrington Memorial Lung Pathology Library.)

are diffusely enlarged. *Distal* (septal, pleural, localized) emphysema affects the periphery of the acinus, most often beneath the pleura; it may be a cause of spontaneous pneumothorax in the young adult. *Irregular* emphysema may be seen in association with a lung scar, such as those due to healed Langerhans cell histiocytosis, granulomatous inflammation, dust deposits, or pulmonary infarcts. Although gross examination of the lungs allows distinction between centriacinar and panacinar emphysema,[158] the surgical biopsy is not a reliable method for diagnosing pulmonary emphysema. Noting the presence of emphysema on surgical wedge biopsies is reasonable, but attempts to grade its severity are not advisable (Fig. 8-55). The associated small-airway and vascular changes may be prominent and include tortuosity.

Neuroendocrine Cell Hyperplasia with Occlusive Bronchiolar Fibrosis (Aguayo-Miller Disease)

Diffuse idiopathic neuroendocrine cell hyperplasia (DIPNECH) of the bronchioles is a primary proliferation of neuroendocrine cells which can be associated with partial or total occlusion of airway lumens by fibrous tissue.[162] DIPNECH is more frequent in women and is not related to cigarette smoke. DIPNECH may be an incidental finding or may present as a symptomatic disease, typically nonproductive cough, dyspnea, which usually is not progressive, and an obstructive lung function profile.[163,164] HRCT scans may reveal evidence of small airway obstruction and coexistence of minute pulmonary nodules. Rare cases have been found in association with multiple endocrine neoplasia (MEN) type 1 syndrome or other

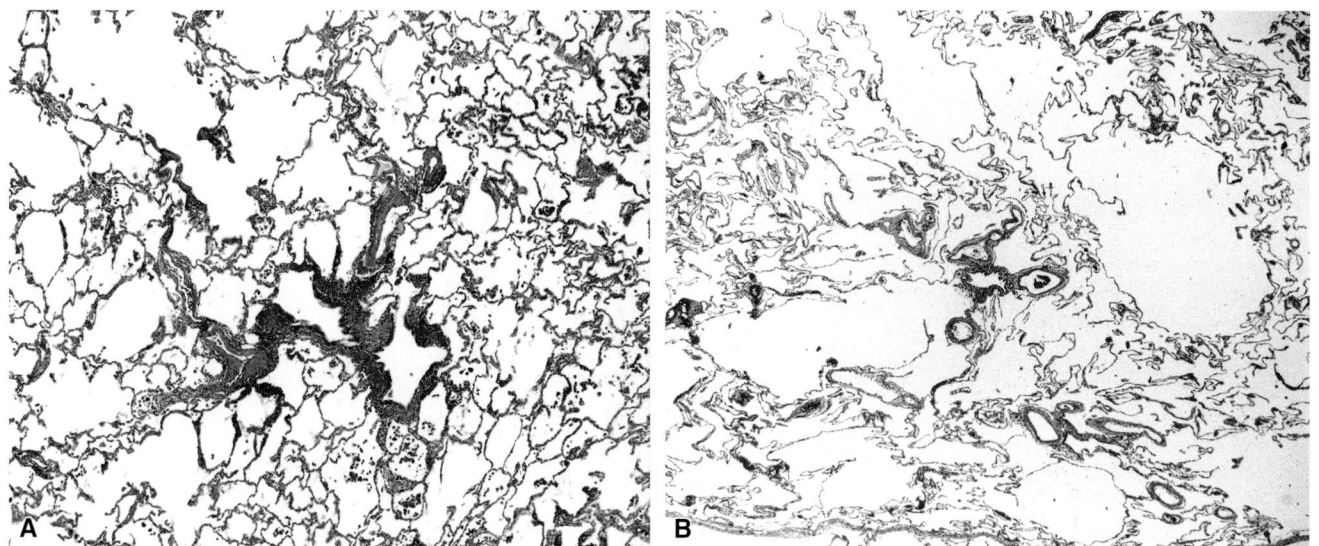

Figure 8-55. Emphysema. The type and severity of emphysema may be difficult or impossible to determine on histopathologic grounds. **A,** Here, centriacinar emphysema is seen with dilatation of the air spaces surrounding the bronchiole. **B,** By contrast, panacinar emphysema features a more diffuse air space dilatation.

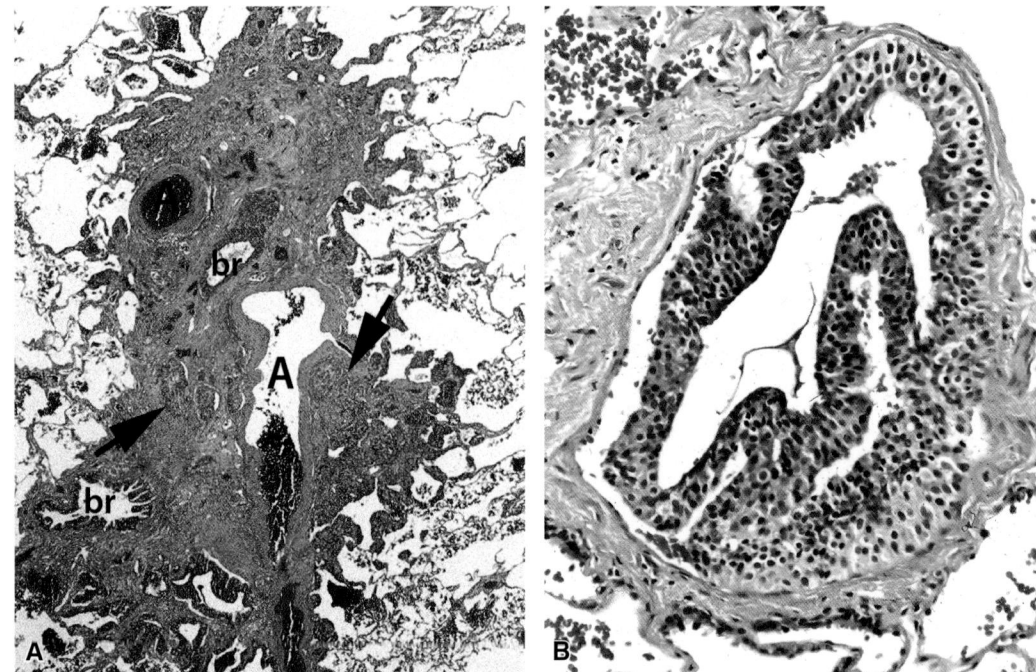

Figure 8-56. Aguayo-Miller disease. These lung preparations are from a 74-year-old woman who presented with dyspnea of recent onset. Multiple pulmonary nodules are easily identified in the low-magnification view of a lung biopsy. **A,** One of the nodules showing fibrosis encasing the pulmonary artery (A). Several neuroendocrine cell aggregations (*arrows*) and tortuous bronchiolar profiles (br) are seen. These nodules are composed of neuroendocrine cells, demonstrable by their immunoreactivity for chromogranin A and synaptophysin. The entrapped airways in the nodule show a narrowed lumen, with neuroendocrine cell aggregates that may bulge into the bronchiolar lumen. **B,** Neuroendocrine cell hyperplasia in Aguayo-Miller disease is not limited to airways associated with the nodules but can also be found in isolated airways.

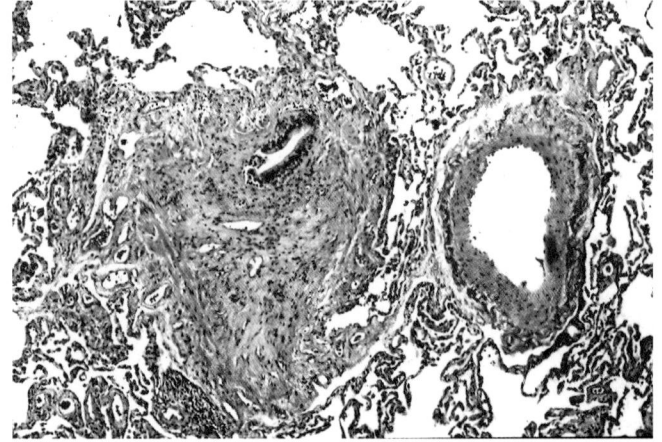

Figure 8-57. Aguayo-Miller disease: Constrictive bronchiolitis. In Aguayo-Miller disease the clinical picture is dominated by obstructive physiology. In this case, besides the neuroendocrine hyperplasia, other bronchioles demonstrated prominent fibrosis with luminal narrowing.

endocrine disorders.[163] Pathologically, the mildest lesions consist of linear zones of neuroendocrine cell hyperplasia with very focal subepithelial fibrosis. More obvious lesions consist of a plaque of eccentric fibrous tissue partially occluding the airway lumen. Sometimes the occlusion can be caused directly by the proliferation of neuroendocrine cells (Figs. 8-56 and 8-57) within the airway epithelium. The most severely involved bronchioles show total occlusion of their lumens by fibrous tissue, with few visible neuroendocrine cells.

Diffuse Panbronchiolitis

Diffuse panbronchiolitis (DPB), first described by Yamanaka and coworkers,[165] is a distinctive inflammatory condition characterized by chronic bronchiolitis associated with prominent interstitial vacuolated or "foamy" histiocytes in a peribronchiolar distribution (Fig. 8-58). DPB is seen more commonly in natives of Japan, Korea, and China, and only rare cases have been described in non-Asian individuals.[166,167] The age range for affected patients is 20 to 60 years. Men are twice as commonly affected as women. Chronic productive cough and dyspnea are the typical presenting complaints, and most patients have sinusitis.[166,168–174] A genetic susceptibility has been well documented over the years, and recently has been identified as a human leukocyte antigen (HLA)-associated major susceptibility gene, probably residing within the HLA-B locus on the short arm of chromosome 6 (6p21.3). HLA-B54 is the haplotype reported in Japanese patients, and HLA-A11 is identified in those of Korean ancestry, suggesting that the DPB susceptibility locus is located between the HLA-B and HLA-A genes.[175,176]

A summary of the key morphologic findings related to diseases of the large and small airways is presented in Table 8-3.

Self-assessment questions related to this chapter can be found online on the Expert Consult site for this title.

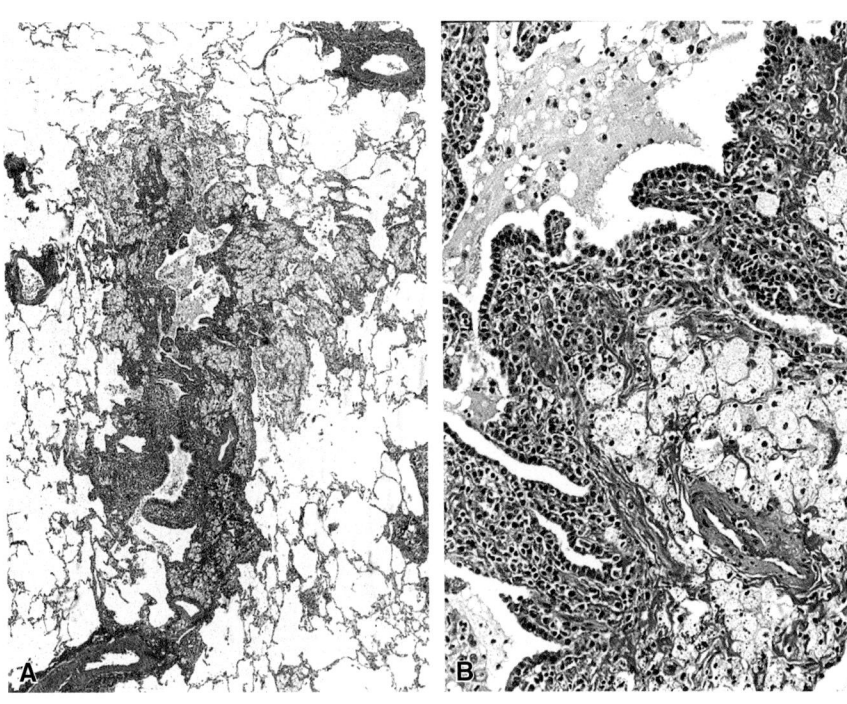

Figure 8-58. Diffuse panbronchiolitis. **A,** Low-magnification view shows a centrilobular nodule, composed of distinctive foamy macrophages distending the peribronchiolar septa, alveolar duct walls, and some alveolar septa. **B,** This infiltration by pale foamy macrophages is more evident at higher magnification, and an associated chronic inflammatory infiltrate can also be appreciated. This biopsy was taken from a Japanese man with a long history of chronic cough, sputum production, and dyspnea. A plain film of the chest showed diffuse disseminated nodular shadows with hyperinflation. Pulmonary function testing indicated an obstructive pattern with hypoxemia.

Table 8-3. Key Morphologic Findings in Diseases of the Large and Small Airways

Observation	Considerations
Small non-necrotizing granulomas in bronchial mucosa	Sarcoidosis, infection, aspiration, berylliosis, tracheobronchial amyloidosis
Small non-necrotizing granulomas around bronchioles	Hypersensitivity pneumonitis, infection, aspiration, Wegener granulomatosis, sarcoidosis, Crohn disease, Sjögren syndrome, primary biliary cirrhosis
Well-formed non-necrotizing granulomas	Sarcoidosis, berylliosis, infection
Well-formed necrotizing granulomas	Infection
Necrosis	Infection, Wegener granulomatosis, bronchocentric granulomatosis, relapsing polychondritis, pyoderma gangrenosum, fume exposure
Lymphoid follicles around bronchioles	Collagen vascular diseases, distal to bronchiectasis, lymphoproliferative diseases, inflammatory bowel diseases, as a minor component of a localized inflammation
Bronchiolar metaplasia	Healed bronchiolitis, chronic hypersensitivity pneumonitis, distal to bronchiectasis, as a component of constrictive bronchiolitis, as a focal incidental finding
Mucostasis	Bronchiolitis (of any cause), distal to bronchiectasis, allergic bronchopulmonary aspergillosis, as part of a localized inflammation, as an incidental finding (in the smoker)
Intra-alveolar foamy macrophages	Distal to bronchial obstruction (of any cause), hypersensitivity pneumonitis, cryptogenic organizing pneumonia, reactions to some drugs (e.g., amiodarone), some metabolic disorders
Interstitial foamy macrophages	Diffuse panbronchiolitis, inflammatory bowel diseases, distal to bronchiectasis
Lightly pigmented alveolar macrophages	Respiratory bronchiolitis (in smokers)
Densely pigmented alveolar macrophages	Chronic hemorrhage, asbestosis (if hemosiderin), dust exposure (when anthracotic with or without refractile material)
Conchoidal calcifications	Sarcoidosis, infection, hypersensitivity pneumonitis, berylliosis, aspiration
Neuroendocrine cell proliferation	Diffuse idiopathic pulmonary neuroendocrine hyperplasia (with or without partial or total occlusion of airway lumens by fibrous tissue), as an incidental finding frequently associated with bronchiectasis
Reduction in airway lumen diameter (sometimes associated with bronchioloectasia)	Constrictive/obliterative bronchiolitis as a consequence of infection, toxic fume inhalation, drug reaction, chemical toxins, connective tissue disease, transplantation
Mucous cell hyperplasia	Asthma
Smooth muscle hyperplasia	Asthma, constrictive bronchiolitis, fibrosing lung disease, localized inflammatory process, bronchiolar scarring/peribronchiolar metaplasia, incidental finding (especially in smoker), DIPNECH with occlusive bronchiolar fibrosis

DIPNECH, diffuse idiopathic pulmonary neuroendocrine cell hyperplasia.

References

1. Al Jahdali H, Bamefleh H, Memish Z, et al. Upper airway obstruction due to rhinoscleroma: case report. *J Chemother*. 2001;13(suppl 1):69–72.

2. Verma G, Kanawaty D, Hyland R. Rhinoscleroma causing upper airway obstruction. *Can Respir J*. 2005;12(1):43–45.

3. Hellmann D, Laing T, Petri M, et al. Wegener's granulomatosis: isolated involvement of the trachea and larynx. *Ann Rheum Dis*. 1987;46(8):628–631.

4. Schokkenbroek AA, Franssen CF, Dikkers FG. Dilatation tracheoscopy for laryngeal and tracheal stenosis in patients with Wegener's granulomatosis. *Eur Arch Otorhinolaryngol*. 2008;265(5):549–555.

5. Berk JL, O'Regan A, Skinner M. Pulmonary and tracheobronchial amyloidosis. *Semin Respir Crit Care Med*. 2002;23(2):155–165.

6. O'Regan A, Fenlon HM, Beamis Jr JF, et al. Tracheobronchial amyloidosis. The Boston University experience from 1984 to 1999. *Medicine (Baltimore)*. 2000;79(2):69–79.

7. Ozyigit LP, Kiyan E, Okumus G, Yilmazbayhan D. Isolated laryngo-tracheal amyloidosis presenting as a refractory asthma and longstanding hoarseness. *J Asthma*. 2009;46(3):314–317.

8. Papla B, Dubiel-Bigaj M. Tracheobronchial amyloidosis. *Pol J Pathol*. 1998;49(1):27–34.

9. Cordier JF, Loire R, Brune J. Amyloidosis of the lower respiratory tract. *Chest*. 1986;90:827–831.

10. Howard ME, Ireton J, Daniels F, et al. Pulmonary presentations of amyloidosis. *Respirology*. 2001;6(1):61–64.

11. Yang S, Chia SY, Chuah KL, Eng P. Tracheobronchial amyloidosis treated with rigid bronchoscopy and stenting. *Surg Endosc*. 2003;17(4):658–659.

12. Kalra S, Utz JP, Edell ES, Foote RL. External-beam radiation therapy in the treatment of diffuse tracheobronchial amyloidosis. *Mayo Clin Proc*. 2001;76(8):853–856.

13. Fukumura M, Mieno T, Suzuki T, Murata Y. Primary diffuse tracheobronchial amyloidosis treated by bronchoscopic Nd-YAG laser irradiation. *Jpn J Med*. 1990;29(6):620–622.

14. Herman DP, Colchen A, Milleron B, et al. The treatment of tracheobronchial amyloidosis using a bronchial laser. Apropos of a series of 13 cases. *Rev Mal Respir*. 1985;2(1):19–23.

15. Carden KA, Boiselle PM, Waltz DA, Ernst A. Tracheomalacia and tracheobronchomalacia in children and adults: an in-depth review. *Chest*. 2005;127(3):984–1005.

16. Loring SH, O'Donnell CR, Feller-Kopman DJ, Ernst A. Central airway mechanics and flow limitation in acquired tracheobronchomalacia. *Chest*. 2007;131(4):1118–1124.

17. Zhang J, Hasegawa I, Hatabu H, et al. Frequency and severity of air trapping at dynamic expiratory CT in patients with tracheobronchomalacia. *AJR Am J Roentgenol*. 2004;182(1):81–85.

18. Masaoka A, Yamakawa Y, Niwa H, et al. Pediatric and adult tracheobronchomalacia. *Eur J Cardiothorac Surg*. 1996;10(2):87–92.

19. Jacobs IN, Wetmore RF, Tom LW, et al. Tracheobronchomalacia in children. *Arch Otolaryngol Head Neck Surg*. 1994;120(2):154–158.

20. Mair EA, Parsons DS. Pediatric tracheobronchomalacia and major airway collapse. *Ann Otol Rhinol Laryngol*. 1992;101(4):300–309.

21. Ghanei M, Moqadam FA, Mohammad MM, Aslani J. Tracheobronchomalacia and air trapping after mustard gas exposure. *Am J Respir Crit Care Med*. 2006;173(3):304–309.

22. Turkstra F, Rinkel RN, Biermann H, et al. Tracheobronchomalacia due to amyloidosis in a patient with rheumatoid arthritis. *Clin Rheumatol*. 2008;27(6):807–808.

23. Nuutinen J. Acquired tracheobronchomalacia. *Eur J Respir Dis*. 1982;63(5):380–387.

24. Letko E, Zafirakis P, Baltatzis S, et al. Relapsing polychondritis: a clinical review. *Semin Arthritis Rheum*. 2002;31(6):384–395.

25. Tsunezuka Y, Sato H, Shimizu H. Tracheobronchial involvement in relapsing polychondritis. *Respiration*. 2000;67(3):320–322.

26. Lee KS, Ashiku SK, Ernst A, et al. Comparison of expiratory CT airway abnormalities before and after tracheoplasty surgery for tracheobronchomalacia. *J Thorac Imaging*. 2008;23(2):121–126.

27. Abu-Hijleh M, Lee D, Braman SS. Tracheobronchopathia osteochondroplastica: a rare large airway disorder. *Lung*. 2008;186(6):353–359.

28. Meyer CN, Dossing M, Broholm H. Tracheobronchopathia osteochondroplastica. *Respir Med*. 1997;91(8):499–502.

29. Vilkman S, Keistinen T. Tracheobronchopathia osteochondroplastica. Report of a young man with severe disease and retrospective review of 18 cases. *Respiration*. 1995;62(3):151–154.

30. Chroneou A, Zias N, Gonzalez AV, Beamis Jr JF. Tracheobronchopathia osteochondroplastica. An underrecognized entity? *Monaldi Arch Chest Dis*. 2008;69(2):65–69.

31. Prakash UB. Tracheobronchopathia osteochondroplastica. *Semin Respir Crit Care Med*. 2002;23(2):167–175.

32. Cowan MJ, Gladwin MT, Shelhamer JH. Disorders of ciliary motility. *Am J Med Sci*. 2001;321(1):3–10.

33. O'Sullivan BP, Freedman SD. Cystic fibrosis. *Lancet*. 2009;373(9678):1891–1904.

34. Javidan-Nejad C, Bhalla S. Bronchiectasis. *Radiol Clin North Am*. 2009;47(2):289–306.

35. Barker AF, Bardana Jr EJ. Bronchiectasis: update of an orphan disease. *Am Rev Respir Dis*. 1988;137(4):969–978.

36. Nicotra MB, Rivera M, Dale AM, et al. Clinical, pathophysiologic, and microbiologic characterization of bronchiectasis in an aging cohort. *Chest*. 1995;108(4):955–961.

37. Barker AF. Bronchiectasis. *N Engl J Med*. 2002;346(18):1383–1393.

38. Tanawuttiwat T, Harindhanavudhi T. Bronchiectasis: Pulmonary manifestation in chronic graft versus host disease after bone marrow transplantation. *Am J Med Sci*. 2009;337(4):292.

39. Kanbay M, Kanbay A, Boyacioglu S. *Helicobacter pylori* infection as a possible risk factor for respiratory system disease: a review of the literature. *Respir Med*. 2007;101(2):203–209.

40. Tsang KW, Lam SK, Lam WK, et al. High seroprevalence of *Helicobacter pylori* in active bronchiectasis. *Am J Respir Crit Care Med*. 1998;158(4):1047–1051.

41. Tsang KW, Lam WK, Kwok E, et al. *Helicobacter pylori* and upper gastrointestinal symptoms in bronchiectasis. *Eur Respir J*. 1999;14(6):1345–1350.

42. Kang EY, Miller RR, Muller NL. Bronchiectasis: comparison of preoperative thin-section CT and pathologic findings in resected specimens. *Radiology*. 1995;195(3):649–654.

43. Lucidarme O, Grenier P, Coche E, et al. Bronchiectasis: comparative assessment with thin-section CT and helical CT. *Radiology*. 1996;200(3):673–679.

44. Young K, Aspestrand F, Kolbenstvedt A. High resolution CT and bronchography in the assessment of bronchiectasis. *Acta Radiol*. 1991;32(6):439–441.

45. Cartier Y, Kavanagh PV, Johkoh T, et al. Bronchiectasis: accuracy of high-resolution CT in the differentiation of specific diseases. *AJR Am J Roentgenol*. 1999;173(1):47–52.

46. Whitwell F. A study of the pathology and pathogenesis of bronchiectasis. *Thorax*. 1952;7(3):213–239.

47. Kwon KY, Myers JL, Swensen SJ, Colby TV. Middle lobe syndrome: a clinicopathological study of 21 patients. *Hum Pathol*. 1995;26(3):302–307.

48. Reich JM, Johnson RE. *Mycobacterium avium* complex pulmonary disease presenting as an isolated lingular or middle lobe pattern. The Lady Windermere syndrome. *Chest*. 1992;101(6):1605–1609.

49. Bhatt SP, Nanda S, Kintzer Jr JS. The Lady Windermere syndrome. *Prim Care Respir J*. 2009;18(4):334–336.

50. Reich JM. Pathogenesis of Lady Windermere syndrome. *Am J Respir Crit Care Med*. 2009;179(12):1165 author reply 1165.

51. Fujita J, Ohtsuki Y, Suemitsu I, et al. Pathological and radiological changes in resected lung specimens in *Mycobacterium avium intracellulare* complex disease. *Eur Respir J*. 1999;13(3):535–540.

52. Priftis KN, Mermiri D, Papadopoulou A, et al. The role of timely intervention in middle lobe syndrome in children. *Chest*. 2005;128(4):2504–2510.

53. Colby TV. Bronchiolar pathology. In: Epler GR, ed. *Diseases of the Bronchials*. New York: Raven Press; 1994:77–100.

54. Couture C, Colby TV. Histopathology of bronchiolar disorders. *Semin Respir Crit Care Med*. 2003;24(5):489–498.

55. Poletti V, Costabel U. Bronchiolar disorders: classification and diagnostic approach. *Semin Respir Crit Care Med*. 2003;24(5):457–464.

56. Lynch DA. Imaging of small airways disease and chronic obstructive pulmonary disease. *Clin Chest Med*. 2008;29(1):165–179, vii.

57. Ryu JH. Classification and approach to bronchiolar diseases. *Curr Opin Pulm Med*. 2006;12(2):145–151.

58. Ryu JH, Myers JL, Swensen SJ. Bronchiolar disorders. *Am J Respir Crit Care Med*. 2003;168(11):1277–1292.

59. Yousem S. Small airways disease. *Pathol Annu*. 1991;26(part 2):109–143.

60. Colby TV. Bronchiolitis. Pathologic considerations. *Am J Clin Pathol*. 1998;109(1):101–109.

61. Becroft DMO. Histopathology of fatal adenovirus infection of the respiratory tract in young children. *J Clin Pathol*. 1967;20:561–569.

62. Becroft DMO. Bronchiolitis obliterans, bronchiectasis and other sequelae of adenovirus type 21 infection in young children. *J Clin Pathol*. 1971;24:72–79.

63. Travis WD, Hoffman GS, Leavitt RY, et al. Surgical pathology of the lung in Wegener's granulomatosis. Review of 87 open lung biopsies from 67 patients. *Am J Surg Pathol*. 1991;15(4):315–333.

64. Colby TV, Leslie KO. Small airway lesions. In: Cagle PT, ed. *Diagnostic Pulmonary Pathology*. New York: Marcel Dekker; 2000:231–249.

65. Howling SJ, Hansell DM, Wells AU, et al. Follicular bronchiolitis: thin-section CT and histologic findings. *Radiology*. 1999;212(3):637–642.

66. Wells AU, du Bois RM. Bronchiolitis in association with connective tissue disorders. *Clin Chest Med*. 1993;14(4):655–666.

67. Nicholson AG, Colby TV, Wells AU. Histopathological approach to patterns of interstitial pneumonia in patients with connective tissue disorders. *Sarcoidosis Vasc Diffuse Lung Dis*. 2002;19(1):10–17.

68. Leslie KO, Trahan S, Gruden J. Pulmonary pathology of the rheumatic diseases. *Semin Respir Crit Care Med*. 2007;28(4):369–378.

69. Lee HK, Kim DS, Yoo B, et al. Histopathologic pattern and clinical features of rheumatoid arthritis–associated interstitial lung disease. *Chest*. 2005;127(6):2019–2027.

70. Nicholson AG, Wotherspoon AC, Diss TC, et al. Reactive pulmonary lymphoid disorders. *Histopathology*. 1995;26(5):405–412.

71. Yousem SA, Colby TV, Carrington CB. Follicular bronchitis/bronchiolitis. *Hum Pathol*. 1985;16(7):700–706.

72. Fiche M, Caprons F, Berger F, et al. Primary pulmonary non-Hodgkin's lymphomas. *Histopathology*. 1995;26(6):529–537.

73. Boag AH, Colby TV, Fraire AE, et al. The pathology of interstitial lung disease in nylon flock workers. *Am J Surg Pathol*. 1999;23(12):1539–1545.

74. Burkhart J, Jones W, Porter DW, et al. Hazardous occupational exposure and lung disease among nylon flock workers. *Am J Ind Med*. 1999;1(suppl):145–146.

75. Eschenbacher WL, Kreiss K, Lougheed MD, et al. Nylon flock–associated interstitial lung disease. *Am J Respir Crit Care Med*. 1999;159(6):2003–2008.

76. Kern DG, Kuhn 3rd C, Ely EW, et al. Flock worker's lung: chronic interstitial lung disease in the nylon flocking industry. *Ann Intern Med*. 1998;129(4):261–272.

77. Kern DG, Kuhn 3rd C, Ely EW, et al. Flock worker's lung: broadening the spectrum of clinicopathology, narrowing the spectrum of suspected etiologies. *Chest*. 2000;117(1):251–259.

78. Romero S, Barroso E, Gil J, et al. Follicular bronchiolitis: clinical and pathologic findings in six patients. *Lung*. 2003;181(6):309–319.

79. Khoor A, Leslie KO, Tazelaar HD, et al. Diffuse pulmonary disease caused by nontuberculous mycobacteria in immunocompetent people (hot tub lung). *Am J Clin Pathol*. 2001;115(5):755–762.

80. Yousem SA. The histological spectrum of chronic necrotizing forms of pulmonary aspergillosis. *Hum Pathol*. 1997;28(6):650–656.

81. Casey MB, Tazelaar HD, Myers JL, et al. Noninfectious lung pathology in patients with Crohn's disease. *Am J Surg Pathol*. 2003;27(2):213–219.

82. Barnes TW, Vassallo R, Tazelaar HD, et al. Diffuse bronchiolar disease due to chronic occult aspiration. *Mayo Clin Proc*. 2006;81(2):172–176.

83. Mukhopadhyay S, Katzenstein AL. Pulmonary disease due to aspiration of food and other particulate matter: a clinicopathologic study of 59 cases diagnosed on biopsy or resection specimens. *Am J Surg Pathol*. 2007;31(5):752–759.

84. Camus P, Piard F, Ashcroft T, et al. The lung in inflammatory bowel disease. *Medicine (Baltimore)*. 1993;72(3):151–183.

85. Camus P, Colby TV. The lung in inflammatory bowel disease. *Eur Respir J*. 2000;15(1):5–10.

86. Kar PM, Aronoff G, Schuette P. Bronchopulmonary disease: an association with ulcerative colitis and pyoderma gangrenosum. *J Ky Med Assoc*. 1993;91(8):320–323.

87. Fukuhara K, Urano Y, Kimura S, et al. Pyoderma gangrenosum with rheumatoid arthritis and pulmonary aseptic abscess responding to treatment with dapsone. *Br J Dermatol*. 1998;139(3):556–558.

88. Wang JL, Wang JB, Zhu YJ. Pyoderma gangrenosum with lung injury. *Thorax*. 1999; 54(10):953–955.

89. Krüger S, Piroth W, Amo Takyi B, et al. Multiple aseptic pulmonary nodules with central necrosis in association with pyoderma gangrenosum. *Chest*. 2001;119(3):977–978.

90. Field S, Powell FC, Young V, Barnes L. Pyoderma gangrenosum manifesting as a cavitating lung lesion. *Clin Exp Dermatol*. 2008;33(4):418–421.

91. Kitagawa KH, Grassi M. Primary pyoderma gangrenosum of the lungs. *J Am Acad Dermatol*. 2008;59(suppl 5):S114–S116.

92. Myers JL, Veal Jr CF, Shin MS, Katzenstein AL. Respiratory bronchiolitis causing interstitial lung disease. A clinicopathologic study of six cases. *Am Rev Respir Dis*. 1987;135:880–884.

93. Yousem S, Colby T, Gaensler E. Respiratory bronchiolitis and its relationship to desquamative interstitial pneumonia. *Mayo Clin Proc*. 1989;64:1373–1380.

94. Moon J, du Bois RM, Colby TV, et al. Clinical significance of respiratory bronchiolitis on open lung biopsy and its relationship to smoking related interstitial lung disease. *Thorax*. 1999;54(11):1009–1014.

95. Fraig M, Shreesha U, Savici D, Katzenstein AL. Respiratory bronchiolitis: a clinicopathologic study in current smokers, ex-smokers, and never-smokers. *Am J Surg Pathol*. 2002;26(5): 647–653.

96. Wells AU, Nicholson AG, Hansell DM, du Bois RM. Respiratory bronchiolitis–associated interstitial lung disease. *Semin Respir Crit Care Med*. 2003;24(5):585–594.

97. Aubry MC, Wright JL, Myers JL. The pathology of smoking-related lung diseases. *Clin Chest Med*. 2000;21(1):11–35, vii.

98. Hartman TE, Tazelaar HD, Swensen SJ, Müller NL. Cigarette smoking: CT and pathologic findings of associated pulmonary diseases. *Radiographics*. 1997;17(2):377–390.

99. Hansell DM, Nicholson AG. Smoking-related diffuse parenchymal lung disease: HRCT-pathologic correlation. *Semin Respir Crit Care Med*. 2003;24(4):377–392.

100. Caminati A, Harari S. Smoking-related interstitial pneumonias and pulmonary Langerhans cell histiocytosis. *Proc Am Thorac Soc*. 2006;3(4):299–306.

101. Yousem SA. Respiratory bronchiolitis–associated interstitial lung disease with fibrosis is a lesion distinct from fibrotic nonspecific interstitial pneumonia: a proposal. *Mod Pathol*. 2006;19(11):1474–1479.

102. Yousem S, Colby T, Gaensler E. Respiratory bronchiolitis–associated interstitial lung disease and its relationship to desquamative interstitial pneumonia. *Mayo Clin Proc*. 1989;64:1373–1380.

103. Vassallo R, Jensen EA, Colby TV, et al. The overlap between respiratory bronchiolitis and desquamative interstitial pneumonia in pulmonary Langerhans cell histiocytosis: high resolution CT, histologic, and functional correlations. *Chest*. 2003;124(4):1199–1205.

104. Kitamura H, Kameda Y, Ito T, Hayashi H. Atypical adenomatous hyperplasia of the lung. Implications for the pathogenesis of peripheral lung adenocarcinoma. *Am J Clin Pathol*. 1999;111(5):610–622.

105. Chapman AD, Kerr KM. The association between atypical adenomatous hyperplasia and primary lung cancer. *Br J Cancer*. 2000;83(5):632–636.

106. Mori M, Rao SK, Popper HH, et al. Atypical adenomatous hyperplasia of the lung: a probable forerunner in the development of adenocarcinoma of the lung. *Mod Pathol*. 2001;14(2):72–84.

107. Nakahara R, Yokose T, Nagai K, et al. Atypical adenomatous hyperplasia of the lung: a clinicopathological study of 118 cases including cases with multiple atypical adenomatous hyperplasia. *Thorax*. 2001;56(4):302–305.

108. Sartori G, Cavazza A, Bertolini F, et al. A subset of lung adenocarcinomas and atypical adenomatous hyperplasia–associated foci are genotypically related: an EGFR, HER2, and K-ras mutational analysis. *Am J Clin Pathol*. 2008;129(2):202–210.

109. Guinee D, Singh R, Azumi N, et al. Multifocal micronodular pneumocyte hyperplasia: a distinctive pulmonary manifestation of tuberous sclerosis. *Mod Pathol*. 1995;8(9):902–906.

110. Muir TE, Leslie KO, Popper H, et al. Micronodular pneumocyte hyperplasia. *Am J Surg Pathol*. 1998;22(4):465–472.

111. Myers JL. Micronodular pneumocyte hyperplasia: the versatile type 2 pneumocyte all dressed up in yet another brand new suit! *Adv Anat Pathol*. 1999;6(1):49–55.

112. Leslie K, Colby T, Swensen S. Anatomic distribution and histopathologic patterns in interstitial lung disease. In: Schwarz M, King TJ, eds. *Interstitial Lung Disease*. Hamilton, ON: BC Decker; 2002:31–50.

113. Lange W. Ueber eine eigenth atumliche erkrankung der kleinen bronchien und bronchiolen (bronchitis et bronchiolitis obliterans). *Dtsch Arch Klin Med*. 1901;70:342–364.

114. Davison AG, Heard BE, McAllister WA, Turner-Warwick ME. Cryptogenic organizing pneumonitis. *Q J Med*. 1983;52:382–394.

115. American Thoracic Society, European Respiratory Society. American Thoracic Society/European Respiratory Society International Multidisciplinary Consensus Classification of the Idiopathic Interstitial Pneumonias. This joint statement of the American Thoracic Society (ATS), and the European Respiratory Society (ERS) was adopted by the ATS board of directors, June 2001 and by the ERS Executive Committee, June 2001. *Am J Respir Crit Care Med*. 2002;165(2):277–304.

116. Epler GR, Colby TV, McLoud TC, et al. Bronchiolitis obliterans organizing pneumonia. *N Engl J Med*. 1985;312(3):152–158.

117. Colby TV, Myers AR. Clinical and histologic spectrum of bronchiolitis obliterans including bronchiolitis obliterans organizing pneumonia. *Semin Respir Med*. 1992;13:113–119.

118. Wright JL, Cagle P, Churg A, et al. Diseases of the small airways. *Am Rev Respir Dis*. 1992;146(1):240–262.

119. Grossman EJ, Shilling RA. Bronchiolitis obliterans in lung transplantation: the good, the bad, and the future. *Transl Res*. 2009;153(4):153–165.

120. Huang HJ, Yusen RD, Meyers BF, et al. Late primary graft dysfunction after lung transplantation and bronchiolitis obliterans syndrome. *Am J Transplant*. 2008;8(11):2454–2462.

121. Cordier JF. Cryptogenic organising pneumonia. *Eur Respir J*. 2006;28(2):422–446.

122. Sato M, Keshavjee S. Bronchiolitis obliterans syndrome: alloimmune-dependent and -independent injury with aberrant tissue remodeling. *Semin Thorac Cardiovasc Surg*. 2008;20(2):173–182.

123. Garg K, Lynch DA, Newell JD, King Jr TE. Proliferative and constrictive bronchiolitis: classification and radiologic features. *AJR Am J Roentgenol*. 1994;162(4):803–808.

124. Myers JL, Colby TV. Pathologic manifestations of bronchiolitis, constrictive bronchiolitis, cryptogenic organizing pneumonia, and diffuse panbronchiolitis. *Clin Chest Med*. 1993;14(4):611–622.

125. Kraft M, Mortenson RL, Colby TV, et al. Cryptogenic constrictive bronchiolitis. A clinicopathologic study. *Am Rev Respir Dis*. 1993;148(4 Pt 1):1093–1101.

126. Chin AC, Stich D, White FV, et al. Paraneoplastic pemphigus and bronchiolitis obliterans associated with a mediastinal mass: a rare case of Castleman's disease with respiratory failure requiring lung transplantation. *J Pediatr Surg*. 2001;36(12):E22.

127. Mann JM, Sha KK, Kline G, et al. World Trade Center dyspnea: bronchiolitis obliterans with functional improvement: a case report. *Am J Ind Med*. 2005;48(3):225–229.

128. Akpinar-Elci M, Travis WD, Lynch DA, Kreiss K. Bronchiolitis obliterans syndrome in popcorn production plant workers. *Eur Respir J*. 2004;24(2):298–302.

129. Ghanei M, Tazelaar HD, Chilosi M, et al. An international collaborative pathologic study of surgical lung biopsies from mustard gas–exposed patients. *Respir Med*. 2008;102(6): 825–830.

130. Shah AP, Xu H, Sime PJ, Trawick DR. Severe airflow obstruction and eosinophilic lung disease after Stevens-Johnson syndrome. *Eur Respir J*. 2006;28(6):1276–1279.

131. White ES, Tazelaar HD, Lynch 3rd JP. Bronchiolar complications of connective tissue diseases. *Semin Respir Crit Care Med*. 2003;24(5):543–566.

132. Wang JS, Tseng HH, Lai RS, et al. *Sauropus androgynus*-constrictive obliterative bronchitis/bronchiolitis—histopathological study of pneumonectomy and biopsy specimens with emphasis on the inflammatory process and disease progression. *Histopathology*. 2000;37(5):402–410.

133. Mauad T, Dolhnikoff M. Histology of childhood bronchiolitis obliterans. *Pediatr Pulmonol*. 2002;33(6):466–474.

134. Fenton ME, Cockcroft DW, Wright JL, Churg A. Hypersensitivity pneumonitis as a cause of airway-centered interstitial fibrosis. *Ann Allergy Asthma Immunol*. 2007;99(5):465–466.

135. Churg A, Myers J, Suarez T, et al. Airway-centered interstitial fibrosis: a distinct form of aggressive diffuse lung disease. *Am J Surg Pathol*. 2004;28(1):62–68.

136. Yousem SA, Dacic S. Idiopathic bronchiolocentric interstitial pneumonia. *Mod Pathol*. 2002;15(11):1148–1153.

137. Takemura T, et al. Pathology of hypersensitivity pneumonitis. *Curr Opin Pulm Med*. 2008;14(5):440–454.

138. Churg A, Muller NL, Flint J, Wright JL. Chronic hypersensitivity pneumonitis. *Am J Surg Pathol*. 2006;30(2):201–208.

139. Churg A, Brauer M, del Carmen Avila-Casado M, et al. Chronic exposure to high levels of particulate air pollution and small airway remodeling. *Environ Health Perspect*. 2003;111(5):714–718.

140. Hogg JC. The pathology of asthma. *APMIS*. 1997;105(10):735–745.

141. Ueda T, Niimi A, Matsumoto H, et al. Role of small airways in asthma: investigation using high-resolution computed tomography. *J Allergy Clin Immunol*. 2006;118(5):1019–1025.

142. Hogg JC. Pathology of asthma. *J Allergy Clin Immunol*. 1993;92(1 Pt 1):1–5.

143. Hogg JC. Bronchiolitis in asthma and chronic obstructive pulmonary disease. *Clin Chest Med*. 1993;14(4):733–740.

8

144. Bergeron C, Al-Ramli W, Hamid Q. Remodeling in asthma. *Proc Am Thorac Soc*. 2009;6(3):301–305.

145. Sumi Y, Hamid Q. Airway remodeling in asthma. *Allergol Int*. 2007;56(4):341–348.

146. Agarwal R. Allergic bronchopulmonary aspergillosis. *Chest*. 2009;135(3):805–826.

147. Cockrill BA, Hales CA. Allergic bronchopulmonary aspergillosis. *Annu Rev Med*. 1999;50:303–316.

148. Sulavik SB. Bronchocentric granulomatosis and allergic bronchopulmonary aspergillosis. *Clin Chest Med*. 1988;9(4):609–621.

149. Aubry MC, Fraser R. The role of bronchial biopsy and washing in the diagnosis of allergic bronchopulmonary aspergillosis. *Mod Pathol*. 1998;11(7):607–611.

150. Martinez S, Heyneman LE, McAdams HP, et al. Mucoid impactions: finger-in-glove sign and other CT and radiographic features. *Radiographics*. 2008;28(5):1369–1382.

151. Katzenstein A, Liebow A, Friedman P. Bronchocentric granulomatosis, mucoid impaction, and hypersensitivity reactions to fungi. *Am Rev Respir Dis*. 1975;111:497–537.

152. Tsai SH, Jenne JW. Mucoid impaction of the bronchi. *Am J Roentgenol Radium Ther Nucl Med*. 1966;96(4):953–961.

153. Sanerkin NG, Seal RM, Leopold JG. Plastic bronchitis, mucoid impaction of the bronchi and allergic broncho-pulmonary aspergillosis, and their relationship to bronchial asthma. *Ann Allergy*. 1966;24(11):586–594.

154. Myers JL. Bronchocentric granulomatosis. Disease or diagnosis? *Chest*. 1989;96(1):3–4.

155. Koss MN, Robinson RG, Hochholzer L. Bronchocentric granulomatosis. *Hum Pathol*. 1981;12(7):632–638.

156. Katzenstein AL, Liebow AA, Friedman PJ. Bronchocentric granulomatosis, mucoid impaction, and hypersensitivity reactions to fungi. *Am Rev Respir Dis*. 1975;111(4):497–537.

157. Ward S, Heyneman LE, Flint JD, et al. Bronchocentric granulomatosis: computed tomographic findings in five patients. *Clin Radiol*. 2000;55(4):296–300.

158. Wright JL, Churg A. Advances in the pathology of COPD. *Histopathology*. 2006;49(1):1–9.

159. Gelb AF, Hogg JC, Müller NL, et al. Contribution of emphysema and small airways in COPD. *Chest*. 1996;109(2):353–359.

160. Jeffery PK. Histological features of the airways in asthma and COPD. *Respiration*. 1992;59 (suppl 1(2)):13–16.

161. Cosio MG, Cosio Piqueras MG. Pathology of emphysema in chronic obstructive pulmonary disease. *Monaldi Arch Chest Dis*. 2000;55(2):124–129.

162. Aguayo SM, Miller YE, Waldron Jr JA, et al. Brief report: idiopathic diffuse hyperplasia of pulmonary neuroendocrine cells and airways disease. *N Engl J Med*. 1992;327:1285–1288.

163. Davies SJ, Gosney JR, Hansell DM, et al. Diffuse idiopathic pulmonary neuroendocrine cell hyperplasia: an under-recognised spectrum of disease. *Thorax*. 2007;62(3):248–252.

164. Adams H, Brack T, Kestenholz P, et al. Diffuse idiopathic neuroendocrine cell hyperplasia causing severe airway obstruction in a patient with a carcinoid tumor. *Respiration*. 2006;73(5):690–693.

165. Yamanaka A, Saiki S, Tamura S, Saito K. [Problems in chronic obstructive bronchial diseases, with special reference to diffuse panbronchiolitis.] *Naika*. 1969;23(3):442–451.

166. Poletti V, Casoni G, Chilosi M, Zompatori M. Diffuse panbronchiolitis. *Eur Respir J*. 2006;28(4):862–871.

167. Aslan AT, Ozcelik U, Talim B, et al. Childhood diffuse panbronchiolitis: a case report. *Pediatr Pulmonol*. 2005;40(4):354–357.

168. Iwata M, Colby T, Kitaichi M. Diffuse panbronchiolitis: diagnosis and distinction from various pulmonary diseases with centrilobular interstitial foam cell accumulations. *Hum Pathol*. 1994;25:357–363.

169. Nishimura K, Kitaichi M, Izumi T, Itoh H. Diffuse panbronchiolitis: correlation of high-resolution CT and pathologic findings. *Radiology*. 1992;184:779–785.

170. Randhawa P, Hoagland M, Yousem S. Diffuse panbronchiolitis in North America. *Am J Surg Pathol*. 1991;15:43–47.

171. Izumi T. Diffuse panbronchiolitis. *Chest*. 1991;100(3):596–597.

172. Kitaichi M. Pathology of panbronchiolitis from the viewpoint of differential diagnosis. In: Grassi C, Rizzato G, Pozzi E, eds. *Sarcoidosis*. Amsterdam: Elsevier Scientific; 1988:741–746.

173. Akira M, Kitatani F, Lee YS, et al. Diffuse panbronchiolitis: evaluation with high-resolution CT. *Radiology*. 1988;168:433–438.

174. Homma H, Yamanaka A, Tanimoto S, et al. Diffuse panbronchiolitis. *Chest*. 1983;83:63–69.

175. Keicho N, Ohashi J, Tamiya G, et al. Fine localization of a major disease-susceptibility locus for diffuse panbronchiolitis. *Am J Hum Genet*. 2000;66(2):501–507.

176. Matsuzaka Y, Tounai K, Denda A, et al. Identification of novel candidate genes in the diffuse panbronchiolitis critical region of the class I human MHC. *Immunogenetics*. 2002;54(5):301–309.

177. Valdivia-Arenas MA, Soriano AO, Arteaga RB. Constrictive bronchiolitis after treatment of colon cancer with 5-fluorouracil. *Chemotherapy*. 2007;53(5):316–319.

178. Radzikowska E, Pawlowski J, Chabowski M, Langfort R. Constrictive bronchiolitis obliterans in patient with Castleman's disease. *Monaldi Arch Chest Dis*. 2005;63(4):226–229.

Pneumoconioses

Kelly J. Butnor, MD, and Victor L. Roggli, MD

Overview and General Considerations

Pneumoconiosis literally means dust in the lung, and the term has come to refer to disease of the lung related to the inhalation of dusts. Pneumoconioses are for the most part due to the inhalation of inorganic dusts in the workplace, and the reaction of the lungs to these dusts is generally fibrosis. These diseases typically evolve over several decades, although there are some exceptions to this rule. The pathologic findings in these conditions can resemble those in other fibrotic and granulomatous disorders of the lung, so the pathologist must be familiar with their diagnostic features. Although no specific treatment is available for most of these disorders, proper diagnosis is crucial for accurate determination of prognosis and, when indicated, compensation.

The toxicity and corresponding fibrogenicity of inorganic particulates are related to both the nature of the dust and the nature of the host response.[1] One important feature of particle toxicity is the aerodynamic diameter, with particles in the size range of 1 to 5 µm having the highest probability of deposition and retention within the respiratory tract. In addition, the total inhaled dose and intrinsic properties of the dust are important determinants of fibrosis. For example, crystalline silica is highly fibrogenic, whereas carbon is an innocuous "nuisance" dust. Host factors include efficiency of clearance mechanisms and individual susceptibility. Many of the dusts have a characteristic reaction pattern or appearance in histologic sections, which permits an accurate diagnosis. The silicotic nodule and the asbestos body are familiar examples. Others are associated with a reaction pattern that may suggest the diagnosis, but a careful occupational history or use of supplemental analytic techniques may be required to confirm the diagnosis, such as with berylliosis, in which the histologic findings closely resemble those in sarcoidosis.

Analytic electron microscopy provides a powerful tool for identification of dusts in lung tissue samples, and these methods are emphasized when appropriate.[2] An analytic electron microscope consists of a scanning or transmission electron microscope equipped with an energy-dispersive spectrometer. Electron microscopic techniques may permit the detection of particles too small to be observed by light microscopy. Furthermore, energy-dispersive x-ray analysis (EDXA) identifies the elemental composition of individual particulates, which can be critical to the identification and, in some cases, the source of the inhaled dust. It must be emphasized, however, that the identification of a particular xenobiotic in lung tissue is in and of itself not proof of disease and must be correlated with the pathologic response (if any) to the dust in routine histologic sections.

Types of Pneumoconiosis

Silicosis

Silicosis results from the inhalation of particles of crystalline silica. It is characterized by circumscribed areas of nodular fibrosis that tend to have the greatest profusion in the upper lung zones. Occupations with exposure to crystalline silica are summarized in Box 9-1.[3] In the past, very heavy exposures occurred from sandblasting. This type of exposure has been banned in most places. Soil in the extreme eastern and western portions of the United States is rich in alpha quartz (the most

Box 9-1. Occupations with Exposure to Crystalline Silica

Abrasive powder maunfacture
Boiler scaling
Farming*
Firebrick manufacture
Foundry work
Mining[†]
Molding and grinding
Pottery and ceramic manufacture
Quarry work
Sandblasting
Stonemasonry

*Soil in extreme eastern and western portions of the United States.
[†]Coal, copper, gold, graphite, lead, mica, and tin.

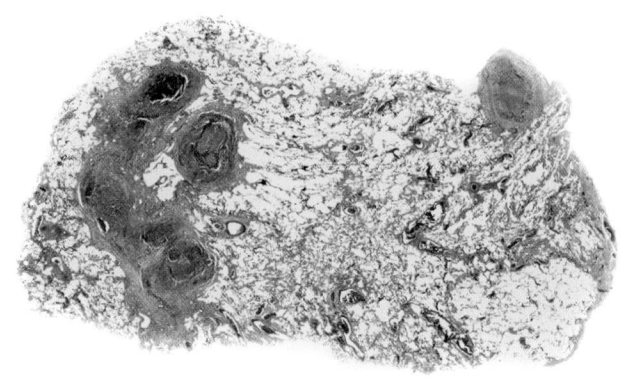

Figure 9-2. Silicosis. At low magnification, silicotic nodules are sharply circumscribed and densely collagenous (Masson trichrome stain).

common form of crystalline silica). Silicotic nodules may be found in the thoracic lymph nodes and even within the lung parenchyma in farmers and agricultural laborers working in these regions.

Clinical Presentation

Patients demonstrate a range of clinical presentations, from asymptomatic with simple silicosis to markedly dyspneic with conglomerate silicosis. In conglomerate silicosis, hypoxemia and cor pulmonale may be fatal.

Pathologic Findings

Silicotic nodules are of firm consistency and typically slate gray in appearance, measuring from a few millimeters to approximately 1 cm in diameter (Figs. 9-1 and 9-2). As the disease progresses in severity, the nodules may become confluent (Figs. 9-3 and 9-4). Areas of confluent fibrosis greater than 2 cm in maximum dimension are the defining feature of conglomerate silicosis. Cavitation may occur within areas of confluent fibrosis and, when present, suggests the possibility of superimposed tuberculosis.

The histologic hallmark of silicosis is the silicotic nodule.[4,5] This lesion is a sharply circumscribed nodule consisting of dense, whorled hyalinized collagen (Fig. 9-5). More loosely arranged collagen bundles

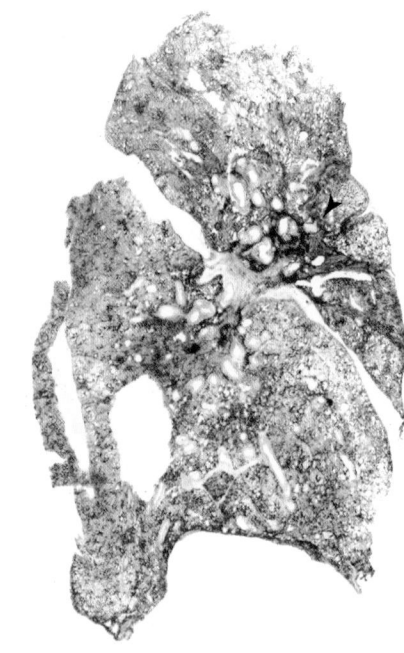

Figure 9-3. Conglomerate silicosis. A Gough-Wentworth section of lung from a tobacco field worker demonstrates confluent fibrosis in the upper lobe (*arrowhead*).

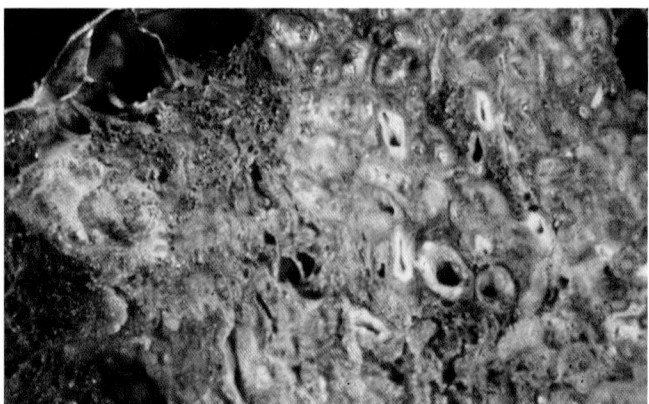

Figure 9-1. Silicosis. In this gross specimen, circumscribed areas of nodular fibrosis are slate gray and of firm consistency.

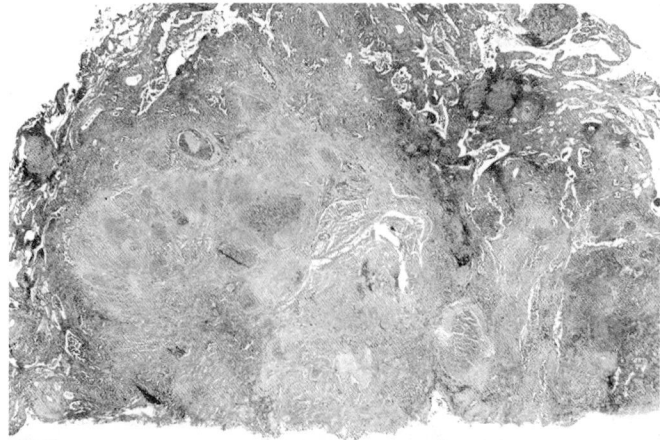

Figure 9-4. Conglomerate silicosis. Multiple silicotic nodules have coalesced, forming an area of confluent fibrosis.

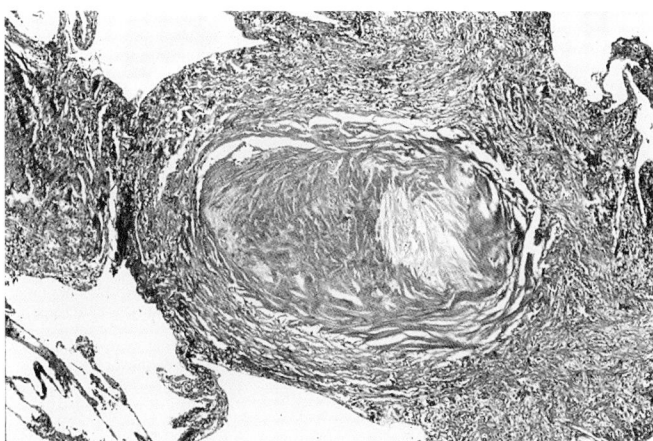

Figure 9-5. Silicosis. This silicotic nodule demonstrates the typical whorled appearance. Macrophages are present at the periphery of the nodule.

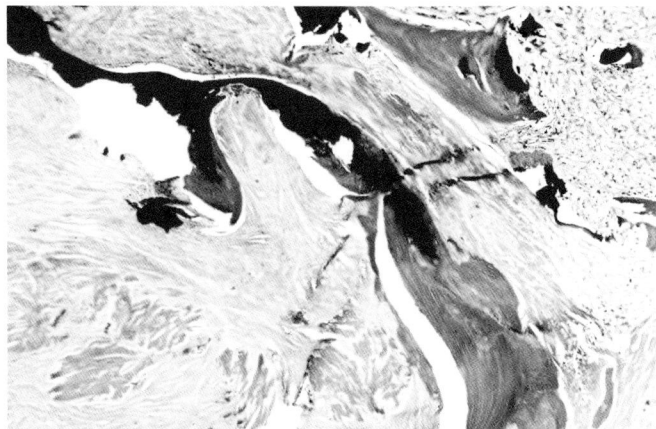

Figure 9-6. Silicosis. A mature silicotic nodule exhibits partial ossification.

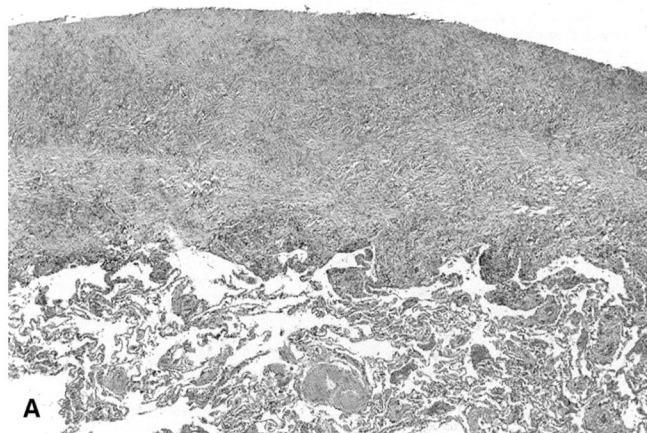

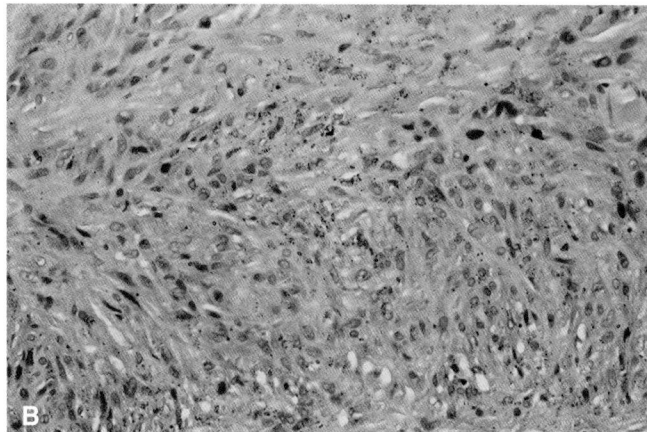

Figure 9-8. Pleural silicosis. **A,** Pleural involvement sometimes manifests as dense fibrosis. **B,** At higher magnification, a cellular area consisting of fibroblasts and histiocytes is evident. Polarizing microscopy showed numerous birefringent particulates.

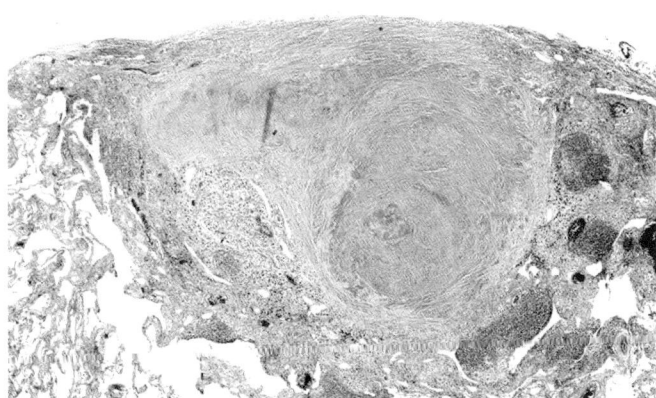

Figure 9-7. Silicosis. The lung parenchyma underlying the pleura is a common location for silicotic nodules.

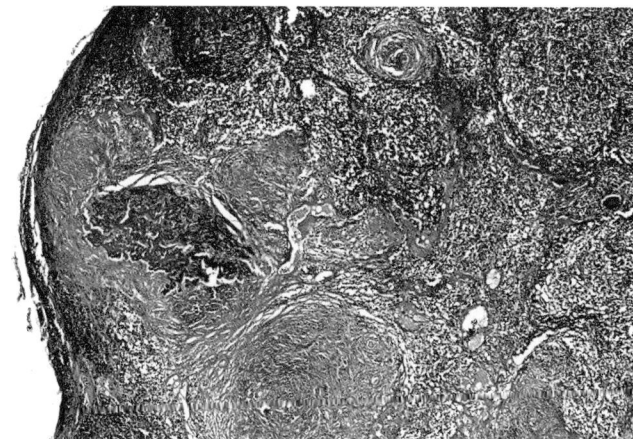

Figure 9-9. Silicosis. Silicotic nodules within a lymph node characteristically contain centrally dense, hyalinized collagen surrounded by concentric whorls of more loosely arranged collagen bundles.

are typically found at the periphery of the nodule. In recently formed lesions, macrophages form a mantle around the fibrotic center. Longstanding lesions may be calcified or even ossified (Fig. 9-6). The nodules may be present anywhere within the lung parenchyma but typically are most numerous in the upper lung zones. Not uncommonly, they are concentrated beneath the pleura (Fig. 9-7). There may also

be extensive pleural fibrosis[6] (Fig. 9-8). Nodules are frequently also present within hilar lymph nodes (Fig. 9-9). In patients with extremely high exposures to very fine silica particles, the pattern of resultant lung injury may closely resemble that in pulmonary alveolar proteinosis, characterized by the presence of granular eosinophilic material filling the alveoli, alveolar ducts, and bronchioles (Fig. 9-10). Cholesterol

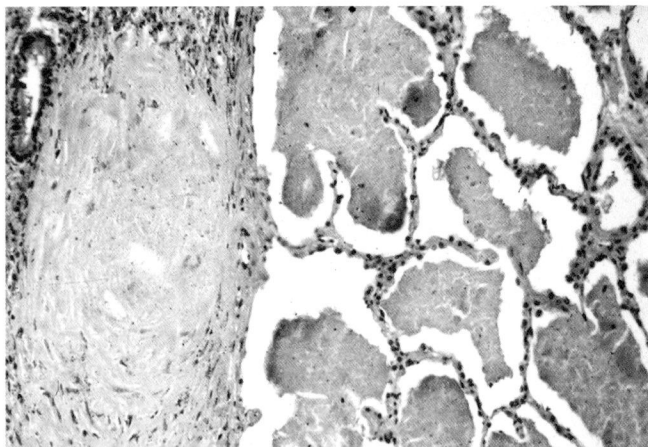

Figure 9-10. Acute silicosis. Granular eosinophilic material fills alveoli, imparting an appearance similar to that in pulmonary alveolar proteinosis. Note the presence of a silicotic nodule at *left*. (From Sporn TA, Roggli VL. Pneumoconioses, mineral and vegetable. In: Tomashefski JF, ed. *Dail and Hammar's Pulmonary Pathology*, vol 1, 3rd ed. New York: Springer-Verlag; 2008:911–949, with permission.)

clefts may be prominent within the intra-alveolar material. The granular proteinaceous exudate typically stains strongly positive with periodic acid/Schiff with diastase (D-PAS).

Examination with polarizing microscopy shows faintly birefringent particulates within the fibrotic nodules (Fig. 9-11). Larger, brightly birefringent particles, which represent silicates, may also be seen, but these should not predominate (see later section on silicatosis).[7] On scanning electron microscopy the particles appear angulated (Fig. 9-12). Analytic electron microscopy with EDXA reveals peaks for silicon only (Fig. 9-13).

Differential Diagnosis
Silicotic nodules must be distinguished from the fibrotic nodules of healed or "burned-out" sarcoidosis, as well as healed mycobacterial or fungal infections, a classic example being the so-called histoplasmoma. The presence of multinucleate giant cells and the absence of significant dust deposits favor sarcoidosis. Sarcoid granulomas may contain fine needle-like or large, platy birefringent particles, which represent

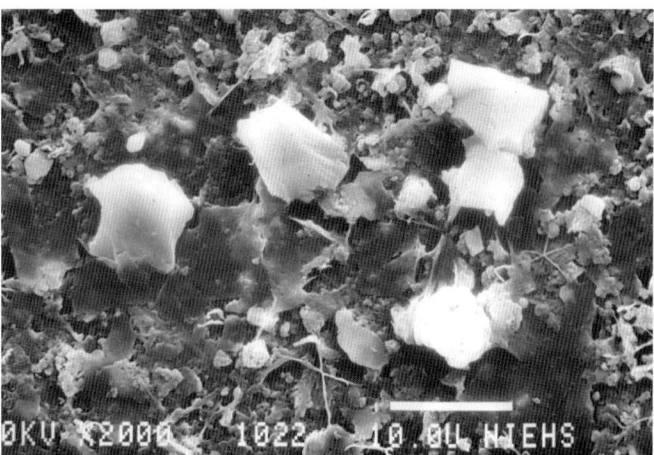

Figure 9-12. Silicosis. Scanning electron microscopy demonstrates angulated silica particles.

endogenous calcium carbonate or oxalate, respectively (Fig. 9-14). These particles should not be confused with the foreign material of pneumoconiosis. The presence of necrosis in association with giant cells favors an infectious etiology. Patients with silicosis are at increased risk for acquiring tuberculosis.[8] Both processes may be present simultaneously. Concurrent tuberculosis infection is most likely to occur with conglomerate silicosis.

Extrathoracic location does not rule out a silicotic origin of a fibrous nodule, because silicotic nodules have been found in the liver, spleen, bone marrow, and abdominal lymph nodes.[9] Extrathoracic involvement, when present, usually occurs in the setting of advanced pulmonary silicosis. The diagnostic yield of transbronchial biopsy in silicosis is low, probably because the firm circumscribed nodules are pushed aside by the biopsy forceps.

Coal Worker's Pneumoconiosis

Coal worker's pneumoconiosis (CWP), also known as "black lung disease," occurs in persons involved in the mining of coal. The nature of the disease is related to the intensity and duration of exposure, host

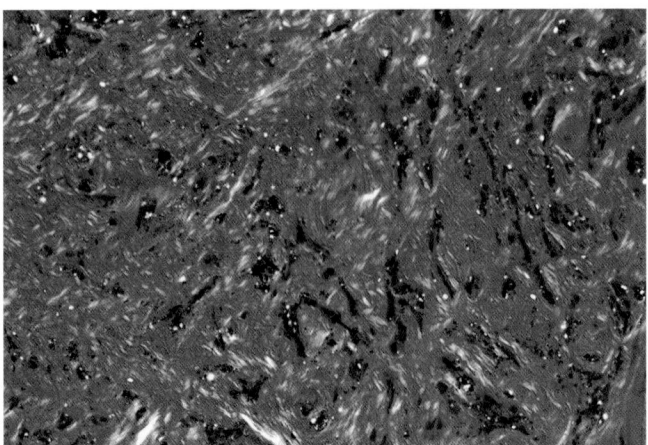

Figure 9-11. Silicosis. Partial polarization of a silicotic nodule demonstrates faintly birefringent silica particles.

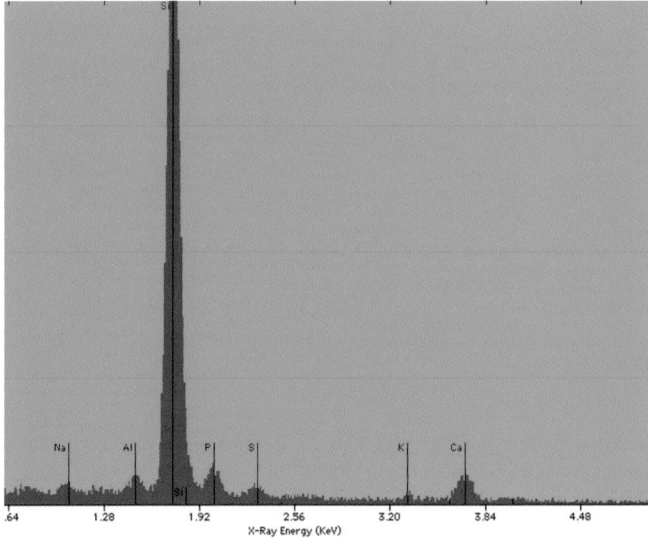

Figure 9-13. Energy-dispersive x-ray analysis (EDXA) spectrum shows a peak for silicon (Si).

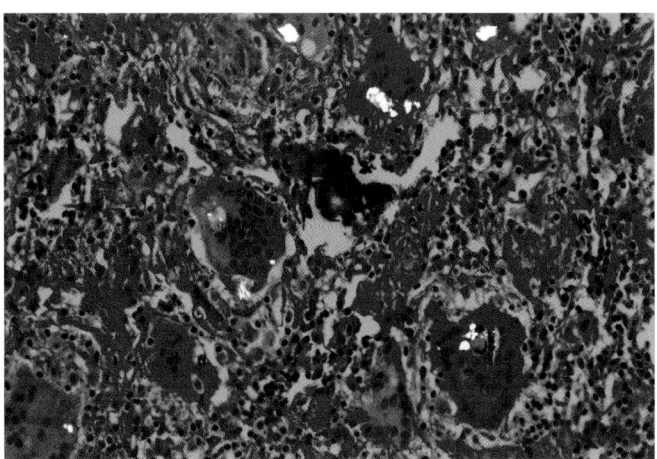

Figure 9-14. Birefringent particles in sarcoidosis. In contrast to silicosis, this example of sarcoidosis contains large platy birefringent particles, typical for endogenous calcium oxalate.

factors, and the specific duties of the miner. Workers involved with drilling in the ceiling of the shaft or constructing communicating shafts are exposed to greater amounts of silica than those working at the coal face. Dust suppression measures have greatly reduced the incidence of progressive massive fibrosis (PMF), the advanced form of CWP.

Clinical Presentation
Patients exhibit a range of clinical presentations, from asymptomatic with simple CWP to markedly dyspneic with PMF. The latter is associated with hypoxemia and cor pulmonale and may be fatal.[10,11]

Pathologic Findings
CWP is characterized by increased pigmentation in the lungs resulting from the deposition of coal dust (Figs. 9-15 to 9-17). Foci of accentuated pigmentation, superimposed on a background of diffusely increased pigment, are present on the pleura and within the lung parenchyma. In some cases, palpable nodules are present within the lung parenchyma and

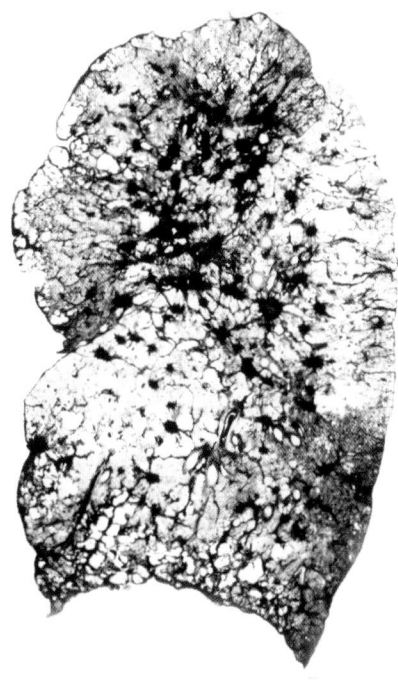

Figure 9-16. Simple coal worker's pneumoconiosis. This thin section of lung demonstrates multiple small, circumscribed black nodules, predominantly in the upper lobe. (From Kleinerman J, Green FHY, Laquer W, et al. Pathology standards for coal workers pneumoconiosis. *Arch Pathol Lab Med*. 1979;103:375–432, with permission.)

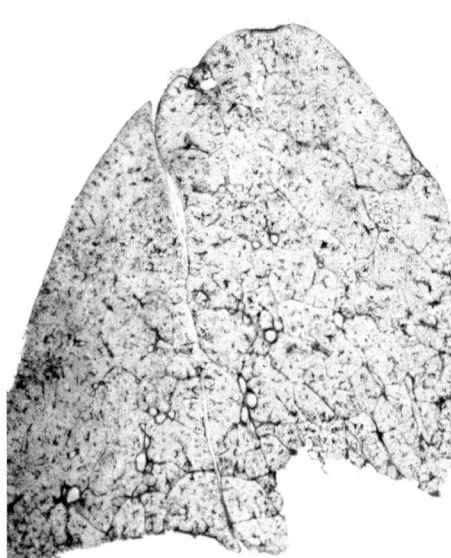

Figure 9-15. Normal lung. A Gough-Wentworth section of normal lung shows scattered minimal accumulations of anthracotic pigment and intact parenchyma. (From Kleinerman J, Green FHY, Laquer W, et al. Pathology standards for coal workers pneumoconiosis. *Arch Pathol Lab Med*. 1979;103:375–432, with permission.)

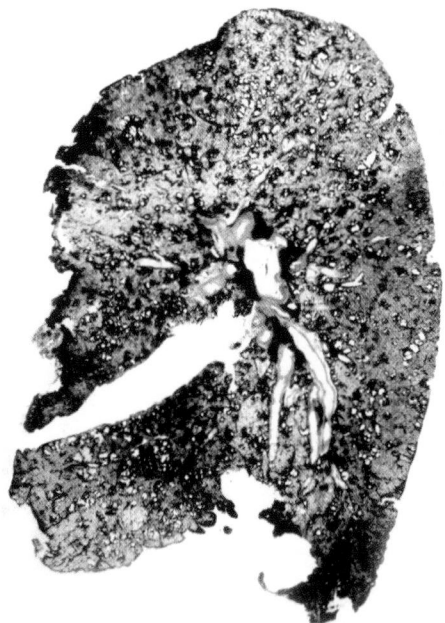

Figure 9-17. Simple coal worker's pneumoconiosis. In contrast to the normal lung, this thin section shows diffusely increased pigment resulting from the deposition of coal dust. (From Kleinerman J, Green FHY, Laquer W, et al. Pathology standards for coal workers pneumoconiosis. *Arch Pathol Lab Med*. 1979;103:375–432, with permission.)

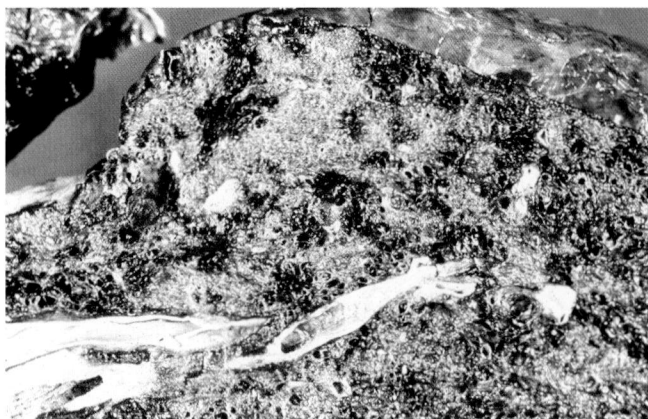

Figure 9-18. Simple coal worker's pneumoconiosis. In addition to diffusely increased pigmentation, the lung parenchyma shows well-demarcated black nodules. Centrilobular emphysematous bullae are also present.

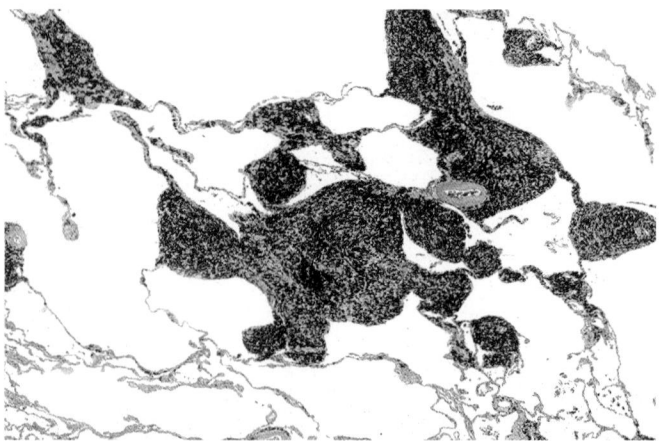

Figure 9-20. Simple coal worker's pneumoconiosis. The coal dust macule is characterized by focal interstitial pigment deposition. In this example, destruction of the adjacent alveolar septa, termed focal emphysema, is also seen.

usually are most numerous in the upper lung zones. These nodules are grossly similar to silicotic nodules, except for being black rather than slate gray (Fig. 9-18). The most advanced cases of CWP feature greater than 2 cm in maximal dimension confluent areas of irregular fibrosis with the consistency of vulcanized rubber, typically in the upper to mid-lung zones (Fig. 9-19). These are the lesions of PMF. Cavitation may occur in areas of PMF and, when present, suggests superimposed tuberculosis.[12]

The histologic hallmark of CWP is the coal dust macule (Fig. 9-20). Coal dust macules consist of discrete collections of interstitial pigment deposition in the vicinity of respiratory bronchioles. Areas of emphysematous destruction, referred to as focal emphysema, are typically present at the periphery of macules. Pigment-laden macrophages may be present within alveolar spaces, and pigment deposits may occur anywhere along the lymphatic routes of the lung, including the secondary lobular septa, as well as in the pleura. Lymph nodes frequently contain numerous pigmented macrophages and may also demonstrate

silicotic nodules. Silicotic nodules may also be present within the lung parenchyma, but unlike cases of pure silicosis, a collarette of pigmented macrophages often surrounds the nodules, imparting a "Medusa head" appearance (Fig. 9-21). Areas of massive fibrosis (Fig. 9-22) consist of collagen bundles that are arranged in a haphazard distribution and intermixed with abundant pigment (Figs. 9-23 and 9-24). Vascular obliteration is common within areas of PMF, and ischemia may be the cause of cavitation in some cases.

Examination with polarizing microscopy typically shows numerous faintly to brightly birefringent particulates within a background of black pigment (Fig. 9-25). This appearance reflects the mixed nature of coal dust, which is composed of amorphous carbon, silicates, and silica. The presence of silica in coal dust is responsible for the formation of silicotic nodules and is an important factor in the pathogenesis of PMF.[13] Ferruginous bodies are sometimes seen in the lungs of coal workers, typically within the alveolar spaces (Fig. 9-26). These may be distinguished from true asbestos bodies by virtue of their black carbonaceous cores[14] (Fig. 9-27). Tuberculosis may also complicate CWP (Fig. 9-28).

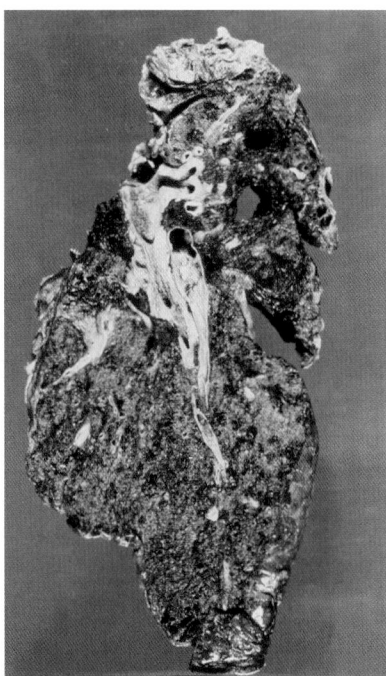

Figure 9-19. Complicated coal worker's pneumoconiosis. The upper lobe contains a confluent irregular area of fibrosis with the consistency of vulcanized rubber. Central cavitation is present.

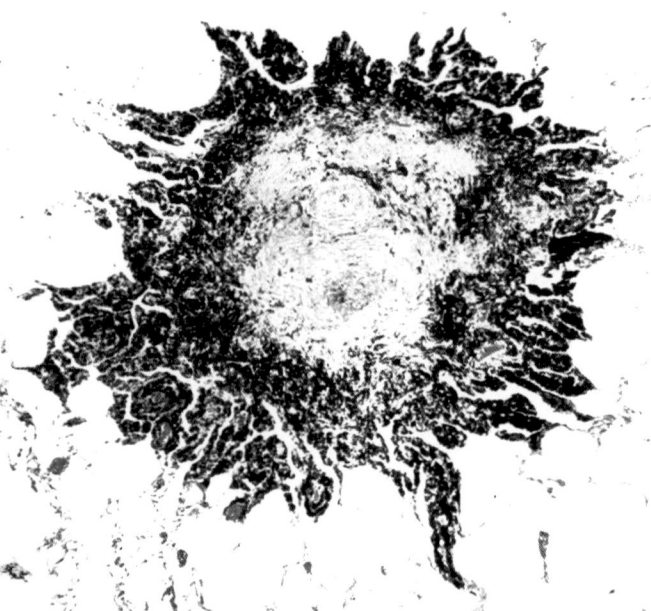

Figure 9-21. Simple coal worker's pneumoconiosis. A collarette of pigmented macrophages gives a "Medusa head" appearance to this intraparenchymal silicotic nodule.

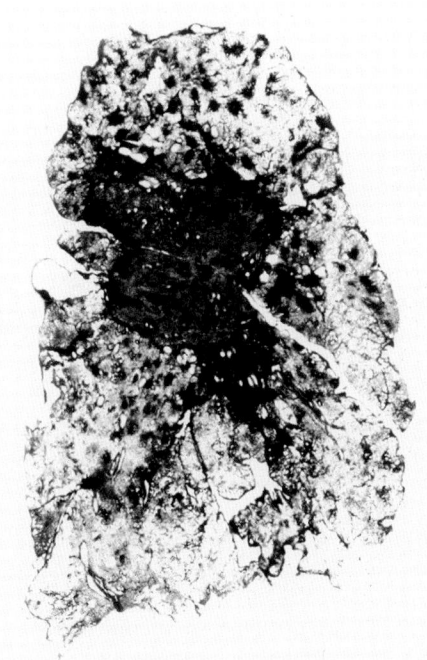

Figure 9-22. Complicated coal worker's pneumoconiosis. A large black irregular fibrotic lesion has destroyed the perihilar lung parenchyma. (From Kleinerman J, Green FHY, Laquer W, et al. Pathology standards for coal workers pneumoconiosis. *Arch Pathol Lab Med.* 1979;103:375–432, with permission.)

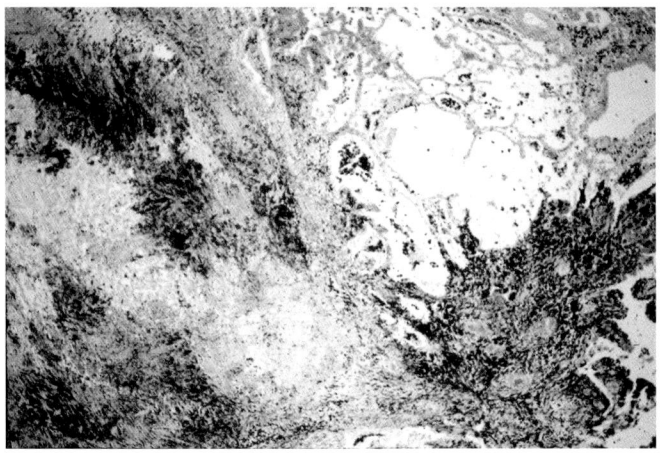

Figure 9-23. Complicated coal worker's pneumoconiosis. In this example of progressive massive fibrosis, haphazardly arranged collagen bundles are interspersed with abundant pigment.

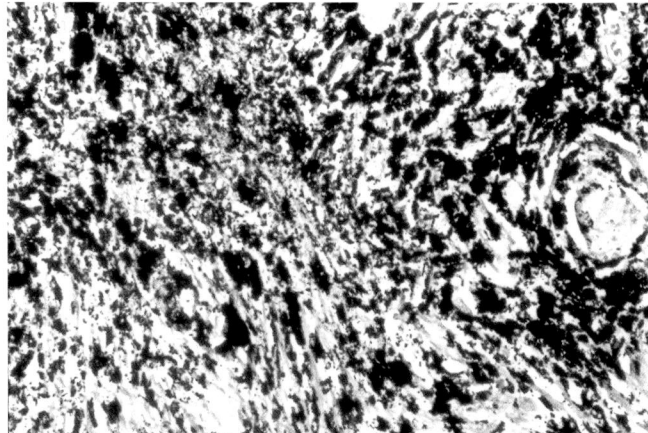

Figure 9-24. Complicated coal worker's pneumoconiosis. A Masson trichrome stain highlights the collagenous composition of a heavily pigmented region of progressive massive fibrosis.

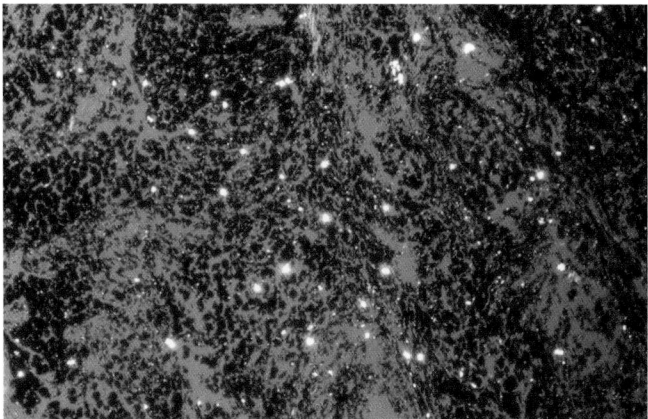

Figure 9-25. Coal worker's pneumoconiosis. Partial polarization shows a mixture of faintly and brightly birefringent particles superimposed on black pigment.

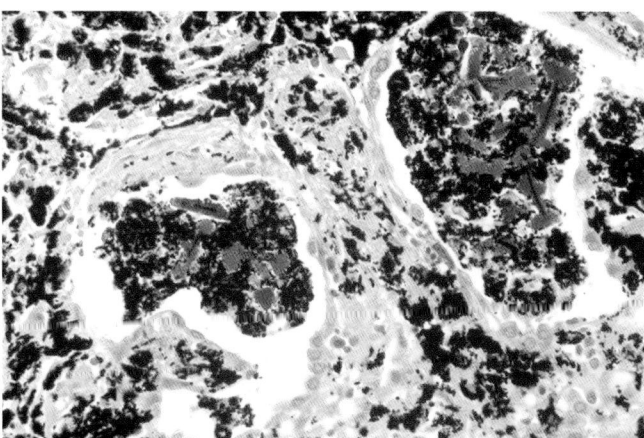

Figure 9-26. Coal worker's pneumoconiosis. Along with pigmented macrophages, this case demonstrates numerous intra-alveolar ferruginous bodies.

Differential Diagnosis

CWP must be distinguished from the anthracotic pigment deposition that occurs in urban dwellers and cigarette smokers, and from graphite worker's pneumoconiosis. The extent of pigmentation in normal persons is a function of environmental exposure to carbon-containing dust and the natural ability of the lung to rid itself of particulates. Distinction from CWP is somewhat a matter of degree, but the presence of true coal dust macules, as described earlier, is indicative of CWP. The finding of anthracotic pigment-laden macrophages within alveoli is also a useful feature, but such macrophages may be absent in miners who have been retired for many years. Graphite worker's pneumoconiosis appears similar to CWP, but graphite is crystalline, whereas the carbon present in coal is amorphous (Fig. 9-29). A giant cell reaction to the crystalline carbon of graphite assists in this distinction.[3] Transbronchial biopsy may be useful in the diagnosis of CWP, showing the typical changes described earlier. However, areas of nodular fibrosis or PMF may be missed by such sampling. Therefore, transbronchial biopsy is not useful for assessing disease severity.

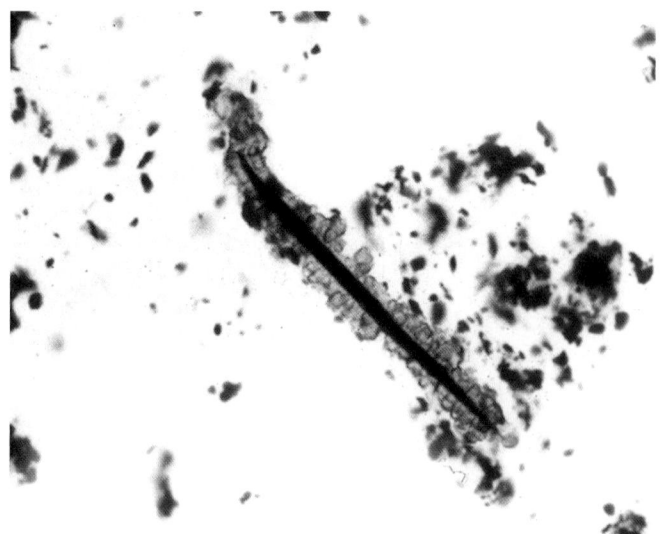

Figure 9-27. Coal worker's pneumoconiosis. At higher magnification, the black carbonaceous core of this ferruginous body (pseudoasbestos body) is evident.

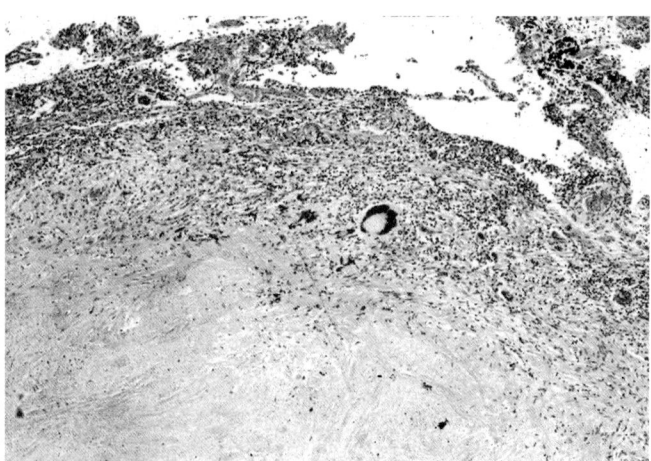

Figure 9-28. Coal worker's pneumoconiosis. A caseous granuloma in this case of coal worker's pneumoconiosis was found to contain acid-fast bacilli.

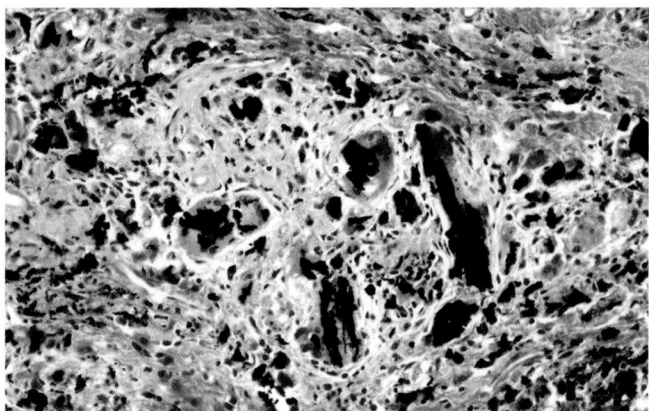

Figure 9-29. Graphite worker's pneumoconiosis. Although somewhat similar in appearance to particulates in coal worker's pneumoconiosis, graphite particles appear crystalline and elicit a giant cell reaction.

Asbestosis

Asbestosis is defined as pulmonary interstitial fibrosis caused by the inhalation of asbestos fibers.[15,16] Substantial and significant exposures to asbestos can occur in a variety of occupational settings, including the mining and milling of asbestos, the manufacture of asbestos-containing products, and the use of products containing asbestos. Occupations that involve the use of asbestos-containing products include insulators, shipyard workers, railroad workers, power plant workers, U.S. Navy or Merchant Marine seamen, oil or chemical refinery workers, construction workers, steel and other molten metal workers, and paper mill workers (Box 9-2). A few cases of asbestosis have also occurred among household contacts of asbestos workers, apparently as a consequence of exposure to asbestos brought home on the workers' clothing.

Clinical Presentation

In patients with asbestosis, the clinical presentation ranges from asymptomatic to severely dyspneic at rest. Hypoxemia and cor pulmonale may prove fatal in these patients. Pulmonary function testing typically shows restrictive changes, and the diffusion capacity is reduced. Patients with asbestosis who smoke cigarettes have a markedly increased risk for developing lung cancer. Pleural plaques in and of themselves are rarely symptomatic, and when present in isolation should not be referred to as "asbestosis." Although the pleural and parenchymal changes caused by asbestos may be recognized on plain films, high-resolution computed tomography (HRCT) is considered to be a more sensitive and specific modality for the radiographic evaluation of asbestosis.

Pathologic Findings

The fibrosis in asbestosis demonstrates a fine, reticular pattern, and the macroscopic appearance of the lungs ranges from normal to severely scarred and shrunken (Fig. 9-30) with evidence of honeycombing.[17,18] Diffuse visceral pleural fibrosis is frequently present and is usually most severe over the lower lung zones. Parietal pleural plaques, which are frequently bilateral (Fig. 9-31), are present in the vast majority of cases and may be calcified. Although diffuse pleural fibrosis and plaques serve as a suggestive indicator of an asbestos etiology of pulmonary fibrosis, the term "asbestosis" should not be applied to these pleural abnormalities when they occur in the absence of parenchymal disease.

Histologically, asbestosis is characterized by discrete foci of fibrosis in the walls of respiratory bronchioles accompanied by asbestos bodies[17] (Box 9-3 and Fig. 9-32). As the fibrotic process progresses, it extends distally to the alveolar ducts and proximally to the membranous (terminal) bronchioles. The fibrosis also extends radially to involve alveolar septa distant from the respiratory bronchiole (Fig. 9-33). In the most advanced cases, honeycomb fibrosis is present (Fig. 9-34), characterized by 0.5- to 1-cm–diameter fibrotic-walled cysts that are lined by bronchiolar epithelium and often contain pools

Box 9-2. Industries/Industrial Facilities with Exposure to Asbestos

Asbestos mining and milling
Asbestos products manufacture
Construction
Glass and ceramic manufacture
Insulation
Oil or chemical refineries
Paper mills
Power plants
Railroad operation/maintenance
Shipbuilding/ship repair
Steel and other molten metal manufacture
U.S. Navy/Merchant Marine

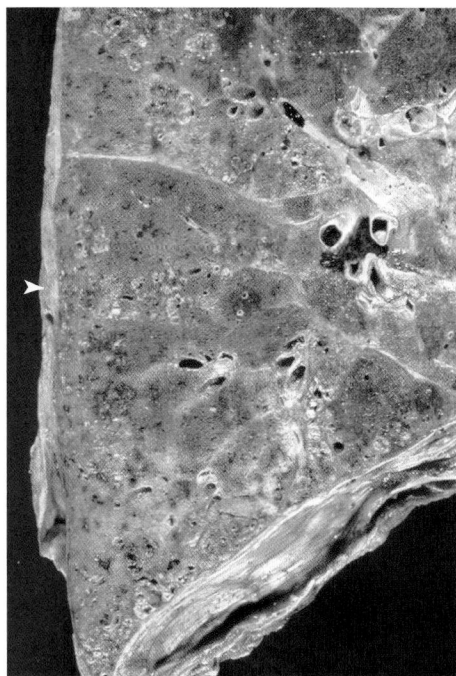

Figure 9-30. Asbestosis. The lower lobe parenchyma shows patchy fibrosis. Visceral pleural thickening also is evident (*arrowhead*). (From Roggli VL, Oury TD, Sporn TA, eds. *Pathology of Asbestos-Associated Diseases*, 2nd ed. New York: Springer; 2004, with permission.)

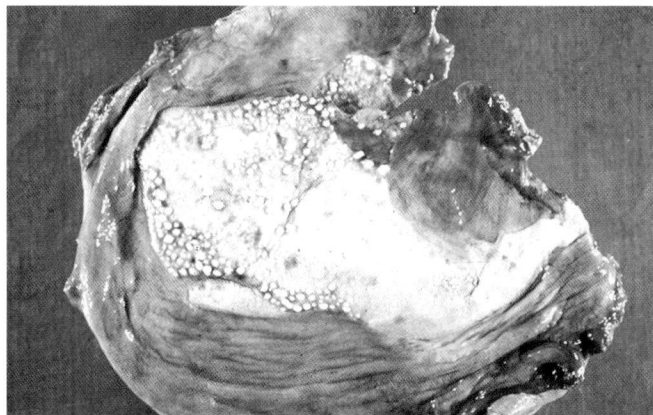

Figure 9-31. Pleural plaque. The gross appearance has been likened to that of candle wax drippings.

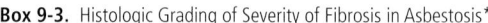

Box 9-3. Histologic Grading of Severity of Fibrosis in Asbestosis*

Grade 0: No appreciable peribronchiolar fibrosis, or fibrosis confined to the bronchiolar walls
Grade 1: Fibrosis confined to the walls of respiratory bronchioles and the first tier of adjacent alveoli
Grade 2: Extension of fibrosis to involve alveolar ducts and/or ≥2 tiers of alveoli adjacent to the respiratory bronchiole, with sparing of at least some alveoli between adjacent bronchioles
Grade 3: Fibrotic thickening of the walls of all alveoli between ≥2 adjacent respiratory bronchioles
Grade 4: Honeycomb changes

*An average score is obtained for an individual case by adding the scores for each slide (0–4), then dividing by the number of slides examined.
From Roggli VL, Gibbs AR, Attanoos R, et al. Pathology of asbestosis—an update of the diagnostic criteria. Report of the Asbestosis Committee of the College of American Pathologists and Pulmonary Pathology Society. *Arch Pathol Lab Med*. 2010;134:462–480.

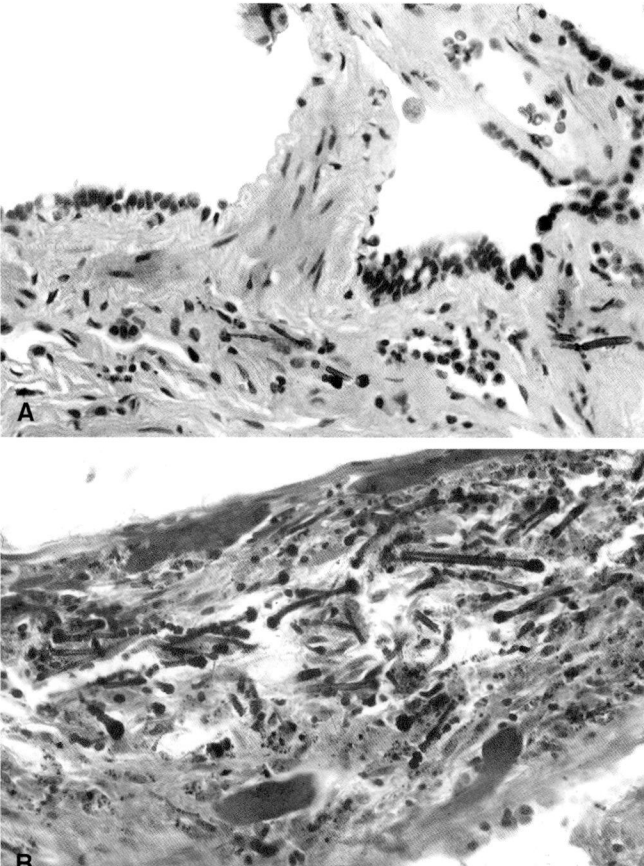

Figure 9-32. Asbestosis. **A,** The histologic hallmarks of asbestosis are peribronchiolar fibrosis accompanied by asbestos bodies. **B,** Numerous asbestos bodies are present within a fibrotic alveolar septum in this case with heavy asbestos exposure. Note the variable beaded, rod-like, and dumbbell shapes.

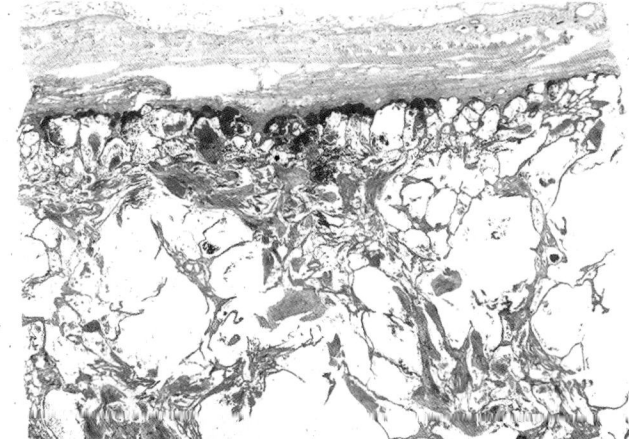

Figure 9-33. Asbestosis. Peribronchiolar fibrosis extends into adjacent alveolar septa. Centrilobular emphysema and visceral pleural fibrosis (*top*) are also seen.

of mucus. Alveolar macrophages are sometimes so prominent as to suggest a diagnosis of desquamative interstitial pneumonia (DIP). In some cases, multinucleate giant cells may be identified, within either the interstitium or the alveolar spaces (Fig. 9-35). Rarely, hyperplastic alveolar type II pneumocytes may contain cytoplasmic hyaline (Fig. 9-36) reminiscent of that found in the cytoplasm of hepatocytes in alcoholic liver disease.

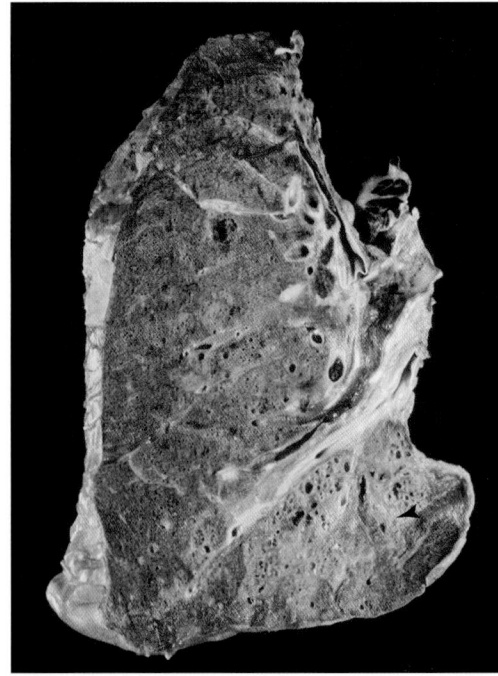

Figure 9-34. Asbestosis. In a more advanced case, honeycombing (*arrowhead*) is seen, in addition to lower lobe fibrosis.

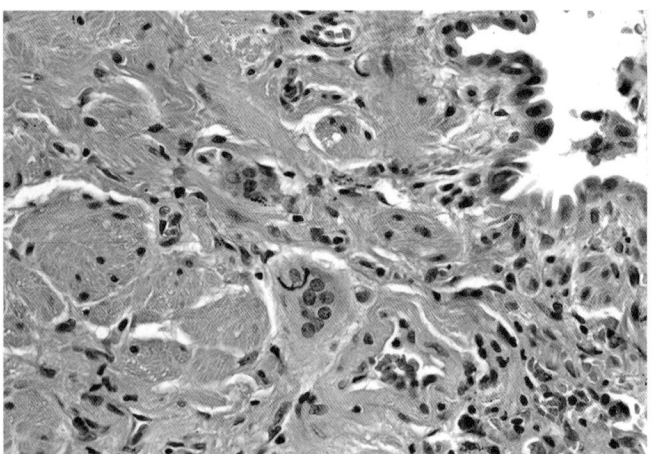

Figure 9-35. Asbestosis. Within an interstitial giant cell lies a curvilinear asbestos body in this transbronchial biopsy specimen.

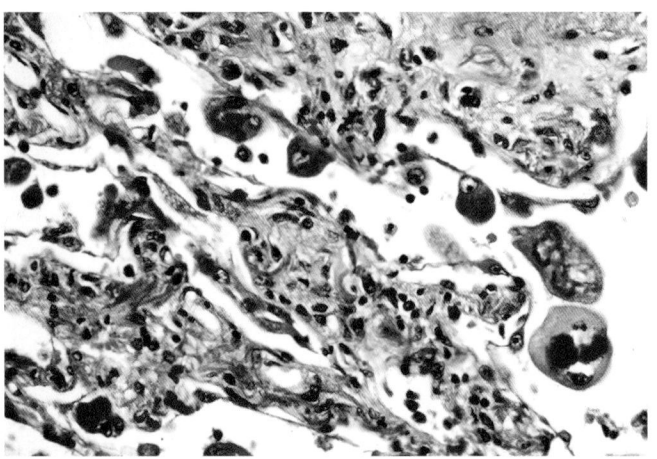

Figure 9-36. Asbestosis. Type II pneumocytes demonstrate cytoplasmic hyaline.

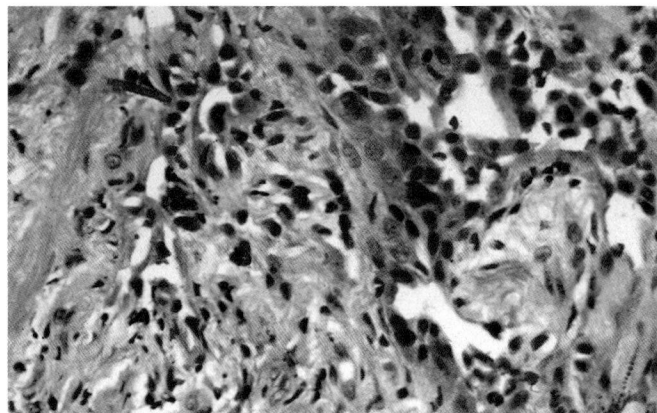

Figure 9-37. Asbestosis. In a transbronchial biopsy, interstitial fibrosis and an asbestos body (*upper left*) can be seen.

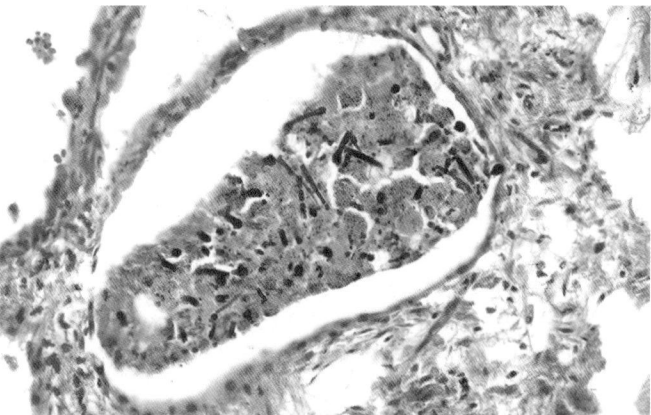

Figure 9-38. Asbestosis. Asbestos bodies are present within an alveolar space in this case of severe asbestosis.

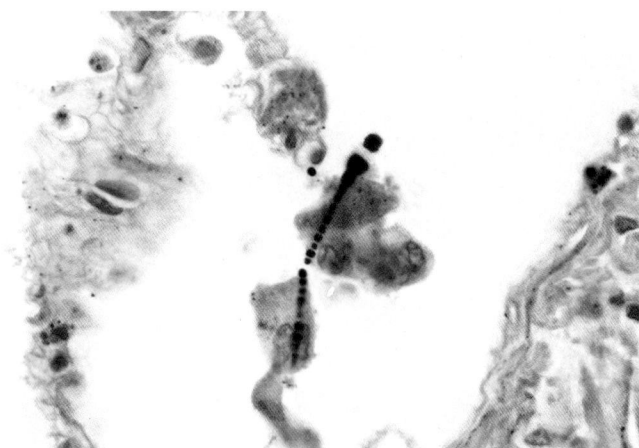

Figure 9-39. Asbestosis. In this iron-stained section of lung, an asbestos body has a characteristic beaded morphology and deep blue color.

The hallmark of asbestos exposure is the asbestos body, a rod-like, beaded, or dumbbell-shaped structure with golden brown coating and a thin, translucent core.[19] Asbestos bodies are typically found in the peribronchiolar interstitium (Fig. 9-37), but, with heavy exposure, may be seen in the alveolar spaces (Fig. 9-38). Detection of asbestos bodies may be facilitated by the use of iron stains, which impart a deep blue color (Fig. 9-39). Asbestos bodies may also be seen in sputum (Fig. 9-40) and in thoracic lymph nodes (Fig. 9-41) of patients with heavy exposure to asbestos. Pleural plaques consist of layers of acellular hyalinized collagen, arranged in a "basketweave" pattern (Fig. 9-42). Visceral pleural fibrosis may show this basketweave pattern or appear as compact layers of collagen. A mild lymphocytic infiltrate sometimes accompanies the fibrosis.

Digestion procedures have been developed for quantifying the content of asbestos in lung tissue (Fig. 9-43). Any of the commercial forms of asbestos (chrysotile and amphiboles) may be identified in lung tissue from patients with asbestosis by means of analytic electron microscopy[20] (Figs. 9-44 and 9-45). In cases in which asbestos bodies are not identified in histologic sections, the fiber burden is typically always more than 2 standard deviations below the mean value in cases with bona fide (histologically confirmed) asbestosis.[21] Polarizing microscopy is not useful for the detection of asbestos in histologic sections.

Differential Diagnosis

Asbestosis must be distinguished not only from usual interstitial pneumonia (UIP) and other forms of diffuse pulmonary fibrosis but also from peribronchiolar fibrosis associated with cigarette smoking. UIP is characterized by honeycomb changes, fibroblastic foci, and the absence of asbestos bodies in histologic sections (see Chapter 7). Honeycomb changes are a rarity in asbestosis, and, in our experience, fibroblastic foci are also uncommon. Pleural changes are much more common in

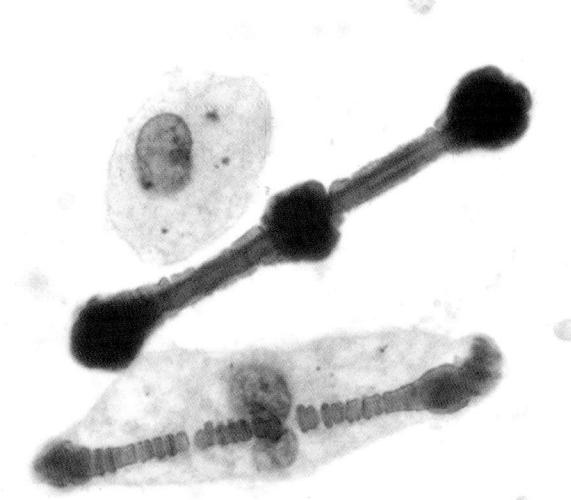

Figure 9-40. Asbestosis. Asbestos bodies in a sputum cytology specimen.

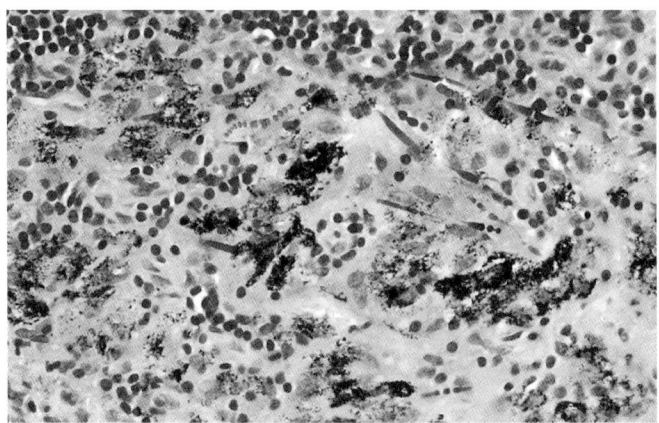

Figure 9-41. Asbestosis. A section from a thoracic lymph node from a heavily exposed individual contains numerous asbestos bodies.

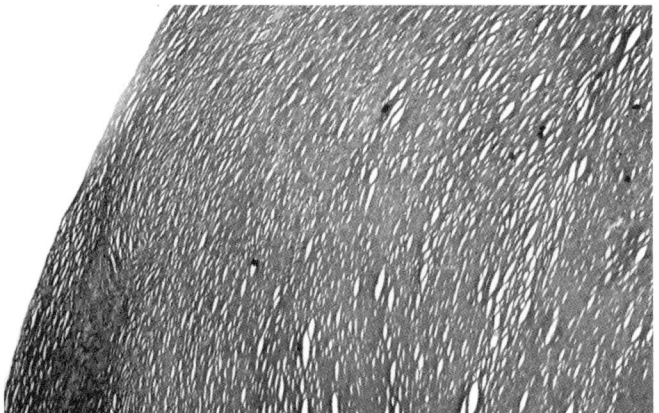

Figure 9-42. Pleural plaque. Pleural plaque showing the typical composition of layers of acellular hyalinized collagen arranged in a "basket-weave" pattern.

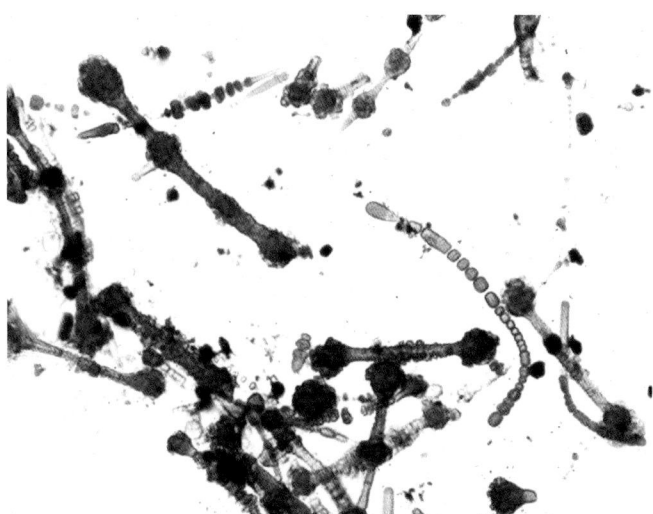

Figure 9-43. Asbestosis. Asbestos bodies from a lung tissue digest on a Nuclepore filter. (From Roggli VL, Oury TD, Sporn TA, eds. *Pathology of Asbestos-Associated Diseases*, 2nd ed. New York: Springer; 2004, with permission.)

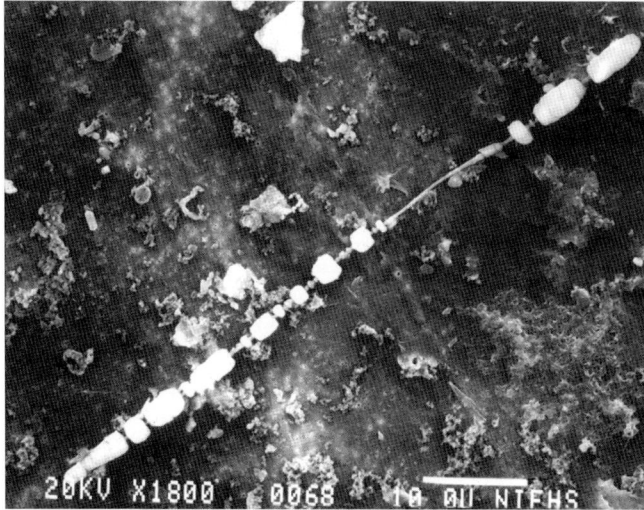

Figure 9-44. Asbestosis. Scanning electron microscopy image of an asbestos body. Note the thin, beaded appearance.

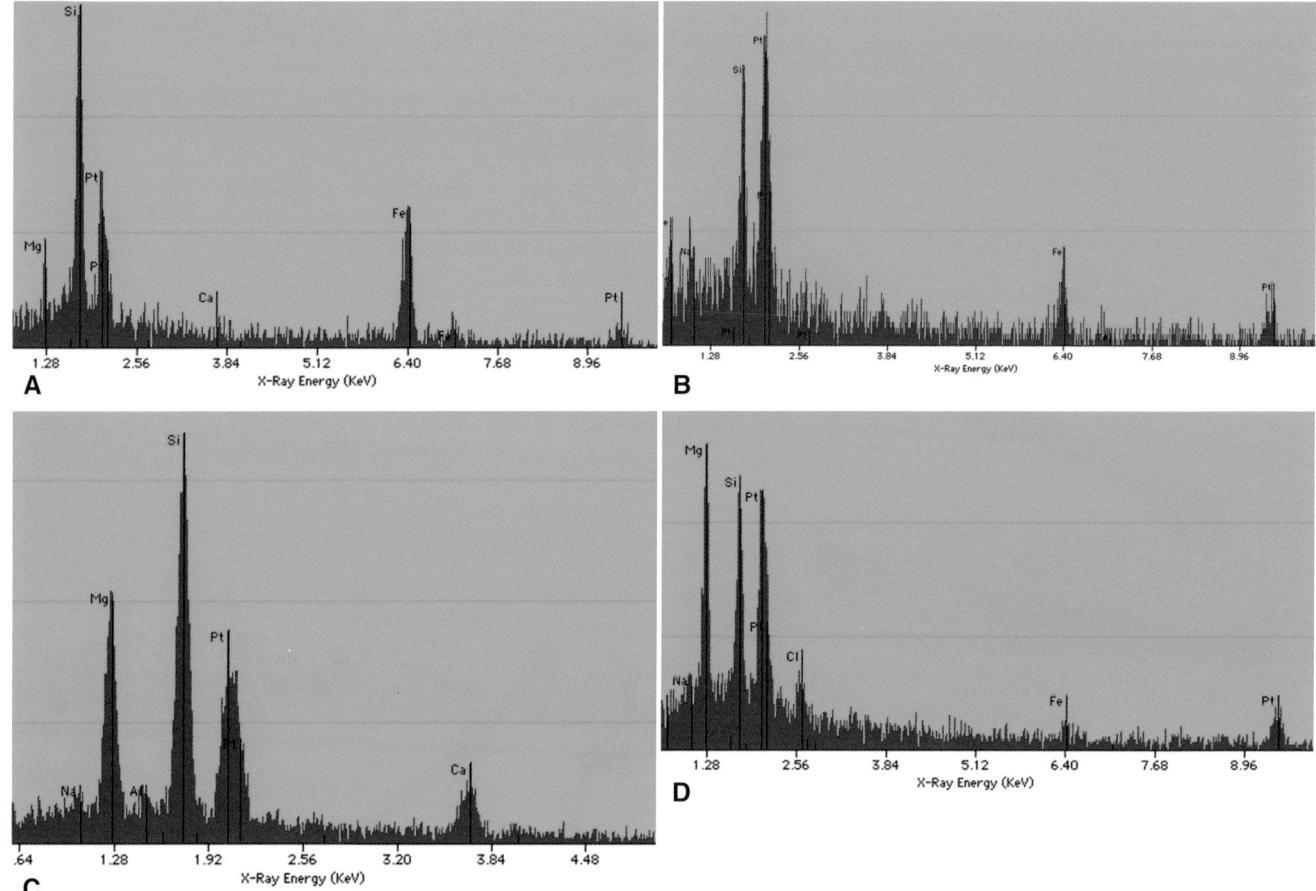

Figure 9-45. Asbestosis. Energy-dispersive x-ray analysis (EDXA) spectra showing characteristic elemental composition of types of asbestos. **A,** Amosite has a prominent peak for silica (Si), as well as peaks for magnesium (Mg) and iron (Fe). **B,** Crocidolite shows a peak for sodium (Na) in addition to silica and iron. **C,** Tremolite demonstrates peaks for silica, magnesium, and calcium (Ca). **D,** Chrysotile exhibits a prominent peak for magnesium with smaller peaks for silica and iron. The peak for platinum (Pt) represents the coating applied to the specimen prior to electron microscopic examination.

individuals with asbestosis than in individuals with UIP. In contrast to asbestosis, the form of small-airway disease known as *respiratory bronchiolitis* that is seen in cigarette smokers and is characterized by peribronchiolar fibrosis and pigmented smokers'-type macrophages tends to involve membranous (terminal) bronchioles and is often accompanied by mucous plugging and goblet cell metaplasia. Asbestos bodies are absent in respiratory bronchiolitis.

Asbestos bodies must be distinguished from non-asbestos ferruginous bodies ("pseudoasbestos bodies") that instead have broad yellow or black central cores (see Fig. 9-27) (also see "Silicatosis" section). The use of transbronchial biopsy in the diagnosis of asbestosis is controversial.[16,20] In our experience, patients with evidence of diffuse pulmonary fibrosis on plain chest films or HRCT scans who have pulmonary fibrosis and asbestos bodies on transbronchial biopsy can be reliably diagnosed as having asbestosis. Conversely, the absence of asbestos bodies on transbronchial biopsy does not exclude the possibility that asbestosis is the cause of pulmonary fibrosis.

Silicatosis (Silicate Pneumoconiosis)

Silicatosis is caused by the inhalation of silicates. A variety of silicate minerals may be encountered in the workplace, usually in the setting of mining and quarry work. Silicates include talc (see section on talcosis), vermiculite, mica, feldspar, kaolinite, bentonite, and fuller's earth.[3,22–25] Mixed dust pneumoconiosis occurs among patients

exposed to a mixture of silica and non-fibrous silicates. Silicate pneumoconiosis has also been described in farm workers in areas with silica-rich soil.[26]

Clinical Presentation

Patients with uncomplicated silicate pneumoconiosis are typically asymptomatic. With extensive fibrosis, patients may be short of breath and demonstrate restrictive changes on pulmonary function testing. In the rare case with massive fibrosis, hypoxemia and cor pulmonale may supervene.

Pathologic Findings

Silicatosis is characterized by irregular deposits of collagen, predominantly in a peribronchiolar and perivascular distribution, associated with numerous birefringent particulates.[5,27] The lungs may be macroscopically normal in mild disease or may be firm and fibrotic (Fig. 9-46). In patients with significant exposure to silica in addition to silicates, silicotic nodules and even massive fibrosis may also be present (Fig. 9-47). Paracicatricial emphysema may sometimes be seen adjacent to areas of fibrosis (Fig. 9-48).

The histologic findings in silicatosis include perivascular and peribronchiolar deposits of dust-laden macrophages (dust macules) (Fig. 9-49). Interstitial fibrosis may also be present, characterized by irregularly contoured, stellate lesions with variable collagenization. Non-asbestos ferruginous bodies with broad yellow sheet silicate-type cores

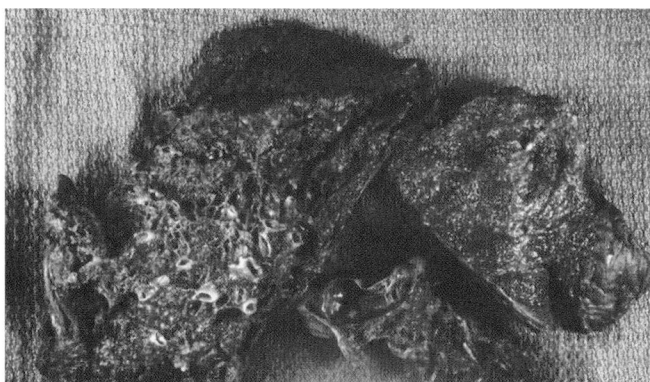

Figure 9-46. Silicatosis. Grossly, this lung from a kaolinite worker shows scattered gray areas of fibrosis in addition to centrilobular emphysema.

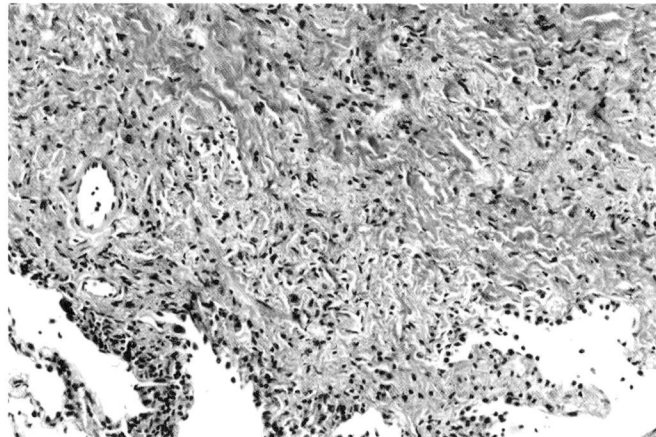

Figure 9-47. Silicatosis. Area of massive fibrosis with deposits of dust-laden macrophages.

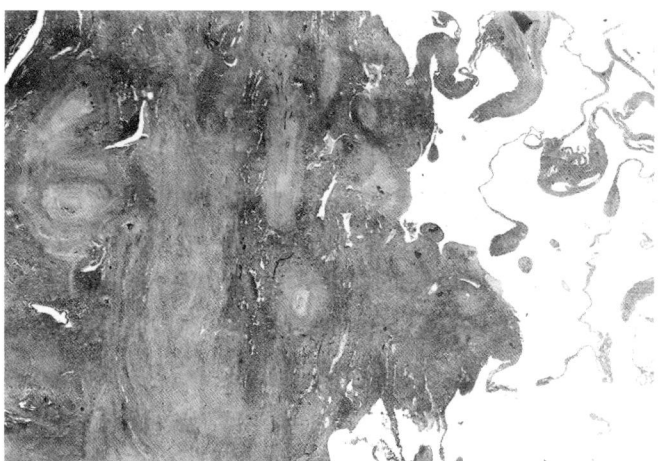

Figure 9-48. Silicatosis. A section of lung from a patient with heavy exposure to kaolin dust demonstrates an area of massive fibrosis with paracicatricial emphysema.

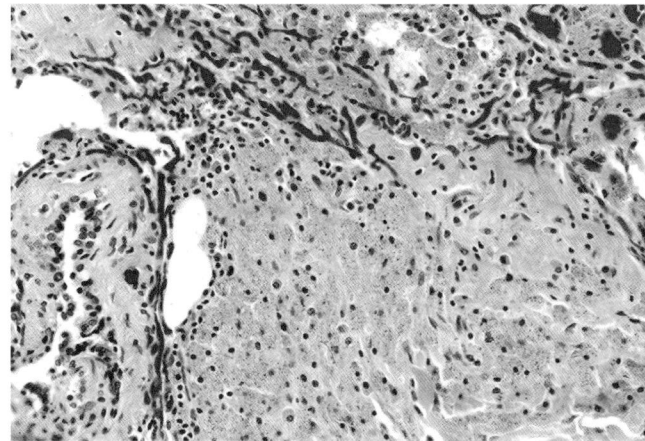

Figure 9-49. Silicatosis. At higher magnification, dust-laden macrophages are apparent.

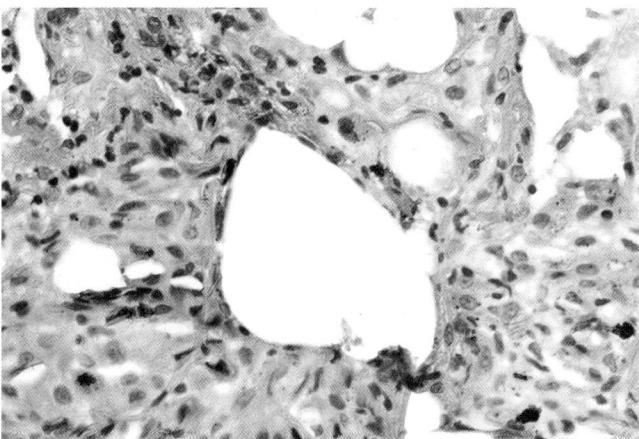

Figure 9-50. Silicatosis. Pseudoasbestos ferruginous bodies accompany interstitial fibrosis in this transbronchial biopsy specimen from a patient who had silicatosis with exposure to feldspar.

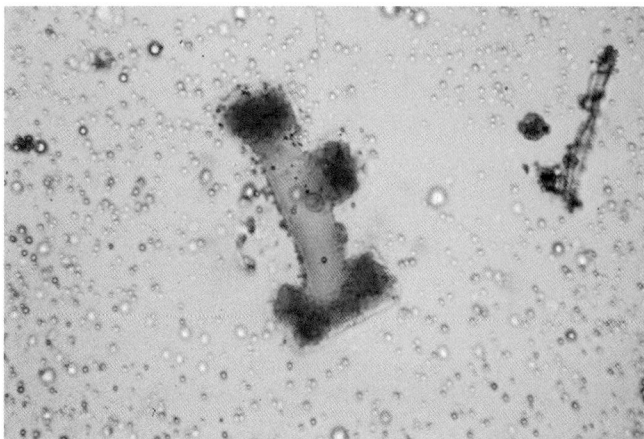

Figure 9-51. Silicatosis. Pseudoasbestos bodies with broad yellow sheet silicate-type cores.

(Figs. 9-50 and 9-51) may be observed in some cases.[14,27] Examination with polarizing microscopy typically demonstrates numerous brightly birefringent particulates (Fig. 9-52) associated with macrophages or within stellate lesions. Analytic electron microscopy shows numerous particulates, most of which consist of silicon combined with other elements, such as magnesium, aluminum, potassium, calcium, or iron.[28]

A special variant of silicatosis is mixed dust pneumoconiosis (MDP), defined as the occurrence of dust macules and stellate lesions producing so-called "mixed dust fibrotic nodules" (Figs. 9-53 and 9-54), with or without accompanying silicotic nodules.[29] For a diagnosis of MDP, the macules and mixed dust fibrotic nodules should outnumber

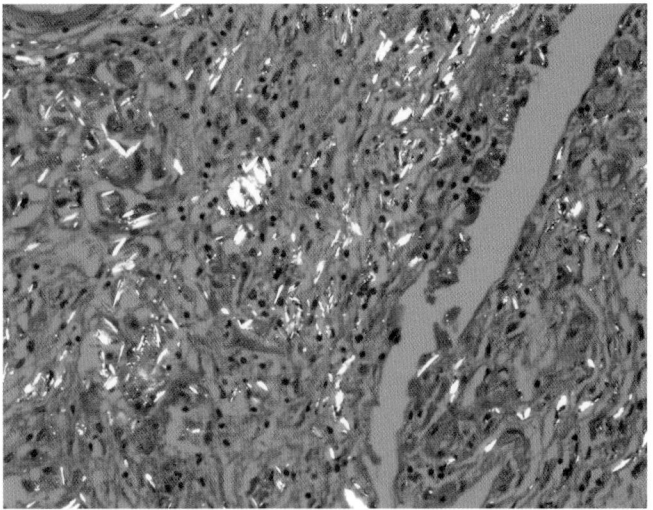

Figure 9-52. Silicatosis. Partial polarization of a fibrotic area demonstrates brightly birefringent silicate particles. (Courtesy of Dr. Thomas V. Colby, Mayo Clinic, Scottsdale, AZ.)

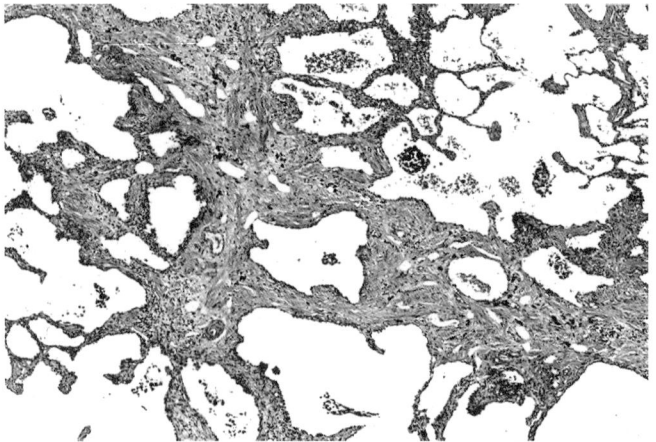

Figure 9-53. Mixed dust pneumoconiosis. The peribronchiolar distribution of fibrosis seen in this case is typical of mixed dust pneumoconiosis.

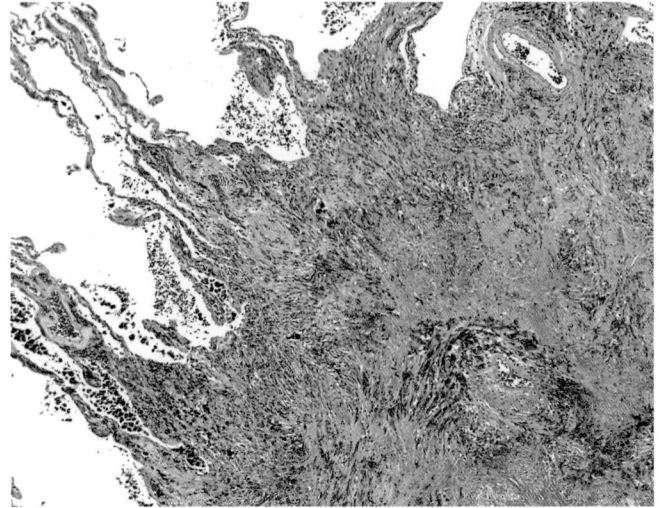

Figure 9-54. Mixed dust pneumoconiosis. Dust deposits are evident in this stellate mixed dust fibrotic nodule. (Courtesy of Dr. Thomas V. Colby, Mayo Clinic, Scottsdale, AZ.)

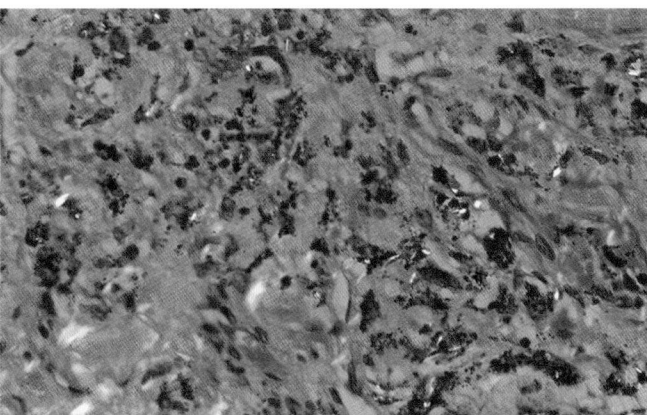

Figure 9-55. Mixed dust pneumoconiosis. Partially polarized photomicrograph of a mixed dust fibrotic nodule showing particles with variable birefringence.

silicotic nodules. If silicotic nodules predominate, the preferred diagnosis is silicosis. MDP can occur in individuals who have worked in the coal mining industry, most typically those involved in the installation of roof bolts in coal mine shafts. Analytic electron microscopy in MDP shows aluminum silicates with varying numbers of silica (SiO_2) particles.

Differential Diagnosis

Silicatosis must be distinguished from silicosis, UIP, and nonspecific interstitial pneumonia (NSIP). In cases with dust macules, mixed dust fibrotic lesions, and silicotic nodules, a diagnosis of silicosis should be made when silicotic nodules predominate. UIP has well-defined features that are not seen in silicate pneumoconiosis (see Chapter 7). It is important to keep in mind that a few scattered birefringent particulates may be found in the lungs of members of the general population, including those with UIP and NSIP. Such findings should not be confused with those in silicate pneumoconiosis, in which numerous brightly birefringent silicate particles are present within dust macules or mixed dust fibrotic lesions (Fig. 9-55).

Talcosis (Talc Pneumoconiosis)

Talcosis, or talc pneumoconiosis, is a type of silicate pneumoconiosis with unique morphologic and clinical features. Talc is used in many industries. Typical exposures include those related to mining and milling, as well as the rubber and steel industries. Exposures may also occur among individuals who use excessive amounts of talcum powder. Talc is a filler in many medications intended for oral consumption. It may reach the lungs by the vascular route in individuals who intravenously inject crushed tablets. Talc is also frequently used for pleurodesis and may be observed in radical extrapleural pneumonectomy or autopsy specimens from patients with malignant mesothelioma.

Clinical Presentation

Patients are often asymptomatic, but fatal pulmonary fibrosis has been reported among talc miners and millers.[30] Intravenous drug abusers may develop pulmonary hypertension, massive fibrosis, or paracicatricial emphysema with spontaneous pneumothorax as a complication of massive intravascular deposition of talc within the lungs.[31,32]

Pathologic Findings

Macroscopically, the lungs in talcosis may be normal or firm in consistency.[33,34] Histologically, patchy peribronchiolar and perivascular fibrosis is associated with abundant dust deposits (Fig. 9-56). The particles within these deposits are needle-like and have a bluish-gray color.

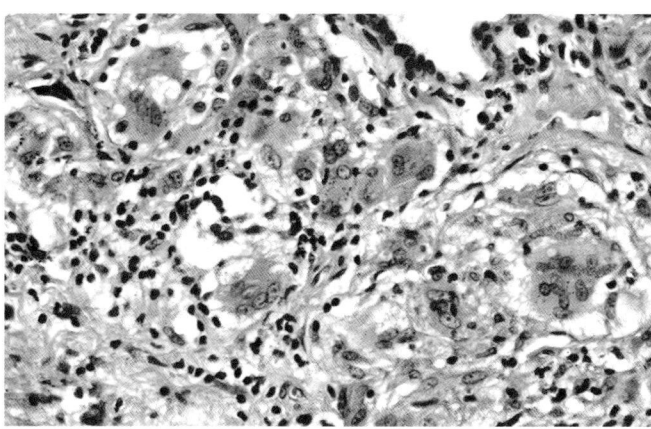

Figure 9-56. Talcosis. In this example, needle-like talc particles are associated with an exuberant giant cell response.

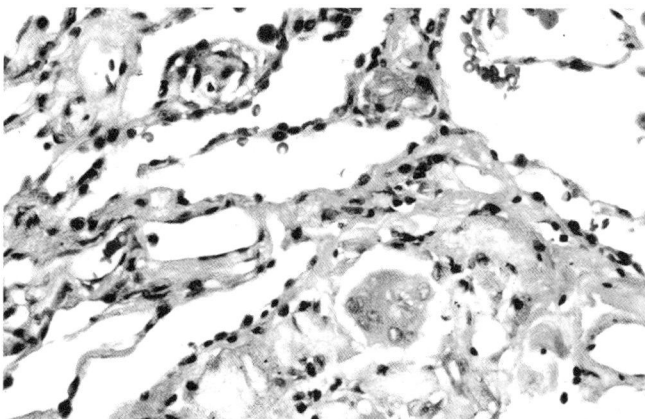

Figure 9-58. Intravenous talcosis. Faintly blue-gray talc particles occupy cleft-like spaces. Note the presence of an asteroid body within a giant cell.

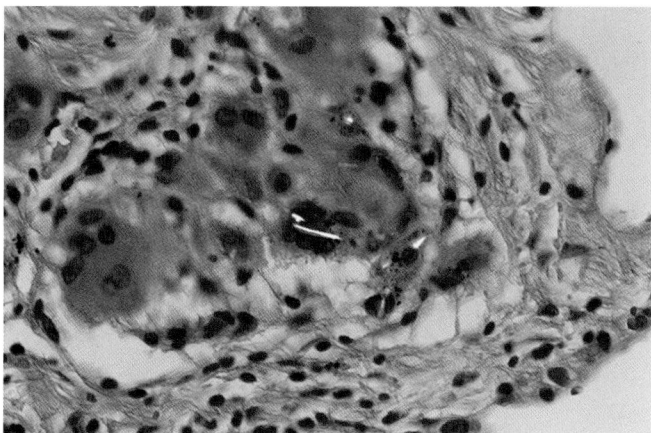

Figure 9-57. Talcosis. Partially polarized view of talc, exhibiting a characteristic needle-like morphology.

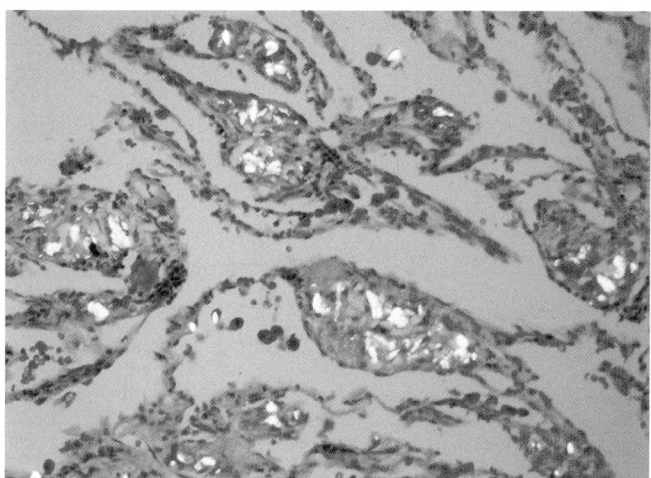

Figure 9-59. Intravenous talcosis. Talc particles appear brightly birefringent under polarized light.

Examination by polarizing microscopy shows numerous brightly birefringent, needle-like particles within giant cells (Fig. 9-57), granulomas, or foci of interstitial fibrosis. Multinucleate giant cells are variably present in talcosis, and in some cases, a granulomatous reaction resembling sarcoidosis is seen. Ferruginous bodies with broad yellow sheet silicate-type cores may also be seen.[14] True asbestos bodies may also be observed in cases in which talc is contaminated with substantial amounts of asbestos (anthophyllite or tremolite). Similarly, silicotic nodules may be seen when there is substantial contamination with quartz.

Intravenous drug abuse talcosis is characterized by the accumulation of numerous talc granulomas within the pulmonary vasculature and alveolar septal walls (Figs. 9-58 and 9-59). Progressive massive fibrosis has been reported in some cases.[31] Concomitant paracicatricial emphysema may be pronounced.[32] Accumulations of talc can also be seen in talc pleurodesis, which is characterized by deposits of talc (Figs. 9-60 and 9-61) within the pleura that are associated with macrophages and are also accompanied by a giant cell reaction.[35]

Analytic electron microscopy in talcosis demonstrates platy particles composed of magnesium and silicon[36] (Figs. 9-62 and 9-63).

Differential Diagnosis

Inhalational talcosis must be distinguished from intravenous talcosis and from sarcoidosis. In inhalational talcosis, the deposits are primarily perivascular and peribronchiolar, and intra-alveolar ferruginous bodies may be observed. In intravenous talcosis, talc deposits are intravascular

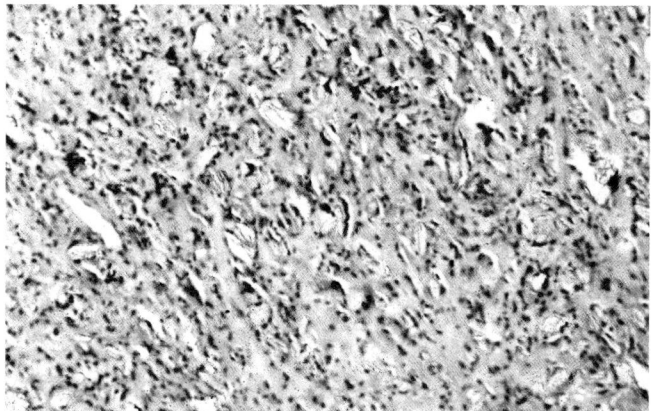

Figure 9-60. Talc pleurodesis. Talc instilled into the pleural space for therapeutic purposes elicited a florid fibrohistiocytic response in this case from a patient with recurrent empyema.

and within alveolar capillary walls. The talc particles in intravenous talcosis are on average larger than those observed with inhalational talcosis. Often they are too large to be deposited by inhalation. Inhalational talcosis producing a prominent granulomatous reaction differs from sarcoidosis in the presence of numerous, long, needle-like birefringent crystals, as compared to the smaller and sparser

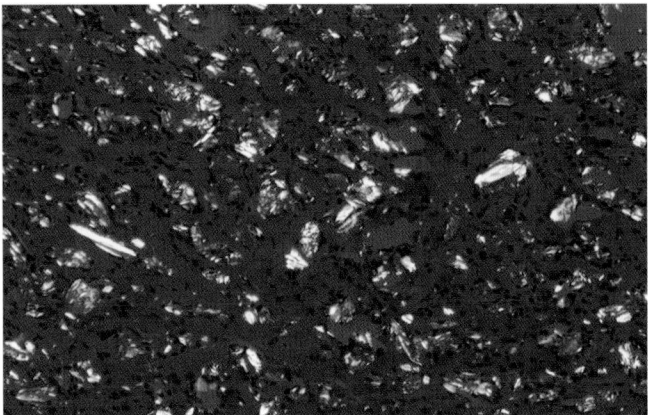

Figure 9-61. Talc pleurodesis. Partial polarization of the case in Figure 9-60 shows numerous platy and needle-shaped birefringent talc particles.

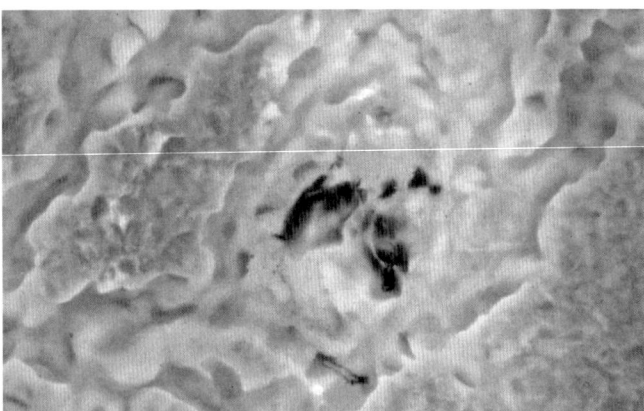

Figure 9-62. Talcosis. In this backscatter microscope electron image, talc has a platy appearance.

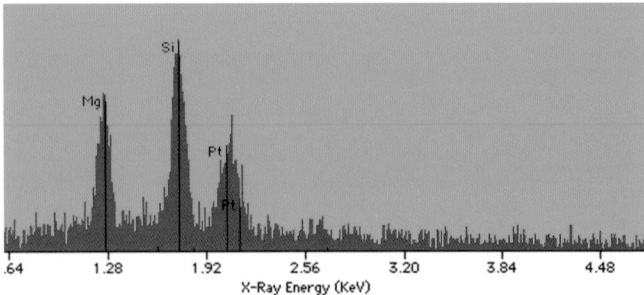

Figure 9-63. Talcosis. Energy-dispersive x-ray analysis (EDXA) spectrum of a talc particle demonstrating peaks for silica (Si) and magnesium (Mg). The peak for platinum (Pt) represents the coating applied to the specimen before electron microscopic examination.

needle-like particles of endogenous calcium carbonate that are sometimes seen in sarcoidosis. In difficult cases, analytic electron microscopy may be required to make the distinction. The fibrohistiocytic reaction to talc pleurodesis may superficially resemble areas of sarcomatoid mesothelioma. The distinction can be made by the observation of foreign body giant cells and numerous platy birefringent particles in talc pleurodesis.

Siderosis

Siderosis refers to the accumulation of exogenous iron particulates within the lung parenchyma. This disease occurs primarily among hematite miners, iron foundry workers, and welders. Miners and foundry workers may be exposed to significant amounts of silica in the workplace, resulting in siderosilicosis, characterized by histologic features of both siderosis and silicosis.

Clinical Presentation

Iron is minimally fibrogenic, so even patients with heavy exposures are typically asymptomatic. Chest x-rays may suggest interstitial fibrosis owing to shadows cast by the deposits of iron pigment.[37] Patients with significant exposures to silica or asbestos in addition to iron may demonstrate clinical features related to the inhalation of such dusts.[38]

Pathologic Findings

Iron pigment imparts a reddish-brown color to the lung parenchyma.[3,39] Because iron is minimally fibrogenic, there is no increase in firmness in pure siderosis. However, in cases in which there is concomitant exposure to significant amounts of silica or asbestos, excess collagen may be deposited (Fig. 9-64).

The histologic hallmark of siderosis is perivascular and peribronchiolar deposition of iron pigment (Fig. 9-65).[40] The pigment, which consists predominantly of iron oxide, typically is dark brown to black, often with a distinctive golden brown halo (Fig. 9-66). The pigment may be found in macrophages or the interstitium, or both, with very little fibrous response. As mentioned earlier, the finding of significant amounts of fibrosis should prompt a search for evidence of exposure to asbestos or silica (Figs. 9-67 and 9-68). Ferruginous bodies may be observed in some cases[14] (Figs. 9-69 and 9-70). These may have black

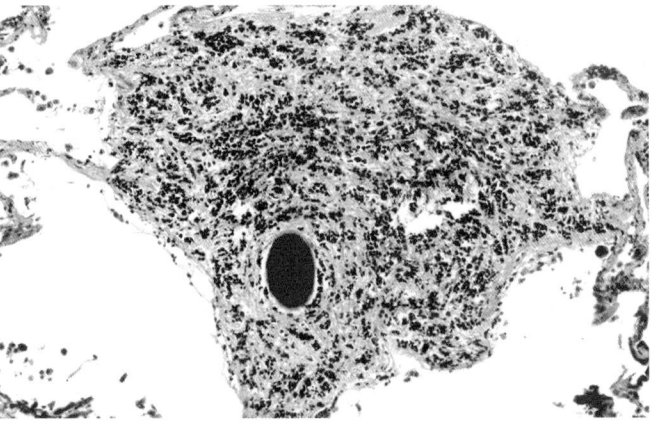

Figure 9-64. Siderosilicosis. This case demonstrates welder's pigment, as well as nodular fibrosis typical of siderosilicosis.

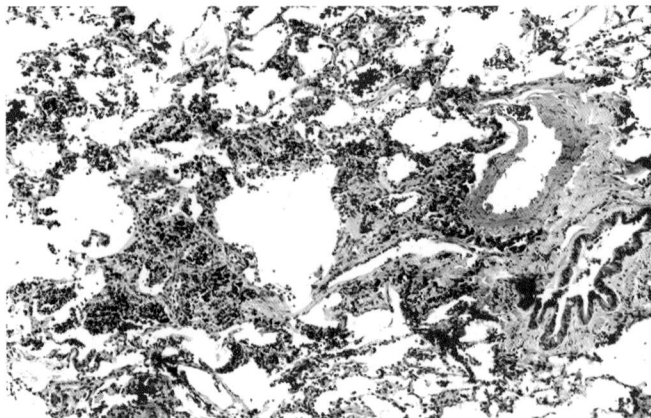

Figure 9-65. Siderosis. Perivascular pigment deposition is seen in this histologic section taken from the lung of a welder.

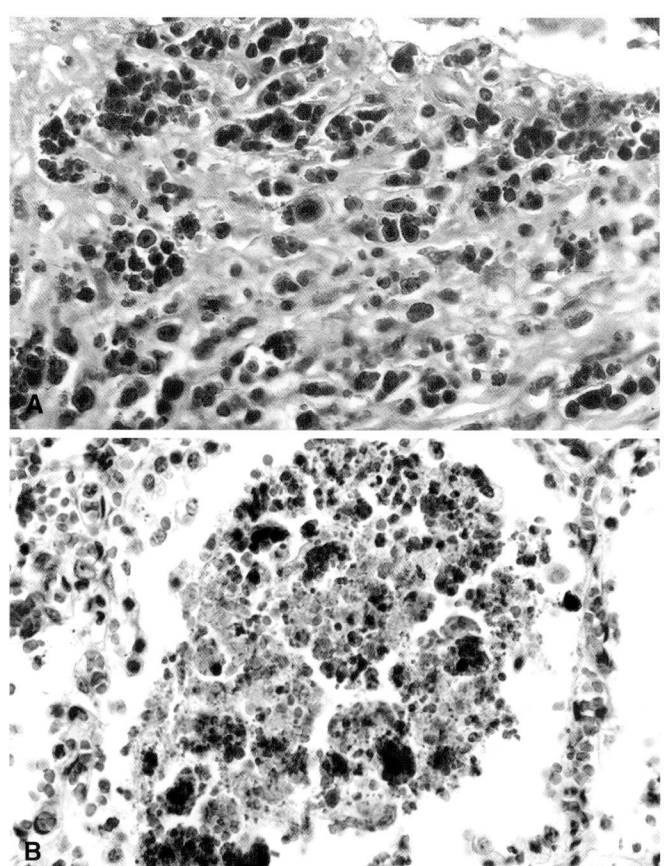

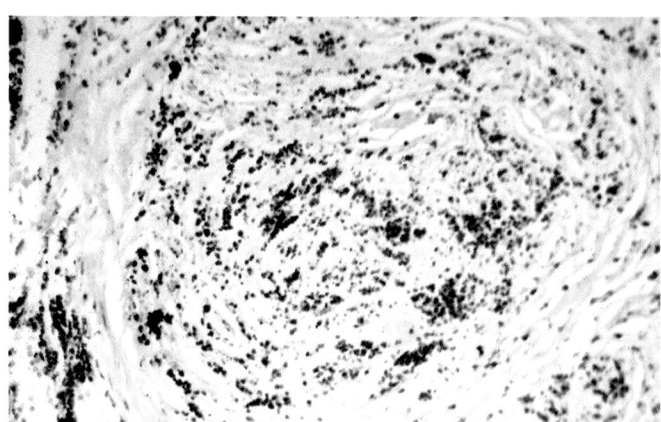

Figure 9-66. Siderosis. **A,** Detail of iron oxide, or welder's pigment, which appears brown-black with a golden-brown halo. **B,** In contrast to welder's pigment, hemosiderin is typically intra-alveolar and lacks black central cores.

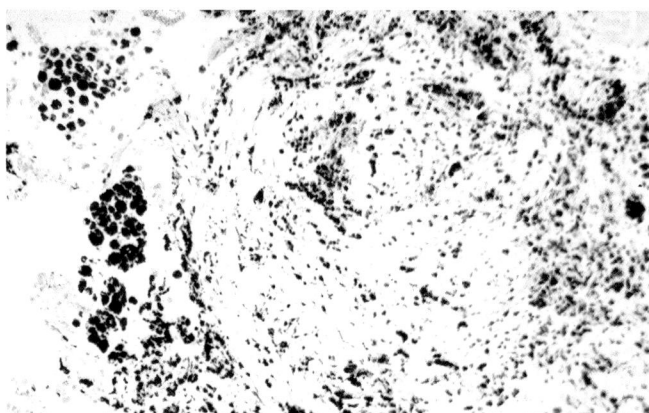

Figure 9-68. Siderosilicosis. The iron pigment appears deep blue in this iron-stained section of the silicotic nodule depicted in Figure 9-67.

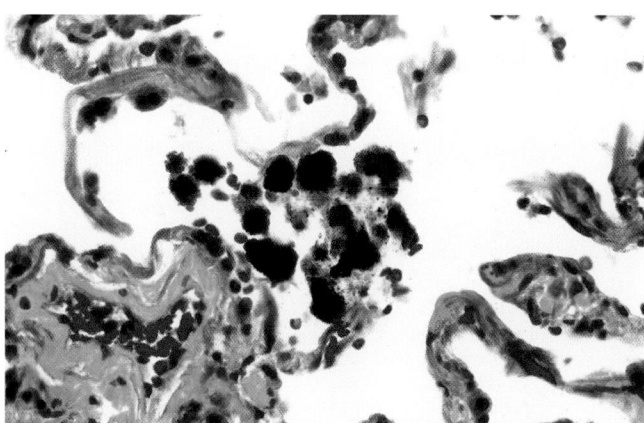

Figure 9-69. Siderosis. Pseudoasbestos bodies with broad yellow sheet silicate cores are seen in this case from a welder.

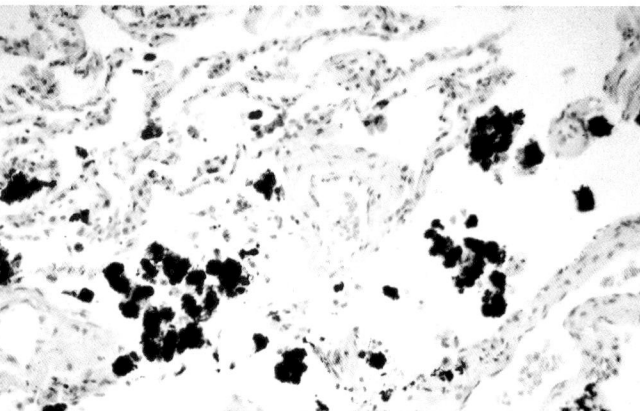

Figure 9-67. Siderosilicosis. A Masson trichrome stain demonstrates the whorled appearance of this heavily pigmented silicotic nodule.

Figure 9-70. Siderosis. Iron stained section of lung from the same patient as in Figure 9-69 demonstrates numerous pseudoasbestos bodies.

Differential Diagnosis

Siderosis must be distinguished from chronic passive congestion of the lungs, and from anthracosis (perivascular and peribronchiolar deposits of anthracotic pigment). Chronic passive congestion manifests as intra-alveolar accumulation of numerous hemosiderin-laden macrophages. Although both hemosiderin and exogenous iron pigment stain with Prussian blue, hemosiderin lacks the dark brown to black centers characteristic of iron oxide. At low magnification, iron oxide deposits may resemble anthracotic pigment. However, anthracotic pigment is black throughout, lacking the golden brown rim characteristic of iron oxide.

iron oxide cores, particularly in iron foundry workers (Fig. 9-71), or broad yellow sheet silicate cores in welders. True asbestos bodies may also be observed if there has been significant exposure to asbestos, as with shipyard welders.

Iron oxide pigment is typically nonrefringent when viewed with polarizing microscopy. Analytic electron microscopy demonstrates spherical particles with prominent peaks for iron (Figs. 9-72 and 9-73).

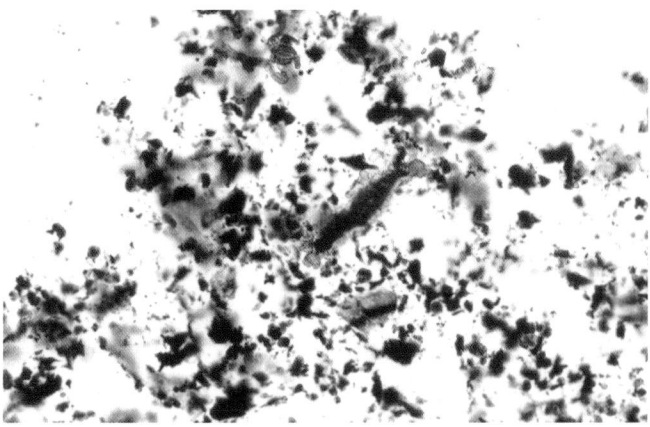

Figure 9-71. Siderosis. Pseudoasbestos body on a tissue digestion filter from the lung of an iron foundry worker. Note the stout, irregularly shaped black iron oxide core.

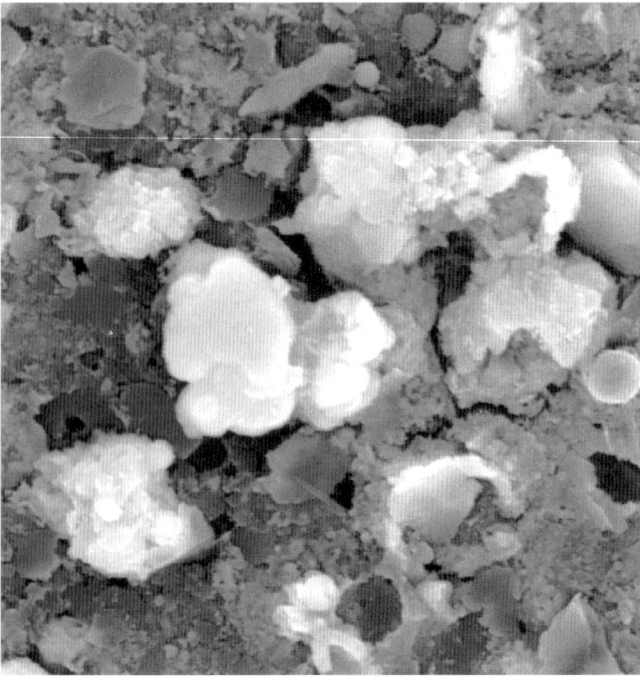

Figure 9-72. Siderosis. Scanning electron micrograph of iron oxide particles from a welder's lung.

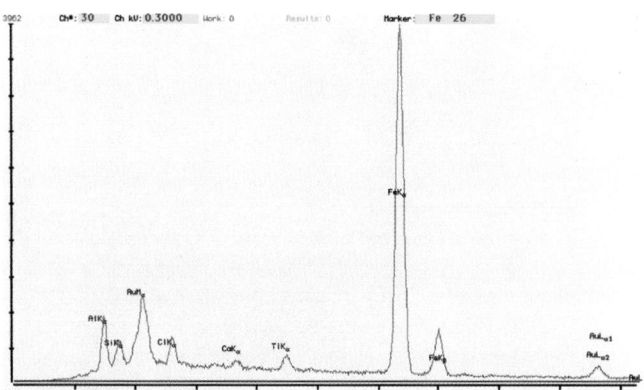

Figure 9-73. Siderosis. Energy-dispersive x-ray analysis (EDXA) spectrum of iron oxide particles, showing predominant peak for iron (Fe).

Aluminosis

Aluminosis is a pneumoconiosis caused by the inhalation of aluminum-containing dusts. Although aluminum is relatively ubiquitous within the environment, aluminosis is a rare disease. Hypersensitivity to aluminum is believed to play a role in the pathogenesis of aluminosis. Substantial exposure to aluminum-containing dust may occur in the setting of aluminum smelting, manufacture of aluminum oxide (corundum) abrasives, aluminum polishing, and aluminum arc-welding.[41–43]

Clinical Presentation

Aluminosis in which interstitial fibrosis is the dominant tissue reaction may manifest as dyspnea on exertion and restrictive changes on pulmonary function testing. Fatal cases with severe interstitial fibrosis have been reported.[43]

Pathologic Findings

Macroscopically, the lung parenchyma in aluminosis ranges from essentially normal to heavy and grayish black with dense fibrotic areas scattered throughout[3] (Fig. 9-74). A metallic sheen, resembling tarnished aluminum, has been described in some cases.

Histologic examination discloses perivascular and peribronchiolar accumulations of dust-laden macrophages (Fig. 9-75). The dust is refractile and gray to brown (Fig. 9-76). Tissue reaction to aluminum ranges in degree from nil to interstitial fibrosis to granulomatous

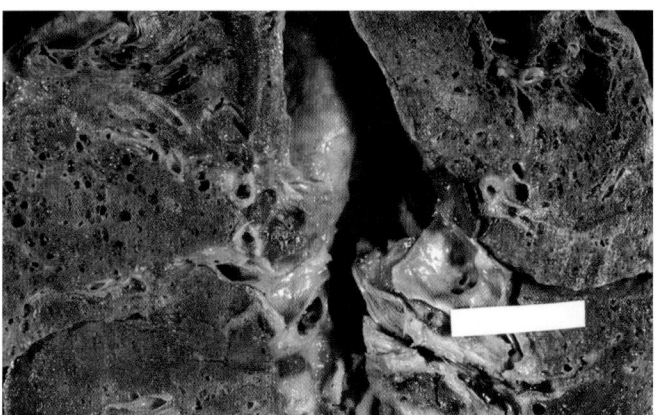

Figure 9-74. Aluminosis. Scattered areas of fibrosis are present in the lungs of this aluminum arc welder.

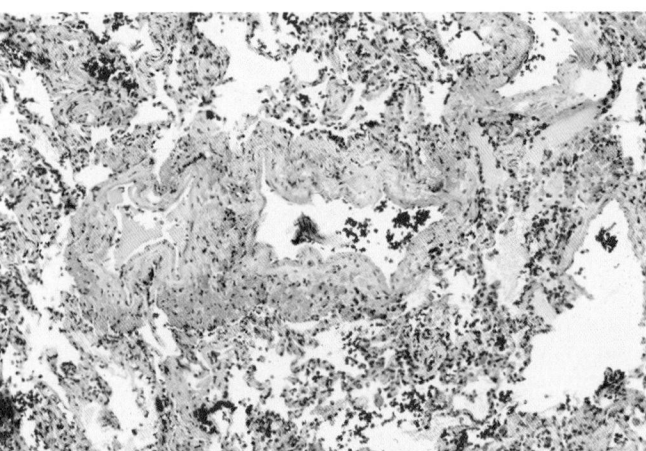

Figure 9-75. Aluminosis. An accumulation of dust-laden macrophages surrounds a pulmonary vessel.

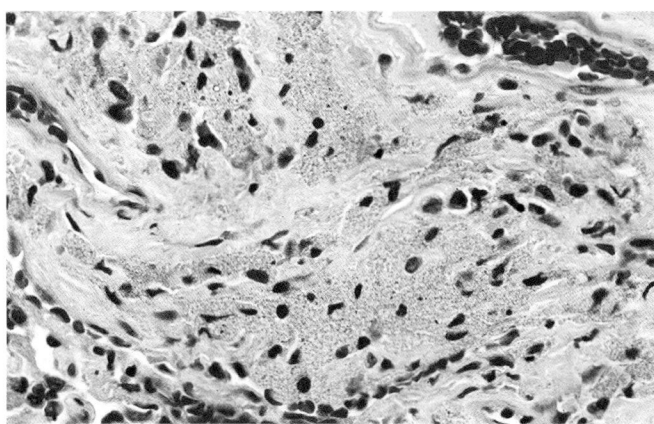

Figure 9-76. Aluminosis. Detail of dust-laden macrophages, showing the gray-brown granular appearance typical of aluminum oxide.

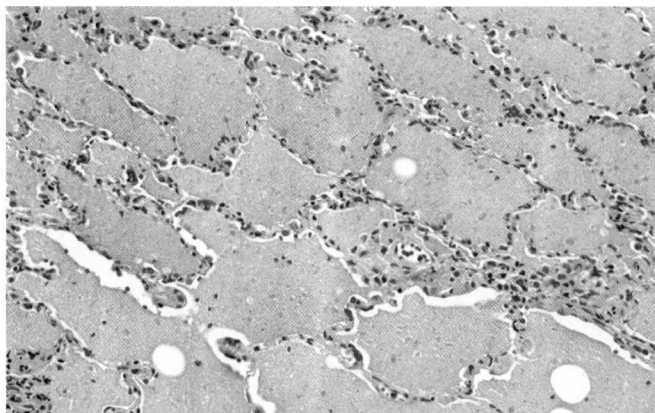

Figure 9-77. Aluminosis. Amorphous eosinophilic material fills the alveoli in a pattern similar to pulmonary alveolar proteinosis. Interstitial accumulations of dust-laden macrophages are also present.

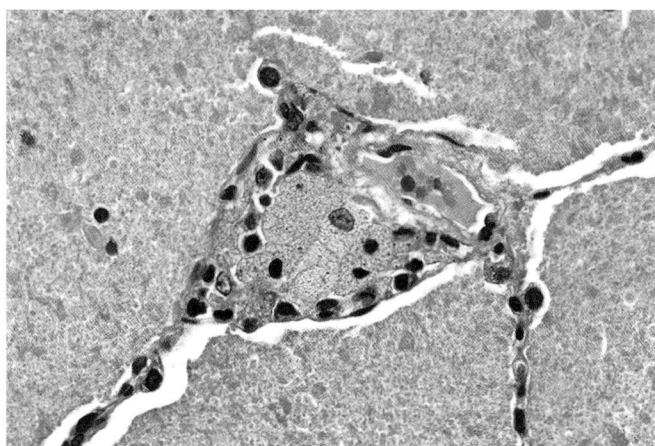

Figure 9-78. Aluminosis. Higher magnification view showing the characteristic granular appearance of aluminum-laden macrophages.

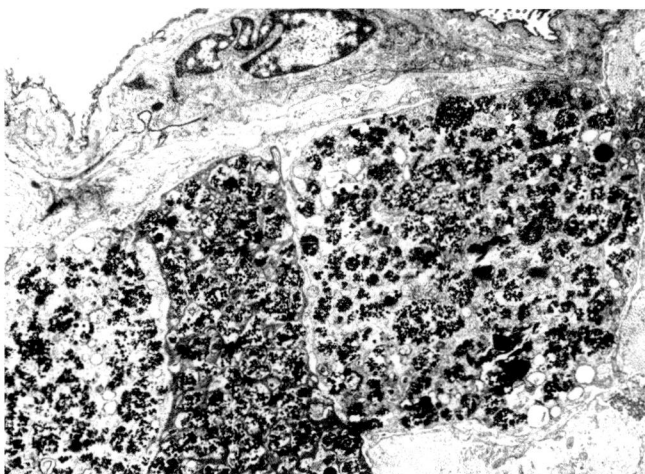

Figure 9-79. Aluminosis. Transmission electron micrograph showing an alveolar type II cell overlying a dust-filled interstitial macrophage.

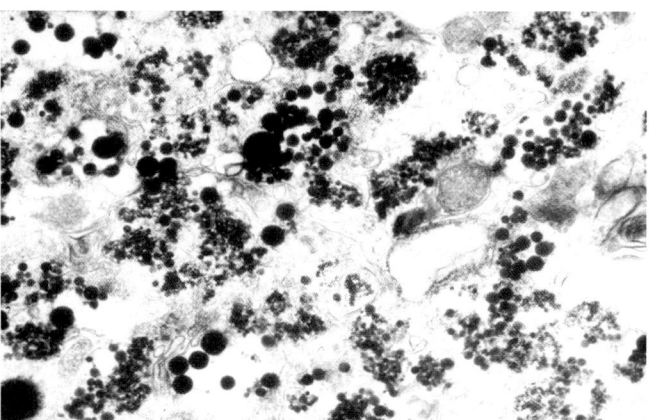

Figure 9-80. Aluminosis. In this transmission electron micrograph of an aluminum-containing macrophage, the aluminum particles appear spherical and electron-dense. (From Roggli VL. Rare pneumoconioses: metalloconioses. In: Saldana MJ, ed. *Pathology of Pulmonary Disease*. Philadelphia: Lippincott; 1994:411–422, with permission.)

Differential Diagnosis

Dust deposits of aluminum must be distinguished from kaolinite (a form of aluminum silicate; see "Silicatosis" section) and smoker's macrophages. The dust deposits in kaolin worker's pneumoconiosis are fine and tan, whereas aluminum is more refractile and gray to brown in color. In difficult cases, analytic electron microscopy may be required to make the distinction. Smoker's macrophages are located primarily within the alveolar spaces and are typically associated with scattered black dot-like carbon particles. Aluminum-induced granulomatosis must be considered in the differential diagnosis for sarcoidosis. In addition, aluminum exposure must be considered in cases with a pulmonary alveolar proteinosis pattern. In such cases, the presence of aluminum dust deposits is a useful differentiating feature.

Hard Metal Lung Disease

Tungsten carbide is used in the manufacture of cutting tools, drilling equipment, armaments, alloys, and ceramics (Box 9-4). Cobalt is used as a binder and may constitute up to 25% of the final product by weight. Hard metal lung disease occurs as a consequence of the inhalation of hard metal dust. Exposure may occur during the manufacturing process of hard metal–containing products or during their use.[48] Cobalt exposure has also been reported in diamond polishers who had no exposure to hard metal dust.[49,50]

inflammation.[43–46] Cases with a prominent granulomatous response may mimic sarcoidosis. Areas resembling DIP may also be observed.[47] Rare cases have been described with an alveolar proteinosis–like pattern (Figs. 9-77 and 9-78) similar to that seen in acute silicoproteinosis.[40]

Aluminum dust is nonrefringent when examined by polarizing microscopy. Analytic electron microscopy shows electron-dense spherical particles (Figs. 9-79 and 9-80) composed of aluminum (Fig. 9-81).

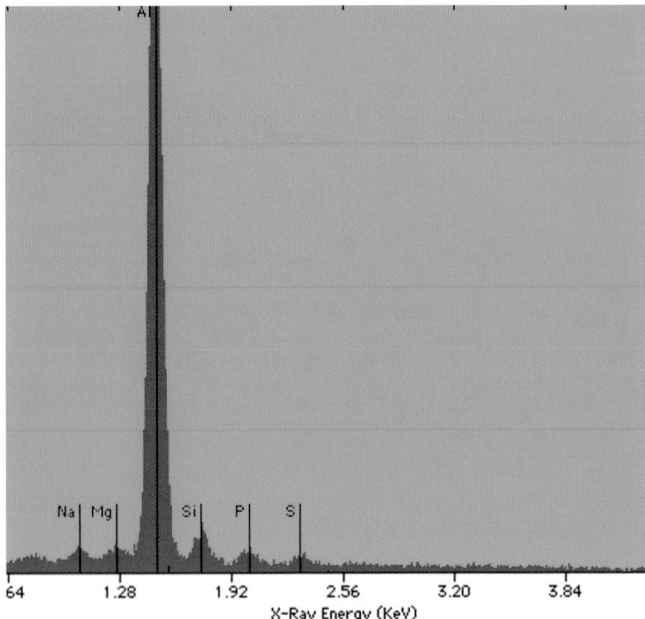

Figure 9-81. Aluminosis. Energy-dispersive x-ray analysis (EDXA) spectrum in a case of aluminosis demonstrates a peak for aluminum only (AL).

Clinical Presentation

Workers with hard metal lung disease present with dyspnea of insidious onset and restrictive changes with small lung volumes on pulmonary function testing. Diffusely increased interstitial markings are observed on plain chest films and CT scans. Disease develops in less than 1% of those exposed, suggesting that hypersensitivity to cobalt is the underlying pathogenic mechanism. Workers may also present with asthma that predates interstitial lung disease by months to years. Hard metal lung disease has been reported to recur after lung transplantation without additional exposure.[51]

Pathologic Findings

Macroscopically, the lungs in hard metal lung disease are small and fibrotic. Microscopically, hard metal lung disease is synonymous with giant cell interstitial pneumonia (GIP),[52] once considered to be one of the "idiopathic" interstitial pneumonias. In this disorder, the alveolar septa are thickened and fibrotic and lined by hyperplastic type II pneumocytes (Figs. 9-82 and 9-83). A moderate chronic inflammatory infiltrate is present. Multinucleate giant cells are a conspicuous feature (Fig. 9-84) and are found both within the alveolar spaces and lining the alveolar septa. Alveolar macrophages are present in increased numbers, and in some cases a pattern reminiscent of DIP is observed (Fig. 9-85). Occasionally, the overall pattern mimics that of UIP, with areas of microscopic honeycombing (Figs. 9-86 and 9-87). The fibrotic and inflammatory reaction may be accentuated around bronchioles.

Dust deposits are not readily identified by either routine or polarizing light microscopy. The individual metal particles can be observed by analytic electron microscopy (Figs. 9-88 and 9-89).[53] Tungsten

Box 9-4. Uses for Tungsten Carbide

Alloys
Armaments
Ceramics
Circular saw blades
Cutting tools
Driling equipment

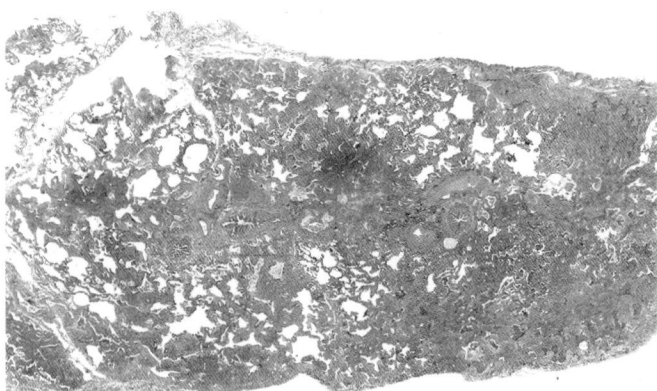

Figure 9-82. Hard metal pneumoconiosis. At low magnification, the interstitium appears widened, accompanied by alveolar filling.

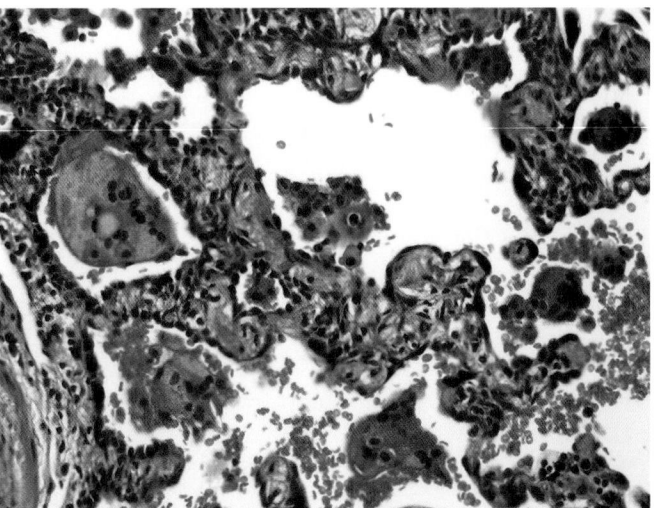

Figure 9-83. Hard metal pneumoconiosis. This example demonstrates interstitial pneumonia with hyperplastic type II pneumocytes and multinucleate giant cells in alveolar spaces. (Courtesy of Dr. Thomas V. Colby, Mayo Clinic, Scottsdale, AZ.)

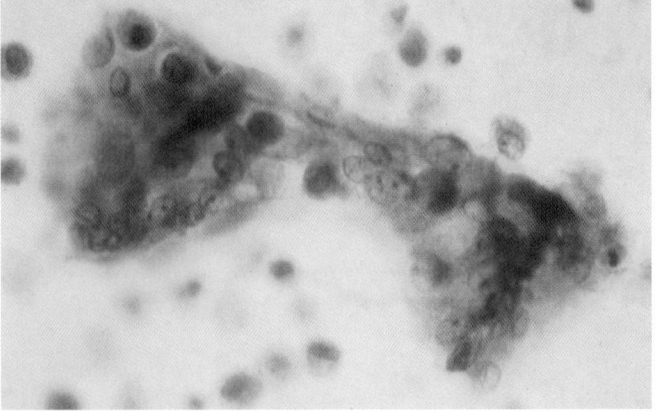

Figure 9-84. Hard metal pneumoconiosis. Bronchoalveolar lavage fluid from a patient with hard metal pneumoconiosis contains multinucleate giant cells. (From Tabatowski K, Roggli VL, Fulkerson WJ, et al. Giant cell interstitial pneumonia in a hard-metal worker: cytologic, histologic and analytical electron microscopic investigation. *Acta Cytol.* 1988;32:240–246, with permission.)

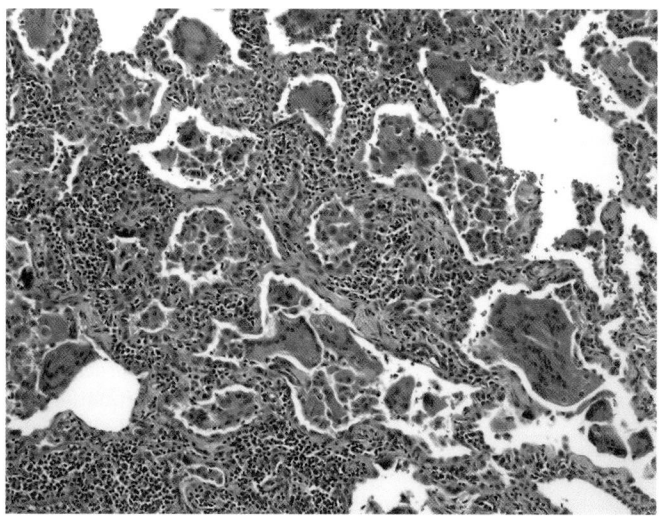

Figure 9-85. Hard metal pneumoconiosis. Along with multinucleate giant cells, macrophages fill alveolar spaces in a pattern resembling desquamative interstitial pneumonia. (Courtesy of Dr. Thomas V. Colby, Mayo Clinic, Scottsdale, AZ.)

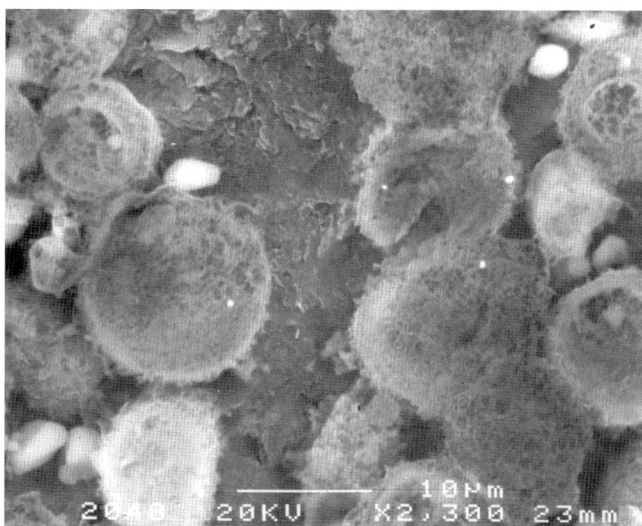

Figure 9-88. Hard metal pneumoconiosis. Scanning electron microscopy image of alveolar macrophages shows small, electron-dense metal particles. (Courtesy of Dr. Frank Johnson and Dr. Jose Centano, Armed Forces Institute of Pathology, Washington, DC.)

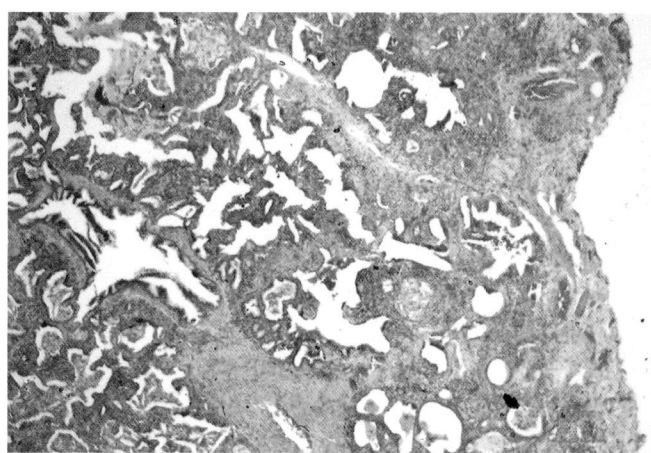

Figure 9-86. Features reminiscent of usual interstitial pneumonia (UIP) in a case of tungsten carbide pneumoconiosis include server interstitial fibrosis and honeycombing.

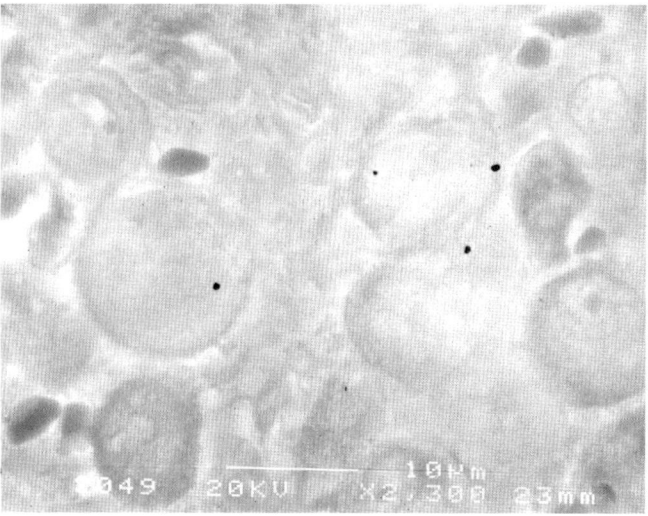

Figure 9-89. Hard metal pneumoconiosis. The metal particles shown in Figure 9-88 appear as dark dots in this backscatter electron microscopic image. (Courtesy of Dr. Frank Johnson and Dr. Jose Centano, Armed Forces Institute of Pathology, Washington, DC.)

particles are most common, followed by titanium and tantalum (Fig. 9-90). Cobalt, the suspected causative agent of the disease, may or may not be identified, because its water solubility makes it susceptible to removal from tissue during fixation and processing.

Differential Diagnosis

Hard metal lung disease must be distinguished from UIP, DIP, and hypersensitivity pneumonitis. The presence of intra-alveolar and alveolar septal giant cells and the absence of honeycomb changes favor hard metal disease. In the absence of giant cells, analytic electron microscopy may be required to confirm the diagnosis. In contrast with hard metal lung disease, DIP has a monotonous pattern with minimal interstitial fibrosis, and lining of the alveolar septa by giant cells is not a feature of DIP. Hypersensitivity pneumonitis is characterized by an interstitial chronic inflammatory infiltrate associated with small clusters of interstitial giant cells that form ill-defined granulomas, as opposed to the intra-alveolar or alveolar septal giant cells of hard metal lung disease.

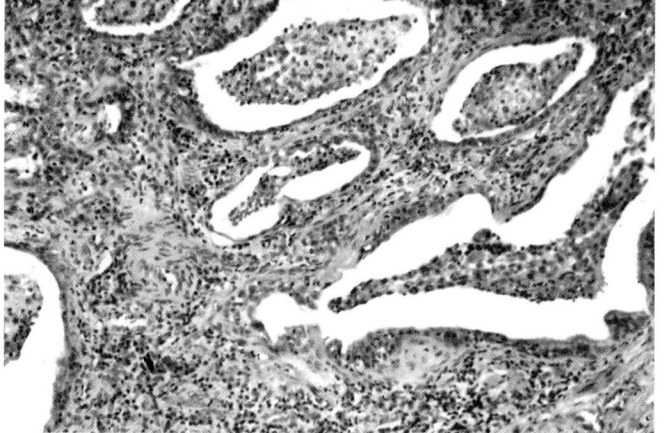

Figure 9-87. Hard metal pneumoconiosis. Detail of the case shown in Figure 9-86, demonstrating honeycomb cysts filled with macrophages.

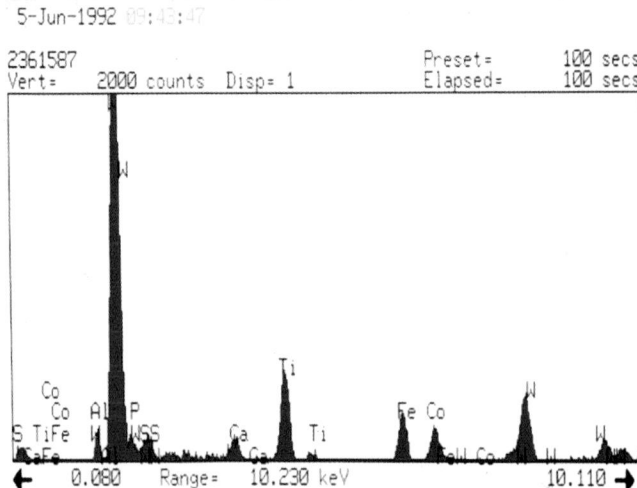

5-Jun-1992 09:43:47

2361587
Vert= 2000 counts Disp= 1   Preset=   100 secs
                                              Elapsed=   100 secs

W

Co
Co   Ti
S Ti Fe Al   P   Fe Co   W
Ca Fe   K Na S S   Ca   Ti   Cu Co   W   W
                    Ca   W

← 0.080   Range= 10.230 keV   10.110 →

Figure 9-90. Hard metal pneumoconiosis. Energy-dispersive x-ray analysis (EDXA) spectrum demonstrates a large peak for tungsten, also known as wolfram (W). A small peak for cobalt (Co) is also present. (Courtesy of Dr. Frank Johnson and Dr. Jose Centano, Armed Forces Institute of Pathology, Washington, DC.)

Transbronchial biopsy and bronchoalveolar lavage may be useful in the diagnosis of hard metal lung disease.[54] Analytic electron microscopy can be performed on either of these types of specimens and may demonstrate the characteristic profile of metallic elements.

Berylliosis

Berylliosis is a granulomatous lung disease caused by the inhalation of beryllium-containing dust.[55,56] Beryllium is used in the aerospace industry in the manufacture of structural materials, guidance systems, optical devices, rocket motor parts, and heat shields. It is also used in the manufacture of ceramic parts, thermal couplings, and crucibles and as a controller in nuclear reactors (Box 9-5). Exposure may occur in any of these industries, as well as in the mining or extraction of beryllium ores.[57-59] Historically, beryllium was used in the manufacture of fluorescent lightbulbs, which accounted for most of the initial reports of berylliosis.

Clinical Presentation

Patients with berylliosis present with insidiously progressive dyspnea. Pulmonary function testing shows restriction with diminished diffusing capacity. Plain films of the chest show a fibronodular process. Only about 1% of patients at risk develop berylliosis. Beryllium hypersensitivity has therefore been postulated as the likely pathogenic mechanism, as in the diseases caused by exposure to aluminum and hard metal. In vitro

Box 9-5. Uses of Beryllium

Aircraft brakes, engines
Ceramics
Electrical components
Inertial guidance systems
Laser tubes
Nuclear reactors
Rocket motors
Spark plugs
Turbine rotor blades
Weapons
X-ray tube windows

reactivity of peripheral blood or bronchoalveolar lavage lymphocytes to beryllium salts has been used as part of the diagnostic workup.[60]

Pathologic Findings

Macroscopically, the lungs in chronic berylliosis are small and fibrotic and may show honeycomb changes.[3] Bilateral hilar lymphadenopathy may be present. Microscopically, there are well-formed non-necrotizing granulomas (Figs. 9-91 and 9-92). A chronic interstitial inflammatory infiltrate typically is present (Fig. 9-93). Granulomas may also be found in hilar lymph nodes. Schaumann bodies (Fig. 9-94) and asteroid bodies (Fig. 9-95) within multinucleate giant cells are observed in some cases.[39,40]

Beryllium is a lightweight metal that has recently become detectable by analytic electron microscopy.[61] Other techniques, such as wet chemical analysis, electron energy loss spectrometry, or ion or laser microprobe mass spectrometry, are also used for detection.[2] Polarizing microscopy is not useful in the diagnosis of berylliosis.

Differential Diagnosis

Berylliosis must be distinguished from sarcoidosis and hypersensitivity pneumonitis. Sarcoidosis closely resembles berylliosis histologically, so a high index of suspicion for exposure to beryllium and a thorough occupational history are necessary in order to arrive at the

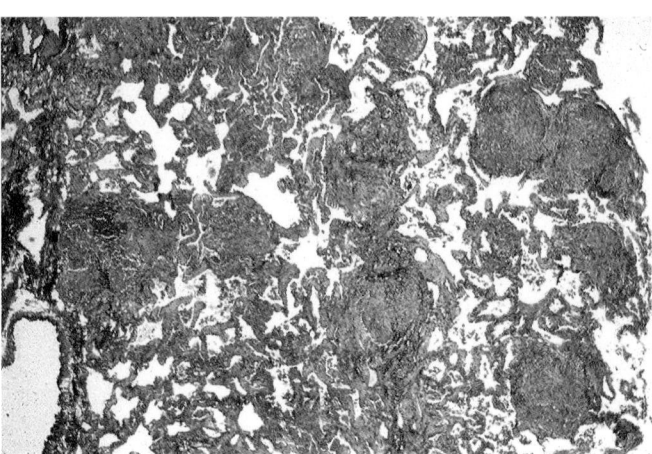

Figure 9-91. Berylliosis. The presence of numerous granulomas is characteristic of berylliosis. (Courtesy of Dr. Fred Askin, Johns Hopkins University, Baltimore, MD.)

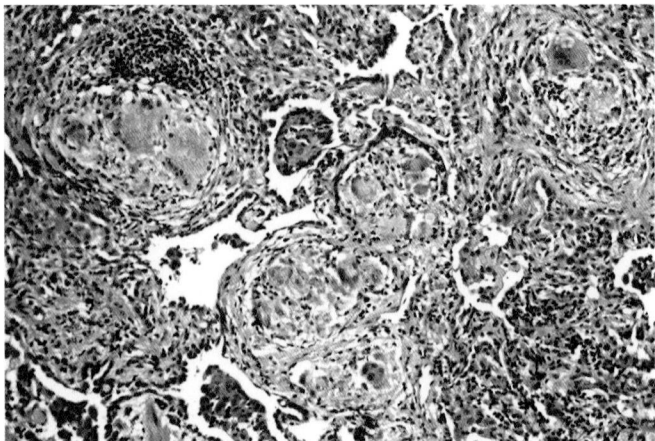

Figure 9-92. Berylliosis. The granulomas in berylliosis are compact and lack necrosis. (From Roggli VL, Shelburne JD. Pneumoconioses, mineral and vegetable. In: Dail DH, Hammar SP, eds. *Pulmonary Pathology*, 2nd ed. New York: Springer-Verlag; 1994: 867–900, with permission.)

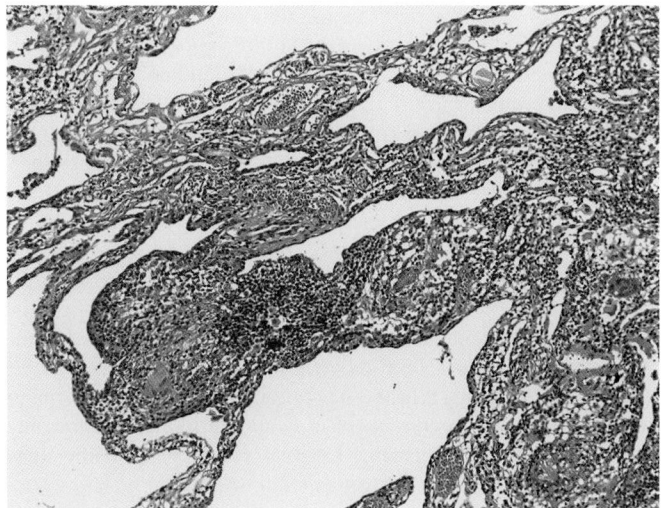

Figure 9-93. Berylliosis. In addition to granulomatous inflammation, a chronic interstitial inflammatory infiltrate is seen. (Courtesy of Dr. Thomas V. Colby, Mayo Clinic, Scottsdale, AZ.)

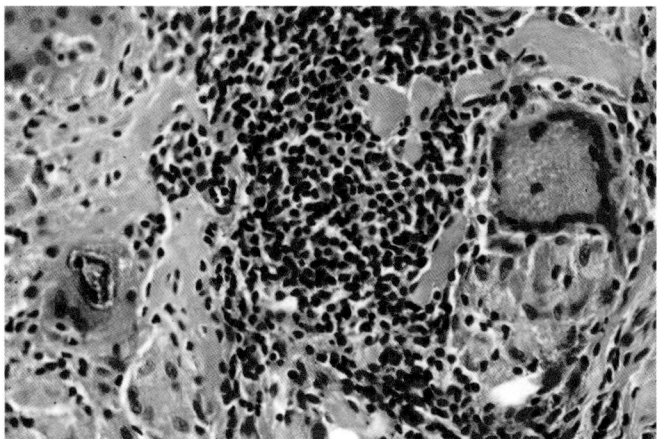

Figure 9-94. Berylliosis. A Schaumann body, with its characteristic basophilic laminations, is observed within a giant cell (*lower left*). (From Roggli VL. Rare pneumoconioses: metalloconioses. In: Saldana MJ, ed. *Pathology of Pulmonary Disease*. Philadelphia: Lippincott; 1994:411–422, with permission.)

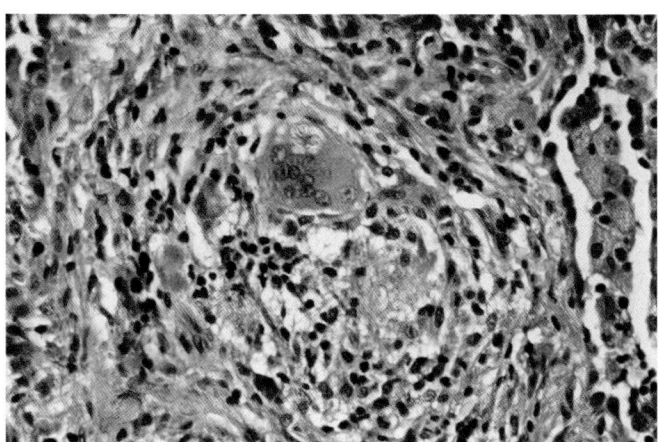

Figure 9-95. Berylliosis. This granuloma features a giant cell containing an asteroid body (*upper center*). (From Roggli VL. Rare pneumoconioses: metalloconioses. In: Saldana MJ, ed. *Pathology of Pulmonary Disease*. Philadelphia: Lippincott; 1994: 411–422, with permission.)

correct diagnosis. Hypersensitivity pneumonitis is associated with a more intense lymphocytic interstitial and peribronchiolar infiltrate and lacks the well-formed granulomas observed in berylliosis.

Rare Earth Pneumoconiosis

Rare earth (or cerium oxide) pneumoconiosis is an uncommon disease caused by the inhalation of rare earth metals, primarily cerium oxide. Only about 20 cases have been reported, and descriptions of the pathologic findings are sparse. Most patients with rare earth pneumoconiosis have been employed in settings in which they were exposed to dust from carbon arc lamps. Two patients were exposed to cerium oxide in an extraction plant, two patients used cerium oxide rouge to polish lenses, and one patient was a producer of glass rubbing polish.[62–65]

Clinical Presentation

The clinical presentation ranges from no symptoms to insidiously progressive dyspnea. Chest films show a diffuse interstitial pattern. Pulmonary function testing shows a restrictive or a mixed restrictive/obstructive pattern and reduced diffusion capacity. The rarity of this disease suggests hypersensitivity to cerium as the pathogenic mechanism.

Pathologic Findings

The spectrum of histopathologic features includes granulomatous disease and interstitial fibrosis.[62] The fibrosis is similar to that observed with UIP or NSIP (Fig. 9-96). Pigmented dust deposits may be observed with light microscopy, although these may be sparse. Cerium oxide is birefringent on polarizing microscopy. Analytic electron microscopy demonstrates rare earth metals, primarily cerium and to a lesser degree lanthanum, samarium, and neodymium (Figs. 9-97 and 9-98).

Differential Diagnosis

Rare earth pneumoconiosis is most readily confused with UIP or NSIP. Sarcoidosis may be considered if there is a prominent granulomatous reaction. The diagnosis can be made on the basis of a thorough occupational history and detection of rare earth compounds in lung tissue by analytic electron microscopy.

Other Pneumoconioses

A myriad of other substances have been implicated as causes of pneumoconiosis. Although an exhaustive list is beyond the scope of this discussion, several uncommon and recently recognized pneumoconioses are presented in this section.

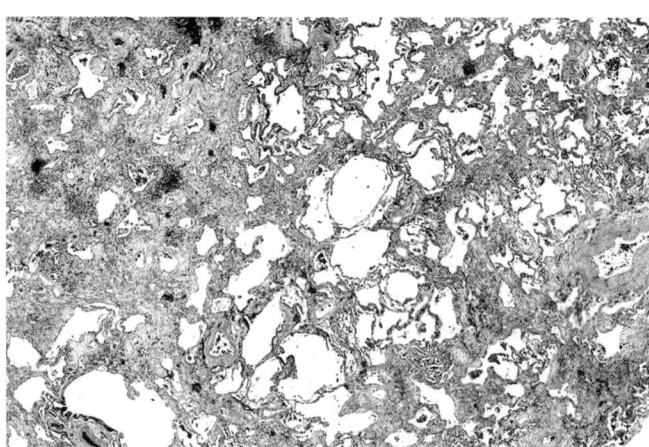

Figure 9-96. Rare earth pneumoconiosis. Diffuse interstitial fibrosis with honeycomb cyst formation in a pattern reminiscent of that seen in usual interstitial pneumonia (UIP).

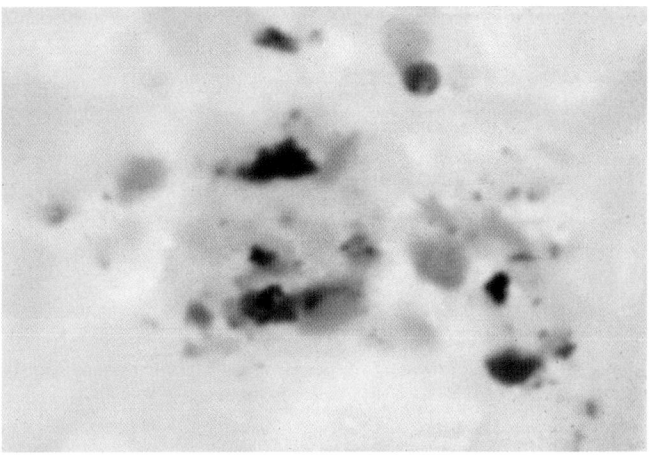

Figure 9-97. Rare earth pneumoconiosis. Backscatter electron microscopy image of electron-dense cerium oxide particles.

Acute high-intensity exposure to cadmium results in acute respiratory distress syndrome, whereas chronic exposure is purported to cause emphysema.[66,67] Most reports on the pulmonary effects of chronic cadmium exposure appear not to have taken smoking as a confounding factor into consideration.[68,69] In addition to being a major cause of emphysema, cigarette smoking is itself a source, albeit small, of cadmium exposure (approximately 2 µg per cigarette).[70–72] One study that reported an increased rate of emphysema in workers exposed to cadmium did control for smoking but unfortunately included only clinicoradiographic data and no histopathologic descriptions.[73]

Granulomatous interstitial inflammation and nodular fibrosis reminiscent of silicosis have been reported in some vineyard workers.[74,75] Vineyard sprayer's lung is believed to be caused by chronic exposure to copper sulfate, a main constituent of fungicidal solutions commonly used in viticulture. Histochemical stains for copper reportedly highlight the dust within macrophages and fibrotic nodules.[74]

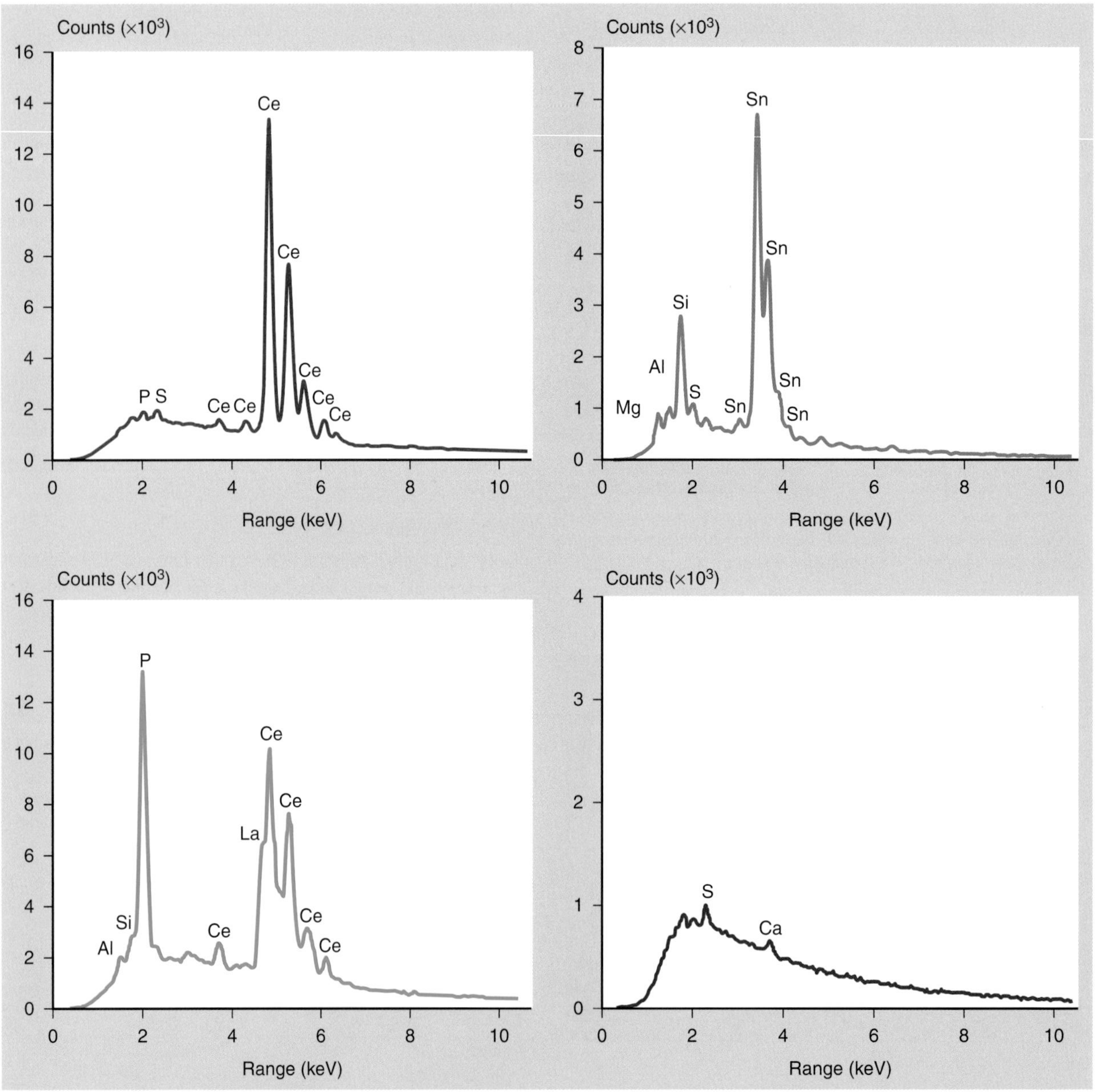

Figure 9-98. Rare earth pneumoconiosis. Energy-dispersive x-ray analysis (EDXA) spectra demonstrate peaks for rare earth metals, including cerium (Ce) (*upper left panel*) and cerium and lanthanum (La) (*lower left panel*). Background is shown in the *lower right panel*, and a tin particle (Sn) in the *upper right panel*. (From McDonald JW, Ghio AJ, Sheehan CE, et al. Rare earth (cerium oxide) pneumoconiosis: analytical scanning electron microscopy and literature review. *Mod Pathol*. 1995;8:859–865.)

Exposure to silicon carbide (carborundum), a synthetic abrasive, has been associated with nodular and diffuse interstitial fibrosis resembling silicosis or mixed dust pneumoconiosis.[76-78] Abundant dust and ferruginous bodies with black silicon carbide cores have been described.

A variety of pathologic features, which in some cases appear to resemble those of silicosis or mixed dust pneumoconiosis, have been reported under the rubric of "dental technician's pneumoconiosis."[77,79-83] The heterogeneity of reported findings is not surprising, in view of the plethora of substances that have been used in dental prostheses, including silica, beryllium, chromium, cobalt, and molybdenum.

Exposure to oil mists or fine sprays in certain machining and engineering applications, particularly oils low in viscosity or high in mineral oil content, has been reported to cause exogenous lipoid pneumonia. The histologic features are similar to those of mineral oil aspiration.[84-87]

Metal-working fluids (MWFs) are used extensively in automotive parts manufacturing and other metal-working industries as coolants, cleaning agents, and anti-corrosives that are sprayed onto the fabrication surfaces during the machining process.[88] Composed of pure petroleum or a mixture of petroleum or synthetic oils and water, MWFs provide a lipid-rich substrate for the growth of microorganisms. Fungal and bacterial antigens in contaminated MWFs have been implicated in outbreaks of hypersensitivity pneumonia in MWF-exposed workers, with recent outbreaks attributed to non-tuberculous mycobacterial antigens[89-91] (Fig. 9-99).

Flock worker's lung derives its name from an interstitial lung disease that has been reported in some individuals employed in the flocking industry. Flocking involves the application of short synthetic fibers, frequently nylon, onto an adhesive backing, resulting in a plush material. Respired shards generated in the process of cutting fibers to length with a rotary cutter are believed to cause a restrictive process characterized histologically by lymphoid hyperplasia, lymphocytic bronchiolitis, and peribronchiolar interstitial inflammation[92-95] (Fig. 9-100). A spectrum of other histologic features and patterns have been reported, including diffuse lymphocytic interstitial inflammation, interstitial fibrosis, fibroblastic foci, bronchiolitis obliterans organizing pneumonia (BOOP), and NSIP.[93]

Initially recognized in former workers at a microwave popcorn plant and thus dubbed *popcorn worker's lung*, a form of lung disease

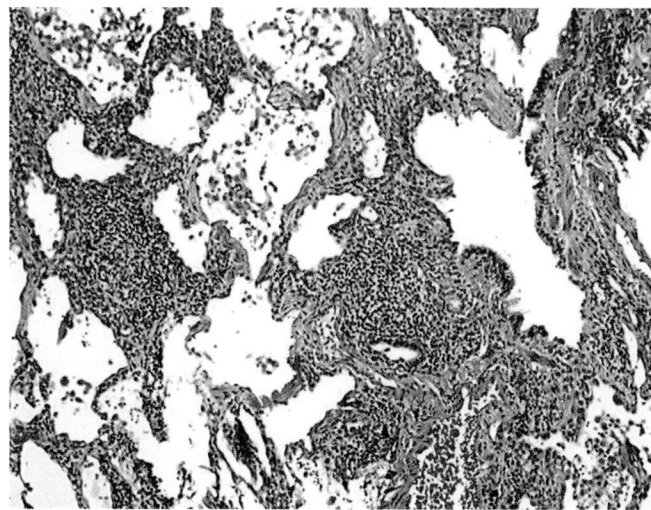

Figure 9-100. Flock worker's lung. Lymphocytic bronchiolitis and lymphoid hyperplasia, sometimes with germinal center formation, as seen in this case, are among the more frequently reported findings in this condition. (Courtesy of Dr. Armando Fraire, University of Massachusetts, Worcester, MA.)

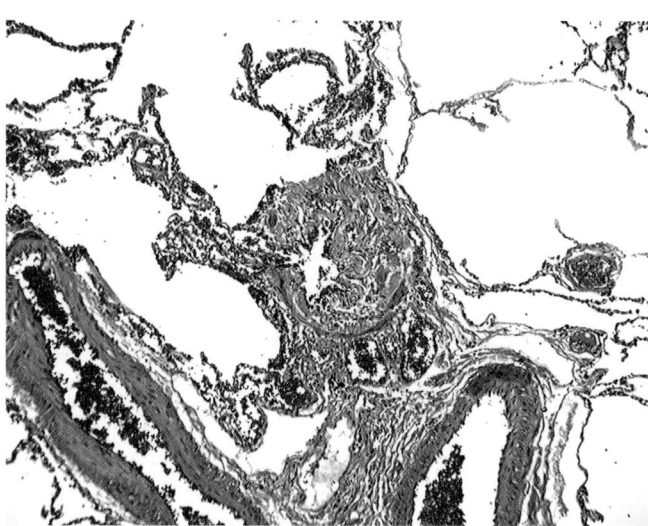

Figure 9-101. Flavorings-related lung disease. Bronchiolitis obliterans, characterized by mural bronchiolar fibrosis, in a microwave popcorn plant worker. (Courtesy of Dr. William Travis, Memorial Sloan-Kettering Cancer Center, New York.)

featuring bronchiolitis obliterans (BO) and occasionally peribronchiolar granulomas has also been reported in workers at food flavorings production plants[96-100] (Fig. 9-101). The broader term *flavorings-related lung disease* has been invoked as a more accurate designation for these recently recognized exposures. Although it is possible that other flavoring agents to which workers at these plants have been exposed contribute to the development of this condition, exposure data and animal inhalational studies suggest that diacetyl (2,3-butanedione), a principal component of butter flavoring, plays a causal role.[101]

Pulmonary disease caused by polluted indoor air is a vastly underrecognized problem.[102-110] Cooking indoors with coal or biomass fuels such as wood, peat, crop residues, or dung in open pit fires or poorly ventilated stoves is commonplace in developing countries. This practice releases numerous particulates, including silicates, into the air. Not

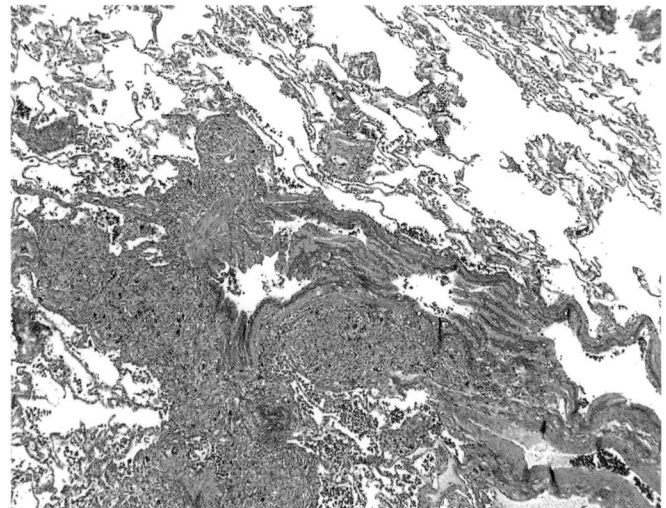

Figure 9-99. Metalworking fluid hypersensitivity pneumonia. Collections of peribronchiolar granulomas are evident. In this example, scattered dust particles are present within the granulomas. (Courtesy of Dr. Thomas V. Colby, Mayo Clinic, Scottsdale, AZ.)

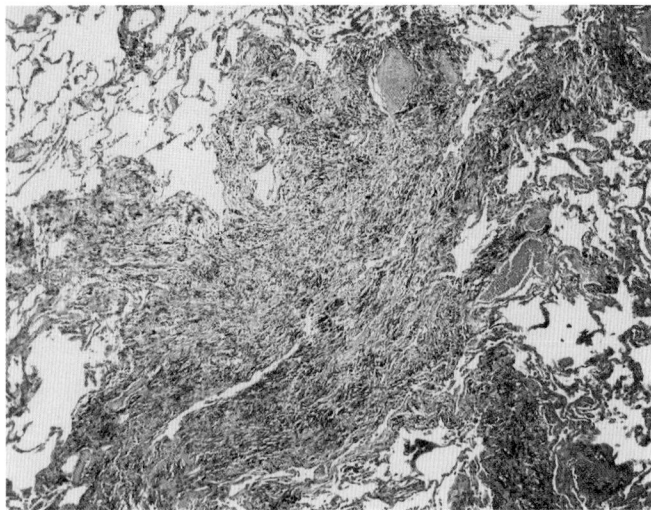

Figure 9-102. "Hut lung." Extensive interstitial fibrosis with abundant entrapped dust particles are seen. This biopsy is from a woman who had recently immigrated to the United States from a developing country, where for many years she cooked with a poorly ventilated indoor stove that used biomass fuels. (Courtesy of Dr. Thomas V. Colby, Mayo Clinic, Scottsdale, AZ.)

surprisingly, most reported cases of this pneumoconiosis, which has been referred to as "hut lung," or *domestically acquired particulate lung disease* (DAPLD), have been in women. The rare cases that have come to biopsy exhibit dust macules, nodular fibrosis, or occasionally, progressive massive fibrosis (Fig. 9-102).

Self-assessment questions related to this chapter can be found online on the Expert Consult site for this title.

References

1. Sporn TA, Roggli VL. Pneumoconioses, mineral and vegetable. In: Tomashefski JF, ed. *Dail and Hammar's Pulmonary Pathology*, vol 1, 3rd ed. New York: Springer-Verlag; 2008;911–949.
2. Ingram P, Shelburne JD, Roggli VL, LeFurgey EA. *Biomedical Applications of Microprobe Analysis*. San Diego: Academic Press; 1999.
3. Spencer H. The pneumoconioses and other occupational lung diseases. In: Spencer H, ed. *Pathology of the Lung*, vol. 1, 4th ed. Oxford: Pergamon Press; 1985:413–510.
4. Churg A, Green FHY. *Pathology of Occupational Lung Disease*. 2nd ed. Baltimore: Williams & Wilkins; 1998.
5. Craighead JE, Kleinerman J, Abraham JL, et al. Diseases associated with exposure to silica and nonfibrous silicate minerals. *Arch Pathol Lab Med*. 1988;112:673–720.
6. Zeren EH, Colby TV, Roggli VL. Silica-induced pleural disease: an unusual case mimicking mesothelioma. *Chest*. 1997;112:1436–1438.
7. McDonald JW, Roggli VL. Detection of silica particles in lung tissue by polarizing light microscopy. *Arch Pathol Lab Med*. 1995;119:242–246.
8. Cowie RL. The epidemiology of tuberculosis in gold miners with silicosis. *Am J Respir Crit Care Med*. 1994;150:1460–1462.
9. Slavin RE, Swedo JL, Brandes D, et al. Extrapulmonary silicosis: a clinical, morphologic, and ultrastructural study. *Hum Pathol*. 1985;16:393–412.
10. Vallyathan V, Brower PS, Green FHY, Attfield MD. Radiographic and pathologic correlation of coal workers' pneumoconiosis. *Am J Respir Crit Care Med*. 1996;154:741–748.
11. Marine WM, Gurr D, Jacobsen M. Clinically important respiratory effects of dust exposure and smoking in British coal miners. *Am Rev Respir Dis*. 1988;137:106–112.
12. Kleinerman J, Green FHY, Laquer W, et al. Pathology standards for coal workers pneumoconiosis. *Arch Pathol Lab Med*. 1979;103:375–432.
13. Pratt PC. Role of silica in progressive massive fibrosis in coal workers' pneumoconiosis. *Arch Environ Health*. 1968;16:734–737.
14. Roggli VL. Asbestos bodies and non-asbestos ferruginous bodies. In: Roggli VL, Oury TD, Sporn TA, eds. *Pathology of Asbestos-Associated Diseases*, 2nd ed. New York: Springer; 2004:34–70.
15. Hammar SP, Dodson RF. Asbestos. In: Dail DH, Hammar SP, eds. *Pulmonary Pathology*, 2nd ed. New York: Springer-Verlag; 1994:901–983.
16. Roggli VL, Oury TD, Sporn TA, eds. *Pathology of Asbestos-Associated Diseases*, 2nd ed. New York: Springer; 2004.
17. Roggli VL, Gibbs AR, Attanoos R, et al. Pathology of asbestosis—an update of the diagnostic criteria. Report of the Asbestosis Committee of the College of American Pathologists and Pulmonary Pathology Society. *Arch Pathol Lab Med*. 2010;134:462–480.
18. Roggli VL. Pathology of human asbestosis: a critical review. In: Fenoglio-Preiser C, ed. *Advances in Pathology*, vol 2. Chicago: Year Book; 1989:31–60.
19. Roggli VL. The pneumoconioses: asbestosis. In: Saldana MJ, ed. *Pathology of Pulmonary Disease*. Philadelphia: Lippincott; 1994:395–410.
20. Churg A. Nonneoplastic disease caused by asbestos. In: Churg A, Green FHY, eds. *Pathology of Occupational Lung Disease*, 2nd ed. Baltimore: Williams & Wilkins; 1998:277–338.
21. Schneider F, Sporn TA, Roggli VL. Asbestos fiber content of lungs with diffuse interstitial fibrosis: an analytical scanning electron microscopic analysis of 249 cases. *Arch Pathol Lab Med*. 2010;134:457–461.
22. Morgan WKC, Donner A, Higgins ITT, et al. The effects of kaolin on the lung. *Am Rev Respir Dis*. 1988;138:813–820.
23. Lapenas D, Gale P, Kennedy T, et al. Kaolin pneumoconiosis: radiologic, pathologic, and mineralogic findings. *Am Rev Respir Dis*. 1984;130:282–288.
24. Wagner JC, Pooley FD, Gibbs A, et al. Inhalation of china stone and china clay dusts: relationship between the mineralogy of dust retained in the lungs and pathologic changes. *Thorax*. 1986;41:190–196.
25. Landas SK, Schwartz DA. Mica-associated pulmonary interstitial fibrosis. *Am Rev Respir Dis*. 1991;144:718–721.
26. Sherwin RP, Barman ML, Abraham JL. Silicate pneumoconiosis of farm workers. *Lab Invest*. 1979;40:576–582.
27. Green FHY, Churg A. Diseases due to nonasbestos silicates. In: Churg A, Green FHY, eds. *Pathology of Occupational Lung Disease*, 2nd ed. Baltimore: Williams & Wilkins; 1998:235–276.
28. Roub LW, Dekker A, Wagenblast HW, Reece GJ. Pulmonary silicatosis: a case diagnosed by needle-aspiration biopsy and energy-dispersive x-ray analysis. *Am J Clin Pathol*. 1979;72:871–875.
29. Honma K, Abraham JL, Chiyotani K, et al. Proposed criteria for mixed dust pneumoconiosis: definition, descriptions, and guidelines for pathological diagnosis and clinical correlation. *Hum Pathol*. 2004;35:1515–1523.
30. Vallyathan NV, Craighead JE. Pulmonary pathology in workers exposed to nonasbestiform talc. *Hum Pathol*. 1981;12:28–35.
31. Crouch E, Churg A. Progressive massive fibrosis of the lung secondary to intravenous injection of talc: a pathologic and mineralogic analysis. *Am J Clin Pathol*. 1983;80:520–526.
32. Pare JP, Cote G, Fraser RS. Long-term follow-up of drug abusers with intravenous talcosis. *Am Rev Respir Dis*. 1989;139:233–241.
33. Bemer A, Gylseth B, Levy F. Talc dust pneumoconiosis. *Acta Pathol Microbiol Scand [A]*. 1981;89:17–21.
34. Vallyathan NV. Talc pneumoconiosis. *Respir Ther*. 1980;10:34–39.
35. Kennedy L, Sahn SA. Talc pleurodesis for the treatment of pneumothorax and pleural effusion. *Chest*. 1994;106:1215–1222.
36. Miller A, Teirstein AS, Bader ME, et al. Talc pneumoconiosis: significance of sublight microscopic mineral particles. *Am J Med*. 1971;50:395–402.
37. Sferlazza SJ, Beckett WS. The respiratory health of welders. *Am Rev Respir Dis*. 1991;143:1134–1148.
38. Stern RM. The assessment of risk: application to the welding industry. Lung Cancer. *The Danish Welding Institute Report*; 1983;83:13.
39. Churg A, Colby TV. Diseases caused by metals and related compounds. In: Churg A, Green FHY, eds. *Pathology of Occupational Lung Disease*, 2nd ed. Baltimore: Williams & Wilkins; 1998:77–128.
40. Roggli VL. Rare pneumoconioses: metalloconioses. In: Saldana MJ, ed. *Pathology of Pulmonary Disease*. Philadelphia: Lippincott; 1994:411–422.
41. Abramson MJ, Wlodarczyk JH, Saunders NA, Hensley MJ. Does aluminum smelting cause lung disease? *Am Rev Respir Dis*. 1989;139:1042–1057.
42. Vallyathan V, Bergeron WN, Robichaux PA, Craighead JE. Pulmonary fibrosis in an aluminum arc welder. *Chest*. 1982;81:372–374.
43. Jederlinic PJ, Abraham JL, Churg A, et al. Pulmonary fibrosis in aluminum oxide workers: investigation of nine workers, with pathologic examination and microanalysis in three of them. *Am Rev Respir Dis*. 1990;142:1179–1184.
44. Gilks B, Churg A. Aluminum-induced pulmonary fibrosis: do fibers play a role? *Am Rev Respir Dis*. 1987;136:176–179.
45. Chen W-J, Monnat RJ, Chen M, Moffet NK. Aluminum induced pulmonary granulomatosis. *Hum Pathol*. 1978;9:705–711.
46. De Vuyst P, Dumortier P, Schandene L, et al. Sarcoidlike lung granulomatosis induced by aluminum dusts. *Am Rev Respir Dis*. 1987;135:493–497.
47. Herbert A, Sterling G, Abraham J, Corrin B. Desquamative interstitial pneumonia in an aluminum welder. *Hum Pathol*. 1982;13:694–699.
48. Sprince NL, Oliver LC, Eisen EA, et al. Cobalt exposure and lung disease in tungsten carbide production: a cross-sectional study of current workers. *Am Rev Respir Dis*. 1988;138:1220–1226.
49. Nemery B, Nagels J, Verbeken E, et al. Rapidly fatal progression of cobalt lung in a diamond polisher. *Am Rev Respir Dis*. 1990;141:1373–1378.
50. Nemery B, Casier P, Roosels D, et al. Survey of cobalt exposure and respiratory health in diamond polishers. *Am Rev Respir Dis*. 1992;145:610–616.
51. Frost AE, Keller CA, Brown RW, et al. Giant cell interstitial pneumonitis: disease recurrence in the transplanted lung. *Am Rev Respir Dis*. 1993;148:1401–1404.
52. Ohori NP, Sciurba FC, Owens GR, et al. Giant-cell interstitial pneumonia and hard-metal pneumoconiosis: a clinicopathologic study of four cases and review of the literature. *Am J Surg Pathol*. 1989;13:581–587.

53. Stettler LE, Groth DH, Platek SF. Automated characterization of particles extracted from human lungs: three cases of tungsten carbide exposure. *Scan Electron Microsc*. 1983;I:439–448.

54. Tabatowski K, Roggli VL, Fulkerson WJ, et al. Giant cell interstitial pneumonia in a hard-metal worker: cytologic, histologic and analytical electron microscopic investigation. *Acta Cytol*. 1988;32:240–246.

55. Meyer KC. Beryllium and lung disease. *Chest*. 1994;106:942–946.

56. Kriebel D, Brain JD, Sprince NL, Kazemi H. The pulmonary toxicity of beryllium. *Am Rev Respir Dis*. 1988;137:464–473.

57. Cullen MR, Kominsky JR, Rossman MD, et al. Chronic beryllium disease in a precious metal refinery. *Am Rev Respir Dis*. 1987;135:201–208.

58. Newman LS, Kreiss K, King TE, Seay S, Campbell PA. Pathologic and immunologic alterations in early stages of beryllium disease: re-examination of disease definition and natural history. *Am Rev Respir Dis*. 1989;139:1479–1486.

59. Kotloff RM, Richman PS, Greenacre JK, Rossman MD. Chronic beryllium disease in a dental laboratory technician. *Am Rev Respir Dis*. 1993;147:205–207.

60. Newman LS, Kreiss K. Nonoccupational beryllium disease masquerading as sarcoidosis: identification by blood lymphocyte proliferative response to beryllium. *Am Rev Respir Dis*. 1992;145:1212–1214.

61. Butnor KJ, Sporn TA, Ingram P, et al. Beryllium detection in human lung tissue using electron probe X-ray microanalysis. *Mod Pathol*. 2003;16:1171–1177.

62. McDonald JW, Ghio AJ, Sheehan CE, Bernhardt PF, Roggli VL. Rare earth (cerium oxide) pneumoconiosis: analytical scanning electron microscopy and literature review. *Mod Pathol*. 1995;8:859–865.

63. Waring PM, Waring RJ. Rare earth deposits in a deceased movie projectionist: a new case of rare earth pneumoconiosis? *Med J Aust*. 1990;153:726–730.

64. Sulotto F, Romano C, Berra A, et al. Rare earth pneumoconiosis: a new case. *Am J Ind Med*. 1986;9:567–575.

65. Husain MH, Dick JA, Kaplan YS. Rare earth pneumoconiosis. *J Soc Occup Med*. 1980;30:15–19.

66. Beton DC, Andrews GS, Davies HJ, et al. Acute cadmium fume poisoning. Five cases with one death from renal necrosis. *Br J Ind Med*. 1966;23:292–301.

67. Yamamoto K, Ueda M, Kikuchi H, et al. An acute fatal occupational cadmium poisoning by inhalation. *Z Rechtsmed*. 1983;91:139–143.

68. Lane RE, Campbell AC. Fatal emphysema in two men making a copper cadmium alloy. *Br J Ind Med*. 1954;11:118–122.

69. Bonnell JA. Emphysema and proteinuria in men casting copper-cadmium alloys. *Br J Ind Med*. 1955;12:181–195.

70. Kelleher P, Pacheco K, Newman LS. Inorganic dust pneumonias: the metal-related parenchymal disorders. *Environ Health Perspect*. 2000;108(suppl 4):685–696.

71. Elinder CG, Kjellstrom T, Lind B, et al. Cadmium exposure from smoking cigarettes: variations with time and country where purchased. *Environ Res*. 1983;32:220–227.

72. Hirst Jr RN, Perry Jr HM, Cruz MG, et al. Elevated cadmium concentration in emphysematous lungs. *Am Rev Respir Dis*. 1973;108:30–39.

73. Davison AG, Fayers PM, Taylor AJ, et al. Cadmium fume inhalation and emphysema. *Lancet*. 1988;1:663–667.

74. Pimentel JC, Marques F. "Vineyard sprayer's lung": a new occupational disease. *Thorax*. 1969;24:678–688.

75. Villar TG. Vineyard sprayer's lung. Clinical aspects. *Am Rev Respir Dis*. 1974;110:545–555.

76. Funahashi A, Schlueter DP, Pintar K, et al. Pneumoconiosis in workers exposed to silicon carbide. *Am Rev Respir Dis*. 1984;129:635–640.

77. Loewen GM, Weiner D, McMahan J. Pneumoconiosis in an elderly dentist. *Chest*. 1988;93:1312–1313.

78. Masse S, Begin R, Cantin A. Pathology of silicon carbide pneumoconiosis. *Mod Pathol*. 1988;1:104–108.

79. Silicosis in dental laboratory technicians—five states, 1994–2000. *MMWR Morb Mortal Wkly Rep*. 2004;53:195–197.

80. De Vuyst P, Vande Weyer R, De Coster A, et al. Dental technician's pneumoconiosis. A report of two cases. *Am Rev Respir Dis*. 1986;133:316–320.

81. Morgenroth K, Kronenberger H, Michalke G, et al. Morphology and pathogenesis of pneumoconiosis in dental technicians. *Pathol Res Pract*. 1985;179:528–536.

82. Rom WN, Lockey JE, Lee JS, et al. Pneumoconiosis and exposures of dental laboratory technicians. *Am J Public Health*. 1984;74:1252–1257.

83. Selden A, Sahle W, Johansson L, et al. Three cases of dental technician's pneumoconiosis related to cobalt-chromium-molybdenum dust exposure. *Chest*. 1996;109:837–842.

84. Cullen MR, Balmes JR, Robins JM, et al. Lipoid pneumonia caused by oil mist exposure from a steel rolling tandem mill. *Am J Ind Med*. 1981;2:51–58.

85. Skorodin MS, Chandrasekhar AJ. An occupational cause of exogenous lipoid pneumonia. *Arch Pathol Lab Med*. 1983;107:610–611.

86. Jarvholm B. Cutting oil mist and bronchitis. *Eur J Respir Dis Suppl*. 1982;118:79–83.

87. Skyberg K, Ronneberg A, Kamoy JI, et al. Pulmonary fibrosis in cable plant workers exposed to mist and vapor of petroleum distillates. *Environ Res*. 1986;40:261–273.

88. Beckett W, Kallay M, Sood A, et al. Hypersensitivity pneumonitis associated with environmental mycobacteria. *Environ Health Perspect*. 2005;113:767–770.

89. Kreiss K, Cox-Ganser J. Metalworking fluid-associated hypersensitivity pneumonitis: a work-shop summary. *Am J Ind Med*. 1997;32:423–432.

90. Bernstein DI, Lummus ZL, Santilli G, et al. Machine operator's lung. A hypersensitivity pneumonitis disorder associated with exposure to metalworking fluid aerosols. *Chest*. 1995;108:636–641.

91. Gupta A, Rosenman KD. Hypersensitivity pneumonitis due to metal working fluids: sporadic or under reported? *Am J Ind Med*. 2006;49:423–433.

92. Eschenbacher WL, Kreiss K, Lougheed MD, et al. Nylon flock–associated interstitial lung disease. *Am J Respir Crit Care Med*. 1999;159:2003–2008.

93. Kern DG, Kuhn 3rd C, Ely EW, et al. Flock worker's lung: broadening the spectrum of clinicopathology, narrowing the spectrum of suspected etiologies. *Chest*. 2000;117:251–259.

94. Kern DG, Crausman RS, Durand KT, et al. Flock worker's lung: chronic interstitial lung disease in the nylon flocking industry. *Ann Intern Med*. 1998;129:261–272.

95. Boag AH, Colby TV, Fraire AE, et al. The pathology of interstitial lung disease in nylon flock workers. *Am J Surg Pathol*. 1999;23:1539–1545.

96. Kanwal R, Kullman G, Piacitelli C, et al. Evaluation of flavorings-related lung disease risk at six microwave popcorn plants. *J Occup Environ Med*. 2006;48:149–157.

97. van Rooy FG, Rooyackers JM, Prokop M, et al. Bronchiolitis obliterans syndrome in chemical workers producing diacetyl for food flavorings. *Am J Respir Crit Care Med*. 2007;176:498–504.

98. Kreiss K, Gomaa A, Kullman G, et al. Clinical bronchiolitis obliterans in workers at a microwave-popcorn plant. *N Engl J Med*. 2002;347:330–338.

99. Akpinar-Elci M, Travis WD, Lynch DA, et al. Bronchiolitis obliterans syndrome in popcorn production plant workers. *Eur Respir J*. 2004;24:298–302.

100. Hendrick DJ. "Popcorn worker's lung" in Britain in a man making potato crisp flavouring. *Thorax*. 2008;63:267–268.

101. Hubbs AF, Battelli LA, Goldsmith WT, et al. Necrosis of nasal and airway epithelium in rats inhaling vapors of artificial butter flavoring. *Toxicol Appl Pharmacol*. 2002;185:128–135.

102. Balakrishnan K, Sankar S, Parikh J, et al. Daily average exposures to respirable particulate matter from combustion of biomass fuels in rural households of southern India. *Environ Health Perspect*. 2002;110:1069–1075.

103. Balakrishnan K, Sambandam S, Ramaswamy P, et al. Exposure assessment for respirable particulates associated with household fuel use in rural districts of Andhra Pradesh, India. *J Expo Anal Environ Epidemiol*. 2004;14(suppl 1):S14–S25.

104. Grobbelaar JP, Bateman ED. Hut lung: a domestically acquired pneumoconiosis of mixed aetiology in rural women. *Thorax*. 1991;46:334–440.

105. Gold JA, Jagirdar J, Hay JG, et al. Hut lung. A domestically acquired particulate lung disease. *Medicine (Baltimore)*. 2000;79:310–317.

106. Dennis RJ, Maldonado D, Norman S, et al. Woodsmoke exposure and risk for obstructive airways disease among women. *Chest*. 1996;109:115–119.

107. Bruce N, Perez-Padilla R, Albalak R. Indoor air pollution in developing countries: a major environmental and public health challenge. *Bull World Health Organ*. 2000;78:1078–1092.

108. Perez-Padilla R, Regalado J, Vedal S, et al. Exposure to biomass smoke and chronic airway disease in Mexican women. A case-control study. *Am J Respir Crit Care Med*. 1996;154:701–706.

109. Ramirez-Venegas A, Sansores RH, Perez-Padilla R, et al. Survival of patients with chronic obstructive pulmonary disease due to biomass smoke and tobacco. *Am J Respir Crit Care Med*. 2006;173:393–397.

110. Diaz JV, Koff J, Gotway MB, et al. Case report: a case of wood-smoke-related pulmonary disease. *Environ Health Perspect*. 2006;114:759–762.

Pulmonary Vasculitis and Pulmonary Hemorrhage

William D. Travis, MD, Kevin O. Leslie, MD, and Mary Beth Beasley, MD

PULMONARY VASCULITIS
Overview of Pulmonary Vasculitis

Inflammation of arteries and veins can occur in many inflammatory lung diseases, including infections. By convention, the diagnostic term *pulmonary vasculitis* is restricted to a relatively limited number of diseases in which vascular inflammation is thought to be a major component of the pathologic process. Most pulmonary vasculitides are believed to be immune-mediated diseases, although their etiology and pathogenesis remain unknown. By best estimates, the overall annual incidence of the major forms of vasculitis is 39 per 1 million.[1]

When pulmonary vasculitis occurs, there is inflammation of the vessel wall, often accompanied by fibrin and sometimes, necrosis. Cuffing of blood vessels by inflammatory cells, a nonspecific finding, must be distinguished from infiltration of inflammatory cells into the media and intima of arteries and veins (Fig. 10-1).

A diagnosis of pulmonary vasculitis carries a strong implication for immediate therapeutic intervention (typically immunosuppression) and therefore should never be made lightly. Furthermore, serologic and clinical correlation with the pathologic findings is essential for a correct diagnosis. Typical histologic examples of pulmonary vasculitis-capillaritis are shown in Figure 10-2.

The general category of pulmonary vasculitis includes a number of different diseases that can be more easily understood by dividing them into three main groups: (1) idiopathic vasculitic syndromes that commonly involve the lung (e.g., Wegener granulomatosis [WG]), (2) vasculitic disorders that rarely involve the lung (a much larger number), and (3) miscellaneous conditions that produce pulmonary vascular inflammation[2,3] (Box 10-1).

WG, Churg-Strauss syndrome (CSS), and microscopic polyangiitis are the idiopathic vasculitis syndromes that commonly affect the lung. The conditions of bronchocentric granulomatosis and lymphomatoid granulomatosis traditionally have been grouped in the category of pulmonary "angiitis and granulomatosis"; however, neither of these entities is currently thought to be a vasculitic condition. Bronchocentric granulomatosis is a morphologic pattern of airway inflammation that occurs in a variety of conditions, especially infection, and lymphomatoid granulomatosis (also known as angiocentric immunoproliferative disorder) is now known to represent a lymphoproliferative disease in which prominent vascular involvement occurs.[4–6]

Idiopathic vasculitis syndromes that rarely affect the lung include such diseases as necrotizing sarcoid granulomatosis, Takayasu arteritis, giant cell arteritis, and Behçet syndrome, among others. Necrotizing sarcoid granulomatosis was formerly regarded as one of the major vasculitic syndromes, but it is very rare and does not typically cause a systemic vasculitis, so it is now grouped with the syndromes that

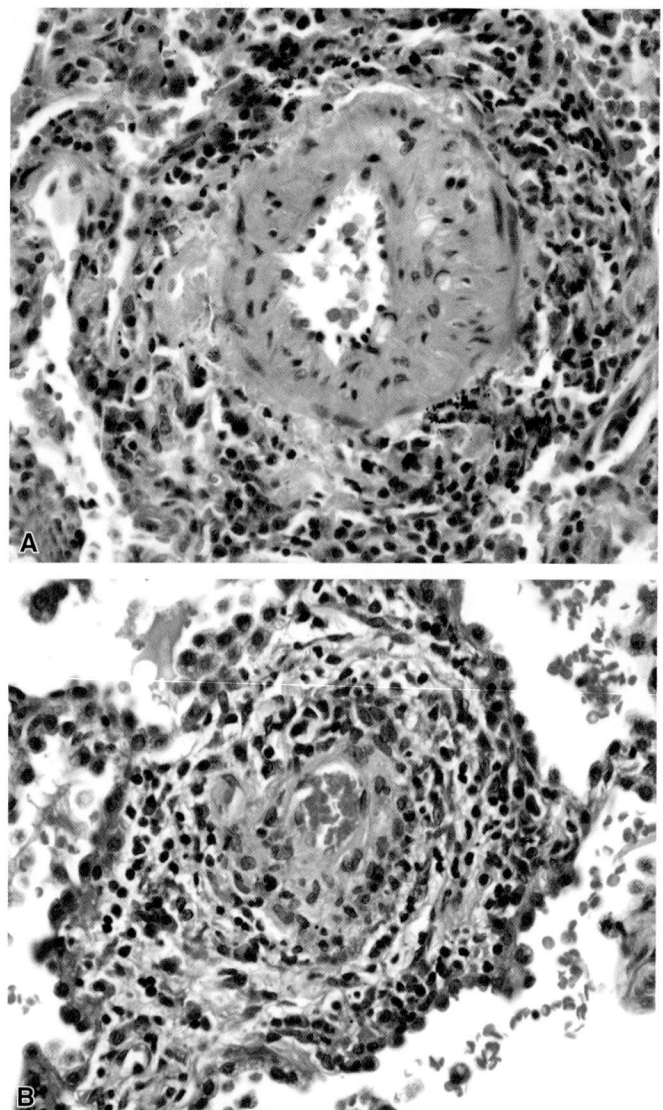

Figure 10-1. Vascular inflammation versus vasculitis. **A,** Vessel-associated inflammation. **B,** True vasculitis. Note the disruption of the media by inflammatory cells in true vasculitis.

Box 10-1. Pulmonary Vasculitis Syndromes

Idiopathic vasculitis syndromes that commonly affect the lung
    Wegener granulomatosis
    Churg-Strauss angiitis and granulomatosis
    Microscopic polyangiitis
Idiopathic vasculitis syndromes that uncommonly affect the lung
    Necrotizing sarcoid granulomatosis
    Polyarteritis nodosa
    Small-vessel vasculitis
    Takayasu arteritis
    Henoch-Schönlein purpura
    Behçet syndrome
    Cryoglobulinemic vasculitis
    Hypocomplementemic vasculitis
    Idiopathic granulomatous arteritis
        Giant cell arteritis
        Disseminated visceral giant cell angiitis
Miscellaneous systemic disorders
    Classic sarcoid
    Collagen vascular disease
    Inflammatory bowel disease
    Malignancy
Diffuse pulmonary hemorrhage syndromes
Secondary or localized vasculitis
    Pulmonary infection
    Bronchocentric granulomatosis
    Pulmonary hypertension
    Interstitial lung diseases
        Chronic eosinophilic pneumonia
        Histiocytosis X
    Inflammatory pseudotumors and pseudolymphomas
    Sequestration
    Embolic material (intravenous drug abuse)
    Drug or toxic substances
    Transplantation
    Radiation
Vascular involvement in lymphoproliferative disorders
    Angiocentric immunoproliferative lesion (lymphomatoid granulomatosis)
    Non-Hodgkin lymphoma
    Intravascular malignant lymphoma

Modified from Travis W, Koss M. Vasculitis. In: Dail D, Hammar S, eds. *Pulmonary Pathology.* New York: Springer-Verlag; 1994:1027–1095.

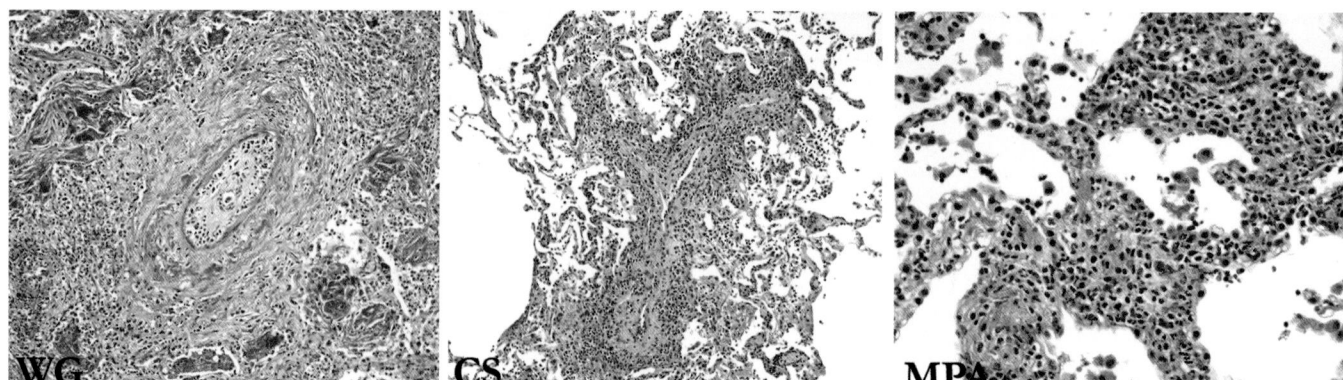

Figure 10-2. Common histopathologic manifestations of pulmonary vasculitis. Histopathologic appearance in three of the most common manifestations of pulmonary vasculitis: Wegener granulomatosis (WG), Churg-Strauss syndrome (CS), and microscopic polyangiitis (MPA).

uncommonly affect the lung. Pulmonary vascular inflammation also occurs in a number of miscellaneous systemic disorders, in diffuse pulmonary hemorrhage syndromes (discussed later), and in a variety of secondary or localized forms.

Vasculitic syndromes pose major challenges to the surgical pathologist. First, as with many non-neoplastic lung diseases, the diagnosis does not rest on pathology alone. Correlation among clinical, radiologic, and pathologic features is required for most of these entities. Second, because these are rare disorders, few pathologists have much experience with their diagnostic subtleties. Third, the pathologic features of these infrequently encountered conditions overlap with those of common inflammatory lesions, including necrotizing infectious granulomas produced by mycobacteria or fungi. Because most vasculitis syndromes are treated with immunosuppressive agents, separation from infectious conditions is essential. With the use of antineutrophil cytoplasmic antibody (ANCA) testing the diagnosis often is suspected early in the course of disease, so biopsies may be obtained before the tissues show all of the classic histologic manifestations. In addition, partial treatment before the biopsy can alter the expected histologic findings. Finally, in many cases, the histopathologic findings may not be "classic," requiring the recognition of subtle clues in order to suspect the diagnosis.

Idiopathic Vasculitic Syndromes That Commonly Affect the Lung

Wegener Granulomatosis

WG is a rare systemic inflammatory disease of unknown etiology that has vasculitis as a major histologic manifestation. WG predominantly affects the upper and lower respiratory tract and the kidneys.[7] Although this pattern of involvement is often referred to as the "classic triad" of WG, more frequently only one or two sites may be involved. In one series reported by DeRemee and associates, involvement of all three sites was seen in only 14 of 50 patients.[8] "Limited WG" historically has been defined as disease involving the lungs without associated glomerular disease,[9] although the term is also used to describe active disease without involvement that threatens the function of a vital organ or the patient's life.[10]

Despite the designation *granulomatosis*, well-defined granulomas without necrosis (sarcoid-like) are not a feature of this disease. The necrotizing lesions of WG have a peripheral zone of palisaded histiocytes, contrasting with the more epithelioid histiocytes seen at the periphery of necrosis produced by mycobacteria or fungi (Fig. 10-3). In fact, when well-formed (sarcoid-like) granulomas without necrosis are present in a potential case of WG, another diagnosis should be considered (usually infection).

Clinical Features

WG affects about 1 in every 3 million people in the United States[11] and 1 in 8.5 million people in the United Kingdom.[12] There is debate as to whether WG occurs more frequently during cold seasons, with some studies suggesting an increased occurrence in winter months.[12] Other studies have disputed these results.[11] Although the etiology of WG remains essentially unknown, several theories have been proposed. One theory is that an inciting inflammatory event invokes a specific immune response leading to the production of ANCAs (also discussed in the "Laboratory Studies" section), with ANCA playing a direct role in inciting tissue damage.[13,14] A potential link between infections and the development of WG is being explored. It has been noted that a subtype of ANCA directed against lysosomal membrane–associated protein 2 (LAMP-2) is found in more than 90% of patients with pauci-immune necrotizing glomerulonephritis and frequently coexists with antiproteinase-3, and antimyeloperoxidase LAMP-2 has been observed to activate neutrophils, as well as causing injury to vascular endothelial cells in the absence of neutrophils. LAMP-2 cross-reacts with the bacterial adhesin FimH, and one study found that infection with bacteria expressing FimH occurred in 69% of patients in whom ANCA-positive glomerulonephritis subsequently developed.[15,16] Although such findings suggest a potential link between infection and the production of ANCA, further study is needed in regard to a link between infection and WG. Similarly, other studies have demonstrated a link between T cells and the development of ANCA and have shown a particular role for T-helper 1 (Th1) lymphocytes, although the role of the Th1 lymphocytic pathway in the development of WG is still being elucidated.[17,18] Genetic factors, toxic exposures, and deficient proteinase-3 clearance are also being explored as potential causes and contributing factors.[11,19]

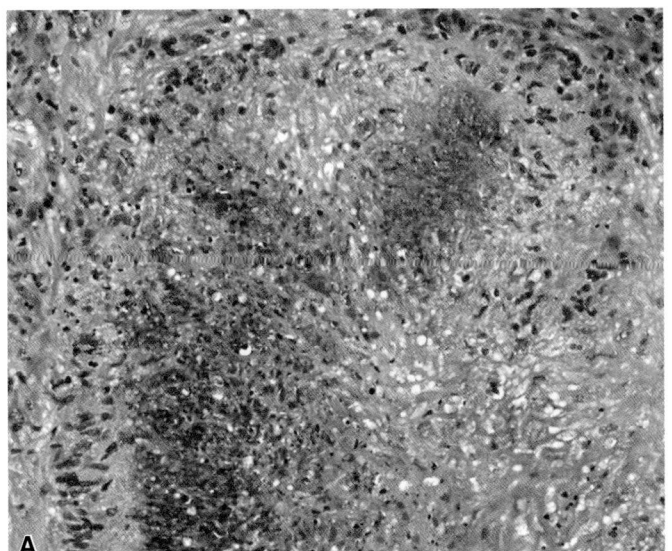
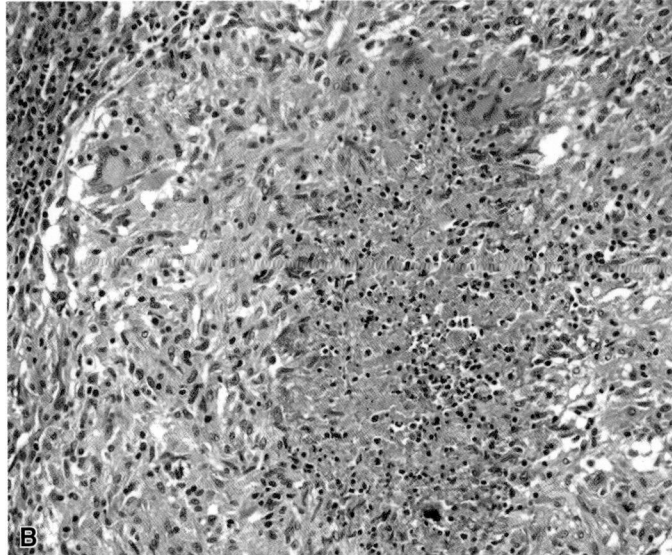

Figure 10-3. The granulomas of Wegener granulomatosis (WG). WG granulomas (**A**) tend to be more "palisaded" than those seen in granulomatous infection (**B**). Also note the *blue* (basophilic) necrosis of WG, compared with the *pink* (eosinophilic) necrosis of infection.

WG occurs at any age but typically is a disease of adults, with a mean age of 50 years.[20-22] A list of the clinical manifestations of WG is presented in Table 10-1. Body sites most commonly affected are the head and neck region, followed by the lung, kidney, and eye.[20,23] Patients may experience a number of other complaints such as

Table 10-1. Wegener Granulomatosis: Clinical Manifestations

Manifestation	At Presentation	During Course of Disease
	Frequency (%)	
Head and neck manifestations	73	92
Sinusitis	51	85
Nasal disease	36	68
Otitis media	25	44
Hearing loss	14	42
Subglottic stenosis	8	16
Ear pain	1	14
Oral lesions	3	10
Pulmonary manifestations	45	85
Infiltrates	23	66
Nodule	22	59
Cough	19	46
Hemoptysis	12	30
Pleuritis	10	28
Renal manifestations	18	77
Eye manifestations	15	52
Conjunctivitis	5	18
Dacryocystitis	1	18
Scleritis	6	16
Proptosis	2	15
Eye pain	3	11
Visual loss	0	8
Retinal lesions	0	4
Corneal ulcers	0	1
Iritis	0	2
Systemic manifestations		
Joints	32	67
Fever	23	50
Skin changes	13	46
Weight loss	15	35
Peripheral nervous system abnormalities	1	15
Central nervous system abnormalities	1	8
Pericarditis	2	6

Data from Hoffman GS, Kerr GS, Leavitt RY, et al. Wegener's granulomatosis: an analysis of 158 patients. *Ann Intern Med.* 1992;116:488–498.

hoarseness, stridor, earache, hearing loss, otorrhea, cough, dyspnea, hemoptysis, or pleuritic pain. Pulmonary symptoms in the absence of upper respiratory tract manifestations are unusual. Destructive inflammation of the nose may result in a saddlenose deformity. In addition, patients may exhibit more generalized systemic signs and symptoms including arthralgias, fever, cutaneous lesions, weight loss, and peripheral neuropathy.[24] Rarely WG may involve the salivary glands, pancreas, breast, mediastinum, gastrointestinal tract, prostate and urethra, vagina and cervix, heart, spleen, or peripheral or central nervous system.[2,25-27]

The most frequent abnormality on pulmonary function testing is airflow obstruction, often associated with a reduced diffusing capacity for carbon monoxide (DLco), but restrictive or mixed patterns can occur. When significant airflow obstruction is identified, patients may be at risk for tracheal obstruction or lobar collapse secondary to bronchial wall damage resulting from the disease.

Laboratory Studies

Nonspecific abnormalities on general laboratory tests are often present in patients with WG. The most common of these include leukocytosis, thrombocytosis (>400,000 cells/µL), marked elevation of the erythrocyte sedimentation rate, and normochromic normocytic anemia. In the past decade, the diagnosis of WG has been dramatically aided by the discovery and use of serum ANCA.[28-32]

Two major immunofluorescence patterns occur as expressions of ANCA (Fig. 10-4): the cytoplasmic or classic type (c-ANCA) and the perinuclear type (p-ANCA).[33] The c-ANCA pattern is associated with WG and is present in the vast majority of patients with active generalized disease. Partial or complete remission of disease is reflected in a lower frequency of a positive test result, but 30% to 40% of patients in complete remission still have identifiable antibodies.[34] The p-ANCA pattern can be seen in a small percentage of patients with WG, but it is more characteristic of idiopathic necrotizing and crescentic glomerulonephritis, microscopic polyangiitis, polyarteritis nodosa, and CSS.[35]

The ANCA immunofluorescence patterns have been shown to correspond to specific antigen immunoreactivities; c-ANCA typically has specificity for proteinase-3, while most p-ANCAs have a specificity for myeloperoxidase. Studies have shown no significant difference in the lung biopsy findings from WG patients with c-ANCAs versus those with p-ANCAs.[36,37] Levels of c-ANCA in the bronchoalveolar lavage fluid have not been shown to be a more specific predictor of WG or of the level of disease.[38] Importantly, the presence or absence of a positive serum test for c-ANCA alone is not sufficiently specific

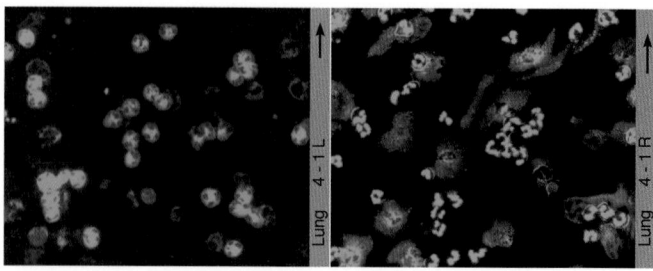

Figure 10-4. Antineutrophilic cytoplasmic antibody (ANCA) immunofluorescence. *Left,* Cytoplasmic staining of neutrophils characterizes the c-ANCA pattern. *Right,* Perinuclear accentuation of staining is seen with the p-ANCA pattern. (From Travis WD, Colby TV, Koss MN, et al, eds. *Non-Neoplastic Disorders of the Lower Respiratory Tract.* In: King DW, ed. *Atlas of Nontumor Pathology.* Washington, DC: American Registry of Pathology and Armed Forces Institute of Pathology; 2002, Figure 4-1.)

to make or exclude the diagnosis of WG, and c-ANCA may occasionally be encountered in patients with other vasculitic syndromes or infection.[39]

Radiologic Features

Most patients with pulmonary disease have multiple opacities (Figs. 10-5 and 10-6) in the form of well-marginated nodules or masses of variable size (0.5–10 cm). Lesions may wax and wane over time. Most occur in the lower lobes.[40–42] Poorly defined or even spiculated nodules may also be seen.[43] Cavitation of nodules occurs in 25% to 50% of cases, with cavity walls typically being thick and

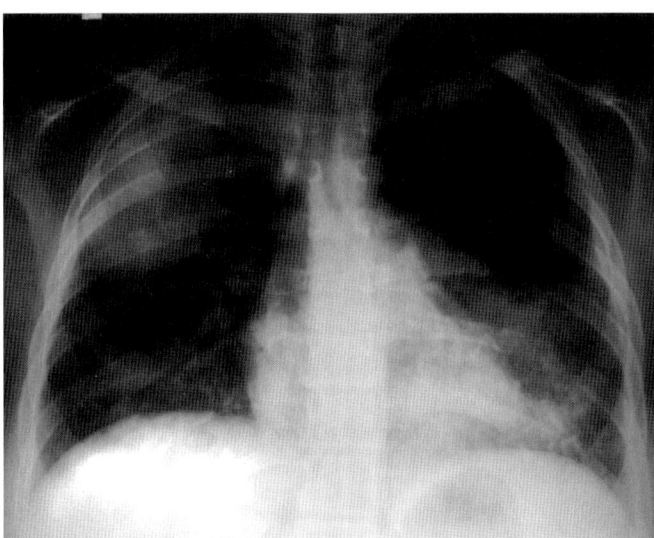

Figure 10-5. Wegener granulomatosis (WG): radiographic features. Posteroanterior chest radiograph from a patient with WG. Note the multifocal nodules, some of which appear cavitated. (From Travis WD, Colby TV, Koss MN, et al, eds. *Non-Neoplastic Disorders of the Lower Respiratory Tract.* In: King DW, ed. *Atlas of Nontumor Pathology.* Washington, DC: American Registry of Pathology and Armed Forces Institute of Pathology; 2002, Figure 4-2.)

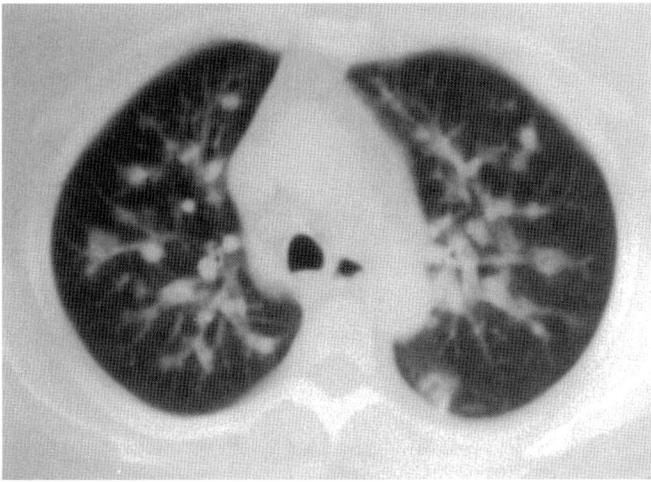

Figure 10-6. Wegener granulomatosis: computed tomography (CT) features. Chest CT scan (lung window) demonstrates multifocal, ill-defined small nodular opacities in close relationship to pulmonary arteries. Note the thick walls of these well-marginated lesions. (From Travis WD, Colby TV, Koss MN, et al, eds. *Non-Neoplastic Disorders of the Lower Respiratory Tract.* In: King DW, ed. *Atlas of Nontumor Pathology.* Washington, DC: American Registry of Pathology and Armed Forces Institute of Pathology; 2002, Figure 4-3.)

irregular. Such lesions may evolve into thin-walled cysts or disappear completely with therapy.[42,44] WG is often included in the differential diagnosis for interstitial lung disease because multifocal, ill-defined parenchymal consolidations can occur (with or without cavitation) and diffuse reticular and nodular interstitial opacities have also been reported.[42,45]

Patients with WG may present initially with pulmonary hemorrhage. In this setting, diffuse infiltrates on chest radiographs and diffuse air space opacities on computed tomograms are observed (see Fig. 10-6). In children, pulmonary hemorrhage is a common presentation of WG, while pulmonary nodules occur less frequently in pediatric patients.[22]

Pleural effusion accompanies WG in 20% to 50% of cases, sometimes with focal pleural thickening. Hilar or mediastinal lymphadenopathy is an unusual finding in WG and, when significant, should raise concern for an alternate diagnosis. On rare occasions, WG occurs as a solitary pulmonary nodule (with or without cavitation), or as an isolated area of consolidation.[46]

Computed tomography (CT) provides optimal visualization of the number, location, and morphologic characteristics of the pulmonary abnormalities in WG. Well-marginated nodules and masses, sometimes with spiculated borders, are typical findings. A "feeding" vessel is seen in 88% of nodules (see Fig. 10-6), consistent with the angiocentric nature of this disorder.[47] Cavitation is identified in 50% of cases. Another very common finding in WG is wedge-shaped peripheral opacities mimicking the CT appearance of infarct. Other, less common radiologic presentations include air bronchograms and the CT halo sign (ground glass opacity surrounding a pulmonary nodule or mass).[47,48] Stenosis of the trachea or large airways may occur in short or long segments and may be complicated by partial or complete lobar collapse.[45,49,50]

Pathologic Features

WG is characterized by the presence of multiple bilateral pulmonary nodules, often with cavitation[51] (Fig. 10-7; see also Fig. 10-6). Solid nodular zones of consolidation with areas of punctate or geographic necrosis are typical findings (Figs. 10-8 and 10-9). WG can rarely present with a solitary lung lesion, but solitary granulomatous disease is more likely to be of infectious origin.[52] When dealing with a solitary granulomatous lung nodule, a combination of both the classical histology and typical clinical or serologic findings of WG should be present before making a diagnosis.[46] Even when special stains for organisms and cultures are negative, most of these solitary lesions represent old fungal or mycobacterial infection. Rarely the lesions of WG may predominantly involve bronchi. When acute lung hemorrhage is prominent, the cut surface of the lung is bloody and dark red.

At scanning magnification, the pulmonary lesions of WG simulate their radiologic appearance (see Fig. 10-8). The classic findings consist of nodular areas of consolidation with variable zones of necrosis. Major diagnostic criteria, presented in Box 10-2, include parenchymal necrosis (see Fig. 10-9), vasculitis (Fig. 10-10), and granulomatous inflammation (Fig. 10-11). Another important feature is a mixed inflammatory infiltrate composed of neutrophils, lymphocytes, plasma cells, macrophages, giant cells, and eosinophils (Fig. 10-12). Parenchymal necrosis can take the form of neutrophilic microabscesses (Fig. 10-13) or large zones of geographic necrosis (see Fig. 10-9). The neutrophilic microabscesses are nearly pathognomonic of the disease and can be found within the mixed inflammatory infiltrate or within fibrous connective tissue including the adventitial collagen of larger arteries and veins and the pleura. Early microabscesses may consist of a small collection of neutrophils surrounding a focus of degenerated, often hypereosinophilic, collagen.[51]

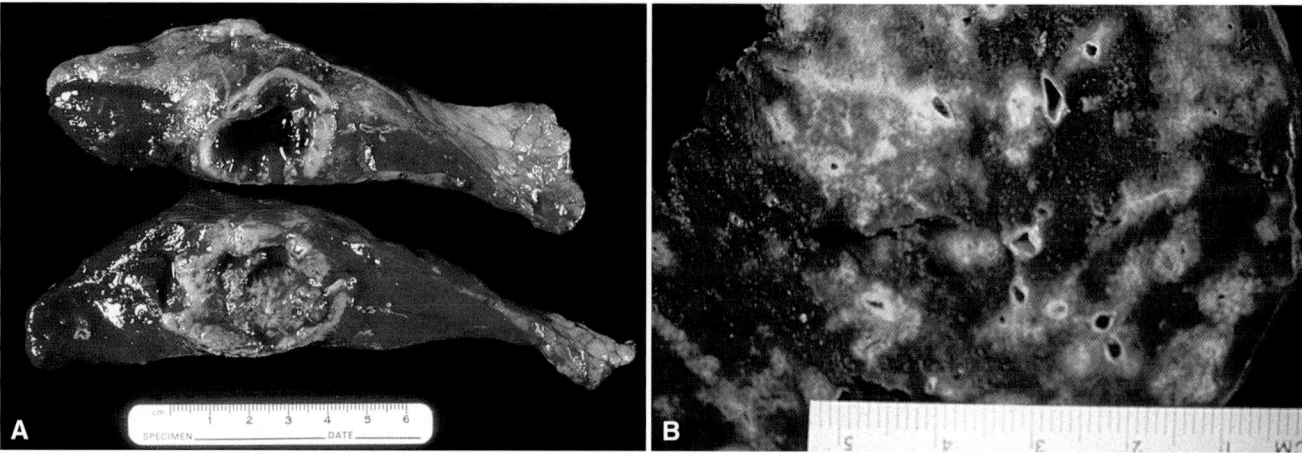

Figure 10-7. Wegener granulomatosis: gross specimen. **A,** This necrotizing granuloma is cavitated with a necrotic center and an inflammatory border. **B,** Multiple scattered nodular foci of consolidation are present. *Yellow-white areas* represent necrosis. (From Travis WD, Colby TV, Koss MN, et al, eds. *Non-Neoplastic Disorders of the Lower Respiratory Tract.* In: King DW, ed. *Atlas of Nontumor Pathology.* Washington, DC: American Registry of Pathology and Armed Forces Institute of Pathology; 2002, Figure 4-5.)

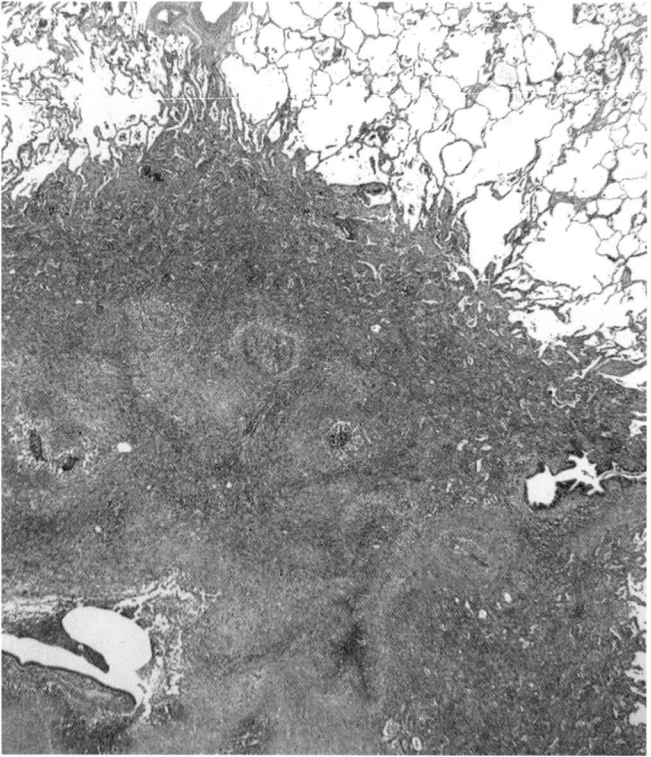

Figure 10-8. Wegener granulomatosis: nodular lesions. A characteristic nodular lesion seen at scanning magnification shows the thick inflammatory wall surrounding irregular zones of basophilic necrosis. Note the airways and arteries visible within the lesion.

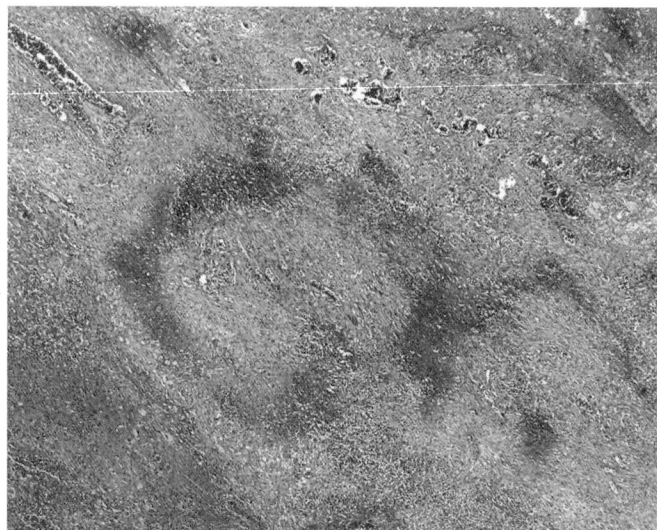

Figure 10-9. Wegener granulomatosis: geographic necrosis. The basophilic necrosis can be appreciated at scanning magnification.

Box 10-2. Wegener Granulomatosis: Major Histopathologic Manifestations (Diagnostic Criteria)

Vasculitis
Arteritis, venulitis, capillaritis*
Six types of inflammation: acute, chronic, necrotizing granulomatous, non-
   necrotizing granulomatous, fibrinoid necrosis, cicatricial changes[†]

Parenchymal Necrosis
Microabscess
Geographic necrosis

Granulomatous Inflammation (and Mixed Inflammatory Infiltrate)
Microabscess surrounded by granulomatous inflammation
Palisading histiocytes
Scattered giant cells
Poorly formed granulomas
Sarcoid-like granulomas (rare)

*Capillaritis was characterized primarily by acute inflammation. Veins and arteries demonstrated all six types of inflammatory changes as listed.
[†]Cicatricial vascular changes are nonspecific and should not be used as a diagnostic criterion.
Data from Travis W, Koss M. Vasculitis. In: Dail D, Hammar S, eds. *Pulmonary Pathology.* New York: Springer-Verlag; 1994:1027–1095; and Travis WD, Hoffman GS, Leavitt RY, et al. Surgical pathology of the lung in Wegener's granulomatosis. Review of 87 open lung biopsies from 67 patients. *Am J Surg Pathol.* 1991;15:315–333.

As illustrated in Figure 10-9, the classic geographic necrosis of WG is typically basophilic, owing to the presence of numerous necrotic neutrophils. The necrotic centers of WG lesions often lack the "ghosted" image of lung structure, a diagnostic clue useful in the case with atypical features (Fig. 10-14). This likely occurs because the necrotic zones of WG generally are not the result of "infarct-like" zonal parenchymal necrosis but rather occur by progressive expansion of collagen necrosis.

The "granulomatous" inflammation of WG typically includes giant cells scattered randomly or in loose aggregates.[10–15] Also commonly observed are palisaded histiocytes (Fig. 10-15), giant cells lining the border of geographic necrosis or microabscesses, and microgranulomas consisting of small foci of palisaded histiocytes arranged in a

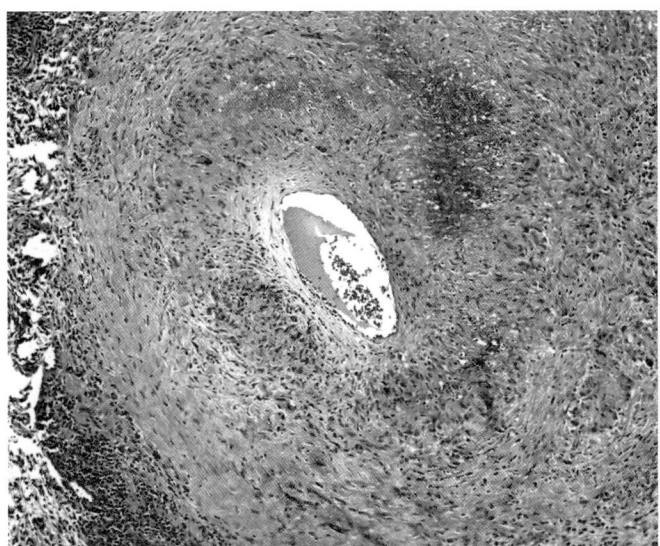

Figure 10-10. Wegener granulomatosis: vasculitis. The vasculitis of Wegener granulomatosis is characterized by necrotizing granulomas involving adventitia and media. This narrowed vessel shows palisaded granulomas with basophilic necrosis accompanied by inflammation and fibrosis of the adventitia.

cartwheel pattern around a central nidus of necrosis[51] (Fig. 10-16). The presence of tightly cohesive, sarcoid-like granulomas is very rare in WG and suggests infection or necrotizing sarcoid. Also, the presence of granulomas without associated necrosis favors an infectious etiology over WG.

The vasculitis of WG typically affects small arteries and veins up to 5 mm in diameter. When vasculitis is seen in the surgical biopsy, it most often occurs within the dense inflammatory infiltrate surrounding nodular or geographic areas of necrosis (Fig. 10-17). Vasculitis in WG may comprise a variety of inflammatory cells including acute or chronic mural inflammation, necrotizing stellate granulomas, non-necrotizing stellate granulomas, and giant cells.[51] Cicatricial changes consisting of mural fibrosis or luminal obliteration may be seen in specimens following therapy. Destruction of the vascular elastic laminae is commonly observed (Fig. 10-18). Sometimes the inflammation is limited to the endothelium (endotheliolitis) and subendothelial aspect

of the vessel wall. Despite these potential vascular changes, if necrotizing vasculitis is held as a requirement for the diagnosis, many cases of WG will be missed.

As mentioned, all types of inflammatory cells may occur in WG, including neutrophils, lymphocytes, plasma cells, eosinophils, histiocytes, and giant cells. Occasionally the inflammatory infiltrate consists mostly of lymphoid cells but this is unusual. In such cases, distinction of WG from lymphomatoid granulomatosis may be difficult.

Another distinctive vascular manifestation of WG is capillaritis (Fig. 10-19). In many cases, capillaritis is only focally evident in the biopsy.[51] When capillaritis is prominent, it is distinctive and easily recognized. In the rare case of WG dominated by capillaritis, a careful search throughout the rest of the biopsy should be made for more typical findings of WG such as granulomas, foci of necrosis (such as neutrophilic microabscesses), multinucleate giant cells, and vasculitis affecting arterioles or veins.

In addition to these major histologic features, a variety of minor histologic features may be encountered (Box 10-3), including alveolar hemorrhage, interstitial fibrosis, lipoid pneumonia, organizing pneumonia, lymphoid hyperplasia, extravascular tissue eosinophils, and xanthomatous lesions. WG can also involve the airways, causing chronic bronchiolitis, acute bronchiolitis or bronchopneumonia, the histologic pattern of organizing pneumonia (see further on), bronchocentric granulomatosis, follicular bronchiolitis, and bronchial stenosis.[51,53] Occasionally one of these minor lesions may be the dominant lung biopsy finding.[51] Diffuse pulmonary hemorrhage is a severe life-threatening manifestation of WG. The pattern of bronchocentric granulomatosis is another rare manifestation of WG encountered in 1% of cases.[51,53] Organizing pneumonia (Fig. 10-20) can be seen in 70% of lung biopsies from patients with WG[51]; rarely, it may be sufficiently dominant that some have referred to this manifestation as the "bronchiolitis obliterans organizing pneumonia" (BOOP) variant of WG.[51,54] This should not be confused with the idiopathic entity of BOOP (cryptogenic organizing pneumonia) but should be recognized as nonspecific secondary organization following alveolar injury related to the underlying lesions of WG.

The lung biopsy findings from patients with WG may not show classical histologic findings, especially if patients are either biopsied very early in the course of disease or following therapy.[51,55] Interstitial fibrosis (sometimes with scattered giant cells, but without necrosis)

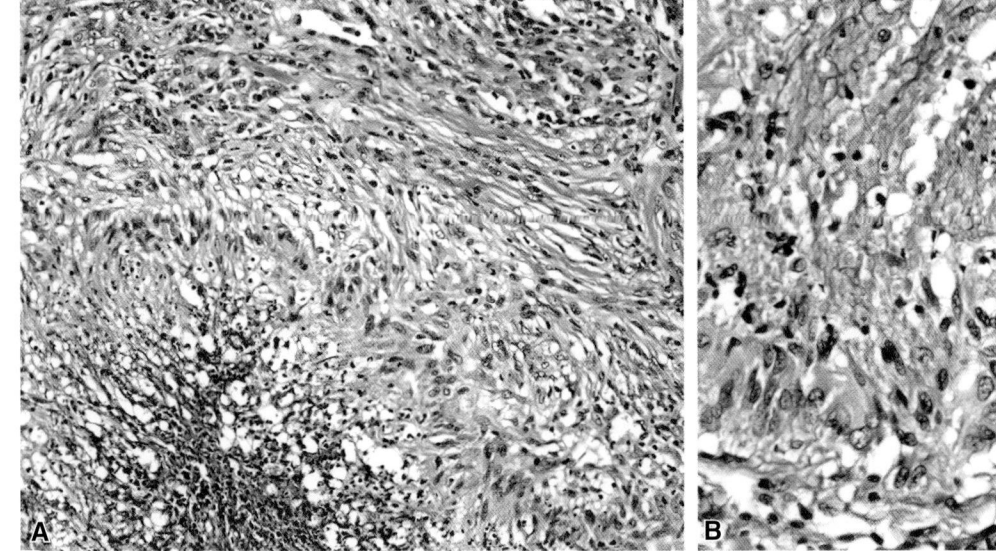

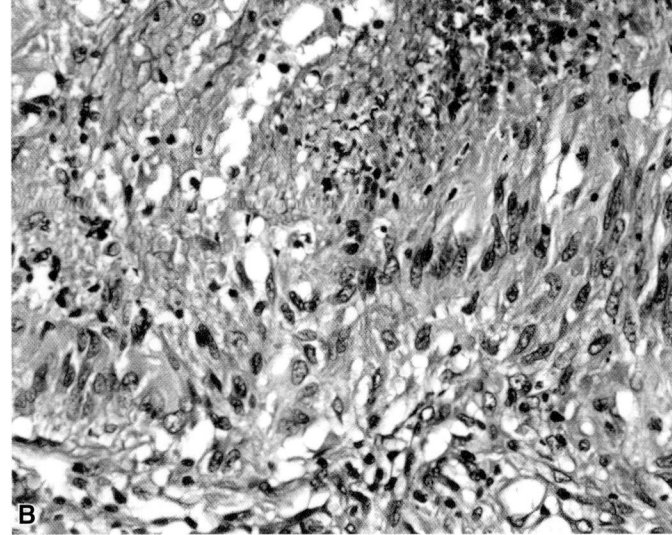

Figure 10-11. Wegener granulomatosis (WG): granulomatous inflammation. **A,** The granulomatous inflammation of WG generally has a palisaded configuration. **B,** A closer view of palisaded histiocytes can be seen bordering basophilic necrosis with nuclear debris.

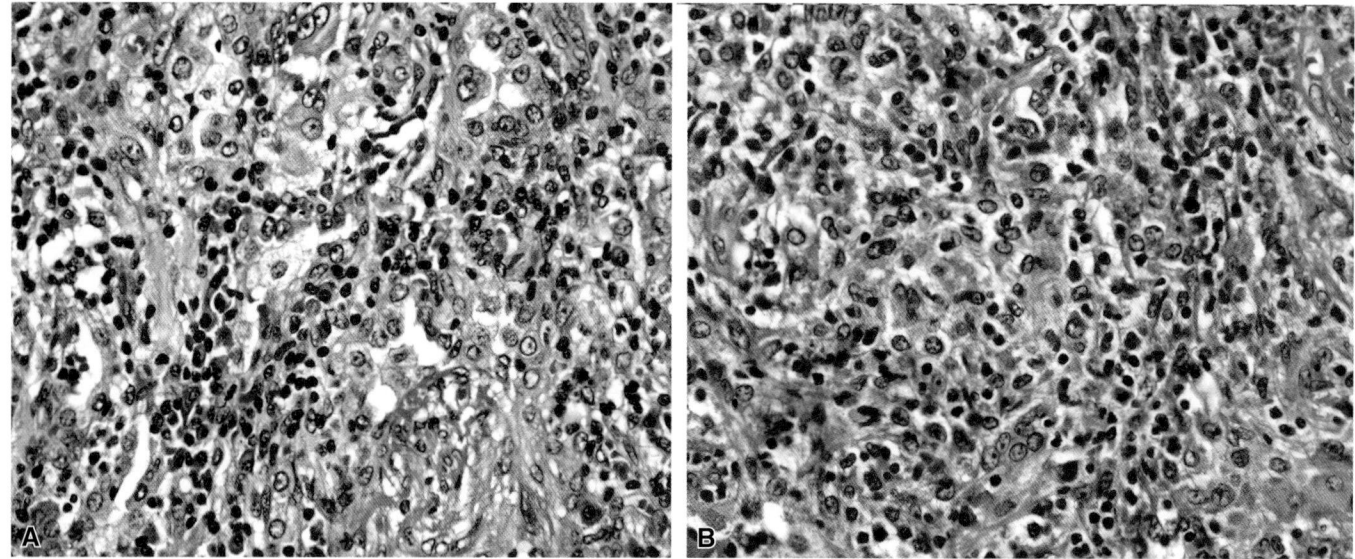

Figure 10-12. Wegener granulomatosis (WG): associated inflammation. Inflammatory infiltrate of WG is generally mixed with plasma cells, lymphocytes (**A**), and a variable number of eosinophils (**B**).

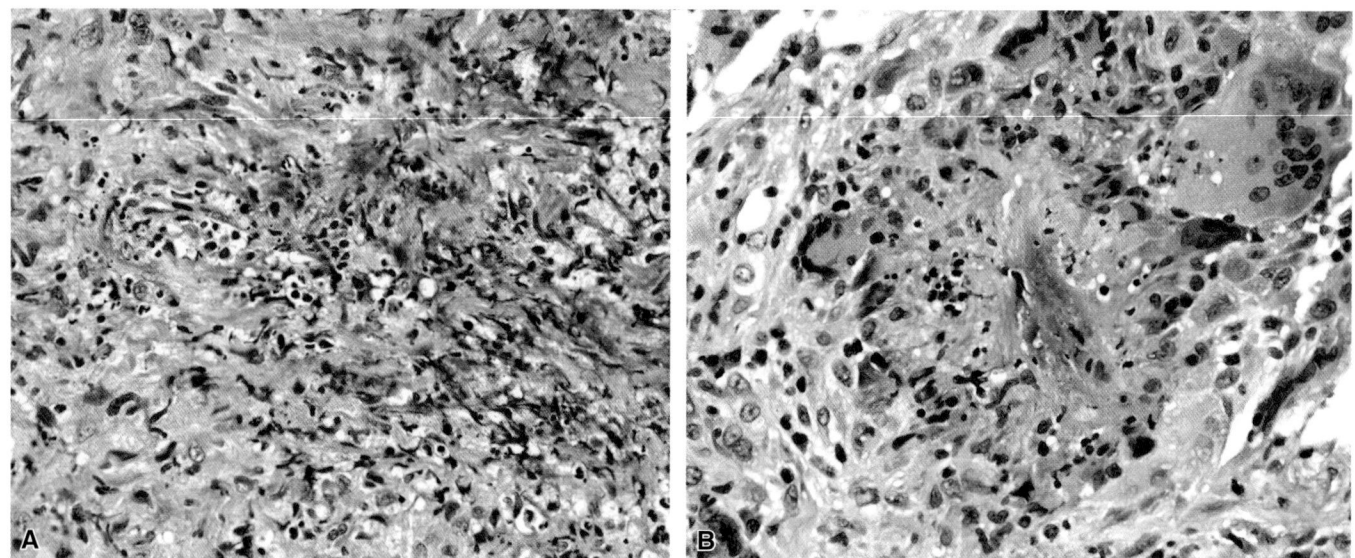

Figure 10-13. Wegener granulomatosis (WG): collagen necrosis. Collagen necrosis is thought to be the primary pathologic event in WG. Zones of collagen necrosis can be vague (**A**) or discrete and associated with giant cells and granulomatosis inflammation (**B**).

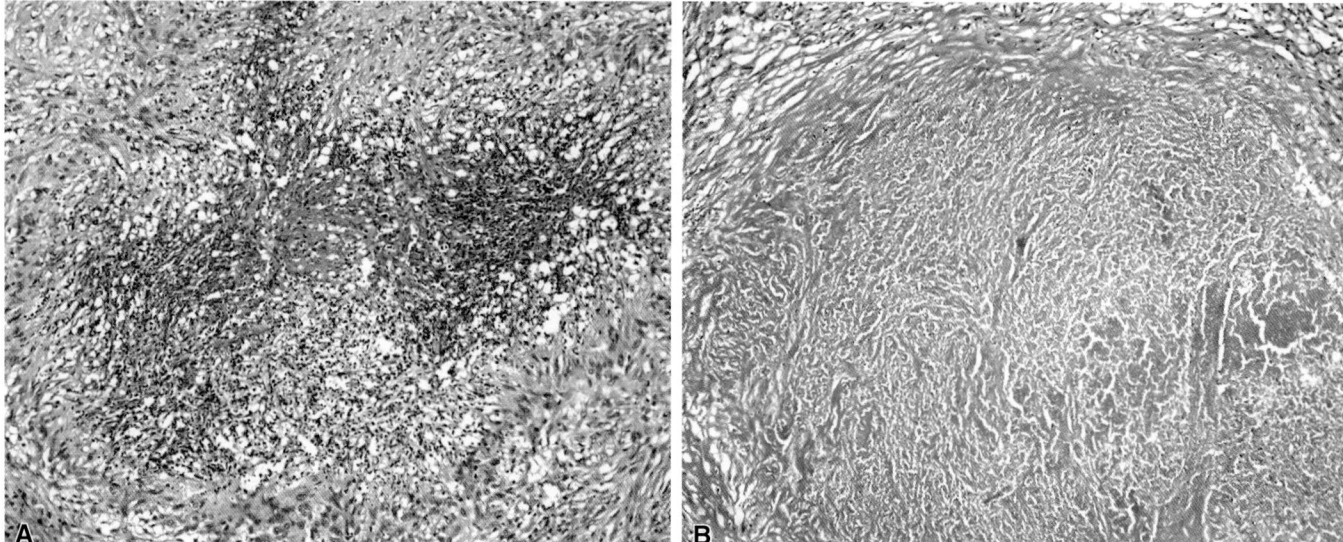

Figure 10-14. Wegener granulomatosis (WG): basophilic necrosis. **A,** The necrosis of WG is basophilic owing to an abundance of nuclear debris. **B,** In necrotizing granulomatous infection, the necrosis typically has an eosinophilic appearance with some preservation of structure in areas of necrosis (this background structure visible within necrosis often is absent in WG).

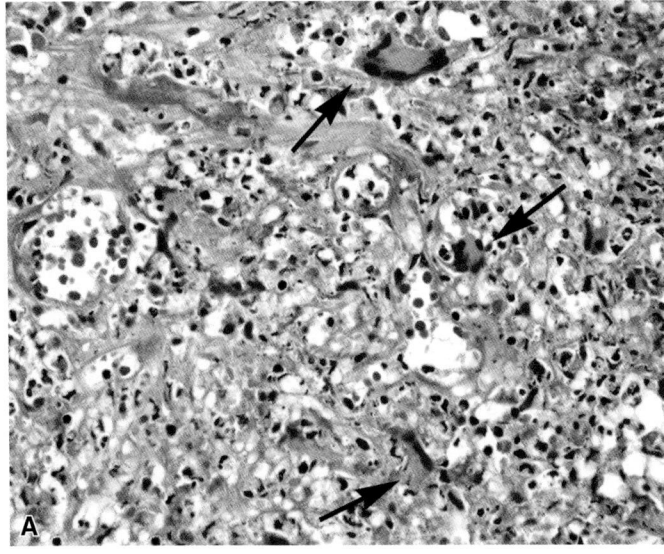

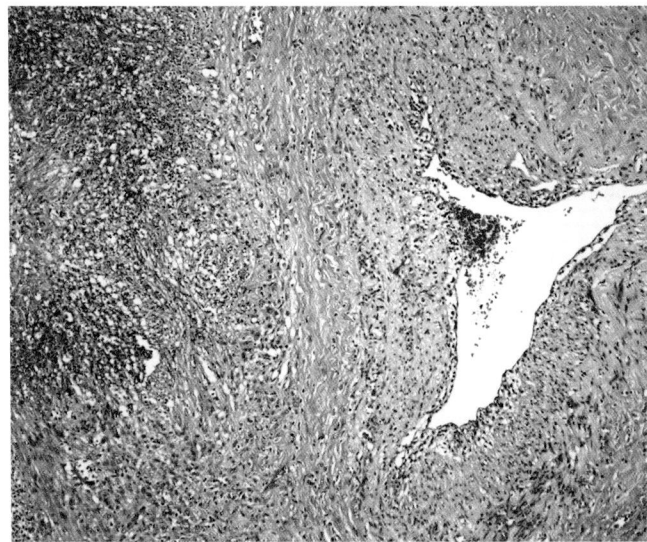

Figure 10-17. Wegener granulomatosis: vasculitis. Vasculitis at the edge of basophilic necrosis. Note the adventitial fibrosis and expansion of the vascular media by inflammatory cells. Multinucleate giant cells can be seen at the interface of muscularis and adventitia in a focal distribution (*lower right*).

(Fig. 10-21), bronchial or bronchiolar scarring, and cicatricial vascular changes (Fig. 10-22) are common in lung biopsies from patients who have received therapy.[51,55] Wedge biopsies provide the best results for an accurate diagnosis of WG. Transbronchial biopsies rarely yield diagnostic information, although in the appropriate clinical context the presence of a few neutrophil microabscesses, giant cells, or capillaritis may be helpful in supporting the diagnosis. Transthoracic needle core biopsies may occasionally show features suggesting a diagnosis of WG.

Differential Diagnosis
The differential diagnosis for WG based on lung biopsy tissue depends somewhat on the constellation of changes present and includes granulomatous infection,[52] lymphomatoid granulomatosis,[56,57] CSS,[58–61] sarcoidosis, necrotizing sarcoid granulomatosis,[56,62,63] rheumatoid nodules,[63] bronchocentric granulomatosis,[53,63,64] and diffuse pulmonary hemorrhage syndromes.[65,66]

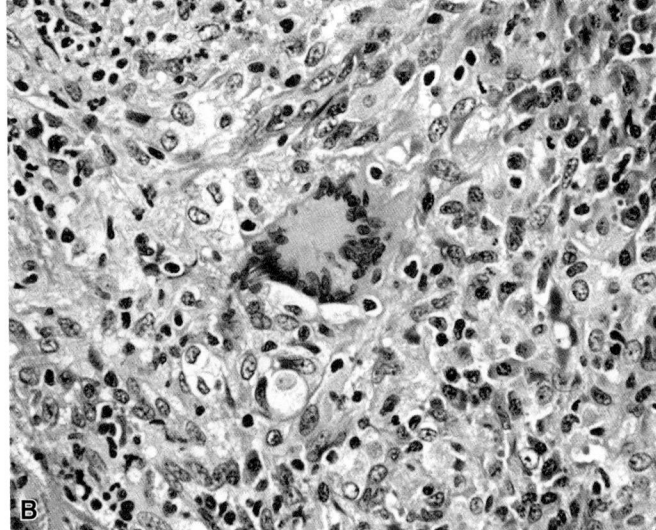

Figure 10-15. Wegener granulomatosis: giant cells. **A,** The characteristic giant cells (*arrows*) have smudged basophilic nuclei, often marginated at the periphery of the cell. **B,** A typical multinucleate giant cell is evident at the periphery of necrosis (*upper left*).

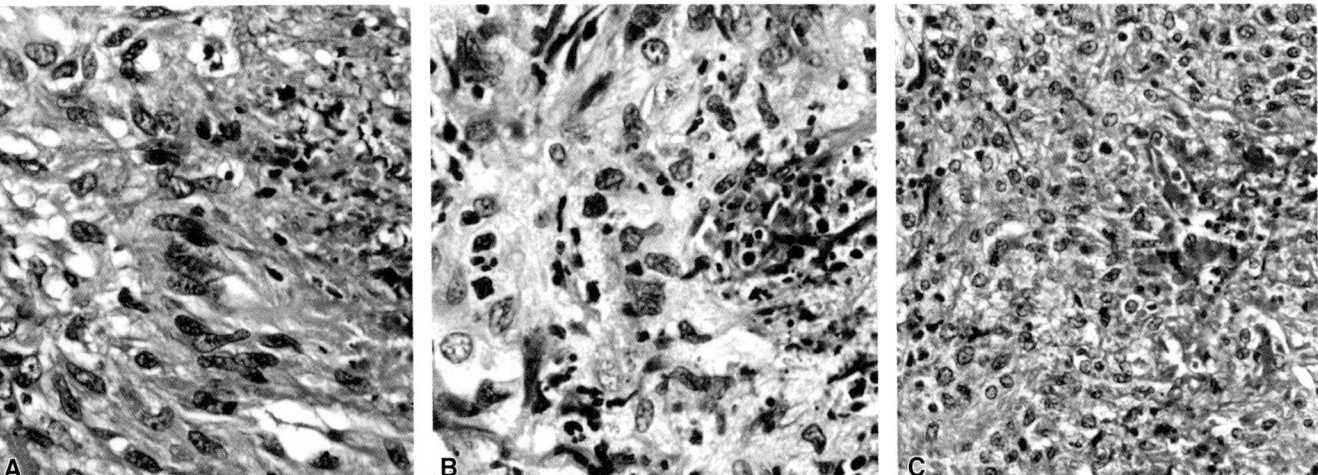

Figure 10-16. Wegener granulomatosis: types of "granulomatous" inflammation. Three examples of granulomatous inflammation at the periphery of necrosis: palisaded histiocytes (**A**); epithelioid histiocytes with little organization (**B**); plump eosinophilic histiocytes (**C**).

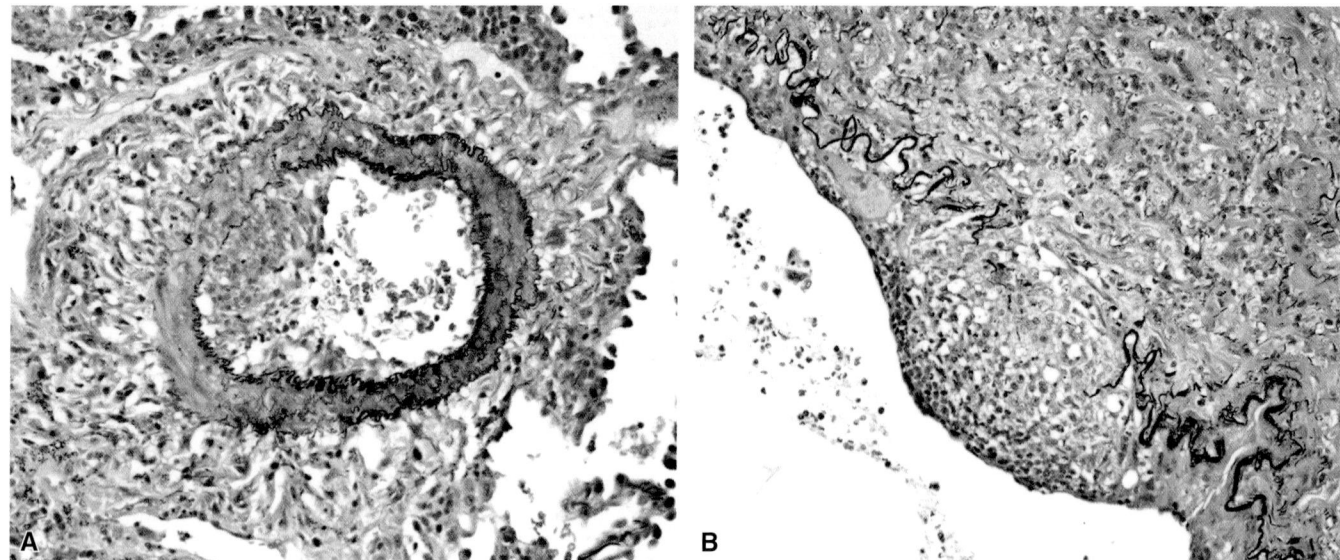

Figure 10-18. Wegener granulomatosis: elastic tissue stains. **A,** Elastic tissue stains demonstrate disruption of the elastic lamina in involved arteries. **B,** Granuloma can be seen displacing elastic lamina and protruding into the vessel lumen.

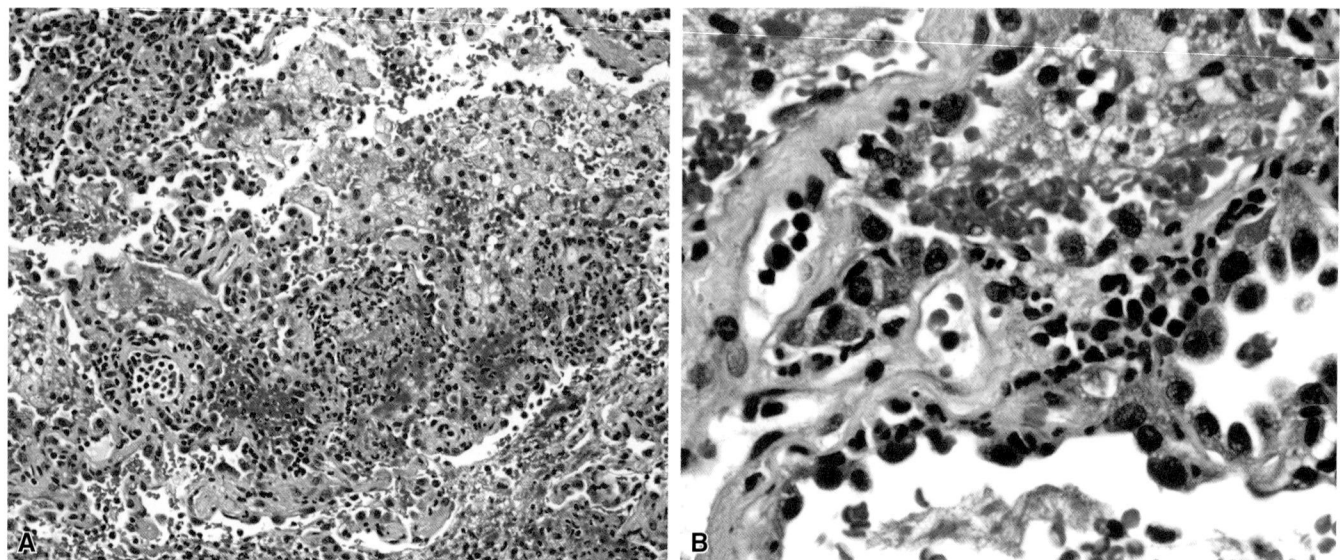

Figure 10-19. Wegener granulomatosis (WG): capillaritis. **A,** Capillaritis can be seen in WG and at times may be the dominant feature. **B,** At higher magnification, an alveolar wall with increased neutrophils and disruption of capillaries is visible. Note the hemosiderin aggregates at *upper right.*

Occasionally, a form of diffuse large B cell malignant lymphoma commonly referred to as *lymphomatoid granulomatosis* (see Chapter 15) can bear a striking resemblance to WG[6] (Fig. 10-23). Like classic WG, this neoplastic process is characterized pathologically by the presence of multiple necrotic pulmonary nodules. In addition to major clinical differences between these diseases, important histopathologic differences become evident at closer inspection. First, the necrotic areas in lymphomatoid granulomatosis typically demonstrate pale shadows of large necrotic cells (dead lymphoma cells). Second, within the necrotic zones, and at the periphery of necrosis, medium-sized blood vessels can be seen whose outline is expanded by an angiocentric infiltration of lymphoid cells. As noted, this is a diffuse large B cell lymphoma in which the atypical B lymphoid cells are infected with Epstein-Barr virus (EBV) and associated with a T lymphocyte–rich inflammatory reaction and vasculitis. In high-grade disease, the vasocentric infiltrate is composed mainly of large atypical B cells. In lower-grade forms, the infiltrate may be polymorphous with more prominent T cells and a mixture of plasma cells, and eosinophils. Immunohistochemistry for CD20 and CD3 highlights the large malignant B cells and background of inflammatory T cells. Immunohistochemistry for EBV latent membrane protein 1 (LMP-1) and in situ hybridization studies for EBV are valuable diagnostic tools in this setting. Third, lymphomatoid granulomatosis is a vasodestructive lymphoid neoplasm, so necrosis and obliteration of vessels are common. WG may show necrosis in vascular adventitia, but wholesale medial necrosis in arteries and veins is unusual. Fourth, the atypical cells of lymphomatoid granulomatosis often contain EBV,[4,67] a finding not expected in WG. Finally, granulomatous inflammation is comparatively rare in lymphomatoid granulomatosis, so the presence of granulomas in nodular lung lesions should suggest a diagnosis other than lymphomatoid granulomatosis (e.g., infection or WG).

Box 10-3. Wegener Granulomatosis: Minor Histopathologic Manifestations*

Parenchymal Changes
Nodular interstitial fibrosis
Endogenous lipoid pneumonia
Alveolar hemorrhage
Organizing intraluminal fibrosis
Lymphoid aggregates
Tissue eosinophils
Xanthogranulomatous lesions
Alveolar macrophage accumulation

Bronchial/Bronchiolar Lesions
Chronic bronchiolitis
Acute bronchiolitis/bronchopneumonia
Bronchiolitis obliterans or a BOOP histologic pattern
Bronchocentric granulomatosis
Follicular bronchiolitis
Bronchial stenosis

*May uncommonly represent a dominant pathologic feature.
BOOP, bronchiolitis obliterans with organizing pneumonia.
Data from Rose A, Sinclair-Smith C. Takayasu's arteritis. A study of 16 autopsy cases. *Arch Pathol Lab Med.* 1980;104:231–237; and Jakob H, Volb R, Stangl G, et al. Surgical correction of a severely obstructed pulmonary artery bifurcation in Takayasu's arteritis. *Eur J Cardiothorac Surg.* 1990;4:456–458.

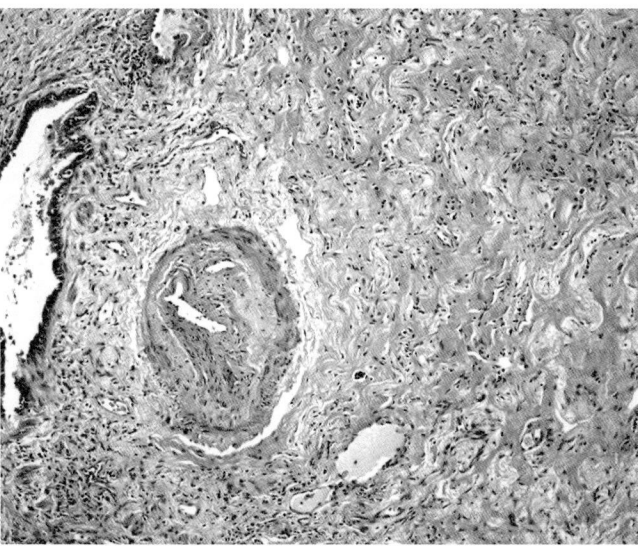

Figure 10-21. Wegener granulomatosis: treatment effect. Areas of lung fibrosis may occur after treatment for this disorder, frequently associated with parenchymal collapse (*right*). Here, a bronchiole and accompanying pulmonary artery show inflammatory sequelae of the disease.

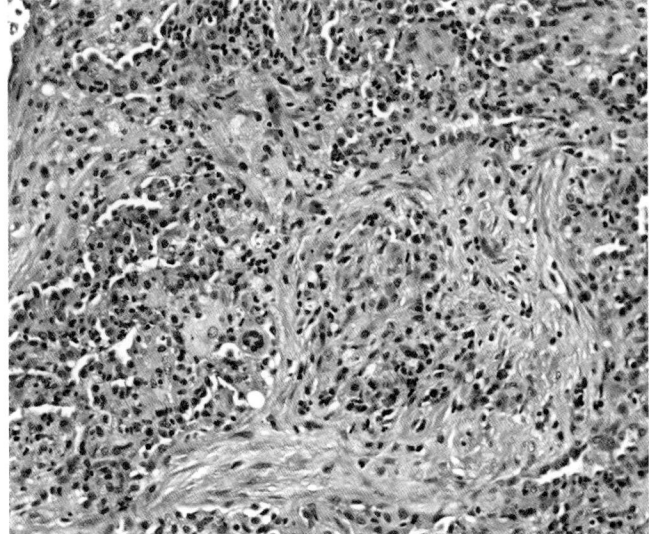

Figure 10-20. Wegener granulomatosis (WG): organizing pneumonia. Organization may be prominent in WG and at times may be the dominant feature. Often capillaritis is evident, as are the "footprints" of previous hemorrhage (hemosiderin at *center*). Scattered multinucleate giant cells may be seen.

Prominent tissue eosinophilia occurs in approximately 5% of cases of WG (Fig. 10-24). With this finding, the differential diagnosis should include CSS (see later), along with fungal or parasitic infection.[58,61,68,69] Peripheral blood eosinophilia is characteristic of CSS and is uncommon in WG.[70] Also, asthma is not a characteristic feature of WG, although rarely, asthmatic individuals may develop WG, presumably at a rate similar to that seen in the general population. The distinction between WG and CSS is usually straightforward, but some cases may require careful assessment of all of the clinical, pathologic, and laboratory data (Table 10-2).

Perhaps the most important, and often problematic, consideration in the diagnosis of WG is the exclusion of infection. Mycobacteria and fungi can cause necrotizing granulomatous inflammation and vasculitis resembling that seen in WG. Solitary necrotizing granulomas can be associated with vasculitis in 87% of mycobacterial lung infections and 57% of fungal lung infections.[52] Also, neutrophilic microabscesses are a feature of certain infections, such as blastomycosis and nocardiosis.

A number of important clues can be helpful in the approach to this differential diagnosis, even before special stains for organisms or culture data (which should be routinely ordered in such cases) are available. First, if the lesion is solitary, a high index of suspicion for infection is appropriate.[46] Second, WG does not tend to make granulomas without central necrosis,[51] except in the rare occurrence of infection superimposed on the necrotic center of a WG lesion. Third, the necrosis of infection may show the "ghosted" outlines of underlying lung parenchyma, a finding uncharacteristic of WG. Fourth, the patient with infection, in whom a bilateral multiple-nodular appearance on radiologic studies may simulate that in WG, is typically quite ill, with generalized systemic symptoms. By contrast, the patient with WG may be relatively asymptomatic, despite numerous necrotic nodules in the lung. Finally, when strictly morphologic assessment fails to clarify the diagnosis, inquiry regarding the presence of sinonasal disease or renal disease and serologic data (c-ANCA and p-ANCA) will usually resolve the quandary.

When WG presents with a predominantly bronchocentric pattern of lung involvement, bronchocentric granulomatosis must be considered in the differential diagnosis.[51,53] Patients with bronchocentric WG should demonstrate other distinguishing features of WG, including renal or sinus involvement and a positive ANCA serology.

Diagnosis
The histologic features of WG can be very suggestive of the diagnosis, but as a general rule, it is extremely important to correlate the histopathology with clinical and serologic findings before making a definitive diagnosis on a lung biopsy specimen. The diagnosis can be impossible to make in cases in which only partial clinical or pathologic criteria are present. In these situations a purely descriptive diagnosis with a differential diagnosis may be necessary. As mentioned earlier, ANCA serology can be helpful, as long as one keeps in mind that ANCAs are not specific for WG.[71] Moreover, when all other clinical and histopathologic findings are compelling for WG, the diagnosis is still possible despite negative ANCA studies.[39]

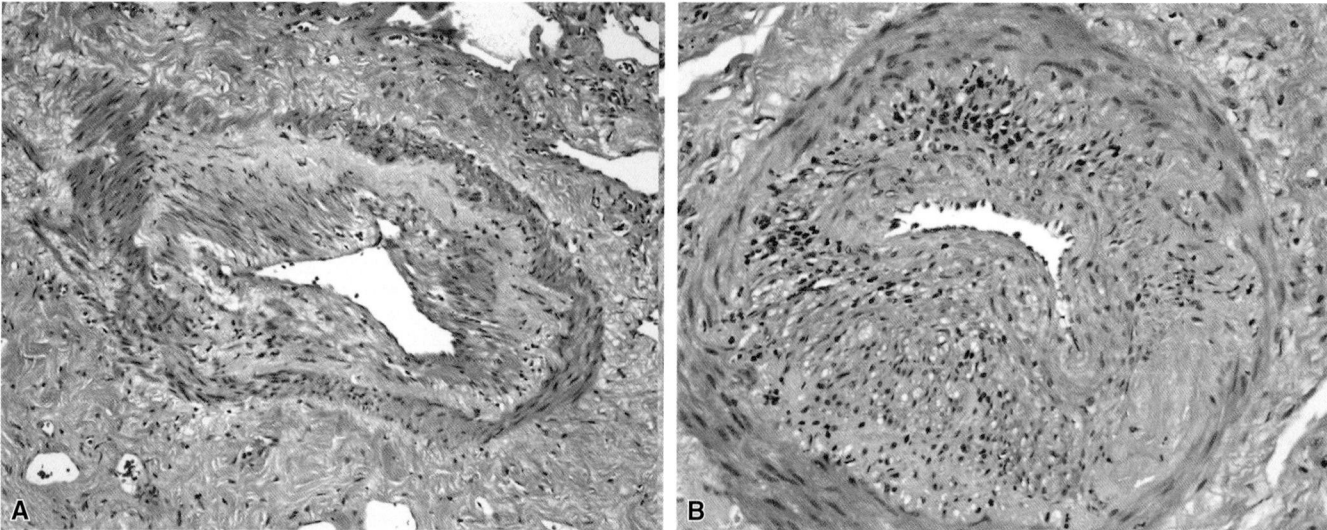

Figure 10-22. Wegener granulomatosis: treatment effect. **A,** Significant vascular scarring consequent to treatment. **B,** Remnants of the inflammatory infiltrate may persist within the vascular media. Note the giant cell within the media (*upper center*).

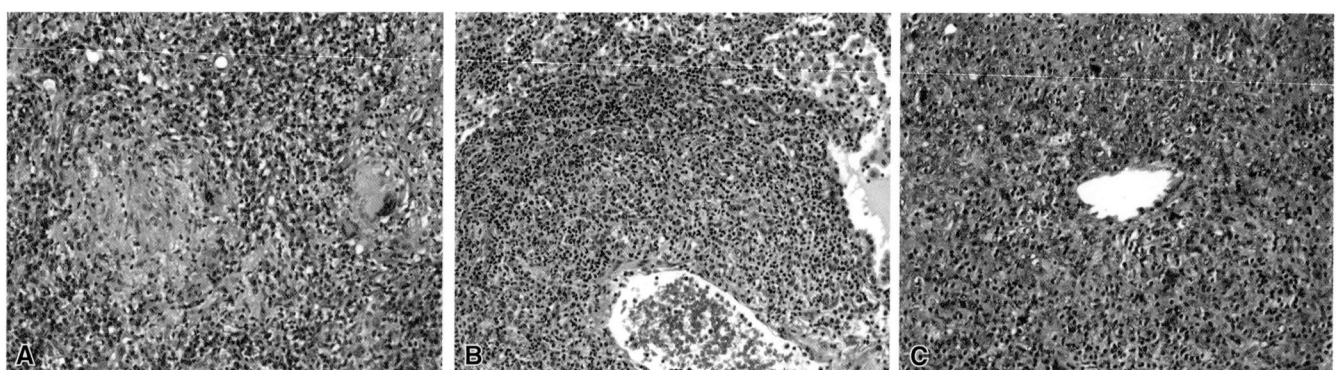

Figure 10-23. Wegener granulomatosis (WG): prominent lymphoid infiltrates. **A,** WG may be dominated by lymphocytes. When this occurs, differentiation from lymphoma (specifically, angiocentric lymphoma) may be difficult. **B** and **C,** Note the expansile appearance of the inflammatory infiltrate with vessel wall destruction. Closer inspection will often reveal a degree of atypia in the lymphoid cells not seen in WG.

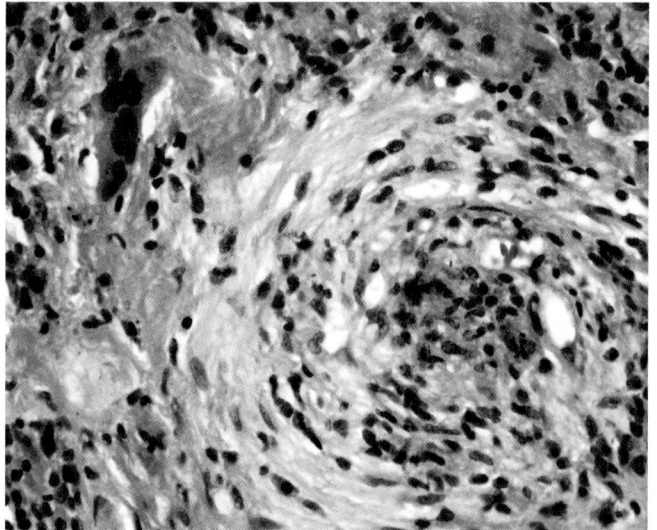

Figure 10-24. Wegener granulomatosis: prominent eosinophils. When eosinophils are a prominent histopathologic feature, the differential diagnosis will include Churg-Strauss syndrome. Here a vessel is obliterated by inflammation and fibroblastic proliferation, and eosinophils are abundant. Note multinucleate giant cell in *upper left*.

Table 10-2. Wegener Granulomatosis versus Churg-Strauss Syndrome: Distinguishing Features

Clinical/Pathologic Feature	Wegener Granulomatosis	Churg-Strauss Syndrome
Asthma	Rare	Characteristic (diagnostic criterion)
Eosinophilia		
Peripheral	Up to 12%	Characteristic*
Tissue	Up to 6%	Characteristic*
Sinus disease	Destructive, often causing saddlenose deformity	Less severe, usually allergic rhinitis
Renal disease	More severe	Usually mild
Cardiac disease	Rare	Common
ANCA	Usually c-ANCA	Usually p-ANCA

*Eosinophilia may be fleeting and may be difficult to demonstrate during steroid therapy.
ANCA (c-ANCA, p-ANCA), antineutrophil cytoplasmic antibodies (cytoplasmic, perinuclear).

Treatment and Prognosis

WG is commonly a fatal disease if left untreated, with up to 90% of patients dying within 2 years of diagnosis, most often from respiratory or renal failure. Fortunately, therapy with cyclophosphamide and prednisone is very effective in achieving remissions, with 85% to 90% of patients responding to therapy and approximately 75% experiencing complete remission.[72] The median time to remission is 12 months, although occasional patients require treatment for more than 2 years before all symptoms resolve. Even in those patients who initially respond to therapy, relapses are common, with up to 50 of initial responders experiencing at least one relapse requiring another course of therapy. Trimethoprim-sulfamethoxazole, pulse cyclophosphamide, and methotrexate are also used to treat WG.[20,73–75] Trimethoprim-sulfamethoxazole may reduce relapses for those patients who are in remission.[76] The mechanism of this protective action is unknown. Rituximab has more recently shown promise in treatment of WG, particularly limited disease refractory to standard therapy.[77] Initial trials of antagonists of tumor necrosis factor-alpha (TNF-α) showed some benefit, but formal trials did not support the initial findings; thus, further study is needed to determine the efficacy of this potential therapy.[78] The outcome with WG seems to be significantly worse for patients older than 60 years of age than for younger patients, despite similar clinical manifestations and treatment regimen. Lung function frequently improves after treatment, but in some patients the diffusing capacity may never return to normal.

Churg-Strauss Syndrome

CSS is a multisystem disorder characterized by the triad of asthma, peripheral blood eosinophilia, and vasculitis.[58,59,61,68–70,79–81] Although CSS was initially described by Churg and Strauss based on a series of autopsy cases,[58] it is now recognized primarily as a clinical entity. Accordingly, most cases today are diagnosed on the basis of clinical findings rather than lung biopsy.[61]

In 1990, the American College of Rheumatology (ACR) proposed two approaches to the diagnosis of CSS (Table 10-3): a traditional format classification and a classification tree.[82,83] According to the *traditional format classification*, six criteria are identified: (1) asthma, (2) eosinophils greater than 10% of the white blood cell differential count, (3) mononeuropathy (including multiplex) or polyneuropathy, (4) non-fixed radiographic pulmonary infiltrates, (5) paranasal sinus abnormalities, and (6) a biopsy containing a blood vessel with extravascular eosinophils.[82] If four of six of these criteria are met, the diagnosis can be established with a sensitivity of 85% and a specificity of 99.7%.[82] The ACR criteria for CSS have been retained in the subsequent 1994 Chapel Hill consensus conference criteria and the more recently proposed Watts criteria.[84]

The major criteria used in the *classification tree* are asthma, eosinophilia with greater than 10% eosinophils, and a history of allergy.[82] According to this method, patients with well-documented systemic vasculitis, but lacking a history of asthma, can be diagnosed with CSS if they have peripheral blood eosinophilia (>10% eosinophils) and a history of allergy other than drug sensitivity.[82] This seems appropriate, since patients without asthma, but with a history of allergic disease, can develop CSS.[85–87] Both classification methods appear to be useful in the diagnosis, with greater sensitivity provided by the classification tree and greater specificity by the traditional approach.[82]

Clinical Features

Despite more than 40 years of study, the incidence and epidemiology of CSS remain unclear. Based on available (although limited) population-based studies, CSS is second only to WG as a major cause of systemic

Table 10-3. Churg-Strauss Syndrome: Clinical Manifestations

Manifestation	Frequency (% of Patients Affected)
Pulmonary infiltrates	72
Mononeuritis multiplex	66
Abdominal pain	59
Arthritis/arthralgias	51
Mild/moderate renal disease	49
Purpura	48
Cardiac failure	47
Myalgia	41
Löffler syndrome	40
Erythema/urticaria	35
Diarrhea	33
Pericarditis	32
Skin nodules	30
Pleural effusion	29
Hypertension	29
Central nervous system abnormalities	27
Gastrointestinal bleeding	18
Renal failure	9

Modified from Lanham J, Churg J. Churg-Strauss syndrome. In: Churg A, Churg J, eds. *Systemic Vasculitides*. New York: Igaku-Shoin; 1991:101–120.

vasculitis, and CSS is the diagnosis in approximately 10% of patients who develop a major vasculitic syndrome.[1] The exact etiology of CSS is unknown, but an autoimmune etiology is most likely.

CSS affects both sexes equally. The mean age at diagnosis is 50 years, but the systemic vasculitic phase is frequently evident in patients in their late 30s. CSS mainly involves the upper respiratory tract, lungs, skin, and peripheral nerves.[59,61,69] Involvement of the heart and kidney also occurs and may be associated with a worse outcome.

CSS often progresses through three distinct phases. In the early or *prodrome phase*, the disease manifests as allergic rhinitis, asthma, peripheral eosinophilia, and/or eosinophilic infiltrative disease.[59,61,69,70] Recurrent episodes of asthma may develop over a period of years before the onset of vasculitis and some data suggest that the interval between the onset of asthma and the subsequent vasculitis phase of the disease has a direct association with prognosis.[58,59,61] In the prodrome phase, tissue infiltration by eosinophils can affect the lungs or the gastrointestinal tract. Pulmonary manifestations may take the form of Löffler syndrome, with fleeting pulmonary infiltrates or even chronic eosinophilic pneumonia.

The prodrome is followed by the *vasculitis phase*. During this phase, patients develop systemic signs and symptoms of vasculitis, such as mononeuritis multiplex and cutaneous leukocytoclastic vasculitis. Results of p-ANCA assay are usually positive. The ACR criteria necessary for diagnosis are present only during this phase.[69] Unfortunately, most of the permanent damage is done by the disease during this phase. For this reason, when eosinophilic pneumonia occurs in an asthmatic patient, CSS should always be raised as a possibility in the differential diagnosis, especially when prominent eosinophilic vasculitis is present in the lung biopsy.

The vasculitis phase is followed by a *postvasculitis phase.* Here, patients may experience neuropathy and hypertension, typically with persistent asthma and allergic rhinitis.[69,88] Proteinuria and gastrointestinal involvement are poor prognostic indicators.[89]

A major difference between CSS and WG is the frequency of cardiac and renal involvement. Although the heart may be involved in both disorders, up to 47% of CSS patients develop cardiac disease.[61,69] CSS can cause cardiac failure, pericarditis, hypertension, and acute myocardial infarction.[58,59,61] Also, while renal disease is characteristic in WG, it is less frequent and less severe in patients with CSS.[59,61,90]

Peripheral neuropathy, often in the form of mononeuritis multiplex, is seen in approximately two thirds of patients with CSS. The most common cutaneous manifestation is leukocytoclastic vasculitis.[91] Sinonasal manifestations include nasal obstruction, nasal polyps, rhinorhea, and thick intranasal crusts.[92] Central nervous system involvement can occur in 25% of cases.[61,69,81] Gastrointestinal hemorrhage and perforation are potential complications.[93] Serologic studies usually show the p-ANCA pattern, although c-ANCA can also be seen (the inverse of ANCA types in WG).[94] Elevated serum IgE is also a characteristic finding in CSS.[59–61,69]

A CSS-like syndrome develops as a rare complication in steroid-dependent asthmatics successfully treated with leukotriene receptor antagonists (e.g., pranlukast).[95–99] This complication probably is related to steroid withdrawal facilitated by the drugs, which unmasks underlying CSS, rather than a manifestation of the drugs. To this point, a similar unmasking of CSS has occurred in asthmatic patients whose withdrawal from oral steroids was facilitated by inhaled steroids.[99] Also, an unusual association between a CSS-like vasculitis and the illicit use of "free base" cocaine has been reported.[100]

There are no laboratory tests specific for CSS. Peripheral blood eosinophilia (eosinophil counts usually 5000–9000/µL) is the most characteristic finding. Other nonspecific laboratory abnormalities include normochromic normocytic anemia, markedly elevated erythrocyte sedimentation rate, leukocytosis, elevated IgE level, and hypergammaglobulinemia. Bronchoalveolar lavage fluid shows a high percentage of eosinophils (usually >33%). Pulmonary function abnormalities most often reflect the patient's underlying asthma.

Radiologic Features

CSS most commonly manifests radiologically as multifocal lung parenchymal infiltrates that change in location and size over time[42,58,101] (Fig. 10-25). The infiltrates may also exhibit a peripheral distribution, thereby mimicking those of chronic eosinophilic pneumonia. Lung involvement by pulmonary consolidation may be widespread. Diffuse miliary nodules have also been reported.[40,101] Cavitation of nodules is rare and when present should suggest superimposed infection.[102] Eosinophilic pleural effusions may be seen in 29% of cases.[42,101] Hilar lymphadenopathy is infrequent. The chest radiograph can be normal in appearance in as many as 25% of patients.[42]

High-resolution CT (HRCT) features of CSS most commonly consist of parenchymal opacifications (consolidation or ground-glass attenuation), followed in frequency by pulmonary nodules, bronchial wall thickening or dilatation, interlobular septal thickening, and normal anatomy.[103] One case report described "stellate-shaped" peripheral pulmonary arteries and peribronchial and septal interstitial thickening. Small patchy opacities were also noted. These HRCT abnormalities correlated with eosinophilic infiltration and foci of eosinophilic pneumonia, respectively.[104]

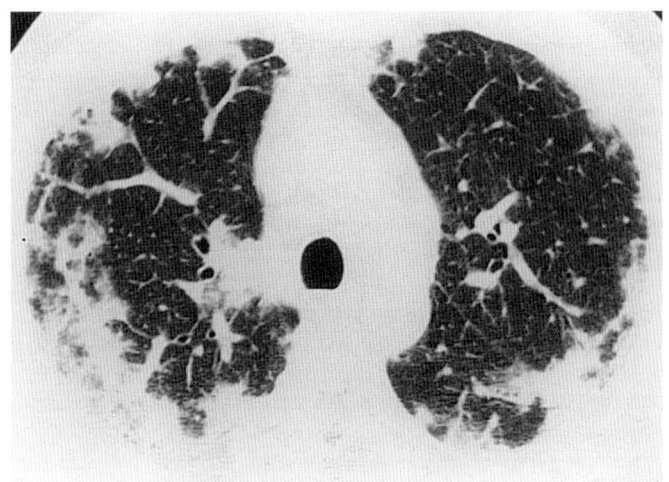

Figure 10-25. Churg-Strauss syndrome (CSS): computed tomography (CT) features. Chest CT scan (lung window) in a patient with a 10-year history of asthma and peripheral eosinophilia demonstrates multifocal peripheral subpleural consolidations. The diagnosis of CSS was confirmed at open lung biopsy. (From Travis WD, Colby TV, Koss MN, et al, eds. *Non-Neoplastic Disorders of the Lower Respiratory Tract.* In: King DW, ed. *Atlas of Nontumor Pathology.* Washington, DC: American Registry of Pathology and Armed Forces Institute of Pathology; 2002, Figure 4-18.)

Pathologic Features

The findings on lung biopsy depend on the stage of the disease during which the biopsy is obtained and whether or not the patient has received therapy, particularly steroids. Lung biopsies from CSS patients in the full blown vasculitic phase may show asthmatic bronchitis, eosinophilic pneumonia (Fig. 10-26), extravascular stellate granulomas (Fig. 10-27), and vasculitis[58,69] (Fig. 10-28). In some cases, the inflammatory lesions extend along the pleura and interlobular septa. The extravascular granulomas have a border of palisaded histiocytes and multinucleate giant cells, surrounding a central necrotic zone replete with eosinophils and eosinophil cellular debris. Such lesions have been called "allergic granulomas."

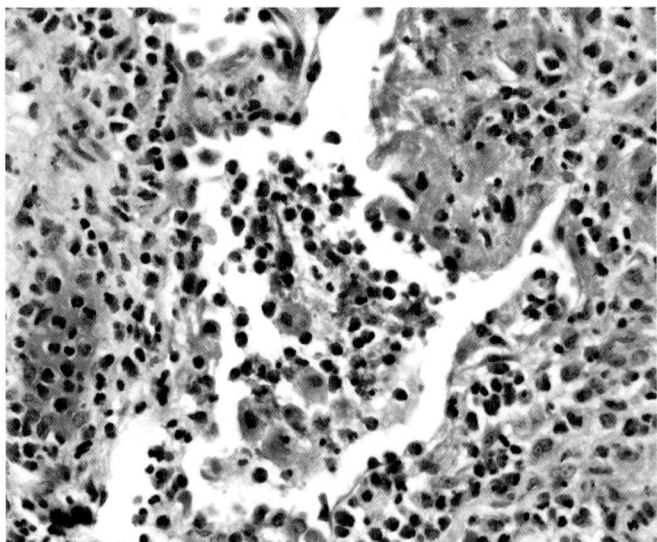

Figure 10-26. Churg-Strauss syndrome (CSS): eosinophilic pneumonia. Eosinophilic pneumonia is the most consistent manifestation of CSS. Here, the triad of air space eosinophils, eosinophilic macrophages with fibrin, and atypical alveolar lining cells can be readily appreciated.

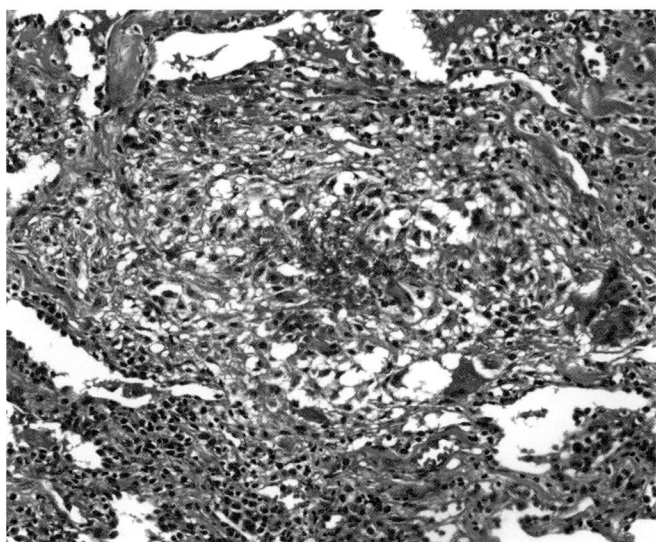

Figure 10-27. Churg-Strauss syndrome: allergic granulomas. Characteristic "allergic granuloma" is readily apparent. Note the vaguely palisaded histiocytes at the periphery of eosinophilic necrosis (*center*). Multinucleate giant cells may be present and typically have a brightly eosinophilic cytoplasm.

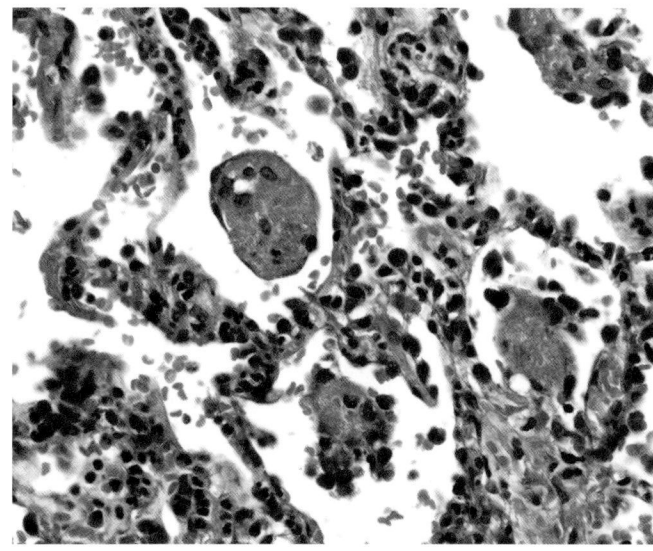

Figure 10-29. Churg-Strauss syndrome (CSS): pulmonary hemorrhage. Diffuse pulmonary hemorrhage with capillaritis can occur in CSS. Capillaritis is demonstrated here, associated with aggregated air space fibrin and eosinophils.

Vasculitis can affect arteries, veins, or capillaries. The vascular inflammatory infiltrates can be composed of chronic inflammatory cells, eosinophils, epithelioid cells, multinucleate giant cells, and neutrophils. Diffuse pulmonary hemorrhage and capillaritis (Fig. 10-29) can be seen.[90,105] In patients who are partially treated, the pathologic (and clinical) features may be incomplete.[101] Lung biopsy is not required for diagnosis, if pulmonary infiltrates are present in association with other systemic findings that fulfill the required diagnostic criteria.

Differential Diagnosis

The differential diagnosis of CSS includes eosinophilic pneumonia from any cause, WG,[51] allergic bronchopulmonary fungal disease (ABPFD),[106] infection (especially parasitic and fungal),[107] Hodgkin disease, and drug-induced vasculitis.[108]

Eosinophilic pneumonia and ABPFD lack systemic vasculitis, although some cases of eosinophilic pneumonia can show a mild non-necrotizing vasculitis, and "allergic granulomas" may be present. Features helpful in distinguishing CSS from WG are summarized in Table 4-5. Pathologic features similar to those of CSS can also be mimicked by certain parasitic infections, such as those caused by *Strongyloides stercoralis*[109] and *Toxocara canis*.[107] Therefore, parasitic infection should be carefully excluded when CSS is in the differential diagnosis on histopathologic grounds. Some fungal infections, especially those due to *Aspergillus* species and *Coccidioides immitis*, may be associated with granulomatous inflammation, prominent eosinophilia, and vasculitis. Rarely, Hodgkin disease with prominent eosinophils and vascular inflammation may be confused with CSS. Drugs such as carbamazepine also can cause a CSS-like syndrome, so attention should be paid to the patient's drug history.[108]

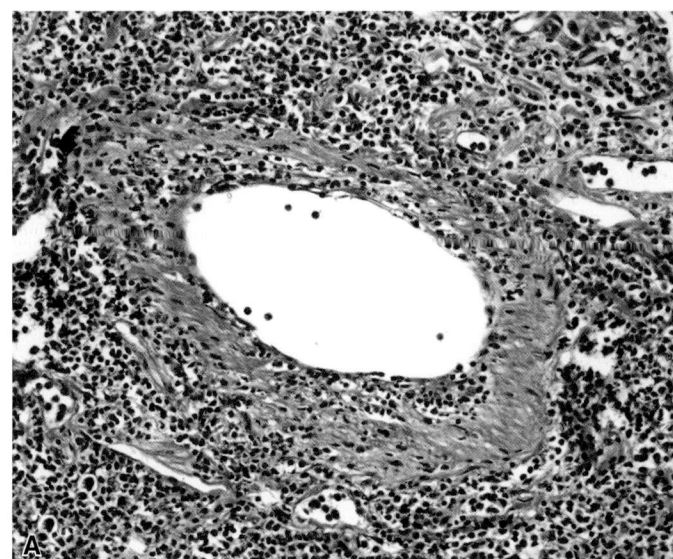

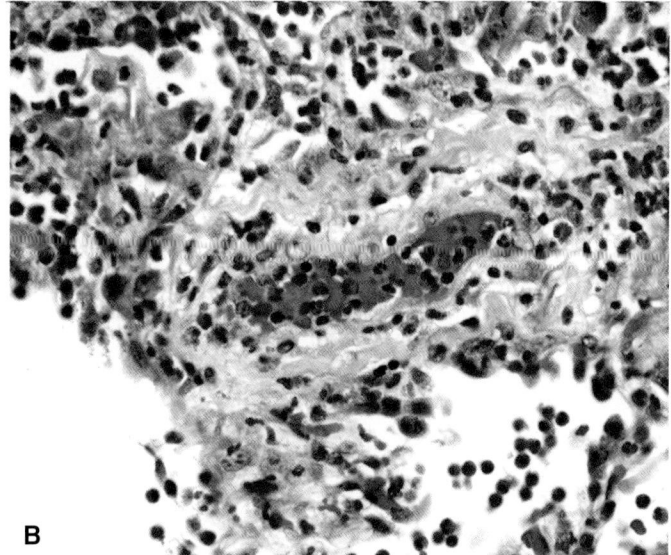

Figure 10-28. Churg-Strauss syndrome (CSS): vasculitis. Vasculitis is characteristic in CSS. **A,** A medium-sized artery infiltrated by eosinophils and scattered lymphocytes. **B,** A venule infiltrated by eosinophils. Note fibrin and eosinophils in surrounding air spaces.

Treatment and Prognosis

Most patients with CSS respond to systemic corticosteroids. In order to avoid irreversible organ injury, some authorities have favored treatment with cytotoxic immunosuppressive agents, such as cyclophosphamide, from the outset.[69] Azathioprine, interferon-α, and high-dose intravenous immune globulin have been used with apparent benefit in patients with severe, fulminant disease or in patients unresponsive to systemic corticosteroids. Plasma exchange occasionally has been used but appears to have no added benefit to that observed with treatment with systemic corticosteroids, with or without the addition of cyclophosphamide.[110]

Patients who die from CSS typically have cardiac complications such as congestive heart failure or myocardial infarction. Other, less common causes of death include renal failure, cerebral hemorrhage, gastrointestinal perforation or hemorrhage, status asthmaticus, and respiratory failure.[69,111]

Microscopic Polyangiitis

Microscopic polyangiitis encompasses the spectrum of vasculitic disorders that previously have been called systemic necrotizing vasculitis, leukocytoclastic vasculitis, and hypersensitivity vasculitis.[112-115] An International Consensus Conference on the Nomenclature of Systemic Vasculitides[116,117] defined microscopic polyangiitis as a vasculitis restricted to arterioles, venules, and capillaries.[116,117] The designation *polyangiitis* was favored over *polyarteritis* because venules are affected as well as arterioles. Microscopic polyangiitis differs from polyarteritis nodosa in that it involves arterioles, venules, and capillaries, as opposed to medium-sized arteries.

Clinical Features

Systemic manifestations of microscopic polyangiitis are more common than pulmonary manifestations and include glomerulonephritis (in 97% of the cases), fever (in 62%), myalgia and arthralgia (in 52%), weight loss (in 45%), ear, nose, and throat symptoms (in 31%), and skin involvement (in 17%) (Table 10-4).[117,118] Approximately 50% of the patients develop pulmonary involvement,[116] and these persons are typically middle-aged or older (average age, 56 ± 17 years) when this occurs. Women are affected slightly more often than men (1.5:1 female-to-male ratio).[118] Onset of symptoms is rapid in most patients, but up to 28% may have symptoms for more than 1 year before diagnosis.

Bronchoalveolar lavage fluid typically shows acute hemorrhage or hemosiderin-laden macrophages when the lungs are involved. Kidney biopsies may show a necrotizing glomerulonephritis.[118] More than 80% of patients have a positive ANCA, most often demonstrating the perinuclear type (p-ANCA).[117] Microscopic polyangiitis is the most common cause of so-called pulmonary hemorrhage renal syndrome.[117]

Radiographic Features

The typical findings in microscopic polyangiitis are manifestations of pulmonary hemorrhage. Bilateral alveolar infiltrates are seen on plain chest films, and ground-glass attenuation is seen on CT scans. The lower lung zones may be most frequently affected.[118]

Pathologic Features

Surgical lung biopsies in microscopic polyangiitis typically show pulmonary hemorrhage, hemosiderin-laden macrophages in alveolar spaces, and neutrophilic capillaritis[37,117] (Fig. 10-30). At scanning magnification, neutrophilic capillaritis often appears as scattered foci of increased alveolar wall cellularity, in a background of alveolar hemorrhage (Fig. 10-31). Closer inspection reveals the presence of neutrophils within the alveolar walls, sometimes spilling over into the surrounding alveolar spaces. In severe cases, the neutrophils may

Table 10-4. Microscopic Polyangiitis: Clinical Features at Presentation

Manifestation	Number of Patients Affected (N = 29)	Frequency (%)
Pulmonary	29	100
Dyspnea	26	90
Cough	26	90
Hemoptysis	23	79
Chest pain	5	17
Crackles	13	45
Renal	28	97
Fever (temperature > 37.5°C)	18	62
Weight loss	13	45
Musculoskeletal	15	52
Arthralgias	13	4
Arthritis	4	14
Myalgia	6	21
Ear, nose, and throat	9	31
Epistaxis	5	17
Sore throat	1	3
Mouth ulcers	2	7
Hearing loss	1	3
Skin	5	17
Purpura	4	14
Nodules	1	3
Erythema elevatum diutinum	1	3
Bullae	1	3
Hypertension	7	25
Ocular	7	25
Episcleritis	5	17
Xerophthlamia	2	7
Peripheral neuropathy	2	7
Gastrointestinal bleeding	1	3

From Lauque D, Cadranel J, Lazor R, et al. Microscopic polyangiitis with alveolar hemorrhage. A study of 29 cases and review of the literature. Groupe d'Etudes et de Recherche sur les Maladies "Orphelines" Pulmonaires (GERM"O"P). *Medicine (Baltimore)*. 2000;79:222–233.

fill the alveoli and focally resemble an acute infectious pneumonia (Fig. 10-32). Identification of distinctive fibrinoid necrosis of capillary walls is often not possible. Alveolar fibrin may accompany the lesions of capillaritis, sometimes in a polypoid fashion (Fig. 10-33). As the lesions of capillaritis heal, polypoid plugs of organizing fibrosis may be seen, sometimes resulting in a organizing pneumonia pattern (Fig. 10-34) (previously referred to as a "BOOP pattern"). The presence of hemosiderin (typically within alveolar macrophages) is essential for an accurate diagnosis, because blood alone may be present in lung biopsies as an artifactual finding.

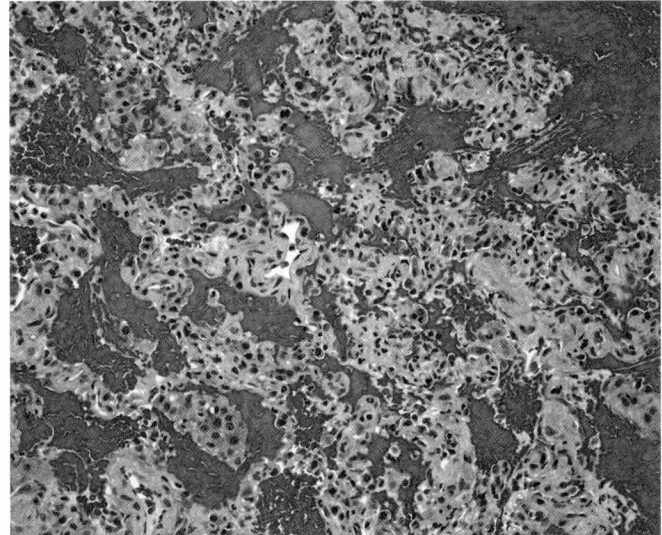

Figure 10-30. Microscopic polyangiitis: pulmonary hemorrhage. Alveolar hemorrhage with capillaritis is a common manifestation of this disorder.

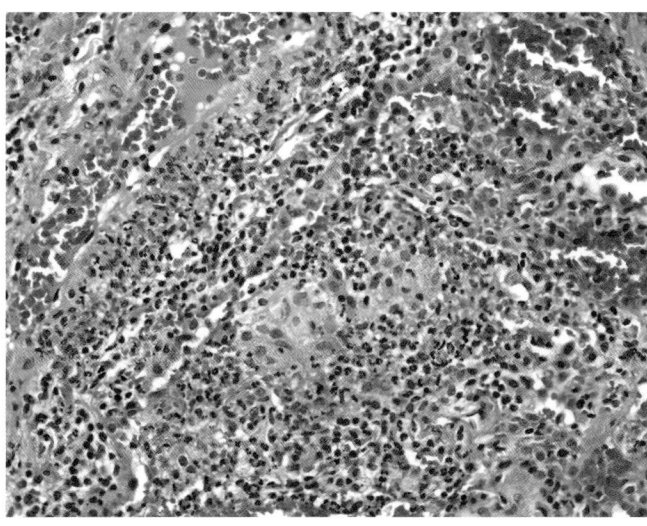

Figure 10-32. Microscopic polyangiitis: pseudobronchopneumonia. Capillaritis may result in shedding of neutrophils into air spaces. When this occurs, neutrophilic acute bronchopneumonia may be simulated.

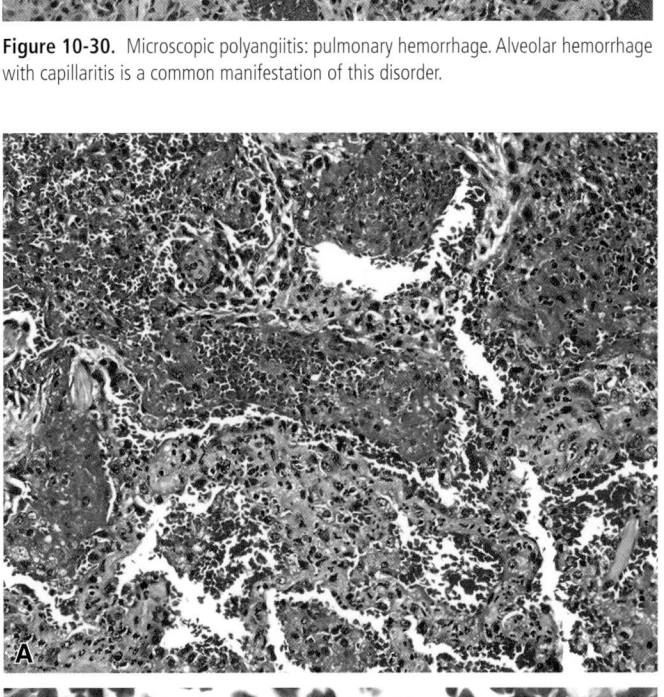

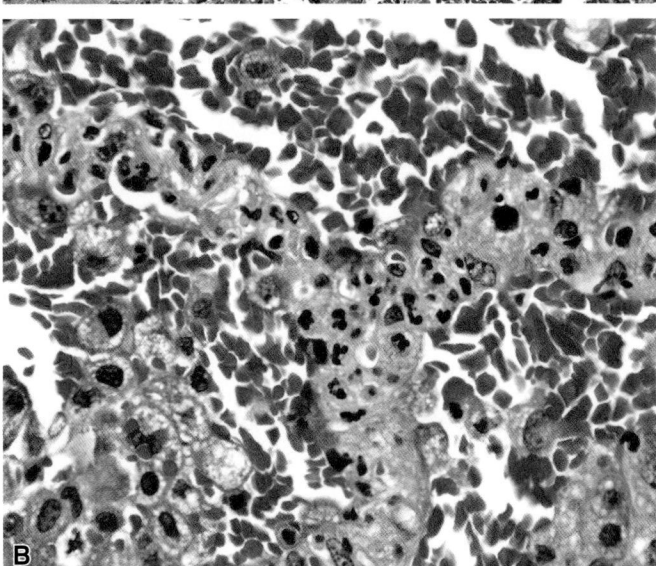

Figure 10-31. Microscopic polyangiitis: capillaritis. **A,** The capillaritis of microscopic polyangiitis can be quite diffuse. **B,** At higher magnification, fibrin and capillary disruption associated with neutrophils can be seen. Note hemosiderin-laden macrophages in adjacent air spaces (*bottom left*).

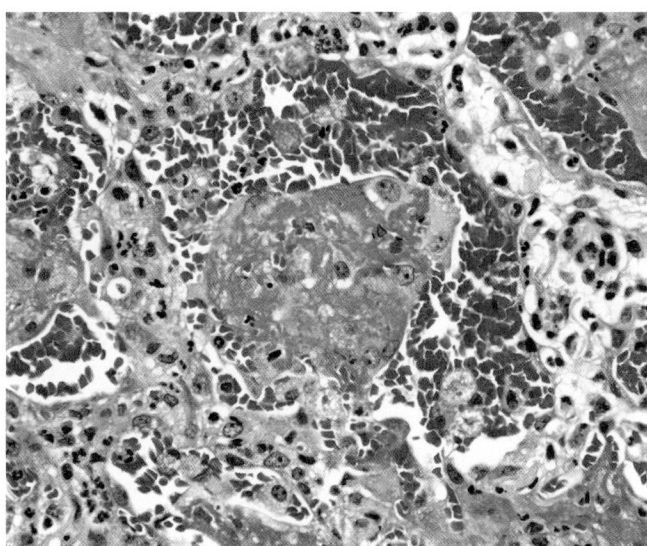

Figure 10-33. Microscopic polyangiitis: classic features. Note the characteristic capillaritis with aggregated air space fibrin and hemosiderin-laden macrophages.

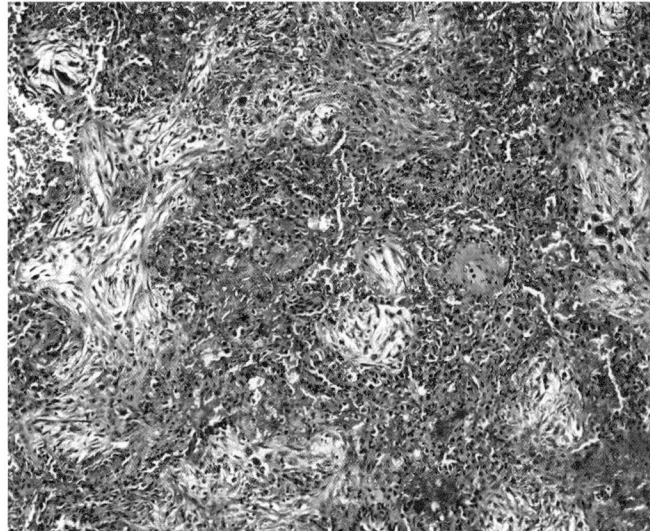

Figure 10-34. Microscopic polyangiitis: fibrin polyps. Polypoid fibrin plugs may resolve with air space organization. Air space fibroblasts fill alveoli in this biopsy section. Note the cellular interstitium replete with neutrophils.

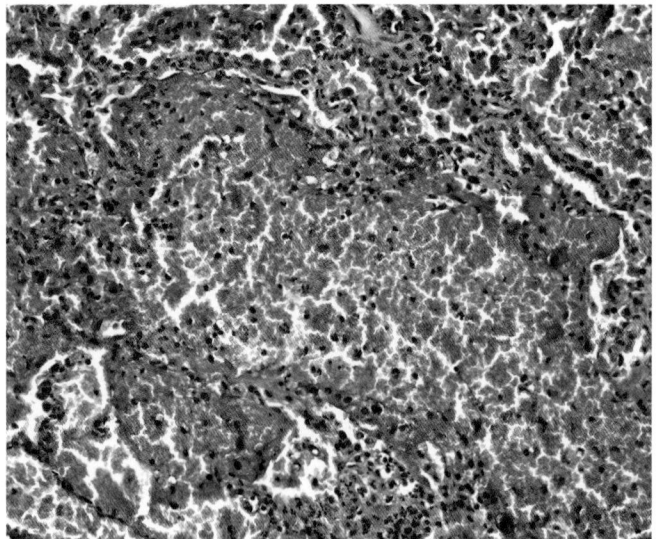

Figure 10-35. Microscopic polyangiitis: hyaline membranes. Hyaline membranes may be a feature of microscopic polyangiitis as well as other diffuse alveolar hemorrhage syndromes. Note the diffuse capillaritis evident here.

Hyaline membranes (Fig. 10-35) identical to those of diffuse alveolar damage (DAD) may also be seen.[37,119] In some cases it may be difficult to distinguish hemorrhagic DAD from a diffuse pulmonary hemorrhage syndrome with capillaritis. Pulmonary fibrosis[36,37] and progressive obstructive airway disease with emphysematous features[120,121] have also been reported in patients with microscopic polyangiitis.

Differential Diagnosis

The differential diagnosis for microscopic polyangiitis includes hemorrhagic lung infections, WG with prominent capillaritis, Goodpasture syndrome, certain systemic collagen vascular diseases (e.g., systemic lupus erythematosus [SLE]) and other small-vessel vasculitides, such as Henoch-Schönlein purpura and cryoglobulinemia, and even certain rare drug reactions (e.g., diphenylhydantoin).[122]

WG typically has granulomatous inflammation often consisting of palisaded histiocytes surrounding necrosis. *Pure capillaritis forms of WG cannot be reliably distinguished from microscopic polyangiitis on histologic grounds.* In most of these instances, some areas of collagen necrosis will be present in WG. Unfortunately, granulomatous inflammation may not be included in the tissue sampled if a conservative approach is taken to obtaining tissue biopsies in patients with WG. Moreover, on occasion granulomas can be absent altogether in WG, or the biopsy may be obtained during a phase of disease in which granulomas are not prominent. In these scenarios, clinical and serologic data are often helpful in separating these two diseases, even when biopsies cannot.

As mentioned earlier, microscopic polyangiitis is distinguished from polyarteritis nodosa by the involvement of vessels smaller than medium-sized arteries in microscopic polyangiitis, such as arterioles, venules, and capillaries[117] (Table 10-5).

Finally, microscopic polyangiitis must be distinguished from a heterogeneous group of vasculitic disorders affecting venules, capillaries, and arterioles, some of which are associated with drugs or other agents[113-115,122,123] (Box 10-4). Microscopic polyangiitis is not associated with immune deposits in lung as are some other types of small-vessel vasculitis, such as Henoch-Schönlein purpura, cryoglobulinemic vasculitis, serum sickness, and lupus vasculitis.[116,117] Other conditions known to produce small-vessel vasculitis (listed in Box 10-4) can typically be excluded on clinical and serologic grounds.

Table 10-5. Microscopic Polyangiitis: Differential Diagnosis

Feature	Microscopic Polyangiitis	Wegener Granulomatosis	Polyarteritis Nodosa
Size of affected vessels			
Medium-sized arteries	Sometimes	Sometimes	Yes (bronchial arteries)
Arterioles, venules, capillaries	Yes	Yes	No
Granulomatous inflammation	No	Yes	No
Lung involvement	Common	Common	Uncommon
ANCA	Mostly p-ANCA	Mostly c-ANCA	Mostly p-ANCA

ANCA (c-ANCA, p-ANCA), antineutrophil cytoplasmic antibodies (cytoplasmic, perinuclear).

Box 10-4. Microscopic Polyangiitis and Other Conditions Associated with Small-Vessel Vasculitis

Idiopathic Microscopic Polyangiitis (Small-Vessel Vasculitis)*
Systemic[117]
Localized pulmonary small-vessel vasculitis[186]

Small-Vessel Vasculitis Associated with Known Conditions
Hypersensitivity vasculitis (drug-induced)[187]
  Penicillin
  Sulfonamides
  Diuretics
  Nonsteroidal anti-inflammatory drugs
  Anticonvulsants
Infection[114,115]
  Hepatitis B
  Upper respiratory tract streptococcal infections
Other diseases
  Collagen vascular diseases[113,123]
  Malignancy[188,189]
  Henoch-Schönlein purpura[190-192]
  Mixed cryoglobulinemia[193-195]
  Pulmonary interstitial fibrosis in elderly patients[196]
  Cystic fibrosis[187]
Bone marrow transplantation[197]

*The terms microscopic polyangiitis, microscopic polyarteritis, and hypersensitivity vasculitis all have been used for idiopathic small-vessel vasculitis syndromes.[112,117]
Data from Calabrese LH, Michel BA, Bloch DA, et al. The American College of Rheumatology 1990 criteria for the classification of hypersensitivity vasculitis. *Arthritis Rheum.* 1990;33:1108–1113; Churg J. Nomenclature of vasculitic syndromes: a historical perspective. *Am J Kidney Dis.* 1991;18:148–153; Swerlick R, Lawley T. Small-vessel vasculitis and cutaneous vasculitis. In: Churg A, Churg J, eds. *Systemic Vasculitides.* New York: Igaku-Shoin; 1991:193–201; Jennette J, Falk R. Small-vessel vasculitis. *N Engl J Med.* 1997;337:1512–1523; and Churg J, Churg A. Idiopathic and secondary vasculitis: a review. *Mod Pathol.* 1989;2:144–160.

Treatment and Prognosis

Microscopic polyangiitis is treated with immunosuppressive agents.[117] Lauque and colleagues treated a group of 29 patients using corticosteroids (in 100%) with cyclophosphamide (in 79%), plasmapheresis (in 24%), dialysis (in 28%), and mechanical ventilation (in 10%).[118] The 5-year survival rate was 68%, with causes of death divided equally between vasculitis and side effects of treatment. Complete recovery occurred in most patients (69%). Pulmonary function abnormalities persisted in 24%, and 11 patients relapsed, 2 of whom died of alveolar hemorrhage.[118]

Vasculitic Syndromes That Uncommonly Affect the Lung

Necrotizing Sarcoid Granulomatosis

Necrotizing sarcoid granulomatosis is a rare granulomatous disease that primarily affects the lungs. Nodular masses of confluent sarcoid-like or epithelioid granulomas are seen in the lung parenchyma, often with extensive areas of necrosis and vasculitis. Debate continues over whether necrotizing sarcoid granulomatosis is a vasculitic syndrome, a variant of sarcoidosis, or simply a manifestation of unusual infection. The principal argument against the disorder's being a vasculitic syndrome is that it is not a systemic vasculitic disorder and the lung pathology is primarily that of necrotizing granulomatous inflammation rather than vasculitis. A case of necrotizing sarcoid was recently reported in a patient who had family members with typical sarcoid, potentially lending further support to the theory of a primary granulomatous disorder.[124]

Clinical Features

Necrotizing sarcoid granulomatosis is typically a disease of adults. A summary of clinical and radiologic features reported in case studies is presented in Table 10-6. The average age for patients who develop the disease is 50, but it can occur from adolescence to late adulthood.[25,79,125] Women are affected twice as often as men.[126,127] The usual presentation includes cough, fever, chest pain, dyspnea, malaise, and weight loss.[62,126,128] Up to one fourth of patients may be asymptomatic at the time of diagnosis. Extrapulmonary manifestations are uncommon, with rare reports of uveitis and hypothalamic insufficiency.[63,129–131] Upper airway disease, glomerulonephritis, and systemic vasculitis are not expected findings. To date, positive ANCAs have not been reported in this disease.

Radiologic Features

Necrotizing sarcoid granulomatosis usually manifests as bilateral, multifocal parenchymal nodular opacities. Nodules may either be well marginated or have ill-defined borders (Fig. 10-36). Like the granulomas of sarcoidosis, lesions typically have a bronchovascular and subpleural

Table 10-6. Necrotizing Sarcoid Granulomatosis: Summary of Reported Clinical-Radiologic Features

Feature	Reported Findings				
	Liebow	Saldana	Churg et al.	Koss et al.	Others
Number of cases	11	30	32	13	8
Male-to-female ratio	~1:1	12:18	1:4	3:10	3:5
Bilateral (%)	82	12	72	62	50
Solitary (%)	18*	88	22	15	25
Hilar adenopathy (%)	9	7	65	8	25
Cavitation (%)	NA	3	0	23	13
Recurrence (%)	25	11	12	15	13
Died (%)	0	0	4†	0	13‡

*Described as "localized, unilateral disease."
†One patient died of pneumonia several months after resection of a solitary nodule.
‡Patient died of oat cell carcinoma.
NA, not available.
Data from Liebow A. The J. Burns Amberson lecture—pulmonary angiitis and granulomatosis. *Am Rev Respir Dis.* 1973;108:1–18; Saldana M. Necrotizing sarcoid granulomatosis: clinicopathologic observations in 24 patients [Abstract]. I 1978;38:364; Churg A, Carrington C, Gupta R. Necrotizing sarcoid granulomatosis. *Chest.* 1979;76:406–413; and Koss MN, Hochholzer L, Feigin DS, et al. Necrotizing sarcoid-like granulomatosis: clinical, pathologic, and immunopathologic findings. *Human Pathol.* 1980;11(suppl):510–519. Other case reports include Beach RC, Corrin B, Scopes JW, Graham E. Necrotizing sarcoid granulomatosis with neurologic lesions in a child. *J Pediatr.* 1980;97:950–953; Singh N, Cole S, Krause PJ, et al. Necrotizing sarcoid granulomatosis with extrapulmonary involvement. Clinical, pathologic, ultrastructural, and immunologic features. *Am Rev Respir Dis.* 1981;124:189–192; Stephen JG, Braimbridge MV, Corrin B, et al. Necrotizing 'sarcoidal' angiitis and granulomatosis of the lung. *Thorax.* 1976;31:356–360; Rolfes D, Weiss M, Sanders M. Necrotizing sarcoid granulomatosis with suppurative features. *Am J Clin Pathol.* 1984;82:602–607; Spiteri MA, Gledhill A, Campbell D, Clarke SW. Necrotizing sarcoid granulomatosis. *Br J Dis Chest.* 1987;81:70–75; Chabalko J. Solitary lung lesion with cavitation due to necrotizing sarcoid granulomatosis. *Del Med J.* 1986;58:15–16; and Fisher M, Christ M, Bernstein J. Necrotizing sarcoid–like granulomatosis: radiologic-pathologic correlation. *J Can Assoc Radiol.* 1984;35:313–315.

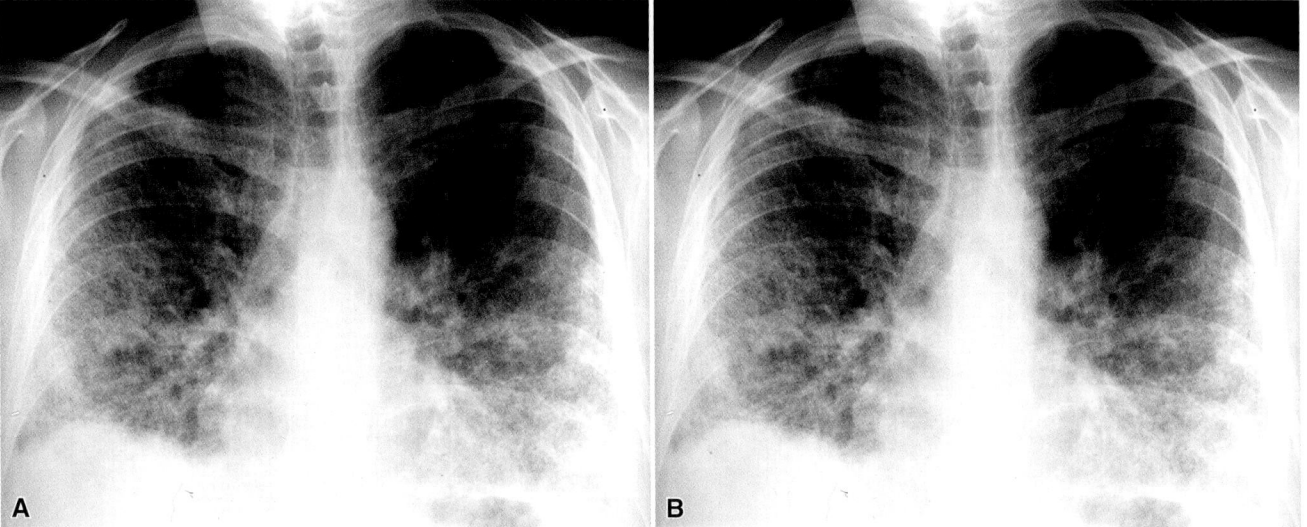

Figure 10-36. Necrotizing sarcoid granulomatosis. Posteroanterior chest radiographs from a 40-year-old man with fatigue, fever, and dyspnea. **A,** At clinical presentation, note diffuse bilateral air space consolidation with a predilection for the bases and the mid lung zones. **B,** After biopsy and steroid therapy, marked improvement is evident, with residual parenchymal consolidation in the lung periphery and lower lobes. (From Travis WD, Colby TV, Koss MN, et al, eds. *Non-Neoplastic Disorders of the Lower Respiratory Tract.* In: King DW, ed. *Atlas of Nontumor Pathology.* Washington, DC: American Registry of Pathology and Armed Forces Institute of Pathology; 2002, Figure 4-24.)

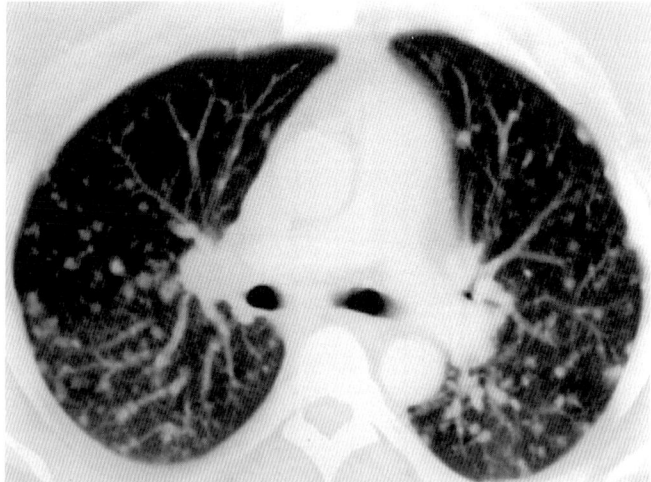

Figure 10-37. Necrotizing sarcoid granulomatosis: computed tomography (CT) features. Chest CT scan (lung window) in a 41-year-old man with cough demonstrates multifocal small nodules. (From Travis WD, Colby TV, Koss MN, et al, eds. *Non-Neoplastic Disorders of the Lower Respiratory Tract.* In: King DW, ed. *Atlas of Nontumor Pathology.* Washington, DC: American Registry of Pathology and Armed Forces Institute of Pathology; 2002, Figure 4-25.)

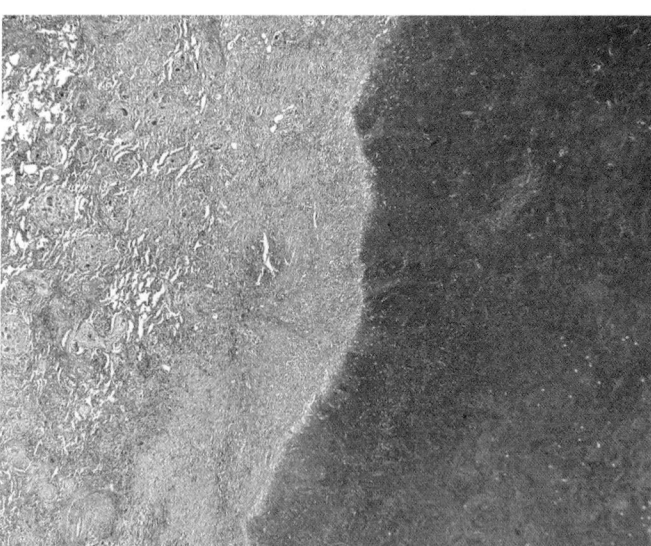

Figure 10-39. Necrotizing sarcoid granulomatosis: large zones of necrosis. Large zones of necrosis are seen at *right*.

distribution, but unlike in sarcoidosis, they may be more numerous in the lower lung zones.[42,62,79,80,132] Solitary lesions and parenchymal consolidations may occur but are unusual manifestations.

On CT scans, cavitation and heterogeneous contrast enhancement of the lesions may be seen (Fig. 10-37), correlating with intralesional necrosis.[129] Pleural involvement with thickening or effusion may also be observed.[132] Hilar lymphadenopathy is variable and not seen as frequently as in sarcoidosis.[56]

Pathologic Features
Confluent non-necrotizing granulomas form large nodules in the lung parenchyma (Fig. 10-38). Large zones of necrosis are present in the nodules (Fig. 10-39), and vasculitis (Fig. 10-40) is typically present. The granulomas in necrotizing sarcoid granulomatosis resemble those of sarcoidosis, except for the presence of necrosis, with tight clusters of giant cells and epithelioid cells (Fig. 10-41). One can also see a sarcoidal pattern of lung involvement with a lymphangitic distribution to the granulomas.[56,62,127] In addition to the large zones of necrosis, smaller foci of necrosis often are present.[56]

The vasculitis of necrotizing sarcoid granulomatosis can affect both arteries and veins. Three patterns of vasculitis can be seen: necrotizing granulomas (Fig. 10-42), giant cell vasculitis (Fig. 10-43), and infiltration by chronic inflammatory cells.[133] Necrotizing granulomas may be present circumferentially along the vascular walls (Fig. 10-44).

Differential Diagnosis
The differential diagnosis for necrotizing sarcoid granulomatosis includes granulomatous infection, nodular sarcoidosis, and WG. The most important of these entities, and the most difficult to exclude, is granulomatous infection,[56,61] especially because granulomatous infections caused by mycobacteria and fungi can produce both vasculitis and sarcoid-like granulomas.[51,52] Some investigators regard necrotizing

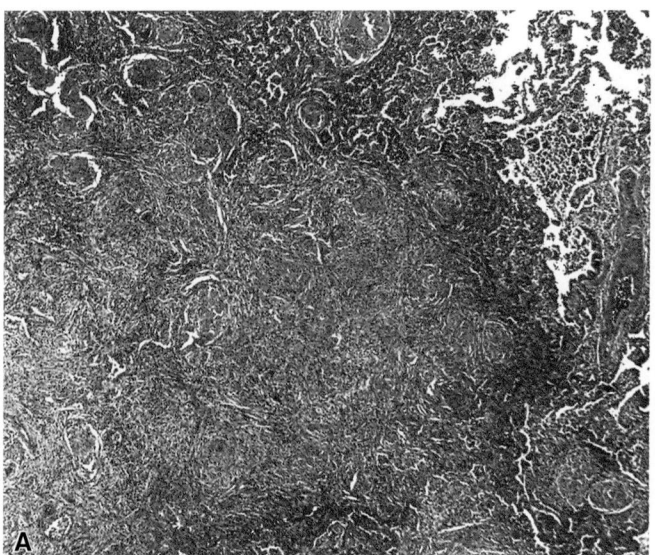
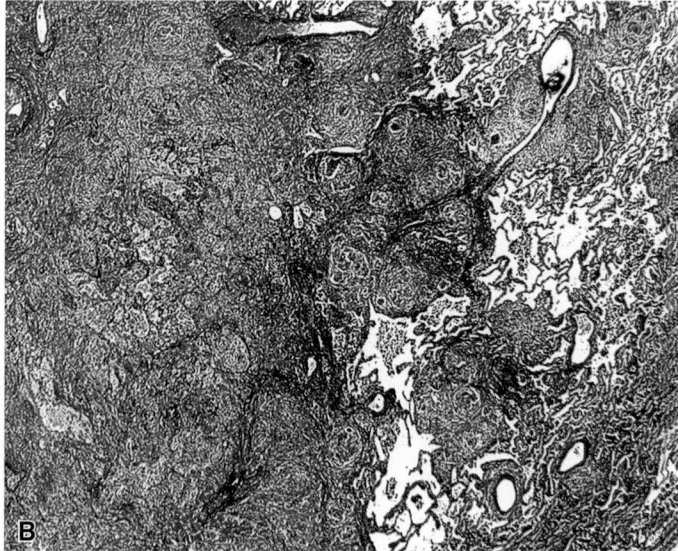

Figure 10-38. Necrotizing sarcoid granulomatosis: large nodules with variable necrosis. Large parenchymal inflammatory nodules with necrosis are typically seen. **A,** Confluent non-necrotizing granulomas are a dominant feature. **B,** Elastic tissue stains help demonstrate vascular involvement within and around nodules (*upper right, off center*).

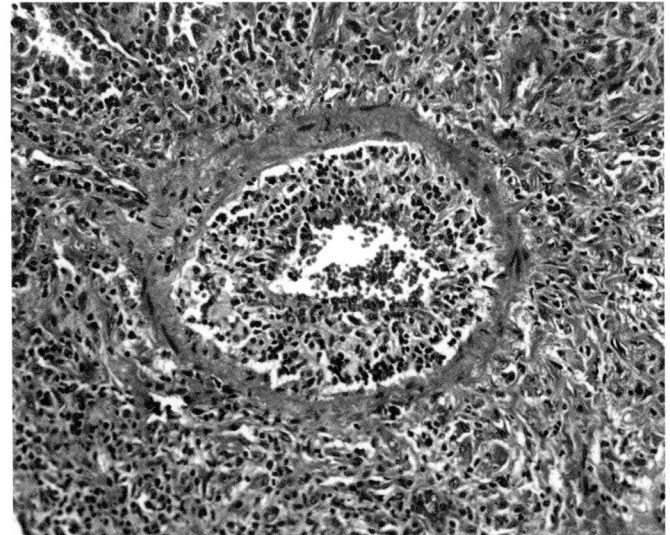

Figure 10-40. Necrotizing sarcoid granulomatosis: vasculitis. Vasculitis is a typical feature of this disorder. Here, lymphocytes and plasma cells infiltrate the media and subintimal region of a pulmonary artery. Note adventitial fibrosis.

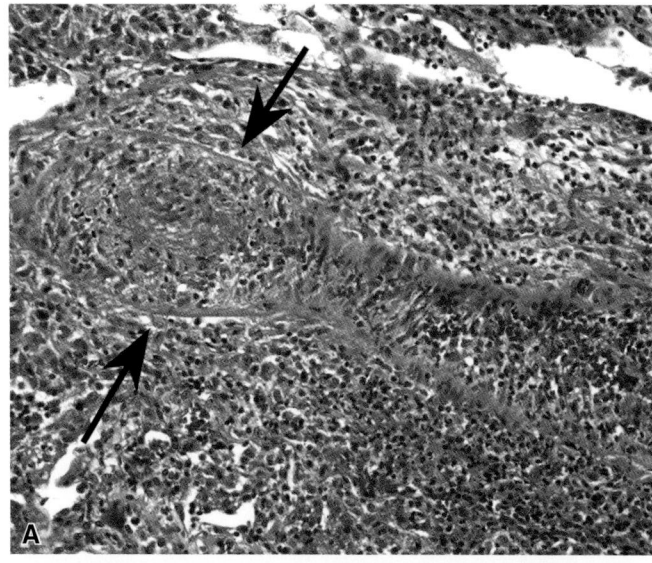

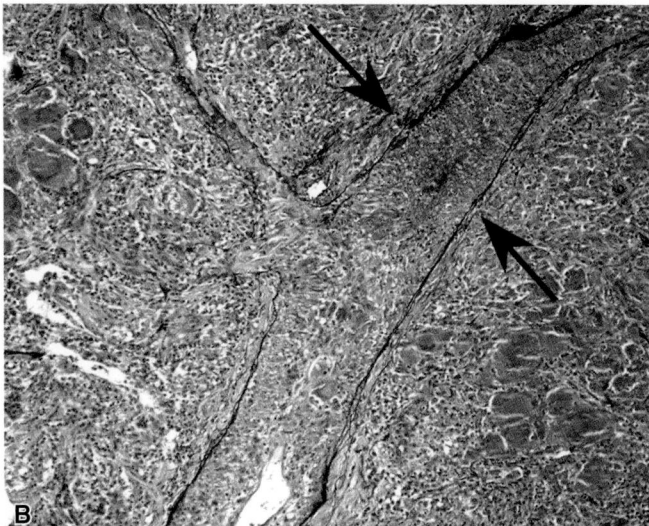

Figure 10-42. Necrotizing sarcoid granulomatosis: granulomatous vasculitis. **A,** Granulomatous vasculitis (*arrows*) is a common pattern in this disorder. **B,** An elastic tissue stain is often helpful in defining distorted arteries (*arrows*) within the inflammatory process.

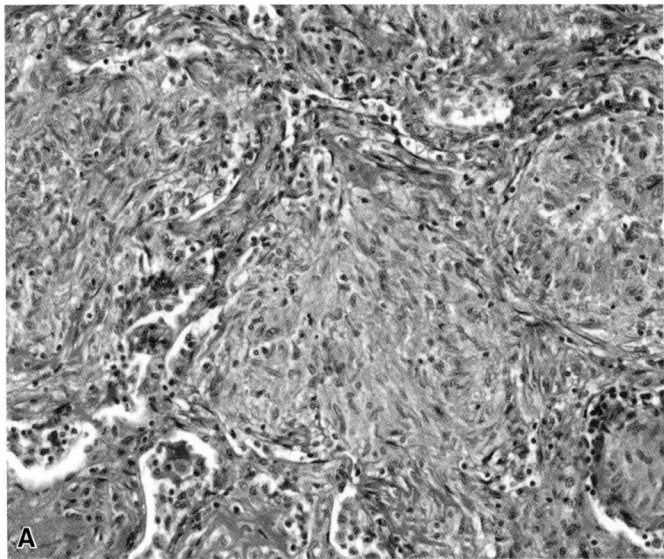

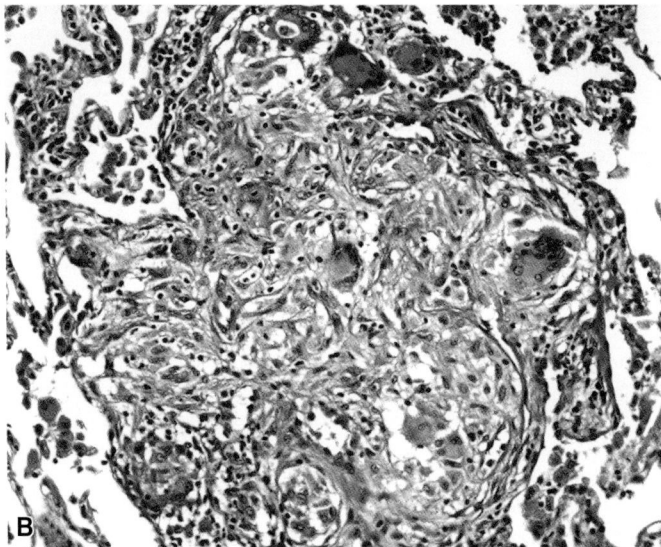

Figure 10-41. Necrotizing sarcoid granulomatosis: sarcoid-like granulomas. **A,** The granulomas in this disorder resemble those of sarcoidosis. **B,** Admixed multinucleate giant cells are typically seen.

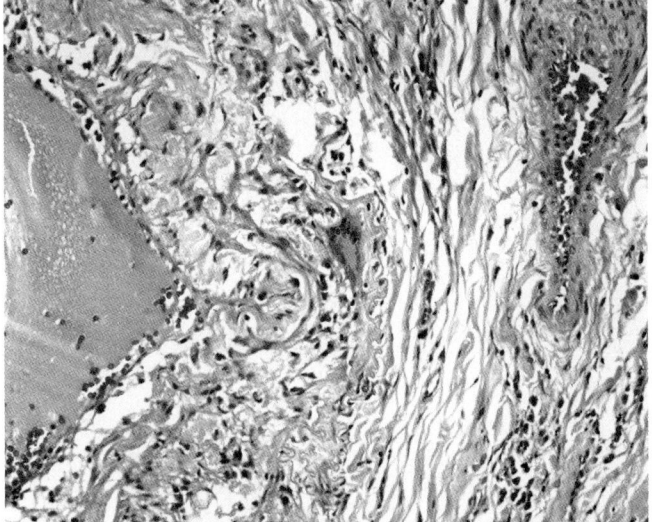

Figure 10-43. Necrotizing sarcoid granulomatosis: giant cells in arteries. Giant cells may be a prominent component of the vasculitis.

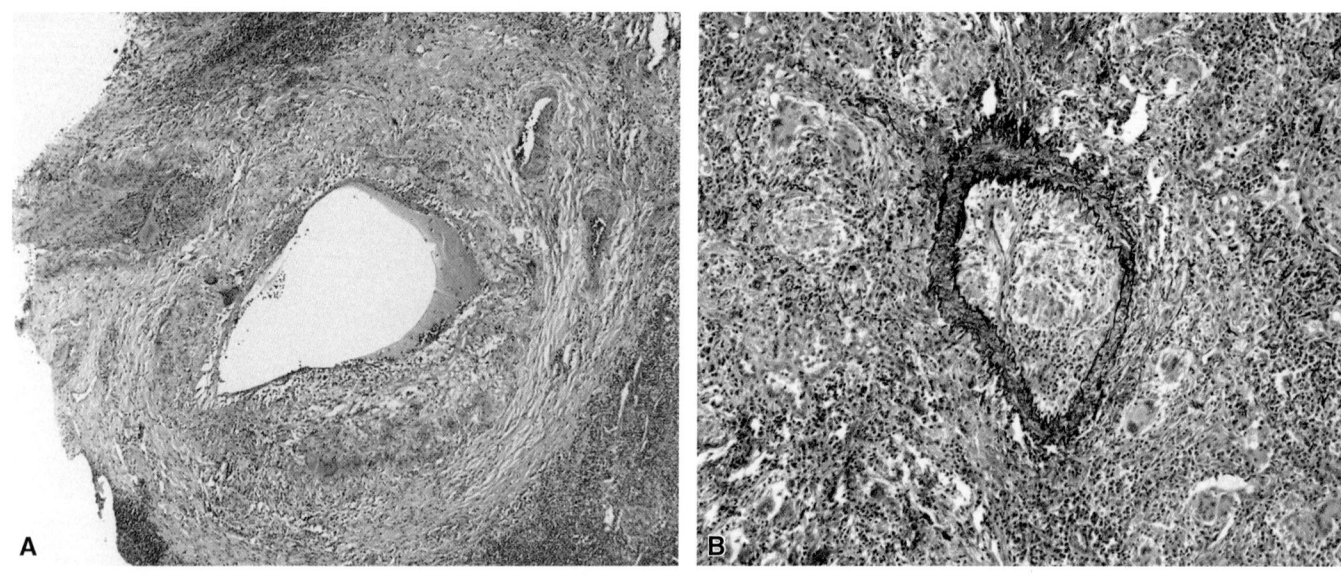

Figure 10-44. Necrotizing sarcoid granulomatosis: circumferential vascular envelopment. **A,** In this disorder, granulomas may envelop arteries in a circumferential fashion. **B,** An elastic tissue stain shows both subintimal granulomas, as well as granulomas involving the adventitia in a circumferential fashion.

sarcoid granulomatosis as representing the subset of sarcoidosis referred to as "nodular sarcoidosis," but true necrosis, as seen in this disorder, is not typically present in the nodular form of sarcoidosis. The key features distinguishing necrotizing sarcoid granulomatosis from WG are summarized in Table 10-7.

Treatment and Prognosis

The prognosis for patients with necrotizing sarcoid granulomatosis is excellent.[127,134] Localized disease can be cured by surgical resection alone. Patients with bilateral opacities or nodules may respond to systemic corticosteroids. A small percentage of patients will have persistent opacities[62,63] or will experience a relapse.[56,135] The only deaths reported in patients with necrotizing sarcoid granulomatosis have been due to opportunistic infections, so cytotoxic immunosuppression generally is not recommended.[62]

Giant Cell (Temporal) Arteritis

Giant cell arteritis is a vasculitis that most commonly involves the temporal arteries in older individuals. Vascular lesions include giant cells, typically centered on the vascular elastic lamina (Fig. 10-45). Lower respiratory tract involvement is extremely rare, although the disease can be associated with upper respiratory tract symptoms in approximately 10% of patients.[88] When the lungs are involved, patients may have nodules,[136,137] interstitial opacities,[138] and unilateral pleural effusions on chest radiographs.[88] Pulmonary arterial involvement is rarer still,[139] but giant cell arteritis can affect the pulmonary trunk and main pulmonary arteries, as well as large and medium-sized intrapulmonary elastic arteries.[139] Histologically the vasculitis shows medial and adventitial chronic inflammation with included giant cells. This causes destruction of the elastic laminae sometimes with focal fibrinoid medial necrosis.[139] Bronchoscopic biopsies may show granulomatous inflammation of pulmonary arteries and fragmented elastic fibers.[136,139] Giant cell arteritis can be distinguished from WG, necrotizing sarcoid granulomatosis, CSS, and granulomatous infections by the absence of parenchymal inflammation.[139] The temporal artery involvement and older age of patients with giant cell arteritis distinguishes them from those with Takayasu arteritis.[139]

A very rare disorder known as "*idiopathic isolated pulmonary giant cell arteritis*" has also been described.[140–142] The disease is limited to the lungs. Dyspnea on exertion may be a presenting manifestation, but patients usually lack hemoptysis, fever, or elevation of the erythrocyte sedimentation rate. The vasculitis is usually an unsuspected finding seen first in a surgical or an autopsy specimen.[140,141] Histologically, organized arterial thrombi with recanalization are identified, and narrowing of large pulmonary arteries is seen. The vasculitis is characterized by a destructive inflammatory infiltrate of giant cells, histiocytes, and lymphocytes causing fragmentation of elastic laminae.[140–142] Peripheral lung infarcts can occur.

Disseminated visceral giant cell angiitis is another rare form of giant cell arteritis that affects extracranial small arteries and arterioles, including those in the lung. This is a very rare condition, with only five reported cases, in males, three of whom had lung involvement.[143,144] In all of these cases, the disorder was recognized as an incidental autopsy finding.[143] Extracranial small arteries and arterioles were affected, and each patient demonstrated involvement of at least three of the following organs: heart, lung, kidneys, liver, pancreas, and stomach. The vasculitis showed prominent multinucleate giant cells of both foreign body and Langerhans types, but most of the inflammatory cells consisted of histiocytes, lymphocytes, and plasma cells. A relationship has

Table 10-7. Wegener Granulomatosis versus Necrotizing Sarcoidosis: Distinguishing Features

Clinical/Pathologic Feature	Wegener Granulomatosis	Necrotizing Sarcoidosis
Lung involvement	66–85%	100%
Extrapulmonary involvement	90–100% ENT, kidney, skin, neurologic	≤10% Ocular, neurologic
ANCA	Yes	No
Histopathologic pattern		
Sarcoidal granulomas	Rare	Characteristic
Vasculitis	Characteristic	Characteristic

ANCA, antineutrophil cytoplasmic antibodies; ENT, ear, nose, and throat.

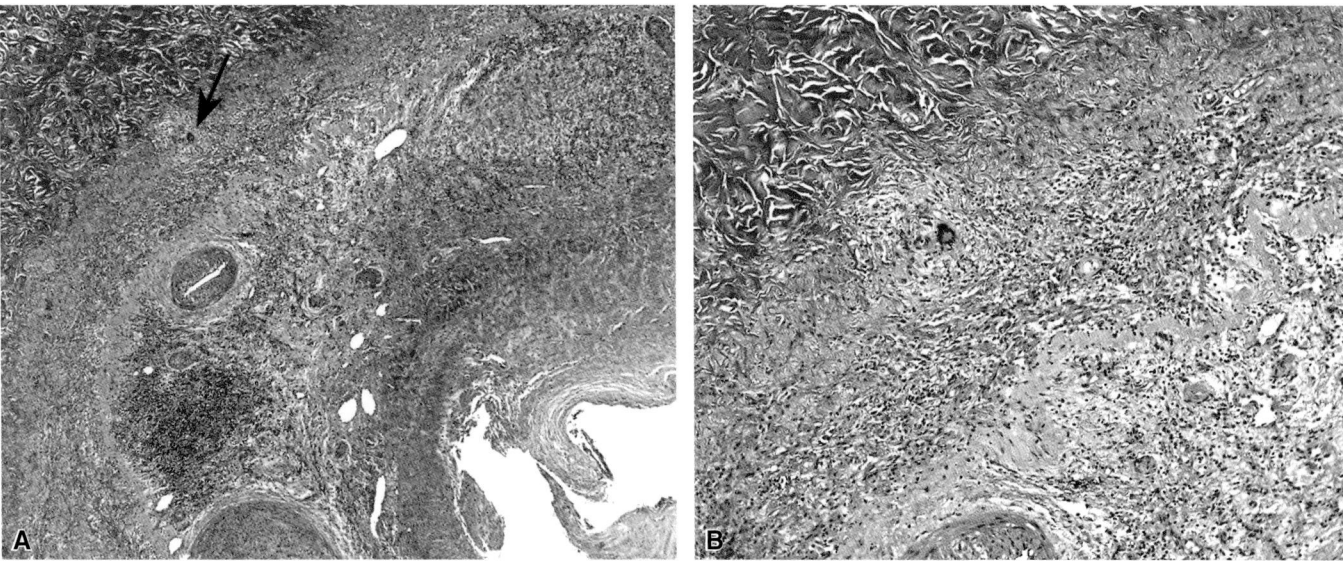

Figure 10-45. Giant cell arteritis: involvement of a large pulmonary artery. **A,** A central pulmonary artery shows extensive medial damage. **B,** The area designated by an *arrow* in part **A** at higher magnification. Note the multinucleate giant cell and inflammation along the elastic lamina of the vessel.

been proposed between sarcoidosis and disseminated visceral giant cell arteritis, but the occurrence of these two manifestations together is so rare that it is difficult to confirm.[145-147]

Polyarteritis Nodosa

Classic polyarteritis nodosa is a vasculitis that involves arteries of medium and small size (Fig. 10-46). It can involve virtually any organ but rarely affects the lungs. Most cases previously reported as polyarteritis nodosa with lung involvement probably were examples of CSS[114,148-150] or possibly small-vessel vasculitis (i.e., microscopic polyangiitis). Polyarteritis nodosa differs from CSS and microscopic polyangiitis in that only arteries are affected. The tissue eosinophilia and extravascular granulomas characteristic of CSS are not seen. Polyarteritis nodosa differs from microscopic polyangiitis in that medium-sized arteries are affected (primarily bronchial arteries),[12,150] whereas in microscopic polyangiitis, smaller arteries, venules and capillaries typically manifest the disease.[116,117]

Takayasu Arteritis

Takayasu arteritis is a vasculitis that primarily affects the aorta and its branches. The arteritis is comprised of lymphocytes, macrophages, and giant cells that infiltrate the adventitia, media, and intima of these vessels.

Clinical Features

Takayasu arteritis most commonly affects women less than 40 years of age.[151] Pulmonary arteries are involved in 12% to 86% of patients with the disease,[151-154] and rarely, pulmonary artery involvement may be the presenting manifestation.[155] Takayasu arteritis may affect the kidneys, heart, skin and gastrointestinal tract.[156] Because it is difficult to obtain tissue biopsy specimens from large vessels such as the aorta or pulmonary artery, the diagnosis is usually established by angiography. Pulmonary artery stenosis, irregular narrowing, and occlusion may be seen.[152,153,157] Fistulas between pulmonary arteries and systemic arteries may occur.[158]

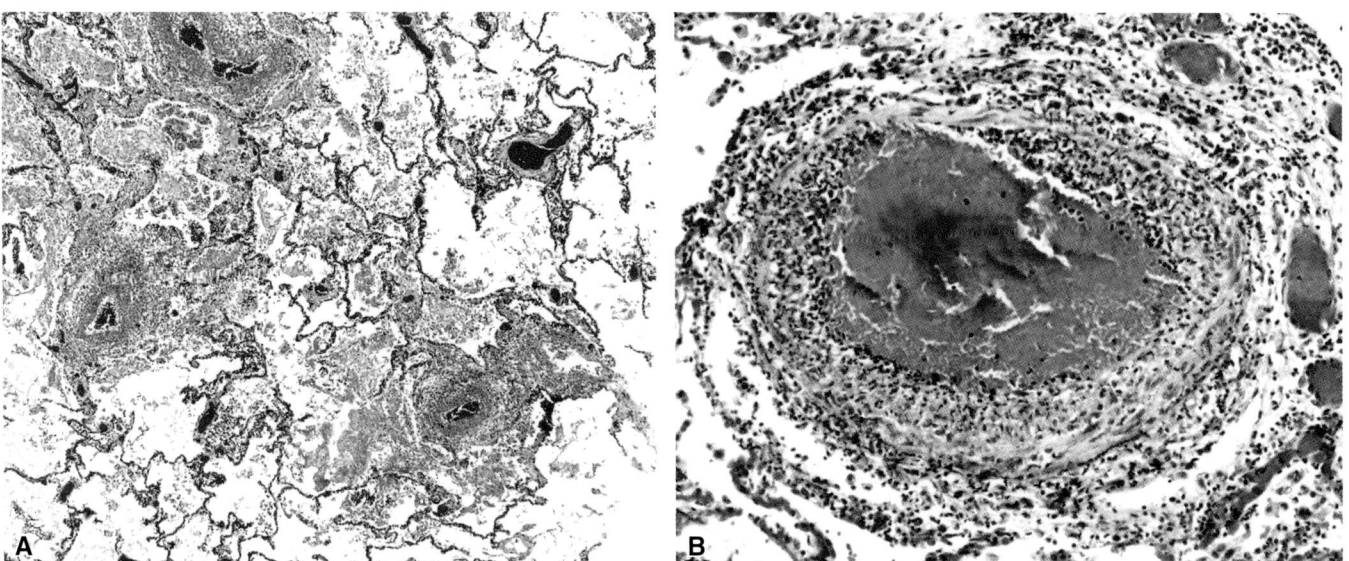

Figure 10-46. Polyarteritis nodosa: arteritis. **A,** Arteries of medium and small size typically are involved. **B,** The vasculitic process at higher magnification.

Radiographic Features

CT scan findings in Takayasu arteritis frequently include areas of low attenuation in the lung, presumably on the basis of regional hypoperfusion related to upstream arteritis.[159] Subpleural linear reticular changes and pleural thickening also occur.[159]

Pathologic Features

Takayasu arteritis involves the adventitia, media, and intima of large elastic pulmonary arteries (Fig. 10-47). Infiltration by lymphocytes, macrophages, and giant cells is characteristic. Thrombi may also be seen. There is progression to diffuse or nodular fibrosis of the artery wall with disintegration or loss of elastic fibers.[160,161] The fibrosis can result in stenosis or obliteration of the vascular lumen and cause aneurysm formation or dilatation of the artery. Matsubara and associates described a stenosis-recanalization phenomenon they called "blood vessels in blood vessels," occurring within the pulmonary elastic and muscular arteries.[161]

Treatment

Corticosteroid therapy is often effective, but some patients with Takayasu arteritis require the addition of a cytotoxic agent (e.g., cyclophosphamide) for management. Stenotic arterial lesions have been successfully corrected by surgical techniques.[162]

Behçet Syndrome

Behçet syndrome is a multisystem inflammatory disorder characterized by skin lesions, oral and genital ulcers, and iridocyclitis. Debate continues over the nature of the disease. The etiology is unknown, but environmental, genetic, viral, bacterial, and immunologic factors have been implicated in its pathogenesis. The lung manifestations are clearly vasculitic, but an immune complex–mediated hypersensitivity reaction has been proposed for the mucocutaneous lesions, and an association with human leukocyte antigen (HLA)-B51 has been identified.[163]

Clinical Features

Behçet syndrome has a worldwide distribution but is most commonly a disease of the Mediterranean basin, the Middle East, and Japan.[164,165] The disease typically affects individuals between adolescence and middle age. The diagnosis is based primarily on clinical criteria (Box 10-5). The

---

Box 10-5. Behçet Syndrome: Diagnostic Clinical Criteria

Recurrent oral aphthosis
and
At least two of the following five clinical manifestations:
    Recurrent genital aphthosis
    Uveitis
    Synovitis
    Cutaneous vasculitis
    Meningoencephalitis
Absence of inflammatory bowel disease or other collagen vascular diseases

---

clinical feature that is common to all patients with Behçet syndrome is recurrent painful aphthous oral or genital ulcers. Oral ulceration occurring more than three times in 1 year is required to meet the diagnostic criteria for the disease. These lesions must be distinguished from ulcers related to viral infection such as herpes simplex, and other diseases such as inflammatory bowel disease or systemic lupus erythematosus.

Symptoms of pulmonary involvement include dyspnea, cough, chest pain, and hemoptysis.[165] Males are more likely to develop lung manifestations, particularly hemoptysis.[165,166] The presence of circulating immune complexes in patients with active pulmonary disease suggests that immune complexes may be important in the pathogenesis of the lung involvement.[166,167]

Radiographic Features

Air space consolidation consistent with pulmonary hemorrhage, lung infarction, and pulmonary artery aneurysms may be seen when the lungs are involved.[168,169] Thoracic involvement in the patient with Behçet syndrome can sometimes be suggested on CT images by the presence of thrombosis in the pulmonary arteries or in the superior vena cava. Characteristic aneurysms of the pulmonary arteries can also occur.[168,169] Pulmonary aneurysms and thromboses can be detected with angiography as well.[165]

Pathologic Features

Pulmonary involvement is characterized by a lymphocytic and necrotizing vasculitis that involves pulmonary arteries of all sizes, veins, and alveolar septal capillaries (Fig. 10-48). Additional findings include aneurysms of elastic pulmonary arteries, arterial and venous thromboses

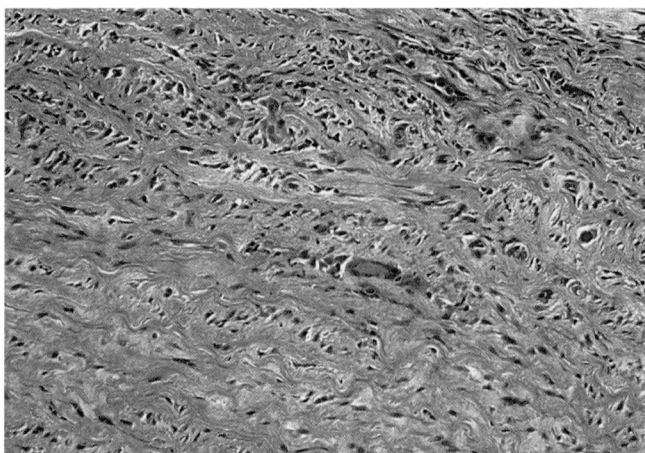

Figure 10-47. Takayasu arteritis. The wall of this pulmonary artery is infiltrated by lymphocytes and giant cells. (From Travis WD, Colby TV, Koss MN, et al, eds. *Non-Neoplastic Disorders of the Lower Respiratory Tract*. In: King DW, ed. *Atlas of Nontumor Pathology*. Washington, DC: American Registry of Pathology and Armed Forces Institute of Pathology; 2002, Figure 4-29.)

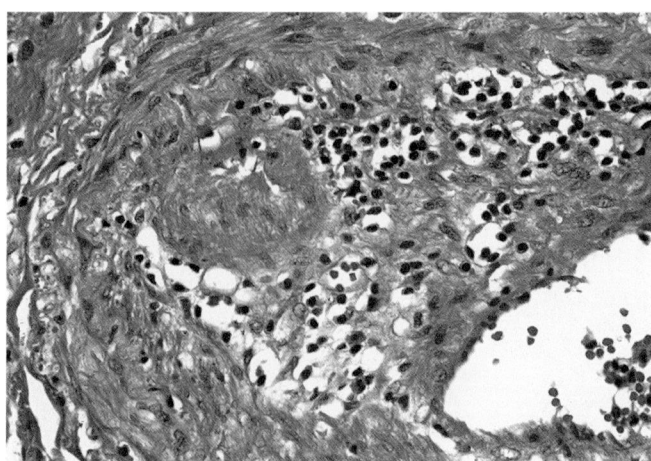

Figure 10-48. Behçet syndrome: vasculitis. The wall of this small artery is infiltrated by lymphocytes. (From Travis WD, Colby TV, Koss MN, et al, eds. *Non-Neoplastic Disorders of the Lower Respiratory Tract*. In: King DW, ed. *Atlas of Nontumor Pathology*. Washington, DC: American Registry of Pathology and Armed Forces Institute of Pathology; 2002, Figure 4-30.)

(Fig. 10-49), pulmonary infarcts (Fig. 10-50), bronchial erosion by pulmonary artery aneurysms, and arteriobronchial fistulas.[165,170,171] Perivascular adventitial fibrosis may be prominent. Collateral vessels lacking elastic lamellae may develop in the periadventitial fibrous tissues around thrombosed arteries and aneurysms (Fig. 10-51). Hemorrhage[172] and acute interstitial pneumonia[173] may occur as life-threatening pulmonary complications.

Treatment

A variety of treatments have been used to address the mucocutaneous manifestations of the disease, including oral colchicine, topical anesthetics, and corticosteroids (topical, intralesional, or systemic). Thalidomide and dapsone have also been shown to be effective. Aggressive immunosuppression with combined systemic corticosteroids and another agent (azathioprine, cyclophosphamide, cyclosporine, chlorambucil) may be necessary when significant ocular, neurologic, gastrointestinal, and vascular manifestations occur. Patients who develop thromboses require anticoagulation.[166] Severe hemoptysis may require surgical intervention.[172] The clinical course of Behçet syndrome is characterized by exacerbations and remissions. Over time, the disease may decrease in severity.

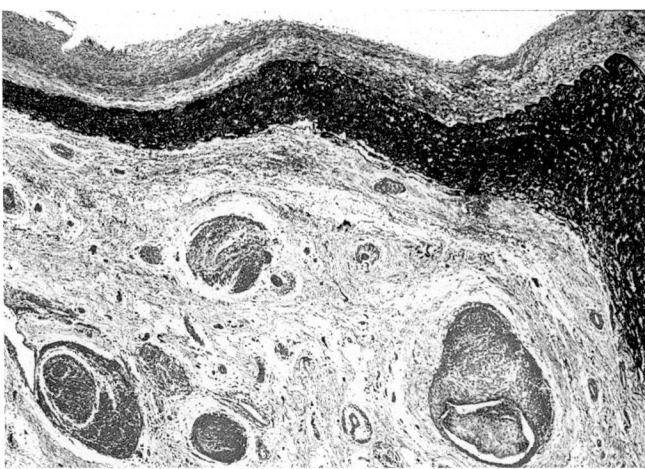

Figure 10-51. Behçet syndrome: collateral vessels. The collateral vessels in the periadventitial tissues surrounding this large elastic artery lack elastic lamellae. (From Travis WD, Colby TV, Koss MN, et al, eds. *Non-Neoplastic Disorders of the Lower Respiratory Tract.* In: King DW, ed. *Atlas of Nontumor Pathology.* Washington, DC: American Registry of Pathology and Armed Forces Institute of Pathology; 2002, Figure 4-33.)

Secondary Vasculitis

Pulmonary Infection and Septic Emboli

When pulmonary vessels are involved by inflammation and necrosis in the setting of infection, secondary vasculitis should always be a strong consideration. Certain bacterial pneumonias, especially those caused by *Pseudomonas aeruginosa*[174] and *Legionella pneumophila*,[175] are well known for their tendency to invade and produce necrosis of blood vessel walls. The necrotizing granulomas produced in response to fungal and mycobacterial infections commonly involve blood vessel walls, causing potential confusion with vascular involvement by WG.[52] Necrotizing vasculitis may also be a consequence of angioinvasive fungal infections in the immunocompromised patient, especially infections due to *Aspergillus* and *Mucor* species. Such vasculitis may be granulomatous and frequently causes pulmonary infarction. Pulmonary vasculitis can also accompany certain parasitic pulmonary infections such as *Dirofilaria immitis*, *Schistosoma*, and *Wuchereria* infections. In HIV-infected patients, vasculitis can even be be a rare complication of *Pneumocystis* pneumonia.[176]

Classic Sarcoidosis

Classic sarcoidosis can produce so-called granulomatous vasculitis (involvement of blood vessel walls by typical sarcoid granulomas) as an incidental histologic finding in surgical lung biopsies (see Chapter 7, Chronic Diffuse Lung Diseases).[177]

In rare instances, a systemic vasculitis can occur in patients with sarcoidosis. Fernandes and colleagues reported 6 cases in which patients exhibited features of both sarcoidosis and systemic vasculitis and reviewed 22 similar cases that had been previously reported.[178] The group included 13 children and 15 adults who developed fever, peripheral adenopathy, hilar adenopathy, rash, pulmonary parenchymal disease, musculoskeletal symptoms, and scleritis or iridocyclitis.[178]

Radiologic Features

Arteriography demonstrated involvement of medium-sized or large arteries in approximately one half of the patients and features of small-vessel disease in the remaining patients.[178]

Pathologic Features

Pathologic findings consisted of sarcoid-like granulomas, sometimes with foci of necrosis, involving vessels in the skin, lymph node, lung, synovium, bone, bone marrow, liver, trachea, or sclera.

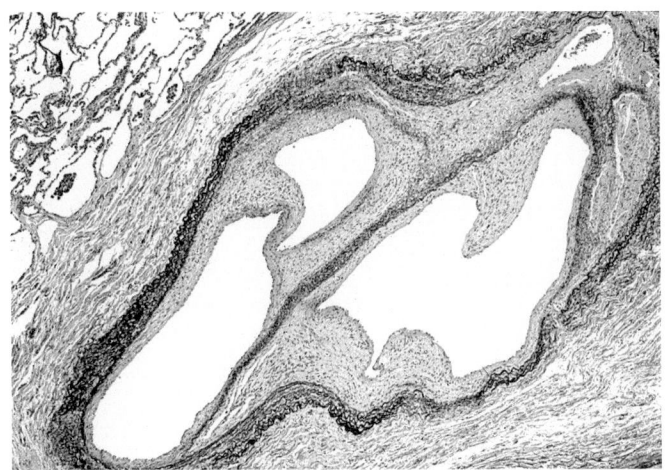

Figure 10-49. Behçet syndrome: organizing thrombus. The web of fibrosis traversing the lumen of this elastic artery is a recanalized thrombus. (From Travis WD, Colby TV, Koss MN, et al, eds. *Non-Neoplastic Disorders of the Lower Respiratory Tract.* In: King DW, ed. *Atlas of Nontumor Pathology.* Washington, DC: American Registry of Pathology and Armed Forces Institute of Pathology; 2002, Figure 4-31.)

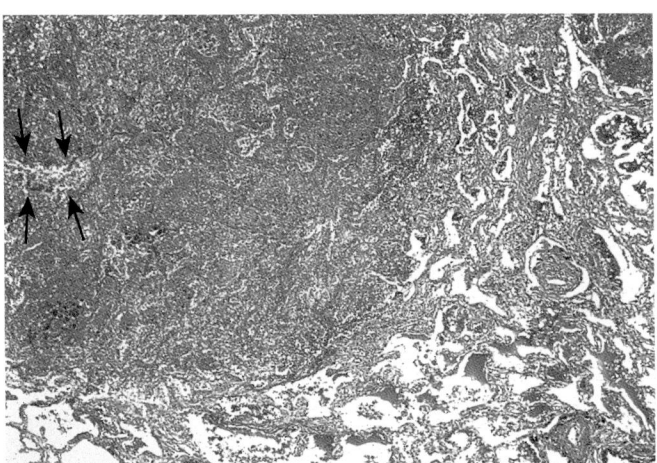

Figure 10-50. Behçet syndrome: pulmonary infarct. A pulmonary infarct can be seen here on elastic tissue stain. The *arrows* designate disrupted elastica of a pulmonary artery at the edge of a lung infarct (*red*).

Therapy and Prognosis

Patients may respond to prednisone alone; as reported by Fernandes and colleagues, however, relapses tended to occur when the medication was tapered or withdrawn.[178]

PULMONARY HEMORRHAGE

Hemorrhage in the lung may occur as a localized phenomenon or as a diffuse disease. Clinically significant hemorrhage is nearly always accompanied by hemoptysis. When blood is identified in the lung biopsy specimen, the question frequently arises as to whether it is a real finding or simply an artifact related to the procedure. Real pulmonary hemorrhage can be caused by a number of unrelated mechanisms. Pulmonary vasculitis and vasculitic syndromes, such as Goodpasture syndrome, are important clinical causes of lung hemorrhage and typically require urgent therapy. Because the differential diagnosis is broad in scope, and the consequences of accurate diagnosis are significant, a diagnostic approach to pulmonary hemorrhage is presented here. A useful algorithm for this exercise is presented in Figure 10-52.

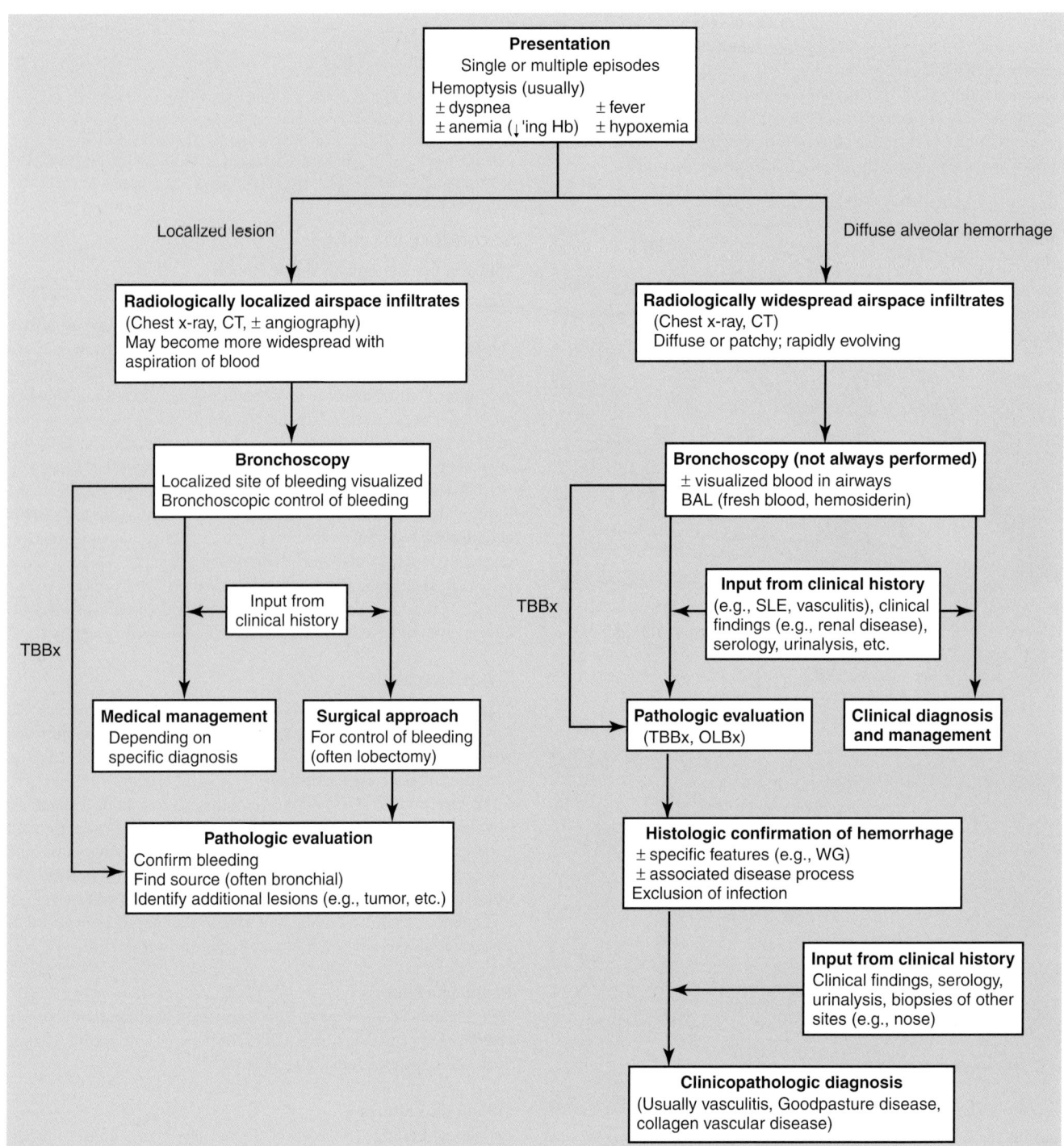

Figure 10-52. Diffuse alveolar hemorrhage. Algorithm. (From Colby TV, Fukuoka J, Ewaskow SP, et al. Pathologic approach to pulmonary hemorrhage. *Ann Diagn Pathol.* 2001;5:309–319.)

Clinical View of Pulmonary Hemorrhage

The occurrence of hemoptysis is alarming to patient and clinician alike. The potential causes of hemoptysis are presented in Box 10-6. The distinction of localized from diffuse hemorrhage is important for management purposes but is not always feasible. With the classic presentation of sudden unilateral chest pain followed by expectoration of bright red blood, pulmonary embolus is usually high on the list of diagnostic possibilities. In most instances, however, the clinician must rely heavily on the radiologic findings in the approach to the patient with hemoptysis, because the physical examination is typically limited in defining the origin or extent of any hemorrhagic event. Bronchoscopy plays an important role as well in defining a potential localized source of bleeding and documenting the presence of hemosiderin-laden macrophages (siderophages) in lavage specimens examined under the microscope. Localized causes of pulmonary hemorrhage are often straightforward and include thromboembolism, tumor, abscess, bronchiectasis, and broncholithiasis. Dieulafoy disease is a rare entity characterized by an abnormal submucosal location of arterial branches. This abnormality is more frequently described in the gastrointestinal tract, but rare bronchial cases have been reported.[179] At times, localized hemorrhage may be life-threatening, requiring lobectomy for control. In this situation, blood may be abundant in the lung parenchyma, but no exact origin for bleeding can be identified (analogous to colectomy for massive hemorrhage associated with diverticulosis). Diffuse pulmonary hemorrhage is more complicated in terms of etiology and will be the main focus here.

Morphologic Approach to Pulmonary Hemorrhage

Not all patients with hemoptysis have histologic evidence of hemorrhage and conversely, not all hemorrhage, or hemosiderin, seen in lung tissue is associated with hemoptysis or other evidence of lung hemorrhage. For the pathologist, the first step in the evaluation of extravascular blood seen in a biopsy specimen is to ascertain the context in which it occurs. Clinically significant hemorrhage rarely is seen in biopsy specimens as blood alone. When intact red cells abound, the most common cause is trauma related to the biopsy procedure, especially in the case of thoracoscopic biopsies because of intraoperative manipulation.[180] In artifactual hemorrhage (Fig. 10-53), fibrin, hemosiderin-laden macrophages, and cellular reactive changes in adjacent alveolar walls typically are lacking. Also, focal areas of organization may be seen within the air spaces in true hemorrhage and may be a useful marker for associated lung injury.

Box 10-6. Causes of Hemoptysis

Infectious Diseases
Bacterial
    Lung abscess*
    Bronchitis*
    Tuberculosis*
    Bronchiectasis (including cystic fibrosis)
    "Chronic pneumonia"
Viral
Fungal
    Mycetoma
Parasitic
    Paragonimiasis (in endemic areas)*

Cardiovascular Diseases
Left ventricular failure*
Pulmonary thromboembolism with infarction*
Mitral stenosis
Tricuspid endocarditis
Pulmonary hypertension
Aneurysms
    Aortic aneurysm
    Subclavian artery aneurysm
    Left ventricular pseudoaneurysm
Vascular prostheses
Arteriovenous malformation
Portal hypertension
Absence of the inferior vena cava
Pulmonary artery agenesis with lung systemic vascularization

Neoplasms
Pulmonary carcinoma*
    Squamous cell carcinoma
    Small cell carcinoma*
Carcinoid tumor
Tracheobronchial gland tumors
Metastatic carcinoma/sarcoma

Trauma
Aortic tear
Lung contusion
Lithotripsy

Ruptured bronchus
Tracheocarotid fistula
Bronchoscopy
Swan-Ganz catheterization
Lung biopsy
Transtracheal aspirate
Lymphangiography
Hickman catheter–induced cavabronchial fistula

Immunologic Conditions
Vasculitides
    Wegener granulomatosis
    Systemic lupus erythematosus
    Microscopic polyangiitis
Goodpasture syndrome
Idiopathic pulmonary hemosiderosis
Other lung-renal syndromes

Drugs and Toxins
Anticoagulants
Cocaine
Penicillamine
Trimellitic anhydride
Solvents
Amiodarone

Miscellaneous Entities
Increased bleeding tendency
    Coagulopathy
    Thrombocytopenia
Amyloidosis
Broncholithiasis
Endometriosis
Thoracic splenosis
Aspirated foreign body
Intralobar sequestration
Radiation
Lymphangiomyomatosis
Factitious
Bronchiolitis obliterans organizing (BOOP)
Lipoid pneumonia

*Most common causes.
From Colby TV, Fukuoka J, Ewaskow SP, et al. Pathologic approach to pulmonary hemorrhage. *Ann Diagn Pathol.* 2001;5:309–319 (data adapted from Fraser R, Müller N, Colman N, Paré P. *Fraser and Paré's Diagnosis of Diseases of the Chest,* 4th ed. Philadelphia: Saunders; 1999).

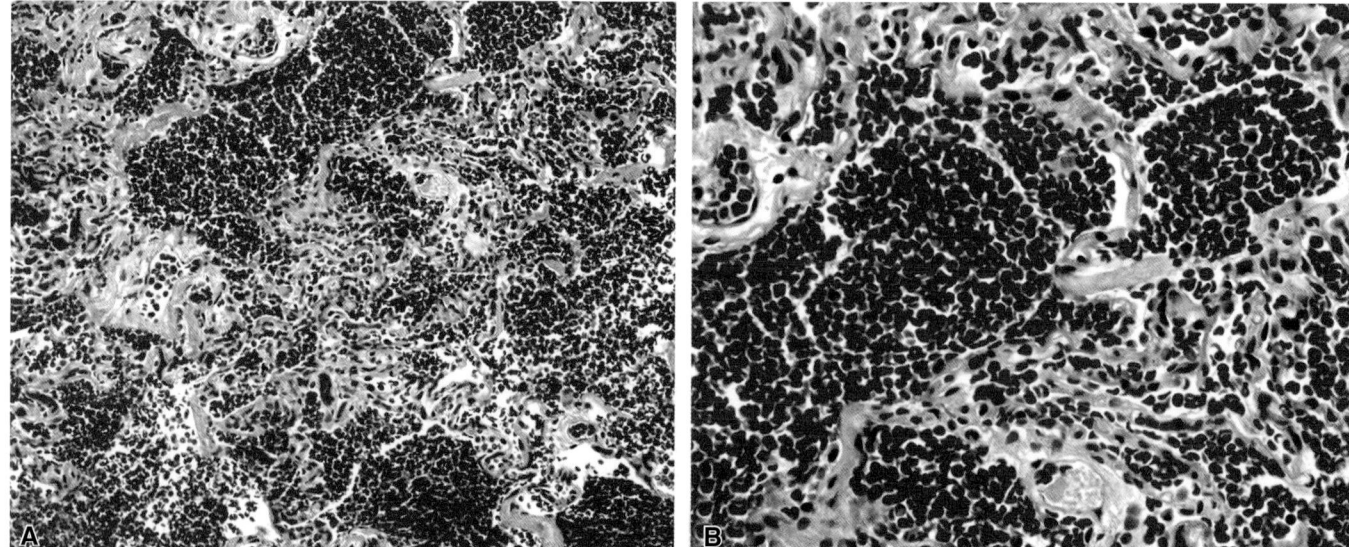

Figure 10-53. Diffuse alveolar hemorrhage: artifactual hemorrhage. The distinction of artifactual hemorrhage into alveolar spaces from true hemorrhage can be difficult at times. **A,** Artifactual hemorrhage in alveolar spaces. **B,** Note the absence of fibrin and hemosiderin-laden macrophages. Also, the interstitium exhibits no evidence of cellular reaction.

Unfortunately, the presence of siderophages alone is not sufficiently specific for active hemorrhage in the absence of other, more acute findings. Siderophages can occur as early as 2 days after an episode of alveolar hemorrhage, but can persist for weeks or even months after the event. Furthermore, the distinction of siderophages caused by hemorrhage from the pigmented macrophages seen in the lungs of cigarette smokers can be difficult on occasion.

The Prussian blue histochemical stain for iron is sometimes cited as a means of distinguishing siderophages from hemorrhage from macrophages seen in smokers (Fig. 10-54), but caution must be exerted, because so-called smoker's macrophages may contain considerable amounts of stainable iron (Fig. 10-55). The pigment in smoker's macrophages tends to be finely granular and light brown, typically admixed with punctate black pigment. True siderophages, on the other hand, are characterized by the presence of coarse, golden brown pigment that is minimally refractile (Fig. 10-56). Also, it is important to keep in mind that the Prussian blue stain reacts with other iron-associated substances in the lung, in addition to hemosiderin. Occupational

dusts may contain iron and simulate siderophages in the patient with pneumoconiosis.

When all of the elements in the biopsy add up to real hemorrhage, and the patient has radiologic evidence of *diffuse* alveolar infiltrates, the differential diagnosis becomes one of DAH. The potential causes of DAH are presented in Box 10-7. It is useful to divide DAH into two forms characterized by the presence or absence of capillaritis, respectively. Rapidly evolving acute DAH is often accompanied by capillaritis and evokes a differential diagnosis of narrow scope.

Diffuse Alveolar Hemorrhage

The histopathology of DAH is stereotypical, regardless of etiology. This fact is important for the surgical pathologist, because a specific diagnosis requires clinical and serologic data.[66] A generic designation such as "[acute] and/or [organizing] pulmonary hemorrhage [with] or [without] capillaritis," followed by a differential diagnosis is often all that is required.

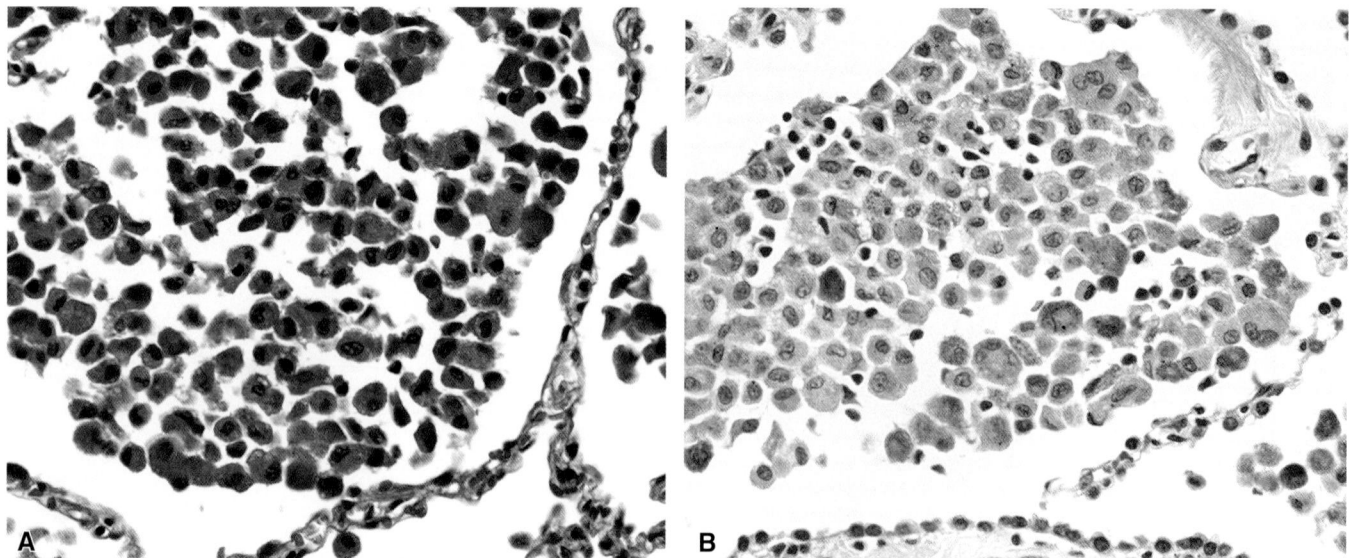

Figure 10-54. Diffuse alveolar hemorrhage: iron in smoker's macrophages. **A,** The pigmented macrophages in the lungs of smokers can contain iron in their cytoplasm, evident as granular brown material. **B,** An iron stain will show this phenomenon.

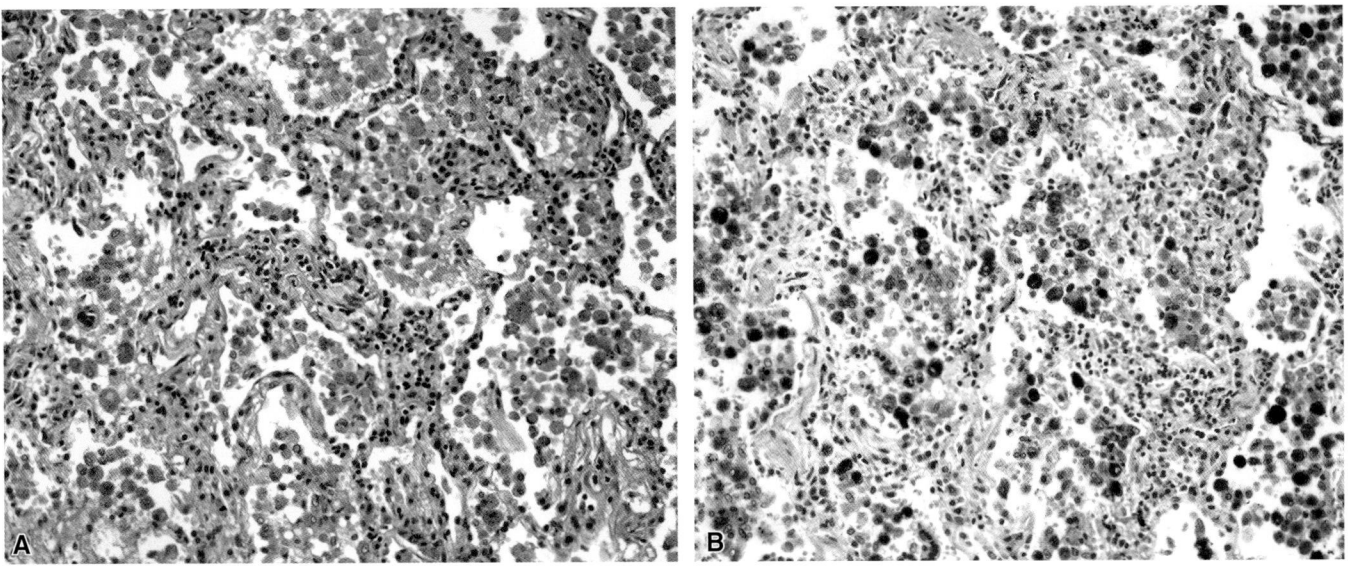

Figure 10-55. Diffuse alveolar hemorrhage: iron in smoker's macrophages. **A,** Caution is advised in interpreting the significance of pigment in macrophages. **B,** Here pigmented macrophages in the lung of a cigarette smoker contain abundant hemosiderin. Other histopathologic features of immunologically mediated hemorrhage are not seen.

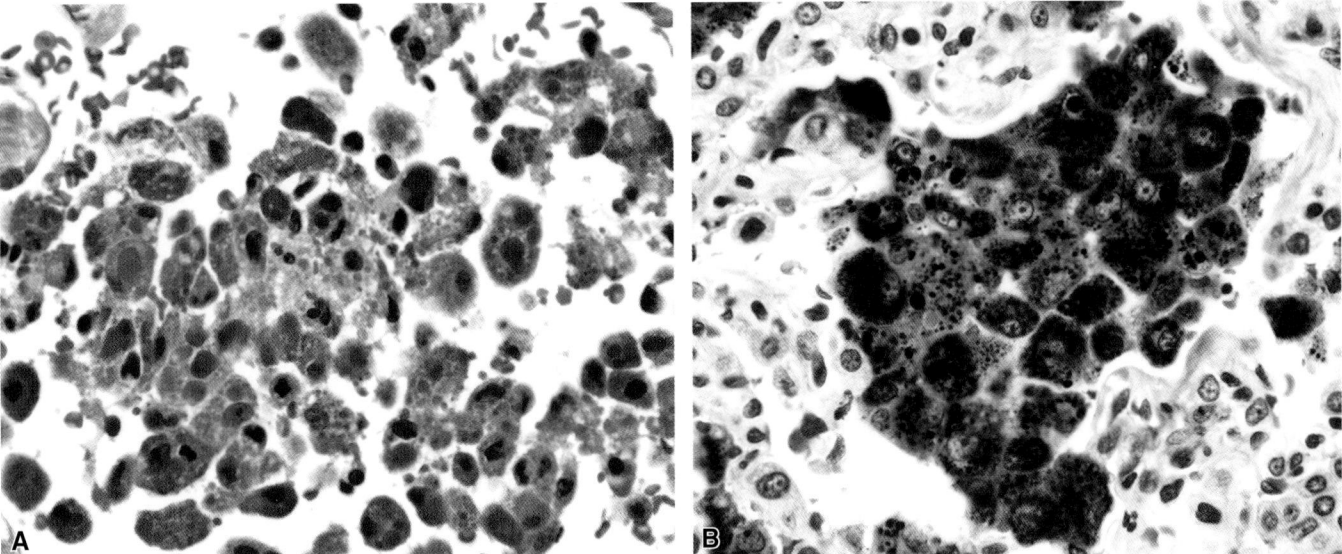

Figure 10-56. Diffuse alveolar hemorrhage: true hemosiderin-laden macrophages of hemorrhage. **A,** In contrast with smoker's macrophages with iron, true siderophages have granular refractile hemosiderin, which aggregates into large and small globular particles. **B,** An iron stain accentuates this distinction.

Box 10-7. Causes of Diffuse Alveolar Hemorrhage

With Pulmonary Capillaritis
Wegener granulomatosis
Microscopic polyangiitis
Isolated pulmonary capillaritis
Connective tissue diseases
Primary antiphospholipid syndrome
Mixed cryoglobulinemia
Behçet syndrome
Henoch-Schönlein purpura
Goodpasture syndrome
Systemic lupus erythematosus
Pauci-immune glomerulonephritis
Immune complex–associated glomerulonephritis
Drug-induced
Acute lung allograft rejection

Without Pulmonary Capillaritis
Idiopathic pulmonary hemosiderosis
Systemic lupus erythematosus
Goodpasture syndrome
Diffuse alveolar damage
Drug-induced: penicillamine, trimellitic anhydride
Mitral stenosis
Coagulation disorders
Pulmonary veno-occlusive disease
Pulmonary capillary hemangiomatosis
Lymphangioleiomyomatosis/tuberous sclerosis
Human immunodeficiency virus infection
Neoplasms (e.g., metastatic angiosarcoma, choriocarcinoma)

From Colby TV, Fukuoka J, Ewaskow SP, et al. Pathologic approach to pulmonary hemorrhage. *Ann Diagn Pathol.* 2001;5:309–319

Most causes of DAH are immunologically mediated. Some of these diseases have specific patterns of immunoglobulin deposition that can be visualized in tissue sections using immunofluorescence staining of a specially prepared portion of the surgical lung biopsy. When such staining is performed correctly, the results can be diagnostically useful and visually striking. Fortunately, in practice today, immunofluorescence staining is rarely necessary for diagnosis because serologic studies are widely available and reasonably specific for the subtypes of DAH. For those forms of DAH mediated by immune complexes, deposits in the lung tissue can also be visualized ultrastructurally. Again, although historically interesting, electron microscopy really plays no role in the diagnosis of DAH today. A comparison of the major defined pulmonary vasculitis syndromes is presented in Table 10-8.

Specific Forms of Diffuse Alveolar Hemorrhage
Goodpasture Syndrome

Goodpasture syndrome (antiglomerular basement membrane antibody disease) affects persons of all ages and both sexes, but the typical patient is a young male smoker.[181] Circulating antibodies directed against the non-collagenous domain of the alpha 3 chain of collagen

Table 10-8. Diffuse Alveolar Hemorrhage Manifestations in Major Pulmonary Vasculitis Syndromes

			Vasculitic Syndrome				
Feature	Pulmonary Capillaritis	HSP	Goodpasture Syndrome	WG	MPA	SLE	Isolated IPH
Laboratory Findings							
AFBA	Yes	No	No	No	No	No	No
c-ANCA	No	Usually	Occasional	No	No	No	NA
p-ANCA	No	Occasional	Usually	No	No	No	NA
ANA	No	No	No	Yes	No	No	NA
Extrapulmonary Involvement							
Kidney	Yes	Often	Often	Often	No	No	Yes
Other organs	No	Often	Often	Sometimes	No	No	Yes
Histopathologic Findings							
Necrotizing capillaritis	Occasional, mild	Yes	Yes	Yes	Yes	Yes	Yes
Immunofluorescence	Linear	No	No	Granular	No	No	Yes
Electron-dense deposits	No	No	No	Yes	No	No	Yes

AFBA, acid-fast bacilli (mycobaterial infection); ANA, antinuclear antibody; c-ANCA/p-ANCA, cytoplasmic/perinuclear antineutrophil cytoplasmic antibodies; HSP, Henoch-Schönlein purpura; IPH, idiopathic pulmonary hemosiderosis; MPA, microscopic polyangiitis; NA, not available [insufficient data]; SLE, systemic lupus erythematosus; WG, Wegener granulomatosis.
Data from Lynch J, Leatherman J. Alveolar hemorrhage syndromes. In: Fishman A, Elias JA, Fishman JA, et al, eds. *Fishman's Pulmonary Diseases and Disorders,* 3rd ed. New York: McGraw-Hill; 1998:1193–1210; Schwarz M, Cherniak P, King T. Diffuse alveolar hemorrhage and other rare infiltrative disorders. In: Murray J, Nadel J, eds. *Textbook of Respiratory Medicine.* Philadelphia: Saunders; 2000:1733–1755; Katzenstein A. Alveolar hemorrhage syndromes. In: Katzenstein A, Askin F, eds. *Surgical Pathology of Non-neoplastic Lung Disease.* Philadelphia: Saunders; 1997:153–159; and Jennette J, Thomas D, Falk R. Microscopic polyangiitis (microscopic polyarteritis). *Semin Diagn Pathol.* 2001;18:3–13.

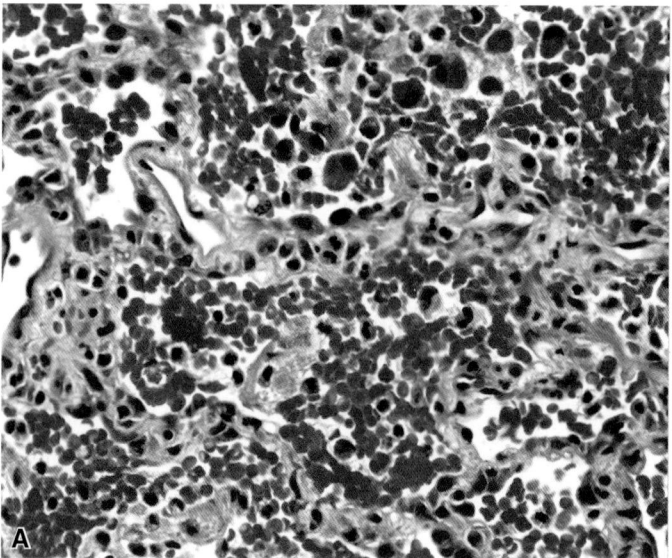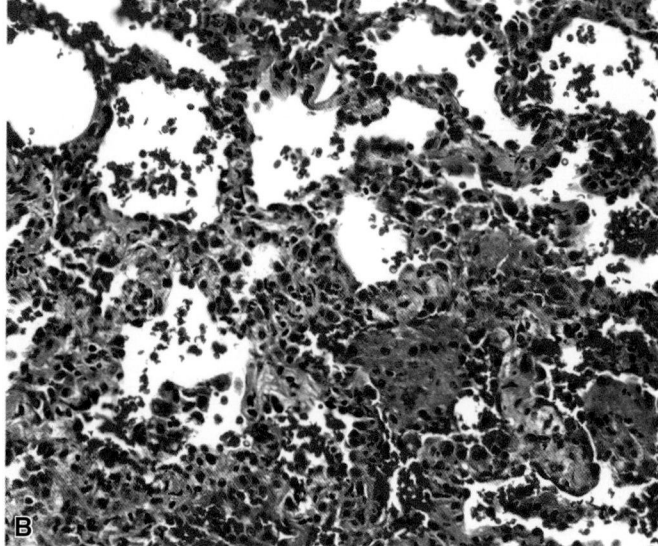

Figure 10-57. Goodpasture syndrome: diffuse alveolar hemorrhage with capillaritis. **A,** Alveolar hemorrhage with capillaritis is a typical finding in Goodpasture syndrome. **B,** In some cases, the capillaritis may be quite cellular and prominent.

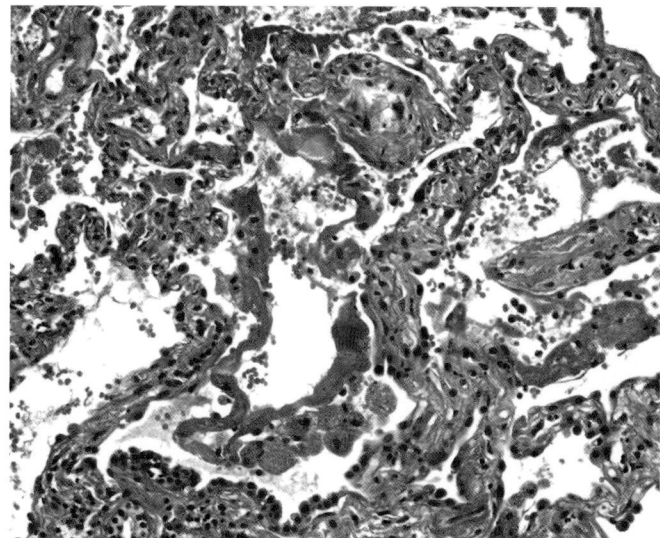

Figure 10-58. Goodpasture syndrome: hyaline membranes. As in other immune-mediated forms of alveolar hemorrhage, hyaline membranes may occur in Goodpasture syndrome.

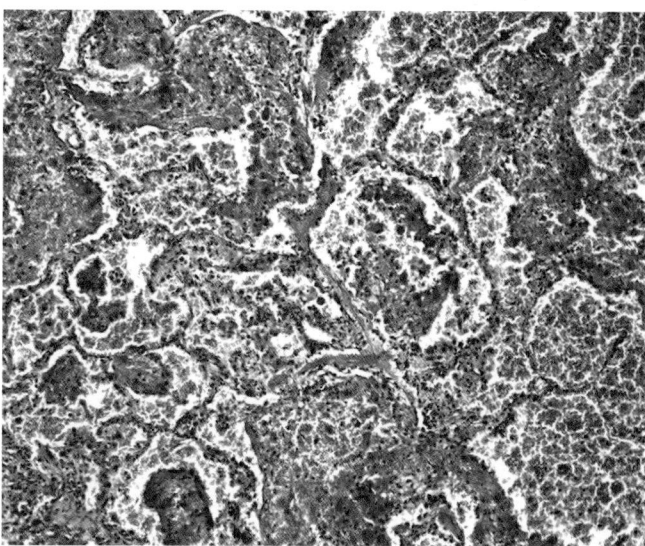

Figure 10-59. Wegener granulomatosis (WG): capillaritis. Diffuse alveolar hemorrhage with capillaritis indistinguishable from other hemorrhage syndromes can be seen in WG. Here, air space hemorrhage, fibrin, hemosiderin-laden macrophages, and capillaritis are all evident.

type IV are identified in patients with Goodpasture syndrome. Using immunolocalization techniques, these antibodies can also be detected in the lung and kidney, where they are deposited in association with basement membranes. The histopathology of Goodpasture syndrome in the lung is not specific and resembles that in other DAH syndromes (Fig. 10-57). Capillaritis may be present but generally is not prominent.[182] Hyaline membranes may accompany the pulmonary hemorrhage of Goodpasture syndrome (Fig. 10-58).

Wegener Granulomatosis

A minority of patients with WG present with pulmonary hemorrhage, although hemorrhage may occur in the course of the disease.[182] The typical systemic and serologic features of WG, as outlined earlier, often accompany DAH, making a clinical diagnosis possible even when the

lung biopsy lacks diagnostic features. DAH in WG is often attended by dramatic capillaritis (Fig. 10-59). A careful search may reveal small foci of collagen necrosis, typically involving the adventitia of pulmonary arteries and the collagen surrounding bronchi and bronchioles. The presence of scattered giant cells may also be helpful in suggesting WG as a possible underlying disorder in DAH.

Microscopic Polyangiitis

Microscopic polyangiitis has been discussed in detail earlier in this chapter. When alveolar hemorrhage dominates the presentation, distinction from WG may be impossible on biopsy findings alone (Fig. 10-60). The frequency of extrathoracic site involvement in the two diseases and the common presence of p-ANCA in microscopic polyangiitis usually suffice to differentiate them.

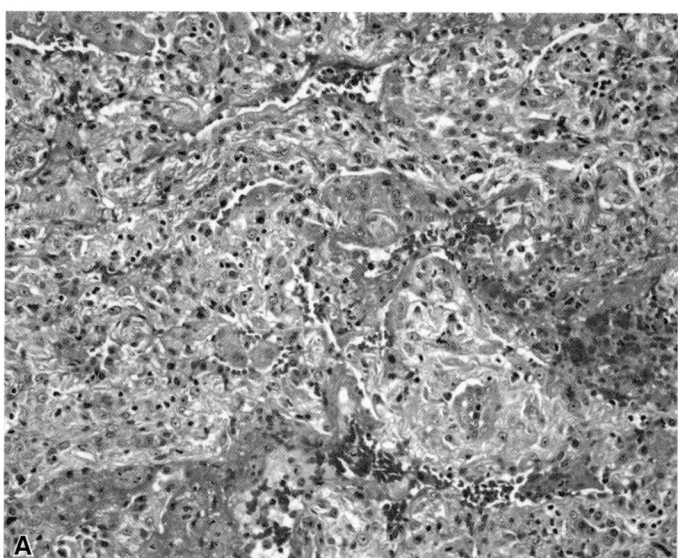

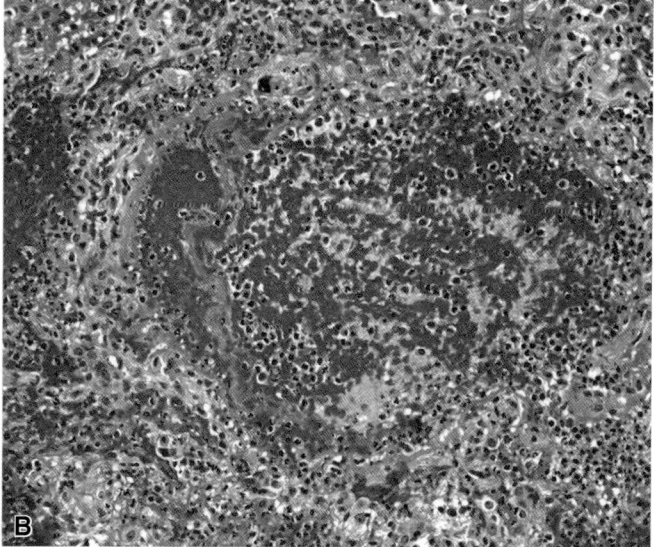

Figure 10-60. Microscopic polyangiitis: capillaritis. **A,** A case of microscopic polyangiitis showing air space fibrin and a cellular interstitium. **B,** Another example showing neutrophils filling alveolar spaces, resembling acute bronchopneumonia.

Systemic Lupus Erythematosus

DAH occurs more commonly in SLE than in any other connective tissue disease. Nevertheless, DAH is the presenting manifestation of the disease in only 11% of patients with SLE.[183] Patients with lupus nephritis are at increased risk for DAH. The histopathology of DAH in SLE is similar to that of other pulmonary hemorrhage syndromes, including the presence of capillaritis (Fig. 10-61).

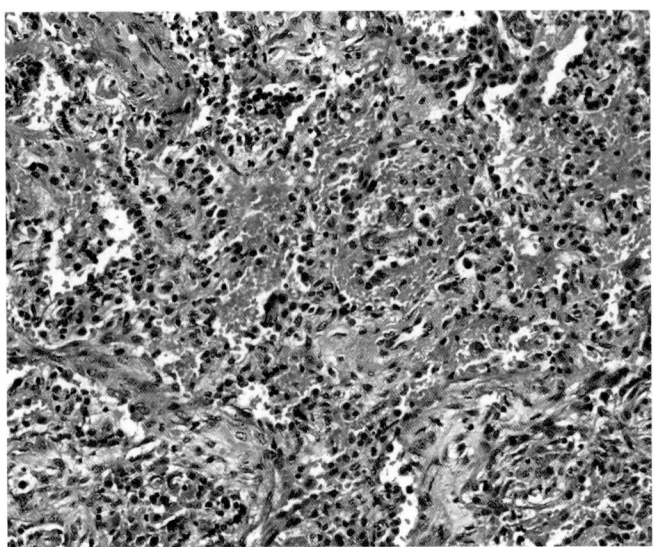

Figure 10-61. Systemic lupus erythematosus (SLE): capillaritis. Alveolar hemorrhage with capillaritis can occur in SLE. Here, the picture is indistinguishable from that seen previously with Goodpasture syndrome, Wegener granulomatosis, and microscopic polyangiitis.

Idiopathic Pulmonary Hemosiderosis

Idiopathic pulmonary hemosiderosis affects children more commonly than adults and is characterized by recurrent episodes of DAH with hemoptysis. Patients are frequently anemic. An immunologic mechanism for the disease has not yet emerged, and capillaritis is not seen. The histopathology of idiopathic pulmonary hemosiderosis is dominated by the presence of hemosiderin (Fig. 10-62). Interstitial widening with collagen deposition occurs over time.[184]

Henoch-Schönlein Purpura

Like idiopathic pulmonary hemosiderosis, Henoch-Schönlein purpura affects children more often than adults.[122,181,183,185] Alveolar hemorrhage is rare and typically overshadowed by other systemic manifestations of the disease—such as involvement of the skin, joints, and kidneys. The histopathologic changes of pulmonary hemorrhage in Henoch-Schönlein purpura are nonspecific and resemble those of other pulmonary hemorrhage syndromes.

Isolated Pulmonary Capillaritis

Isolated pulmonary capillaritis is a rare form of DAH in which no associated immunologic or systemic manifestations are found. There may be overlap between this disorder, idiopathic pulmonary hemosiderosis in adults, and the group of diseases designated by Travis and coworkers as "idiopathic pulmonary hemorrhage."[66] The histopathology of isolated pulmonary capillaritis is similar to that in other alveolar hemorrhage syndromes that include capillaritis.

Self-assessment questions related to this chapter can be found online on the Expert Consult site for this title.

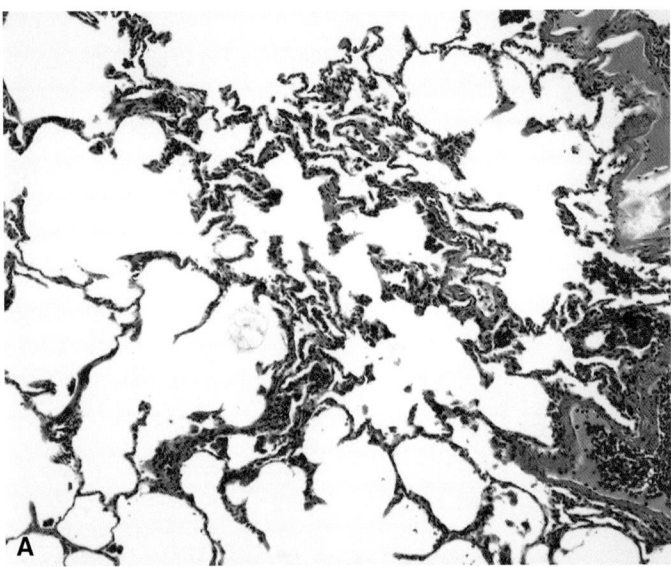
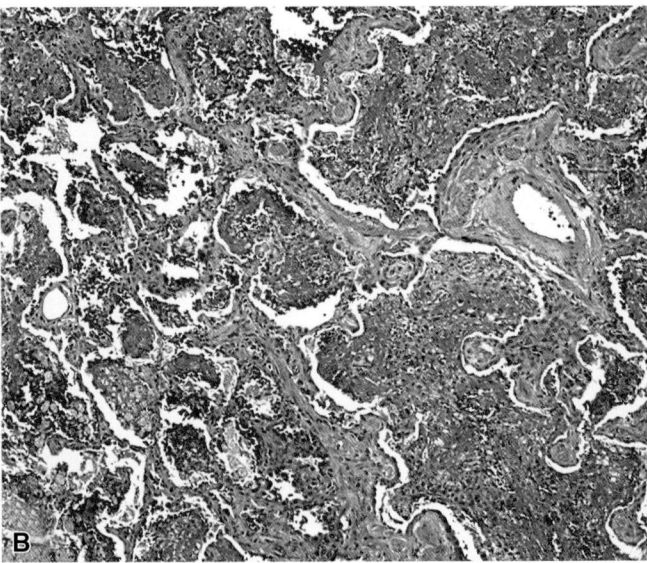

Figure 10-62. Idiopathic pulmonary hemosiderosis: mild hemosiderosis to fibrosis. The hemosiderin deposition can be mild (**A**) or prominently associated with interstitial thickening and air space fibrin (**B**). Capillaritis and vasculitis are not expected findings in this disorder.

References

1. Watts RA, Scott DG. Epidemiology of the vasculitides. *Curr Opin Rheumatol*. 2003; 15(1):11–16.
2. Travis WD. Vasculitis. In: Tomashefski JF, Cagle PT, Farver CF, Fraire AE, eds. *Dail and Hammar's Pulmonary Pathology*, 3rd ed. New York: Springer; 2008:1088–1138.
3. Travis WD, et al. Pulmonary vasculitis. In: Travis WD, Colby TV, Koss MN, et al., eds. *Non-Neoplastic Disorders of the Lower Respiratory Tract*. In: King DW, ed: *Atlas of Nontumor Pathology*. Washington, DC: American Registry of Pathology and Armed Forces Institute of Pathology; 2002:233–264.
4. Guinee Jr D, Jaffe E, Kingma D, et al. Pulmonary lymphomatoid granulomatosis. Evidence for a proliferation of Epstein-Barr virus infected B-lymphocytes with a prominent T-cell component and vasculitis. *Am J Surg Pathol*. 1994;18:753–764.
5. Nicholson AG, Wotherspoon AC, Diss TC, et al. Lymphomatoid granulomatosis: evidence that some cases represent Epstein-Barr virus–associated B-cell lymphoma. *Histopathology*. 1996;29:317–324.
6. Travis WD, et al. Pathology and genetics. In: Travis WD, Brambilla E, Müller-Hermelink HK, Harris CC, eds. *Tumours of the Lung, Pleura, Thymus and Heart*. Lyon: IARC Press; 2004.

7. Wegener F. Generalized septic vascular diseases [Translation]. *Verh Dtsch Path Ges*. 1936;29:202–210.

8. DeRemee RA, McDonald TJ, Harrison Jr EG, Coles DT. Wegener's granulomatosis. Anatomic correlates, a proposed classification. *Mayo Clin Proc*. 1976;51:777–781.

9. Carrington CB, Liebow AA. Limited forms of angiitis and granulomatosis of Wegener's type. *Am J Med*. 1966;41:497–527.

10. Stone JH. Limited versus severe Wegener's granulomatosis: baseline data on patients in the Wegener's granulomatosis etanercept trial. *Arthritis Rheum*. 2003;48:2299–2309.

11. Cotch MF, Hoffman GS, Yerg DE, et al. The epidemiology of Wegener's granulomatosis. Estimates of the five-year period prevalence, annual mortality, and geographic disease distribution from population-based data sources. *Arthritis Rheum*. 1996;39:87–92.

12. Carruthers DM, Watts RA, Symmons DP, Scott DG. Wegener's granulomatosis—increased incidence or increased recognition? *Br J Rheumatol*. 1996;35:142–145.

13. Pallan L, Savage CO, Harper L. ANCA-associated vasculitis: from bench research to novel treatments. *Nat Rev Nephrol*. 2009;5:278–286.

14. Savage CO. The evolving pathogenesis of systemic vasculitis. *Clin Med*. 2002;2(5):458–464.

15. Kain R, Exner M, Brandes R, et al. Molecular mimicry in pauci-immune focal necrotizing glomerulonephritis. *Nat Med*. 2008;14:1088–1096.

16. Kain R, Matsui K, Exner M, et al. A novel class of autoantigens of anti-neutrophil cytoplasmic antibodies in necrotizing and crescentic glomerulonephritis: the lysosomal membrane glycoprotein h-lamp-2 in neutrophil granulocytes and a related membrane protein in glomerular endothelial cells. *J Exp Med*. 1995;181(2):585–597.

17. Lúdvíksson BR, Sneller MC, Chua KS, et al. Active Wegener's granulomatosis is associated with HLA-DR+ CD4+ T cells exhibiting an unbalanced Th1-type T cell cytokine pattern: reversal with IL-10. *J Immunol*. 1998;160:3602–3609.

18. Marinaki S, Kälsch AI, Grimminger P, et al. Persistent T-cell activation and clinical correlations in patients with ANCA-associated systemic vasculitis. *Nephrol Dial Transplant*. 2006;21:1825–1832.

19. Beaudreuil S, Lasfargues G, Lauériere L, et al. Occupational exposure in ANCA-positive patients: a case-control study. *Kidney Int*. 2005;67(5):1961–1966.

20. Hoffman GS, Kerr GS, Leavitt RY, et al. Wegener's granulomatosis: an analysis of 158 patients. *Ann Intern Med*. 1992;116:488–498.

21. Roberti I, Reisman L, Churg J. Vasculitis in childhood. *Pediatr Nephrol*. 1993;7:479–489.

22. Wadsworth D, Siegel M, Day D. Wegener's granulomatosis in children: chest radiographic manifestations. *AJR Am J Roentgenol*. 1994;163:901–904.

23. Langford C, Hoffman G. Rare diseases. 3: Wegener's granulomatosis. *Thorax*. 1999;54:629–637.

24. Colby T, Specks U. Wegener's granulomatosis in the 1990s—a pulmonary pathologist's perspective. In: Churg A, Katzenstein A-L, eds. *The Lung: Current Concepts*. Baltimore: Williams & Wilkins; 1993:195–218.

25. Travis W. Common and uncommon manifestations of Wegener's granulomatosis. *Cardiovasc Pathol*. 1994;3:217–225.

26. Goulart R, Mark E, Rosen S. Tumefactions as an extravascular manifestation of Wegener's granulomatosis. *Am J Surg Pathol*. 1995;19:145–153.

27. Travis WD, Colby TV, Koss MN, et al., eds. *Non-Neoplastic Disorders of the Lower Respiratory Tract*. In: King DW, ed. *Atlas of Nontumor Pathology*. Washington, DC: American Registry of Pathology and Armed Forces Institute of Pathology; 2002.

28. Gross W, Csernok E. Immunodiagnostic and pathophysiologic aspects of antineutrophil cytoplasmic antibodies in vasculitis. *Curr Opin Rheumatol*. 1995;7:11–19.

29. Jennette J, Falk R, Wilkman A. Anti-neutrophilic antibodies—a serologic marker for vasculitides. *Ann Acad Med Singapore*. 1995;24:248–253.

30. Specks U. Pulmonary vasculitis. In: Schwarz M, King T, eds. *Interstitial Lung Disease*. Hamilton, ON: BC Decker; 1998:507–534.

31. Gross WL, Schnabel A, Trabandt A. New perspectives in pulmonary angiitis. From pulmonary angiitis and granulomatosis to ANCA associated vasculitis. *Sarcoidosis Vasc Diffuse Lung Dis*. 2000;17:33–52.

32. Schultz D, Diego J. Antineutrophil cytoplasmic antibodies (ANCA) and systemic vasculitis: update of assays, immunopathogenesis, controversies, and report of a novel de novo ANCA-associated vasculitis after kidney transplantation. *Semin Arthritis Rheum*. 2000;29:267–285.

33. Davenport A, Lock R, Wallington T. Clinical relevance of testing for antineutrophil cytoplasm antibodies (ANCA) with a standard indirect immunofluorescence ANCA test in patients with upper or lower respiratory tract symptoms. *Thorax*. 1994;49:213–217.

34. Nölle B, Specks U, Lüdemann J, et al. Anticytoplasmic autoantibodies: their immunodiagnostic value in Wegener's granulomatosis. *Ann Intern Med*. 1989;111:28–40.

35. Jennette J, Charles L, Falk R. Anti-neutrophil cytoplasmic autoantibodies: disease associations, molecular biology, and pathophysiology. *Int Rev Exp Pathol*. 1991;32:193–221.

36. Gal A, Salinas F, Staton GJ. The clinical and pathological spectrum of antineutrophil cytoplasmic autoantibody-related pulmonary disease. A comparison between perinuclear and cytoplasmic antineutrophil cytoplasmic autoantibodies. *Arch Pathol Lab Med*. 1994;118:1209–1214.

37. Gaudin PB, Askin FB, Falk RJ, Jennette JC. The pathologic spectrum of pulmonary lesions in patients with anti-neutrophil cytoplasmic autoantibodies specific for anti-proteinase 3 and anti-myeloperoxidase. *Am J Clin Pathol*. 1995;104:7–16.

38. Schnabel A, Reuter M, Csernok E, et al. Subclinical alveolar bleeding in pulmonary vasculitides: correlation with indices of disease activity. *Eur Respir J*. 1999;14(1):118–124.

39. Jennings CR, Jones NS, Dugar J, et al. Wegener's granulomatosis—a review of diagnosis and treatment in 53 patients. *Rhinology*. 1998;36(4):188–191.

40. Feigin D. Vasculitis in the lung. *J Thorac Imaging*. 1988;3:33–48.

41. Cordier JF, Valeyre D, Guillevin L, et al. Pulmonary Wegener's granulomatosis. A clinical and imaging study of 77 cases. *Chest*. 1990;97:906–912.

42. Fraser RS, et al. Diseases of altered immunologic activity. In: Fraser RS, Paré J, Fraser RG, Paré P, eds. *Synopsis of Diseases of the Chest*, 2nd ed. Philadelphia: WB Saunders; 1994:392–443.

43. Staples C. Pulmonary angiitis and granulomatosis. *Radiol Clin North Am*. 1991;29:973–982.

44. Farrelly C. Wegener's granulomatosis: a radiological review of the pulmonary manifestations at initial presentation and during relapse. *Clin Radiol*. 1982;33:545–551.

45. Aberle D, Gamsu G, Lynch D. Thoracic manifestations of Wegener granulomatosis: diagnosis and course. *Radiology*. 1990;174:703–709.

46. Katzenstein A, Locke W. Solitary lung lesions in Wegener's granulomatosis. Pathologic findings and clinical significance in 25 cases. *Am J Surg Pathol*. 1995;19:545–552.

47. Kuhlman J, Hruban R, Fishman E. Wegener granulomatosis: CT features of parenchymal lung disease. *J Comput Assist Tomogr*. 1991;15:948–952.

48. Primack SL, Hartman TE, Lee KS, Müller NL. Pulmonary nodules and the CT halo sign. *Radiology*. 1994;190:513–515.

49. Daum TE, Specks U, Colby TV, et al. Tracheobronchial involvement in Wegener's granulomatosis. *Am J Respir Crit Care Med*. 1995;151:522–526.

50. Maguire R, Fauci AS, Doppman JL, Wolff SM. Unusual radiographic features of Wegener's granulomatosis. *AJR Am J Roentgenol*. 1978;130:233–238.

51. Travis WD, Hoffman GS, Leavitt RY, et al. Surgical pathology of the lung in Wegener's granulomatosis. Review of 87 open lung biopsies from 67 patients. *Am J Surg Pathol*. 1991;15:315–333.

52. Ulbright T, Katzenstein A. Solitary necrotizing granulomas of the lung: differentiating features and etiology. *Am J Surg Pathol*. 1980;4:13–28.

53. Yousem SA. Bronchocentric injury in Wegener's granulomatosis: a report of five cases. *Hum Pathol*. 1991;22:535–540.

54. Uner A, Rozum-Slota B, Katzenstein A. Bronchiolitis obliterans—organizing pneumonia (BOOP)-like variant of Wegener's granulomatosis. A clinicopathologic study of 16 cases. *Am J Surg Pathol*. 1996;20:794–801.

55. Mark E, Flieder D, Matsubara O. Treated Wegener's granulomatosis: distinctive pathological findings in the lungs of 20 patients and what they tell us about the natural history of the disease. *Hum Pathol*. 1997;28:450–458.

56. Koss MN, Hochholzer L, Feigin DS, et al. Necrotizing sarcoid-like granulomatosis: clinical, pathologic, and immunopathologic findings. *Human Pathol*. 1980;11(suppl):510–519.

57. Lipford Jr EH, Margolick JB, Longo DL, et al. Angiocentric immunoproliferative lesions: a clinicopathologic spectrum of post-thymic T-cell proliferations. *Blood*. 1988;72:1674–1681.

58. Churg J, Strauss L. Allergic granulomatosis, allergic angiitis and periarteritis nodosa. *Am J Pathol*. 1951;27:277–294.

59. Chumbley L, Harrison Jr E, DeRemee R. Allergic granulomatosis and angiitis (Churg-Strauss syndrome). Report and analysis of 30 cases. *Mayo Clin Proc*. 1977;52:477–484.

60. Koss M, Antonovych T, Hochholzer L. Allergic granulomatosis (Churg-Strauss syndrome). *Am J Surg Pathol*. 1981;5:21–28.

61. Lanham JG, Elkon KB, Pusey CD, Hughes GR. Systemic vasculitis with asthma and eosinophilia: a clinical approach to the Churg-Strauss syndrome. *Medicine (Baltimore)*. 1984;63:65–81.

62. Churg A, Carrington C, Gupta R. Necrotizing sarcoid granulomatosis. *Chest*. 1979;76:406–413.

63. Churg A. Pulmonary angiitis and granulomatosis revisited. *Hum Pathol*. 1983;14:868–883.

64. Koss M, Robinson R, Hochholze L. Bronchocentric granulomatosis. *Hum Pathol*. 1981;12:632–638.

65. Mark E, Ramirez J. Pulmonary capillaritis and hemorrhage in patients with systemic vasculitis. *Arch Pathol Lab Med*. 1985;109:413–418.

66. Travis WD, Colby TV, Lombard C, Carpenter HA. A clinicopathologic study of 34 cases of diffuse pulmonary hemorrhage with lung biopsy confirmation. *Am J Surg Pathol*. 1990;14:1112–1125.

67. Myers JL, Kurtin PJ, Katzenstein AL, et al. Lymphomatoid granulomatosis. Evidence of immunophenotypic diversity and relationship to Epstein-Barr virus infection. *Am J Surg Pathol*. 1995;19:1300–1312.

68. Churg J. Allergic granulomatosis and granulomatous-vascular syndromes. *Ann Allergy*. 1963;21:619–628.

69. Lanham J, Churg J. Churg-Strauss syndrome. In: Churg A, Churg J, eds. *Systemic Vasculitides*. New York: Igaku-Shoin; 1991:101–120.

70. Specks U, DeRemee R. Granulomatous vasculitis. Wegener's granulomatosis and Churg-Strauss syndrome. *Rheum Dis Clin North Am*. 1990;16:377–397.

71. Fienberg R, Mark EJ, Goodman M, et al. Correlation of antineutrophil cytoplasmic antibodies with the extrarenal histopathology of Wegener's (pathergic) granulomatosis and related forms of vasculitis. *Hum Pathol*. 1993;24:160–168.

72. Fauci AS, Haynes BF, Katz P, Wolff SM. Wegener's granulomatosis: prospective clinical and therapeutic experience with 85 patients over 21 years. *Ann Intern Med*. 1983;98:76–85.

73. DeRemee R, McDonald T, Weiland L. Wegener's granulomatosis: observations on treatment with antimicrobial agents. *Mayo Clin Proc*. 1985;60:27–32.

74. Langford C, Sneller M. New developments in the treatment of Wegener's granulomatosis, polyarteritis nodosa, microscopic polyangiitis, and Churg-Strauss syndrome. *Curr Opin Rheumatol*. 1997;9:26–30.

75. Langford C, Sneller M. Update on the diagnosis and treatment of Wegener's granulomatosis. *Adv Intern Med*. 2001;46:177–206.

76. Stegeman CA, Tervaert JW, de Jong PE, Kallenberg CG. Trimethoprim-sulfamethoxazole (co-trimoxazole) for the prevention of relapses of Wegener's granulomatosis. Dutch Co-Trimoxazole Wegener Study Group. *N Engl J Med*. 1996;335:16–20.

77. Seo P, Specks U, Keogh KA. Efficacy of rituximab in limited Wegener's granulomatosis with refractory granulomatous manifestations. *J Rheumatol*. 2008;35:2017–2023.

78. Lee RW, D'Cruz DP. Novel therapies for anti-neutrophil cytoplasmic antibody–associated vasculitis. *Drugs*. 2008;68:747–770.

79. Travis W, Koss M. Vasculitis. In: Dail D, Hammar S, eds. *Pulmonary Pathology*. New York: Springer-Verlag; 1994:1027–1095.

80. Travis W, Koss M. Pulmonary angiitis and granulomatosis: necrotizing sarcoid granulomatosis and Churg-Strauss syndrome. In: Saldana M, ed. *Pathology of Pulmonary Disease*. Philadelphia: JB Lippincott; 1994:803–809.

81. Sehgal M, Swanson JW, DeRemee RA, Colby TV. Neurologic manifestations of Churg-Strauss syndrome. *Mayo Clin Proc*. 1995;70:337–341.

82. Masi AT, Hunder GG, Lie JT, et al. The American College of Rheumatology 1990 criteria for the classification of Churg-Strauss syndrome (allergic granulomatosis and angiitis). *Arthritis Rheum*. 1990;33:1094–1100.

83. Lie J. Illustrated histopathologic classification criteria for selected vasculitis syndromes. American College of Rheumatology Subcommittee on Classification of Vasculitis. *Arthritis Rheum*. 1990;33:1074–1087.

84. Liu LJ, et al. Evaluation of a new algorithm in classification of systemic vasculitis. *Rheumatology (Oxf)*. 2008;47:708–712.

85. Sasaki A, Hasegawa M, Nakazato Y, et al. Allergic granulomatosis and angiitis (Churg-Strauss syndrome). Report of an autopsy case in a nonasthmatic patient. *Acta Pathol Jpn*. 1988;38:761–768.

86. Gambari PF, Ostuni PA, Lazzarin P, et al. Eosinophilic granuloma and necrotizing vasculitis (Churg-Strauss syndrome?) involving a parotid gland, lymph nodes, liver and spleen. *Scand J Rheumatol*. 1989;18:171–175.

87. Lipworth B, Slater DN, Corrin B, et al. Allergic granulomatosis without asthma: a rare 'forme fruste' of the Churg-Strauss syndrome. *Respir Med*. 1989;83:249–250.

88. Larson T, Hall S, Hepper NG, Hunder GG. Respiratory tract symptoms as a clue to giant cell arteritis. *Ann Intern Med*. 1984;101:594–597.

89. Guillevin L, Lhote F, Gayraud M, et al. Prognostic factors in polyarteritis nodosa and Churg-Strauss syndrome. A prospective study in 342 patients. *Medicine (Baltimore)*. 1996;75:17–28.

90. Clutterbuck E, Pusey C. Severe alveolar hemorrhage in Churg-Strauss syndrome. *Eur J Respir Dis*. 1987;71:158–163.

91. Gibson L. Granulomatous vasculitides and the skin. *Dermatol Clin*. 1990;8:335–345.

92. Olsen KD, Neel 3rd HB, Deremee RA, Weiland LH. Nasal manifestations of allergic granulomatosis and angiitis (Churg-Strauss syndrome). *Otolaryngol Head Neck Surg*. 1980;88(1):85–89.

93. Fraioli P, Barberis M, Rizzato G. Gastrointestinal presentation of Churg Strauss syndrome. *Sarcoidosis*. 1994;11:42–45.

94. Harrison DJ, Simpson R, Kharbanda R, et al. Antibodies to neutrophil cytoplasmic antigens in Wegener's granulomatosis and other conditions. *Thorax*. 1989;44:373–377.

95. Churg J, Churg A. Zafirlukast and Churg-Strauss syndrome [Letter]. *JAMA*. 1998;279:1949–1950.

96. Green R, Vayonis A. Churg-Strauss syndrome after zafirlukast in two patients not receiving systemic steroid treatment [Letter]. *Lancet*. 1999;353:725–726.

97. Holloway J, Ferriss J, Groff J, et al. Churg-Strauss syndrome associated with zafirlukast. [Published erratum appears in *J Am Osteopath Assoc* 1998;98(12):676]. *J Am Osteopath Assoc*. 1998:98:275–278.

98. Frosi A, Foresi A, Bozzoni M, et al. Churg-Strauss syndrome and antiasthma therapy [Letter]. *Lancet*. 1999;353:1102.

99. Wechsler ME, Finn D, Gunawardena D, et al. Churg-Strauss syndrome in patients receiving montelukast as treatment for asthma. *Chest*. 2000;117:708–713.

100. Orriols R, Muñoz X, Ferrer J, et al. Cocaine-induced Churg-Strauss vasculitis. *Eur Respir J*. 1996;9:175–177.

101. Churg A, Brallas M, Cronin SR, Churg J. Formes frustes of Churg-Strauss syndrome. *Chest*. 1995;108:320–323.

102. Amundson D. Cavitary pulmonary cryptococcosis complicating Churg-Strauss vasculitis. *South Med J*. 1992;85:700–702.

103. Worthy SA, Müller NL, Hansell DM, Flower CD. Churg-Strauss syndrome: the spectrum of pulmonary CT findings in 17 patients. *AJR Am J Roentgenol*. 1998;170:297–300.

104. Buschman D, Waldron Jr J, King TJ. Churg-Strauss pulmonary vasculitis. High-resolution computed tomography scanning and pathologic findings. *Am Rev Respir Dis*. 1990;142:458–461.

105. Lai RS, Lin SL, Lai NS, Lee PC. Churg-Strauss syndrome presenting with pulmonary capillaritis and diffuse alveolar hemorrhage. *Scand J Rheumatol*. 1998;27:230–232.

106. Travis WD, Kwon-Chung KJ, Kleiner DE, et al. Unusual aspects of allergic bronchopulmonary fungal disease: report of two cases due to *Curvularia* organisms associated with allergic fungal sinusitis. *Hum Pathol*. 1991;22:1240–1248.

107. Brill R, Churg J, Beaver J. Allergic granulomatosis associated with visceral larva migrans. *Am J Clin Pathol*. 1953;23:1208–1215.

108. Imai H, Nakamoto Y, Hirokawa M, et al. Carbamazepine-induced granulomatous necrotizing angiitis with acute renal failure. *Nephron*. 1989;51:405–408.

109. Strazzella W, Safirstein B. Asthma due to parasitic infestation. *N J Med*. 1989;89:947–949.

110. Guillevin L, Cohen P, Gayraud M, et al. Churg-Strauss syndrome. Clinical study and long-term follow-up of 96 patients. *Medicine (Baltimore)*. 1999;78:26–37.

111. Abu-Shakra M, Smythe H, Lewtas J, et al. Outcome of polyarteritis nodosa and Churg-Strauss syndrome. An analysis of twenty-five patients. *Arthritis Rheum*. 1994;37:1798–1803.

112. Calabrese LH, Michel BA, Bloch DA, et al. The American College of Rheumatology 1990 criteria for the classification of hypersensitivity vasculitis. *Arthritis Rheum*. 1990;33:1108–1113.

113. Churg J. Nomenclature of vasculitic syndromes: a historical perspective. *Am J Kidney Dis*. 1991;18:148–153.

114. Leavitt R, Travis W, Fauci A. Vasculitis. In: Shelhamer J, Pizzo P, Parrillo JE, Masur H, eds. *Respiratory Disease in the Immunosuppressed Host*. Philadelphia: JB Lippincott; 1991:703–727.

115. Swerlick R, Lawley T. Small-vessel vasculitis and cutaneous vasculitis. In: Churg A, Churg J, eds. *Systemic Vasculitides*. New York: Igaku-Shoin; 1991:193–201.

116. Jennette J, Falk RJ, Andrassy K, et al. Nomenclature of systemic vasculitis. *Arthitis Rheum*. 1994;37:187–192.

117. Jennette J, Falk R. Small-vessel vasculitis. *N Engl J Med*. 1997;337:1512–1523.

118. Lauque D, Cadranel J, Lazor R, et al. Microscopic polyangiitis with alveolar hemorrhage. A study of 29 cases and review of the literature. Groupe d'Etudes et de Recherche sur les Maladies "Orphelines" Pulmonaires (GERM"O"P). *Medicine (Baltimore)*. 2000;79:222–233.

119. Akikusa B, Kondo Y, Irabu N, et al. Six cases of microscopic polyangiitis exhibiting acute interstitial pneumonia. [Published erratum appears in *Pathol Int*. 1995;45:901]. *Pathol Int*. 1995;45:580–588.

120. Brugiere O, Raffy O, Sleiman C, et al. Progressive obstructive lung disease associated with microscopic polyangiitis. *Am J Respir Crit Care Med*. 1997;155:739–742.

121. Schwarz MI, Mortenson RL, Colby TV, et al. Pulmonary capillaritis. The association with progressive irreversible airflow limitation and hyperinflation. *Am Rev Respir Dis*. 1993;148:507–511.

122. Green RJ, Ruoss SJ, Kraft SA, et al. Pulmonary capillaritis and alveolar hemorrhage. Update on diagnosis and management. *Chest*. 1996;110(5):1305–1316.

123. Churg J, Churg A. Idiopathic and secondary vasculitis: a review. *Mod Pathol*. 1989;2:144–160.

124. Lazzarini LC, de Fatima do Amparo Teixeira M, Souza Rodrigues R, Marcos Nunes Valiante P: Necrotizing sarcoid granulomatosis in a family of patients with sarcoidosis reinforces the association between both entities. *Respiration*. 2008;76(3):356–360.

125. Tauber E, Wojnarowski C, Horcher E, et al. Necrotizing sarcoid granulomatosis in a 14-yr-old female. *Eur Respir J*. 1999;13:703–705.

126. Beach RC, Corrin B, Scopes JW, Graham E. Necrotizing sarcoid granulomatosis with neurologic lesions in a child. *J Pediatr*. 1980;97:950–953.

127. Singh N, Cole S, Krause PJ, et al. Necrotizing sarcoid granulomatosis with extrapulmonary involvement. Clinical, pathologic, ultrastructural, and immunologic features. *Am Rev Respir Dis*. 1981;124:189–192.

128. Stephen JG, Braimbridge MV, Corrin B, et al. Necrotizing 'sarcoidal' angiitis and granulomatosis of the lung. *Thorax*. 1976;31:356–360.

129. Niimi H, Hartman T, Muller N. Necrotizing sarcoid granulomatosis: computed tomography and pathologic findings. *J Comput Assist Tomogr*. 1995;19:920–923.

130. Le Gall F, Loeuillet L, Delaval P, et al. Necrotizing sarcoid granulomatosis with and without extrapulmonary involvement. *Pathol Res Pract*. 1996;192:306–313.

131. Dykhuizen RS, Smith CC, Kennedy MM, et al. Necrotizing sarcoid granulomatosis with extrapulmonary involvement. *Eur Respir J*. 1997;10:245–247.

132. Chittock DR, Joseph MG, Paterson NA, McFadden RG. Necrotizing sarcoid granulomatosis with pleural involvement. Clinical and radiographic features. *Chest*. 1994;106:672–676.

133. Liebow A. The J. Burns Amberson lecture—pulmonary angiitis and granulomatosis. *Am Rev Respir Dis*. 1973;108:1–18.

134. Rolfes D, Weiss M, Sanders M. Necrotizing sarcoid granulomatosis with suppurative features. *Am J Clin Pathol*. 1984;82:602–607.

135. Spiteri MA, Gledhill A, Campbell D, Clarke SW. Necrotizing sarcoid granulomatosis. *Br J Dis Chest*. 1987;81:70–75.

136. Rodat O, Buzelin F, Weber M, et al. Bronchopulmonary manifestations of Horton's disease. Apropos of a case. *Rev Med Interne*. 1983;4:225–230.

137. Bradley JD, Pinals RS, Blumenfeld HB, Poston WM. Giant cell arteritis with pulmonary nodules. *Am J Med*. 1984;77:135–140.

138. Karam G, Fulmer J. Giant cell arteritis presenting as interstitial lung disease. *Chest*. 1982;82:781–789.

139. Ladanyi M, Fraser R. Pulmonary involvement in giant cell arteritis. *Arch Pathol Lab Med*. 1987;111:1178–1180.

140. Wagenaar S, Westermann C, Corrin B. Giant cell arteritis limited to large elastic pulmonary arteries. *Thorax*. 1981;36:876–877.

141. Wagenaar SS, van den Bosch JM, Westermann CJ, et al. Isolated granulomatous giant cell vasculitis of the pulmonary elastic arteries. *Arch Pathol Lab Med*. 1986;110:962–1924.

142. Okubo S, Kunieda T, Ando M, et al. Idiopathic isolated pulmonary arteritis with chronic cor pulmonale. *Chest*. 1988;94:665–666.

143. Lie J. Disseminated visceral giant cell arteritis. Histopathologic description and differentiation from other granulomatous vasculitides. *Am J Clin Pathol*. 1978;69:299–305.

144. Morita T, Kamimura A, Koizumi F. Disseminated visceral giant cell arteritis. *Acta Pathol Jpn*. 1987;37:863–870.

145. Marcussen N, Lund C. Combined sarcoidosis and disseminated visceral giant cell vasculitis. *Path Res Pract*. 1989;184:325–330.

146. Shintaku M, Mase K, Ohtsuki M, et al. Generalized sarcoidlike granulomas with systemic angiitis, crescentic glomerulonephritis, and pulmonary hemorrhage. Report of an autopsy case. *Arch Pathol Lab Med*. 1989;113:1295–1298.

147. Lie J. Combined sarcoidosis and disseminated visceral giant cell angiitis: a third opinion [Letter]. *Arch Pathol Lab Med*. 1991;115:210–211.

148. DeRemee R, Weiland L, McDonald T. Respiratory vasculitis. *Mayo Clin Proc*. 1980;55:492–498.

149. Leavitt R, Fauci A. Pulmonary vasculitis. *Am Rev Respir Dis*. 1986;134:149–166.

150. Rosen S, Falk R, Jennette J. Polyarteritis nodosa, including microscopic form and renal vasculitis. In: Churg A, Churg J, eds. *Systemic Vasculitides*. New York: Igaku-Shoin; 1991:57–77.

151. Arend W, Michel BA, Bloch DA, et al. The American College of Rheumatology 1990 criteria for the classification of Takayasu arteritis. *Arthritis Rheum*. 1990;33:1129–1134.

152. He NS, Liu F, Wu EH, et al. Pulmonary artery involvement in aorto-arteritis. An analysis of DSA. *Chin Med J (Engl)*. 1990;103:666–672.

153. Sharma S, Kamalakar T, Rajani M, et al. The incidence and patterns of pulmonary artery involvement in Takayasu's arteritis. *Clin Radiol*. 1990;42:177–181.

154. Sharma S, Rajani M, Shrivastava S, et al. Non-specific aorto-arteritis (Takayasu's disease) in children. *Br J Radiol*. 1991;64:690–698.

155. Nakabayashi K, Kurata N, Nangi N, et al. Pulmonary artery involvement as first manifestation in three cases of Takayasu arteritis. *Int J Cardiol*. 1996;54(suppl):S177–S183.

156. Sharma B, Jain S, Sagar S. Systemic manifestations of Takayasu arteritis: the expanding spectrum. *Int J Cardiol*. 1997;54(suppl):S149–S154.

157. Lie J. Takayasu's arteritis. In: Churg A, Churg J, eds. *Systemic Vasculitides*. New York: Igaku-Shoin; 1991:159–179.

158. Horimoto M, Igarashi K, Aoi K, et al. Unilateral diffuse pulmonary artery involvement in Takayasu's arteritis associated with coronary-pulmonary artery fistula and bronchial-pulmonary artery fistula: a case report. *Angiology*. 1991;42:73–80.

159. Takahashi K, Honda M, Furuse M, et al. CT findings of pulmonary parenchyma in Takayasu arteritis. *J Comput Assist Tomogr*. 1996;20:742–748.

160. Rose A, Sinclair-Smith C. Takayasu's arteritis. A study of 16 autopsy cases. *Arch Pathol Lab Med*. 1980;104:231–237.

161. Matsubara O, Yoshimura N, Tamura A, et al. Pathological features of the pulmonary artery in Takayasu arteritis. *Heart Vessels Suppl*. 1992;7:18–125.

162. Jakob H, Volb R, Stangl G, et al. Surgical correction of a severely obstructed pulmonary artery bifurcation in Takayasu's arteritis. *Eur J Cardiothorac Surg*. 1990;4:456–458.

163. Direskeneli H. Behçet's disease: infectious aetiology, new autoantigens and HLA-B51. *Ann Rheum Dis*. 2001;60(11):996–1002.

164. Fairley C, Wilson J, Barraclough D. Pulmonary involvement in Behçet's syndrome. *Chest*. 1989;96:1428–1429.

165. Raz I, Okon E, Chajek-Shaul T. Pulmonary manifestations in Behçet's syndrome. *Chest*. 1989;95:585–589.

166. Efthimiou J, Johnston C, Spiro SG, Turner-Warwick M. Pulmonary disease in Behçet's syndrome. *Q J Med*. 1986;58:259–280.

167. Gamble CN, Wiesner KB, Shapiro RF, Boyer WJ. The immune complex pathogenesis of glomerulonephritis and pulmonary vasculitis in Behçet's disease. *Am J Med*. 1979;66:1031–1039.

168. Ahn JM, Im JG, Ryoo JW, et al. Thoracic manifestations of Behçet syndrome: radiographic and CT findings in nine patients. *Radiology*. 1995;194:199–203.

169. Tunaci A, Berkmen Y, Gokmen E. Thoracic involvement in Behcet's disease: pathologic, clinical, and imaging features. *AJR Am J Roentgenol*. 1995;164:51–56.

170. Slavin R, de Groot W. Pathology of the lung in Behçet's disease. Case report and review of the literature. *Am J Surg Pathol*. 1981;5:779–788.

171. Lakhanpal S, Tani K, Lie JT, et al. Pathologic features of Behçet's syndrome: a review of Japanese autopsy registry data. *Hum Pathol*. 1985;16:790–795.

172. Salamon F, Weinberger A, Nili M, et al. Massive hemoptysis complicating Behçet's syndrome: the importance of early pulmonary angiography and operation. *Ann Thorac Surg*. 1988;45:566–567.

173. Corren J. Acute interstitial pneumonia in a patient with Behcet's syndrome and common variable immunodeficiency [clinical conference]. *Ann Allergy*. 1990;64:15–20.

174. Soave R, Murray H, Litrenta M. Bacterial invasion of pulmonary vessels. *Pseudomonas* bacteremia mimicking pulmonary thromboembolism with infarction. *Am J Med*. 1978;65:864–867.

175. Winn W, Myerowitz R. The pathology of the *Legionella* pneumonias. A review of 74 cases and the literature. *Hum Pathol*. 1981;12:401–422.

176. Travis WD, Pittaluga S, Lipschik GY, et al. A typical pathologic manifestations of *Pneumocystis carinii* pneumonia in the acquired immune deficiency syndrome. Review of 123 lung biopsies from 76 patients with emphasis on cysts, vascular invasion, vasculitis, and granulomas. *Am J Surg Pathol*. 1990;14:615–625.

177. Takemura T, Matsui Y, Saiki S, Mikami R. Pulmonary vascular involvement in sarcoidosis: a report of 40 autopsy cases. *Hum Pathol*. 1992;23:1216–1223.

178. Fernandes S, Singsen B, Hoffman G. Sarcoidosis and systemic vasculitis. *Semin Arthritis Rheum*. 2000;30:33–46.

179. Sweerts M, Nicholson AG, Goldstraw P, Corrin B: Dieulafoy's disease of the bronchus. *Thorax*. 1995;50:697–698.

180. Kadokura M, Colby T, Myers J. Pathologic comparison of video-assisted thoracic surgical biopsy with traditional open lung biopsy. *J Thorac Cardiovasc Surg*. 1995;109:494–498.

181. Lynch J, Leatherman J. Alveolar hemorrhage syndromes. In: Fishman A, Elias JA, Fishman JA, et al., eds. *Fishman's Pulmonary Diseases and Disorders*, 3rd ed. New York: McGraw-Hill; 1998:1193–1210.

182. Lombard C, Colby T, Elliott C. Surgical pathology of the lung in antibasement membrane antibody–asociated Goodpasture's syndrome. *Hum Pathol*. 1989;20:445–451.

183. Specks U. Diffuse alveolar hemorrhage syndromes. *Opin Rheumatol*. 2001;13:12–17.

184. Cutz E. Idiopathic pulmonary hemosiderosis and related disorders in infancy and childhood. *Perspect Pediatr Pathol*. 1987;11:47–81.

185. Schwarz M, Cherniak P, King T. Diffuse alveolar hemorrhage and other rare infiltrative disorders. In: Murray J, Nadel J, eds. *Textbook of Respiratory Medicine*. Philadelphia: Saunders; 2000:1733–1755.

186. Jennings CA, King Jr TE, Tuder R, et al. Diffuse alveolar hemorrhage with underlying isolated, pauciimmune pulmonary capillaritis. *Am J Respir Crit Care Med*. 1997;155:1101–1109.

187. Finnegan MJ, Hinchcliffe J, Russell-Jones D, et al. Vasculitis complicating cystic fibrosis. *Q J Med*. 1989;72:609–621.

188. Fortin P, Esdaile J. Vasculitis and malignancy. In: Churg A, Churg J, eds. *Systemic Vasculitides*. New York: Igaku-Shoin; 1991:327–341.

189. Komadina K, Houck R. Polyarteritis nodosa presenting as recurrent pneumonia following splenectomy for hairy-cell leukemia. *Semin Arthritis Rheum*. 1989;18:252–257.

190. Fiegler W, Siemoneit K. Pulmonary manifestations in anaphylactoid purpura (Henoch-Schönlein syndrome). *ROFO Fortschr Geb Rontgenstr Nuklearmed*. 1981;134:269–272.

191. Marandian MH, Ezzati M, Behvad A, et al. Pulmonary involvement in Schönlein-Henoch's purpura. *Arch Fr Pediatr*. 1982;39:255–257.

192. White R. Henoch-Schönlein purpura. In: Churg A, Churg J, eds. *Systemic Vasculitides*. New York: Igaku-Shoin; 1991:203–217.

193. Bombardieri S, Paoletti P, Ferri C, et al. Lung involvement in essential mixed cryoglobulinemia. *Am J Med*. 1979;66:748–756.

194. Churg J. Cryoglobulinemic vasculitis. In: Churg A, Churg J, eds. *Systemic Vasculitides*. New York: Igaku-Shoin; 1991:293–298.

195. Monti G, Galli M, Cereda UG, et al. Mycosis fungoides with mixed cryoglobulinemia and pulmonary vasculitis. A case report. *Boll Ist Sieroter Milan*. 1987;66:324–328.

196. Nada AK, Torres VE, Ryu JH, et al. Pulmonary fibrosis as an unusual clinical manifestation of a pulmonary-renal vasculitis in elderly patients. *Mayo Clin Proc*. 1990;65:847–856.

197. Seiden MV, O'Donnell WJ, Weinblatt M, Licht J. Vasculitis with recurrent pulmonary hemorrhage in a long-term survivor after autologous bone marrow transplantation. *Bone Marrow Transplant*. 1990;6:345–347.

Pulmonary Hypertension

Andrew Churg, MD, and Joanne L. Wright, MD

Biopsy for evaluation of pulmonary hypertension is relatively uncommon, in part because of the dangers of fatal arrhythmias in such patients, and has sometimes been viewed as offering little therapeutic benefit. As argued by Wagenvoort,[1] however, biopsy in patients with pulmonary hypertension serves three purposes:

1. It can establish the nature of the underlying lesion. This is potentially important information, because patients with purely thrombotic lesions appear to have a much better prognosis than patients with plexogenic arteriopathy or veno-occlusive disease.[2]
2. Occasionally, the lung lesions shed light on the type of underlying congenital cardiac abnormality.
3. The lesions seen in the lung biopsy specimen provide an indication of potential reversibility.

This information is important in deciding whether to perform corrective surgery in congenital heart disease[1] and appears to be of value in predicting response to vasodilator therapy.[3]

Morphologic Features of the Pulmonary Vasculature

Pulmonary Arteries

Any diagnosis of pulmonary hypertension requires recognition of the different types of vessels seen in the lung. This is aided by the use of elastic tissue stains, which should be a routine approach when a biopsy or larger specimen shows potential vascular disease. Knowledge of the structure of the normal pulmonary vascular bed is important in assessing biopsy material.[4,5] Branches of the *pulmonary artery* run with the bronchi and then the bronchioles. Arteries associated with the bronchi are typically larger than 1 mm in diameter and have a fairly extensive elastic fiber meshwork in their walls. *Muscular pulmonary arteries* (Fig. 11-1) are usually associated with bronchioles and measure between 100 and 1000 μm. They are frequently abnormal in pulmonary hypertension. Elastic stain (Fig. 11-2) shows that they have both an internal and an external elastic lamina. In the normal lung the diameter of a muscular pulmonary artery and its accompanying airway should be about the same. Below a diameter of about 100 μm, the pulmonary artery

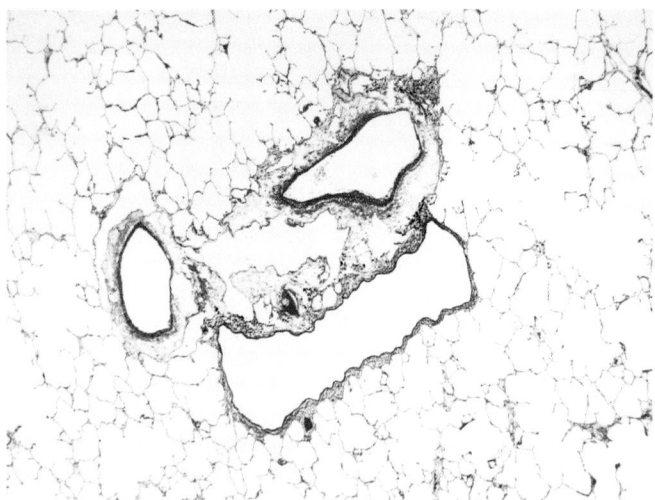

Figure 11-1. Normal muscular pulmonary artery branches accompanying a bronchiole.

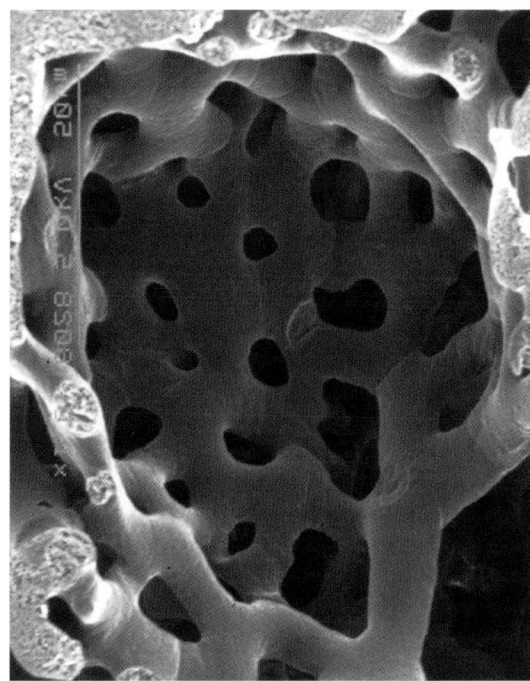

Figure 11-3. Scanning electron micrograph showing a methacrylate vascular cast of an alveolus showing the mesh of capillaries.

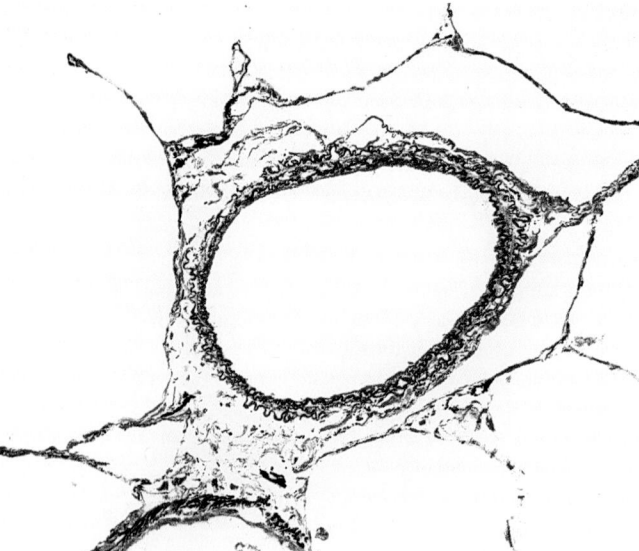

Figure 11-2. Elastic stain of a normal small muscular pulmonary artery showing double elastic laminae surrounding a fairly thin muscular layer. The intima is unobtrusive.

branches lose the internal elastica and are termed *arterioles*. Arterioles run adjacent to the alveolar ducts and can be found as a corner vessel by the alveolar saccules, but should not be found in alveolar walls. A well-defined mesh of capillaries arranged in a single layer of rings and spokes forms the gas exchange system in the alveoli[6] (Fig. 11-3).

Pulmonary Veins

Normal *pulmonary veins* have only a single elastica and a thin layer of muscle. Veins are best identified by anatomic location. Larger pulmonary veins run in the interlobular septa (Fig. 11-4). Smaller veins are found associated with the alveolar saccules and are indistinguishable by morphology from pulmonary arterioles; thus, the identification of a small vessel as a vein often requires tracing it back through several sections until it joins a definite vein in an interlobular septum. Of note, in pulmonary venous hypertension, the larger veins may acquire both a double elastica and additional muscle and resemble muscular arteries, but the location in the septa indicates their true nature.

Bronchial Arteries

Bronchial arteries are found in the walls of the larger bronchi. They usually are heavily muscularized and have a prominent internal elastica and a less well defined external elastica. Bronchial arteries may develop

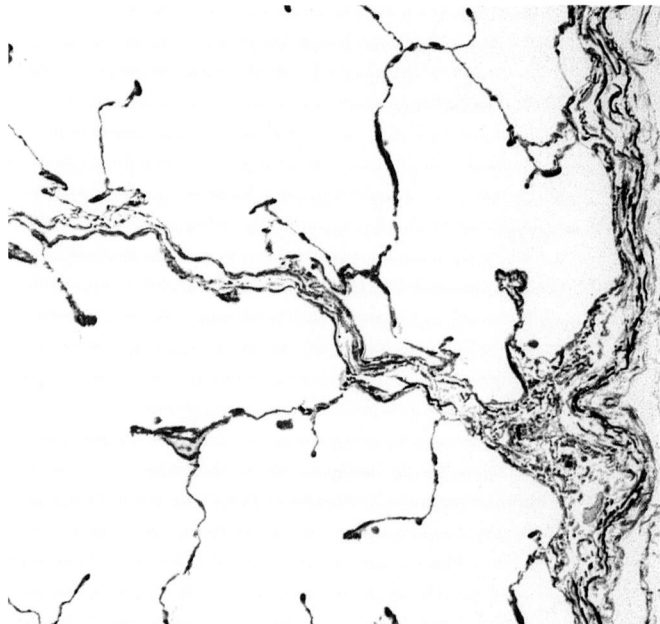

Figure 11-4. Elastic stain of a normal pulmonary vein running in the interlobular septum. Note the single elastica, a characteristic finding of pulmonary veins.

longitudinal muscle bands, a feature helpful in identification. Bronchial arteries are systemic vessels at systemic pressure, and areas where they anastomose with the pulmonary circulation (around bronchiectatic foci, in plexogenic arteriopathy) may be foci of hemorrhage.

Recognition of Right Ventricular Hypertrophy

Significant degrees of pulmonary hypertension are usually associated with right ventricular hypertrophy. A quick, but relatively inaccurate, determination of ventricular hypertrophy can be made by simple measurement of the right ventricular wall muscle thickness (Fig. 11-5). Wall thickness in the normal adult population should be approximately 2 to 3 mm, with measurements greater than 5 mm thought to represent hypertrophy.[7]

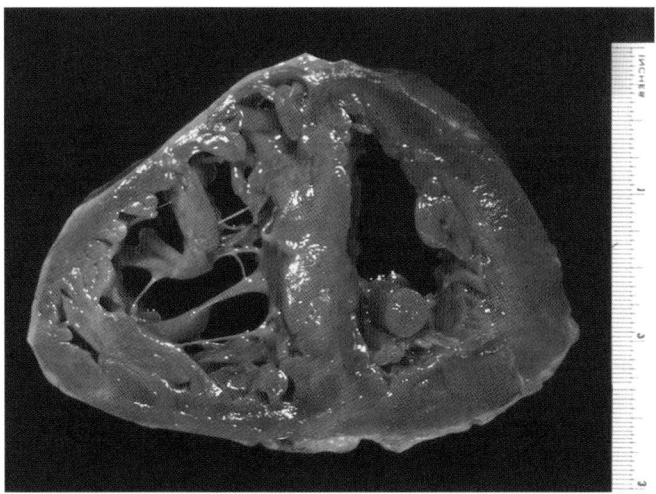

Figure 11-5. Cross section of heart at autopsy from a patient with pulmonary hypertension secondary to fenfluramine-phentermine use. Note the markedly thickened right ventricle.

Partitioning of the heart into right ventricle and left ventricle plus septum[8] provides a sensitive estimation of ventricular hypertrophy, with a right ventricular weight of 65 g or greater considered abnormal.[7] Although a portion of the septum will enlarge with the right ventricle, a ratio of left ventricular weight to right ventricular weight of less than 1.9 is considered to represent right ventricular hypertrophy. Obviously, such ratios are only useful if there is no enlargement of the left ventricle.

Microscopic examination of the right ventricle does not show the generalized increase of fibrosis that can be found in left ventricular hypertrophy. Detailed measurement of the myocardiocytes will demonstrate enlarged fiber diameters,[9] but this finding may be too subtle to recognize visually.

Classification of Pulmonary Hypertension

The normal pressure in the pulmonary artery is 20/12 mm Hg (mean, 15 mm Hg) at sea level and 38/14 mm Hg (mean, 25 mm Hg) at approximately 15,000-feet altitude. In general, a mean arterial pressure of 20 mm Hg at sea level is considered abnormal, whereas at 15,000 feet, a pressure of 25 mm Hg is considered abnormal. Pulmonary hypertension is defined clinically as a mean pulmonary artery pressure at rest of greater than 25 mm Hg, or a mean pressure greater than 30 mm Hg during exercise.[10] Pulmonary hypertension may be a manifestation of a primary pulmonary vascular disease, or may be secondary to other (nonvascular) diseases in the lung, but the morphologic patterns seen in the vessels in pulmonary hypertension are fairly limited, and, thus, clinical correlation is required for a specific diagnosis.

A variety of schemes for classification of pulmonary hypertension have been proposed.[2,11–17] Box 11-1 shows a recent clinical classification, commonly called the 2003 Venice classification.[17] This classification has replaced the older term *primary pulmonary hypertension* with the terms *idiopathic* and *familial* to recognize the occurrence of genetic mutations in the bone morphogenetic protein receptor 2 (*BMPR2*) gene in many cases. A problematic aspect of this classification is the inclusion of pulmonary veno-occlusive disease (PVOD) and pulmonary capillary hemangiomatosis (PCH) in the general category of pulmonary arterial hypertension on the basis of dubious claims that these entities can show all the changes of classic idiopathic pulmonary arterial hypertension, including plexiform lesions (see the sections "Pulmonary Veno-Occlusive Disease" and "Pulmonary Capillary Hemangiomatosis" later in the chapter), and on the basis of a handful of reports of cases with

Box 11-1. The Venice 2003 Clinical Classification of Pulmonary Hypertension

1. Pulmonary arterial hypertension
    1.1. Idiopathic (IPAH)
    1.2. Familial (FPAH)
    1.3. Associated with other systemic conditions
        1.3.1. Collagen vascular disease
        1.3.2. Congenital systemic to portal shunts
        1.3.3. Portal hypertension
        1.3.4. HIV infection
        1.3.5. Drugs and toxins
        1.3.6. Miscellaneous uncommon causes including thyroid disorders, glycogen storage diseases, hereditary hemorrhagic telangiectasia, hemoglobinopathies, myeloproliferative disorders, splenectomy
    1.4. Associated with significant venous or capillary involvement
        1.4.1. Pulmonary veno-occlusive disease (PVOD)
        1.4.2. Pulmonary capillary hemangiomatosis (PCH)
2. Pulmonary hypertension associated with left heart disease
    2.1. Left-sided atrial or ventricular disease
    2.2. Left-sided valvular disease
3. Pulmonary hypertension associated with lung diseases and/or hypoexemia
    3.1. Chronic obstructive pulmonary disease
    3.2. Interstitial lung disease
    3.3. Sleep-disordered breathing
    3.4. Alveolar hypoventilation disorders
    3.5. Chronic exposure to high altitude
    3.6. Developmental abnormalities
4. Pulmonary hypertension due to chronic thrombotic and/or embolic disease
    4.1. Thromboembolic obstruction of proximal pulmonary arteries
    4.2. Thromboembolic obstruction of distal pulmonary arteries
    4.3. Non-thrombotic pulmonary embolism (tumor, parasites, foreign material)
5. Miscellaneous: sarcoidosis, Langerhans cell histiocytosis, lymphangiomatosis, compression of pulmonary vessels by adenopathy, tumor, fibrosing mediastinitis

From Simonneau G, Galiè N, Rubin LJ, et al. Clinical classification of pulmonary hypertension. *J Am Coll Cardiol*. 2004;43(12 suppl):5S–12S.

BMPR2 mutations.[18] Since PVOD and PCH patients often develop pulmonary edema after vasodilator therapy and have a worse outcome than patients in Venice categories 1.1 to 1.3,[18] we believe there is considerable logic in maintaining PVOD and PCH in a separate group (see the section "Treatment of Pulmonary Hypertension" later in the chapter).

Partly for these reasons, we have not adopted the new pathologic classification of pulmonary hypertension arising from the 2003 Venice meeting,[19] but prefer the older and more generally accepted scheme shown in Box 11-2. Some authors have argued that there is no real difference between thrombotic and plexogenic arteriopathy, largely because thrombotic lesions may be found in both.[14] However, we believe, as Wagenvoort and Mulder[20] have argued, there are generally clear clinical and morphologic differences among the entities shown in Box 11-2, and that thrombosis is a secondary phenomenon in most types of pulmonary hypertension (see later on).

Plexogenic Arteriopathy

Clinical Features

The features of pulmonary hypertension in general are very nonspecific. Patients typically describe progressive shortness of breath, which is particularly marked during exercise. Syncopal episodes, presumably related to cardiac arrhythmias, may occur. Chest pain is usually a sign of right-sided cardiac ischemia and is seen late in the course in those who develop cor pulmonale. Similarly, abdominal discomfort is a sign of right-sided heart failure with progressive liver congestion.

In pulmonary hypertension associated with anorectic agents, the pulmonary vascular lesions are associated with cardiac valvular lesions, predominantly on the left side of the heart.[21,22] In those patients who

Box 11-2. Pathologic Classification of Pulmonary Hypertension

Plexogenic arteriopathy
   Idiopathic ("primary") or familial (*BMPR2* mutation)
   Associated with congenital heart disease with left-to-right shunts
   Associated with collagen vascular disease
   Associated with cirrhosis (portal hypertension)
   Secondary to drug use
      Dexfenfluramine, fenfluramine-phentermine ("fen-phen")
      Aminorex
   Associated with HIV infection
   Associated with thyroid disorders, glycogen storage diseases, and other uncommon causes of pulmonary hypertension in 1.4 of the Venice 2003 classification
Thrombotic and embolic pulmonary hypertension
   Associated with recurrent thromboemboli or in situ thromboses
      Affecting proximal pulmonary arteries
      Affecting distal pulmonary arteries
   Associated with sickle cell disease
   Associated with IV drug abuse (injection of insoluble foreign particles)
   Associated with tumor emboli
   Pulmonary tumor thrombotic microangiopathy
Associated with interstitial lung disease, emphysema, or other intrinsic lung diseases
Associated with chronic hypoxia
Pulmonary venous hypertension
   Left-sided cardiac disease, especially mitral stenosis
   Atrial myxomas
   Sclerosing mediastinitis
   Congenital cardiac malformations affecting venous outflow
   Pulmonary veno-occlusive disease
   Pulmonary capillary hemangiomatosis

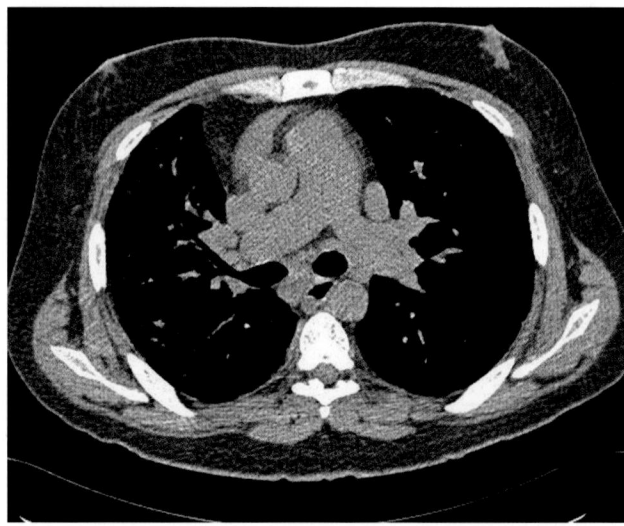

Figure 11-6. Computed tomography scan from a patient with scleroderma and pulmonary hypertension. Note the markedly dilated main pulmonary artery and left and right branches.

develop their pulmonary hypertension in association with human immunodeficiency virus (HIV) disease, the majority can be directly related to HIV infection; other cofactors include liver disease and coagulation abnormalities. There is a wide age range of the affected population. The interval between HIV infection and clinical presentation of pulmonary hypertension may be up to 3 years, but after presentation the prognosis is poor.[23,24]

Radiologic Features

Plain chest film early in the disease may be totally normal in appearance; with more advanced disease, enlarged pulmonary arteries become apparent, and with the development of cor pulmonale, the right ventricle may be visibly enlarged. With long-standing pulmonary hypertension, calcification of the large arteries, presumably representing atherosclerosis, can be seen. Computed tomography (CT) scanning allows measurements of the diameters of the main pulmonary artery; in general, if the diameter of the pulmonary artery is larger than that of the ascending aorta—strictly speaking, if the diameter of the main pulmonary artery at the level of its bifurcation is greater than 29 mm (Fig. 11-6)—there is a high probability of pulmonary hypertension.[25] Angiography classically demonstrates vascular "pruning," in which the vessels have a simplified branching pattern.

Morphologic Features

Plexiform lesions were first clearly characterized by Heath and Edwards.[16] The term *plexogenic pulmonary arteriopathy* was coined by Wagenvoort[11] to describe a morphologic response pattern that sometimes, but not always, is characterized by the formation of peculiar thrombi with multiple small channels—"plexiform lesions." Such lesions are the end result of a series of vascular changes, however, and a given case of plexogenic arteriopathy may show only the lower-grade changes without formation of plexiform lesions.

Plexogenic arteriopathy primarily affects muscular arteries and arterioles, but larger arteries may demonstrate increased atherosclerosis, a finding that may be seen in pulmonary hypertension of any cause or in the absence of hypertension. Statistically, however, the most common cause of atherosclerosis in the pulmonary artery is severe systemic atherosclerosis.[26]

The vascular changes in the muscular arteries and arterioles in plexogenic arteriopathy appear to reflect, in general, the level of pulmonary artery pressure and, to a lesser extent, the length of time hypertension has been present; thus, in a broad sense, higher-grade lesions (see later on) are found in individuals with higher pulmonary artery pressures. The correlations are not exact, however, and only lower-grade lesions may be found in some patients with quite marked pulmonary hypertension. There is also some controversy about the order in which different lesions develop.[2,13,14,16] It is our belief that the original Heath and Edwards classification[16] is incorrect and that the actual sequence of changes is that proposed by Wagenvoort and Wagenvoort,[11] as follows.

Grade I: Muscular Hypertrophy

Muscular hypertrophy appears as thickening of the walls of muscular arteries, often with obvious narrowing of the lumina (Fig. 11-7). Elastic stain shows that the space between the internal and external elastica has become widened by the new muscle. Normal preacinar muscular pulmonary arteries should have, in the fully distended state, a medial thickness that is 1% to 2% of the vessel diameter, although in the smaller muscular arteries (30–100 μm in external diameter), the medial thickness may be up to 5%.[24] However, these values are based on arteries fixed by inflation, and in ordinary specimens, some allowance needs to be made for the fact that uninflated vessels will normally have thicker-appearing walls than inflated vessels.

Muscular hypertrophy in small arteries is often accompanied by *muscularization of arterioles*, such that the arteriole acquires both a double elastica and muscle between the elasticas (Fig. 11-8). Thus, muscularized arterioles come to resemble ordinary muscular arteries but are found in the lung parenchyma; this finding is a clue to the correct diagnosis because arteries are normally present only next to accompanying airways.

Grade II: Intimal Proliferation

In this stage, proliferation of intimal cells leads to a thickened intima superimposed on a thickened muscular media (Fig. 11-9). The intimal cells do not show any special organization.

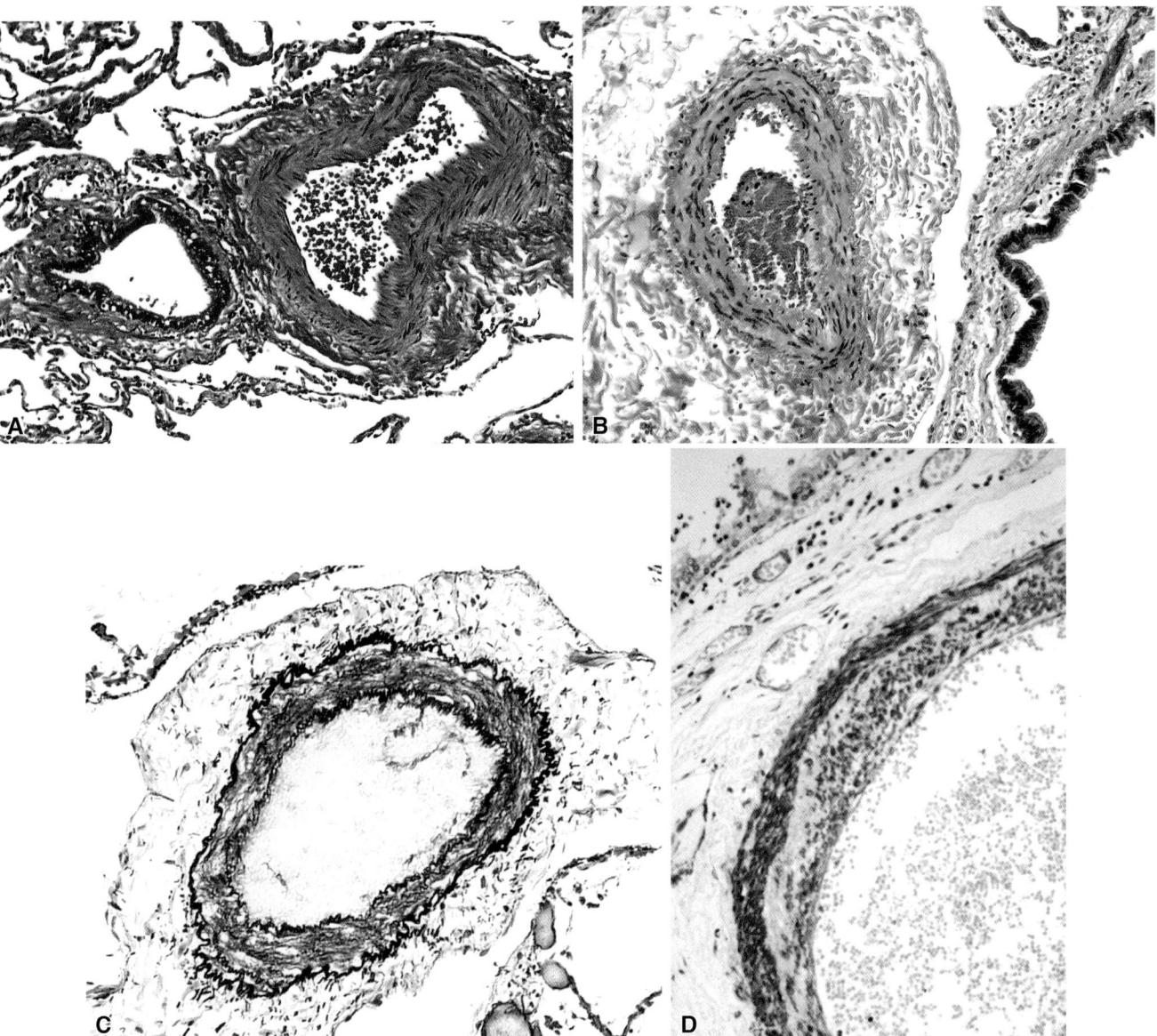

Figure 11-7. Muscular hypertrophy in pulmonary hypertension. **A,** Muscular pulmonary artery branches showing muscular hypertrophy. In normal bronchovascular bundles, airways and vessels are about the same size; here, the vessel is larger and very thick-walled. Note the obviously increased muscle area on the elastic stain (**C**). Muscular hypertrophy of this type may be seen in pulmonary hypertension of any cause and by itself does not indicate a diagnosis of plexogenic arteriopathy. **B,** Thickened muscular media is very obvious at higher magnification. **C,** Increase in muscle well demonstrated on elastic stain. **D,** Occasionally smooth muscle proliferation occurs in the intima in pulmonary hypertension; when this occurs the muscle bundles run longitudinally, as here (smooth muscle actin stain).

Grade III: Concentric Laminar Intimal Fibrosis

In this stage, the intima is markedly thickened and organized in a series of concentric bands of collagen and spindle-shaped cells, which lend a whorled appearance (Fig. 11-10). The lumen is often dramatically narrowed.

Grade IV: Necrotizing Vasculitis

As a result of markedly increased pressure, the arterial wall may become necrotic. The typical pattern is that of *fibrinoid necrosis* with eosinophilic granular necrotic material replacing the normal arterial wall (Fig. 11-11). Inflammatory cells, usually polymorphonuclear leukocytes but sometimes eosinophils, may be present. Elastic stains show that, typically, the internal elastic is destroyed.

Grade V: Plexiform Lesions

Plexiform lesions are typically found in small muscular arteries at branch points. The artery immediately proximal to the plexiform lesion often shows marked muscular hypertrophy and intimal hyperplasia. In the

plexiform lesion itself the vessel is often dilated and the lumen is characteristically filled with capillary channels that very much resemble a fairly cellular organizing thrombus (Fig. 11-12). However, in contradistinction to most thrombi, where the elastic laminae are intact,[2] elastic stains show that the inner elastica is typically destroyed in the region of the plexiform lesion (see Fig. 11-12B), and this feature is useful when a question of thrombotic versus plexogenic arteriopathy arises. This set of findings reflects the fact that plexiform lesions are actually the result of fibrinoid necrosis of the vessels, with subsequent thrombosis and organization. The acute plexiform lesions may show small fibrin thrombi and small numbers of inflammatory cells in the capillary channels; as the lesions age, they scar and become paucicellular. Plexiform lesions are usually not very numerous and can be widely scattered within the lung parenchyma; thus, a certain amount of hunting may be required to demonstrate them. It has been suggested that in plexogenic arteriopathy associated with congenital left-to-right shunts, the plexiform lesions occur in arteries 100

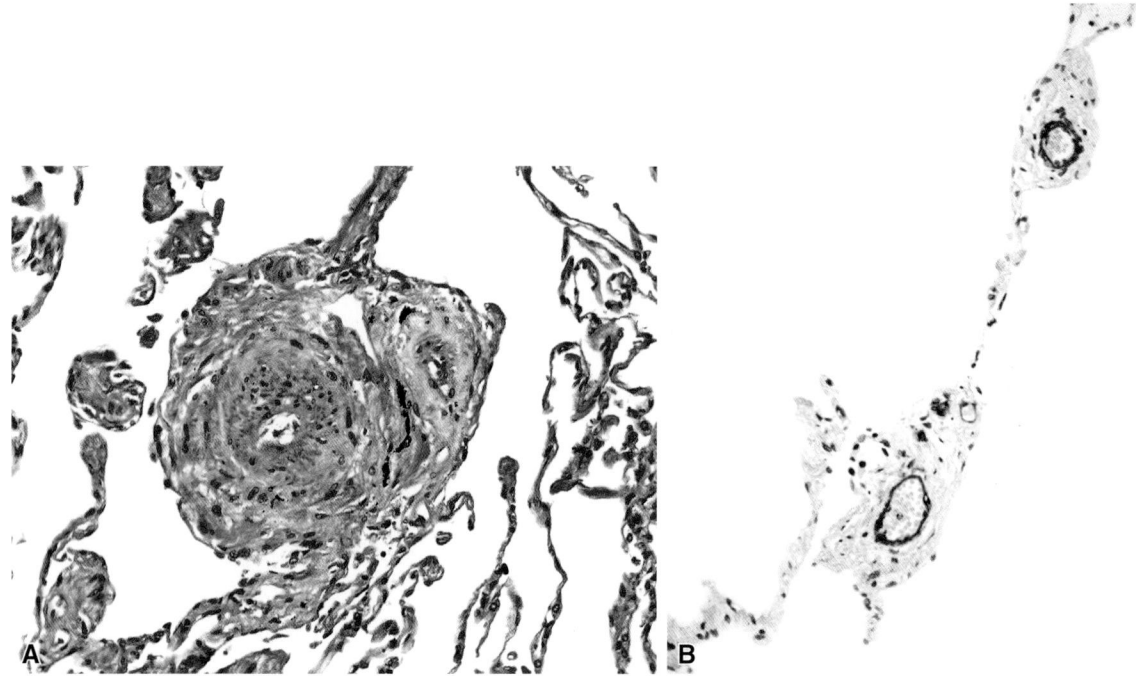

Figure 11-8. A, Severe muscular hypertrophy in a very small arterial branch. **B,** Smooth muscle actin stain of alveolar corner arterioles, showing complete muscular media in a case of pulmonary hypertension. Ordinarily these vessels do not have a complete muscular media.

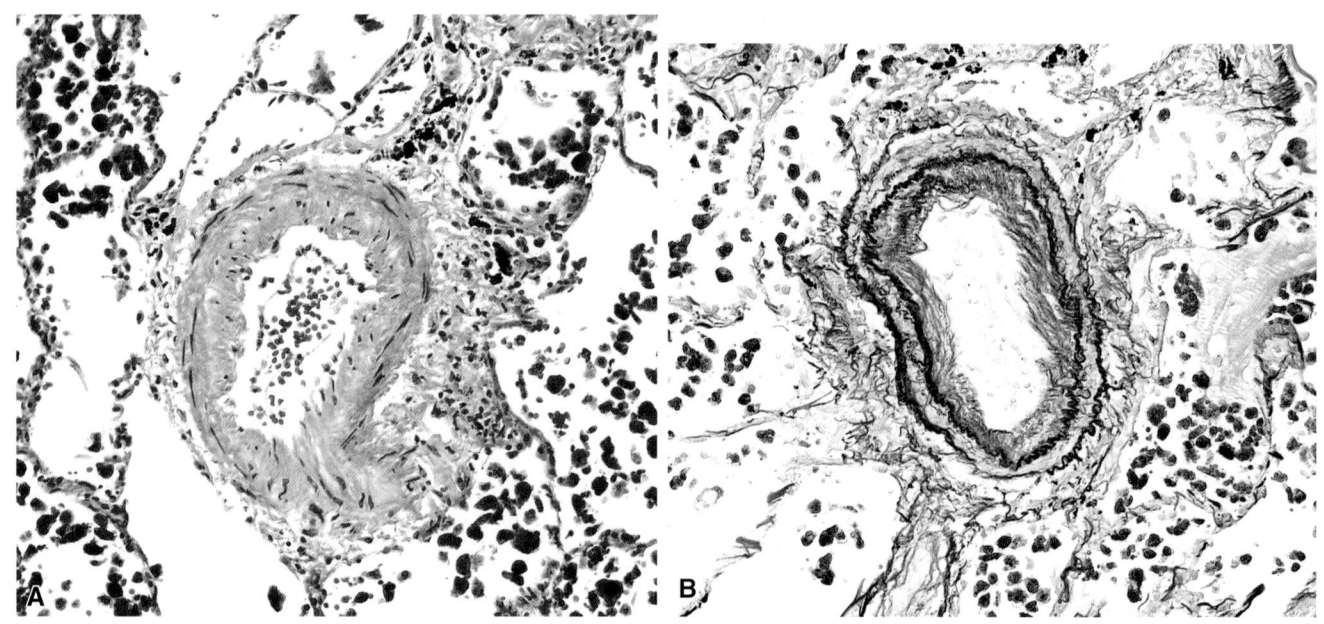

Figure 11-9. A and **B,** Mild intimal proliferation. The elastic stain (**B**) is required to separate this process from muscular hypertrophy.

to 200 µM in external diameter; whereas in idiopathic (primary) pulmonary hypertension, the lesions occur in arteries smaller than 100 µM.[19]

Grade VI: Dilatation and Angiomatoid Lesions

These arterial lesions are located distal to plexiform lesions and probably are related to changes in flow produced by the plexiform lesions. They consist of thin-walled, often dilated and tortuous, channels with a single elastica; these channels are not of obvious arterial structure, but their origin can be proved by tracing back through serial sections (Fig. 11-13). Dilatation and angiomatoid lesions may rupture with resulting pulmonary hemorrhage, and in some instances these lesions appear to anastomose with the bronchial circulation, thus exposing these relatively weak structures to systemic arterial pressures.

Clinical Correlations

As noted earlier, assessment of reversibility or potential for response to treatment is an important reason for performing lung biopsies in patients with pulmonary hypertension. However, the question of what features actually predict reversibility is controversial. As a first approximation, lesions can be separated as shown in Box 11-3.

Wagenvoort[12,13] and Palevsky and associates[3] have more recently suggested that simple qualitative assessment of the types of lesions present is inadequate by itself for predicting response, and that quantitative measurements are required, particularly measurements of intimal proliferation. For example, Palevsky's group[3] found that an average intimal area of more than 18% of the vascular cross section

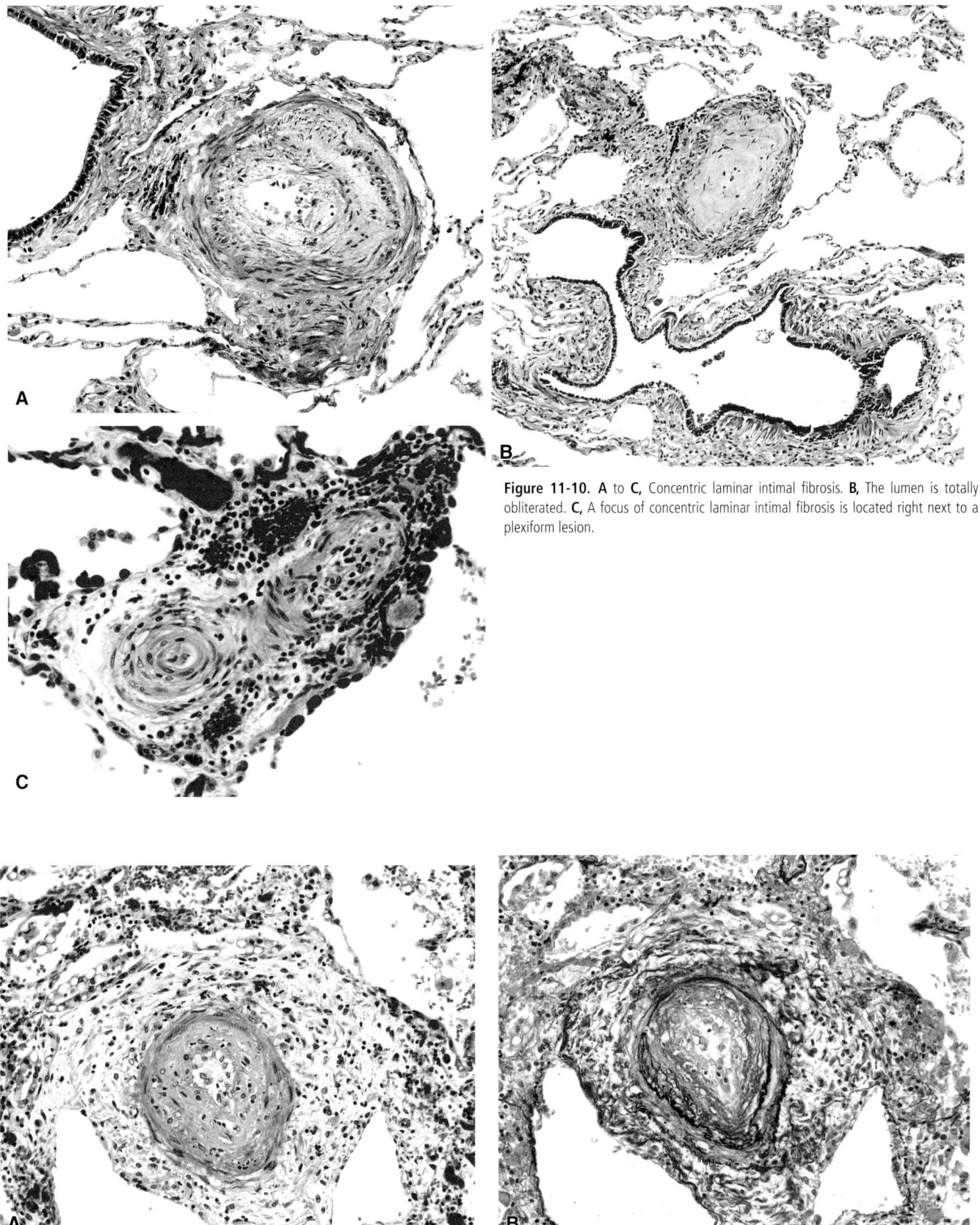

Figure 11-10. **A** to **C,** Concentric laminar intimal fibrosis. **B,** The lumen is totally obliterated. **C,** A focus of concentric laminar intimal fibrosis is located right next to a plexiform lesion.

Figure 11-11. Necrotizing vasculitis. **A,** Note the combination of inflammatory cells and pink material (fibrinoid necrosis) in the vessel wall. **B,** The partial loss of the internal elastica in the matching section.

Continued

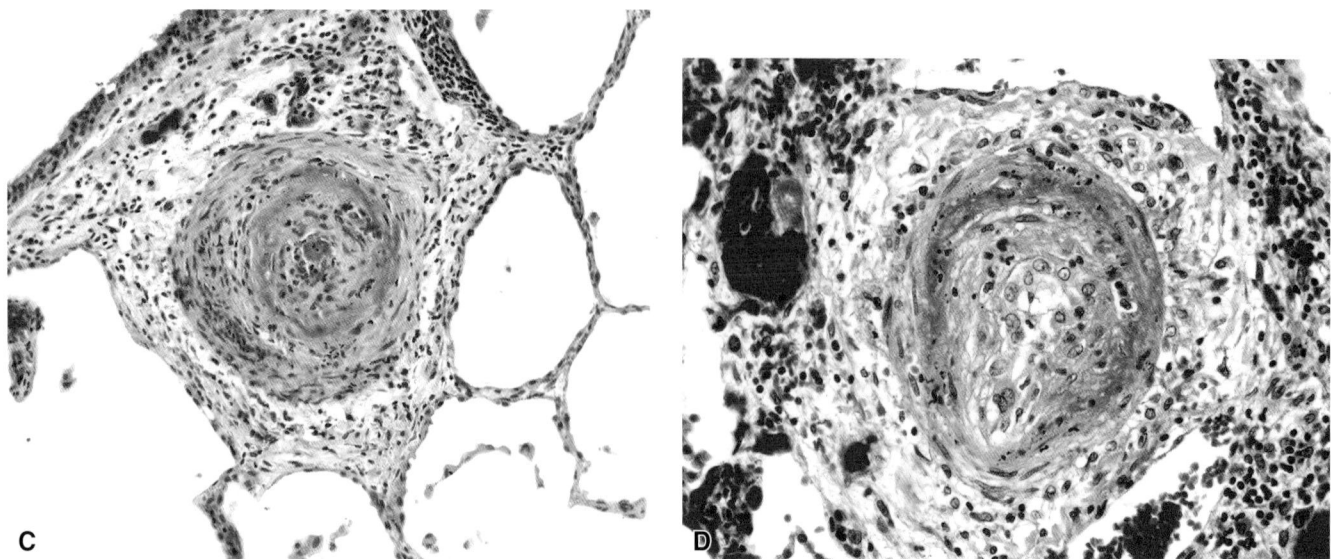

Figure 11-11—cont'd. C, A small thrombus is present in the lumen. **D,** The process is shown at higher magnification.

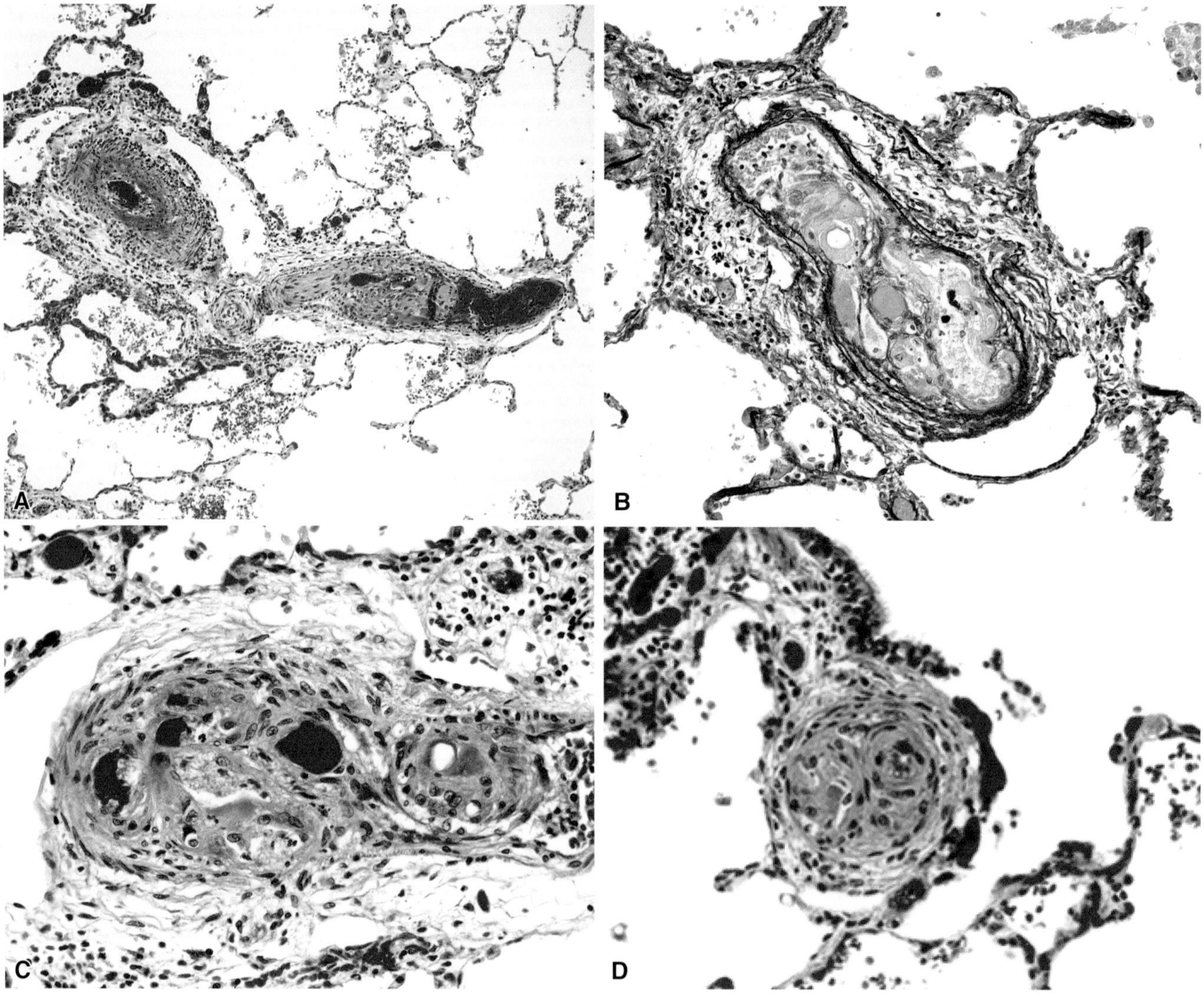

Figure 11-12 Plexiform lesions. **A,** Low-power view showing fibrinoid necrosis in one branch of the artery, concentric laminar intimal fibrosis best seen in the middle of the field, and a plexiform lesion cut in longitudinal section. **B,** Elastic stain of plexiform lesion showing the typical combination of multiple small capillary channels and loss of the internal elastica. **C,** Similar image on hematoxylin and eosin (H&E) stain. **D,** Plexiform lesion seen in cross section. The plexiform lesion appears to represent organization and thrombosis in arteries that have developed necrotizing vasculitis.

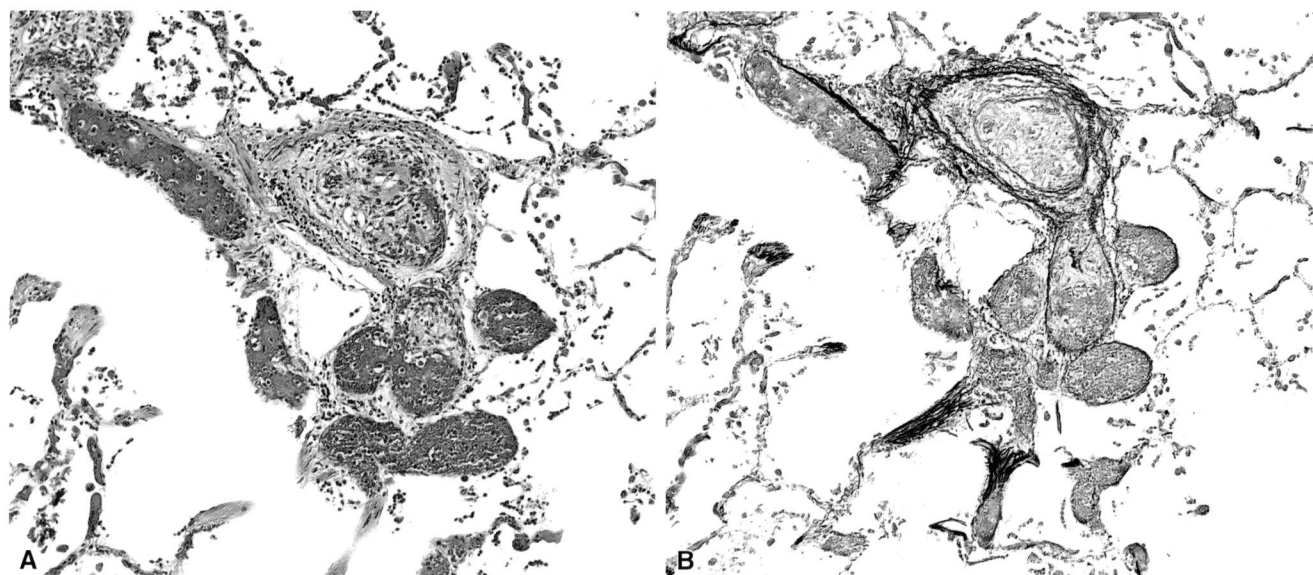

Figure 11-13. Dilatation lesions. **A** and **B,** The dilatation lesions appear as thin-walled, blood-filled channels. Dilatation lesions develop distal to plexiform lesions, shown here at the top of the field. **B,** Elastic stain.

Box 11-3. Reversibility and Morphologic Findings in Plexogenic Arteriopathy

Potentially Reversible
Muscular hypertrophy
Intimal proliferation
Mild concentric lamellar fibrosis

Not Reversible
Marked concentric lamellar fibrosis
Fibrinoid necrosis
Plexiform lesions
Dilatation and angiomatoid lesions

predicted a poor response to therapy. Interested readers should consult the appropriate references.[2,3,13,27]

The long-term outlook for patients with pulmonary hypertension associated with plexogenic arteriopathy tends to be poor, with deaths from cor pulmonale or sudden arrhythmias (see the section "Treatment of Pulmonary Hypertension" later in the chapter). In some forms of congenital heart disease, hypertension may be reversed by repair of the cardiac defect.

Differential Diagnosis

Higher-grade lesions in the plexogenic arteriopathy group are distinctive and not easily confused with other diseases. Systemic necrotizing vasculitis (microscopic polyangiitis, Wegener granulomatosis) may produce fibrinoid necrosis of vessels, but is not associated with lower-grade vascular changes or with plexiform lesions.

It should be remembered that some degree of muscular arterial hypertrophy is seen in virtually all forms of pulmonary hypertension, including veno-occlusive disease, pulmonary capillary hemangiomatosis, and venous hypertension secondary to mitral stenosis or other cardiac lesions.[2,28,29] Thus, the finding of muscular hypertrophy as the only vascular abnormality does not necessarily mean that the patient has plexogenic arteriopathy. Equally important, low-grade morphologic changes, especially isolated muscular hypertrophy, are not necessarily predictors of the degree of pulmonary hypertension; some patients with only muscular hypertrophy, nonetheless, can have quite high pulmonary artery pressures.

A further problem in interpretation is that thrombotic lesions, presumably reflecting in situ thromboses caused by abnormal flow, are now recognized as a finding in many different morphologic types of pulmonary hypertension[2,3,20] (see morphologic description in the next section) and certainly may be found in plexogenic arteriopathy. This does not invalidate the notion that plexogenic arteriopathy is morphologically separate from thrombotic hypertension.[20]

Thrombotic and Embolic Hypertension

Clinical Features

Typically, this form of hypertension is characterized by the insidious onset of shortness of breath without clinical evidence of pulmonary emboli (hence, thrombotic hypertension is sometimes included in the differential diagnosis for "primary" pulmonary hypertension). However, there may be a history of prior events that suggest the diagnosis—for example, recurrent sickle crises, a history of intravenous drug abuse, or known episodes of thromboembolism.

Radiologic Features

The radiologic features are not specific, but angiography or CT with contrast enhancment may reveal large emboli or sometimes evidence of multiple small thrombi, with apparent abrupt ending of the vessels.

Pathologic Findings

Pathologic findings vary with the type of underlying lesion. In classic thrombotic or thromboembolic hypertension, thrombi in various stages of organization, mostly old, are seen in branches of the small muscular pulmonary arteries. Of note, both elastic laminae are usually intact in thrombotic disease, as opposed to the destruction of the internal elastic in plexiform lesions.[2] Larger arteries may show "webs" (Fig. 11-14), which are simply organized thrombi with channels large enough to be seen grossly. In some cases of thrombotic or embolic hypertension, thrombi are only found in the main branches of the pulmonary artery, sometimes with webs as well; these patients often have underlying (nonhypertensive) lung disease or left-sided cardiac disease, as well as peripheral vascular thromboses.[29]

A helpful feature that should alert the pathologist to the presence of thrombi and emboli is the finding of *eccentric* intimal proliferation or intimal fibrosis in arterial vessels (Fig. 11-15); these lesions sometimes represent old small organizing thrombi. Both eccentric lesions and recanalized thrombi may be seen in pulmonary hypertension of other causes.[20]

Patients with sickle cell disease may develop thrombi in their distal pulmonary arterial branches during sickle crises, and recurrent episodes can lead to a form of thrombotic pulmonary hypertension. The lesions look like organizing thrombi, but close examination reveals the presence of sickled cells (Fig. 11-16).

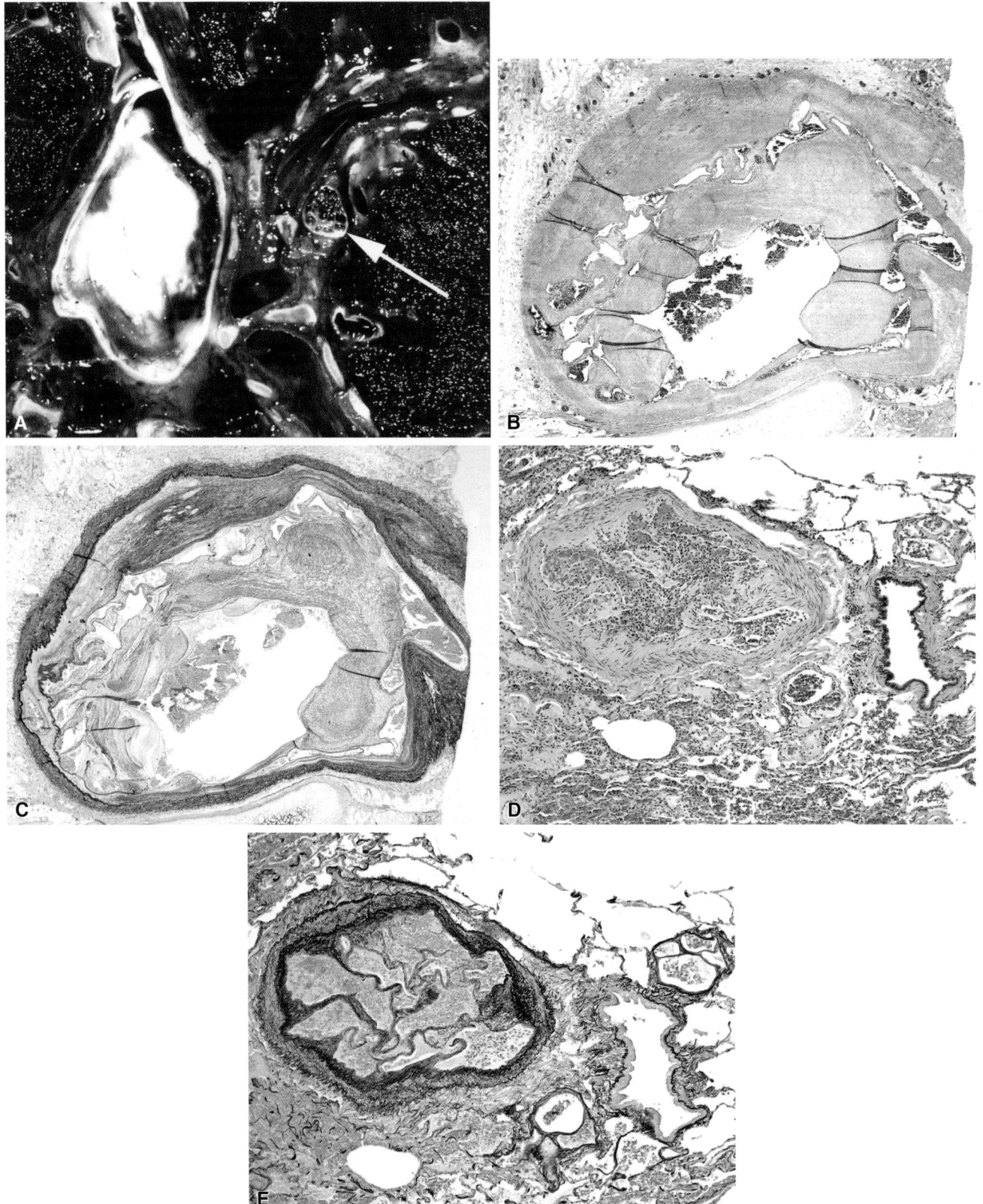

Figure 11-14. Appearance of organized thrombi. **A,** Gross appearance of a web (*arrow*) in a large pulmonary artery. The main pulmonary artery also contains an organized thrombus. **B** and **C,** H&E and elastic stains of another web in a large pulmonary artery branch. Note that the original elastic lamellae of the artery are intact. **D** and **E,** Organized thrombus in a muscular pulmonary artery showing numerous channels. Note again the preservation of the normal elastic structure in the arterial wall. Most thrombi do not disturb the arterial wall structure, as opposed to the destructive process that leads to plexiform lesions.

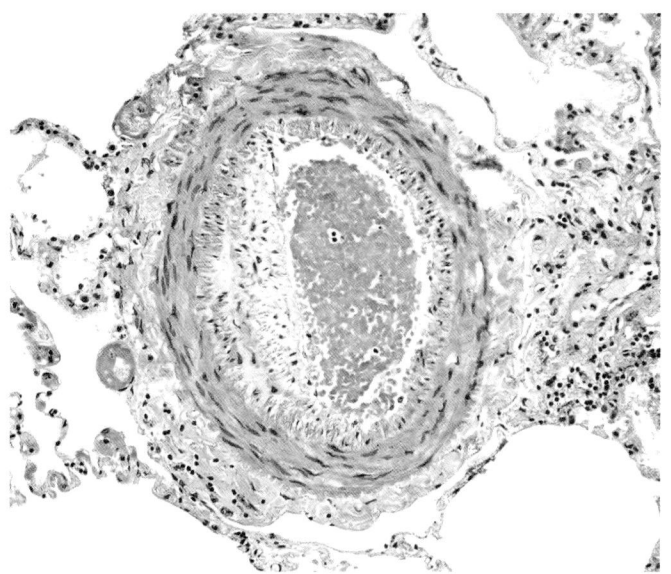

Figure 11-15. Eccentric intimal proliferation representing an old thrombus. Compare with the concentric intimal proliferation of plexogenic arteriopathy in Figures 11-10C and 11-12A.

Intravenous injection of licit drugs intended for oral use, or sometimes of illicit drugs such as heroin or cocaine,[30,31] tends to produce deposits of insoluble filler material from the drug in the small muscular arteries. In mild disease, small numbers of birefringent particles are seen in the lumina or in the arterial walls (Fig. 11-17), presumably having been incorporated into organizing thrombi. With injection of large amounts of drug, the inflammatory and thrombotic reaction to the particles leads to formation of thrombus-like formations with capillary channels called *angiothrombotic lesions*.[31] These are probably just peculiar in situ thrombi caused by large numbers of particles. They more or less completely obstruct the arterial branch, and accumulation of such lesions leads to pulmonary hypertension. Polarized light examination is often useful in demonstrating the particulate matter. Under polarizing light, starch appears as Maltese cross–like images; talc, as brightly birefringent plates; and microcrystalline cellulose, as periodic acid/Schiff–positive rectangular crystals that are also birefringent. For illicit drugs, exact identification of the filler may not be possible.

Pulmonary hypertension may develop as a result of filling of the small arterial branches with tumor emboli (Fig. 11-18). Radiographically or pathologically visible metastases may or may not be present. Pulmonary

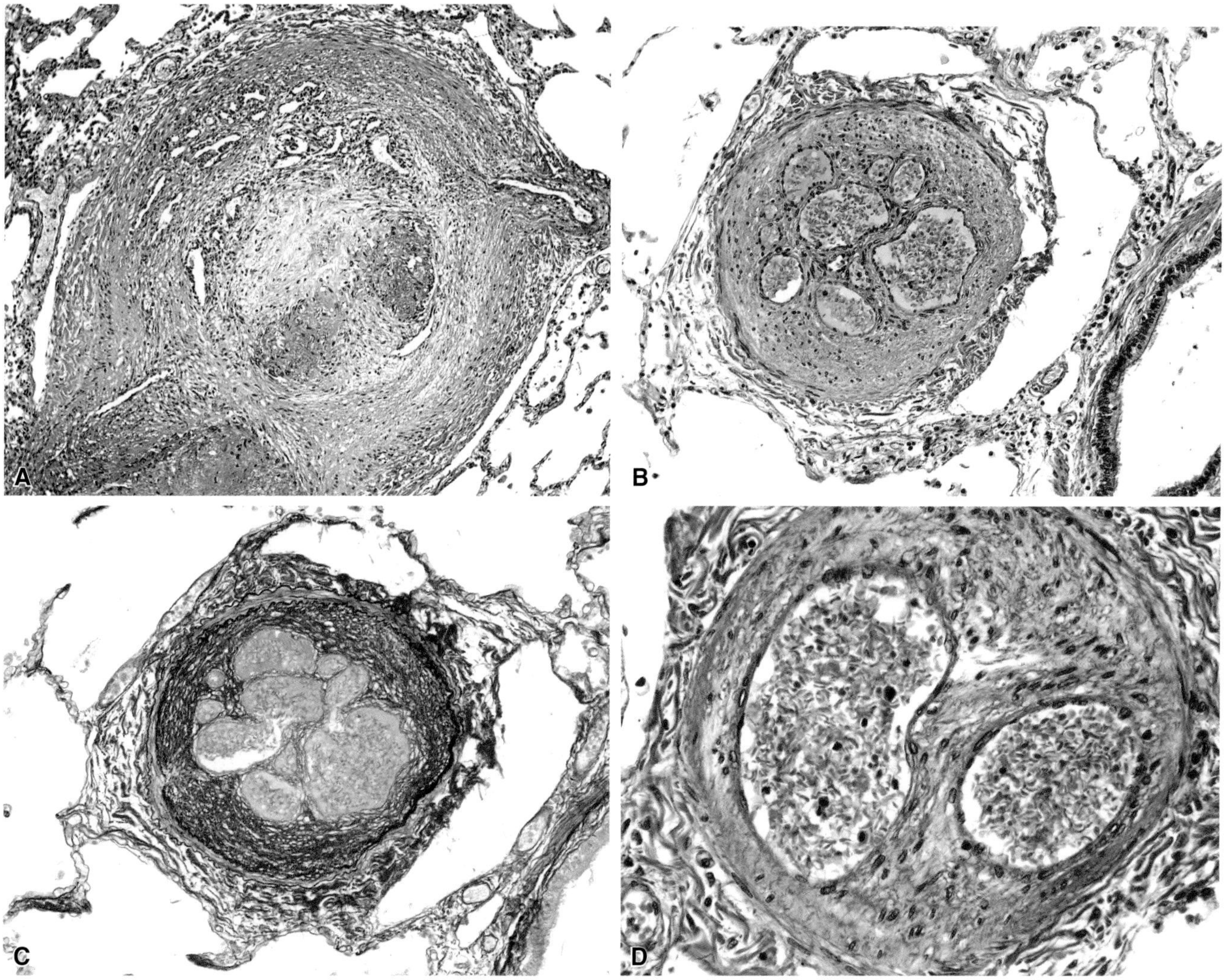

Figure 11-16. Thrombosis in a patient with sickle cell disease. **A,** Acute thrombus. **B** and **C,** Organized thrombus showing multiple channels. This appearance in itself is not specific for etiology, but sickle cells are seen at high power in part **D**.

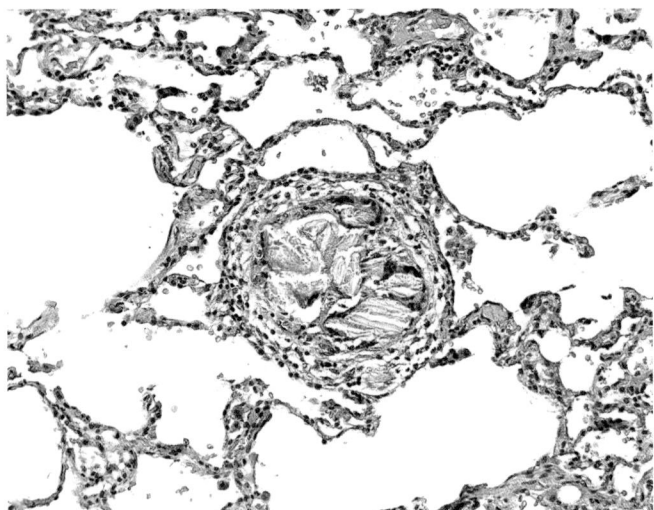

Figure 11-17. Organized thrombus and birefringent particles in a muscular pulmonary artery from an intravenous drug abuser.

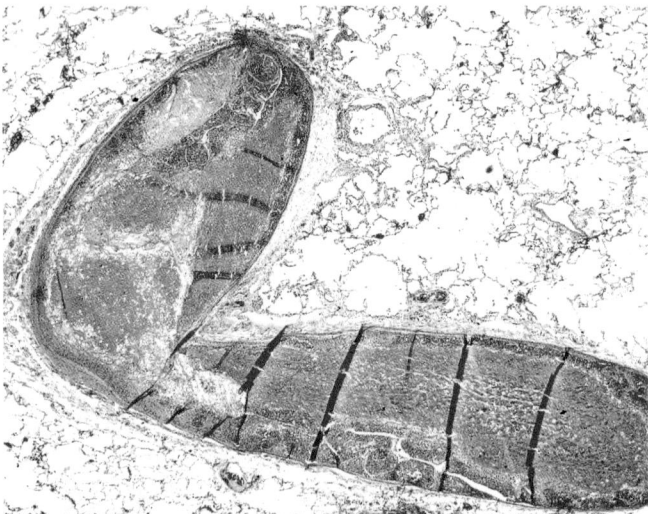

Figure 11-18. Filling of pulmonary artery branches by tumor emboli from a hepato-cellular carcinoma.

hypertension in this setting has been most commonly reported with lung, breast, stomach, ovarian, and hepatocellular carcinomas.[29] An unusual form of tumor-associated pulmonary hypertension is pulmonary tumor thrombotic microangiopathy[32] in which the tumor elicits a marked intimal proliferation with only small numbers of tumor cells present.

Clinical Correlations

In most of these conditions, there is no specific therapy. However, when pulmonary hypertension is caused by large vessel, especially main pulmonary artery, thrombi without significant small vessel thrombi, surgical removal of the thrombi may reverse the hypertension.

Differential Diagnosis

As noted, scattered thrombi are fairly common in other types of pulmonary hypertension, such as plexogenic arteriopathy, and the presence of thrombi or eccentric intimal lesions does not automatically indicate a diagnosis of thrombotic and embolic hypertension. Although it has been claimed that plexiform lesions can, rarely, be seen in thrombotic and embolic hypertension, including sickle cell disease,[17,33] we believe that most such cases, in fact, represent plexogenic arteriopathy with more than the usual number of thrombi. Thus, it is important to be sure that typical plexogenic lesions are not present and to demonstrate the presence of *multiple* thrombi or emboli when making a diagnosis of thrombi or embolic hypertension.

Pulmonary Veno-Occlusive Disease and Other Types of Pulmonary Venous Hypertension

Clinical Features

Like other forms of pulmonary hypertension, PVOD is characterized by the insidious onset of shortness of breath, often associated with a nonproductive cough. Clubbing has been identified in some patients. There is a wide age range of affected subjects, with a mean age of less than 50 years, and including a significant proportion of children. Patients with PVOD do not have clinical evidence of thrombotic or embolic disease, but may have small hemoptyses.

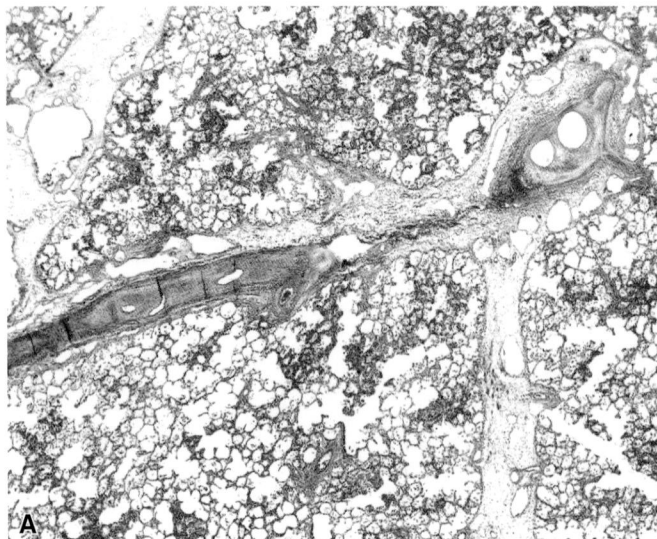
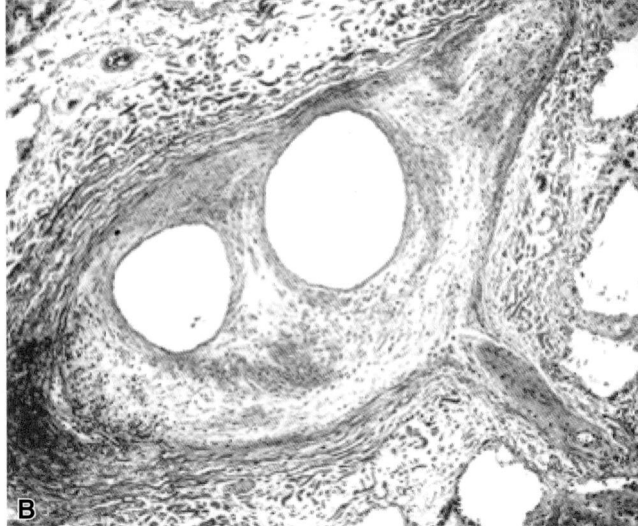

Figure 11-19. Pulmonary veno-occlusive disease. **A,** Low-power view showing thrombosed veins in the interlobular septa and intense congestion in the parenchyma, along with hemosiderin pigment. The interlobular septa also are edematous. **B,** Higher-power view of an organized thrombus in a large vein.

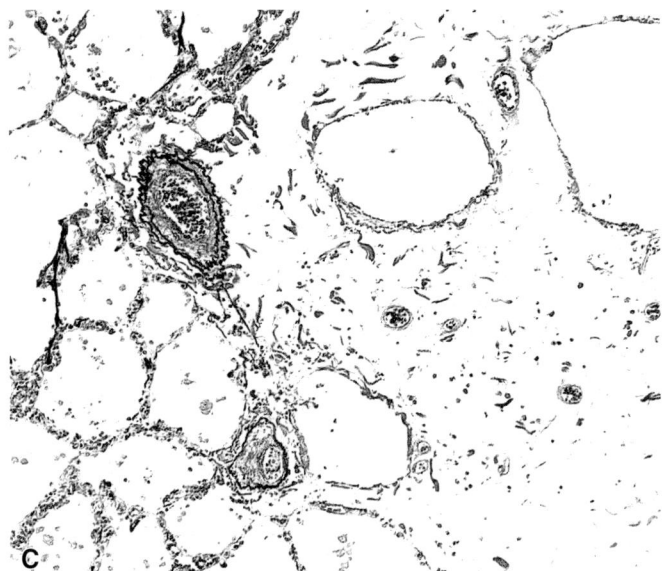

Figure 11-19—cont'd. C, Elastic stain demonstrating arterialized veins and marked edema in the interlobular septa.

Radiologic Features

On plain films, patients with advanced disease show pulmonary artery enlargement and, with cor pulmonale, right ventricular hypertrophy. A helpful finding in PVOD is the presence of prominent Kerley B lines and mild to moderate interstitial infiltrates. The CT scan shows distinctly thickened interlobular septa.[34]

Pathologic Findings

The fundamental lesion in PVOD is thrombosis, typically old thrombosis, of small pulmonary veins and venules, although a recent report documented venulitis in a small proportion of cases.[35] Thrombosis is most easily seen in veins in the interlobular septa (Fig. 11-19) where the location ensures that the structure is indeed a vein. With increasing pressure, such veins may become arterialized, that is, they develop a double elastic lamina and a distinct layer of muscle (see Fig. 11-19C), and are, thus, distinguishable from arteries only by their location.

The venules in PVOD are often thrombosed as well, but this may be difficult to document. Venous hypertension of any cause is associated with intimal fibrosis and luminal narrowing of the veins and venules, but in PVOD the lumen of small venules may simply be obliterated by fibrous tissue (Fig. 11-20). Use of elastic stains is mandatory to find

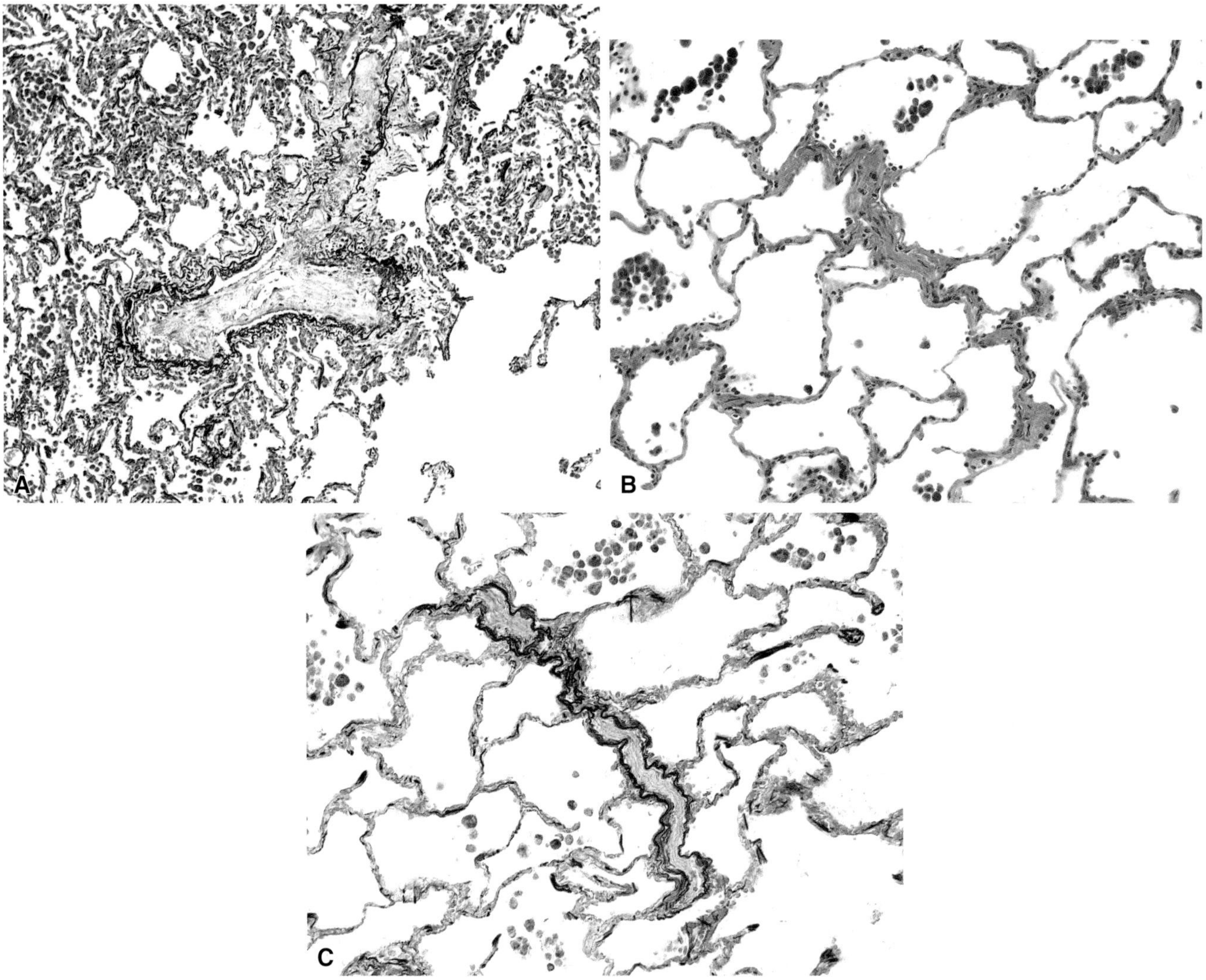

Figure 11-20. Pulmonary veno-occlusive disease. Obliteration of small veins by fibrous tissue. Elastic staining (**A** and **C**) is crucial to the diagnosis; in some instances, obliterated veins do not even appear to be vascular channels on H&E stain (**B**). Compare the same image with elastic staining in part **C**.

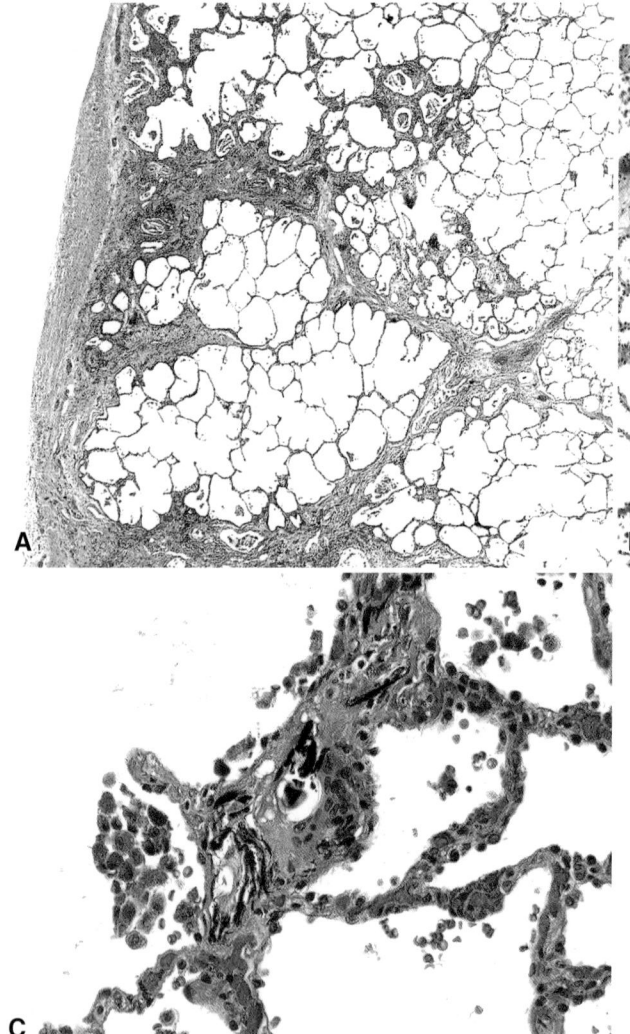

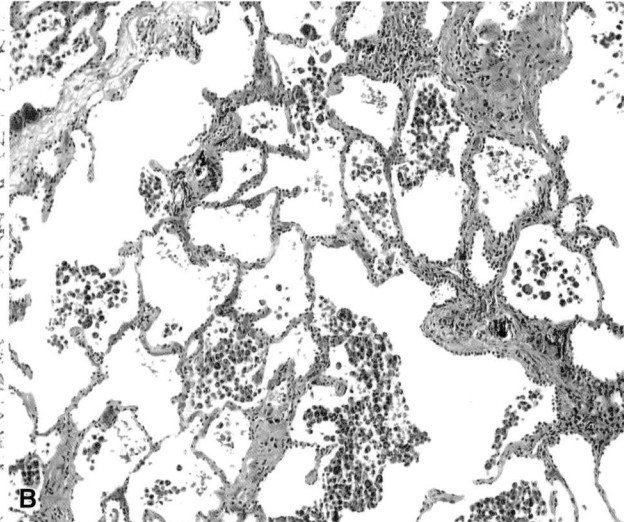

Figure 11-21. Pulmonary veno-occlusive disease. **A,** Low-power view showing peripheral irregular interstitial fibrosis. **B,** Fine fibrosis and hemosiderin-laden macrophages are visible in the higher-power view. **C,** So-called endogenous pneumoconiosis—encrustation of elastic fibers by iron and calcium and reactive multinucleated giant cells. This lesion may be seen in any type of chronic pulmonary hemorrhage.

such vessels, and once small vessels with apparent luminal obliteration are found, they may need to be traced back through several sections until they connect with a vein in an interlobular septum, thus proving their nature. The diagnosis of PVOD can be exceedingly difficult when only small venules are affected.

The vascular changes in PVOD do not occur in isolation. The interlobular septa are generally edematous and the lymphatics prominently dilated (see Fig. 11-19). A peculiar, usually mild, form of interstitial fibrosis that tends to be more marked in the very periphery of the lung under the pleura (Fig. 11-21) is common in PVOD (47% of cases in a recent large series[35]). The fibrosis is fairly homogeneous, typically paucicellular, and raises the morphologic question of a chronic interstitial pneumonia. Accompanying the fibrosis are usually very small foci of acute or old hemorrhage with hemosiderin-laden macrophages (see Fig. 11-21B). The combination of mild, homogeneous fibrosis and small hemorrhages should bring the diagnosis of PVOD to mind and prompt examination of the veins in the interlobular septa.

Arterial changes may be present in PVOD and consist of muscular hypertrophy and sometimes mild intimal fibrosis. Although it has been claimed that plexiform lesions can be seen in PVOD,[19] in our experience this is not true, and plexiform lesions were not seen in 30 patients reported by Lantuéjoul.[35]

Another change that may be seen in PVOD, but also in any disease characterized by repeated pulmonary hemorrhage, is so-called *endogenous pneumoconiosis*, in which elastic fibers are coated by iron and calcium, with a resulting appearance that resembles a ferruginous body (see Fig. 11-21C) of the type seen in asbestosis. Foci of dystrophic ossification also may be present but are a fairly nonspecific marker of venous hypertension (see later discussion).

Clinical Correlations

In most cases, PVOD has no known cause, but it has been reported in a small number of patients given chemotherapeutic agents[36] and patients with autoantibodies against platelets or anticardiolipin antibodies.[35] In general, the prognosis is poor, and, at present, transplantation offers the only hope of cure. Vasodilator therapy must be approached with caution because it may induce severe pulmonary edema.

Differential Diagnosis

PVOD is the most dramatic and severe form of *pulmonary venous hypertension*. Venous hypertension may also be seen in patients with left-sided heart disease, especially mitral stenosis, and, rarely, atrial myxomas; in conditions such as sclerosing mediastinitis, in which the pulmonary veins are obliterated or narrowed in the mediastinum; in some types of congenital cardiac malformations, in which the major

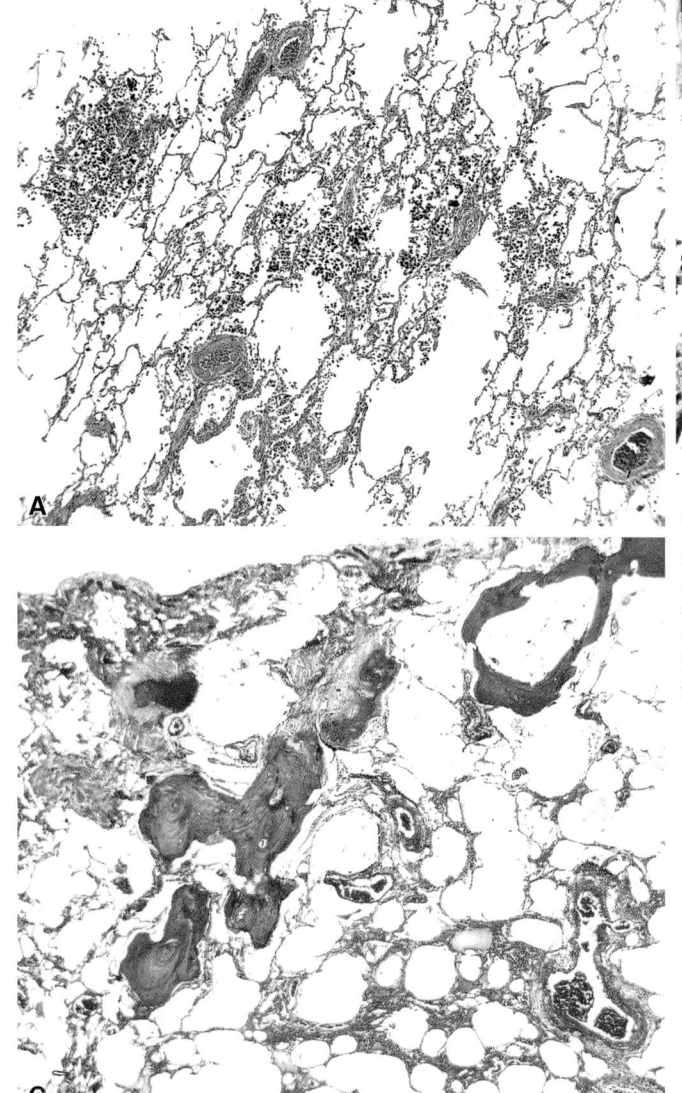

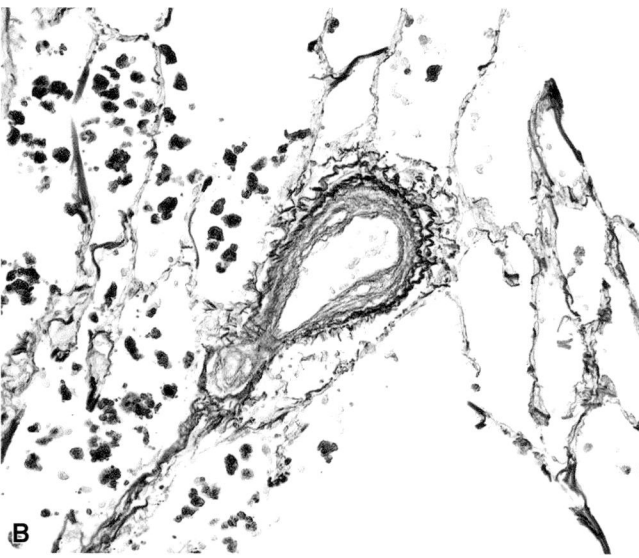

Figure 11-22. Chronic passive congestion. **A,** Low-power view shows numerous foci of microscopic hemorrhages and hemosiderin-laden macrophages. Pulmonary arteries exhibit mild muscular hyperplasia. **B,** Elastic staining of a small vein demonstrates intimal proliferation. This nonspecific finding can be seen in venous hypertension but also is commonly observed as an aging effect. **C,** Ossification in the parenchyma, a common finding with venous stasis.

pulmonary veins are abnormal or absent; and in some patients with collagen vascular diseases.[37] Intimal fibrosis in the small pulmonary veins and venules, mild interstitial inflammation and edema, small hemorrhages, "endogenous pneumoconiosis," and dystrophic ossification are common in all these conditions, and muscular hypertrophy in the small pulmonary arterial branches may be present as well (Fig. 11-22). However, true venous obliteration, the hallmark of PVOD, is absent. Idiopathic interstitial pneumonias and even real pneumoconioses come into the differential diagnosis, as indicated previously.

Pulmonary Capillary Hemangiomatosis

We are treating PCH as a distinct entity, but PCH is a controversial lesion that may or may not be different from PVOD; changes of PCH are sometimes seen in other diseases as well (see later discussion).

Clinical and Radiologic Features

PCH is a very rare disease, mostly seen in adults. The usual nonspecific signs of pulmonary hypertension are present and small hemoptyses may occur. Chest radiography demonstrates interstitial infiltrates with thickened interlobular septa.[38]

Pathologic Findings

PCH is characterized by proliferation of dilated capillary-sized channels along and in the alveolar walls (Fig. 11-23). In this it resembles a very severe form of passive congestion, but careful examination shows that there appears to be duplicate or multiple capillary channels in an alveolar wall, something not present in passive congestion.[39] The proliferating capillary channels extend into arterioles and venules, producing a peculiar pattern of capillary proliferation within the walls of the larger vessel with resulting luminal narrowing or obliteration; it is this involvement of larger vessels that is thought to produce pulmonary hypertension. Often there is an admixture of very abnormal areas of lung with extensive capillary proliferation combined with perfectly normal-appearing lung, again a helpful finding in separating capillary hemangiomatosis from passive congestion (the latter should be more homogeneous). Small acute and old hemorrhages may be present, as may muscular hypertrophy in small pulmonary arteries.

It has recently been suggested that most cases of PCH are really examples of PVOD.[35] Thrombotic occlusion of small veins can be found in PCH, along with small foci of hemorrhage and areas of interstitial fibrosis; conversely, PCH-like foci can be demonstrated in many cases

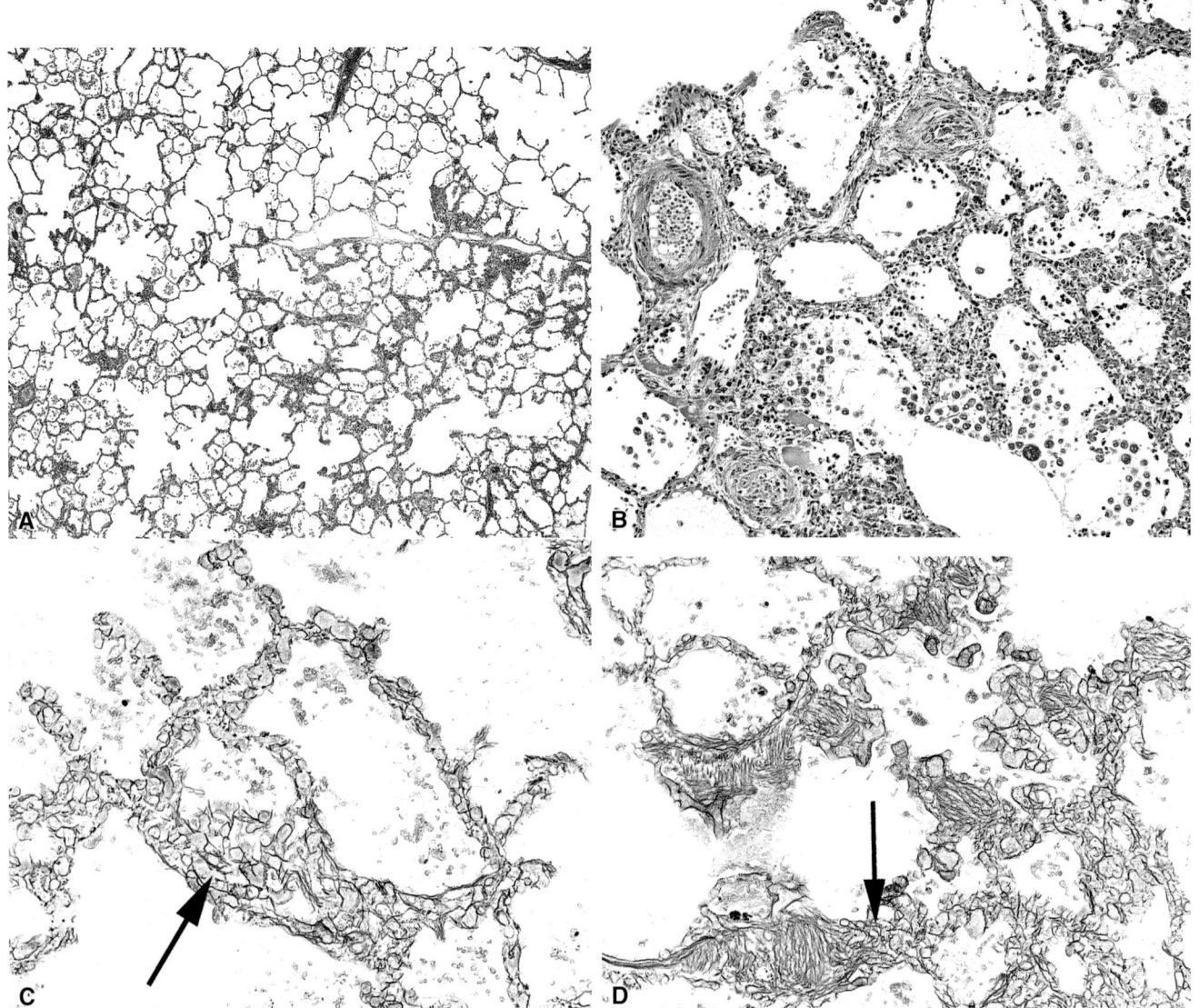

Figure 11-23. Pulmonary capillary hemangiomatosis. **A,** Low-power view showing what at first glance appears to be marked congestion. **B,** Higher-power image demonstrates thickened alveolar walls caused by proliferating capillaries. **C,** Proliferating capillary channels, better demonstrated by reticulin staining, are invading the walls of a small vein (*arrow*). **D,** Reticulin staining shows capillaries invading wall of airway (*arrow*).

of PVOD as well as other forms of pulmonary venous hypertension and also in patients who do not have pulmonary hypertension.[35]

Clinical Correlations

The etiology of PCH, assuming it is an entity different from PVOD, is not known. Some patients have been treated with transplantation.

Pulmonary Hypertension Secondary to Other Forms of Intrinsic Lung Disease

Pulmonary hypertension is commonly found associated with different forms of nonvascular intrinsic lung disease, including emphysema, bronchiectasis, usual interstitial pneumonia, and any other conditions that produce extensive scarring of the parenchyma or that produce chronic hypoxia. In emphysema, claims have been made that hypertension is secondary to loss of capillary bed, although this may not be correct, and vascular changes may be caused by direct effects of cigarette smoke on the vasculature or by local hypoxic vasoconstriction.[40]

Pulmonary hypertension is increasingly being recognized as an important complication of usual interstitial pneumonia; it was seen in 46% of a large series of patients with usual interstitial pneumonia awaiting transplantation.[41] With pulmonary hypertension, the development of cor pulmonale is common in all of these diseases and may be the cause of death.

In all of these settings, the vascular changes consist of muscular hypertrophy of the small pulmonary arteries, often with extension of muscle into the arterioles. Sometimes, mild intimal proliferation is present.

Morphologic Mimics of Pulmonary Hypertension

In our experience, biopsies from patients with interstitial lung disease frequently show muscular arterial hypertrophy, even when cardiac catheterization shows normal pressures (Fig. 11-24). Intimal fibrosis also increases as a normal function of age.[35] Thus, considerable caution should be exercised in the individual case when interpreting what

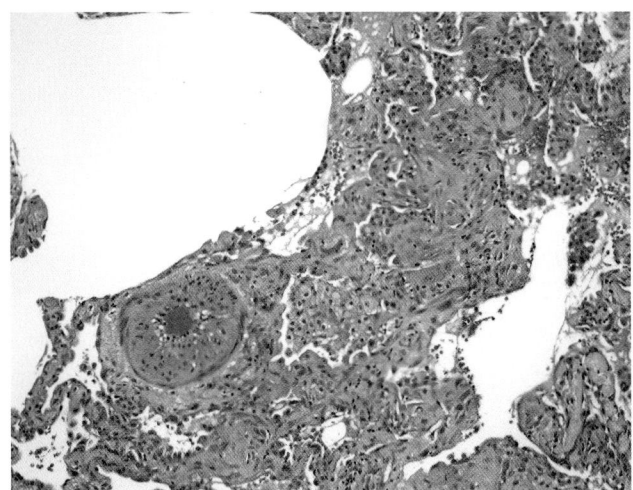

Figure 11-24. Thick-walled pulmonary artery branch from a case of bronchiolitis obliterans organizing pneumonia mimicking changes of pulmonary hypertension. Changes of this type are common in lungs with interstitial lung disease and do not necessarily indicate that pulmonary hypertension is present.

appear to be low-grade hypertensive changes when the morphologic changes occur in a clinical or pathologic setting not suggestive of pulmonary hypertension.

Treatment of Pulmonary Hypertension

The pathophysiology of pulmonary hypertension is complex and involves multiple pathways, including the endothelin (vasoconstriction), protacyclin, and nitric oxide (vasodilation) cascades. Various therapies have been directed toward vasodilation by antagonism or enhancement of the above pathways, in addition to the supportive therapies of diuretics and oxygen; these have shown some benefit.[42,43]

Self-assessment questions related to this chapter can be found online on the Expert Consult site for this title.

References

1. Wagenvoort CA. Lung biopsy specimens in the evaluation of pulmonary vascular disease. *Chest*. 1980;77:614–625.
2. Pietra GG, Edwards WD, Kay JM, et al. Histopathology of primary pulmonary hypertension. *Circulation*. 1989;80:1198–1206.
3. Palevsky HI, Schloo BL, Pietra GG, et al. Primary pulmonary hypertension. Vascular structure, morphometry, and responsiveness to vasodilator agents. *Circulation*. 1989;80: 1207–1220.
4. Wagenvoort CA, Wagenvoort N. Pulmonary vascular bed: normal anatomy and responses to disease. In: Moser KM, ed. *Pulmonary Vascular Diseases: Lung Biology in Health and Disease*. New York: Marcel Dekker; 1979:1–110.
5. Rabinovitch M. Morphology of the developing pulmonary bed: pharmacologic implications. *Pediatr Pharm*. 1985;5:31–48.
6. Schraufnagel DE. Corrosion casting of the lung for scanning electron microscopy. In: Lenfant C, ed. *Electron Microscopy of the Lung*. New York: Marcel Dekker; 1990:257–297.
7. Murphy ML, Bone RC. *Cor Pulmonale in Chronic Bronchitis and Emphysema*. New York: Future Publishing; 1984.
8. Fulton RM, Hutchinson EC, Jones AM. Ventricular weight in cardiac hypertrophy. *Br Heart J*. 1952;14:413–420.
9. Ishikawa S, Fattal GA. Functional morphometry of myocardial fibres in cor pulmonale. *Am Rev Respir Dis*. 1972;105:358–367.
10. Fishman AP. Pulmonary hypertension and cor pulmonale. In: Fishman AP, ed. *Pulmonary Diseases and Disorders*, 2nd ed. New York: McGraw-Hill; 1988.
11. Wagenvoort CA, Wagenvoort N. *Pathology of Pulmonary Hypertension*. New York: John Wiley & Sons; 1977.
12. Wagenvoort CA. Lung biopsies in the differential diagnosis of thromboembolic versus primary pulmonary hypertension. *Prog Resp Res*. 1980;13:16–21.
13. Wagenvoort CA. Grading of pulmonary vascular lesions—a reappraisal. *Histopathology*. 1981;5:595–598.
14. Pietra GG, Ruttner JR. Specificity of pulmonary vascular lesions in primary pulmonary hypertension. A reappraisal. *Respiration*. 1982;52:81–85.
15. Burke AP, Farb A, Virmani R. The pathology of primary pulmonary hypertension. *Mod Pathol*. 1991;4:269–277.
16. Heath D, Edwards JE. The pathology of hypertensive pulmonary vascular disease. *Circulation*. 1958;18:533–543.
17. Simonneau G, Galiè N, Rubin LJ, et al. Clinical classification of pulmonary hypertension. *J Am Coll Cardiol*. 2004;43(12 Suppl S):5S–12S.
18. Montani D, Achouh L, Dorfmüller P, et al. Pulmonary veno occlusive disease: clinical, functional, radiologic, and hemodynamic characteristics and outcome of 24 cases confirmed by histology. *Medicine (Baltimore)*. 2008;87:220–233.
19. Pietra GG, Capron F, Stewart S, et al. Pathologic assessment of vasculopathies in pulmonary hypertension. *J Am Coll Cardiol*. 2004;43(12 Suppl S):25S–32S.
20. Wagenvoort CA, Mulder RGH. Thrombotic lesion in primary plexogenic arteriopathy: similar pathogenesis or complication? *Chest*. 1993;103:844–849.
21. Abenhaim L, Moride UY, Brenot F, et al. Appetite-suppressant drugs and the risk of primary pulmonary hypertension. *N Engl J Med*. 1996;335:609–616.
22. Fishman AP. Aminorex to fen/phen: an epidemic foretold. *Circulation*. 1999;99:156–161.
23. Mehta NJ, Khan LA, Mehta RN, Sepkowitz DA. HIV-related pulmonary hypertension: analytic review of 131 cases. *Chest*. 2000;118:1133–1141.
24. Pellicelli AM, Barbaro G, Palmieri F, et al. Primary pulmonary hypertension in HIV patients: a systematic review. *Angiology*. 2001;51:31–41.
25. Ng CS, Wells AU, Padley SP. A CT sign of chronic pulmonary arterial hypertension: the ratio of main pulmonary artery to aortic diameter. *J Thorac Imaging*. 1999;14:270–278.
26. Moore GW, Smith RR, Hutchins GM. Pulmonary artery atherosclerosis: correlation with systemic atherosclerosis and hypertensive pulmonary vascular disease. *Arch Pathol Lab Med*. 1982;106:378–380.
27. Yamaki S, Wagenvoort CA. Plexogenic pulmonary arteriopathy: significance of medial thickness with respect to advanced pulmonary vascular lesions. *Am J Pathol*. 1981;105:70–75.
28. Fernie JM, Lamb D. Effects of age and smoking on intima of muscular pulmonary arteries. *J Clin Pathol*. 1986;39:1204–1208.
29. Katzenstein ABL. Pulmonary hypertension and other vascular disorders. In: Katzenstein ABL, ed. *Katzenstein and Askin's Surgical Pathology of Non-Neoplastic Lung Disease*, 3rd ed. Philadelphia: WB Saunders; 1997:322–360.
30. Yakel DL, Eisenberg MJ. Pulmonary artery hypertension in chronic intravenous cocaine users. *Am Heart J*. 1995;130:398–399.
31. Tomashefski JF, Hirsch CS. The pulmonary vascular lesions of intravenous drug abuse. *Hum Pathol*. 1980;11:133–145.
32. von Herbay A, Illes A, Waldherr R, Otto HF. Pulmonary tumor thrombotic microangiopathy with pulmonary hypertension. *Cancer*. 1990;66:587–592.
33. Moser KM, Bloor CM. Pulmonary vascular lesions occurring in patients with chronic major vessel thromboembolic pulmonary hypertension. *Circulation*. 1981;210:507–511.
34. Holcomb BS, Loyd JE, Ely W, et al. Pulmonary veno-occlusive disease. *Chest*. 2000;118: 1671–1679.
35. Lantuéjoul S, Sheppard MN, Corrin B, et al. Pulmonary veno-occlusive disease and pulmonary capillary hemangiomatosis: a clinicopathologic study of 35 cases. *Am J Surg Pathol*. 2006;30:850–857.
36. Lombard C, Churg A, Winokur A. Pulmonary veno-occlusive disease following therapy for malignant neoplasms. *Chest*. 1987;92:871–876.
37. Dorfmüller P, Humbert M, Perros F, et al. Fibrous remodeling of the pulmonary venous system in pulmonary arterial hypertension associated with connective tissue diseases. *Hum Pathol*. 2007;38:893–902.
38. Al Fawaz IM, Al Mobiareek KF, Al-Suhaibani M, Ashour M. Pulmonary capillary hemangiomatosis. *Pediatr Pulmonol*. 1995;19:243–248.
39. Tron V, Magee F, Wright J, et al. Pulmonary capillary hemangiomatosis. *Hum Pathol*. 1986;17:1144–1150.
40. Wright JL, Levy RD, Churg A. Pulmonary hypertension in chronic obstructive pulmonary disease: current theories of pathogenesis and their implications for treatment. *Thorax*. 2005;60: 605–609.
41. Shorr AF, Wainright JL, Cors CS, et al. Pulmonary hypertension in patients with pulmonary fibrosis awaiting lung transplant. *Eur Respir J*. 2007;30:715–721.
42. Badesch DB, Abman SH, Simonneau G, et al. Medical therapy for pulmonary arterial hypertension: updated ACCP evidence based clinical practice guidelines. *Chest*. 2007;131:1917–1928.
43. Humbert M, Sitbon O, Simonneau G. Treatment of pulmonary arterial hypertension. *N Engl J Med*. 2004;351:1425–1436.

Pathology of Lung Transplantation

Andras Khoor, MD, and Samuel A. Yousem, MD

Lung transplantation may offer longer survival and improved quality of life to patients with end-stage lung disease. Common indications for single lung, bilateral (double) lung, and heart-lung transplantation are listed in Table 12-1. Bilateral lung transplantation is the norm for cystic fibrosis, but of interest, the proportion of bilateral lung transplantation procedures has been rising for other major indications as well.[1] Living donor single lobe transplantation may be a viable alternative to cadaveric lung transplantation for selected patients.[2] Benchmark survival rates for adult lung transplant recipients are 88% at 3 months, 78% at 1 year, 63% at 3 years, 51% at 5 years, and 28% at 10 years after transplantation.[1]

Unfortunately, the number of patients who can benefit from lung transplantation is limited by the availability of donor organs. Historically, waiting time was the main determinant of donor lung allocation in the United States. In 2005, a lung allocation score (LAS) was implemented, dramatically changing the way donor lungs are distributed.[3] Under the new system, priority for transplantation is determined by medical urgency and expected outcome. Early evaluations of the new system indicate that the waiting time and waitlist mortality rate are decreased, the number of transplants is increased, and the post-transplantation survival is unchanged.[4]

Complications of lung transplantation may be related to (1) the operation itself (primary graft dysfunction, anastomotic complications), (2) the host's immunologic response to the allograft (rejection), and (3) the immunosuppressive therapy used to prevent rejection (infection, post-transplantation lymphoproliferative disorders [PTLDs]). Other complications, such as organizing pneumonia and recurrence of the original disease, may also occur. To aid the differential diagnosis, post-transplant time intervals can be divided arbitrarily into immediate (within 4 days), early (4 days to 1 month), and late (beyond 1 month) post-transplantation periods.[5] Differential diagnostic possibilities for each of these periods are listed in Table 12-2.

Post-transplantation transbronchial biopsy may be performed for a specific clinical indication or for surveillance of acute rejection. The role of surveillance biopsy in lung transplant patients remains controversial.[6,7] At least five pieces of well-expanded alveolated lung parenchyma are required for the assessment of acute rejection.[8] The histopathologic findings most commonly encountered in a post-transplantation transbronchial biopsy include acute rejection, cytomegalovirus infection, airway-centered inflammation, pneumonia, bronchiolitis obliterans, harvest injury, invasive aspergillosis, and PTLDs.[6,9]

Table 12-1. Most Common Indications for Lung Transplant Procedures

Transplant Procedure	Most Common Indications
Adult single lung	Chronic obstructive pulmonary disease Idiopathic pulmonary fibrosis α_1-Anti-trypsin deficiency emphysema
Adult bilateral/double lung	Cystic fibrosis Chronic obstructive pulmonary disease Idiopathic pulmonary fibrosis α_1-Anti-trypsin deficiency emphysema Idiopathic pulmonary arterial hypertension
Adult heart-lung	Congenital heart disease Idiopathic pulmonary arterial hypertension Cystic fibrosis
Pediatric lung	Cystic fibrosis "Primary pulmonary hypertension" Congenital heart disease "Interstitial pneumonitis" Surfactant protein B deficiency

Operation-Related Complications

Primary Graft Dysfunction

Despite many advances in organ preservation, surgical technique, and perioperative care, primary graft dysfunction, also known as harvest injury, ischemia-reperfusion injury, early graft dysfunction, and reimplantation response, contributes significantly to both the morbidity and mortality for lung transplantation. Primary graft dysfunction affects an estimated 10% to 25% of pulmonary allografts and can range in clinical severity from transient decrease in oxygenation to complete graft failure.[10] The International Society for Heart and Lung Transplantation (ISHLT) has proposed a definition and a grading scheme based on the chest film and Pao_2/Fio_2 ratio.[11]

Time Period

Primary graft dysfunction becomes apparent within 72 hours after transplantation.

Clinical Presentation

Primary graft dysfunction has many features in common with other forms of acute lung injury, including severe hypoxemia and pulmonary edema.

Radiologic Findings

Chest radiographs show panlobar alveolar infiltrates.

Diagnosis

The diagnosis of primary graft dysfunction is based on the radiographic and Pao_2/Fio_2 criteria as well as on exclusion of clinically similar conditions such as acute antibody-mediated rejection, venous anastomotic obstruction, cardiogenic pulmonary edema, and pneumonia.[11] In selected cases, a lung biopsy may be helpful.[12]

Pathologic Findings

Mild cases may show alveolar and interstitial edema with scattered neutrophils.[13] The histologic correlate of severe primary graft dysfunction is diffuse alveolar damage.[12] The acute phase of diffuse alveolar damage is characterized by hyaline membranes, interstitial edema, occasional fibrin thrombi, and scattered neutrophils in the alveolar septa (Fig. 12-1). In the organizing phase, hyaline membranes are incorporated into the alveolar septa, which become thickened by fibroblast-rich connective tissue (Fig. 12-2).

Histologic Differential Diagnosis

Diffuse alveolar damage is a nonspecific histologic pattern that can be elicited by various insults in the post-transplantation setting (Box 12-1). Immunofluorescent studies are helpful in separating primary graft dysfunction from acute antibody-mediated rejection. Acute antibody-mediated rejection is characterized by alveolar septal deposits of IgG and complement (particularly C4d), which are absent in primary graft dysfunction. Acute rejection is not a major concern during the immediate post-transplantation period. Any infection can manifest as diffuse alveolar damage in an immunocompromised patient; therefore, it is always prudent to perform special stains to rule out acid-fast bacilli and fungal organisms.

Treatment, Prognosis, and Prevention

The treatment is supportive and may include mechanical ventilation. A retrospective analysis by Christie and associates showed that in patients with and those without primary graft dysfunction, 30-day mortality rates are 42.1% and 6.1%, respectively.[14] Primary graft dysfunction is also associated with an increased risk of obliterative bronchiolitis.[15] For prevention of primary graft dysfunction, research studies have focused on improving lung preservation techniques by optimizing the volume, temperature, pressure and components of preservation solutions, and inflation and ventilation parameters of the organs during transport.[10] So far, these studies have had modest clinical impact.

Table 12-2. Complications of Lung Transplantation

Post-Transplantation Period	Operation-Related Complications	Rejection	Immunosuppression-Related Complications	Other Complications
Immediate (within 4 days)	Primary graft dysfunction Arterial anastomotic obstruction Venous anastomotic obstruction Airway dehiscence	Acute antibody-mediated rejection	Bacterial pneumonia	
Early (4 days to 1 month)	Arterial anastomotic obstruction Venous anastomotic obstruction Airway dehiscence Large airway stenosis	Acute rejection	Infection (bacterial, viral, fungal, *Pneumocystis jiroveci*)	
Late (beyond 1 month)	Large airway stenosis	Acute rejection Chronic airway rejection	Infection (bacterial, viral, fungal, *Pneumocystis jiroveci*) Post-transplantation lymphoproliferative disorders	Organizing pneumonia Recurrence of the primary disease

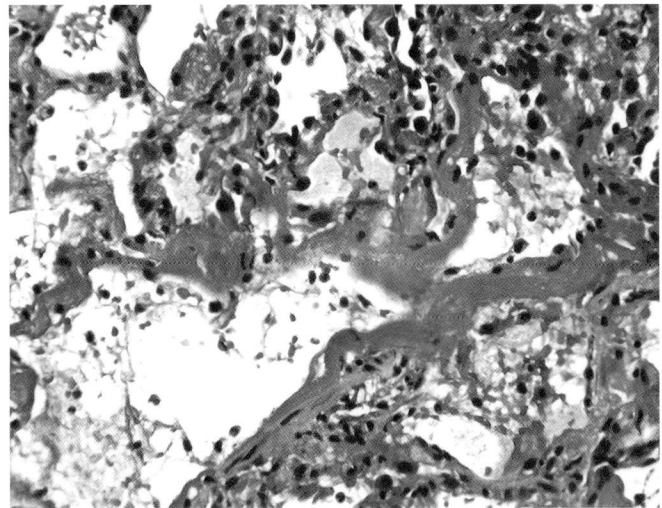

Figure 12-1. Acute diffuse alveolar damage due to harvest injury. The key to the diagnosis is the presence of hyaline membranes.

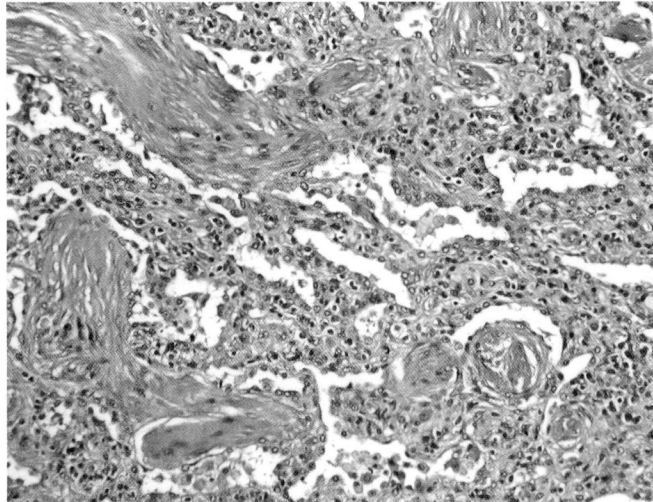

Figure 12-2. Organizing diffuse alveolar damage resulting from harvest injury. In the absence of residual hyaline membranes, the history can aid the diagnosis.

Box 12-1. Common Causes of Diffuse Alveolar Damage in the Pulmonary Allograft

Harvest injury
Acute antibody-mediated rejection
Severe acute rejection
Infection

Arterial Anastomotic Obstruction

The incidence of pulmonary arterial anastomotic obstruction after lung transplantation is relatively low.[16] Causes include narrowed anastomosis, with or without thrombus formation resulting from suboptimal surgical anastomoses and excessive length of donor or recipient pulmonary artery with kinking or torsion of the anastomosis.[16]

Time Period

Arterial anastomotic obstruction usually occurs during the first week after transplantation.

Clinical Presentation

Signs and symptoms include dyspnea, hypoxemia, and elevated pulmonary arterial pressure.

Diagnosis

The diagnosis is suggested by reduced perfusion in the allograft by ventilation-perfusion (V/Q) scan and can be confirmed by echocardiogram or pulmonary angiography. Large areas of infarction may be present. Pathologic confirmation is usually not required.

Venous Anastomotic Obstruction

Minor abnormalities of the pulmonary venous anastomosis are relatively common complications of lung transplantation.[17] Occlusive thrombus formation is relatively rare but may have catastrophic consequences, including allograft failure and stroke.

Time Period

Venous anastomotic obstruction usually presents in the immediate post-transplantation period but has been reported to occur as late as the eighth postoperative day.[16]

Clinical Presentation

Pulmonary venous obstruction after lung transplantation should be suspected in every case of persistent pulmonary edema in the first postoperative days, often associated with a frothy blood-stained secretion from the endotracheal tube.[18]

Radiologic Findings

Chest radiograph reveals diffuse unilateral interstitial edema.

Diagnosis

Transesophageal echocardiography with color-flow Doppler imaging is virtually diagnostic, demonstrating a marked reduction of the flow in the affected pulmonary vein.[18]

Pathologic Findings

The specimen from the surgical revision may include a thrombus. Biopsy of the lung obtained at the same time may show congestion and venous engorgement.

Treatment

Venous anastomotic obstruction is considered a surgical emergency, and revision of the anastomosis with removal of any associated thrombus is required to prevent irreversible injury to the lung allograft.

Airway Dehiscence

In the early years of lung transplantation, airway dehiscence due to ischemia of the donor bronchus was a major cause of morbidity and death. Improved surgical techniques, reduced immunosuppression, and better allograft preservation have reduced the incidence of airway complications.[19] Currently, most centers report a 7% to 18% complication rate with a related mortality rate of 2% to 4%.[19]

Time Period

Airway dehiscence may develop in the first few weeks after transplantation.

Diagnosis

Ischemia and necrosis of the bronchus can be diagnosed by direct visualization with a bronchoscope.

Pathologic Findings

Biopsies show coagulation necrosis of the bronchial mucosa, submucosa, and cartilage. Superimposed bacterial or fungal infection may produce neutrophilic infiltrates, thereby enhancing necrosis and dehiscence of the anastomosis.

Treatment

Surgical options are limited, but may include anastomotic revision, retransplantation, or stent placement.

Large Airway Stenosis

Large airway (bronchial) stenosis is the most common airway complication. The incidence is estimated to be between 1.6% and 32%.[19] It is usually seen after necrosis or dehiscence or in healing or treated infections. "Telescoped" anastomosis is associated with a 7% incidence of airway stenosis.

Nonanastomotic large airway stenosis has also been described.[20,21] The pathogenesis of this lesion is unclear, but it may represent a response to ischemic damage, alloreactive injury, or infection.

Time Period

Bronchial stenosis usually occurs a few months after the transplantation procedure but has been described as early as 8 days.[22]

Clinical Presentation

Clinical findings include dyspnea, retained secretions, recurrent pneumonia, and decline in spirometry, all of which can mimic chronic airway rejection.

Diagnosis

Bronchoscopic examination provides the diagnosis, with biopsies providing confirmatory histology.

Pathologic Findings

Common findings include prominent granulation tissue, fibrosis, and squamous metaplasia.

Treatment

Airway stenting is often used as the primary management option for airway complications after lung transplantation.[23]

Rejection

With the exception of monozygotic twins, donors and recipients are genetically different and express different histocompatibility antigens. As a result, allografts are rejected by the recipient's immune system. Multiple immunologic processes are involved, creating a spectrum of rejection responses. A "working formulation for the classification of pulmonary allograft rejection" was introduced by the ISHLT in 1990.[24] The working formulation was first revised in 1996.[25] The currently accepted scheme for grading pulmonary allograft rejection was approved by the ISHLT board of directors in 2007 (Box 12-2).[8] The differences between the 1996 and 2007 schemes are relatively minor and are related to airway inflammation and chronic airway rejection. Acute antibody-mediated rejection is a controversial subject and is not included in the 2007 working formulation. For the sake of completeness, however, it is discussed at the end of this section.

Acute (Cellular) Rejection

The term *acute rejection* without a qualifier is used to describe acute cellular rejection. This is a cell-mediated process, in contrast to the antibody-mediated process of acute antibody-mediated (humoral)

Box 12-2. 2007 Revised Working Formulation for Classification and Grading of Pulmonary Allograft Rejection

A. Acute rejection
　Grade 0: none
　Grade 1: minimal
　Grade 2: mild
　Grade 3: moderate
　Grade 4: severe
B. Airway inflammation
　Grade 0: none
　Grade 1R: low grade
　Grade 2R: high grade
　Grade X: ungradable
C. Chronic airway rejection—obliterative bronchiolitis
　0: absent
　1: present
D. Chronic vascular rejection—accelerated graft vascular sclerosis

rejection. Most lung transplant recipients experience episodes of acute rejection.

Time Period

Acute rejection may occur as early as 3 days and as late as several years after transplantation. The majority of acute rejection episodes begin within the first 3 months after transplantation.

Clinical Presentation

Clinical features may include low-grade fever, cough, dyspnea, crackles, and adventitious sounds on auscultation. Features suspicious for rejection include a more than 10% decrease in the forced expiratory volume in 1 minute (FEV_1) and hypoxemia.

Radiologic Findings

Radiologic abnormalities include perihilar or lower lung zone alveolar and interstitial infiltrates, septal lines, subpleural edema, peribronchial cuffing, and pleural effusion. In cases of a single-lung transplant, the V/Q lung scan will show decreased perfusion to the allograft.

Diagnosis

Clinical features may suggest acute rejection, but a transbronchial biopsy usually is required to confirm the diagnosis and rule out infection. If biopsy from multiple sites is technically impossible, lower lobe biopsies are preferred because they appear to be more informative.[26]

Pathologic Findings

The hallmark of acute rejection is the presence of perivascular mononuclear cell infiltrates. If small airway inflammation is present, it should be noted (see later discussion).

Acute rejection is graded according to the density and extent of the perivascular infiltrates and the presence or absence of secondary pneumocyte damage (Table 12-3). Rejection-type infiltrates usually involve more than one vessel, but a single perivascular infiltrate should be evaluated by the same criteria as for multiple infiltrates, as follows:

1. Minimal acute rejection (grade A1) is characterized by infrequent two- to three-cell-thick perivascular mononuclear cell infiltrates (Fig. 12-3).

2. In mild acute rejection (grade A2), the perivascular mononuclear cell infiltrates become thicker, denser, and usually more frequent (Fig. 12-4).

Table 12-3. Grading Acute Rejection

Grade of Acute Rejection	Histologic Criteria	Cellular Composition	Comments
A0—none	Normal pulmonary parenchyma		
A1—minimal	Perivascular mononuclear cell infiltrates, 2–3 cells thick (not obvious at low magnification)	Small round, plasmacytoid, and transformed lymphocytes	The perivascular infiltrates are usually infrequent
A2—mild	Perivascular mononuclear cell infiltrates, >3 cells thick (easily seen at low magnification)	Same as A1, with macrophages, and eosinophils	The perivascular infiltrates are usually frequent Endothelialitis and airway inflammation are often present
A3—moderate	Perivascular mononuclear cell infiltrates, similar to A2, with extension into alveolar septa and air spaces	Same as A2, with occasional neutrophils	Endothelialitis and airway inflammation are usually present
A4—severe	Diffuse mononuclear cell infiltrates, similar to A3, with prominent pneumocyte damage	Same as A3	The pneumocyte damage is commonly associated with hyaline membranes

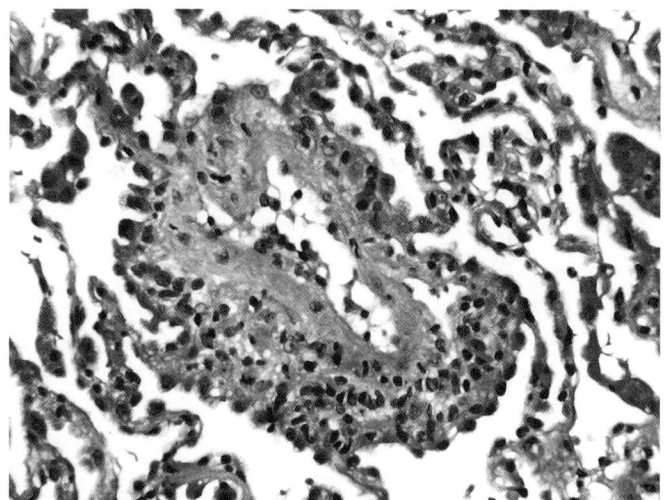

Figure 12-3. Minimal acute rejection (A1) with sparse perivascular mononuclear cell infiltrate.

3. In moderate acute rejection (grade A3), the infiltrates extend into the alveolar septa and air spaces (Fig. 12-5).
4. In severe acute rejection (grade A4), the mononuclear cell infiltrates are associated with pneumocyte damage. The latter often manifests as diffuse alveolar damage with hyaline membranes (Fig. 12-6).

The composition of the cellular infiltrates also changes with increasing severity of rejection. In minimal acute rejection, the perivascular infiltrates are composed predominantly of small, round, plasmacytoid, and transformed lymphocytes. As the rejection advances in intensity, the infiltrates contain more activated lymphocytes, macrophages, eosinophils, and neutrophils. Subendothelial and peribronchiolar infiltrates become more pronounced.

In higher-grade rejection, the inflammatory cells permeate through the vessels with extension to the endothelium, giving rise to endothelialitis. In 30% of mild and 60% of moderate acute rejection, there is also associated airway inflammation.

A rare form of acute rejection also exists, characterized by abundant eosinophils, which may obscure the mononuclear cells in the perivascular infiltrates.

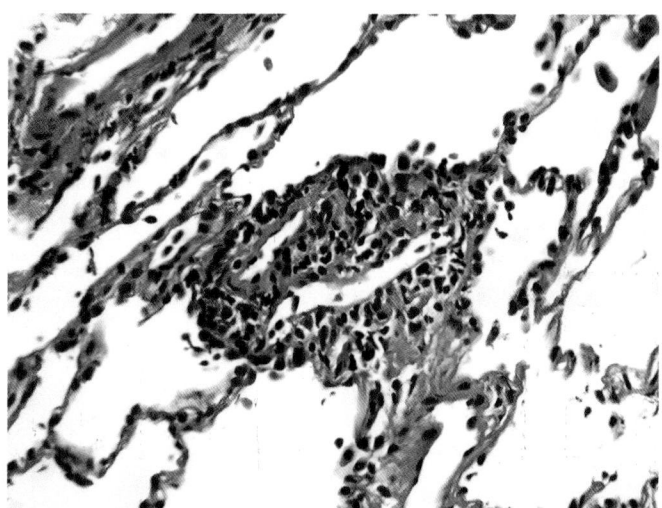

Figure 12-4. In mild acute rejection (A2), the mononuclear cell infiltrate is denser and is more than three cell layers thick. However, it is limited to the perivascular area.

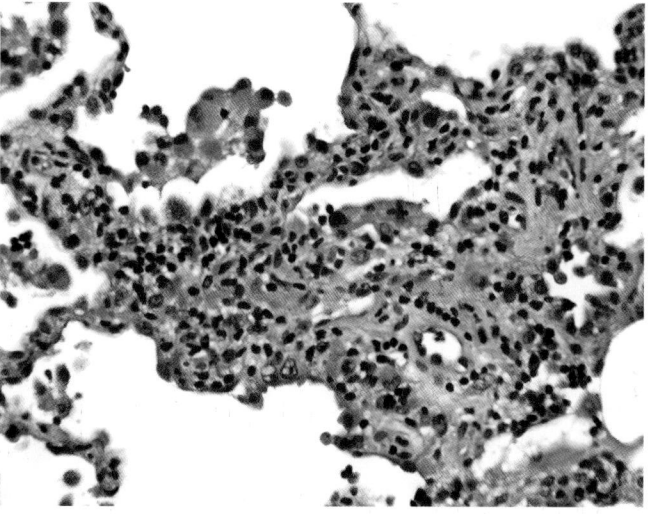

Figure 12-5. In moderate acute rejection (A3), the perivascular infiltrate extends into the alveolar septa.

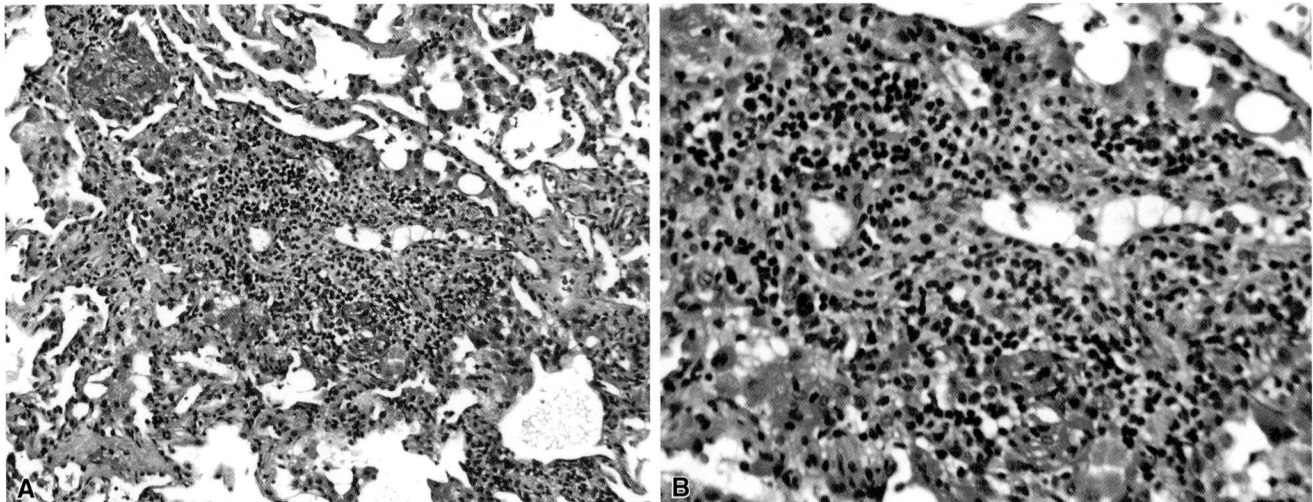

Figure 12-6. In severe acute rejection (A4), the perivascular infiltrates lead to lung injury. The latter manifests as fibrinous exudates and hyaline membranes in this case. **A,** Lower magnification. **B,** Higher magnification.

Histologic Differential Diagnosis

Perivascular and interstitial mononuclear cell infiltrates are not specific for acute rejection.[8] Differential diagnostic considerations include infections, especially cytomegalovirus pneumonia and *Pneumocystis jiroveci* pneumonia,[27-29] and PTLDs.[30] Some histologic features may favor infection over acute rejection (Table 12-4). Cultures and special stains may be helpful in the diagnosis of mycobacterial, fungal, and *Pneumocystis jiroveci* infections. Viral pneumonias can be confirmed by cultures as well as serologic, immunohistochemical, or molecular hybridization techniques.

In some cases, histologic features of acute rejection and infection coexist. In these cases, the pathologist should attempt to decide which is dominant and guide the clinician by favoring one over the other. Follow-up biopsy after appropriate antimicrobial therapy is also recommended so that any acute rejection component can be reassessed.[8] The differential diagnosis between acute rejection and PTLDs is discussed later.

Table 12-4. Histologic Features Favoring Infection over Acute Rejection

Histologic Features	Infection Favored
Predominant alveolar septal infiltrates as compared with perivascular infiltrates	Any infection
Abundant neutrophils	Bacterial pneumonia, CMV pneumonia, or candidiasis
Abundant eosinophils	Fungal infection
Nuclear or cytoplasmic inclusions	Viral pneumonia
Multinucleation	Respiratory syncytial virus or parainfluenza virus pneumonia
Punctate zones of necrosis	Herpes simplex virus, varicella-zoster virus, or CMV pneumonia
Granulomatous inflammation	Mycobacterial, fungal, or *Pneumocystis jiroveci* infection
Frothy intra-alveolar exudates	*Pneumocystis jiroveci* pneumonia

CMV, cytomegalovirus.

Treatment and Prognosis

The treatment of acute rejection typically consists of bolus therapy with intravenous steroids, which may be supplemented by temporary increases in the maintenance immunosuppression regimen. In at least 80% of the cases, acute rejection is successfully treated. However, 15% to 20% of acute rejection episodes persist or recur, presenting a particularly difficult management problem for the clinician. When this occurs, intensified immunosuppression with one or more agents is usually attempted. However, it has been shown that patients with persistent, recurrent, or late (occurring at least 3 months after transplantation) acute rejection are at increased risk for developing chronic airway rejection.[31] Recent studies have indicated that an increased risk may exist even with minimal acute rejection.[32,33]

Airway Inflammation: Lymphocytic Bronchiolitis

The 2007 working formulation has collapsed the four previous B grades into two (grade 1R—low grade and grade 2R—high grade) and has retained B0 (no airway inflammation) and BX (ungradable). Another change from the previous working formulation is that the B grade designation applies only to small airways (bronchioles). Airway inflammation may be a harbinger of chronic airway rejection.[34,35]

Pathologic Findings

Criteria for grading airway inflammation are listed in Table 12-5.

Histologic Differential Diagnosis

Infection, particularly that caused by viral, bacterial, mycoplasmal, fungal, and chlamydial organisms, may mimic the airway inflammation related to acute rejection.[28]

Chronic Airway Rejection: Obliterative Bronchiolitis

Obliterative bronchiolitis is the most significant long-term complication of lung transplantation, with a prevalence of 30% to 50% and an associated mortality rate of 25%.[36] The terminology is somewhat confusing, because obliterative bronchiolitis of chronic airway rejection is sometimes referred to as bronchiolitis obliterans or bronchiolitis obliterans syndrome in the clinical lung transplantation literature. It is important to recognize that obliterative bronchiolitis or bronchiolitis obliterans of chronic airway rejection is both clinically and histologically distinct from the (sub)acute lung injury

Table 12-5. Grading Airway Inflammation

Grade	Airway Inflammation
B0—no airway inflammation	None
B1R—low-grade small airway inflammation	Mononuclear cells in the submucosa (can be infrequent and scattered or forming band-like infiltrates) Occasional eosinophils may be seen
B2R—high-grade small airway inflammation	Mononuclear cells in the submucosa with greater numbers of eosinophils Epithelial damage and intraepithelial lymphocytic infiltration Ulceration and fibrinopurulent exudates may occur
BX—ungradable	Sampling problems, infection, tangential cutting, other problems

pattern once known as bronchiolitis obliterans organizing pneumonia (BOOP). To make this distinction clear, the nomenclature has been changed, and the currently preferred term for BOOP is *organizing pneumonia*.[37]

Time Period
Obliterative bronchiolitis is most frequently diagnosed between 9 and 15 months after transplantation.[38] It rarely develops during the first 3 months but has been reported as early as 2 months after transplantation.[38]

Clinical Presentation
Obliterative bronchiolitis often develops insidiously with vague general symptoms, and nonproductive cough. Later, progressive dyspnea on exertion becomes the dominant complaint. At this later stage, pulmonary function tests show a decline in the FEV_1 as compared to a previously established post-transplantation baseline.

Radiologic Findings
Chest radiographs are typically unremarkable until later in the disease, when a variable pattern of bronchiectasis is accompanied by airway tapering/obliteration and zones of hyperinflation. These changes reflect the peculiar nature of chronic airway rejection—proximal bronchiectasis (dilatation) with distal obliterative bronchiolitis (constriction).

Diagnosis
Transbronchial biopsy is an insensitive method for the detection of obliterative bronchiolitis.[8] An ad hoc ISHLT working group has concluded that FEV_1 is the most reliable and consistent indicator of chronic airway rejection.[39]

Pathologic Findings
The term *obliterative bronchiolitis* refers to hyalinized fibrous plaques present in the submucosa of small airways.[8,13] They lead to partial or complete luminal compromise (Fig. 12-7). The scar tissue may be concentric or eccentric and may be associated with destruction of the smooth muscle wall. The 1996 working formulation retained the designation of active versus inactive obliterative bronchiolitis, depending on the presence and degree of accompanying inflammation.[25] However, the consensus in 2007 was that the distinction between active and inactive is no longer useful, and the condition should be designated merely as C0, indicating a biopsy with no evidence of obliterative bronchiolitis, and C1, indicating that obliterative bronchiolitis is present in the biopsy.[8] Obliterative bronchiolitis often produces mucostasis or postobstructive (endogenous lipid) pneumonia.[8,13]

Histologic Differential Diagnosis
Transplant-related obliterative bronchiolitis involves the small airways. Large airway fibrosis is a nonspecific finding and should not be considered as evidence of chronic airway rejection. Organizing pneumonia pattern is manifested as fibromyxoid connective tissue plugs within the lumina of bronchioles and alveoli.[40] These loose edematous airspace-filling plugs should be distinguished from the densely eosinophilic submucosal scars of transplant bronchiolitis obliterans.

Treatment and Prognosis
Augmented immunosuppression appears to be of some benefit in treating bronchiolitis obliterans, but it is far from optimal. Avoiding this complication of lung transplantation may require better use of current immunosuppressive medications, or the development of novel immunosuppressive strategies.[38]

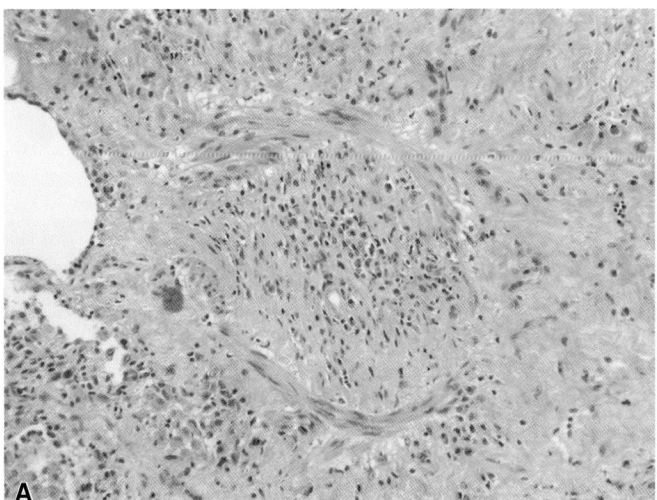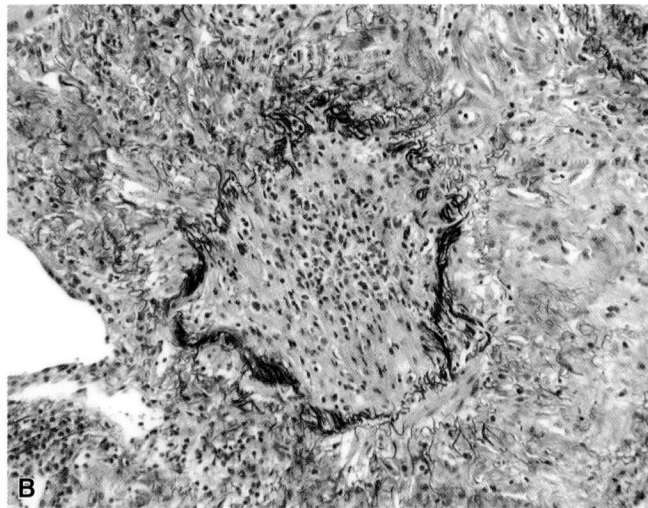

Figure 12-7. Bronchiolitis obliterans. Scar tissue obliterates the lumen of a bronchiole, which can be recognized by the presence of smooth muscle and elastic fibers in the wall. **A,** Hematoxylin-eosin stain. **B,** Elastic–van Gieson stain.

Chronic Vascular Rejection: Accelerated Graft Vascular Sclerosis

The clinicopathologic significance of chronic vascular rejection is not entirely clear. However, chronic vascular changes may coincide with the presence of obliterative bronchiolitis in lung transplant recipients and with the presence of accelerated coronary artery disease in combined heart-lung transplant recipients.[41,42]

Diagnosis

Chronic vascular rejection is not applicable with transbronchial biopsies but may be noted in surgical lung samples.[8]

Pathologic Findings

In chronic vascular rejection, there is fibrointimal thickening in arteries and veins (Fig. 12-8). There may also be an "active" inflammatory component consisting of subendothelial, intimal, or medial, predominantly lymphoid, mononuclear cell infiltrates.

Acute Antibody-Mediated (Humoral) Rejection

Acute antibody-mediated (humoral) rejection is mediated by antibodies specific for donor antigens, particularly those of the human leukocyte antigen (HLA) system. These antibodies, which may develop before and after transplantation, bind to target antigens and activate the complement system, leading to tissue injury.[43,44] Improvements in anti-HLA antibody detection have increased recognition of antibody-mediated rejection following renal, heart, and lung transplantation.[43,45,46] Early observations of acute antibody-mediated rejection were based on the phenomenon of hyperacute rejection, in which pre-existent antibodies lead to complement activation and rapid graft loss. With improved cross-matching before transplantation, the incidence of hyperacute rejection has decreased.

Time Period

Hyperacute rejection is noticeable within minutes to hours after transplantation. However, humoral sensitization and acute antibody-mediated rejection may also occur beyond the immediate post-transplantation period.

Clinical Presentation

Clinical findings include progressive respiratory failure.

Radiologic Findings

In hyperacute rejection, complete opacification of the pulmonary allograft is seen.

Diagnosis

The presence of donor-specific anti-HLA antibodies in the context of vascular C4d deposition and refractory acute rejection fulfills the criteria for antibody-mediated rejection.[47] Assays used for HLA antibody screening and identification include complement-dependent cytotoxicity (CDC) and solid-phase technologies such as enzyme-linked immunosorbent assay (ELISA), flow cytometry, and Luminex analysis.[43]

Pathologic Findings

The recent ISHLT report remains very cautious in discussing the pathologic appearance of acute antibody-mediated rejection.[8] The consensus is that capillaritis, along with immunofluorescent or immunohistochemical staining for C4d, should raise clinical suspicion for acute antibody-mediated rejection.[48,49] Histologic features of hyperacute rejection also include diffuse alveolar damage.[50-52]

Histologic Differential Diagnosis

Capillaritis is a nonspecific histologic finding that may occur in infection, diffuse alveolar damage, and severe acute cellular rejection.[8] However, the presence of capillaritis and C4d staining as well as anti-HLA antibodies should be seen as strong evidence for acute antibody-mediated rejection.

Prevention, Treatment, and Prognosis

One of the major goals in donor selection is to avoid HLA antigens against which the potential recipient has preformed antibodies.[43]

Optimal treatment of acute antibody-mediated rejection remains uncertain. Intravenous immunoglobulin (IVIG) is one of the most common therapies used to decrease antibody-mediated immunity.[53] Rituximab, an anti-CD20 monoclonal antibody that causes B cell depletion, has been proved effective in the treatment of presensitized renal transplant recipients in conjunction with IVIG.[43] Plasmapheresis has been shown to lead to clinical improvement in lung transplant recipients with pulmonary capillaritis unresponsive to steroids.[48] However, it is usually reserved for severe cases of suspected acute antibody-mediated rejection, given the side effects and difficulties of administration.

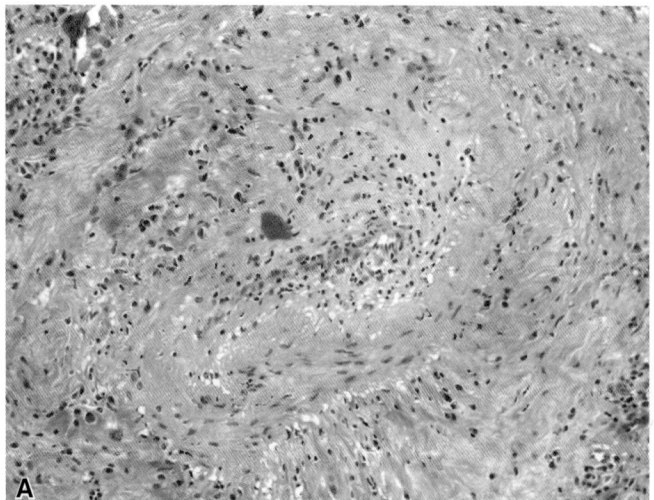
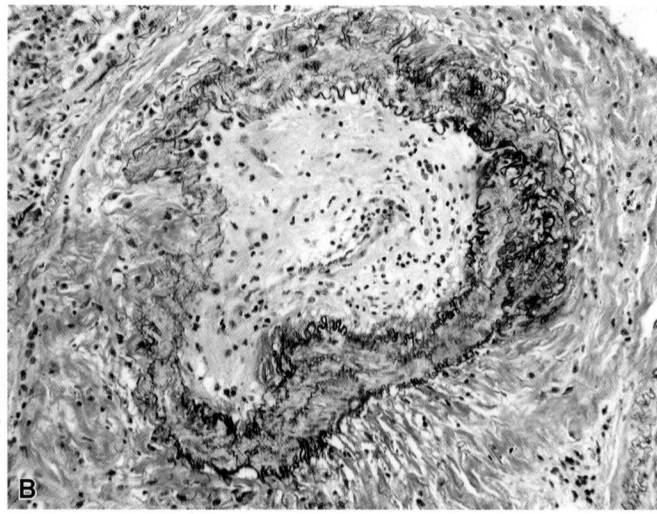

Figure 12-8. Chronic vascular rejection (accelerated vascular sclerosis). Intimal proliferation occludes the lumen of a muscular pulmonary artery, which can be recognized by the presence of two elastic laminae. **A,** Hematoxylin-eosin stain. **B,** Elastic–van Gieson stain.

Infection

Pulmonary infections are the most common cause of morbidity in the lung transplant population. Prompt recognition and treatment are necessary to prevent poor outcomes.

Bacterial Infections

Cystic fibrosis patients frequently show airway colonization with gram-negative bacteria both before and after lung transplantation. Recent data suggest that colonization with gram-negative bacteria may play a role in the pathogenesis of chronic airway rejection.[54]

Bacterial infections of the lower respiratory tract may manifest as acute bronchitis or bronchopneumonia. Gram-negative infections, especially those caused by *Pseudomonas* species, account for about 75% of bacterial pneumonias. Other reported bacterial pathogens include a wide range of nosocomial organisms. Legionellosis is rarely reported.[55]

Time Period
Bacterial infections can occur shortly after transplantation presumably due to transmission of bacteria from the donor. Nevertheless, the risk of bacterial infection persists throughout the lifetime of the allograft.

Clinical Presentation
The clinical findings include fever, cough, purulent sputum, shortness of breath, rales on auscultation, hypoxemia, leukocytosis, and decline in spirometry.

Radiologic Findings
New or increasing infiltrates on chest radiograph are common manifestations of bacterial pneumonias.

Diagnosis
Most of the clinical features of transplant-associated pneumonia are nonspecific and largely modified by the patient's immunocompromised status. Bronchoalveolar lavage (BAL) and transbronchial biopsy are often performed in the evaluation of new infiltrates. Culture results are often an important part of the diagnostic workup.

Pathologic Findings
In acute bronchitis, neutrophils infiltrate the bronchial mucosa. This pathologic change may be associated with mucosal ulceration and intraluminal neutrophils. As in the normal host, acute pneumonia is recognized by the presence of neutrophils within the alveolar spaces (Fig. 12-9).

Histologic Differential Diagnosis
The composition of inflammatory infiltrates distinguishes bacterial infection from acute rejection. Bacterial infection is characterized by the presence of neutrophils, whereas mononuclear cells (mainly lymphoid cells) are seen predominantly in acute rejection.

Treatment and Prognosis
Organism-specific management is essential. Any regimen of broad-spectrum antibiotics instituted before identification of an organism should include agents effective against *Pseudomonas* species.

Viral Infections

Cytomegalovirus (CMV) infection remains a serious problem in lung transplant recipients. Donor-recipient mismatch, with the donor being seropositive and the recipient seronegative for CMV, poses the highest risk for the development of CMV pneumonia. Seropositive

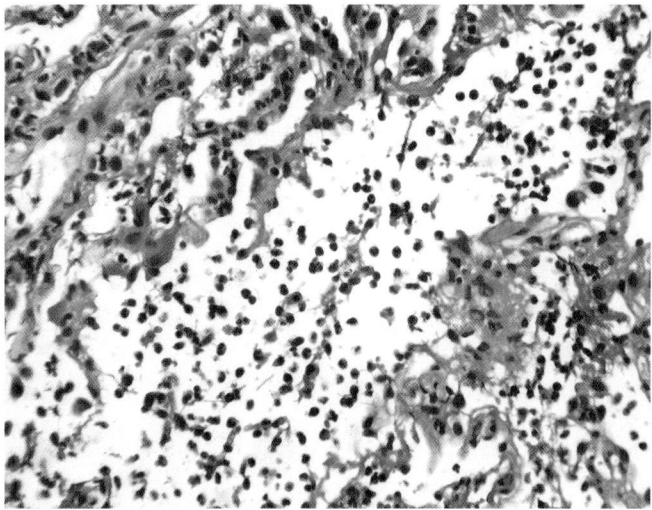

Figure 12-9. Acute pneumonia. Neutrophil granulocytes are present in the alveolar spaces.

recipients of a seropositive or seronegative donor are at intermediate risk of acquiring active CMV pneumonia, and seronegative recipients of a seronegative donor are at lowest risk. Universal ganciclovir prophylaxis is a strategy aimed at reducing CMV infection and delaying the development of obliterative bronchiolitis. However, the optimal duration of ganciclovir prophylaxis remains unclear. If the prophylaxis is discontinued, the incidence of CMV pneumonia is around 57%.[56] A recent study has suggested that indefinite ganciclovir prophylaxis may prevent CMV pneumonia in 98% of lung transplant recipients.[56]

Herpes simplex virus (HSV) infections are also a potential problem in lung transplantation. The frequency of HSV infections has also been reduced remarkably with the routine use of ganciclovir prophylaxis.

Other viruses responsible for respiratory infections include adenovirus, respiratory syncytial virus, influenzavirus, parainfluenza virus, and varicella-zoster virus.[57,58]

Time Period
Before universal ganciclovir prophylaxis, CMV infection generally occurred between 2 weeks and 4 months after transplantation. HSV infection typically began as oral ulcers or tracheitis during the first month after transplantation.

Clinical Presentation
Fever, malaise, myalgias, chills, abdominal discomfort, cough, and shortness of breath are frequent symptoms of CMV pneumonia. Physical examination may reveal crackles or may be normal. Other features include hypoxemia and decline in spirometry values. Fortunately, pneumonia caused by HSV is now rare, thanks to routine prophylaxis. The clinical features are similar to those of CMV pneumonia.

Radiologic Findings
Chest radiographs may show reticular or reticulonodular infiltrates but may be clear in up to two thirds of patients.

Diagnosis
The diagnosis of viral pneumonia is often impossible on clinical grounds alone. BAL and transbronchial biopsy play important roles in establishing the diagnosis.

Pathologic Findings

Recognizing tissue responses and cytopathic effects may help in identifying viral infections (see Chapter 6). Tissue responses to viral pathogens range from minimal nonspecific inflammation to diffuse alveolar damage. Most cases of CMV infection show interstitial pneumonia with a mixed lymphocytic and polymorphonuclear cell infiltrate[27] (Figs. 12-10 and 12-11). Zonal necrosis may be seen with herpes simplex, varicella-zoster, and CMV pneumonia (Figs. 12-12 and 12-13). CMV may also be associated with neutrophilic microabscesses. Necrotizing bronchiolitis may be a feature of adenovirus, influenzavirus, and respiratory syncytial virus infections. Some characteristic viral cytopathic effects are listed in Table 12-6. These cytopathic effects, however, can be sparse or absent.

Immunohistochemistry, in situ hybridization, and polymerase chain reaction (PCR) techniques can be used to identify many viruses and have largely replaced electron microscopy in this role (Fig. 12-14).

Histologic Differential Diagnosis

The histologic differential diagnosis of viral pneumonia includes acute rejection.[27] Both processes can exhibit perivascular and interstitial mononuclear cell infiltrates. However, perivascular infiltrates

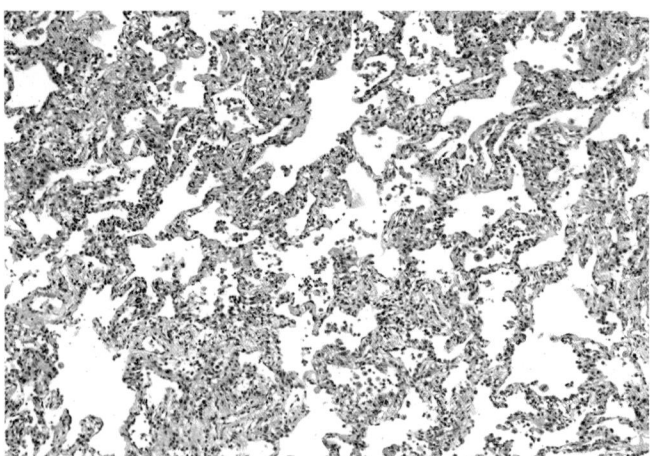

Figure 12-10. Cytomegalovirus pneumonia. Mononuclear cells infiltrate the alveolar septa diffusely, with no perivascular accentuation.

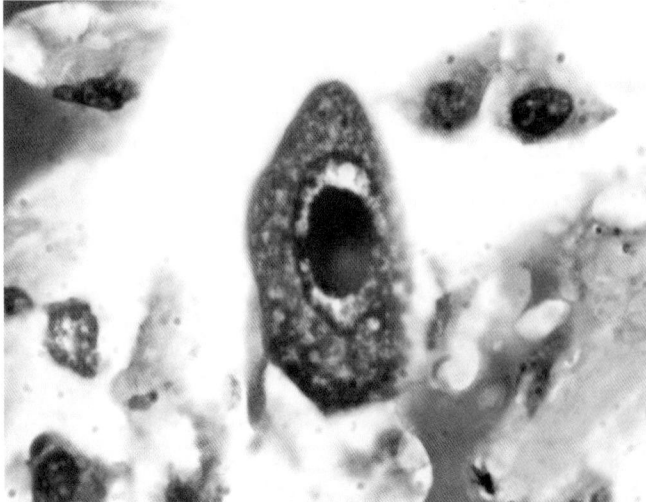

Figure 12-11. Cytopathic effects characteristic of cytomegalovirus infection. Both nuclear and cytoplasmic inclusions are present, but the latter are less apparent.

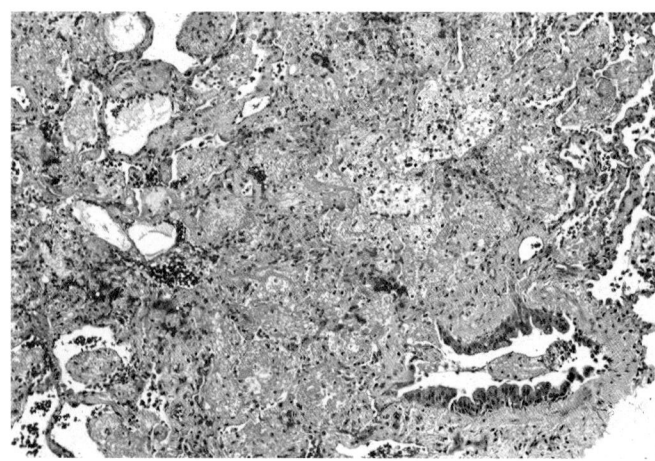

Figure 12-12. Herpes simplex virus pneumonia with an area of necrosis.

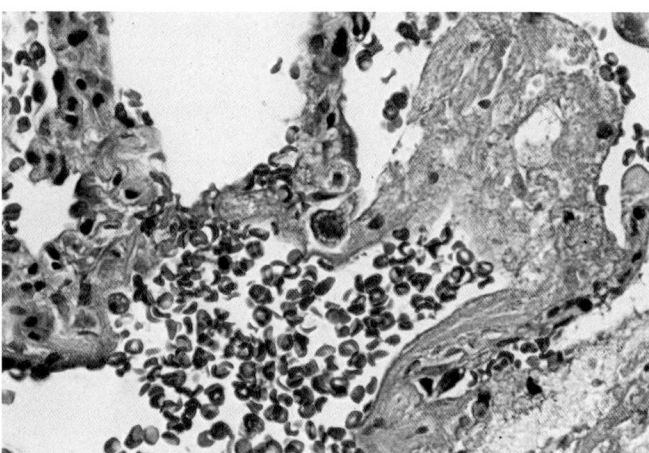

Figure 12-13. Higher-power view of involved lung in herpes simplex pneumonia showing a nuclear inclusion.

Table 12-6. Viruses and Their Cytopathic Effects

Virus	Cytopathic Effects
Cytomegalovirus	Cytomegaly, nuclear and cytoplasmic inclusions
Herpes simplex virus	Nuclear inclusions
Varicella-zoster virus	Nuclear inclusions
Adenovirus	Smudge cells, nuclear inclusions
Respiratory syncytial virus	Occasional multinucleation, cytoplasmic inclusions
Influenzavirus	None
Parainfluenza virus	Occasional multinucleation, cytoplasmic inclusions

predominate in acute rejection, and alveolar septal infiltrates are more prominent in viral infection (see Table 12-4). The presence of CMV inclusions is indicative of CMV pneumonia, but attention to other histologic details is necessary to exclude concurrent acute rejection and bronchiolitis obliterans, which are frequently associated with CMV infection.

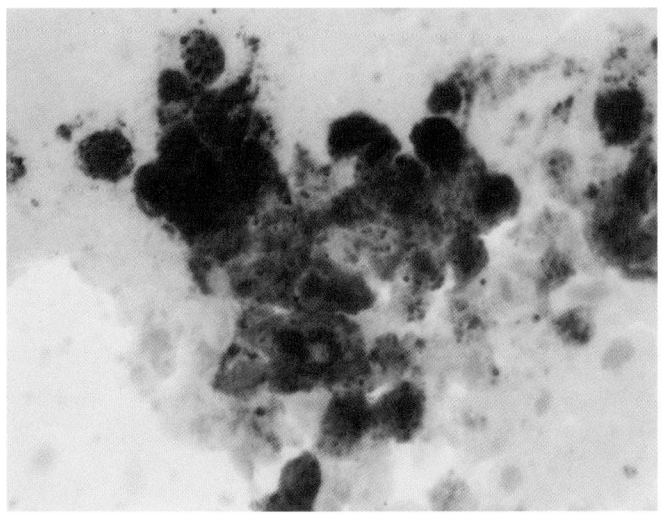

Figure 12-14. Herpes simplex virus infection. Paraffin immunoperoxidase studies reveal herpes simplex virus–positive cells.

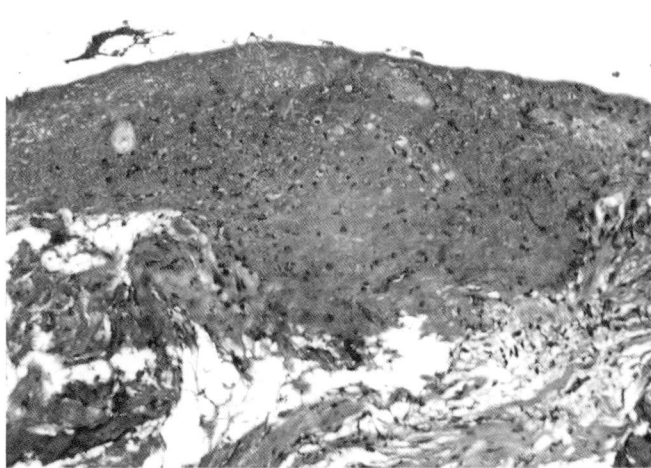

Figure 12-15. Bronchial mucosal necrosis and associated *Aspergillus* infection. There is no significant inflammation.

Fungal Infections

Fungal infections are less frequent than other infections in the transplant recipient but carry a high mortality rate when they do occur. The fungal species most commonly encountered in lung transplant biopsies include *Aspergillus* and *Candida*.[59] Cryptococcosis, histoplasmosis, coccidioidomycosis, and mucormycosis have also been reported.[59,60] Fungal organisms may colonize the respiratory tract or cause overt infection.[60] Prolonged antibiotic therapy predisposes patients to disseminated candidiasis.

Time Period

Fungal infections have a bimodal presentation: early onset between 2 weeks and 2 months after transplantation, secondary to difficult postsurgical periods and prior colonizations; and late onset, primarily secondary to chronic rejection and terminal renal insufficiency.[60]

Clinical Presentation

The clinical picture is not specific. Fungal pneumonias may manifest with fever, leukocytosis, and hypoxemia.

Radiologic Findings

Radiographically, pulmonary infiltrates with consolidation or cavitary nodules may be seen.

Diagnosis

The diagnosis is most often made by a combination of clinical features and the recovery of fungal organisms from BAL, transbronchial biopsy, blood, or other body fluids.

Pathologic Findings

Fungal species may be a source of bronchial anastomotic infections (Figs. 12-15 and 12-16). Aspergillus pneumonia is characterized by hemorrhagic infarction, and sparse inflammatory cell infiltrates (Figs. 12-17 and 12-18). Long, septate hyphae, with 45-degree branching points, invade blood vessels and permeate alveolar septa. Candida infection produces neutrophilic infiltrates and is associated with abscess formation. Clusters of pseudohyphae and yeast forms are often found in the center of abscesses.

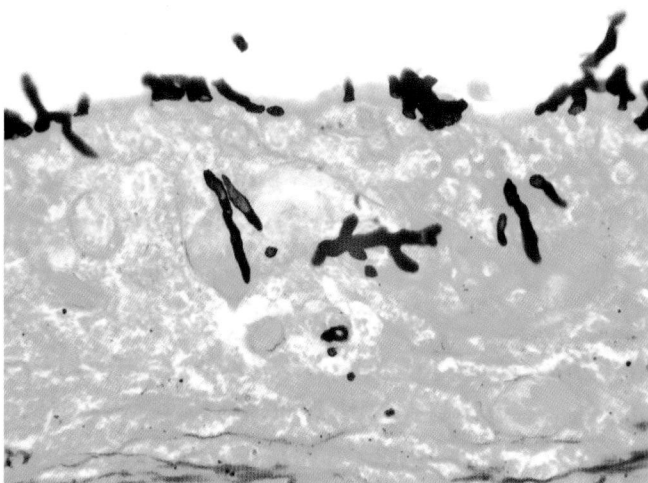

Figure 12-16. Grocott methenamine silver stain of material from the same case as in Figure 12-15 reveals fungal organisms compatible with *Aspergillus* species.

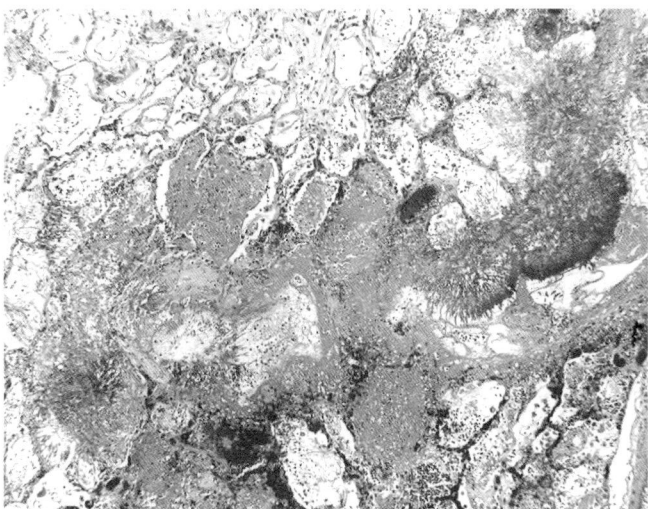

Figure 12-17. *Aspergillus* pneumonia with an area of infarction.

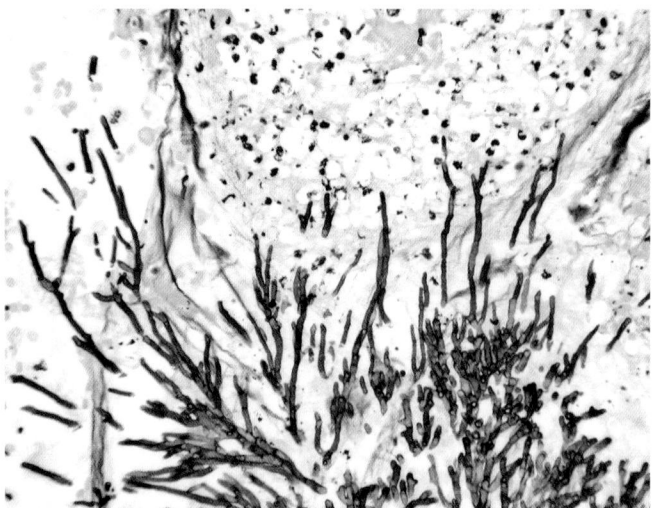

Figure 12-18. Grocott methenamine silver stain of material from the same case as in Figure 12-17 shows vasoinvasive fungal elements compatible with *Aspergillus* species.

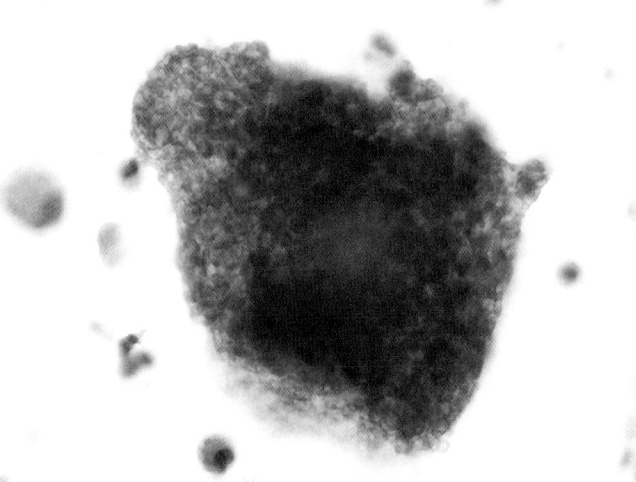

Figure 12-19. *Pneumocystis jiroveci* pneumonia, bronchoalveolar lavage. Frothy exudate can be seen.

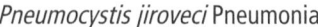

Pneumocystis jiroveci Pneumonia

Although recent studies have strongly suggested that *Pneumocystis jiroveci* (formerly known as *Pneumocystis carinii*) is a fungus, we discuss *Pneumocystis jiroveci* pneumonia separately from other fungal infections for didactic purposes. Without prophylaxis, *Pneumocystis jiroveci* pneumonia occurs in nearly all lung transplant recipients.[61] Thanks to the routine use of prophylaxis, it is rarely seen today in this patient population.

Time Period

Historically, infections were most common around the seventh post-transplantation week.

Clinical Presentation

The clinical presentation is nonspecific and includes cough, fever, dyspnea, and hypoxemia.

Radiologic Findings

Radiographically, diffuse pulmonary infiltrates are seen.

Diagnosis

Because *Pneumocystis jiroveci* cannot be grown in culture, the diagnosis is usually made by identification of the organisms in lavage fluid. Rarely, transbronchial lung biopsy is required.

Pathologic Findings

The classic histologic picture of interstitial pneumonia with frothy intra-alveolar exudates, seen in patients with acquired immunodeficiency syndrome, is rarely encountered in lung transplant recipients (Figs. 12-19 and 12-20). In these patients, *Pneumocystis jiroveci* pneumonia more often manifests as diffuse alveolar damage and the organisms are typically embedded in the prominent hyaline membranes (Fig. 12-21). Granulomatous inflammation is a less common manifestation of infection with *Pneumocystis jiroveci*.

Post-Transplantation Lymphoproliferative Disorders

PTLD lesions are lymphoid or plasmacytic proliferations that develop as a consequence of immunosuppression in an allograft recipient.[62] Characteristics of PTLDs vary somewhat with allograft types and

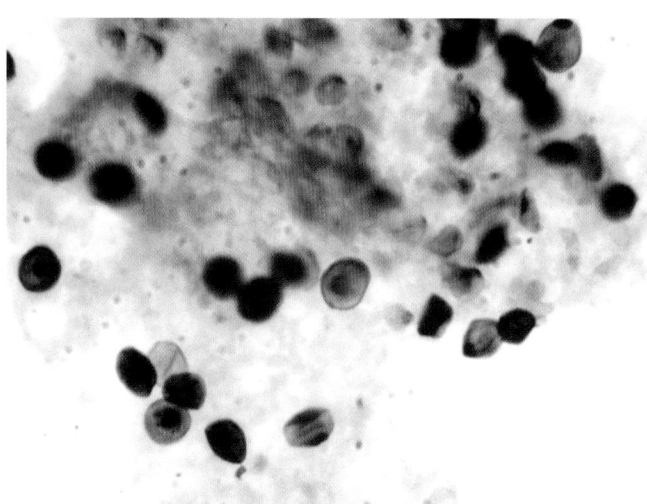

Figure 12-20. Grocott methenamine silver stain of material from the same case as in Figure 12-19 reveals *Pneumocystis jiroveci* organisms.

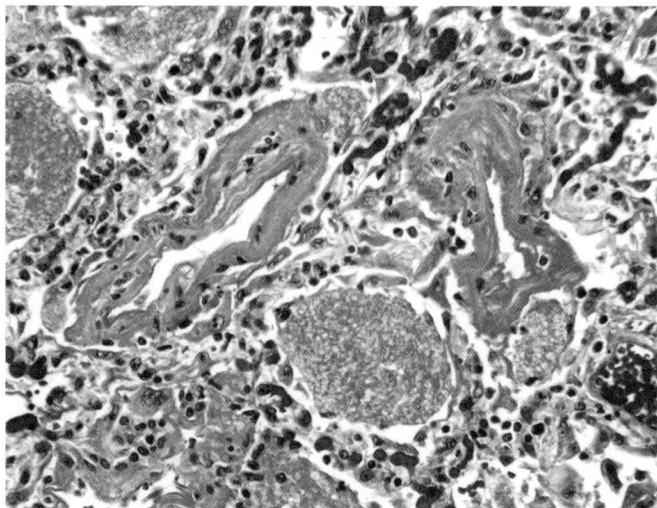

Figure 12-21. *Pneumocystis jiroveci* pneumonia. Both frothy intra-alveolar exudates and hyaline membranes are visible.

with immunosuppressive regimens. PTLDs are relatively more common among pulmonary allograft recipients as a result of higher levels of immunosuppression.[30] In this population, the occurrence rate for PTLDs may be as high as 5%.

A majority of PTLDs are associated with primary or reactivated Epstein-Barr virus (EBV) infection and appear to represent EBV-induced B cell or rarely T cell proliferations. EBV-seronegative recipients who develop primary EBV infection have a higher incidence of PTLD. Approximately 20% of patients with PTLDs are EBV-seronegative. The etiology of EBV-negative cases is unknown, but the fact that some of them respond to decreased immunosuppression suggests that they are also related to decreased immune competence.

Time Period

PTLD most commonly develops in the first year after lung transplantation.[63]

Clinical Presentation

Primary EBV infection often presents as a mononucleosis-like illness with fever and sore throat. Pulmonary involvement by PTLD may cause shortness of breath or may be discovered incidentally on a routine chest radiograph. Simultaneous involvement of extrapulmonary sites may result in diarrhea, due to involvement of the gastrointestinal tract, and dysphagia, due to involvement of the tonsils. Physical examination may reveal lymphadenopathy, enlarged tonsils, splenomegaly, and crackles on chest auscultation. In some cases, the physical examination may be entirely normal.

Radiologic Findings

Thoracic abnormalities are present in most lung transplant recipients with PTLD.[64] The most common radiologic finding is multiple pulmonary nodules. Other manifestations include a solitary nodule, multifocal alveolar infiltrates, and hilar or mediastinal adenopathy.

Diagnosis

The diagnosis is usually suspected on the basis of the clinical and radiologic findings, but histologic diagnosis is required.

Pathologic Findings

The spectrum of PTLDs ranges from early lesions to polymorphic PTLD to lymphomas.[65,66] Several classification schemes have been proposed, but the World Health Organization (WHO) Classification is now widely accepted and is presented in Box 12-3.[62]

Box 12-3. Classification of Post-Transplantation Lymphoproliferative Disorders (PTLDs)

1. Early lesions
   Plasmacytic hyperplasia
   Infectious mononucleosis–like lesion
2. Polymorphic PTLD
3. Monomorphic PTLDs (classify according to lymphoma they resemble)
   B cell neoplasms
   • Diffuse large B cell lymphoma
   • Burkitt lymphoma
   • Plasma cell myeloma
   • Plasmacytoma-like lesions
   • Other
   T cell neoplasms
   • Peripheral T cell lymphoma, not otherwise specified
   • Hepatosplenic T cell lymphoma
   • Other
4. Classic Hodgkin lymphoma–type PTLD

Specimen evaluation for the diagnosis of PTLD should include routine morphologic examination, immunophenotyping, preservation of tissue for potential molecular genetic studies, and detection of EBV infection.[62,67] Flow cytometry or frozen section immunohistochemistry is more useful in determining cell lineage and clonality than paraffin section immunohistochemistry. If immunophenotyping studies show polytypic immunoglobulin, clonality can be further assessed by molecular genetic studies that are capable of identifying polyclonal or monoclonal gene rearrangement. EBV infection can be detected using immunohistochemistry for latent membrane protein (LMP-1), but in situ hybridization for EBV-encoded nuclear RNA (EBER) is considered the gold standard.

Early Lesions

Early lesions of PTLD include plasmacytic hyperplasia and infectious mononucleosis–like lesions. These lesions usually arise in lymph nodes or Waldeyer's ring and only rarely involve true extranodal sites such as the lung. They are characterized by some degree of architectural preservation of the involved tissue,[62] but they differ from typical reactive follicular hyperplasia in having a diffuse proliferation of plasma cells. Plasmacytic hyperplasia is distinguished by numerous plasma cells and rare immunoblasts, and infectious mononucleosis–like lesion has the typical morphologic features of infectious mononucleosis in the lymph node, namely paracortical expansion and numerous immunoblasts in a background of T cells and plasma cells.

Immunophenotypic studies show an admixture of polyclonal B cells, plasma cells, and T cells. EBV-positive immunoblasts are typically present.

Polymorphic PTLDs

Polymorphic PTLDs are destructive lesions that efface the architecture of lymph nodes or form destructive extranodal masses.[62] In contrast with most lymphomas, polymorphic PTLDs show the full extent of B cell maturation and are composed of immunoblasts, plasma cells, small and intermediate-sized lymphocytes, and centrocyte-like cells. Scattered large, bizarre cells (atypical immunoblasts) and areas of necrosis may also be present. Polymorphic PTLDs were at one time subdivided into "polymorphic B cell hyperplasia" and "polymorphic B cell lymphoma." Today this separation is not deemed necessary, because both have similar clinical features. Immunophenotyping studies typically show a mixture of B and T cells. Most of the cases are monoclonal, at least by molecular genetic studies. EBV-positive immunoblasts are present in a majority of the cases.

Monomorphic B Cell PTLDs

Monomorphic B cell PTLDs are characterized by nodal architectural effacement or tumoral growth in extranodal sites, with confluent sheets of large, transformed cells.[62] These tumors should be diagnosed as B cell lymphomas and should be classified according to lymphoma classification guidelines. However, PTLD should also appear in the differential diagnosis. A majority of B cell PTLDs have morphologic features of diffuse large B cell lymphoma (Figs. 12-22 to 12-24). A minority may be classified as Burkitt lymphoma, plasma cell myeloma, or plasmacytoma-like lesions. Immunophenotyping studies of monomorphic B cell PTLD show B cell–associated antigen expression (CD19, CD20, CD79a). Many cases co-express antigens usually associated with T cells (CD43, CD45RO). A majority of cases are monoclonal and EBV-positive. Monomorphic B cell PTLDs often contain oncogene or tumor suppressor gene alterations (N-ras gene codon 61 point mutation, p53 gene mutation, or c-myc gene rearrangement).[68,69]

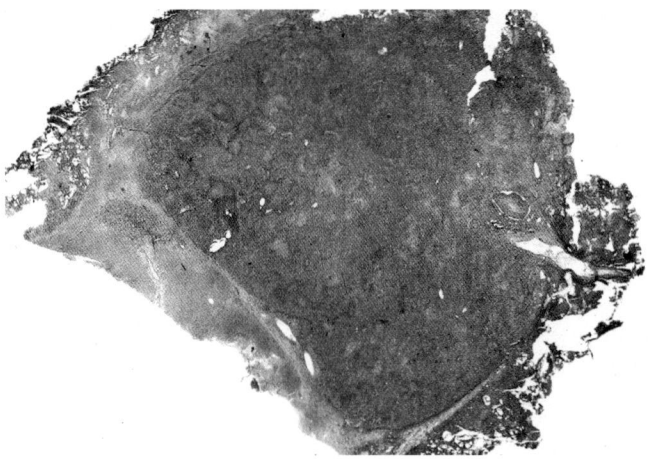

Figure 12-22. Panorama view of monomorphic B cell post-transplantation lymphoproliferative disorder showing a mass-like lesion in the pulmonary parenchyma.

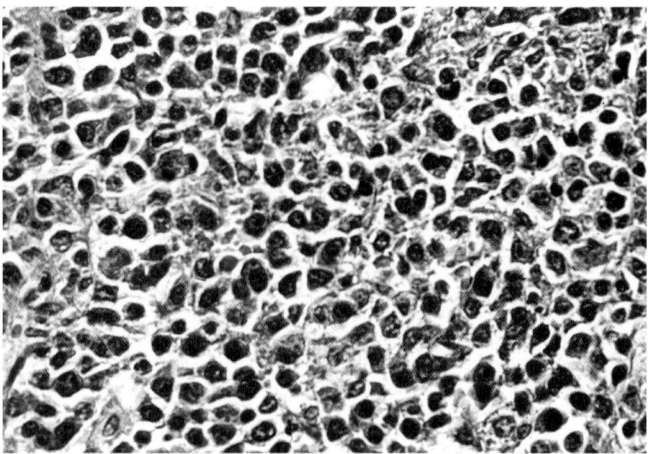

Figure 12-23. Higher magnification of involved lung in B cell post-transplantation lymphoproliferative disorder showing morphologic features of a diffuse large B cell lymphoma.

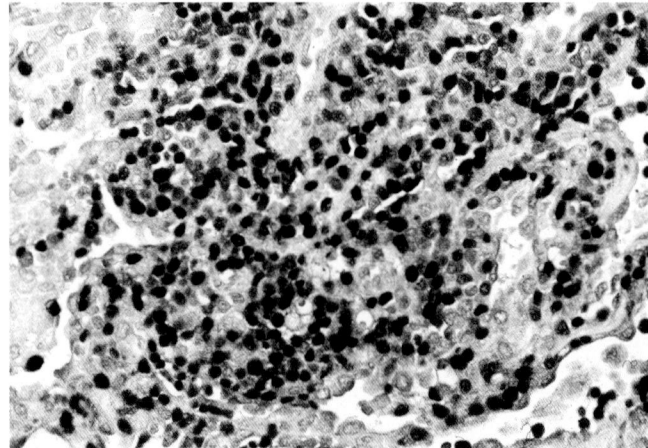

Figure 12-24. In situ hybridization studies performed on involved lung in B cell post-transplantation lymphoproliferative disorder reveal numerous cells that are positive for Epstein-Barr virus–encoded nuclear RNA.

Monomorphic T Cell PTLDs

T cell lymphomas have been reported in allograft recipients. Similar to monomorphic B cell PTLDs, monomorphic T cell PTLDs have sufficient atypia to be recognized as neoplastic and should be classified according to the standard lymphoma classification. Monomorphic T cell PTLDs express pan–T cell antigens. Most of the reported cases are EBV-negative.

Classic Hodgkin Lymphoma–Type PTLD

Classic Hodgkin lymphoma–type PTLD is the least common form of PTLD.[62] The diagnosis is based on classic morphologic and immunophenotypic features, preferably including both CD15 and CD30 expression. This type of PTLD is almost always EBV-positive. Because Reed-Sternberg–like cells may also be seen in some polymorphic and monomorphic PTLDs, the distinction between classic Hodgkin lymphoma–type PTLD and Hodgkin lymphoma–like PTLD may be difficult in some cases. However, the latter are better categorized as either polymorphic or monomorphic PTLDs.

Histologic Differential Diagnosis

Acute rejection may be considered in the differential diagnosis for PTLDs, especially in small biopsy samples. Detection of EBV infection is very helpful in this respect. A sheet-like monomorphous infiltrate with a mononuclear composition of more than 25% B cells and more than 30% large lymphoid cells also favors PTLD over acute rejection.[70]

Treatment and Prognosis

Therapy of PTLD must be tailored to the individual patient. Newer modalities such as anti-CD20 monoclonal antibody therapy (with rituximab) complement the standard stepwise approach that begins with a reduction of immunosuppression.[71] The role of chemotherapy continues to be defined, and in some cases early recourse to this approach may be desirable. Survival varies by age and extent of disease, with pediatric patients and those with localized disease tending to fare better.

Other Complications

Cryptogenic Organizing Pneumonia

Cryptogenic organizing pneumonia, previously known as idiopathic BOOP, occurs as a response to acute lung injury. In lung transplant recipients, it is commonly associated with aspiration, infection, and acute rejection.[40,72-74] However, organizing pneumonia is not a component of, and does not necessarily predispose to, chronic airway rejection (obliterative bronchiolitis).

Time Period

The time from transplantation to onset of cryptogenic organizing pneumonia ranges from 2 to 43 months.

Clinical Presentation

The clinical findings are nonspecific and may include cough, dyspnea, fever, hypoxemia, and a decline in pulmonary function.

Radiologic Findings

The chest film may be normal in appearance or show localized or diffuse infiltrates.

Diagnosis

Cryptogenic organizing pneumonia is a clinical diagnosis that requires histopathologic confirmation by transbronchial or surgical lung biopsy (i.e., the presence of organizing pneumonia).

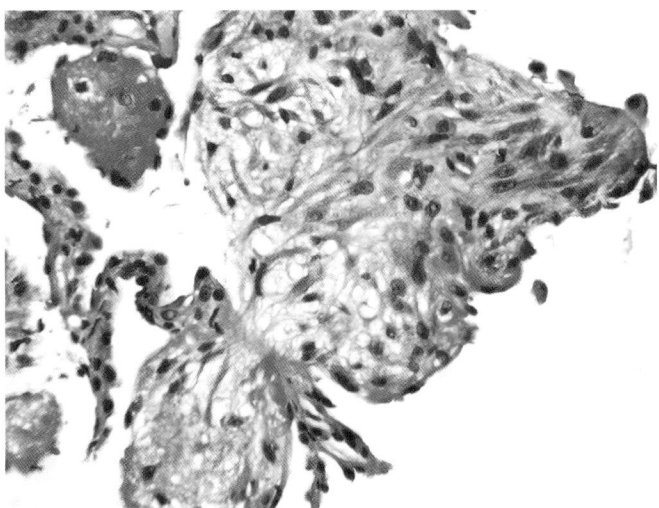

Figure 12-25. Organizing pneumonia with intra-alveolar fibroblastic plugs.

Pathologic Findings

Fibromyxoid plugs of granulation tissue are seen within small airways and airspaces, typically in a patchy distribution (Fig. 12-25).

Histologic Differential Diagnosis

In organizing diffuse alveolar damage, the fibroblastic proliferation involves the interstitium rather than the airspaces and remnants of hyaline membranes may be seen.[40] However, organizing pneumonia and diffuse alveolar damage are both acute lung injury patterns and features of both may be present in a given case. Airspace fibromyxoid tissue can also be seen in organizing infectious pneumonia and healing rejection, especially higher-grade rejection following steroid therapy. Separation of organizing pneumonia from transplant obliterative bronchiolitis has been discussed earlier.

Recurrence of the Primary Disease

A relatively small percentage of transplant patients are at risk for recurrence of their primary disease following lung transplantation. Sarcoidosis is the most common disease to recur.[75] Other reported cases include recurrence of lymphangioleiomyomatosis,[76-78] diffuse panbronchiolitis,[79] giant cell interstitial pneumonia,[80] desquamative interstitial pneumonia,[72] intravenous talc granulomatosis,[81] and bronchioloalveolar carcinoma.[82]

Clinical Features

Recurrence of the primary disease is usually an incidental finding on transbronchial biopsy or autopsy. However, symptomatic cases have also been described.

Diagnosis

The diagnosis depends on transbronchial or other biopsy samples.

Self-assessment questions related to this chapter can be found online on the Expert Consult site for this title.

References

1. Christie JD, Edwards LB, Aurora P, et al. Registry of the International Society for Heart and Lung Transplantation: Twenty-fifth official adult lung and heart/lung transplantation report—2008. *J Heart Lung Transplant.* 2008;27(9):957–969.

2. Yamane M, Date H, Okazaki M, et al. Long-term improvement in pulmonary function after living donor lobar lung transplantation. *J Heart Lung Transplant.* 2007;26(7):687–692.

3. Egan TM, Murray S, Bustami RT, et al. Development of the new lung allocation system in the United States. *Am J Transplant.* 2006;6(5 Pt 2):1212–1227.

4. Hachem RR, Trulock EP. The new lung allocation system and its impact on waitlist characteristics and post-transplant outcomes. *Semin Thorac Cardiovasc Surg.* 2008;20(2):139–142.

5. Nizami I, Frost AE. Clinical diagnosis of transplant-related problems. In: Cagle PT, ed. *Diagnostic Pulmonary Pathology.* New York: Marcel Dekker; 2000:485–499.

6. McWilliams TJ, Williams TJ, Whitford HM, Snell GI. Surveillance bronchoscopy in lung transplant recipients: Risk versus benefit. *J Heart Lung Transplant.* 2008;27(11):1203–1209.

7. Valentine VG, Gupta MR, Weill D, et al. Single-institution study evaluating the utility of surveillance bronchoscopy after lung transplantation. *J Heart Lung Transplant.* 2009;28(1):14–20.

8. Stewart S, Fishbein MC, Snell GI, et al. Revision of the 1996 working formulation for the standardization of nomenclature in the diagnosis of lung rejection. *J Heart Lung Transplant.* 2007;26(12):1229–1242.

9. Hopkins PM, Aboyoun CL, Chhajed PN, et al. Prospective analysis of 1,235 transbronchial lung biopsies in lung transplant recipients. *J Heart Lung Transplant.* 2002;21(10):1062–1067.

10. Lee JC, Christie JD. Primary graft dysfunction. *Proc Am Thorac Soc.* 2009;6(1):39–46.

11. Christie JD, Carby M, Bag R, et al. Report of the ISHLT Working Group on Primary Lung Graft Dysfunction part II: Definition. A consensus statement of the International Society for Heart and Lung Transplantation. *J Heart Lung Transplant.* 2005;24(10):1454–1459.

12. Meyers BF, de la Morena M, Sweet SC, et al. Primary graft dysfunction and other selected complications of lung transplantation: a single-center experience of 983 patients. *J Thorac Cardiovasc Surg.* 2005;129(6):1421–1429.

13. Tazelaar HD, Yousem SA. The pathology of combined heart-lung transplantation: an autopsy study. *Hum Pathol.* 1988;19(12):1403–1416.

14. Christie JD, Kotloff RM, Ahya VN, et al. The effect of primary graft dysfunction on survival after lung transplantation. *Am J Respir Crit Care Med.* 2005;171(11):1312–1316.

15. Daud SA, Yusen RD, Meyers BF, et al. Impact of immediate primary lung allograft dysfunction on bronchiolitis obliterans syndrome. *Am J Respir Crit Care Med.* 2007;175(5):507–513.

16. Clark SC, Levine AJ, Hasan A, et al. Vascular complications of lung transplantation. *Ann Thorac Surg.* 1996;61(4):1079–1082.

17. Schulman LL, Anandarangam T, Leibowitz DW, et al. Four-year prospective study of pulmonary venous thrombosis after lung transplantation. *J Am Soc Echocardiogr.* 2001;14(8):806–812.

18. Ruffini E, Maggi G, Actis-Dato G, et al. Successful bilobectomy for pulmonary venous obstruction after bilateral lung transplantation. *J Thorac Cardiovasc Surg.* 1998;116(4):648–649.

19. Santacruz JF, Mehta AC. Airway complications and management after lung transplantation: ischemia, dehiscence, and stenosis. *Proc Am Thorac Soc.* 2009;6(1):79–93.

20. Hasegawa T, Iacono AT, Orons PD, Yousem SA. Segmental nonanastomotic bronchial stenosis after lung transplantation. *Ann Thorac Surg.* 2000;69(4):1020–1024.

21. Yousem SA, Paradis IL, Dauber JA, et al. Large airway inflammation in heart-lung transplant recipients—its significance and prognostic implications. *Transplantation.* 1990;49(3):654–656.

22. Griffith BP, Magee MJ, Gonzalez IF, et al. Anastomotic pitfalls in lung transplantation. *J Thorac Cardiovasc Surg.* 1994;107(3):743–753 discussion 753–754.

23. Kapoor BS, May B, Panu N, et al. Endobronchial stent placement for the management of airway complications after lung transplantation. *J Vasc Interv Radiol.* 2007;18(5):629–632.

24. Berry GJ, Brunt EM, Chamberlain D, et al. A working formulation for the standardization of nomenclature in the diagnosis of heart and lung rejection: Lung Rejection Study Group. The International Society for Heart Transplantation. *J Heart Transplant.* 1990;9(6):593–601.

25. Yousem SA, Berry GJ, Cagle PT, et al. Revision of the 1990 working formulation for the classification of pulmonary allograft rejection: Lung Rejection Study Group. *J Heart Lung Transplant.* 1996;15(1 Pt 1):1–15.

26. Hasegawa T, Iacono AT, Yousem SA. The anatomic distribution of acute cellular rejection in the allograft lung. *Ann Thorac Surg.* 2000;69(5):1529–1531.

27. Nakhleh RE, Bolman 3rd RM, Henke CA, Hertz MI. Lung transplant pathology. A comparative study of pulmonary acute rejection and cytomegaloviral infection. *Am J Surg Pathol.* 1991;15(12):1197–1201.

28. Stewart S. Pulmonary infections in transplantation pathology. *Arch Pathol Lab Med.* 2007;131(8):1219–1231.

29. Tazelaar HD. Perivascular inflammation in pulmonary infections: implications for the diagnosis of lung rejection. *J Heart Lung Transplant.* 1991;10(3):437–441.

30. Randhawa PS, Yousem SA, Paradis IL, et al. The clinical spectrum, pathology, and clonal analysis of Epstein-Barr virus–associated lymphoproliferative disorders in heart-lung transplant recipients. *Am J Clin Pathol.* 1989;92(2):177–185.

31. Valentine VG, Robbins RC, Wehner JH, et al. Total lymphoid irradiation for refractory acute rejection in heart-lung and lung allografts. *Chest.* 1996;109(5):1184–1189.

32. Hachem RR, Khalifah AP, Chakinala MM, et al. The significance of a single episode of minimal acute rejection after lung transplantation. *Transplantation.* 2005;80(10):1406–1413.

33. Khalifah AP, Hachem RR, Chakinala MM, et al. Minimal acute rejection after lung transplantation: a risk for bronchiolitis obliterans syndrome. *Am J Transplant.* 2005;5(8):2022–2030.

34. Yousem SA. Lymphocytic bronchitis/bronchiolitis in lung allograft recipients. *Am J Surg Pathol.* 1993;17(5):491–496.

35. Girnita AL, Duquesnoy R, Yousem SA, et al. HLA-specific antibodies are risk factors for lymphocytic bronchiolitis and chronic lung allograft dysfunction. *Am J Transplant.* 2005;5(1):131–138.

36. Bando K, Paradis IL, Similo S, et al. Obliterative bronchiolitis after lung and heart-lung transplantation. An analysis of risk factors and management. *J Thorac Cardiovasc Surg.* 1995;110(1):4–13.

37. American Thoracic Society/European Respiratory Society International Multidisciplinary Consensus Classification of the Idiopathic Interstitial Pneumonias. This joint statement of the American Thoracic Society (ATS), and the European Respiratory Society (ERS) was adopted by the

ATS board of directors, June 2001 and by the ERS Executive Committee, June 2001. *Am J Respir Crit Care Med*. 2002;165(2):277–304.

38. Paradis I, Yousem S, Griffith B. Airway obstruction and bronchiolitis obliterans after lung transplantation. *Clin Chest Med*. 1993;14(4):751–763.

39. Cooper JD, Billingham M, Egan T, et al. A working formulation for the standardization of nomenclature and for clinical staging of chronic dysfunction in lung allografts. International Society for Heart and Lung Transplantation. *J Heart Lung Transplant*. 1993;12(5):713–716.

40. Yousem SA, Duncan SR, Griffith BP. Interstitial and airspace granulation tissue reactions in lung transplant recipients. *Am J Surg Pathol*. 1992;16(9):877–884.

41. Yousem SA, Paradis IL, Dauber JH, et al. Pulmonary arteriosclerosis in long-term human heart-lung transplant recipients. *Transplantation*. 1989;47(3):564–569.

42. Martinu T, Howell DN, Davis RD, et al. Pathologic correlates of bronchiolitis obliterans syndrome in pulmonary retransplant recipients. *Chest*. 2006;129(4):1016–1023.

43. Martinu T, Chen DF, Palmer SM. Acute rejection and humoral sensitization in lung transplant recipients. *Proc Am Thorac Soc*. 2009;6(1):54–65.

44. Morrell MR, Patterson GA, Trulock EP, Hachem RR. Acute antibody-mediated rejection after lung transplantation. *J Heart Lung Transplant*. 2009;28(1):96–100.

45. Gloor J, Cosio F, Lager DJ, Stegall MD. The spectrum of antibody-mediated renal allograft injury: implications for treatment. *Am J Transplant*. 2008;8(7):1367–1373.

46. Reed EF, Demetris AJ, Hammond E, et al. Acute antibody-mediated rejection of cardiac transplants. *J Heart Lung Transplant*. 2006;25(2):153–159.

47. Girnita AL, McCurry KR, Yousem SA, et al. Antibody-mediated rejection in lung transplantation: case reports. *Clin Transpl*. 2006;508–510.

48. Astor TL, Weill D, Cool C, et al. Pulmonary capillaritis in lung transplant recipients: treatment and effect on allograft function. *J Heart Lung Transplant*. 2005;24(12):2091–2097.

49. Badesch DB, Zamora M, Fullerton D, et al. Pulmonary capillaritis: a possible histologic form of acute pulmonary allograft rejection. *J Heart Lung Transplant*. 1998;17(4):415–422.

50. Choi JK, Kearns J, Palevsky HI, et al. Hyperacute rejection of a pulmonary allograft. Immediate clinical and pathologic findings. *Am J Respir Crit Care Med*. 1999;160(3):1015–1018.

51. Frost AE, Jammal CT, Cagle PT. Hyperacute rejection following lung transplantation. *Chest*. 1996;110(2):559–562.

52. Masson E, Stern M, Chabod J, et al. Hyperacute rejection after lung transplantation caused by undetected low-titer anti-HLA antibodies. *J Heart Lung Transplant*. 2007;26(6):642–645.

53. Appel 3rd JZ, Hartwig MG, Davis RD, Reinsmoen NL. Utility of peritransplant and rescue intravenous immunoglobulin and extracorporeal immunoadsorption in lung transplant recipients sensitized to HLA antigens. *Hum Immunol*. 2005;66(4):378–386.

54. Gottlieb J, Mattner F, Weissbrodt H, et al. Impact of graft colonization with gram-negative bacteria after lung transplantation on the development of bronchiolitis obliterans syndrome in recipients with cystic fibrosis. *Respir Med*. 2009;103(5):743–749.

55. Marchevsky A, Hartman G, Walts A, et al. Lung transplantation: the pathologic diagnosis of pulmonary complications. *Mod Pathol*. 1991;4(2):133–138.

56. Valentine VG, Weill D, Gupta MR, et al. Ganciclovir for cytomegalovirus: a call for indefinite prophylaxis in lung transplantation. *J Heart Lung Transplant*. 2008;27(8):875–881.

57. Holt ND, Gould FK, Taylor CE, et al. Incidence and significance of noncytomegalovirus viral respiratory infection after adult lung transplantation. *J Heart Lung Transplant*. 1997;16(4):416–419.

58. Ohori NP, Michaels MG, Jaffe R, et al. Adenovirus pneumonia in lung transplant recipients. *Hum Pathol*. 1995;26(10):1073–1079.

59. Kramer MR, Marshall SE, Starnes VA, et al. Infectious complications in heart-lung transplantation. Analysis of 200 episodes. *Arch Intern Med*. 1993;153(17):2010–2016.

60. Sole A, Salavert M. Fungal infections after lung transplantation. *Curr Opin Pulm Med*. 2009;15(3):243–253.

61. Gryzan S, Paradis IL, Zeevi A, et al. Unexpectedly high incidence of *Pneumocystis carinii* infection after lung-heart transplantation. Implications for lung defense and allograft survival. *Am Rev Respir Dis*. 1988;137(6):1268–1274.

62. Swerdlow SH, Webber SA. Post-transplant lymphoproliferative disorders. In: Swerdlow SH, Campo E, Harris NL, et al, eds. *WHO Classification of Tumours of Haematopoietic and Lymphoid Tissues*. Lyon: IARC Press; 2008:343–349.

63. Paranjothi S, Yusen RD, Kraus MD, et al. Lymphoproliferative disease after lung transplantation: comparison of presentation and outcome of early and late cases. *J Heart Lung Transplant*. 2001;20(10):1054–1063.

64. Borhani AA, Hosseinzadeh K, Almusa O, et al. Imaging of posttransplantation lymphoproliferative disorder after solid organ transplantation. *Radiographics*. 2009;29(4):981–1000; discussion 1000–1002.

65. Lewin KJ. Post-transplant lymphoproliferative disorders. *Pathol Oncol Res*. 1997;3(3):177–182.

66. Tsao L, Hsi ED. The clinicopathologic spectrum of posttransplantation lymphoproliferative disorders. *Arch Pathol Lab Med*. 2007;131(8):1209–1218.

67. Harris NL, Ferry JA, Swerdlow SH. Posttransplant lymphoproliferative disorders: summary of Society for Hematopathology Workshop. *Semin Diagn Pathol*. 1997;14(1):8–14.

68. Chadburn A, Cesarman E, Knowles DM. Molecular pathology of posttransplantation lymphoproliferative disorders. *Semin Diagn Pathol*. 1997;14(1):15–26.

69. Knowles DM, Cesarman E, Chadburn A, et al. Correlative morphologic and molecular genetic analysis demonstrates three distinct categories of posttransplantation lymphoproliferative disorders. *Blood*. 1995;85(2):552–565.

70. Rosendale B, Yousem SA. Discrimination of Epstein-Barr virus–related posttransplant lymphoproliferations from acute rejection in lung allograft recipients. *Arch Pathol Lab Med*. 1995;119(5):418–423.

71. Nalesnik MA. Clinicopathologic characteristics of post-transplant lymphoproliferative disorders. *Recent Results Cancer Res*. 2002;159:9–18.

72. Keller CA, Cagle PT, Brown RW, et al. Bronchiolitis obliterans in recipients of single, double, and heart-lung transplantation. *Chest*. 1995;107(4):973–980.

73. Chaparro C, Chamberlain D, Maurer J, et al. Bronchiolitis obliterans organizing pneumonia (BOOP) in lung transplant recipients. *Chest*. 1996;110(5):1150–1154.

74. Siddiqui MT, Garrity ER, Husain AN. Bronchiolitis obliterans organizing pneumonia-like reactions: a nonspecific response or an atypical form of rejection or infection in lung allograft recipients? *Hum Pathol*. 1996;27(7):714–719.

75. Collins J, Hartman MJ, Warner TF, et al. Frequency and CT findings of recurrent disease after lung transplantation. *Radiology*. 2001;219(2):503–509.

76. O'Brien JD, Lium JH, Parosa JF, et al. Lymphangiomyomatosis recurrence in the allograft after single-lung transplantation. *Am J Respir Crit Care Med*. 1995;151(6):2033–2036.

77. Collins J, Müller NL, Kazerooni EA, et al. Lung transplantation for lymphangioleiomyomatosis: Role of imaging in the assessment of complications related to the underlying disease. *Radiology*. 1999;210(2):325–332.

78. Chen F, Omasa M, Kondo N, et al. Sirolimus treatment for recurrent lymphangioleiomyomatosis after lung transplantation. *Ann Thorac Surg*. 2009;87(1):6–7.

79. Baz MA, Kussin PS, Van Trigt P, et al. Recurrence of diffuse panbronchiolitis after lung transplantation. *Am J Respir Crit Care Med*. 1995;151(3 Pt 1):895–898.

80. Frost AE, Keller CA, Brown RW, et al. Giant cell interstitial pneumonitis. Disease recurrence in the transplanted lung. *Am Rev Respir Dis*. 1993;148(5):1401–1404.

81. Cook RC, Fradet G, English JC, et al. Recurrence of intravenous talc granulomatosis following single lung transplantation. *Can Respir J*. 1998;5(6):511–514.

82. Garver Jr RI, Zorn GL, Wu X, et al. Recurrence of bronchioloalveolar carcinoma in transplanted lungs. *N Engl J Med*. 1999;340(14):1071–1074.

Neuroendocrine Lesions of the Lung

Mark R. Wick, MD, Timothy C. Allen, MD, JD, Kevin O. Leslie, MD,
Jon H. Ritter, MD, and Stacey E. Mills, MD

The concept of a "diffuse neuroendocrine system" (DNS) is not a new one. Feyrter[1] developed this paradigm in 1938, in a philosophical attempt to unify tumors in several anatomic locations that had potential secretory functions and similar morphologic characteristics. Pearse[2] refined and renamed the cellular network in question 35 years later, coining the designation of "APUD" system (for amine precursor uptake and decarboxylation) to describe its shared biochemical attributes. Inherent in the latter scheme was the presumption that all "APUD" cells—and tumors deriving from them ("APUDomas")—emanated from the remnants of the neural crest. In light of these and other observations, continuing nosologic revisionism over the last 10 years has pushed many pathologists away from such traditional diagnostic terms as "carcinoid" and "islet cell tumor" in describing certain potentially malignant but low-grade neoplasms of the neuroendocrine system,[3,4] although "traditionalists" remain.[5] The classification of poorly differentiated lesions has changed as well. This chapter outlines the current foundations of existing classification schemes for neuroendocrine tumors. The reader should come away with a simplified—and therefore practical—understanding of this confusing area of oncology.

Terminology Pertaining to Neuroendocrine Neoplasms

There is perhaps no other single aspect of neuroendocrine neoplasia that is as perplexing as the pathologic terminology that has been used to describe it. Such terms as "bronchial adenoma," "carcinoid," "atypical carcinoid," "Kulchitsky cell carcinoma," "argentaffinoma," "APUDoma," "atypical endocrine carcinoma," "oat cell carcinoma," "medullary thyroid carcinoma," "islet cell tumor," and "cutaneous Merkel cell carcinoma" (group 1) have all been employed historically in this context, in addition to "neuroblastoma," "esthesioneuroblastoma," "olfactory neuroblastoma," "medulloblastoma," "pineoblastoma," "retinoblastoma," "paraganglioma," "pheochromocytoma," "chemodectoma," and "glomus jugulare tumor" (group 2).[6-10]

This diverse lexicon reflects a basic division of neuroendocrine tumors into two broad categories—epithelial (group 1) and neural (group 2).[6] With that piece of information in hand, one can then go on to structure a much more user-friendly and straightforward classification scheme that has made significant inroads in the pathology literature.

Another crucial concept in understanding the categorization and clinical behavior of neuroendocrine neoplasms is that all of them are at least potentially malignant tumors, regardless of whether they belong to group 1 or group 2.[9] Moreover, in selected subgroups (e.g., classic "carcinoid" tumor, extra-adrenal paraganglioma [PG], and pheochromocytoma [intra-adrenal PG]), one cannot reliably use the gross or microscopic characteristics of the tumors to predict whether they will behave innocuously or aggressively. Therefore, it follows logically that the modifier "benign" should not be applied in conjunction with any of the diagnostic terms noted earlier. For example, even with regard to appendiceal or classic bronchial "carcinoids"—generally regarded as defining the "low" end of the spectrum of biologic behavior in this context[11-13]—there are many well-documented examples of metastasizing lesions that can be found in the literature.

Current terminological recommendations are, therefore, different from those that might have pertained even 10 years ago, or from those with which some practitioners may feel "comfortable." The designation of "neuroendocrine carcinoma" (NEC) has been proposed as a replacement for all of the various group 1 terms discussed earlier, with modifiers of "well-differentiated" (grade I/III); "moderately differentiated" (grade II/III); and "poorly differentiated" (grade III/III) being appended as appropriate.[9,12,14] In contrast, most of the traditional rubric has been retained with reference to group 2 tumors, such that the recommended terms for the categorization of this constellation of lesions are "extra-adrenal PG," "intra-adrenal PG" (pheochromocytoma), "sympatheticoadrenal neuroblastoma (NB)" (and congeners [e.g., ganglioneuroblastoma]), "olfactory NB," "retinoblastoma," and "primitive neuroectodermal tumor" (PNET).[9] In reporting on a biopsy or resection specimen, the pathologist can then work within this framework—using further descriptive comments and summaries of the aggregate literature on each tumor—to provide the clinician with an outline of expected behavior for each neoplasm based on its nuances.

There are two notable exceptions to this paradigm. Pituitary adenomas and parathyroid adenomas are, of course, completely benign in the vast majority of cases, and it would be a mistake to label them as "grade 1 NECs." With that said, however, it must be acknowledged that aggressive pituitary adenomas exist, and rare carcinomas also may be encountered in each location.

Distribution and Pathogenesis of Neuroendocrine Neoplasia

If one refers to basic textbooks on human embryogenesis, a common theme that is seen in all anatomic sites is that of a neuroendocrine or neuroectodermal stage of differentiation during early organ development.[6,15,16] Because it is currently thought that oncogenesis partially (and aberrantly) recapitulates normal embryologic development, this information is central to our understanding of why neuroendocrine and neuroectodermal neoplasms have been reported in virtually every topographic location. Some of the latter are, by far, more commonly hosts to such tumors, for unknown reasons. For example, the lung is the most common site of neuroendocrine carcinogenesis, where the process is clearly related etiologically to cigarette smoking and is associated with partial deletion of the short arm of chromosome 3.[17] However, identical sporadic primary neoplasms in other organs have not been linked with any definitive pathogenetic factors.[18] Group 2 neoplasms in the "peripheral primitive neuroectodermal" category similarly demonstrate a uniform balanced translocation between chromosomes 11 and 22,[19,20] with synthesis of a unique gene product (p30/32 glycoprotein) that is recognized by a particular set of monoclonal antibodies (e.g., 12E7 and O13).[20]

Other NECs and group 2 tumors (especially NB and retinoblastoma) occur in definite Mendelian-heritable—typically autosomal dominant—patterns, as seen in multiple endocrine neoplasia (MEN) type 1 (pancreatic and thymic group 1 tumors) and MEN2 (medullary thyroid carcinoma and also group 2 tumors [pheochromocytomas]).[9,11,21,22] Ongoing work has elucidated the locations of at least some operative aberrant gene complexes in such disorders (e.g., the MEN2A locus on chromosome 10 and deletion of the Rb-1 "antioncogene" on chromosome 13 in heritable bilateral retinoblastoma).[17,19,23] However, sporadic examples of the tumors discussed earlier do not necessarily exhibit the same karyotypic or gene sequence abnormalities.[24] Clearly, more work is needed to provide a complete picture of the molecular disturbances at play,[14,25] but this is an exciting area for current and future development because it may yield clinical tests that could be used in early diagnosis and treatment.

Other Pathologic Aspects of Neuroendocrine Neoplasia

Up to this point, this discussion has focused on "pure" neuroendocrine and neuroectodermal neoplasms. Increasingly in recent years, however, it has been recognized that human malignancies much more often show combined or "divergent" differentiation than was appreciated in the past. Accordingly, oncologists are now faced with such diagnoses as "adenocarcinoma/squamous carcinoma/transitional cell carcinoma with neuroendocrine features" or, more simply, "combined adenocarcinoma–small cell NEC."[26-33] In the former scenario, the pathologist is attempting to convey the concept that the tumor looks like conventional squamous carcinoma, adenocarcinoma, or transitional cell carcinoma with a routine hematoxylin and eosin stain, but that additional studies (e.g., ultrastructural or immunohistochemical) have demonstrated submicroscopic neuroendocrine differentiation in the neoplastic cells. In some organ systems, such as the lung, it is believed that such a constellation of findings portends a more aggressive course of certain tumor types (e.g., "large cell anaplastic pulmonary carcinoma with neuroendocrine features").[34] However, generic extrapolation of this model to other tissues would not be scientifically justified at this time and appears to be definitely invalid in some specific settings.[31,33] When a truly combined carcinoma is seen at a light microscopic level, pathologists are describing the juxtaposition and admixture of two distinct histologic patterns, such as adenocarcinoma and small cell carcinoma (SCC).[29,30] Again, using tumors of the lung as examples, it would be expected that the responses to therapy and the behavior of such combined lesions would also be a hybrid of those attending each component (i.e., adenocarcinoma or SCC) in pure form.[35-38] Nonetheless, uniform validation of that premise and delineation of optimal therapeutic approaches for each of these "amalgam" tumors have yet to occur.

Pathologic Recognition of Neuroendocrine Differentiation

Several techniques are available that allow the pathologist to diagnose neuroendocrine differentiation in poorly differentiated malignant neoplasms of the lung and other sites. These methods are considered in the following sections.

Standard Morphologic Examination

Because of the histologic appearance of some tumors, a neuroendocrine phenotype is obvious. Ready examples include classic pulmonary SCC and central bronchial "carcinoid" tumor. The standard cytomorphologic features of SCC are well known and include hyperchromatic nuclei with dispersed chromatin, inconspicuous nucleoli, and a tendency for the nuclei to mold to one another (Fig. 13-1). The cells are oval or carrot-shaped, with scant cytoplasm, and often there is marked crush artifact. Extensive necrosis is often observed, with either a geographic pattern or dropout of individual cells (i.e., apoptosis). Likewise, bronchial "carcinoid" features include stippled nuclear chromatin and a distinctly organoid growth pattern, with formation of rosettes, trabeculae, or ribbons ("festoons")[39] (Fig. 13-2).

In such cases, special stains, electron microscopy, and other adjunctive diagnostic techniques are merely confirmatory. In fact, because SCCs often do not exhibit ultrastructural or immunohistologic markers of endocrine differentiation because of sampling artifacts and other factors, confusion on the part of clinicians may occur when negative results on those studies are obtained. Our practice in dealing with endobronchial biopsy specimens showing groups of small round cells with crush artifact is simply to obtain immunostains for cytokeratin and leukocyte common antigen (CD45; discussed later). This approach

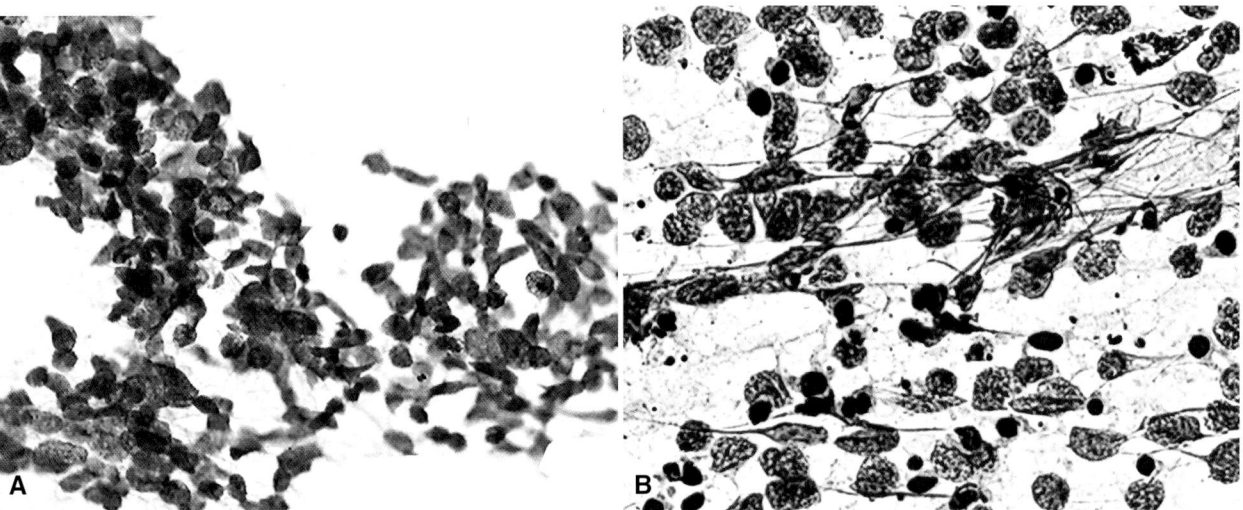

Figure 13-1. A, Fine-needle aspiration biopsy specimen of small cell carcinoma of the lung, showing characteristic crush artifact, nuclear "molding," high nucleocytoplasmic ratios, and a relative lack of nucleoli. The chromatin of small cell carcinoma has a pale powdery appearance, a very helpful feature in distinguishing this neoplasm from others cytologically. **B,** Nuclear "molding" and dispersed nuclear chromatin can be seen in this image of the same tumor. The chromatin appears slightly coarser here, likely related to preservation.

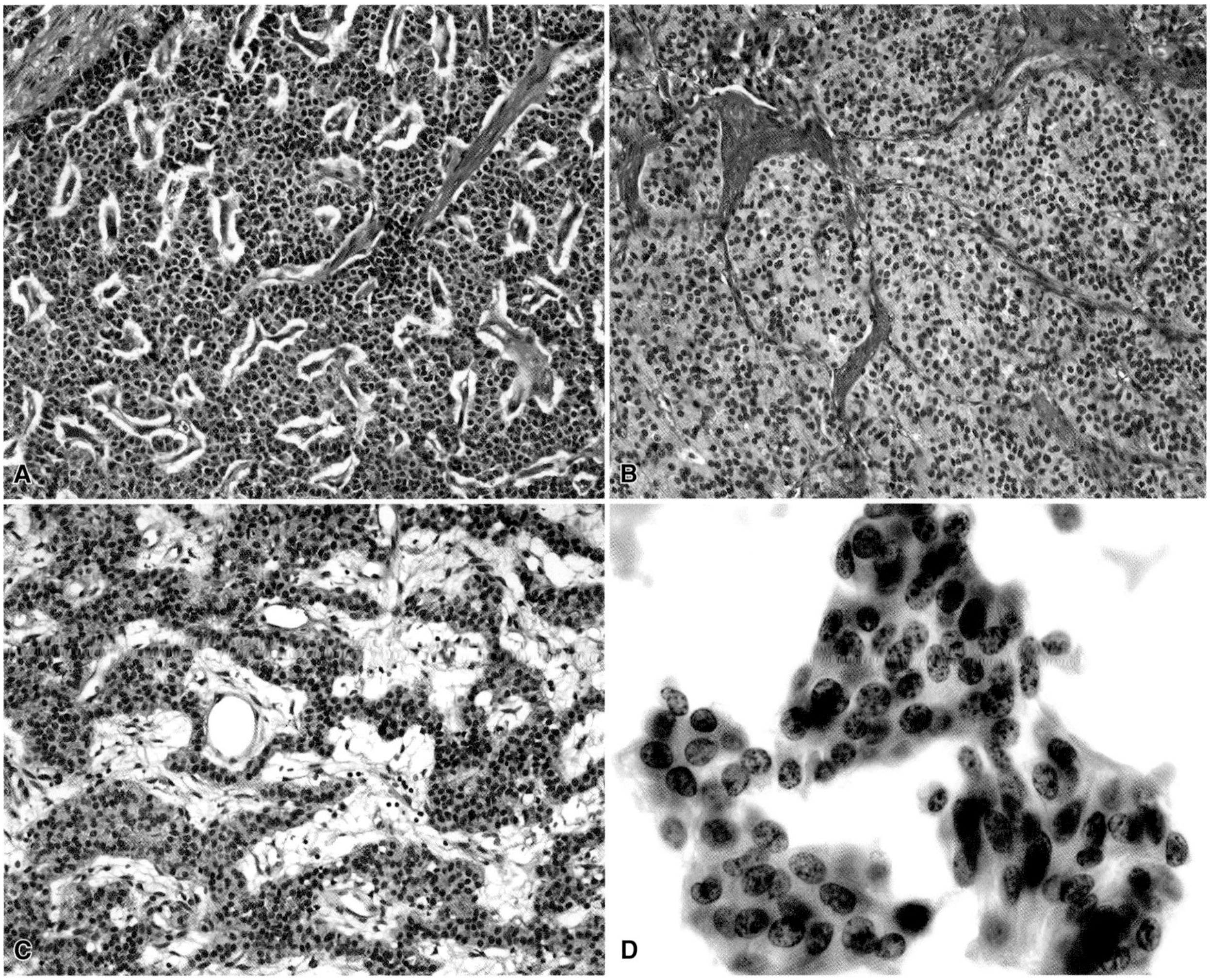

Figure 13-2. Characteristic growth patterns in neuroendocrine carcinoma, including insular cellular arrangement (**A** and **B**) and insular and ribboning growth (**C**). **D,** Insulae are seen in fine-needle aspiration biopsy specimens as well.

simply addresses generic cellular lineage, with the conclusion that small cell epithelial lesions with the specified characteristics represent SCCs. Adjunctive procedures become more valuable when one encounters large cell pulmonary malignancies that do not have prototypical neuroendocrine characteristics.

Histochemical Methods

Histochemical techniques are still valuable in selected settings, although in current practice, they have been supplanted by newer technologies. With reference to neuroendocrine lesions, such techniques rely on the ability of endocrine cells to reduce silver solutions and form insoluble precipitates in tissue sections. Available methods are broadly subdivided into two groups—argentaffin and argyrophil stains.[40–42]

Argentaffin techniques depend on endogenous cellular reducing agents. The most widely used is the Fontana–Masson stain, which is only variably reactive with pulmonary neuroendocrine neoplasms. Argyrophilic methods are those in which an exogenous reducing agent is added, such as in the Grimelius or Churukian–Schenk procedure. They are typically positive in the majority of well-differentiated neuroendocrine tumors of the lung (Fig. 13-3), with much lesser reactivity in high-grade carcinomas, such as SCC.[42]

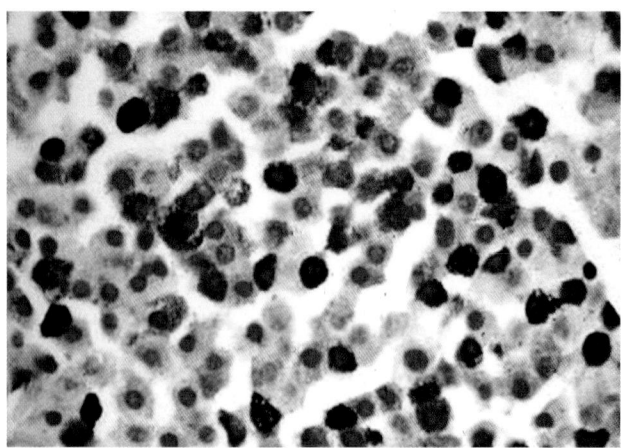

Figure 13-3. Argyrophil reactivity of neuroendocrine carcinoma with the Churukian–Schenck method.

Electron Microscopy

The ultrastructural hallmark of neuroendocrine neoplasms in the lung and elsewhere is the presence of cytoplasmic neurosecretory granules. These are rounded structures that consist of a central dense core, a peripheral lucent halo, and a single delimiting outer membrane. They vary from 30 to 300 nm in diameter, and may occur singly or in clusters[42–55] (Fig. 13-4). Budding of neurosecretory granules from prominent Golgi apparatus is occasionally observed. One drawback of electron microscopy is that the number of granules and the number of cells containing granules tend to be greatest in well-differentiated tumors and lowest in poorly differentiated lesions (where they are most needed for diagnosis). Also, electron microscopy can examine only relatively few cells in any given tumor. However, it is still a highly useful technique if sufficient time and care are invested in a thorough search for dense core granules. In a study by Nagle and colleagues,[40] ultrastructural analysis documented neuroendocrine differentiation in all of 41 putative neuroendocrine lesions, whereas a significant percentage of lesions were negative for endocrine markers using immunohistochemical techniques.

Immunohistology

Advances in immunohistochemistry over the last 15 years have yielded powerful tools for the pathologist in recognizing neuroendocrine differentiation.[44,50,54–60] Advantages of this approach include a relatively low cost, rapid turnaround time, the ability to perform studies on routinely processed tissue, and the capacity to screen a large number of cells rapidly as opposed to the limited number that can be evaluated with electron microscopy. The following markers have the greatest utility in this context.

Intermediate Filament Proteins

Group I neuroendocrine neoplasms manifest uniform immunoreactivity for keratin, especially keratin classes 8 and 18.[61] To a lesser extent, keratin 19 is also observed in NECs in general. Pulmonary NECs may label for keratin 20 as well, but only in fewer than 10% of cases.[62] Keratin proteins are generally well recognized by several commercial monoclonal antibodies, especially CAM5.2 and MFN116. Monospecific reagents directly against only one keratin class polypeptide are also available, but are not necessary in this specific context. In our opinion, the optimal approach to the detection of keratin in

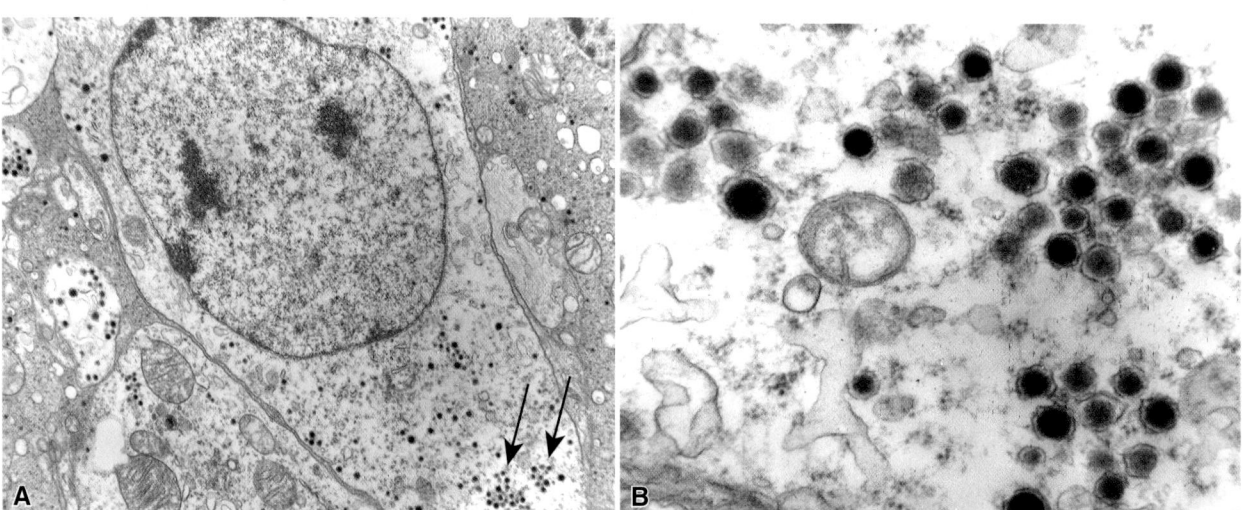

Figure 13-4. A, Electron micrograph of neuroendocrine carcinoma of the lung, demonstrating numerous cytoplasmic dense-core (neurosecretory) granules (*arrows*). **B,** These inclusions are demonstrable even in specimens retrieved from paraffin blocks.

any poorly differentiated neoplasm, neuroendocrine or otherwise, is to prepare a mixture of monoclonal antikeratin antibodies with partially overlapping and partially distinctive keratin class specificities. When reagents of this type are used on paraffin sections, together with properly performed proteolytic digestion or microwave (heat)-mediated epitope "retrieval" methods, the detectability of keratin in NECs should approximate 100%, even in essentially "undifferentiated" tumors (e.g., SCC).[63] Another feature of keratin reactivity in many NECs is a distinctive punctate or globoid perinuclear zone of positivity.[64] This result (Fig. 13-5) is simultaneously diagnostic of both epithelial and neuroendocrine differentiation in a small cell malignancy, and it obviates the need for other "neuroendocrine markers." Keratin is not typically expected in group II neuroendocrine neoplasms, although some lesions in that group have shown its presence in an "aberrant" manner.[65–68] The foremost example of that phenomenon is represented by PNET with "divergent" differentiation (also known as "polyphenotypic small cell tumor"), an example of which is the "desmoplastic small round cell tumor."[69–71] In most cases of keratin expression in more nondescript PNETs, reactivity for that protein is focal, unlike its pattern in NECs; in addition, vimentin expression tends to be mutually exclusive in PNETs and NECs. Nonetheless, problems in differential diagnosis may arise between those classes of neuroendocrine tumors, sometimes necessitating cytogenetic evaluation to distinguish between them.[72]

Neurofilament protein is variably coexpressed by NECs,[73–76] but that determinant is seen as the sole intermediate filament in the majority of differentiated group II neuroendocrine tumors, such as PGs and pheochromocytomas, as well as some NBs.[77–79] Unfortunately, neurofilament protein is not well visualized in paraffin sections, even with epitope retrieval technology, and it is most reliably evaluated in frozen material. Vimentin also may be evident in the cells of PGs in approximately 50% of cases,[79] and it is the only intermediate filament that can be detected in primitive group II tumors, such as NB and PNET.[68] That is also true in Ewing sarcoma, a tumor that is in the same family as PNETs. Vimentin is only exceptionally present in NECs, as stated earlier. Eusebi and coworkers[80] recently described three NECs that coexpressed keratin and desmin as a reflection of divergent (sarcomatoid) rhabdomyoblastic differentiation. This same proclivity is regularly seen in desmoplastic small round cell tumors, in which keratin, desmin, and vimentin are commonly present concomitantly in the same neoplastic cells.[69–71]

Glial fibrillary acidic protein is not an expected reactant in either NEC or PNET. In the central nervous system, therefore, this marker is helpful in the differential diagnosis with small cell malignant gliomas,[81] most of which are reactive for glial fibrillary acidic protein. That fact is all the more important because a proportion of glial tumors manifest aberrant keratin reactivity[82] and also express vimentin.

Chromogranins

Chromogranins are matrical proteins that are associated with neurosecretory granules and are absolutely specific for neuroendocrine differentiation.[83–85] These polypeptides have been subdivided biochemically into two groups, A and B,[86,87] with the latter being synonymous with secretogranin-I. Conceptually, every cell that packages peptides into neurosecretory granules must synthesize either chromogranin-A (CGA) or chromogranin-B (CGB); hence, a screening reagent incorporating antibodies to both of those proteins would be extremely useful diagnostically. Unfortunately, reliable commercial anti-CGB products have not been introduced. The most widely used anti-CGA antibody is clone LK2H10.[88] This reagent was raised against pheochromocytoma cells and shows excellent reactivity with paraffin sections (Fig. 13-6). The major shortcoming of anti-CGA is twofold. First, because neuroendocrine cells or tumors may preferentially synthesize CGB, CGA obviously cannot be regarded as a "universal" marker of such elements. Secondly, the detectability of both CGA and CGB is directly related to the number of neurosecretory granules in any given neuroendocrine cell population. If one is dealing with poorly differentiated malignancies that have only scant numbers of such organelles, immunostains for CGA and CGB will be predictably negative in the majority of cases. Therefore, one may legitimately conclude that a tumor has neuroendocrine properties if it can be labeled for a chromogranin, but negative results do not exclude that possibility, particularly in high-grade neoplasms.

Synaptophysin

Synaptophysin is a 38 kDa molecule that is associated with the synaptic vesicles of neurons and cells with neuroendocrine or neuroectodermal characteristics.[78,89–92] Monoclonal antibodies to this marker have been used widely in diagnostic surgical pathology and cytopathology, with good success, particularly in conjunction with epitope retrieval techniques (Fig. 13-7). In light of its subcellular associations, one might

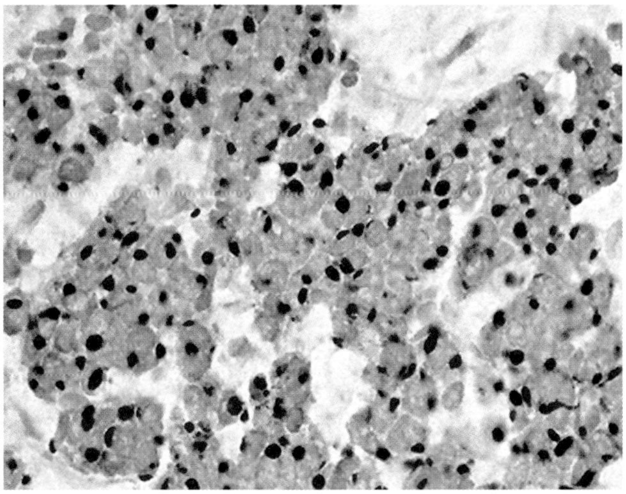

Figure 13-5. Paranuclear "dot"-like immunoreactivity for keratin in small cell pulmonary neuroendocrine carcinoma. This pattern concurrently establishes the epithelial and the neuroendocrine nature of the tumor.

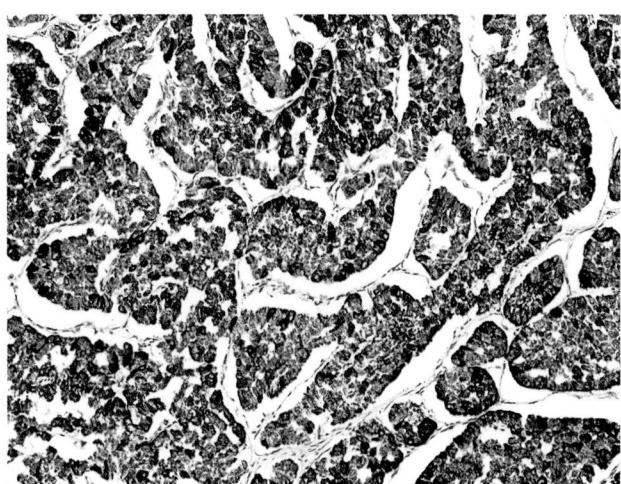

Figure 13-6. Immunoreactivity for chromogranin-A in neuroendocrine carcinoma of the lung.

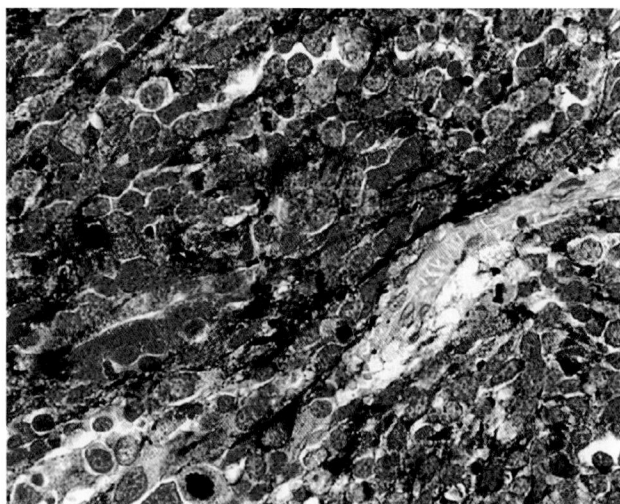

Figure 13-7. Immunolabeling for synaptophysin in pulmonary neuroendocrine carcinoma.

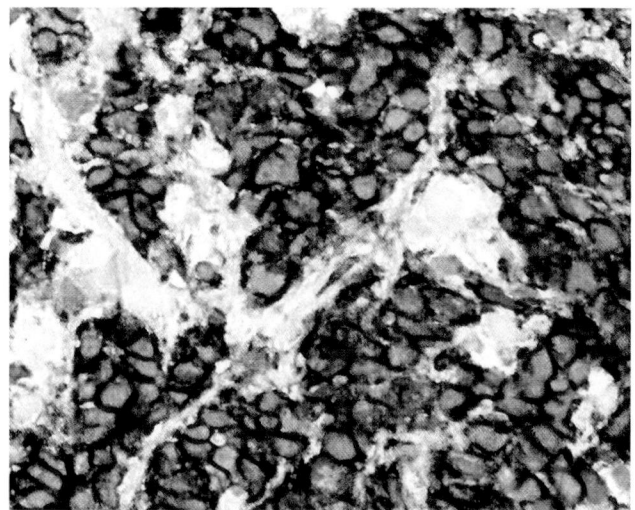

Figure 13-8. Immunoreactivity for CD56 (neural cell adhesion molecule) in neuroendocrine carcinoma of the lung.

assume that synaptophysin would have a synonymous tissue distribution to that of the chromogranins; however, in practicality, that is not true. Thus, a sizable proportion of neuroendocrine neoplasms label for CGA or CGB, but not synaptophysin; the converse also applies.[93] Thus, anti-synaptophysins and anti-chromogranins should be conceptualized as complementary reagents.

Loy and colleagues[59] have challenged the specificity of chromogranins and synaptophysin as markers of neuroendocrine lineage, in a study using ultrastructure as the standard for definition of that lineage. However, in our opinion, the concept behind that analysis was flawed. Sampling bias (a significant problem in fine structural evaluations) probably accounted for those cases in which immunoreactivity was observed for the specified endocrine markers, but no neurosecretory granules were identified by electron microscopy.

CD57 (Leu-7)
CD57 was originally characterized as a marker for natural killer lymphocytes, and it is recognized by monoclonal antibody HNK-1,[94] among others. Subsequently, shared epitopes of this molecule have been detected immunohistochemically in normal constituents and tumors of the brain, peripheral nervous system, soft tissues, prostate gland, thymus, and DNS.[95-101] With specific reference to neuroendocrine neoplasms, CD57 appears to bind to a matrical component of neurosecretory granules that is distinct from both CGA and CGB.[102] It both corroborates and extends the sensitivity of chromogranin immunostains in many clinical settings. Nonetheless, because of the imperfect specificity of Leu-7, it cannot be used as confidently as a "standalone" neuroendocrine marker. Moreover, it has the same failings in sensitivity as CGA and CGB that relate to the density of neurosecretory granules in poorly differentiated tumors.

Neural Cell Adhesion Molecule (NCAM; CD56)
The monoclonal antibodies 123C3 and JLP5B9 recognize formalin-preserved epitopes of CD56, or neural cell adhesion molecule, a cell membrane protein that has a role in the cohesiveness of cells in the peripheral and central nervous systems.[103-109] Like synaptophysin, NCAM is distributed among neuroendocrine and neuroectodermal cells and tumors (Fig. 13-8). Several studies have shown that NCAM is a sensitive marker of endocrine lineage in SCC of the lung as well as extrapulmonary sites.[106-108] Nonetheless, it is not absolutely specific for neuroendocrine differentiation; a minority (up to 25%) of ovarian

surface carcinomas, renal cell carcinomas, nonendocrine lung cancers, and endometrial carcinomas demonstrate CD56 immunoreactivity.[108] Despite this caveat, antibodies to NCAM are useful additions to diagnostic panels for endocrine tumors. Reagents raised against the polysialylated form of CD56 are considered the most sensitive among this group.[105]

Neuron-Specific (Gamma-Dimer) Enolase
"Neuron-specific" enolase (NSE) is a gamma-dimeric form of 14-3-2 protein, a glycolytic enzyme that is present in neurons and cells of the DNS.[110] It is thought to be associated with the formation of intercellular synapses in the nervous system. NSE was one of the first markers to be used in diagnostic immunohistochemistry as a general indicator of putative neuroendocrine differentiation.[110-112] Heteroantisera to NSE are very sensitive in that regard, labeling virtually all neuronal and neuroendocrine proliferations, regardless of the level of cellular differentiation.[112] Nevertheless, the specificity of those reagents is poor, owing to cross-reactivity between gamma-dimers and heterodimers (e.g., alpha-gamma, alpha-beta) of NSE that are expressed by non-neuroendocrine neoplasms of many types.[113] In reaction to that problem, monoclonal antibodies to NSE have been developed and tested,[114] but these have generally manifested a low degree of sensitivity and have not enjoyed widespread usage. An alternative approach to lessening the cross-reactivity of anti-NSE heteroantisera is to absorb them with acetone-fixed, pulverized human tissues known to contain high levels of the alpha or beta form of the molecule. However, that approach is time-consuming and somewhat demanding technically, and for this reason, has not been embraced in clinical practice. Currently, antibodies to NSE are primarily used as "screens" for endocrine differentiation,[115-117] and reactivity with them is usually pursued further by applying other neuroendocrine immunostains, as described elsewhere in this chapter.

Protein Gene Product 9.5 (PGP9.5)
PGP9.5 is a protein that removes ubiquitin (an intermediate filament) from other proteins and protects them from degradation by proteases. It is expressed widely within cells and tumors of the DNS and therefore has been applied as an immunohistochemical marker of neuroendocrine differentiation.[118-120] Nevertheless, the general distribution of PGP9.5 in human neoplasms has shown that it is not particularly specific for an endocrine lineage; in particular, non–small cell carcinomas of the lung that lack neuroendocrine morphologic patterns and

contain no neurosecretory granules on ultrastructural analysis have been PGP9.5-positive in approximately 55% of cases in some series.[121] Thus, the practical utility of this marker is similar to that of NSE.

Specific Neuropeptides

Specific neuropeptides, such as adrenocorticotropic hormone, gastrin, insulin, somatostatin, calcitonin, "whole" bombesin and its C-terminal flanking peptide, leu- and met- enkephalins, were the initial molecular moieties that were evaluated immunohistochemically in an effort to substantiate the neuroendocrine nature of selected epithelial human neoplasms.[93] Today, these markers have been largely relegated to a secondary role in the pathologic assessment of tumors in the DNS. Antibodies to such peptides are of academic interest in correlating clinical endocrinopathies with histopathologic findings, but are not nearly sensitive enough to serve as screening reagents. Another potential but limited application is in the delineation of "occult" (non–endocrinopathy-related) peptide production by neuroendocrine tumors, which may serve as the basis for serologic monitoring of tumor growth and activity.

CD99 (MIC2; p30/32 Protein)

The membranocytoplasmic protein known as "CD99" in the hematopoietic antigen cluster designation is the same molecule that has been called "MIC2" or "p30/32 protein."[122] The function of this moiety is uncertain, but it is empirically known to be expressed in virtually all PNETs and Ewing sarcomas[122,123] (Fig. 13-9). The specificity of CD99 antibodies for a neuroectodermal lineage is not absolute, however, because they may also label a minority (<15%) of alveolar rhabdomyosarcomas as well as the overwhelming majority (90%) of lymphoblastic lymphomas.[124] CD99 is observed in up to 20% of NECs in some body sites as well.[125,126] This is important because it may obscure the difference between NEC and PNET in selected instances; this is particularly true in light of the potential for keratin reactivity that both lesions have. On the other hand, differentiated group II neuroendocrine tumors, such as PGs, are nonreactive for this determinant.

Other Reagents

Several other antibodies have been developed that have immunohistochemical properties that overlap those of LK2H10 (anti-CGA).

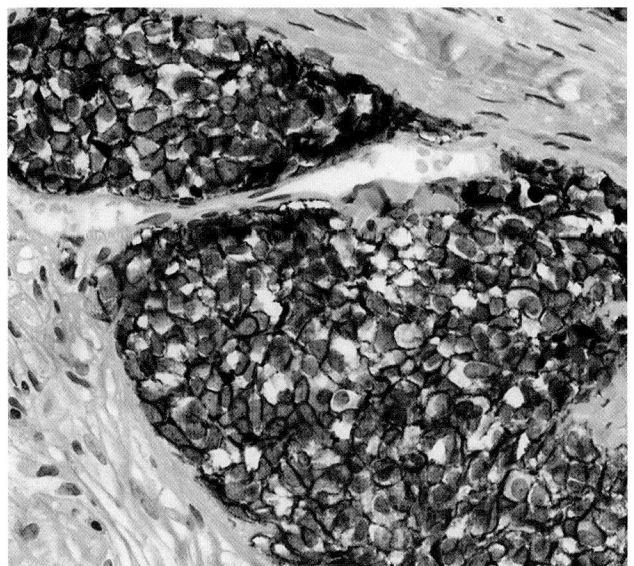

Figure 13-9. Immunolabeling for CD99 (MIC2 protein) in primitive neuroectodermal tumor. This marker can also be observed in neuroendocrine carcinomas.

These include both polyclonal and hybridoma reagents. A monoclonal antibody designated "HISL-19" by Krisch and coworkers[127] is believed to manifest neuroendocrine specificity. The determinant that it recognizes is proteinaceous, but seems to be nonidentical to chromogranin. This statement is based on the relative strength of reactivity of HISL-19 with several neuroendocrine tissues, which is dissimilar to that of LK2H10. Moreover, some nonendocrine tissues and tumors, such as the gallbladder epithelium and adenocarcinomas of the lung, stomach, and endometrium, are labeled by the former reagent but not by the latter. These differences notwithstanding, HISL-19 appears to bind to a neurosecretory granule-related moiety, and neoplasms with few of these granules (parathyroid adenoma, melanoma, NB, and oat cell lung cancer) are only weakly stained, but others with numerous granules (pituitary adenoma, pheochromocytoma, medullary thyroid carcinoma, carcinoid, and islet cell tumor) are labeled intensely. Western immunoblot analyses have shown that the target of HISL-19 is not neuron-specific enolase.[127]

Lloyd and colleagues[128] employed monoclonal antibodies to adrenaline (epinephrine) and noradrenaline (norepinephrine) in the study of similar neuroendocrine neoplasms. In general, pheochromocytomas displayed adrenaline alone, but extra-adrenal PGs exhibited reactivity for adrenaline and noradrenaline, or noradrenaline only. NBs, carcinoids, pituitary adenomas, pancreatic endocrine tumors, and parathyroid adenomas also showed positivity for noradrenaline. These authors emphasized that catecholamine-positive neoplasms also expressed reactivity with LK2H10, implying that stains for adrenaline and noradrenaline did not add appreciably to the diagnostic information obtained with antichromogranin.

Haspel and colleagues[129] found that mice infected with reovirus type I often had autoimmune syndromes featuring polyendocrinopathies. Spleen cells from such animals were used as the substrates for hybridoma production, and two of the resulting monoclonal antibodies (5B5 and 5B8) showed reactivity with human anterior pituitary cells in frozen and Bouin's-fixed specimens.[129] Further immunostaining results in normal and neoplastic human tissues were not provided, but it was believed that 5B5 and 5B8 recognized discrete hormonal products, such as growth hormone, based on competitive inhibition studies.

The absence of discussion of S-100 protein may seem surprising because of the still-common belief that this marker is associated with neuroendocrine tumors. In reality, that is not so. The only endocrine neoplasm that reproducibly contains cells positive for S-100 protein is PG, and the immunoreactive elements therein are actually "sustentacular" cells rather than tumor cells.[79] It has been contended that sustentacular elements decrease in density when PGs undergo malignant change,[130] but that is an uncertain tenet in reference to individual cases.

Several markers have been assessed with regard to their associations with neuroendocrine tumor grade; SOX2, PAX5, and CD117 are the principal analytes. Each demonstrates a tendency for greater reactivity in this context as the histologic grade increases, such that grade III lesions show the highest level of immunolabeling.[131–133]

Yet another applicable reagent is antithyroid transcription factor-1 (TTF1).[134–140] This intranuclear protein is expressed not only by thyroid epithelium but also by glandular cells of the lung, pulmonary adenocarcinomas, and NECs of the lung (Fig. 13-10). Among the last of these lesional groups, SCC and large cell NECs have the highest incidence of reactivity (in approximately 85% to 90% of cases). Interestingly, however, extrapulmonary high-grade NECs show a tendency to be TTF1-positive in many organ sites (bladder, uterine cervix, prostate, gastrointestinal tract), and therefore this marker can be considered to represent an "adjunct" neuroendocrine determinant, if additional studies for thyroid-related and lung-associated labels are negative.

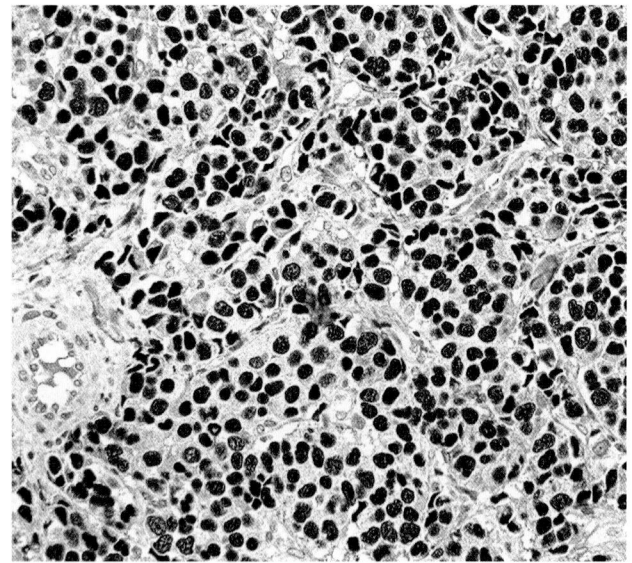

Figure 13-10. Nuclear immunoreactivity for thyroid transcription factor-1 in pulmonary neuroendocrine carcinoma.

Obviously, then, TTF1 cannot be employed reliably to distinguish metastatic NEC of the lung from other neuroendocrine malignancies.

Specific Features of Pulmonary Neuroendocrine Proliferations

Before further discussion of specific neuroendocrine proliferations in the lung, a general consideration of the current nosology is in order. Travis et al.[141,142] recently provided a classification scheme for pulmonary neoplasms in general through the auspices of the World Health Organization (WHO; Box 13-1).

As discussed earlier, we believe that all neuroendocrine proliferations of the lung are at least potentially malignant. The only exceptions are pulmonary tumorlets and neuroepithelial bodies, which are considered hyperplastic rather than neoplastic. As others have done,[143] we espoused

---

Box 13-1. World Health Organization Classification of Pulmonary Neuroendocrine Lesions

Submacroscopic Pulmonary Neuroendocrine Lesions
Tumorlet
Neuroendocrine body

Common Tumors with a Light Microscopic Neuroendocrine Appearance
Carcinoid tumor
Atypical carcinoid/well-differentiated neuroendocrine carcinoma
Large cell neuroendocrine carcinoma (intermediate cell neuroendocrine carcinoma)
Small cell carcinoma
   Pure small cell carcinoma (oat cell and intermediate variants)
   Small cell/large cell neuroendocrine carcinoma
   Combined small cell/non–small cell carcinoma

Non–Small Cell Carcinoma with Neuroendocrine Features (Neuroendocrine Differentiation Detected Only by Immunostaining or Electron Microscopy)

Uncommon Primary Tumors with Neuroendocrine Differentiation
Amphicrine neoplasms
Blastoma with neuroendocrine differentiation
Primitive neuroectodermal tumors

From Travis WD, Colby TV, Corrin B, et al: *Histological Typing of Lung & Pleural Tumours: International Histological Classification of Tumours.* Geneva: World Health Organization; 1999:1–55.

Box 13-2. Alternative Classification of Neuroendocrine Proliferations of the Lung

Neuroendocrine hyperplasias: microscopic tumorlet, neuropeithelial body
Type I neoplastic lesions (neuroendocrine carcinomas [NECs])
   Grade I NEC (formerly called "classic carcinoid")
   Grade II NEC (formerly called "atypical carcinoid" or "well-differentiated neuroendocrine carcinoma")
   Grade III NEC (further characterized by cell size as small cell NEC or large cell NEC, or mixtures thereof)
   Mixed neuroendocrine/non-neuroendocrine carcinomas
   Non–small cell carcinoma with occult neuroendocrine differentiation
Type II neoplastic lesions (paraganglioma, primitive neuroectodermal tumor, and neuroblastoma)

---

the scheme shown in Box 13-2 as more appropriate than the WHO paradigm in the general categorization of neuroendocrine lesions.

The following points constitute our rationale for this type of classification:

1. From 5% to 15% of classic bronchial "carcinoids" may metastasize to regional lymph nodes, and at least 1% to 2% may be fatal.[5] These tumors, thus, have low-grade biologic attributes and can usually be cured by complete resection, but their malignant potential is not nil. However, these data clearly escape many observers, who equate the term "carcinoid" with a benign process.

2. The term "atypical carcinoid" is fraught with interpretative problems because it is still regarded erroneously as a variant of classic carcinoid by many clinicians. This is a reflection of the fact that many pathologists tend to use the term "atypical," particularly in cytopathology, to describe benign but morphogically abnormal cells. By contrast, "atypical carcinoid" (grade II NEC) is an undeniably aggressive malignancy, with a 5-year mortality rate of at least 35%.[5] The term "atypical carcinoid" has taken on a nebulous quality, with a general lack of agreement on the necessary criteria for that diagnosis. Some use the term for any neuroendocrine lesion of the lung that is not a central classic "carcinoid" or a SCC.

4. Large cell NECs appear to be unquestionably high-grade tumors, behaviorally and histologically. Referring to these neoplasms as "moderately differentiated" or "intermediate"[12] underestimates their biologic potential. In addition, use of the term "intermediate" is confounding in this specific context because it has been employed in the past in reference to variants of SCC of the lung.[35]

5. The time has probably come to reexamine the venerated dichotomy of surgical or nonsurgical treatment of non–small cell and SCCs of the lung, respectively. Although they are rare, pathologic stage I SCCs are surgically treatable lesions[143]; conversely, high-grade large cell NECs could benefit from chemotherapeutic approaches that are usually applied for SCC.[4] However, these issues are unresolved and are likely to remain so as long as the traditional small cell/non–small cell carcinoma paradigm is rigidly followed.

6. The argument is often made that clinicians understand only the "traditional" terms for neuroendocrine neoplasms; therefore, these terms should remain in the lexicon of pathologists. In contrast, our sense is that clinical physicians do not understand well the biologic potential of pulmonary neuroendocrine proliferations, and that several terms that have been used for years serve only to perpetuate myths.

At this time, we make the diagnosis of "NEC," followed by its grade, for all type I (epithelial) neuroendocrine tumors of the lung.[144] Parenthetically, the traditional terminology is usually used as well to facilitate transitions in nomenclature.[145] At some point, it should be possible to omit the older terminology altogether.

Grade I Neuroendocrine Carcinoma ("Classic Carcinoid")

Bronchopulmonary "carcinoid" (grade I NEC) was initially considered an "adenoma" of the bronchus,[146] a term that unfortunately persists in the lexicon of some individuals. The similarity of this lesion to gastrointestinal carcinoids, or "carcinoma-like tumors," described 30 years earlier, was noted. Although the majority of classic carcinoids are centrally located, approximately 10% to 20% are found in the periphery (Fig. 13-11) of the lung.[11,12,15,45,147–152] An anatomic landmark that is commonly used to distinguish central and peripheral tumors is the cartilaginous airways; neoplasms associated with such structures are considered central, and others without that relationship are considered peripheral.[148]

Clinical Features

Grade I NECs with typical histologic features are rarely diagnostic problems. They usually grow as polypoid intraluminal masses with an intact overlying epithelium (Fig. 13-12) or one demonstrating squamous metaplasia.[45,147,148] This pattern explains a common clinical presentation, which is localized airway obstruction. Patients manifest with wheezing,

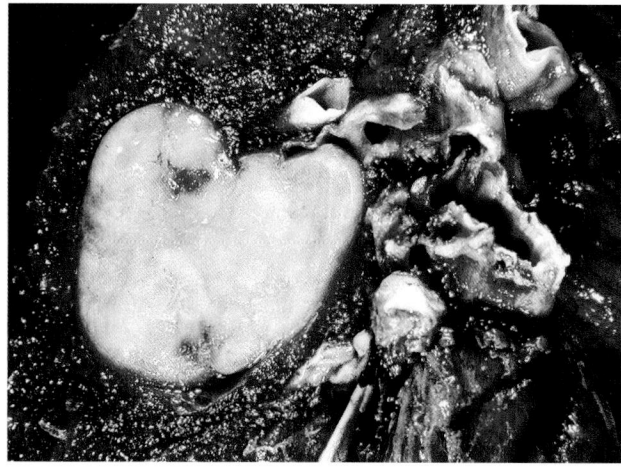

Figure 13-11. This yellow-white mass in the peripheral pulmonary parenchyma had the histologic image of a grade I neuroendocrine carcinoma ("classic carcinoid").

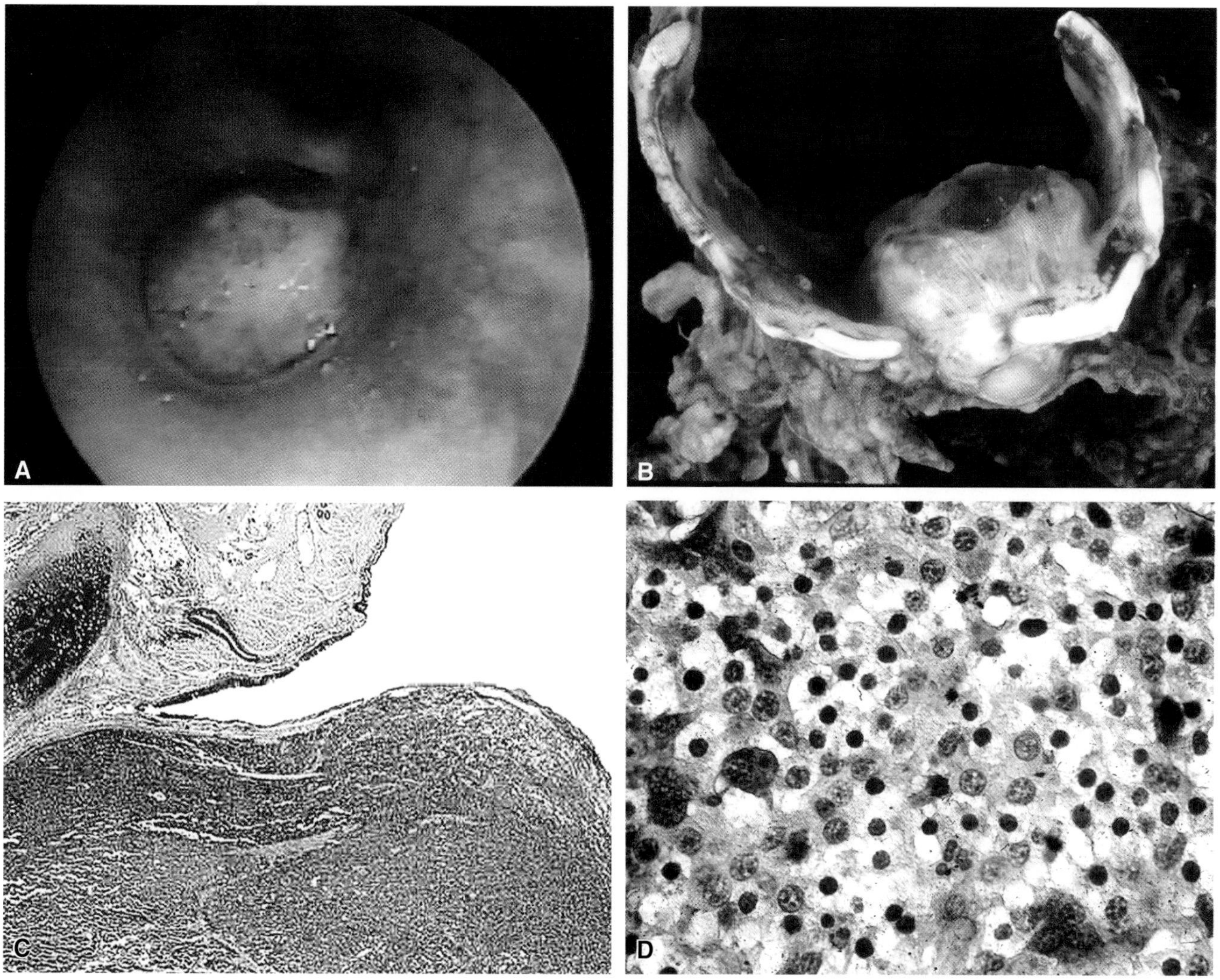

Figure 13-12. A, Endoscopic photograph of low-grade neuroendocrine carcinoma, protruding as a polypoid mass into the bronchial lumen. **B,** Gross photograph of grade I neuroendocrine carcinoma of the lung, straddling the bronchial cartilage. **C,** Photomicrograph of low-grade neuroendocrine carcinoma, protruding into the bronchial lumen. **D,** Immunoreactivity for adrenocorticotrophic hormone in this low-grade pulmonary neuroendocrine carcinoma. The patient had Cushing syndrome.

cough, or pneumonia. Carcinoid syndrome almost never develops, presumably because the tumors in question are incapable of synthesizing the biochemical substances responsible for its pathogenesis. Rare individuals with grade I NEC have associated Cushing syndrome or other endocrinopathies as a result of ectopic neuropeptide production by the neoplasm (see Fig. 13-12D).[153-159] A proposed association between pulmonary carcinoids and sarcoidosis has also been made.[160]

Localized obstruction also dominates the radiographic picture, with evidence of obstructive pneumonia or atelectasis (Fig. 13-13). Occasionally, a central mass with a dumbbell-like configuration is seen on plain films, and computed tomography usually demonstrates a lesion within and adjacent to a large airway.[161]

Men and women are approximately equally affected by pulmonary "carcinoids." Although all age groups may have grade I pulmonary NECs, young to middle-aged adults account for the majority of cases. The lesions therefore appear at substantially lower ages than those associated with other pulmonary carcinomas.

Peripheral carcinoids are subpleural, small, and well circumscribed.[148,151,152] They often present as incidental findings, lacking the propensity to produce the obstructive changes of their central counterparts. Instead, the differential diagnosis of a "coin lesion" is encountered. Radiographically, such entities as granulomas, hamartomas, or peripheral adenocarcinomas enter consideration. Some studies have shown a predominance of peripheral grade I NECs in the right middle lobe, and a greater number of women have those tumors compared with central NECs of the lung.[151,152]

Rarely, grade I NECs may be synchronously multifocal.[162,163] That eventuality is troublesome because of the possibility of metastasis to the lung from an extrapulmonary source. Extensive clinical evaluations and appropriate immunohistologic studies (discussed later) are usually required.

Gross and Microscopic Pathologic Findings
"Classic carcinoids" are typically 2 to 4 cm in maximum dimension. The lesions vary in color from tan-yellow to dark red, and they lack obvious internal necrosis and hemorrhage. Central tumors display diverse growth patterns, including trabecular, ribboning, insular, and

solid sheet-like configurations[11,147,148] (Fig. 13-14). A delicate fibrovascular stroma is present, sometimes with associated matrical amyloid deposition.[164] Rare lesions may contain metaplastic bone or cartilage.[11] The latter findings are postulated to reflect the production of factors related to tumor growth factor beta or various bone morphogenetic proteins.[148] Tumor cell cytoplasm is relatively abundant, and it may be strikingly granular and oncocytic or even clear.[165-169] Eccentricity of the nuclei can yield a plasmacytoid cellular image, particularly in fine-needle aspiration biopsy specimens (Fig. 13-15). A papillary configuration has also been reported.[11,170] Other variants of grade I NEC produce melanin,[171,172] and some are said to contain sustentacular cells immunoreactive to S-100 protein, as is more typically seen in PGs.[173] An exceptional case presented by Skinner and Ewen[174] featured diffuse replacement of the lung parenchyma by carcinoid tumor cells.

Peripheral carcinoids may be morphologically identical to central tumors, in which case the diagnosis is usually made without difficulty. Nonetheless, peripheral grade I NECs often demonstrate a prominent spindle cell growth pattern, which is associated with a somewhat different set of diagnostic alternatives (discussed later)[151,152,175] (Fig. 13-16).

Differential Diagnostic Considerations
The intraluminal growth pattern of grade I pulmonary NEC can be simulated by salivary gland-like tumors, such as mucoepidermoid carcinoma; mesenchymal lesions, including peripheral nerve sheath tumors and rare inflammatory pseudotumors; and some metastatic neoplasms. Most of these possibilities present little difficulty histologically. Nonetheless, problems may arise occasionally in differentiating carcinoids from well-differentiated adenocarcinomas, higher-grade NECs, primary pulmonary PGs, and "solid" adenoid cystic carcinomas, particularly in small transbronchial biopsy specimens, which may demonstrate significant artifactual distortion. Distinction from "atypical" carcinoids is discussed in more detail later. However, uniform nuclear features, the lack of significant mitotic activity, abundant cytoplasm, and the absence of necrosis are all indicative of grade I NEC rather than a grade II tumor.[3,5,149] Because of the well-differentiated nature of classic carcinoids, one can expect almost all of them to be diffusely reactive for keratin, CGA, synaptophysin, and CD57,[4,173] whereas the other diagnostic alternatives do not show that immunophenotypic profile. The p53 gene, as studied by immunohistochemical or genetic analysis, is infrequently mutated in grade I NEC,[176] as opposed to higher-grade neuroendocrine tumors.[177]

Another differential diagnostic consideration in this specific context is metastatic grade I neuroendocrine NEC from a source outside the lungs. Srivastava and Hornick[178] immunohistologically compared pulmonary with nonpulmonary well-differentiated NECs, finding that the presence of thyroid transcription factor 1 was restricted to primary tumors of the lung. Classic pulmonary carcinoids also lacked reactivity for CDX2 and PDX1, both of which are alimentary tract–related markers.

Spindle cell growth in grade I NECs raises a dissimilar set of differential diagnostic considerations. These include fibrous and smooth muscle neoplasms, fibrous pseudotumors, primary or metastatic spindle cell melanomas, and metastatic medullary thyroid carcinomas. Careful attention to nuclear detail in spindle cell carcinoids shows retention of the typical stippled chromatin pattern, and nucleoli are small and inconspicuous. The lesions also express the majority of immunohistologic markers seen in central carcinoids, as discussed earlier. A combination of morphologic and adjunctive studies should be capable of excluding most of the differential diagnostic considerations mentioned earlier, but metastatic medullary thyroid carcinoma is virtually indistinguishable from grade I pulmonary NEC on pathologic grounds.[164] Likewise, Eyden and coworkers[179] have shown that metastatic melanomas sometimes exhibit partial neuroendocrine differentiation in ultrastructural or immunohistochemical studies.

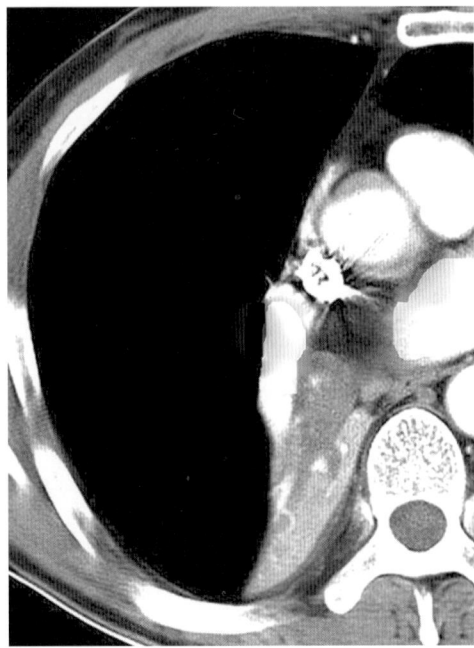

Figure 13-13. Bronchial obstruction by central low-grade neuroendocrine carcinoma caused segmental atelectasis of the right upper lobe, as seen in this computed tomogram of the thorax.

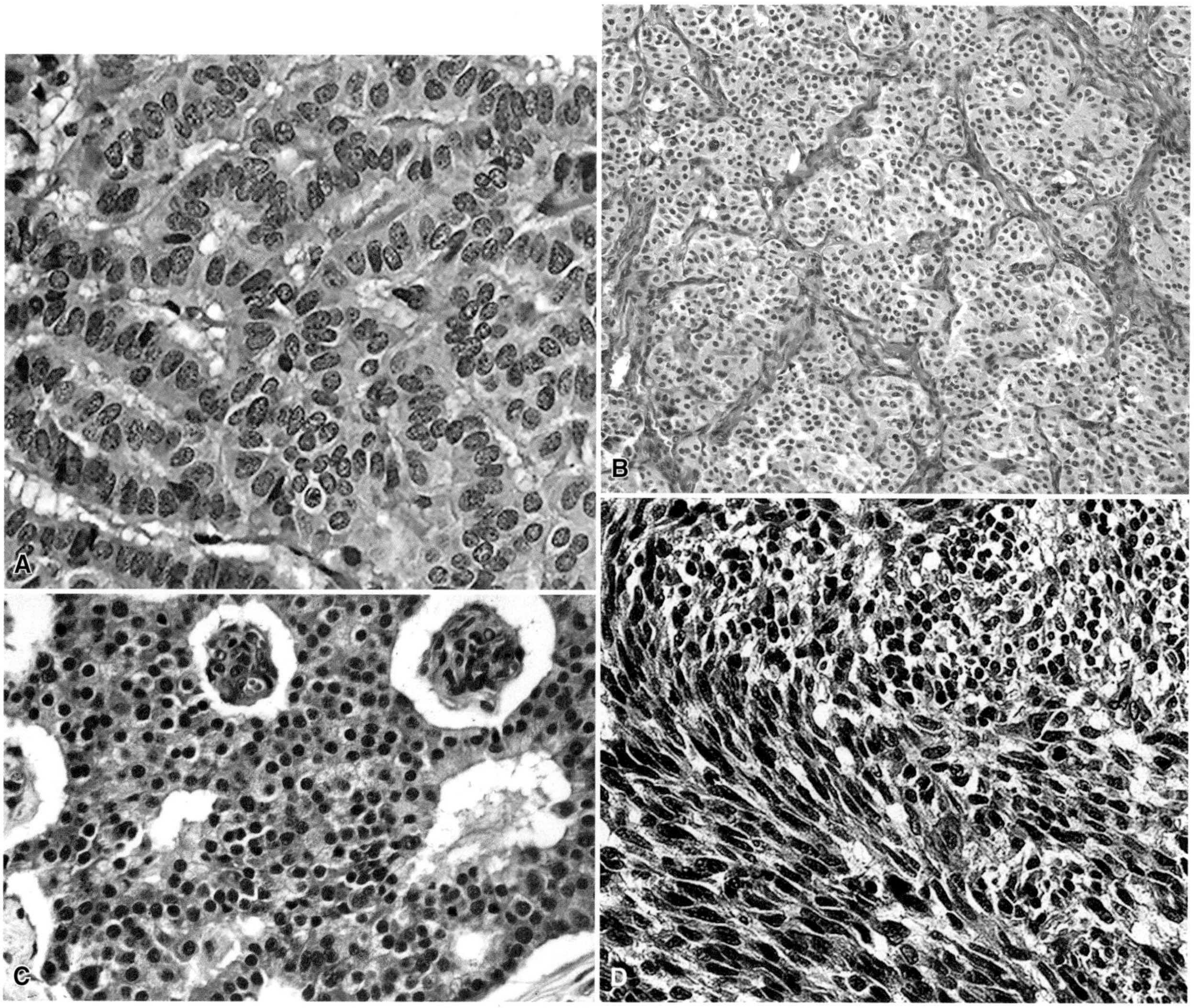

Figure 13-14. Grade I neuroendocrine carcinoma (classic carcinoid) may assume several growth patterns, including trabecular (**A**), insular (**B**), pseudoglandular (**C**), and spindle cell (**D**; in a cell block from a fine-needle aspiration biopsy specimen).

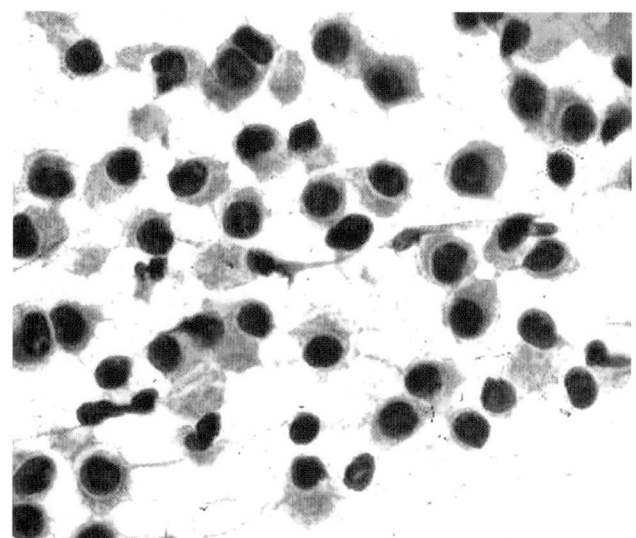

Figure 13-15. Fine-needle aspirates of low-grade neuroendocrine carcinomas may show dyshesive cells with plasmacytoid configurations, causing potential confusion with hematopoietic proliferations.

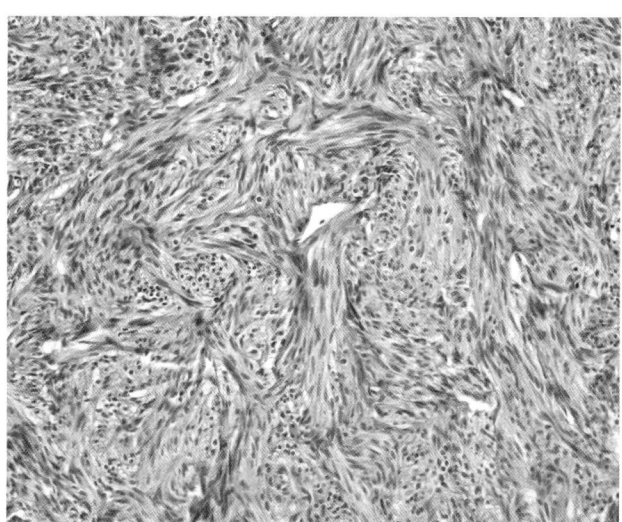

Figure 13-16. Spindle cell growth in a peripheral low-grade neuroendocrine carcinoma of the lung.

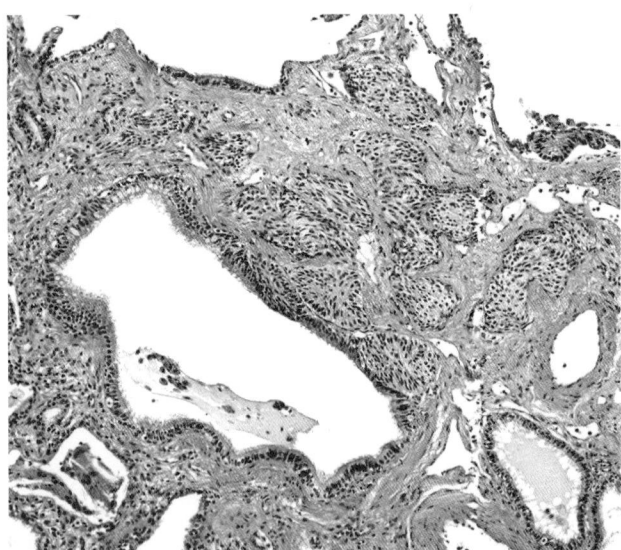

Figure 13-17. This neuroendocrine tumorlet (NT) has the same cytologic features as those of low-grade neuroendocrine carcinoma of the lung; however, NTs are microscopic, are associated with chronic airway disease, and tend to grow in packets separated by fibrous tissue (carcinoid tumors have a more sheet-like growth pattern).

A similar issue is the separation of tumorlets (Fig. 13-17) from peripheral carcinoids. This is an arbitrary distinction because immunohistochemical and ultrastructural studies indicate that the cells of these two lesions are essentially identical.[180-182] Also, there is debate over whether tumorlets represent true neoplasms or are instead hyperplasias of respiratory neuroendocrine cells.[15,181,183] They generally occur within and around small bronchioles, and they typically have a spindle cell composition. The small nests of tumor cells in a neuroendocrine tumorlet tend to be divided by a fibrous stroma into small packets, and this feature helps to differentiate neuroendocrine tumorlets from small peripheral carcinoid tumors, where tumor cell growth is more sheetlike, with variable fibrous stands interlaced. Although such tumorlets, which may number in the hundreds in some cases, are said to occur most often in diseased lungs with such associated lesions as bronchiectasis or pulmonary fibrosis,[180-184] they also may arise in otherwise normal lungs.[162] Rizvi and colleagues[185] and Ferolla and colleagues[186] have also shown that neuroendocrine hyperplasia is much more common in patients with pulmonary NECs than in others with non-neuroendocrine neoplasms. In any event, an arbitrary size of 4 mm or less has been suggested for tumorlets; larger lesions are considered peripheral carcinoids.[181] A continuum for such proliferations was suggested by Miller and Muller,[187] who found that peripheral carcinoid tumors were often associated with diffuse neuroendocrine cell hyperplasia and airway obstruction. A particular pitfall associated with tumorlets is that they may be misdiagnosed as much more aggressive lesions in small biopsy specimens, especially when clinical data are ignored or unavailable.[188,189]

Treatment and Outcome

The clinical outcome in cases of central grade I NECs of the lung is generally excellent.[5,11,45] Complete excision is the treatment of choice, possibly necessitating lobectomy or sleeve resection.[190] Conservative endobronchial excision is generally associated with an unacceptable rate of local recurrence.[190-193]

A peripheral location or a spindle cell growth pattern does not, in and of itself, equate with "atypical" morphology in grade I NECs of the lung. The prognosis for low-grade spindle cell peripheral lesions is equivalent to that of their central relatives, despite a slightly higher rate of lymph node metastasis in some series.[45,151,152]

Figures for the incidence of metastasis differ widely and depend on two major variables. These include the definition of peribronchial lymph node metastasis (i.e., direct invasion of nodes vs. embolic metastatic involvement) and the histologic purity of the primary lesion. Some studies with high rates of metastasis for classic "carcinoid" have improperly included higher-grade neuroendocrine lesions. Quoted metastasis rates vary from 1% to 20%; a figure of approximately 5% to 10% is probably closest to the actual incidence, and most secondary implants involve adjacent peribronchial or hilar lymph nodes.[5,192-196] It is this behavioral attribute that leads us, as well as others, to consider central pulmonary carcinoids irrefutable carcinomas.[143] Distant metastases also occur rarely, and there is a tendency for spread to the bones, liver, skin, or brain.[45,193,194] Interestingly, osseous metastases are typically blastic.[197] Flow cytometric measurement of DNA content in grade I NECs is not helpful in predicting their metastatic potential.[149,198]

The overall survival rate for patients with grade I NEC of the lung is greater than 95% at 5 years.[5,45,148,192-196,199] Metastatic disease may be palliated with interleukin or somatostatin analogs,[38,200] and surgical excision of secondary implants can be considered, given the slow growth of this tumor type.

Grade II Neuroendocrine Carcinoma ("Atypical Carcinoid")

The term "atypical carcinoid" was first used by Arrigoni and coworkers in 1972.[201] Those authors reviewed 216 bronchial carcinoids treated at the Mayo Clinic and found 23 with unusual features, including pleomorphism, mitotic activity, nuclear hyperchromatism with increased nucleocytoplasmic ratios, and evidence of spontaneous necrosis or hemorrhage. In the original series, 70% of the lesions metastasized and seven patients (30%) died of their tumors. Several terms have subsequently entered the literature on this lesion, including "Kulschitzky cell carcinoma"[202] and "well-differentiated NEC,"[12,15,194,202-209] and the criteria for their definition are still being debated.[3,5,35]

Clinical Findings

"Atypical carcinoids" of the lung are usually greater than 3 cm in maximum dimension. Other characteristics include an etiologic link to cigarette smoking, differing from the epidemiologic features of grade I NECs.[5,201-216] Grade II NECs are more likely to be peripherally located in the lung (Fig. 13-18) compared with "classic" carcinoids; the former lesions have been so situated in the majority of cases in several studies.[201-216] Potential associations with Cushing syndrome[217] and Eaton-Lambert syndrome also apply to these lesions.

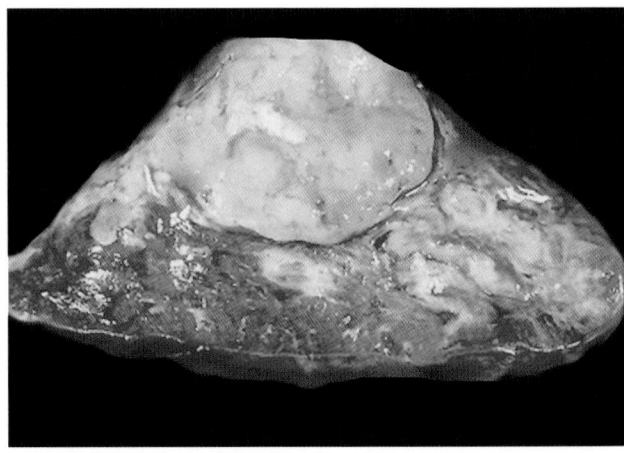

Figure 13-18. Grade II neuroendocrine carcinoma (atypical carcinoid) is usually peripherally located in the lung parenchyma and may contain areas of hemorrhage or necrosis, as seen in this gross photograph.

Pathologic Findings

With the exception of the possible gross identification of hemorrhage or necrosis and a tendency to be slightly larger, the lesions were difficult, if not impossible, to distinguish from typical carcinoids by clinical, radiographic, or gross pathologic evaluation (Fig. 13-19). The

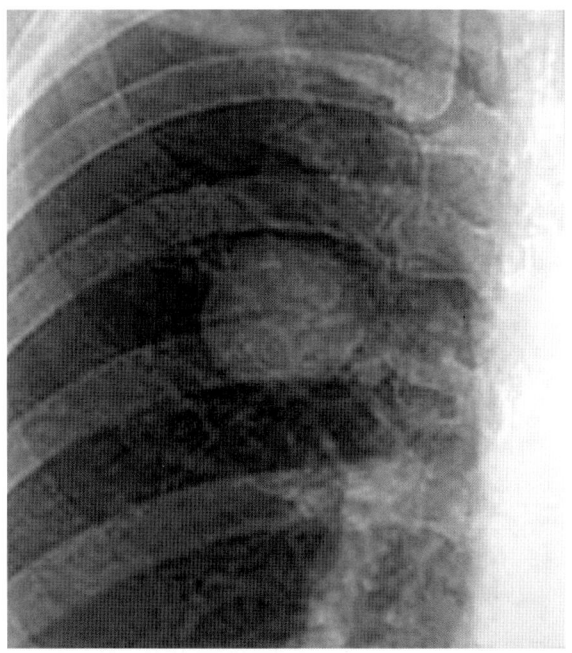

Figure 13-19. Chest radiograph of grade II neuroendocrine carcinomas of the lung (atypical carcinoids) shows features that are essentially identical to those associated with grade I tumors.

pathologic requirements for a diagnosis of "atypical carcinoid" have varied from study to study, but most have included mitotic activity and necrosis. We currently use the criteria of El-Naggar and colleagues[149] to define grade II NEC of the lung (Fig. 13-20), preferring that term to "atypical carcinoid," but stipulating that the two are conceptually synonymous. Those requirements center on the following points:

- Mitotic rate of five or more division figures per 10 high-power (×400) fields
- Discernible nuclear pleomorphism
- At least focal necrosis, brisk apoptosis, or both
- At least focal loss of an organoid growth pattern

Spindle cell change in grade II NECs of the lung is potentially seen but uncommon.[215] As observed by Yousem and Taylor,[3,218] a requirement for at least two of these criteria is more reasonable than basing the diagnosis of grade II NEC on only one feature in a lesion that is otherwise a classic carcinoid of the lung.

Immunohistochemical studies show some differences between grade I NEC and grade II NEC of the lung. As expected of more poorly differentiated tumors, "atypical carcinoids" tend to express fewer markers of neuroendocrine differentiation or to demonstrate more focal labeling for them; such markers as synaptophysin, CGA, and CD57 are usually less impressive in grade II lesions.[92,117,120,219,220] Reactivity for specific neuropeptides—such as bombesin, calcitonin, and adrenocorticotropic hormone (ACTH)—is relatively uncommon.[221] Mutant p53 protein is demonstrable by immunostaining in some atypical carcinoids, as opposed to its absence in the great majority of typical carcinoids but like its presence in most SCCs.[176,222,223]

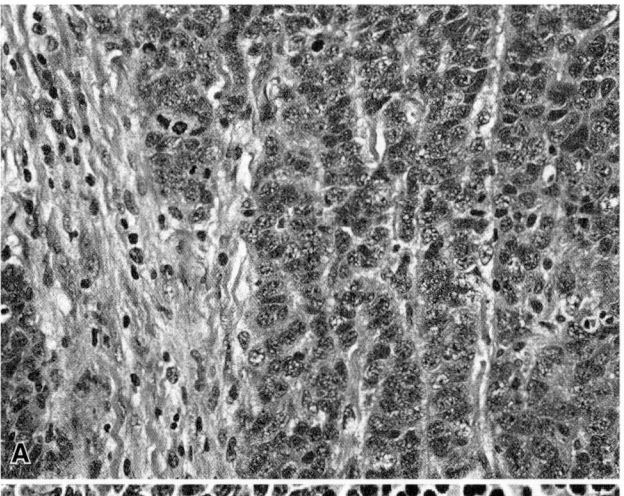

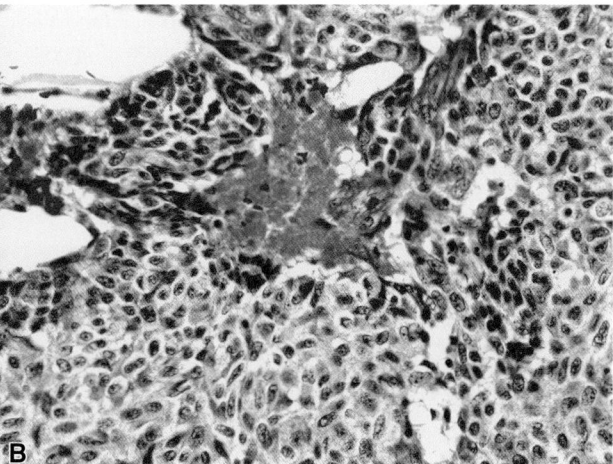

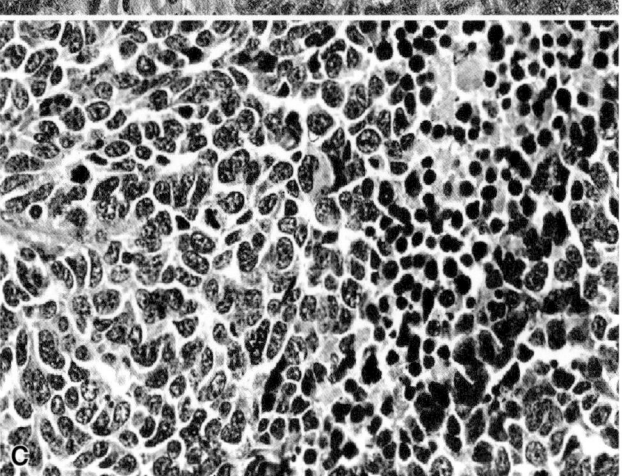

Figure 13-20. A to **C,** Grade II neuroendocrine carcinomas exhibit organoid growth patterns but show notable mitotic activity and areas of spontaneous necrosis, unlike grade I tumors.

Ultrastructural analysis of grade II NEC shows fewer neurosecretory granules compared with grade I neuroendocrine neoplasms.[207] Cytogenetic analysis also has demonstrated multiple karyotypic abnormalities in grade II NEC but not in classic carcinoid,[224–227] paralleling the flow cytometric incidences of aneuploidy in the two tumor types.[149,218,228]

Differential Diagnosis

In addition to its distinction from other neuroendocrine lesions, the differential diagnosis of grade II NEC includes poorly differentiated non-neuroendocrine carcinomas of the lung.[44,50,53,210] In particular, selected examples of high-grade adenocarcinoma may simulate the microscopic configuration of "atypical carcinoids," and "basaloid carcinoma" (basaloid squamous cell carcinoma)[229] is regularly confused with grade II NEC. The nuclear characteristics of those lesions differ from one another in that non-neuroendocrine tumors do not manifest the dispersed chromatin seen in "atypical carcinoids," instead showing more vesicular nuclei with often-prominent nucleoli (Fig. 13-21). Immunohistochemical studies may assist with the differential diagnosis in this context, but because some grade II NECs lack reactivity for endocrine markers and conversely selected non-neuroendocrine carcinomas of the lung demonstrate their presence, this technique is problematic. Electron microscopy is still probably the surest technique for differentiating grade II NEC from its non-neuroendocrine diagnostic simulators.

Treatment and Clinical Outcome

A vexing problem is which diagnostic label to assign a neuroendocrine pulmonary tumor with only one indicator of potentially aggressive behavior, such as angiolymphatic invasion, brisk mitotic activity, aneuploidy, or large size. None of these features independently appears to warrant adjuvant therapy, but it is probably prudent to suggest that they may be associated with an adverse outcome and to monitor the patient carefully for recurrence. Special techniques may provide additional information. In a flow cytometric analysis by El-Naggar and colleagues,[149] approximately 80% of "atypical carcinoids" were aneuploid, whereas 80% of classic carcinoids were diploid. Also, grade II lesions were more likely to have an S-phase fraction of greater than 7%. Both of these factors were statistically linked to a worse outcome. However, in that analysis,

the most significant predictor was accurate morphologic separation into grade I and grade II categories. Rush and colleagues,[206] Jackson-York and coworkers,[228] and Travis and colleagues[230] concluded that accurate classification of these tumors is more important in the prognosis than DNA content. Other factors said to significantly decrease survival rates in cases of "atypical carcinoid" include lymph node metastases, vascular invasion, and overall tumor size of greater than 3 cm.[5,148,201–209,210–216,230]

Lymph node metastases are found at diagnosis in 30% to 50% of cases, and approximately 25% of patients with grade II NEC of the lung have remote metastatic disease at presentation.[5,215,216,231] As in cases of SCC, the brain is a common site for metastasis and recurrence. Importantly, the mortality rate for this neoplasm is 30% to 50% at 2 years.[5,148,201–209,210–215] Rush and colleagues[206] have reported 5- and 10-year survival rates of 60% and 40%, respectively. Obviously, these figures reflect a different biologic potential than those of classic carcinoid and SCC. The use of adjunctive therapy in the management of grade II NEC of the lung is unresolved.[232,233] Some researchers have suggested that chemotherapy, irradiation, or both can be beneficial in this setting, but there has been no consensus on that point, much less on which pharmacologic agents to use. The difficulty in securing diagnostically "pure" study populations for treatment evaluations has likely contributed to this uncertainty.

Grade III Neuroendocrine Carcinoma, Small Cell Type

Small cell carcinoma is probably the best recognized neuroendocrine neoplasm in this discussion, accounting for approximately 25% of all lung carcinomas.[32] That diagnostic entity is generally traced to Barnard's 1926 description of "oat cell carcinoma"[234]; although the tumor had been believed to represent a lymphoma or sarcoma before that time, he accurately recognized its epithelial nature. In 1959, Azzopardi refined the pathologic description of SCC.[235]

Clinical Features

Small cell carcinoma of the lung has many potential modes of clinical presentation. These include symptoms and signs similar to those of other common carcinomas of the lung, such as cough, hemoptysis, weight loss, anorexia, fatigue, and the syndrome of hypertrophic osteoarthropathy.[236,237] In addition, however, unusual findings, such

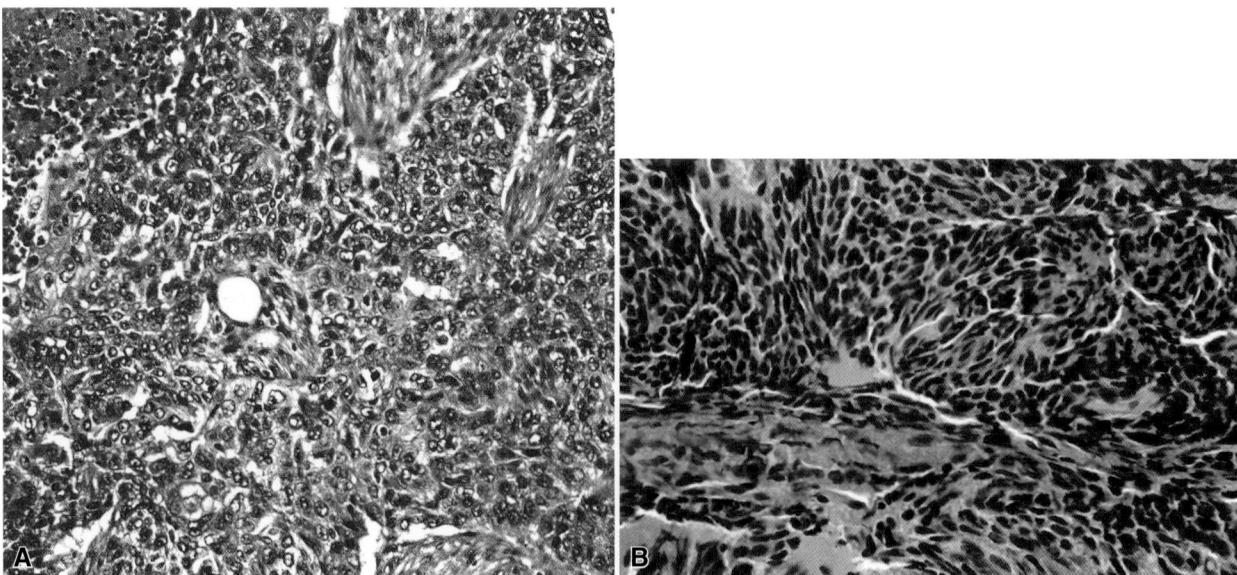

Figure 13-21. Basaloid squamous carcinoma of the lung is also composed of polygonal (**A**) and spindle-shaped (**B**) tumor cells, potentially like those of neuroendocrine carcinomas, but the former tumors have more vesicular nuclear chromatin and prominent nucleoli. Their immunophenotypes also lack positivity for endocrine markers, and no neurosecretory granules are present on electron microscopy.

as hyponatremia, hypercalcemia, or Cushing syndrome, may emanate from ectopic production by the tumor of antidiuretic hormone, parathyroid hormone-like peptides, and ACTH, respectively.[155,159,236,238,239] Rarely, individuals with SCC manifest Eaton-Lambert (pseudomyasthenia) syndrome owing to paraneoplastic interference with neuromuscular function.[240,241] Retinopathy, central and peripheral neuropathies, encephalitis, glomerulonephritis, cutaneous reactions, sarcoid-like granulomatous lesions, and systemic vasculitis also have been reported in this context.[241-248] Massive hepatomegaly with liver failure,[249] myelophthisic anemia,[250,251] or seizure activity and headaches[252] are additional clinical constellations related to the effects of distant visceral metastases at initial diagnosis.

Chest radiographic findings may be relatively unremarkable or may demonstrate a central hilar (or, more rarely, a peripheral intrapulmonary) mass (Fig. 13-22). Obstructive pneumonia is a potential complication; bulky peribronchial or mediastinal lymphadenopathy is common and may be massive.[161,236] Pleural effusions typically signify serosal metastases of SCC, and rarely, the tumor may so markedly involve the pleura that it produces a peripulmonary "rind" similar to that seen in association with mesotheliomas.[253]

Pathologic Findings

The gross features of SCC are such that the tumor bears more resemblance to a lymphoma than to other carcinomas. The cut section of the lesion is typically uniformly gray-tan and fleshy, with possible small areas of necrosis or hemorrhage.

Microscopically, SCC exhibits a spectrum of morphologic appearances.[235,254-263] Classic "oat cell" tumors are relatively rare, accounting for only 10% to 20% of cases.[254,255] Oat cell morphology (Fig. 13-23), with bluntly fusiform, carrot-shaped cells, nuclear molding, and crush artifact, is more often seen in bronchial biopsy specimens or fine-needle aspiration biopsy specimens than in resected neoplasms or lymph node metastases. Tumor cell size is in the range of 1.5 to 3 times the diameter of non-neoplastic lymphocytes.[263] The now defunct term "intermediate cell variant" of SCC (Fig. 13-24) accounts for approximately 75% of cases, and may be combined with oat cell areas.[256-259] Cell size in the former subtype is more variable, but may be as much as twice that seen in oat cell SCC. Nuclear molding and crush artifact are less conspicuous; the tumor cells also may show small nucleoli, but they maintain the marked hyperchromatism and granular chromatin that are seen in other forms of SCC. There may be blunt spindle cell change, and the cells may show pseudorosette formation or may grow in distinct ribbons. Other recognized types are combined small cell and large cell NEC[260,264,265] and mixtures of SCC with either adenocarcinoma or squamous carcinoma (Fig. 13-25).[27] All variations share the tendency to show prominent apoptosis, brisk mitotic activity, scant amphophilic cytoplasm, and the "Azzopardi phenomenon," which is the accretion of basophilic nucleic acid around intratumoral blood vessels[254,255] (Fig. 13-26). Interestingly,

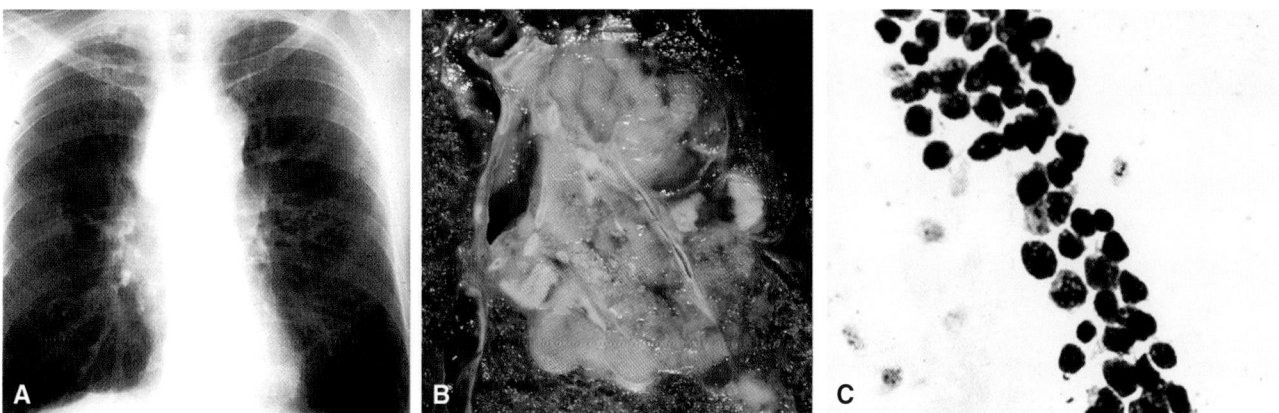

Figure 13-22. A, Chest radiograph of small cell neuroendocrine carcinoma of the lung, showing a right hilar mass with mediastinal widening. **B,** Gross photograph of small cell neuroendocrine carcinoma. The tumor has a "fish-flesh" appearance, as is more often seen in lymphomas or sarcomas. **C,** This sputum cytology specimen demonstrates an aggregate of tumor cells from small cell neuroendocrine carcinoma on the left; their sizes can be contrasted with that of a benign squamous cell in the photograph.

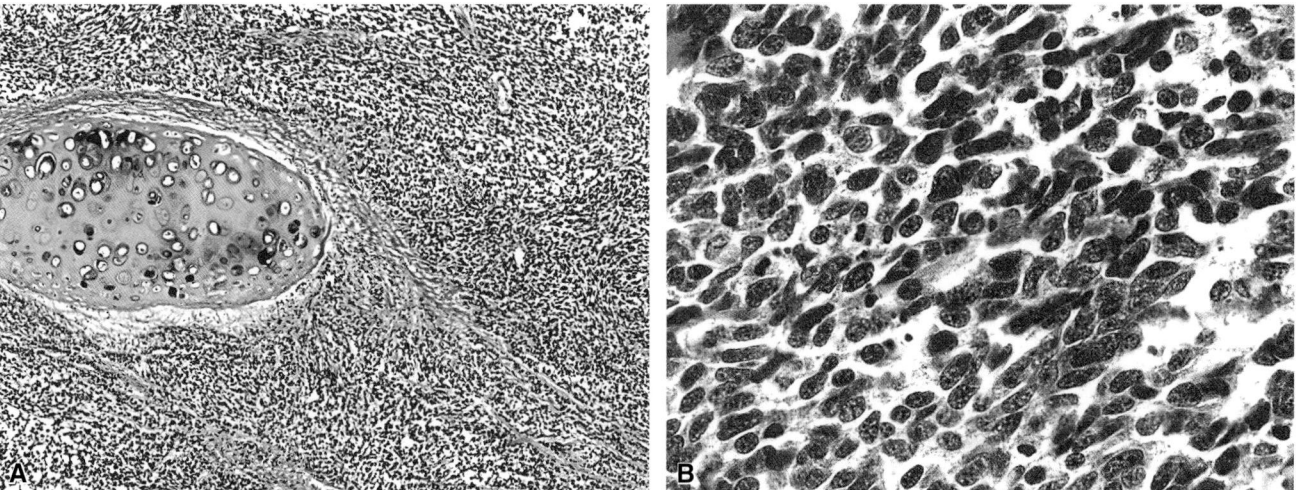

Figure 13-23. A, Small cell carcinoma of the lung, engulfing a fragment of bronchial wall. **B,** Numerous mitoses and abundant apoptosis are seen in this small cell carcinoma.

Figure 13-24. "Intermediate" variant of grade III neuroendocrine carcinoma, small cell type. The tumor cells grow in a discernibly organoid fashion (**A**) and are more regular in shape and size (**B**) than those of the oat cell subtype. However, the distinction between histologic variants of small cell neuroendocrine carcinoma has no clinical importance and poor reproducibility. These variants have been eliminated from the current World Health Organization classification.

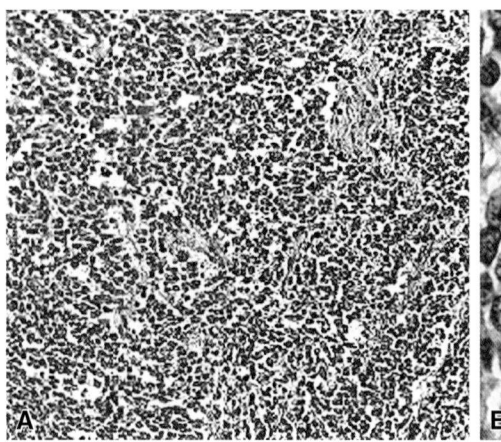 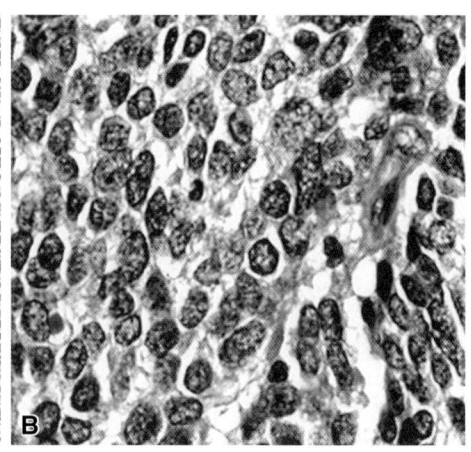

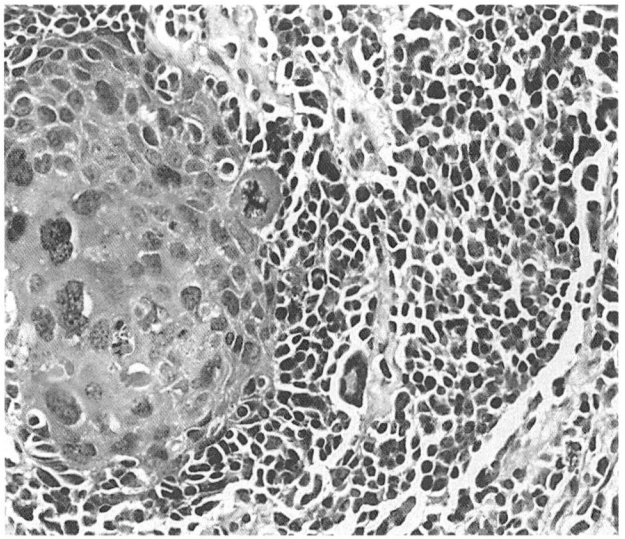

Figure 13-25. Divergent squamous differentiation is apparent in this small cell neuroendocrine carcinoma (*left upper center*).

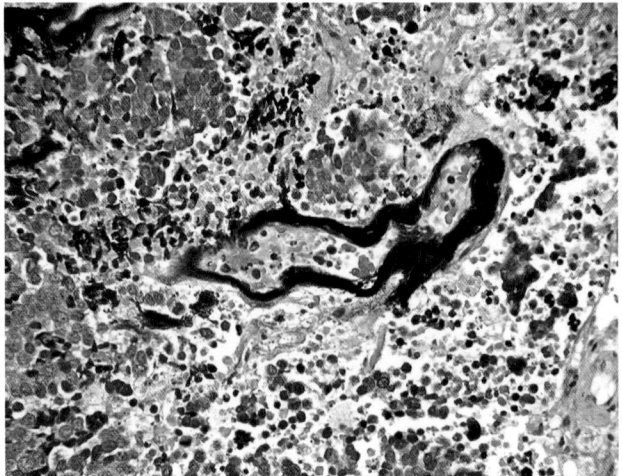

Figure 13-26. The "Azzopardi phenomenon" is represented by accretion of densely basophilic, smudgy nucleic acid material adjacent to intratumoral blood vessels in small cell carcinoma.

D'Adda and coworkers[266] found that both neoplastic components were genetically homologous in tumors showing a combination of SCC and large cell NEC.

In our opinion, differences in cytomorphology in SCC have little or no prognostic importance, based on a synthesis of the aggregated literature.[236,256–259,267,268] Instead, it is necessary to be familiar with the microscopic subtypes to avoid misdiagnosis. Some variation in nuclear size, small nucleoli, and a modest amount of cytoplasm should not prevent one from making a diagnosis of SCC, recognizing that these features are seen regularly in the intermediate variant of SCC, especially in cytologic preparations.[265] This is particularly true in fine-needle aspirate material.[262,269–271]

Another difficulty that one may face is the identification of SCC in biopsy specimens of peripheral lung nodules, as seen in approximately 10% of cases.[272] In that setting, the fear among many pathologists is that the lesion may represent a lower-grade neuroendocrine lesion. This difficulty is best resolved by paying close attention to cytologic details. Marked nuclear hyperchromatism, brisk apoptosis, and scanty cytoplasm usually allow one to comfortably exclude a lower-grade lesion. Secondly, and more importantly, evidence has emerged that suggests that surgical therapy is appropriate for peripheral high-grade but low-stage NECs of the lung.[272–278] As stated earlier, rigid adherence to the dogma of "surgery for non–small cell carcinoma; no surgery for SCC" is probably improperly restrictive. Smit and colleagues[275] studied 20 patients with resected SCC of stages I, II, and III. The median survival in that series was 29 months for stage I and II tumors and 20 months for stage III lesions. Another review of this topic was published by Mentzer and colleagues.[274] Other contextual topics of debate include whether surgery should precede or follow chemotherapy or be accompanied by irradiation.[236,279,280] Nonetheless, we believe that sufficient data are available to suggest that all low-stage NECs of the lung should be resected, regardless of grade.

Another conundrum in fine-needle aspirates, limited biopsy specimens, or frozen sections is the distinction between SCC and high-grade large cell NEC of the lung.[281,282] The two forms of grade III may coexist in the same tumor mass, yielding the neoplastic variant known as "combined SCC."[263–265,283] As discussed earlier, the separation of these two forms of high-grade NEC has dubious significance, in our opinion, with regard to the suitability of surgical management. Use of the designation "high-grade NEC" is an equitable solution; whether the lesion is then excised should be decided by the clinical stage rather than by cytologic details.

Differential Diagnosis

The diagnosis of SCC in biopsy material involves the exclusion of lymphoid infiltrates as well as other types of carcinoma that may be composed of small basaloid cells.[254,255,284–286] As stated previously, broadly reactive keratin antibody mixtures label essentially all SCCs, in many cases with a characteristic dot-like pattern of cytoplasmic staining. Hence, a simple two-antibody panel for cytokeratin and CD45 is effective in showing that a morphologically indeterminate small cell tumor is epithelial.[56] Extremely rare reports of apparent CD45 reactivity in SCC[287] underscore the inadvisability of relying on one immunostain diagnostically. In our experience, a more difficult question is the exclusion of basaloid squamous cell carcinoma, particularly in a small biopsy specimen.[229] The keratin labeling pattern described earlier may be helpful, and an extended panel of antibodies to CGA, neural cell adhesion molecule (NCAM; CD56), synaptophysin (Fig. 13-27), and CD57 can be applied as well. That set of reagents will identify approximately 80% of all SCCs.[56,219] Incidentally, we do not subscribe to the premise that there are "small cell neuroendocrine" and "small cell undifferentiated" carcinomas, but rather believe that some poorly differentiated tumors simply do not express overt neuroendocrine differentiation to a degree detectable by current methods.[56,288] Again, clinical stage is the best determinant of whether surgery is advisable, and in that framework, it becomes less crucial to separate SCC from basaloid squamous carcinoma in biopsy specimens.

Treatment and Clinical Outcome

Over the years, SCC has emerged as a clinically distinctive entity. As virtually all physicians are aware, long-term survival of patients with this neoplasm is rare; it is reported in fewer than 5% of cases in most centers,[233,236,279,280,289,290] with rare exceptions.[291] A staging system centered on the terms "limited" and "extensive" SCC has been supplanted by American Joint Committee on Cancer staging, in which stages I, II, and III correspond to the old "limited" stages and "extensive" disease is stage IV.[236] Staging is a powerful parameter and is virtually the only reliable indicator of clinical outcome for pulmonary SCC. As we have stated repeatedly, low-stage tumors are potentially resectable[272–278]; chemotherapy with or without irradiation can be given postoperatively as "consolidation" treatment.[236]

Naturally, many factors have been investigated as possible prognostic indicators in SCC. As stated earlier, we do not believe that cytologic subdivision into "oat cell" and "intermediate cell" SCC is prognostically contributory, despite the claims of some other authors.[268] Combined

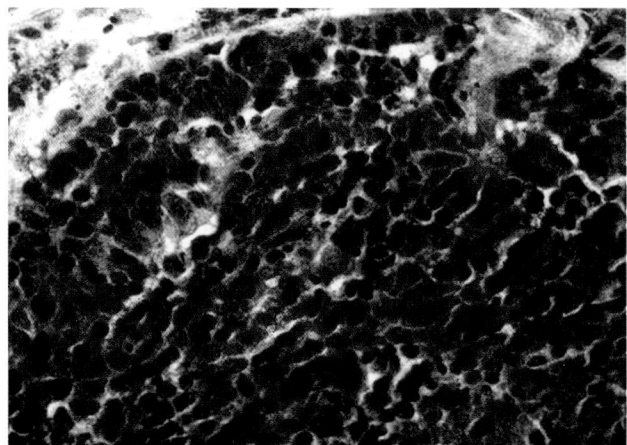

Figure 13-27. Diffuse immunoreactivity for synaptophysin in grade III neuroendocrine carcinoma of the lung, small cell type.

SCC (e.g., SCC admixed with squamous carcinoma, adenocarcinoma) and combined SCC (SCC admixed with large cell NEC) do, however, appear to be more refractory to therapy.[236,292] Vollmer and colleagues[263] have suggested that an ultrastructural loss of desmosomes was associated with more aggressive behavior in SCC, but that observation has not been the focus of practical application. DNA ploidy analysis similarly does not seem to contribute significant information. Numerous cytogenetic abnormalities are now reported in SCC of the lung; one of the most common is a deletion of 3p,[293–296] suggesting that that area may harbor potential tumor suppressor loci. Other abnormalities that have commonly been seen include deletions of 5q, 9p, 11p, 13q, and 17p.[296,297] Proto-oncogenes implicated include c-myc, n-myc, myb, c-kit, c-src, and c-jun.[294,296] At least two tumor suppressor genes—p53 and the retinoblastoma gene—may play a role in the carcinogenesis of SCC.[25,294,296] As mentioned in the discussion of grade I and grade II NECs of the lung, the *p53* gene is more often mutated in SCC than it is in lower-grade lesions. Other molecules, including p-glycoprotein (the multidrug resistance protein), CD99, and bcl-2 protein have likewise been investigated as possible prognosticators.[294,296] Duncavage and coworkers[298] have shown that tumor cells in primary and metastatic SCC of the lung lack the Merkel cell polyoma virus, separating it biologically from primary SCC of the skin. Conversely, Ralston and colleagues[299] found nuclear MASH1 immunoreactivity in more than 80% of cases of pulmonary SCC, but that marker was not apparent in primary cutaneous NECs.

Grade III Neuroendocrine Carcinoma, Large Cell Type (Large Cell Neuroendocrine Carcinoma)

The diagnosis of "large cell neuroendocrine carcinoma" (LCNC) is a relatively new addition to the nomenclature pertaining to pulmonary carcinomas. Travis and coworkers[230] proposed that this term be used for tumors that show morphologically overt features of neuroendocrine differentiation by light microscopy, but do not fit into the categories of grade I NEC, grade II NEC, or SCC. Thus, LCNCs are, by definition, different lesions than non–small cell lung cancers that demonstrate evidence of neuroendocrine differentiation only by immunohistochemical or ultrastructural studies[26,34]; those are discussed later. LCNC is also synonymous with neoplasms that have been called "intermediately differentiated NEC" by Warren and coworkers.[12,55] As we have already stated, we believe that use of the modifier "intermediate" for these cases is ill-chosen because it introduces confusion with the "intermediate" cellular variant of SCC. We prefer the term "grade III NEC, large cell type" to refer to LCNC, for reasons that are specified later. Other authors have endorsed that usage.

Clinical Features

The clinical attributes of LCNCs are hybrids of those attending adenocarcinoma of the lung and SCC. In series by Travis and colleagues[5,230] and others,[233,289,290,297,300–303] LCNCs almost always occur in heavy smokers, as does SCC. Symptoms and signs are generally most like those of non-neuroendocrine carcinoma; however, as in SCC, examples of Eaton-Lambert syndrome[304] and paraneoplastic retinopathy[305] also have been reported in connection with grade III large cell NEC. Although a minority of cases of LCNC present as central masses, they tend to be situated in the mid-to-peripheral lung fields (Fig. 13-28). Oddly, despite a high histologic grade, most LCNCs present as T1 or T2 tumors without lymph node metastases or evidence of systemic spread.[5,300]

Pathologic Findings

Grossly, pulmonary grade III NEC of the large cell type varies in maximum dimension from 1 to more than 10 cm and often demonstrates central necrosis, with or without dystrophic calcification.[5,297,300]

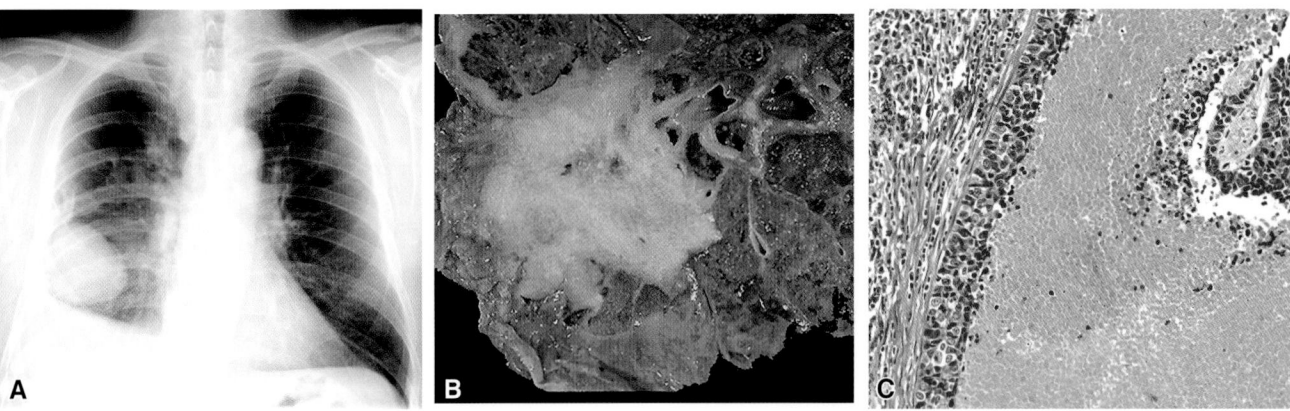

Figure 13-28. **A,** A large mass is seen in the lower right lung field, representing a large cell neuroendocrine carcinoma (LCNC). **B,** The gross appearance of LCNC is much like that of small cell neuroendocrine carcinoma (see Fig. 13-22B). **C,** Prominent infarct-like necrosis is a common finding in large cell neuroendocrine carcinoma of the lung.

Microscopically, it typically shows extensive coagulative necrosis that is obvious on low-power examination (see Fig. 13-28). At slightly higher magnification, one often sees an insular or ribboning growth pattern in the tumor between the necrotic zones. The individual neoplastic cells are larger than those of grade II lesions, with moderate-to-abundant amphophilic cytoplasm. In some instances, tumor cells are granular and eosinophilic; Chetty and coworkers[306] have reported rare examples with "rhabdoid" cytologic features, in which globular hyaline cytoplasmic inclusions were apparent in the tumor cells, and Khalifa and colleagues[307] documented an example of LCNC with divergent sarcomatoid (pleomorphic and spindle cell) differentiation. Nuclei in LCNC are more heterogeneous than those in SCC or grade II NEC; nucleoli are variable in prominence and nuclear chromatin is more heterogeneous, varying from granular to vesicular (Fig. 13-29). The mitotic rate in LCNC is brisk, usually measuring in excess of 10 division figures per 10 high-power microscopic fields, and sometimes being in the range of 50 to 100.[5] All cases show reactivity for cytokeratin, and immunoreactivity for at least one neuroendocrine determinant is observed in almost all cases.[5,297] Nevertheless, we believe that a diagnosis of LCNC can be made confidently, even if all such markers are absent. In those instances, the cytomorphologic attributes of the tumor are so classically those of a neuroendocrine neoplasm that no interpretative doubt exists. Electron microscopy shows dense core granules in large cell grade III NEC.[5,230,302]

Differential Diagnosis

These lesions may be challenging to recognize. In the past, examples of LCNC were probably assigned to one of three other diagnostic categories: "atypical carcinoid"; "non–small cell carcinoma, not further specified"; or "large cell undifferentiated carcinoma." A distinction from grade II NEC can usually be made by paying attention to several features. First, the cells of LCNC tend to be larger, and there is more nuclear pleomorphism. Chromatin in "atypical carcinoid" tends to be granular and nucleoli are small[308]; in contrast, the chromatin of LCNC is not uncommonly vesicular, and nucleoli are often prominent. Nucleocytoplasmic ratios in grade II tumors are actually higher than those of LCNCs. Necrosis in the latter tumor type is generally extensive and infarct-like, in contrast to grade II NEC, in which more punctate or limited confluent necrosis is seen. Mitotic activity is another key feature in this diagnostic comparison. As outlined by Travis and colleagues,[5,230,308] LCNC has a high mitotic rate (>50/10 high-power fields). Accordingly, those authors suggested that cases with more than 10 mitoses per 10 high-power fields probably represent LCNC, whereas "atypical carcinoid" is more likely to show a figure of 10 or

fewer. However, we prefer to assess the overall microscopic configuration of the lesion in making that distinction, rather than relying on one pathologic parameter. Despite that caveat, some examples of pulmonary neuroendocrine tumors are still encountered in which it is virtually impossible to assign a label of grade II NEC versus LCNC with certainty.

Differentiation of LCNC from non-neuroendocrine non–small cell carcinomas depends first and foremost on endocrine morphologic features, enumerated earlier. As referenced earlier, we believe that the low-power appearance of grade III large cell NEC is one of the most helpful indicators of the proper diagnosis. Extensive zonal necrosis, producing a "jigsaw puzzle" pattern, is often visible. Prompted by this feature, which, of course, can be mimicked by the appearance of necrotic squamous cell carcinoma or poorly differentiated adenocarcinoma, one then examines the lesion for organoid growth and neuroendocrine nuclear features. In contrast to our discussion of SCC, special techniques sometimes play an important part in the diagnosis of LCNC of the lung, and ultrastructural studies are useful in demonstrating neurosecretory granules.[5,309] By immunohistochemical analysis, all cases of grade III large cell NEC should demonstrate keratin reactivity and many are carcinoembryonic antigen-positive.[5,230,297] Virtually all LCNCs react with antibodies to NSE and CD56; among more "specific" markers, CGA is the most consistently detected antigen. Antibodies to CD57 and synaptophysin stain fewer cases. Rossi and coworkers[310] showed that a three-marker panel comprising synaptophysin, CGA, and CD56 was effective in separating LCNC from nonendocrine tumors; if any two of those determinants were seen, the diagnosis was secure.

This discussion raises several points. First, given the vagaries of immunohistochemistry and neoplasia, one could predict that cases will be encountered with morphologic features that are consistent with—but not diagnostic of—LCNC, but do not demonstrate any "neuroendocrine" markers. Electron microscopic examination can be used in such cases (Fig. 13-30A and B). It is advisable to provide some corroborating evidence of neuroendocrine differentiation before making a diagnosis of LCNC in this specific context, because some basaloid squamous cell carcinomas[229] and other non-neuroendocrine large cell carcinomas may closely mimic LCNC.[26,34] Conversely, however, if no light microscopic features support the diagnosis of LCNC, immunostaining results and ultrastructural analysis should not be used to make the diagnosis. It has been well documented that generic non–small cell lung neoplasms may contain cells with endocrine characteristics,[26,34] as considered subsequently.

Even though they are both forms of grade III NEC, LCNC and SCC can usually be distinguished from one another readily in surgical

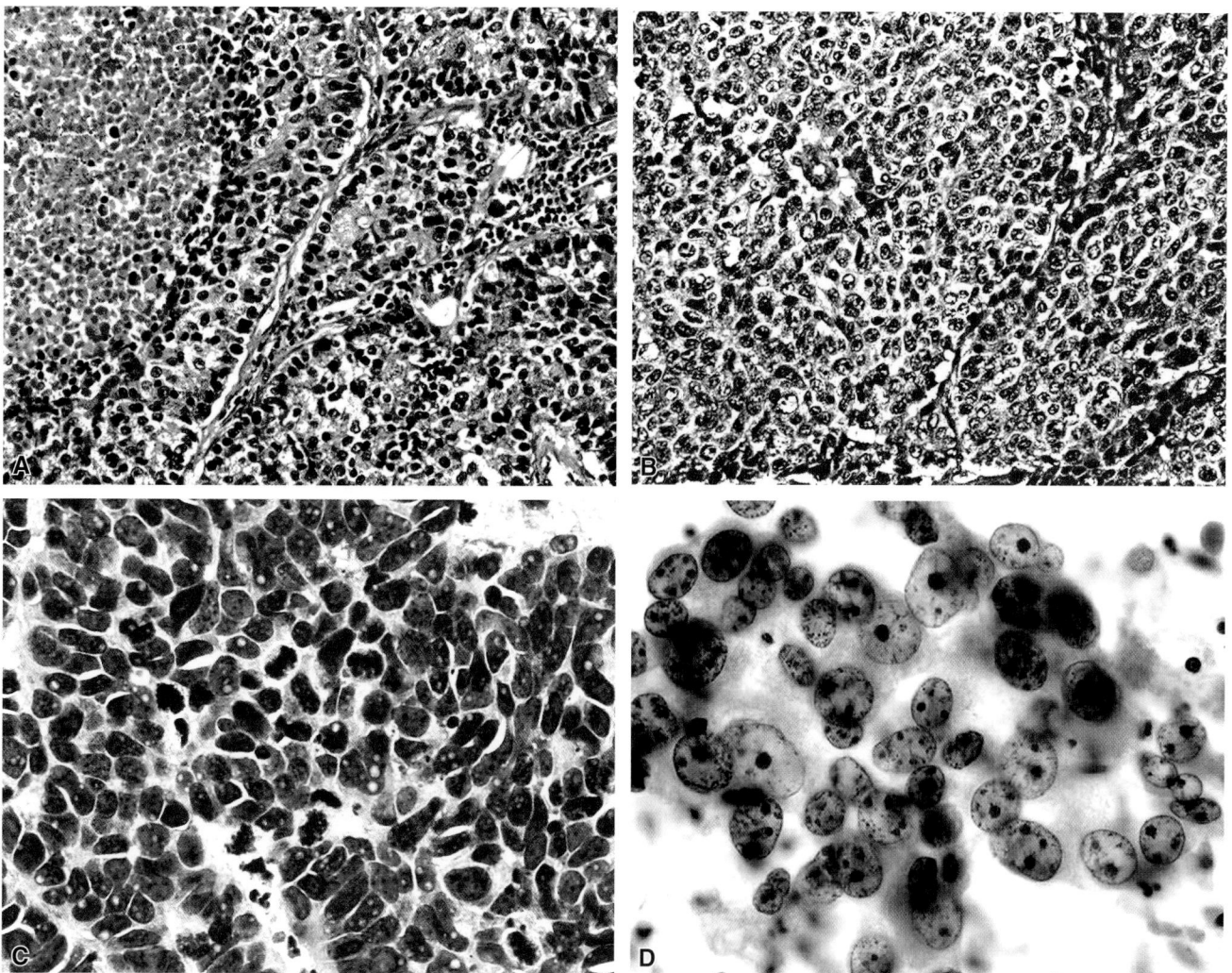

Figure 13-29. A to **C,** Foci of geographic necrosis and relatively prominent nucleoli are seen in large cell neuroendocrine carcinoma (LCNC). **D,** This fine-needle aspiration biopsy specimen of LCNC shows nuclear molding by the tumor cells as well as dispersed chromatin.

material. The fact that they are different tumor entities is supported by the observations of Ullmann and colleagues,[311] showing that LCNC and SCC have dissimilar genotypes. The larger cell size, polygonal shape, lower nucleocytoplasmic ratios, nucleolation, and more irregular chromatin in LCNCs should make this distinction relatively straightforward in most cases. Nevertheless, the two cytologic forms of high-grade NEC occasionally coexist in "combined SCCs."[35,263,264] Moreover, in cytologic material, the cited distinction between SCC and LCNC is sometimes very challenging.[312] Yang and coworkers[269] have described three potential images of LCNC in fine-needle aspiration specimens, one of which closely simulates SCC. The presence of prominent nucleoli is a helpful clue to the recognition of LCNC in that setting.[269,270]

Treatment and Clinical Outcome

The aggressive behavior of grade III large cell NECs of the lung cannot be overstated[313–317] (see Fig. 13-30C and D). Of 10 patients studied by Warren and colleagues,[12] only 1 was alive at 2 years' follow-up, despite the fact that all of the cases were stage I (T1 or 2/N0/M0). All of the patients in series by Travis and colleagues[5,230] had either died of their tumors or were likely to do so at the same time point. Another report by Rush and coworkers[206] quoted respective 5- and 10-year survival rates of 33% and 11% for LCNC. Dresler and colleagues[300] studied a series of 40 non–small cell NECs, including 23 LCNC as defined here.

The survival rate for stage I cases in that series was 18% at 40 months, significantly worse than that for those with similarly staged adenocarcinomas or squamous carcinomas. Surprisingly, the survival of patients with resected low-stage SCCs,[272–278] which are usually peripheral, is better than that of patients with LCNC. Likewise, the latter tumor type is more aggressive than "atypical carcinoid."[5,206,230,300]

Travis and colleagues[5] and Rush and co-workers[206] performed flow cytometric DNA analysis on cases of grade III large cell NEC of the lung. Both groups found no prognostic value in those studies.

The optimal therapy for these lesions is still in evolution, in large part because there has been a frustrating tendency for both pathologists and clinicians to push LCNC inappropriately into generic non–small cell carcinoma treatment protocols rather than evaluating them as a separate tumor entity. Because LCNCs tend to present as low-stage lesions,[300–303,318] most can—and should—be surgically resected.[315–317,319,320] However, there have been few randomized trials to address the value of specific chemotherapy regimens or irradiation. In most patients with grade III large cell NEC, therapy appears to fail, with either distant metastases or intrathoracic recurrence occurring.[5,230,297,300] Therefore, the use of adjunctive treatment modalities would appear to have merit.[315–317] Nonetheless, accrued experience suggests that LCNCs respond relatively unimpressively to standard chemotherapy regimens used for SCC.[321] With selected exceptions, tumors representing

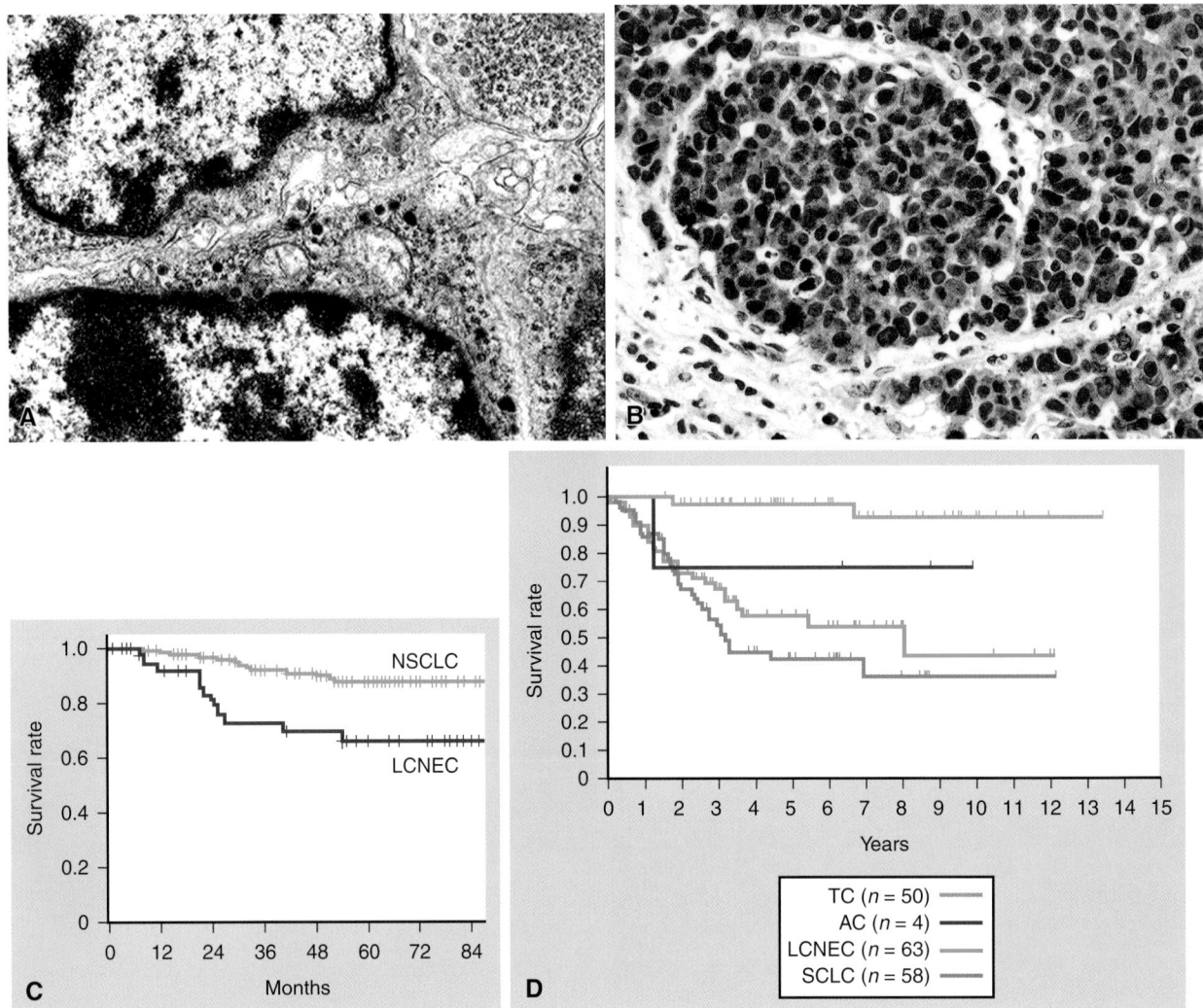

Figure 13-30. A, Large cell grade III neuroendocrine carcinomas of the lung may require ultrastructural study to document their endocrine nature. This example shows scattered neurosecretory granules (*center*). **B,** Immunoreactivity for chromogranin-A is present in this large cell neuroendocrine carcinoma (LCNEC) of the lung. **C,** This figure contrasts the survival of patients with LCNEC with that of those with nonendocrine lung cancers. **D,** This graph depicts the relative survival rates of patients with grade 1 (TC), grade 2 (AC), and grade 3 small cell neuroendocrine carcinoma (SCLC) and LCNEC neuroendocrine carcinomas. The data for SCLC and LCNEC are similar.

"combined SCCs" (SCC/LCNC in the same tumor mass) have also had only a modest response to such treatment.[35,236,263,264] In that regard, it is intriguing that expression of the multidrug resistance protein seems to be relatively common in grade III large cell NECs.[322] Unfortunately, pulmonary NECs do not appear to manifest mutations in the epidermal growth factor receptor gene. Therefore, they are not likely to respond to epidermal growth factor receptor inhibitors.[323] Faggiano and colleagues[324] have found that a high mitotic count (>10 mitoses/high-power [×400] microscopic field), an absence of immunohistologic neuroendocrine markers, and an immunohistochemical bcl-2/bax ratio of greater than 1 were adverse prognosticators for LCNC at a pathologic level of evaluation.

Composite (Combined) Neuroendocrine/Non-Neuroendocrine Carcinomas

The concept of overtly "combined" or "divergent" differentiation has been recognized increasingly in the last few years, using conventional light microscopy.[27,325] Although this pattern is perhaps most frequently encountered in the gut and the lung,[258,325,326] composite epithelial tumors with a partial neuroendocrine phenotype have been observed in a wide variety of organ sites. The biologic significance of composite tumors with neuroendocrine differentiation is still being studied, but it appears to depend on the location of the particular neoplasm being considered as well as the level of cytologic anaplasia inherent in that tumor.[282,325]

A bewildering array of terms has been used to describe these neoplasms, and many are still in use. These include "stem cell carcinoma," "amphicrine carcinoma," "composite carcinoma (SCC/adenocarcinoma or squamous cell carcinoma)," and "carcinoid with glandular differentiation."[325,327-338] Needless to say, many people are confused by this diverse lexicon and are uncertain as to how to treat the neoplasms. In our view, because mixtures of NEC (with variable levels of differentiation, including high-grade tumors) and squamous cell carcinoma, adenocarcinoma, transitional carcinoma, or spindle cell carcinoma have been documented in malignant epithelial neoplasms of the lung, pancreas, stomach, duodenum, small bowel, colon, rectum, pancreas, liver, biliary tree, urinary bladder, prostate, uterine cervix and endometrium, ovaries, breast, skin, thyroid, salivary glands, and larynx,[51,327-338] it would seem most straightforward to use descriptive terminology diagnostically, such as "combined NEC–adenocarcinoma" (Fig. 13-31) or "combined NEC–squamous cell carcinoma," along with comments in

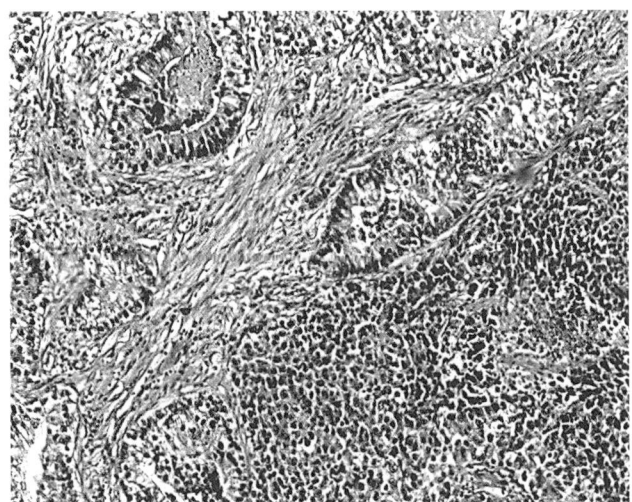

Figure 13-31. Combined adenocarcinoma (*left*) and grade II neuroendocrine carcinoma (*right*) of the lung.

surgical pathology reports that summarize the morphologic details and expected behavioral attributes of the lesion.

Clinical Findings

Virtually any carcinoma in the lung can potentially have a neuroendocrine component, which can be grade I, II, or III NEC. Hence, there are no specific clinical features that can be ascribed to "combined" neuroendocrine/non-neuroendocrine tumors. Nonetheless, mixtures of squamous carcinoma or adenocarcinoma with NEC are most commonly seen in biopsy specimens that are taken after therapy,[339] suggesting that effective treatment of the neuroendocrine cell population may allow for "overgrowth" of a minor nonendocrine component.

Pathologic Features

Unlike poorly differentiated carcinomas in which neuroendocrine differentiation is "occult," and therefore discernible only by application of immunohistology or electron microscopy,[340] the tumors considered in this section are recognizable as mixed by conventional microscopy. All of the neuroendocrine tumor types (i.e., grade I NEC, grade II NEC, small cell or large cell grade III NEC) that have been discussed up to this point may be components of combined carcinomas in the lung.

Special studies are likely to lead to a spectrum of findings. Some tumors demonstrate truly bifid differentiation—exhibiting, for example, true glandular and neuroendocrine features in the same neoplastic cells.[325,327] Others display admixtures of cellular elements with mutually exclusive ultrastructural or immunophenotypic properties. These differences do not appear to have any meaning from mechanistic or clinical points of view. There are discussions in the literature about whether divergent neuroendocrine lesions are "collision" tumors.[325] Because virtually all neoplasms derive from transformed stem cells, regardless of anatomic site, it would appear much more logical to conclude that divergent growth simply emanates from dissimilar (and largely unknown) post-transformational modulators of differentiation.[341,342]

Differential Diagnosis

Because of the unique histologic appearance of combined carcinomas with neuroendocrine elements, differential diagnostic considerations are limited. These generally concern making a distinction between poorly differentiated NEC components and high-grade portions of "pure" adenocarcinomas or squamous cell carcinomas with variable microscopic patterns that simulate neuroendocrine differentiation.[284]

Ultrastructural and immunohistochemical markers of neuroendocrine differentiation should be pursued if that question arises.

Treatment and Clinical Outcome

Combined neuroendocrine/non-neuroendocrine carcinomas generally have more adverse prognoses than histologically "pure" tumors,[27,236,292,337,343] including lesions with grade I NEC components, which are very rare.[338] Thus, therapy must be chosen to address all of the cellular elements in these composite neoplasms, but with the expectation that response to treatment will likely be blunted and survival will be worse than that of patients with pathologically homogeneous lesions.

Non–Small Cell Lung Carcinomas with Occult Neuroendocrine Differentiation

Beginning in the 1980s, several investigators have noted neuroendocrine features (e.g., neurosecretory granules, immunoreactivity for endocrine peptides) in lung tumors that otherwise had the microscopic appearance of poorly differentiated squamous cell carcinoma and adenocarcinoma or large cell "undifferentiated" carcinoma.[26,340,344-355] With those observations, controversies began over diagnostic terms that should be appended to such neoplasms, as well as their behavioral attributes.

The notion that there may be a variety of cell types in any given neoplasm has steadily gained recognition over the last decade. Tumors of the skin, genitourinary tract, gastrointestinal tract, lung, and many other sites all share this potential, which is best termed "multidirectional differentiation."[325] "Occult" neuroendocrine lesions are no different than others with glandular or squamous differentiation in this context, in the sense that very poorly differentiated neoplasms may not show light microscopic patterns that indicate any of these cellular lineages.[356] Their "hidden" characteristics can only be detected by adjunctive pathologic techniques; as stated previously, that practical point of difference nosologically separates LCNC (which has microscopically overt neuroendocrine features) and "large cell carcinoma with occult neuroendocrine differentiation" (which does not).

Clinical Findings

Pulmonary carcinomas with occult neuroendocrine differentiation (OND) are not substantially different clinically than "pure" non-neuroendocrine malignancies of the lung in the symptoms and signs they produce. The only exceptional aspect of lung cancer with OND is the occasional paraneoplastic phenomenon that can be ascribed to the production of an endocrine substance. For example, we have observed several examples of poorly differentiated adenocarcinoma of the lung associated with watery diarrhea–hypokalemia syndrome, in which immunoreactivity for vasoactive intestinal polypeptide was found in the tumor cells. Similarly, hypercalcemia or hypercortisolism may relate to ectopic production of parathyroid hormone–related peptides or ACTH by such neoplasms.

Pathologic Features

As discussed earlier, pulmonary squamous cell carcinomas and adenocarcinomas with OND are no different grossly or histologically than their counterparts that lack endocrine features.[340,345-347,357] With specific reference to large cell "anaplastic" carcinomas of the lung with OND,[26,34,341,350,351] the tumor cells are at least twice as large as those of SCC. By definition, those lesions lack overt glandular or squamous differentiation and have rather monomorphic nuclei with dispersed or vesicular chromatin and prominent nucleoli. Small foci of necrosis may be seen, but these lesions lack the infarct-like configuration seen in LCNC. Similarly, manifestations of organoid growth (e.g., insulae, ribbons, cords, rosettes) are absent in large cell carcinomas with OND. Still other tumors with occult neuroendocrine elements may show more unusual histologic patterns, such as sarcomatoid differentiation[273] or a blastomatous configuration (e.g., as in "well-differentiated adenocarcinoma simulating fetal lung").[358,359]

There is some debate over the "best" method to document OND in lung carcinomas.[59,360] Some observers argue that ultrastructure should be the standard technique,[59] but as discussed earlier, sampling problems interfere with the reliability of that procedure. Putative nonspecificity of neuroendocrine determinants, such as chromogranin and synaptophysin, is not a problem in our view, because we believe that publications that raised such concerns[59] contained conceptual flaws. They were based on electron microscopy as the "validating" technology, ignoring the effects of sampling just cited. In our view, positivity for either of these two immunomarkers (Fig. 13-32) reliably predicts neuroendocrine differentiation. With reference to the *incidence* of neuroendocrine reactivity in nonendocrine carcinomas, Sørhaug and coworkers[361] have posited that it is steadily increasing as immunohistochemical techniques become more sensitive.

Differential Diagnosis
The differential diagnosis of squamous cell carcinomas or adenocarcinomas with OND principally includes similar tumors that lack endocrine features. On the other hand, large cell carcinoma with OND must be distinguished from both large cell "undifferentiated" lung carcinoma and LCNC, primarily by electron microscopy and immunohistology.[34] In addition, large cell carcinomas may be sufficiently nebulous morphologically that metastatic melanoma, poorly differentiated sarcoma with epithelioid features, and large cell lymphoma enter into diagnostic consideration. Again, adjunctive pathologic studies are usually required.[362]

Treatment and Clinical Outcome
Some investigators have concluded that neuroendocrine differentiation justifies the use of modified therapeutic approaches, such as those employed in SCC, whereas other authors have demurred on that point.[363-367] Similarly, there is no consensus as to whether any prognostic value may be derived from the identification of "occult" neuroendocrine differentiation in lung cancers of various pathologic types, with contradictions in published studies.[365-369] Currently, all that can be said with confidence is that surgical excision is still the foundation of treatment in low-stage cases.[34,367]

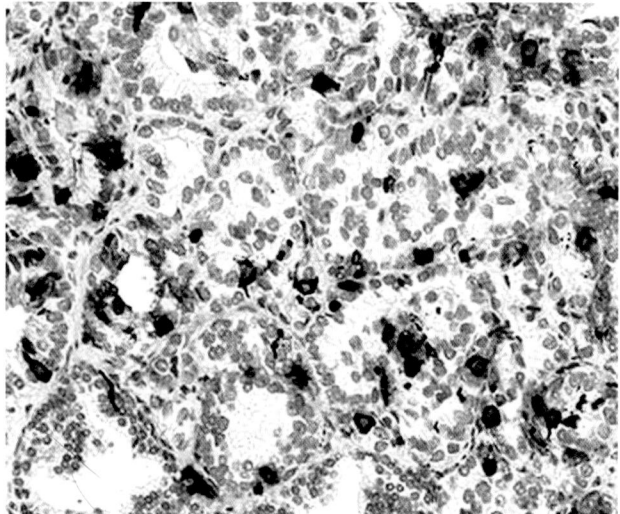

Figure 13-32. "Occult" neuroendocrine differentiation in adenocarcinoma of the lung, manifested by immunoreactivity for chromogranin-A.

Primary Intrapulmonary Paraganglioma

Paraganglioma is a distinctly uncommon lesion in the population at large,[370] and it is vanishingly rare as a primary pulmonary tumor, with fewer than 25 reported cases in the world literature.[371-381] The demographic profiles of patients with this neoplasm are variable, depending on the topographic location of the lesion and its possible occurrence in genetic syndrome complexes.

Clinical Features
In sporadic cases of PG in the lung and elsewhere, men predominate and usually come to diagnostic attention in middle life (40–50 years of age).[370-380] In contrast, women outnumber men in the context of the MEN type 2 syndromes, and they are recognized as having a PG approximately 15 years earlier.[370] The latter observation may simply reflect the fact that family members in kindreds with MEN are usually regularly screened for constituent tumors from childhood onward.[382] PGs have been described in virtually all organ sites, including the orbits, nasal cavity, thyroid, heart, urinary bladder, gallbladder, liver, biliary system, kidneys, prostate, urethra, spermatic cord, uterus, ovaries, vagina, vulva, cauda equina, and lungs; primary pulmonary tumors are among the rarest.[371]

Functionality of PGs in these diverse locations is sporadic. Biosynthetic tumors may present with episodic or sustained hypertension; hypertensive crisis or "malignant hyperthermia" on induction of general anesthesia; episodic nausea, weakness, cardiac arrhythmias, pallor, flushing, headache, diaphoresis, anxiety, or localized pain; or cardiovascular decompensation with heart failure. Reflections of neuropeptide production may include Cushing syndrome with PGs that synthesize ACTH or watery diarrhea–hypokalemia complex (Verner-Morrison syndrome) with neoplasms that manufacture vasoactive intestinal polypeptide. Occasional examples also have apparently produced a parathyroid hormone–related peptide, with associated hypercalcemia, or an erythropoietin-like moiety in linkage with paraneoplastic polycythemia. Finally, rare patients with PG and associated systemic abnormalities may have von Recklinghausen disease (neurofibromatosis) or Beckwith-Wiedemann syndrome (hemihypertrophy and macroglossia).[370]

Nonfunctional tumors become manifest only through the appearance of a steadily enlarging mass, with other symptoms and signs dependent on the anatomic location of the lesion. In the lung, PGs that impinge on large airways produce symptoms related to obstruction (e.g., cough or stridor), but peripheral nonfunctional lesions are typically found incidentally on screening chest radiographs[371-380] (Fig. 13-33). Rarely, multiple synchronous intrapulmonary PGs may be encountered,[381] simulating metastases on chest radiographs.

Pathologic Features
Grossly, PGs are typically spherical or slightly lobulated masses that range from a few millimeters to several centimeters in greatest dimension. They may be either centrally or peripherally located in the lung. Their cut surfaces are bloody in most cases because of dense intralesional vascularity, and the tumor tissue itself may be gray, pink, lavender, brown, or mottled (Fig. 13-34). Characteristically, immersion of fresh tissue in Bouin's fixative or another picric acid–containing solution causes the specimen to assume a brownish appearance. In general, PG is a circumscribed lesion with a partial or complete fibrous capsule; hence, the surgeon will report that the lesion was relatively easy to dissect from contiguous structures. However, approximately 10% to 20% of tumors demonstrate local infiltration of adjacent tissues,[371] and these may be submitted to the surgical pathology laboratory in a fragmented state or with adherent structures attached to their peripheral aspects. An important step in the initial pathologic evaluation of PG is not only

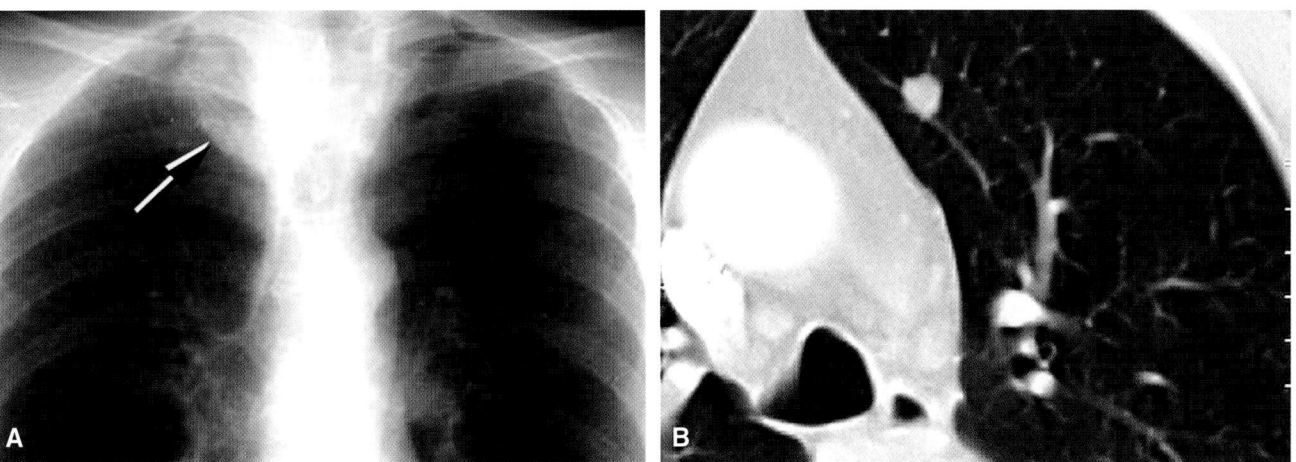

Figure 13-33. A, Chest radiograph of intrapulmonary paraganglioma, represented by a right apical mass (*arrow*). **B,** Computed tomography of the chest; the lesions represent synchronous multifocal paragangliomas.

to perform standard three-dimensional measurement of the lesion but also to weigh it after dissection of attached extraneous soft tissue. Secondly, one should pay special attention to whether a PG appears to be multinodular or multifocal. Multicentricity of such neoplasms correlates well with a syndromic association.

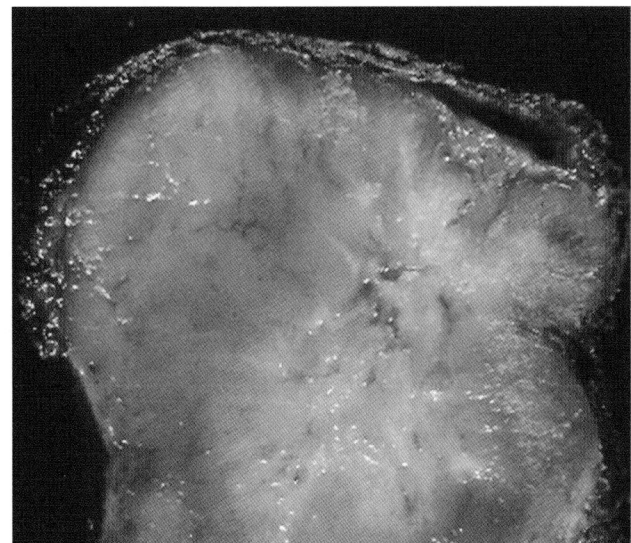

Figure 13-34. Gross photograph of a resected intrathoracic paraganglioma, showing a relatively nondescript reddish-yellow lobulated tumor.

The histopathologic characteristics of pulmonary PGs are also variable. The peculiar nesting configuration of the tumor cells, separated by prominent fibrovascular stromal septa ("zellballen"; Fig. 13-35) is poorly developed in many of these lesions. In the lung in particular, this feature leads to considerable difficulty in distinguishing PG from carcinoid tumors (which, of course, are far more common). Aside from the organoid growth pattern of PGs, they are marked by a tendency toward nuclear pleomorphism, the common presence of intranuclear "pseudoinclusions" (invaginations of cytoplasm), intercellular hyaline globules, accumulations of intercellular proteinaceous material resembling thyroid colloid, potential spindle cell or oncocytic change, and elements resembling ganglion cells[383,384] (Fig. 13-36). Mitotic figures are seen in approximately 45% of benign PGs and 65% of malignant lesions, regardless of location; hence, they are not useful in and of themselves in predicting tumor behavior. Similarly, although vascular invasion is apparent in one-fifth of malignant PGs, it is also evident in 5% to 6% of benign tumors.[384] Thus, requests for a definitive diagnosis of PG in the frozen section laboratory are impossible to satisfy, particularly with reference to pulmonary tumors.

Relatively few PGs have been subjected to fine-needle aspiration and cytologic assessment.[385-387] However, a report on this topic by Gonzalez-Campora and colleagues[386] showed that such tumors commonly exhibited marked anisokaryosis, a tendency to form acini or follicles, and intranuclear invaginations of cytoplasm similar to those seen in papillary thyroid carcinoma. Nuclear pleomorphism has not been correlated with adverse behavior; in fact, malignant PGs have tended to display less nuclear variability than did their benign counterparts.[384]

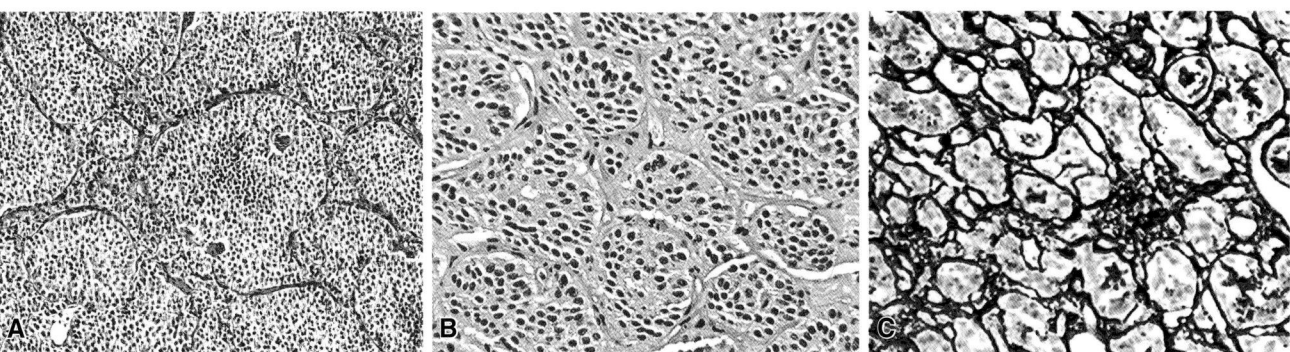

Figure 13-35. The formation of distinct cell groups ("zellballen") may be conspicuous (**A**) or relatively vague (**B**) in paraganglioma. **C,** A reticulin stain highlights the organoid growth pattern of paraganglioma.

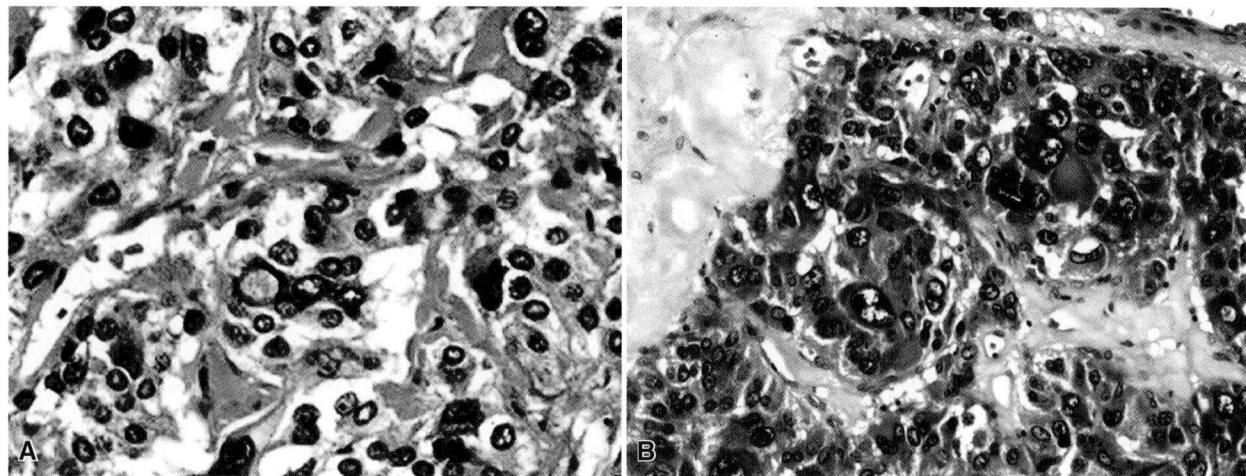

Figure 13-36. Intranuclear pseudoinclusions (**A**) and nuclear pleomorphism with eosinophilic cytoplasmic inclusions (**B**) in paraganglioma.

Differential Diagnosis

Special studies are typically needed to bolster the histologic diagnosis of PG in visceral locations, especially the lung. Other considerations in pulmonary cases center on NEC as well as metastatic malignant PG originating at another site. Electron microscopy is still a useful modality in this context, and the neurosecretory granules of paraganglion cell tumors generally differ from those of other neuroendocrine cells and neoplasms.[370] They feature an unusual "blister"-like configuration, where the internal submembranous "halos" of the granules are obviously eccentric and appear to emanate from the dense core in a bubble-like fashion. Otherwise, the cells of PGs are similar to those of the dispersed neuroendocrine system, showing prominent Golgi complexes and rough endoplasmic reticulum, macular intercellular junctions, and incomplete pericellular basal lamina.[388]

Immunohistologically, most examples of PG have a distinctive intermediate filament protein profile that is not shared by other neoplasms except for NBs.[76,389] This features neurofilament protein, with or without vimentin, to the exclusion of other intermediate filament proteins. Neurofilament protein may be difficult to demonstrate in formalin-fixed, paraffin-embedded tissues, so in practical terms, the majority of routinely processed PGs do not manifest detectable intermediate filament protein.[389] This observation is useful in making the distinction between PG (and other "type 2" [neural] neuroendocrine tumors) and "type 1" (epithelial) neoplasms that often are considered in the differential diagnosis and that uniformly exhibit keratin positivity.[56] We have not found keratin proteins in PGs, in the lung or elsewhere. This is in stark contrast to the rate of 30% that has been cited by some authors for keratin positivity in PG[66]—a rate we believe to be a reflection of procedural shortcomings. Occasional examples of PG may also show focal immunoreactivity for glial fibrillary acidic protein, but they uniformly lack desmin.[76] Virtually all PGs are diffusely and intensely positive for chromogranin-A and synaptophysin, whereas beta-tubulin and microtubule-associated protein are only focally seen in such lesions and are instead characteristic of neuroblastic and ganglioneuromatous neoplasms.[56,83,89,90] Other immunodeterminants that can be detected in PGs include ACTH (approximately 30%), vasoactive intestinal polypeptide (40%), Leu- or Met-enkephalins (50% to 60%), calcitonin (<5%), CD56 (90%), CD57 (50%), and beta-endorphin (10%).[75,79,93]

A word is in order regarding "minute pulmonary chemodectoma" as a differential diagnostic consideration in this context. "Chemodectoma" is a term that was formerly used in reference to PG.[370] In fact, minute pulmonary chemodectomas have no relationship to the paraganglion system. They are small peripheral pulmonary parenchymal aggregations of polygonal or bluntly fusiform cells, often with a concentric configuration. Immunohistochemical studies of minute pulmonary chemodectomas have demonstrated a similarity to meningothelial rather than neuroendocrine tissues, with reactivity for vimentin and epithelial membrane antigen.[390] Moreover, analyses of cellular clonality in such lesions have demonstrated that they are polyclonal and probably reactive,[391] rather than neoplastic, as is true of PGs.

One other recent development should be mentioned in reference to PGs. It has now been shown conclusively that both familial (MEN2-related) and selected sporadic examples of this tumor demonstrate mutations in the *ret* gene on chromosome 10.[382] These take the form of (Cys634 → Arg) in MEN2A and (Met918 → Thr) in MEN2B. Whether this information enters the diagnostic sphere in the near future must await further technical developments and clinical correlation.

Treatment and Clinical Outcome

The most contentious aspect of PGs is the prediction of their often-capricious behavior. In the lung, the great majority of primary paraganglionic tumors have been benign biologically, but occasional examples have metastasized to regional lymph nodes or other viscera.[371–380]

At one extreme, some authors have stated that a diagnosis of malignant PG can only be made after metastasis has occurred; others have claimed that other findings can be correlated with aggressive behavior. These include pathologic mitotic figures or vascular invasion,[384] decreased immunoreactivity for selected neuropeptides (particularly neuropeptide Y),[392] and loss of intratumoral sustentacular cells positive for S-100 protein.[130,393] These concepts are admittedly still in evolution. Some reports concerning the biology of PG have provided additional useful information. Based on the results of logistical regression analyses, mitotic activity, nuclear atypia, and vascular or capsular invasion are of little or no use as individual parameters in the prognostication of PGs.[384] Similarly, Lack,[370] Linnoila and colleagues,[384] and Gonzalez-Campora and colleagues[394] found no statistically significant association between static or flow cytometric DNA aneuploidy and behavior in paraganglion cell tumors, with only Pang and Tsao[395] demurring on the latter point. Multiparametric assessment of 16 nonmicroscopic and histologic features by Linnoila and associates[384] showed that 4 of them were the most predictively useful. These included extra-adrenal location, coarse gross nodularity of the tumor, confluent tumor necrosis on microscopic examination, and absence of intercellular hyaline globules. Among 120 PGs in that series, 71% of the biologically malignant lesions showed two or three of the four specified features, whereas 89% of the benign tumors manifested zero or one of them. Accordingly, there was a greater than 95% probability that more than 70% of PGs could be correctly classified using this paradigm.[384] In our opinion, such an approach is recommended. It can be used by any pathologist and does not require special equipment.

Primary Primitive Neuroectodermal Tumors of the Lung

Primitive neuroectodermal tumors are small round cell neoplasms that are most commonly seen as primary soft tissue tumors. In the thorax, they typically affect the pleura and chest wall and are known as "Askin tumors" (Figs. 13-37 and 13-38). In the lung, only a few examples of PNET have been well documented as primary tumors by Imamura and coworkers,[396] Mikami and coworkers,[397] Verfaillie and colleagues,[398] Suárez Antelo and coworkers,[399] Lee and coworkers,[400] and Takahashi and colleagues.[401] Accordingly, specific clinicopathologic information on primary intrapulmonary lesions is anecdotal. These neoplasms have been seen in patients between 17 and 67 years of age who presented with nodular intrapulmonary masses. Characteristic t(11;22) chromosomal translocations and expression of CD99 or FLI-1[402,403] (Fig. 13-39) were observed in each neoplasm, and they lacked immunoreactivity for

keratin, myogenic markers, and S-100 protein. After surgical excision and appropriate chemotherapy, three of the patients were alive and free of disease; the others were lost to follow-up or were still being treated.

The differential diagnosis principally involves SCC—which should be uniformly keratin-positive[56] and lack t(11;22)—and metastatic PNET arising in other locations and involving the lung secondarily. Another possibility is small cell primary or metastatic pulmonary synovial sarcoma, which is a particular interpretative trap because it shares potential immunoreactivity for CD99 and FLI-1[402] with PNET.[398] However, the cytogenetic profiles of those lesions are mutually exclusive; synovial sarcoma lacks t(11;22) and consistently exhibits a t(X;18) chromosomal translocation. Those genotypes can be identified using either in situ hybridization techniques or polymerase chain reaction–based assays.[404]

Primary Neuroblastoma of the Lung

Neuroblastoma continues to represent an important neoplasm in pediatric oncology. It is the fourth most frequently encountered malignancy in children, behind leukemia, lymphoma, and aggressive central nervous system tumors.[370,405,406] The majority of NBs (and congeners

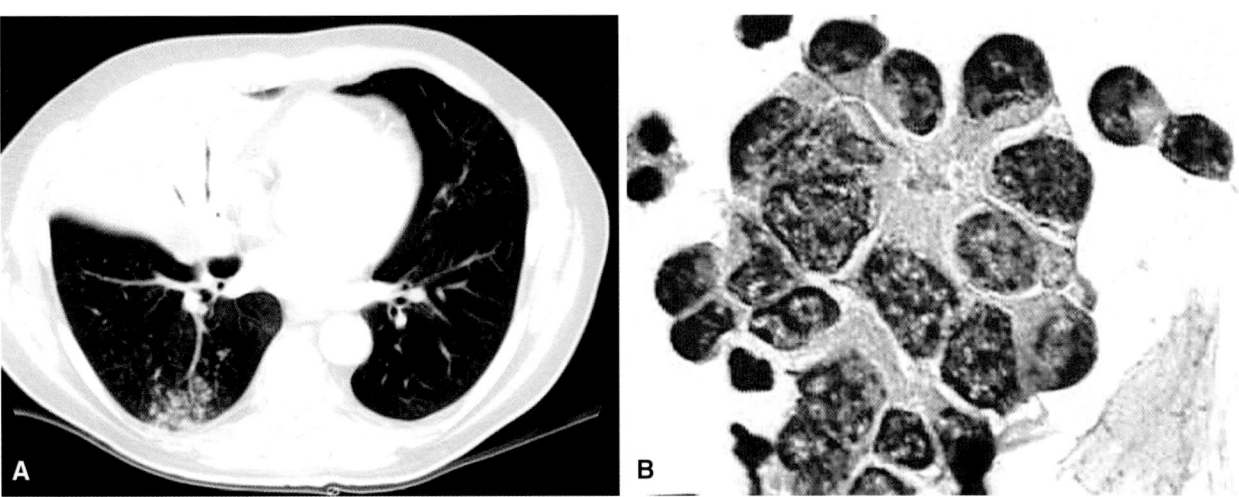

Figure 13-37. A, This computed tomogram of the chest demonstrates a large right-sided mass that abuts the pleura in a 17-year-old boy. The lesion represents a primitive neuroectodermal ("Askin") tumor. **B,** This fine-needle aspiration biopsy specimen of an Askin tumor shows monomorphous, loosely aggregated cells with dispersed chromatin. The image may easily be mistaken for a high-grade neuroendocrine carcinoma.

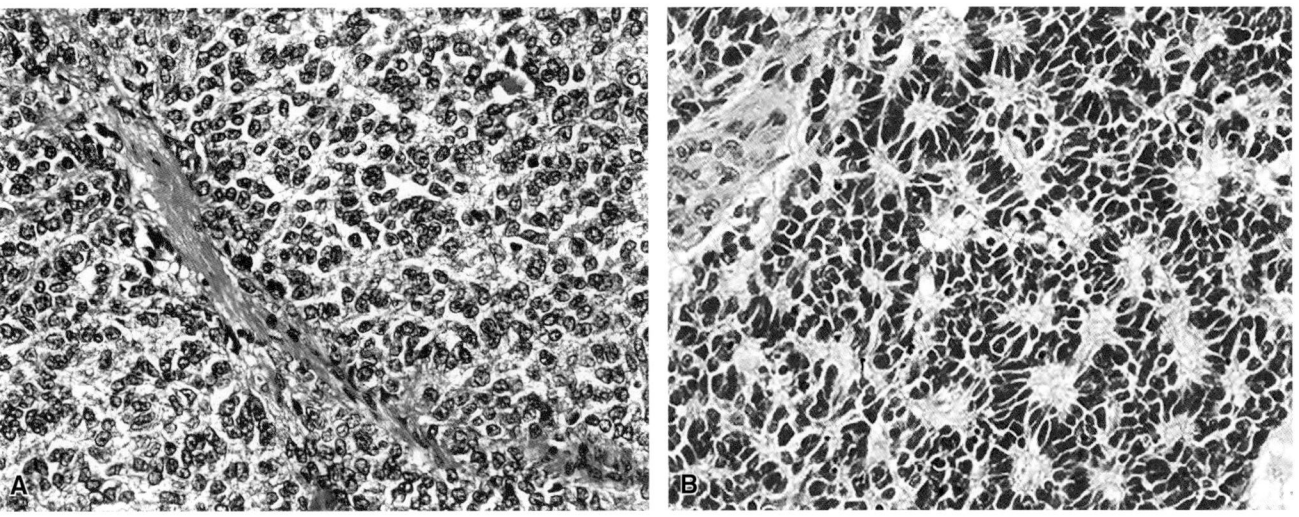

Figure 13-38. Primitive neuroectodermal tumor (**A**) comprises monomorphic small round cells (**B**), which may focally form rosettes.

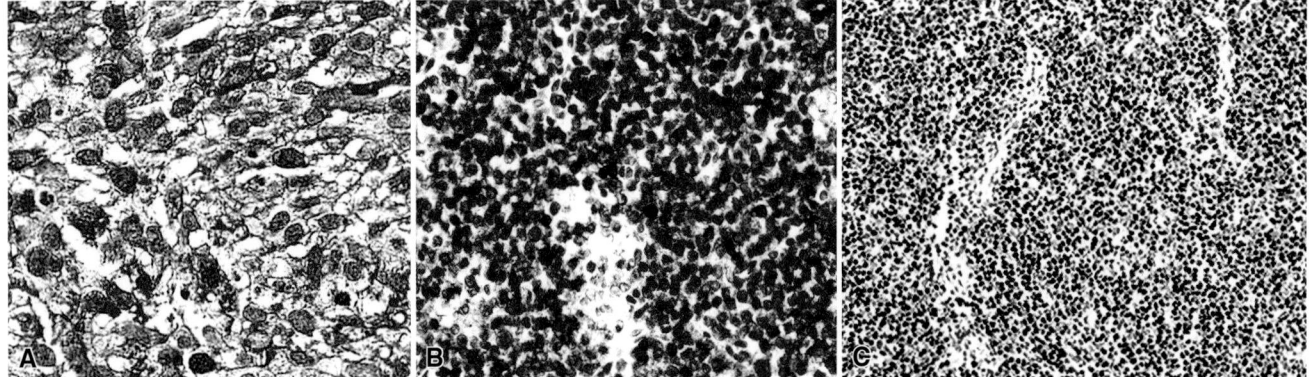

Figure 13-39. A, Periodic acid/Schiff stain shows glycogen in the cells of an Askin tumor. **B,** CD99 immunoreactivity is present in primitive neuroectodermal tumor. **C,** Nuclear immunoreactivity for FLI-1 is present in an Askin tumor.

thereof) are encountered in the first decade of life, with no particular predilection for either sex and only rare cases in adults.[407,408] Paradoxically, however, the only examples of primary intrapulmonary NB that have thus far been reported have been in three patients older than 20 years of age.[409,410]

Clinical Features

Symptoms and signs of these neoplasms typically relate to the presence of an enlarging mass (Fig. 13-40). In the lung, they are therefore most closely allied to interference with the function of structures on which the lesions impinge, such as the major bronchi. In unusual instances, paraneoplastic phenomena such as those seen with more differentiated autonomic neural tumors—i.e., PGs—may be seen at presentation in association with NBs.[411–413] In one case of pulmonary ganglioneuroblastoma reported by Hochholzer and associates,[410] signs of a MEN syndrome were also observed.

Pathologic Findings

The gross pathologic attributes of neuroblastic tumors are variable. Undifferentiated NB has a prototypical gray-white, encephaloid appearance. In lesions with partial ganglionic differentiation, nodules of more "fleshy" tissue are noted as discrete foci in the cut surfaces of the lesion. Other potential gross features of neuroblastic neoplasms include a hemangioma-like image because of extreme intratumoral hemorrhage, extensive cystic change, and diffuse or localized calcification that is often readily apparent on sectioning the mass.[414]

The microscopic characteristics of these tumors likewise form a continuum.[414–418] At one pole, one encounters classic undifferentiated small round cell tumors with little or no discernible stroma and no attempts at neural rosette formation (Fig. 13-41). Further along the spectrum of differentiation, the next group of NBs begins to exhibit background "neuropil," a fibrillary eosinophilic matrix that represents the elaboration of numerous cytoplasmic extensions by the tumor

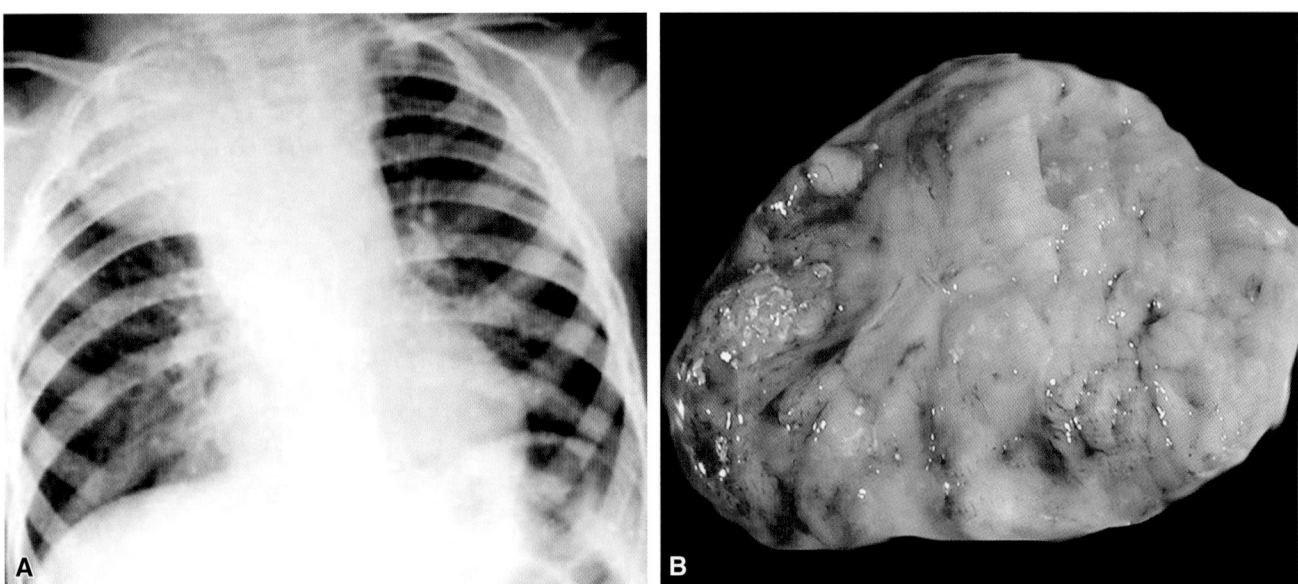

Figure 13-40. A, An apical right pulmonary mass is present in this 4-year-old boy, representing a neuroblastoma. **B,** Gross photograph of neuroblastoma, demonstrating a homogeneous, "fleshy," white-tan cut surface.

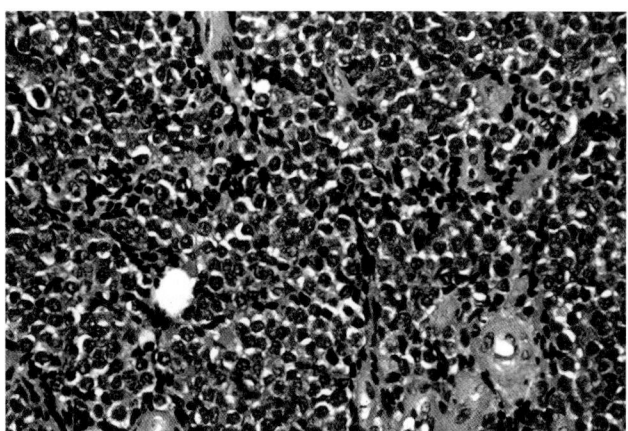

Figure 13-41. Solid, undifferentiated growth of small round anaplastic tumor cells in neuroblastoma. This appearance is similar to that of high-grade neuroendocrine carcinoma.

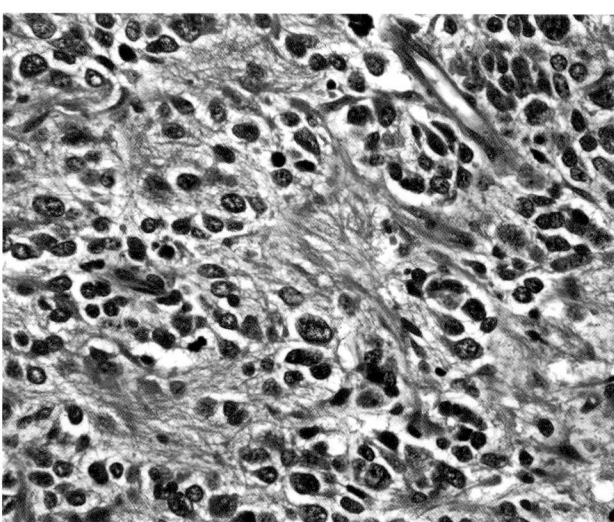

Figure 13-42. Differentiating neuroblastoma, exhibiting the formation of fibrillar eosinophilic cytoplasmic extensions (neuropil).

cells (Fig. 13-42). Often, Homer Wright rosettes—having a fibrillary nonluminal center—are also encountered. The separation between NB and ganglioneuroblastoma requires definable ganglion cell differentiation in the latter neoplasms, but determining where they begin and "differentiating NB" ends is more art than science. This statement is limited to "diffuse ganglioneuroblastomas" ("differentiating stromal-poor NBs" reported by Shimada and colleagues[418]) because, as noted earlier, stromal-rich tumors look most like ganglioneuromas (composed of mature ganglion cells and spindled Schwann cell–like elements) rather than predominantly small cell proliferations. Stromal-rich neoplasms that are not nodular (i.e., composite ganglioneuroblastoma) are further subdivided into "well-differentiated" lesions, with only a few randomly dispersed neuroblastic cells punctuating the image of a ganglioneuroma and "intermixed" tumors that contain small nests of neuroblasts having sharp interfaces with the surrounding ganglionic/Schwannian tissue.

Rarely, primitive NBs exhibit a striking degree of nuclear pleomorphism; those lesions have been termed "anaplastic NBs."[419] Whether the pleomorphic appearance of such neoplasms correlates with a worse prognosis is uncertain.

Differential Diagnosis

The differential diagnosis with other small round cell tumors is principally a problem in "undifferentiated" NB.[414] In that setting, electron microscopy demonstrates characteristically elongated cell processes containing microtubular complexes in neuroblastic tumors, with or without presynaptic vesicles or dense-core granules as well[420] (Fig. 13-43).

Immunohistologically, most neuroblastic neoplasms express only neurofilament protein among all of the intermediate filament types. Because that marker is usually not well preserved in formalin-fixed tissues, no intermediate filaments are demonstrable in the majority of cases.[421] In contrast, SCC, an important consideration in adults, is uniformly keratin-positive.[63,64] Synaptophysin is usually present in NB, ganglioneuroblastomas, and ganglioneuromas,[89,90] but CGA is uncommonly observed in those neoplasms.[83] Neuron-specific enolase and CD56 are sensitive markers for NB (and may have limited utility in

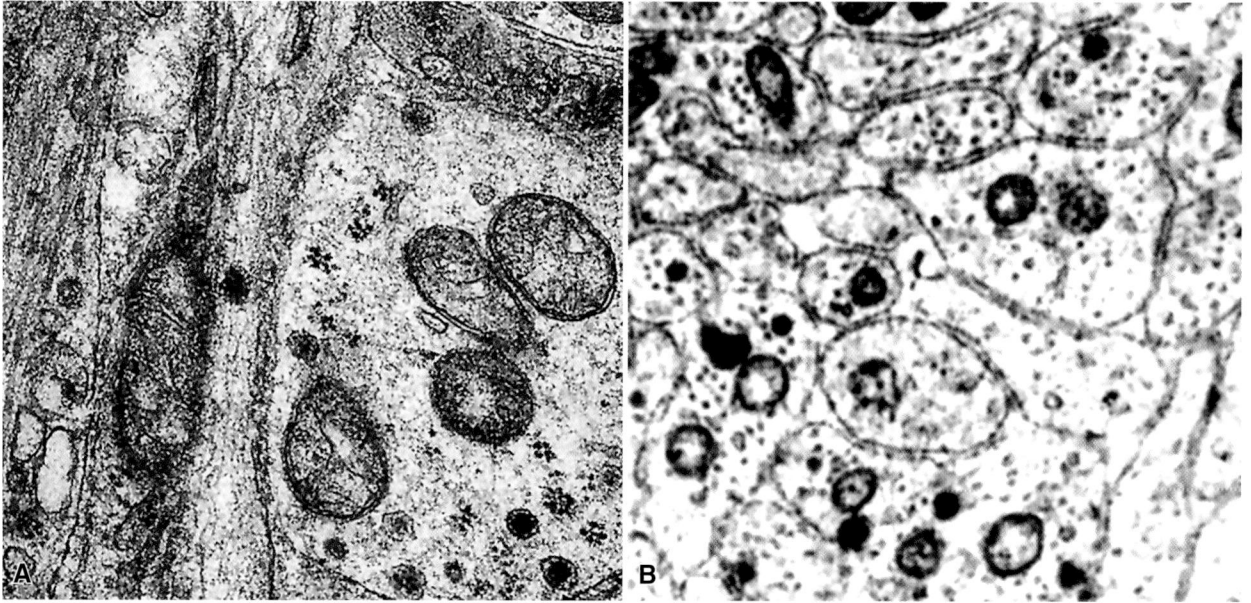

Figure 13-43. Electron photomicrograph of neuroblastoma, demonstrating interdigitating cytoplasmic extensions, each of which contains microtubules (**A**), synaptic-neurosecretory granules (**B**), or both. This constellation of findings would not be expected in epithelial neuroendocrine neoplasms.

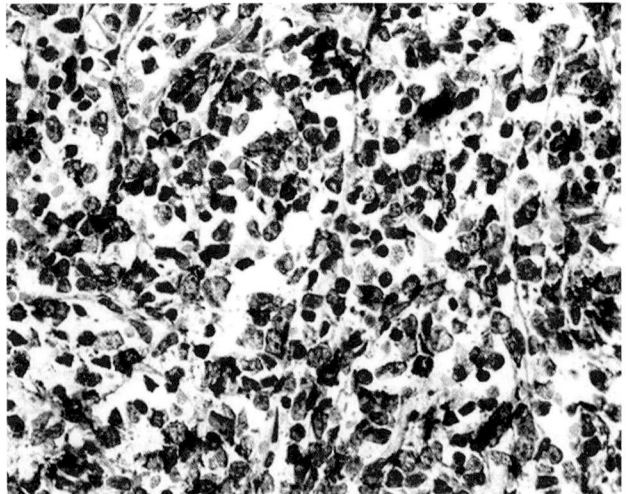

Figure 13-44. Immunoreactivity is present in this neuroblastoma with the antibody known as NB84.

identifying bone marrow micrometastases[422]), but they have a lack of specificity and may also be seen in PNETs as well as some cases of rhabdomyosarcoma.[112] NB84 is another marker showing selective reactivity with NB and PNET, to the exclusion of other small cell tumors[423] (Fig. 13-44). The once-difficult distinction between NB and PNET has been facilitated by the availability of antibodies to CD99 and beta-2-microglobulin, both of which are seen in PNET but not NB.[362] Likewise, immunoreactivity for muscle-specific actin or desmin characterizes rhabdomyoblastic neoplasms and is not expected in NB.[362] This observation principally comes into play in examples of "anaplastic" NB that may resemble embryonal rhabdomyosarcoma on conventional microscopy.[424]

Treatment and Clinical Outcome

With reference to the three reported cases of primary intrapulmonary NB, two patients were alive and well 1 and 2.5 years, respectively, after surgical resection and chemotherapy.[410,411] The other patient died shortly after admission to the hospital.

In much more general terms, two histologic parameters with prognostic significance should be additionally recorded in evaluating neuroblastic neoplasms. These include the level of ganglionic differentiation (<5% or ≥5%)[414–418] and the "mitotic-to-karyorrhectic index" (MKI).[418,425,426] The MKI is the number of mitotic or karyorrhectic nuclei counted in an evaluation of 5000 tumor cells in "neuropil-free" areas of any given tumor. The daunting prospect of assessing that many cells has dissuaded many pathologists from embracing the Shimada system with enthusiasm. However, common practice has shown that a reasonable estimation of the MKI can be obtained with simple pattern-matching approaches. With data on differentiation and MKI, prognostic substratification of stromal-poor neoplasms can be accomplished within appropriately age-, location-, and stage-matched tumor groups.[427]

Accurate classification and prognostication of neuroblastic tumors mandates the availability of detailed data on clinical, gross, and histologic levels. Moreover, biochemical observations—as derived from the clinical chemistry laboratory—may provide additional nuances in this context.[428] The presence of vanillacetic acid in the urine (as opposed to homovanillic acid or vanillyolmandelic acid) worsens the clinical outlook, as do elevated serum levels of ferritin, lactate dehydrogenase, NSE, CGA, and creatine kinase isozyme BB.[428] On the other hand, elevated somatostatin levels in serum or tumor tissue have been linked to a better prognosis.[429]

With regard to other adjunctive modalities of pathologic evaluation as applied to neuroblastic tumors, three have been used increasingly in the last decade. Cytogenetic assessment (requiring submission of fresh tissue, although current fluorescence–in situ hybridization methods may change that) has shown aberrations (deletions and rearrangements) in chromosome 1p in most cases of NB and ganglioneuroblastoma,[430] possibly aiding in the differential diagnosis with other small cell tumors that lack such abnormalities. Prognostically, aneuploidy, hyperdiploidy, and near-tetraploidy in neuroblastic neoplasms correlate with improved prognosis, in contrast to the norm for most other malignant tumors.[414,425] Conversely, DNA diploid lesions tend to behave aggressively. Likewise, increased copy numbers of the oncogene N-myc are also biologically detrimental in NBs.[431–434] This marker can be assessed directly by the Southern blot method or indirectly by Northern/Western blot or in situ hybridization. Immunohistology for the protein product of N-myc can also be performed on fresh tissue, with generally acceptable results. The *RET* gene, which is important in the prognosis of other neuroendocrine tumors, also appears to correlate with neuronal differentiation in NBs and, therefore, roughly with prognosis.[435] Lastly, the immunolabeling index for Ki-67 (an indicator of cell replication) is inversely correlated with the length of survival in NB[436]; further, loss of expression of the *Trk-A* gene or CD44 by the tumor cells is associated with high stage at diagnosis and a poor outcome.[434]

Self-assessment questions related to this chapter can be found online on the Expert Consult site for this title.

References

1. Feyrter F. *Uber diffuse endokrine epitheliale organe*. Leipzig: JA Barth; 1938.
2. Pearse AGE. The APUD cell concept and its implications in pathology. *Pathol Annu*. 1974;9:27–41.
3. Yousem SA. Pulmonary carcinoid tumors and well-differentiated neuroendocrine carcinomas: is there room for an atypical carcinoid? *Am J Clin Pathol*. 1991;95:763–764.
4. Hasleton PS, Bostanci G. Pulmonary carcinoid and related tumors. *Rocz Akad Med Bialymst*. 1997;42(suppl 1):28–42.
5. Travis WD, Rush W, Flieder DB, et al. Survival analysis of 200 pulmonary neuroendocrine tumors with clarification of criteria for atypical carcinoid and its separation from typical carcinoid. *Am J Surg Pathol*. 1998;22:934–944.
6. Lloyd RV. *Endocrine Pathology*. New York: Springer-Verlag; 1990.
7. Lee JE, Evans DB. Advances in the diagnosis and treatment of gastrointestinal neuroendocrine tumors. *Cancer Treat Res*. 1997;90:227–238.
8. Warner RR. Gut neuroendocrine tumors. *Curr Ther Endocrinol Metab*. 1997;6:606–614.
9. Mendelsohn G. *Diagnosis and Pathology of Endocrine Diseases*. Philadelphia: JB Lippincott; 1988.
10. Argani P, Erlandson RA, Rosai J. Thymic neuroblastoma in adults: report of three cases with special emphasis on its association with the syndrome of inappropriate secretion of antidiuretic hormone. *Am J Clin Pathol*. 1997;108:537–543.
11. Hasleton PS, Al-Saffar N. The histological spectrum of bronchial carcinoid tumors. *Appl Pathol*. 1989;7:205–218.
12. Warren WH, Faber LP, Gould VE. Neuroendocrine neoplasms of the lung: a clinicopathologic update. *J Thorac Cardiovasc Surg*. 1989;98:321–332.
13. Glasser CM, Bhagavan BS. Carcinoid tumors of the appendix. *Arch Pathol Lab Med*. 1980;104:272–275.
14. Rusch VW, Klimstra DS, Venkatraman ES. Molecular markers help characterize neuroendocrine lung tumors. *Ann Thorac Surg*. 1996;62:798–809.
15. Gould VE, Linnoila RI, Memoli VA, Warren WH. Neuroendocrine components of the bronchopulmonary tract. *Lab Invest*. 1983;49:519–537.
16. Shackney SE, Shankey TV. Common patterns of genetic evolution in human solid tumors. *Cytometry*. 1997;29:1–27.
17. Yunis JJ. Genes and chromosomes in the pathogenesis and prognosis of human cancers. *Adv Pathol Lab Med*. 1989;2:147–188.
18. Galanis E, Frytak S, Lloyd RV. Extrapulmonary small cell carcinoma. *Cancer*. 1997;79:1729–1736.
19. Fletcher JA. Cytogenetic aberrations in malignant soft tissue tumors. *Adv Pathol Lab Med*. 1991;4:235–246.
20. Dehner LP. Primitive neuroectodermal tumor and Ewing's sarcoma. *Am J Surg Pathol*. 1993;17:1–13.
21. Simpson NE, Kidd KK, Goodfellow PJ, et al. Assignment of multiple endocrine neoplasia type 2A to chromosome 10 by linkage. *Nature*. 1987;328:528–530.
22. Komminoth P. Multiple endocrine neoplasia type 1 and 2: 1997 diagnostic guidelines & molecular pathology. *Pathologe*. 1997;18:286–300.

23. Komminoth P. Multiple endocrine neoplasia type 1 & 2: from morphology to molecular pathology 1997. *Verh Dtsch Ges Pathol*. 1997;81:125–138.

24. Eng C, Mulligan LM. Mutations of the RET protooncogene in the multiple endocrine neoplasia type 2 syndromes, related sporadic tumors, & Hirschsprung's disease. *Hum Mutat*. 1997;9:97–109.

25. Cagle PT, El-Naggar AK, Xu HJ, et al. Differential retinoblastoma protein expression in neuroendocrine tumors of the lung: potential diagnostic implications. *Am J Pathol*. 1997;150:393–400.

26. McDowell EM, Wilson TS, Trump BF. Atypical endocrine tumors of the lung. *Arch Pathol Lab Med*. 1981;105:20–28.

27. Adelstein DJ, Tomashefski JF. Mixed small-cell and non-small-cell lung cancer. *Chest* 1986;89:699–704.

28. Hishima T, Fukayama M, Hayashi Y, et al. Neuroendocrine differentiation in thymic epithelial tumors, with special reference to thymic carcinoma & atypical thymoma. *Hum Pathol*. 1998;29:330–338.

29. Usuda H, Emura I, Naito M, Hirono T. Peripheral lung carcinomas associated with central fibrosis and mixed small cell and other histologic components. *Pathol Int*. 1995;45:940–946.

30. Robertson NJ, Rahamim J, Smith ME. Carcinosarcoma of the esophagus showing neuroendocrine, squamous, and glandular differentiation. *Histopathology*. 1997;31:263–266.

31. McWilliam LJ, Manson C, George NJ. Neuroendocrine differentiation and prognosis in prostatic adenocarcinoma. *Br J Urol*. 1997;80:287–290.

32. Leslie KO, Colby TV. Pathology of lung cancer. *Curr Opin Pulm Med*. 1997;3:252–256.

33. Bosman FT. Neuroendocrine cells in non-endocrine tumors: what does it mean? *Verh Dtsch Ges Pathol*. 1997;81:62–72.

34. Wick MR, Berg LC, Hertz MI. Large cell carcinoma of the lung with neuroendocrine differentiation. *Am J Clin Pathol*. 1992;97:796–805.

35. Radice PA, Matthews MJ, Ihde DC, et al. The clinical behavior of mixed small cell/large cell bronchogenic carcinoma compared to pure small cell subtypes. *Cancer*. 1982;50:2894–2902.

36. Fushimi H, Kikui M, Morino H, et al. Histologic changes in small cell lung carcinoma after treatment. *Cancer*. 1996;77:278–283.

37. Wiseman GA, Kvols LK. Therapy of neuroendocrine tumors with radiolabeled MIBG and somatostatin analogues. *Semin Nucl Med*. 1995;25:272–278.

38. DiBartolomeo M, Bajetta E, Buzzoni R, et al. Clinical efficacy of octreotide in the treatment of metastatic neuroendocrine tumors: a study by the Italian Trials in Medical Oncology group. *Cancer*. 1996;77:402–408.

39. Saldiva PHN, Capelozzi VL, Battlehner CN. Neuroendocrine tumors of the lung. In: Corrin B, ed. *Pathology of Lung Tumors*. New York: Churchill-Livingstone; 1997:55–70.

40. Nagle RB, Payne CM, Clark VA. Comparison of the usefulness of histochemistry and ultrastructural cytochemistry in the identification of neuroendocrine neoplasms. *Am J Clin Pathol*. 1986;85:289–296.

41. Samsonov VA. Carcinoid lung tumors: clinicomorphologic characteristics and diagnosis. *Arkh Patol*. 1995;57:20–24.

42. Kogan EA, Sekamova SM, Mazurenko NN, Bogatyrev VN. Peripheral small cell carcinoma, atypical and typical lung carcinoids. *Arkh Patol*. 1991;53:42–48.

43. Erlandson RA. *Diagnostic Transmission Electron Microscopy of Tumors*. New York: Raven Press; 1994:123–125.

44. Carey FA, Save VE. Neuroendocrine differentiation in lung cancer. *J Pathol*. 1997;182:9–10.

45. Soga J, Yakuwa Y. Bronchopulmonary carcinoids: an analysis of 1875 reported cases with special reference to a comparison between typical carcinoids and typical varieties. *Ann Thorac Cardiovasc Surg*. 1999;5:211–219.

46. Dardick I, Christensen H, Stratis M. Immunoelectron microscopy for chromogranin A in small cell neuroendocrine carcinoma of lung. *Ultrastruct Pathol*. 1996;20:361–368.

47. Yang GC. Mixed small cell/large cell carcinoma of the lung: report of a case with cytologic features and ultrastructural correlation. *Acta Cytol*. 1995;39:1175–1181.

48. Taccagni GL, Rovere E, Terreni MR, et al. Divergent differentiative histogenetic lines in lung tumors: identification of histotypes with pure and mixed ultrastructural phenotype and their prognostic significance. *Ultrastruct Pathol*. 1995;19:61–73.

49. Mount SL, Taatjes DJ, von Turkovich M, et al. Diagnostic immunoelectron microscopy in surgical pathology: assessment of various tissue fixation and processing protocols. *Ultrastruct Pathol*. 1993;17:547–556.

50. Przybylowski P, Mlynarczyk W, Blotna-Filipiak M, Biczysko W. Application of electron microscopy and immunocytochemistry in lung cancer diagnosis. *Folia Morphol*. 1993;52:191–200.

51. Tsubota YT, Kawaguchi T, Hoso T, et al. A combined small cell and spindle cell carcinoma of the lung: report of a unique case with immunohistochemical and ultrastructural studies. *Am J Surg Pathol*. 1992;16:1108–1115.

52. Pilotti S, Patriarca C, Lombardi L, et al. Well-differentiated neuroendocrine carcinoma of the lung: a clinicopathologic and ultrastructural study of 10 cases. *Tumori*. 1992;78:121–129.

53. Dardick I, Yazdi HM, Brosko C, et al. A quantitative comparison of light and electron microscopic diagnoses in specimens obtained by fine needle aspiration biopsy. *Ultrastruct Pathol*. 1991;15:105–129.

54. Muller KM, Fisseler-Eckhoff A. Small cell bronchial cancer – pathologic anatomy. *Langenbecks Arch Chir Suppl Kongressbd*. 1991;534–543.

55. Warren WH, Gould VE. Neuroendocrine tumors of the bronchopulmonary tract: a reappraisal of their classification after 20 years. *Surg Clin North Am*. 2002;82:525–540.

56. Wick MR: Immunohistology of neuroendocrine and neuroectodermal tumors. *Semin Diagn Pathol*. 19(4):207–218.

57. Brambilla E, Veale D, Moro D, et al. Neuroendocrine phenotype in lung cancers: comparison of immunohistochemistry with biochemical determination of enolase isoenzymes. *Am J Clin Pathol*. 1992;98:88–97.

58. Broers JL, Mijnheere EP, Rot MK, et al. Novel antigens characteristic of neuroendocrine malignancies. *Cancer*. 1991;67:619–633.

59. Loy TS, Darkow GVD, Quesenbery JT. Immunostaining in the diagnosis of pulmonary neuroendocrine carcinomas. An immunohistochemical study with ultrastructural correlations. *Am J Surg Pathol*. 1995;19:173–182.

60. Tome Y, Hirohashi S, Noguchi M, et al. Immunocytologic diagnosis of small-cell lung cancer in imprint smears. *Acta Cytologica*. 1991;35:485–490.

61. Miettinen M. Keratin immunohistochemistry: update of applications and pitfalls. *Pathol Annu*. 1993;28(2):113–143.

62. Chan JKC, Suser S, Wenig BM, et al. Cytokeratin 20 immunoreactivity distinguishes Merkel cell (primary cutaneous neuroendocrine) carcinomas and salivary gland small cell carcinomas from small cell carcinomas of various sites. *Am J Surg Pathol*. 1997;21:226–234.

63. Battifora H. Diagnostic uses of antibodies to keratins: a review and immunohistochemical comparison of seven monoclonal and three polyclonal antibodies. *Prog Surg Pathol*. 1988;8:1–16.

64. Battifora H, Silva EG. The use of antikeratin antibodies in the immunohistochemical distinction between neuroendocrine (Merkel cell) carcinoma of the skin, lymphoma, and oat cell carcinoma. *Cancer*. 1986;58:1040–1046.

65. Labrousse F, Leboutet MJ, Petit B, et al. Cytokeratin expression in paragangliomas of the cauda equina. *Clin Neuropathol*. 1999;18:208–213.

66. Chetty R, Pillay P, Jaichand V. Cytokeratin expression in adrenal pheochromocytomas and extra-adrenal paragangliomas. *J Clin Pathol*. 1998;51:477–478.

67. Marley EF, Liapis H, Humphrey PA, et al. Primitive neuroectodermal tumor of the kidney – another enigma: a pathologic, immunohistochemical, and molecular diagnostic study. *Am J Surg Pathol*. 1997;21:354–359.

68. Moll R, Lee I, Gould VE, et al. Immunocytochemical analysis of Ewing's tumors: patterns of expression of intermediate filaments and desmosomal proteins indicate cell type heterogeneity and pluripotential differentiation. *Am J Pathol*. 1987;127:288–304.

69. Thorner P. Intraabdominal polyphenotypic tumor. *Pediatr Pathol Lab Med*. 1996;16:161–169.

70. Gerald WL, Ladanyi M, de Alava E, et al. Clinical, pathologic, and molecular spectrum of tumors associated with t(11;22)(p13;q12): desmoplastic small round cell tumor and its variants. *J Clin Oncol*. 1998;16:3028–3036.

71. Ordonez NG. Desmoplastic small round cell tumor. II. An ultrastructural and immunohistochemical study with emphasis on new immunohistochemical markers. *Am J Surg Pathol*. 1998;22:1314–1327.

72. Winters JL, Geil JD, O'Connor WN. Immunohistology, cytogenetics, and molecular studies of small round cell tumors of childhood: a review. *Ann Clin Lab Sci*. 1995;25:66–78.

73. Broers JL, Carney DN, de Ley L, et al. Differential expression of intermediate filament proteins distinguishes classic from variant small-cell lung cancer cell lines. *Proc Natl Acad Sci U S A*. 1985;82:4409–4413.

74. Merot Y, Margolis RJ, Dahl D, et al. Coexpression of neurofilament and keratin proteins in cutaneous neuroendocrine carcinoma cells. *J Invest Dermatol*. 1986;86:74–77.

75. Moran CA, Suster S, Fishback N, Koss MN. Mediastinal paragangliomas: a clinicopathologic and immunohistochemical study of 16 cases. *Cancer*. 1993;72:2358–2364.

76. Kimura N, Nakazato Y, Nagura H, Sasano N. Expression of intermediate filaments in neuroendocrine tumors. *Arch Pathol Lab Med*. 1990;114:506–510.

77. Hirose T, Scheithauer BW, Lopes MB, et al. Olfactory neuroblastoma: an immunohistochemical, ultrastructural, and flow cytometric study. *Cancer*. 1995;76:4–19.

78. Miettinen M. Synaptophysin and neurofilament proteins as markers for neuroendocrine tumors. *Arch Pathol Lab Med*. 1987;111:813–818.

79. Johnson TL, Zarbo RJ, Lloyd RV, Crissman JD. Paragangliomas of the head and neck: immunohistochemical neuroendocrine and intermediate filament typing. *Mod Pathol*. 1988;1:216–223.

80. Eusebi V, Damiani S, Pasquinelli G, et al. Small cell neuroendocrine carcinoma with skeletal muscle differentiation. *Am J Surg Pathol*. 2000;24:223–230.

81. Friede RL, Janzer RC, Roessmann U. Infantile small cell gliomas. *Acta Neuropathol*. 1982;57:103–110.

82. Oh D, Prayson RA. Evaluation of epithelial and keratin markers in glioblastoma multiforme: an immunohistochemical study. *Arch Pathol Lab Med*. 1999;123:917–920.

83. Wilson RS, Lloyd RV. Detection of chromogranin in neuroendocrine cells with a monoclonal antibody. *Am J Pathol*. 1984;115:458–468.

84. Settleman J, Fonseca R, Nolan J, Angeletti RH. Relationship of multiple forms of chromogranin. *J Biol Chem*. 1985;260:1645–1651.

85. O'Connor DT. Chromogranin: widespread immunoreactivity in polypeptide hormone-producing tissues and in serum. *Regul Pept*. 1983;6:263–280.

86. Eriksson B, Arnberg H, Oberg K, et al. A polyclonal antiserum against chromogranin A and B – a new sensitive marker for neuroendocrine tumors. *Acta Endocrinol*. 1990;122:145–155.

87. Woussen-Colle MC, Gourlet P, Vandermeers A, et al. Identification of a new chromogranin B fragment (314–365) in endocrine tumors. *Peptides*. 1995;16:231–236.

88. Lloyd RV, Wilson RS. Specific endocrine marker defined by a monoclonal antibody. *Science*. 1983;222:628–630.

89. Gould VE, Lee I, Wiedenmann B, et al. Synaptophysin: a novel marker for neurons, certain neuroendocrine cells, and their neoplasms. *Hum Pathol*. 1986;17:979–983.

90. Buffa R, Rindi G, Sessa F, et al. Synaptophysin immunoreactivity and small clear vesicles in neuroendocrine cells and related tumors. *Mol Cell Probes*. 1987;1:367–381.

91. Stridsberg M. The use of chromogranin, synaptophysin, and islet amyloid polypeptide as markers for neuroendocrine tumors. *Ups J Med Sci*. 1995;100:169–199.

92. Poola I, Graziano SL. Expression of neuron-specific enolase, chromogranin A, synaptophysin, and Leu-7 in lung cancer cell lines. *J Exp Clin Cancer Res*. 1998;17:165–173.

93. Erlandson RA, Nesland JM. Tumors of the endocrine/neuroendocrine system: an overview. *Ultrastruct Pathol*. 1994;18:149–170.

94. Lipinski M, Braham K, Caillaud JM, et al. HNK-1 antibody detects an antigen expressed on neuroectodermal cells. *J Exp Med*. 1983;158:1775–1780.

95. Tsutsumi Y. Leu-7 immunoreactivity as a histochemical marker for paraffin-embedded neuroendocrine tumors. *Acta Histochem Cytochem*. 1984;17:15–21.

96. Bunn Jr PA, Linnoila I, Minna JD, et al. Small cell lung cancer, endocrine cells of the fetal bronchus, and other neuroendocrine cells express the Leu-7 antigenic determinant present on natural killer cells. *Blood*. 1985;65:764–768.

97. Perentes E, Rubinstein LJ. Immunohistochemical recognition of human nerve sheath tumors by anti-Leu 7 (HNK-1) monoclonal antibody. *Acta Neuropathol*. 1985;68:319–324.

98. Abenoza P, Manivel JC, Swanson PE, Wick MR. Synovial sarcoma: ultrastructural study and immunohistochemical analysis by a combined PAP/ABC procedure. *Hum Pathol*. 1986;17:1107–1115.

99. Rusthoven JJ, Robinson JB, Kolin A, Pinkerton PH. The natural killer cell associated HNK-1 (Leu-7) antibody reacts with hypertrophic and malignant prostatic epithelium. *Cancer*. 1985;56:289–293.

100. May EE, Perentes E. Anti-Leu 7 immunoreactivity with human tumors: its value in the diagnosis of prostatic adenocarcinoma. *Histopathology*. 1987;11:295–304.

101. Kodama T, Watanable S, Sato Y, et al. An immunohistochemical study of thymic epithelial tumors. I. Epithelial component. *Am J Surg Pathol*. 1986;10:26–33.

102. Tischler AS, Mobtaker H, Mann K, et al. Anti-lymphocyte antibody Leu-7 (HNK-1) recognizes a constituent of neuroendocrine granule matrix. *J Histochem Cytochem*. 1986;34:1213–1216.

103. Lantuejoul S, Moro D, Michalides RJ, et al. Neural cell adhesion molecules (NCAM) and NCAM-PSA expression in neuroendocrine lung tumors. *Am J Surg Pathol*. 1998;22:1267–1276.

104. Kaufmann O, Georgi T, Dietel M. Utility of 123C3 monoclonal antibody against CD56 (NCAM) for the diagnosis of small cell carcinomas on paraffin sections. *Hum Pathol*. 1997;28:1373–1378.

105. Del Rio M, Demoly P, Koros AM, et al. JLP5B9: new monoclonal antibody against polysialylated neural cell adhesion molecule is of value in phenotyping lung cancer. *J Immunol Meth*. 2000;233:21–31.

106. Hage R, Elbers HR, Brutel de la Riviere A, van den Bosch JM. Neural cell adhesion molecule expression: prognosis in 889 patients with resected non-small cell lung cancer. *Chest*. 1998;114:1316–1320.

107. Jaques G, Auerbach B, Pritsch M, et al. Evaluation of serum neural cell adhesion molecule as a new tumor marker in small cell lung cancer. *Cancer*. 1993;72:418–425.

108. Seldeslagh KA, Lauweryns JM. NCAM expression in the pulmonary neural and diffuse neuroendocrine cell system. *Microsc Res Tech*. 1997;37:69–76.

109. Kwa HB, Verheijen MG, Litvinov SV, et al. Prognostic factors in resected non-small cell lung cancer: an immunohistochemical study of 39 cases. *Lung Cancer*. 1996;16:35–45.

110. Tapia FJ, Barbosa AJA, Marangos PJ, et al. Neuron-specific enolase is produced by neuroendocrine tumors. *Lancet*. 1981;2:808–811.

111. Wick MR, Scheithauer BW, Kovacs K. Neuron-specific enolase in neuroendocrine tumors of the thymus, bronchus, and skin. *Am J Clin Pathol*. 1983;79:703–707.

112. Carlei F, Polak JM. Antibodies to neuron-specific enolase for the delineation of the entire diffuse neuroendocrine system in health and disease. *Semin Diagn Pathol*. 1984;1:59–70.

113. Haimoto H, Takahashi Y, Koshikawa T, et al. Immunohistochemical localization of gamma-enolase in normal human tissues other than nervous and neuroendocrine tissues. *Lab Invest*. 1985;52:257–263.

114. Thomas P, Battifora H, Manderino GL, Patrick J. A monoclonal antibody against neuron-specific enolase: immunohistochemical comparison with a polyclonal antiserum. *Am J Clin Pathol*. 1987;88:146–152.

115. Vinores SA, Bonnin JM, Rubinstein LJ, Marangos PJ. Immunohistochemical demonstration of neuron-specific enolase in neoplasms of the CNS and other tissues. *Arch Pathol Lab Med*. 1984;108:536–540.

116. DeLellis RA. Endocrine tumors. In: Colvin RB, Bhan AK, McCluskey RT, eds. *Diagnostic Immunopathology*, 1st ed. New York: Raven Press; 1988:301–338.

117. Said JW, Vimadalal S, Nash G, et al. Immunoreactive neuron-specific enolase, bombesin, and chromogranin-A as markers for neuroendocrine lung tumors. *Hum Pathol*. 1985;16:236–240.

118. Rode J. PGP 9.5 – a new marker for vertebrate neurons and neuroendocrine cells. *Brain Res*. 1983;278:224–228.

119. Gosney JR, Gosney MA, Lye M, Butt SA. Reliability of commercially available immunocytochemical markers for identification of neuroendocrine differentiation in bronchoscopic biopsies of bronchial carcinoma. *Thorax*. 1995;50:116–120.

120. Addis BJ, Hamid Q, Ibrahim NB, et al. Immunohistochemical markers of small cell carcinoma and related neuroendocrine tumors of the lung. *J Pathol*. 1987;153:137–150.

121. Hibi K, Westra WH, Borges M, et al. PGP9.5 as a candidate tumor marker for non-small cell lung cancer. *Am J Pathol*. 1999;155:711–715.

122. Amann G, Zoubek A, Salzer-Kuntschik M, et al. Relation of neurological marker expression and EWS gene fusion types in MIC2/CD99-positive tumors of the Ewing family. *Hum Pathol*. 1999;30:1058–1064.

123. Dehner LP. Primitive neuroectodermal tumors and Ewing's sarcoma. *Am J Surg Pathol*. 1993;17:1–13.

124. Soslow RA, Bhargava V, Warnke RA. MIC2, TdT, bcl-2, and CD34 expression in paraffin-embedded high-grade lymphoma/acute lymphoblastic leukemia distinguishes between distinct clinicopathologic entities. *Hum Pathol*. 1997;28:1158–1165.

125. Lumadue JA, Askin FB, Perlman EJ. MIC2 analysis of small cell carcinoma. *Am J Clin Pathol*. 1994;102:692–694.

126. Nicholson SA, McDermott MB, Swanson PE, Wick MR. CD99 and cytokeratin-20 in small-cell and basaloid tumors of the skin. *Appl Immunohistochem Mol Morphol*. 2000;8(1):37–41.

127. Krisch K, Buxbaum P, Horvat G, et al. Monoclonal antibody HISL-19 as an immunocytochemical probe for neuroendocrine differentiation. Its application in diagnostic pathology. *Am J Pathol*. 1986;123:100–108.

128. Lloyd RV, Sisson JC, Shapiro B, Verhofstad AA. Immunohistochemical localization of epinephrine, norepinephrine, catecholamine-synthesizing enzymes, and chromogranin in neuroendocrine cells and tumors. *Am J Pathol*. 1986;125:45–64.

129. Haspel MV, Onodera T, Prabhakar BS, et al. Multiple organ-reactive monoclonal autoantibodies. *Nature*. 1983;304:73–76.

130. Unger P, Hoffman K, Pertsemlidis D, et al. S100 protein-positive sustentacular cells in malignant and locally aggressive adrenal pheochromocytomas. *Arch Pathol Lab Med*. 1991;115:484–487.

131. Sholl LM, Long KB, Hornick JL. Sox2 expression in pulmonary non-small cell and neuroendocrine carcinomas. *Appl Immunohistochem Mol Morphol*. 2010;18:55–61.

132. Sica G, Vazquez MF, Altorki N, et al. PAX-5 expression in pulmonary neuroendocrine neoplasms: its usefulness in surgical and fine-needle aspiration biopsy specimens. *Am J Clin Pathol*. 2008;129:556–562.

133. LaPoint RJ, Bourne PA, Wang HL, Xu H. Coexpression of c-kit and bcl-2 in small cell carcinoma and large cell neuroendocrine carcinoma of the lung. *Appl Immunohistochem Mol Morphol*. 2007;15:401–406.

134. Sturm N, Rossi G, Lantuejoul S, et al. Expression of thyroid transcription factor-1 in the spectrum of neuroendocrine cell lung proliferations with special interest in carcinoids. *Hum Pathol*. 2002;33:175–182.

135. Oliveira AM, Tazelaar HD, Myers JL, et al. Thyroid transcription factor-1 distinguishes metastatic pulmonary from well-differentiated neuroendocrine tumors of other sites. *Am J Surg Pathol*. 2001;25:815–819.

136. Ordonez NG. Value of thyroid transcription factor-1 immunostaining in distinguishing small cell lung carcinomas from other small cell carcinomas. *Am J Surg Pathol*. 2000;24:1217–1223.

137. Kaufmann O, Dietel M. Expression of thyroid transcription factor-1 in pulmonary and extrapulmonary small cell carcinomas and other neuroendocrine carcinomas of various primary sites. *Histopathology*. 2000;36:415–420.

138. Agoff SN, Lamps LW, Philip AT, et al. Thyroid transcription factor-1 is expressed in extrapulmonary small cell carcinomas but not in other extrapulmonary neuroendocrine tumors. *Mod Pathol*. 2000;13:238–242.

139. Folpe AL, Gown AM, Lamps LW, et al. Thyroid transcription factor-1: immunohistochemical evaluation in pulmonary neuroendocrine tumors. *Mod Pathol*. 1999;12:5–8.

140. Zamecnik J, Kodet R. Value of thyroid transcription factor-1 and surfactant apoprotein A in the differential diagnosis of pulmonary carcinomas: a study of 109 cases. *Virchows Arch A*. 2002;440:353–361.

141. Travis WD, Colby TV, Corrin B, et al. In: *Histological Typing of Lung and Pleural Tumours (International Histological Classification of Tumours)*. Geneva, Switzerland: World Health Organization; 1999:1–55.

142. Travis WD. Lung tumours with neuroendocrine differentiation. *Eur J Cancer*. 2009;45(Suppl 1):251–266.

143. Hofler H. Neuroendocrine tumors of the lung. *Verh Dtsch Ges Pathol*. 1997;81:118–124.

144. Moran CA, Suster S, Coppola D, Wick MR. Neuroendocrine carcinomas of the lung: a critical analysis. *Am J Clin Pathol*. 2009;131:206–221.

145. Franks TJ, Galvin JR. Lung tumors with neuroendocrine morphology: essential radiologic and pathologic features. *Arch Pathol Lab Med*. 2008;132:1055–1061.

146. Kramer R. Adenoma of the bronchus. *Ann Otol Rhinol Laryngol*. 1930;39:689–695.

147. Carter D, Eggleston JC. Tumors of the lower respiratory tract. In: *Atlas of Tumor Pathology*, series 2, fascicle 17. Washington, DC: Armed Forces Institute of Pathology; 1995:162–188.

148. Colby TV, Koss MN, Travis WD. Tumors of the lower respiratory tract. In: *Atlas of Tumor Pathology*, series 2, fascicle 13. Washington, DC: Armed Forces Institute of Pathology; 1995:287–318.

149. El-Naggar AK, Ballance W, Abdul Karim FW, et al. Typical and atypical bronchopulmonary carcinoids. *Am J Clin Pathol*. 1991;95:828–834.

150. McCaughan BC, Martini N, Bains MS. Bronchial carcinoids: review of 124 cases. *J Thorac Cardiovasc Surg*. 1985;89:8–17.

151. Abdi EA, Goel R, Bishop S, Bain GO. Peripheral carcinoid tumours of the lung: a clinicopathologic study. *J Surg Oncol*. 1988;39:190–196.

152. Ranchod M, Levine GD. Spindle cell carcinoid tumors of the lung: a clinicopathologic study of 35 cases. *Am J Surg Pathol*. 1980;4:315–331.

153. Zarate A, Kovacs K, Flores M, et al. ACTH and CRF-producing bronchial carcinoid associated with Cushing's syndrome. *Clin Endocrinol*. 1986;24:523–529.

154. Findling JW, Tyrrell JB. Occult ectopic secretion of corticotropin. *Arch Intern Med*. 1986;146:929–933.

155. Ankotche A, Raffin-Sanson ML, Mosnier-Pudard H, et al. Ectopic ACTH secretion: a heterogeneous entity. *Presse Med*. 1997;26:1330–1333.

156. Shrager JB, Wright CD, Wain JC, et al. Bronchopulmonary carcinoid tumors associated with Cushing's syndrome: a more aggressive variant of typical carcinoid. *J Thorac Cardiovasc Surg*. 1997;114:367–375.

157. Oliaro A, Filosso PL, Casadio C, et al. Bronchial carcinoid associated with Cushing's syndrome. *J Cardiovasc Surg*. 1995;36:511–514.

158. White A, Clark AJ. The cellular and molecular basis of the ectopic ACTH syndrome. *Clin Endocrinol*. 1993;39:131–141.

159. Liu TH, Liu HR, Lu ZL, et al. Thoracic ectopic ACTH-producing tumors with Cushing's syndrome. *Zentrabl Pathol*. 1993;139:131–139.

160. Levy NT, Rubin J, DeRemee RA, et al. Carcinoid tumors and sarcoidosis – does a link exist? *Mayo Clin Proc*. 1997;72:112–116.

161. Flieder DB, Vazquez VF. Lung tumors with neuroendocrine morphology: a perspective for the new millenium. *Radiol Clin North Am*. 2000;38:563–577.

162. Aubry MC, Thomas Jr CF, Jett JR, et al. Significance of multiple carcinoid tumors and tumorlets in surgical lung specimens: analysis of 28 patients. *Chest*. 2007;131:1635–1643.

163. Davies SJ, Gosney JR, Hansell DM, et al. Diffuse idiopathic pulmonary neuroendocrine cell hyperplasia: an under-recognised spectrum of disease. *Thorax*. 2007;62:248–252.

164. Al-Kaisa N, Abdul-Karim FW, Mendelsohn G, Jacobs G. Bronchial carcinoid tumor with amyloid stroma. *Arch Pathol Lab Med*. 1988;112:211–214.

165. Scharifker D, Marchevsky A. Oncocytic carcinoid tumor of lung: an ultrastructural analysis. *Cancer*. 1981;47:530–532.

166. Sklar JL, Churg A, Bensch KG. Oncocytic carcinoid tumor of the lung. *Am J Surg Pathol*. 1980;4:287–292.

167. Ritter JH, Nappi O. Oxyphilic proliferations of the respiratory tract and paranasal sinuses. *Semin Diagn Pathol*. 1999;16:105–116.

168. Gaffey MJ, Mills SE, Frierson Jr HF, et al. Pulmonary clear cell carcinoid tumor: another entity in the differential diagnosis of pulmonary clear cell neoplasia. *Am J Surg Pathol*. 1998;22:1020–1025.

169. Arora R, Mathur SR, Aron M, et al. Oncocytic carcinoid tumor of the lung: a case report of diagnostic pitfall in filter membrane preparation of bronchial washings. *Acta Cytol*. 2007;51:907–910.

170. Mark EJ, Quay SC, Dickerson GR. Papillary carcinoid tumor of the lung. *Cancer*. 1981;48:316–324.

171. Grazer R, Cohen SM, Jacobs JB, Lucas P. Melanin-containing peripheral carcinoid tumor of the lung. *Am J Surg Pathol*. 1982;6:73–78.

172. Carlson JA, Dickersin GR. Melanotic paragangliod carcinoid tumor: a case report and review of the literature. *Ultrastruct Pathol*. 1993;17:353–372.

173. Al-Khafaji B, Noffsinger AE, Miller MA, et al. Immunohistologic analysis of gastrointestinal and pulmonary carcinoid tumors. *Hum Pathol*. 1998;29:992–999.

174. Skinner C, Ewen SWB. Carcinoid lung: diffuse pulmonary infiltration by a multifocal bronchial carcinoid. *Thorax*. 1976;31:212–219.

175. Fulciniti F, La Vecchia F, Staiano M, et al. Spindle cell neuroendocrine carcinoma of the lung: report of a case with fine needle aspiration cytology and differential diagnostic considerations. *Acta Cytol*. 2007;51:227–230.

176. Lohmann DR, Fesseler B, Putz B, et al. Infrequent mutations of the p53 gene in pulmonary carcinoid tumors. *Cancer Res*. 1993;53:5797–5801.

177. Jiang SX, Kameya T, Shinada J, Yoshimura H. The significance of frequent and independent p53 and bcl-2 expression in large cell neuroendocrine carcinoma of the lung. *Mod Pathol*. 1999;12:362–369.

178. Srivastava A, Hornick JL. Immunohistochemical staining for CDX-2, PDX-1, NESP-55, and TTF-1 can help distinguish gastrointestinal carcinoid tumors from pancreatic endocrine and pulmonary carcinoid tumors. *Am J Surg Pathol*. 2009;33:626–632.

179. Eyden B, Pandit D, Banerjee SS. Malignant melanoma with neuroendocrine differentiation: clinical, histological, immunohistochemical and ultrastructural features of three cases. *Histopathology*. 2005;47:402–409.

180. Pelosi G, Zancanaro C, Sbabo L, et al. Development of innumerable neuroendocrine tumorlets in pulmonary lobe scarred by intralobar sequestration: immunohistochemical and ultrastructural study of an unusual case. *Arch Pathol Lab Med*. 1992;116:1167–1174.

181. Canessa PA, Santini D, Zanelli M, Capecchi V. Pulmonary tumorlets and microcarcinoids in bronchiectasis. *Monaldi Arch Chest Dis*. 1997;52:138–139.

182. Ramon-Capilla M, Arnau-Obrer A, Navarro-Ibanez R, et al. Pulmonary tumorlet: report of 5 cases. *Arch Bronchopneumorol*. 1996;32:489–491.

183. Zanetta G, Zanoni M, Colombo F. Argentaffin pulmonary tumorlets. *Tumori*. 1979;65:761–766.

184. Watanabe H, Kobayashi H, Honma K, et al. Diffuse panbronchiolitis with multiple tumorlets: a quantitative study of the Kultschitzky cells and the clusters. *Acta Pathol Jpn*. 1985;35:1221–1231.

185. Rizvi SM, Goodwill J, Lim E, et al. The frequency of neuroendocrine cell hyperplasia in patients with pulmonary neuroendocrine tumours and non-neuroendocrine cell carcinomas. *Histopathology*. 2009;55:332–337.

186. Ferolla P, Daddi N, Urbani M, et al. Regional Multidisciplinary Group for the Diagnosis and Treatment of Neuroendocrine Tumors, CRO, Umbria Region Cancer Network, Italy. Tumorlets, multicentric carcinoids, lymph-nodal metastases, and long-term behavior in bronchial carcinoids. *J Thorac Oncol*. 2009;4:383–387.

187. Miller RR, Muller NL. Neuroendocrine cell hyperplasia and obliterative bronchiolitis in patients with peripheral carcinoid tumors. *Am J Surg Pathol*. 1995;19:653–658.

188. Satoh Y, Fujiyama J, Ueno M, Ishikawa Y. High cellular atypia in a pulmonary tumorlet: report of a case with cytologic findings. *Acta Cytol*. 2000;44:242–246.

189. Higashiyama M, Doi O, Kodama K, et al. A case of pulmonary tumorlet with tuberculoma misdiagnosed as small cell lung carcinoma by transbronchial lung biopsy. *Kyobu Geka*. 1995;48:165–168.

190. Shah R, Sabanathan S, Mearns J, et al. Carcinoid tumor of the lung. *J Cardiovasc Surg*. 1997;38:187–189.

191. DiGiorgio A, Tocchi A, Puntillo G, et al. Tracheobronchial carcinoids: current therapeutic trends. *Ann Ital Chir*. 1990;61:405–409.

192. Huwer H, Kalweit G, Kruger B, et al. Bronchopulmonary carcinoids: surgical therapy and prognosis. *Pneumonologie*. 1996;50:786–789.

193. Ferguson MK, Landreneau RJ, Hazelrigg SR, et al. Long-term outcome after resection for bronchial carcinoid tumors. *Eur J Cardiothorac Surg*. 2000;18:156–161.

194. Warren WH, Gould VE, Faber LP, et al. Neuroendocrine neoplasms of the bronchopulmonary tract: a classification of the spectrum of carcinoid to small cell carcinoma and intervening variants. *J Thorac Cardiovasc Surg*. 1985;89:819–825.

195. Skov BG, Krasnik M, Lantuejoul S, et al. Reclassification of neuroendocrine tumors improves the separation of carcinoids and the prediction of survival. *J Thorac Oncol*. 2008;3:1410–1415.

196. Gustafsson BI, Kidd M, Chan A, et al. Bronchopulmonary neuroendocrine tumors. *Cancer*. 2008;113:5–21.

197. Ashraf MH. Bronchial carcinoid with osteoblastic metastases. *Thorax*. 1977;32:509–511.

198. Padberg BC, Woenckhaus J, Hilger G, et al. DNA cytophotometry and prognosis in typical and atypical bronchopulmonary carcinoids: a clinicomorphologic study of 100 neuroendocrine lung tumors. *Am J Surg Pathol*. 1996;20:815–822.

199. Daddi N, Urbani M, Semeraro A, et al. Surgical treatment of well differentiated neuroendocrine tumours of the lung. *G Chir*. 2008;29:246–249.

200. Lissoni P, Barni S, Tacini G, et al. Immunoendocrine therapy with low-dose subcutaneous interleukin-2 plus melatonin of locally advanced or metastatic endocrine tumors. *Oncology*. 1995;52:163–166.

201. Arrigoni MG, Woolner LB, Bernatz PE. Atypical carcinoid tumors of the lung. *J Thorac Cardiovasc Surg*. 1972;64:413–421.

202. Paladugu RR, Benefield JR, Pak HY, et al. Bronchopulmonary Kulchitzky cell carcinomas: a new classification scheme for typical and atypical carcinoids. *Cancer*. 1985;55:1303–1311.

203. Lequaglie C, Patriarca C, Cataldo I, et al. Prognosis of resected well-differentiated neuroendocrine carcinoma of the lung. *Chest*. 1991;100:1053–1056.

204. Memoli V. Well-differentiated neuroendocrine carcinoma: a designation comes of age. *Chest*. 1991;100:892.

205. Garcia-Yuste M, Matilla JM, Alvarez-Gago F, et al. Prognostic factors in neuroendocrine lung tumors. *Ann Thorac Surg*. 2000;70:258–263.

206. Rush W, Zeren H, Griffin JL, et al. Histologic subtypes of neuroendocrine carcinoma: prognostic correlations [abstract]. *Lab Invest*. 1995;153A:72.

207. Warren WH, Memoli VA, Gould VE. Immunohistochemical and ultrastructural analysis of bronchopulmonary neuroendocrine neoplasms. II. Well-differentiated neuroendocrine carcinomas. *Ultrastruct Pathol*. 1984;7:185–199.

208. Warren WH, Memoli VA, Gould VE. Well differentiated and small cell neuroendocrine carcinomas of the lung: two related but distinct clinicopathologic entities. *Virch Arch B Cell Pathol*. 1988;55:299–310.

209. Warren WH, Memoli VA, Jordan AG, et al. Re-evaluation of pulmonary neoplasms resected as small cell carcinomas: significance of distinguishing between well-differentiated and small cell neuroendocrine carcinomas. *Cancer*. 1990;65:1003–1010.

210. Carter D, Yesner R. Carcinomas of the lung with neuroendocrine differentiation. *Semin Diagn Pathol*. 1985;2:235–254.

211. Oliaro A, Donati G, Filosso PL, Ruffini E. Neuroendocrine tumors of the lung. *Minerva Chir*. 2000;66:7–16.

212. Slodkowska J, Langfort R, Rudzinski P, Kupis W. Typical and atypical pulmonary carcinoids: pathologic and clinical analysis of 77 cases. *Pneumonol Alergol Pol*. 1998;66:297–303.

213. Pareja E, Arnau A, Aartigues E, et al. Bronchial carcinoid tumors: a prospective study. *Arch Bronchopneumorol*. 1998;34:71–75.

214. Balli M, Fabris GA, Dewar A. Atypical carcinoid tumor: a study of 33 cases with prognostic features. *Histopathology*. 1994;24:363–369.

215. Mills SE, Walker AN, Cooper PH, et al. Atypical carcinoid tumor of the lung: a clinicopathologic study of 17 cases. *Am J Surg Pathol*. 1982;6:643–654.

216. Grote TH, Macon WR, Davis B, et al. Atypical carcinoid of the lung: a distinct clinicopathologic entity. *Chest*. 1988;93:370–375.

217. Burns TM, Juel VC, Sanders DB, Phillips LH. Neuroendocrine lung tumors and disorders of the neuromuscular junction. *Neurology*. 1999;52:1490–1491.

218. Yousem SA, Taylor SR. Typical and atypical carcinoid tumors of lung. A clinicopathologic and DNA analysis of 20 tumors. *Modern Pathol*. 1990;3:502–507.

219. Guinee Jr DG, Fishback NF, Koss MN, et al. The spectrum of immunohistochemical staining of small cell lung carcinoma in specimens from transbronchial and open-lung biopsies. *Am J Clin Pathol*. 1994;102:406–414.

220. Slodkowska J. The value of immunohistochemical identification of neuroendocrine differentiation in non-small cell lung carcinoma. *Rocz Akad Med Bialymst*. 1997;42(suppl 1):23–27.

221. Al-Saffar N, White A, Moore M, Hasleton PS. Immunoreactivity of various peptides in typical and atypical bronchopulmonary carcinoid tumors. *Br J Cancer*. 1988;58:762–766.

222. Couce ME, Bautista D, Costa J, Carter D. Analysis of K-ras, N-ras, H-ras, and p53 in lung neuroendocrine neoplasms. *Diagn Mol Pathol*. 1999;8:71–79.

223. Roncalli M, Doglioni C, Springall DR, et al. Abnormal p53 expression in lung neuroendocrine tumors. Diagnostic and prognostic implications. *Diag Molec Pathol*. 1992;1:129–135.

224. Anbazhagan R, Tihan T, Bornman DM, et al. Classification of small cell lung cancer and pulmonary carcinoid by gene expression profiles. *Cancer Res*. 1999;59:5119–5122.

225. Onuki N, Wistuba II, Travis WD, et al. Genetic changes in the spectrum of neuroendocrine lung tumors. *Cancer*. 1999;85:600–607.

226. Ullmann R, Schwendel A, Klemen H, et al. Unbalanced chromosomal aberrations in neuroendocrine lung tumors as detected by comparative genomic hybridization. *Hum Pathol*. 1998;29:1145–1149.

227. Johansson M, Heim S, Mandahl N, et al. Cytogentic analysis of six bronchial carcinoids. *Cancer Gen Cytogen*. 1993;66:33–38.

228. Jackson-York GL, David BH, Warren WH, et al. Flow cytometric DNA content analysis in neuroendocrine carcinoma of the lung. *Cancer*. 1991;68:374–379.

229. Brambilla E, Moro D, Veale D, et al. Basal cell (basaloid) carcinoma of the lung: a new morphologic and phenotypic entity with separate prognostic significance. *Hum Pathol*. 1992;23:993–1003.

230. Travis WD, Linnoila RI, Tsokos MG, et al. Neuroendocrine tumors of the lung with proposed criteria for large-cell neuroendocrine carcinoma: an ultrastructural, immunohistochemical, and flow cytometric study of 35 cases. *Am J Surg Pathol*. 1991;15:529–553.

231. McBurney RP, Kirklin JW, Woolner LB. Metastasizing bronchial adenomas. *Surg Gynecol Obstet*. 1953;96:482–492.

232. Marty-Ane CH, Costes V, Pujol JL, et al. Carcinoid tumors of the lung: do atypical features require aggressive management? *Annu Thorac Surg*. 1995;59:78–83.

233. Carretta A, Ceresoli GL, Arrigoni G, et al. Diagnostic and therapeutic management of neuroendocrine lung tumors: a clinical study of 44 cases. *Lung Cancer*. 2000;29:217–225.

234. Barnard WG. The nature of the "oat cell sarcoma" of the mediastinum. *J Pathol Bacteriol*. 1926;29:241–244.

235. Azzopardi JG. Oat cell carcinoma of the bronchus. *J Pathol Bacteriol*. 1959;78:513–519.

236. Cook RM, Miller YE, Bunn Jr PA. Small cell lung cancer: etiology, biology, clinical features, staging, and treatment. *Curr Probl Cancer*. 1993;17:69–141.

237. Perkins PJ. Delayed onset of secondary hypertrophic osteoarthropathy. *Am J Roentgenol*. 1978;130:561–562.

238. Johnson BE, Chute JP, Rushin J, et al. A prospective study of patients with lung cancer and hyponatremia of malignancy. *Am J Respir Crit Care Med*. 1997;156:1669–1678.

239. Takai E, Yano T, Iguchi H, et al. Tumor-induced hypercalcemia and parathyroid hormone-related protein in lung carcinoma. *Cancer*. 1996;78:1384–1387.

240. Ferroir JP, Milleron B, Ropert A, et al. Atypical paraneoplastic myasthenic syndrome: Lambert–Eaton syndrome or myasthenia? *Rev Pneumonol Clin*. 1999;55:168–170.

241. Posner JB. Paraneoplastic syndromes: a brief review. *Ann N Y Acad Sci*. 1997;835:83–90.

242. Thirkill CE. Lung cancer-induced blindness. *Lung Cancer*. 1996;14:253–264.

243. Usalan C, Emri S. Membranoproliferative glomerulonephritis associated with small cell lung carcinoma. *Int Urol Nephrol*. 1998;30:209–213.

244. Brenner S, Golan H, Gat A, Bialy-Golan A. Paraneoplastic subacute cutaneous lupus erythematosus: report of a case associated with cancer of the lung. *Dermatology*. 1997;194:172–174.

245. Hsu CW, Wang HC, Lu JY. Small cell lung carcinoma associated with paraneoplastic limbic encephalitis. *J Formos Med Assoc*. 1999;18:368–371.

246. Kamiyoshihara M, Hirai T, Kawashima O, et al. Sarcoid reactions in primary pulmonary carcinoma: report of seven cases. *Oncol Rep*. 1998;5:177–180.

247. Conejo-Mir JS, Casals M, Carciandia C, et al. Cutaneous sarcoid granulomas with oat cell carcinoma of the lung. *Dermatology*. 1995;191:59–61.

248. Ponge T, Boutoille D, Moreau A, et al. Systemic vasculitis in a patient with small-cell neuroendocrine bronchial cancer. *Eur Respir J*. 1998;12:1228–1229.

249. Krauss EA, Ludwig PW, Sumner HW. Metastatic carcinoma presenting as fulminant hepatic failure. *Am J Gastroenterol*. 1979;72:651–654.

250. Horlyck A, Henriques U, Jakobsen A. The value of bone marrow examination in small cell carcinoma. *Acta Oncol*. 1994;33:909–911.

251. Tritz DB, Doll DC, Ringenberg QS, et al. Bone marrow involvement in small cell lung cancer: clinical significance and correlation with routine laboratory values. *Cancer*. 1989;63:763–766.

252. Nguyen LN, Maor MH, Oswald MJ. Brain metastases as the only manifestation of an undetected primary tumor. *Cancer*. 1998;83:2181–2184.

253. Falconieri G, Zanconati F, Bussani R, DiBonito L. Small cell carcinoma of lung simulating pleural mesothelioma: report of 4 cases with autopsy confirmation. *Pathol Res Pract*. 1995;191:1147–1152.

254. Yesner R. Small cell tumors of the lung. *Am J Surg Pathol*. 1983;7:775–785.

255. Carter D. Small cell carcinoma of the lung. *Am J Surg Pathol*. 1983;7:787–795.

256. Aisner SC, Finkelstein DM, Ettinger DS, et al. The clinical significance of variant morphology small cell carcinoma of the lung. *J Clin Oncol*. 1990;8:402–408.

257. Bepler G, Neumann K, Holle R, et al. Clinical relevance of histologic subtyping in small cell lung cancer. *Cancer*. 1980;45:74–79.

258. Hirsch FR, Matthews MJ, Aisner SC, et al. Histopathologic classification of small cell lung cancer: changing concepts and terminology. *Cancer*. 1988;62:973–977.

259. Hirsch FR, Matthews MJ, Yesner R. Histopathologic classification of small cell carcinoma of the lung: comments based on an interobserver examination. *Cancer*. 1982;50:1360–1366.

260. Magum MD, Greco FA, Hainsworth JD, et al. Combined small cell and non-small cell lung cancer. *J Clin Oncol*. 1989;7:607–612.

261. Sehested M, Hirsch FR, Osterlind K, et al. Morphologic variations of small cell lung cancer: a histopathologic study of pretreatment and posttreatment specimens in 104 patients. *Cancer*. 1986;57:805–807.

262. Thomas JS, Lamb D, Ashcroft T, et al. How reliable is the diagnosis of lung cancer using small biopsy specimens? Report of a UKCCCR Lung Cancer Working Party. *Thorax*. 1993;48:1135–1139.

263. Vollmer RT. The effect of cell size on the pathologic diagnosis of small and large cell carcinomas of the lung. *Cancer*. 1982;50:1380–1383.

264. Fushimi H, Kukui M, Morino H, et al. Detection of large cell component in small cell lung carcinoma by combined cytologic and histologic examinations and its clinical implication. *Cancer*. 1992;70:599–605.

265. Nicholson SA, Beasley MB, Brambilla E, et al. Small cell lung carcinoma (SCLC): a clinicopathologic study of 100 cases with surgical specimens. *Am J Surg Pathol*. 2002;26:1184–1197.

266. D'Adda T, Pelosi G, Lagrasta C, et al. Genetic alterations in combined neuroendocrine neoplasms of the lung. *Mod Pathol*. 2008;21:414–422.

267. Facilone F, Cimmino A, Assennato G, et al. What is the prognostic significance of histomorphology in small cell lung carcinoma? *Pathologica*. 1993;85:387–393.

268. Fraire AE, Johnson EH, Yesner R, et al. Prognostic significance of histopathologic subtype and stage in small cell lung cancer. *Hum Pathol*. 1992;23:520–528.

269. Yang YJ, Steele CT, Ou XL, et al. Diagnosis of high-grade pulmonary neuroendocrine carcinoma by fine-needle aspiration biopsy: nonsmall-cell or small-cell type? *Diagn Cytopathol*. 2001;25:292–300.

270. Nicholson SA, Ryan MR. A review of cytologic findings in neuroendocrine carcinomas including carcinoid tumors with histologic correlation. *Cancer*. 2000;90:148–161.

271. Tome Y, Hirohashi S, Noguchi M, et al. Immunocytologic diagnosis of small cell lung cancer in imprint smears. *Acta Cytol*. 1991;35:485–490.

272. Gephardt GN, Grady KJ, Ahmad M, et al. Peripheral small cell undifferentiated carcinoma of the lung: clinicopathologic features of 17 cases. *Cancer*. 1988;61:1002–1008.

273. Hamzik J, Vrastyak J, Janik M, et al. Surgical treatment of small cell pulmonary carcinoma. *Rozhledy V Chir*. 1994;73:106–109.

274. Mentzer SJ, Reilly JJ, Sugarbaker DJ. Surgical resection in the management of small cell carcinoma of the lung. *Chest*. 1993;103(suppl):349S–351S.

275. Smit EF, Croen HJ, Timens W, et al. Surgical resection for small cell carcinoma of the lung: a retrospective study. *Thorax*. 1994;49:20–22.

276. Ishida T, Nishino T, Oka T, et al. Surgical treatment of patients with small cell carcinoma of the lung: a histochemical and immunohistochemical study. *J Surg Oncol*. 1989;40:188–193.

277. Shepherd FA, Ginsberg RJ, Feld R, et al. Surgical treatment for limited small-cell lung cancer: the University of Toronto Lung Oncology Group experience. *J Thorac Cardiovasc Surg*. 1991;101:385–393.

278. Shepherd FA, Ginsberg RJ, Patterson GA, et al. Is there ever a role for salvage operations in limited small cell lung cancer? *J Thorac Cardiovasc Surg*. 1991;101:196–200.

279. Bunn Jr PA, Carney DN. Overview of chemotherapy for small cell lung cancer. *Semin Oncol*. 1997;24(2 suppl 7):S69–S74.

280. Comis RL. Developments in therapy for extensive disease small cell lung cancer. *Semin Oncol*. 1992;19(6 suppl 13):45–50.

281. Marchevsky AM, Gal AA, Shah S, Koss MN. Morphometry confirms the presence of considerable nuclear size overlap between "small cells" and "large cells" in high-grade pulmonary neuroendocrine neoplasms. *Am J Clin Pathol*. 2001;116:466–472.

282. Wiatrowska BA, Krol J, Zakowski MF. Large-cell neuroendocrine carcinoma of the lung: proposed criteria for cytologic diagnosis. *Diagn Cytopathol*. 2001;24:58–64.

283. Brambilla E, Lanteujoul S, Sturm N. Divergent differentiation in neuroendocrine lung tumors. *Semin Diagn Pathol*. 2000;17:138–148.

284. Warren WH, Gould VE. Differential diagnosis of small cell neuroendocrine carcinoma of the lung. *Chest Surg Clin N Am*. 1997;7:49–63.

285. Brambilla E, Travis WD, Colby TV, et al. The new World Health Organization classification of lung tumors. *Eur Respir J*. 2001;18:1059–1068.

286. Hammar SP. Approach to the diagnosis of neuroendocrine lung neoplasms: variabilities and pitfalls. *Semin Thorac Cardiovasc Surg*. 2006;18:183–190.

287. Nandedkar MA, Palazzo J, Abbondanzo SL, et al. CD45 (leukocyte common antigen) immunoreactivity in metastatic undifferentiated and neuroendocrine carcinoma: a potential diagnostic pitfall. *Mod Pathol*. 1998;11:1204–1210.

288. Copple B, Wright SE, Moatamed F. Electron microscopy in small cell lung carcinomas: clinical correlations. *J Clin Oncol*. 1984;2:910–916.

289. Garcia-Yuste M, Matilla JM, Alvarez-Gago T, et al. Prognostic factors in neuroendocrine lung tumors: a Spanish multicenter study. Spanish Multicenter Study of neuroendocrine tumors of the lung of the Spanish Society of Pneumonology and Thoracic Surgery (EMETNE-SEPAR). *Ann Thorac Surg*. 2000;70:258–263.

290. Cooper WA, Thourani VH, Gal AA, et al. The surgical spectrum of pulmonary neuroendocrine neoplasms. *Chest*. 2001;119:14–18.

291. Huang Q, Muzitansky A, Mark EJ. Pulmonary neuroendocrine carcinomas: a review of 234 cases and a statistical analysis of 50 cases treated at one institution using a simple clinicopathologic classification. *Arch Pathol Lab Med*. 2002;126:545–553.

292. Cakir E, Demirag E, Aydin M, Unsal E. Clinicopathologic features and prognostic significance of lung tumours with mixed histologic patterns. *Acta Chir Belg*. 2009;109:489–493.

293. Hosoe S, Shigedo Y, Ueno K, et al. Detailed deletion mapping of the short arm of chromosome 3 in small cell and non-small cell carcinoma of the lung. *Lung Cancer*. 1994;20:297–305.

294. Vuitch F, Sekido Y, Fong K, et al. Neuroendocrine tumors of the lung: pathology and molecular biology. *Chest Surg Clin N Am*. 1997;7:21–47.

295. Kovatich A, Friedland DM, Druck T, et al. Molecular alterations to human chromosome 3q loci in neuroendocrine lung tumors. *Cancer*. 1998;83:1109–1117.

296. Williams CL. Basic science of small cell lung cancer. *Chest Surg Clin N Am*. 1997;7:1–19.

297. Jiang SX, Kameya T, Shoji M, et al. Large cell neuroendocrine carcinoma of the lung: a histologic and immunohistochemical study of 22 cases. *Am J Surg Pathol*. 1998;22:526–537.

298. Duncavage EJ, Le BM, Wang D, Pfeifer JD. Merkel cell polyomavirus: a specific marker for Merkel cell carcinoma in histologically similar tumors. *Am J Surg Pathol*. 2009;33:1771–1777.

299. Ralston J, Chiriboga L, Nonaka D. MASH1: a useful marker in differentiating pulmonary small cell carcinoma from Merkel cell carcinoma. *Mod Pathol*. 2008;21:1357–1362.

300. Dresler CM, Ritter JH, Patterson GA, et al. Clinical-pathologic analysis of 40 patients with large cell neuroendocrine carcinoma of the lung. *Ann Thorac Surg*. 1997;63:180–185.

301. Takei H, Asamura H, Maeshima, et al. Large cell neuroendocrine carcinoma of the lung: a clinicopathologic study of eighty-seven cases. *J Thorac Cardiovasc Surg*. 2002;124:285–292.

302. Jung KJ, Lee KS, Han J, et al. Large cell neuroendocrine carcinoma of the lung: clinical, CT, and pathologic findings in 11 patients. *J Thorac Imaging*. 2001;16:156–162.

303. Iyoda A, Hiroshima K, Toyozaki T, et al. Clinical characterization of pulmonary large-cell neuroendocrine carcinoma and large-cell carcinoma with neuroendocrine morphology. *Cancer*. 2001;91:1992–2000.

304. Demirer T, Ravits J, Aboulafia D. Myasthenic (Eaton–Lambert) syndrome associated with pulmonary large cell neuroendocrine carcinoma. *South Med J*. 1994;87:1186–1189.

305. Stanford MR, Edelstein CE, Hughes JD, et al. Paraneoplastic retinopathy in association with large cell neuroendocrine bronchial carcinoma. *Br J Ophthalmol*. 1995;79:617–618.

306. Chetty R, Bhana B, Batitang S, Govender D. Lung carcinoma composed of rhabdoid cells. *Eur J Surg Oncol*. 1997;23:432–434.

307. Khalifa M, Hruby G, Ehrlich L, et al. Combined large cell neuroendocrine carcinoma and spindle cell carcinoma of the lung. *Ann Diagn Pathol*. 2001;5:240–245.

308. Oliaro A, Filosso PL, Donati G, Ruffini E. Atypical bronchial carcinoids: review of 46 patients. *J Cardiovasc Surg*. 2000;41:131–135.

309. Franklin WA. Diagnosis of lung cancer: pathology of invasive and preinvasive neoplasia. *Chest*. 2000;117(4 suppl 1):80S–89S.

310. Rossi G, Marchioni A, Milani M, et al. TTF-1, cytokeratin 7, 34betaE12, and CD56/NCAM immunostaining in the subclassification of large cell carcinomas of the lung. *Am J Clin Pathol*. 2004;122:884–893.

311. Ullmann R, Petzmann S, Sharma A, et al. Chromosomal aberrations in a series of large-cell neuroendocrine carcinomas: unexpected divergence from small-cell carcinoma of the lung. *Hum Pathol*. 2001;32:1059–1063.

312. Hiroshima K, Abe S, Ebihara Y, et al. Cytological characteristics of pulmonary large cell neuroendocrine carcinoma. *Lung Cancer*. 2005;48:331–337.

313. Sun L, Sakurai S, Sano T, et al. High-grade neuroendocrine carcinoma of the lung: comparative clinicopathological study of large cell neuroendocrine carcinoma and small cell lung carcinoma. *Pathol Int*. 2009;59:522–529.

314. Asamura H, Kameya T, Matsuno Y, et al. Neuroendocrine neoplasms of the lung: a prognostic spectrum. *J Clin Oncol*. 2006;24:70–76.

315. Fernandez FG, Battafarano RJ. Large-cell neuroendocrine carcinoma of the lung: an aggressive neuroendocrine lung cancer. *Semin Thorac Cardiovasc Surg*. 2006;18:206–210.

316. Battafarano RJ, Fernandez FG, Ritter J, et al. Large cell neuroendocrine carcinoma: an aggressive form of non-small cell lung cancer. *J Thorac Cardiovasc Surg*. 2005;130:166–172.

317. Veronesi G, Morandi U, Alloisio M, et al. Large cell neuroendocrine carcinoma of the lung: a retrospective analysis of 144 surgical cases. *Lung Cancer*. 2006;53:111–115.

318. Shin AR, Shin BK, Choi JA, et al. Large-cell neuroendocrine carcinoma of the lung: radiologic and pathologic findings. *J Comput Assist Tomogr*. 2000;24:567–573.

319. García-Yuste M, Matilla JM, González-Aragoneses F. Neuroendocrine tumors of the lung. *Curr Opin Oncol*. 2008;20:148–154.

320. Iyoda A, Hiroshima K, Nakatani Y, Fujisawa T. Pulmonary large cell neuroendocrine carcinoma: its place in the spectrum of pulmonary carcinoma. *Ann Thorac Surg*. 2007;84:702–707.

321. Saji H, Tsuboi M, Matsubayashi J, et al. Clinical response of large cell neuroendocrine carcinoma of the lung to perioperative adjuvant chemotherapy. *Anticancer Drugs*. 2010;21:89–93.

322. Lai SL, Goldstein LJ, Gottesman MM, et al. MDR1 gene expression in lung cancer. *J Natl Cancer Inst USA*. 1989;81:1144–1150.

323. Sartori G, Cavazza A, Sgambato A, et al. EGFR and K-ras mutations along the spectrum of pulmonary epithelial tumors of the lung and elaboration of a combined clinicopathologic and molecular scoring system to predict clinical responsiveness to EGFR inhibitors. *Am J Clin Pathol*. 2009;131:478–489.

324. Faggiano A, Sabourin JC, Ducreux M, et al. Pulmonary and extrapulmonary poorly differentiated large cell neuroendocrine carcinomas: diagnostic and prognostic features. *Cancer*. 2007;110:265–274.

325. DeLellis RA, Tischler AS, Wolfe HJ. Multidirectional differentiation in neuroendocrine neoplasms. *J Histochem Cytochem*. 1984;32:899–904.

326. Gaffey MJ, Mills SE, Lack EE. Neuroendocrine carcinoma of the colon and rectum. *Am J Surg Pathol*. 1990;14:1010–1023.

327. Chejfec G, Capella C, Solcia E, et al. Amphicrine cells, dysplasias, and neoplasias. *Cancer*. 1985;56:2683–2690.

328. Eusebi V, Capella C, Bondi A, et al. Endocrine-paracrine cells in pancreatic exocrine carcinomas. *Histopathology*. 1981;9:599–613.

329. Groben P, Reddick R, Askin FB. The pathologic spectrum of small cell carcinoma of the cervix. *Int J Gynecol Pathol*. 1985;4:42–47.

330. Hales M, Rosenau W, Okerlund MD, Galante M. Carcinoma of the thyroid with a mixed medullary and follicular pattern. *Cancer*. 1982;50:1352–1359.

331. Lewin K. Carcinoid tumors and the mixed (composite) glandular-endocrine cell carcinomas. *Am J Surg Pathol*. 1987;11(suppl 1):71–76.

332. Manivel JC, Wick MR, Sibley RK. Neuroendocrine differentiation in Mullerian neoplasms. *Am J Clin Pathol*. 1986;86:438–443.

333. McCluggage WG, Napier SS, Primrose WJ, et al. Sinonasal neuroendocrine carcinoma exhibiting amphicrine differentiation. *Histopathology*. 1995;27:79–82.

334. Mills SE, Wolfe JT, Weiss MA, et al. Small cell undifferentiated carcinoma of the urinary bladder. *Am J Surg Pathol*. 1987;11:606–617.

335. Reid JD, Yuh SL, Petrelli M, Jaffe R. Ductoinsular tumors of the pancreas. *Cancer*. 1982;49:908–915.

336. Silva EG, Mackay B, Goepfert H, et al. Endocrine carcinoma of the skin (Merkel cell carcinoma). *Pathol Annu*. 1984;19(1):1–30.

337. Brambilla E, Lanteujoul S, Sturm N. Divergent differentiation in neuroendocrine lung tumors. *Semin Diagn Pathol*. 2000;17:138–148.

338. Sen F, Borczuk AC. Combined carcinoid tumor of the lung: a combination of carcinoid and adenocarcinoma. *Lung Cancer*. 1998;21:53–58.

339. Frank GA, Trakhtenberg AK, Boguslavskii VM. The prognosis of small cell carcinoma and malignant carcinoid of the lung. *Vopr Onkol*. 1989;35:192–198.

340. Mooi WJ, Dewar A, Springall D, et al. Non-small cell lung carcinomas with neuroendocrine features: a light microscopic, immunohisto-chemical, and ultrastructural study of 11 cases. *Histopathology*. 1988;13:329–337.

341. Otto WR. Lung stem cells. *Int J Exp Pathol*. 1997;78:291–310.

342. Huang J, Behrens C, Wistuba II, et al. Clonality of combined tumors. *Arch Pathol Lab Med*. 2002;126:437–441.

343. Cakir E, Demirag E, Aydin M, Unsal E. Clinicopathologic features and prognostic significance of lung tumours with mixed histologic patterns. *Acta Chir Belg*. 2009;109:489–493.

344. Piehl MR, Gould VE, Warren WH, et al. Immunohistochemical identification of exocrine and neuroendocrine subsets of large cell lung carcinomas. *Pathol Res Pract*. 1988;183:675–682.

345. Neal MH, Kosinski R, Cohen P, et al. Atypical endocrine tumors of the lung: a histologic, ultrastructural, and clinical study of 19 cases. *Hum Pathol*. 1986;17:1264–1277.

346. Visscher DW, Zarbo RJ, Trojanowski JQ, et al. Neuroendocrine differentiation in poorly differentiated lung carcinomas: a light microscopic and immunologic study. *Mod Pathol*. 1990;3:508–512.

347. Skov BG, Sorenson JB, Hirsch FR, et al. Prognostic impact of histologic demonstration chromogranin A and neuron specific enolase in pulmonary adenocarcinoma. *Ann Oncol*. 1991;2:355–360.

348. Linnoila RI, Gazdar AF. Non-small cell lung carcinoma with neuroendocrine features. *Anat Pathol*. 1990;18:1–5.

349. Linnoila RI, Mulshine JL, Steinberg SM, et al. Neuroendocrine differentiation in endocrine and nonendocrine lung carcinomas. *Am J Clin Pathol*. 1988;90:641–652.

350. Hammond ME, Sause WT. Large cell neuroendocrine tumors of the lung: clinical significance and histopathologic definition. *Cancer*. 1985;56:1624–1629.

351. Berendsen HH, Deleij L, Poppema S. Clinical characterization of non-small cell lung cancer tumors showing neuroendocrine differentiation features. *J Clin Oncol*. 1989;7:1614–1629.

352. Hiroshima K, Iyoda A, Shibuya K, et al. Prognostic significance of neuroendocrine differentiation in adenocarcinoma of the lung. *Ann Thorac Surg*. 2002;73:1732–1735.

353. Carnaghi C, Rimassa L, Garassino I, Santoro A. Clinical significance of neuroendocrine phenotype in non-small-cell lung cancer. *Ann Oncol*. 2001;12(suppl 2):S119–S123.

354. Baldi A, Groger AM, Esposito V, et al. Neuroendocrine differentiation in non-small-cell lung carcinomas. *In Vivo*. 2000;14:109–114.

355. Fresvig A, Qvigstad G, Halvorsen TB, et al. Neuroendocrine differentiation in bronchial carcinomas of classic squamous cell type: an immunohistochemical study of 29 cases applying the tyramide signal amplification technique. *Appl Immunohistochem Mol Morphol*. 2001;9:9–13.

356. Churg A. The fine structure of large cell undifferentiated carcinoma of the lung: evidence for its relation to squamous cell carcinomas and adenocarcinomas. *Hum Pathol*. 1978;9:143–156.

357. Baldi A, Groger AM, Esposito Y, et al. Neuroendocrine differentiation in non-small cell lung carcinomas. *In Vivo*. 2000;14:109–114.

358. Nakatani Y, Kitamura H, Inayama Y, et al. Pulmonary adenocarcinoma of the fetal lung type: a clinicopathologic study indicating differences in histology, epidemiology, and natural history of low-grade and high-grade forms. *Am J Surg Pathol*. 1998;22:399–411.

359. Chetritt J, Fiche M, Cassagnau E, et al. Pulmonary endodermal tumor resembling fetal lung: low grade adenocarcinoma of the fetal lung type. *Ann Pathol*. 1999;19:116–118.

360. Abbona G, Papotti M, Viberti L, et al. Chromogranin A gene expression in non-small cell lung carcinomas. *J Pathol*. 1998;186:151–156.

361. Sørhaug S, Steinshamn S, Haaverstad R, et al. Expression of neuroendocrine markers in non-small cell lung cancer. *APMIS*. 2007;115:152–163.

362. Leong ASY, Wick MR, Swanson PE. *Immunohistology and Electron Microscopy of Anaplastic and Pleomorphic Tumors*. Cambridge, UK: Cambridge University Press; 1997:161–208.

363. Graziano SL, Mazid R, Newman N, et al. The use of neuroendocrine immunoperoxidase markers to predict chemotherapy response in patients with non-small-cell lung cancer. *J Clin Oncol*. 1989;7:1398–1406.

364. Hainsworth JD, Johnson DH, Greco FA. Poorly-differentiated neuroendocrine carcinoma of unknown primary site: a newly recognized clinicopathologic entity. *Ann Intern Med*. 1988;109:364–371.

365. Hainsworth JD, Wright EP, Johnson DH, et al. Poorly differentiated carcinoma of unknown primary site: clinical usefulness of immunoperoxidase staining. *J Clin Oncol*. 1991;9:1931–1938.

366. Schleusener J, Tazelaar H, Jung S. Neuroendocrine differentiation correlates with survival in chemotherapy treated non-small cell lung cancer [abstract]. *Lab Invest*. 1995;72:153A.

367. Wertzel H, Grahmann PR, Bansbach S, et al. Results after surgery in undifferentiated large cell carcinoma of the lung: the role of neuroendocrine expression. *Eur J Cardiothorac Surg*. 1997;12:698–702.

368. Segawa Y, Takata S, Fujii M, et al. Immunohistochemical detection of neuroendocrine differentiation in non-small-cell lung cancer and its clinical implications. *J Cancer Res Clin Oncol*. 2009;135:1055–1059.

369. Sterlacci W, Fiegl M, Hilbe W, et al. Clinical relevance of neuroendocrine differentiation in non-small cell lung cancer assessed by immunohistochemistry: a retrospective study on 405 surgically resected cases. *Virchows Arch*. 2009;455:125–132.

370. Lack EE. *Pathology of Adrenal and Extraadrenal Paraganglia*. Philadelphia: WB Saunders; 1994:1–350.

371. Goodman ML, Laforet EG. Solitary primary chemodectomas of the lung. *Chest*. 1972;61:48–60.

372. Siingh G, Lee RE, Brooks DH. Primary pulmonary paraganglioma: report of a case and review of the literature. *Cancer*. 1977;40:2286–2289.

373. DeLuise VP, Holman CW, Gray GF. Primary pulmonary paraganglioma. *N Y State J Med*. 1977;77:2270–2271.

374. Hangartner JR, Loosemore TM, Burke M, Pepper JR. Malignant primary pulmonary paraganglioma. *Thorax*. 1989;44:154–156.

375. Dusseldorf M, Straaten HG. Primary pulmonary paraganglioma. *Zentralbl Chir*. 1990;115:1575–1578.

376. Lemonick DM, Pai PB, Hines GL. Malignant primary pulmonary paraganglioma with hilar metastasis. *J Thorac Cardiovasc Surg*. 1990;99:563–564.

377. Vuorela AL, Anttinen J. Primary chemodectoma of the lung. *Am J Roentgenol*. 1993;161:1111–1112.

378. Hagemeyer O, Gabius HJ, Kayser K. Paraganglioma of the lung—developed after exposure to nuclear radiation by the Tschernobyl atomic reactor accident? *Respiration*. 1994;61:236–239.

379. Skodt V, Jacobsen GK, Helsted M. Primary paraganglioma of the lung: report of two cases and review of the literature. *APMIS*. 1995;103:597–603.

380. Saeki T, Akiba T, Joh K, et al. An extremely large solitary primary paraganglioma of the lung: report of a case. *Surg Today*. 1999;29:1195–1200.

381. Sattar HA, Yang DL, Husain AN, et al. Multiple paragangliomata of the lungs and temporal bone. *Ear Nose Throat J*. 2008;87:E4–E6.

382. Rossel M, Pasini A, Chappuis S, et al. Distinct biological properties of two RET isoforms activated by MEN2A and MEN2B mutations. *Oncogene*. 1997;14:265–275.

383. Hironaka M, Fukayama M, Takayashiki N, et al. Pulmonary gangliocytic paraganglioma: case report and comparative immunohistochemical study of related neuroendocrine neoplasms. *Am J Surg Pathol*. 2001;25:688–693.

384. Linnoila RI, Keiser HR, Steinberg SM, Lack EE. Histopathology of benign versus malignant sympathoadrenal paragangliomas: clinicopathologic study of 120 cases including unusual histologic features. *Hum Pathol*. 1990;21:1168–1180.

385. Engzell V, Franzen S, Zajicek J. Aspiration biopsy of tumors of the neck. II. Cytologic findings in 13 cases of carotid body tumors. *Acta Cytol*. 1971;15:25–30.

386. Gonzalez-Campora R, Otal-Salaverri C, Panea-Flores P, et al. Fine needle aspiration cytology of paraganglionic tumors. *Acta Cytol*. 1988;32:386–390.

387. Hood IC, Qizilbash AH, Young JEH, Archibald SD. Fine needle aspiration biopsy cytology of paragangliomas. *Acta Cytol*. 1983;27:651–657.

388. Fournel P, Boucheron S, Baril A, et al. Intrapulmonary chemodectoma: a new case with ultrastructural study. *Rev Pneumonol Clin*. 1986;42:250–253.

389. Trojanowski JQ. Neurofilament and glial filament proteins. In: Wick MR, Siegal GP, eds. *Monoclonal Antibodies in Diagnostic Immunohistochemistry*. New York: Marcel Dekker; 1988:115–146.

390. Gaffey MJ, Mills SE, Askin FB. Minute pulmonary meningothelial-like nodules: a clinicopathologic study of so-called minute pulmonary chemodectoma. *Am J Surg Pathol*. 1988;12:167–175.

391. Niho S, Yokose T, Nishiwaki Y, Mukai K. Immunohistochemical and clonal analysis of minute pulmonary meningothelial-like nodules. *Hum Pathol*. 1999;30:425–429.

392. Helman LJ, Cohen PS, Averbuch SD, et al. Neuropeptide Y distinguishes benign from malignant pheochromocytoma. *J Clin Oncol*. 1989;7:720–725.

393. Schroder HD, Johannsen L. Demonstration of S100 protein in sustentacular cells of pheochromocytomas and paragangliomas. *Histopathology*. 1986;10:1023–1033.

394. Gonzalez-Campora R, Diaz-Cano S, Lerma-Puertas E, et al. Paragangliomas: static cytometric studies of nuclear DNA patterns. *Cancer*. 1993;71:820–824.

395. Pang LC, Tsao KC. Flow cytometric DNA analysis for the determination of malignant potential in adrenal and extra-adrenal pheochromocytomas or paragangliomas. *Arch Pathol Lab Med*. 1993;117:1142–1147.

396. Imamura F, Funakoshi T, Nakamura S, et al. Primary primitive neuroectodermal tumor of the lung: report of two cases. *Lung Cancer*. 2000;27:55–60.

397. Mikami Y, Nakajima M, Hashimoto H, et al. Primary pulmonary primitive neuroectodermal tumor (PNET): a case report. *Pathol Res Pract*. 2001;197:113–119.

398. Verfaillie G, Hoorens A, Lamote J. Primary primitive neuroectodermal tumour of the lung. *Acta Chir Belg*. 2009;109:381–384.

399. Suárez Antelo J, Rodríguez García C, Montero Martínez C, Verea Hernando H. Pulmonary Ewing sarcoma/primitive neuroectodermal tumor: a case report and a review of the literature. *Arch Bronconeumol*. 2010;46:44–46.

400. Lee YY, Kim do H, Lee JH, et al. Primary pulmonary Ewing's sarcoma/primitive neuroectodermal tumor in a 67-year-old man. *J Korean Med Sci*. 2007;22(suppl):S159–S163.

401. Takahashi D, Nagayama J, Nagatoshi Y, et al. Primary Ewing's sarcoma family tumors of the lung a case report and review of the literature. *Jpn J Clin Oncol*. 2007;37:874–877.

402. Rossi S, Orvieto E, Furlanetto A, et al. Utility of the immunohistochemical detection of FLI-1 expression in round cell and vascular neoplasm using a monoclonal antibody. *Mod Pathol*. 2004;17:547–552.

403. Llombart-Bosch A, Machado I, Navarro S, et al. Histological heterogeneity of Ewing's sarcoma/PNET: an immunohistochemical analysis of 415 genetically confirmed cases with clinical support. *Virchows Arch*. 2009;455:397–411.

404. Jambhekar NA, Bagwan IN, Ghule P, et al. Comparative analysis of routine histology, immunohistochemistry, reverse transcriptase polymerase chain reaction, and fluorescence in situ hybridization in diagnosis of Ewing family of tumors. *Arch Pathol Lab Med*. 2006;130:1813–1818.

405. Jaffe N. Neuroblastoma: review of the literature and an examination of factors contributing to its enigmatic character. *Cancer Treat Rev*. 1976;3:61–82.

406. Young Jr JL, Miller RW. Incidence of malignant tumors in children. *J Pediatr*. 1975;86:254–258.

407. Kilton LJ, Aschenbrener C, Burns CP. Ganglioneuroblastoma in adults. *Cancer*. 1976;37:974–983.

408. Nagashima Y, Miyagi Y, Tanaka Y, et al. Adult ganglioneuroblastoma of the anterior mediastinum. *Pathol Res Pract*. 1997;193:727–732.

409. Cooney TP. Primary pulmonary ganglioneuroblastoma in an adult: maturation, involution, and the immune response. *Histopathology*. 1981;5:451–463.

410. Hochholzer L, Moran CA, Koss MN. Primary pulmonary ganglioneuroblastoma: a clinicopathologic and immunohistochemical study of two cases. *Ann Diagn Pathol*. 1998;2:154–158.

411. Kaplan SJ, Holbrook CT, McDaniel HG, et al. Vasoactive intestinal peptide secreting tumors of childhood. *Am J Dis Childhood*. 1980;134:21–24.

412. Kenny FM, Stavrides A, Voorhess ML, Klein R. Cushing's syndrome associated with adrenal neuroblastoma. *Am J Dis Childhood*. 1967;113:611–615.

413. Ikuno N, Shimokawa I, Nakamura T, et al. RET oncogene expression correlates with neuronal differentiation of neuroblastic tumors. *Pathol Res Pract*. 1995;191:92–99.

414. Dehner LP. Pathologic anatomy of classic neuroblastoma, including prognostic factors and differential diagnosis. In: Pochedly C, ed. *Neuroblastoma: Tumor Biology and Therapy*. Boca Raton: CRC Press; 1990:111–143.

415. Hughes M, Marsden HB, Palmer MK. Histologic patterns of neuroblastoma related to prognosis and clinical stage. *Cancer*. 1974;34:1706–1711.

416. Makinen J. Microscopic patterns as a guide to prognosis of neuroblastomas in childhood. *Cancer*. 1972;29:1637–1646.

417. McLaughlin JE, Urich H. Maturing neuroblastoma and ganglioneuroblastoma: a study of four cases with long survival. *J Pathol*. 1977;121:19–26.

418. Shimada H, Chatten J, Newton Jr WA, et al. Histopathologic prognostic factors in neuroblastic tumors. *J Natl Cancer Inst*. 1984;73:405–416.

419. Abramowsky CR, Katzenstein HM, Alvarado CS, Shehata BM. Anaplastic large cell neuroblastoma. *Pediatr Dev Pathol*. 2009;12:1–5.

420. Hicks MJ, Mackay B. Comparison of ultrastructural features among neuroblastic tumors: maturation from neuroblastoma to ganglioneuroma. *Ultrastruct Pathol*. 1995;19:311–322.

421. Molenaar WM, Baker DL, Pleasure D, et al. The neuroendocrine and neural profiles of neuroblastomas, ganglioneuroblastomas, and ganglioneuromas. *Am J Pathol*. 1990;136:375–382.

422. Crary GS, Singleton TP, Neglia JP, et al. Detection of metastatic neuroblastoma in bone marrow biopsy specimens with an antibody to neuron-specific enolase. *Mod Pathol*. 1992;5:308–314.

423. Miettinen M, Chatten J, Paetau A, Stevenson A. Monoclonal antibody NB84 in the differential diagnosis of neuroblastoma and other small round cell tumors. *Am J Surg Pathol*. 1998;22:327–332.

424. Cozzutto C, Carbone A. Pleomorphic (anaplastic) neuroblastoma. *Arch Pathol Lab Med*. 1988;112:621–625.

425. Berthold F, Trechow R, Utsch S, Zieschang J. Prognostic factors in metastatic neuroblastoma: a multivariate analysis of 182 cases. *Am J Pediatr Hematol Oncol*. 1992;14:207–215.

426. Joshi VV, Chatten J, Sather HN, Shimada H. Evaluation of the Shimada classification in advanced neuroblastoma with a special reference to the mitosis-karyorrhexis index. *Mod Pathol*. 1991;4:139–147.

427. Coldman AJ, Fryer CJH, Elwood JM, Sonley MJ. Neuroblastoma: influence of age at diagnosis, stage, tumor site, and sex on prognosis. *Cancer*. 1980;46:1896–1901.

428. Gitlow SE, Dziedzic LB, Strauss L, et al. Biochemical and histologic determinants in the prognosis of neuroblastoma. *Cancer*. 1973;32:898–905.

429. Kogner P, Borgstrom P, Bjellerup P, et al. Somatostatin in neuroblastoma and ganglioneuroma. *Eur J Cancer*. 1997;33:2084–2089.

430. Hayashi Y, Kanda N, Inaba T, et al. Cytogenetic findings and prognosis in neuroblastoma with emphasis on marker chromosome 1. *Cancer*. 1989;63:126–132.

431. Berthold F, Sahin K, Hero B, et al. The current contribution of molecular factors to risk estimation in neuroblastoma patients. *Eur J Cancer*. 1997;33:2092–2097.

432. Brodeur GM, Seeger RC, Sather H, et al. Clinical implications of oncogene activation in human neuroblastomas. *Cancer*. 1986;58:541–545.

433. Hashimoto H, Daimaru Y, Enjoji M, Nakagawara A. N-myc gene product expression in neuroblastoma. *J Clin Pathol*. 1989;42:52–55.

434. Kramer K, Cheung NK, Gerald WL, et al. Correlation of myc-N amplification, Trk-A and CD44 expression with clinical stage in 250 patients with neuroblastoma. *Eur J Cancer*. 1997;33:2098–2100.

435. Ikuno N, Shimokawa I, Nakamura T, et al. RET oncogene expression correlates with neuronal differentiation of neuroblastic tumors. *Pathol Res Pract*. 1995;191:92–99.

436. Graham D, Magee H, Kierce B, et al. Evaluation of Ki-67 reactivity in neuroblastoma using paraffin-embedded tissue. *Pathol Res Pract*. 1995;191:87–91.

13

Sarcomas and Sarcomatoid Neoplasms of the Lungs and Pleural Surfaces

Mark R. Wick, MD, Timothy C. Allen, MD, JD, Kevin O. Leslie, MD, and Mark H. Stoler, MD

Primary malignant pleuropulmonary tumors showing sarcomatoid features are exceedingly uncommon. Overwhelmingly, such lesions are typically epithelial in nature; neoplasms with a mesenchymal lineage in the lung and pleura are most often proven to be secondary, emanating from deep soft tissue sites or the female genital tract. In fact, because of the rarity of this category of pleuropulmonary malignancies, relatively few data exist in the literature regarding the morphologic or clinical details of such lesions. Hence, one can correctly anticipate that most pulmonologists, oncologists, radiologists, and pathologists are unfamiliar with intrathoracic tumors composed of spindled and pleomorphic cells.

This chapter summarizes the clinicopathologic information pertaining to such lesions. It devotes exclusive attention to malignant lesions; benign mesenchymal neoplasms of the lung and pleura are discussed in Chapter 19. Pseudotumors are likewise considered in another portion of this book. Nevertheless, those pathologic categories and other lesions will indeed be mentioned here in the context of differential diagnosis. The entities that are discussed are arranged in order of frequency, to give the reader a sense of their relative incidences.

Sarcomatoid Carcinoma of the Lung

Recent changes in the classification of lung tumors have included sarcoma-like tumors. Five subtypes of those lesions are now codified; pleomorphic carcinoma, spindle cell carcinoma, giant cell carcinoma, carcinosarcoma, and pulmonary blastoma are predicated on the particulars of their microscopic appearances.[1,2] We consider all of these neoplasms to be part of the same tumor family, that of sarcomatoid carcinomas (SCs), as discussed in more detail subsequently. Although SCs are rare in an absolute sense, they represent the most common mesenchymal-like malignancies of the airways.[3,4] True sarcomas are very infrequently seen in the tracheobronchial tree.[4–13] Therefore, one usually considers a cytologically atypical spindle cell tumor of the lung to be an SC unless thorough immunohistological and ultrastructural studies indicate otherwise.[5] This review will discuss neoplasms in this general category, using information taken from the pertinent literature as well as the personal experience of the authors.

Historical and Terminologic Considerations

Controversy has existed for some time concerning the mechanisms through which obvious foci of carcinoma of the lung are admixed with malignant but nondescript spindle cell elements or tissues with a "committed" sarcomatous differentiation pattern. Also, purely spindle cell and pleomorphic pulmonary carcinomas are recognized nosologically but are incompletely characterized at a molecular level.

Over time, morphologically similar tumors have been given a variety of designations in the upper and lower respiratory tracts. These diagnostic terms have included *blastoma, sarcomatoid carcinoma, spindle cell carcinoma, squamous cell carcinoma with pseudosarcomatous stroma, pseudosarcoma,* and *carcinosarcoma,* based largely on the specific microscopic attributes of the lesions in question and the conceptual leanings of the authors describing them.[14-43]

More than 70 years ago, Saphir and Vass[44] assessed the literature then extant on carcinosarcomas and concluded that they represented primary epithelial malignancies that had undergone divergent differentiation (tumor metaplasia). Their paper cited several lesions of the lung. Thereafter, opposing publications on histogenesis espoused the opinion that biphasic neoplasms of the airways were "collision" tumors, or that they reflected the proliferation of non-neoplastic mesenchymal tissue components that were induced by the carcinomatous elements.[45-47] At the turn of the last century, Krompecher[48] and others[49] had held to the same theories as those of Saphir and Vass. In the past two decades, results of studies using electron microscopy, immunohistology, and "molecular" assays of clonality have tended to support the latter foresighted views of those pioneers convincingly. Hence, it is believed currently that blastomas, carcinosarcomas, carcinomas with pseudosarcomatous stroma, and SCs comprise a single morphological spectrum of basically epithelial tumors, regardless of their anatomic locations.[34-36] *Biphasic sarcomatoid carcinoma* and *monophasic sarcomatoid carcinoma* have been proposed as replacements for the former designations of carcinosarcoma and spindle cell carcinoma, respectively.[33,34,37] In the penultimate iteration of the World Health Organization nosologic scheme, such lesions were included in the category designated "carcinoma with pleomorphic, sarcomatoid, or sarcomatous elements."[36]

Clinicopathologic Features of Pulmonary Sarcomatoid Carcinomas

Clinical Attributes

SCs arise in the large bronchi and peripheral lung fields much more often than in the trachea, although the authors have indeed seen some lesions that originated above the carina. The majority of individuals with pulmonary SC are men, and most have a history of heavy smoking.[14,23,24] The average patient is 60 years of age.[33] Clinical signs and symptoms produced by these tumors are directly associated with the tumor's specific location. Endoluminal lesions in large tubular airways characteristically cause refractory or recurrent pneumonia in the corresponding distal parenchyma, or they are associated with progressive dyspnea, cough, hemoptysis, and audible expiratory rhonchi over the affected lung field.[14-17,23,45-47,50,51] In contrast, SC in the peripheral lung often manifests no symptoms or, alternatively, leads to chest pain caused by invasion of the pleura and extrapulmonary soft tissue.[23] As might be expected, central endobronchial tumors are smaller than peripheral SCs; their average sizes are 6 cm and greater than 10 cm, respectively[46,52] (Fig. 14-1).

Despite their anaplastic nature, SCs of the lung are surgically resectable in roughly 90% of cases,[23,33] and approximately one half of patients with such neoplasms present with stage I disease. Paradoxically, however, the prognosis of pulmonary SC is still dismal. Overall 5-year survival is 20%, with a slightly better figure being associated with small, central endobronchial lesions.[23,33,52] Metastatic SC of the lung involves the same organ sites that are affected by more usual forms of lung cancer: namely, the opposite lung, liver, bones, adrenal glands, and brain.[46,51] The metastases may exhibit either carcinomatous or sarcoma-like histologic configurations, or both.[46] Adjuvant radiation treatment and chemotherapy have been used in many cases of pulmonary SC, but these measures have provided little benefit in general.[14,33,38]

Macroscopic Features

Grossly, the lesions of pulmonary SC that are greater than 5 cm in size tend to exhibit central necrosis and hemorrhage, and they also demonstrate irregular permeation of the surrounding lung parenchyma[33,34] (Fig. 14-2). Tumors that are smaller and located within bronchial confines often exhibit a polypoid appearance and are attached to the subjacent mucosa by a relatively narrow stalk of tissue.[52] SCs in the peripheral lung parenchyma may have the gross appearance of conventional adenocarcinomas.[34]

Histologic Characteristics

Biphasic SCs of the lung can be divided into two subgroups, based on the nature of the stromal elements in each lesion. These variants may be called homologous and heterologous SCs.

Homologous Biphasic Sarcomatoid Carcinoma
Variants of SC that are also called spindle cell carcinomas are constituted microscopically by a predominance of nondescript spindled and pleomorphic cells, admixed with a minor, obviously carcinomatous, component. The latter portion of such lesions is generally

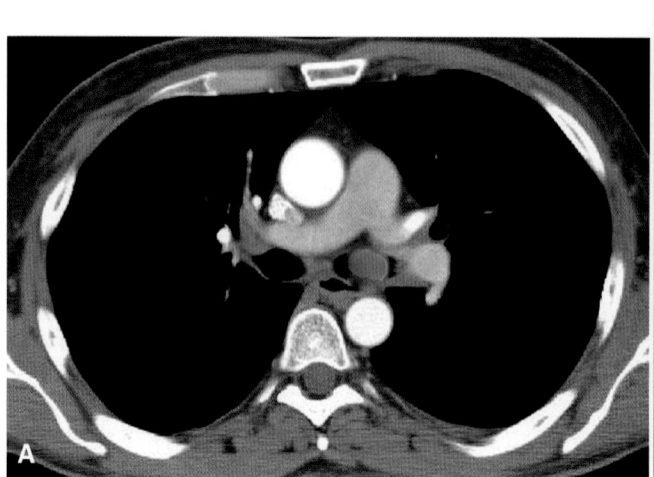
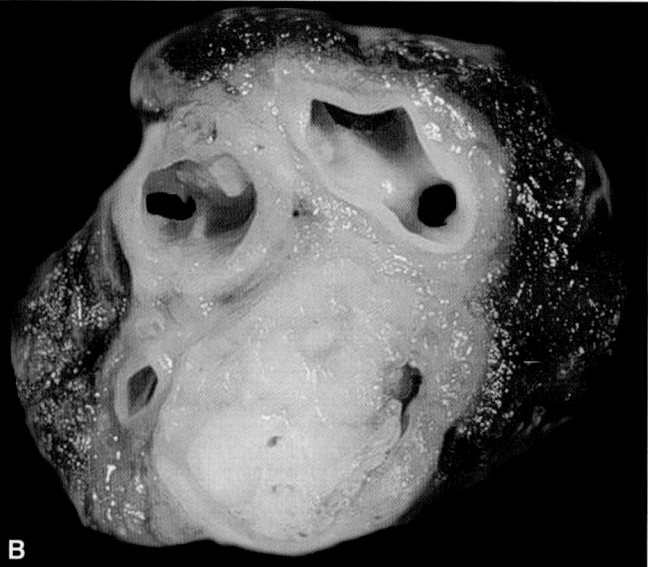

Figure 14-1. A, Computed tomogram showing an endobronchial mass in the left mainstem bronchus. **B,** Resection of the lung demonstrated an endoluminal neoplasm that proved to be a sarcomatoid carcinoma.

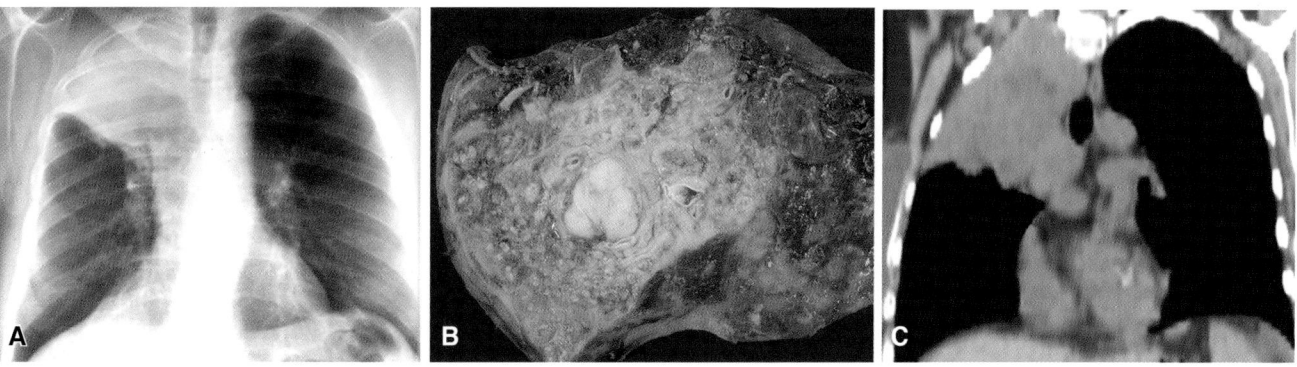

Figure 14-2. Peripheral sarcomatoid carcinoma of the right lung, as seen in a plain chest film (**A**) and in a lobectomy specimen (**B**). A reconstructed computed tomography image (**C**) demonstrates a Pancoast tumor.

inconspicuous and variably distributed; in roughly 40% of cases, such foci are very rare and require extensive sampling to document their presence. The general appearance of the carcinomatous elements is that of a well- to moderately differentiated squamous malignancy in most instances, whereas adenosquamous, adenocarcinomatous, large cell undifferentiated, or neuroendocrine carcinoma is seen in a minority of cases[14,53-56] (Fig. 14-3). Rare examples of this tumor type show mixtures of several carcinoma morphotypes.[54] Zones of transition between epithelial and sarcoma-like components are usually evident, at least focally.

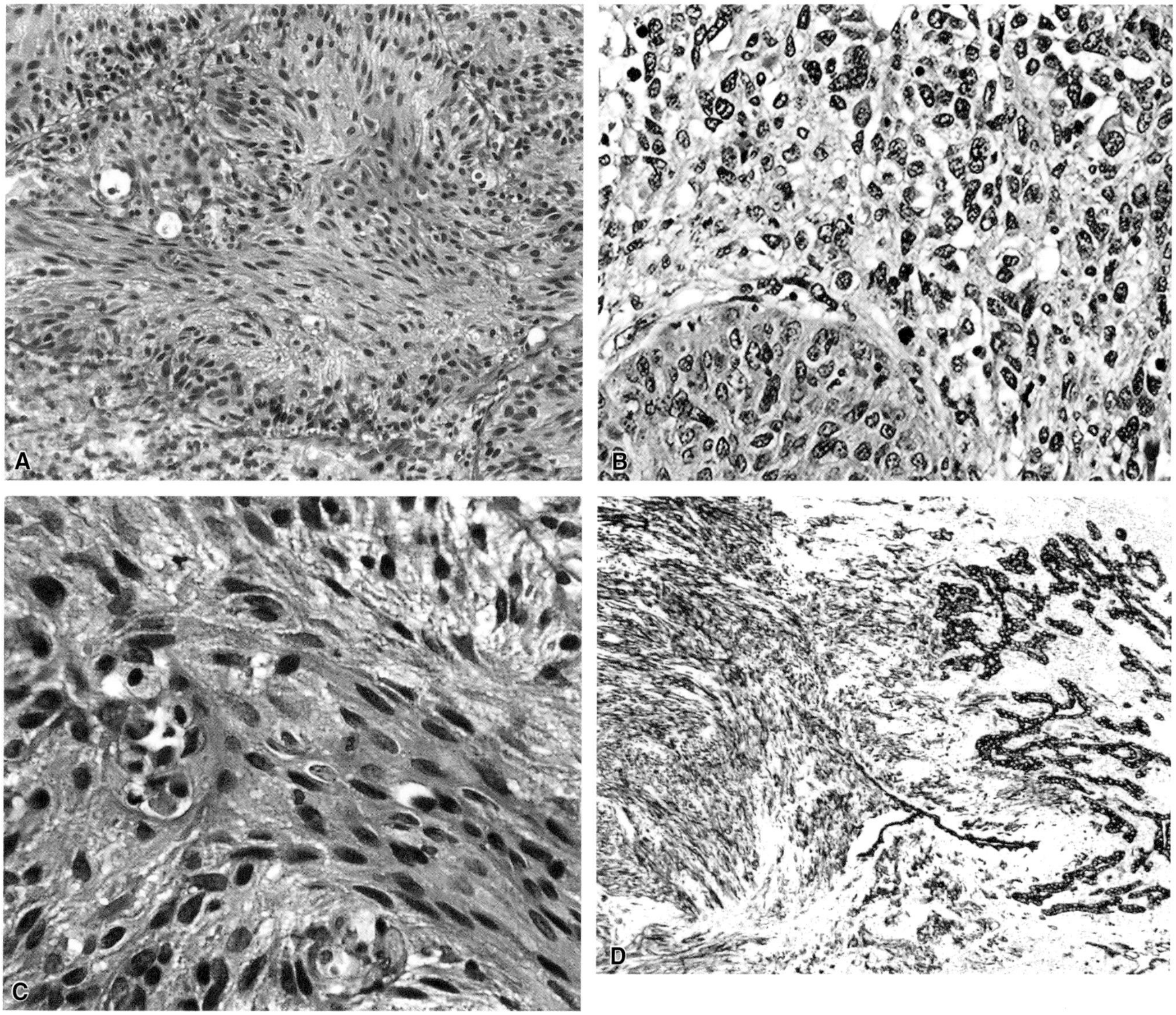

Figure 14-3. **A** to **C,** Homologous biphasic sarcomatoid carcinoma of the lung, showing overtly epithelial growth apposed to sarcoma-like pleomorphic elements. **D,** An immunostain for keratin demonstrates reactivity in both neoplastic components. Cytokeratin expression can be highly variable, with some tumors expressing only scant cytokeratin immunoreactivity.

The sarcomatoid elements of this subtype of SC lack specialized differentiation into identifiable myogenic, chondro-osseous, or vasoformative tissues by standard light microscopy, and, as such, are homologous (organ-appropriate) to the lung. They are composed of markedly heterogeneous cells with nuclear atypia and variable growth patterns. The corresponding microscopic images range from those of fibromatosis-like or low-grade fibrosarcoma-like areas, with relatively bland nuclear features, sparse mitoses, moderate-to-rich matrical collagen deposition, and a "herringbone" pattern, to others in which pleomorphic giant cells are mixed with fusiform elements showing dense cellularity, coarse chromatin, prominent nucleoli, and numerous mitoses[14–16,23,33,45] (Fig. 14-4). The last of these descriptions is closely similar to that attending spindle cell–pleomorphic malignant fibrous histiocytoma (MFH) of the soft tissues.[54] Neoplastic spindle cells often infiltrate the submucosa of small- and medium-sized bronchi, which nonetheless tend to retain their mural cartilage plates and mucosal integrity.[33,34]

Sarcoma-like elements in some biphasic spindle cell carcinomas may include cytologically bland, osteoclast-like giant cells[52,57,58] (Fig. 14-5). The latter are admixed with atypical fusiform cells or more uniform polygonal tumor cells. Another variant histologic pattern is that in which bluntly fusiform tumor cells surround discrete zones of necrosis, producing a necrotizing granuloma-like image. Rare examples of SC may demonstrate extravasated erythrocytes between relatively bland spindled tumor cells, simulating the characteristics of Kaposi sarcoma (KS) or even nodular fasciitis.[33]

Heterologous Biphasic Sarcomatoid Carcinoma
Other biphasic sarcomatoid neoplasms differ from the descriptions just given, in regard to their content of focal myogenous, vasogenic, chondro-osseous, or lipogenic differentiation.[59] Thus, they are analogous to the heterologous form of malignant mixed müllerian tumors of the uterus, ovaries, and other female genital sites.[60,61] Those neoplasms may exhibit microscopic foci that simulate embryonal or adult-type pleomorphic rhabdomyosarcoma, which contain proliferations of closely apposed compact round cells with a slightly myxoid background, or large "strap" cells with cytoplasmic eosinophilia and cross-striations, respectively[14–16,33,34,46,52] (Fig. 14-6). Other heterologous SCs contain components that closely imitate the histologic features of osteosarcoma or chondrosarcoma.[23,34] In light of this information, it is easy to understand why lesions with such microscopic features were believed to be carcinosarcomas in the past and are still so designated by some observers today. The obviously carcinomatous elements in these lesions usually take the form of squamous carcinoma, but lesions with glandular or neuroendocrine differentiation have also been reported.[14,54,55] Transitional zones between obvious epithelial foci, nondescript sarcomatoid areas, and myosarcoma-like components are often evident.

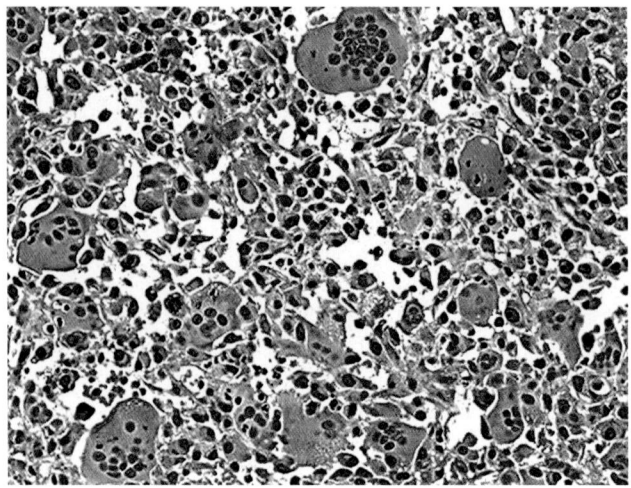

Figure 14-5. Osteoclast-like giant cells may be identified in sarcomatoid lung carcinoma.

With regard to the relationship between biologic behavior and histologic appearance, there is no difference in the clinical evolution of homologous and heterologous biphasic pulmonary SCs. A distinction is made between those lesions only to reflect their synonymity with sarcomatoid epithelial tumors in other body sites.[60,61]

Monophasic Sarcomatoid Carcinomas
Some SCs display no conventional light microscopic evidence of epithelial differentiation whatsoever. A carcinomatous nature for these neoplasms is discerned only after immunohistochemical or ultrastructural evaluations have been done, but it is usually suspected beforehand because of the clinical and gross characteristics of the lesions.[33]

Most tumors in this category are constituted exclusively of cell populations like those in the sarcoma-like components of biphasic SCs. These potentially include foci that have an unremarkable spindle cell or pleomorphic image (Fig. 14-7) as well as areas imitating rhabdomyosarcoma, osteosarcoma, or other morphologic appearances that do not correspond to native tissues in the non-neoplastic lung. Because of the monomorphic nature of the tumor variants under discussion here, which lack any attributes of conventional lung carcinomas histologically, the corresponding diagnosis suggested by the World Health Organization criteria for pulmonary neoplasms[62] (based only on hematoxylin and eosin stains and conventional histologic examination) would be that of a primary pulmonary sarcoma. The latter point has made the existence of monophasic SC of the lung somewhat

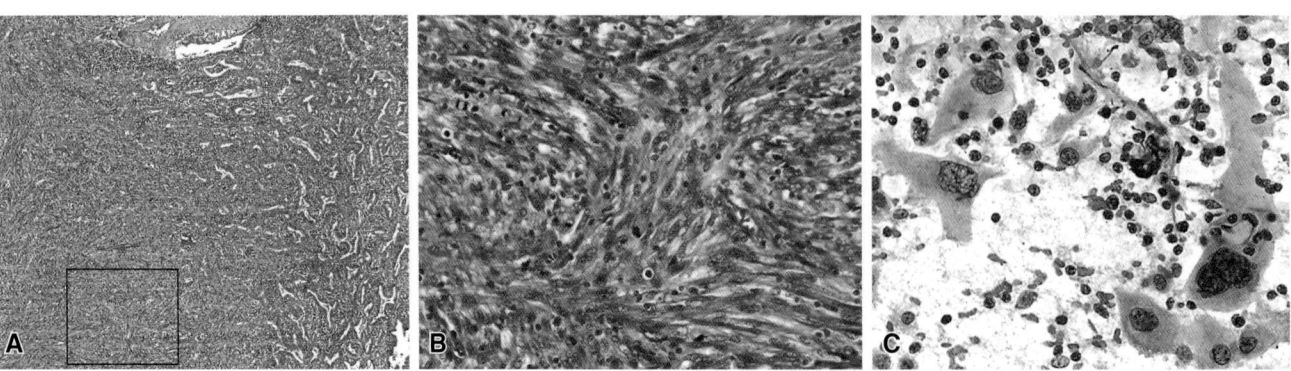

Figure 14-4. Sarcomatoid carcinoma of the lung simulating malignant fibrous histiocytoma (**A**) with storiform growth of neoplastic fusiform and pleomorphic cells (**B**; *boxed area* in part **A**). **C**, Fine needle aspiration biopsy of sarcomatoid carcinoma showing dyshesive and pleomorphic malignant cells, such as those seen in true sarcomas.

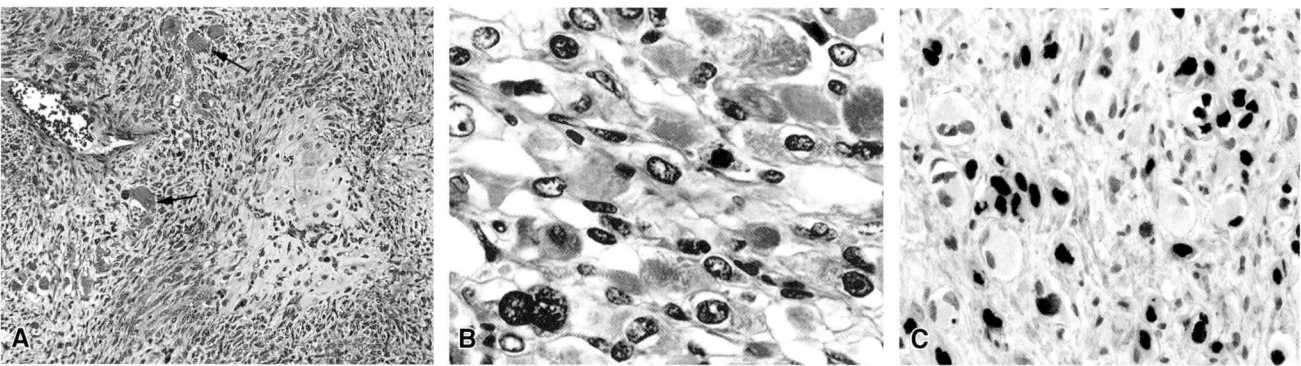

Figure 14-6. A, Heterologous biphasic sarcomatoid carcinoma of the lung, showing obviously epithelial elements juxtaposed to rhabdomyosarcoma (RMS)-like elements with cytoplasmic cross-striations (*arrows*). **B,** Cytoplasmic eosinophilia is present in the RMS-like cells. **C,** Immunoreactivity is seen for myogenin in the RMS-like foci.

contentious. Nevertheless, we have no doubt of its validity as a reproducible pathologic entity, and other authors appear to concur.[35]

Indeed, one might go so far as to state that virtually all malignant pulmonary tumors that are exclusively composed of heterologous (organ-inappropriate) elements—such as osteoblastic tissues[63,64]—are, in reality, monophasic SCs. That statement pertains even if no immunohistochemical evidence of epithelial differentiation can be found, because the ultimate biological evolution of such lesions is identical to that of conventional lung cancers.

Special Variants of Sarcomatoid Carcinoma of the Lung

There are three subtypes of SC of the lung that deserve additional discussion. These include the tumors known as pulmonary blastoma, pseudoangiosarcomatous (pseudovascular) carcinoma, and inflammatory SC.

Pulmonary Blastoma

Since its initial description by Barnett and Barnard[65] and a later discussion by Spencer,[66] pulmonary blastoma (PB) has been regarded by some observers as the pulmonary counterpart of primitive childhood tumors of other organs.[67–73] This view has been fostered in part by confusion of PB with pleuropulmonary blastoma (PPB; discussed subsequently), the latter of which is primarily seen in adolescent patients.[74–80] PB is a biphasic neoplasm, containing a mixture of tubular epithelial cell profiles and compact groupings of nondescript bluntly fusiform cells with a blastema-like configuration[39,74,77] (Fig. 14-8). These

resemble the elements of renal Wilms tumors.[81] On the other hand, PPB altogether lacks epithelial differentiation and may instead show divergent mesenchymal differentiation into myogenous or chondroosseous tissues.[77] Moreover, PB shows no particular disease associations, whereas PPB is linked in a familial fashion to a number of other malignant neoplasms and non-neoplastic disorders.[79]

If one carefully excludes examples of PPB from consideration, it becomes clear that PB is seen overwhelmingly in adults, and its clinical characteristics are superimposable on those of ordinary lung cancers and other pulmonary SCs. This realization allows one to more easily embrace an alternative view of the nature of PB that was advanced in the past by Souza and colleagues,[82] Stackhouse and associates,[14] and Millard,[83] among others. Those authors held the opinion that PB is merely a special, usually peripheral form of pulmonary SC (carcinosarcoma), rather than a blastemal neoplasm that contains truly embryonal tissues. We also espouse the latter premise.

Returning to the particular microscopic attributes of PB, it should be noted that this tumor may demonstrate the same range of epithelial and mesenchymoid differentiation that is seen in other biphasic pulmonary SCs.[39,69,84] The epithelial elements in PB resemble fetal pulmonary pseudoglands (a misnomer), composed of stratified columnar cells with glycogen-rich clear cytoplasm and high nuclear-to-cytoplasmic ratios.[69,84–86] Luminal mucin may be present in those cellular arrays, and squamous morules are sometimes also evident.[69] Interestingly, "occult" neuroendocrine differentiation is a rather common finding

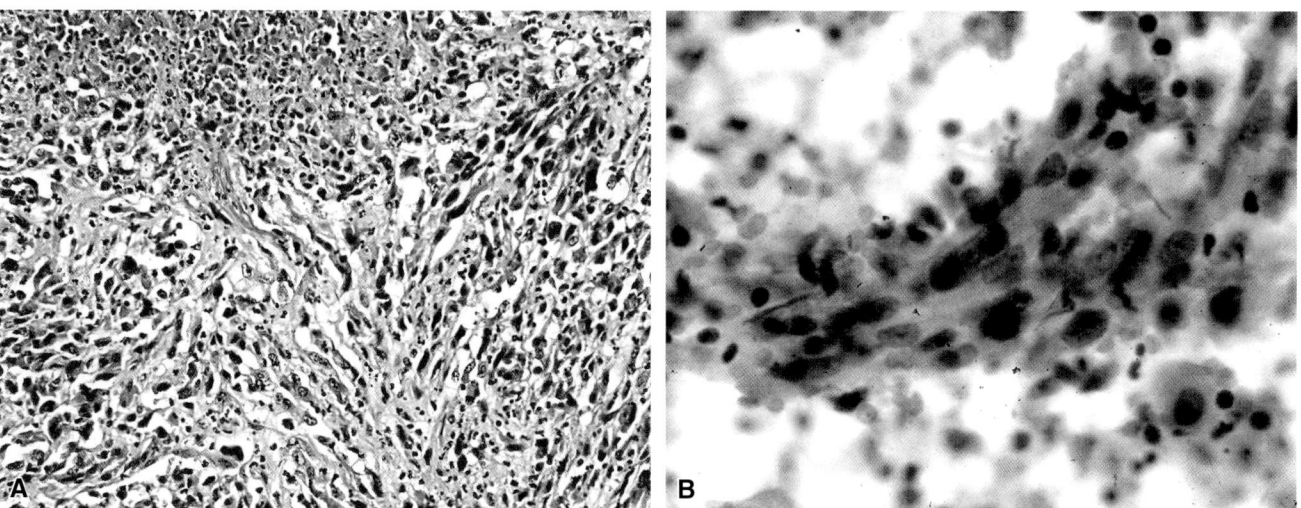

Figure 14-7. A, Monophasic spindle cell sarcomatoid carcinoma of the lung, simulating fibrosarcoma or monophasic synovial sarcoma. **B,** Fine needle aspiration specimens from this case demonstrate loosely cohesive aggregates of the spindle cells and may be viewed as generic images for all lesions discussed in this chapter.

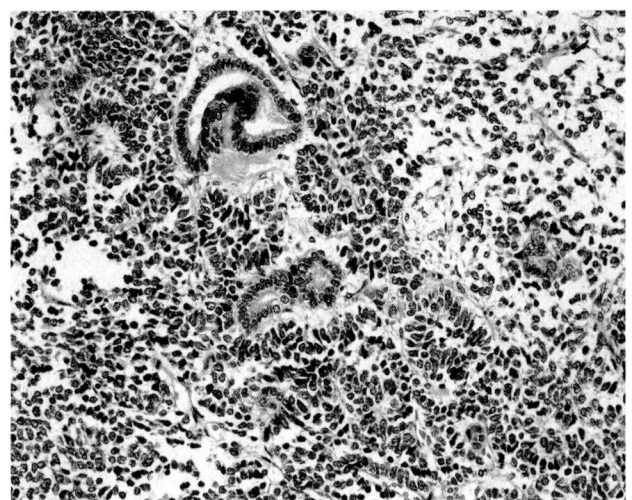

Figure 14-8. Adult-type pulmonary blastoma (carcinosarcoma), showing an admixture of fetal-type primitive glands and undifferentiated spindle cell elements. This tumor is a special morphologic form of sarcomatoid carcinoma, and it occurs preferentially in adults (not to be confused with pleuropulmonary blastoma, which occurs in childhood).

in the epithelial components of PB, with potential histochemical argyrophilia and immunoreactivity for neuroendocrine markers.[87,88] There is a significant sharing of microscopic features between classic PB and the tumor described as "pulmonary endodermal tumor resembling fetal lung" or alternatively as "well-differentiated adenocarcinoma simulating fetal lung" (Fig. 14-9). It differs in its relative lack of a malignant stromal component and more frequent synthesis of a particular oncofetal polypeptide—α-fetoprotein.[39,85,87-90]

The elements of PB showing mesenchymoid differentiation are, as stated earlier, usually nondescript morphologically and blastema-like or fibroblast-like. However, examples of this tumor have been documented in which heterologous rhabdomyoblastoid, leiomyosarcomatoid, or apparent chondro-osseous tissues were present.[69,84] This observation serves to further solidify the linkage of PB to other sarcomatoid pulmonary carcinomas, as do reports of some tumors in which "typical" PB was admixed with homologous or heterologous biphasic SC, as described earlier.[82,91-93]

The clinical behavior of PB is difficult to determine with certainty, because of the aforementioned contamination of some series with cases of PPB. However, mortality figures of 30% to 70% have been reported, with death usually being due to distant metastases.[67,69,84] Secondary

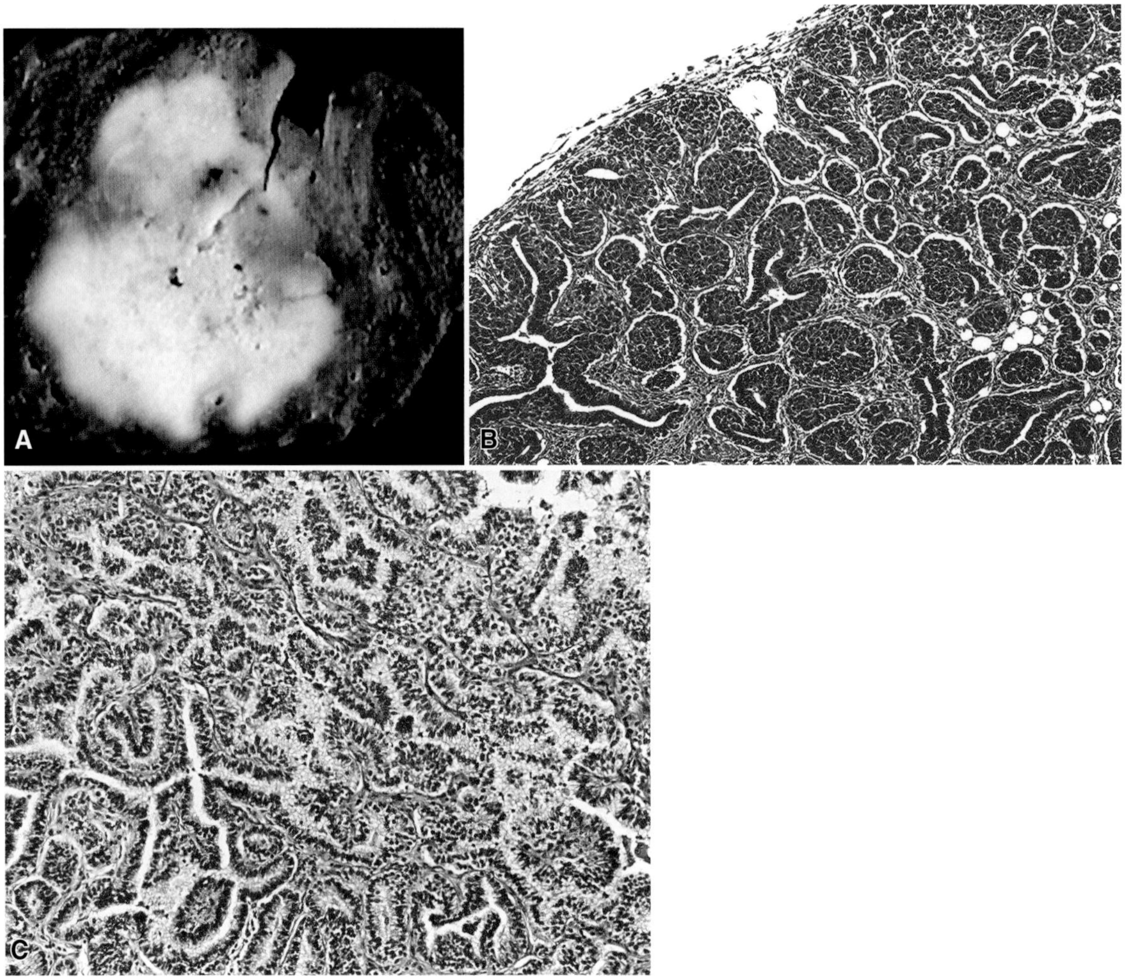

Figure 14-9. Gross (**A**) and microscopic (**B** and **C**) images of fetal-type adenocarcinoma of the lung, representing a monophasic epithelial variant of pulmonary blastoma. (**A,** Courtesy of Dr. Samuel A. Yousem, Pittsburgh, PA.)

deposits of PB may have a purely epithelial, purely mesenchymal-like, or biphasic appearance, as is true of other SCs.

Pseudoangiosarcomatous (Pseudovascular) Carcinoma

The authors have studied several lung tumors in which obvious squamous cell carcinoma was admixed with areas demonstrating interanastomosing channels mantled by anaplastic, plump, epithelioid cells, focally grouped into pseudopapillae. Because the open spaces in these areas contained erythrocytes and focally formed blood lakes, the histologic appearance was that of biphasic SC in which an angiosarcomatoid component was admixed with overt squamous carcinoma.[94] (Fig. 14-10). These neoplasms are believed to represent the pulmonary counterparts of pseudovascular adenoid squamous cell carcinoma, as seen in the skin, breast, thyroid gland, and other organs.[34,94-99] This is a tumor type that is known to simulate true angiosarcoma but lacks actual endothelial differentiation. Thus, pseudoangiosarcomatous carcinoma (PASC) would be an apt synonym.[96]

Primary pulmonary angiosarcoma is, comparatively, a very rare lesion, comprising only 10% of true sarcomas of the lung in one report from the Mayo Clinic.[2] Mainly anecdotal reports of this tumor exist in the remaining literature, and not all of them satisfy rigorous diagnostic criteria.[100-108] Metastases to the lung from angiosarcomas arising in extrapulmonary sites are much more common, including examples that have originated in the heart, great vessels, or extrathoracic viscera.[100]

Similar to reports on previously cited pseudovascular carcinomas in other body sites, two publications have specifically considered squamous cell carcinomas of the lung that imitated angiosarcomas. The first, by Banerjee and coworkers,[96] showed that such tumors produced clinical symptoms and signs resembling those of ordinary types of lung cancer. They presented in the fifth to seventh decades of life; were associated with cigarette smoking, complaints of cough, weight loss, and dyspnea; and were visible on chest radiographs as well-defined central or peripheral parenchymal masses. In another series by Nappi and colleagues,[94] the tumors were essentially identical microscopically to pseudovascular squamous carcinomas of the

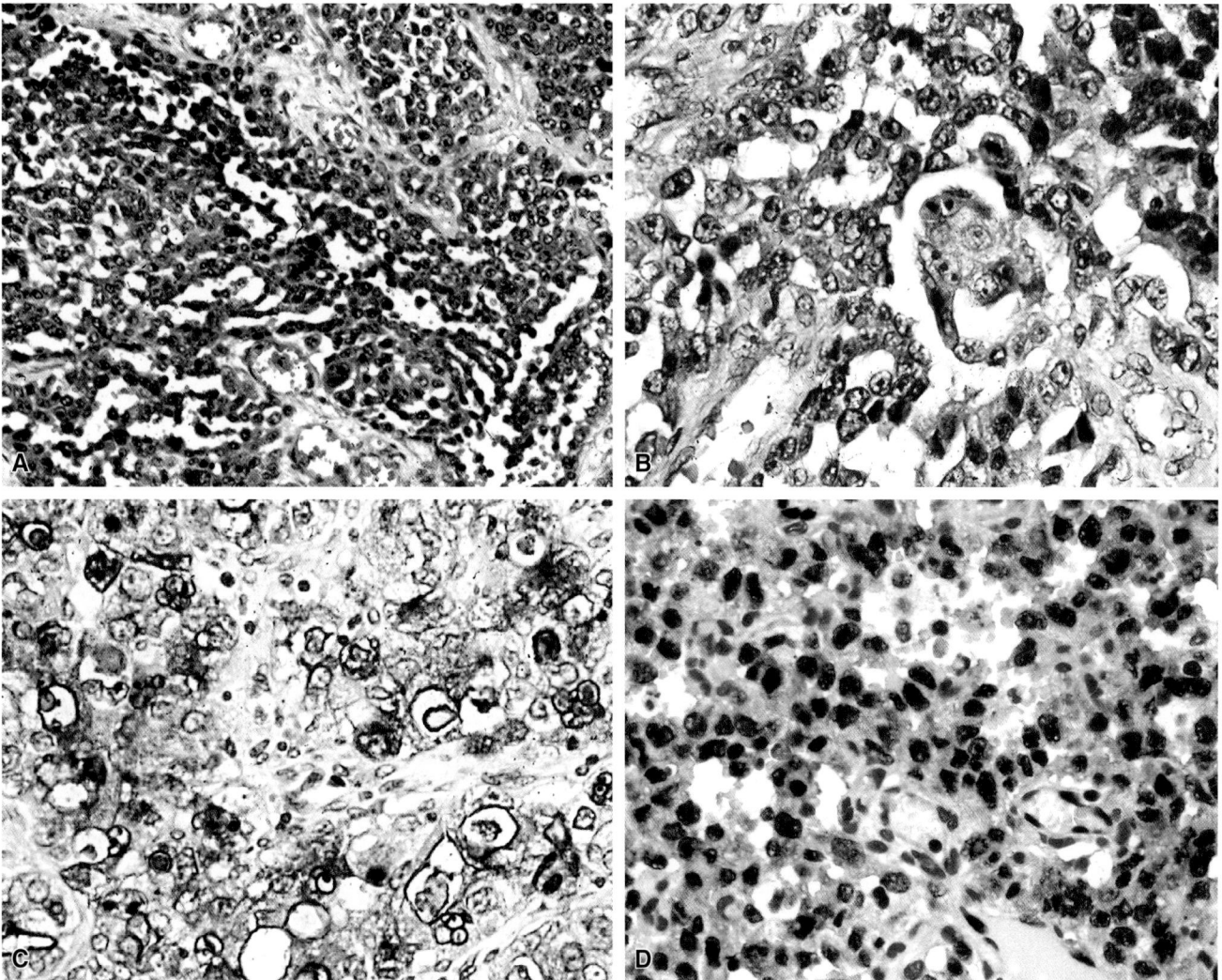

Figure 14-10. A, Pseudoangiosarcomatous sarcomatoid carcinoma of the lung demonstrating dyscohesion of the neoplastic cells in a fashion simulating the image of angiosarcoma. **B,** A focus of more obviously carcinomatous growth is apparent in the center of this figure. **C** and **D,** Immunoreactivity for epithelial membrane antigen and for p63 protein confirm the carcinomatous nature of the tumor.

breast and skin. Important differences between PASCs and true pleuropulmonary angiosarcomas include an absence of atypical endothelial cells in stromal blood vessels surrounding the tumor mass in PASCs; less infiltrative growth through the interstitium of the lung; and, perhaps most importantly, the presence of small foci of morphologically obvious squamous cell carcinoma in most PASCs.[94]

The behavioral features of PASCs are similar to those of other sarcomatoid pulmonary carcinomas. The patients studied by Nappi and colleagues developed distant metastases to the bones, liver, adrenal glands, and contralateral lung, and they died after follow-up periods of 5 to 34 months.

Inflammatory Sarcomatoid Carcinoma

Much attention has been given to a group of space-occupying lesions in the lung that carry the popular but inaccurate designation of *inflammatory pseudotumors* (IPs).[101-114] These proliferations may occur in children or adults and have been divided into fibrohistiocytic, plasma cell granulomatous, and focal organizing pneumonia types, based on their individual clinicopathological features. The nomenclature used for this group of lesions has been well summarized by Koss[114] and Matsubara and associates.[106] There is still some controversy over whether all such lesions are neoplastic, or whether some might be reactive in nature.[115] However, the bulk of available information indicates that IPs are relatively innocuous clinical imitators of overtly malignant neoplasms.[114] Occasional cases have been linked causally to specific infectious organisms,[116,117] but the etiologic factors associated with most pulmonary IPs are uncertain.

In contrast, primary SC is generally regarded as a neoplasm that may simulate pleuropulmonary mesenchymal malignancies, and it is typically not mentioned in discussions on the pathologic differential diagnosis of IPs. This is so because SC usually demonstrates obvious cytologic anaplasia and lacks a significant component of inflammatory cells. Indeed, the morphologic distinction between IPs and all bronchogenic carcinomas (including SC) has been portrayed by some authors as an uncomplicated process.[105,108] However, we have observed several examples of pulmonary SC that exhibited surprisingly bland morphologic appearances, and which, as a result, were separable from IP only by thorough study and adjunctive pathologic techniques. These have been designated as examples of inflammatory sarcomatoid carcinoma (ISC).[118,119]

Examples of ISC are composed of variably densely apposed spindle cells with only modest pleomorphism, arranged haphazardly or in fascicular and storiform patterns. The stroma is at least partially myxoid in some cases and may be prominently so. The tumors demonstrate an irregular, spiculated interface with the surrounding lung. The adjacent parenchyma exhibits interstitial fibrosis, and small nodular infiltrates of mature lymphocytes are admixed with dense collagenous tissue at the periphery of ISCs (Fig. 14-11). Focally hyalinized, keloidal-type collagen is admixed with the tumor cells in the central portions of some of these tumors, with or without small foci of central necrosis. Vascular invasion and luminal obliteration by neoplastic cells may be apparent. Similarly, bronchial submucosal infiltration is another potential observation. ISCs do not contain appreciable stromal neutrophils, eosinophils, or xanthoma cells, but a moderate number of lymphocytes and plasma cells can be seen.

Cytologically, the nuclei of the tumor cells in ISCs are relatively uniform in size and spindle-shaped, with coarse chromatin and occasional small nucleoli (Fig. 14-12). Cytoplasm is moderate in amount and amphophilic. Generally, there are no more than 2 mitoses per 10 high-power fields (×400) on average, and pathologic division figures are absent. Thorough sampling of the tumor tissue in cases of ISC typically demonstrates minute foci of cohesive epithelioid cells, suggesting the diagnosis of squamous carcinoma on conventional histologic grounds. However, some ISCs lack such foci and are recognizable as carcinomas only with special pathologic evaluations (see Fig. 14-12B).[118]

Pleurotropic (Pseudomesotheliomatous) Sarcomatoid Carcinoma

Occasional examples of SC are distinctive not because of their histologic attributes but because of their macroscopic appearances. In particular, a small subset of these neoplasms arises in the very periphery of the pulmonary parenchyma and grows preferentially into the pleura that encases the lungs.[120,121] This produces clinical symptoms and signs that are indistinguishable from those of malignant mesothelioma; hence, the names pleurotropic or pseudomesotheliomatous carcinoma.[121,122] Moreover, the microscopic features of pleurotropic SC are basically superimposable with those of biphasic or sarcomatoid mesotheliomas.

Even though there is no pragmatic clinical value in making the distinction between pleurotropic SC and mesothelioma, with regard to the efficacy of treatment or prognosis, legal ramifications of these

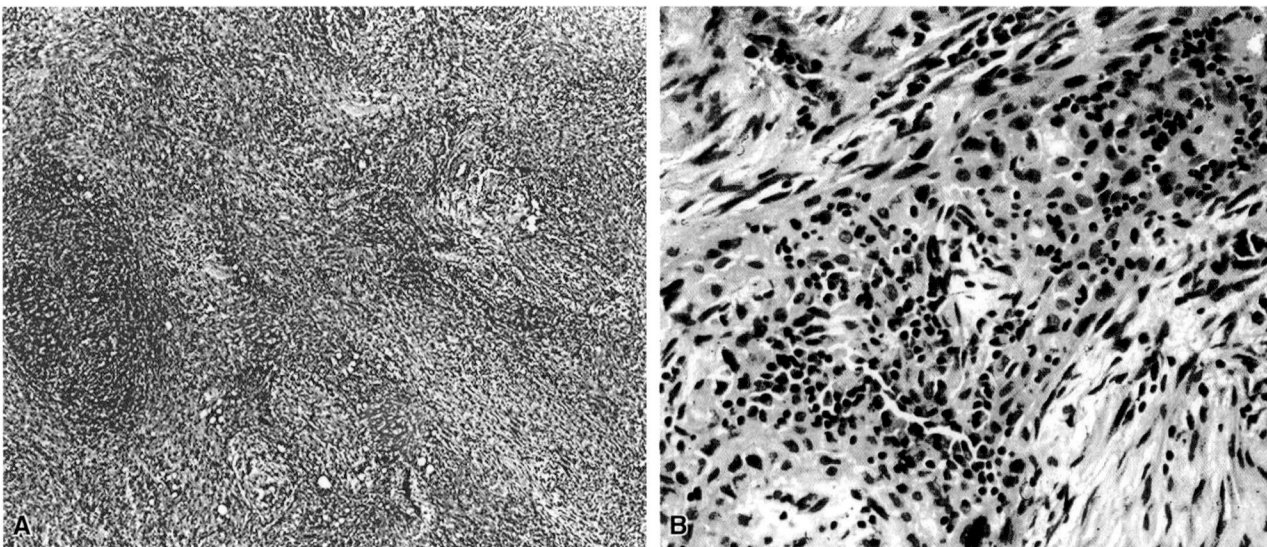

Figure 14-11. A, Inflammatory sarcomatoid carcinoma of the lung showing brisk intratumoral and peritumoral chronic inflammation. **B,** Bland proliferation of fibroblast-like cells at the periphery.

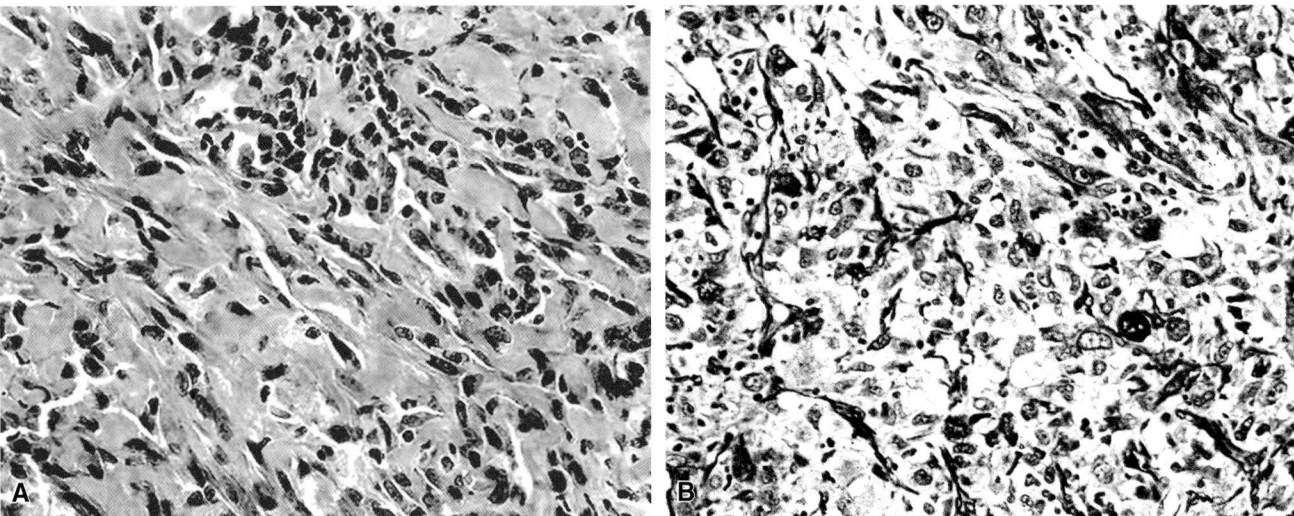

Figure 14-12. A, Higher magnification of the tumor shown in Figure 14-11 reveals nuclear atypia in the spindle cells. **B,** The tumor cells are all keratin-reactive immunohistologically.

diagnoses are worthy of comment. Because of the potential causal linkage of mesothelioma with occupational-level amphibole asbestos exposure, some patients with that tumor are eligible for monetary compensation. However, there is no convincing evidence to link pleurotropic SC with asbestos, and its etiology appears to be identical to that of "routine" forms of lung cancer.

Results of Adjunctive Pathologic Studies

Accounts of the electron microscopic and immunohistologic characteristics of pulmonary SC have not been altogether uniform. Some authors have preferred the view that such data in fact confirm the existence of true carcinosarcomas,[123–125] whereas others have thought that this information instead supports the concept of a pathologic continuum that is predicated on carcinoma in pure form.[15,17,38,126–130] We strongly prefer the second of these opinions.

It is true that the sarcoma-like elements in SC of the airways do not uniformly exhibit the ultrastructural presence of intercellular junctions and tonofibrils, or immunoreactivity for keratin or epithelial membrane antigen (EMA) in fusiform and pleomorphic tumor cells. In fact, these generic markers of epithelial differentiation may be seen only extremely focally in such neoplastic components, and we have even seen isolated examples in which cell membrane–based EMA reactivity was obvious, but keratin positivity was altogether absent. Humphrey and coworkers observed cytoplasmic tonofibrils or keratin positivity in the sarcomatoid elements of only three of eight pulmonary SCs.[15] However, it should be noted that the latter study was performed with a single heteroantiserum to high-molecular-weight keratin, representing a relatively insensitive means of immunodetection. In our previously published experience with SCs of the respiratory tract,[33] 81% were ultrastructurally or immunohistochemically proven (with a mixture of monoclonal antikeratin antibodies [AE1/AE3/CAM5.2/MAK-6]) to be wholly epithelial in nature, and other authors have recorded similar findings at immunohistochemical and genetic levels of investigation.[126–132]

The fact that features of epithelial differentiation are present at all in the sarcomatoid elements of these neoplasms strongly supports the premise that respiratory tract SC is a basically carcinomatous lesion "in transition."[133] This concept has been well-accepted in reference to dedifferentiated sarcomas of the soft tissue, in which clonal evolution is thought to account for a change in the morphology as well as the immunophenotype of the progenitor lesion.[134] Lessons learned in the latter sphere—as well as molecular biologic

assessments of clonality in SCs[135]—have direct corollaries in the context under discussion here. We have observed the coexpression of vimentin (a "primordial" intermediate filament) in all examples of keratin-positive SC of the airways, and a minority of these lesions are additionally labeled for desmin (the intermediate filament of myogenous cells) and muscle-specific actin in the same cells that contain the other two filament proteins (Fig. 14-13).[33] Collagen type IV is also seen surrounding individual tumor cells in most instances. Markers of neuroendocrine differentiation, such as chromogranin-A, CD57, and synaptophysin, likewise may be seen in selected lesions in their overtly epithelial components,[53,55] and S100 protein is apparent in foci resembling chondroid tissue by conventional microscopy.[4] In contrast, Friend leukemia-virus integration protein-1 (FLI-1) and CD31 are typically absent in PASC, whereas one or both of those endothelial determinants would be expected in true pleuropulmonary angiosarcomas.[95,136]

These accrued observations coincide with ultrastructural findings reported by Battifora in two cases of SC, which demonstrated the coincidence of desmosomes, tonofibrils, and collagen production in the same neoplastic cells, implying the presence of multilinear differentiation.[137]

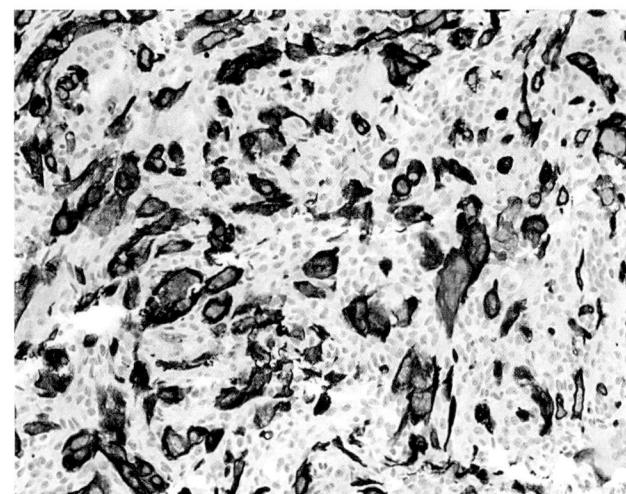

Figure 14-13. Muscle-specific actin immunostain in pulmonary sarcomatoid carcinoma. This tumor coexpressed vimentin, pancytokeratin, and desmin.

Thus, SC can be viewed basically as an epithelial neoplasm with divergent mesenchymal differentiation, in which carcinoma cells acquire the potential to express a mesenchymal phenotype at light microscopic, ultrastructural, and immunohistologic levels. The pathogenetic bases for this peculiarity are currently unknown, but the practical deduction to be gleaned from this construct is that all SCs of the respiratory tract should be treated clinically as poorly differentiated carcinomas.

Wakely has reviewed the characteristics of pulmonary spindle cell tumors as seen in fine needle aspiration biopsy specimens[138] (see Fig. 14-7). He concluded that adjunctive pathologic studies, such as those discussed above, were virtually mandatory before definitive diagnoses could be reached in that context.

Differential Diagnosis of Sarcomatoid Carcinoma

The differential diagnosis of SCs of the airways principally centers on the exclusion of true sarcomas, which are discussed later in this chapter. As a particular word of caution, it should be noted that synovial sarcoma (SS) and sarcomatoid mesothelioma may be very closely similar to SC as seen with the electron microscope or in immunophenotypic evaluations. The marked propensity for SS to affect children, adolescents, and young adults, its typical t(X;18) (p11.2;q11.2) cytogenetic aberration,[139,140] and nuclear labeling for transducin-like enhancer [of Split]-1 (TLE1) protein[141-144] (not seen in carcinomas) are crucial points in its distinction from SC of the upper airways. Of course, nuances of histologic appearances and radiographic characteristics are also valuable in this specific differential diagnostic setting. Similarly, roentgenologic findings are more helpful than morphologic observations in making the distinction between SC and spindle cell or biphasic mesothelioma. The ultrastructural profiles of the latter two lesions are again very similar,[1,4,145] and, aside from selective reactivity for calretinin and podoplanin[146] in mesotheliomas, the same comment applies to their immunophenotypes.

True Primary Sarcomas of the Lung

Kaposi Sarcoma

The natural history of KS is a sad testimony to the global impact of acquired immunodeficiency syndrome (AIDS). Before the 1980s, KS was a relatively rare neoplasm outside of Africa and the Mediterranean basin. Moreover, with relatively uncommon exceptions, this lesion was a cutaneous proliferation that uncommonly involved the viscera.[147]

However, today, with particular regard to the intrathoracic organs, KS is—in most large metropolitan areas of the world—the most common of all pulmonary sarcomas.[148] Whereas initial presentation of this tumor in the bronchopulmonary tract was an almost-unknown phenomenon prior to the advent of AIDS, it is currently a well-recognized variation of the latter disease.[149]

Clinical Summary

In the context just mentioned, many patients with KS of the lung are homosexual men,[150-156] but they also include other high-risk groups for AIDS such as intravenous drug abusers. Most individuals with KS generally have other symptoms and signs of AIDS, such as weight loss, fever, night sweats, fatigue, lymphadenopathy, and opportunistic infections. However, fever may be directly caused by KS in the lungs. There has been a case report of an AIDS patient with persistent pyrexia for which no source of infection was found but that finally resolved after radiation therapy.[157] Cutaneous KS is usually detected early in its clinical evolution, but identical tumors of the bronchial mucosa and lung parenchyma typically have grown to a volume sufficient to produce symptoms and therefore are relatively advanced at the time of diagnosis.[158] Presenting complaints specific to the neoplasm include dyspnea, stridor (when endobronchial lesions are present), cough, and hemoptysis, which may be massive.[149]

On bronchoscopic examination, nodular or flat bluish-red discolorations in the mucosa are seen, some of which may be actively bleeding. This bronchoscopic appearance is usually considered diagnostic, and endobronchial lesions are not generally biopsied. The diagnostic yield of transbronchial biopsies is usually low, and unless they are deep enough, KS of the lung will be missed because the mucosa itself is uninvolved.[159] Open lung biopsies are more productive, but they are not absolutely sensitive.

Radiographic findings on chest x-rays may be nonspecific, showing only ill-defined interstitial infiltrates (Fig. 14-14). An alveolar filling pattern is usually evident only if the patient has suffered hemoptysis and aspirated blood, but pleural effusions or pneumothorax may be seen in cases where the lesion involves the serosal surfaces as well as the lung parenchyma.[160,161] Mediastinal adenopathy is not common, but, if it is present, this can be very helpful in separating KS from *Pneumocystis jiroveci* infection, because the latter does not cause adenopathy. Computed tomography (CT) scans and magnetic resonance imaging (MRI) generally provide no more information than chest radiography. In summary, the presence of bilateral pleural effusions and bilateral interstitial infiltrates with ill-defined nodularity is suggestive of pulmonary KS, especially in a patient with known tumor elsewhere.[150,151]

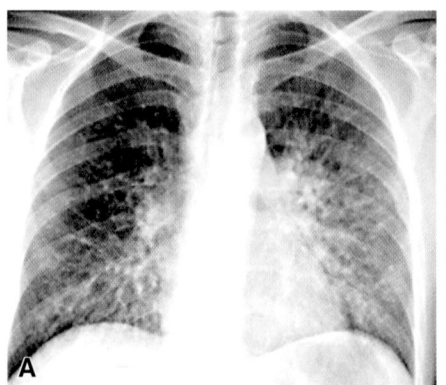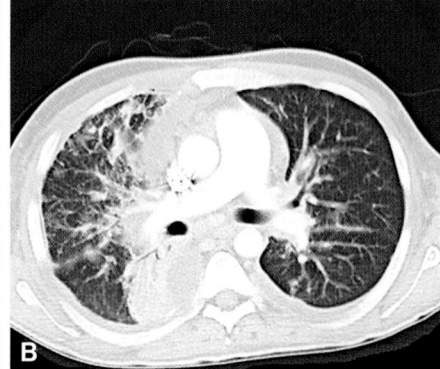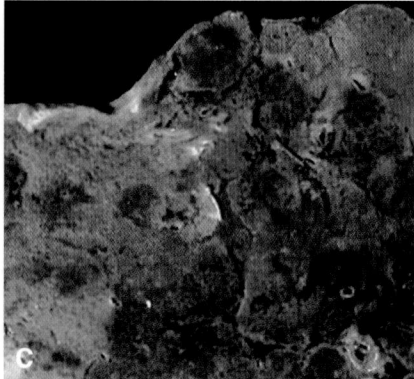

Figure 14-14. A relatively nondescript reticulonodular interstitial infiltrate is seen on a conventional chest radiograph (**A**) and computed tomogram (**B**) in a patient with acquired immunodeficiency syndrome. The clinical differential diagnosis of such a pattern would include infection as well as neoplasia, but pulmonary Kaposi sarcoma was the ultimate interpretation in this case. **C,** An autopsy example of this condition shows irregularly consolidated and hemorrhagic parenchyma.

Pathologic Findings

As alluded to above, it is distinctly uncommon for the pathologist to be able to make a definitive diagnosis of KS of the lung on a transbronchial biopsy specimen. Usually, a wedge biopsy is necessary, as obtained via video-guided thoracoscopy or a limited thoracotomy.[159] On gross examination, this type of specimen exhibits numerous hemangiomatoid or ecchymosis-like zones of bluish-red discoloration in the parenchyma, with ill-defined borders.

In the lung, KS shows a tendency to grow along pre-existing fibrous intrapulmonary septa, and it also concentrates around small tubular airways and blood vessels (Fig. 14-15). The tumor comprises a mixture of ectatic, thin-walled blood vessels that "dissect" or push through the pulmonary interstitial collagen, together with haphazardly arranged fascicles of spindle cells that show only modest nuclear atypia and may contain cytoplasmic vacuoles.[149,159] Extravasated erythrocytes and hemosiderin pigment are common in and around the tumor masses (Fig. 14-16). Pleural KS "layers" itself over the submesothelial mantle of connective tissue, effacing the mesothelium itself in doing so.

Mitotic activity is variable in primary KS of the lung, but it is usually detectable. If it is present at all, necrosis is limited in scope and visible only on microscopy.

The differential diagnosis of KS from vascular granulation tissue and other spindle cell proliferations in the lung is greatly enhanced by immunohistochemical analyses. KS is reactive for latent nuclear antigen-1 of human herpesvirus-8 in approximately 85% of cases[162] (Fig. 14-17). It also labels for FLI-1[163] and podoplanin.[164]

Therapy and Prognosis

Regardless of its occurrence in AIDS or in non–human immunodeficiency virus (HIV)-related cases, the presence of KS in the lung is prognostically ominous. Virtually all patients with visceral disease die within 2 years, from infection if not from KS itself.[148,154,156] Because of the multiplicity of KS, surgical resection is not a realistic option in the management of patients with this neoplasm. Chemotherapy is considered the treatment of choice, with a relatively good response rate and relatively rapid improvement within 2 to 4 weeks.[25] Chemotherapy regimens in the few published therapeutic trials designed specifically for pulmonary KS have primarily included adriamycin, bleomycin, and vincristine.[149,165–167] Gill and colleagues found an 85% response with combination chemotherapy in a group of 13 patients.[166] Patients who benefited from this treatment included those who achieved at least partial responses. Complete response is defined by the following three criteria:

- Direct bronchoscopy revealing complete disappearance of KS lesions in the tracheobronchial tree
- A normal chest x-ray
- Resolution of all other sites of disease

A partial response is characterized by the same three points, except that the degree of resolution is not total.[165,166]

Despite fairly good results with combination chemotherapy, patients with pulmonary KS do not show long survival. In the trial reported by Gill and colleagues, the median survival for responders was slightly but significantly longer than that of nonresponders (10 versus 6 months, respectively). However, considerable overlap between the two groups was present.[166]

Other more experimental (and inconclusive) approaches have included the administration of zidovudine, interferon, and other antiviral compounds.[147,153,154] Radiotherapy may provide palliation of symptoms but is noncurative. The most important piece of data in prognosticating cases of KS of the lung is the serologic HIV status of the patient, inasmuch as AIDS is currently a uniformly lethal, albeit chronic, illness.

Fibrosarcoma

Primary fibrosarcoma of the lung (FSL), like its soft tissue counterpart, is defined as a fibroblastic spindle cell neoplasm without any evidence of specialized cellular differentiation. Although it has been cited in the past—along with leiomyosarcoma—as the most common primary pulmonary sarcoma,[168] FSL was, and probably still is, overdiagnosed.[169] Two separate studies from the Mayo Clinic cited two different time-dependent incidence figures for FSL. From 1950 to 1978, it constituted 50% of all primary pulmonary sarcomas[170] but only 20% in the decade 1980 to 1990.[171] As considered previously, it is our belief that the great majority of pulmonary "fibrosarcomas" are actually SCs. Only those tumors that have been subjected to rigorous and specialized pathologic examination should be accepted as bona fide examples of this rare sarcoma variant.

Clinical Summary

Guccion and Rosen studied 13 cases of FSL, which were divided into endobronchial and intrapulmonary types.[168] This classification scheme was said to have clinical and prognostic importance.

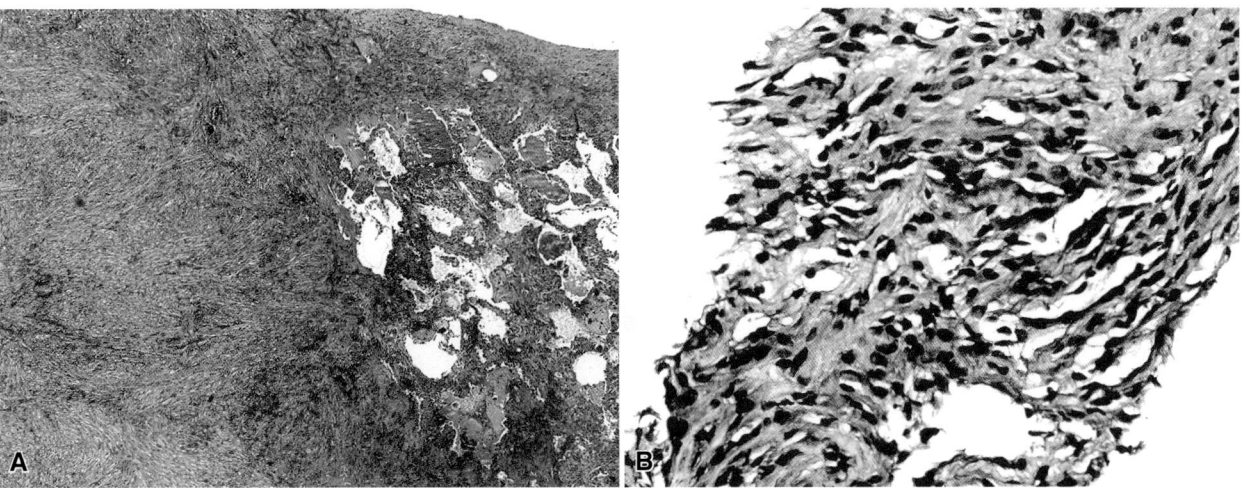

Figure 14-15. A, Low-magnification image of pulmonary Kaposi sarcoma (KS), showing a nodular proliferation of spindle cells and neovascular spaces (*left*) that permeates the pulmonary interstitium (*right*). **B,** A transbronchial biopsy specimen of KS shows a spindle cell proliferation and interanastomosing vascular channels.

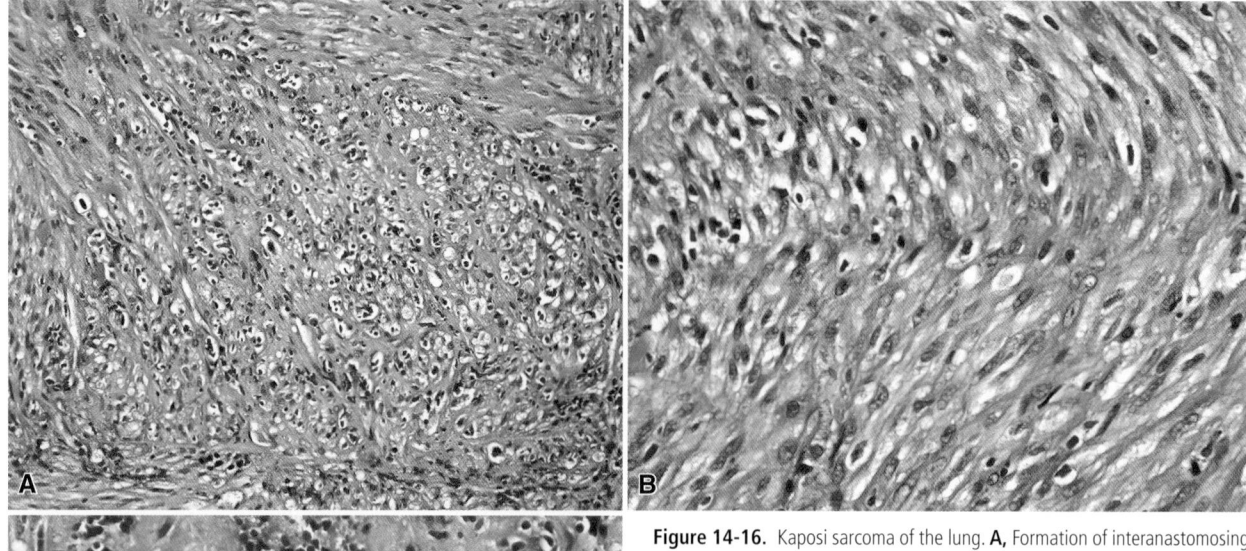

Figure 14-16. Kaposi sarcoma of the lung. **A,** Formation of interanastomosing vascular channels. **B,** Foci of solid spindle cell growth. **C,** Areas with extravasation of erythrocytes into the stroma and deposition of hemosiderin pigment.

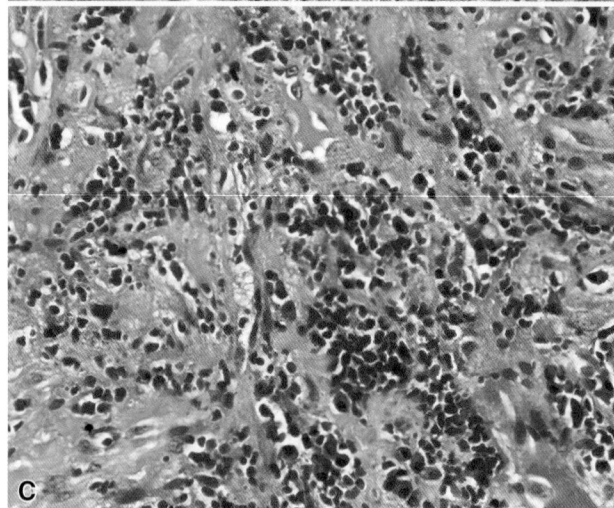

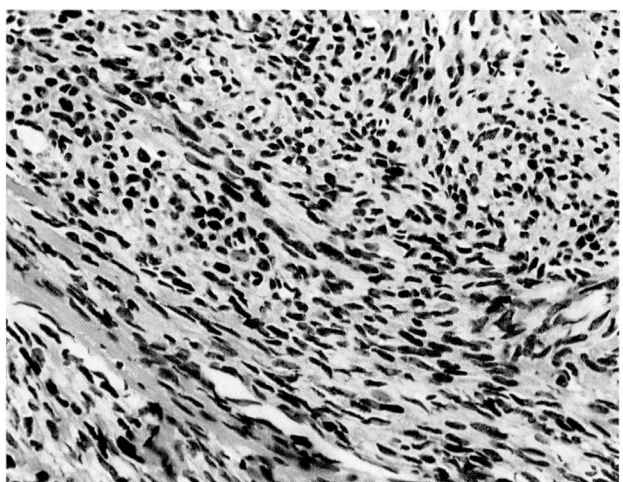

Figure 14-17. Diffuse immunoreactivity is seen for herpesvirus-8–latent nuclear antigen-1 in Kaposi sarcoma of the lung.

In conjunction with a review of 48 reported cases in the literature, the authors just cited found that the majority of endobronchial FSLs occurred in children and young adults, whereas parenchymal tumors predominated in middle-aged and elderly patients. In contrast, Pettinato and associates reported three parenchymal tumors in two newborns and a 6-month old infant.[172] There was roughly an equal distribution by gender among endobronchial lesions; however, most intraparenchymal neoplasms occurred in men. All cases of endobronchial FSL in a series reported from the Armed Forces Institute of Pathology (AFIP) had symptoms of cough, hemoptysis, or chest pain; some of the parenchymal cases did as well.[168] Thoracic imaging studies of FSL usually show discrete, homogenous masses. However, one reported pulmonary fibrosarcoma simulated a bronchogenic cyst clinically and radiographically.[173] Gladish and coworkers[13] have observed that fibrosarcoma is much more likely to arise in the soft tissue of the chest wall and secondarily involve the lung than it is to show the converse of that relationship.

Pathologic Findings
Endobronchial fibrosarcomas are smaller than microscopically similar tumors in the parenchyma; the former variants usually measure less than 3 cm, and the latter range from 3.5 to 23 cm in greatest dimension. Parenchymal masses are typically well-delimited and lobulated, with frequent areas of necrosis and hemorrhage.

FSL is histologically identical to its soft tissue counterparts and characteristically shows sheets and intertwining fascicles of spindle-shaped cells with a typical interdigitating growth pattern and discernible stromal collagenogenesis (Fig. 14-18). The tumor cells contain oval to elongated, hyperchromatic nuclei, and scant amphophilic cytoplasm with ill-defined cellular borders. In addition, some areas may have a slightly epithelioid appearance, in which the tumor cells are

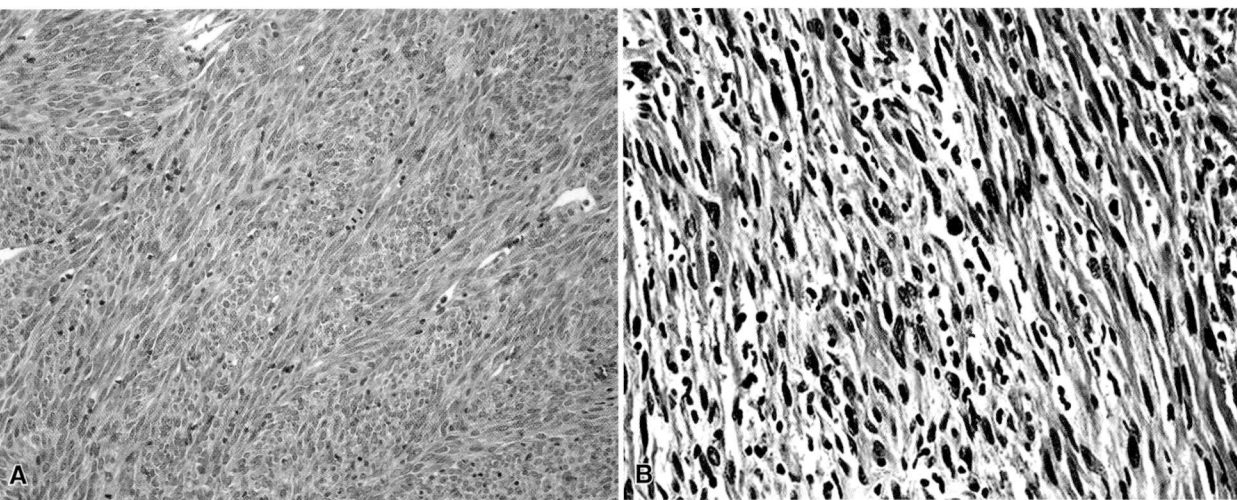

Figure 14-18. A, Pulmonary fibrosarcoma represented by a cellular proliferation of atypical spindle cells. **B,** Nuclear anaplasia is apparent on high magnification.

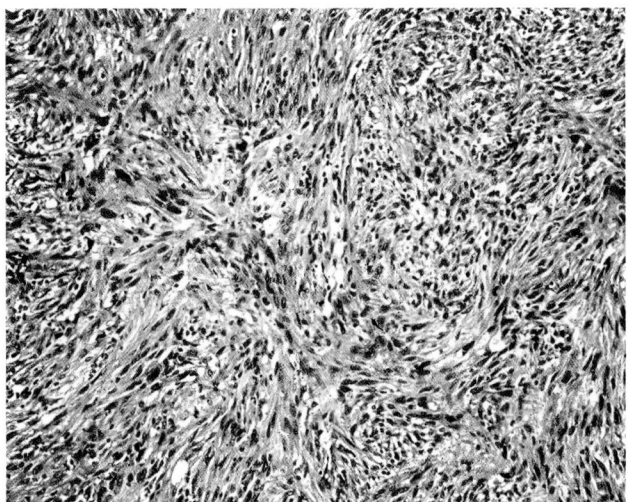

Figure 14-19. This image from another case of high-grade intrapulmonary fibrosarcoma shows more nuclear pleomorphism in the tumor cells, overlapping the appearance of malignant fibrous histiocytoma.

more ovoid than spindled, and others may show significant pleomorphism that merges with the image of MFH (Fig. 14-19). Mitotic activity is variable.

Electron microscopic and immunohistochemical studies are required to confirm the fibroblastic nature of these neoplasms. The tumor cells in FSL are characterized by abundant rough endoplasmic reticulum and free ribosomes, as well as the production of extracellular collagen fibers that may be aligned at right angles to the tumor cell membranes. There should be no detectable myofilaments, pericellular basal lamina, or intercellular junctions in lesions thought to represent FSL. Because there are no specific immunologic markers for fibroblasts, the diagnosis of fibrosarcoma is one of ultimate immunohistologic exclusion. Tumor cells in FSL generally stain only for vimentin, a primitive intermediate filament protein, and they lack all epithelial, myogenous, neural, and endothelial markers.[172,174,175]

Therapy and Prognosis

Although resection is the treatment of choice, many surgically treated fibrosarcomas of the lungs do recur, and survival after this event is short, with patient fatality usually occurring within 2 years.[168] Three

cases seen at the Mayo Clinic between 1980 and 1990 occurred in young women whose lesions all recurred within 15 months following surgical excision.[171] In contrast, primary bronchopulmonary fibrosarcomas in children appear to have a relatively favorable prognosis and behave only as low-grade malignancies.[172,173] The five patients with pediatric FSL reported by Pettinato and colleagues all had complete surgical removal of their tumors, and four were disease-free after 4 to 9 years. The fifth case in that series had insignificant follow-up.[172] The efficacy of adjunctive chemotherapy and irradiation has not yet been proven.

Primary Pulmonary Hyalinizing Spindle Cell Tumor with Giant Rosettes

A rare lesion that is probably biologically related to FSL is one called *hyalinizing spindle cell tumor with giant rosettes* (HSCT). This entity was originally documented as a low-grade sarcoma in the deep soft tissues of adults,[176] but at least two cases have been reported as primary pulmonary examples.[177,178] HSCT has a distinctive morphologic appearance, featuring the multifocal presence of large rosette-like structures amid a bland spindle cell proliferation (Fig. 14-20). The lesion has infiltrative borders, with no necrosis and only limited mitotic activity.

HSCT has a partial kinship with Evans tumor (low-grade fibromyxoid sarcoma)[179] of soft tissue, on behavioral, morphologic, and cytogenetic grounds. Both of those tumors manifest a t(7;16)(q33;p11) chromosomal translocation, producing fusion of the *FUS* and *CREB3L2* genes.[178] Unlike FSL, HSCT demonstrates some immunophenotypic variability, often labeling for alpha-isoform actin in its spindle cell population. The cells in the giant rosettes may manifest immunoreactivity for S100 protein and CD45RO,[176] the latter of which is more typically a hematopoietic determinant. The precise biologic potential of HSCT in the lung is uncertain, because of the anecdotal nature of reported cases.

Primary Pulmonary Leiomyosarcoma

The most common anatomic locations for leiomyosarcomas in general are the uterus, gastrointestinal tract, and soft tissue, in order of relative frequency. The extremely uncommon primary pulmonary leiomyosarcoma (PPLMS) presumably originates from bronchial or pulmonary vascular smooth muscle. Only three cases of leiomyosarcoma were found among roughly 10,000 primary malignancies of the lung at one large American medical center between 1980 and 1990.[171] Because

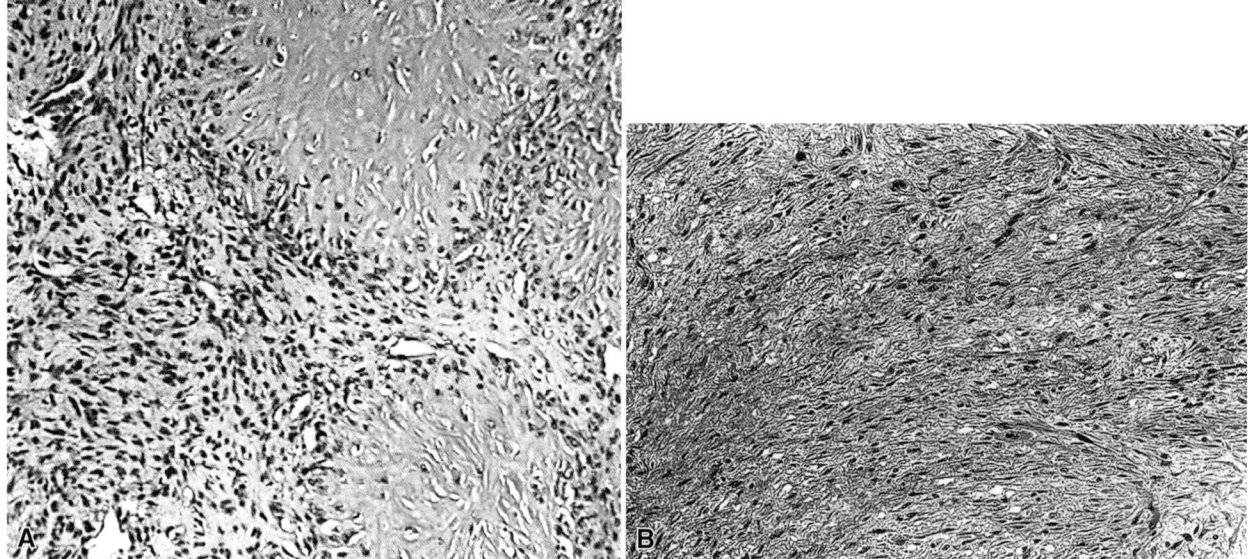

Figure 14-20. A, So-called spindle cell tumor (low-grade fibrosarcoma) with giant rosettes primarily arising in the lung. **B,** Other areas of this neoplasm show a virtual identity to fibromyxoid sarcoma of Evans, and those two tumor types have an identical cytogenetic profile.

secondary pulmonary involvement by malignant smooth muscle tumors is a relatively frequent event, the diagnosis of PPLMS absolutely requires exclusion of an occult extrathoracic neoplasm presenting with a single "herald" metastasis to the lung.

Clinical Summary

A series of 19 PPLMSs seen at the AFIP was divided into those neoplasms that were predominantly endobronchial and others that were intraparenchymal, in analogy to pulmonary fibrosarcomas.[168] The majority of these tumors in children are endobronchial in nature,[180,181] whereas those in adults are not. In contrast to leiomyosarcomas of the soft tissue, which occur most commonly in women, patients in the aforementioned report from the AFIP were almost exclusively men. However, another survey that reviewed 92 cases of PPLMS in the literature found a male-to-female ratio of 2.5, suggesting that the paramilitary study just cited was biased demographically by its affiliation with the armed services.[182] In contrast to carcinoma of the lung, leiomyosarcoma is not associated with cigarette smoking or other potential inhalant carcinogens. Most patients with PPLMS (particularly its endobronchial form) are symptomatic, often complaining of cough, hemoptysis, or chest pain. However, intraparenchymal lesions may be discovered incidentally on chest radiographs. Roentgenographically, PPLMS usually takes the form of a discrete mass (Fig. 14-21), sometimes with cavitation or cyst formation that is best seen by CT of the thorax.[168,183,184]

Pathologic Findings

Parenchymal tumors range from 3 to 15 cm in maximum dimension. They are well circumscribed, white to yellowish tan, and variably firm. Cut surfaces of these neoplasms commonly show hemorrhagic and necrotic areas. Endobronchial tumors are often smaller than the intraparenchymal lesions, presumably because of confinement by the bronchial walls.[185]

Microscopy discloses histologic features that mirror those of leiomyosarcomas elsewhere in the body. On low-power magnification, there are interlacing fascicles of spindled cells arranged haphazardly, yielding a "whorled" appearance (Fig. 14-22). The neoplastic cells have cigar-shaped nuclei with blunt ends, a moderate amount of cytoplasm, and indistinct cell borders (Fig. 14-23). Fascicles cut in cross section demonstrate characteristic intracellular perinuclear lucencies.[185–188] Prominent myxoid stromal change may be observed.[189]

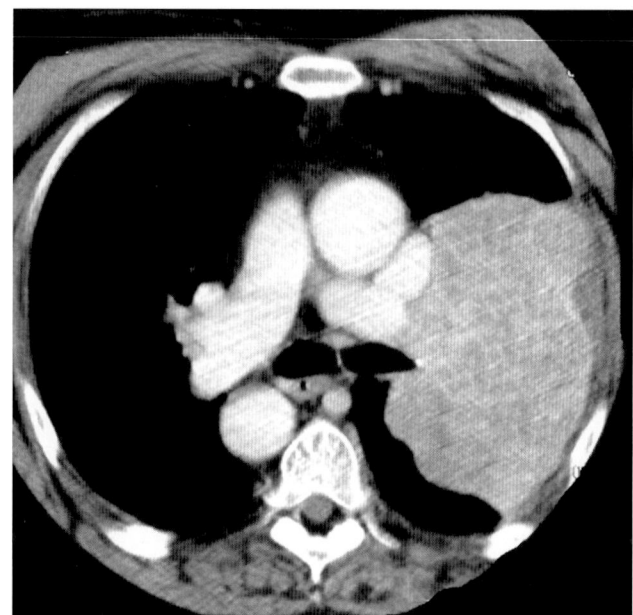

Figure 14-21. Computed tomogram of the thorax showing primary leiomyosarcoma of the lung.

The differential diagnosis of PPLMS includes fibrosarcoma and malignant peripheral nerve sheath tumor, as well as SC. Electron microscopy and immunohistochemistry are again helpful in confirming the smooth muscle nature of a spindle cell neoplasm.[187] Ultrastructural features of leiomyogenous differentiation include cytoplasmic dense bodies punctuating skeins of thin filaments, subplasmalemmal dense plaques, plasmalemmal pinocytotic vesicles, and pericellular basal lamina (Fig. 14-24). Immunoreactivity for desmin, muscle-specific actin, calponin, caldesmon, or smooth muscle actin is also characteristic of the tumor cells in PPLMS.[190]

Transthoracic fine needle aspiration of possible PPLMS can be attempted if the lesion is large and peripherally located. The cytologic preparations from that procedure typically show a dyshesive population of relatively monotonous spindle cells, with blunt-ended fusiform nuclei.

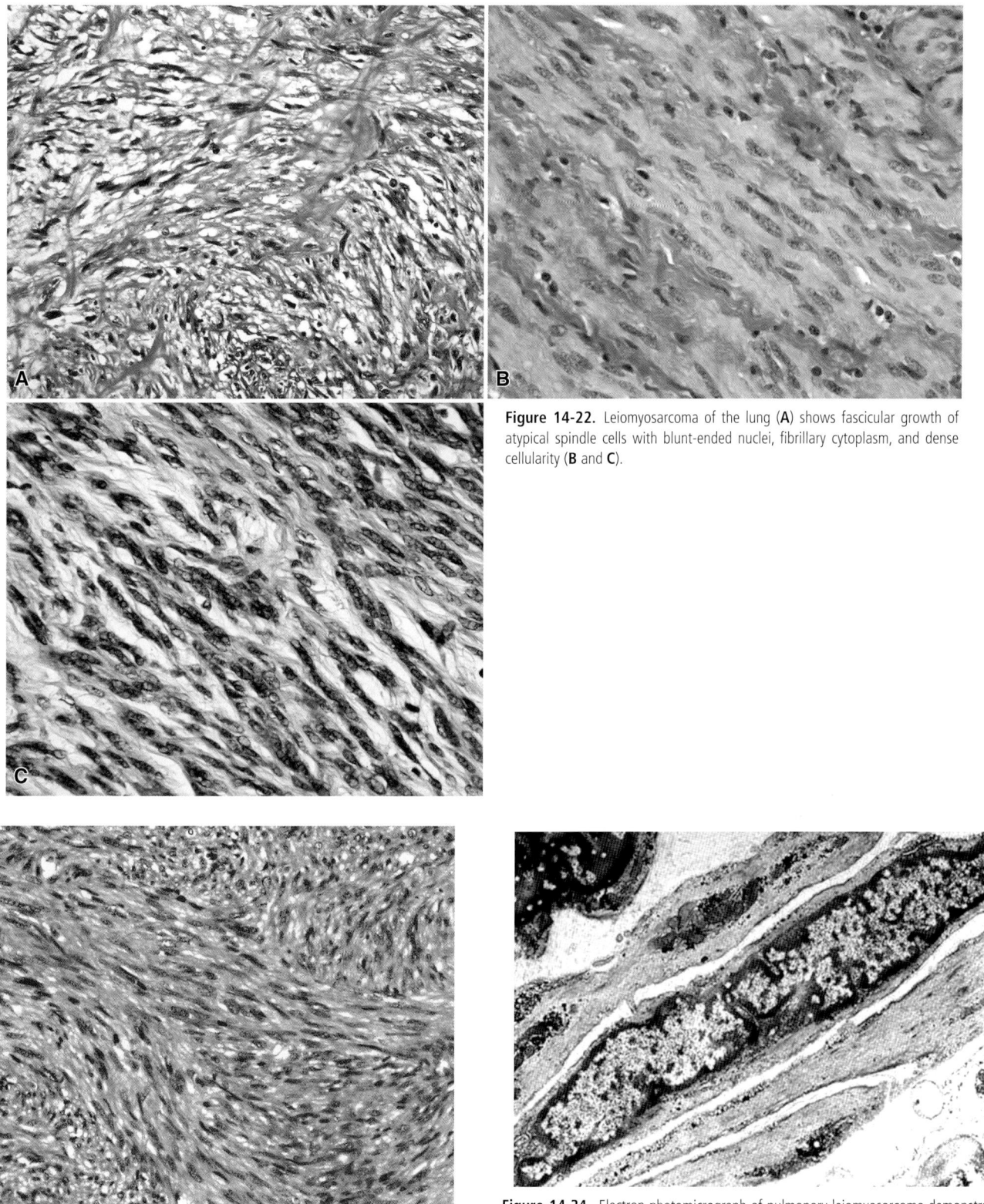

Figure 14-22. Leiomyosarcoma of the lung (**A**) shows fascicular growth of atypical spindle cells with blunt-ended nuclei, fibrillary cytoplasm, and dense cellularity (**B** and **C**).

Figure 14-23. Cytologic details are clearly seen in this primary pulmonary leiomyosarcoma.

Figure 14-24. Electron photomicrograph of pulmonary leiomyosarcoma demonstrating cytoplasmic thin filaments, pericellular basal lamina, and cytoplasmic dense bodies.

Mitotic figures and nuclear pleomorphism are variably seen; some lesions also may exhibit a more epithelioid cytologic image[191–193] (Fig. 14-25).

Therapy and Prognosis
The natural history of PPLMS and its responses to various therapeutic regimens are difficult to predict because of the rarity of this neoplasm.

However, there is generally a consensus that surgical resection is the treatment of choice[182,185–187] and that it produces a survival rate of 45% to 50% at 5 years. Survival for as long as 15 to 30 years has been documented in PPLMS cases.[168,170] However, pulmonary leiomyosarcomas appear to be relatively resistant to irradiation and chemotherapy.[182,188] Various prognostic variables have been discussed in connection with

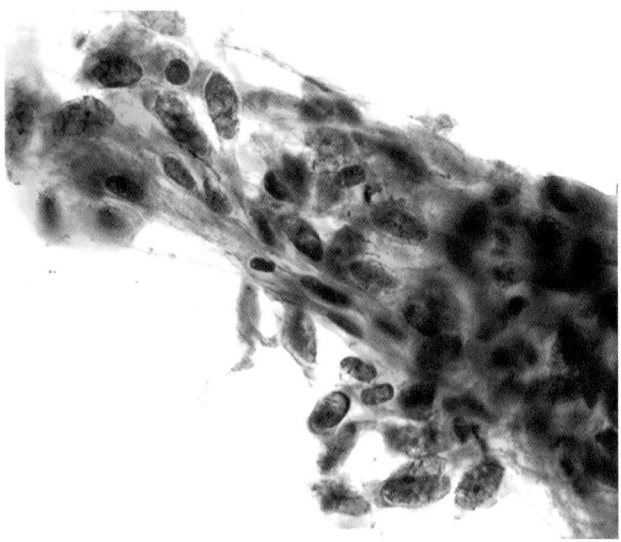

Figure 14-25. Fine needle aspiration biopsy of primary pulmonary leiomyosarcoma showing loosely cohesive tumor cells with blunt-ended fusiform nuclei.

these lesions.[168,170] Endobronchial tumors are thought to be less aggressive than parenchymal neoplasms, largely because the former tend to be smaller and are diagnosed earlier. It follows, therefore, that tumor size is an important indicator of biologic behavior for all pulmonary leiomyosarcomas. The scope of mitotic activity may affect prognosis as well. In an AFIP series on PPLMS, a mitotic rate of 8 or less per 10 high-power fields was associated with infrequent metastasis and a generally favorable clinical outcome.[168]

Epithelioid Hemangioendothelioma

In 1975, Dail and Liebow reported the first cases of an unusual pulmonary neoplasm that they termed *intravascular bronchioloalveolar tumor* (IVBAT). This name reflected their original hypothesis that the lesion in question was an epithelial tumor—specifically, a bronchioloalveolar carcinoma variant showing prominent vascular invasion.[194,195] Four years thereafter, Corrin and associates alternatively proposed an endothelial origin for this tumor based on the results of ultrastructural studies.[196] Subsequent evaluations by other authors have confirmed the vascular histogenesis of the IVBAT. Indeed, in 1982, Weiss and Enzinger described a series of soft tissue tumors that were histologically identical to IVBAT, and these authors were the first to use the term *epithelioid hemangioendothelioma* (EH) to emphasize their distinctively epithelioid (or histiocytoid) cytologic features.[197] In addition to the lungs and soft tissues, EH also primarily occurs in the bone and liver.[198]

Clinical Summary

EH of the lung is a neoplasm that arises predominantly in female patients; women account for roughly 80% of all cases.[195,199,200] It primarily occurs in young adults, with approximately 50% of affected individuals being younger than 40 years of age; only 10% are older than 50 years of age at diagnosis.[198,201] Many affected persons are asymptomatic, and their tumors are detected incidentally on chest radiographs. Patients who have tumor-related complaints usually present with pleuritic pain, dyspnea, and cough. Case reports have also documented alveolar hemorrhage as a presenting sign of pulmonary EH,[202,203] and it may simulate thromboembolic disease symptomatically as well.[204] Chest radiographs commonly show numerous, small nodular lesions throughout both lung fields (Fig. 14-26).

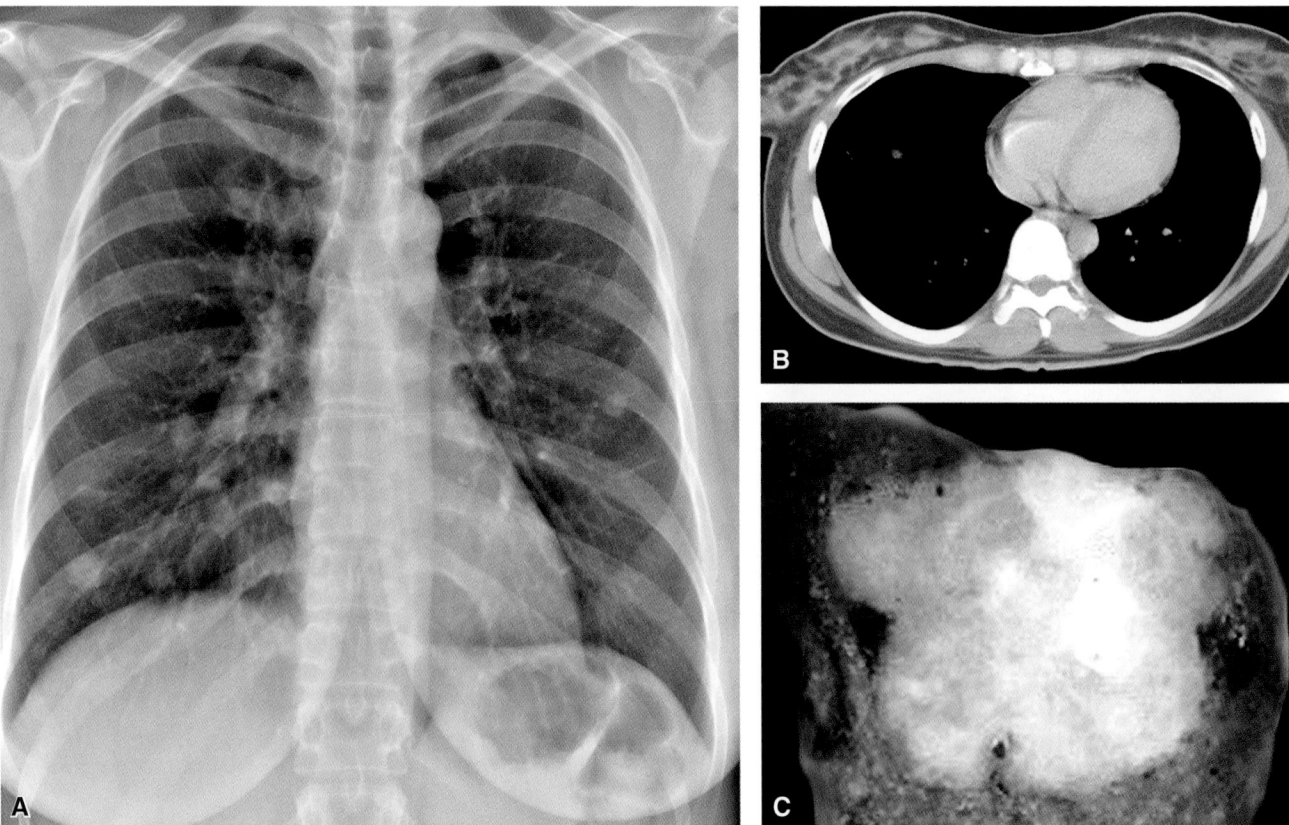

Figure 14-26. Multiple nodular densities are seen throughout both lung fields on plain film radiography (**A**) and computed tomography (**B**) in this case of primary pulmonary epithelioid hemangioendothelioma. **C,** Gross photograph of epithelioid hemangioendothelioma of the lung, in a wedge-excision specimen.

Therefore, EH enters the roentgenographic differential diagnosis of multiple pulmonary nodules in asymptomatic young women, together with metastatic germ cell tumors, chondroid pulmonary hamartomas, multiple arteriovenous malformations of the lung, deposits of "benign metastasizing leiomyoma," and malignant lymphoma.[205]

Pathologic Findings

The pathologic diagnosis of EH is almost always made by open lung biopsy, inasmuch as transbronchial biopsy is usually ineffectual because of sampling constraints. Most nodules of EH are discrete and usually measure less than 2 cm. They are grayish-white to tan and have a chondroid macroscopic consistency. More nodules are typically seen on histologic examination than are apparent grossly. Microscopically, EH is typified by multiple oval or round nodules with hypocellular, sclerotic, or necrotic centers[195,199] (Fig. 14-27). These are surrounded by rims of viable, more cellular tissue that is associated with a myxohyaline fibrous stroma; exceptionally, metaplastic bone formation may be apparent.[206] The neoplastic cell population is composed of plump, epithelioid cells, which are the histologic hallmark of EH (Fig. 14-28). They have centrally located, round-to-oval nuclei, with ample amounts of eosinophilic cytoplasm. Often, intracytoplasmic vacuoles are evident, which should raise the possibility of endothelial differentiation on light microscopy. Saqi and colleagues have described "rhabdoid" cellular differentiation in EH as well.[207]

Tumoral involvement of arterioles, venules, and lymphatics is variable within the tumor nodules as well as other distant sites. EH commonly shows an intra-alveolar pattern of growth secondary to tumor extension through the pores of Kohn, and surgical margins may be, therefore, difficult to ascertain on gross examination if a limited resection of the lesion is attempted.

Ultrastructural and immunohistochemical evaluation can be of great assistance in confirming the endothelial origin of EH.[196,198,208–211] Briefly, ultrastructural features of this tumor include cytoplasmic vacuoles, Weibel-Palade bodies (Fig. 14-29), cell membranous pinocytotic vesicles, and pericellular basal lamina.[210] Histochemical and immunologic markers of endothelial differentiation—such as *Ulex europaeus* I lectin, anti-CD31, anti-FLI-1, and anti-CD34—are helpful in labeling the neoplastic cells in virtually all examples of EH.[206,212] Weinreb and coworkers have also described labeling for CD10 in a majority of EH cases.[213]

Fine needle aspiration biopsy of EH yields a loosely cohesive population of epithelioid cells that may be binucleated or multinucleated. Variably sized cytoplasmic vacuoles are demonstrable in a proportion of the tumor cells (Fig. 14-30).[214]

Therapy and Prognosis

Surgery is usually not feasible as effective treatment for EH because of its tendency to show intrapulmonary multicentricity. Unfortunately, irradiation and chemotherapy likewise have been of little benefit.[195,199]

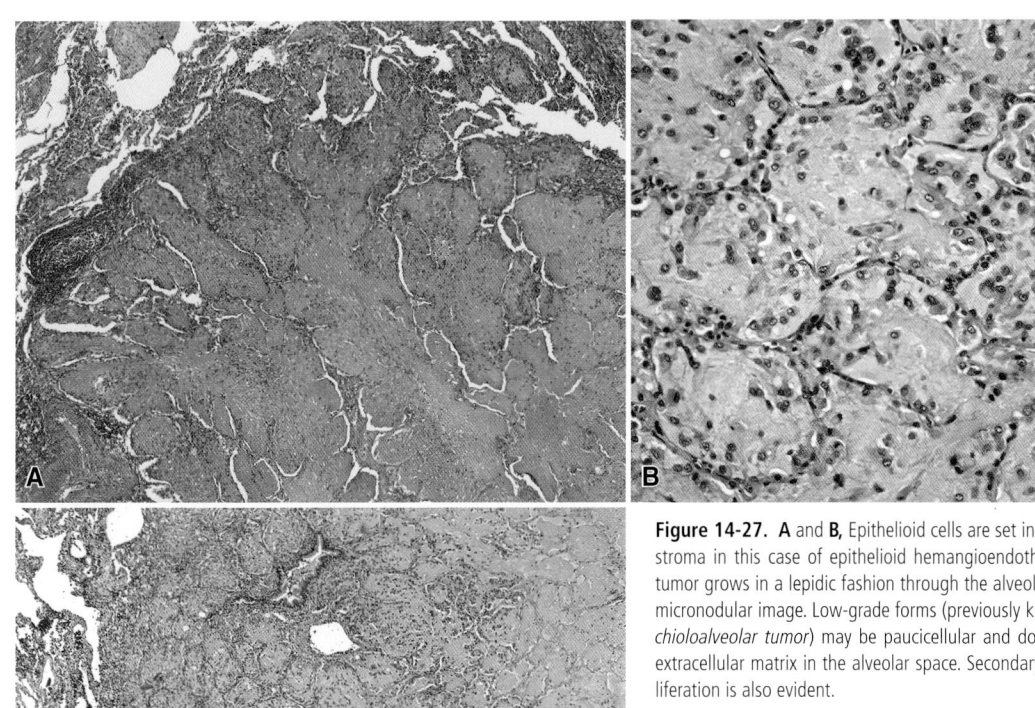

Figure 14-27. A and **B**, Epithelioid cells are set in a sclerotic and myxofibrous stroma in this case of epithelioid hemangioendothelioma of the lung. **C**, The tumor grows in a lepidic fashion through the alveolar pores of Kohn, yielding a micronodular image. Low-grade forms (previously known as *intravascular bronchioloalveolar tumor*) may be paucicellular and dominated by an eosinophilic extracellular matrix in the alveolar space. Secondary alveolar pneumocytic proliferation is also evident.

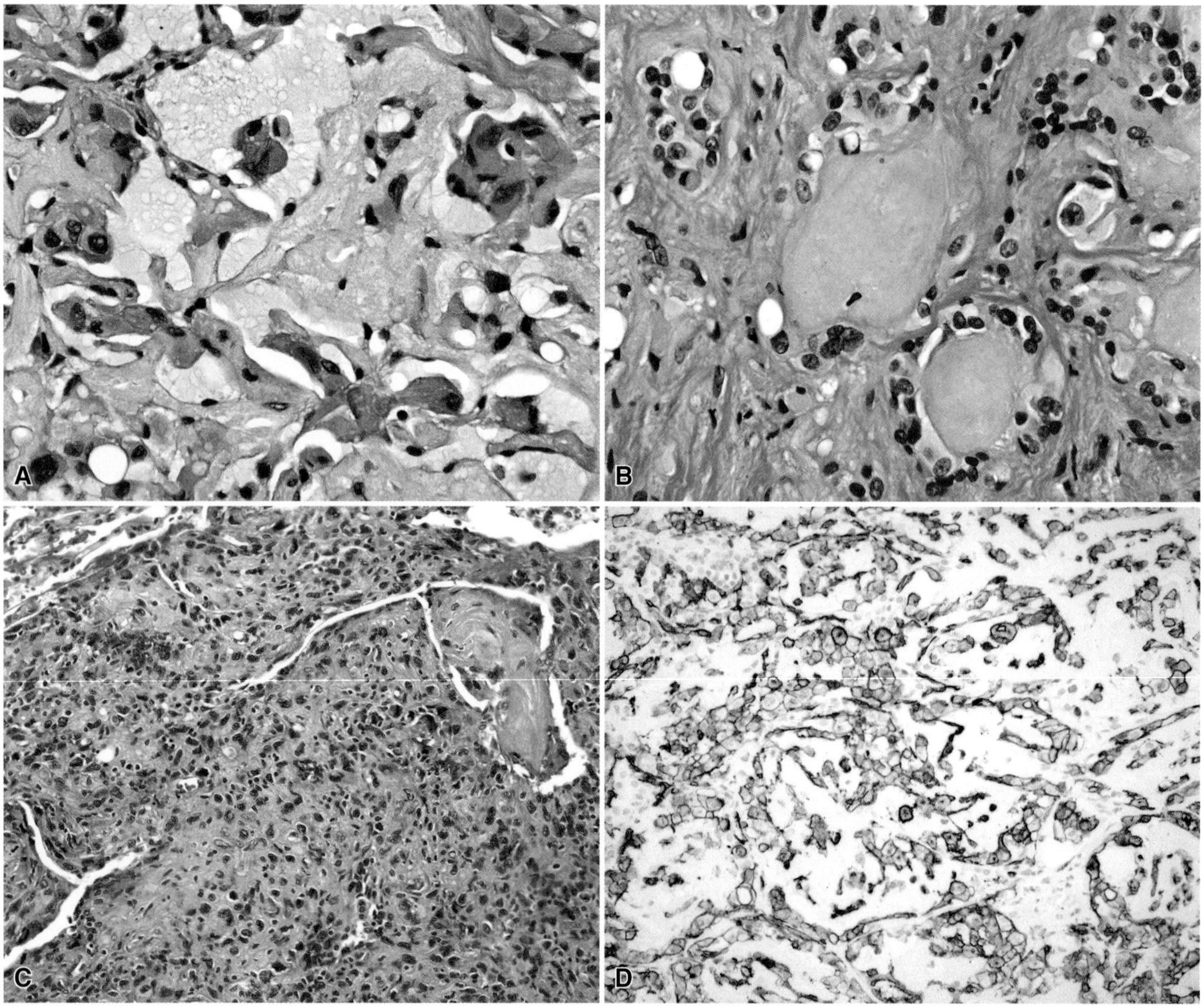

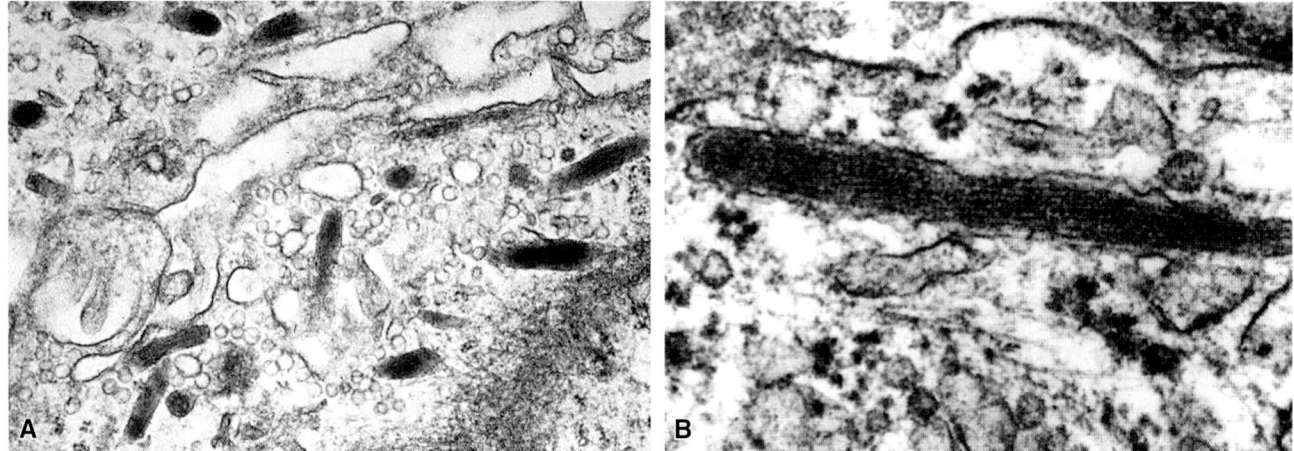

Figure 14-28. A, The epithelioid nature of the tumor cells in pulmonary epithelioid hemangioendothelioma (PEH), as well as the myxofibrous stroma, is clearly seen in these photographs. **B,** The neoplastic cells in PEH are bland cytologically, and some have intracytoplasmic lumina. **C,** This example of PEH demonstrates a greater degree of nuclear atypia. Such tumors may show mitotic activity as well. **D,** Immunoreactivity for CD31 indicating the endothelial nature of PEH.

Figure 14-29. A and **B,** Numerous Weibel-Palade bodies, which have the appearance of lysosomal-like inclusions with internal striations, are present in epithelioid hemangioendothelioma in these electron photomicrographs. These organelles are the intracellular packaging sites for von Willebrand factor.

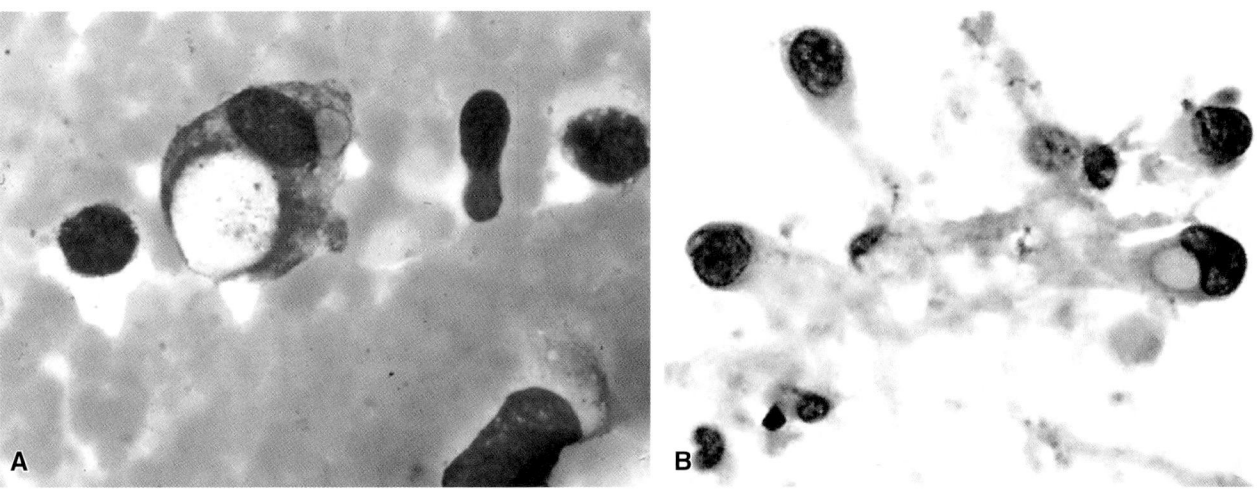

Figure 14-30. Fine needle aspiration biopsy of epithelioid hemangioendothelioma shows dispersed polygonal tumor cells (**A**), some of which contain cytoplasmic vacuoles (**B**).

Nevertheless, EH is generally an indolent neoplasm that is classified as a borderline malignancy. It is associated with a protracted clinical course and potential survival of several years after diagnosis.[208] Most patients do eventually succumb to the tumor and die of respiratory failure secondary to progressive parenchymal replacement; in one series reported by Einsfelder and Kuhnen, 36% of patients were dead or likely to die of their tumors after 52 months' follow-up.[206] Adverse prognostic factors that predict a more rapid decline in pulmonary function include prominent symptoms at the time of presentation; radiographic demonstration of extensive intravascular, endobronchial, or pleural spread of the tumor;[195] and the presence of fusiform tumor cells.[200]

A particularly vexing clinical problem is represented by those patients who have EH synchronously in several organs, including the lungs. In such cases, one is never certain whether tumor multifocality or metastasis is operative. Pragmatically, each involved organ is usually treated as if it harbors an independent primary tumor in this scenario.[215]

The general predilection of EH for women, a reported association of primary hepatic EH with oral contraceptives, and the lack of effective therapy for this tumor have prompted some investigators to explore the possibility of treatment involving hormonal modulation. These tumors have been examined for possible expression of estrogen and progesterone receptor proteins as well as other estradiol-binding moieties. Ohori and colleagues analyzed five cases of pulmonary EH for steroid hormone receptors by immunohistochemical methods, using paraffin-embedded material.[216] Only one case showed apparent binding of estradiol. Our own unpublished experience with the immunohistologic characteristics of pulmonary EH has disclosed no reactivity with monoclonal antibodies against estrogen and progesterone receptor proteins. Thus, we believe that hormonal therapies are unlikely to produce significant results in this setting.

Hemangiopericytoma and Intrapulmonary Solitary Fibrous Tumor

As first described in 1942 by Stout and Murray,[217] hemangiopericytoma (HPC) is an uncommon, potentially malignant neoplasm that shows apparent differentiation toward the phenotype of pericytes. These are cells with long cytoplasmic processes that surround capillaries and serve a vasoregulatory function. HPC occurs most commonly in the deep muscles of the thigh, the pelvic fossa, and the retroperitoneum. However, 5% to 10% of all hemangiopericytomas are said to present

as primary pulmonary tumors.[185,218] It must be remembered that the lungs and the bones are the anatomic sites that most frequently harbor metastases of HPC,[219] and therefore a primary extrapulmonary tumor must be excluded before a diagnosis of a primary HPC can be rendered safely.

It should also be understood that the currently recommended classification scheme for mesenchymal neoplasms has merged HPC with solitary fibrous tumor (SFT).[220,221] Hence, for all intents and purposes, the two entities are considered to be closely related if not identical, and the abbreviation of HPC-SFT will be used in reference to that tumor group.

Clinical Summary

Pulmonary HPC-SFT affects men and women equally, and most commonly arises in middle adulthood. The peak incidence of this lesion is in the fifth decade of life, although individuals as young as 4 years of age and as old as 73 years of age have been reported.[222,223] Some tumors are detected incidentally on radiographic studies without causing pulmonary symptoms; 6 of 18 cases in one series fit this scenario.[224] Alternatively, presenting symptoms may include hemoptysis, chest pain, cough, and dyspnea, and, more rarely, pulmonary osteoarthropathy.[224]

Various radiographic imaging studies have been used in studying this neoplasm. Although angiography has usually not been performed, vascular contrast studies of HPC-SFT generally show a characteristic intralesional "blush."[225] No other pathognomonic features are evident in chest x-rays, CT scans, and MRIs of the lung.[223,226] Plain film x-rays typically show a discrete, homogeneously dense mass with lobulated contours. On CT images, however, HPC-SFT is heterogeneous. Central low-density areas are evident that correspond to necrotic foci, and an apparent capsule may be seen at the interface with surrounding lung parenchyma. MRIs also show intratumoral heterogeneity with respect to tissue density and are apparently more sensitive in depicting intralesional hemorrhage. These images were found to be the most useful in delineating the potential plane of surgical separation between an HPC-SFT and surrounding soft tissue in one report.[227] In summary, a radiologic diagnosis of pulmonary HPC-SFT may be suspected in a middle-aged person lacking pulmonary symptoms, but whose radiographic imaging studies reveal a large, lobulated, sharply marginated, variably dense mass (Fig. 14-31) that does not cause compression atelectasis.[226]

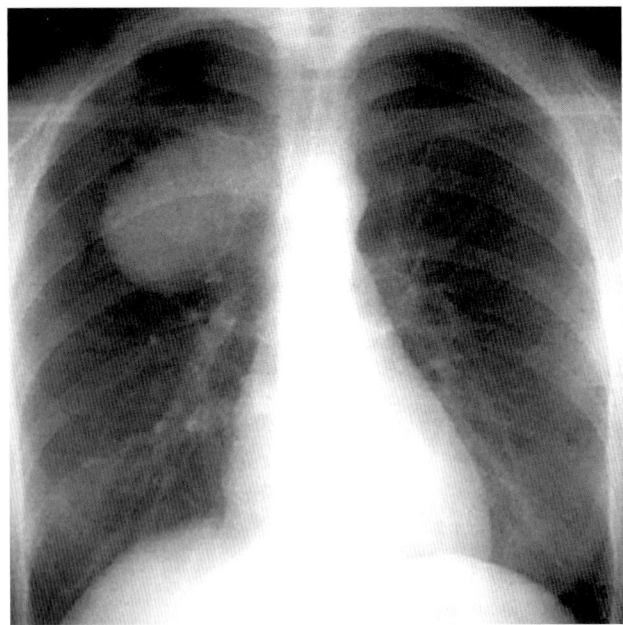

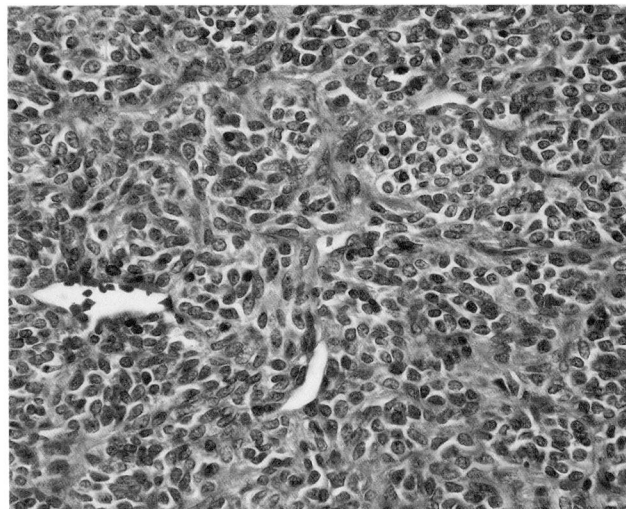

Figure 14-32. Pulmonary hemangiopericytoma showing ill-defined clusters of bluntly fusiform tumor cells and prominent stromal blood vessels.

Figure 14-31. Chest radiograph of primary pulmonary hemangiopericytoma/solitary fibrous tumor, represented by a nondescript large globoid mass in the right upper lung field.

Pathologic Findings

HPC-SFTs of the lung can attain large sizes, and lesions measuring up to 18 cm have been documented. The typical gross appearance of this tumor is that of a well-circumscribed, yellow to tan-brown mass with a pseudocapsule, as well as areas of internal necrosis and hemorrhage. Histologic sections typically show a relatively monomorphous cellular proliferation surrounding thin-walled, anastomosing vascular channels lined by a single endothelial layer. These blood vessels often (but not always) assume gaping, "staghorn," or "antler-like" configurations (Figs. 14-32 and 14-33). The population of neoplastic cells is uniform, with oval compact nuclei and ill-defined cytoplasm.[185] Mitotic activity and areas of necrosis and hemorrhage are noted frequently. Vascular invasion of large pulmonary vessels, however, is uncommon. With regard to the latter features, some pathologists have, in the past, rendered a diagnosis of benign hemangiopericytoma if necrosis, hemorrhage, and

mitoses were absent. In our view, this approach is highly inadvisable. We have seen cases of pulmonary HPC-SFT with exceedingly bland histologic profiles in which metastasis nonetheless supervened. Accordingly, it is advised that each report on this tumor should carry the statement that HPC-SFT is at least *potentially* malignant behaviorally.[219,224]

Pulmonary HPC-SFT has sometimes been overdiagnosed because other neoplasms may show foci that resemble the former lesion. In this regard, it is notable that in their seminal report, Stout and Murray admonished others to make the diagnosis of hemangiopericytoma by ultimate exclusion.[217] The histologic differential diagnosis includes SC, SS, fibrous histiocytomas, leiomyosarcoma, and mesenchymal chondrosarcoma.[219] Distinctions among these neoplasms are best made by ancillary studies.

Electron microscopy can confirm the pericytic nature of HPC through the demonstration of polygonal cells with cytoplasmic processes, pinocytotic vesicles, basal lamina, and a paucity of other organelles.[174,219] HPC-SFT is a neoplasm that demonstrates a relatively restricted group of immunoreactants; these include vimentin, collagen type IV, CD34, CD99, CD57, and bcl-2 protein[54,228] (Fig. 14-34). Endothelial stains such as *Ulex europaeus* I, CD31, and FLI-1 highlight

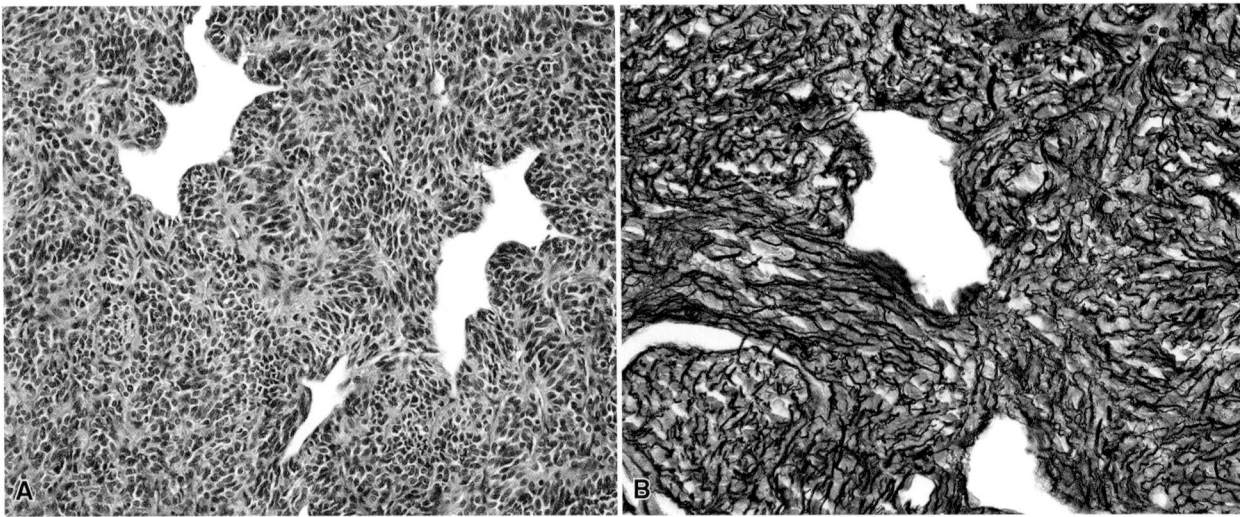

Figure 14-33. A, "Staghorn"-shaped blood vessels in primary pulmonary hemangiopericytoma (HPC). **B,** Individual tumor cells are invested by reticulin fibers in HPC (reticulin stain method).

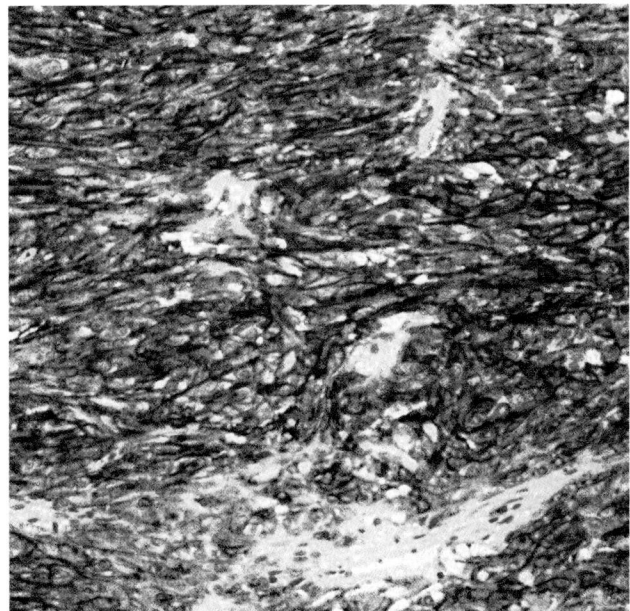

Figure 14-34. Immunoreactivity for CD99 is seen in pulmonary hemangiopericytoma-solitary fibrous tumor. CD34 and *bcl*-2 protein are usually present in this tumor as well.

the lining of intralesional vascular spaces but do not label the surrounding tumor cells. Silver impregnation techniques highlight a complex reticulin matrix with individual cell investment.

Therapy and Prognosis

As in the management of soft tissue HPC-SFT, complete surgical excision is the mainstay of therapy for primary pulmonary tumors of this type. However, it is known that intraoperative rupture of pulmonary HPC-SFT may occur (especially those tumors that are adherent to the chest wall). As expected, this complication results in early local recurrence, as reported by Van Damme and associates, and should therefore be avoided at all costs.[223] Chemotherapy and irradiation have not been shown to be consistently effective adjuvant modalities, but they may have some role to play in management.[229,230] A study by Jha and coworkers on the general role of radiation therapy in treating HPC-SFT showed that postoperative irradiation was useful for local tumor control, salvage therapy after local recurrence, and palliation.[231] Tumors less than 5 cm in maximum dimension exhibit a better response than those that are larger than 10 cm.[232]

As mentioned above, hemangiopericytomas in general are well known for their unpredictable biologic behavior. Postoperative survival has ranged from 10 weeks to 18 years.[223,232] Even with apparently complete surgical resection, HPC-SFT recurs locally within 2 years in approximately 50% of cases,[224,227,233] and later recurrences are seen as well; distant metastasis, however, is uncommon.[228]

Clinical and histologic features that have been cited as prognostically useful[219,222,227] include the presence of symptoms at presentation, mitotic activity of four or more mitoses per 10 high-power microscopic fields, spontaneous tumor necrosis, vascular invasion, and tumor size greater than 5 cm. In one series, metastases were seen in one third of tumors that measured greater than 5 cm, and in two thirds of those greater than 10 cm.[222] However, Yousem and Hochholzer did not find any single histologic or clinical feature that was statistically significant in reliably predicting the clinical course of primary pulmonary HPC-SFT.[224]

Malignant Fibrous Histiocytoma

MFH (now commonly called *pleomorphic sarcoma, not further specified*) is a common, extensively studied soft tissue sarcoma of older adults that develops most frequently in the extremities and the retroperitoneum. In a series of 200 cases by Weiss and Enzinger,[234] the lungs were the most common site of metastases. Thus, exclusion of an occult soft tissue tumor is once again necessary before a diagnosis of primary pulmonary malignant fibrous histiocytoma (PPMFH) can be made. A review of Mayo Clinic cases found only four examples among 10,134 tumors arising in the lung.[171] Currently, there are fewer than 75 reported cases of PPMFH in the English literature.[234–245]

Clinical Summary

In general, MFH is a neoplasm of patients who are in late middle age, with a median of 54 years. However, its occasional occurrence in children and young adults has also been reported.[235,244] No consistent predilection for either gender is seen. Previous irradiation is a pathogenetic risk factor for tumors arising in soft tissue, and the literature similarly contains sporadic reports of PPMFH presenting in patients who have received radiation therapy previously. Clinical and radiographic features of this tumor are nonspecific, and a distinction from the much more common epithelial tumors of the lungs absolutely requires tissue examination. The majority of patients present with symptoms of cough, chest pain, hemoptysis, or dyspnea. Chest x-rays generally show a solitary mass with a nondescript appearance and a relatively homogeneous density on CT or MRI studies.[243]

Pathologic Findings

Most examples of PPMFH are intraparenchymal, but occasional endobronchial lesions have also been observed.[235] There is apparently no predilection for any particular lobe of either lung. These tumors are usually large, ranging up to 25 cm in maximum dimension,[246] with an average size of 6 to 7 cm. They are well circumscribed, lobular, and white-tan, and not uncommonly they contain central necrosis or cavitation on macroscopic examination.

Histologically, PPMFH is characterized by fusiform and pleomorphic elements that are arranged in storiform, fascicular, or medullary patterns (Fig. 14-35). As the name "MFH" implies, this tumor was originally thought to be composed of malignant fibroblast-like and the histiocytoid cells; however, it now appears that there is little if any relationship between the neoplastic elements and true histiocytes. Fusiform tumor cells contain elongated nuclei and relatively scant cytoplasm, and the histiocytoid cells have round-to-oval nuclei with a moderate quantity of amphophilic cytoplasm (Fig. 14-36). A hallmark of most lesions in this category is the presence of large, bizarre, often multinucleated cells with irregular contours. Mitoses, including atypical forms, are easily found and number from 5 to 30 per 10 high-power microscopic fields.[174]

The differential diagnosis of PPMFH by light microscopy includes primary or secondary pleomorphic sarcomas (e.g., dedifferentiated leiomyosarcoma and pleomorphic rhabdomyosarcoma), metastatic malignant melanoma, and SC.[13] Immunohistochemical and electron microscopic studies can be used to separate these pathologic entities.[236–240,246] Ultrastructurally, PPMFH shows fibroblastic and histiocyte-like differentiation, with abundant rough endoplasmic reticulum, numerous lysosomes, and a variable number of small cytoplasmic lipid droplets. Desmosomes, tonofibrils, elongated cell processes, myogenous filament skeins, and cytoplasmic dense bodies are absent. PPMFH expresses vimentin but is devoid of other specialized markers of myogenous, neural, or epithelial differentiation on immunohistologic analyses.[174]

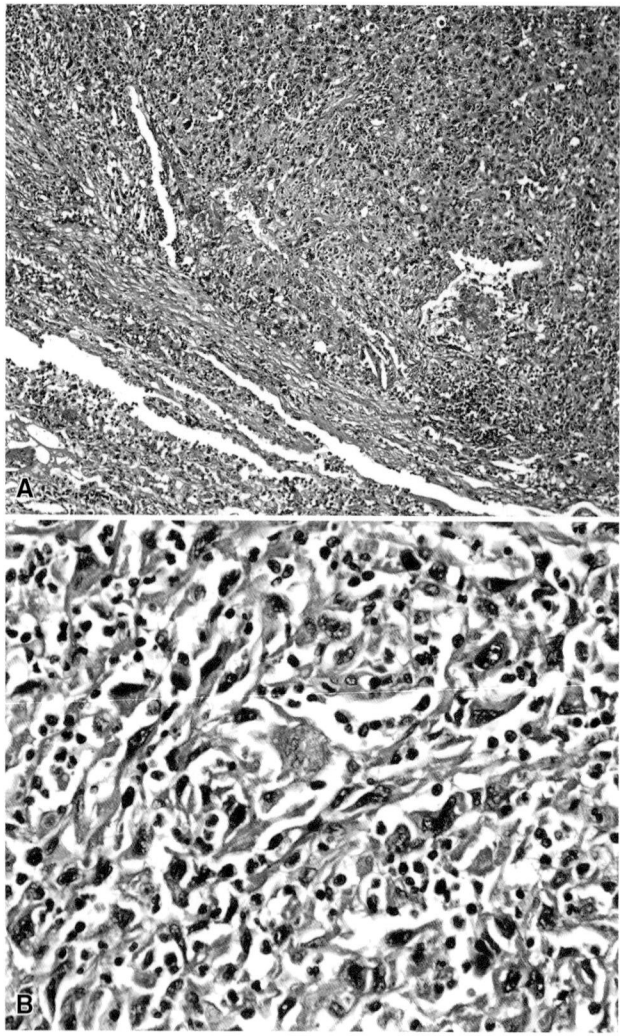

Figure 14-35. A, Primary pulmonary malignant fibrous histiocytoma showing a disorganized proliferation of atypical spindle cells and pleomorphic elements that entraps alveolar airspaces. **B,** Marked nuclear pleomorphism and multinucleation are focally present in the lesion.

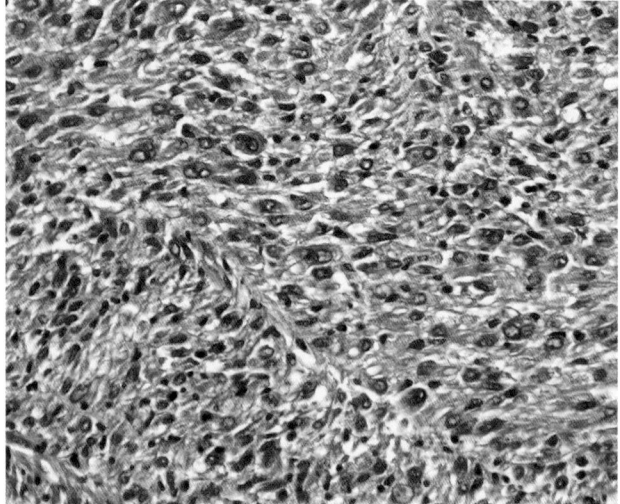

Figure 14-36. This example of primary pulmonary malignant fibrous histiocytoma shows a more epithelioid cell population that could cause diagnostic confusion with poorly differentiated carcinoma.

Therapy and Prognosis

The rarity of PPMFH again serves as an impediment to assessments of optimal treatment for this tumor. Surgical resection is currently the recommended treatment of choice, even if the lesion in question shows limited extrapulmonary spread to the intrathoracic great vessels or soft tissue.[247] Adjunctive chemotherapy and irradiation have not proven to be effective in the few published cases of PPMFH in which these treatments have been used.[235,245,246] In one series of 22 examples,[235] 7 of 15 patients who underwent radical surgical resection suffered relapses and died from metastatic disease. There was recurrence in the lungs and pleura, as well as metastasis to the liver and brain; almost all of these events occurred within 12 months of diagnosis. However, survival for as long as 5 to 10 years has been documented in a few patients with PPMFH.[235,237]

Potential adverse prognostic factors include an advanced clinical or pathologic stage at presentation (with mediastinal, chest wall, or carinal involvement), prominent symptoms at diagnosis, incompleteness of excision, and tumor recurrence. Histologic findings have not been found to affect behavior.

Rhabdomyosarcoma

For practical purposes, primary rhabdomyosarcoma of the lung (RMSL) is a tumor that is confined to the pediatric population. In adults, tumors resembling rhabdomyosarcoma are almost invariably examples of SC,[1,4] and this fact should be borne in mind in interpreting all but the most recent literature on this topic. Moreover, this is another sarcoma type that much more commonly arises outside of the lungs, and the probability that one is dealing with metastasis to the pulmonary parenchyma is therefore important to remember.

Clinical Summary

To date, there are less than 30 well-documented examples of bona fide, "pure" intrapulmonary rhabdomyosarcoma in the pertinent literature. They all occurred in patients who were in the first two decades of life, and most were in children younger than 10 years of age.[248–251] At least one lesion, documented by Choi and colleagues, was seen in a child with neurofibromatosis.[252] Symptoms and signs of RMSL may be nonspecific, including cough, wheezing, and dyspnea, or the patient may present with spontaneous pneumothorax.[253] The latter relates to a peculiar tendency of RMSL to associate itself with cystic lesions of the lungs, particularly as one component of a PPB (see subsequent discussion).[249,250,254] When these cysts rupture, pneumothorax results. The underlying lesions in such cases of RMSL have included not only PPB, but also congenital cystic adenomatoid malformations and peripheral bronchogenic cysts.[254]

Roentgenographic studies may demonstrate a single, nondescript, intraparenchymal mass that is homogeneous on CT or MRI analysis, or they may reveal the presence of a mass in the wall of a cyst. The second of these scenarios is much more likely to result in a correct diagnosis by the radiologist.

Pathologic Findings

As mentioned above, RMSL may be associated with preexisting cystic lesions of the lung. Hence, the cyst walls should always be examined microscopically for a malignant component, despite the contextual rarity of the latter complication.

Pulmonary rhabdomyosarcomas have most often assumed an embryonal or an alveolar growth pattern[249,250] (Figs. 14-37 and 14-38), although pleomorphic tumors, which are usually encountered in the soft tissues of adults, have been reported in the lung as well.[255] These neoplasms are typically composed of small round cells that are configured in one of three ways. These include "solid"

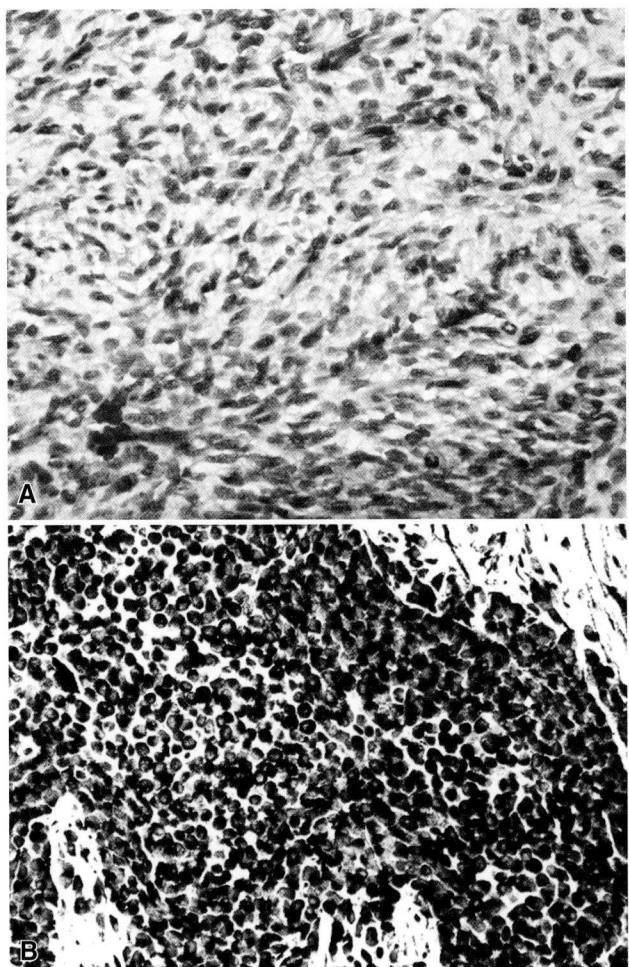

Figure 14-37. A, Embryonal rhabdomyosarcoma (ERMS) of the lung, which presented as an endobronchial lesion in a child. The tumor comprises hyperchromatic small cells with modestly irregular nuclear outlines, set in a myxoid stroma. **B,** Immunoreactivity for desmin is intense in another example of ERMS.

sheetlike clusters with no further distinguishing morphologic attributes, dyscohesive groups with internal pseudolumina or alveoli, and "botryoid" proliferations in which a polypoid lesion (usually within a bronchial lumen) shows a zonation into hypocellular and hypercellular cellular strata (so-called "cambium" layers).[256] In contradistinction to other small round cell tumors of children, RMSL demonstrates a moderate degree of cellular pleomorphism and anisonucleosis. Nuclear chromatin is usually coarse and clumped, cytoplasm is scanty and amphophilic or eosinophilic, and mitoses and apoptotic cells are easily found. Small foci of spontaneous necrosis are also present.

Particularly in those lesions that have an embryonal "solid" appearance histologically, special pathologic studies are nearly always necessary to procure a definitive diagnosis. Moreover, these analyses should also be done in all putative cases in adults, for reasons mentioned earlier. Histochemical stains show that striated muscle tumors contain abundant glycogen, as determined with the periodic acid/Schiff (PAS) method with and without diastase digestion. Electron microscopically, rhabdomyosarcoma is characterized by the focal presence of intermediate filament whorls in the cytoplasm, sometimes with the addition of thick filaments in aggregates that resemble primitive muscular Z-bands (Fig. 14-39). Furthermore, cytoplasmic glycogen

is present, and pericellular basal lamina can be visualized. This constellation of fine structural attributes excludes other small cell tumors from diagnostic consideration.[257] By immunohistology, RMSL is found to express one or more myogenous determinants, such as desmin, tropomyosin, titin, muscle-specific actin, "fast" myosin, myo-D1, myogenin (Fig. 14-40), or Z-band protein.[258–260] Vimentin is also uniformly found, but markers of epithelial differentiation, such as keratin and EMA, must be absent in order to make the diagnosis of RMSL.

Therapy and Prognosis

The great majority of reported cases of RMSL have been treated surgically, with the usual addition of postoperative irradiation and standard chemotherapy such as that used by the InterGroup Rhabdomyosarcoma Study.[248–255] However, there are no controlled studies to determine whether this protocol is the optimal approach to management. Once again, the extreme rarity of the lesion in question interferes with the design of the most efficacious therapeutic regimen.

Prognostically, the fact that RMSL is a visceral manifestation of rhabdomyosarcoma is an adverse clinical variable, along with the probability that such tumors may attain a size of several centimeters before coming to clinical attention. Pathologic features that have been associated with unfavorable tumoral behavior include the focal or global presence of an alveolar growth pattern and the existence of areas that resemble adult-type pleomorphic rhabdomyosarcoma.[261]

Chondrosarcoma of the Respiratory Tract

Chondrosarcomas are uncommon but well-documented in the supporting tissues of both the upper and lower airways. Indeed, although cartilaginous malignancies are usually observed in the proximal long bones of adults, visceral lesions of this type have been reported in a variety of locations. As one would expect, there are few if any examples of primary pulmonary chondrosarcoma (PPCS) that involve the most distal portion of the respiratory tract, because cartilaginous support for the bronchi ends at the level of subsegmental bronchi.[262–264] Accordingly, most of these lesions affect the trachea and major bronchial divisions,[265–267] and chondrosarcomas that are seen in the peripheral lung fields should be carefully examined radiologically to make certain that they are not extensions of contiguous bony lesions in the sternum, vertebral bodies, or ribs.

In contrast to statements pertaining to other sarcoma morphotypes in the lung, the metastasis of chondroid malignancies while they are still occult in peripheral osseous or soft tissue sites is virtually unknown. Thus, once a pathologic diagnosis of chondrosarcoma has been established for a lesion that clearly involves the airway, it may safely be considered to have arisen at that location.

Clinical Summary

Patients with PPCS are adults, with no predilection of the tumor for either gender. They may present with slowly evolving stridor, wheezing, cough, vague chest pain, or episodes of hemoptysis.[264,265] Systemic complaints are not encountered. Tracheobronchoscopy usually demonstrates a smooth, nodular, glistening mass that stretches and attenuates the overlying mucosa but does not ulcerate it. Attempted biopsy of the mass through the bronchoscope is usually unsuccessful because of the firm consistency of the tumor and difficulty of sampling submucosal lesions in general.[262]

Radiographically, there may be no visible abnormalities on plain films if the neoplasm is predominantly or exclusively intraluminal in a large airway. Other examples of PPCS are manifested simply as sharply circumscribed, lobulated masses (Fig. 14-41) that may contain flecks of central calcification or cystic change.[267] The latter findings are more graphically displayed in CT or MRI studies.[265]

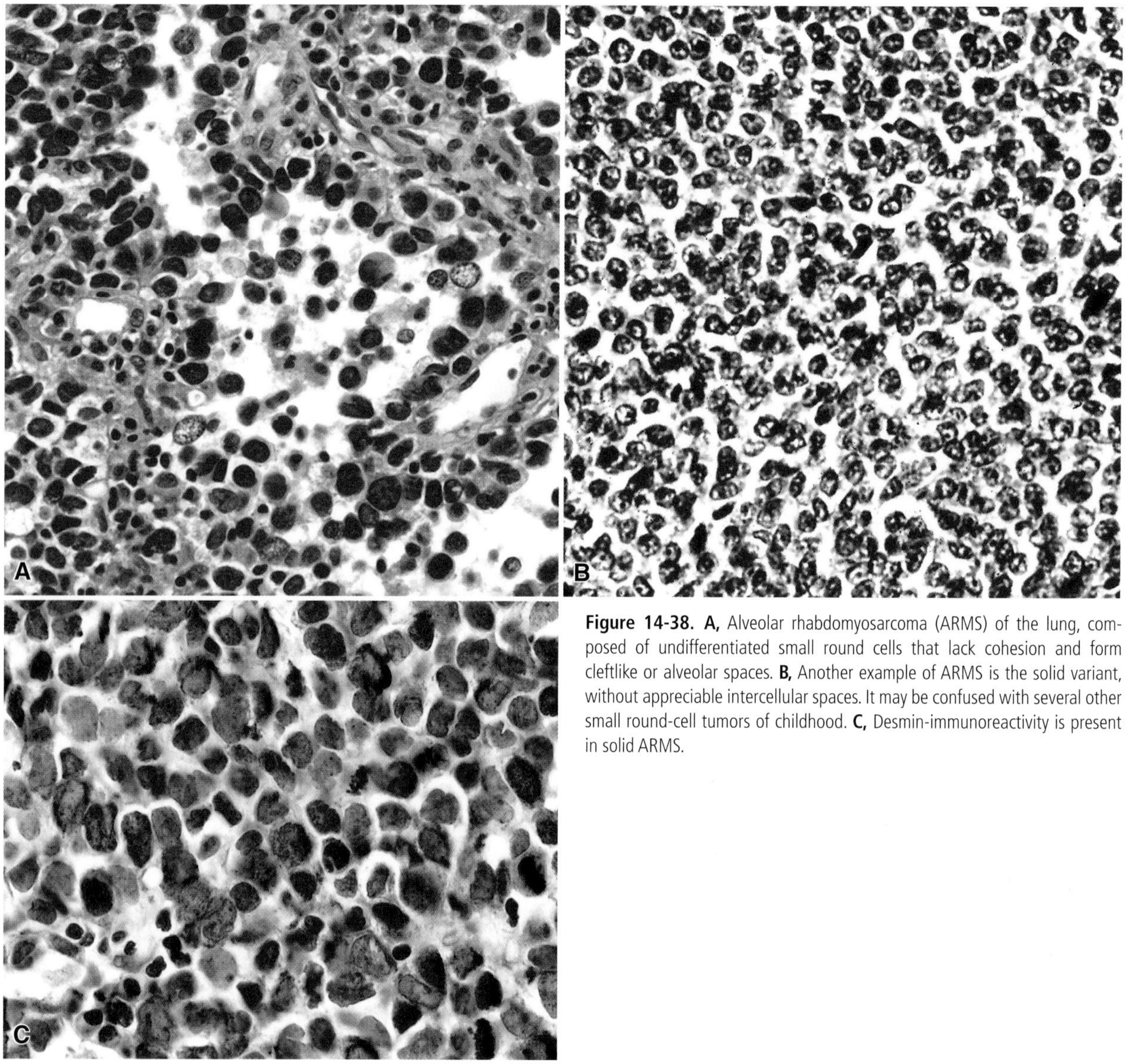

Figure 14-38. A, Alveolar rhabdomyosarcoma (ARMS) of the lung, composed of undifferentiated small round cells that lack cohesion and form cleftlike or alveolar spaces. B, Another example of ARMS is the solid variant, without appreciable intercellular spaces. It may be confused with several other small round-cell tumors of childhood. C, Desmin-immunoreactivity is present in solid ARMS.

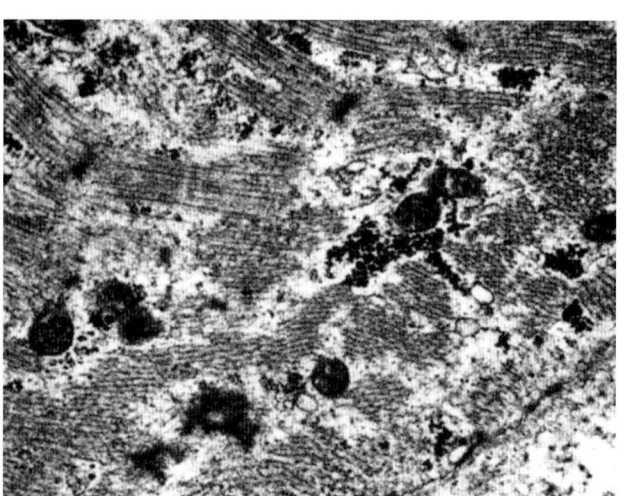

Figure 14-39. Electron photomicrograph of pulmonary rhabdomyosarcoma showing cytoplasmic sarcomeric differentiation with formation of Z-bands.

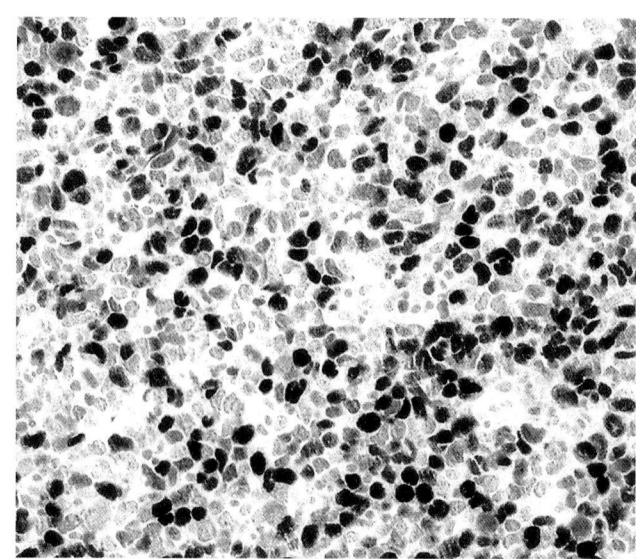

Figure 14-40. Nuclear immunoreactivity for Myo-D1, shown here, is another general feature of rhabdomyosarcoma.

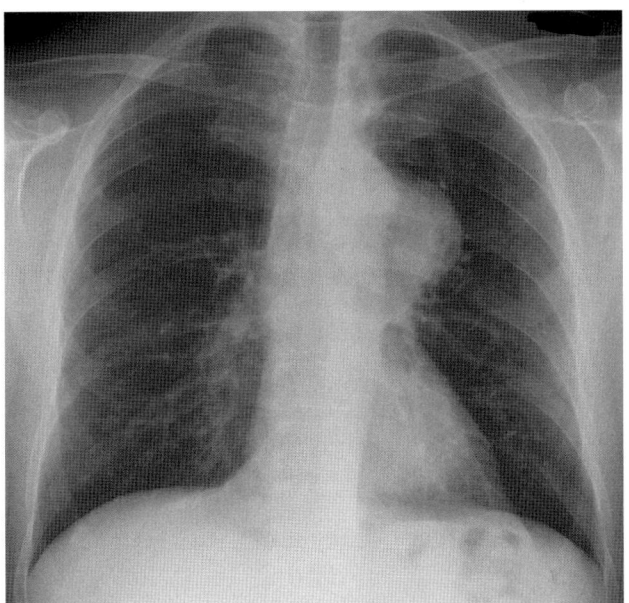

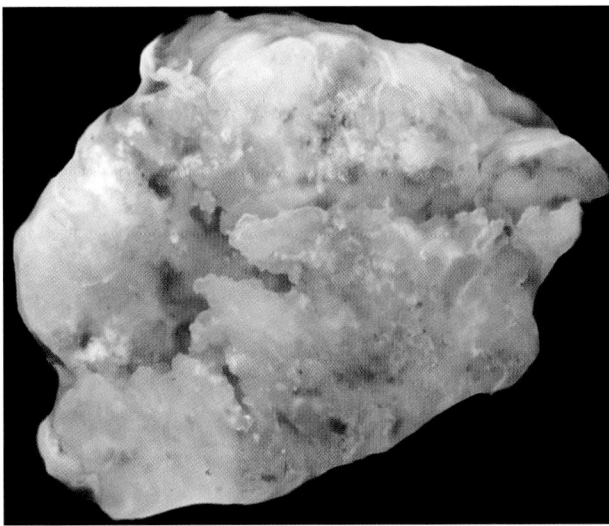

Figure 14-42. Excisional gross specimen of carinal chondrosarcoma demonstrating obvious bluish foci of cartilaginous differentiation.

Figure 14-41. Plain chest film showing chondrosarcoma arising from the carina represented by a rounded mass that projects into the left lung field.

Pathologic Findings

Chondrosarcomas of the lung differ significantly from pulmonary chondroid hamartomas on macroscopic and microscopic grounds. The latter of those two lesions are sharply marginated grossly; they typically entrap small tubular airways and are composed of extremely well-differentiated chondrocytes. In contrast, a PPCS has an irregular peripheral macroscopic interface with the lung (Fig. 14-42); it exhibits at least modest nuclear pleomorphism, nuclear crowding, and cellular binucleation; and it does not contain respiratory epithelial profiles[262,264] (Fig. 14-43). Despite the statements just made, most chondrosarcomas of the lung are well-differentiated tumors. Hence, a striking degree of nondescript spindle cell growth or cellular anaplasia in a cartilage-forming tumor should instead invoke concerns over a probable diagnosis of SC with divergent chondroid areas.[1,4] Mesenchymal chondrosarcomas,[263] represented by small cell neoplasms of childhood with a resemblance to Ewing sarcoma (see later discussion) (Fig. 14-44) are rare and special variants that differ from the descriptions just given. They comprise sheets of small lymphocyte-like cells, often punctuated by hemangiopericytoid blood vessels, with interposed islands of embryonal-type cartilage. Another singular subtype of chondrosarcoma is the dedifferentiated form, in which low-grade chondroid tissue is juxtaposed to a highly anaplastic pleomorphic tumor component (Fig. 14-45). It has been reported only rarely as a primary pulmonary lesion.[268,269]

With these features in mind, there are few other differential diagnostic considerations in cases of PPCS. Thus, special histochemical, ultrastructural, and immunohistochemical assessments are not usually needed to establish a confident diagnosis.

Therapy and Prognosis

Primary chondrosarcomas of the airway are best treated by surgical ablation. Because these are, in most cases, slowly growing and generally low-grade malignancies, such intervention carries with it a good chance of long-term survival if the tumor can be completely extirpated.[265] Chemotherapy and irradiation are ineffectual in treating PPCS and probably incur more morbidity than is acceptable in the treatment

of an indolent sarcoma. On the other hand, those interventions would be appropriate to consider for examples of dedifferentiated PPCS.

In extrapolation from bone tumor pathology, there are only three features that correlate with a risk of recurrence or metastasis of chondrosarcoma: tumor size greater than 5 cm, vascular invasion by the neoplastic cells, and a dedifferentiated microscopic image. There is no evidence that preemptive adjuvant treatment of patients with the first two risk factors in any way improves the clinical outlook. Indeed, it is our opinion that reoperation to remove any recurrent masses is the most sensible approach to patient management in this context.

Primary Pulmonary Synovial Sarcoma

Although SS is primarily a peripheral soft tissue tumor, it is also potentially seen as a primary pleuropulmonary lesion. Published reports of approximately 100 cases have now attested to that fact.[190,270–278] Because of the range of histologic and radiographic appearances associated with SS, it enters into differential diagnosis with several other neoplasms in the lung and pleura.

Clinical Findings

The basic symptoms and signs that are associated with primary pulmonary SS are no different than those attending bronchogenic carcinomas, except they are seen in a younger age group (mean, 38.5 years). Chest pain, cough, shortness of breath, and hemoptysis may be encountered, but, in one series, one fourth of all patients were asymptomatic.[270] Men and women are relatively equally likely to develop SS of the lung. Roentgenographically, there is usually little to point the radiologist toward a specific diagnosis of SS in the lung (Fig. 14-46), which may arise in any segment of any pulmonary lobe. However, some cases show flocculent or particulate calcification on plain film radiographs or CT scans. Cystic change may also be noted, and a minority of lesions is clearly associated with a major bronchus.[270–277]

Pathologic Findings

The gross and microscopic spectrum of SS of the lung parallels that seen in similar tumors of peripheral soft tissue.[279] Macroscopically, one sees a fleshy, ill-circumscribed mass in virtually any intrapulmonary location (Fig. 14-47). Classically, biphasic SS is composed of fascicles of compact spindle cells arranged in interweaving or "herringbone"

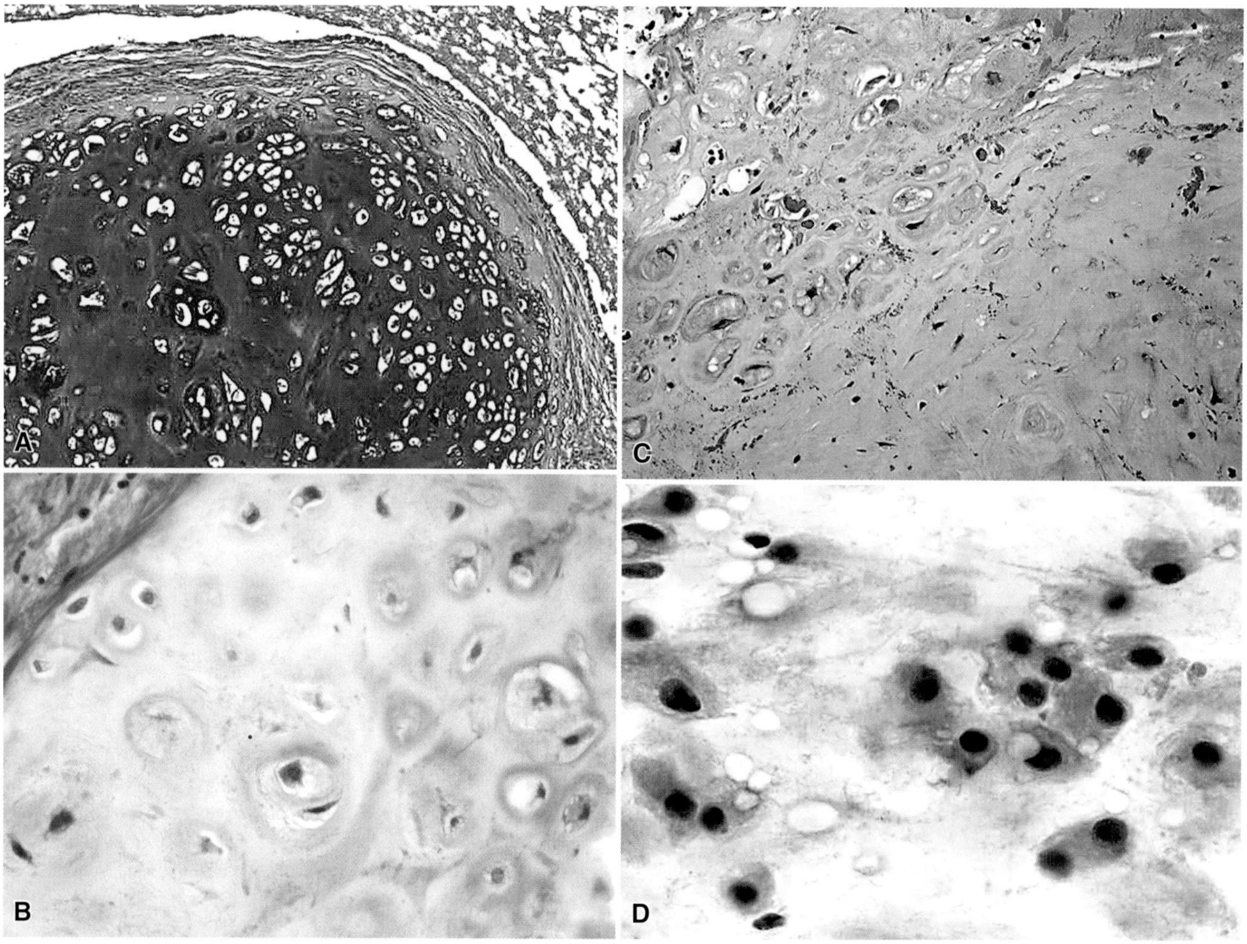

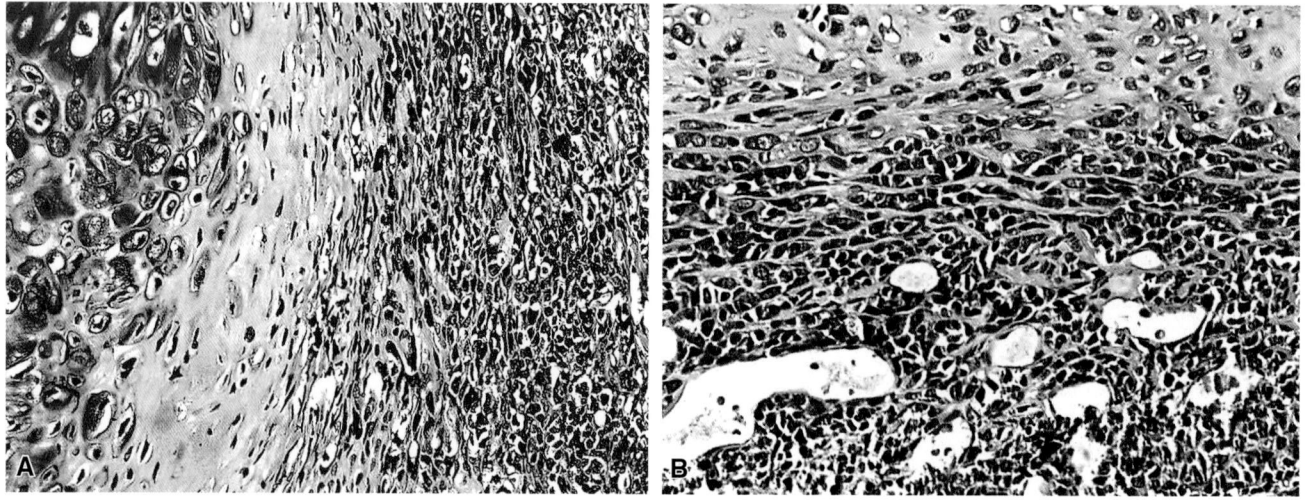

Figure 14-43. Low-grade chondrosarcoma of the carina. **A** to **C,** The constituent neoplastic chondrocytes are minimally atypical, but this particular lesion grossly demonstrated obvious destruction of the wall of the airway and justified a malignant diagnosis. **D,** Fine needle aspiration biopsy of the tumor shows dyshesive ovoid cells, some of which contain cytoplasmic vacuoles. The stroma is amorphous.

Figure 14-44. A and **B,** Mesenchymal chondrosarcoma of the lung showing a juxtaposition of chondroid islands and undifferentiated small round tumor cells.

fascicles, punctuated by clefts or overtly glandlike spaces that are lined by cuboidal to low columnar tumor cells (Fig. 14-48). The latter inclusions may contain mucoid matrical material and may also demonstrate squamous or goblet cell metaplasia. Nuclei of the neoplastic cells in both components are generally monomorphic, with dispersed chromatin and inconspicuous nucleoli. Cytoplasm is sparse in the fusiform cellular elements. In contrast, a moderate quantity of amphophilic, eosinophilic, or vacuolated cytoplasm is apparent in glandlike foci. Mitotic activity is greatly variable, may be surprisingly scant, and only rarely features the presence of "atypical" division figures. Intercellular

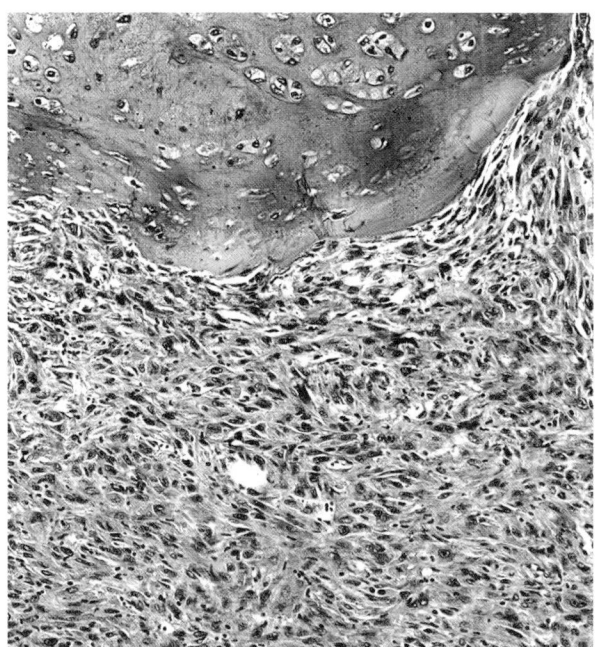

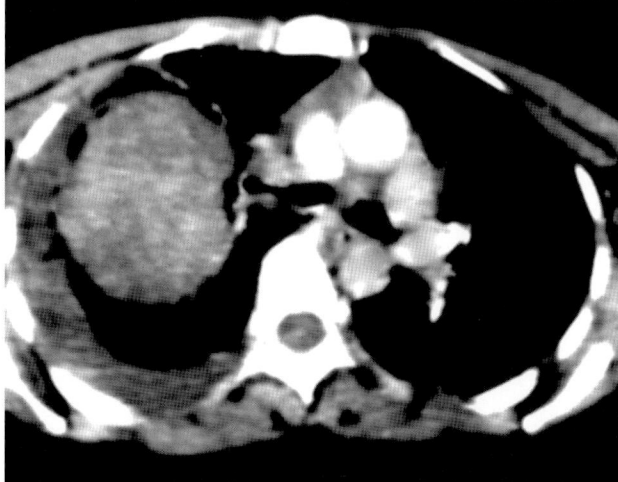

Figure 14-46. Computed tomography scan of primary pulmonary synovial sarcoma showing a large mass in the right hemithorax.

Figure 14-45. Dedifferentiated chondrosarcoma of the lung demonstrating a low-grade "parent" component (*top*) and an abruptly juxtaposed anaplastic sarcomatous derivative thereof (*bottom*).

calcifications (sometimes with a psammomatous configuration) may be scattered randomly throughout the tumor (Fig. 14-49), be clustered in discrete foci, or be lacking altogether. The finding of necrosis is likewise highly variable. Tumoral stroma can be overtly collagenous, delicate and fibrovascular, or myxoid. Besides the prototypic form of biphasic SS, another with an admixture of solid polygonal cell clusters and spindle cell zones (Fig. 14-50) is recognized.[279]

The existence of monophasic SS is now undeniable. This variant may be composed entirely of fusiform elements, epithelioid polygonal cells that may or may not demonstrate obvious glandlike differentiation, or sheets of small round cells.[270] Monophasic spindle cell SS is more common by far (Fig. 14-51), and recognition of it as a distinct entity has resulted in reclassification of many fibrosarcomas of the soft tissues and other sites. It is now realized that the great majority

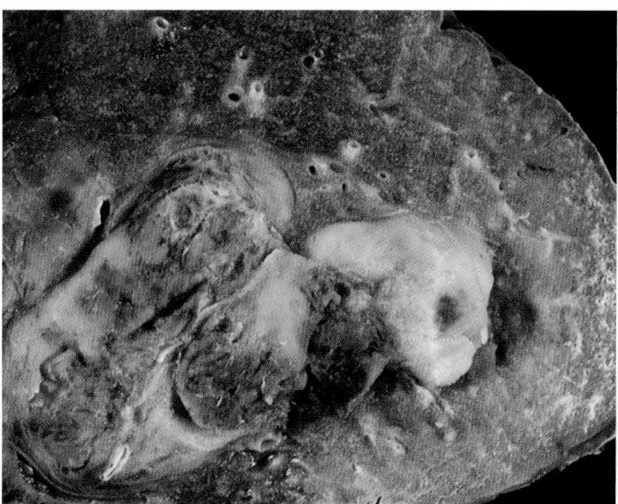

Figure 14-47. Grossly, primary pulmonary synovial sarcoma exhibits a fleshy tan-gray cut surface.

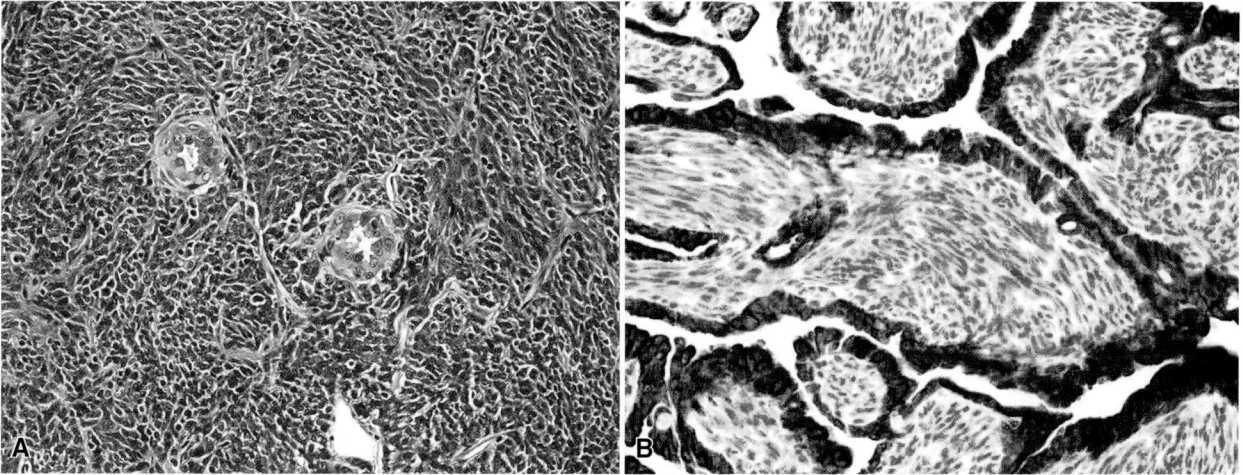

Figure 14-48. A, Photomicrograph of biphasic synovial sarcoma of the lung. The tumor contains glandlike epithelial structures punctuating a neoplastic spindle cell proliferation. Diagnostic confusion with biphasic sarcomatoid carcinoma is possible. **B,** Immunostaining for pankeratin highlights the overtly epithelial glandular component of this neoplasm.

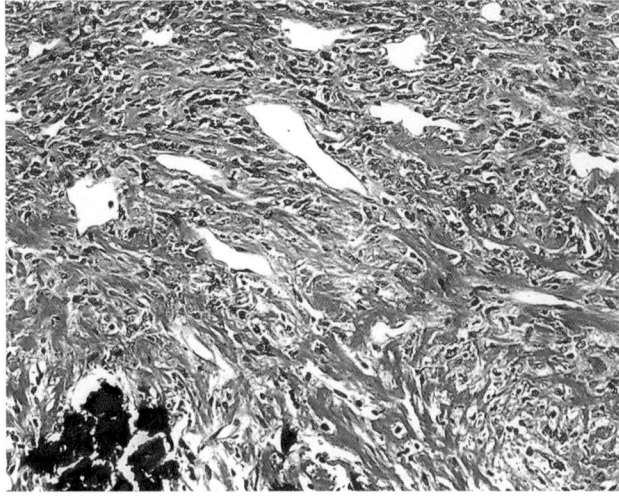

Figure 14-49. Stromal calcification is present in this pulmonary synovial sarcoma.

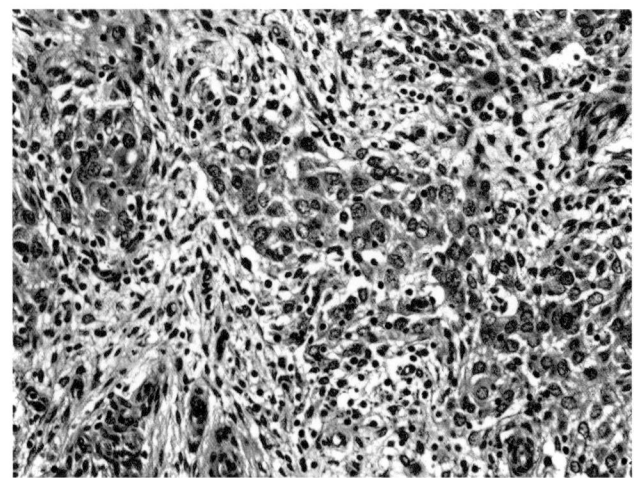

Figure 14-50. Another variant of biphasic synovial sarcoma of the lung contains solid epithelial cell nests, admixed with spindle cell areas.

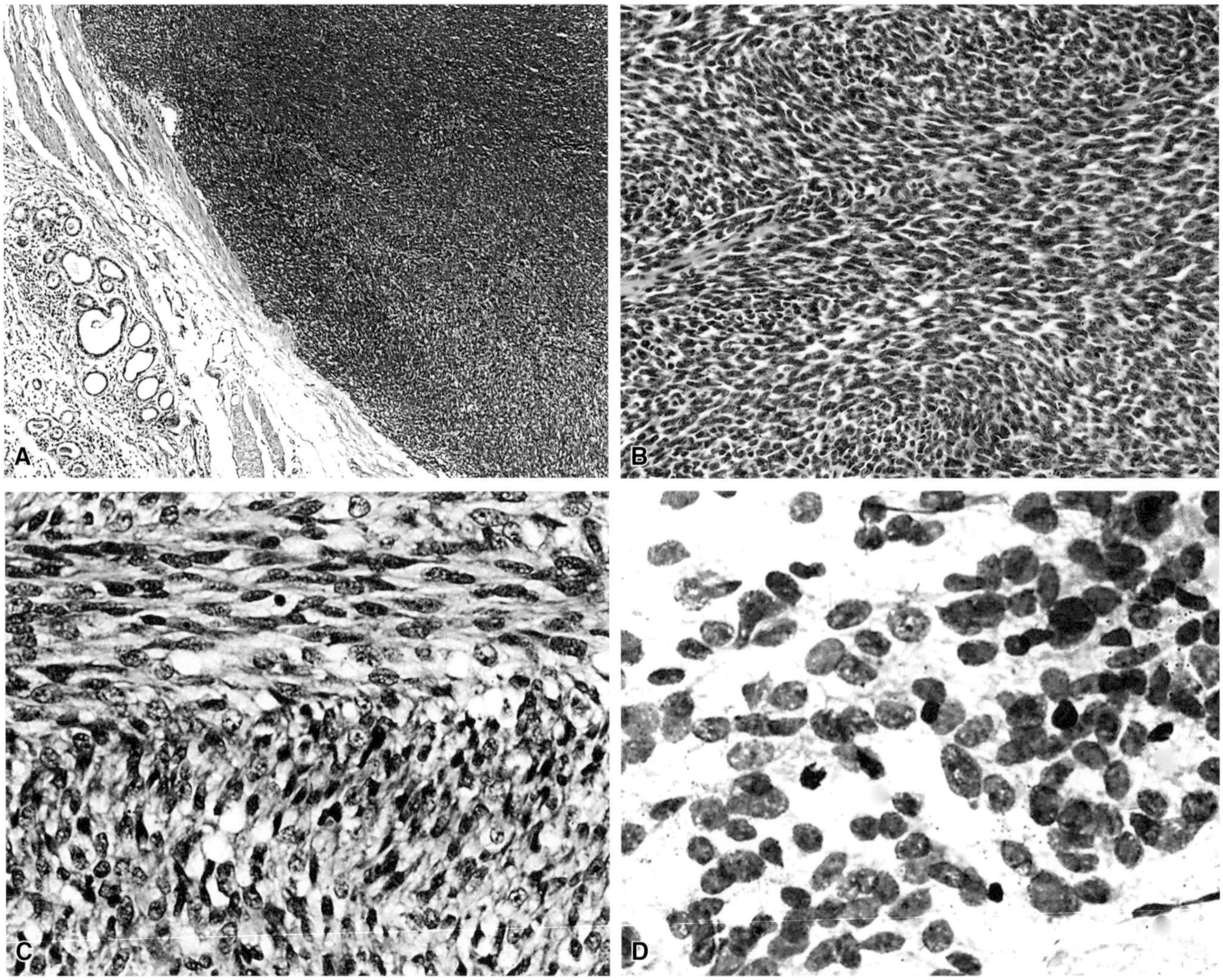

Figure 14-51. **A** to **C,** Monophasic spindle cell synovial sarcoma (MSS). The images shown here overlap with those of sarcomatoid carcinomas as well as other sarcoma morphotypes. **D,** Fine needle aspiration biopsy of MSS shows loosely cohesive and blunt-ended spindle cells with no other distinguishing cytologic features.

of sarcomas with a "herringbone" spindle cell constituency are actually synovial rather than fibroblastic, as traditionally taught.[258] Another key feature to the recognition of monophasic spindle cell SS is the presence of a "staghorn" pattern of intratumoral vascularity.[279] Divergent differentiation, simulating osteogenic, neural, or squamous lesions, is another pathologic facet of monophasic SS that may cause diagnostic consternation.[270]

Electron microscopy and immunohistology have shown that SS is actually an epithelial proliferation, with ultrastructurally well-formed junctional complexes between the tumor cells.[258,279] Reticulin stains are often useful in outlining epithelioid cell clusters when they are present but indistinct. Immunostains for keratin and EMA (Fig. 14-52) can be used to similar advantage; these determinants are also commonly seen together with vimentin in the spindle cells of biphasic or monophasic SS. CD99, calretinin, and bcl-2 protein are often observed in SS as well.[279] Another extremely useful marker is TLE-1; it is a nuclear protein that is observed in virtually all cases of SS[141-144] (Fig. 14-53); there is some sharing of reactivity for TLE1 with neural neoplasms,[143] but, when used in an immunohistochemical panel setting, that should not pose a diagnostic problem. It is clear that SS shows a characteristic t(X;18) (p11.2;q11.2) chromosomal translocation (Fig. 14-54), which can be assessed using traditional cytogenetic techniques or fluorescence or chromogenic in situ hybridization.[272,273] This karyotypic aberration produces a selective fusion transcript known as SYT-SSX, and the polymerase chain reaction can be used to detect it diagnostically, using suitable primer pairs of nucleotides.[144,277]

The major differential diagnostic alternatives to primary SS in the lung are metastatic SS from soft tissue sites, HPC-SFT, fibrosarcoma, mesothelioma, and SC. Among these possibilities, only SS shows the aforementioned t(X;18) chromosomal abnormality, making cytogenetic evaluation, with or without other adjunctive studies, highly desirable in this context. A decision tree that can be used in the differential diagnosis of SS is shown in Figure 14-55.

Therapy and Prognosis

The long-term outlook for patients with SS of the lung is guarded at best. In a series reported by Zeren and associates, 14 of 18 patients had died of their tumors or were likely to do so at a mean follow-up period of 12.5 years.[270] In general, this neoplasm has the ability to recur locally or demonstrate distant metastasis many years after its initial diagnosis; indeed, follow-up shows that tumor-related mortality continues to accrue up to 20 years after presentation.[279]

Essary and coworkers[280] also reported that primary pulmonary SS is a more aggressive lesion than its soft tissue counterpart. They posited that this was due to its usual large size at diagnosis and because of a common difficulty in resecting the tumor completely.

Recommended therapy for primary pulmonary SS is predicated on radical surgical extirpation. The efficacy of adjuvant radiation treatment and chemotherapy is somewhat controversial.

Other Primary Pulmonary Sarcomas

In addition to those tumors that have been previously considered, other sarcoma morphotypes may be encountered in the lungs. These include liposarcoma[281-283] (Fig. 14-56), angiosarcoma,[245,284] malignant peripheral nerve sheath tumor,[185,190,285,286] osteosarcoma,[245,287] angiomatoid fibrous histiocytoma[288] (Fig. 14-57), and alveolar soft parts sarcoma[289-292] (Fig. 14-58). Fewer than 20 cases each of these neoplasms have been documented in the literature, making it impossible to present their clinicopathologic attributes as if they were thoroughly studied and well-characterized.

However, a few generalizations do appear to be appropriate. First, liposarcomas and malignant schwannomas of the lung have usually

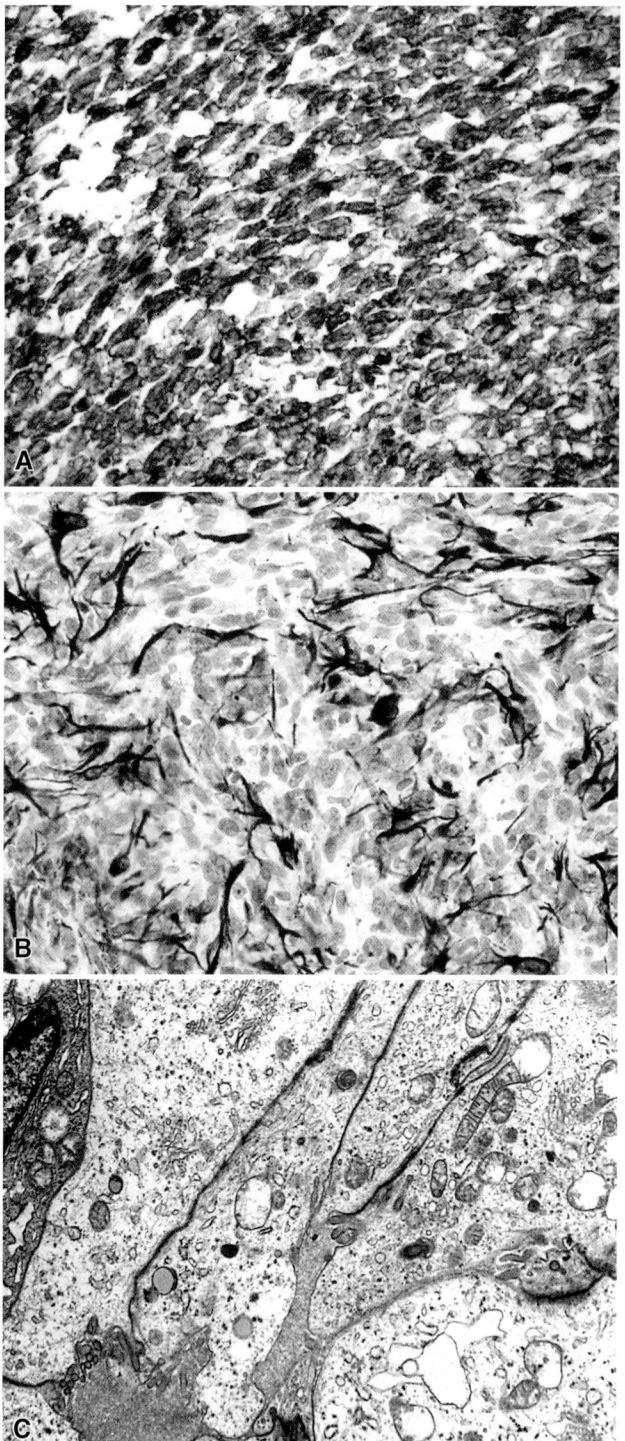

Figure 14-52. Immunoreactivity for epithelial membrane antigen (**A**) and pankeratin (**B**) is potentially seen in monophasic synovial sarcoma (MSS). **C,** Electron microscopy of MSS demonstrates well-formed junctional complexes between the fusiform tumor cells, consistent with their epithelial nature.

been documented as tumors that have an endobronchial component, potentially producing airway obstruction. In contrast, this feature is not part of the profile of either angiosarcoma or osteosarcoma. Secondly, both angiosarcoma-like and osteosarcoma-like epithelial neoplasms are vastly more common in the respiratory tract than true sarcomas with those respective microscopic patterns.[4] Thus, the pathologist

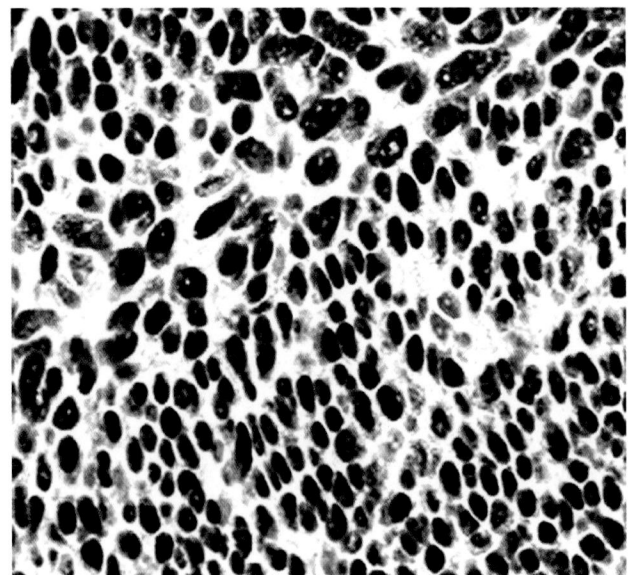

Figure 14-53. Nuclear immunoreactivity for TLE1 is a selective marker for synovial sarcoma of both monophasic and biphasic types, among all sarcoma morphotypes.

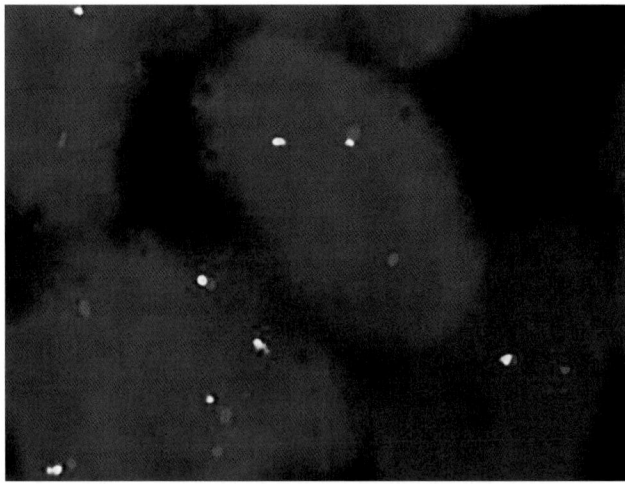

Figure 14-54. Fluorescent in situ hybridization preparation from primary pulmonary synovial sarcoma showing the t(X;18) chromosomal translocation that typifies this neoplasm. The green signal (white in this image) corresponds to a segment of chromosome 18; the red signal corresponds to a segment on the X chromosome.

must be certain to address the likelihood of SC under such circumstances. Finally, therapy for those rare lesions in this category that have proven to be primary in the lungs is completely anecdotal and has been based on extrapolation from treatment used for histologically similar neoplasms in osseous and soft tissue sites.

Primary Malignant Melanomas of the Lung

Melanomas arising primarily in the lung are extraordinarily rare; the literature contains sparse reports on this topic.[293–303] The largest series is from the AFIP, consisting of eight cases seen over a period of many years.[293] Although rigorous criteria have been proposed for primary malignant melanoma of the lung (PMML), this interpretation cannot be established with absolute certainty because of the well-known capacity for spontaneous regression of primary melanomas in mucosal or cutaneous sites. To consider a diagnosis of PMML seriously, there obviously must be no prior history of a potentially malignant pigmented tumor of the skin or ocular uveal tract. Moreover, clinical examination for possibly occult melanomas in the integument, nail beds, eyes, nasal cavity, paranasal sinuses, oral cavity, esophagus, anus, rectum, vulva, and leptomeninges should not show any extrapulmonary lesions. In fact, some authors have suggested that a case of PMML can be regarded as bona fide only retrospectively, after a postmortem examination has excluded another source of a primary melanoma.[294–296] Hence, it is self-evident that this diagnosis can never be considered irrefutable during life.

As to the fundamental question of the origin of primary melanoma in the respiratory tract, some have stressed that the tracheobronchial

Figure 14-55. Decision tree for the immunohistochemical diagnosis of synovial sarcoma. (+), positive; (–), negative; EMA, epithelial membrane antigen; Indeterm, immunohistologically indeterminate category (requires molecular characterization for diagnosis); Meso, mesothelioma; Sarc CA, sarcomatoid carcinoma; SFT, solitary fibrous tumor; Syn Sarc, synovial sarcoma.

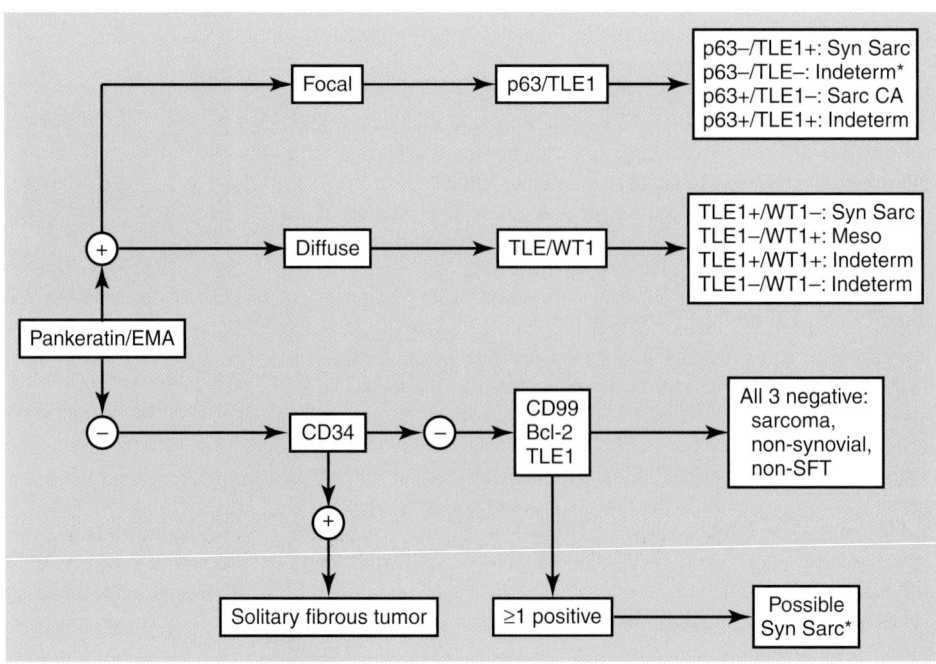

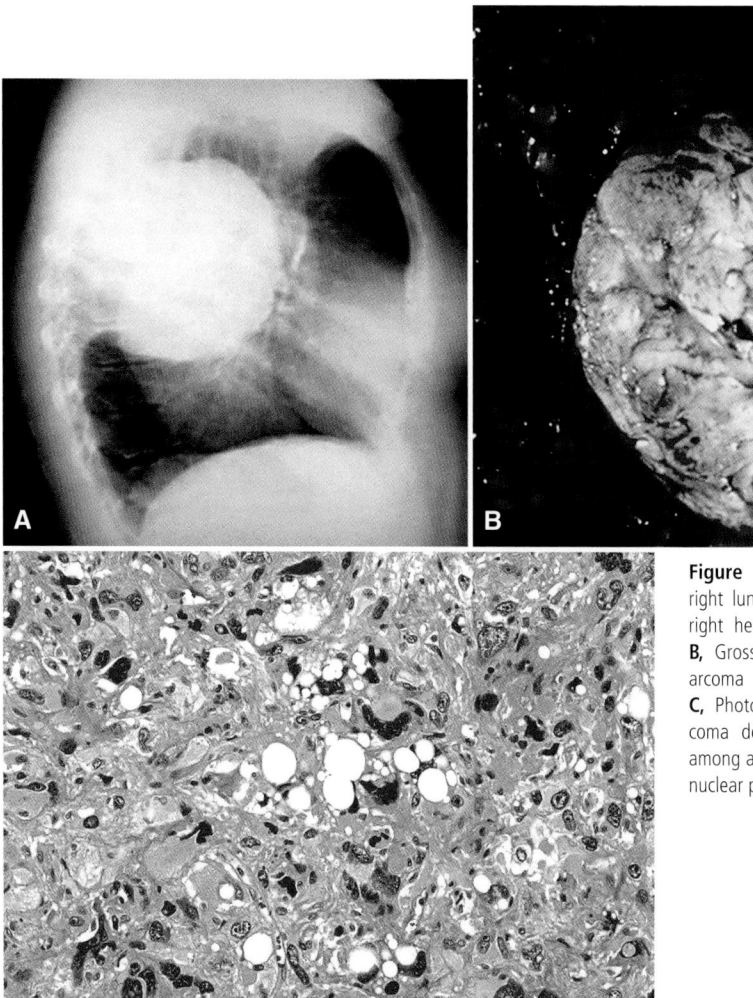

Figure 14-56. A, Pleomorphic liposarcoma of the right lung represented by a large rounded mass in the right hemithorax on this lateral plain film radiograph. **B,** Gross photograph of pleomorphic pulmonary liposarcoma showing a yellow-white, lobulated cut surface. **C,** Photomicrograph of pleomorphic pulmonary liposarcoma demonstrating obvious lipoblastic differentiation among a population of cells with markedly heterogeneous nuclear profiles.

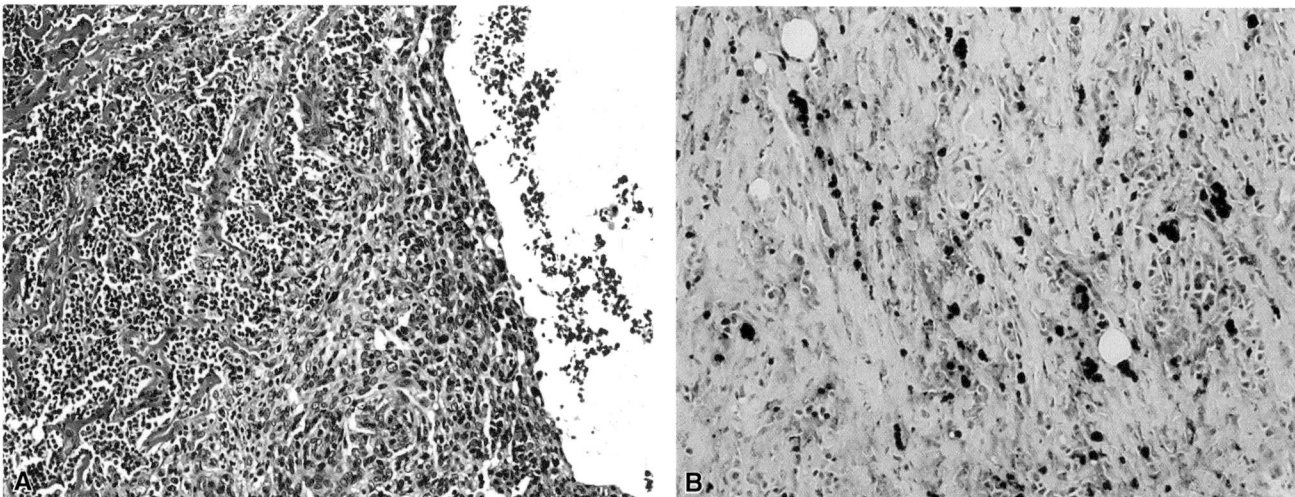

Figure 14-57. A, Angiomatoid (malignant) fibrous histiocytoma (AFH) of the lung showing a central blood lake (*right*), a zone of relatively monomorphic spindle cells, and a cuff of mature lymphocytes (*left*). This tumor manifests either a t(12;16)(q13;p11) or a t(12;22)(q13;p12) chromosomal translocation, yielding *FUS-ATF1* and *EWSR1-ATF1* fusion genes, respectively. **B,** Perls staining of AFH shows abundant deposits of hemosiderin amid the tumor cells, providing a potentially helpful finding in differential diagnosis with other spindle cell lesions.

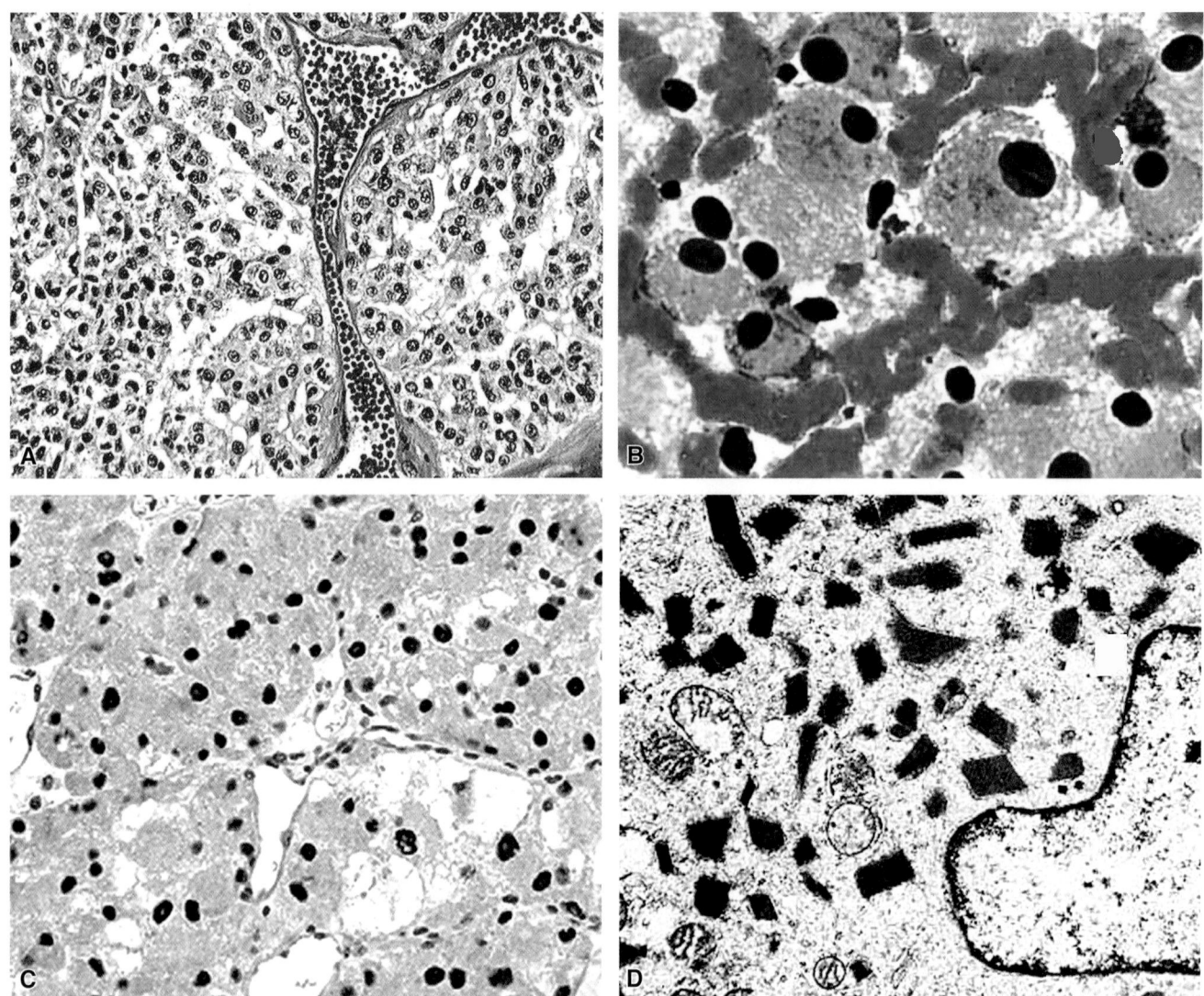

Figure 14-58. A, Alveolar soft part sarcoma (ASPS), primary in the lung, comprising well-defined nests of loosely-apposed epithelioid cells with prominent nucleoli and eosinophilic cytoplasm. This tumor exhibits a recurrent der(17) chromosomal aberration, related to a nonreciprocal t(X;17)(p11.2;q25) translocation. **B,** Fine needle aspiration biopsy of ASPS showing dyshesive large round cells with fluffy amphophilic cytoplasm. **C,** Nuclear immunoreactivity for the TFE3 protein is present in ASPS, related to the t(X;17) translocation. **D,** ASPS contains crystalloid cytoplasmic inclusions by electron microscopy. These structures are thought to represent aggregates of myogenous proteins. (**B,** Courtesy of Dr. Paul Wakely, Columbus, OH.)

tree is, in fact, of endodermal derivation—similar to the oral cavity and the esophagus—where well-documented primary melanomas have originated.[296] Nonetheless, these tumors are generally thought to be neuroectodermal, and their presence in endodermal or mesodermal sites is therefore problematic with reference to classic histogenetic theory. We instead subscribe to the "stem cell" theory of neoplasia, wherein embryologic constructs are essentially irrelevant, to explain the phenomenon under discussion here. In that vein, it is interesting that some benign proliferations of the lung also demonstrate partial or global melanocytic differentiation—namely, clear-cell "sugar" tumor, angiomyolipoma, and lymphangioleiomyomatosis.[304–308]

Clinical Summary
The ages of reported patients with PMML have ranged from 29 to 80 years. Because of the rarity of this lesion, no meaningful statements can be made regarding gender-related incidence figures. Some patients with bronchopulmonary melanoma have been asymptomatic, whereas others have presented with hemoptysis, dyspnea, or cough.[293–301] A location in the lumen of the trachea may be associated with asthma-

like symptoms. Plain film radiographic examinations generally have shown abnormalities only if the tumors were in the pulmonary parenchyma; in other words, endobronchial tumors are visible only on CT or MRI.

Pathologic Findings
In several reported cases of PMML, the lesions have been centered in large airways, including the trachea and major bronchi.[293,299,301,309–311] Grossly, these tumors are generally polypoid, endoluminal masses that are partially or completely obstructing, or they present as nodules within the lung parenchyma, which range from 1 to 4.5 cm in greatest dimension. In addition, they are characteristically colored, in shades of brown or black, but may occasionally be amelanotic (tan-gray).

Histologically, PMMLs are composed of heterogeneously pigmented and variably pleomorphic cells that range from epithelioid to fusiform in configuration with occasional gigantiform figures; overtly sarcoma-like lesions are certainly part of the repertoire of these neoplasms (Fig. 14-59). Indeed, divergent differentiation into chondro-osseous–like tissue has been reported in melanomas.[312]

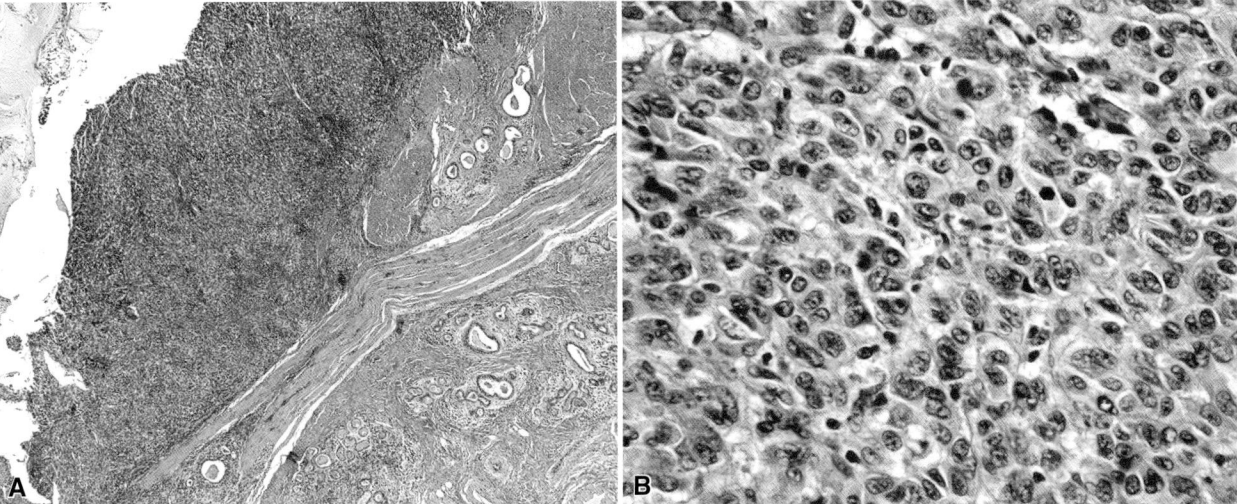

Figure 14-59. A and **B,** Apparently primary malignant melanoma of the lung represented by an amelanotic proliferation of pleomorphic tumor cells within a bronchus. Immunohistologic studies were necessary to support the presence of melanocytic differentiation in this case.

Several times over the years, we have made mistakes in the microscopic interpretation of melanoma (usually metastatic) in the lungs. If pigment is absent or sparse in the tumor cells, no meaningful historical data are supplied by the surgeon, and the lesion being studied is solitary; the stage is set for a possible error. Maeda and colleagues[313] and Yamada and associates[314] have discussed the particular resemblance of amelanotic melanoma to large cell undifferentiated lung carcinoma, and we concur with their conclusions. It is certainly not a necessary step to subject all undifferentiated pulmonary neoplasms to immunohistologic evaluations. Nonetheless, if such studies are obtained, and there is no reactivity in the tumor cells for pankeratin (often used as an "internal control" in carcinoma cases), the alternative possibility of melanoma should be considered.

An important microscopic feature that supports a primary origin in the respiratory tract is the presence of a cytologically atypical in situ melanocytic proliferation in adjacent bronchial mucosa, which may be metaplastic[293,296] (Fig. 14-60). To confirm the presence of melanocytic differentiation[293] and exclude the differential diagnoses of anaplastic carcinoma or sarcoma, electron microscopic studies showing the presence of cytoplasmic premelanosomes (Fig. 14-61)

or immunohistochemical negativity for keratin and labeling for S100 protein, HMB-45 antigen, Melan-A/MART-1, PNL2, or tyrosinase are useful.

Therapy and Prognosis

Before assigning a diagnosis of probable PMML, one must undertake a thorough dermatologic examination, as well as extensive radiologic and endoscopic assessments.[315-317] Those measures are designed to detect an occult primary mucocutaneous melanoma in another location. De Wilt and coworkers also have considered the scenario in which pathologists confront a possible diagnosis of intrapulmonary melanoma in intraoperative consultation.[318] If the tumor being analyzed is amelanotic, it will likely resemble a high-grade carcinoma in frozen sections and touch preparations. Even if the patient has a known history of melanoma, the surgeon should be counseled to perform

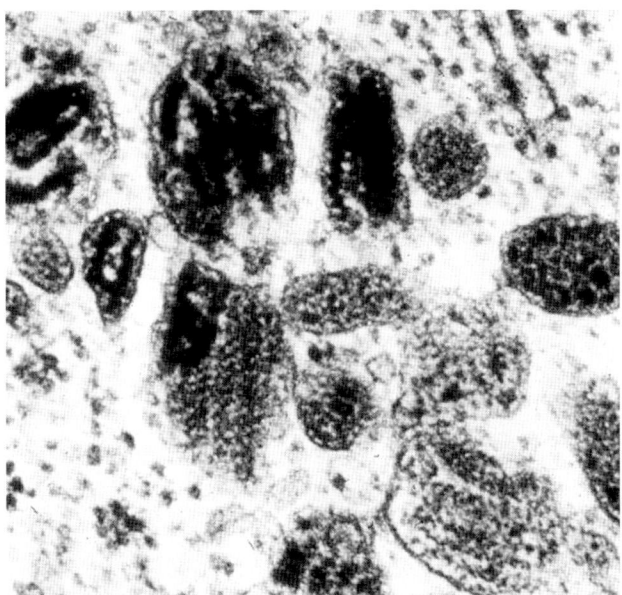

Figure 14-60. In situ malignant melanoma of the bronchial mucosa. The tumor cells are scattered throughout the epithelium randomly.

Figure 14-61. Electron photomicrograph of malignant melanoma demonstrating the presence of cytoplasmic premelanosomes. These inclusions are diagnostic.

a conservative—but adequate—excisional procedure that would be appropriate for primary lung cancer under those circumstances.

In most documented cases of PMML, patients have fared extremely poorly, with the majority dying within 1 year of diagnosis.[293,296–298,300] Reid and Mehta reported one individual who survived 11 years after surgery[299]; however, there was no mention in the latter study of clinical evaluations that were designed to exclude other primary sites of origin, and no in situ melanocytic proliferation was found in the pulmonary resection specimen. Thus, the latter case is doubtful as a verifiable PMML. Most patients have undergone surgical resections of their tumors, although a few have received irradiation or chemotherapy.[294] In extension of therapeutic results obtained in cases of other primary melanomas of the viscera, it must be concluded that long-term survival of patients with PMML is an idiosyncratic and unlikely event.

Sarcomas of the Pulmonary Arterial Trunk

Although it is technically not part of the respiratory tract, the pulmonary arterial trunk is an appropriate topic for this discussion that centers on intrathoracic mesenchymal malignancies. For more than 75 years, it has been known that this vascular segment may serve as the point of origin for sarcomas with diverse histologic features and clinical manifestations that are just as variable.[319] To date, approximately 200 cases of pulmonary trunk sarcoma (PTS) have been documented.[13,319–322]

Clinical Summary

Patients with PTS are adults in middle life or beyond, with no predilection for either gender. They present with a panoply of potential symptoms and signs, the most common of which simulate the findings of right-sided cardiac failure or pulmonary thromboembolic disease.[323] Patients often complain of intractable cough, progressive dyspnea, and dull chest pain that may increase with exertion; cardiac tamponade has rarely been observed.[321] Neck veins may be distended, a loud precordial systolic heart murmur may be audible at the upper left sternal border, and the patient may manifest the complete clinical scenario of anasarca.[324,325] However, cardiac imaging studies demonstrate no evidence of ventricular hypokinesis or perfusion abnormalities.[309]

In the era before modern angiography, echocardiography, CT, and specialized radionuclide scans, the diagnosis of PTS was usually made for the first time at autopsy.[319] However, current imaging modalities are now capable of revealing the tumor in question rather easily[309] (Fig. 14-62). It takes the form of a partially obstructing, endoluminal mass at the level of the right ventricular outlet or above it, and it may extend over a span of several centimeters. Attachment of the lesion to the arterial wall is variable in character and may be sessile or pedunculated. The neoplasm is typically somewhat heterogeneous in density and greatly heterogeneous in size, from case to case.

Pathologic Findings

The preoperative diagnosis of PTS is typically one that may not involve the pathologist, inasmuch as biopsy of an intravascular mass in the right ventricular outlet is a challenging procedure. Thus, his or her first encounter with such lesions may be in the frozen section laboratory during a definitive surgical procedure. In this context, it is important to realize that a firm diagnosis of a particular sarcoma type (or even of a malignancy) may not be an easy proposition. Some PTSs take the form of rather paucicellular myxoid proliferations with surprisingly bland cytologic characteristics (Fig. 14-63), whereas others are anaplastic tumors that defy easy classification under the microscope[319]

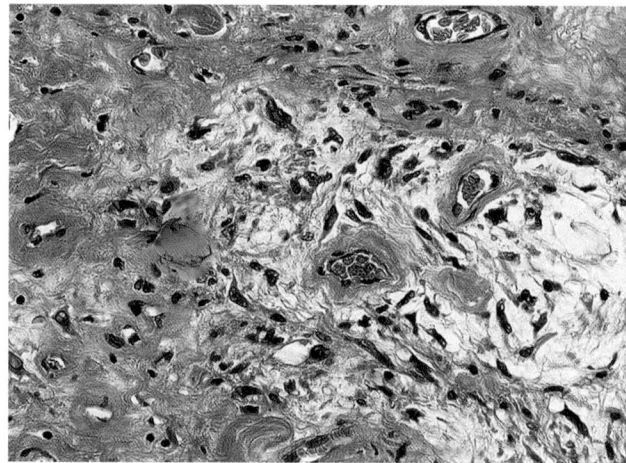

Figure 14-63. This pulmonary trunk sarcoma has a low-grade fibromyxoid image.

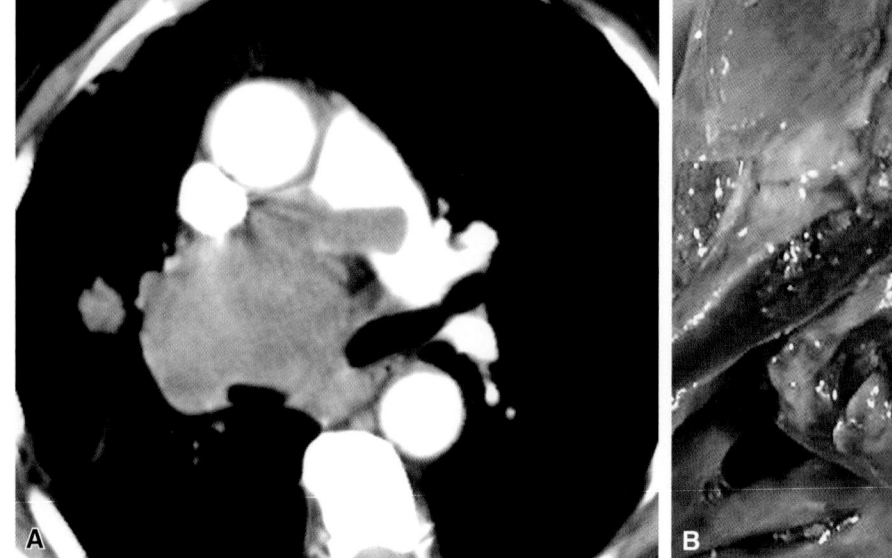 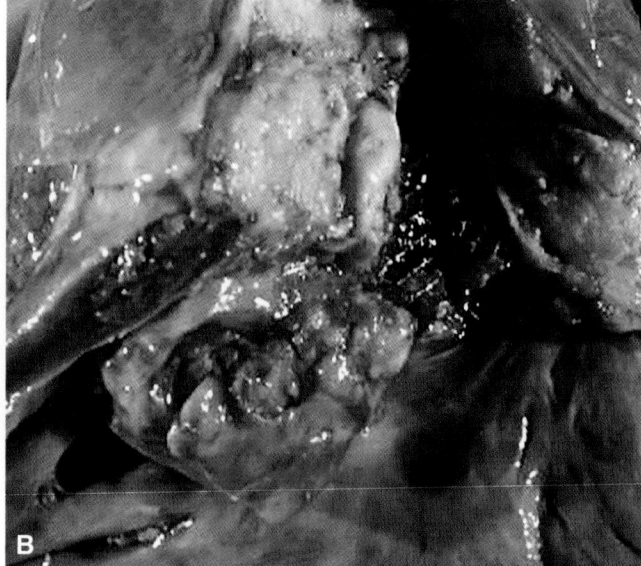

Figure 14-62. A, Computed tomogram showing a mass within the pulmonary trunk, representing pulmonary trunk sarcoma. **B,** Another pulmonary trunk sarcoma, as seen at autopsy.

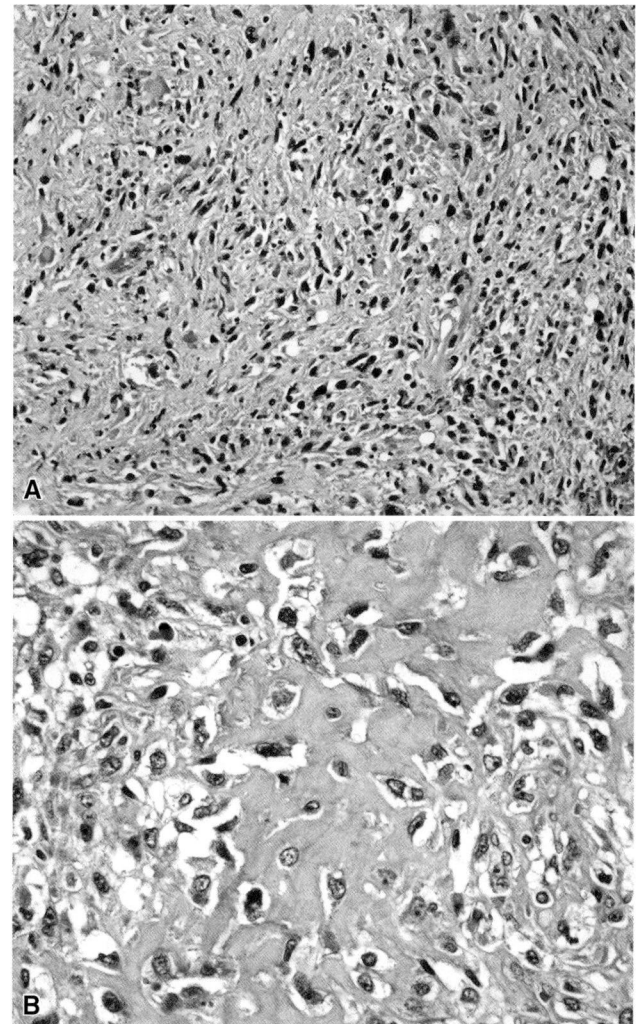

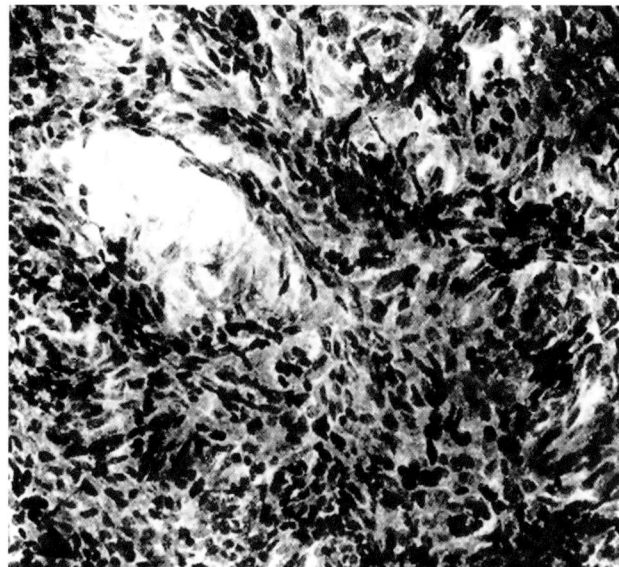

Figure 14-65. Generic fine needle aspiration biopsy image of a spindle cell sarcoma.

Figure 14-64. These microscopic images of a case of pulmonary trunk sarcoma demonstrate one area (**A**) that resembles malignant fibrous histiocytoma histologically, whereas another focus in the lesion (**B**) shows obvious formation of osteoid. The exact nosologic classification of such tumors is often difficult.

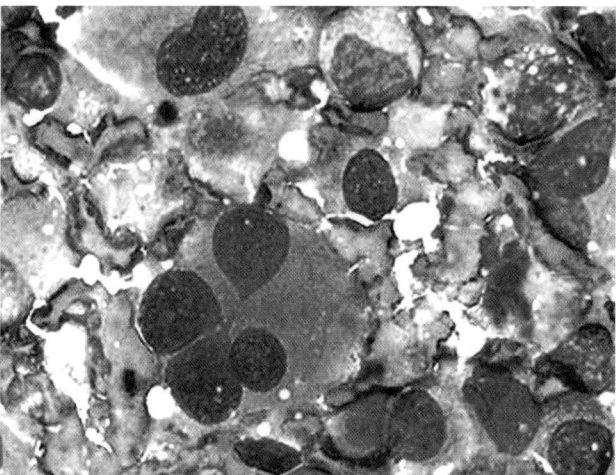

Figure 14-66. Generic fine needle aspiration biopsy image of a pleomorphic sarcoma.

(Fig. 14-64). The proffered pathologic interpretations in the literature on PTS include such diagnoses as undifferentiated sarcoma, angiosarcoma, leiomyosarcoma, rhabdomyosarcoma, fibromyxosarcoma, fibrosarcoma, chondrosarcoma, osteosarcoma, hemangioendothelioma, malignant fibrous histiocytoma, and malignant mesenchymoma. [325-335] What one is able to glean from this apparently confusing list is that the histologic spectrum and pathologic grades of PTS are broadly distributed, such that no two individual lesions look quite the same under the microscope. Beyond that, pathologists take a great deal of interest in speculating on the mechanistic reasons for this diversity, but this issue has admittedly little clinical import at the present time.

With respect to differential diagnosis, the majority of PTSs have the characteristics of high-grade spindle cell or pleomorphic sarcomas, which, in current parlance, would usually be grouped together under the rubric "MFH." However, some low-grade fibromyxoid variants can closely simulate an intracardiac myxoma or organizing mural thrombus.[319] Close attention to morphologic detail is the only certain method for distinguishing between such possibilities.

With particular regard to cytologic preparations of thoracic sarcomas, including PTS, the relative lack of architectural detail seen in fine needle aspiration biopsies has an "equalizing" effect. With the exception of biphasic synovial sarcoma, spindle cell sarcomas of various lineages (Fig. 14-65), pleomorphic sarcomas (Fig. 14-66), and small round cell tumors (Fig. 14-67) have superimposable microscopic images in such preparations. Thus, ancillary diagnostic methods are necessary to make specific diagnoses in those neoplastic categories.

Therapy and Prognosis

Because of the dominance of autopsy reports in the earliest literature on PTS, the recommended therapy for this tumor must still be considered evolutionary. At the present time, providing that a firm radiologic diagnosis can be made or a frozen section interpretation of sarcoma can be rendered, the surgeon may perform an en bloc resection of the pulmonary trunk and its luminal tumor contents, followed by interposition of a synthetic graft.[310] This is probably the most definitive approach to operative therapy, inasmuch as it is difficult to determine the boundaries of intramural tumor growth by visual inspection. The latter point makes more limited vascular resections and reconstructions a tenuous enterprise.

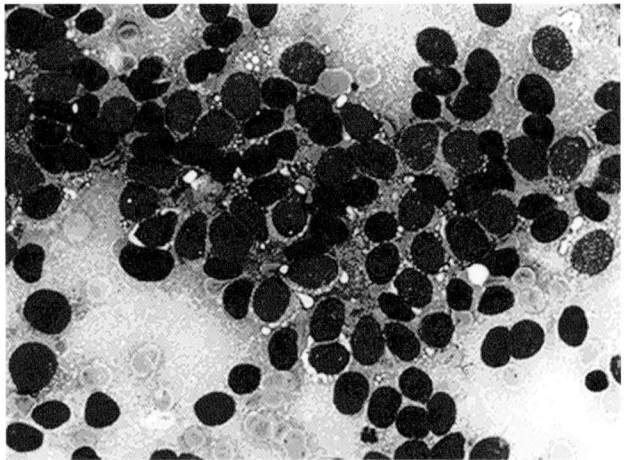

Figure 14-67. Generic fine needle aspiration biopsy image of a small round cell sarcoma.

Extension of the tumor through the wall of the pulmonary artery is the single most important piece of pathologic information in cases of PTS, inasmuch as histologic grading generally does not appear to correlate with tumor behavior in a consistent fashion.[319,325] An exception to the latter statement is embodied in a report by Tavora and colleagues, who suggested that low-grade myofibroblastic PTS had a distinctly better prognosis than other histotypes.[336] In addition, the surgeon's or radiologist's estimation of whether the lesion is pedunculated or sessile has considerable importance. Tumors with a narrow stalk tend to "flutter" in the stream of ejected blood in the ventricular outflow tract, and pieces of the neoplasm may be embolized into the lungs.[337] This phenomenon is not as common with lesions that assume a broadly based sessile macroscopic growth pattern.

Cases demonstrating metastasis or obvious extravascular spread of PTS may be managed with irradiation or chemotherapy. However, there are no unified recommendations for the use of these treatments, and their implementation has produced discouraging results thus far.

Tumors of the Pleura

Sarcomatoid Malignant Mesothelioma (see also Chapter 20)

Clinical Summary

Regardless of histologic subtype—sarcomatoid or otherwise—the clinical features of intrathoracic mesothelioma are the same.[338–340] Malignant mesothelioma (MM) of the pleura typically affects adult

men, although women and children are certainly represented in the patient population with this neoplasm.[340,341] The most common presenting symptoms and signs are pleuritic-type chest pain and progressive shortness of breath, with a pleural effusion on chest radiographs. An influenza-like syndrome is occasionally reported in association with pleural mesothelioma. The lesion most commonly takes the form of multiple nodules and plaques in the serosal surfaces but may occasionally be represented by a solitary localized mass (Fig. 14-68). Later in the clinical course, encasement of the lung by confluent neoplastic tissue is seen (Fig. 14-69).

Like examples of peritoneal mesothelioma that have been linked causally to chronic recurrent peritonitis in the context of familial Mediterranean fever,[342] the authors have observed several pleural tumors that arose in the background of chronic pleuritis in patients with a connective tissue disease (e.g. lupus erythematosus). Roughly

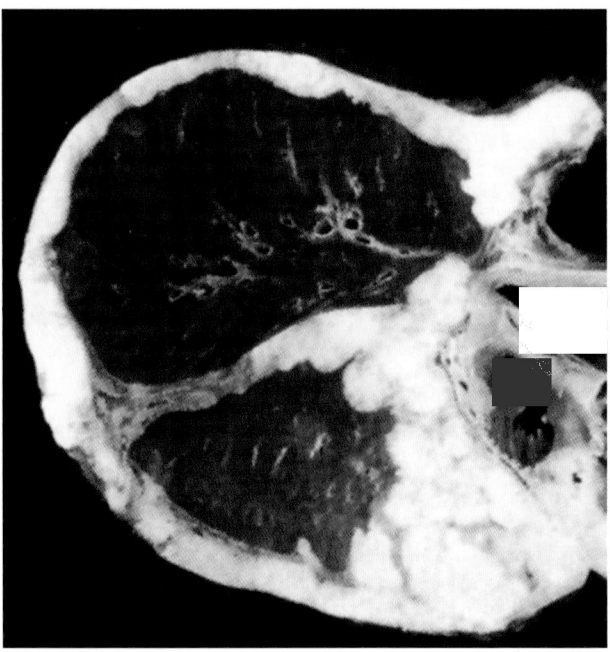

Figure 14-69. In this case, an extrapleural pneumonectomy specimen demonstrates circumferential encasement of the lung by tumor tissue, as well as extension into the interlobar septa.

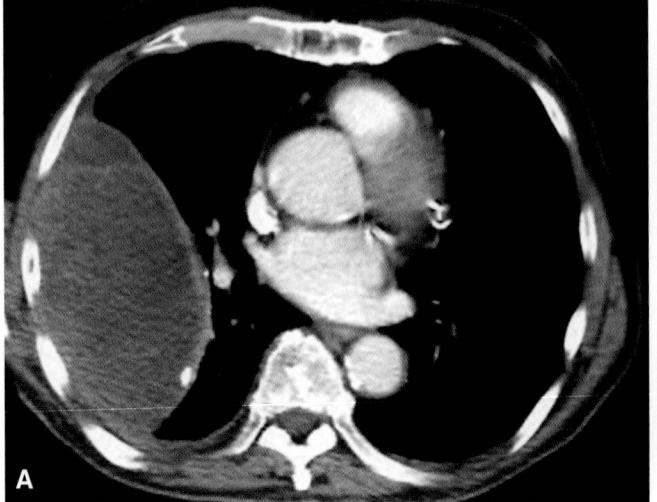

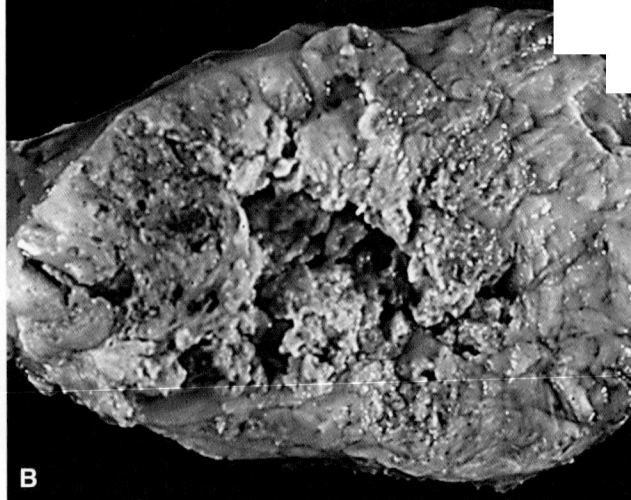

Figure 14-68. Computed tomogram (**A**) and gross photograph (**B**) of localized sarcomatoid mesothelioma.

50% to 70% of pleural mesotheliomas can be objectively related to prior occupational-level asbestos exposure.[343] In those instances, 85% to 90% of patients show the presence of (1) pleural plaques or pleural calcifications or (2) quantitative pulmonary asbestos fiber burdens clearly in excess of the background, serving as tangible markers of such exposure.[344–350] Those findings are vastly more reliable than patients' historical accounts of occupational conditions and should be sought in all instances before concluding objectively that a given mesothelioma is indeed asbestos-related etiologically.

Other accepted pathogenetic factors in mesothelioma cases include inhalation exposure to erionite, chronic infection of the pleural spaces (e.g., in tuberculous pleuritis), and prior therapeutic irradiation of the thorax.[351,352] Substantial recent interest has centered on the potential role of simian virus-40 in this setting,[353] but conclusions about whether this agent is indeed causative in any way are premature. At least 30% of pleural mesotheliomas are idiopathic.[343]

Pathologic Findings

In considering the pathologic appearances of overtly malignant mesothelial tumors, a surprising variety of patterns has emerged over time, and these have expanded the traditional categorical outline, which previously included "epithelioid," "biphasic," and "sarcomatoid" mesotheliomas.[340,354,355] The epithelioid subgroup has now been enlarged to include mesothelial malignancies that have a wholly clear cell, oncocytoid ("deciduoid") or granular cell, tubulopapillary, large polygonal cell, polyhedral stromal mucin-producing, "medullary" epithelioid, or even small cell appearance (see Chapter 20).[354] The differential diagnostic potentialities raised by such images are numerous, including metastatic non–small cell carcinomas of various primary origins, metastatic melanoma, pleural sarcomas with an epithelioid or small round cell appearance, and even metastatic small cell neuroendocrine carcinoma. In reference to biphasic MM—with epithelioid and sarcoma-like elements—primary SS of the pleura is an important diagnostic alternative.[356] Indeed, in the absence of data showing the characteristic t(X;18) chromosomal translocation of SS, which is associated with production of SYT-SSX fusion transcripts,[357] or immunoreactivity for TLE1 (see earlier discussion), its separation from MM can be extremely challenging. This is so because the immunophenotypes of the two tumors are so similar.[358]

Monophasic sarcomatoid mesothelioma potentially simulates a range of spindle cell sarcoma morphotypes that may affect the pleura (Figs. 14-70 and 14-71), again including monophasic SS, but also

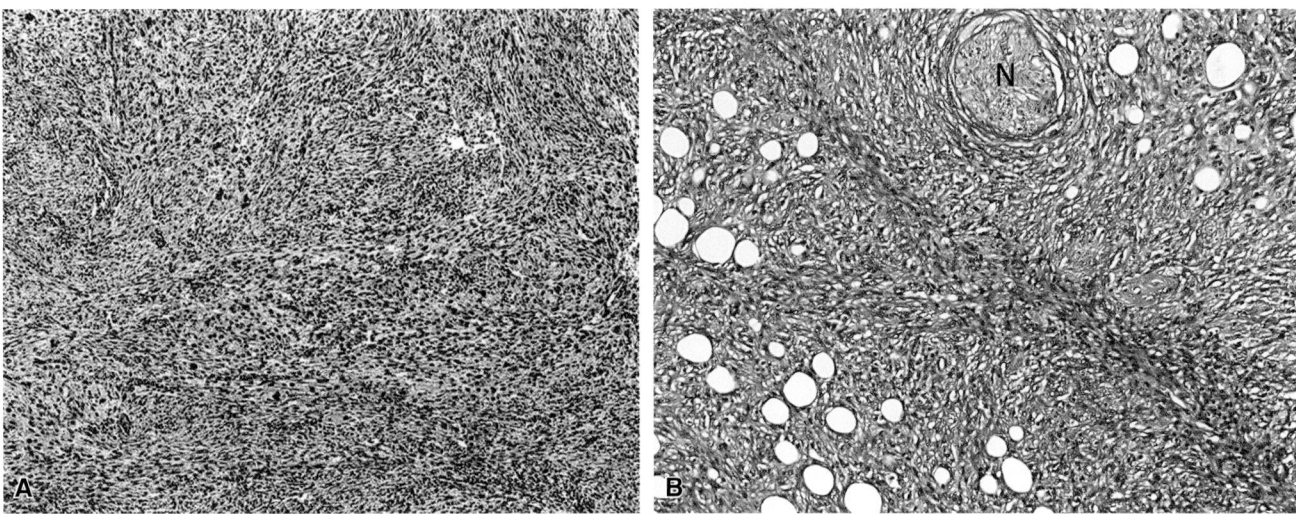

Figure 14-70. A and **B,** Microscopic images of sarcomatoid malignant mesothelioma showing a disorganized proliferation of highly atypical spindle cells, surrounding a nerve (N). Metastatic or pleurotropic sarcomatoid carcinoma and true sarcomas of the pleura are differential diagnostic alternatives.

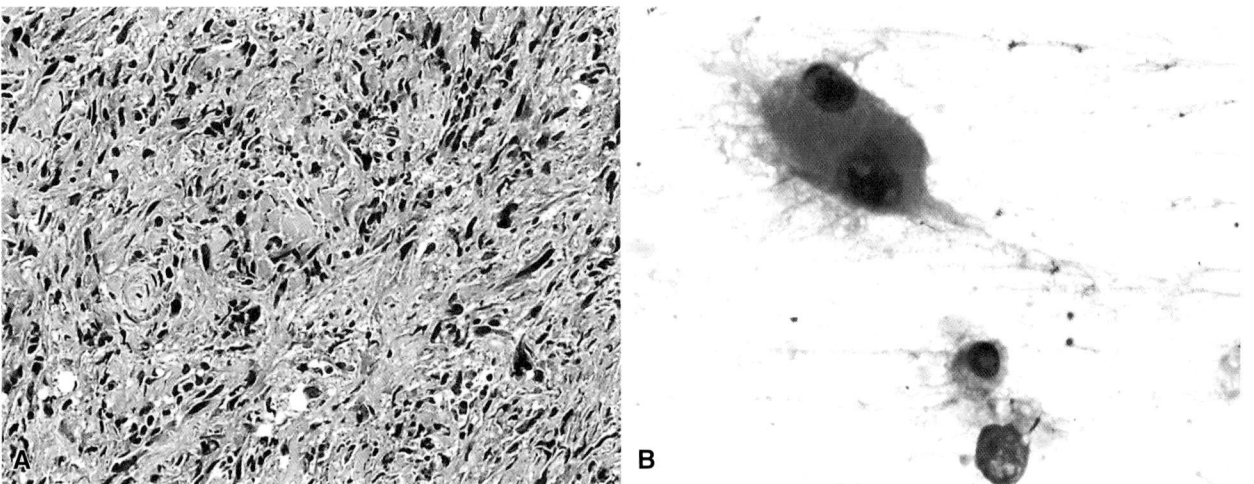

Figure 14-71. Another example of sarcomatoid mesothelioma is more anaplastic cytologically (**A**), simulating the appearance of pleomorphic sarcomas. This attribute is also visible in a fine needle aspiration biopsy specimen (**B**).

fibrosarcoma, MFH, rhabdomyosarcoma, chondrosarcoma, osteosarcoma, leiomyosarcoma, and malignant peripheral nerve sheath tumor.[1,359-363] Pseudomesotheliomatous secondary pleural carcinomas with a sarcomatoid phenotype also enter the differential diagnosis in a meaningful fashion, as referenced earlier in this discussion. The histomorphologic findings in that particular differential diagnostic group of tumors have been summarized previously.

In specific reference to sarcomatoid mesotheliomas, the basic histologic image of such lesions is virtually identical to that associated with SC of the lung.[364-369] Indeed, cases in which a tumor mass involves both the peripheral lung and the pleura require immunohistologic or molecular evaluation in order for a distinction to be made with definition between those tumor types.[370] As such, sarcomatoid mesotheliomas are composed exclusively by overtly malignant spindle cells and pleomorphic elements, with or without such heterotopic tissue as osteoid, cartilage, muscle, or osteoclast-like giant cells.

Lymphohistiocytic mesothelioma[371,372] was formerly classified as a sarcomatoid subtype, but that lesion is now generally considered to be a form of epithelioid mesothelioma with a lymphoepithelioma-like image. Another special variant of sarcomatoid mesothelioma merits further consideration: namely, desmoplastic mesothelioma.[373-379] That tumor is characterized by relatively bland neoplastic spindle cells that are set in a densely collagenized fibrohyaline matrix with a so-called "patternless pattern" of growth (Fig. 14-72). Differential diagnosis of that tumor type is with fibrous (or fibrohyaline) pleuritis ("fibrous pleurisy"); the presence of focally dense and atypical cellular growth, necrosis, obvious invasion of lung or soft tissue, or metastasis points to a diagnosis of mesothelioma.[378] On the other hand, lymphohistiocytoid mesotheliomas may be confused with malignant lymphoma, inflammatory myofibroblastic (pseudo)tumor of the pleura, or metastatic lymphoepithelioma-like carcinoma.[371,372]

This information brings one to a consideration of adjunctive pathologic studies in the objectification of a diagnosis of MM. In regard to this important topic, it should be remembered that there are definite roles for a number of laboratory analyses, including but not limited to histochemistry, immunohistology, electron microscopy, fluorescent or chromogenic in situ hybridization, the polymerase chain reaction using appropriately chosen primers, and traditional cytogenetic evaluations.[338-350,380,381]

Although most attention has been paid in recent years to the immunohistochemical separation of epithelioid MM from metastatic adenocarcinoma,[382,383] the panel of markers used for that purpose is generally not helpful in the differential diagnosis of nonepithelioid (i.e., sarcomatoid) MM variants, with selected exceptions. Standard approaches to separating MM from adenocarcinoma include immunostains for keratin (either "pankeratin," or keratin 5/6, or both), EMA, thrombomodulin, HBME-1, calretinin, Wilms tumor gene product 1 (WT1), podoplanin,[146] tumor-associated glycoprotein-72 (recognized by B72.3), carcinoembryonic antigen, CD15, Ber-EP4, BG8, and MOC-31, with expected reactivity in MM primarily including any of the first seven of those determinants.[384] Electron microscopy is still extremely useful in this particular context, inasmuch as the long, branching, bushy microvilli that one associates with mesothelial cells are best represented in epithelioid MM.[385]

Neither immunohistology nor electron microscopy is nearly as helpful in the realm of biphasic or sarcomatoid tumors, and an entirely different set of morphologic and immunophenotypic variables must be assessed in those lesions. For example, keratin, WT1, podoplanin, and calretinin assume much greater value in the differential diagnosis of sarcomatoid MM (Fig. 14-73).[146,384,386] The principal interpretative

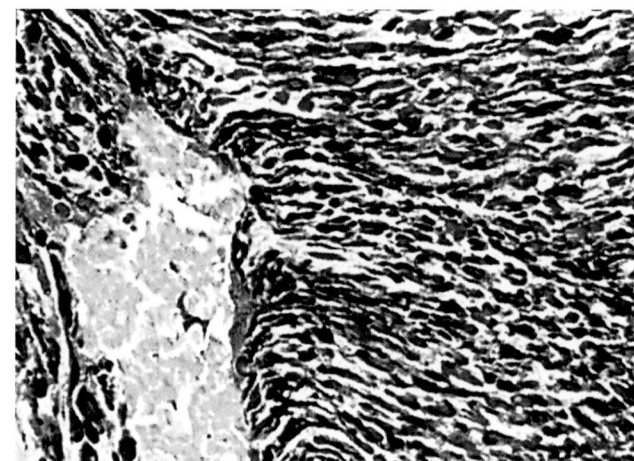

Figure 14-73. Diffuse immunoreactivity is seen in this sarcomatoid mesothelioma for podoplanin, with antibody D2-40.

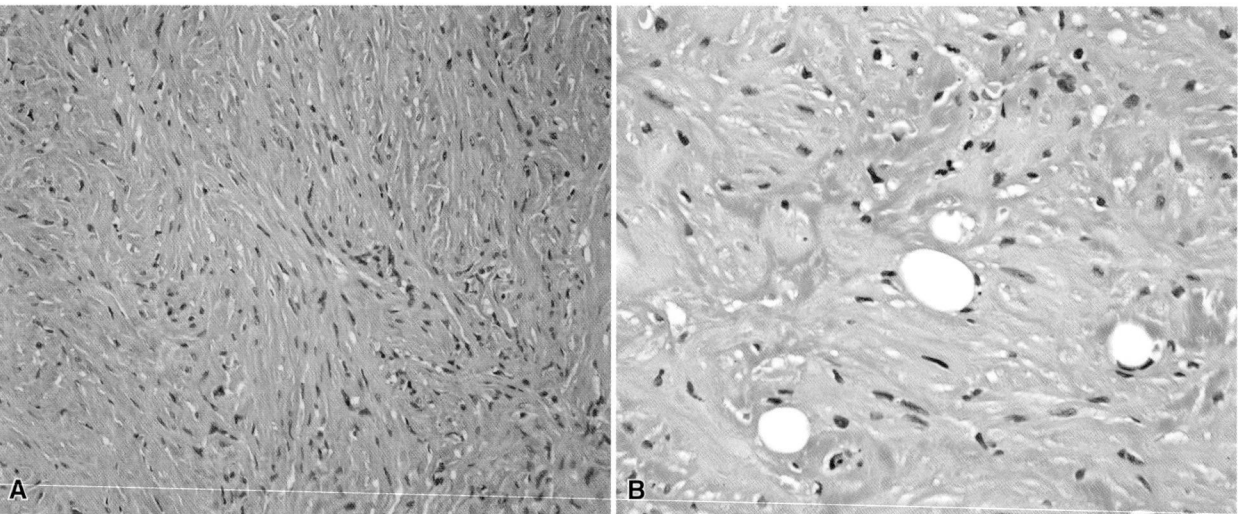

Figure 14-72. A and **B,** Desmoplastic sarcomatoid malignant mesothelioma composed of minimally atypical spindle cells set in a densely hyalinized collagenous stroma. A distinction from fibrous pleurisy is often difficult.

14

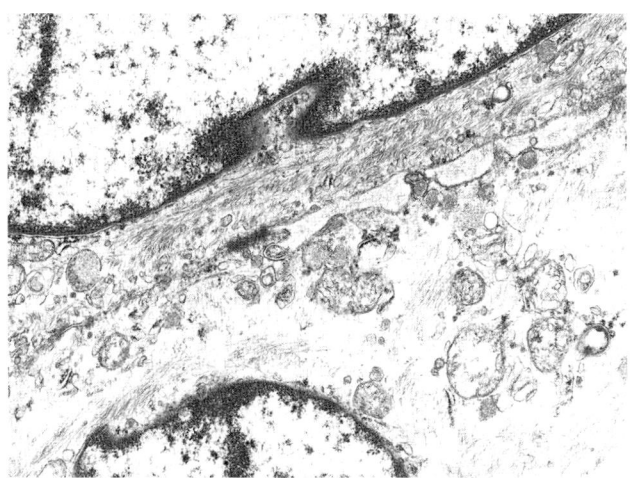

Figure 14-74. This electron photomicrograph of sarcomatoid mesothelioma shows an intercellular attachment plaque (*left center*), but there are otherwise no specialized markers of epithelial differentiation.

alternatives are those of true sarcoma, sarcomatoid pseudomesotheliomatous carcinoma, or malignant solitary fibrous tumor; sarcoma-like mesothelioma differs from the latter two entities in that it may divergently express specialized mesenchymal markers such as desmin and muscle actin isoforms.[387,388]

Fluorescent in situ hybridization or polymerase chain reaction for SYT-SSX transcripts may be necessary to separate some examples of SS (which are also reactive for keratin and potentially for calretinin) from MM with certainty.[357,358] Electron microscopic analyses are likewise not very helpful in the differential diagnosis of sarcomatoid MM, because that variant of mesothelioma tends to lose specialized ultrastructural features of epithelial cells (Fig. 14-74).[369,389] Rarely, localized sarcomatoid mesotheliomas also may resemble solitary fibrous tumors of the pleura[390]; in those cases, immunoreactivity for CD34, or CD99, or both, tends to exclude a diagnosis of MM.[391]

Therapy and Prognosis

The natural history of malignant pleural mesothelioma is an adverse one. The usual survival of patients with that tumor is less than 15 months, with death occurring because of cardiorespiratory embarrassment or pulmonary superinfection.[338,339,392] A peculiarity of this neoplasm is its tendency to grow through surgical defects in the chest wall, either represented by thoracotomy incisions or thoracostomy sites. Metastases outside the thorax are relatively rare, although they have been reported in a small minority of cases in such sites as liver, bones, and skin.[393] Treatment is generally supportive, inasmuch as irradiation and chemotherapy produce little survival benefit.[394] Extrapleural pneumonectomy is still a controversial surgical approach to mesothelioma; its proponents claim a definite decrease in mortality in the operative group compared with stage-matched and age-matched controls managed by other means.[395] However, those observations have not been supported by other studies.[396]

Primary Pleural Sarcoma

Sarcomas are as rare in the pleura as they are in the lungs. Most neoplasms that take the generic appearance of malignant mesenchymal tumors in the serosae of the thorax are, in actuality, epithelial lesions. They may either represent metastatic SCs or variants of MM, as considered earlier. In addition, there are only a limited number of definable clinicopathologic entities to consider in this specific anatomic location. These include fibrosarcoma, malignant solitary (localized) fibrous tumor of the pleura, leiomyosarcoma, SS, Askin

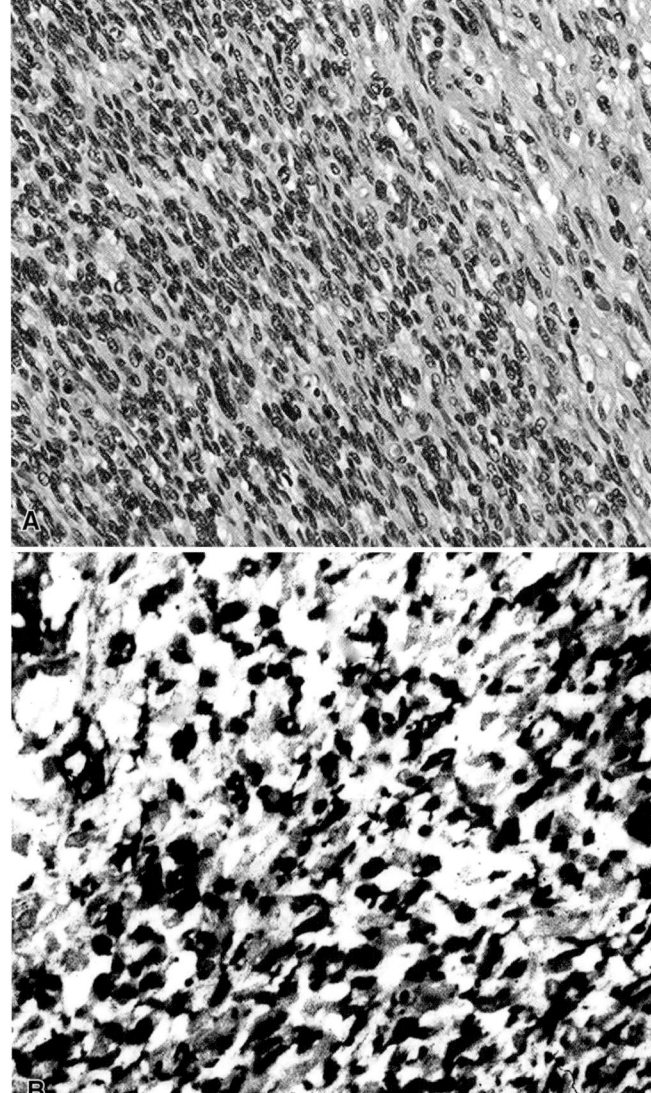

Figure 14-75. A, Malignant peripheral nerve sheath tumor of the pleura showing variation in cellular density and a tendency for nuclei to align themselves in parallel. **B,** The tumor is immunoreactive for CD56.

malignant thoracopulmonary small round cell tumor, PPB, KS, EH, and angiosarcoma. Extraordinarily rare examples of granulocytic sarcoma (extramedullary tumefactive acute myeloid leukemia),[397] malignant peripheral nerve sheath tumor (Fig. 14-75),[362] mesenchymal chondrosarcoma,[398] extraskeletal myxoid chondrosarcoma (Fig. 14-76),[399] liposarcoma,[400,401] and extraosseous osteosarcoma[402,403] have been documented as apparently primary pleural tumors, but information on such lesions is anecdotal.

Pleural Fibrosarcoma and Malignant Solitary (Localized) Fibrous Tumor

A review of the literature on serosal neoplasms reveals few examples of well-documented primary pleural fibrosarcoma (PPFS).[404,405] The latter is only arbitrarily distinguished from malignant solitary (localized) fibrous tumor (MSFT) of the pleura[406,407] by its clinical growth pattern, which is diffuse rather than localized. However, in other respects, these two tumor entities are virtually identical to one another; in fact, some examples of PPFS have apparently evolved from solitary fibrous

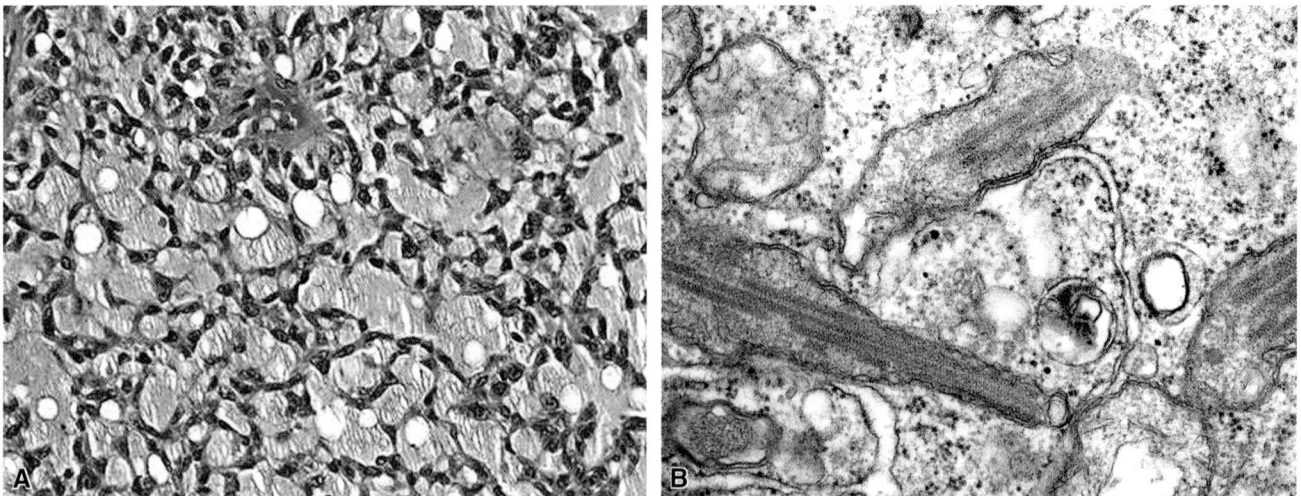

Figure 14-76. A, Extraskeletal myxoid chondrosarcoma (EMCS) of the pleura resembling epithelioid mesothelioma. Cords of tumor cells are set in a myxoid stroma. **B,** The tumor cells contain intrareticular microtubules, a singular finding in EMCS.

tumors of the pleura.[408–413] Although some authors prefer to separate malignant fibrous tumors of the pleura into "true" fibrosarcoma and MFH-like tumors,[414] all of these lesions will herein be considered as a single group because of their closely similar clinicopathologic attributes.

Clinical Summary

Pleural fibrosarcoma and MSFT arise in adult patients over a wide range of ages (15–75 years), with a male-to-female ratio of 3:1. They may be associated with dull or pleuritic chest pain, dyspnea, cough, systemic flu-like symptoms, and digital clubbing.[414,415] In addition, a small proportion of patients may manifest paraneoplastic hypoglycemia (Doege-Potter syndrome) because of the production of an insulin-like peptide by the tumor cells.[415,416] It appears that pleural sarcomas have no association with prior asbestos exposure (in contradistinction to a proportion of MMs).[367] Other potential etiologies of these lesions are unsettled at the present time, but some authors have reported a putative pathogenetic linkage to chronic tuberculous pleuritis and prior pyothorax.[417,418]

Radiographic studies in cases of PPFS commonly demonstrate the presence of a unilateral pleural effusion, which may be massive.[415,419] In addition, a dominant mass and diffuse but irregular thickening of the pleura are usually evident, and are especially visible with CT or MRI studies.[419] Based on clinical data, it is not possible to distinguish PPFS from diffuse MM, and tissue procurement is mandatory for this purpose. On the other hand, MSFT are typically well-circumscribed, pleural-based masses on chest x-rays; they usually show rounded contours, but may occasionally be lobulated[415] (Fig. 14-77). Most measure between 1 and 10 cm in maximal dimension. In contrast to benign solitary fibrous pleural tumors, MSFTs are less often pedunculated and usually attain a larger size. Moreover, the latter lesion has a higher likelihood of involving the parietal pleura or mediastinum, or of demonstrating "inverting" growth into the subjacent lung parenchyma.[408,415]

Pathologic Findings

The macroscopic appearance of PPFS is virtually identical to that of diffuse MM (i.e., as a "rind" of solid tissue that encases the lung and restricts its movement). These tumors commonly extend into interlobar fissures and intrapulmonary interstitial septa as well.[404–416] On the other hand, MSFTs are sessile or pedunculated localized masses

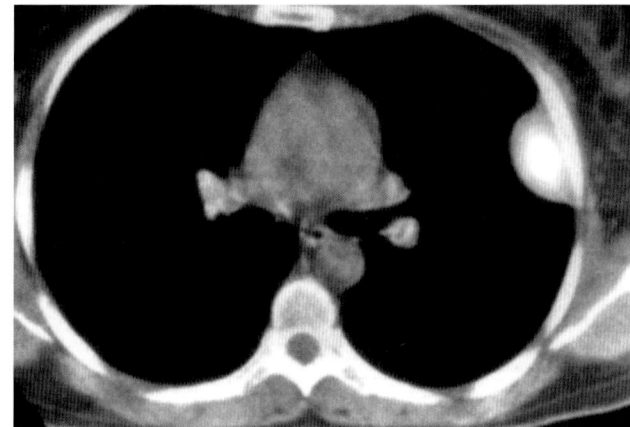

Figure 14-77. Computed tomogram showing a left pleural-based mass, which proved to be a malignant solitary fibrous tumor.

that are most often seen in the upper portions of either hemithorax. They have bosselated, fleshy, tan-gray cut surfaces, usually with foci of spontaneous necrosis and hemorrhage[408,415] (Fig. 14-78).

Microscopically, one sees a dense proliferation of spindle cells with high nuclear-to-cytoplasmic ratios, coarse chromatin, nuclear irregularity, and prominent nucleoli. Mitotic activity is typically brisk, and foci of spontaneous hemorrhage and necrosis may be evident as well (Fig. 14-79). The neoplastic cells may be arranged in a storiform fashion and show moderate-to-marked pleomorphic cytologic features, calling to mind the histologic attributes of MFH (see earlier discussion).[404,415] In other cases, they are aligned in a fascicular "herringbone" configuration, as in pulmonary fibrosarcomas (Fig. 14-80). The subjacent lung is involved by tumor only if it extends downward from the pleura via the intrasegmental fibrous septa, and there is no association with pleural fibrohyaline plaques, the presence of intraparenchymal asbestos fibers, or asbestosis. MSFT may contain areas that resemble benign solitary fibrous pleural tumors, in which more bland spindle cell aggregates are enmeshed in hyalinized, keloidal-type collagen.[415] A "staghorn" stromal vascular pattern is common in such areas as well.

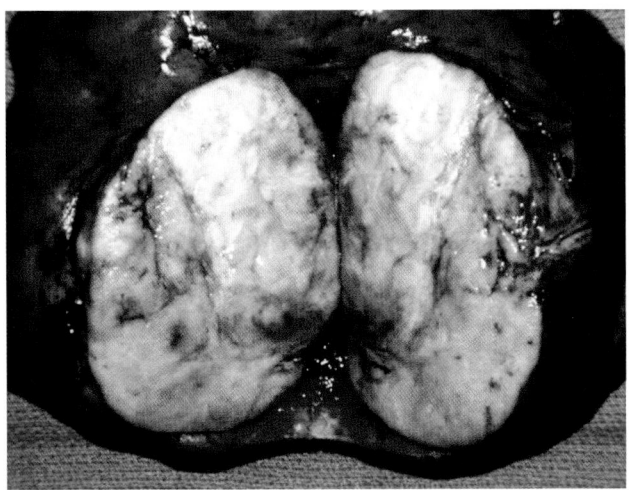

Figure 14-78. Gross photograph of excised malignant solitary fibrous tumor of the pleura demonstrating internal foci of necrosis.

Electron microscopy shows only primitive, fibroblast-like characteristics of the neoplastic cells. They are loosely apposed and surrounded in part by collagen fibers. Cytoplasmic contents are rudimentary and include the basic metabolic organelles as well as abundant free polyribosomes and rough endoplasmic reticulum (Fig. 14-81). There is no ultrastructural evidence of epithelial or myogenous differentiation. Similarly, immunohistologic assessment of PPFS and MSFT demonstrates reactivity for vimentin alone, to the exclusion of actin, desmin, keratin, and EMA.[404–409] In contrast, true mesotheliomas (including sarcomatoid variants) uniformly express epithelial markers.[386] In contrast to benign SFTs, some MSFTs may lack immunoreactivity for CD34, bcl-2 protein, and CD99.[413]

Therapy and Prognosis

PPFS is not often treatable by surgical means because of its diffuse nature. The only operative procedure that can be attempted in such circumstances is extrapleural pneumonectomy, which generally is associated with a very high level of morbidity and mortality. Radiotherapy and chemotherapy (including intrapleural instillation of pharmaceuticals) may play a role in palliation of symptoms, but

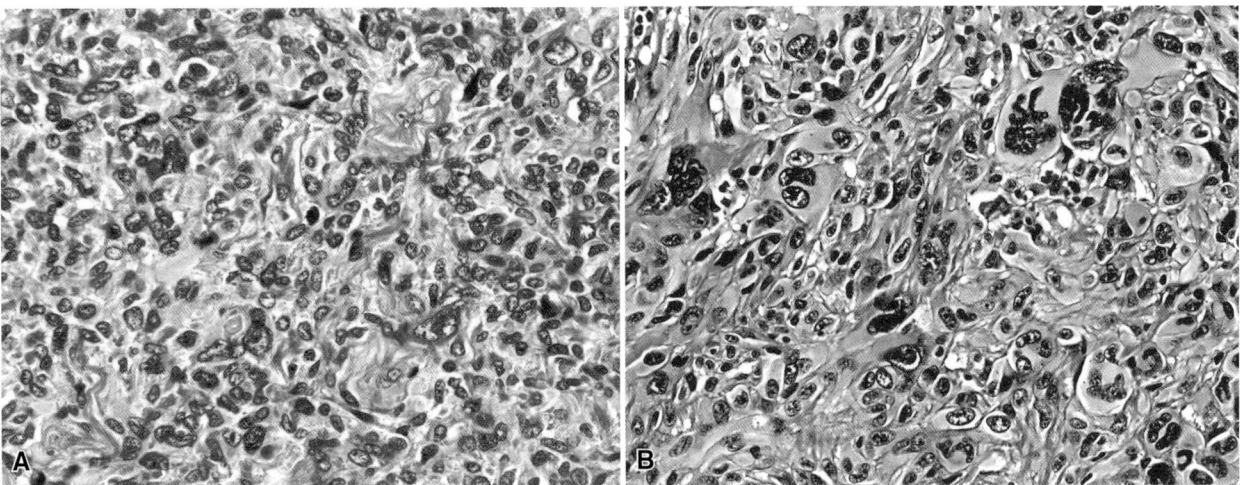

Figure 14-79. A, Microscopic image of malignant solitary fibrous tumor (MSFT) of the pleura showing an atypical spindle cell proliferation. **B,** Another MSFT is more pleomorphic in appearance.

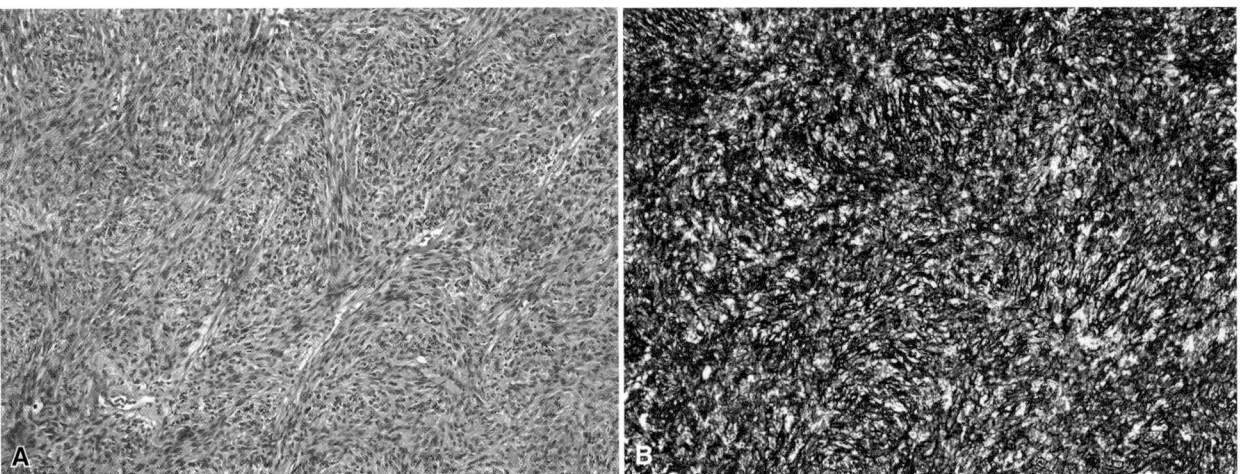

Figure 14-80. A, A "herringbone" pattern of densely cellular growth and mitotic activity are present in this malignant solitary (localized) fibrous tumor (MSFT) of the pleura. **B,** The lesion is immunoreactive for CD34, although a proportion of MSFTs lose that marker.

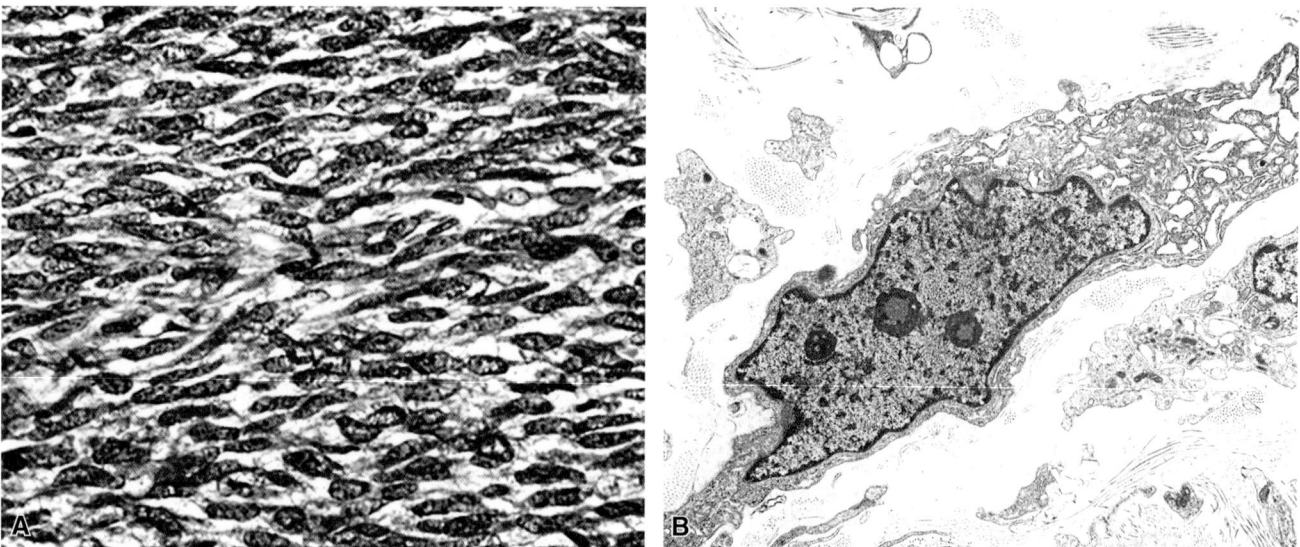

Figure 14-81. Fibrosarcoma-like malignant solitary fibrous tumor of the pleura (**A**), comprising cells that ultrastructurally resemble fibroblasts (**B**).

unfortunately they are not curative treatments. Death is due to progressive respiratory compromise, and PPFS also may involve the pericardium and produce cardiac embarrassment.[420] Actuarial 1-year survival was only 39% in one series where multimodality therapy was used.[414]

MSFT, on the other hand, is amenable to complete surgical resection in a high proportion of cases; in a series from the AFIP, 45% of such lesions were cured by excision alone.[415] Most of these were pedunculated, well-localized masses that involved only a small area of the pleural surface, and the authors of the latter report therefore suggested that resectability was the single most favorable prognostic feature in MSFT cases. Those lesions that do go on to recur may seed the ipsilateral pleural surfaces or involve the contralateral pleura, the lung parenchyma, and other viscera. Interestingly, relapses often still take the form of localized masses, and even patients with persistent tumor may go on to survive for extended periods of time.[367] Irradiation and chemotherapy do not appear to offer any benefits in this setting, and they may even shorten the survival of patients with MSFT.[415]

Primary Pleural Leiomyosarcoma

Leiomyosarcomas are extremely rare as primary pleural neoplasms, with fewer than 25 well-documented cases in the literature.[421,422] Only one series of such tumors has been reported, by Moran and associates.[421]

Clinical Summary

Patients with primary pleural leiomyosarcoma present in a similar fashion to those with mesothelioma, except that a greater proportion have had asymptomatic lesions. Radiographically, pleural effusions have not been observed consistently in association with such tumors, the majority of which appeared as solitary, solid, unilateral masses measuring up to 18 cm in greatest dimension (Fig. 14-82).[423] Some examples have encased the lung completely, simulating malignant mesothelial tumors.[421]

Pathologic Findings

As in other anatomic sites, pleural leiomyosarcomas are characterized by fascicles and whorls of atypical spindle cells, featuring fusiform nuclei, fibrillary eosinophilic cytoplasm, nuclear pleomorphism, and

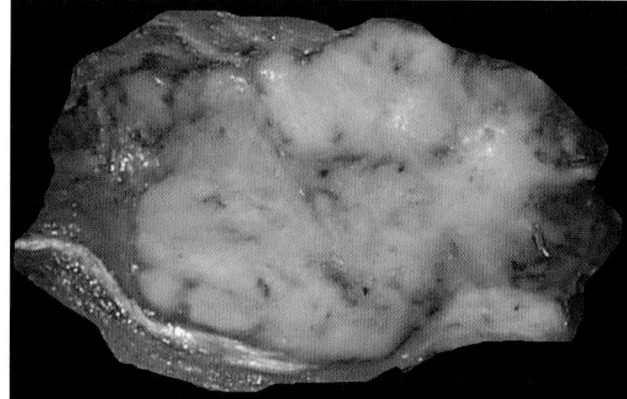

Figure 14-82. Gross photograph of primary pleural leiomyosarcoma showing a localized lesion with a "fleshy," white-gray cut surface.

mitotic activity (Fig. 14-83). Necrosis is also frequently encountered as well. The tumors invade the lung parenchyma, or the soft tissues of the chest wall, or both.

Ultrastructural analyses have shown typical findings of smooth muscle differentiation in such tumors, including plasmalemmal dense plaques, pinocytotic vesicles, cytoplasmic thin filaments punctuated by dense bodies, and pericellular basal lamina (Fig. 14-84). Immunohistologically, pleural leiomyosarcomas are reactive for vimentin, desmin, muscle-specific actin, caldesmon, calponin, and alpha-isoform actin (Fig. 14-85),[421] yielding potential immunophenotypic overlap with SC or mesothelioma. However, in our experience, keratin, EMA, and calretinin are uniformly absent, providing points of difference from the latter two epithelial tumors.

Therapy and Prognosis

Because of the rarity of these lesions, only anecdotal information is available on the biology of primary pleural leiomyosarcomas. Moran and associates advocated surgical ablation but found that two of five such lesions they studied could not be resected completely.[421] The merits of adjuvant therapeutic modalities are as yet unstudied.

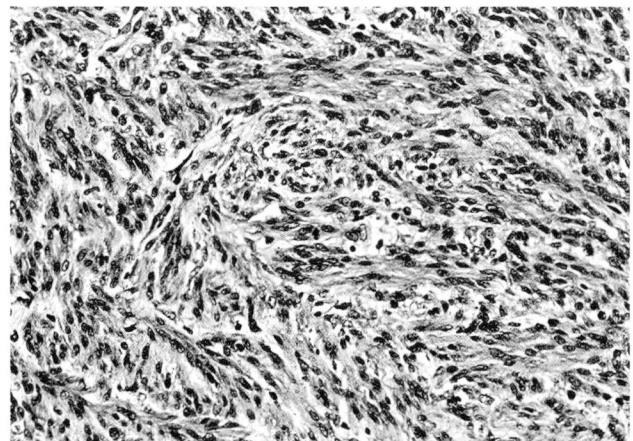

Figure 14-83. Fascicular spindle cell growth is evident in this primary pleural leiomyosarcoma.

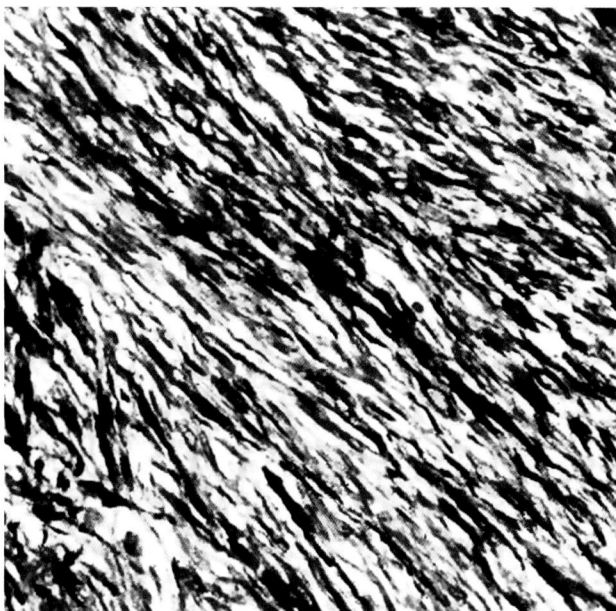

Figure 14-85. Immunoreactivity for caldesmon is apparent in primary pleural leiomyosarcoma.

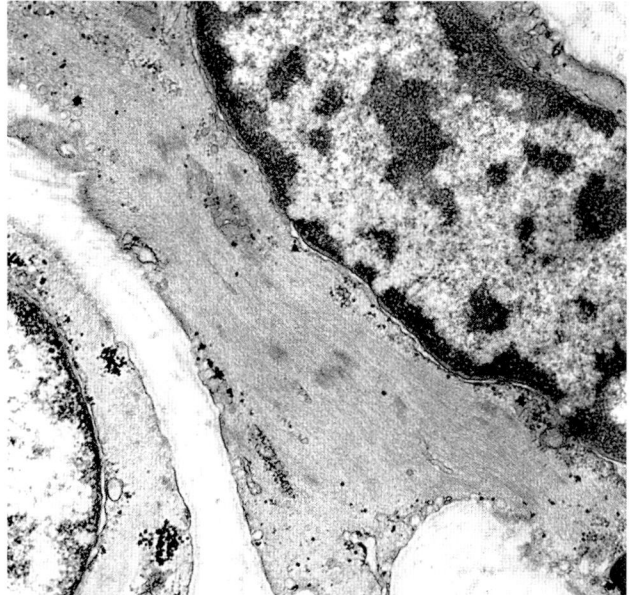

Figure 14-84. Cytoplasmic skeins of thin filaments, punctuated by dense bodies, are seen in this electron photomicrograph of primary pleural leiomyosarcoma.

Askin Tumor (Primitive Neuroectodermal Tumor) and Desmoplastic Small Round Cell Tumor

In 1979, Askin and colleagues described a peculiar thoracic neoplasm that was seemingly limited to children, adolescents, and young adults.[424] This lesion arises from the pleura or the extrapleural intercostal soft tissue and was originally named the *malignant small cell tumor of the thoracopulmonary region*. Since then, it has become known more simply as *Askin tumor*, or, alternatively—because the neoplasm has been shown to exhibit neuroepithelial differentiation—*thoracopulmonary primitive neuroectodermal tumor* (TPNET).[425-436] Prior to its seminal description, it is likely that this lesion was included among cases of Ewing sarcoma of the thorax or peripheral neuroblastoma.[437] Primary primitive neuroectodermal tumor of the lung is considered elsewhere in this monograph, but Askin tumor is technically considered to be separate from that entity and will therefore be discussed at this point. A related neoplasm is known as desmoplastic small round cell tumor (DSRCT)

of the serosal surfaces. It was originally described in the peritoneum and is more common there by far, but several examples have been described in the pleura as well.[438-440]

Clinical Summary

Askin tumor and DSRCT demonstrate a peak incidence during the second decade of life (mean age, 15 years), and they show a slight male predilection. Isolated cases of TPNETs in infants and in older adults have also been documented.[438-443] These neoplasms may present as asymptomatic masses in the chest wall or produce symptoms of cough, unilateral chest pain, and dyspnea or tachypnea. Pleural effusion is a common complication and may be detected on physical examination or by radiography of the thorax.[425] Although Askin tumors and DSRCTs have been confused with classic neuroblastoma in some reports, they are not associated with elevations of catecholamine metabolite levels in the urine or blood, and they do not produce the opsoclonus-myoclonus syndrome.[433,441]

Chest x-rays and other imaging studies typically show a large mass that may be pleural-based or centered in the thoracic soft tissue, with secondary extension into the pleural space (Fig. 14-86). TPNETs and DSRCTs often reach greater than 10 cm at the time of initial diagnosis, and they demonstrate ill-defined interfaces with the subjacent lung or surrounding tissues.[444]

Pathologic Findings

Askin tumor is one of the prototypical small round cell neoplasms of children and may be confused with several other tumor entities by the pathologist.[433] At a macroscopic level, TPNET is lobulated with fleshy, relatively soft, tan-gray cut surfaces (Fig. 14-87) that may show foci of hemorrhage and necrosis.[424] Microscopically, it exhibits cellular monomorphism, with round-to-oval nuclei, even distribution of chromatin, indistinct nucleoli, and variable mitotic activity (Fig. 14-88). Stromal blood vessels are numerous and form a discernible network within the tumor mass; matrical hemorrhage also may be manifest.[424-441] One of the most characteristic findings of TPNET on conventional microscopy is the presence of neural-type cellular "rosettes," wherein tumor cells are disposed radially around

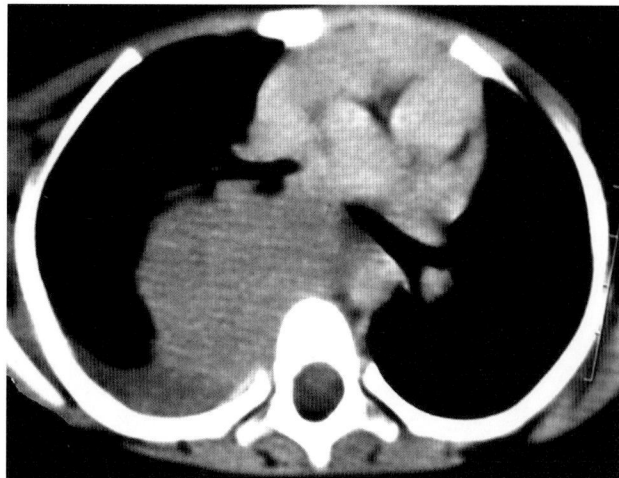

Figure 14-86. Askin tumor (primitive neuroectodermal tumor) of the right hemithorax in a young child, as seen in a computed tomography scan.

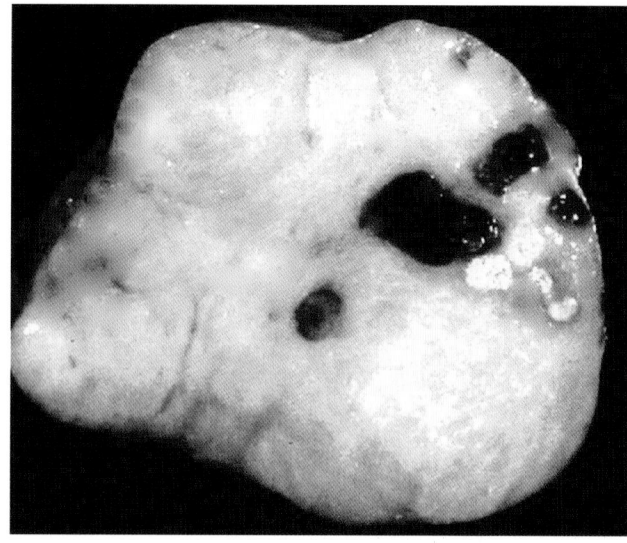

Figure 14-87. Partial excision of the lesion yielding a fleshy mass demonstrating internal foci of necrosis.

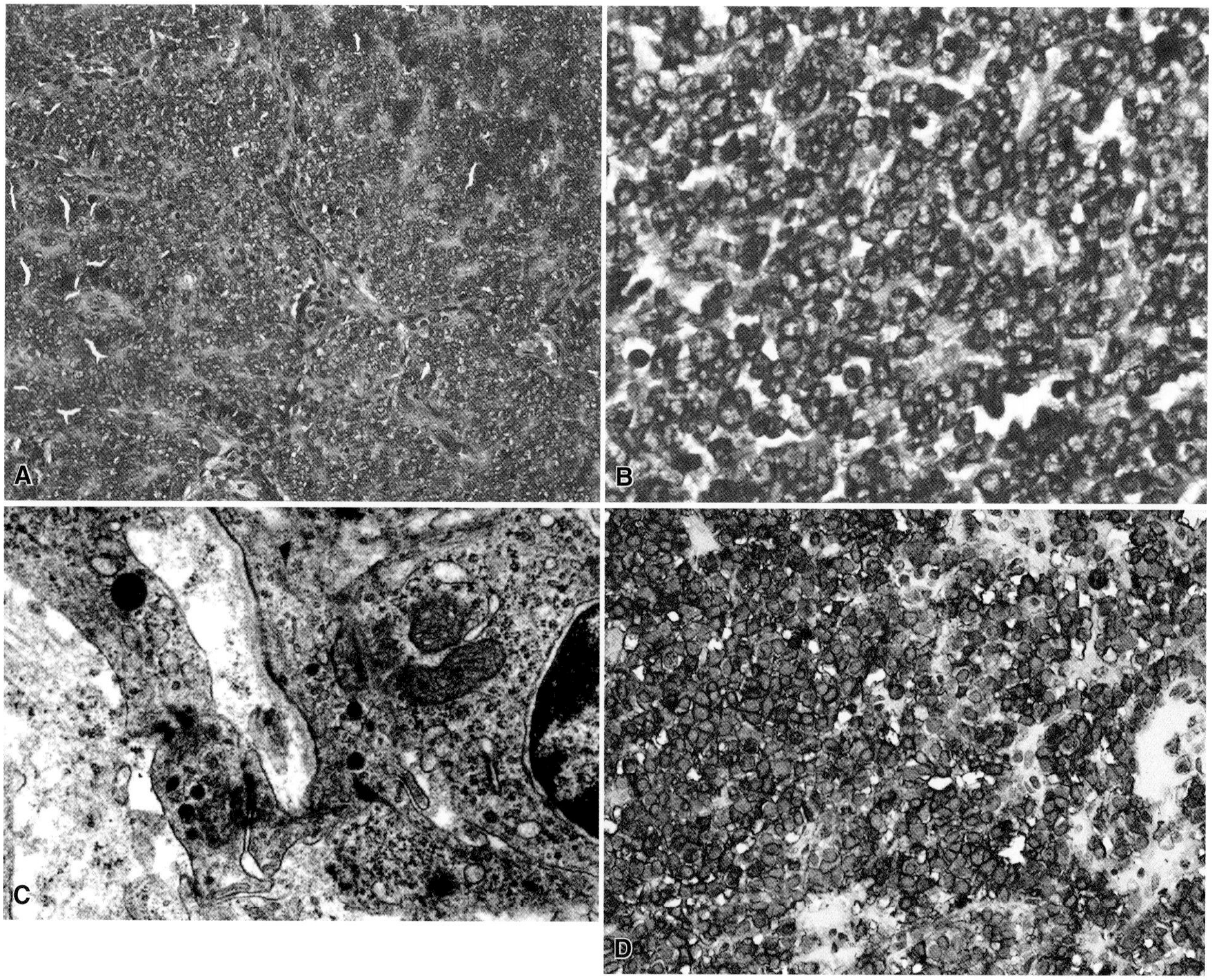

Figure 14-88. A, Microscopic image of primitive neuroectodermal tumor showing a densely cellular proliferation of monomorphic small round cells. **B,** The neoplastic cells have scant cytoplasm and dispersed nuclear chromatin. **C,** An electron micrograph of the lesion showing primitive cytoplasmic extensions that contain neurosecretory-type or synaptic vesicles. **D,** Immunoreactivity for CD99 (MIC2 protein) is also present.

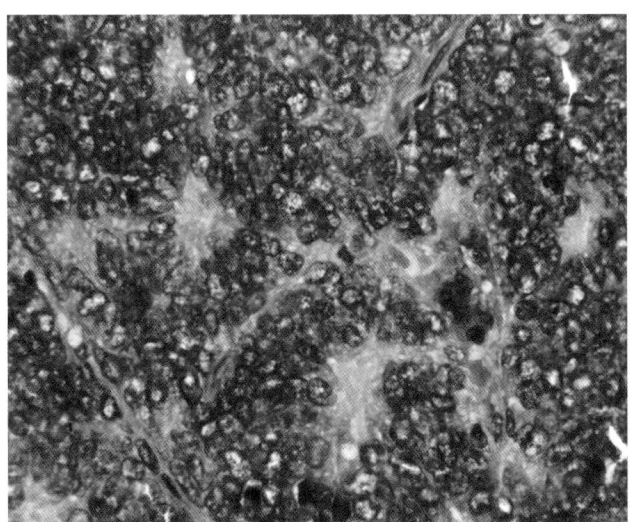

Figure 14-89. Primitive intercellular rosettes are present in this Askin tumor (primitive neuroectodermal tumor).

small virtual tissue spaces[424,425] (Fig. 14-89). Histochemically, Askin tumor may or may not contain abundant glycogen with the PAS method (Fig. 14-90), although in the original series on this lesion, only PAS-negative neoplasms were accepted to facilitate separation from classic Ewing sarcoma.

DSRCT differs from the description just given in that it features aggregates of small monomorphic tumor cells that are set in a much more fibrogenic stroma than that seen in Askin tumor (Fig. 14-91). The growth pattern is also more organoid than in conventional TPNET.[438–440] Although no obvious evidence of myogenous differentiation is apparent at a conventional morphologic level, immunostains typically show coreactivity for vimentin, desmin, and keratin in DSRCT (Fig. 14-92),[439] and ultrastructural studies also support the presence of bifid epithelial-myogenic differentiation.

Special studies of biopsy or resection specimens are mandatory to recognize TPNET and DSRCT properly and exclude other diagnostic possibilities. Those include mesenchymal chondrosarcoma, small cell

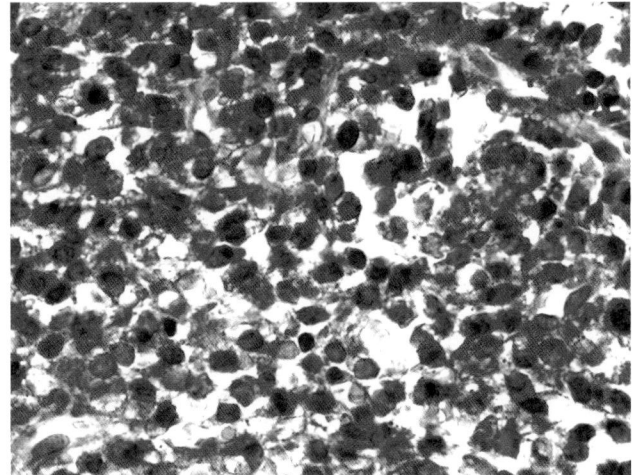

Figure 14-90. Diffuse reactivity is seen with the periodic acid/Schiff stain in the Askin tumor, reflecting the presence of abundant cytoplasmic glycogen.

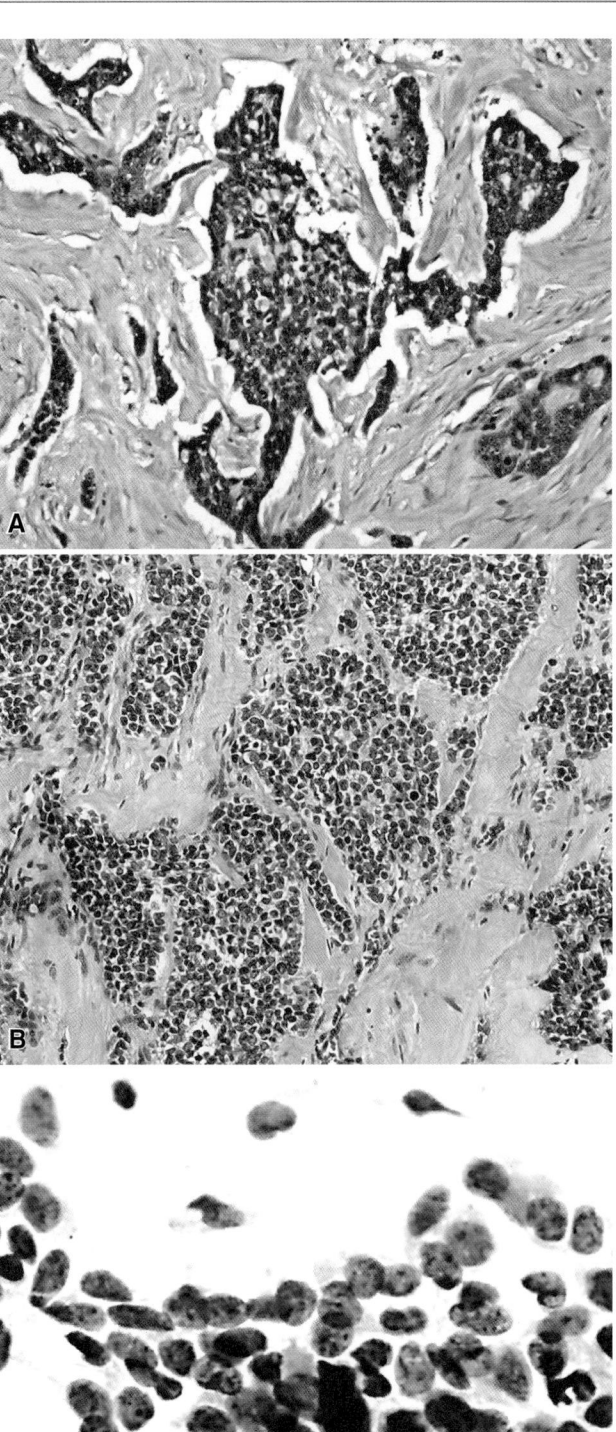

Figure 14-91. A and **B,** Desmoplastic small round cell tumor of the pleura, in which angular cell groups composed of cells like those of "ordinary" primitive neuroectodermal tumor (see Figs. 14-88 and 14-89) are set in a markedly fibrous stroma. They are dyshesive and monomorphic in a fine needle aspiration biopsy specimen (**C**).

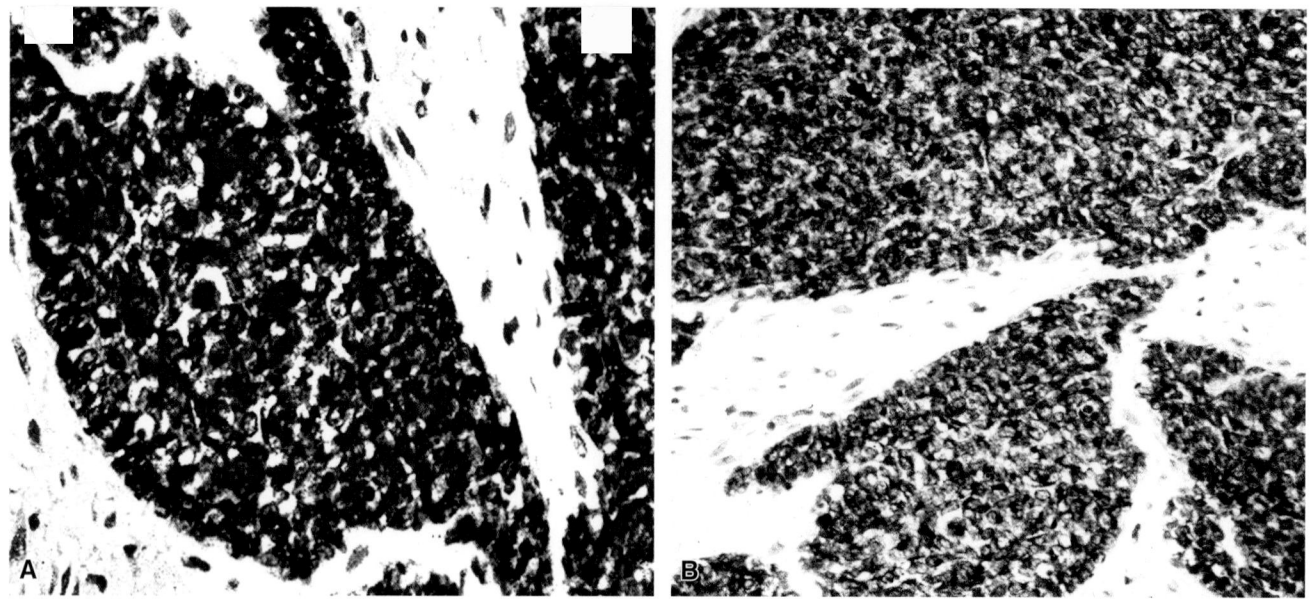

Figure 14-92. The neoplastic cells in desmoplastic small round cell tumor of the pleura are concurrently immunoreactive for keratin (**A**) and desmin (**B**).

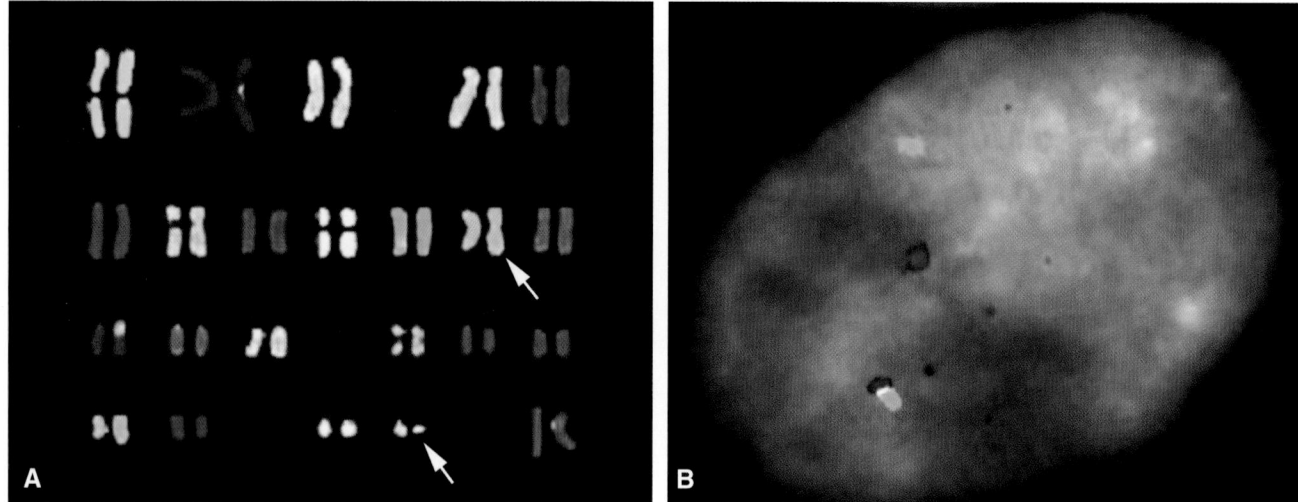

Figure 14-93. The characteristic t(11;22) chromosomal translocation of primitive neuroectodermal tumor is seen in a spectral karyotypic preparation (**A**) and a fluorescent in situ hybridization preparation, using "break-apart" probes (**B**).

synovial sarcoma, hemangiopericytoma, and metastatic small cell neuroendocrine carcinoma; the last of these possibilities is unlikely in the usual patient group with TPNET. Along with other peripheral neuroepithelial neoplasms, TPNET and DSRCT demonstrate characteristic t(11;22) chromosomal translocations[425,445] (Fig. 14-93). By electron microscopy, they demonstrate blunt cytoplasmic processes that contain dense-core granules or microtubules; these characteristics are seen in classic neuroblastoma as well, but not in other small round cell tumors.[433]

Immunohistochemically, TPNET is related to classic Ewing tumor–PNET in that it shows consistent reactivity for synaptophysin as well as for CD99.[446] DSRCT is more variable with regard to its positivity for both of those markers.[447,448] Askin tumor may be distinguished from classic neuroblastoma immunophenotypically; the former lesion is reactive for both beta$_2$-microglobulin and CD99,[439] whereas the latter tumor is not. Among primitive neuroectodermal tumor, DSRCT, and neuroblastoma, only DSRCT labels for WT1 (Fig. 14-94).[449,450]

Therapy and Prognosis

The most important prognostic procedure in cases of TPNET or DSRCT is that of accurate staging. Using a scheme devised by the National Cancer Institute, stage I tumors are defined as those measuring less than 5 cm in maximum diameter that can be completely excised, stage II lesions are less than 5 cm and are grossly resectable but show positive microscopic margins, stage III neoplasms are greater than 5 cm and are nonresectable, and stage IV primitive neuroectodermal tumors have metastasized to extrapleural sites.[425] Low stage

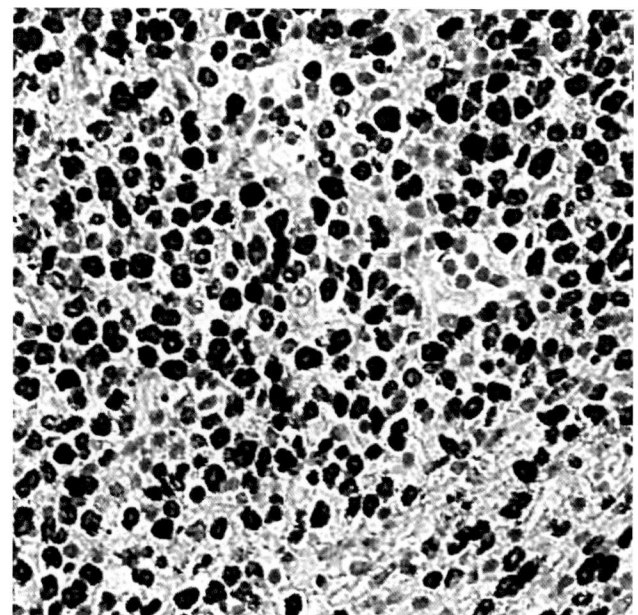

Figure 14-94. Nuclear immunoreactivity for Wilms tumor gene product 1 protein is apparent in pleural desmoplastic small round cell tumor.

has shown a direct correlation with long-term survival after surgical removal and intensive cyclical postoperative treatment with irradiation and chemotherapy, using protocols similar to those used for Ewing sarcoma.[426,451] Stage III and IV TPNETs and DSRCTs are probably best managed nonsurgically, because there are no data to support a role for debulking surgery in such circumstances.[425]

A sobering aspect of the therapy for TPNET and DSRCT is that it undeniably subjects patients who become survivors to the risk of a second malignancy. Intensive radiation to the chest wall may be followed years later by a postradiation sarcoma (or mesothelioma) in approximately 1% of cases, and Farhi and coworkers have described several examples of postchemotherapy myelodysplastic syndrome and acute leukemia in this context.[452]

Pleuropulmonary Blastoma

Until 1988, a group of anaplastic mesenchymal tumors of the peripheral lung and pleura in children had been grouped together under the rubric "pediatric pulmonary blastoma." Nonetheless, Manivel and colleagues[74] showed that such lesions differed from typical PBs in adults, which comprise a subset of SCs. The childhood tumors were found to be more often primary in the pleura; they also showed a histologic resemblance to soft tissue sarcomas. Because of these important points of difference from adult PBs, the pediatric lesions were reclassified as PPBs.

Clinical Summary

PPBs arise most often in the first decade of life, without a distinct preference for males or females. However, isolated examples have been reported in adult patients as well.[74–80,453–463] Cough, chest pain, weight loss, dyspnea or tachypnea, and spontaneous pneumothorax are the most common presenting complaints.[74,459] Evidence of a pleural effusion may also be found on physical examination, and a small subset of patients present with acute, rapidly progressive respiratory embarrassment.[464] It is clear that this neoplasm may be part of certain "cancer families," in which other soft tissue sarcomas, variants of Wilms tumor, and cystic nephromas may be seen in other members of the

kindred.[78,79,459,460] Other familial and patient-specific associations have been noted between PPB and sex-cord stromal tumors of the gonads, seminomatous germ cell tumors, intestinal polyps, and thyroid hyperplasia.[465] The operative gene defect that ultimately yields PPB has now been identified. It is represented by a constitutive mutation in the DICER1 gene on chromosome 12, which encodes an endoribonuclease that is critical to the generation of small regulatory ribonucleic acid molecules.[466]

Radiologic studies typically demonstrate the presence of a large, irregularly outlined mass in the thorax, which may have its epicenter in the pleura, the mediastinal soft tissue, or the peripheral lung parenchyma. These lesions can be massive—sometimes effacing an entire hemithorax—and they demonstrate internal variation in density on CT or MRI (Fig. 14-95). Some examples may show focal internal calcification, and types I and II PPB (see subsequent discussion) demonstrate obvious internal cyst formation (Fig. 14-96).[74,459,461,462]

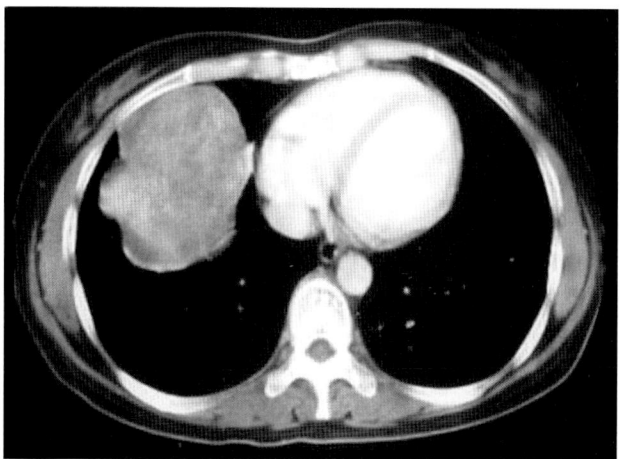

Figure 14-95. Computed tomogram of pleuropulmonary blastoma in a young adult showing partial effacement of the right hemithorax.

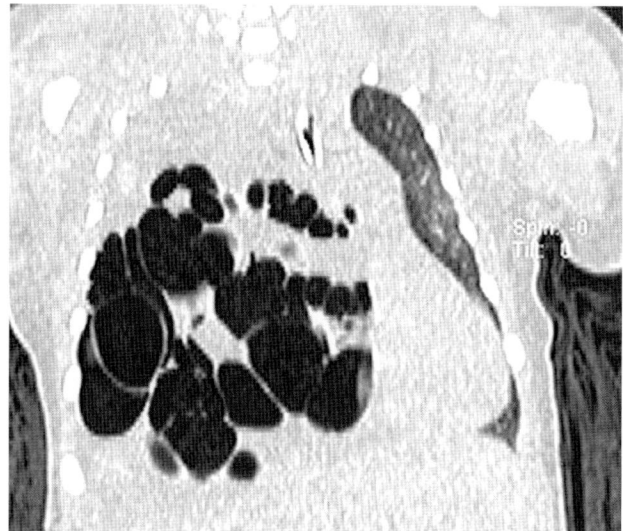

Figure 14-96. Multilocular internal cystic change is apparent in this pleuropulmonary blastoma, as seen in a high-resolution computed tomography scan.

Pathologic Findings

PPB is grossly cystic or fleshy and tan-pink-gray on prosection, with frequent foci of internal hemorrhage and punctate necrosis; overt cystification is also seen in many cases. Chondroid areas may be apparent on macroscopic examination of the mass, and areas of calcification may be manifest as "grittiness" that is encountered when sectioning the lesion.

Dehner and associates[77,459] have subclassified PPBs into three groups, based on the extent of cystic change that they demonstrate. Type I tumors are predominantly cystic, type II lesions are mixed solid and cystic, and type III PPBs are predominantly solid (Figs. 14-97 to 14-99). Cystic foci are lined by modified respiratory epithelium that is typically bland cytologically, and the surrounding stroma is variably myxoid and relatively hypocellular. It is now believed that PPB

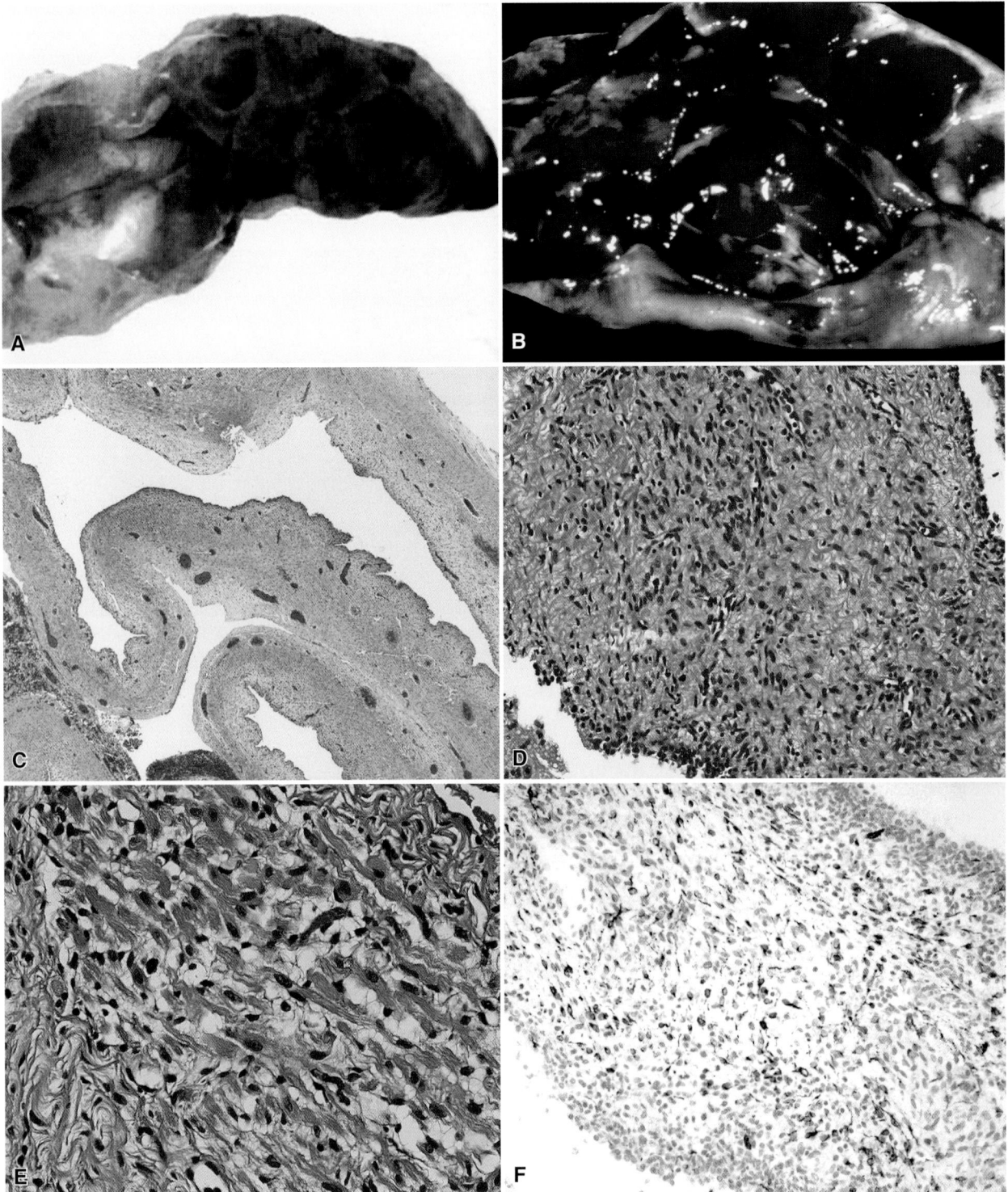

Figure 14-97. A and **B,** Gross photographs of type I pleuropulmonary blastoma demonstrating extensive cystic change in the lesions. The cyst walls contain primitive mesenchymal tissue (**C**), as well as elements with rhabdomyoblastic features (**D** and **E**), which are immunoreactive for desmin (**F**).

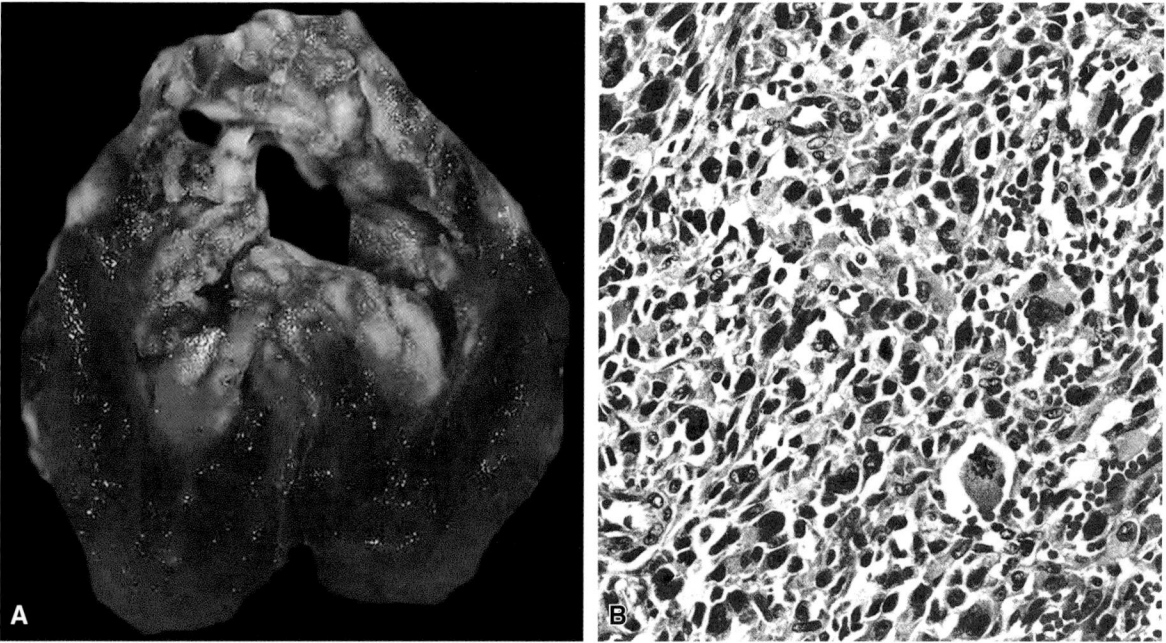

Figure 14-98. Gross photograph of type II pleuropulmonary blastoma (**A**), the solid areas of which (**B**) resemble the microscopic image of pleomorphic sarcoma.

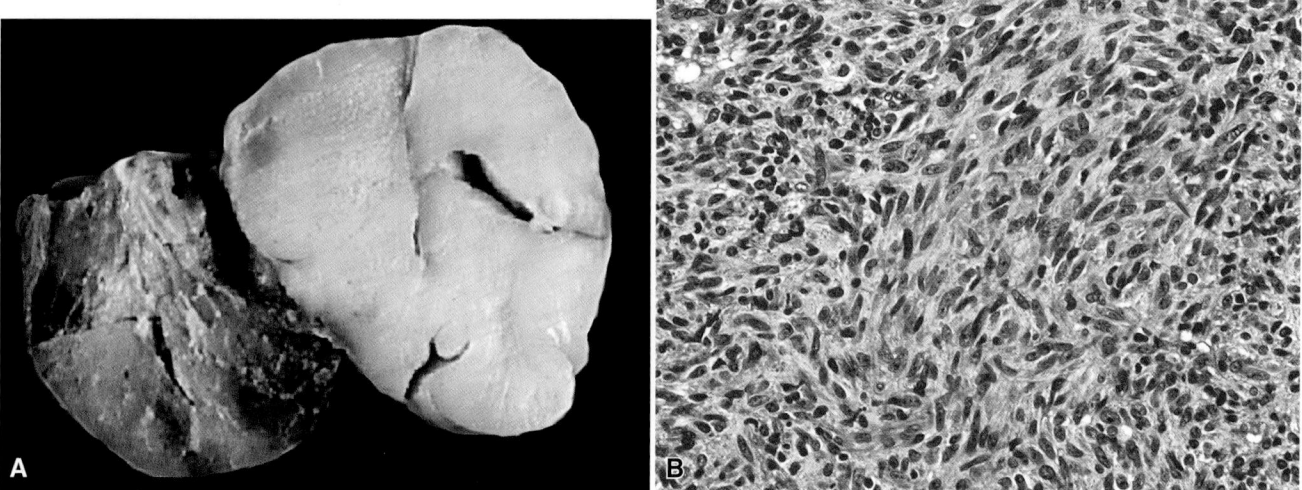

Figure 14-99. A, Type III pleuropulmonary blastoma, represented by a solid mass. **B,** This particular tumor has a nondescript spindle cell constituency. (Courtesy of Dr. D. Ashley Hill, Washington, DC.)

is associated with "type 4" cystic congenital adenomatoid malformations (CCAMs) of the lung, whereas bronchioloalveolar carcinoma of the lung in children is linked to CCAM type 1[467,468] (see Chapter 4).

Microscopically, one sees a heterogeneous mixture of growth patterns that are admixed with one another in various solid regions of these tumors. Some foci resemble MFH (Fig. 14-100); others take on a rhabdomyosarcomatous appearance; and still other areas have the features of fibrosarcoma, liposarcoma, chondrosarcoma, or osteosarcoma.[74,459] In the past, some observers applied the term "malignant mesenchymoma" to PPB, but such a designation has generally fallen from favor in current nosology. Importantly, epithelial foci are absent in PPB, in contrast to their dominance in so-called "adult pulmonary blastoma."[74,77,459] Immunohistochemical and ultrastructural studies demonstrate findings that are in accord with the aforementioned microscopic features, and they again fail to reveal epithelial characteristics in these lesions.[74,469]

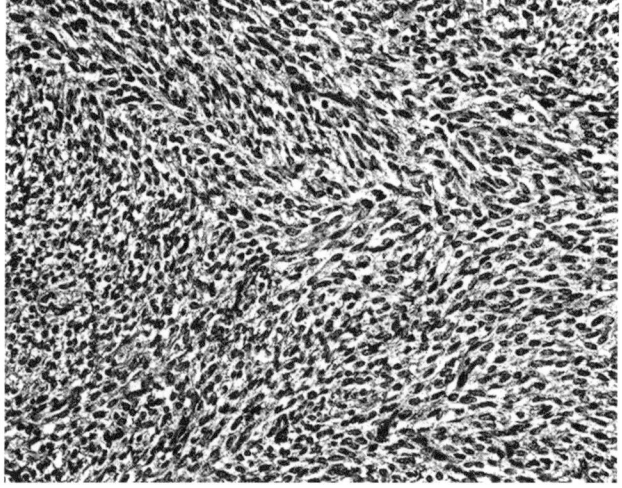

Figure 14-100. Another type III pleuropulmonary blastoma.

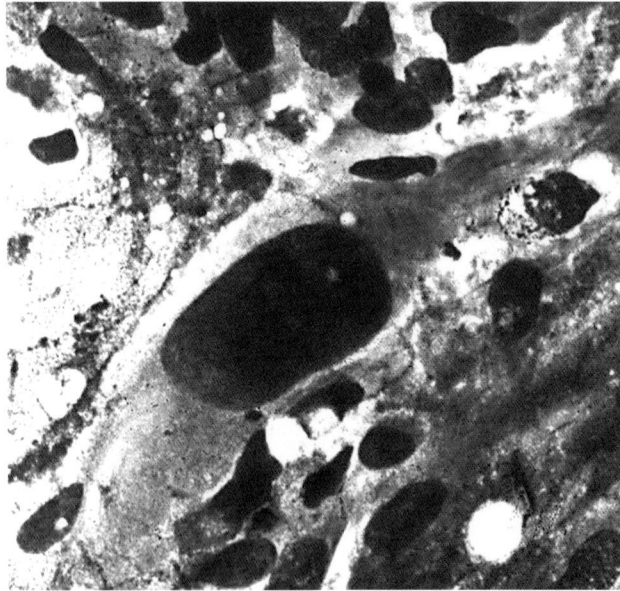

Figure 14-101. Bizarre, large, dyshesive spindle cells are seen in this fine needle aspiration biopsy specimen of type III pleuropulmonary blastoma.

Figure 14-103. A chondroid area is present in this pleuropulmonary blastoma.

Fine needle aspiration biopsies typically show dyshesive, pleomorphic cells from PPBs (Fig. 14-101). Immunohistologic studies are required to assess the presence of lineage-related markers in such elements.

Hill and coworkers have suggested that cystic type I PPB evolves into types II or III over time in a sizable proportion of cases. Type I tumors show the presence of primitive mesenchymal tissues mantling intralesional cysts, beneath a cytologically bland lining of respiratory epithelium. Rhabdomyosarcoma-like and chondrosarcoma-like elements are present in 49% and 40% of cases, respectively (Figs. 14-102 and 14-103). The latter elements become even more common in types II and III PPB.[470]

The pathologic differential diagnosis of PPB concerns SC of the lung and pleura, sarcomatoid mesothelioma with divergent differentiation, and rhabdomyosarcoma arising in congenital pulmonary cysts or teratoid tumors involving the pleura. The absence of keratin in PPB excludes pulmonary blastoma, other forms of carcinoma, mesothelioma, and germ cell tumors from further consideration.

Therapy and Prognosis

PPB is a rare tumor; therefore, organized protocol studies of therapy are still in evolution. In general, however, it is obvious that this neoplasm is a highly aggressive lesion that requires every effort at surgical extirpation, followed by intensive radiation and chemotherapy.[459,465] Because of the histologic characteristics of the tumor, which are like those of de novo soft tissue sarcomas, it would seem appropriate to use drug combinations that are directed toward the various histologic components of PPB (e.g., rhabdomyosarcoma, MFH, osteosarcoma). Surgical debulking of the tumor mass should also be considered in individual cases where complete resection is not thought to be feasible. Dehner and colleagues have related morphologic findings in PPBs to prognosis; predominantly cystic lesions have the best outlook, whereas type II and type III neoplasms are aggressive and often prove fatal

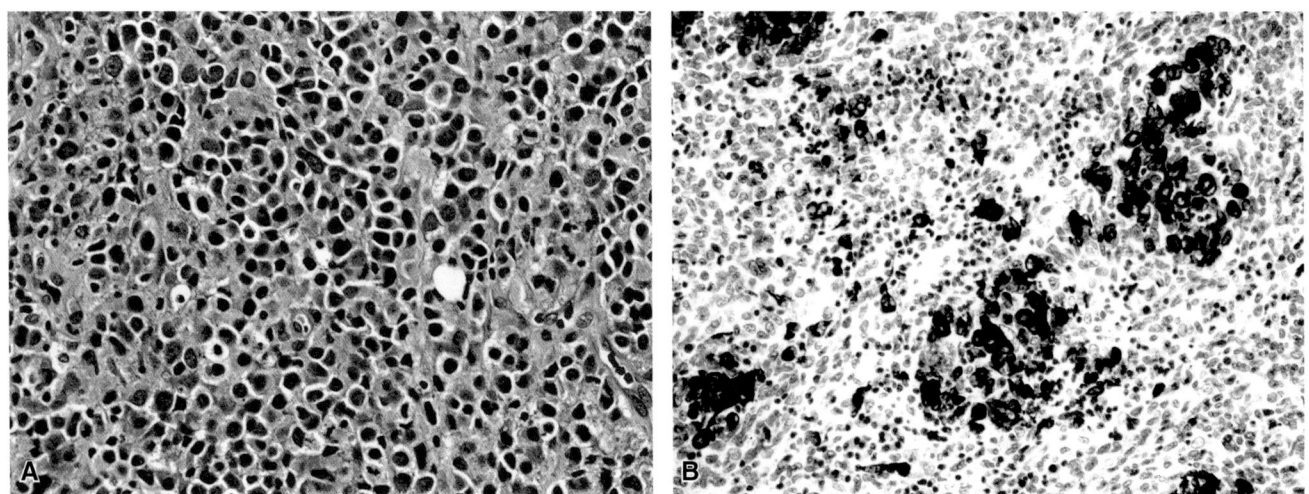

Figure 14-102. Solid, alveolar rhabdomyosarcoma-like growth in type III pleuropulmonary blastoma (**A**), showing immunoreactivity for fast muscle myosin (**B**).

within 2 years of diagnosis.[459] Interestingly, Wright has also reported a case wherein successive recurrences of a PPB showed progressive transformation from type I to type III morphology.[463] Priest and associates have reported a singular tendency for PPB to demonstrate metastases to the brain (Fig. 14-104). That complication is observed in 11% of type II cases and 54% of type III cases.[471]

Vascular Sarcomas of the Pleura

As mentioned previously, angiosarcoma, KS, and EH may take origin in the pleura as well as in the pulmonary parenchyma. The general clinicopathologic attributes of these lesions have been described above. It is notable that the most common initial sign of angiosarcoma and KS of the pleura is the presence of a bloody pleural effusion (Fig. 14-105).[284] Gross examination of the tumor at thoracotomy or thoracoscopy shows multiple soft, hemorrhagic, red-violet, nodular pleural implants in examples of angiosarcoma and KS. On the other hand, EH is virtually identical to MM at a macroscopic level (Fig. 14-106), and histologic study is necessary to distinguish between them.[472,473] As is true of their intrapulmonary counterparts, KS and angiosarcoma of the pleura are associated with a dismal prognosis,[474,475] whereas patients with EH may survive for prolonged periods.[472]

Self-assessment questions related to this chapter can be found online on the Expert Consult site for this title.

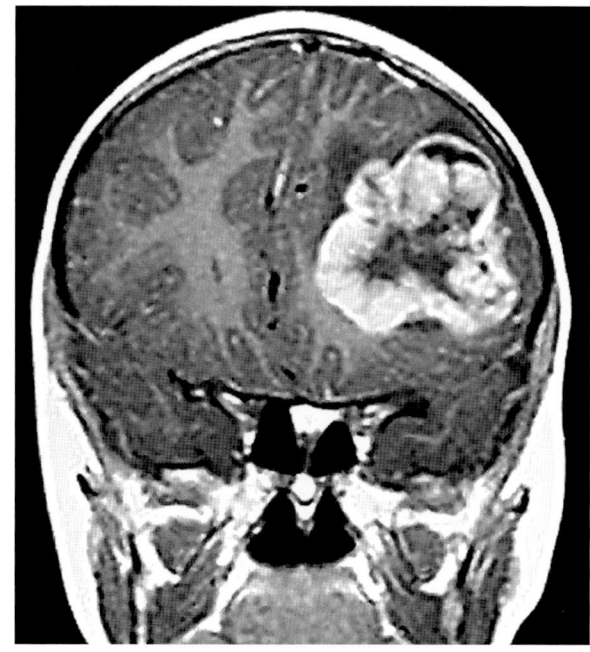

Figure 14-104. Metastasis of pleuropulmonary blastoma to the brain, as seen in a magnetic resonance image of the head.

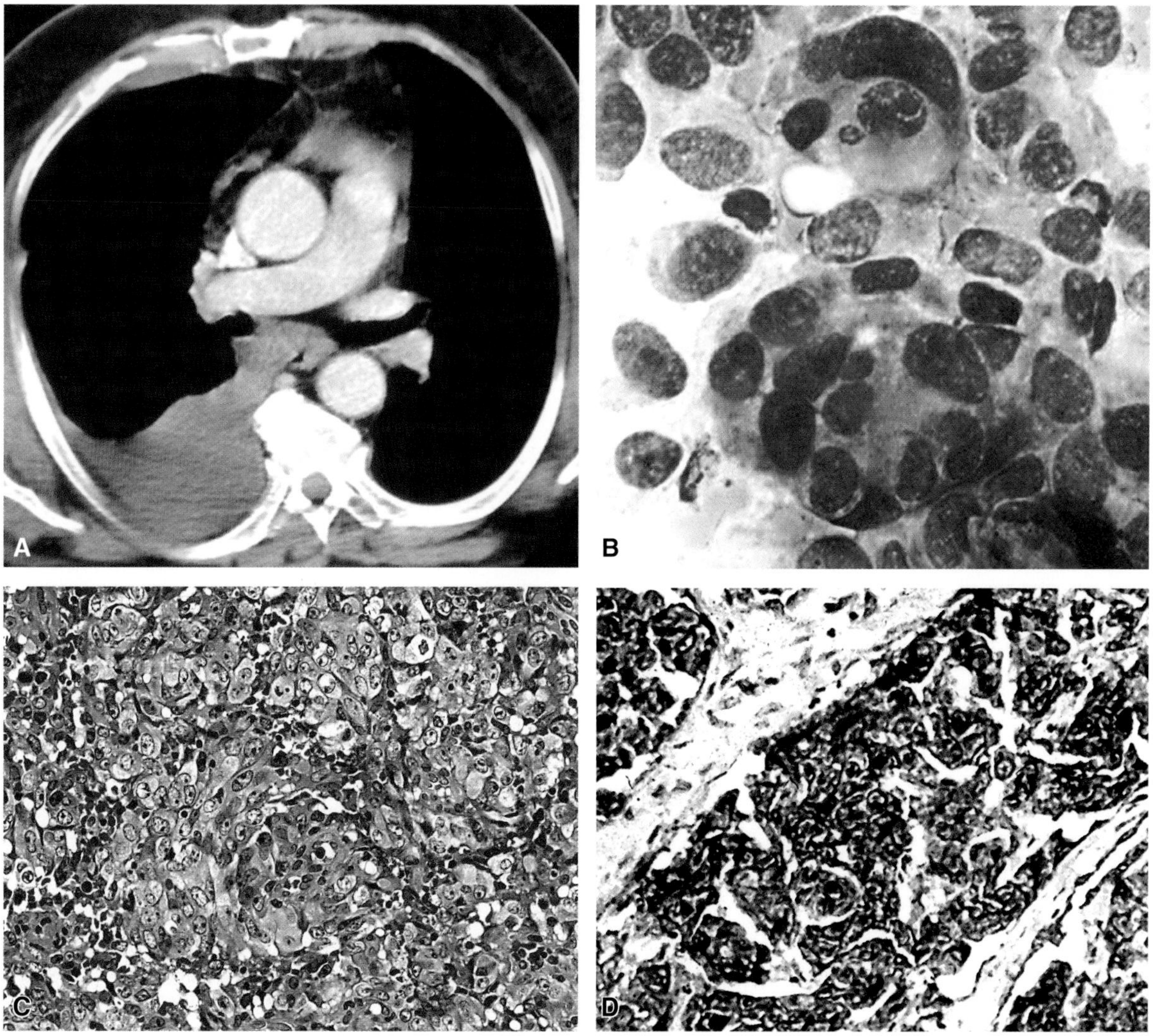

Figure 14-105. A, A pleural tumor is seen in the right hemithorax on this computed tomography scan, with an associated pleural effusion. **B,** Fine needle aspiration biopsy of the lesion shows modestly cohesive malignant epithelioid cells. **C,** A concurrent biopsy yields the same results as the fine needle aspiration biopsy. **D,** Immunoreactivity for CD31 establishes the diagnosis of epithelioid angiosarcoma of the pleura.

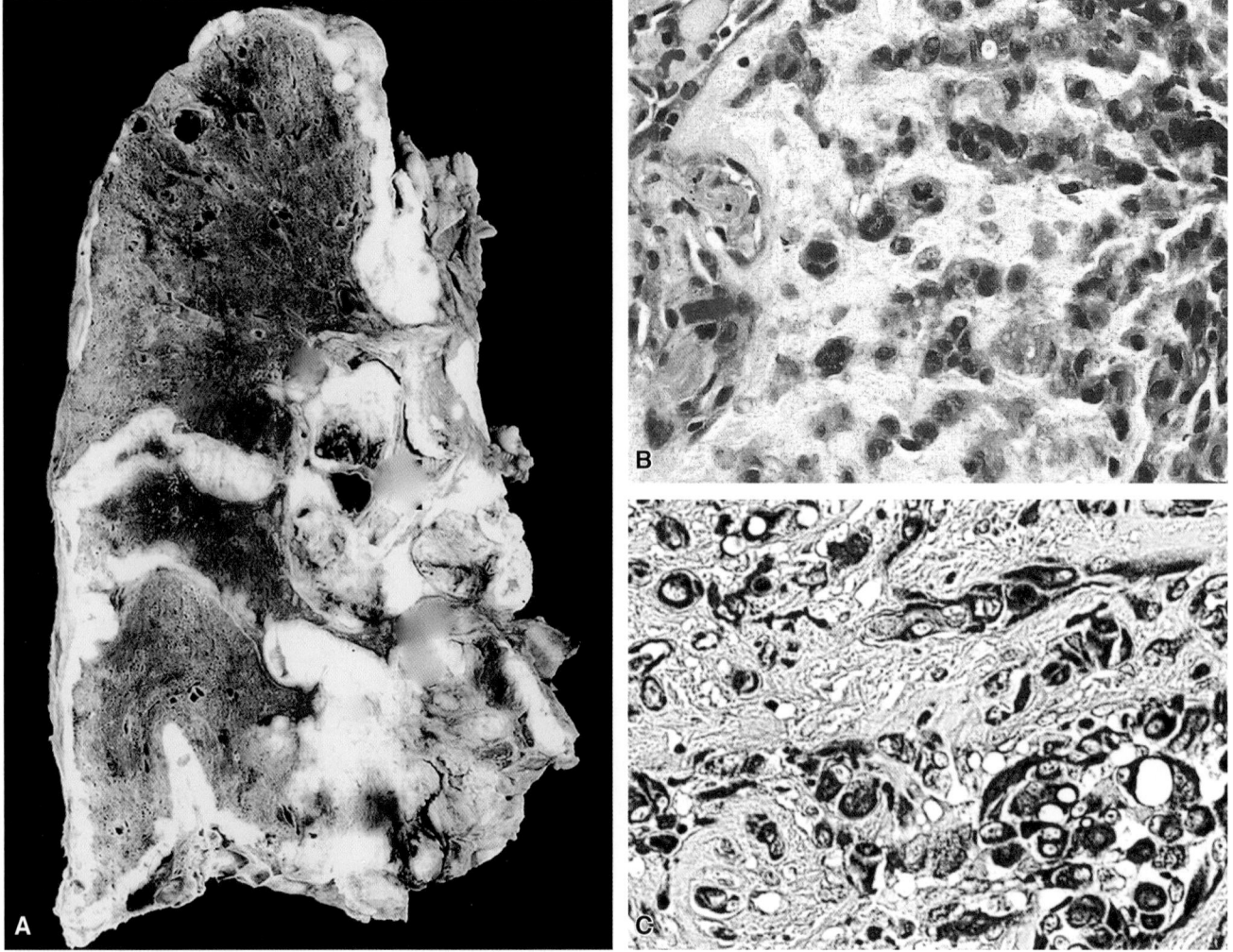

Figure 14-106. Gross (**A**) and microscopic (**B** and **C**) images of primary epithelioid hemangioendothelioma (EH) of the pleura, closely resembling those of epithelioid mesothelioma. However, EH is immunoreactive for CD31, unlike mesothelioma. (**A,** Courtesy of Dr. Victor Roggli, Durham, NC.)

References

1. Huang JC, Ritter JH, Wick MR. Malignant nonepithelial neoplasms of the lungs and pleural surfaces. In: Aisner J, et al., eds. *Comprehensive Textbook of Thoracic Oncology.* Baltimore: Williams & Wilkins; 1996:815–849.
2. Franks TJ, Galvin JR. Sarcomatoid carcinoma of the lung: histologic criteria and common lesions in the differential diagnosis. *Arch Pathol Lab Med.* 2010;134:49–54.
3. Pelosi G, Sonzogni A, De Pas T, et al. Pulmonary sarcomatoid carcinomas: a practical overview. *Int J Surg Pathol.* 2010;18:103–120.
4. Wick MR, Ritter JH, Humphrey PA. Sarcomatoid carcinomas of the lung: a clinicopathologic review. *Am J Clin Pathol.* 1997;108:40–53.
5. Litzky LA. Pulmonary sarcomatous tumors. *Arch Pathol Lab Med.* 2008;132:1104–1117.
6. Steele RH. Lung tumors: a personal review. *Diagn Histopathol.* 1983;6:119–123.
7. Nascimento AG, Unni KK. Sarcomas of the lung. *Mayo Clin Proc.* 1982;57:355–359.
8. Guccion JG, Rosen SH. Bronchopulmonary leiomyosarcomas and fibrosarcomas: a study of 32 cases and review of the literature. *Cancer.* 1972;30:835–847.
9. Przygodzki RM, Moran CA, Suster S, Koss MN. Primary pulmonary rhabdomyosarcomas: a clinicopathologic and immunohistochemical study of three cases. *Mod Pathol.* 1995;8:658–661.
10. Suster S. Primary sarcomas of the lung. *Semin Diagn Pathol.* 1995;12:140–157.
11. Zeren H, Moran CA, Suster S, et al. Primary pulmonary sarcomas with features of monophasic synovial sarcoma: a clinicopathological, immunohistochemical, and ultrastructural study of 25 cases. *Hum Pathol.* 1995;26:474–480.
12. Gaertner E, Zeren EH, Fleming MV, et al. Biphasic synovial sarcomas arising in the pleural cavity: a clinicopathologic study of five cases. *Am J Surg Pathol.* 1996;20:36–45.
13. Gladish GW, Sabloff BM, Munden RF, et al. Primary thoracic sarcomas. *Radiographics.* 2002;22:621–637.
14. Stackhouse EM, Harrison Jr EG, Ellis Jr FH. Primary mixed malignancies of lung: carcinosarcoma and blastoma. *J Thorac Cardiovasc Surg.* 1969;57:385–399.
15. Humphrey PA, Scroggs MW, Roggli VL, et al. Pulmonary carcinoma with a sarcomatoid element. *Hum Pathol.* 1988;19:155–165.
16. Ishida T, Tatsishi M, Kaneko S, et al. Carcinosarcoma and spindle-cell carcinoma of the lung. *J Thorac Cardiovasc Surg.* 1990;100:844–852.
17. Matsui K, Kitagawa M. Spindle cell carcinoma of the lung: a clinicopathologic study of three cases. *Cancer.* 1991;67:2361–2367.
18. Leventon GS, Evans HL. Sarcomatoid squamous cell carcinoma of the mucous membranes of the head and neck. *Cancer.* 1981;48:994–1003.
19. Piscioli F, Aldovini D, Bondi A, et al. Squamous cell carcinoma with sarcoma-like stroma of the nose and paranasal sinuses: report of two cases. *Histopathology.* 1984;8:633–639.
20. Lane N. Pseudosarcoma (polypoid sarcoma-like masses) associated with squamous cell carcinoma of the mouth, fauces, and larynx: report of ten cases. *Cancer.* 1957;10:19–41.
21. Lasser KH, Naeim F, Higgins J, et al. "Pseudosarcoma" of the larynx. *Am J Surg Pathol.* 1979;3:397–404.
22. Lambert PR, Ward PH, Berci G. Pseudosarcoma of the larynx: a comprehensive analysis. *Arch Otolaryngol.* 1980;106:700–708.
23. Davis MP, Eagan RT, Weiland LH, et al. Carcinosarcoma of the lung: Mayo Clinic experience and response to chemotherapy. *Mayo Clin Proc.* 1984;59:598–603.
24. Chang YL, Lee YC, Shih JY, et al. Pulmonary pleomorphic (spindle) cell carcinoma: peculiar clinicopathologic manifestations different from ordinary non-small-cell carcinoma. *Lung Cancer.* 2001;34:91–97.
25. Fung CH, Lo JW, Yonan TN, et al. Pulmonary blastoma: an ultrastructural study with brief review of literature and discussion of pathogenesis. *Cancer.* 1977;39:153–163.
26. Heffner DK, Hyams VJ. Teratocarcinosarcoma (malignant teratoma?) of the nasal cavity and paranasal sinuses: a clinicopathologic study of 20 cases. *Cancer.* 1984;53:2140–2154.
27. Patterson SD, Ballard RW. Nasal blastoma: a light and electron microscopic study. *Ultrastruct Pathol.* 1980;1:487–494.
28. Minckler DS, Meligro CH, Norris HT. Carcinosarcoma of the larynx. *Cancer.* 1970;26:195–200.

29. Goellner JR, Devine KD, Weiland LH. Pseudosarcoma of the larynx. *Am J Clin Pathol*. 1973;59:312–326.

30. Farrell DJ, Cooper PN, Malcolm AJ. Carcinosarcoma of the lung associated with asbestosis. *Histopathology*. 1995;27:484–486.

31. Berho M, Moran CA, Suster S. Malignant mixed epithelial/mesenchymal neoplasms of the lung. *Semin Diagn Pathol*. 1995;12:123–139.

32. Reynolds S, Jenkins G, Akosa A, et al. Carcinosarcoma of the lung: an unusual cause of empyema. *Respir Med*. 1995;89:73–75.

33. Nappi O, Glasner SD, Swanson PE, et al. Biphasic and monophasic sarcomatoid carcinomas of the lung: a reappraisal of "carcinosarcomas" and "spindle cell carcinomas". *Am J Clin Pathol*. 1994;102:331–340.

34. Nappi O, Wick MR. Sarcomatoid neoplasms of the respiratory tract. *Semin Diagn Pathol*. 1993;10:137–147.

35. Nakajima M, Kasai T, Hashimoto H, et al. Sarcomatoid carcinoma of the lung: a clinicopathologic study of 37 cases. *Cancer*. 1999;86:608–616.

36. Brambilla E, Travis WD, Colby TV, et al. The new World Health Organization classification of lung tumors. *Eur Respir J*. 2001;18:1059–1068.

37. Terzi A, Gorla A, Piubello Q, et al. Biphasic sarcomatoid carcinoma of the lung: report of 5 cases and review of the literature. *Eur J Surg Oncol*. 1997;23:457.

38. Ro JY, Chen JL, Lee JS, et al. Sarcomatoid carcinoma of the lung: immunohistochemical and ultrastructural studies of 14 cases. *Cancer*. 1992;69:376–386.

39. Koss MN. Pulmonary blastomas. *Cancer Treat Res*. 1995;72:349–362.

40. Miller RR, Champagne K, Murray RC. Primary pulmonary germ cell tumor with blastomatous differentiation. *Chest*. 1994;106:1595–1596.

41. Huwer H, Kalweit G, Straub U, et al. Pulmonary carcinosarcoma: diagnostic problems and determinants of prognosis. *Eur J Cardiothorac Surg*. 1996;10:403–407.

42. Melissari M, Giordano G, Gabrielli M. Immunohistochemical and ultrastructural study of a case of carcinosarcoma (biphasic sarcomatoid carcinoma) of the lung with rhabdomyoblastic differentiation. *Pathologica*. 1997;89:412–419.

43. Pankowski J, Grodzki T, Janowski H, et al. Carcinosarcoma of the lung: report of three cases. *J Cardiovasc Surg*. 1998;39:121–125.

44. Saphir O, Vass A. Carcinosarcoma. *Am J Cancer*. 1938;33:331–359.

45. Sarma DP, Deshotels Jr SJ. Carcinosarcoma of the lung. *J Surg Oncol*. 1982;19:216–218.

46. Bergmann M, Ackerman LV, Kemler RL. Carcinosarcoma of the lung: review of the literature and report of two cases treated by pneumonectomy. *Cancer*. 1951;4:919–929.

47. Kakos GS, Williams Jr TE, Assor D, et al. Pulmonary carcinosarcoma: etiologic, therapeutic, and prognostic considerations. *J Thorac Cardiovasc Surg*. 1971;61:777–783.

48. Krompecher E. Der drusernartige Oberflachen-Epitheliakrebscarcinom epitheliale Adenoides. *Beitr Pathol*. 1900;28:1–41.

49. Herxheimer G, Reinke F. Carcinoma sarcomatodes: pathologie des Krebses. *Ergeb Allg Pathol Pathol Anat*. 1912;16:280–282.

50. Moore TC. Carcinosarcoma of the lung. *Surgery*. 1961;50:886–893.

51. Cabarcos A, Gomez-Dorronsoro M, Lobo-Beristain JL. Pulmonary carcinosarcoma: a case study and review of the literature. *Br J Dis Chest*. 1985;79:83–90.

52. Ludwigsen E. Endobronchial carcinosarcoma. *Virchows Arch A Pathol Anat*. 1977;373:293–302.

53. Rainosek DE, Ro JY, Ordonez NG, et al. Sarcomatoid carcinoma of the lung: a case with atypical carcinoid and rhabdomyosarcomatous components. *Am J Clin Pathol*. 1994;102:360–364.

54. Fishback NF, Travis WD, Moran CA, et al. Pleomorphic (spindle/giant cell) carcinoma of the lung: a clinicopathologic correlation of 78 cases. *Cancer*. 1994;73:2936–2945.

55. Tsubota YT, Kawaguchi T, Hoso T, et al. A combined small cell and spindle cell carcinoma of the lung: report of a unique case with immunohistochemical and ultrastructural studies. *Am J Surg Pathol*. 1992;16:1108–1115.

56. Khalifa M, Hruby G, Ehrlich L, et al. Combined large cell neuroendocrine carcinoma and spindle cell carcinoma of the lung. *Ann Diagn Pathol*. 2001;5:240–245.

57. Oyasu R, Battifora HA, Buckingham WB, et al. Metaplastic squamous cell carcinoma of bronchus simulating giant cell tumor of bone. *Cancer*. 1977;39:1119–1128.

58. Love GL, Droca PJ. Bronchogenic sarcomatoid squamous cell carcinoma with osteoclast-like giant cells. *Hum Pathol*. 1983;14:1004–1006.

59. Kitazawa R, Kitazawa S, Nishimura Y, et al. Lung carcinosarcoma with liposarcoma element: autopsy case. *Pathol Int*. 2006;56:449–452.

60. Colombi RP. Sarcomatoid carcinomas of the female genital tract (malignant mixed müllerian tumors). *Semin Diagn Pathol*. 1993;10:169–175.

61. George E, Manivel JC, Dehner LP, et al. Malignant mixed müllerian tumors: an immunohistochemical study of 47 cases with histogenetic considerations and clinical correlation. *Hum Pathol*. 1991;22:215–223.

62. Travis WD, Colby TV, Corrin B, et al. In: *Histological Typing of Lung and Pleural Tumours (International Histological Classification of Tumours)*. Geneva, Switzerland: World Health Organization; 1999:1–55.

63. Wagner MS, Reyes CV. Primary chondroblastic osteosarcoma of the lung. *Sarcoma*. 1999;3:193–195.

64. Niimi R, Matsumine A, Kusuzaki K, et al. Primary osteosarcoma of the lung: a case report and review of the literature. *Med Oncol*. 2008;25:251–255.

65. Barnett NR, Barnard WG. Some unusual thoracic tumors. *Br J Surg*. 1945;32:447–457.

66. Spencer H. Pulmonary blastoma. *J Pathol Bacteriol*. 1961;82:161–165.

67. Francis D, Jacobsen M. Pulmonary blastoma. *Curr Top Pathol*. 1983;73:265–294.

68. Ohtomo K, Araki T, Yashiro N, et al. Pulmonary blastoma in children. *Radiology*. 1983;147:101–104.

69. Gal AA, Marchevsky AM, Koss MN. Unusual tumors of the lung. In: Marchevsky AM, ed. *Surgical Pathology of Lung Neoplasms*. New York: Marcel Dekker; 1990:325–388.

70. Jetley NK, Bhatnagar V, Krishna A, et al. Pulmonary blastoma in a neonate. *J Pediatr Surg*. 1988;23:1009–1010.

71. Jimenez JF. Pulmonary blastoma in childhood. *J Surg Oncol*. 1987;334:87–93.

72. Senac Jr MO, Wood BP, Isaacs H, et al. Pulmonary blastoma: a rare childhood malignancy. *Radiology*. 1991;179:743–746.

73. Cohen M, Emms M, Kaschula ROC. Childhood pulmonary blastoma: a pleuropulmonary variant of the adult pulmonary blastoma. *Pediatr Pathol*. 1991;11:737–739.

74. Manivel JC, Priest JR, Watterson J, et al. Pleuropulmonary blastoma: the so-called pulmonary blastoma of childhood. *Cancer*. 1988;62:1516–1526.

75. Hachitanda Y, Aoyama C, Sato JK, et al. Pleuropulmonary blastoma in childhood: a tumor of divergent differentiation. *Am J Surg Pathol*. 1993;17:382–391.

76. Seballos RM, Klein RL. Pulmonary blastoma in children: report of two cases and review of the literature. *J Pediatr Surg*. 1994;29:1553–1556.

77. Dehner LP. Pleuropulmonary blastoma is the pulmonary blastoma of childhood. *Semin Diagn Pathol*. 1994;11:144–151.

78. Delahunt B, Thomson KJ, Ferguson AF, et al. Familial cystic nephroma and pleuropulmonary blastoma. *Cancer*. 1993;71:1338–1342.

79. Sciot R, Dal-Cin P, Brock P, et al. Pleuropulmonary blastoma (pulmonary blastoma of childhood): genetic link with other embryonal malignancies? *Histopathology*. 1994;24:559–563.

80. Schmaltz C, Sauter S, Opitz O, et al. Pleuropulmonary blastoma: a case report and review of the literature. *Med Pediatr Oncol*. 1995;25:479–484.

81. Re GG, Hazen-Martin DJ, Sens DA, et al. Nephroblastoma (Wilms' tumor): a model system of aberrant renal development. *Semin Diagn Pathol*. 1994;11:125–135.

82. Souza RC, Peasley ED, Takaro T. Pulmonary blastomas: a distinctive group of carcinosarcomas of the lung. *Ann Thorac Surg*. 1965;1:259–268.

83. Millard M. Lung, pleura, and mediastinum. In: Anderson WAD, ed. *Pathology*, vol. 2, 6th ed. St. Louis: CV Mosby; 1971:875–997.

84. Koss MN, Hochholzer L, O'Leary T. Pulmonary blastomas. *Cancer*. 1991;67:2368–2381.

85. Takahasi H, Tanaka K, Uchida Y, et al. A case of pulmonary blastoma composed of histological features of both pulmonary blastoma and pulmonary endodermal tumor resembling fetal lung. *J Jpn Assn Thorac Surg*. 1995;43:1217–1222.

86. Babycos PB, Daroca Jr PJ. Polypoid pulmonary endodermal tumor resembling fetal lung: report of a case. *Mod Pathol*. 1995;8:303–306.

87. Kodama T, Shimosato Y, Watanabe S, et al. Six cases of well-differentiated adenocarcinoma simulating fetal lung tissues in pseudoglandular stage: comparison with pulmonary blastoma. *Am J Surg Pathol*. 1984;8:735–744.

88. Kradin RL, Young RH, Dickersin RG, et al. Pulmonary blastoma with argyrophil cells lacking sarcomatous features (pulmonary endodermal tumor resembling fetal lung). *Am J Surg Pathol*. 1982;6:165–172.

89. Manning JT, Ordonez NG, Rosenberg HS, et al. Pulmonary endodermal tumor resembling fetal lung. *Arch Pathol Lab Med*. 1985;109:48–50.

90. Muller-Hermelink HK, Kaiserling E. Pulmonary adenocarcinoma of fetal type: alternating differentiation argues in favor of a common endodermal stem cell. *Virchows Arch A*. 1986;409:195–210.

91. Olenick SJ, Fan CC, Ryoo JW. Mixed pulmonary blastoma and carcinosarcoma. *Histopathology*. 1994;25:171–174.

92. Roth JA, Elquezabel A. Pulmonary blastoma evolving into carcinosarcoma: a case study. *Am J Surg Pathol*. 1978;2:407–413.

93. Jacobsen M, Francis D. Pulmonary blastoma: a clinicopathologic study of eleven cases. *Acta Pathol Microbiol Immunol Scand [A]*. 1980;88:151–160.

94. Nappi O, Swanson PE, Wick MR. Pseudovascular adenoid squamous cell carcinoma of the lung: clinicopathologic of three cases and comparison with true pleuropulmonary angiosarcoma. *Hum Pathol*. 1994;25:373–378.

95. Ritter JH, Mills SE, Nappi O, et al. Angiosarcoma-like neoplasms of epithelial organs: true endothelial tumors or variants of carcinoma? *Semin Diagn Pathol*. 1995;12:270–282.

96. Banerjee SS, Eyden BP, Wells S, et al. Pseudoangiosarcomatous carcinoma: a clinicopathological study of seven cases. *Histopathology*. 1992;21:13–23.

97. Nappi O, Wick MR, Pettinato G, et al. Pseudovascular adenoid squamous cell carcinoma of the skin: a neoplasm that may be mistaken for angiosarcoma. *Am J Surg Pathol*. 1992;16:429–438.

98. Eusebi V, Lamovec J, Cattani MG, et al. Acantholytic variant of squamous cell carcinoma of the breast. *Am J Surg Pathol*. 1986;10:855–861.

99. Mills SE, Gaffey MJ, Watts JC, et al. Angiomatoid carcinoma and "angiosarcoma" of the thyroid gland: a spectrum of endothelial differentiation. *Am J Clin Pathol*. 1994;102:322–330.

100. Umiker W, Iverson L. Postinflammatory "tumors" of the lung. *J Thorac Surg*. 1954;28:55–63.

101. Titus J, Harrison Jr EG, Clagett O, et al. Xanthomatous and inflammatory pseudotumors of the lung. *Cancer*. 1962;15:522–538.

102. Mandelbaum I, Brashear RE, Hull MT. Surgical treatment and course of pulmonary pseudotumor (plasma cell granuloma). *J Thorac Cardiovasc Surg*. 1981;82:77–82.

103. Berardi RS, Lee SS, Chen HP, et al. Inflammatory pseudotumors of the lung. *Surg Gynecol Obstet*. 1983;156:89–96.

104. Chen HP, Lee SS, Berardi RS. Inflammatory pseudotumor of the lung: ultrastructural and light microscopic study of a myxomatous variant. *Cancer*. 1984;54:861–865.

105. Maples MD, Adkins Jr RB, Graham BS, et al. Pseudotumor of the lung. *Am Surg*. 1985;51:84–88.

106. Matsubara O, Tan-Liu NS, Kenney RM, et al. Inflammatory pseudotumors of the lung: progression from organizing pneumonia to fibrous histiocytoma or to plasma cell granuloma in 32 cases. *Hum Pathol*. 1988;19:807–814.

107. Machicao CN, Sorensen K, Abdul KF, et al. Transthoracic needle aspiration biopsy in inflammatory pseudotumors of the lung. *Diagn Cytopathol*. 1989;5:400–403.

108. Ishida T, Oka T, Nishino T, et al. Inflammatory pseudotumor of the lung in adults: radiographic and clinicopathological analysis. *Ann Thorac Surg*. 1989;48:90–95.

109. Barbareschi M, Ferrero S, Aldovini D, et al. Inflammatory pseudotumor of the lung: immunohistochemical analysis on four new cases. *Histol Histopathol*. 1990;5:205–211.

110. Kobzik L. Benign pulmonary lesions that may be misdiagnosed as malignant. *Semin Diagn Pathol*. 1990;7:129–138.

111. Vujanic GM, Dojcinov D. Inflammatory pseudotumor of the lung in children. *Pediatr Hematol Oncol*. 1991;8:121–129.

112. Daudi FA, Lees GM, Higa TE. Inflammatory pseudotumors of the lung: two cases and a review. *Can J Surg*. 1991;34:461–464.

113. Nonomura A, Mizukami Y, Matsubara F, et al. Seven patients with plasma cell granuloma (inflammatory pseudotumor) of the lung, including two with intrabronchial growth: an immunohistochemical and electron microscopic study. *Intern Med*. 1992;31:756–765.

114. Koss MN. Tumor-like conditions of lung. *Adv Pathol Lab Med*. 1994;7:123–150.

115. Pettinato G, Manivel JC, DeRosa N, et al. Inflammatory myofibroblastic tumor (plasma cell granuloma): clinicopathologic study of 20 cases with immunohistochemical and ultrastructural observations. *Am J Clin Pathol*. 1990;94:538–546.

116. Lipton JH, Fong TC, Gill MJ, et al. Q fever inflammatory pseudotumor of the lung. *Chest*. 1987;92:756–757.

117. Bishopric GA, D'Agay MF, Schlemmer B, et al. Pulmonary pseudotumor due to *Corynebacterium equi* in a patient with the acquired immunodeficiency syndrome. *Thorax*. 1988;43:486–487.

118. Wick MR, Ritter JH, Nappi O. Inflammatory sarcomatoid carcinoma of the lung: report of three cases and clinicopathologic comparison with inflammatory pseudotumors in adult patients. *Hum Pathol*. 1995;26:1014–1021.

119. Antic T, Kapur U, Vigneswaran WT, et al. Inflammatory sarcomatoid carcinoma: a case report and discussion of a malignant tumor with benign appearance. *Arch Pathol Lab Med*. 2005;129:1334–1337.

120. Hartmann CA, Schutze H. Mesothelioma-like tumors of the pleura: a review of 72 autopsy cases. *Cancer Res Clin Oncol*. 1994;120:331–347.

121. Shah IA, Salvatore JR, Kummet T, et al. Pseudomesotheliomatous carcinoma involving pleura and peritoneum: a clinicopathologic and immunohistochemical study of three cases. *Ann Diagn Pathol*. 1999;3:148–159.

122. Inomata M, Kawagishi Y, Yamada T, et al. Two cases of pulmonary sarcomatoid carcinoma mimicking malignant mesothelioma. *J Jpn Resp Soc*. 2010;48:33–38.

123. Huszar M, Herczeg E, Lieberman Y, et al. Distinctive immunofluorescent labeling of epithelial and mesenchymal elements of carcinosarcoma with antibodies specific for different intermediate filaments. *Hum Pathol*. 1984;15:532–538.

124. Zimmerman KG, Sobonya RE, Payne CM. Histochemical and ultrastructural features of an unusual pulmonary carcinosarcoma. *Hum Pathol*. 1981;12:1046–1051.

125. Koss MN, Hochholzer L, Frommelt RA. Carcinosarcomas of the lung: a clinicopathologic study of 66 patients. *Am J Surg Pathol*. 1999;23:1514–1526.

126. Yousem SA, Wick MR, Randhawa P, et al. Pulmonary blastoma: an immunohistochemical comparison to fetal lung in its pseudoglandular stage. *Am J Clin Pathol*. 1990;93:167–175.

127. Matsui K, Kitagawa M, Miwa A. Lung carcinoma with spindle cell components: sixteen cases examined by immunohistochemistry. *Hum Pathol*. 1992;23:1289–1297.

128. Addis BJ, Corrin B. Pulmonary blastoma, carcinosarcoma, and spindle-cell carcinoma: an immunohistochemical study of keratin intermediate filaments. *J Pathol*. 1985;147:291–301.

129. Suster S, Huszar M, Herczeg E. Spindle-cell carcinoma of the lung: immunocytochemical and ultrastructural study of a case. *Histopathology*. 1987;11:871–878.

130. Berean K, Truong LD, Dudley Jr AW, et al. Immunohistochemical characterization of pulmonary blastoma. *Am J Clin Pathol*. 1988;89:773–777.

131. Pelosi G, Scarpa A, Manzotti M, et al. K-ras gene mutational analysis supports a monoclonal origin of biphasic pleomorphic carcinoma of the lung. *Mod Pathol*. 2004;17:538–546.

132. Hountis P, Moraitis S, Dedeilias P, et al. Sarcomatoid lung carcinomas: a case series. *Cases J*. 2009;2:7900–7910.

133. Wick MR, Swanson PE. Carcinosarcomas—current perspectives and a historical review of nosological concepts. *Semin Diagn Pathol*. 1993;10:118–127.

134. Brooks JJ. The significance of double phenotypic patterns and markers in human sarcomas. *Am J Pathol*. 1986;125:113–123.

135. Thompson L, Chang B, Barsky SH. Monoclonal origins of malignant mixed tumors (carcinosarcomas). *Am J Surg Pathol*. 1996;20:277–287.

136. Rossi S, Orvieto E, Furlanetto A, et al. Utility of the immunohistochemical detection of FLI-1 expression in round cell and vascular neoplasm using a monoclonal antibody. *Mod Pathol*. 2004;17:547–552.

137. Battifora H. Spindle-cell carcinoma: ultrastructural evidence of squamous origin and collagen production by the tumor cells. *Cancer*. 1976;37:2275–2282.

138. Wakely Jr PE. Pulmonary spindle cell lesions: correlation of aspiration cytopathology and histopathology. *Ann Diagn Pathol*. 2001;5:216–228.

139. Roberts CA, Seemayer TA, Neff JR, et al. Translocation (X;18) in primary synovial sarcoma of the lung. *Cancer Genet Cytogenet*. 1996;88:49–52.

140. Kaplan MA, Goodman MD, Satish J, et al. Primary pulmonary sarcoma with morphologic features of monophasic synovial sarcoma and chromosome translocation t(X;18). *Am J Clin Pathol*. 1996;105:195–199.

141. Terry J, Saito T, Subramanian S, et al. TLE1 as a diagnostic immunohistochemical marker for synovial sarcoma emerging from gene expression profiling studies. *Am J Surg Pathol*. 2007;31:240–246.

142. Jagdis A, Rubin BP, Tubbs RR, et al. Prospective evaluation of TLE1 as a diagnostic immunohistochemical marker in synovial sarcoma. *Am J Surg Pathol*. 2009;33:1743–1751.

143. Kosemehmetoglu K, Vrana JA, Folpe AL. TLE1 expression is not specific for synovial sarcoma: a whole section study of 163 soft tissue and bone neoplasms. *Mod Pathol*. 2009;22:872–878.

144. Knösel T, Heretsch S, Altendorf-Hofmann A, et al. TLE1 is a robust diagnostic biomarker for synovial sarcomas and correlates with t(X;18): analysis of 319 cases. *Eur J Cancer*. 2010;46:1170–1176.

145. Kung IT, Thallas V, Spencer EJ, et al. Expression of muscle actins in diffuse mesotheliomas. *Hum Pathol*. 1995;26:565–570.

146. Padgett DM, Cathro HP, Wick MR, et al. Podoplanin is a better immunohistochemical marker for sarcomatoid mesothelioma than calretinin. *Am J Surg Pathol*. 2008;32:123–127.

147. Wick MR. Kaposi's sarcoma unrelated to the acquired immunodeficiency syndrome: a review. *Curr Opin Oncol*. 1991;3:377–383.

148. Ognibene FP, Shelhamer JH. Kaposi's sarcoma. *Clin Chest Med*. 1988;9:459–465.

149. Garay SM, Belenko M, Fazzini E, et al. Pulmonary manifestations of Kaposi's sarcoma. *Chest*. 1987;91:39–43.

150. White DA, Matthay RA. Noninfectious pulmonary complications of infection with the human immunodeficiency virus. *Am Rev Respir Dis*. 1989;140:1763–1787.

151. Meduri GU, Stover DE, Lee M, et al. Pulmonary Kaposi's sarcoma in the acquired immune deficiency syndrome: clinical, radiographic, and pathologic manifestations. *Am J Med*. 1986;81:11–18.

152. Purdy LJ, Colby TV, Yousem SA, et al. Pulmonary Kaposi's sarcoma: premortem histologic diagnosis. *Am J Surg Pathol*. 1986;10:301–311.

153. Cadranel J, Naccache J, Wislez M, et al. Pulmonary malignancies in the immunocompromised patient. *Respiration*. 1999;66:289–309.

154. Katariya K, Thurer RJ. Malignancies associated with the immunocompromised state. *Chest Surg Clin N Am*. 1999;9:63–77.

155. Smith C, Lilly S, Mann KP, et al. AIDS-related malignancies. *Ann Med*. 1998;30:323–344.

156. Hannon FB, Easterbrook PJ, Padley S, et al. Bronchopulmonary Kaposi's sarcoma in 106 HIV-1-infected patients. *Int J STD AIDS*. 1998;9:518–525.

157. Bach MC, Bagwell SP, Fanning JP. Primary pulmonary Kaposi's sarcoma in the acquired immunodeficiency syndrome: a cause of persistent pyrexia. *Am J Med*. 1988;85:274–275.

158. Hanno R, Owen LG, Callen JP. Kaposi's sarcoma with extensive silent internal involvement. *Int J Dermatol*. 1979;18:718–721.

159. Gal AA, Koss MN, Hartmann B, et al. A review of pulmonary pathology in the acquired immune deficiency syndrome. *Surg Pathol*. 1988;1:325–346.

160. O'Brien RF, Cohn DL. Serosanguineous pleural effusions in AIDS-associated Kaposi's sarcoma. *Chest*. 1989;96:460–466.

161. Floris C, Sulis ML, Bernascani M, et al. Pneumothorax in pleuropulmonary Kaposi's sarcoma related to acquired immune deficiency syndrome. *Am J Med*. 1989;87:123–124.

162. Cheuk W, Wong KO, Wong CS, et al. Immunostaining for human herpesvirus 8 latent nuclear antigen-1 helps distinguish Kaposi sarcoma from its mimickers. *Am J Clin Pathol*. 2004;121:335–342.

163. Folpe AL, Chand EM, Goldblum JR, et al. Expression of Fli-1, a nuclear transcription factor, distinguishes vascular neoplasms from potential mimics. *Am J Surg Pathol*. 2001;25:1061–1066.

164. Weninger W, Partanen TA, Breiteneder-Geleff S, et al. Expression of vascular endothelial growth factor receptor-3 and podoplanin suggests a lymphatic endothelial cell origin of Kaposi's sarcoma tumor cells. *Lab Invest*. 1999;79:243–251.

165. Ireland-Gill A, Espina BM, Akil B, et al. Treatment of acquired immunodeficiency syndrome-related Kaposi's sarcoma using bleomycin-containing combination chemotherapy regimens. *Semin Oncol*. 1992;19(2 suppl 5):32–37.

166. Gill PS, Akil B, Colletti P, et al. Pulmonary Kaposi's sarcoma: clinical findings and results of therapy. *Am J Med*. 1989;87:57–61.

167. Ognibene FP, Steis RG, Macher AM, et al. Kaposi's sarcoma causing pulmonary infiltrates and respiratory failure in the acquired immunodeficiency syndrome. *Ann Intern Med*. 1985;102:471–475.

168. Guccion JG, Rosen SH. Bronchopulmonary leiomyosarcoma and fibrosarcoma: a study of 32 cases and review of the literature. *Cancer*. 1972;30:836–847.

169. Enzinger FM, Weiss SW. Fibrosarcoma. In: *Soft Tissue Tumors*, 2nd ed. St. Louis: CV Mosby; 1988:201–222.

170. Nascimento AG, Unni KK, Bernatz PE. Sarcomas of the lung. *Mayo Clin Proc*. 1982;57:355–359.

171. Miller DL, Allen MS. Rare pulmonary neoplasms. *Mayo Clin Proc*. 1993;68:492–498.

172. Pettinato G, Manivel JC, Saldana MJ, et al. Primary bronchopulmonary fibrosarcoma of childhood and adolescence: reassessment of a low-grade malignancy. *Hum Pathol*. 1989;20:463–471.

173. Goldthorn JF, Duncan MH, Kosloske AM, et al. Cavitating primary pulmonary fibrosarcoma in a child. *J Thorac Cardiovasc Surg*. 1986;91:932–934.

174. Wick MR, Manivel JC. Primary sarcomas of the lung. In: Williams CJ, Krikorian JG, Green MR, Raghavan D, eds. *Textbook of Uncommon Cancer*. New York: John Wiley & Sons; 1988:335–381.

175. Logrono R, Filipowicz EA, Eyzaguirre EJ, et al. Diagnosis of primary fibrosarcoma of the lung by fine needle aspiration and core biopsy. *Arch Pathol Lab Med*. 1999;123:731–735.

176. Lane KL, Shannon RJ, Weiss SW. Hyalinizing spindle cell tumor with giant rosettes: a distinctive tumor closely resembling low-grade fibromyxoid sarcoma. *Am J Surg Pathol*. 1997;21:1481–1488.

177. Magro G, Fraggetta F, Manusia M, et al. Hyalinizing spindle cell tumor with giant rosettes: a previously undescribed lesion of the lung. *Am J Surg Pathol*. 1998;22:1431–1433.

178. Kim L, Yoon YH, Choi SJ, et al. Hyalinizing spindle cell tumor with giant rosettes arising in the lung: report of a case with FUS-CREB3L2 fusion transcripts. *Pathol Int*. 2007;57:153–157.

179. Vernon SE, Bejarano PA. Low-grade fibromyxoid sarcoma: a brief review. *Arch Pathol Lab Med*. 2006;130:1358–1360.

180. Beluffi G, Bertolotti P, Mietta A, et al. Primary leiomyosarcoma of the lung in a girl. *Pediatr Radiol*. 1986;16:240–244.

181. Jimenez JF, Uthman EO, Townsend JW, et al. Primary bronchopulmonary leiomyosarcoma in childhood. *Arch Pathol Lab Med*. 1986;110:348–351.

182. Yellin A, Rosenman Y, Lieberman Y. Review of smooth muscle tumours of the lower respiratory tract. *Br J Dis Chest*. 1984;78:337–351.

183. Lillo-Gil R, Albrechtsson U, Jakobsson B. Pulmonary leiomyosarcoma appearing as a cyst: report of one case and review of the literature. *Thorac Cardiovasc Surg*. 1985;33:250–252.

184. Yu H, Ren H, Miao Q, et al. Pulmonary leiomyosarcoma: report of three cases. *Chin Med J*. 1996;11:191–194.

185. Attanoos RL, Appleton MA, Gibbs AR. Primary sarcomas of the lung: a clinicopathological and immunohistochemical study of 14 cases. *Histopathology*. 1996;29:29–36.

186. Morgan PGM, Ball J. Pulmonary leiomyosarcomas. *Br J Dis Chest*. 1980;74:245–252.

187. Wick MR, Scheithauer BW, Piehler JM, et al. Primary pulmonary leiomyosarcomas: a light and electron microscopic study. *Arch Pathol Lab Med*. 1982;106:510–514.

188. Chaudhuri MR. Primary leiomyosarcoma of the lung. *Br J Dis Chest*. 1973;67:75–80.

189. Koizumi H, Fukuda T, Ohnishi Y, et al. Pulmonary myxoid leiomyosarcoma. *Pathol Int*. 1995; 45:879–884.

190. Keel SB, Bacha E, Mark EJ, et al. Primary pulmonary sarcoma: a clinicopathologic study of 26 cases. *Mod Pathol*. 1999;12:1124–1131.

191. Yu H, Ren H, Miao Q, et al. Pulmonary leiomyosarcoma—report of three cases. *Chin Med Sci J*. 1996;11:191–194.

192. Hummel P, Cangiarella JF, Cohen JM, et al. Transthoracic fine-needle aspiration biopsy of pulmonary spindle cell and mesenchymal lesions: a study of 61 cases. *Cancer*. 2001;93:187–198.

193. Yamaguchi T, Imamura Y, Nakayama K, et al. Primary pulmonary leiomyosarcoma. Report of a case diagnosed by fine needle aspiration cytology. *Acta Cytol*. 2002;46:912–916.

194. Dail DH, Liebow AA. Intravascular bronchioloalveolar tumor. *Am J Pathol*. 1975;78:6a [abstract].

195. Dail DH, Liebow AA, Gmelich JT, et al. Intravascular, bronchiolar, and alveolar tumor of the lung (IVBAT). *Cancer*. 1983;51:452–464.

196. Corrin B, Manners B, Millard M, et al. Histogenesis of so-called "intravascular bronchioloalveolar tumour". *J Pathol*. 1979;128:163–167.

197. Weiss SW, Enzinger FM. Epithelioid hemangioendothelioma: a vascular tumor often mistaken for a carcinoma. *Cancer*. 1982;50:970–981.

198. Schattenberg T, Kam R, Klopp M, et al. Pulmonary epithelioid hemangioendothelioma: report of three cases. *Surg Today*. 2008;38:844–849.

199. Weiss SW, Ishak KG, Dail DH, et al. Epithelioid hemangioendothelioma and related lesions. *Semin Diagn Pathol*. 1986;3:259–287.

200. Kitaichi M, Nagai S, Nishimura K, et al. Pulmonary epithelioid hemangioendothelioma in 21 patients, including three with partial spontaneous regression. *Eur Respir J*. 1998;12:89–96.

201. Rock MJ, Kaufman RA, Lobe TE, et al. Epithelioid hemangioendothelioma of the lung (intravascular bronchioloalveolar tumor) in a young girl. *Pediatr Pulmonol*. 1991;11:181–186.

202. Carter EJ, Bradburne RM, Jhung JW, et al. Alveolar hemorrhage with epithelioid hemangioendothelioma: a previously unreported manifestation of a rare tumor. *Am Rev Respir Dis*. 1990;142:700–701.

203. Briens E, Caulet-Maugendre S, Desrues B, et al. Alveolar hemorrhage revealing epithelioid hemangioendothelioma. *Respir Med*. 1997;91:111–114.

204. Yi ES, Auger WR, Friedman PJ, et al. Intravascular bronchioloalveolar tumor of the lung presenting as pulmonary thromboembolic disease and pulmonary hypertension. *Arch Pathol Lab Med*. 1995;119:255–260.

205. Ross GJ, Violi L, Friedman AC, et al. Intravascular bronchioloalveolar tumor: CT and pathologic correlation. *J Comput Assist Tomogr*. 1989;13:240–243.

206. Einsfelder B, Kuhnen C. Epithelioid hemangioendothelioma of the lung (IVBAT)—clinicopathological and immunohistochemical analysis of 11 cases. *Pathologe*. 2006; 27(2):106–115.

207. Saqi A, Nisbet L, Gagneja P, et al. Primary pleural epithelioid hemangioendothelioma with rhabdoid phenotype: report and review of the literature. *Diagn Cytopathol*. 2007;35:203–208.

208. Bhagavan BS, Murthy MSN, Dorfman HD, et al. Intravascular bronchiolo-alveolar tumor (IVBAT): a low-grade sclerosing epithelioid angiosarcoma of lung. *Am J Surg Pathol*. 1982;6:41–52.

209. Corrin B, Harrison WJ, Wright DH. The so-called intravascular bronchioloalveolar tumour of lung (low grade sclerosing angiosarcoma). *Diagn Histopathol*. 1983;6:229–237.

210. Corrin B, Dewar A, Simpson CG. Epithelioid hemangioendothelioma of the lung. *Ultrastruct Pathol*. 1996;20:345–347.

211. Buggage RR, Soudi N, Olson JL, et al. Epithelioid hemangioendothelioma of the lung: pleural effusion cytology, ultrastructure, and brief literature review. *Diagn Cytopathol*. 1995;13:54–60.

212. Bollinger BK, Laskin WB, Knight CB. Epithelioid hemangioendothelioma with multiple site involvement: literature review and observations. *Cancer*. 1994;73:610–615.

213. Weinreb I, Cunningham KS, Perez-Ordoñez B, et al. CD10 is expressed in most epithelioid hemangioendotheliomas: a potential diagnostic pitfall. *Arch Pathol Lab Med*. 2009;133:1965–1968.

214. Carretero A, Elmberger PG, Sköld CM, et al. Pulmonary epithelioid hemangioendothelioma: report of a case with fine needle aspiration biopsy. *Acta Cytol*. 2006;50:455–459.

215. Celikel C, Yumuk PF, Basaran G, et al. Epithelioid hemangioendothelioma with multiple organ involvement. *APMIS*. 2007;115:881–888.

216. Ohori NP, Yousem SA, Sonmez-Alpan E, et al. Estrogen and progesterone receptors in lymphangioleiomyomatosis, epithelioid hemangioendothelioma, and sclerosing hemangioma of the lungs. *Am J Clin Pathol*. 1991;96:529–535.

217. Stout AP, Murray MR. Hemangiopericytoma: a vascular tumor featuring Zimmerman's pericytes. *Ann Surg*. 1942;116:26–33.

218. Meade JB, Whitwell F, Bickford BJ, et al. Primary haemangiopericytoma of lung. *Thorax*. 1974;29:1–15.

219. Murphey MD. World Health Organization classification of bone and soft tissue tumors: modifications and implications for radiologists. *Semin Musculoskelet Radiol*. 2007;11:201–214.

220. Sakurai H, Tanaka W, Kaji M, et al. Intrapulmonary localized fibrous tumor of the lung: a very unusual presentation. *Ann Thorac Surg*. 2008;86:1360–1362.

221. Enzinger FM, Weiss SW, eds. Hemangiopericytoma. In: *Soft Tissue Tumors*. 2nd ed. St. Louis: CV Mosby; 1988:596–613.

222. Shin MS, Ho KJ. Primary hemangiopericytoma of lung: radiography and pathology. *AJR*. 1979;133:1077–1083.

223. Van Damme H, Dekoster G, Creemers E, et al. Primary pulmonary hemangiopericytoma: early local recurrence after perioperative rupture of the giant tumor mass (two cases). *Surgery*. 1990;108:105–109.

224. Yousem SA, Hochholzer L. Primary pulmonary hemangiopericytoma. *Cancer*. 1987;59: 549–555.

225. Yaghmai I. Angiographic manifestations of soft-tissue and osseous hemangiopericytomas. *Radiology*. 1978;126:653–659.

226. Halle M, Blum U, Dinkel E, et al. CT and MR features of primary pulmonary hemangiopericytomas. *J Comput Assist Tomogr*. 1993;17:51–55.

227. Rusch VW, Shuman WP, Schmidt R, et al. Massive pulmonary hemangiopericytoma: an innovative approach to evaluation and treatment. *Cancer*. 1989;64:1928–1936.

228. Liu CC, Wang HW, Li FY, et al. Solitary fibrous tumors of the pleura: clinicopathological characteristics, immunohistochemical profiles, and surgical outcomes with long-term follow-up. *Thorac Cardiovasc Surg*. 2008;56:291–297.

229. Kiefer T, Wertzel H, Freudenberg N, et al. Long-term survival after repetitive surgery for malignant hemangiopericytoma of the lung with subsequent systemic metastases: case report and review of the literature. *Thorac Cardiovasc Surg*. 1997;45:307–309.

230. Wong PP, Yagoda A. Chemotherapy of malignant hemangiopericytoma. *Cancer*. 1978;41:1256–1260.

231. Jha N, McNeese M, Barkley HT, et al. Does radiotherapy have a role in hemangiopericytoma management? Report of 14 new cases and a review of the literature. *Int J Radiat Oncol Biol Phys*. 1987;13:1399–1402.

232. Mira JG, Chu FCH, Fortner JG. The role of radiotherapy in the management of malignant hemangiopericytoma: report of eleven new cases and review of the literature. *Cancer*. 1977;39:1254–1259.

233. Hansen CP, Francis D, Bertelsen S. Primary hemangiopericytoma of the lung: case report. *Scand J Thorac Cardiovasc Surg*. 1990;24:89–92.

234. Weiss SW, Enzinger FM. Malignant fibrous histiocytoma: an analysis of 200 cases. *Cancer*. 1978;41:2250–2266.

235. Yousem SA, Hochholzer L. Malignant fibrous histiocytoma of the lung. *Cancer*. 1987;60: 2532–2541.

236. McDonnell T, Kyriakos M, Roper C, et al. Malignant fibrous histiocytoma of the lung. *Cancer*. 1988;61:137–145.

237. Lee JT, Shelburne JD, Linder J. Primary malignant fibrous histiocytoma of the lung: a clinicopathologic and ultrastructural study of five cases. *Cancer*. 1984;53:1124–1130.

238. Bedrossian CW, Verani R, Unger KM, et al. Pulmonary malignant fibrous histiocytoma: light and electron microscopic studies of one case. *Chest*. 1979;75:186–189.

239. Kern WH, Hughes RK, Meyer BW, et al. Malignant fibrous histiocytoma of the lung. *Cancer*. 1979;44:1793–1801.

240. Chowdhury LN, Swerdlow MA, Jao W, et al. Postirradiation malignant fibrous histiocytoma of the lung: demonstration of alpha-1-antitrypsin-like material in neoplastic cells. *Am J Clin Pathol*. 1980;74:820–826.

241. Kimizuka G, Okuzawa K, Yarita T. Primary giant cell malignant fibrous histiocytoma of the lung: a case report. *Pathol Int*. 1999;49:342–346.

242. Barbas CS, Capelozzi VL, Takagaki TY, et al. Primary malignant fibrous histiocytoma of the lung: report of a case with bronchial brushing cytologic features. *Acta Cytol*. 1997;41:919–923.

243. Halyard MY, Camoriano JK, Culligan JA, et al. Malignant fibrous histiocytoma of the lung: report of four cases and review of the literature. *Cancer*. 1996;78:2492–2497.

244. Shah SJ, Craver RD, Yu LC. Primary malignant fibrous histiocytoma of the lung in a child: a case report and review of literature. *Pediatr Hematol Oncol*. 1996;13:531–538.

245. Corpa-Rodríguez ME, Mayoralas-Alises S, García-Sánchez J, et al. Postoperative course in 7 cases of primary sarcoma of the lung. *Arch Bronconeumol*. 2005;41:634–637.

246. Juettner FM, Popper H, Sommersgutter K, et al. Malignant fibrous histiocytoma of the lung: prognosis and therapy of a rare disease: report of two cases and review of the literature. *Thorac Cardiovasc Surg*. 1987;35:226–231.

247. Higashiyama M, Doi O, Kodama K, et al. Successful surgery of malignant fibrous histiocytoma in the lung with gross extension into the right main pulmonary artery. *Thorac Cardiovasc Surg*. 1993;41:73–76.

248. McDermott VG, MacKenzie S, Hendry GM. Case report: primary intrathoracic rhabdomyosarcoma: a rare childhood malignancy. *Br J Radiol*. 1993;66:937–941.

249. Schiavetti A, Dominici C, Matrunola M, et al. Primary pulmonary rhabdomyosarcoma in childhood: clinicobiologic features in two cases with review of the literature. *Med Pediatr Oncol*. 1996;26:201–207.

250. Noda T, Todani T, Watanabe Y, et al. Alveolar rhabdomyosarcoma of the lung in a child. *J Pediatr Surg*. 1995;30:1607–1608.

251. Hancock BJ, DiLorenzo M, Youssef S, et al. Childhood primary pulmonary neoplasms. *J Pediatr Surg*. 1993;28:1133–1136.

252. Choi JS, Choi JS, Kim EJ. Primary pulmonary rhabdomyosarcoma in an adult with neurofibromatosis-1. *Ann Thorac Surg*. 2009;88:1356–1358.

253. Allan BT, Day DL, Dehner LP. Primary pulmonary rhabdomyosarcoma of the lung in children: report of two cases presenting with spontaneous pneumothorax. *Cancer*. 1987;59:1005–1011.

254. Murphy JJ, Blair GK, Fraser GC, et al. Rhabdomyosarcoma arising within congenital pulmonary cysts: report of three cases. *J Pediatr Surg*. 1992;27:1364–1367.

255. Lee SH, Rengaciary SS, Paramesh J. Primary pulmonary rhabdomyosarcoma: a case report and review of the literature. *Hum Pathol*. 1981;12:92–96.

256. Eriksson A, Thunell M, Lundquist G. Pedunculated endobronchial rhabdomyosarcoma with fatal asphyxia. *Thorax*. 1982;37:390–391.

257. Triche TJ, Askin FB, Kissane JM. Neuroblastoma, Ewing's sarcoma, and the differential diagnosis of small round blue cell tumors. In: Finegold M, ed. *Pathology of Neoplasia in Children and Adolescents*. Philadelphia: WB Saunders; 1986:145–195.

258. Wick MR, Swanson PE, Manivel JC. Immunohistochemical analysis of soft tissue sarcomas: comparisons with electron microscopy. *Appl Pathol*. 1988;6:169–196.

259. Stock N, Chibon F, Binh MB, et al. Adult-type rhabdomyosarcoma: analysis of 57 cases with clinicopathologic description, identification of 3 morphologic patterns and prognosis. *Am J Surg Pathol*. 2009;33:1850–1859.

260. Morgenstern DA, Rees H, Sebire NJ, et al. Rhabdomyosarcoma subtyping by immunohistochemical assessment of myogenin: tissue array study and review of the literature. *Pathol Oncol Res*. 2008;14:233–238.

261. Dehner LP. Soft tissue, peritoneum, and retroperitoneum. In: Dehner LP, ed. *Pediatric Surgical Pathology*, 2nd ed. Baltimore: Williams & Wilkins; 1987:869–938.

262. Sun CCJ, Kroll M, Miller JE. Primary chondrosarcoma of the lung. *Cancer*. 1982;50:1864–1866.

263. Kurotaki H, Tateoka H, Takeuchi M, et al. Primary mesenchymal chondrosarcoma of the lung: a case report with immunohistochemical and ultrastructural studies. *Acta Pathol Jpn*. 1992;42:364–371.

264. Hayashi T, Tsuda N, Iseki M, et al. Primary chondrosarcoma of the lung: a clinicopathologic study. *Cancer*. 1993;72:69–74.

265. Morgan AD, Salama FD. Primary chondrosarcoma of the lung: case report and review of the literature. *J Thorac Cardiovasc Surg*. 1972;64:460–466.

266. Fallahnejad M, Harrell D, Tucker J, et al. Chondrosarcoma of the trachea: report of a case and five-year followup. *J Thorac Cardiovasc Surg*. 1973;65:210–213.

267. Parker LA, Molina PL, Bignault AG, et al. Primary pulmonary chondrosarcoma mimicking bronchogenic cyst on CT and MRI. *Clin Imaging*. 1996;20:181–183.

268. Boueiz A, Abougergi MS, Noujeim C, et al. Primary dedifferentiated chondrosarcoma of the lung. *South Med J*. 2009;102:861–863.

269. Steurer S, Huber M, Lintner F. Dedifferentiated chondrosarcoma of the lung: case report and review of the literature. *Clin Lung Cancer*. 2007;8:439–442.

270. Zeren H, Moran CA, Suster S, et al. Primary pulmonary sarcomas with features of monophasic synovial sarcoma: a clinicopathological, immunohistochemical, and ultrastructural study of 25 cases. *Hum Pathol*. 1995;26:474–480.

271. Yoon GS, Park SY, Kang GH, et al. Primary pulmonary sarcoma with morphologic features of biphasic synovial sarcoma: a case report. *J Korean Med Sci*. 1998;13:71–76.

272. Kaplan MA, Goodman MD, Satish J, et al. Primary pulmonary sarcoma with morphologic features of monophasic synovial sarcoma and chromosome translocation t(X;18). *Am J Clin Pathol*. 1996;105:195–199.

273. Roberts CA, Seemayer TA, Neff JR, et al. Translocation t(X;18) in primary synovial sarcoma of the lung. *Cancer Genet Cytogenet*. 1996;88:49–52.

274. Sekeres M, Vasconcelles MJ, McMenamin M, et al. Two patients with sarcoma. Case 1: Synovial cell sarcoma of the lung. *J Clin Oncol*. 2000;18:2341–2342.

275. Zaring RA, Roepke JE. Pathologic quiz case: pulmonary mass in a patient presenting with a hemothorax. Diagnosis: primary pulmonary biphasic synovial sarcoma. *Arch Pathol Lab Med*. 1999;123:1287–1289.

276. Bacha EA, Wright CD, Grillo HC, et al. Surgical treatment of primary pulmonary sarcomas. *Eur J Cardiothorac Surg*. 1999;15:456–460.

277. Hisaoka M, Hashimoto H, Iwamasa T, et al. Primary synovial sarcoma of the lung: report of two cases confirmed by molecular detection of SYT-SSX fusion gene transcripts. *Histopathology*. 1999;34:205–210.

278. Béguéret H, Galateau-Salle F, Guillou L, et al. Primary intrathoracic synovial sarcoma: a clinicopathologic study of 40 t(X;18)-positive cases from the French Sarcoma Group and the Mesopath Group. *Am J Surg Pathol*. 2005;29:339–346.

279. Fisher C. Synovial sarcoma. *Ann Diagn Pathol*. 1998;2:401–421.

280. Essary LR, Vargas SO, Fletcher CD. Primary pleuropulmonary synovial sarcoma: reappraisal of a recently described anatomic subset. *Cancer*. 2002;94:459–469.

281. Sawamura K, Hashimoto T, Nanjo S, et al. Primary liposarcoma of the lung. *J Surg Oncol*. 1982;19:243–246.

282. Achir A, Ouadnouni Y, Smahi M, et al. Primary pulmonary liposarcoma—a case report. *Thorac Cardiovasc Surg*. 2009;57:119–120.

283. Loddenkemper C, Pérez-Canto A, Leschber G, et al. Primary dedifferentiated liposarcoma of the lung. *Histopathology*. 2005;46:710–712.

284. Yousem SA. Angiosarcoma presenting in the lung. *Arch Pathol Lab Med*. 1986;110:112–115.

285. Bartley TD, Arean VM. Intrapulmonary neurogenic tumors. *J Thorac Cardiovasc Surg*. 1965;50:114–123.

286. Manabe H, Umemoto T, Takagi H, et al. Primary neurogenous sarcoma of the lung; report of a case. *Jpn J Thorac Surg*. 2005;58:337–340.

287. Reingold IM, Amromin GD. Extraosseous osteosarcoma of the lung. *Cancer*. 1971;28:491–498.

288. Ren L, Guo SP, Zhou XG, et al. Angiomatoid fibrous histiocytoma: first report of primary pulmonary origin. *Am J Surg Pathol*. 2009;33:1570–1574.

289. Trabelsi A, Ben Abdelkrim S, Taher Yacoubi M, et al. Primary alveolar soft part sarcoma of the lung. *Rev Mal Respir*. 2009;26:329–332 [article in French].

290. Kim YD, Lee CH, Lee MK, et al. Primary alveolar soft part sarcoma of the lung. *J Korean Med Sci*. 2007;22:369–372.

291. Wakely Jr PE, McDermott JE, Ali SZ. Cytopathology of alveolar soft part sarcoma: a report of 10 cases. *Cancer Cytopathol*. 2009;117:500–507.

292. Ladanyi M, Lui MY, Antonescu CR, et al. The der(17)t(X;17)(p11;q25) of human alveolar soft part sarcoma fuses the TFE3 transcription factor gene to ASPL, a novel gene at 17q25. *Oncogene*. 2001;20:48–57.

293. Wilson RW, Moran CA. Primary melanoma of the lung: a clinicopathologic and immunohistochemical study of eight cases. *Am J Surg Pathol*. 1997;21:1196–1202.

294. Ost D, Joseph C, Sogoloff H, et al. Primary pulmonary melanoma: case report and literature review. *Mayo Clin Proc*. 1999;74:62–66.

295. Jensen OA, Egedorf J. Primary malignant melanoma of the lung. *Scand J Respir Dis*. 1967;48:127–135.

296. Salm R. A primary malignant melanoma of the bronchus. *J Pathol Bacteriol*. 1963;85:121–126.

297. Bagwell SP, Flynn SD, Cox PM, et al. Primary malignant melanoma of the lung. *Am Rev Respir Dis*. 1989;139:1543–1547.

298. Carstens PHB, Kuhns JG, Ghazi C. Primary malignant melanomas of the lung and adrenal. *Hum Pathol*. 1984;15:910–914.

299. Reid JD, Mehta VT. Melanoma of the lower respiratory tract. *Cancer*. 1966;19:627–631.

300. Robertson AJ, Sinclair DJM, Sutton PP, et al. Primary melanocarcinoma of the lower respiratory tract. *Thorax*. 1980;35:158–159.

301. Reed RJ, Kent EM. Solitary pulmonary melanomas: two case reports. *J Thorac Cardiovasc Surg*. 1964;48:226–231.

302. Gephardt GN. Malignant melanoma of the bronchus. *Hum Pathol*. 1981;12:671–673.

303. Ozdemir N, Cangir AK, Kutlay H, et al. Primary malignant melanoma of the lung in an oculocutaneous albino patient. *Eur J Cardiothorac Surg*. 2001;20:864–867.

304. Hashimoto T, Oka K, Hakozaki H, et al. Benign clear cell tumor of the lung. *Ultrastruct Pathol*. 2001;25:479–483.

305. Gaffey MJ, Mills SE, Askin FB, et al. Clear cell tumor of the lung: a clinicopathologic, immunohistochemical, and ultrastructural study of eight cases. *Am J Surg Pathol*. 1990;14:248–259.

306. Kuhnen C, Preisler K, Muller KM. Pulmonary lymphangioleiomyomatosis: morphologic and immunohistochemical findings. *Pathologe*. 2001;22:197–204 [article in German].

307. Ferrans VJ, Yu ZX, Nelson WK, et al. Lymphangioleiomyomatosis (LAM): a review of clinical and morphological features. *J Nippon Med Sch*. 2000;67:311–329.

308. Ito M, Sugamura Y, Ikari H, et al. Angiomyolipoma of the lung. *Arch Pathol Lab Med*. 1998;122:1023–1025.

309. Hynes JK, Smith HC, Holmes DR. Pulmonary artery sarcoma: preoperative diagnosis noninvasively by two-dimensional echocardiography. *Circulation*. 1983;67:459–477.

310. Lyerly HK, Reves JG, Sabiston DC. Management of primary sarcomas of the pulmonary artery and reperfusion intrabronchial hemorrhage. *Surg Gynecol Obstet*. 1986;163:291–298.

311. Gaissert HA, Mark EJ. Tracheobronchial gland tumors. *Cancer Control*. 2006;13:286–294.

312. Banerjee SS, Eyden B. Divergent differentiation in malignant melanomas: a review. *Histopathology*. 2008;52:119–129.

313. Maeda R, Isowa N, Onuma H, et al. Primary malignant melanoma of the lung with rapid progression. *Gen Thorac Cardiovasc Surg*. 2009;57:671–674.

314. Yamada G, Tanaka Y, Otsuka M, et al. Metastatic malignant melanoma mimicking primary lung adenocarcinoma. *Intern Med*. 2006;45:1255–1256.

315. Saint-Blancard P, Vaylet F, Jancovici R. A rare pulmonary tumour, primary malignant melanoma. *Rev Mal Respir*. 2009;26:57–61.

316. Reddy VS, Mykytenko J, Giltman LI, et al. Primary malignant melanoma of the lung: review of literature and report of a case. *Am Surg*. 2007;73:287–289.

317. Kundranda MN, Clark CT, Chaudhry AA, et al. Primary malignant melanoma of the lung: a case report and review of the literature. *Clin Lung Cancer*. 2006;7:279–281.

318. de Wilt JH, Farmer SE, Sarah EJ, et al. Isolated melanoma in the lung where there is no known primary site: metastatic disease or primary lung tumor? *Melanoma Res*. 2005;15:531–537.

319. McGlennen RC, Manivel JC, Stanley SJ, et al. Pulmonary artery trunk sarcoma: a clinicopathologic, ultrastructural, and immunohistochemical study of four cases. *Mod Pathol*. 1989;2:486–494.

320. Tanaka I, Masuda R, Inoue M, et al. Primary pulmonary artery sarcoma: report of a case with complete resection and graft replacement, and review of 47 surgically-treated cases reported in the literature. *Thorac Cardiovasc Surg*. 1994;42:64–68.

321. Al-Robaish A, Lien DC, Slatnik J, et al. Sarcoma of the pulmonary artery trunk: report of a case complicated with hemopericardium and cardiac tamponade. *Can J Cardiol*. 1995;11:707–709.

322. Timmers L, Bové T, De Pauw M. Intimal sarcoma of the pulmonary artery: a report of two cases. *Acta Cardiol*. 2009;64:677–679.

323. Austin BA, Griffin BP. Pulmonary artery intimal sarcoma: a brief case series. *J Am Soc Echocardiogr*. 2008;21:978.e5–978.e7.

324. Sethi GK, Slaven JE, Kepes JJ. Primary sarcoma of the pulmonary artery. *J Thorac Cardiovasc Surg*. 1972;63:587–596.

325. Baker PB, Goodwin RA. Pulmonary artery sarcoma. *Arch Pathol Lab Med*. 1985;109:35–40.

326. Weijmer MC, Kummer JA, Thijs LG. Case report of a patient with an intimal sarcoma of the pulmonary trunk presenting as a pulmonary embolism. *Neth J Med*. 1999;55:80–83.

327. Pagni S, Passik CS, Riordan C, et al. Sarcoma of the main pulmonary artery: an unusual etiology for recurrent pulmonary emboli. *J Cardiovasc Surg*. 1999;40:457–461.

328. Babatasi G, Massetti M, Agostini D, et al. Leiomyosarcoma of the heart and great vessels. *Ann Cardiol Angiol*. 1998;47:451–458.

329. Fujii H, Osako M, Otani H, et al. Primary pulmonary artery sarcoma. *Jpn Circ J*. 1998;62:379–381.

330. Babatasi G, Massetti M, Galateau F, et al. Pulmonary artery trunk leiomyosarcoma. *Thorac Cardiovasc Surg*. 1998;46:45–47.

331. Mazzucco A, Luciani GB, Bertolini P, et al. Primary leiomyosarcoma of the pulmonary artery: diagnostic and surgical implications. *Ann Thorac Surg*. 1994;57:222–225.

332. Johansson L, Carien B. Sarcoma of the pulmonary artery: report of four cases with electron microscopic and immunohistochemical examinations, and review of the literature. *Virchows Arch A*. 1994;424:217–224.

333. Ramp U, Gerharz CD, Iversen S, et al. Sarcoma of the pulmonary artery: report of two cases and a review of the literature. *J Cancer Res Clin Oncol*. 1992;118:551–556.

334. Mayer F, Aebert H, Rudert M, et al. Primary malignant sarcomas of the heart and great vessels in adult patients—a single-center experience. *Oncologist*. 2007;12:1134–1142.

335. Huo L, Moran CA, Fuller GN, et al. Pulmonary artery sarcoma: a clinicopathologic and immunohistochemical study of 12 cases. *Am J Clin Pathol*. 2006;125:419–424.

336. Tavora F, Miettinen M, Fanburg-Smith J, et al. Pulmonary artery sarcoma: a histologic and follow-up study with emphasis on a subset of low-grade myofibroblastic sarcomas with a good long-term follow-up. *Am J Surg Pathol*. 2008;32:1751–1761.

337. Bleisch VR, Kraus FT. Polypoid sarcoma of the pulmonary trunk. *Cancer*. 1980;46:314–321.

338. Law MR, Gregor A, Hodson ME, et al. Malignant mesothelioma of the pleura: a study of 52 treated and 54 untreated patients. *Thorax*. 1984;39:25–259.

339. Adams VI, Unni KK, Muhm JR, et al. Diffuse malignant mesothelioma of pleura: diagnosis and survival in 92 cases. *Cancer*. 1986;58:1540–1551.

340. Grondin SC, Sugarbaker DJ. Malignant mesothelioma of the pleural space. *Oncology*. 1999;13:919–932.

341. Coffin CM, Dehner LP. Mesothelial and related neoplasms in children and adolescents: a clinicopathologic and immunohistochemical analysis of eight cases. *Pediatr Pathol*. 1992;12:333–347.

342. Gentiloni N, Febbraro S, Barone C, et al. Peritoneal mesothelioma in recurrent familial peritonitis. *J Clin Gastroenterol*. 1997;24:276–279.

343. Walz R, Koch HK. Malignant pleural mesothelioma: some aspects of epidemiology, differential diagnosis, and prognosis. Histological and immunohistochemical evaluation and followup of mesotheliomas diagnosed from 1964 to January 1985. *Pathol Res Pract*. 1990;186:124–134.

344. Bianchi C, Brollo Ramani L, Zuch C. Pleural plaques as risk indicators for malignant pleural mesothelioma: a necropsy-based study. *Am J Ind Med*. 1997;32:445–449.

345. Sanden A, Jarvholm B. A study of possible predictors of mesothelioma in shipyard workers exposed to asbestos. *J Occup Med*. 1991;33:770–773.

346. Hasan FM, Nash G, Kazemi H. The significance of asbestos exposure in the diagnosis of mesothelioma: a 28-year experience from a major urban hospital. *Am Rev Respir Dis*. 1977;115:761–768.

347. Hasan FM, Nash G, Kazemi H. Asbestos exposure and related neoplasia: the 28-year experience of a major urban hospital. *Am J Med*. 1978;65:649–654.

348. Grant DC, Seltzer SE, Antman KH, et al. Computed tomography of malignant pleural mesothelioma. *J Comput Assist Tomogr*. 1983;7:626–632.

349. Kishimoto T, Ono T, Okada K, et al. Relationship between number of asbestos bodies in autopsy lung and pleural plaques on chest x-ray film. *Chest*. 1989;95:549–552.

350. Navratil M, Trippe F. Prevalence of pleural calcification in persons exposed to asbestos dust, and in the general population in the same district. *Environ Res*. 1972;5:210–216.

351. Peterson JT, Greenberg SD, Buffler P. Non-asbestos-related malignant mesothelioma: a review. *Cancer*. 1984;54:951–960.

352. Cavazza A, Travis LB, Travis WD, et al. Post-irradiation malignant mesothelioma. *Cancer*. 1996;77:1379–1385.

353. Strickler HD, Goedert JJ, Fleming M, et al. Simian virus 40 and pleural mesothelioma in humans. *Cancer Epidemiol Biomarkers Prev*. 1996;5:473–475.

354. Wick MR, Mills SE. Mesothelial proliferations: an increasing morphological spectrum. *Am J Clin Pathol*. 2000;113:619–622.

355. Law MR, Hodson ME, Heard BE. Malignant mesothelioma of the pleura: relation between histological type and clinical behavior. *Thorax*. 1982;37:810–815.

356. Gaertner E, Zeren EH, Fleming MV, et al. Biphasic synovial sarcomas arising in the pleural cavity: a clinicopathologic study of five cases. *Am J Surg Pathol*. 1996;20:36–45.

357. Argani P, Zakowski MF, Klimstra DS, et al. Detection of the SYT-SSX chimeric RNA of synovial sarcoma in paraffin-embedded tissue and its application in problematic cases. *Mod Pathol*. 1998;11:65–71.

358. Miettinen M, Limon J, Niezabitowski A, et al. Calretinin and other mesothelioma markers in synovial sarcoma: analysis of antigenic similarities and differences with malignant mesothelioma. *Am J Surg Pathol*. 2001;25:610–617.

359. Attanoos RL, Biggs AR. Pathology of malignant mesothelioma. *Histopathology*. 1997; 30:403–418.

360. Andrion A, Mazzuco G, Bernardi P, et al. Sarcomatous tumor of the chest wall with osteochondroid differentiation: evidence of mesothelial origin. *Am J Surg Pathol*. 1989;13:707–712.

361. Yousem SA, Hochholzer L. Malignant mesothelioma with osseous and cartilaginous differentiation. *Arch Pathol Lab Med*. 1987;111:62–66.

362. Okamoto T, Yokota S, Shinkawa K, et al. Pleural malignant mesothelioma with osseous, cartilaginous, and rhabdomyogenic differentiation. *Nihon Kokyuki Gakkai Zasshi*. 1998; 36:696–701.

363. Ordonez NG, Tornos C. Malignant peripheral nerve sheath tumor of the pleura with epithelial and rhabdomyoblastic differentiation: report of a case clinically simulating mesothelioma. *Am J Surg Pathol*. 1997;21:1515–1521.

364. Corson JM. Pathology of diffuse malignant pleural mesothelioma. *Semin Thorac Cardiovasc Surg*. 1997;9:347–355.

365. Avellini C, Alampi G, Cocchi V, et al. Malignant sarcomatoid mesothelioma of the pleura: a histological and immunohistochemical study of a case. *Pathologica*. 1991;83:335–340.

366. Cagle PT, Truong LD, Roggli VL, et al. Immunohistochemical differentiation of sarcomatoid mesotheliomas from other spindle cell neoplasms. *Am J Clin Pathol*. 1989;92:566–571.

367. Carter D, Otis CN. Three types of spindle cell tumors of the pleura: fibroma, sarcoma, and sarcomatoid mesothelioma. *Am J Surg Pathol*. 1988;12:747–753.

368. Montag AG, Pinkus GS, Corson JM. Keratin protein immunoreactivity of sarcomatoid and mixed types of diffuse malignant mesothelioma: an immunoperoxidase study of 30 cases. *Hum Pathol*. 1988;19:336–342.

369. Hammar SP, Bolen JW. Sarcomatoid pleural mesothelioma. *Ultrastruct Pathol*. 1985;9:337–343.

370. Weinbreck N, Vignaud JM, Begueret H, et al. SYT-SSX fusion is absent in sarcomatoid mesothelioma allowing its distinction from synovial sarcoma of the pleura. *Mod Pathol*. 2007;20:617–621.

371. Khalidi HS, Medeiros LJ, Battifora H. Lymphohistiocytoid mesothelioma: an often misdiagnosed variant of sarcomatoid malignant mesothelioma. *Am J Clin Pathol*. 2000;113(5):649–654.

372. Henderson DW, Attwood HD, Constance TJ, et al. Lymphohistiocytoid mesothelioma: a rare lymphomatoid variant of predominantly sarcomatoid mesothelioma. *Ultrastruct Pathol*. 1988;12:367–384.

373. Mangano WE, Cagle PT, Churg A, et al. The diagnosis of desmoplastic malignant mesothelioma and its distinction from fibrous pleurisy: a histologic and immunohistochemical analysis of 31 cases including p53 immunostaining. *Am J Clin Pathol*. 1998;110:191–199.

374. Wilson GE, Hasleton PS, Chatterjee AK. Desmoplastic malignant mesothelioma: a review of 17 cases. *J Clin Pathol*. 1992;45:295–298.

375. Crotty TB, Colby TV, Gay PC, et al. Desmoplastic malignant mesothelioma masquerading as sclerosing mediastinitis: a diagnostic dilemma. *Hum Pathol*. 1992;23:79–82.

376. Epstein JI, Budin RE. Keratin and epithelial membrane antigen immunoreactivity in nonneoplastic fibrous pleural lesions: implications for the diagnosis of desmoplastic mesothelioma. *Hum Pathol*. 1986;17:514–519.

377. Cantin R, Al-Jabi M, McCaughey WT. Desmoplastic diffuse mesothelioma. *Am J Surg Pathol*. 1982;6:215–222.

378. Colby TV. The diagnosis of desmoplastic malignant mesothelioma. *Am J Clin Pathol*. 1998;110:135–136.

379. Colby TV. Malignancies in the lung and pleura mimicking benign processes. *Semin Diagn Pathol*. 1995;12:30–44.

380. Center R, Lukeis R, Dietzsch E, et al. Molecular deletion of 9p sequences in non-small cell lung cancer and malignant mesothelioma. *Genes Chromosomes Cancer*. 1993;7:47–53.

381. Cheng JQ, Jhanwar SC, Lu YY, et al. Homozygous deletions within 9p21-p22 identify a small critical region of chromosomal loss in human malignant mesotheliomas. *Cancer Res*. 1993;53:4761–4763.

382. Brown RW, Clark GM, Tandon AK, et al. Multiple-marker immunohistochemical phenotypes distinguishing malignant pleural mesothelioma from pulmonary adenocarcinoma. *Hum Pathol*. 1993;24:347–354.

383. Riera JR, Astengo-Osuna C, Longmate JA, et al. The immunohistochemical diagnostic panel for epithelial mesothelioma: a reevaluation following heat-induced epitope retrieval. *Am J Surg Pathol*. 1997;21:1409–1419.

384. Ordonez NG. Role of immunohistochemistry in differentiating epithelial mesothelioma from adenocarcinoma: review and update. *Am J Clin Pathol*. 1999;112:75–89.

385. Burns TR, Greenberg D, Mace ML, et al. Ultrastructural diagnosis of epithelial malignant mesothelioma. *Cancer*. 1985;56:2036–2040.

386. Cury PM, Butcher DN, Corrin B, et al. The use of histological and immunohistochemical markers to distinguish pleural malignant mesothelioma and in situ mesothelioma from reactive mesothelial hyperplasia and reactive pleural fibrosis. *J Pathol*. 1999;189:251–257.

387. Kung IT, Thallas V, Spencer EJ, et al. Expression of muscle actins in diffuse mesotheliomas. *Hum Pathol*. 1995;26:565–570.

388. Hurliman J. Desmin and neural marker expression in mesothelial cells and mesotheliomas. *Hum Pathol*. 1994;25:753–757.

389. Klima M, Bossart MI. Sarcomatous type of malignant mesothelioma. *Ultrastruct Pathol*. 1983;4:349–358.

390. Allen TC, Cagle PT, Churg AM, et al. Localized malignant mesothelioma. *Am J Surg Pathol*. 2005;29:866–873.

391. Flint A, Weiss SW. CD34 and keratin expression distinguishes solitary fibrous tumor (fibrous mesothelioma) of pleura from desmoplastic mesothelioma. *Hum Pathol*. 1995;26:428–431.

392. Huncharek M, Kelsey K, Mark EJ, et al. Treatment and survival in diffuse malignant pleural mesothelioma: a study of 83 cases from the Massachusetts General Hospital. *Anticancer Res*. 1996;16(3A):1265–1268.

393. Machin T, Mashiyama ET, Henderson JA, et al. Bony metastases in desmoplastic pleural mesothelioma. *Thorax*. 1988;43:155–156.

394. Chahinian AP, Antman K, Goutsou M, et al. Randomized phase II trial of cisplatin with mitomycin or doxorubicin for malignant mesothelioma by the Cancer & Leukemia Group B. *J Clin Oncol*. 1993;11:1559–1565.

395. Sugarbaker DJ, Garcia JP, Richards WG, et al. Extrapleural pneumonectomy in the multimodality therapy of malignant pleural mesothelioma results in 120 consecutive patients. *Ann Surg*. 1996;224:288–296.

396. DaValle MJ, Faber LP, Kittle CF, et al. Extrapleural pneumonectomy for diffuse malignant mesothelioma. *Ann Thorac Surg*. 1986;42:612–618.

397. Lee MJ, Grogan L, Meehan S, et al. Pleural granulocytic sarcoma: CT characteristics. *Clin Radiol*. 1991;43:57–59.

398. Luppi G, Cesinaro AM, Zoboli A, et al. Mesenchymal chondrosarcoma of the pleura. *Eur Respir J*. 1996;9:840–843.

399. Goetz SP, Robinson RA, Landas SK. Extraskeletal myxoid chondrosarcoma of the pleura: report of a case clinically simulating mesothelioma. *Am J Clin Pathol*. 1992;97:498–502.

400. Okby NT, Travis WD. Liposarcoma of the pleural cavity: clinical and pathologic features of 4 cases with a review of the literature. *Arch Pathol Lab Med*. 2000;124:699–703.

401. Wong WW, Pluth JR, Grado GL, et al. Liposarcoma of the pleura. *Mayo Clin Proc*. 1994;69:882–885.

402. Stark P, Smith DC, Watkins GE, et al. Primary intrathoracic extraosseous osteogenic sarcoma: report of three cases. *Radiology*. 1990;174:725–726.

403. Matono R, Maruyama R, Ide S, Kitagawa D, et al. Extraskeletal osteosarcoma of the pleura: a case report. *Gen Thorac Cardiovasc Surg*. 2008;56:180–182.

404. Moran CA, Suster S, Koss MN. The spectrum of histologic growth patterns in benign and malignant fibrous tumors of the pleura. *Semin Diagn Pathol*. 1992;9:169–180.

405. Kim SY, Kim MY, Hwang YJ, et al. Low-grade fibromyxoid sarcoma: CT, sonography, and MR findings in 3 cases. *J Thorac Imaging*. 2005;20:294–297.

406. Miyoshi N, Takami K, Okami J, et al. Extrapleural pneumonectomy for relapsed solitary fibrous tumors of the pleura with pleural dissemination. *Jpn J Thorac Surg*. 2007;60:800–805.

407. Krishnadas R, Froeschle PO, Berrisford RG. Recurrence and malignant transformation in solitary fibrous tumour of the pleura. *Thorac Cardiovasc Surg*. 2006;54:65–67.

408. Ali SZ, Hoon V, Hoda S, et al. Solitary fibrous tumor: a cytologic–histologic study with clinical, radiologic, and immunohistochemical correlations. *Cancer*. 1997;81:116–121.

409. Hanau CA, Miettinen M. Solitary fibrous tumor: histological and immuno histochemical spectrum of benign and malignant variants presenting at different sites. *Hum Pathol*. 1995;26:440–449.

410. Mezzetti M, Augusti A. Fibrosarcoma of the pleura: circumscribed primary pleural neoplasms. *Arch Ital Chir*. 1969;95:544–555.

411. Meyer M, Krause U. Solitary fibrous tumors of the pleura. *Chirurg*. 1999;70:979–1952.

412. Vallat-Decouvelaere AV, Dry SM, Fletcher CDM. Atypical and malignant solitary fibrous tumors in extrathoracic locations: evidence of their comparability to intrathoracic tumors. *Am J Surg Pathol*. 1998;22:1501–1511.

413. Yokoi T, Tsuzuki T, Yatabe Y, et al. Solitary fibrous tumor: significance of p53 and CD34 immunoreactivity in its malignant transformation. *Histopathology*. 1998;32:423–432.

414. Myoui A, Aozasa K, Iuchi K, et al. Soft tissue sarcoma of the pleural cavity. *Cancer*. 1991;68:1550–1554.

415. England DM, Hochholzer L, McCarthy MJ. Localized benign and malignant fibrous tumors of the pleura. *Am J Surg Pathol*. 1989;13:640–658.

416. Fukasawa Y, Takada A, Tateno M, et al. Solitary fibrous tumor of the pleura causing recurrent hypoglycemia by secretion of insulin-like growth factor II. *Pathol Int*. 1998;48:47–52.

417. Theegarten D, Meisel M. Malignant fibrous histiocytoma of the thoracic wall in the area of a tuberculous pleural callosity. *Pneumologie*. 1993;47:458–460.

418. Watanabe S, Hitomi S, Nakamura T, et al. A clinical study of six surgically-treated patients with malignant tumors arising from chronic pleuritis and pyothorax. *Nippon Kyobu Geka Gakkai Zasshi*. 1989;37:281–286.

419. Saiffudin A, DaCosta P, Chalmers AG, et al. Primary malignant localized fibrous tumors of the pleura: clinical, radiological, and pathological features. *Clin Radiol*. 1992;45:13–17.

420. Toochika H, Kiminok K, Tagawa Y, et al. Malignant fibrous histiocytoma of the chest cavity: report of four resected cases. *Nippon Kyobu Geka Gakkai Zasshi*. 1990;38:647–653.

421. Moran CA, Suster S, Koss MN. Smooth muscle tumors presenting as pleural neoplasms. *Histopathology*. 1995;27:227–234.

422. Gibbs AR. Smooth muscle tumors of the pleura. *Histopathology*. 1995;27:295–296.

423. Al-Daraji WI, Salman WD, Nakhuda Y, et al. Primary smooth muscle tumor of the pleura: a clinicopathological case report with ultrastructural observations and a review of the literature. *Ultrastruct Pathol*. 2005;29:389–398.

424. Askin FB, Rosai J, Sibley RK, et al. Malignant small cell tumor of the thoracopulmonary region in childhood. *Cancer*. 1979;43:2438–2451.

425. Israel MA. Peripheral neuroepithelioma. In: Williams CJ, Krikorian JG, Green MR, Rhagavan D, eds. *Textbook of Uncommon Cancer*. New York: John Wiley & Sons; 1988:683–690.

426. Jurgens H, Bier V, Harms D, et al. Malignant peripheral neuroectodermal tumors. *Cancer*. 1988;61:349–357.

427. Dang NC, Siegel SE, Phillips JD. Malignant chest wall tumors in children and young adults. *J Pediatr Surg*. 1999;34:1773–1778.

428. Promnitz S, Petri F, Schulz HJ, et al. Askin's tumor: a rare entity. Case report with references to the literature. *Pneumologie*. 1999;53:393–399.

429. Liptay MJ, Fry WA. Malignant bone tumors of the chest wall. *Semin Thorac Cardiovasc Surg*. 1999;11:278–284.

430. Kabiri H, El-Fakir Y, Mahassini N, et al. Malignant small cell thoracic pulmonary tumor. *Rev Pneumonol Clin*. 1999;55:21–25.

431. Taneli C, Genc A, Erikci V, et al. Askin tumors in children: a report of four cases. *Eur J Pediatr Surg*. 1998;8:312–314.

432. Sallustio G, Pirronti T, Lasorella A, et al. Diagnostic imaging of primitive neuroectodermal tumor of the chest wall (Askin tumor). *Pediatr Radiol*. 1998;28:697–702.

433. Askin FB, Perlman EJ. Neuroblastoma and peripheral neuroectodermal tumors. *Am J Clin Pathol*. 1998;109(4 suppl 1):S23–S30.

434. Sabate JM, Franquet T, Parellada JA, et al. Malignant neuroectodermal tumor of the chest wall (Askin tumor): CT and MR findings in eight patients. *Clin Radiol*. 1994;49:634–638.

435. Shamberger RC, Tarbell NJ, Perez-Atayde AR, et al. Malignant small round cell tumor (Ewing's-PNET) of the chest wall in children. *J Pediatr Surg*. 1994;29:179–185.

436. Winer-Muram HT, Kauffman WM, Gronemeyer SA, et al. Primitive neuroectodermal tumors of the chest wall (Askin tumors): CT and MR findings. *Am J Roentgenol*. 1993;161:265–268.

437. Dehner LP. Soft tissue sarcomas of childhood. *Natl Cancer Inst Monogr*. 1981;56:43–59.

438. Sapi Z, Szentirmay Z, Orosz Z. Desmoplastic small round cell tumor of the pleura: a case report with further cytogenetic and ultrastructural evidence of "mesothelioblastemic" origin. *Eur J Surg Oncol*. 1999;25:633–634.

439. Parkash V, Gerald WL, Parma A, et al. Desmoplastic small round cell tumor of the pleura. *Am J Surg Pathol*. 1995;19:659–665.

440. Bian Y, Jordan AG, Rupp M, et al. Effusion cytology of desmoplastic small round cell tumor of the pleura: a case report. *Acta Cytol*. 1993;37:77–82.

441. Sarkar MR, Bahr R. The Askin tumor. *Chirurg*. 1992;63:973–976.

442. Contesso G, Llombart-Bosch A, Terrier P, et al. Does malignant small round cell tumor of the thoracopulmonary region (Askin tumor) constitute a clinicopathologic entity? *Cancer*. 1992;69:1012–1020.

443. Takahashi K, Dambara T, Uekusa T, et al. Massive chest wall tumor diagnosed as Askin tumor: successful treatment by intensive combined modality therapy in an adult. *Chest*. 1993;104:287–288.

444. Fitzgibbons JF, Feldhaus SJ, McNamara LF, et al. Diagnostic features and treatment of the Askin tumor—malignant small cell tumor of the thoracopulmonary region: a case report. *Nebr Med J*. 1993;78:2–6.

445. Kushner BH, LaQuaglia MP, Cheung NK, et al. Clinically critical impact of molecular genetic studies in pediatric solid tumors. *Med Pediatr Oncol*. 1999;33:530–535.

446. Dehner LP. Peripheral neuroectodermal tumor and Ewing's sarcoma. *Am J Surg Pathol*. 1993;17:1–13.

447. Lae ME, Roche PC, Jin L, Lloyd RV, et al. Desmoplastic small round cell tumor: a clinicopathologic, immunohistochemical, and molecular study of 32 tumors. *Am J Surg Pathol*. 2002;26:823–835.

448. Gautam U, Srinivasan R, Rajwanshi A, et al. Comparative evaluation of flow-cytometric immunophenotyping and immunocytochemistry in the categorization of malignant small round cell tumors in fine-needle aspiration cytologic specimens. *Cancer*. 2008;114:494–503.

449. Barnoud R, Sabourin JC, Pasquier D, et al. Immunohistochemical expression of WT1 by desmoplastic small round cell tumor: a comparative study with other small round cell tumors. *Am J Surg Pathol*. 2000;24:830–836.

450. Hill DA, Pfeifer JD, Marley EF, et al. WT1 staining reliably differentiates desmoplastic small round cell tumor from Ewing sarcoma/primitive neuroectodermal tumor. An immunohistochemical and molecular diagnostic study. *Am J Clin Pathol*. 2000;114:345–353.

451. Miser JS, Kinsella TJ, Triche TJ, et al. Treatment of peripheral neuroepithelioma in children and young adults. *J Clin Oncol*. 1987;5:1752–1758.

452. Farhi DC, Odell CA, Shurin SB. Myelodysplastic syndrome and acute myeloid leukemia after treatment for solid tumor of childhood. *Am J Clin Pathol*. 1993;100:270–275.

453. Cohen M, Kaschula RO. Primary pulmonary tumors in childhood: a review of 31 years' experience and the literature. *Pediatr Pulmonol*. 1992;14:222–232.

454. Hill DA, Sadeghi S, Schultz MZ, et al. Pleuropulmonary blastoma in an adult: an initial case report. *Cancer*. 1999;85:2368–2374.

455. Szczesny T, Hussein N, Szczesna A. Pulmonary blastoma and related primary malignant pulmonary neoplasms. *Pneumonol Alergol Pol*. 1999;67:263–270.

456. Romeo C, Impellizzeri P, Grosso M, et al. Pleuropulmonary blastoma: long-term survival and literature review. *Med Pediatr Oncol*. 1999;33:372–376.

457. Benouachane T, El-Khorassani M, Nachef MN, et al. Pleuropulmonary blastoma: report of 4 cases. *Rev Mal Respir*. 1999;16:390–394.

458. Baraniya J, Desai S, Kane S, et al. Pleuropulmonary blastoma. *Med Pediatr Oncol*. 1999;32:52–56.

459. Priest JR, McDermott MB, Bhatia S, et al. Pleuropulmonary blastoma: a clinicopathologic study of 50 cases. *Cancer*. 1997;80:147–161.

460. Priest JR, Watterson J, Strong L, et al. Pleuropulmonary blastoma: a marker for familial disease. *J Pediatr*. 1996;128:220–224.

461. Lopez-Andreu JA, Ferris-Tortajada J, Gomez J. Pleuropulmonary blastoma and congenital cystic malformations. *J Pediatr*. 1996;129:773–775.

462. Tagge EP, Mulvihill D, Chandler JC, et al. Childhood pleuropulmonary blastoma: caution against nonoperative management of congenital lung cysts. *J Pediatr Surg*. 1996;31:187–190.

463. Wright JR. Pleuropulmonary blastoma: a case report documenting transition from type I (cystic) to type III (solid). *Cancer*. 2000;88:2853–2858.

464. Piastra M, Ruggiero A, Caresta E, et al. Critical presentation of pleuropulmonary blastoma. *Pediatr Surg Int*. 2005;21:223–226.

465. Priest JR, Williams GM, Hill DA, et al. Pulmonary cysts in early childhood and the risk of malignancy. *Pediatr Pulmonol*. 2009;44:14–30.

466. Hill DA, Ivanovich J, Priest JR, et al. DICER1 mutations in familial pleuropulmonary blastoma. *Science*. 2009;325(5943):965.

467. MacSweeney F, Papagiannopoulos K, Goldstraw P, et al. An assessment of the expanded classification of congenital cystic adenomatoid malformations and their relationship to malignant transformation. *Am J Surg Pathol*. 2003;27:1139–1146.

468. Papagiannopoulos K, Hughes S, Nicholson AG, et al. Cystic lung lesions in the pediatric and adult population: surgical experience at the Brompton Hospital. *Ann Thorac Surg*. 2002;73:1594–1598.

469. Dehner LP. Pleuropulmonary blastoma is THE pulmonary blastoma of childhood. *Semin Diagn Pathol*. 1994;11:144–151.

470. Hill DA, Jarzembowski JA, Priest JR, et al. Type I pleuropulmonary blastoma: pathology and biology study of 51 cases from the international pleuropulmonary blastoma registry. *Am J Surg Pathol*. 2008;32:282–295.

471. Priest JR, Magnuson J, Williams GM, et al. Cerebral metastasis and other central nervous system complications of pleuropulmonary blastoma. *Pediatr Blood Cancer*. 2007;49:266–273.

472. Lin BT, Colby TV, Gown AM, et al. Malignant vascular tumors of the serous membranes mimicking mesothelioma: a report of 14 cases. *Am J Surg Pathol*. 1996;20:1431–1439.

473. Crotty EJ, McAdams HP, Erasmus JJ, et al. Epithelioid hemangioendothelioma of the pleura: clinical and radiologic features. *Am J Roentgenol*. 2000;175:1545–1549.

474. Del Frate C, Mortele K, Zanardi R, et al. Pseudomesotheliomatous angiosarcoma of the chest wall and pleura. *J Thorac Imaging*. 2003;18:200–203.

475. Kurtz JE, Serra S, Duclos B, et al. Diffuse primary angiosarcoma of the pleura: a case report and review of the literature. *Sarcoma*. 2004;8:103–106.

Hematolymphoid Disorders

Madeleine D. Kraus, MD, and Mark R. Wick, MD

In the interval since the first edition of this textbook, there have been clinically significant revisions to the classification of lymphomas that affect the approach to diagnosing hematolymphoid proliferations. These include the identification of new "phenotypic" entities, such as the anaplastic large B cell lymphoma associated with ALK translocations,[1-5] plasmablastic microlymphoma,[6,7] cyclin D1+ large B cell lymphomas,[8] and new "cytogenetic" entities, such as "double-hit" diffuse large B cell lymphomas.[9] Other changes include the subdivision of old entities, such as diffuse large B cell lymphoma into genetic "activated" and "germinal center" subtypes.[10-12] Diagnostic categories, such as atypical Burkitt lymphoma and Hodgkin-like anaplastic large T cell lymphoma, have been retired. This is evident in the revisions of the World Health Organization (WHO) publication on the pathology and genetics of hematopoietic and lymphoid tissues,[5] which increasingly represents a clinicopathologic touchstone for oncology.

The disease-defining characteristics of benign processes require recognition of both the specific patterned immunoarchitectural disturbance and the full range of nonspecific hyperplasia With respect to B lineage lymphomas, the orienting principle of classification remains ontology, with each lymphoma having a close molecular and immunophenotypic resemblance to specific stages of normal B cell development. By contrast, T lineage lymphomas remain a collection of distinct entities with no apparent ontogenic mimicry. With respect to myeloid neoplasms, cytogenetics is central to the definition of specific disease categories.

Twenty-first-century care requires both the generalist and the specialist to be familiar with the indications for the full range of molecular tests available, the specimen requirements for each, and their suitability and relevance to specific differential diagnostic setting. When presented with hematologic proliferations in the lung, pathologists must use an expanding array of special studies to formulate and resolve the differential diagnosis and provide the results of tests that aid in risk stratification.[11] Microarray technology is an established method for both class discovery and class definition[13,14] and in the not-too-distant future may become a part of the diagnostic and prognostic workup of patients with lymphoma.[15] This chapter describes the tests and techniques of hematopathology and the diagnoses that these tests enable.

Special Studies

Immunohistochemistry

Indications

Testing is performed to define the architecture of lymphoid neoplasms and their relationship to the tissue's infrastructure (e.g., alveoli, bronchiolar epithelium, vessels), to correlate the phenotype of specific cell populations with morphologic findings, and to identify clinically significant phenotypic variants of certain lymphomas.

Specimen Requirements

Well-fixed tissue that has been in formalin for at least 6 hours is required. Some hematologic markers yield weak or nonreactive results in B5-, Bouin-, and Hollande-fixed tissue, even though the stain works well on formalin-fixed tissue from the same patient. Acidified zinc-formalin preparations (AZF) perform exceptionally well with most hematologic markers, and they may be the best choice for laboratories wishing to work without mercury and picrate.

Immunophenotypic analysis of tissue sections is an essential part of the evaluation of hematolymphoid proliferations in both nodal and extranodal sites. The range of antibodies and the increase in the number of rabbit monoclonal antibodies available for paraffin-embedded material continues to expand,[16-19] but most differential challenges can be resolved with a handful of markers. Table 15-1 lists markers that cover all of the entities described in this chapter.

Table 15-1. Antibodies Useful in the Paraffin Section Evaluation of Hematolymphoid Proliferations

Marker	Description
B Cell Lineage Markers	
CD10	Positive in follicle center cell non-Hodgkin lymphoma (not lineage-specific; also present on some epithelial and stromal tumors)
CD19	Early B cell marker (also present on B-LBL; not present on plasma cells)
CD20	Mature B cell marker (not present on B-LBL; most plasma cells negative)
CD23	Activated B cells
CD79a	Immature and mature B cells (present on B-LBL as well as plasma cells)
PAX5	Immature B cells, including lymphoblasts, mature B cells; negative in plasma cells; also positive in some neuroendocrine tumors, including small cell carcinoma
CD138	Plasma cells, some cases of classic Hodgkin lymphoma
MUM1	In the proper context, postfollicular B cells and plasma cells
IgD	Immunoglobulin heavy-chain delta, present in benign mantle cells, some lymphomas
κ, λ	Immunoglobulin light chains (cell surface expression assessed by flow; cytoplasmic expression by immunohistochemistry)
T Cell Lineage Markers	
CD1a	Some immature T cells (thymocytes), Langerhans cells
CD2	Pan T cell marker; may also be present on natural killer cells by flow cytometry
CD3	T cells
CD4	Helper/suppressor T cells
CD5	Preferential T cell marker (also positive in some B cell neoplasms)
CD7	T cells, some natural killer cells
CD8	Cytotoxic T cells
CD43	Preferential T cell marker (also positive in some B cell neoplasms and granulocytic proliferations)
CD56	Natural killer cells and some T cells; also positive in some neuroendocrine tumors
CD57	Natural killer cells and some T cells; also expressed on some neuroendocrine tumors
Monocyte/Macrophage/Accessory Cell Markers	
CD1a	Langerhans cells, some T cells (thymocytes)
CD14	Monocytes (paraffin markers available, not widely used)
CD15	Granulocytes, also positive in Hodgkin lymphoma and adenocarcinoma
CD21	Follicular dendritic cells, some B cells
CD31	PECAM-1; marks vascular endothelium and monocytes, macrophages, and histiocytes
CD33	Granulocytes (paraffin marker available, not yet widely used)
CD68	Macrophages, monocytes (two clones; KP1 and PGM1 have slightly different specificities)
CD163	Hemoglobin scavenger receptor; expressed on macrophages and histiocytes, including histiocytic malignancies
Langerin	Langerhans cells, both in Langerhans cell histiocytosis and Langerhans cell sarcoma

Table 15-1. Antibodies Useful in the Paraffin Section Evaluation of Hematolymphoid Proliferations—continued

Marker	Description
Miscellaneous Markers	
ALK1	Positive in some peripheral T cell lymphomas, also in some inflammatory myofibroblastic tumors
bcl6	Transcriptional regulator positive in germinal center B cells as well as some lymphoblasts; may be positive in the lesional cells of some T cell neoplasms
bcl2	Anti-apoptosis protein positive in virtually all lymphoid proliferations *except* benign germinal center B cells and Burkitt lymphoma
Cyclin D1	Cell cycle regulator positive in mantle cell lymphoma, myeloma, and rare cases of large B cell lymphoma
CD45	Leukocyte common antigen present on lymphocytes, blasts, monocytes, and L&H type Reed-Sternberg cells
Oct2	Transcription factor in some B and T cells; also present in L&H type Reed-Sternberg cells
TdT	Terminal deoxynucleotidyl transferase, a marker of the blastic stage
EMA	Epithelial membrane antigen (positive in some large cell lymphomas and some plasmacytomas)
Ki67	Proliferation marker that helps to identify proliferation centers in chronic lymphocytic lymphoma/small lymphocytic leukemia and is also useful in the multiparameter distinction of high-grade large B cell lymphoma and Burkitt lymphoma

B-LBL, B cell lymphoblastic lymphoma: L&H, lymphocytic and histiocytic; PECAM, platelet-endothelial cell adhesion molecule.

Boxes 15-1 and 15-2 describe panels and the manner in which they might be used.

The judicious and cost-effective use of immunostains is maximized if the pathologist puts each marker ordered to specific purpose.[20–23] In the workup of hematolymphoid lesions of the lung, there are four principal goals:

1. *Define the lineage.* Is the lesional cell population of T lineage? B lineage? Histiocytic? Myeloid?[19,23,24]
2. *Identify immunoarchitectural landmarks.* Is the follicular dendritic meshwork in its normal compacted state, or are the edges frayed and the cell bodies more widely dispersed than usual? Is the mantle zone present or overrun? In the lymph nodes, are sinuses present but compressed, or are they entirely effaced?[22,25,26]
3. *Document the aberrant phenotype that is indicative of neoplasia.* Is the CD20+ cell population also positive for CD5 or CD43? Is there a restricted pattern of immunoglobulin light-chain expression? Is there a double-positive or double-negative CD4/CD8 profile on the T cells?[22]
4. *Distinguish clinically different but morphologically similar entities.*[27] Is this a B lineage or a T lineage anaplastic lymphoma? Is this Burkitt lymphoma or a high-grade large cell lymphoma?[27] Is this a cyclin D1+ large cell lymphoma or a mantle cell lymphoma?[17,28,29] Does this T cell lymphoma express ALK protein?[30]

In working up hematologic tumors in the lung, the pathologist needs to be aware of certain pitfalls.[20] It has long been recognized that CD138 (syndecan 1) marks both plasma cells and a range of epithelial tumors. More recently, PAX-5 has been shown in a broad range of neuroendocrine tumors,[31] including small cell carcinoma and Merkel cell carcinoma.[32] These studies show that, especially in the evaluation of lung tumors, no one marker should be the sole basis on which the B cell nature of a lung process is defined.[33] Other pitfalls were reviewed recently by Yaziji and Barry.[20]

Requesting that immunohistochemical stains be performed in a specific sequence on sequentially obtained serial sections can be of immeasurable help. Performing semiquantitative assessment of cytoplasmic light-chain expression is easier if the kappa and lambda stains are performed on two sequential sections with essentially the same population of plasma cells. Similarly, if an assessment for follicular colonization is the goal, requesting that the CD20, CD3, bcl2, bcl6, and CD21 stains be performed on sequential serial sections usually allows evaluation of these markers in the same follicle/germinal center to be made.

Box 15-1. Immunophenotypic Profiles Associated with Lymphoid Neoplasia

Phenotypic Findings Indicative of Lymphoid Neoplasia

Aberrant Gain of a Preferential T Cell Marker on a Proliferation of B Cells

Aberrant expression of CD5 in CD20+ B cells is the hallmark of chronic lymphocytic leukemia/small lymphocytic leukemia and mantle cell lymphoma

Aberrant expression of CD43 in CD20+ B cells is often seen in small lymphocytic leukemia, sometimes in MCL, and seldom in other lymphomas (e.g., follicular lymphoma, marginal zone lymphoma)

Restricted Pattern of a Single Immunoglobulin Light Chain

A profoundly skewed k:l ratio (e.g., 10:1 or 1:10) of kappa-positive or lambda-positive cells provides strong support for the presence of a monoclonal population of B cells (considered definitional of B cell neoplasia)

Aberrant Loss or Gain of a Maturation or Stage-Specific Marker

Absence of CD2, CD5, or CD7 on T cells is abnormal and is common in peripheral T cell lymphomas

Absence of both CD4 and CD8 is abnormal outside of the thymus and is commonly seen in T gamma-delta lymphomas

Presence of both CD4 and CD8 is abnormal outside of the thymus and may be seen in peripheral T cell lymphomas

Phenotypic Findings Helpful in Classifying Neoplastic Small Lymphoid Proliferations

TdT Expression*

Supports classification as a lymphoblastic lymphoma

Cyclin D1 Expression

Supports classification as mantle cell lymphoma (may also be seen in large B cell lymphoma and in plasma cell myeloma, and so should not be the sole basis for classification)

bcl6 Expression

Supports classification as a lymphoma of follicle center cell origin

CD21 Expression

When it highlights a disrupted follicular dendritic cell meshwork indicative of colonization, can assist in diagnosing marginal zone lymphomas of the lung

MUM1 Expression

When other features suggest follicular colonization (bcl6–, bcl2+, CD20+ B cells inside a disrupted follicular dendritic cell meshwork), the presence of MUM1+ cells within such follicles strengthens the interpretation (i.e., an aid in excluding the possibility that the bcl2+, bcl6– cells are of B lineage and are not intrafollicular T cells)

*Because benign cortical and medullary thymocytes are TdT+, great care should be taken in evaluating small biopsy specimens of hilar or midline intrathoracic masses.

Box 15-2. A Panel Approach to Immunophenotypic Analysis of Hematolymphoid Proliferations in the Lung

Small round blue cell proliferations with blastic nuclear features (fine or evenly dispersed chromatin, indistinct nucleoli, scant cytoplasm) for which the differential diagnosis may include LBL (B, T, or natural killer cell lineage), myeloid leukemia, small cell carcinoma, and merkel cell carcinoma
TdT, CD34, PAX5, CD20, CD10, kappa and lambda, CD2, CD3, CD56, CD57, CD14, CD33, myeloperoxidase, lysozyme, cytokeratin, CK20, chromogranin, synaptophysin
Small lymphoid proliferations with a diffuse architecture in the lung for which the differential diagnosis may include CLL/SLL, MCL, FL, and MaZL
CD3, CD20, CD5, CD10, CD23, CD21, CD43, cyclin D1, cytokeratin; Ki67 and MUM1 may be informative in some cases
Small lymphoid proliferations with a nodular component in the lung for which the differential diagnosis may include MCL, FL, and MaZL
CD3, CD20, CD5, CD10, CD23, CD21, CD43, bcl2, bcl6, cytokeratin; IgD MUM1 and cyclin D1 may be informative in some cases
Small lymphoid proliferations with any degree of plasmacytic differentiation in the lung for which the differential diagnosis may include CLL/SLL, LPL, MaZL, WM, and plasma cell myeloma
CD3, CD20, CD5, CD10, CD23, CD21, CD138, cIg k/l, cytokeratin; IgD, EMA, and MUM1 may be informative in some cases.
Large lymphoid proliferations with or without plasmacytic differentiation for which the differential diagnosis may include LCL, plasma cell myeloma, progressed/transformed FL, and MaZL
CD3, CD20, CD5, CD10, bcl6, CD138, CD45, kappa, lambda; CD21 and CD23 may be helpful if there is a concern about progressed (rather than de novo) BLCL
High-grade nonblastic lymphomas for which the differential diagnosis may include high-grade BLCL and BL
CD3, CD20, CD10, bcl2, bcl6, CD138, Ki67, CD30
Bimorphic small-cell and very large–cell populations ("Hodgkin panel")
CD3, CD20, CD45, CD30, CD15, PAX5, CD57; may add Oct2/BOB1, ALK1, CD21, CD2

BL, Burkitt lymphoma; BLCL, large B cell lymphoma; CLL, chronic lymphocytic leukemia; FL, follicular lymphoma; LBL, lymphoblastic lymphoma; LCL, large cell lymphoma; LPL, lymphoplasmacytic leukemia/lymphoma; MaZL, marginal zone lymphoma; MCL, mantle cell lymphoma; SLL, small lymphocytic leukemia; WM, Waldenström macroglobulinemia.

Flow Cytometry

Indications

Flow cytometry is performed to define the light-chain status (monotypic/restricted or polytypic/nonrestricted expression) of B cells, to assess for aberrant coexpression of certain markers on specific B cell populations, to assess for aberrant loss of certain markers on specific T cell populations, and to identify and characterize myeloid and monocytic lineage cell populations.

Specimen Requirements

Fresh (nonfixed) tissue is held in tissue culture media (e.g., RPMI) if not processed immediately. The quantity varies according to how tightly the lesional cells are held in a fibrotic or reticulin meshwork. In a cellular, nonfibrotic lymph node, as little as a 0.5-cm cube may suffice, but in sclerotic mediastinal tissue a $2 \times 1 \times 1$-cm piece of tissue may be needed. As a guide in individual cases, in general, if a touch preparation makes a richly cellular slide, the lower limit may suffice, but if only few cells adhere to the slide, attempting flow cytometry may be a fruitless expenditure of tissue.

An advantage of flow cytometry over tissue section immunophenotyping is that three or four markers can be evaluated simultaneously on specific small- and large-cell populations. Through this detailed multiparameter profile, many lymphoproliferative disorders can be classified more accurately.[34-37] However, flow cytometric phenotyping does not allow for visualization of the immunoarchitecture of the proliferation, which can be an important element of accurate classification of lymphomas, particularly in the lung, where marginal zone lymphoma (MaZL) is so common. In tissue section-based immunophenotyping, the pathologist can readily identify situations in which the lesional foci have disappeared from the sections used for the stains. In flow cytometric immunophenotyping, however, the pathologist must ensure that the lesional cells are present on a cytospin made from the disaggregated cells.

With the rise of reference laboratories and the ease in sending out fresh tissue for flow cytometry, some pathologists without specialty training in hematopathology may be asked to interpret the histograms and data from such analyses. Attempting to simply "call it by the numbers" extracted from the histograms by the technician may misrepresent the data. The pathologist should first check to see that the cytospin contains the cells of interest, and then determine from the histograms whether they have been appropriately selected ("gated") for analysis. For instance, blasts, invariably very dimly CD45+, will not be present in the CD45-bright lymphocyte gate, and will be missed if only the CD45-bright region data are analyzed. If the lesional cells are large, the *low* forward scatter CD45-bright *small* lymphocyte gate contains a polytypic population of B cells, and the only clue to clonality is present in the *high* forward scatter, CD45-bright *large* cell gate.

Flow cytometry yields continuous data that may be reported relative to the *gated* population ("32% of the gated cells are CD34+ blasts") or relative to the *total cellularity* of the specimen (32% of the gated cells are CD34+ blasts, and the gate contains 2.4% of the total cellularity, so CD34+ blasts account for 0.6% of the total cellularity). If the pathologist is not personally extracting the numbers from the histograms, care should be taken to understand and clearly state which type of result is being presented. The difference between 32% blasts and 0.6% blasts in the example would, for instance, lead to different diagnoses.

Most reference laboratories performing flow cytometry have established panels for specific clinical scenarios (lymphoma panel, adult leukemia panel, pediatric leukemia panel, expanded T cell panel) that are tailored to efficiently identify the classic immunophenotypic profiles characteristic of common disease entities.[38-41] The appropriate panel should be used to address the diagnostic question. Perhaps 10% to 15% of the time, however, a particular lymphoma or leukemia will have a variant phenotype.[41,42] Examples include a lack of CD10 in a lymphoma of follicular origin, acquisition of CD10 in hairy cell leukemia, CD5 expression in large cell lymphoma, CD19 expression in acute myeloid leukemia, apparent dim CD23 expression in mantle cell lymphoma, and a lack of CD23 expression in chronic lymphocytic leukemia. For this reason and because the immunoarchitecture is an important part of the disease definition for some lymphomas, both flow cytometry and immunohistochemistry may need to be performed in some cases, and the diagnostician should not be shy about doing both.

Cytogenetics

Indications

Cytogenetic testing is indicated whenever preliminary assessment suggests a high-grade lymphoma (tumoral necrosis with a brisk mitotic rate), a blastic process, or a myeloid disorder, and for all pediatric biopsy specimens in which lymphoma or leukemic involvement is possible or likely.

Specimen Requirements

Classic cytogenetic testing requires fresh (nonfixed) tissue, taken sterilely (preferably in the operating room with a sterile scalpel and forceps) and transported in sterile tissue culture media to the laboratory performing the testing. Fluorescence in situ hybridization (FISH) can be performed on disaggregated cells left over from flow cytometry (if kept refrigerated) or on formalin-fixed, paraffin-embedded tissues.

Many leukemias and lymphomas have recurring chromosomal translocations that can be identified with FISH and classic cytogenetic testing.[43-53] These tests are widely available at many referral laboratories, but they are expensive and time-consuming. Therefore, the pathologist must be aware of their indications, applications, and limitations and also must make the clinician aware of the time frame between biopsy and final results.

One of the most important applications of cytogenetics is in distinguishing between morphologically similar tumors with widely different aggressiveness or treatment protocols. The distinction between small lymphocytic lymphoma and mantle cell lymphoma is an example of the first type, and the distinction between Burkitt lymphoma and high-grade B cell lymphoma is an example of the second type. Although some translocations are characteristic of certain diseases, not all are as specific for a particular entity as once believed. For instance, *c-myc*–related translocations were once believed to be specific for Burkitt lymphoma, but are now known to be present in some large B cell lymphomas and in some lymphomas that populate the new WHO category of "B cell lymphoma unclassifiable with features intermediate between high-grade large B cell lymphoma and Burkitt lymphoma"[5,48] (discussed later). The most common and clinically relevant karyotypic changes related to leukemias and lymphomas are enumerated in Table 15-2.

Molecular Genetics

Indications

Molecular genetic testing is performed to document clonality in B or T lineage proliferations, to identify specific disease-defining rearrangement events (translocations), and to assess for genetic abnormalities that distinguish among chronic myeloproliferative disorders.

Specimen Requirements

The use of formalin-fixed, paraffin-embedded material is standard, although if peripheral blood or bone marrow is also involved, these

Table 15-2. Cytogenetic Analyses Associated with Lymphoid Lymphomas and Leukemias That May Primarily or Secondarily Involve the Lung

Disease	Abnormality	Implicated Loci	Percentage of Affected Cases
B cell lymphoblastic lymphoma	t(9;22)(q34;q11.2)	bcr/ABL1	
	t(V;11q23)	MLL	
	t(12;21)(p13;122)	TEL/AML1	
	t(1;19)(q23;p13.3)	E2A/PBX1	
	t(5;14)(q31;q32) hyperdiploidy	IL3/IgH	
T cell lymphoblastic lymphoma	t(14;10)(q11.2;q24)	TcR delta/HOX11	
	t(14;5)(q11.2;q35)	TcR delta/HOX11L2	
B cell chronic lymphocytic leukemia	Trisomy 12		20% of cases
	del (13)(q14.3)		~15% of cases
	del (11)(q22-q23)	ATM	~15% of cases
	del (17)(p13)(p53)		~10% of cases
T cell prolymphocytic leukemia	inv 14(q11;q32)	TCL1	
	t(14;14)(q11;q32)		
Follicle center cell lymphoma	t(14;18)(q32;q21)	IgH-bcl2	Common
	t(2;18)(p11;q21)	IgL-bcl2	Rare
	t(18;22)(q21;q11)	IgL-bcl2	Rare
	t(3;14)(q27;q32)	bcl6-IgH	Rare
Mantle cell lymphoma	t(11;14)(q13;q32)	bcl1-IgH	
Mucosa-associated lymphoid tissue/marginal zone lymphoma	Trisomy 3		20% of cases
	Trisomy 18		5–10% of cases
	t(11;18)(q21;q21)	API2-MLT	30–50% cases
	t(14;18)(q32;q21)	IgH-MLT1	5–10% cases
	t(1;14)(p22q32)		5% of cases
Large B cell lymphoma	t(3q27;V)	bcl6—variable partners	
"Double-hit B-cell diffuse large cell lymphoma"	(14;18)(q32;q21) with t(8;14)(q24;q32)		
High-grade B large cell lymphoma, not otherwise classified	Complex karyotypes including *c-myc* translocations		See text
ALK+ large B cell lymphoma	t(2;17)(p23;q23)	ALK/clathrin	
Burkitt lymphoma	t(2;8)(p12;q24)	IgL-c-myc	Almost always an isolated karyotypic abnormality
	t(8;14)(q24;q32)	c-myc-IgH	
	t(8;22)(q24;q11)	c-myc-IgL	
T γ/δ hepatosplenic lymphoma	iso7q10		
T cell anaplastic large cell lymphoma	t(2;5)(p23;q35)	NPM1-ALK (80% of cases)	
	t(1;2)(q25;p23)	TPM3/ALK (10–15% cases)	

tissues may be suitable alternatives; some referral laboratories can also use fresh cells if they remain viable during transport and if the quality of DNA and RNA remains high. Some non-formalin fixatives are acceptable (e.g., Histochoice, Amresco, Solon, OH), but B5, Hollande, and Bouin fixatives denature the DNA and are not suitable for polymerase chain reaction (PCR) analysis.

Over the last decade, molecular genetic analysis has gone from being an expensive test seldom ordered by non-hematopathologists to one routinely ordered when an atypical lymphoid infiltrate is encountered and flow cytometry was not performed or the results were not informative.[36] General pathologists must be familiar with the range of molecular tests available, their applications and limits, and the small but real risk of misleading results. Although B5, Bouin, and Hollande fixatives yield excellent cytologic detail, they also denature DNA to the point that tissues fixed in these solutions are not usable for molecular analysis.[54-57] Therefore, care should be taken during prosection to include sufficient tissue in formalin to allow for molecular studies if preliminary findings on touch preparations or frozen section suggest an hematolymphoid process.[58]

Polymerase chain reaction analysis may be used on formalin-fixed, paraffin-embedded material or archived snap-frozen tissue to document clonality,[59-62] define lineage, evaluate for translocation events, and assess for the presence of infectious agents. PCR may also be used to speciate mycobacterial organisms. Clonality is assessed by examination of areas of the immunoglobulin heavy- and light-chain loci or the T cell receptor α/β or γ loci that are rearranged during normal lymphoid development.[54] Specially designed primer sets that flank certain gene loci are used for PCR-based evaluations for certain translocations, a helpful solution when there are no commercially available FISH probes or if tissue suitable for FISH is not available.

As "objective" as they are, molecular genetic tests do not replace the thought process of diagnosis. These test results are adjunctive data that point in one direction or another, but the final diagnosis must be made by the pathologist.[63] The results of molecular studies must be integrated into the "big picture" painted by the clinical setting, the morphologic findings, and the immunophenotypic results. Although clonality is used to define neoplasia, lack of clonality does not prove that a lesion is reactive. The finding of an oligoclonal band is meaningless to the treating physician unless the pathologist puts the result into the context of the morphologic and clinical data. Low tumor cell numbers in Hodgkin lymphoma, lymphomatoid granulomatosis, and T cell–rich B cell lymphoma may yield nonclonal results because of the dilutional effect of reactive cells. Similarly, non–B, non–T cell malignancies, such as natural killer cell lymphomas and myeloid leukemias, yield a polyclonal smear because the lesional cells are of neither B cell nor T cell lineage.

Frozen Section Issues

Because of the timeliness of diagnosis and the completeness of classification of hematolymphoid proliferations, special handling of the tissue is required. Put another way, what works for a fibroid uterus does not work for lymphomatous tissues. Routinely handled formalin-fixed tissue is often all that is necessary, but occasionally lack of fresh tissue for flow cytometry or cytogenetic testing can delay the diagnosis or even prevent classification. By chance or design, those affected are often the sickest patients, and delay in diagnosis introduced by a lack of tissue appropriate for ancillary testing can be frustrating to both the clinician and the pathologist.

Under ideal circumstances, therefore, it is important to talk to the patient's pulmonologist as well as the surgeon. If a patient with known or suspected hematologic disease is undergoing thoracoscopic

or open-lung biopsy, tissue should be set aside sterilely in the operating room for culture, cytogenetic testing, or both, and the remainder should be sent to the frozen section room for immediate evaluation of the quantitative adequacy and distribution of tissue for all appropriate ancillary studies. Touch imprints stained with hematoxylin and eosin or Diff-Quik (Dade Behring, Newark, DE) can quickly discriminate among necrotizing, granulomatous, and neoplastic infiltrates, and are fine means of addressing the difficult differential diagnosis of lymphoblastic, Burkitt, Burkitt-like, and high-grade large B cell lymphomas. Air-dried or alcohol-fixed imprints can be used for enzyme histochemistry (myeloperoxidase, the various esterases) as well as for FISH, and most clinical microbiology laboratories have established protocols for pneumocystis, fungal, and acid-fast stains on smears.

If the lesion is cellular and lymphoid, and if at least 1 cm^3 of tissue is available, half of the tissue should be sent to the flow laboratory for analysis and the other half fixed in formalin or AZF fixative. The flow laboratory should retain unstained, unfixed disaggregated cells in tissue culture media so that it can be sent for FISH analysis if initial studies warrant. If there is more than 1 cm^3 of lesional tissue, taking some for non-formalin fixation (AZF, B5, B1, Hollande) allows for assessment of nuanced cytologic detail, although because this type of fixative has an adverse effect on DNA- and RNA-based studies, it should not be used as the sole fixative.

If there is more than 1 cm^3 of lesional tissue, a frozen section can be considered, but the thawed frozen section remnant is not ideal for detailed morphologic assessment and introduces background into some immunohistochemical stains. Unless there is a compelling clinical question requiring resolution in the next 24 hours, frozen sections of hematolymphoid proliferations should be performed only when touch imprints do not provide sufficient information for triaging tissue. Important questions include: Of what value to the patient is this frozen section diagnosis likely to be? Am I ready to confidently diagnose or exclude lymphoma (or, for that matter, acute leukemia) from the diagnosis based on a hematoxylin and eosin frozen section? Can I distinguish MaZL from follicular lymphoma with marginal zone differentiation or an unusual hyperplasia without the help of flow cytometry? Am I ready to make a definitive distinction among a necrotizing infection, lymphomatoid granulomatosis, and high-grade lymphoma? If not, then the frozen tissue has not advanced the patient's care significantly, but it has rendered a portion of the specimen suboptimal for permanent section histology and immunohistochemistry.

Normal Lymphoid Tissue in the Lung and the Concept of MALT

The lung contains an extensive lymphatic network that channels antigen-rich lymph centripetally toward the parenchymal, septal, hilar, and mediastinal lymph nodes. Organized lymphoid tissue in the periphery of the normal lung is limited to sparse submucosal aggregates of lymphocytes and intrapulmonary lymph nodes, but can be more substantial centrally and along bronchiolar branch points.[64] Inhaled particulate matter is trapped in the mucus layer of the proximal airways, and some passes across patches of specialized epithelium, where it initiates primary and secondary immune responses. Inhaled *irritants* stimulate a principally monocyte/macrophage response, whereas inhaled *immunogens* promote a lymphocytic (or lymphoplasmacytic) response. In practice, inhalational exposures are seldom purely one or the other, and so the tissue response tends to be mixed and is not infrequently masked by fibrinous exudates and actively phagocytic macrophages. The lymphoid tissue proliferates as a result of nonexogenous stimuli as well. In autoimmune conditions and immunodeficiency states, there is an intrinsic dysregulation of lymphoid proliferation, and the lymphoid hyperplasia—"acquired mucosa-associated lymphoid tissue" (MALT) or "bronchus-associated lymphoid tissue"[36,65-67] is less masked by acute-phase mucosal changes. Intrapulmonary lymph nodes, also a part of the pulmonary immune surveillance system, are uncommon, but when found, they are more often solitary, peripherally located, and located in the lower lung field. Their structure and immunoarchitectural compartments—and the diseases that affect them—are no different from those of extrapulmonary lymph nodes.

In addition, MALT has a close and specific relationship to the adjacent alveolar and bronchiolar epithelium, the "lymphoepithelium," where antigen processing and presentation occur. Benign MALT has a distinctive immunoarchitecture, with discrete compartments: the B cell–rich follicles, the mantle, and the T cell–rich interfollicular regions. In some cases and in some areas, a marginal zone of intermediate-sized cells with moderate to abundant amounts of cytoplasm may be interposed between the mantle and the interfollicular regions, although this marginal zone is never as well developed as it is where MALT was originally recognized, in the spleen and Peyer patches (Fig. 15-1). The lymphocytes in these structures shuttle between the mucosa and the circulation to provide ongoing immune surveillance and response to antigens that diffuse through the airways. Between follicles, lymphocytes range from small and resting to intermediate in size and somewhat activated. Plasma cells may be commingled, none with Dutcher bodies. Where immunoblasts are present, their regular size, round nuclear shape, and smooth nuclear contour support a benign interpretation.

Very limited foci of lymphocytes likely have no clinical or radiologic correlate and may not require recognition with a diagnostic line in the report. However, lymphoid accumulations that either have a radiologic correlate or clearly associate with distortions of airways or air spaces should be mentioned (Box 15-3 and Table 15-3).

Reactive Lymphoid Proliferations

Clinicopathologic Patterns of Pulmonary Lymphoid Hyperplasia

Sustained hyperplasia of the MALT of the lung occurs in the setting of autoimmune or altered immune conditions (e.g., acquired immunodeficiency, connective tissue disorders, congenital immunodeficiency). Biopsy is performed to distinguish among superimposed infection, treatment-related pneumotoxicity, and lymphoma.

Box 15-3. Hyperplasia of Mucosa-Associated Lymphoid Tissue: General Features

What Should Be Present
Small discontinuous foci of lymphoid cells often near bronchiolar branch points
One or several germinal centers, with at least partial IgD+ mantle, with light zone/dark zone polarization
bcl6+, bcl2– CD20+ B cells within but not between germinal centers
A tight meshwork of CD21+ follicular dendritic cells with sharp borders

What Should Be Absent
Destruction of lung parenchyma, alveolar walls, and bronchiolar walls
Dutcher bodies
Follicular colonization
Monoclonal plasma cells
No aggregations of monocytoid or plasmacytoid cells within follicles
Compression of the bronchiolar lumen (which suggests follicular bronchiolitis)
Grossly identifiable nodules (which suggests non-Hodgkin lymphoma)
Significant extension into the alveolar walls (which suggests lymphoid interstitial pneumonia)

The three main patterns of lymphoid hyperplasia—follicular bronchiolitis (FB), nodular lymphoid hyperplasia (NLH), and diffuse lymphoid hyperplasia (lymphoid interstitial pneumonia [LIP])—may be seen in isolation or may coexist in the same specimen.[67,68] Much of the work in identifying specific benign and malignant lymphoid proliferations requires the diagnostician to recognize the intactness or the patterned disruption of the morphologic and immunologic landmarks of normal MALT (Fig. 15-2; see also Box 15-3 and Table 15-3).

Follicular Bronchiolitis

Follicular bronchiolitis is slightly more common in males than in females, involves the lungs bilaterally, and produces a centrilobular reticulonodular pattern of involvement on radiologic studies.[69,70] In exceptional cases, opacities up to 1 cm in size may be seen. FB is most commonly seen in patients with congenital or acquired immunodeficiency (HIV, common variable immunodeficiency, or immunoglobulin A deficiency), collagen vascular disease (especially rheumatoid arthritis), or chronic obstructive pulmonary disease,[70–73] and it may also be seen at the periphery of localized infectious processes of the lung.

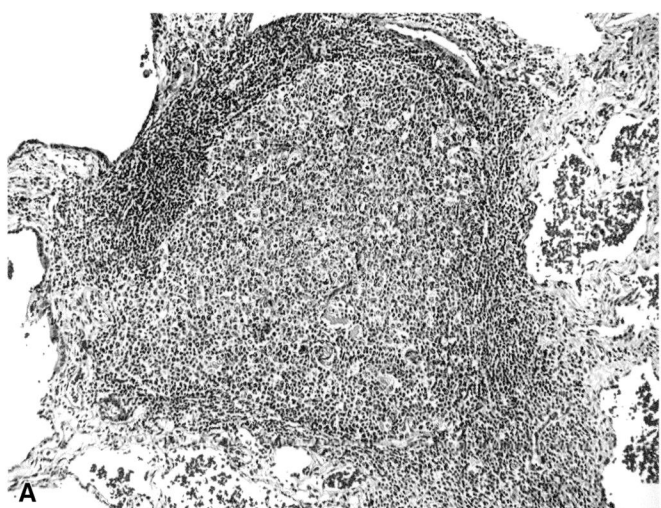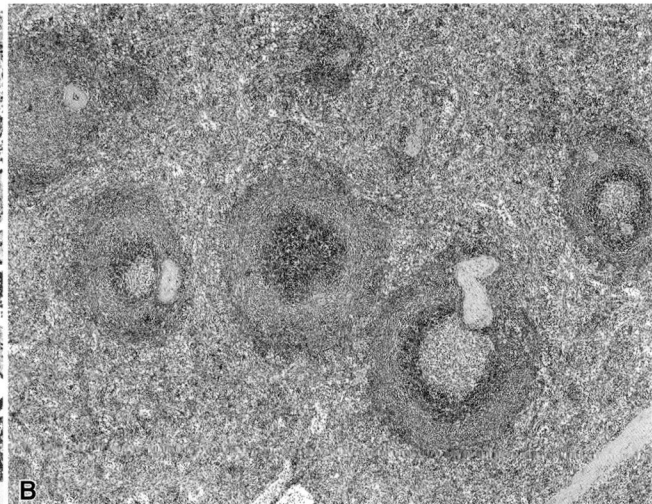

Figure 15-1. A, Benign mucosa-associated lymphoid tissue accumulates adjacent to the airways after exposure to immunogenic material. The proliferation represents a mixture of B and T lineage lymphocytes, with a structure that loosely recapitulates germinal centers. The marginal zone is seldom so well developed as it is in the spleen. **B,** When it is developed, consideration should be given to an evolving lymphoproliferative disorder.

Table 15-3. Comparison of Marginal Zone Lymphoma with Benign Lymphoid Proliferations in the Lung

	Nodular Lymphoid Hyperplasia	Lymphoid Interstitial Pneumonia	Marginal Zone Lymphoma
Clinical features	Adults > children ± altered immune state	Common in children, association with immunodeficiency	Adults > children, association with immunodeficiency
Location of infiltrates	Peribronchiolar, septal patchy, may be multifocal	Interstitial, patchy, may be multifocal	Masslike or patternless, typically unifocal
	A few intraepithelial lymphocytes may be present	A few intraepithelial lymphocytes may be present	Destructive lymphoepithelial lesions are present
Architecture	Diffuse effacement of lung parenchymal structures	Expansion of tissue planes by lymphoid infiltrate	Complete effacement of the normal lung parenchyma
	Germinal centers are often present and sharply defined	Germinal centers may be present and if so are sharply defined	Germinal centers are often present and usually frayed and disrupted (follicular colonization; discussed later)
Cellular composition	Polymorphous array of lymphocytes, plasma cells	Polymorphous array of lymphocytes, plasma cells	Germinal centers are surrounded by a broad marginal zone with variable proportions of centrocytoid, monocytoid, and plasmacytoid cells
	No Dutcher bodies	No Dutcher bodies	Plasma cells with Dutcher bodies may be present
Immunophenotype	Polytypic	Polytypic	Monotypic; clonal B cells are negative for CD5, CD10, CD23
			Follicular colonization is present (influx of CD20+, bcl2+, bcl6– B cells into a network of dendritic cells defined by CD21)

Microscopically, the key feature is multiple foci of eccentric peribronchiolar accumulations of lymphoid tissue that distort and may narrow the bronchiolar lumen[71,74-76] (Box 15-4 and Fig. 15-3). Confluent nodule-forming infiltrates larger than 1 cm should raise concern about lymphoma. The structure of benign MALT is preserved, with bcl2– germinal centers that are crisply demarcated by an immunoglobulin D–positive mantle zone and a polymorphous lymphocytic and histiocytic component at the interface with normal lung parenchyma. The proliferation may compress the airways, leading to postobstructive bronchiectasis in distal parenchyma. There is no interstitial involvement in the alveolar walls away from the bronchioles, and the air spaces are uninvolved (Fig. 15-4), a feature that distinguishes FB from LIP.[69,70,75-77]

Immunophenotypic findings in FB are identical to those seen in NLH (discussed later). In the vast majority of cases of FB, no special stains are required. However, in unusual cases, a useful immunohistochemical panel would include CD20, CD3, bcl2, bcl6, MUM1, and immunoglobulin D. The expected findings include a crisp immunoglobulin

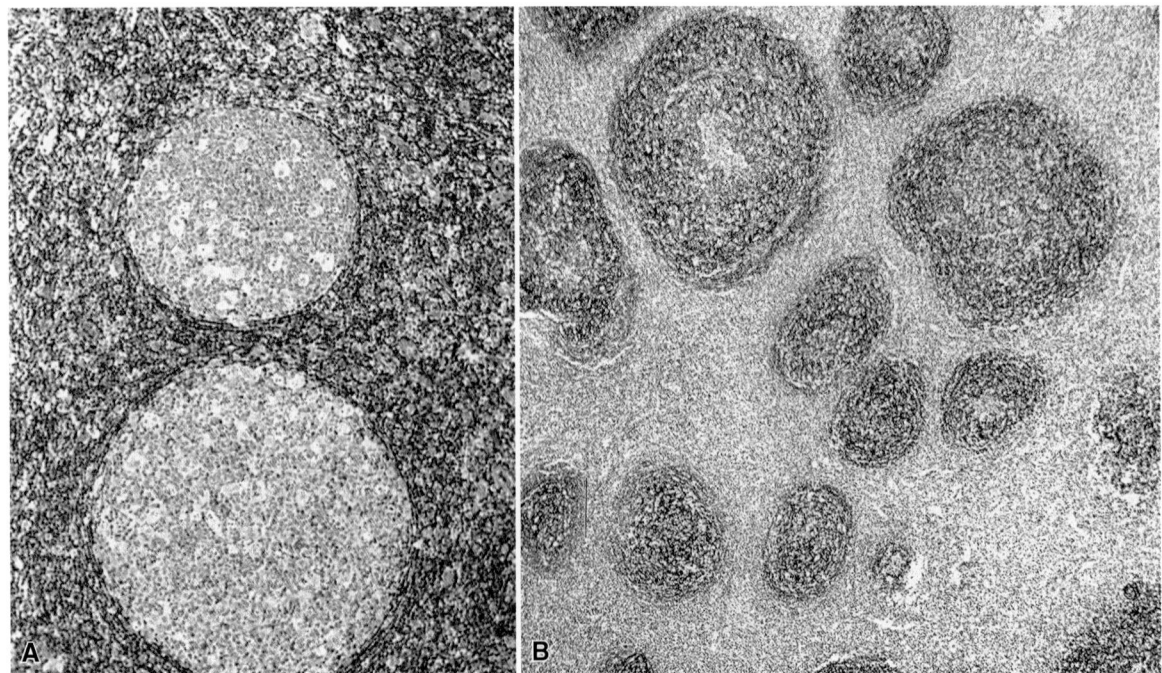

Figure 15-2. The normal immunoarchitecture of bronchiolar lymphoid tissue follows that seen elsewhere. Germinal centers are negative for bcl2 (**A**) and rich in CD21+ follicular dendritic cells (**B**) and bcl6+ centrocytes and centroblasts (**C**). *Continued*

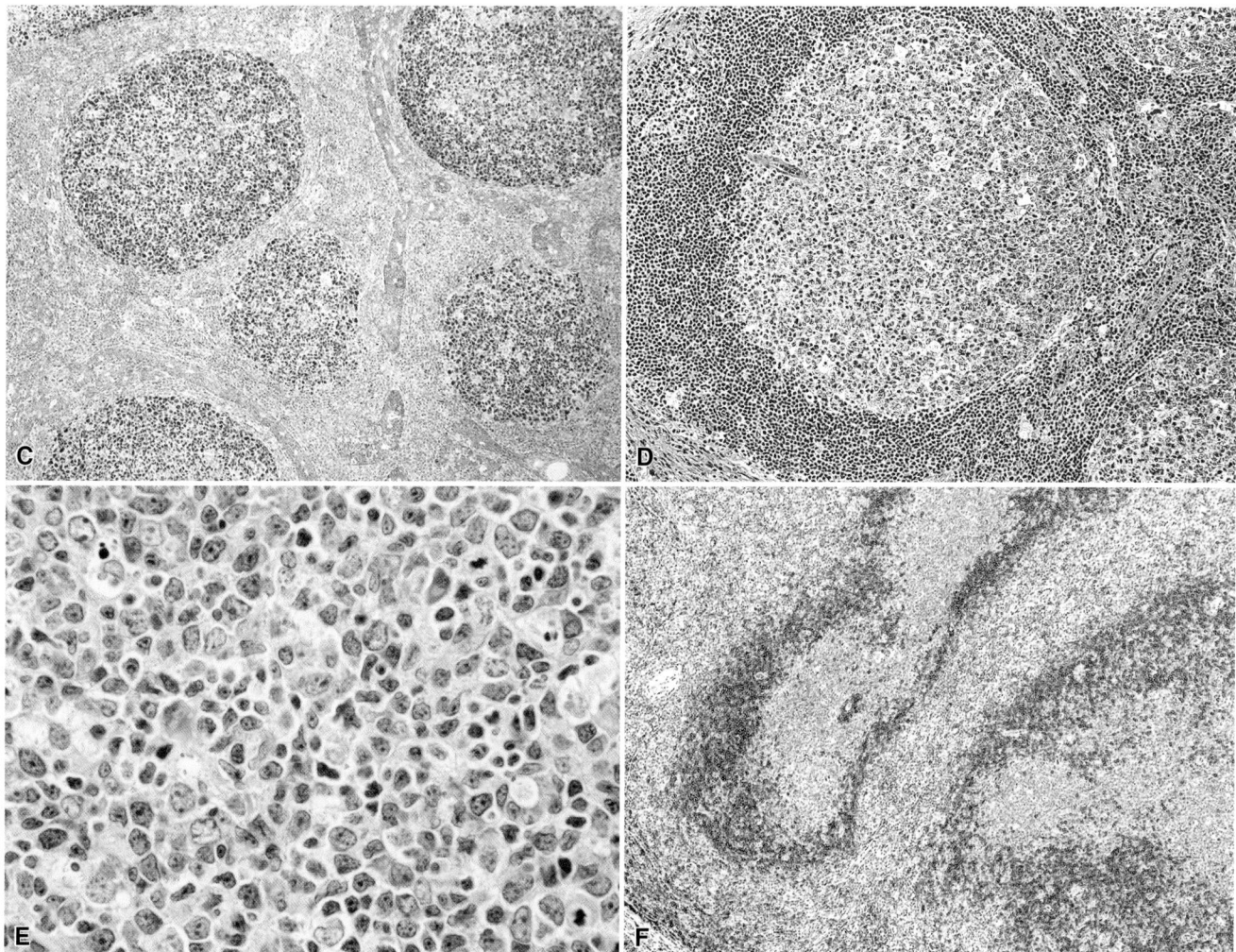

Figure 15-2—cont'd. D, At low power, some of the follicles are polarized into light and dark zones. **E,** At high power there is a rich and heterogenous mix of centrocytes and centroblasts, without a discernible increase in plasma cells or monocytoid cells. **F,** It may be irregular in contour, but an immunoglobulin D–positive mantle is often present.

Box 15-4. Features of Follicular Bronchiolitis

What Should Be Present
Germinal centers with crisp mantles located beside bronchioles along the pathway of bronchovascular bundles
At least partial IgD+ mantle
Bcl2 negativity within follicles

What Might Be Present
Compression of bronchiolar lumina
Distal bronchiectasis
Other features associated with a specific causative condition (e.g., cysts in Sjögren syndrome, rheumatoid nodules and pleuritis in rheumatoid arthritis)

What Should Be Absent
Size > 1 cm
Destruction of lung parenchyma, including lymphoepithelial lesions
Extension along the alveolar septae
Dutcher bodies in plasma cells
Cytologic monotony
Follicular colonization
Monoclonal plasma cells
MUM1+ cells in follicles

What Should Be Communicated in the Report
Findings are benign
A connective tissue disease should be investigated clinically if the patient does not have an established diagnosis

D–positive mantle at least partway around the germinal centers and germinal centers rich in bcl2–, bcl6+, MUM1– B cells, all enmeshed within a compact array of CD21+ follicular dendritic cells. A cytokeratin stain may be added to assess for destructive lymphoepithelial lesions. If even a modest degree of plasmacytic differentiation is evident on hematoxylin and eosin, kappa and lambda staining will mark enough cells to aid in assessing for clonality.

Differential diagnostic considerations include *nonspecific chronic inflammation,*[78,79] which is not organized or airway-centered, and which usually extends into alveolar walls. NLH may enter into the differential diagnosis, and the distinction is as much quantitative as it is a perception of a mass-forming process that compresses adjacent normal lung parenchyma.[80] *Constrictive bronchiolitis* may be associated with lymphocytic accumulations around the bronchioles, but the cue to the correct diagnosis is concomitant peribronchiolar fibrosis with reduction in lumen size such that the bronchiole is significantly smaller in diameter than its accompanying arteriole. An elastin stain may be helpful in defining the architecture in such circumstances.

On transthoracic and transbronchial biopsy specimens, it can be difficult to distinguish a florid focus of FB from *lymphoma,* largely because of the limited nature of the specimen. Monocytoid morphologic features, Dutcher bodies, monotypic plasma cells or lymphoplasmacytoid forms, and molecular testing for clonality may suggest lymphoma in amply sampled cases, but full diagnosis with classification is probably best reserved for wedge biopsy.

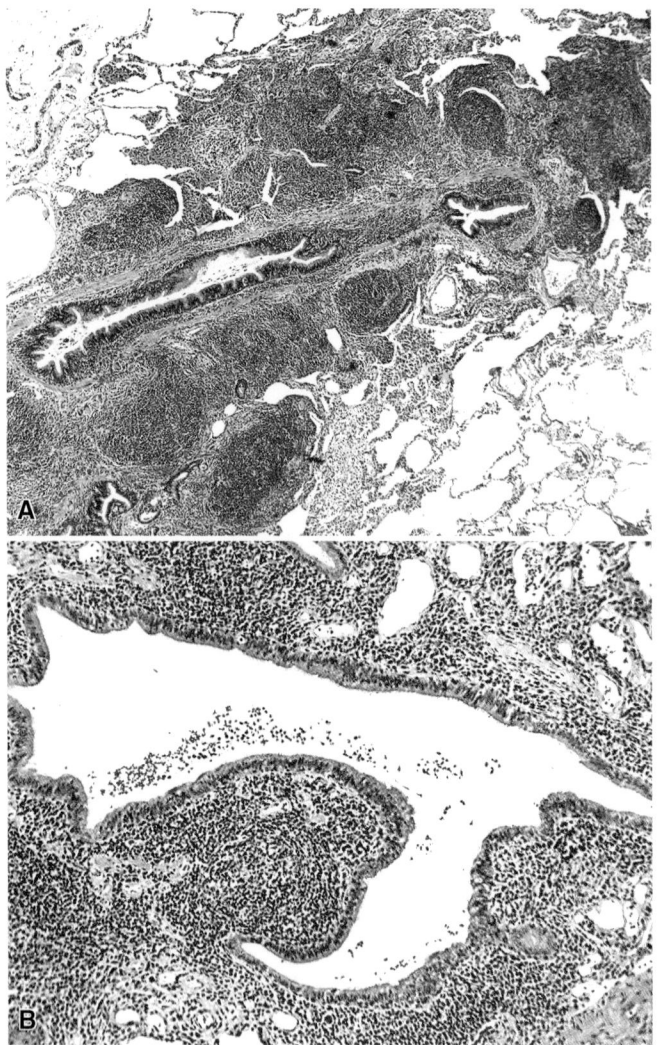

Figure 15-3. **A,** Eccentric accumulation of lymphocytes around airways is the principal morphologic finding in follicular bronchiolitis. **B,** The proliferation may protrude into the lumen, causing symptoms.

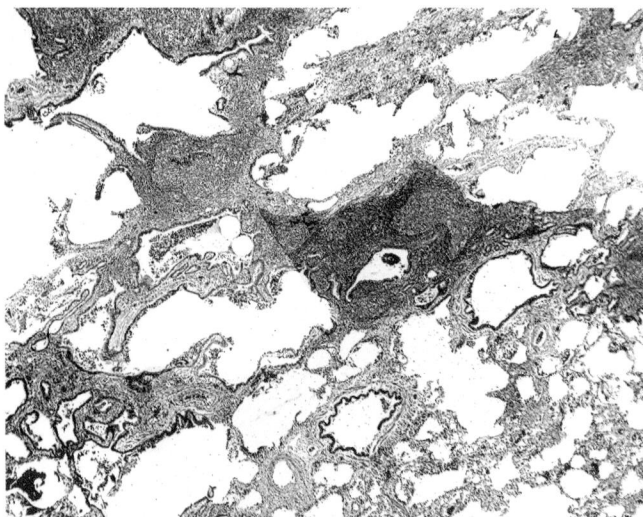

Figure 15-4. In follicular bronchiolitis, there is abrupt termination and a discrete boundary of the proliferation, which does not track along alveolar septa as lymphoid interstitial pneumonitis often does.

Nodular Lymphoid Hyperplasia

Nodular lymphoid hyperplasia is an extremely rare condition, with only one large series published, representing the Armed Forces Institute of Pathology experience over a decade. In older literature, "NLH" has been used synonymously with "pseudolymphoma," an outdated and confusing term that should be discarded.[80] It is a proliferation that is most commonly seen in adults, reported in the second to ninth decade. Whereas there are reports of NLH in patients with an altered immune state, such as autoimmune disorders, collagen vascular disease, or acquired immunodeficiency, in the Armed Forces Institute of Pathology series there was no special relationship with those conditions.[80–82]

Patients come to clinical attention because of cough or reasons unrelated to respiratory symptoms. One or several discrete subpleural or peripheral nodules are detected on radiography.[81] If there is a reticulonodular pattern in the remaining lung, clinical concern for lymphoma as well as infectious etiologies is greater. In contrast to the lymphoid lesions of FB, the nodules of NLH are typically larger than 0.5 cm, but seldom larger than 5 cm.

The lymphoid infiltrate of NLH forms a circumscribed nodule of lymphoid tissue (Box 15-5 and Fig. 15-5), with intact architecture, including germinal centers, a discrete mantle, and a preserved "paracortical" interfollicular zone. The process is not pleurally based, and there should not be a bronchiolar distribution.

Within the mass, follicular architecture predominates.[80,83] Cells within nodules retain centrocytic and centroblastic morphologic features, and the mantle zone retains its population of small cells with deeply basophilic round nuclei and scant cytoplasm. Small resting lymphocytes, stromal elements, and plasma cells fill the interfollicular zone, which may also contain patchy accumulations of histiocytes. Lesional foci of NLH remain sharply circumscribed from the surrounding lung parenchyma, with at least a partial immunoglobulin D–positive mantle (Fig. 15-6), without significant extension along the lobar septa or into the alveolar walls, in contrast to LIP. Plasma cells with Russell bodies and Mott cells may be present, but destructive lymphoepithelial lesions, Dutcher bodies, and follicular colonization[84] should not be identified.

If the nodule was not sampled for flow cytometry, a useful immunohistochemical panel includes CD20, CD21, CD3, *bcl2*, *bcl6*, and immunoglobulin D, as well as kappa, lambda, MUM1, and cytokeratin. The immunoglobulin D–positive mantle should be present and fairly

Box 15-5. Features of Nodular Lymphoid Hyperplasia

What Should Be Present
A discrete usually solitary nodule, typically 1–2 cm, seldom >5 cm
Follicles with light zone/dark zone polarization, sharp IgD+ mantle, and bcl2 and MUM1 negativity in the germinal center

What Might Be Present
Interfollicular plasmacytosis

What Should Be Absent
Extension along the alveolar septae
Dutcher bodies in plasma cells
Cytologic monotony
Follicular colonization
Monoclonal plasma cells
Pleural infiltration
MUM1+ cells in follicles

What Should Be Communicated in the Report
Connective tissue disease and other altered immune states should be investigated clinically
The pattern is benign, but even molecular studies are not 100% sensitive, so the patient should be observed for the appearance of additional lung nodules or adenopathy, with biopsy if the clinical findings warrant

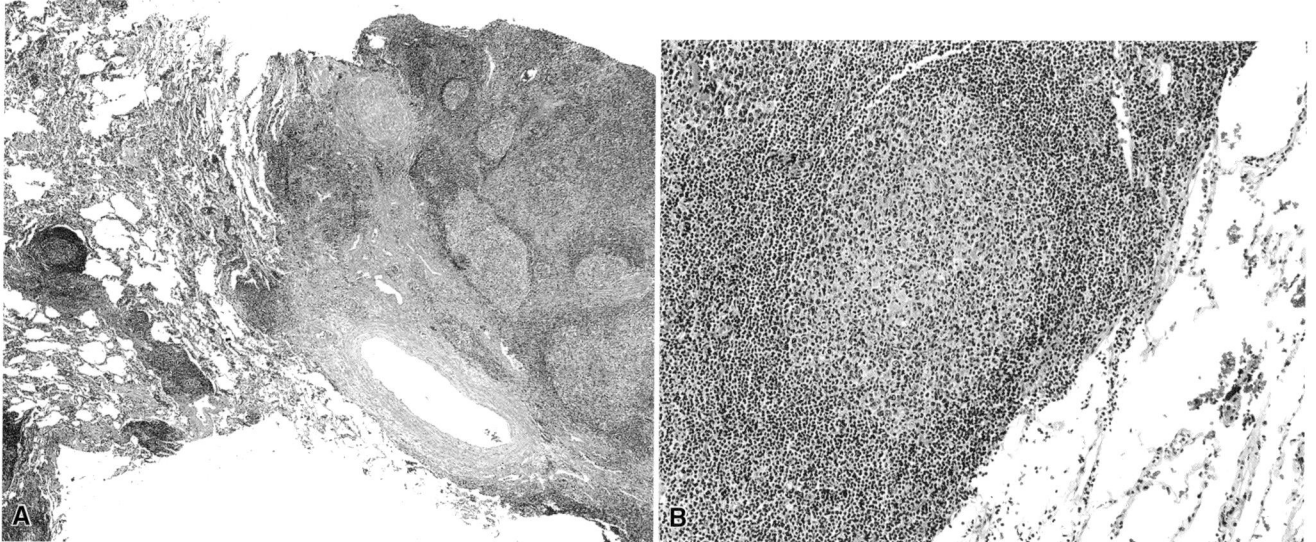

Figure 15-5. Nodular lymphoid hyperplasia is a discrete mass-forming lymphoid proliferation that is spherical or ovoid, in contrast to the linear parabronchial distribution of follicular bronchiolitis. **A,** Germinal centers are widely spaced, vary in size, and maintain the benign immunoarchitectural landmarks seen in Figure 15-2. **B,** Pale-staining monocytoid cells seen in marginal zone lymphoma are not present.

crisply demarcated from the immunoglobulin D–negative germinal center inside and the immunoglobulin D–negative paracortex beyond. The germinal center cells should have a bcl2–, bcl6+ phenotype. The bcl6+, CD20+ B lymphocytes within the follicles are definitionally polytypic, as are the plasma cells and immunoglobulin D–positive mantle cells. The interfollicular areas are rich in CD3+ T cells. CD21 staining in NLH highlights the compact nature of the follicular dendritic cell network (Fig. 15-7). A disrupted appearance, particularly if associated with a significant bcl2+, bcl6–, or MUM1+ population of B cells within the follicles or an increase in the number of interfollicular B cells, suggests the diagnosis of MaZL (see Table 15-3).[82]

Because of its rarity, NLH is a diagnosis that should be approached with caution and made only after all necessary studies to exclude lymphoma are performed. In practice, if neither flow cytometry nor immunohistochemistry yields a secure diagnosis, molecular studies are a reasonable final step. Principal microscopic differential considerations

in transbronchial or transthoracic biopsy specimens may include a particularly robust FB, LIP, and various low-grade lymphomas. In contrast to *FB*, NLH is mass-forming and displaces significant amounts of lung parenchyma.[80] *LIP* is readily excluded by radiologic correlation because it is generally diffuse and bilateral and is not mass-forming, and it is primarily interstitial, with extensive infiltration of the alveolar walls, whereas NLH displaces normal lung tissue as a mass.

In contrast to follicular lymphoma, the germinal centers of NLH are widely spaced, vary in size, exhibit light zone/dark zone polarity, and are demarcated by a distinct immunoglobulin D–positive mantle zone composed of cytologically bland small lymphocytes.[5] The finding of bcl2 positivity within nodules in excess of what CD3+ intrafollicular T cells would yield, or the finding of significant numbers of bcl6+, CD20+ B cells outside of the germinal centers should raise concern about follicular lymphoma. If flow cytometry is not available, molecular assessment for clonality and disease-defining translocations should

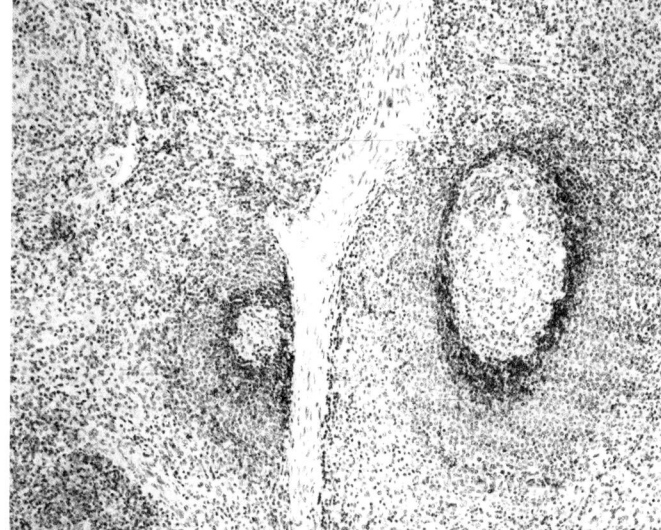

Figure 15-6. A thin immunoglobulin D–positive mantle zone is seen in nodular lymphoid hyperplasia. Because of the close overlap with marginal zone lymphoma, even when the immunoarchitecture is reassuringly intact, flow cytometry or molecular studies are needed to confirm the polyclonal nature of the process.

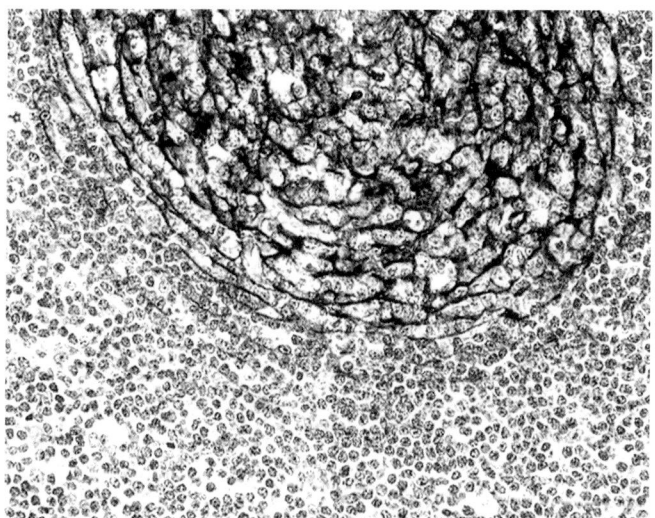

Figure 15-7. The CD21+ follicular dendritic meshwork of nodular lymphoid hyperplasia is sharply circumscribed, in contrast to the ragged appearance of the network in marginal zone lymphoma, which is seen in Figure 15-17B.

be pursued (PCR, FISH). MUM1 immunostaining may be helpful in distinguishing follicular lymphoma from MaZL.

Marginal zone lymphoma is the most challenging element of the differential diagnosis. Because MaZL is much more common than NLH, it can be argued that molecular studies should be pursued in all cases before a benign diagnosis is rendered. The architecture may be identical to that of NLH, or there may be some blurring of the mantle zone separating the germinal centers from the intervening cellularity. A significant population of mono*cytoid* cells (intermediate size, round or reniform nucleus, sufficient quantities of pale cytoplasm that nuclei are widely spaced on routine sections), either within or between nodules, favors MaZL. The nodules may exhibit "follicular colonization" by MaZL,[84] which is seen as displacement of the CD20+, bcl6+, bcl2–, MUM1– centrocytes and centroblasts of the normal follicle by the MaZL cells (CD20+, bcl6–, bcl2+, MUM1+; discussed later). The mantle zone in MaZL is eroded or distorted on immunoglobulin D stain, and the follicular dendritic cell meshwork is diffused through the dilutional effects of the infiltrating MaZL cells. Although they are not diagnostic of MaZL, destructive lymphoepithelial lesions should be sought on cytokeratin stain.

Lymphoid Interstitial Pneumonia and Diffuse Lymphoid Hyperplasia

The pattern of LIP may be seen in both children and adults, and up to 40% of cases are eventually attributable to a specific underlying condition. It is more common in the setting of altered immune states, such as autoimmune conditions and connective tissue disorders (especially Sjögren syndrome[85]), AIDS,[86,87] and congenital immunodeficiency states,[88] and after bone marrow transplant. It may also be a tissue response pattern to infections such as mycoplasma, chlamydia, Epstein-Barr virus (EBV), and legionella.[89] In some series, females are affected disproportionately,[69] perhaps because of the common collagen vascular disease association. Older literature doubtless includes cases of MALT lymphoma, which may skew both outcome and the clinicopathologic parameters that have been associated with LIP.

Patients with LIP present with a cough and slow but progressive shortness of breath, and radiologic studies usually show bilateral basilar patchy opacities or reticulonodular infiltrates.[69,87,89–91] Cysts have been reported in LIP,[92] but correlation with clinical findings suggests that the cysts are more likely a manifestation of the underlying condition (Sjögren syndrome) than of LIP. Some patients have systemic symptoms, such as fever and weight loss, and many (70%) have

Box 15-6. Features of Diffuse Lymphoid Hyperplasia/Lymphoid Interstitial Pneumonia

What Should Be Present
Alveolar wall expansion by mixed lymphoplasmacytic proliferation
Blending and gradual transition from more heavily involved areas to normal lung parenchyma
Occasional germinal centers with sharply defined mantle zones and some light zone/dark zone polarization
Predominance of T cells in alveolar walls; polyclonality in the plasma cells

What Might Be Present
Patchy accumulations of histiocytes, multinucleated giant cells, or small noncaseating granulomas
Clustered intraepithelial T lymphocytes ("lymphoepithelium" of bronchus-associated lymphoid tissue)
Cysts (discussed in the text)
Depending on the underlying condition, some degree of interstitial fibrosis

What Should Be Absent
Destruction of the lung architecture
Evidence of follicular colonization
Intranuclear accumulations of immunoglobulin (Dutcher bodies) in plasma cells
Cytologic monotony or monocytoid morphologic features in B cell–rich zones
Lymphoplasmacytic undermining of the vascular endothelium
Organizing pneumonia

What Should Be Communicated in the Report
Clinical evidence of connective tissue disease, HIV, and other altered immune states should be investigated if these diagnoses are not already established
The pattern is benign, but even molecular studies are not 100% sensitive, so the patient should be evaluated clinically and radiologically for the appearance of additional lung nodules, which should be sampled if clinical or other features suggest heightened concern about lymphoma

polyclonal hypergammaglobulinemia; both the clinical and laboratory abnormalities likely reflect the underlying altered immune state.

In contrast to FB and NLH, the infiltrate of LIP has a dominant interstitial pattern of distribution, although the constituent cellular components are otherwise similar. Small, cytologically bland lymphocytes and intermingled plasma cells distend the alveolar walls, with accentuation along the bronchovascular bundles and lobular septae (Box 15-6 and Fig. 15-8). Aggregates of histiocytes or poorly formed granulomas may be present, but neutrophils and eosinophils are scarce. A few germinal centers may be present.[69,87,90] An intraepithelial component mimicking the lymphoepithelial lesions of MALT lymphoma and a coalescence

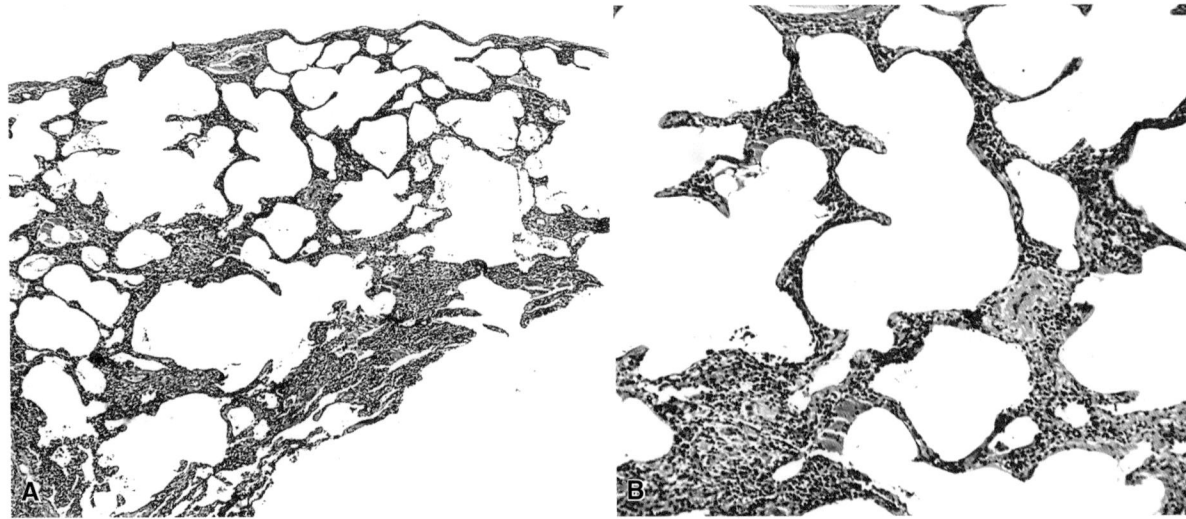

Figure 15-8. A, Lymphoid interstitial pneumonia lacks the mass-forming qualities of nodular lymphoid hyperplasia as well as the nodularity of the latter condition. **B** and **C,** The proliferation expands the interalveolar septa and focally forms microaggregates of constituent lymphocytes. *Continued*

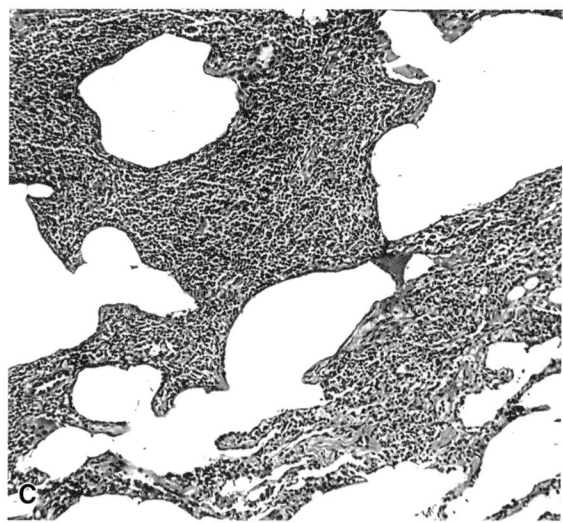

Figure 15-8—cont'd.

in and around the microvasculature have been described, but truly destructive changes are not part of LIP (Fig. 15-9).

An LIP-like pattern has been described in the lung in the setting of atypical infectious mononucleosis.[53,93,94] In these few reports, the alveolar walls and interstitium were expanded by a mixture of lymphocytes, plasma cells, and transformed lymphocytes (immunoblasts), and there was a patchy alveolar exudate. In situ hybridization for EBV-encoded ribonucleotides (EBERs) is the most sensitive and specific means of identifying the virally mediated nature of the process. Immunosuppressed patients are at increased risk for EBV-related lymphoid proliferations, and biopsy is usually undertaken to assess for a specific infectious process. In the transplant setting, the terminology of post-transplant lymphoproliferative disorders (PTLDs) should be used (discussed later).

The cellular phase of *nonspecific interstitial pneumonitis* may be a differential consideration in patients with fibroblasts and an extracellular matrix as well as a lymphoplasmacytic infiltrate in the alveolar walls. *Hypersensitivity pneumonitis* may lead to cellular interstitial infiltrates, but on scanning view, the process should show bronchocentricity, and

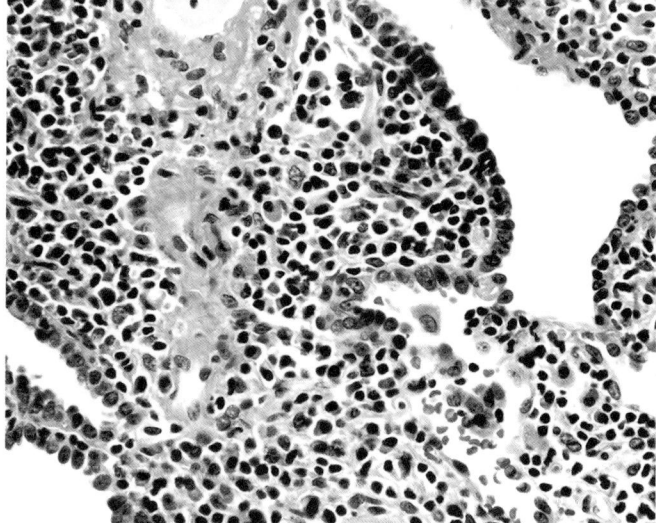

Figure 15-9. Lymphoid interstitial pneumonia shows composition by morphologically mature lymphocytes. Most are CD3+ T cells, a helpful feature in distinguishing this condition from marginal zone lymphoma. Lymphocytes may abut the epithelium of the distal airways, but they do not form destructive aggregations, as seen in marginal zone lymphoma and in Figure 15-15.

loosely formed granulomas or at least multinucleated giant cells are likely to be more prominent. Organizing pneumonia would be less typical of LIP, and if more than an occasional focus is noted, a descriptive diagnosis of chronic interstitial pneumonia with organizing pneumonia might be most appropriate.

Occasional germinal centers and focal intraepithelial accumulations of lymphocytes may prompt consideration of MaZL/*MALT lymphoma*, but the bilateral and interstitial (rather than unifocal and mass-forming) nature of LIP, as well as the lack of a dominant B cell population in the interfollicular areas, provides a strong and objective means of excluding this possibility. Because of the interstitial distribution, dominant T cell population, and cytologic heterogeneity of LIP, distinction from pulmonary presentation of systemic lymphomas, such as small lymphocytic lymphoma, mantle cell lymphoma, or follicle center cell lymphoma is seldom an issue. In difficult cases, or when diagnostic material is limited, immunohistochemistry (CD20, CD3) usually permits a definite diagnosis (discussed later; see Box 15-3 and Table 15-3).

Outcome for patients with an LIP pattern of lung disease is variable and relates largely to the underlying condition. Some patients may have spontaneous resolution, and others achieve a good response to a trial of steroids. Morbidity and mortality are most often seen in patients with superimposed infection or other comorbid conditions, such as renal failure. A subset of patients, generally with a difficult-to-control connective tissue disease, progress to end-stage fibrosis with honeycombing, and so in some cases the prognosis is worse than that of its neoplastic lookalike, MaZL. The reported increased risk of lymphoma likely relates at least in part to the fact that some cases previously diagnosed as LIP were in fact lymphoma ab initio.

Castleman Disease

Castleman disease includes two distinct conditions. One, the "hyaline vascular variant," is almost invariably presents via mass effect of a solitary mediastinal mass or central lymphadenopathy in otherwise asymptomatic individuals and is cured by complete resection. The other, the "plasma cell variant," often manifests with systemic symptoms and multifocal disease, and has significant associated morbidity and mortality. What brings them together[95] is that, first, the two histologies may coexist in the same lymph node, and second, they were characterized in separate publications by the same individual, Benjamin Castleman.

Hyaline Vascular Variant

The hyaline vascular variant of Castleman disease (HVCD) arises in axial node groups of the mediastinum and abdomen, although it may extend along the hilum to involve peribronchial lymph nodes. Most patients have no systemic symptoms and present because of mass effect (e.g., airway compression or superior vena cava syndrome) or have mediastinal adenopathy detected during radiologic studies performed for other reasons.[96-98] A patient who has "B" symptoms and diffuse adenopathy likely has a mixed type of Castleman disease, in which the histologic features of the plasma cell variant are present elsewhere (discussed later). In contrast to the plasma cell variant of Castleman disease (PCCD), there is no consistent abnormality in laboratory findings.

At low power, the architecture is nodular, composed of small and involuted germinal centers with expansive immunoglobulin D–positive mantles formed of small lymphocytes, often in a laminated or "onion skinning" array. Multiple germinal centers may be found in the boundaries of a single mantle zone, and in opportune sections, the lymphoid depletion in the germinal centers unmasks the radially penetrating high endothelium—the "lollipop" motif (Box 15-7 and Fig. 15-10). Sinuses between the regressed follicles are imperceptible usually because they are absent. At high power, the germinal centers are depleted of lymphocytes

Box 15-7. Features of Castleman Disease, Hyaline Vascular Type

What Should Be Present
Regressed germinal centers
Broadened, laminated mantle zones
High endothelial venules with plump endothelium and a variable increase in the
    adjacent extracellular matrix
Pockets of plasmacytoid monocytes in interfollicular regions

What Might Be Present
Mixed histologic features of the hyaline vascular variant and the plasma cell variant
Regressed follicles with radially penetrating high endothelial venules

What Should Be Absent
Clearly patent sinuses
Monoclonality in the mantle cells

What Should Be Communicated in the Report
If the pattern of the hyaline vascular variant is seen in isolation in nodal structures,
    excision is likely to be curative
If, however, there is an admixed plasma cell variant pattern, or if the patient has "B"
    symptoms, organomegaly, or unexplained cytopenias, a diagnosis of multicentric
    Castleman disease is favored and the patient may need systemic therapy

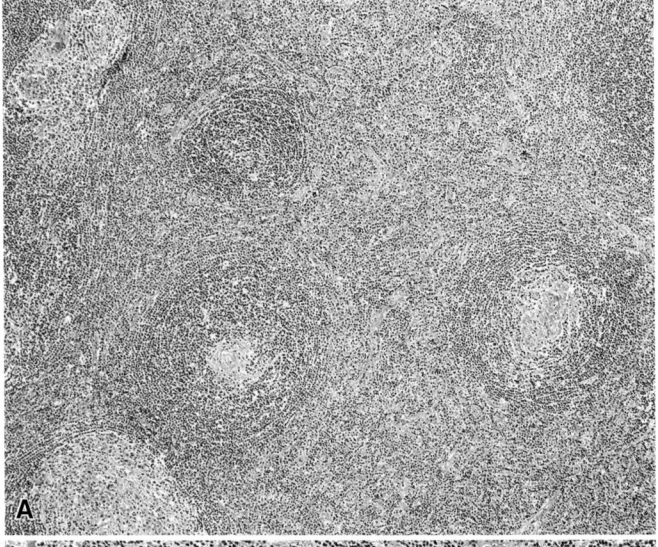

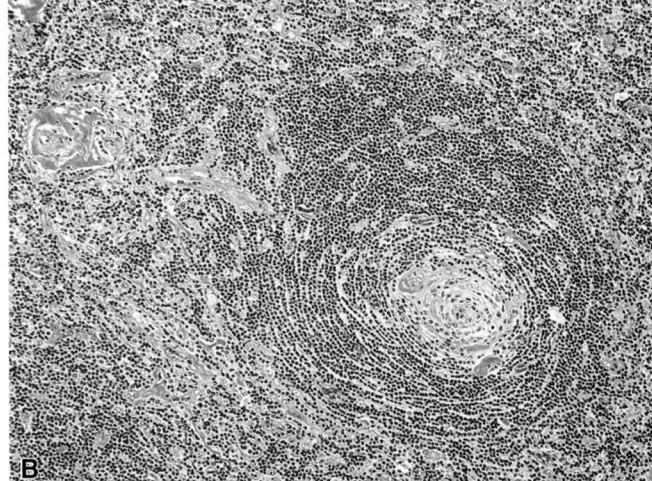

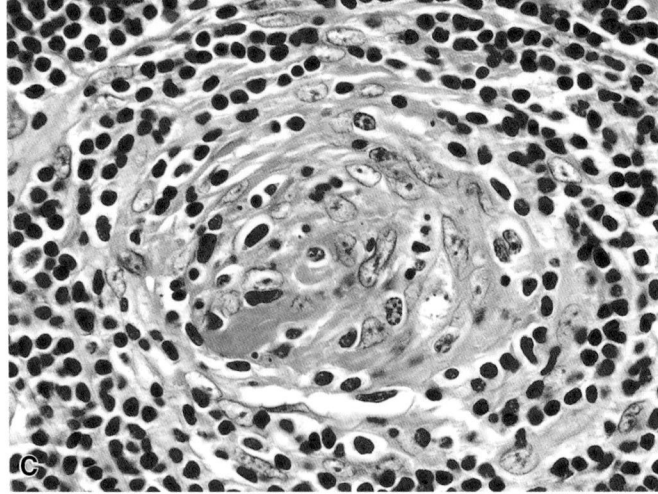

Figure 15-10. A, One of the subtle and least appreciated histologic findings in the hyaline vascular variant of Castleman disease is the absence of the sinuses that weave in between follicles. **B,** The hypervascular nature of the intervening tissues, often creating the radially penetrating "lollipop motif," is the classic feature of Castleman disease. **C,** It is also seen in other settings in which there are regressed germinal centers (e.g., HIV-related changes).

and contain both extracellular matrix and abundant follicle dendritic cells. The interfollicular zone includes plasmacytoid monocytes, stromal myoid cells, histiocytes, dendritic cells, and lymphocytes.[99–101]

Follicle dendritic cells within the germinal centers are CD21+ and S-100–, and are distributed as dense aggregates rather than as circumscribed meshworks with intermingled centrocytes and centroblasts. Their processes extend in a laminar array beyond the germinal center border such that the mantle cells align along them. The lymphocytes of the mantle zone represent a mixture of CD20+ B cells, and the plasmacytoid monocytes are both CD4+ (but CD3–) and CD68+.[99,100,102] Plasmacytoid monocytes aggregate in clusters between regressed follicles, and are demonstrable on HECA-452 (Fig. 15-11).

Differential diagnostic considerations may include a *Castleman-like reaction to tumor*[103,104] and a variety of non-Hodgkin lymphomas. Mantle cell lymphoma is clonal and positive for cyclin D1, and in partially involved nodes, the sinuses may be compressed but still present. Follicular lymphoma rarely (if ever) has an immunoglobulin D–positive mantle zone that is broader than the follicle within, and the nodules are cellular and rich in bcl6+ B cells, rather than depleted. *HIV-related lymph node changes,* particularly the depleted form, which has regressed germinal centers, may enter into the differential diagnosis and may be difficult to exclude, but the laminated array of mantle cells is generally undeveloped, plasmacytoid monocytes are few or absent, and sinuses are present and generally congested with histiocytes. The *angioimmunoblastic lymphadenopathy (AILD) type of peripheral T cell lymphoma* is discussed in the differential diagnosis with HVCD because both have abnormal follicular structures, but in AILD-PTCL the follicles are generally enlarged and fragmented, not regressed, and flow cytometry may show the loss of a pan T cell antigen on T cells. Immunohistochemistry shows *bcl6* expression in CD3+ T cells. Molecular studies often document at least a clonal T cell population and sometimes also a clonal B cell population. Double antibody immunostains highlight a special population of *bcl6*+ T cells in perivascular areas. If there is cytoatypia or a mass-forming coalescence of follicular dendritic cells, consideration should be given to an evolving follicular dendritic cell tumor (discussed later).

Outcome is excellent in patients with fully resected localized HVCD.[105]

Plasma Cell Variant

The plasma cell variant of Castleman disease is most frequently encountered in HIV-positive patients and the elderly, and presenting pulmonary symptoms include shortness of breath, productive cough, and fevers. When it involves the chest structures, PCCD is more often found in the central lymph nodes, with secondary extension into the centrilobular regions of lung tissue. Radiologic studies may show adenopathy alone or concurrent with bilateral interstitial infiltrates.[106] Laboratory

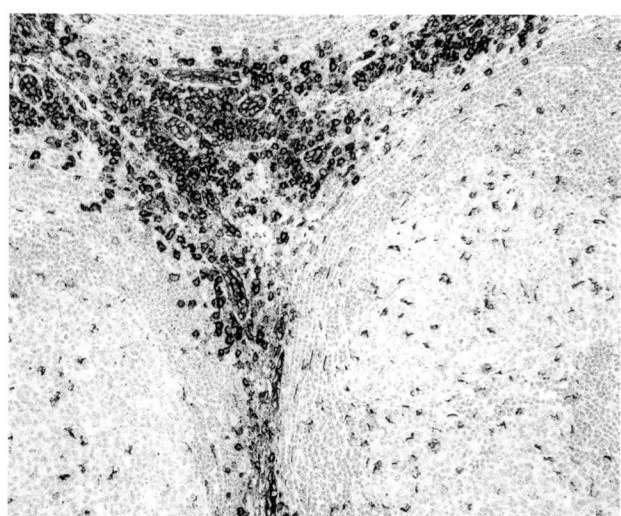

Figure 15-11. Plasmacytoid monocytes, which appear as pale lavender aggregates of cells between regressed follicles in the hyaline vascular variant of Castleman disease, are easiest to see on HECA-452 stain.

Box 15-8. Features of Castleman Disease, Plasma Cell and Multicentric Types

What Should Be Present
Robust follicular hyperplasia
Extensive interfollicular plasmacytosis
Sinuses are evident, but may be compressed and inconspicuous
Polytypic small plasma cells

What Might Be Present
Monotypic IgM-lambda–positive large lymphoid cells or immunoblasts in the perifollicular mantle; these are HHV8+ when present
Extrathoracic disease, particularly in the spleen or axial lymph nodes in the abdomen

What Should Be Absent
Clonality in the small plasma cells and lymphocytes
Bcl2 expression in the follicles or other features of follicular colonization

What Should Be Communicated in the Report
Although the diagnosis is not "malignant" in the strictest sense, the patient may need the attention and care of an oncologist

studies may show cytopenia, an elevated erythrocyte sedimentation rate, and hypergammaglobulinemia—"hyper-IL-6 syndrome."[107,108]

Both localized and multicentric expressions of PCCD occur. Taken together, they are far less common than HVCD. When localized, the adenopathy is typically axial (mediastinum or abdomen and, less commonly, in the neck) and node-based. When the disease is multicentric, patients typically have generalized lymphadenopathy and hepatosplenomegaly, and may have symptoms fitting POEMS syndrome (polyneuropathy, organomegaly, endocrinopathy, "M" spike, skin disorder[109]).

The low-power appearance is that of follicular hyperplasia with marked interfollicular plasmacytosis (Box 15-8 and Fig. 15-12). In contrast to HVCD, the subcapsular and medullary sinuses remain patent; the germinal centers are hyperplastic and large and contain amorphous eosinophilic material and have a discrete, if thinned, mantle zone.[99] Because the potential for lymph nodes to be involved by more than one process (e.g., Castleman disease and Hodgkin lymphoma or plasmablastic non-Hodgkin lymphoma), a careful search for a second diagnosis should be made before the solo diagnosis of PCCD is rendered.

Flow cytometric analysis identifies only polytypic B lymphocytes and phenotypically normal T cells. Routine immunostaining shows a polytypic population of plasma cells. Careful scrutiny of the lambda light-chain stain may show a population of immunoblasts in the perifollicular region. These, all immunoglobulin M-lambda, may be monoclonal on PCR and part of a "microlymphoma" or polyclonal at the genetic level.[99,110,111]

In lymph nodes, the differential diagnosis includes *rheumatoid arthritis*-related lymphadenitis, *syphilitic* lymphadenitis, *lymphoplasmacytic lymphoma, HIV-related* lymphadenitis, and reactive lymph nodes *draining sites of carcinoma. In the lung parenchyma itself,* PCCD may closely mimic the LIP pattern, and *MALT lymphoma* is also an important element of the differential diagnosis. Clinical correlation, good histologic sections, and sufficient tissue to assess for follicular colonization and perform clonality studies are key to resolving this set of differential considerations.

Clinically, PCCD may be smouldering or aggressive, but it is inexorable and is associated with a high rate of morbidity and mortality as a result of infection and progressive renal, hepatic, or immune system dysfunction.[112-114] Median survival time is 2 to 3 years for patients with multicentric disease. A subset of patients has Kaposi sarcoma (approximately 10%), large cell B cell lymphoma, Hodgkin disease, plasmacytoma, myeloma, or POEMS syndrome (up to 20% in HIV-positive patients).

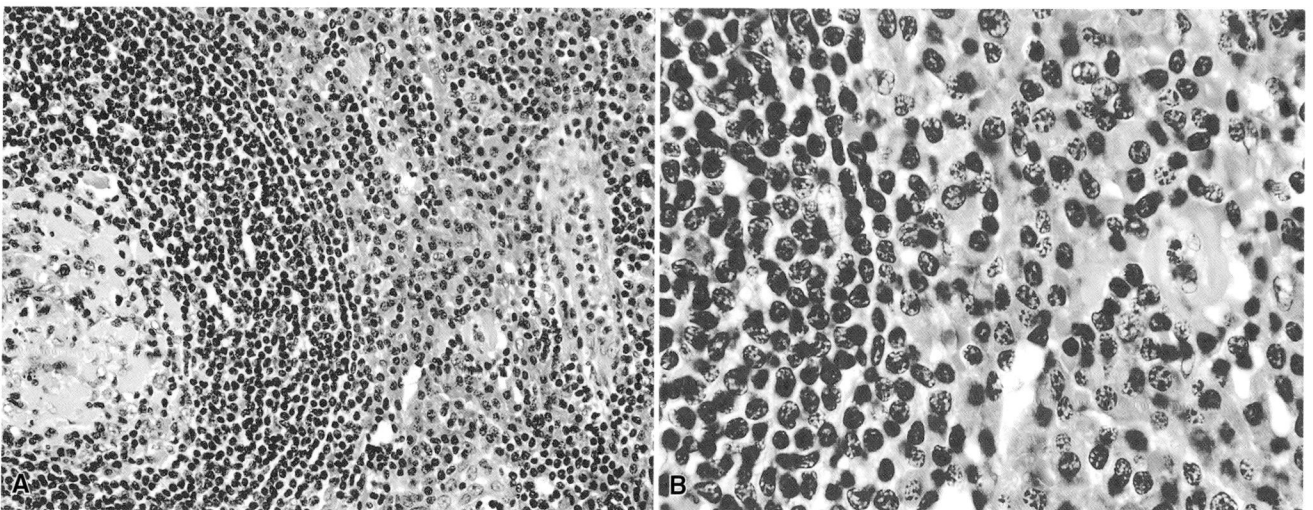

Figure 15-12. Although the germinal centers in the plasma cell variant of Castleman disease may be depleted of lymphocytes (**A**), the interfollicular regions are rich in plasma cells (**B**) and the sinuses are preserved.

Neoplastic and Malignant Lymphoid Proliferations

Classification of extranodal B lineage lymphomas involves an assessment of both patterned architectural disruptions and phenotypic parameters, some of which relate the lesional cells to normal stages of B cell and T cell development. By this paradigm, for instance, the characteristic features used to diagnose follicular *lymphoma* (a monotypic mixture of centrocytes and centroblasts, usually with CD10 and *bcl6* expression) resemble those of the cells of benign follicular *hyperplasia* (a polytypic mixture of centrocytes and centroblasts, usually with CD10 and *bcl6* expression). In contrast, those of mantle cell lymphoma and MaZL recapitulate specific aspects of mantle cell and marginal zone lymphocytes of normal tissues, respectively. No such developmental principle provides structure to the classification of T lineage lymphomas, which remain more of a "laundry list" of ontogenically unrelated entities.

Primary Lung Lymphomas

Regardless of the histologic type, adults are most commonly affected, and primary pulmonary lymphoma is quite rare in the pediatric population.[115,116] The designation of *primary pulmonary lymphoma* is restricted to *de novo* lymphomas that present with lung-limited disease. Other than hilar node involvement, no evidence of extrapulmonary disease is evident on staging at presentation or on restaging studies repeated after a period of observation. The historical definition of disease that remains localized to the lung over the course of a several-month period of observation[117] was likely overinclusive: Up to 40% of patients whose disease was defined in this way progress to stage IV systemic disease or even die of disease within 6 months of initial diagnosis.[118] With the routine use of positron emission tomography scans, initial radiologic staging may replace this approach. Strictly defined, patients with primary pulmonary lymphoma should have little disease-related morbidity and mortality[119,120] unless the disease acquires systemic manifestations or progresses to involve extrathoracic sites.

Mucosa-Associated Lymphoid Tissue Lymphoma

Although it was not recognized as a distinct and separate type of lymphoma until the early 1990s, MaZL of MALT type is the most common type of primary pulmonary lymphoma. Unlike MaZL of the stomach, thyroid, and salivary gland, however, it has an inconstant association with infectious agents or specific autoimmune conditions.[121-123] Recent studies have shown that 40% of cases contain a t(11;18) involving API2 and MALT1.[124] In contrast, other nongastric MALT-type lymphomas rarely harbor this translocation and arise much more often in the setting of an autoimmune condition. Although some patients are entirely asymptomatic, many present with cough, fever, or unexplained weight loss,[121-123] and radiologic studies most commonly show solitary or multiple discrete nodules.[125,126] Findings of serum protein electrophoresis are positive in up to 30% of patients, and staging shows extrathoracic disease in one third of patients. The disease is almost entirely restricted to adults. Occasionally, the tumor starts in the thymus.[127]

Following the paradigm of benign MALT, MaZL is composed of cells that morphologically and phenotypically resemble the mature B cells that form the outer rim of the malpighian corpuscles of the spleen and their counterpart in the organized lymphoid tissue of Peyer patches in the terminal ileum.[121,128-130] At low power, MaZL may have a nodular or diffuse pattern, and at the periphery, the lesion may extend along intact alveolar walls in discontinuous fashion (Fig. 15-13), occasionally with a low-power beading motif. Nodularity may be inconspicuous, but where it is present, it corresponds to residual benign germinal centers that have been infiltrated ("colonized") to a greater or lesser degree by tumor cells.[84] Much of the neoplastic proliferation is present between the nodules and is composed of a mixture of small, resting

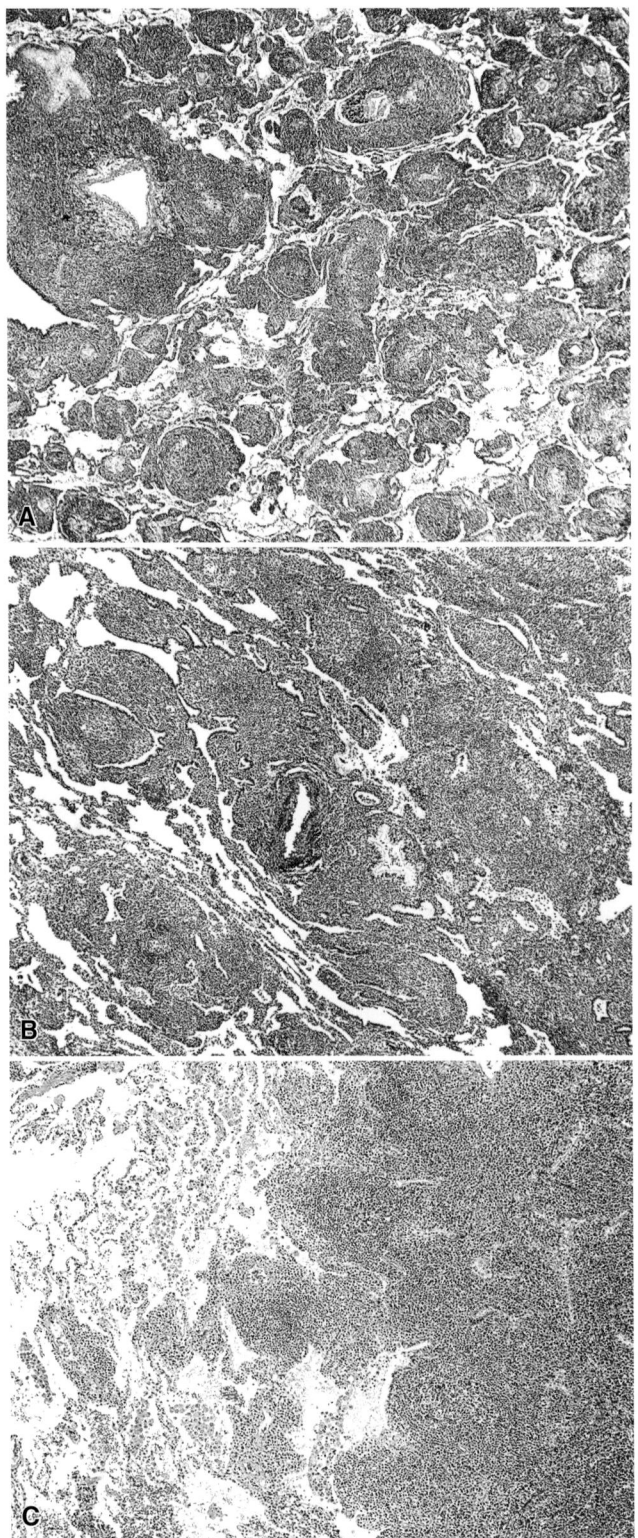

Figure 15-13. **A** and **B**, Marginal zone lymphoma may involve the lung in a reticulonodular pattern within the interstitium. **C**, These generally coalesce centrally in larger lesions to form a diffuse mass.

lymphocytes, monocytoid cells (oval or reniform nuclei, condensed chromatin, and moderate amounts of pale-staining cytoplasm), and plasmacytoid forms (Box 15-9 and Fig. 15-14).

Because of their ontogenic relationship to lymphocytes that home to mucosal surfaces, tumor cells in MaZL have a tendency to form

Box 15-9. Features of Low-Grade Mucosa-Associated Lymphoid Tissue Lymphoma

What Should Be Present
Mixture of centrocytoid, monocytoid, or plasmacytoid cells
Follicular colonization
Evidence of light-chain monotypia by flow, IHC, or both
Destructive lymphoepithelial lesions

What Might Be Present
Clustering of a few large cells
Striking plasmacytosis
Histiocytes filled with crystalline immunoglobulin
Histologic evidence of an underlying condition that predisposes to mucosa-
   associated lymphoid tissue lymphoma (e.g., Sjögren syndrome)

What Should Be Absent
Cyclin D1 expression
CD43 expression
Syncytia of large cells that fill a high-power field

What Should Be Communicated in the Report
If there is a striking degree of plasmacytosis, it may be beneficial to evaluate the
   patient for systemic evidence of an immunoproliferative disorder (SPEP, UPEP),
   which may lead to complications separate from the lymphoma
Although mucosa-associated lymphoid tissue lymphomas are commonly primary
   in the lung, the patient should be fully staged to assess for lymphoma involving
   multiple mucosal sites

IHC, immunohistochemistry; SPEP, serum protein electrophoresis; UPEP, urine protein
electrophoresis.

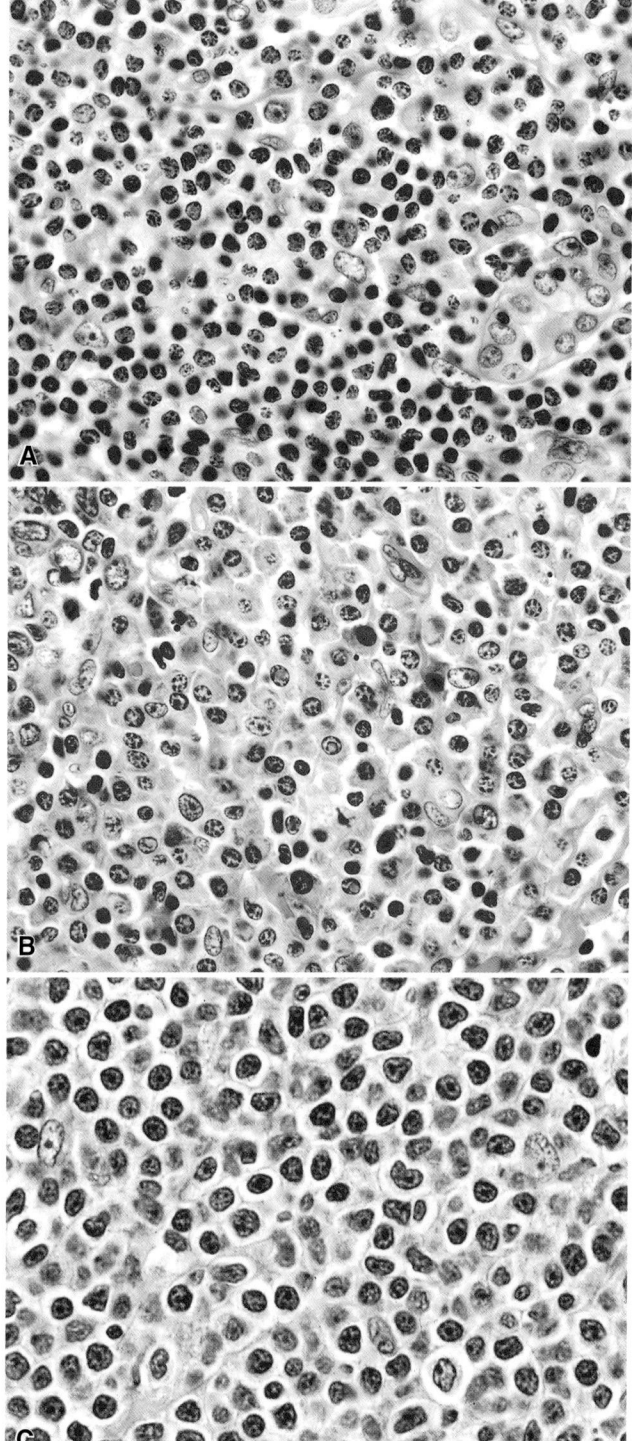

Figure 15-14. Although the histologic features of marginal zone lymphoma are often described as "heterogenous," in any given high-power field, a fairly uniform population of cells is present. In some areas, this is "centrocytoid" (**A**); in others it is plasmacytoid, with Dutcher bodies (**B**); and in yet others it is monocytoid (**C**). In all of these patterns, even the "centrocytoid" pattern, the heterogenous mix of centrocytes, centroblasts, dendritic cells, and tingible body macrophages of normal germinal centers (as seen in Fig. 15-2E) is not present.

destructive lymphoepithelial lesions (Fig. 15-15), a characteristic feature of this disease, although one that is not independently diagnostic of neoplasia in general or MALToma in particular.[68] In some cases, monocytoid morphologic features dominate, whereas in others, the cells more closely resemble centrocytes within germinal centers. Transbronchial biopsy should be approached cautiously because plasmacytoid differentiation may be so striking superficially that the differential diagnosis includes plasmacytoma[131] (Fig. 15-16). With fuller representation (e.g., on wedge biopsy), a concomitant lymphoid component is often identified, however, permitting accurate classification. Occasional cases may have a few cells with intracytoplasmic crystalline immunoglobulin[132-135] or amyloid deposits.[136-140]

The lesional cells of MaZL are CD19+ and CD20+ and do not coexpress CD5, CD10, or CD23, Tdt, cyclin D1, or *bcl6*. In small biopsy specimens, a cytokeratin stain may help to identify lymphoepithelial lesions, and the combination of CD21, *bcl2*, and *bcl6* stains highlights germinal centers colonized and overrun by tumor cells[68,121,130] that are *bcl2+, bcl6–* and have a disrupted network of follicular dendritic cells[84] (Fig. 15-17). Bcl10 protein expression has been shown to correlate with the presence of the t(11;18)(API2/MALT1) translocation, and a positive result by paraffin section immunohistochemistry can be a helpful adjunct to classification.[124]

Although MaZL resembles *NLH*, the latter has a polymorphous population of lymphocytes and histiocytes in the interfollicular areas. In addition, it contains benign, "uncolonized" germinal centers with a CD20+, *bcl2–, bcl6+* phenotype and has interfollicular areas rich in T cells, not B cells[68] (see Box 15-3 and Table 15-3). Importantly, there is no evidence of a monotypic population of B cells on flow cytometry, and NLH is nonclonal on PCR-based molecular studies. Small biopsy specimens of MaZL may have some degree of morphologic overlap with *LIP*, but MaZL tends to overrun normal structures and the process does not have the predominant interstitial localization associated with LIP. Distinction from other lymphomas rests on the findings of immunophenotyping studies[5] (see Boxes 15-2 and 15-3 and Table 15-3), although colonization of the germinal centers and heterogeneity of the lesional infiltrate are two features that favor MaZL. Distinction from *follicular lymphoma with florid*

marginal zone differentiation[141] requires careful attention to immunohistochemical assessment for follicular colonization and may also require FISH for the t(14;18) and t(11;18) translocations. It is important to be attentive to the possibility that the biopsy specimen contains more than one lymphoma, because "collisions" occur.[142]

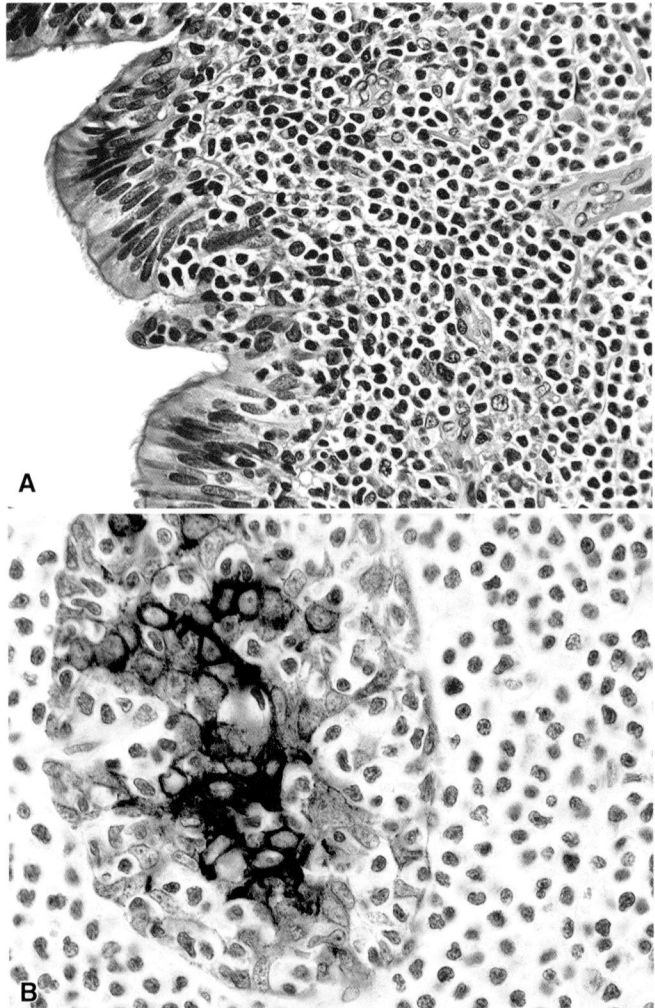

Figure 15-15. Although they are not diagnostic of marginal zone lymphoma, destructive lymphoepithelial lesions are often present and appear as aggregations of 5 to 10 small lymphocytes with sufficient cytoplasm that the nuclei stand apart (**A**). These can be highlighted with cytokeratin stain (**B**).

Diffuse Large B Cell Lymphoma, Variants, and Subtypes

Large cell lymphoma of B cell type (B-LCL) is the second most common type of primary pulmonary lymphoma[5,143,144] and most commonly affects older adults in the sixth and seventh decades. Patients present with cough or dyspnea; hemoptysis is rare. Most lesions are solitary, solid, and off-white, and have a discrete border with adjacent normal lung parenchyma. A subset of B-LCL arises in patients with a preexisting or concurrent low-grade lymphoma, such as MaZL, small lymphocytic lymphoma, or follicular lymphoma. Rapidly proliferating tumors may have central cavitation on computed tomography, as a result of tumoral necrosis.

The neoplastic nature of B-LCL is readily evident from the dominant population of large cells as well as the destructive manner in which it obliterates the lung parenchyma. The lesional cells are large (20–30 microns) and form confluent, discohesive sheets of cells. Cytologic features vary from case to case, although usually the tumor cells have coarse chromatin, distinct nucleoli, and abundant cytoplasm (Fig. 15-18). Essentially all are CD19+, CD20+, and CD79a, and those with a follicle center cell origin also express CD10 and *bcl6*.[5]

Differential diagnostic considerations can include primary or metastatic carcinoma, metastatic melanoma, and other epithelioid malignancies (especially large cell neuroendocrine carcinoma), all

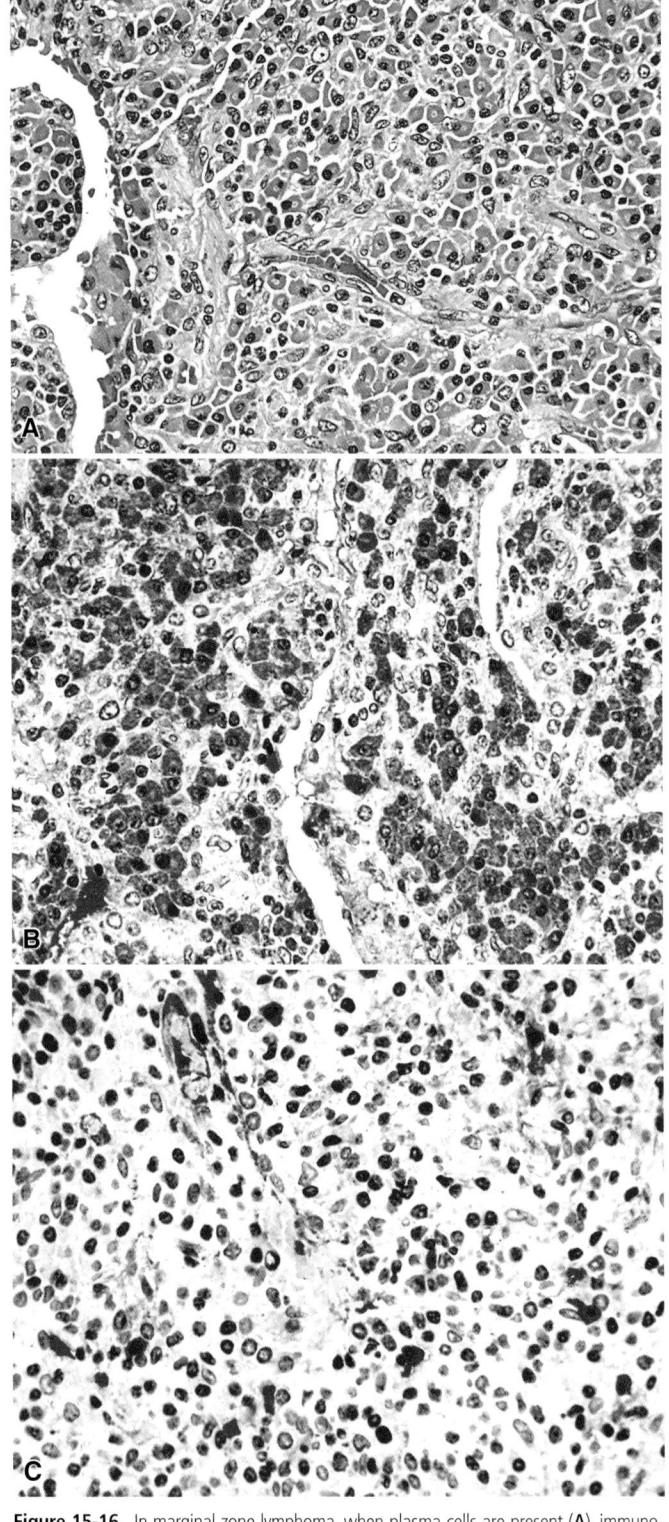

Figure 15-16. In marginal zone lymphoma, when plasma cells are present (**A**), immunohistochemical studies for kappa and lambda light chains should be performed. **B** and **C**, In this case, the kappa-to-lambda ratio is greater than 10:1, a compelling documentation of the clonality of the proliferation.

resolvable on phenotypic analysis. Some cases of B-LCL may have a high content of reactive T cells or histiocytes ("T cell–rich large B cell lymphoma" [TcRBCL])[145] (Fig. 15-19) and may be impossible to distinguish from metastatic lymphoepithelioma-type nasopharyngeal carcinoma or even Hodgkin lymphoma without immunohistochemical studies.

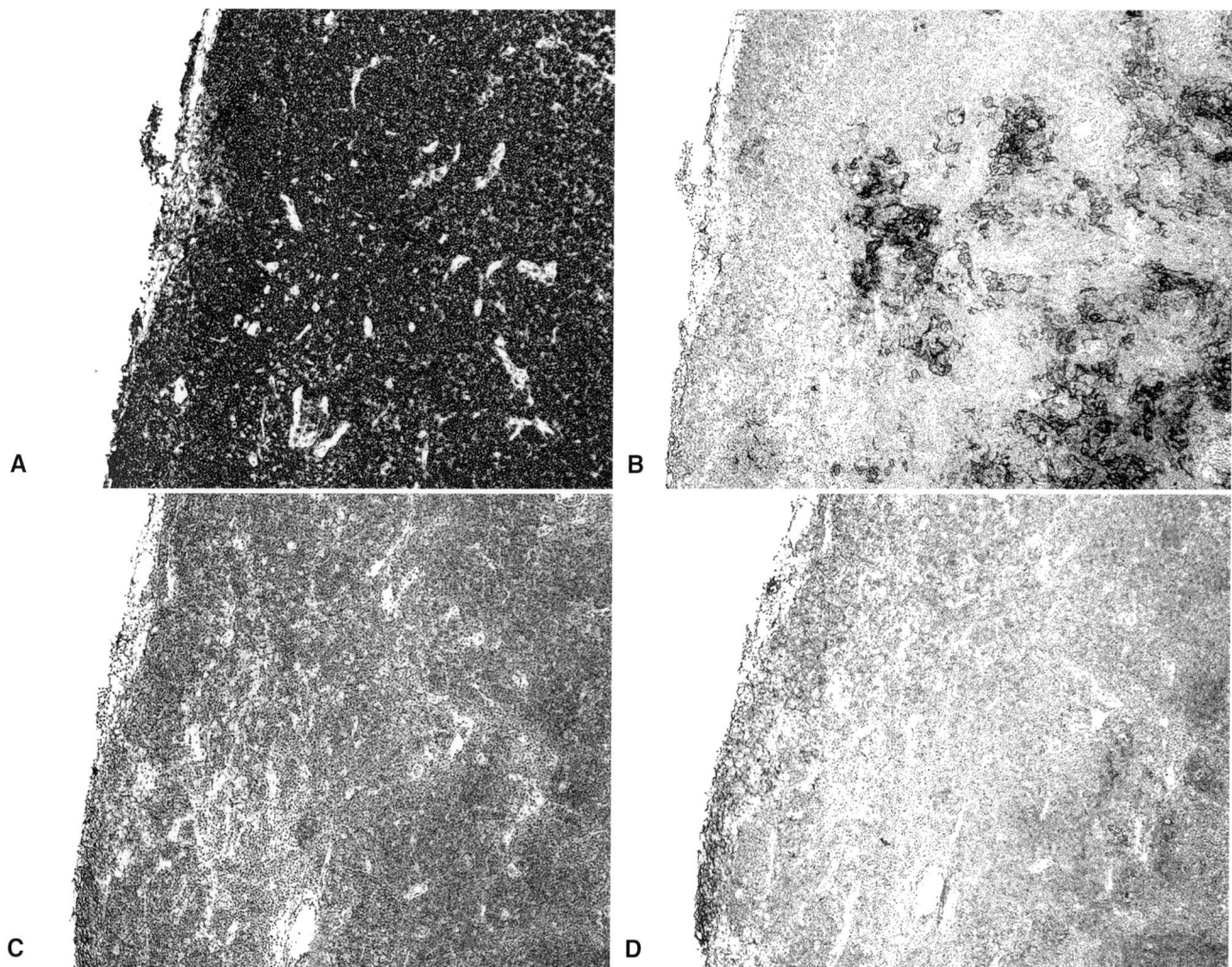

Figure 15-17. Flow cytometry in marginal zone lymphoma shows the nonspecific CD5–, CD10–, CD23– profile. The finding of follicular colonization on immunohistochemical studies helps in classification. The process is composed of CD20+ B cells (**A**) that are present both within and between CD21+ dendritic cell aggregates (**B**). The latter have ragged and "moth-eaten" borders, and there is no evidence of retained bcl2–, bcl6+ benign centrocytes within (**C** representing bcl2 stain and **D** representing bcl6 stain).

Several histologic and immunophenotypic variants bear mentioning because of specific differential considerations. Although most have been reported first in lymph nodes, there is no reason why the same tumor could not involve the lung. The *immunoblastic variant* of B-LCL has vesicular chromatin, thick nuclear membrane, a prominent and centrally placed eosinophilic nucleolus, and abundant amphophilic cytoplasm. A morphologic variant may confer a worse prognosis[5] (Fig. 15-20) and may mimic anaplastic myeloma, plasmablastic lymphoma,[146] carcinoma, and melanoma as well as some dendritic cell tumors. A panel including CD138, cytoplasmic immunoglobulin (cIg), pancytokeratin, CD45, MART1, S-100, and CD21 may be helpful in such cases. The presence of *CD5+ B-cell diffuse large cell lymphoma (B-DLCL)*[147] is rare but recognized, and where this phenotype occurs, cyclin D1 staining and well-prepared slides of well-fixed tissue can be helpful in excluding mantle cell lymphoma. *ALK+ B-DLCL,* although rare, is now well characterized[3] (Fig. 15-21), and like the T cell counterpart, may mimic carcinoma, histiocytic malignancy, and melanoma. These rare variants are usually negative for CD20, CD30 (unlike their T cell counterpart!), CD45, and PAX5, and positive for epithelial membrane antigen. Negative pancytokeratin results help to exclude carcinoma, and positive results for CD138, MUM1, cytoplasmic ALK1, and cytoplasmic immunoglobulin light chains point toward the correct diagnosis. FISH or PCR for the t(2;17)(ALK/clathrin) translocation is confirmatory.

In some cases, a substantial reactive population of T cells or histiocytes may disperse the lesional large B cells such that flow cytometry and molecular studies do not identify a B cell clone. *T cell/histiocyte-rich large B cell lymphoma* is the prototype in this category,[145] and consideration can be given to lymphoepithelioma, metastatic nasopharyngeal carcinoma, and Hodgkin lymphoma of either the classic or the nodular lymphocyte-predominance type. Pancytokeratin, CD30, CD21, CD57, PAX5, and Oct2 can be used to identify such cases. Believed to reflect clonal escape of virally infected cells in older patients with age-related deterioration of immunity, *EBV+ DLCL of the elderly*[148,149] also includes a mix of small and large cells. A cue to this diagnosis is the finding of a polymorphous spectrum of large immunoblasts, Reed-Sternberg (RS)-like cells, and medium-sized transitional lymphoplasmacytoid forms, all diluted by small, reactive lymphocytes in a patient older than 70 years. CD30 findings may be positive, making the exclusion of classic Hodgkin lymphoma difficult, although EBER/EBV-ISH positivity and strong expression of CD20 or CD79a in the large cells help to secure the diagnosis. *Lymphomatoid granulomatosis* is another special subtype of EBV-related B-LCL, described later.

There are also several subtypes of B-DLCL with distinctive clinical aspects that should be addressed. An *intravascular ("angiotrophic") variant* of B-LCL[150] presents without adenopathy, organomegaly, or mass-forming lesions in solid organs, and may only be recognized

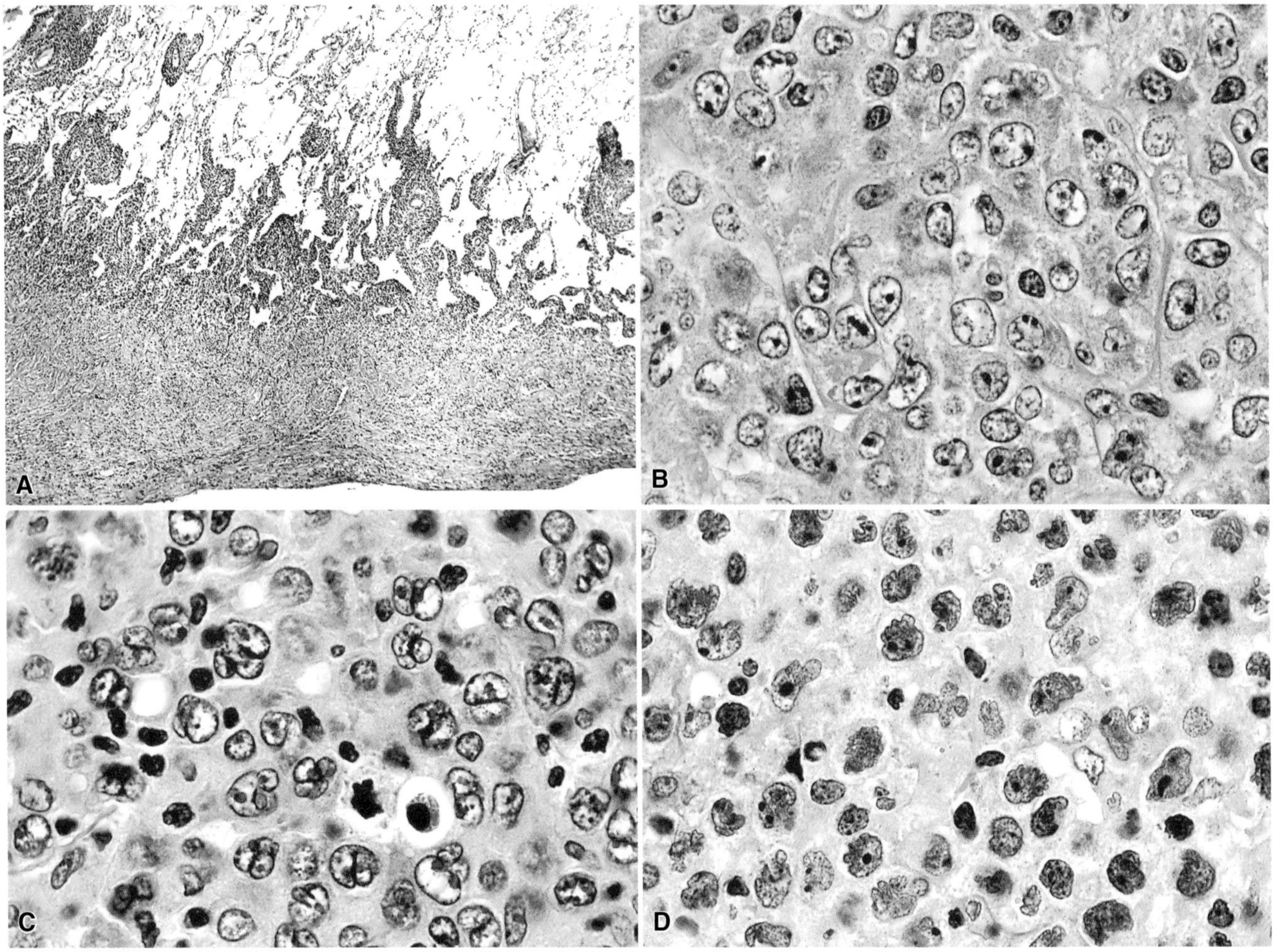

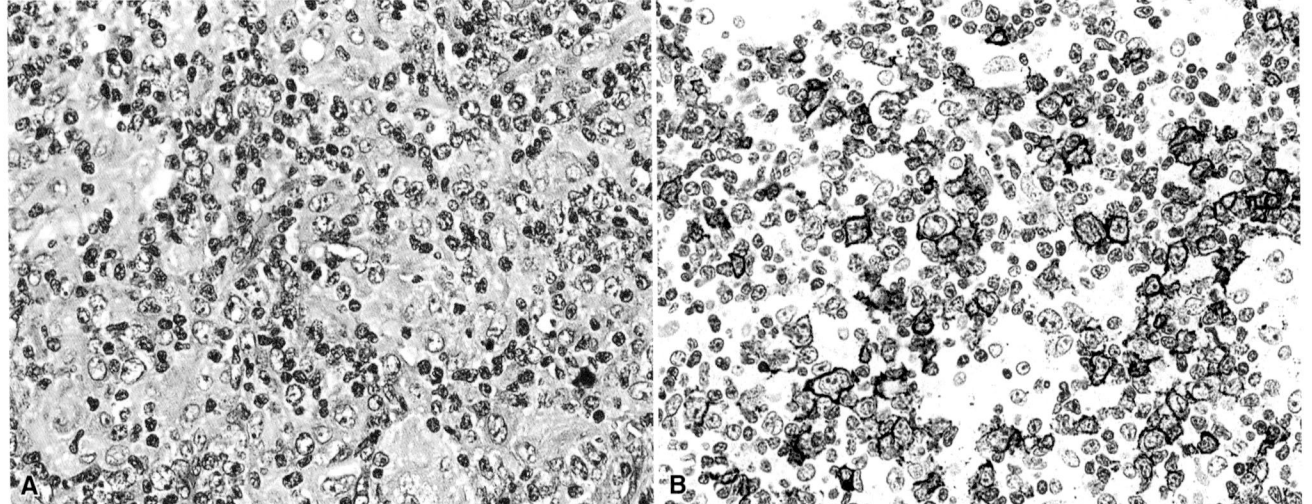

Figure 15-18. Although large B cell lymphoma most often involves the lung in a mass-forming nodular manner, on occasion, it may also have a selectively pleural distribution (**A**). As in the lymph nodes, pulmonary diffuse large B cell lymphomas may have centroblastic (**B**), polylobated (**C**), or large cleaved (**D**) histologic features.

Figure 15-19. T cell–rich large B cell lymphoma forms masses rich in histiocytes and relatively poor in neoplastic cells. **A,** Well-prepared sections are necessary to avoid misinterpreting such lesions as granulomas. **B,** CD20 immunostaining shows large lymphoma cells.

when the patient undergoes biopsy of sites without clinical evidence of lymphomatous involvement, including the lung (Figs. 15-22 and 15-23). The vessels are filled with aggregations of large cells with coarse chromatin and a high nucleus-to-cytoplasm ratio, clearly different from resting lymphocytes or monocytes. *Although it may have a prominent*

pulmonary component, the disease is never restricted to the lung and should be regarded as an aggressive, systemic lymphoma from the outset.

Primary thymic/mediastinal large B cell lymphoma usually presents with mass-related symptoms (e.g., superior vena cava syndrome) in young patients, and when it disseminates, it tends to involve extranodal

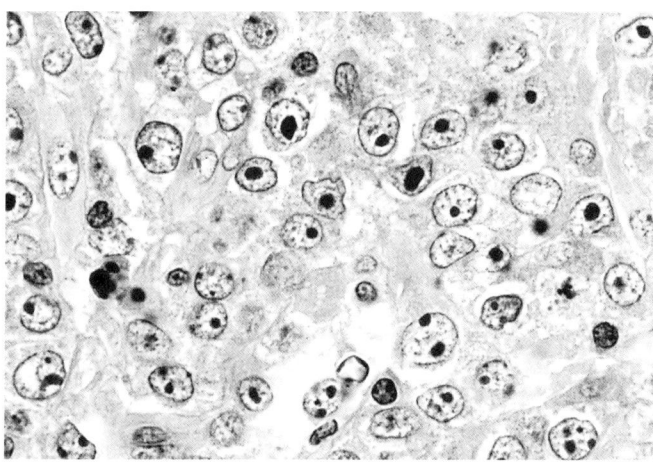

Figure 15-20. The immunoblastic variant of large B cell lymphoma mimics both carcinoma and melanoma.

sites (kidney, adrenal, liver) as much as or more than the development of generalized adenopathy with marrow involvement. The tumor can closely mimic classic Hodgkin lymphoma.[150,151] Because of tumor-related fibrosis (Fig. 15-24), the inherent fragility of cells, and the known lack of surface immunoglobulin display in these tumor cells, flow cytometry findings are often negative. Because many patients with primary

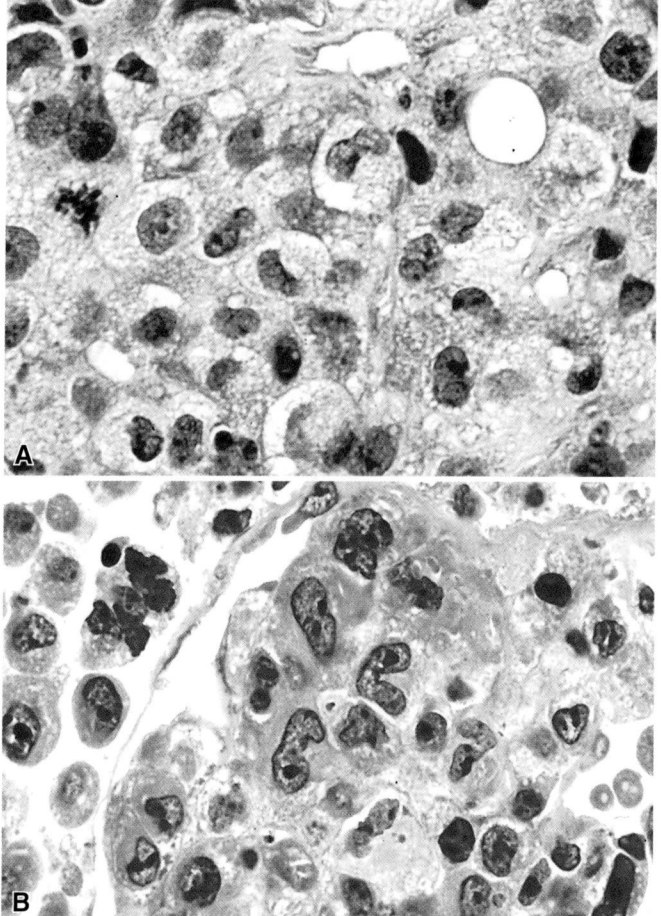

Figure 15-21. Anaplastic large B cell lymphoma is rare and can be distinguished from conventional diffuse large B cell lymphoma by the presence of hallmark cells with eccentrically placed horseshoe-shaped nuclei (**A** and **B**) and ALK expression in large CD20+ B cells.

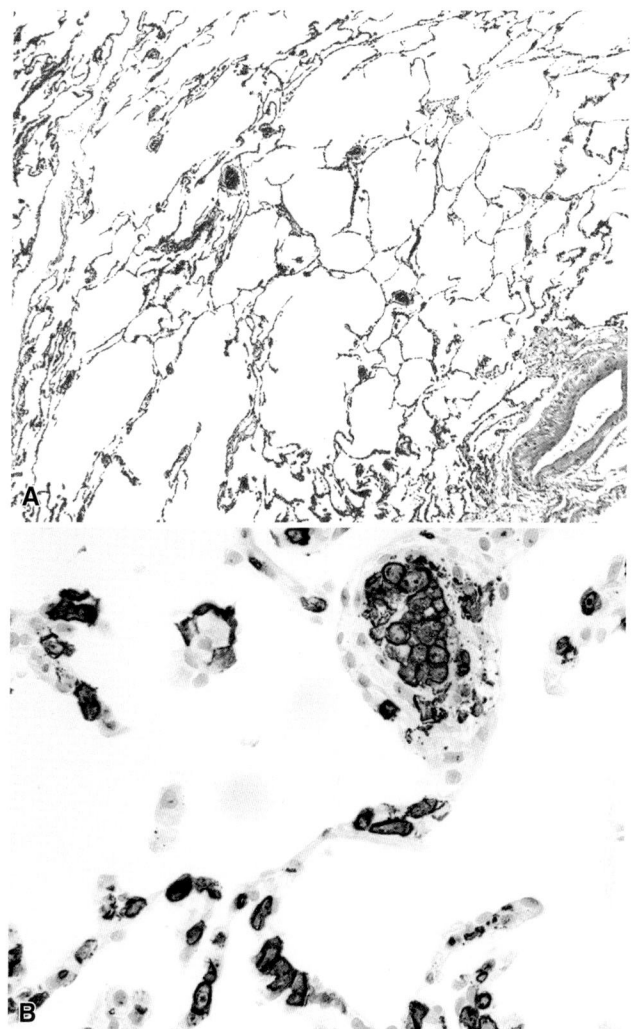

Figure 15-22. Intravascular lymphoma is an aggressive systemic large B cell lymphoma that may present with a confusing array of signs and symptoms, including shortness of breath. The radiologic findings may be normal or may show accentuated interstitial markings. **A,** Histologically, at low power, the lung may appear entirely normal. **B,** At high power, and especially on immunohistochemical staining, numerous CD20+ large B cells are seen plugging the vasculature.

thymic/mediastinal large B cell lymphoma express CD30, exclusion of classic Hodgkin lymphoma relies on assessment of the expression of Oct2, PAX5, CD20, CD79a, and CD23, and on identifying the packeting of tumor cells within long, thin slips of collagenous fibrosis (Fig. 15-25). Treatment for DLCL and treatment for classic Hodgkin lymphoma are fundamentally different, so when there is any degree of ambiguity, gene rearrangements can be pursued. This adjunctive study may not allow for complete clarity in all cases, leaving some in a "gray zone" that the WHO Classification refers to as *"B cell lymphoma unclassifiable with features intermediate between B-DLCL and classic Hodgkin lymphoma."*[5]

Lymphomatoid Granulomatosis

Although the vast majority of the cellularity of lymphomatoid granulomatosis (LyG, also known as "angiocentric immunoproliferative lesions," "polymorphic reticulosis," or "midline lethal granuloma") is of T lineage, studies have shown that the *neoplastic* cells in this process are a clonal population of EBV-infected B cells.[152–154] Consequently, LyG belongs in the category of B lineage lymphoproliferative disorders. It affects primarily

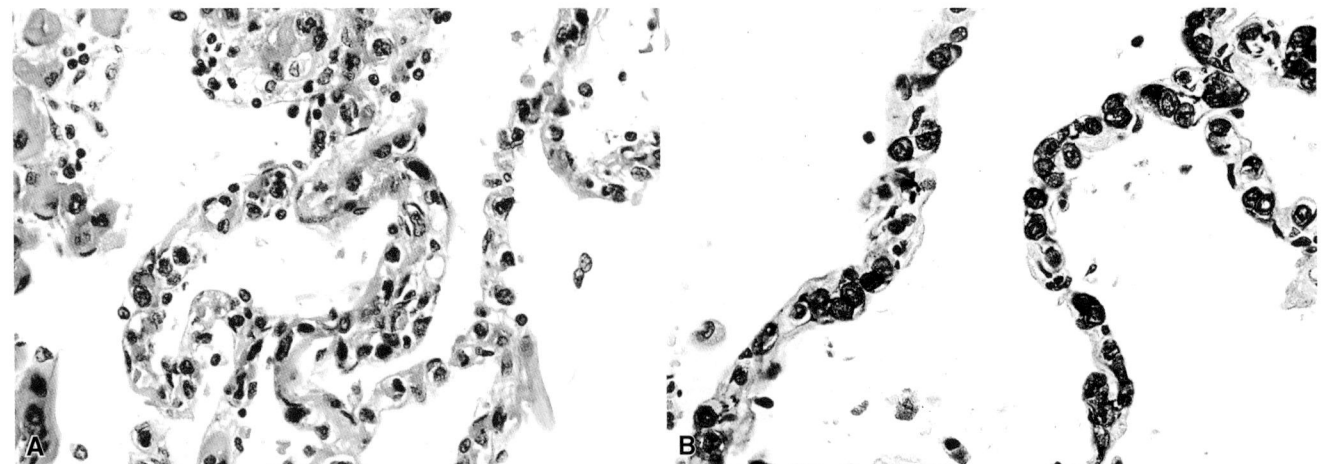

Figure 15-23. Some cases of intravascular lymphoma expand the interstitium, and although the findings of hematoxylin and eosin staining may be less than compelling (**A**), immunostaining for CD20 shows the neoplastic cells (**B**).

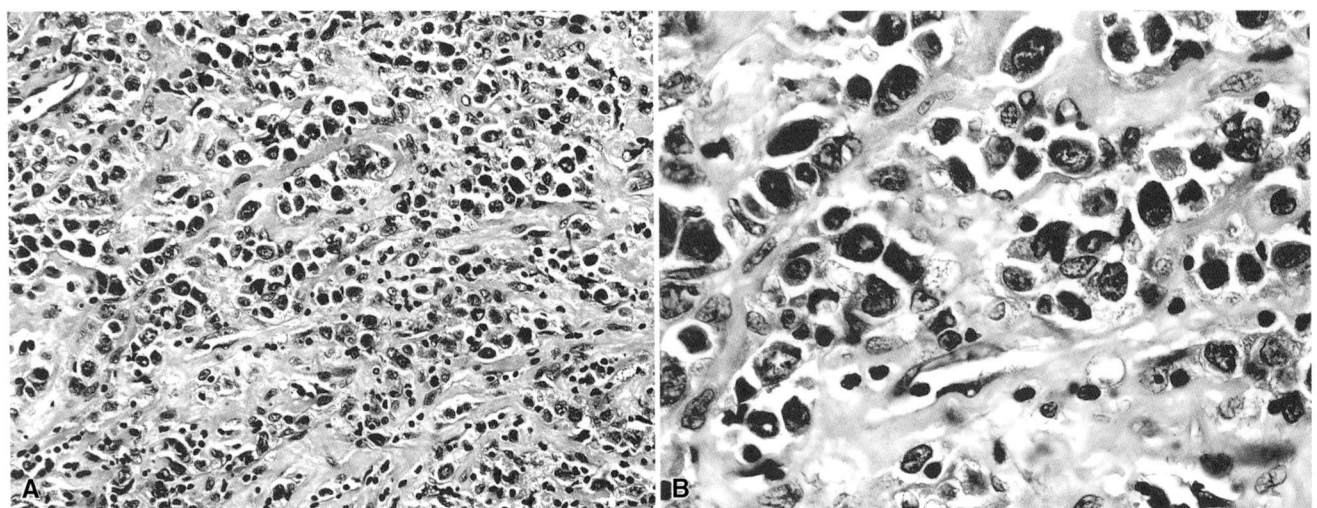

Figure 15-24. A, In primary mediastinal large B cell lymphoma, the lymphoma cells are enmeshed within slips of collagenous fibrosis. **B,** The lesional cells are large, with coarse chromatin and scant cytoplasm.

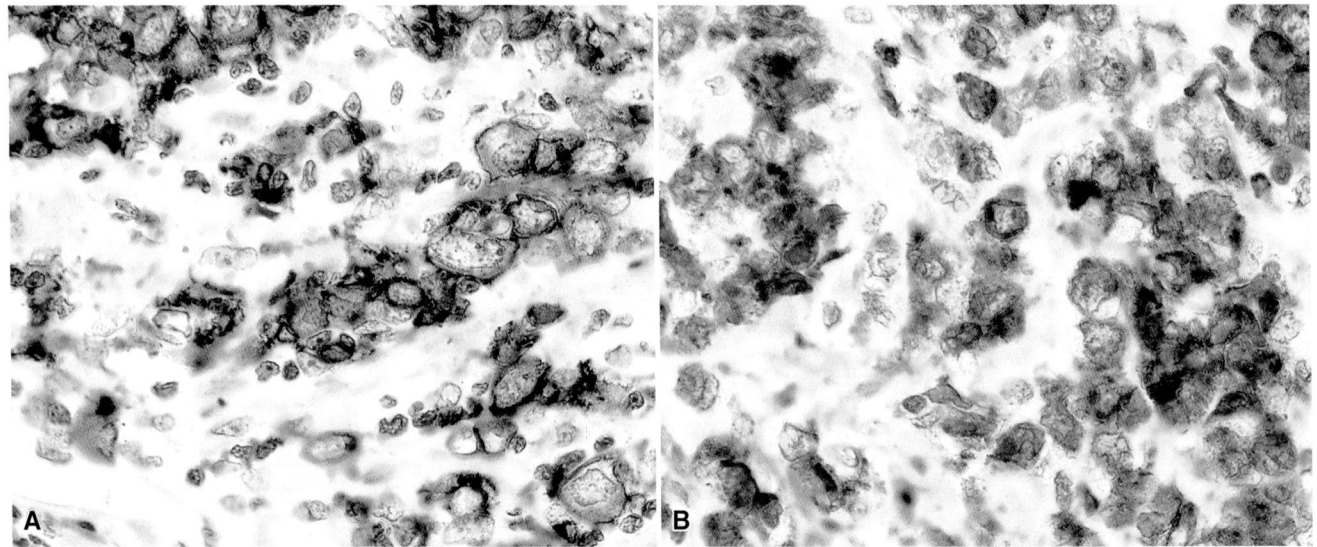

Figure 15-25. Because of the fibrosis and delicate nature of lymphoma cells, flow cytometry may yield false negative results in primary mediastinal large B cell lymphoma. Fortunately, the necessary stains for diagnosis can be performed on paraffin sections. These include positive results for both CD20 (**A**) and CD23 (**B**).

adults, and many cases arise in the setting of immunodeficiency.[155] Most patients have a prodromal phase of fever and nonspecific symptoms that may relate to pulmonary or sinonasal disease (cough, epistaxis). Skin, subcutaneous tissues, and the central nervous system may also be involved,[156] yielding nonpulmonic signs and symptoms that may suggest the correct diagnosis. Radiologic studies usually show multiple opacities and nodules, with or without cavitation,[157] and mediastinal adenopathy is rare. In resection specimens, the tumoral masses are centrally located within the lung and have an homogenous off-white appearance on cut section.

Transbronchial and transthoracic biopsy specimens usually yield insufficient diagnostic material to secure the diagnosis, and a wedge biopsy is usually required. Extensive necrosis, angio-occlusion, and vascular damage (Box 15-10 and Fig. 15-26) in the context of a mixed lymphohistiocytic infiltrate are the histologic hallmarks of LyG.[152,156] The lymphoid component includes small cytotoxic T lymphocytes,[158] intermediate-size activated forms, and large neoplastic B cells that closely resemble centroblasts or immunoblasts. The large lesional B cells are diffusely dispersed and have coarse chromatin, distinct or prominent nucleoli, and moderate amounts of cytoplasm. The process is both angiocentric (accumulations of viable cells around the arterioles and venules) and angiodestructive (mural invasion, lumenal occlusions, and disruption of vessel walls), and the endothelial cells are plump and activated. Necrosis may be present and is usually focal. Diagnostic RS cells are not present, although some cells may have features reminiscent of mononuclear variants.

Three categories, or "grades" have been described according to the density of large lesional B cells. At the low end of the spectrum, in *grade I LyG*, the proliferation is polymorphous and is composed of cytologically bland small lymphocytes, plasma cells, histiocytes, and very rare large lesional cells that may be evident only on CD20 stains (Fig. 15-27) and EBER-ISH. Koss[119] proposed objective boundaries of fewer than five EBV+ cells per high-power field for grade I LyG, although the WHO Classification of hematologic malignancies does not include this recommendation.

Greater numbers of large lesional cells (in the range of 5–20 cells) and more abundant levels of necrosis (Fig. 15-28) are the primary

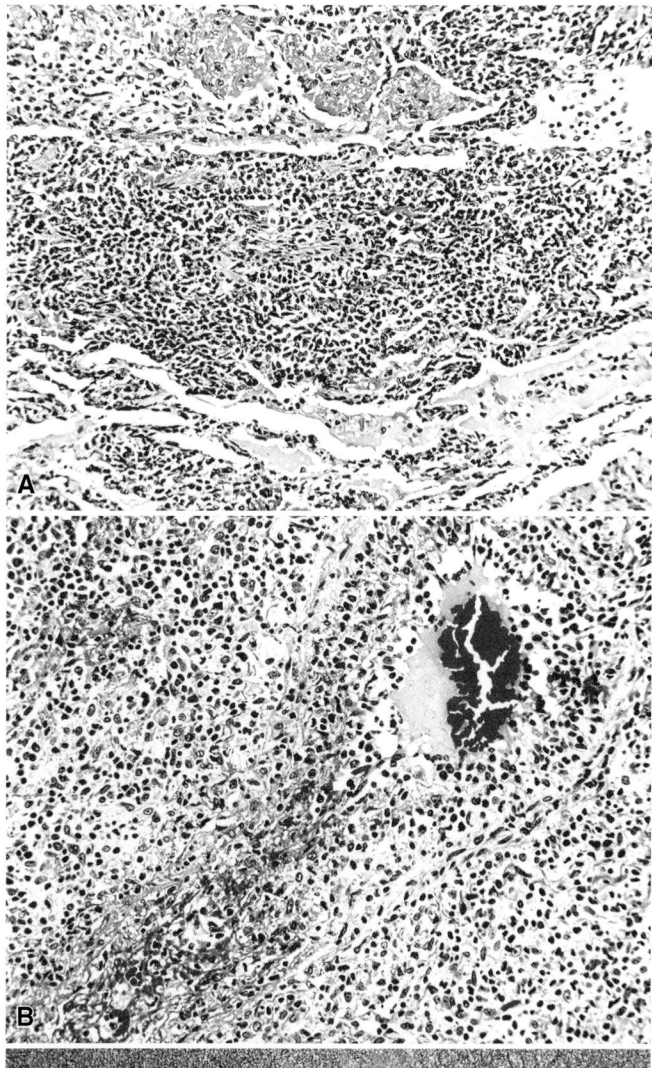

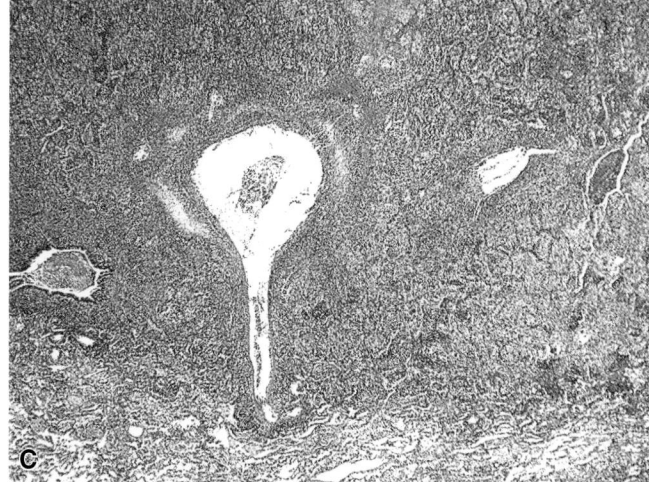

Figure 15-26. A, The lymphoid infiltrate in lymphomatoid granulomatosis engulfs and infiltrates small- and medium-caliber vessel walls. **B,** The media and intima are both expanded by small lymphocytes, with relatively few large neoplastic cells apparent in low-grade lesions. **C,** As the process progresses, it becomes mass-like.

Box 15-10. Features of Lymphomatoid Granulomatosis

What Should Be Present
Predominant population of small resting and activated lymphocytes
At least rare CD20+, EBV+ large cells
Necrosis
Vascular damage mediated by lymphocytes

What Might Be Present
Clustering or syncytia of large lesional cells
CD30 expression in large cells

What Should Be Absent
Antineutrophil cytoplasmic antibody positivity
Sinonasal disease
Diagnostic Reed-Sternberg cells
CD15 expression in large cells
Abundant CD56+ natural killer cells
Well-formed granulomas
A significant number of eosinophils or neutrophils in the background infiltrate

What Should Be Communicated in the Report
Although low-grade lymphomatoid granulomatosis may pursue a more indolent course, higher-grade lymphomatoid granulomatosis has the potential to behave aggressively
If the patient has multiple sites of disease, low-grade histologic features at one site do not exclude the possibility of higher-grade disease at another site
The patient should be monitored for the development of central nervous system disease

findings that distinguish *grade II LyG* from grade I LyG, although the large centroblastic/immunoblastic cells remain widely dispersed and may be difficult to find on routine stains. According to Koss's[119] proposal, EBV+ B cells are present at a density of 5 to 20 per high-power field, on average. *Grade III LyG* has all of the hallmark features of a high-grade

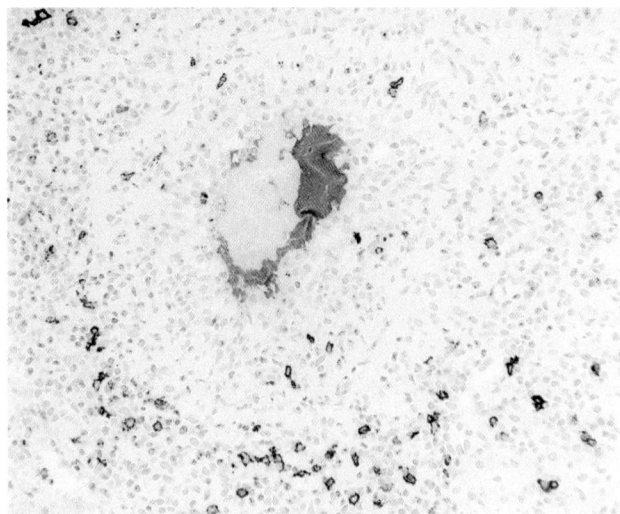

Figure 15-27. CD20+ neoplastic large B cells are more abundant outside of vessel walls than within the walls. In this case, overall, there were sufficient numbers of large cells to warrant the diagnosis of grade II/III disease.

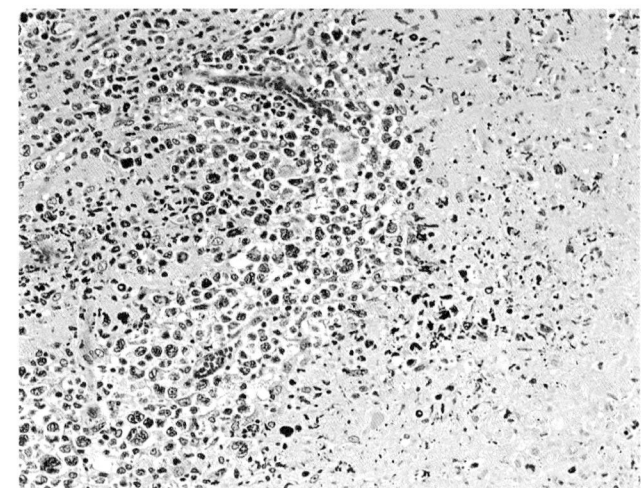

Figure 15-29. Grade III lymphomatoid granulomatosis has both necrosis and an abundance of large cells that are evident even on routine stains.

lymphoma—high content of mitotically active large atypical cells and necrosis (Fig. 15-29), often in sheets and syncitia—although the small lymphoid component persists. When the angiocentric component takes on a monomorphic quality and moderate or marked atypia is noted in the small lymphocytes, the process is best classified as grade III.[70,93,94]

The majority of the small lymphoid component is composed of CD2+, CD3+, and CD4+ T helper cells, with lesser numbers of CD8+ T killer cells and CD16/CD56+ natural killer cells. CD79a and CD20 staining is present in the large-cell component only, and it helps to identify lesional cells that may not be readily evident on hematoxylin and eosin stains. Latent membrane expression and EBERs are present in the lesional large B cells but not the T cells of LyG (Fig. 15-30).[157–159] CD30 may be expressed, and in difficult cases, CD15, PAX5, Oct2 and other markers may be helpful in excluding classic Hodgkin lymphoma. Because lung involvement by classic Hodgkin lymphoma is exceptionally rare without mediastinal involvement, radiologic correlation may also be helpful.

Differential considerations include a range of reactive processes, including poorly confined fungal or bacterial *infection,* necrotizing viral infections such as varicella zoster or herpes infection in immunosuppressed patients, and systemic vasculitic processes such as polyarteritis nodosa and Wegener granulomatosis. *Wegener granulomatosis* shows a degree of morphologic overlap with LyG, but it lacks the large CD20+ B cells and has neutrophil-rich necrosis with histiocyte-rich granuloma-like formations and multinucleated giant cells. Other inflammatory conditions that resemble LyG include *bronchocentric granulomatosis,* although the latter lacks the vasocentric and lymphocyte-rich, neutrophil/eosinophil-poor qualities that typify all grades of LyG. Because of the bimorphic population of large cells set within a polymorphous background lymphoid population, *classic Hodgkin lymphoma* and *T cell/histiocyte-rich large B cell lymphoma* should also be considered in the differential diagnosis with LyG. TcRBCL rarely has necrosis and does not exhibit angiocentricity with angiodestruction. The lung is an unusual site for primary presentation of Hodgkin disease, and radiologic correlation, reactivity for CD15 and CD30 in the large cell population, and lack of Oct2 expression are helpful cues to the correct diagnosis.

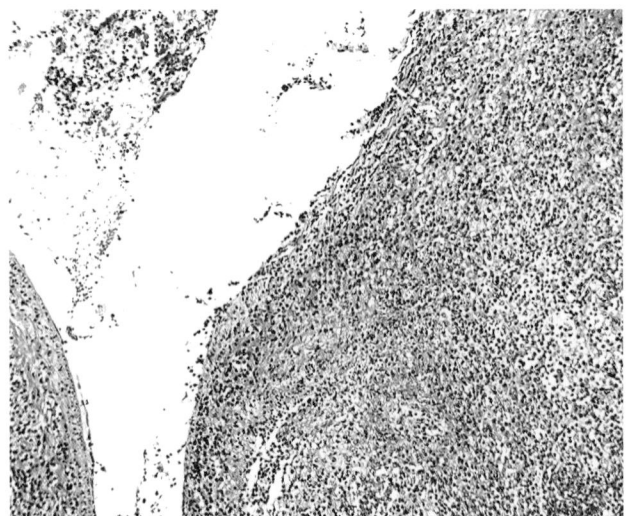

Figure 15-28. Even at the point at which lymphomatoid granulomatosis is mass-forming, there are no "granulomatous" foci.

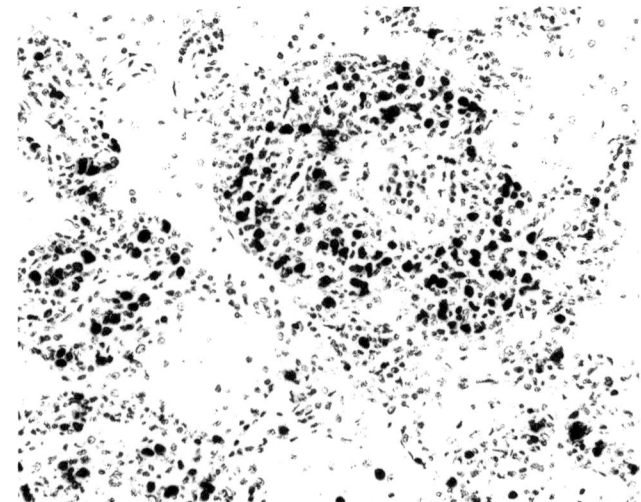

Figure 15-30. The lesional large cells of lymphomatoid granulomatosis are positive for Epstein-Barr virus, best evaluated by in situ hybridization for Epstein-Barr-encoded ribonucleotides.

In contrast to LyG, *peripheral T cell lymphoma* lacks the atypical large CD20+ cells and instead has significant cytologic atypia of small, intermediate, and large cells; patches of cells with small nuclei and abundant pale-staining cytoplasm; tissue eosinophilia; aberrant loss of a stage-specific pan T cell marker (CD2, CD3, CD5, or CD7) (Box 15-11; see also Box 15-2); and usually clonal T cell gene rearrangements by PCR analysis. If there is sinonasal disease, *T/natural killer (NK) cell lymphomas of the "nasal type"* enter into the differential diagnosis. Because these T/NK lymphomas can be angiocentric and angiodestructive as well as EBV+, the presence of CD20+ lesional large cells is the distinguishing feature. An abundance of CD56+ natural killer cells and an absence of CD20+ large cells would favor natural killer cell lymphomas of the non-nasal type.

Hodgkin Lymphoma

Hodgkin lymphoma is a tumor of lymphoid lineage[160,161] in which the neoplastic cells are in the vast numeric minority. The 2008 edition of the WHO Classification of hematologic malignancy includes two diagnostic categories—classic Hodgkin disease and lymphocyte-predominance Hodgkin lymphoma (LPHL). The distinction is based on the phenotype of the lesional cells as well as the nature of the background infiltrate. Most patients with pulmonary Hodgkin lymphoma present with concomitant node-based or mediastinal disease, and the diagnosis is established by lymph node biopsy. In rare cases, however, clinical, pathologic, and radiologic staging shows only pulmonary involvement, invariably mass-forming rather than interstitial (Box 15-12 and Fig. 15-31).[161]

Distinguishing RS cells from mimics can be difficult, and when the cells are few in number, serial sections to find diagnostic forms may be necessary. The cell itself should be six- to eightfold larger than a resting lymphocyte, and the nucleus should be four- to fivefold larger than a small resting lymphocyte. In addition, it should have a thick nuclear membrane and a bilobed, multilobated, or wreath-shaped configuration. The nucleolus approaches or exceeds the size of the whole nucleus of resting lymphocytes and is often rimmed by a halo of pale nonstaining chromatin[162,163] (Fig. 15-32). Cytoplasm is abundant and may be homogenously eosinophilic or feathered and retracted (the latter being the "lacunar variant") (Fig. 15-33). RS-*like* cells may be seen in other clinical contexts, including primary mediastinal large B cell lymphoma, small lymphocytic lymphoma/chronic lymphocytic leukemia, and acute infectious mononucleosis, and so their presence cannot be the *only* criterion for diagnosis.

The milieu of Hodgkin lymphoma varies from area to area and from case to case, and in classic Hodgkin lymphoma, the background infiltrate ranges from a monotony of cytologically bland small T lymphocytes to a polymorphous mixture of lymphocytes, histiocytes, plasma cells, eosinophils, and neutrophils. When sclerosis is present, it consists of broad bands of collagenized fibrosis that encases cellular nodules and is evident grossly and microscopically (Fig. 15-34) rather that the delicate slips of collagen that encircle packets of cells in primary mediastinal large B cell lymphoma. In the lung, the mixed inflammatory milieu of Hodgkin lymphoma may overlap substantially with reactive conditions, such as hypersensitivity pneumonitis, collagen vascular disease, and infection. Apart from infection, however,

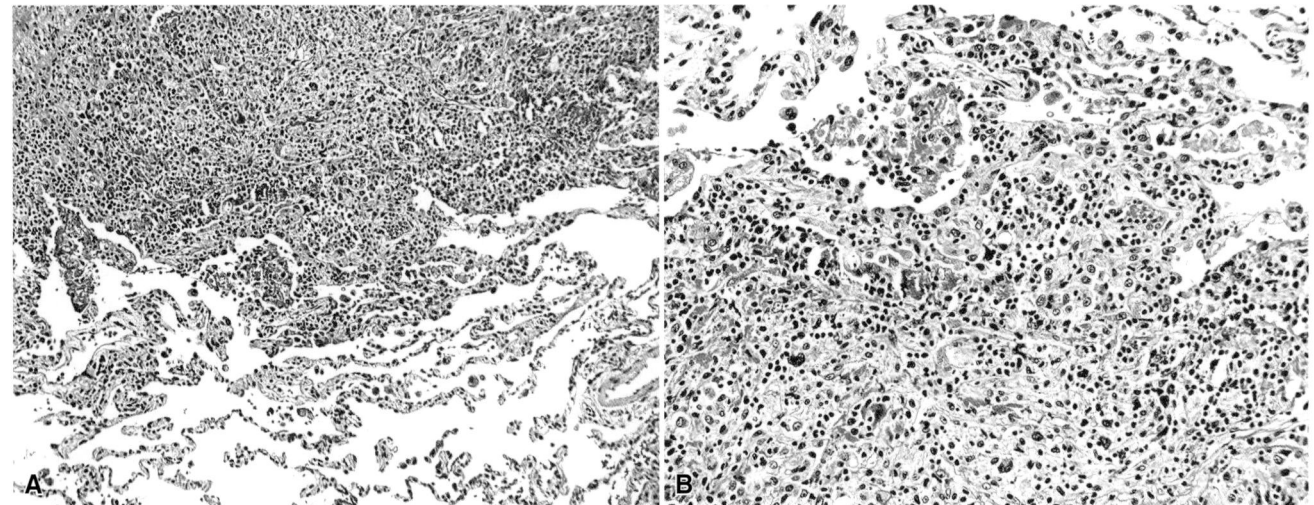

Figure 15-31. A, At low power, this example of pulmonary Hodgkin lymphoma has overlap with both marginal zone lymphoma and lymphomatoid granulomatosis. **B,** The suggestion of a bimorphic population of small and large cells (e.g., the large cell just to the right of the center) may be the only cue to the correct diagnosis.

these conditions are not mass-forming, and none of them contain diagnostic RS cells.

Immunophenotypic staining of RS cells typically yields a CD30+, CD20–, LCA– Oct2–, BOB.1– phenotype (Fig. 15-35). CD15 expression is reported in 60% to 70% of cases, depending on the series, and so is not an essential finding to establish the diagnosis. Weak and granular CD20 reactivity may be present in some cases[162-165] (Table 15-4), as is weak nuclear staining for PAX5. CD79a expression, however, should be lacking. In the lung, differential diagnostic considerations for classic Hodgkin lymphoma with abundant sclerotic stroma include inflamed solitary fibrous tumors of the pleura, inflammatory myofibroblastic tumor, sclerosing mediastinitis, and infection. Without the sclerosis (particularly if the patient has a known cause of immunity), consideration should be given to senile EBV+ B-LCL of the elderly, LyG, and potentially reversible lymphoproliferative disorders arising in the setting of methotrexate therapy and transplantation.

The "nonclassic" or lymphocyte-*predominance* subtype of Hodgkin lymphoma, LPHL, has not been reported as a primary lung tumor or as primary localized mediastinal disease. This disease is often restricted to a single lymph node at presentation, and it pursues an indolent clinical course. In the vast majority of patients, survival is similar to that of age-matched individuals without LPHL.[128] Great care should be taken in evaluating lung biopsy specimens with features suggestive of LPHL: The phenotype of the lymphocytic-histiocytic ("L&H") RS cell variants in LPHL (CD15–, CD30–, CD20+, PAX5+, CD45+ Oct2+, BOB.1+; see Table 15-4) is identical to that seen in the more aggressive TcRBCL.[129,130,166,167] A large specimen is essential in resolving such a differential diagnosis because the B cell–rich milieu is as much a part of the disease definition as the nature of the lesional cells (Fig. 15-36).

Systemic Lymphoproliferative Disorders That May Secondarily Involve the Lung, Pleura, or Mediastinum

Secondary pulmonary lymphoma is a lymphoma diagnosed in the lung of a patient who either has a previous or concurrent nodal diagnosis of lymphoma or has evidence of systemic lymphoma during a relatively short interval after presentation. The diagnostic criteria for lymph node biopsies should be applied.[5,168]

In the United States, follicular lymphoma, systemic large B cell lymphoma, small lymphocytic lymphoma, and mantle cell lymphoma (Fig. 15-37) are the most common systemic lymphomas to secondarily

involve extranodal sites. Careful attention to cytologic detail, a broad immunohistochemistry panel, and above all, the clinical history, should permit complete diagnosis in most cases (Table 15-5). Although all of these lymphomas may remain localized for a period, all have a significant risk of disseminating to other sites. Cues to the diagnosis of *follicular lymphoma* include a mixture of small, intermediate, and large cleaved cells, including cells with irregular, cleaved, elongated "twisted towel," and gourd-shaped nuclei. *Mantle cell lymphoma*, by contrast, is composed of uniform small lymphocytes with condensed chromatin and a minimally irregular nuclear profile. Pink histiocytes are often evenly commingled. *Small lymphocytic lymphoma* is usually composed of small cells with round nuclei with a smooth nuclear contour. Some patients have a greater degree of nuclear contour irregularity ("atypical" chronic lymphocytic leukemia) that is similar to mantle cell lymphoma cytologically. However, the cue to the correct classification is a second cell population of paraimmunoblasts and immunoblasts, which often accumulate together in pale-staining areas ("proliferation centers").[169-171] *MaZL* (discussed in detail earlier) not infrequently involves the lung secondarily after presentation in other mucosal sites. As in *secondary B-LCL,* MaZL cannot be distinguished from a primary lung lymphoma on purely morphologic grounds and diagnosis requires correlation with clinical history and full radiologic staging. Immunohistochemical studies are central to the accurate diagnosis and classification of all of these conditions (see Table 15-5).

High-Grade Lymphomas

As challenging as the differential diagnosis of small lymphoid proliferations is, a subset of aggressive lymphomas is equally difficult to identify, and the diagnosis is usually far more clinically pressing. These are clinically high-grade lymphomas, and there are obvious frozen section and specimen triaging issues. A timely diagnosis requires excellent histologic material and adequate material for immunohistochemistry (flow cytometry seldom has sufficient viable cells for accurate results) and cytogenetic analysis.

The histologic features characteristic of *Burkitt lymphoma* include uniform, intermediate cell size; uniformly round or ovoid nuclei, with coarse chromatin and dispersed, often peripheral, small nucleoli; and a rim of amphophilic cytoplasm with crisp separation from the adjacent cells (sometimes called "squaring off" of cytoplasm).[172-174] The proliferation is uniform, with no commingled small cells (Fig. 15-38).

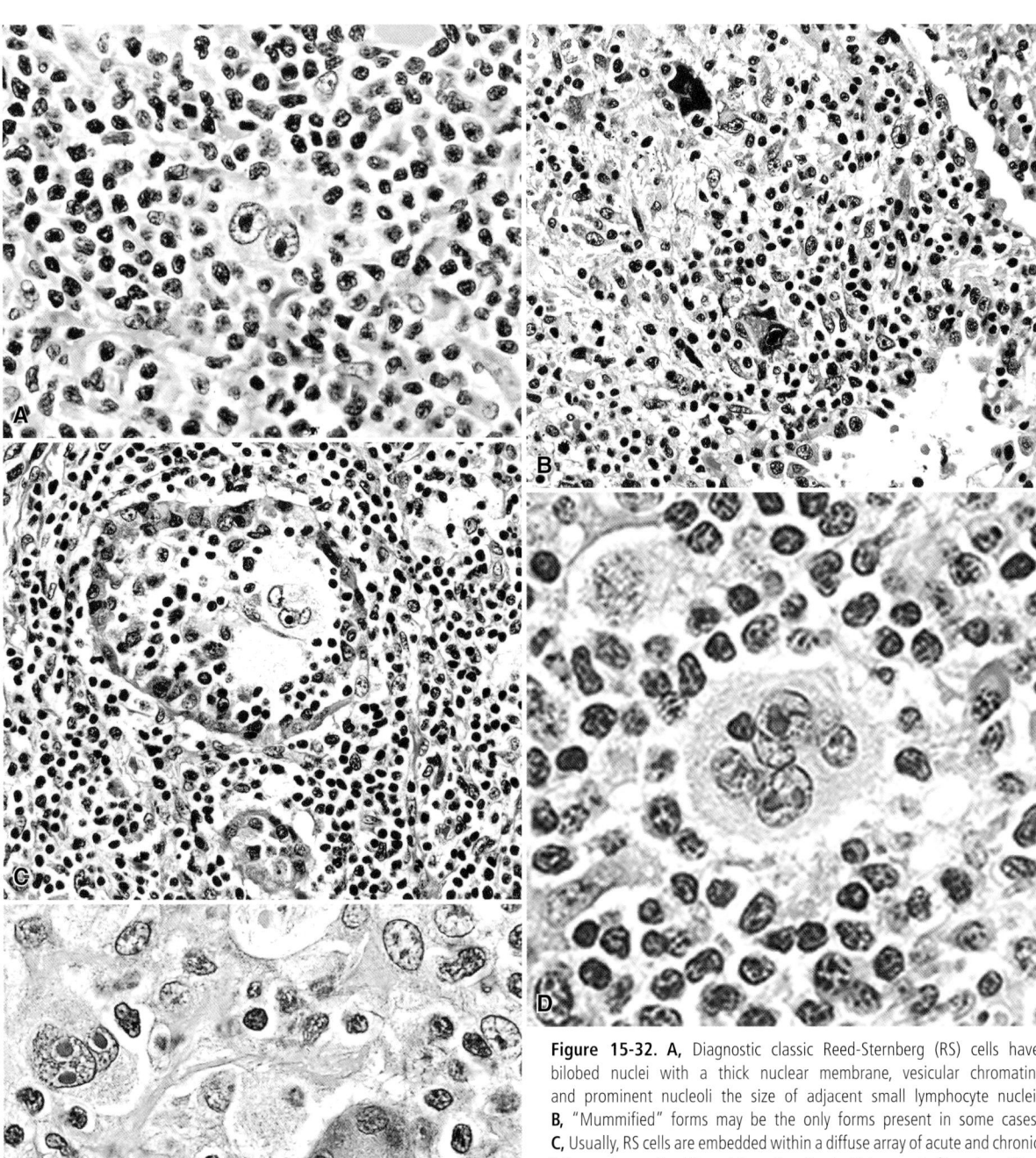

Figure 15-32. A, Diagnostic classic Reed-Sternberg (RS) cells have bilobed nuclei with a thick nuclear membrane, vesicular chromatin, and prominent nucleoli the size of adjacent small lymphocyte nuclei. **B,** "Mummified" forms may be the only forms present in some cases. **C,** Usually, RS cells are embedded within a diffuse array of acute and chronic inflammatory cells, although here they float within a nest of lymphoepithelium. **D,** Variants of the diagnostic RS cells include polylobated forms, which also have the thick nuclear membrane and macronucleoli seen in part **A. E,** In well-fixed, well-prepared sections, a paranucleolar clear zone is often evident around the nucleoli.

Either apoptotic single-cell necrosis or geographic tumoral necrosis may be present, often accompanied by dispersed tingible body macrophages. Exceptional cases may show *"tumoral pneumonia,"* a consolidative picture radiologically because of alveolar filling by tumor cells, extravasated serum, and fibrin.[67] This can also introduce confounding background staining into immunostains. A CD20+, CD10+, bcl6+, bcl2– profile with more than 95% of tumor cells exhibiting nuclear positivity for Ki68 is characteristic. In some cases, CD10 expression may be weak or absent, but bcl6 expression confirms the follicular stage of maturation. When an other-than-characteristic immunophenotype is

obtained, cytogenetic testing should direct the final classification. The outdated term "atypical Burkitt lymphoma" should be avoided.

"B cell lymphoma, unclassifiable with features intermediate between DLBCL and BL" (BCL-U) is a heterogeneous category proposed by the WHO Classification.[5] This category includes cases that have the characteristic morphologic features of Burkitt lymphoma and a phenotype that is not characteristic of BL. It also includes cases with morphologic features closer to those of large B cell lymphoma (greater degree of variation in cell size and nuclear contour irregularity; Fig. 15-39) and high-grade histologic features with a phenotype that is

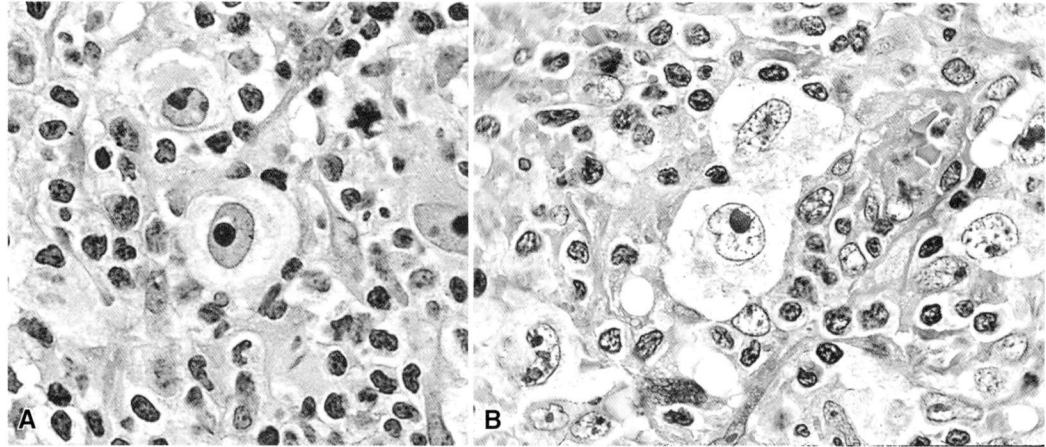

Figure 15-33. Mononuclear variants of diagnostic RS cells are most common in the mixed cellularity subtype of classic Hodgkin lymphoma (**A**), whereas the lacunar variants are most commonly found in the nodular sclerosis type (**B**).

consistent with BL. Patients with either of these two patterns should be further evaluated with cytogenetics. An isolated *c-myc* translocation with either immunoglobulin H or immunoglobulin L loci supports a BL diagnosis, but the finding of a complex karyotype or a *c-myc* translocation with a gene other than immunoglobulin H or immunoglobulin L should prompt the use of BCL-U with a comment about why further classification is not possible or reconsideration of the diagnosis of B-DLCL with a clear delineation of the histologically high-grade nature of the process (Table 15-6).

High-grade large B cell lymphoma, in contrast to BL, is more heterogeneous, with a minor population of commingled small cells. In the lesional cell population there is wide variation in cell size, including cells three to four times the size of small resting lymphocytes; cells with irregular, notched, bilobed, or polylobated nuclei; and usually a blurring of cell borders (no "squaring off") (Fig. 15-40). An additional cue to the diagnosis is commingled small resting lymphocytes among the large lymphoma cells. More variable results for CD10 and *bcl6* are reported in this setting, and at least 20% of the tumor cells are *bcl2*+. The majority of these cases have translocations involving either the *bcl2* or *bcl6*

gene or a complex karyotype, and they only rarely have isolated *c-myc* translocation[175] (see Table 15-6).

Immunoproliferative Disorders

Plasmacytoma

Extraosseous plasmacytoma is uncommon and usually involves the upper (rather than lower) aerodigestive tract.[176] Primary pulmonary plasmacytomas, which are far less common than secondary pulmonary involvement by a disseminated plasma cell dyscrasia (i.e., multiple myeloma), have discretely demarcated edges and are brown or dark tan on cut section.[177–180] Amyloid deposition may be evident grossly as white nodules or streaks in large tumors. Microscopically, the typical plasmacytoma is composed of syncitia of plasma cells with no residual germinal centers and with negligible numbers of intermingled small lymphocytes. Occasionally, lesional cells of plasmacytomas have a pleomorphic or anaplastic appearance (Fig. 15-41A) and may mimic bronchogenic carcinoma or metastatic melanoma. The amphophilic cytoplasm and paranuclear clear zone are preserved in sufficient numbers of cells to suggest the correct diagnosis in most cases.

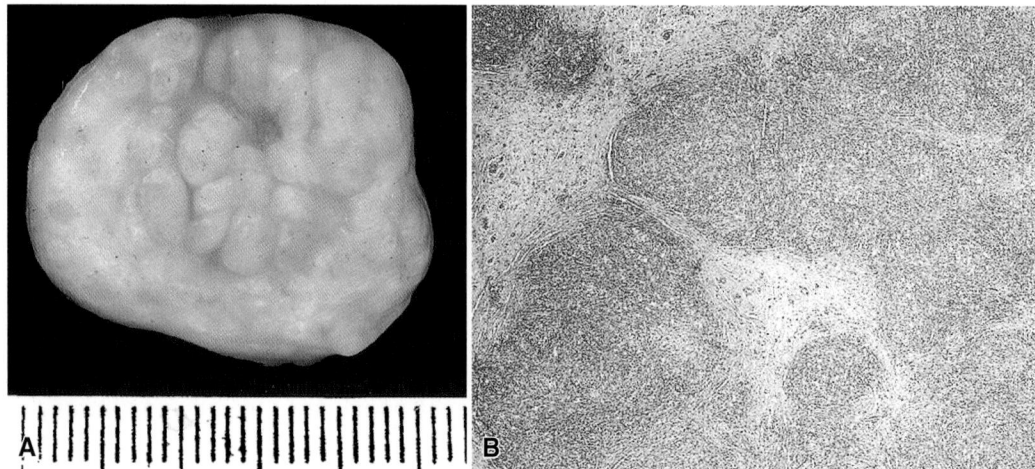

Figure 15-34. Tissues involved by the nodular sclerosis type of classic Hodgkin lymphoma have a nodular architecture grossly (**A**) as well as microscopically (**B**).

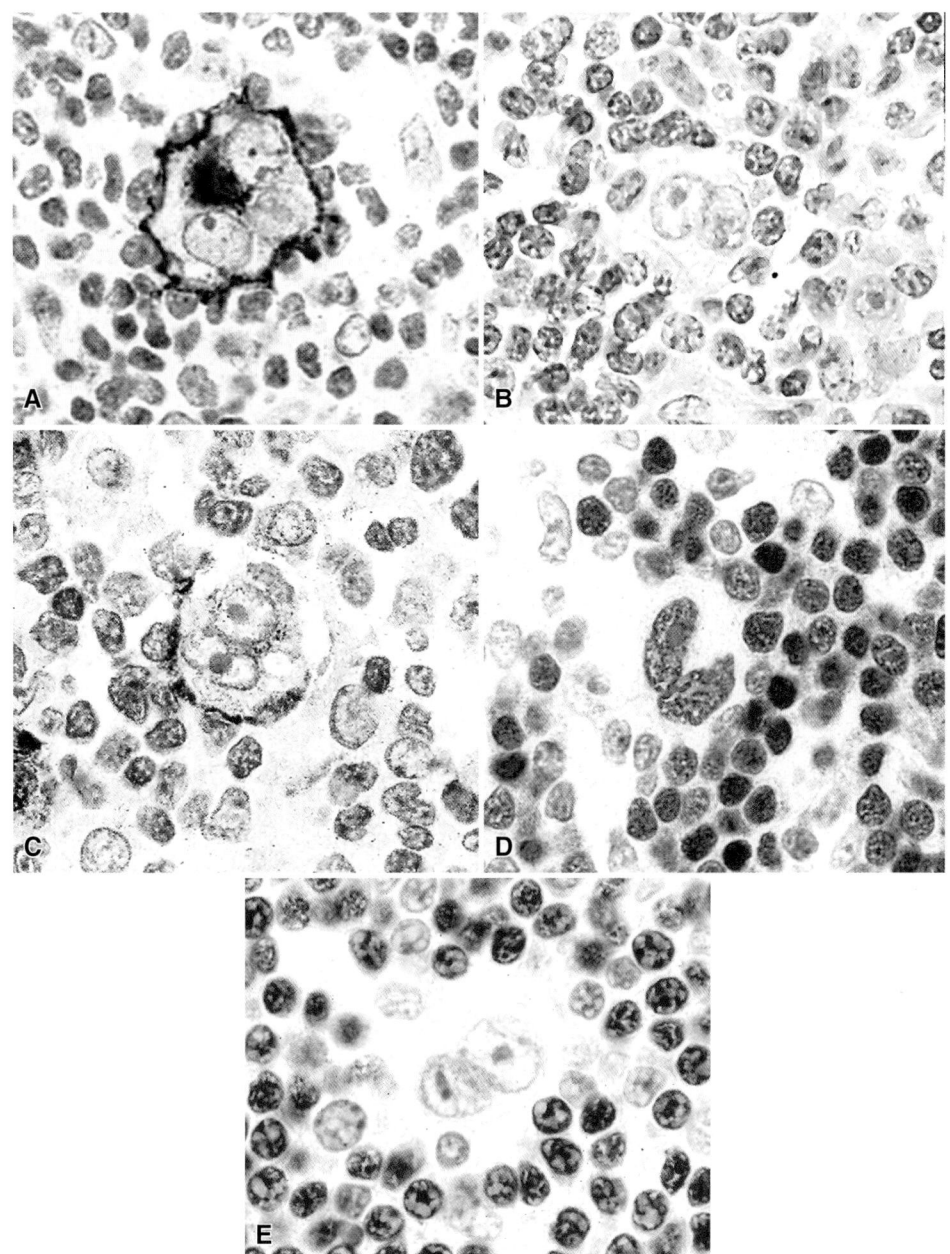

Figure 15-35. A, Although the classic phenotype associated with Reed-Sternberg (RS) cells is CD30+, CD15+, CD20–, the *sine qua non* is CD30 expression. Between 30% and 40% of classic Hodgkin lymphoma cases are negative for CD15 (**B**), and 10% to 20% may express CD20 (**C**) in a weak and partial granular manner. PAX5 expression is expected in RS cells (**D**), although Oct2 is not (**E**). The latter is a helpful means of distinguishing classic Hodgkin lymphoma from T cell–rich large B cell lymphoma.

Flow cytometric analysis of plasmacytomas yields confusing "false negative" results. These terminally differentiated B cells are usually negative for CD45 (leukocyte common antigen) and the B cell markers PAX5, CD19, and CD20, and they do not have sufficient quantities of surface immunoglobulin expression to appear positive on flow cytometry (see Box 15-11). The diagnosis rests on the finding of CD138 expression (see Fig. 15-41B) and a restricted pattern of cytoplasmic immunoglobulin expression, which is easiest to show on paraffin sections. Other markers that may be positive include CD30 and epithelial membrane antigen, but neither is lineage-specific, and both should be interpreted in the context of cytokeratin, S-100 protein, and other marker results.

When more than 20% to 30% of a plasmacytic proliferation is composed of small lymphocytes, consideration should be given to *small*

lymphocytic lymphoma, lymphoplasmacytic lymphoma (Fig. 15-42), and *MaZL.*[181-183] All have a CD45+, CD20+, surface immunoglobulin (sIg+) profile for the lymphoid population, whereas plasmacytomas are negative for these markers (see Table 15-5). Findings that favor MaZL include colonized germinal centers and a polymorphous array of monocytoid, centrocytoid, and plasmacytoid cells. If residual germinal centers are detected in the setting of extreme plasmacytosis, consideration should be given not only to the possibility of MaZL but also to *PCCD.* Because it is impossible to distinguish between a solitary plasmacytoma and pulmonary involvement by a systemic plasma cell dyscrasia (multiple myeloma), all patients with biopsy-proven pulmonary plasmacytoma should be fully evaluated with serum and urine protein electrophoresis, skeletal survey, and bone marrow biopsy.

Table 15-4. Immunophenotypical Comparison of Classic Hodgkin Lymphoma and Differential Considerations

	CD30	CD45	CD15	CD20	CD79a	PAX5	cIg	Oct2	EBV	EMA	ALK1	CD138
cHL	+	0	±	w, f, g	0	w, d	0	0	±	0	0	±
LPHL	0	+	0	++	++	++	±	+	0	±	0	0
TcRBcL	0	+	0	++	++	++	±	+	0	0	0	0
LyG	±	+	±	++	++	++	±	+	+	0	0	0
PMBL	+	+	0	++	++	++	0	0	0	0	0	0
B-ALCL	0	+	0	0	0	0	+	0	0	+	+	+
T-ALCL	+	±	0	0	0	0	0	0	0	±	±	0

B-ALCL, B cell anaplastic large cell lymphoma; cHL, classic Hodgkin lymphoma; d, diffuse (present in >80% of lesional cells); f, focal (present in <20% of lesional cells); g, granular (noncontinuous beaded staining along the membrane or in the cytoplasm); LPHL, lymphocyte-predominance Hodgkin lymphoma; LyG, lymphomatoid granulomatosis; PMBL, primary mediastinal large B cell lymphoma; T-ALCL, T and null cell anaplastic large cell lymphoma; TcRBcL, T cell–rich large B cell lymphoma; w, weak (clearly faint relative to the intensity of nuclear staining in benign small lymphocytes).

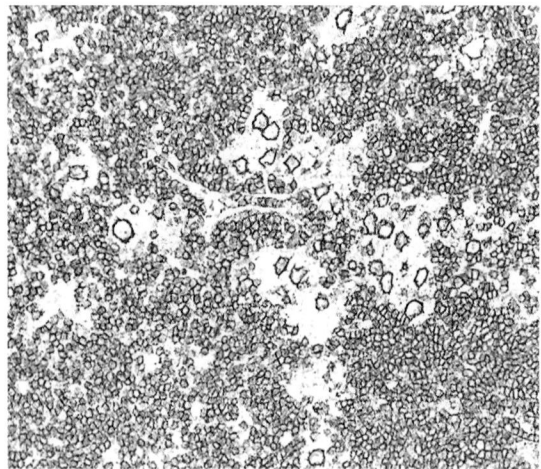

Figure 15-36. The CD30–, CD15–, CD20+ immunophenotype of the lesional cells in the lymphocyte-predominance form of Hodgkin lymphoma (LPHL) helps to distinguish it from classic Hodgkin lymphoma, but is identical to that seen in T cell–rich large B cell lymphoma. Because the latter is not uncommonly seen in the lung, whereas LPHL is vanishingly rare, a large biopsy or resection specimen to assess the milieu is essential for making the correct diagnosis.

Patients with a previously diagnosed plasma cell dyscrasia (or MaZL) may have nodular deposits of amyloid within the lung. These may be solitary or multiple on chest radiograph, and the patient is usually asymptomatic. The material is homogenously eosinophilic and non-fibrillary, and it may contain intermingled lymphocytes, plasma cells, and transitional lymphoplasmacytoid forms. Congo red stain shows orangeophilia in regular light and green birefringence in polarized light in most cases, although noncongophilic amyloidosis occurs (Fig. 15-43). Although accumulations of amyloid are most closely associated with plasma cell dyscrasias, such as multiple myeloma, they also may be seen in association with MaZL and lymphoplasmacytic lymphoma as well as in benign settings.[136–140]

Crystal storing histiocytosis is a rare but distinctive manifestation of immunoglobulin deposition that mimics adult rhabdomyoma. Bone, spleen, lymph node, stomach, thymus, and sinonasal mucosa as well as lung have all been sites of infiltration by this mass-forming proliferation of large polygonal histiocytes that contain large periodic acid/Schiff–positive, phosphotungstic acid-hematoxylin–positive crystalloids (Figs. 15-44 and 15-45). The tumor can be distinguished from rhabdomyoma and plasmacytoma phenotypically by its CD68+, SMA–, CD138– phenotype; the cytoplasmic crystalloids are positive for immunoglobulin light-chain stains, usually of the kappa type (Fig. 15-46).[132–135]

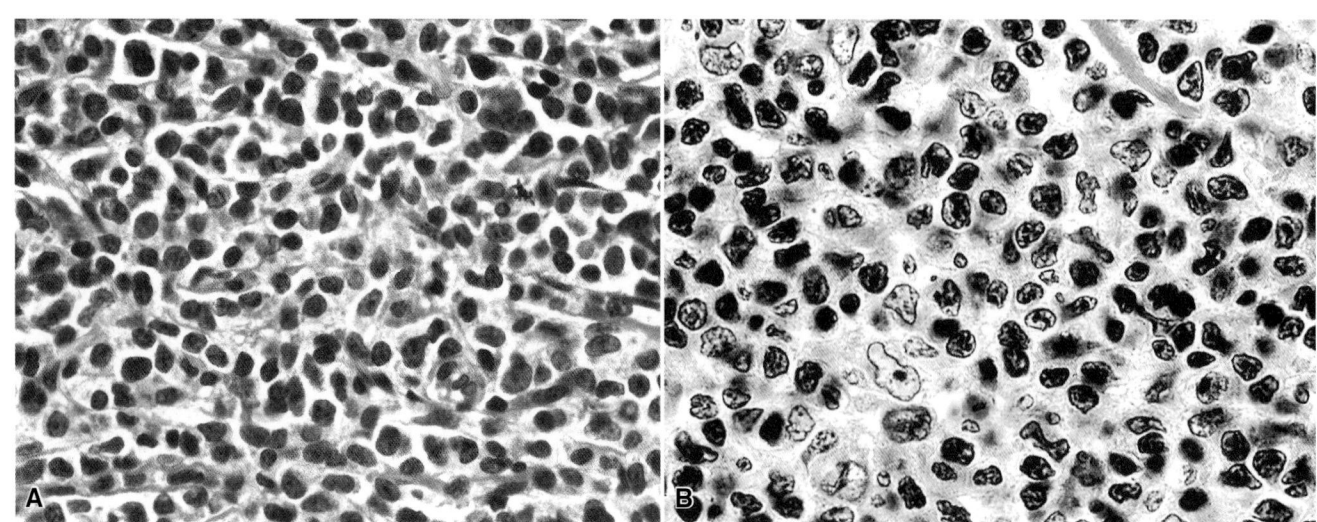

Figure 15-37. **A,** The lung may be secondarily involved by any type of B cell lymphoma. Follicular lymphoma is seen, in which the tumor cells have folded or twisted nuclear profiles. **B,** Another example of intrapulmonary follicular lymphoma, showing irregular nuclear contours.

Continued

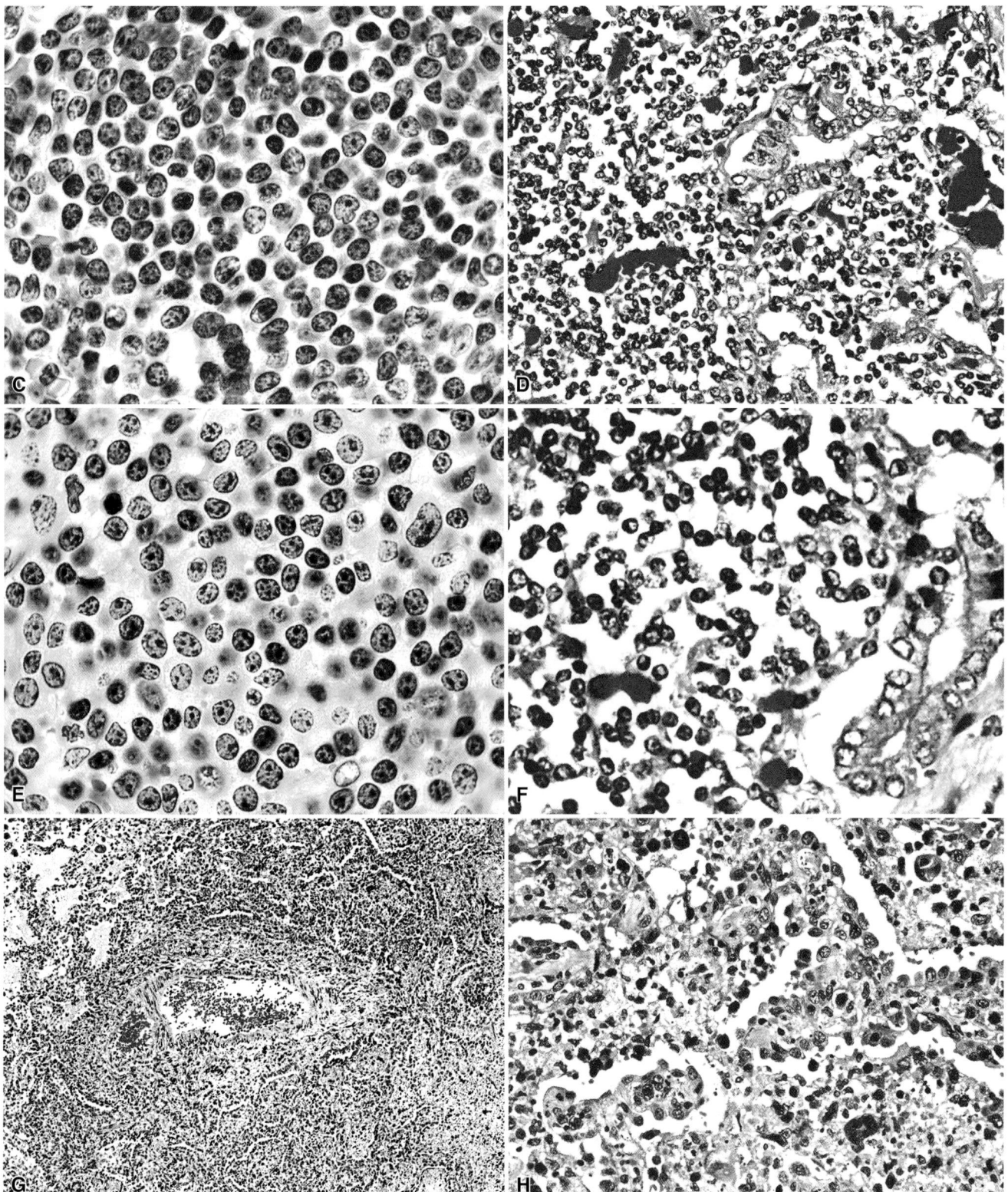

Figure 15-37—cont'd. C, Mantle cell lymphoma of the lung, showing composition by relatively mature and monomorphic small lymphoid cells. This tumor has also been known as "centrocytic lymphoma" or "lymphocytic lymphoma with intermediate differentiation." A chromosomal translocation t(11;14) in mantle cell lymphoma involves the bcl1 locus on chromosome 11 and the immunoglobulin heavy-chain locus on chromosome 14. It leads to overexpression of the *PRAD-1* gene, which encodes cyclin D1. Hence, nuclear immunolabeling for the latter protein is a reproducible diagnostic marker for mantle cell lymphoma. **D,** Small lymphocytic lymphoma (SLL) is shown involving the lung. It is morphologically similar to mantle cell lymphoma but is often accompanied by a leukemic component. Moreover, SLL lacks cyclin D1 immunoreactivity and instead shows labeling for CD5, CD20, and CD43. Flow cytometric studies of SLL also should show positivity for CD23. **E and F,** The similarity of tumor cells in SLL to mature non-neoplastic B lymphocytes is well shown. **G,** Peripheral T cell lymphoma of the lung, growing in an interstitial pattern with a tendency to confluence. **H,** Interalveolar septa are expanded and distorted by obviously atypical lymphoid cells in peripheral cell lymphoma of the lung.

Continued

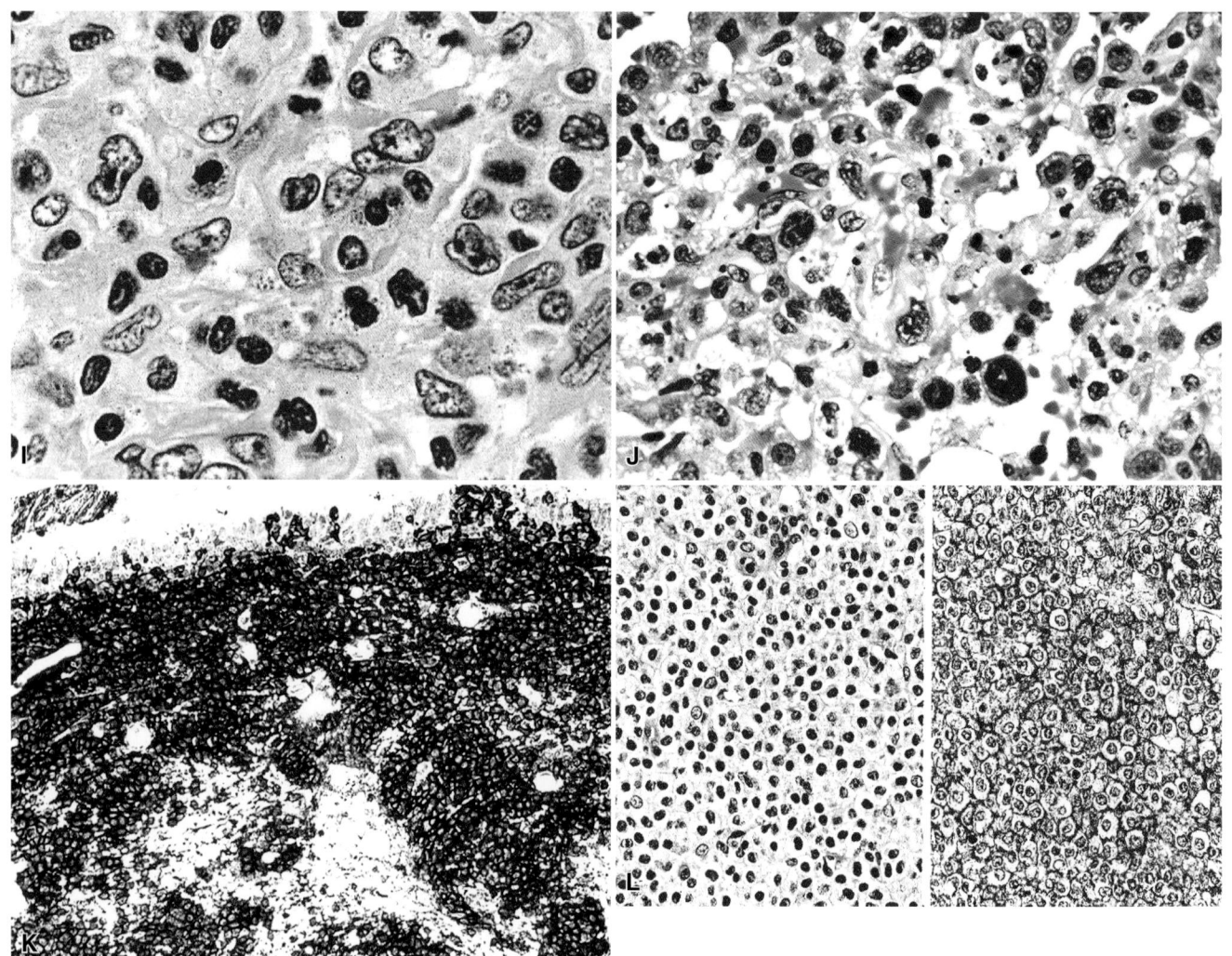

Figure 15-37—cont'd. I, The morphologic triad of a spectrum of small, intermediate, and large atypical cells with pale cytoplasm; hypervascularity; and eosinophilia is often present in peripheral T cell lymphoma, as shown. **J,** Markedly irregular nuclear contours and nuclear hyperchromasia are present in the tumor cells of this intrapulmonary peripheral T cell lymphoma. **K,** Expression of the pan T cell marker CD3 is present in the vast majority of tumor cells in this intrapulmonary peripheral T cell lymphoma. **L,** Many cases of peripheral T cell lymphoma show a selective loss of one or more pan T cell markers, as detected in paraffin section immunostains. CD7 is lacking in the tumor cells (*left*), but CD5 is present (*right*).

Table 15-5. Immunophenotypical Comparison of B Cell Lymphomas Composed of Small Cells

	TdT	CD19	CD20	CD79a	bcl2	bcl6	cyD1	CD5	CD10	CD23	Other*
B-LBL	+	+	0	+	+	0	0	0	±	0	FISH
B-SLL/CLL	0	+	dim	+	+	0	0	+	0	+, d	FISH
MCL	0	+	+	+	+	0	+	+	0	0	FISH
FL	0	+	+	+	+	+	0	0	+	var	FISH
BL	0	+	+	+	0	+	0	0	+	0	Ki67 > 95%
MaZL	0	+	+	+	+	0	0	0	0	0	foll col
HCL	0	+	+	+	0	0	0	0	0	0	CD103, DBA
LPL	0	+	+	+	+	0	0	0	0	0	clg, CD138
PCY	0	0	0	+	±	0	±	0	0	0	clg, CD138

*CD103, lesional cells are CD103+; CD138, lesional cells are CD138+; clg, plasma cells have monotypic cytoplasmic kappa or lambda; DBA, lesional cells are DBA.44+; FISH, in situ hybridization may be helpful in classifying difficult cases or may provide clinically relevant prognostic information (see text); foll col, follicular colonization present (see text); Ki67, proliferation index > 95%.
BL, Burkitt lymphoma; B-LBL, B cell lymphoblastic lymphoma; B-SLL/CLL, B cell small lymphocytic lymphoma/chronic lymphocytic leukemia; cyD1, cyclin D1; FISH, fluorescence in situ hybridization; FL, follicular lymphoma; HCL, hairy cell leukemia; LPL, lymphoplasmacytic leukemia; MaZL, marginal zone lymphoma; MCL, mantle cell lymphoma; PCY, plasmacytoma; var, variable results; some cases may be positive.

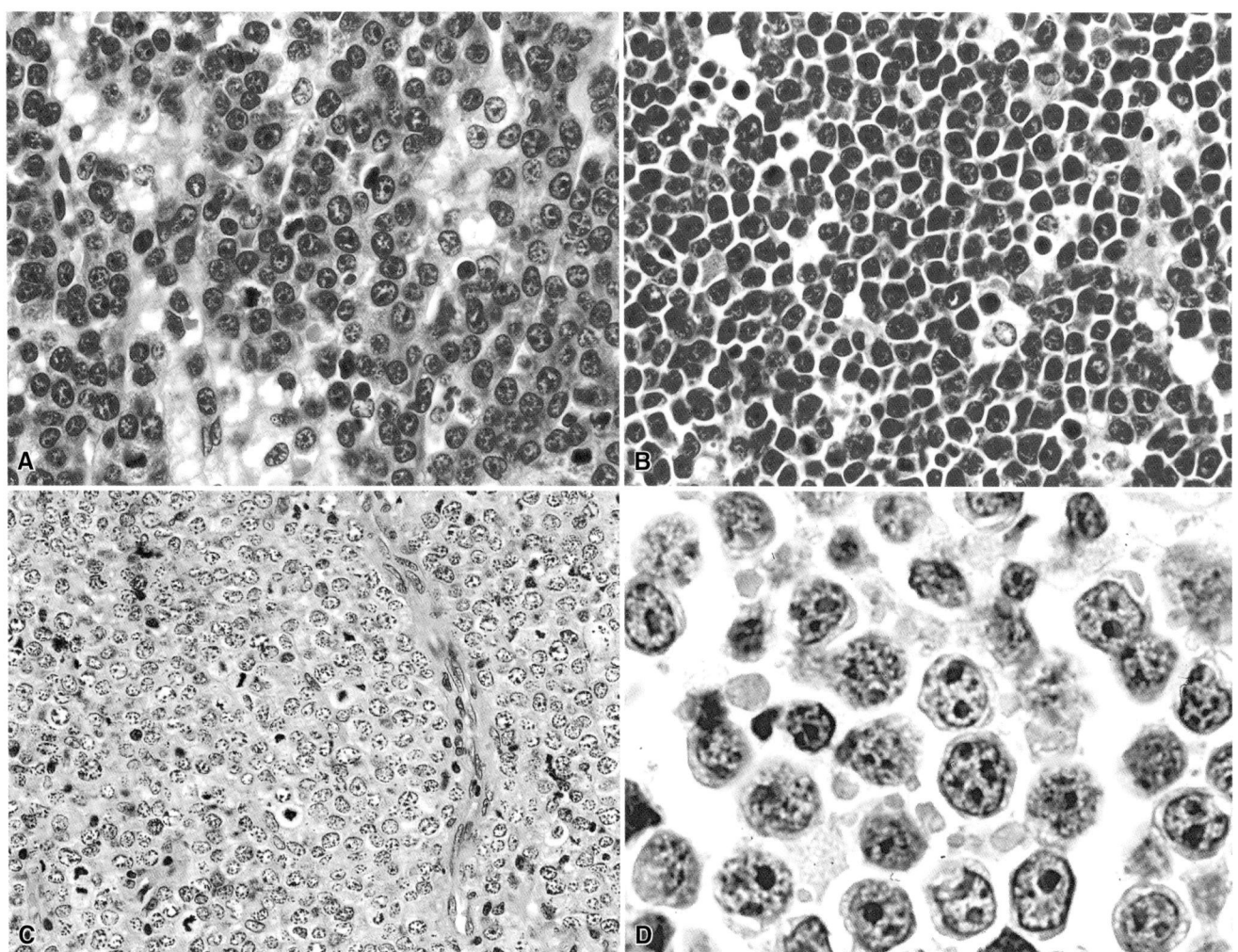

Figure 15-38. Burkitt lymphoma (BL) may involve the lung, usually secondarily. **A,** The key features of BL include intermediate cell size, coarse chromatin with multiple peripherally located small nucleoli, and scant deeply basophilic cytoplasm. **B,** The cells are not especially adherent to one another, creating a sense of dyscohesion and a squaring off of cell borders. **C,** The mitotic rate is brisk, and there is apoptotic single-cell necrosis. **D,** Nuclei are monotonously round and smooth.

Immunodeficiency-Related Lymphoproliferative Disorders

Post-transplant Lymphoproliferative Disorders

The immunosuppressed post-transplant state predisposes solid-organ transplant recipients to the development of lymphoid proliferations, often EBV-related and of B lineage[184,185] (Table 15-7). For most patients, the disease is systemic at the time it is detected clinically, but for many patients who undergo lung transplant, PTLD arises in and remains localized to the graft. Radiographic findings vary from bilateral reticulonodular infiltrates to discrete single or multiple nodules or masses, with the latter most common in patients with high-grade histologic features.[186]

Classification of PTLDs integrates morphologic, phenotypic, and genetic data[186] (see Table 15-7). *Polymorphous PTLD* is composed of a mixture of lymphocytes, plasma cells, and transitional lymphoplasmacytoid forms (Fig. 15-47). In this setting, a polytypic pattern of light-chain expression and the lack of clonality on Southern blot analysis are compatible with classification as "polymorphous B cell hyperplasia" or "nonclonal polymorphous PTLD." With these early lesions, the lymph node architecture is preserved and the disease is usually more localized, so dissemination with lung involvement is uncommon. If there is a monotypic population of B cells seen on flow cytometry, or if gene rearrangement studies identify a clonal population, the proliferation is best diagnosed as "polymorphous B cell lymphoma" or "clonal polymorphous PTLD." Clonal processes are more commonly associated with architectural distortion of the lymph node architecture and may be more likely to involve the lung. *Monomorphous PTLDs* have a uniform appearance and histologic features identical to those of large cell lymphoma, Burkitt lymphoma, or plasmacytoma occurring in an immunocompetent patient (Fig. 15-48). Most cases contain EBV, which can be detected with either immunohistochemistry or in situ hybridization. T lineage PTLDs with no relationship to EBV also occur, and a number have been shown to be of a special T γ/δ hepatosplenic type.

Polymorphic PTLDs are, in general, more likely than their monomorphic counterparts to regress if immunosuppression is reduced. The same can be said of polytypic or polyclonal proliferations relative to monotypic or monoclonal tumors. Therefore, classification plays an important role in initial treatment planning, and it is also an important indicator of prognosis.[186] Transplant patients can have PTLDs in multiple sites, and whereas one might be polymorphous, there may be a monomorphous PTLD elsewhere. For this reason, therapeutic planning requires an integration of pathologic findings with clinical parameters of disease aggressiveness, which may not always be available to the pathologist in a timely manner.

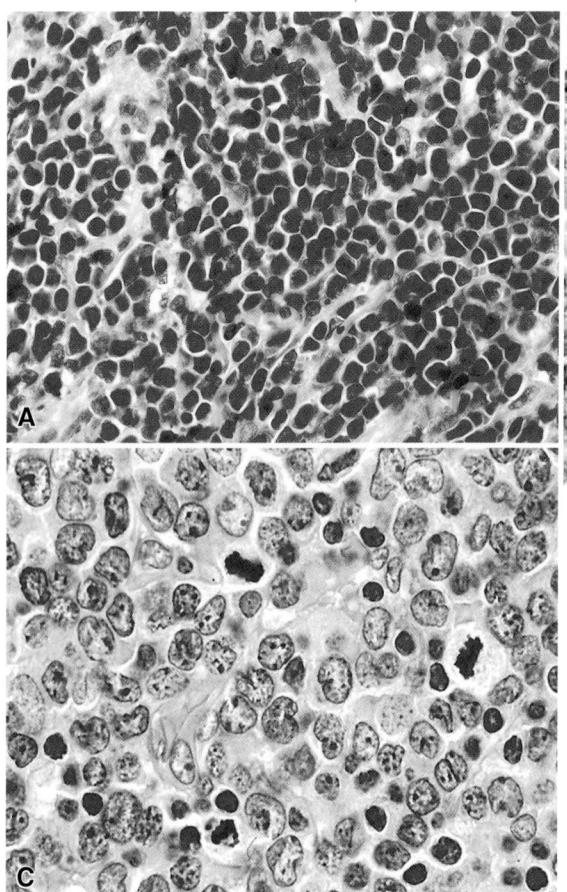

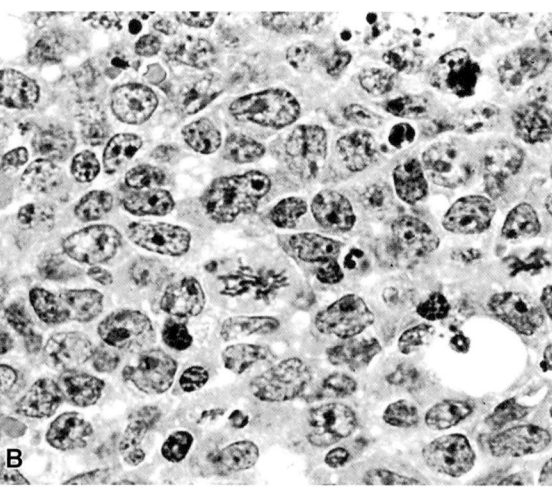

Figure 15-39. Some high-grade lymphomas have morphologic features that fall between those of Burkitt lymphoma and those of diffuse large B cell lymphoma. In these cases, cell size is usually more variable, with both small and large cells present, and nuclear configurations are more irregular, with notched and folded forms (**A** and **B**). Some cases of lymphoblastic lymphoma may overlap with Burkitt lymphoma (**C**), but the latter are TdT+, CD20–, the opposite of Burkitt lymphoma.

Table 15-6. Correlation of the Morphologic Features, Phenotype, and Cytogenetics in Burkitt and Burkitt-like High-Grade Lymphomas

	Phenotype				
	bcl2	bcl6	CD10	Ki-67	**Cytogenetics**
Burkitt morphologic features with bcl2 expression	+	+	+	>90%	Isolated IgH or IgL translocation with c-myc should prompt classification as Burkitt lymphoma A c-myc translocation involving a non-Ig partner or a complex karyotype including a c-myc translocation and other translocations (e.g., t[14;18], t[3q27;V]) should prompt classification as high-grade B-NHL-UC
Burkitt morphologic features without CD10 expression (the same may be applied to a patient with Burkitt morphologic features without bcl6 expression)	0	+	0	>90%	Isolated IgH or IgL translocation with c-myc should prompt classification as Burkitt lymphoma A c-myc translocation involving a non-Ig partner or a complex karyotype including a c-myc translocation and other translocations (e.g., t[14;18], t[3q27;V]) should prompt classification as high-grade B-NHL-UC
Intermediate morphologic features	±	±	±	>90%	Isolated IgH or IgL translocation with c-myc should prompt classification as Burkitt lymphoma; because treatment planning differs, if the pathologist remains unsure, sending the patient for external consultation is always appropriate Patients with a complex karyotype, including a c-myc translocation, a "double hit" of a c-myc translocation with either t(14;18) or t(3q27;V), or an isolated t(14;18) or t(3q27;V) should be diagnosed as having B-NHL-UC or DLCL
Large-cell morphologic features	+	±	±	<80%	If the patient has clear-cut morphologic features of large-cell lymphoma, it should be classified as B-DLCL, regardless of the results of cytogenetic testing; cytogenetic testing may be of clinical use in treatment planning because patients with "double-hit" B-DLCL do worse than those with B-DLCL without this abnormality

Burkitt morphology: Uniformly intermediate-sized cells without nuclear contour irregularity; homogenous eosinophilic cytoplasm with clear-cut edges between cells ("squaring off"); several peripheral small nucleoli. Classic Burkitt phenotype: bcl2–, bcl6+, CD10+.

Intermediate morphology: Mixture of intermediate-sized and larger cells, with mild or moderate nuclear contour irregularity in some; prominent solitary centrally placed nucleoli in some cells; commingled small, resting lymphocytes may be present.

Large-cell morphology: Mixture of large and very large cells with moderate or striking nuclear contour irregularity, or cells with immunoblastic or polylobated nuclei; indistinct cell borders; commingled small lymphocytes with either resting cytology or features of centrocytes.

B-DLCL, B-cell diffuse large cell lymphoma; B-NHL-UC, B-cell non-Hogkin lymphoma, not otherwise classified; DLCL, diffuse large cell lymphoma.

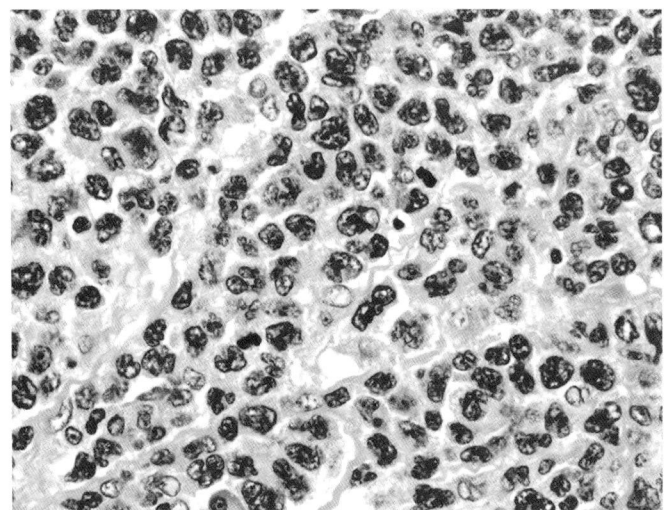

Figure 15-40. Diffuse large B cell lymphoma can have histologic features indicative of high grade, including a brisk mitotic rate, apoptotic or tumoral cell necrosis, and cytoplasmic amphophilia. However, careful scrutiny of viable, well-preserved areas shows the fundamentally large cell size and the irregular nuclear shape of the tumor.

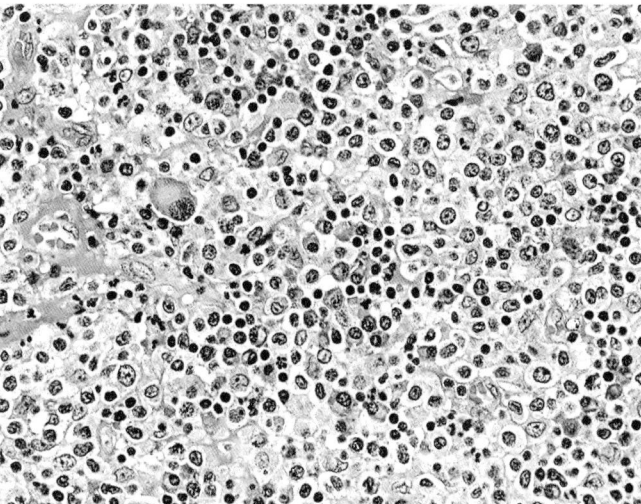

Figure 15-42. In lymphoplasmacytic lymphoma, there is a heterogenous mix of clonal small B lymphocytes, transitional lymphoplasmacytoid forms, and plasma cells. Because of the lymphoid component, flow cytometry findings are positive, and because of the plasmacytic component, paraffin section studies for clonality are also positive.

Differential diagnostic considerations are few because the lymphoid nature of the proliferation is readily apparent histologically, and immunophenotypic studies rarely yield ambiguous results. Difficulty may arise if a transbronchial biopsy specimen has been obtained: The quantity of lesional infiltrate may be too limited to allow a meaningful histologic classification into polymorphic or monomorphic categories, or to fully exclude other diseases, such as lymphomatoid granulomatosis (discussed earlier), Hodgkin lymphoma, or non-neoplastic disorders, such as cytomegalovirus (or other viral) pneumonia.

T Lineage Lymphoid Malignancies

Most patients with peripheral T cell lymphoma (PTCL) are clinically ill with disseminated disease at presentation, and they may have features such as spiking fevers, rash, and lung infiltrates.[187] Radiologic findings may show bilateral miliary nodules or reticulonodular infiltrates simulating interstitial disease, although the finding of one or more masses is most common. There is a systemic distribution of disease at presentation, and the initial diagnosis is usually based on lymph node biopsy.[187] Lung

biopsy may be performed at any point during presentation or treatment to distinguish among infection, treatment-resistant lymphomatous infiltrates, and medication-related interstitial lung disease. The histologic hallmark of most cases of PTCL is the following triad: (1) a spectrum of atypical small, intermediate, and large cells with irregular nuclear shapes and clear cytoplasm; (2) hypervascularity; and (3) tissue eosinophilia[188,189] (Fig. 15-49). Phenotypically, there may be an aberrant loss of a pan T cell marker (CD2, CD3, CD5, or CD7), which may be easiest to detect on flow cytometry, where the tumor cells can be studied for three or four markers at the same time. However, immunohistochemistry on serial sections from paraffin blocks can also show this phenotypic alteration.[188,189]

Specific T lineage lymphomas have distinctive clinicopathologic profiles (Box 15-13), some principally marrow-based and others principally nodal and parenchymally based, but primary or predominant lung or mediastinal involvement is uncommon. Of these, T cell lymphoblastic lymphoma and T-ALCL are the only two malignancies encountered in chest or lung biopsy specimens with any frequency.

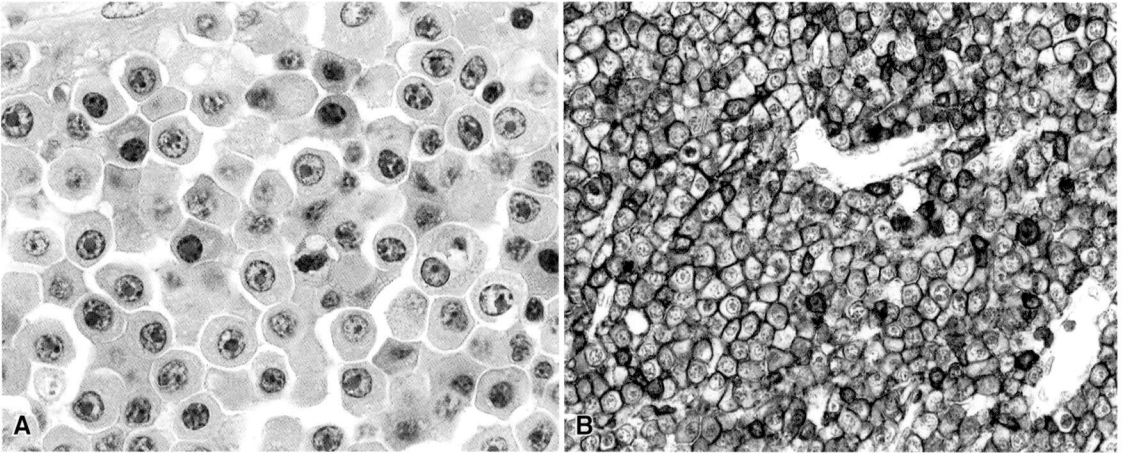

Figure 15-41. A, Plasma cell neoplasms can closely mimic carcinoma, although cellular dyshesion is a clue to the hematologic nature of the process, as is the presence of a prominent Golgi zone in some of the lesional cells. **B,** Although CD45– in most cases, plasmacytomas are strongly CD138+.

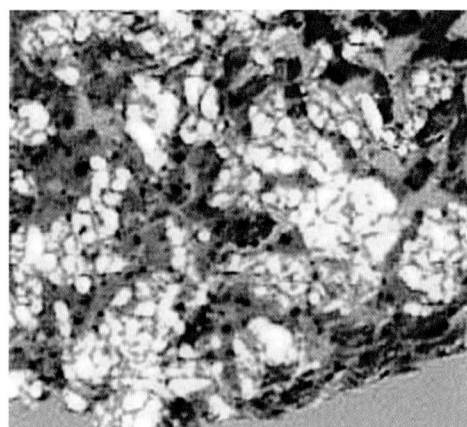

Figure 15-43. Amyloid deposition in the lung may be nodular and mass-forming, as in this case, or may be more subtle and restricted to the alveolar septal walls.

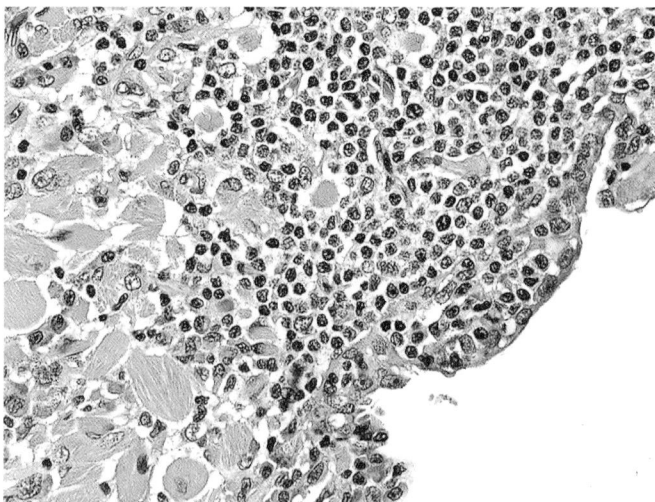

Figure 15-45. Marginal zone lymphoma with crystal-storing histiocytosis.

T Cell Lymphoblastic Lymphoma/T Cell Acute Lymphoblastic Leukemia

T cell LBL often presents in adolescent boys with a mediastinal mass, hepatosplenomegaly, and generalized lymphadenopathy. The liver, spleen, marrow, and blood are often involved.[5]

In fully involved tissues, the architecture is diffuse and the blasts are intermediate in size (approximately 1.5 times the size of a benign lymph node), although there may be a surprising degree of variation in cell size, with some blasts approximatley twice the size of a benign lymph node. The nuclear contours may be smooth or convoluted, and the blasts may have fine or evenly condensed chromatin, often with a distinct nucleolus (Fig. 15-50). With good fixation and thinly sectioned slides, the neoplastic and blastic nature of the infiltrate is seldom in doubt, although with therapy, necrosis and apoptosis may make the diagnosis more difficult.

In most cases, the leukemic cells are positive for TdT, CD2, and CD7, with variable expression of CD34, CD5, CD1a, and CD10 (Box 15-14 and Fig. 15-51). Surface expression of CD3 may be slight to absent, so the cells may appear to be negative on flow cytometry, although immunohistochemical stains show cytoplasmic positivity. There are few to no cytokeratin-positive cells commingled with the blastic infiltrate, and no lobulation is seen on routine or special stains.

Differential diagnostic considerations for T-LBL in the mediastinum include *benign thymus* and lymphocyte-rich *thymoma,* and an adequate sample size is the only way to assess for effacement of the thymic architecture, which would favor T-LBL. Because benign thymic tissues can have an identical phenotype, attempting an initial diagnosis of T-LBL based on the findings of cytology or needle-core biopsy alone can be treacherous. Cytokeratin stains show an intact lobulated array of thymic epithelial elements in benign thymus and lymphocyte-rich thymomas, but these are absent or rare in T-LBL (Fig. 15-52). *Neuroendocrine carcinomas,* including carcinoids and small cell carcinoma, can mimic T-LBL, although immunophenotypic studies readily show the correct diagnosis. *B lineage lymphoblastic lymphoma and acute myeloid leukemia* are histologically indistinguishable, but the former are positive for PAX5, CD19, CD79a, or CD22, and the latter are positive for CD13, CD33, and myeloperoxidase.

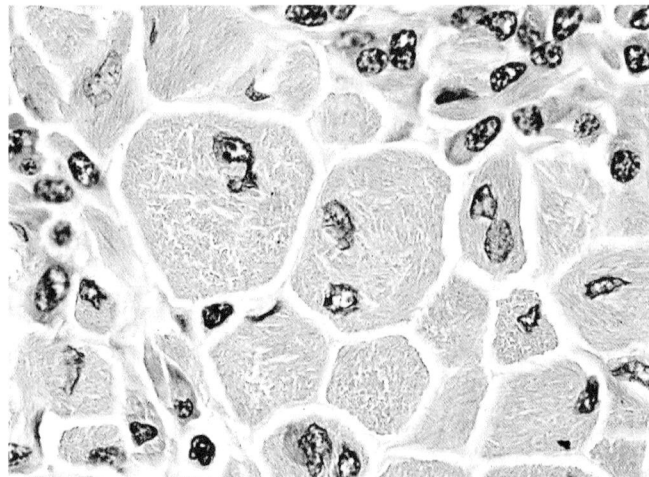

Figure 15-44. The lesional cells of crystal-storing histiocytes are massively enlarged because of the phagocytosis of needle-like shards of crystalline immunoglobulin. When no history of lymphoma or myeloma is given, unusual epithelial malignancies and adult rhabdomyoma are differential considerations.

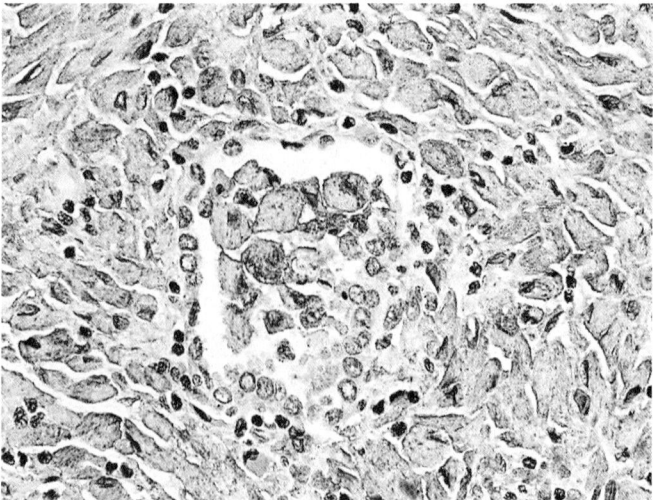

Figure 15-46. Immunoglobulin in crystal-storing histiocytosis is more often of the kappa subtype than chance would allow, as shown in this immunostain for kappa light chains.

Table 15-7. Histologic, Phenotypic, and Genetic Characteristics of Post-transplant Lymphoproliferative Disorders

	P-BCH	P-BCL	M-BLCL	M-BL	M-BPCY
Cellular composition	Mixture of small lymphocytes, plasma cells, and occasional large centroblastic and immunoblastic cells	Mixture of small lymphocytes, plasma cells, and occasional large centroblastic and immunoblastic cells	Uniform population of centroblastic or immunoblastic large cells and moderate quantities of eosinophilic or amphophilic cytoplasm	Uniform population of intermediate-sized cells with coarse chromatin, multiple distinct nucleoli, moderate or abundant quantities of amphophilic cytoplasm	Uniform population of plasmacytic or plasmablastic cells with coarse chromatin
Histologic grade	Low (occasional mitoses, no necrosis)	Low (occasional mitoses, no necrosis)	High (increased mitoses); necrosis may be present	High (numerous mitoses); necrosis often present	May be low or high (no necrosis)
sIg expression	Polytypic	Monotypic	Monotypic	Most cases sIg–	Some cases sIg–
cIg expression	Polytypic	Monotypic	Usually cIg–	Usually cIg–	Monotypic
Clonal IgH/IgL loci rearrangements	None	Present	Present	Present	Present
Outcome	May resolve spontaneously with reduced immunosuppression	May resolve spontaneously with reduced immunosuppression	Less likely to resolve without systemic chemotherapy	Unlikely to resolve without systemic chemotherapy; often fatal	Unlikely to resolve without systemic chemotherapy

cIg, cytoplasmic immunoglobulin; M-BL, monomorphous Burkitt lymphoma; M-BLCL, monomorphous B cell large-cell lymphoma; M-BPCY, monomorphous B cell plasmacytoma; P-BCH, polymorphous B cell hyperplasia; P-BCL, polymorphous B cell lymphoma; sIg, surface immunoglobulin.

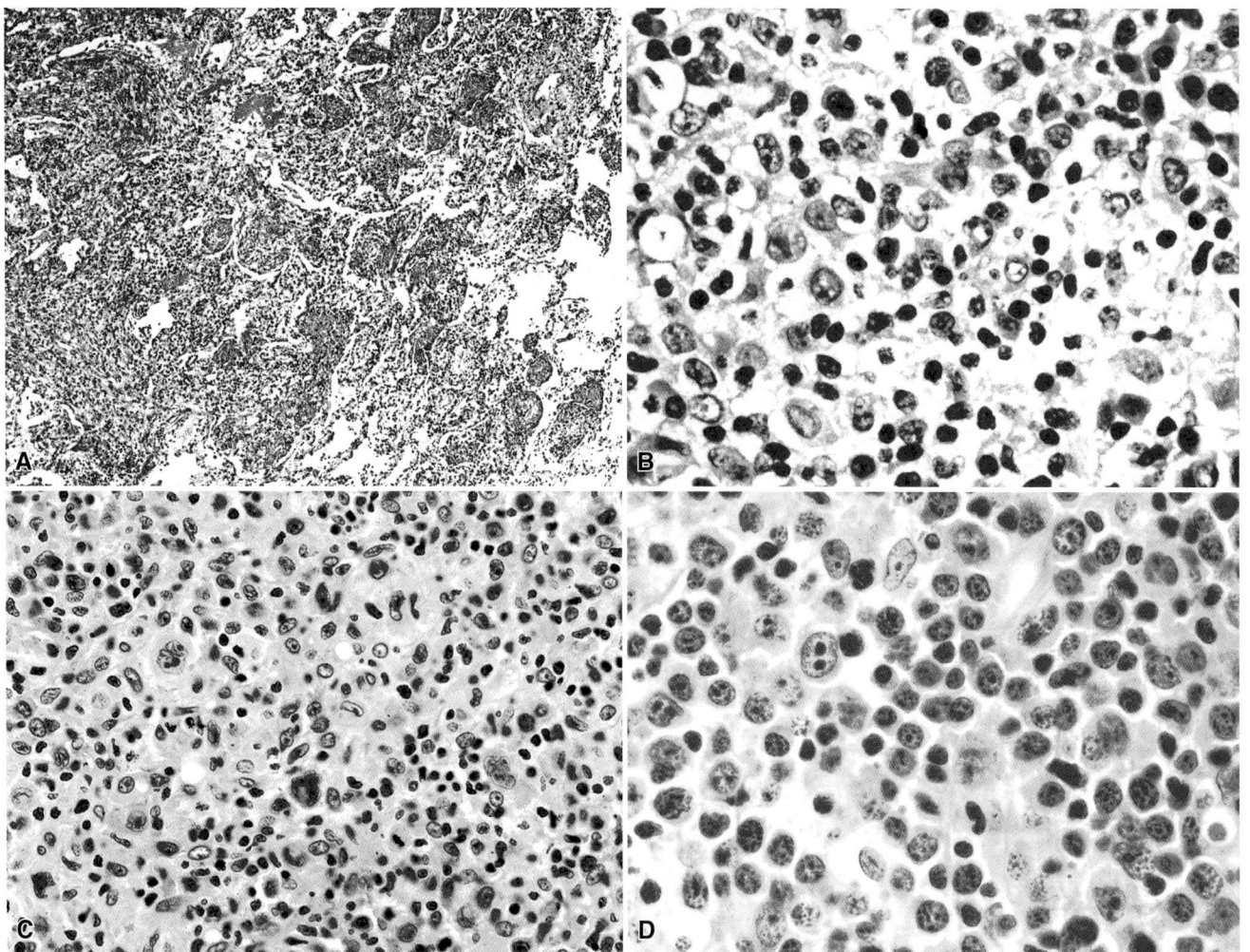

Figure 15-47. Polymorphous post-transplant lymphoproliferative disorder (PTLD) in the lung, showing an alveolar (**A**) and interstitial infiltrate of hematopoietic elements with lymphoplasmacytic features (**B**). **C,** Polymorphous PTLD may show an admixture of atypical mononuclear cells, plasma cells, and Reed-Sternberg cell–like elements, or a prominent histiocytic component together with lymphocytes and plasma cells (**D**). This process is driven by infection with Epstein-Barr virus; it is polyclonal and is not associated with mutations of proto-oncogenes, such as *c-myc*.

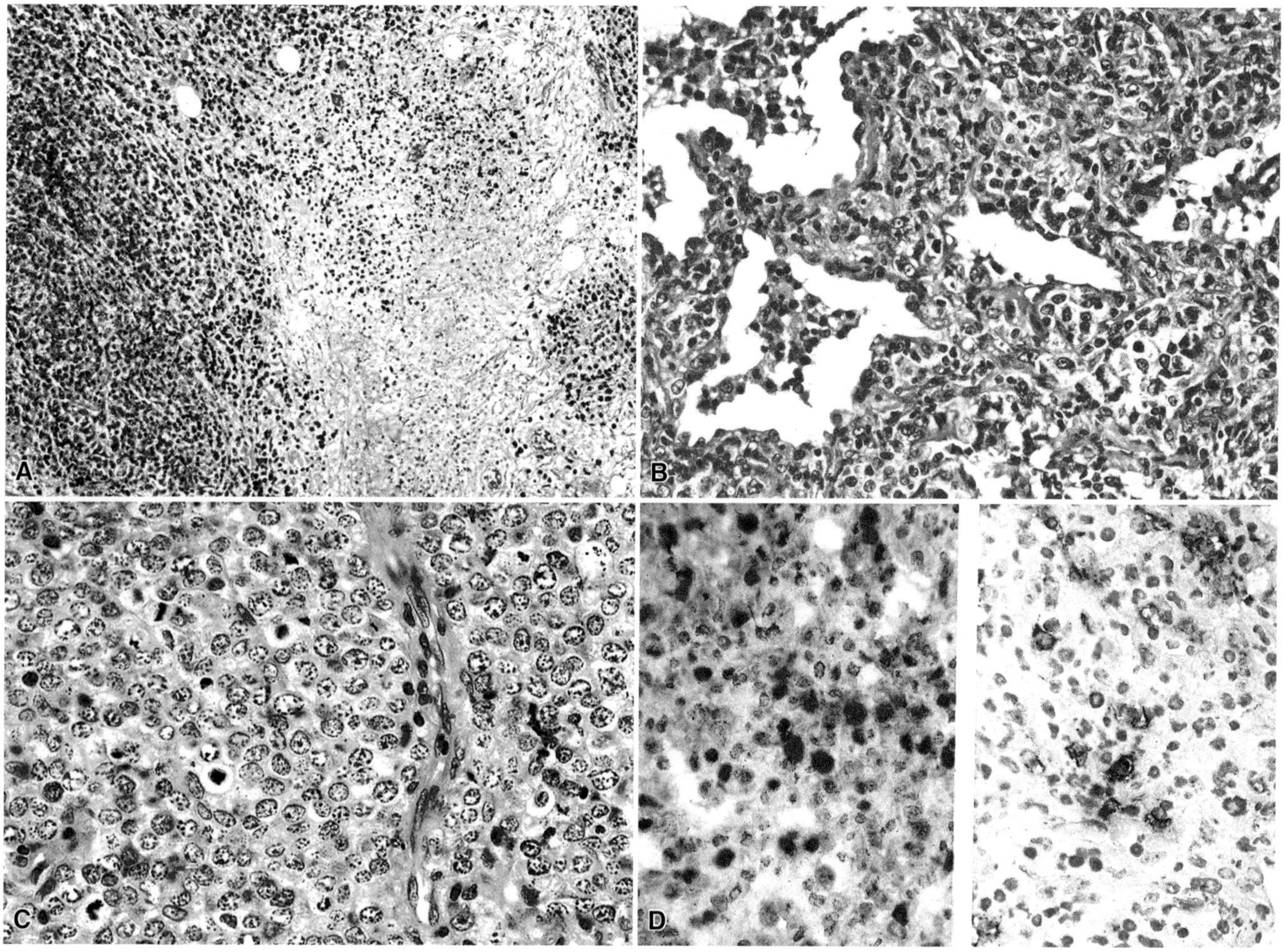

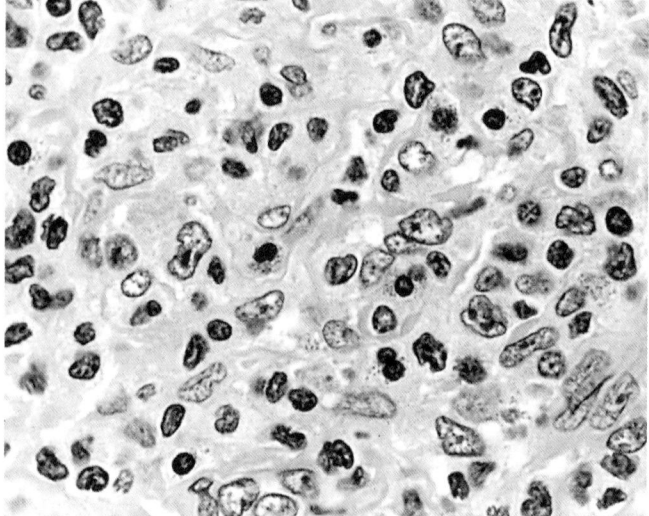

Figure 15-48. **A,** High-grade monotypic post-transplant lymphoproliferative disorder (PTLD) in the lung showing an infiltrate of atypical larger cells in a field of geographic necrosis. **B,** The lesional cells of high-grade monotypic PTLD expand and distort the interalveolar septa. **C,** They show obvious nuclear anaplasia and were monoclonal genotypically and immunophenotypically. **D,** In situ hybridization for Epstein-Barr virus–related ribonucleic acid (*left*) or immunostaining for Epstein-Barr virus latent membrane protein (*right*) usually yields positive results in PTLD of the lung.

Figure 15-49. The morphologic triad of a spectrum of small, intermediate, and large atypical cells with pale cytoplasm; hypervascularity; and eosinophilia is often present in peripheral T cell lymphoma, as shown here.

T Cell Anaplastic Large Cell Lymphoma

The lung is a common site of secondary involvement by systemic T cell anaplastic large cell lymphoma (T-ALCL), and several cases of primary pulmonary ALCL of T or null cell type have also been reported.[190-195] Presentation is via mass effect, with cough, hemoptysis, or symptoms referable to pleural effusions.[195-197]

Box 15-13. T Lineage Malignancies

Principally Leukemic/Bone Marrow–Based
T cell lymphoblastic lymphoma/T cell acute lymphoblastic leukemia
T cell large granular lymphocytic leukemia
T cell prolymphocytic leukemia
Human T cell lymphotropic virus-1–related adult T cell leukemia/lymphoma

Principally Lymphomatous/Mass-Forming
T cell anaplastic large cell lymphoma
Angioimmunoblastic type of peripheral T cell lymphoma
T gamma-delta hepatosplenic lymphoma
Nasal-type extranodal T/natural killer cell lymphoma
Enteropathy-associated T cell lymphoma
Subcutaneous panniculitic T cell lymphoma
Peripheral T cell lymphoma, not otherwise classified

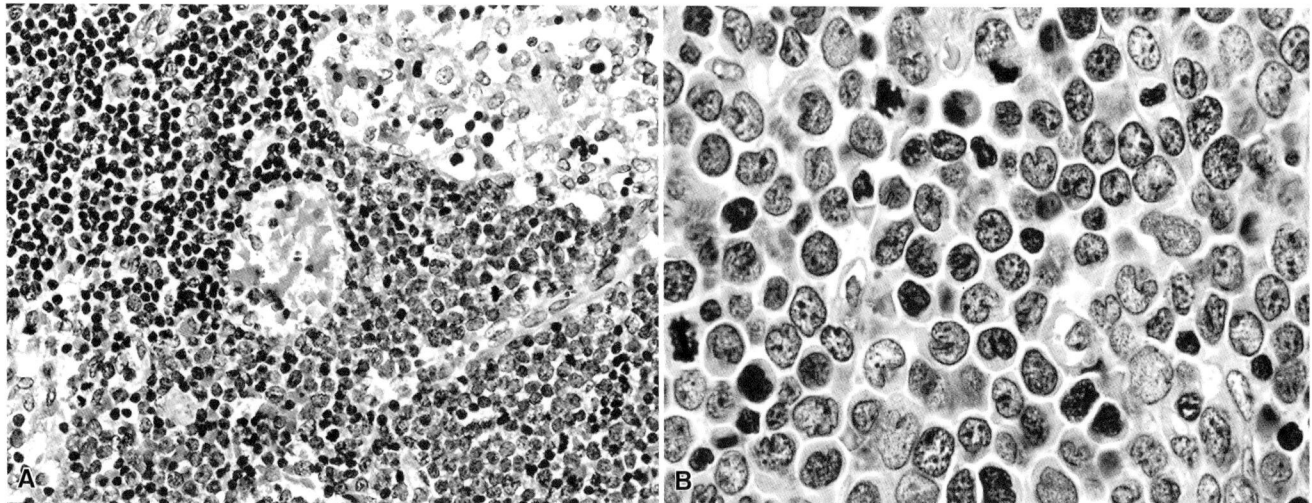

Figure 15-50. A, Lymphoblastic lymphoma creates diffuse proliferations of small cells that leave the tissue planes intact. **B,** The cells have evenly dispersed or fine chromatin, with indistinct nucleoli, irregular ("convoluted") nuclear shapes, and scant agranular cytoplasm.

Microscopically, ALCL is formed of diffuse sheets of large and very large cells with pleomorphic nuclei and abundant cytoplasm, and the similarity to carcinoma or melanoma may be striking. Careful attention to the periphery may show a dishesive array of intra-alveolar tumor cells, a helpful cue that the disease may be of hematolymphoid origin (Box 15-15 and Fig. 15-53). There are multiple histopathologic variants or patterns (Box 15-16), and more than one pattern can be seen in a single patient or a single biopsy specimen. The uniting elements are the very large hallmark cells (Fig. 15-54), which are especially numerous in the common or pleomorphic form.[197] Hallmark cells have reniform, or U-shaped, nuclei, and abundant amounts of cytoplasm compared with other lymphomas. In some cases, the nuclear indentation is in the plane of view, such that the nucleus appears as an O (donut cells). Nucleoli are distinct but generally are not the size of a small lymphocyte and lack the perinucleolar halo characteristic of RS cells. The remainder of the cellularity includes medium and large cells with round, irregular, lobated, and folded nuclear shapes, dispersed chromatin, distinct nucleoli, and moderate or abundant amounts of glassy eosinophilic cytoplasm[193,195,197] (Fig. 15-55).

In general, ALCL is reliably CD30+ (Fig. 15-56A), and the majority of these cases are positive for a pan T cell marker, such as CD2, CD3, or betaF1, although some may be negative for all of these antigens ("null cell phenotype") or negative for leukocyte common antigen. ALK expression can be documented immunohistochemically in many but not all cases of ALCL, and it correlates with the presence of the t(2;5) translocation involving the *nucleophosmin* and ALK genes.[198] Although there are exceptions,[199] ALK expression is associated with better overall survival[5,198] and should be tested in every lymphoma that shows anaplastic morphologic features. B cell lineage and Hodgkin markers, including PAX5, are negative (see Fig. 15-56B).

Differential considerations may include metastatic *carcinoma,* *melanoma,* and epithelioid *sarcoma,* and so a panel of stains including pancytokeratin, S-100, MART1, actin, desmin, and vimentin will be helpful. Some cases have a degree of morphologic overlap with *classic Hodgkin lymphoma,* and PAX5, which has weak to moderate intensity relative to small resting B cells, helps to resolve this gray zone

Box 15-14. Features of T Cell Lymphoblastic Lymphoma

Should Be Present
Diffuse proliferation of small to intermediate cells with fine, evenly dispersed chromatin

May Be Present
"Starry sky" motif
Coarse or condensed chromatin
Cytoplasmic vacuoles
Cytoplasm granules (rare)
Eosinophilia
Rare CK+ thymic epithelial cells

Should Be Lacking
Atypical cells with twisted floret or "banana bunch" nuclei
Macronucleoli
Lobulated architecture or densely distributed epithelial cells
Nuclear molding

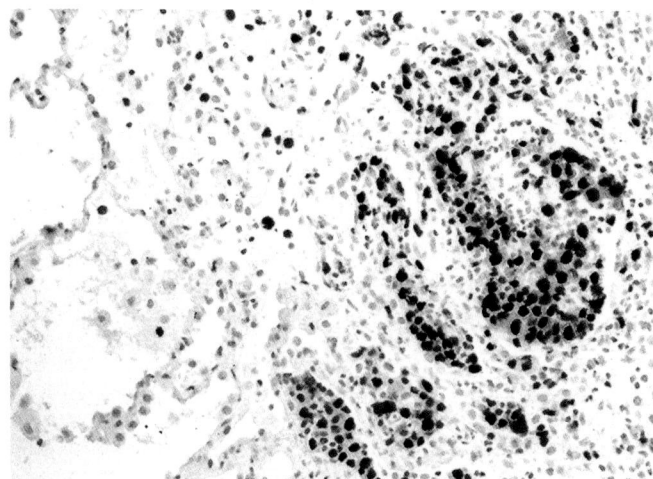

Figure 15-51. TdT stain is the most important stain in evaluating a lymphoid proliferation for the possibility of lymphoblastic lymphoma. In this case, the lymphoma cells distend the alveolar walls (TdT stain).

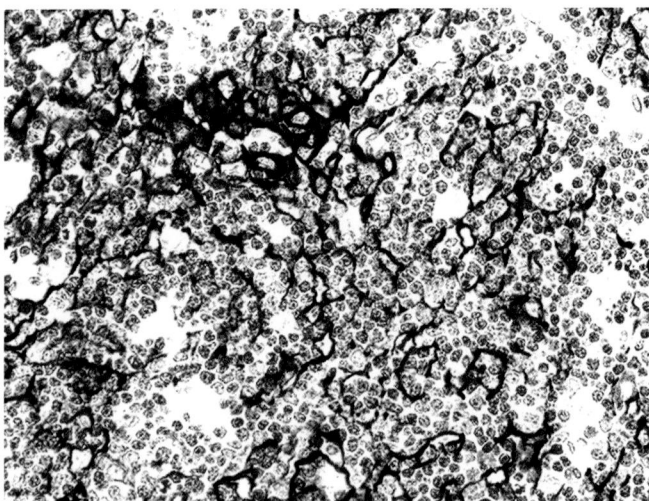

Figure 15-52. The differential diagnosis for blast-like proliferations in the mediastinum includes both lymphoblastic lymphoma and lymphocyte-rich thymoma. The latter, seen here, has abundant cytokeratin-positive thymic epithelial cells that form a network among the thymocytes, whereas lymphoblastic lymphoma is free of this native cell population (cytokeratin stain).

Box 15-15. Features of T Cell Anaplastic Lymphoma

Should Be Present
Hallmark cells (discussed in the text)
CD30 expression (membrane and Golgi)

May Be Present
Reed-Sternberg–like cells
Sinusoidal localization
"Small cell" morphologic features
Inflammatory background or abundant histiocytes
EMA expression

May Be Absent
ALK expression
CD45 expression
CD3 expression

Should Be Lacking
CD20, CD79a, and PAX5 expression
CD15 expression

Box 15-16. Histopathologic Variants of Anaplastic Large Cell Lymphoma

Pleomorphic, 80%
Monomorphic, 5%
Lymphohistiocytic, 5%
Hodgkin-like, 5%
Small cell, <1%
Sarcomatoid, <1%
Neutrophil-rich, 5%
Giant cell–rich, <1%
Signet ring cell, <1%

differential. Exceptional cases of T-ALCL are rich in neutrophils, raising a differential with suppurative inflammation; the presence of CD30+ large cells effectively excludes a reactive process. There is also the potential for morphologic overlap with *true histiocytic malignancies,* which are negative for CD3, CD30, and ALK, and positive for CD68, CD31 (PECAM-1), and CD163. The rare *B lineage ALCL,* which tends to be negative for CD20, enters into differential consideration, but most cases are negative for CD30, a helpful cue, and are positive for CD138 or MUM1.[200] Despite ALK expression, these cases of B lineage ALCL have a more aggressive clinical course than ALK+ T and null cell ALCL, and should therefore be distinguished with the appropriate stains.

Myeloid Proliferations

Extramedullary Myeloid Tumors

Extramedullary myeloid tumors (EMTs; "granulocytic sarcomas") are masses composed of neoplastic (clonal) precursors of the granulocytic lineaege. Cell types include blasts, promyelocytes, and myelocytes, as well as monocytes and precursor monocytoid forms. Myeloid malignancies, such as idiopathic myelofibrosis (agnogenic myeloid metaplasia), may, instead of producing discrete tumefactive masses, produce a radiologic picture similar to that of interstitial lung disease.[201–203] Both the clinical context and the histologic composition are important: In the pediatric setting, most extramedullary accumulations of hematopoiesis are benign and arise because peripheral demand for red cells and neutrophils is in excess of what the marrow space can provide.[204] However, in an adult with an established diagnosis of a chronic myeloproliferative disorder,

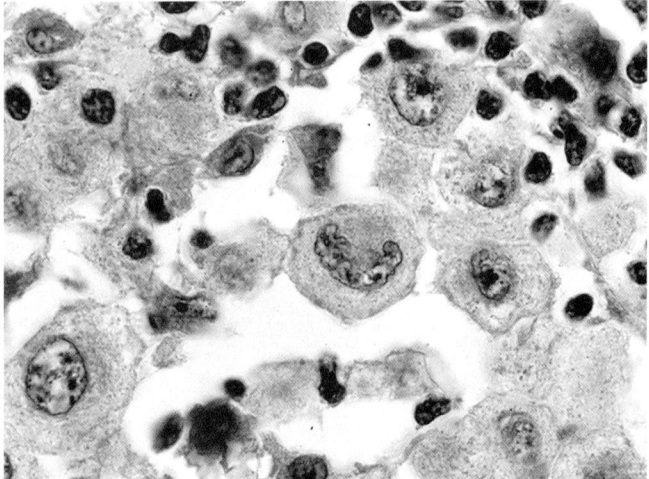

Figure 15-53. Anaplastic large T cell lymphoma can mimic carcinoma, melanoma, or even sarcoma. The cue to the correct diagnosis is often found at the edges of the tumor or within open spaces, where the discohesive nature of the tumor is seen.

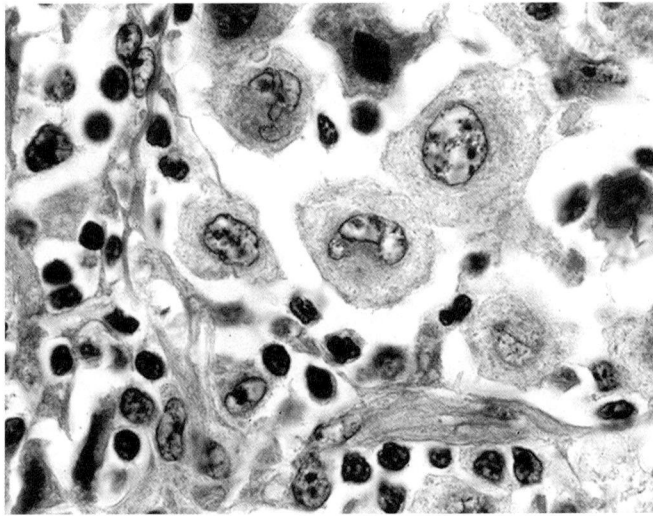

Figure 15-54. The hallmark cells of T cell anaplastic large-cell lymphoma are large and have centrally placed, reniform nuclei.

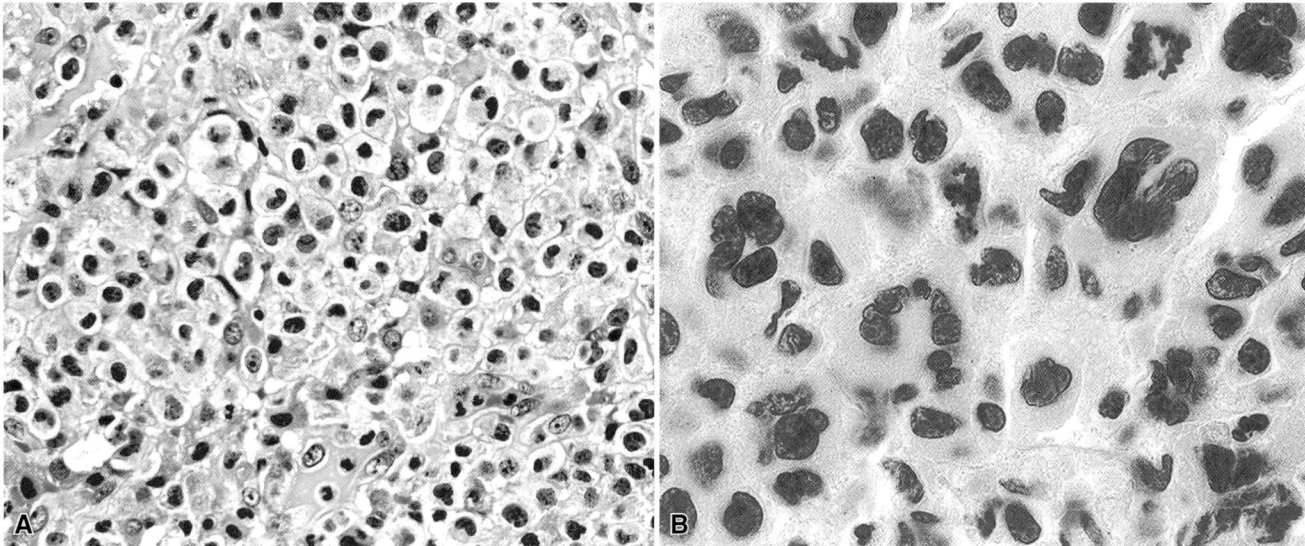

Figure 15-55. Many variants of T cell anaplastic large-cell lymphoma (T-ALCL) have been reported, including a "small-cell variant." The cells are small relative to the usual size for typical ALCL, but are large overall. **A,** Hallmark cells are the key to the diagnosis. **B,** Reed-Sternberg–like cells may also be present in T-ALCL, and although CD30+, they are PAX5+ and ALK–.

the same histologic features suggest a neoplasm and should raise concern that the disease is progressing to a more aggressive phase.[205–207]

By definition, EMTs arise outside the bone marrow. Although they usually develop during the course of systemic myeloproliferative disease, either as a complication or as a transformation from the chronic to the acute phase,[201,202,208] on occasion, they are a presenting sign or the first sign of relapse.[206,207] The underlying condition may be myelodysplasia or acute or chronic leukemia, including hyereosinophilic syndrome/chronic eosinophilic leukemia.[208–215] Therefore, examination of the peripheral blood is a necessary part of the workup (Fig. 15-57). When the peripheral blood is free of blasts but the bone marrow meets the criteria for acute leukemia, the process is often referred to as "aleukemic leukemia."[209,210]

The demographic features of EMTs match those of myeloid malignancy in general. Most patients with both of those conditions are adults, with a median age of 60 years at presentation, simply because nonlymphocytic leukemia is uncommon in pediatric practice. The overall incidence of EMT is estimated at 0.7 cases per million children in the general population per year and 2 cases per million adults per year.[208] Organs that normally harbor hematopoietic cells (bone, spleen, and lymph nodes) are often involved, but a significant proportion of EMTs occur elsewhere—including the lungs.[209,211] Associated pulmonary symptoms and signs include pleural effusions, chest pain, and cough. Gross examination of some excised EMTs shows a greenish color that formed the basis for one of the earliest names for such lesions, "chloroma." The greenish color occurs when these tumors are exposed to room air and is caused by the breakdown of cytoplasmic enzymes, including myeloperoxidase. Otherwise, the gross appearance of EMT is that of a soft tan or off-white lesion, indistinguishable from non-Hodgkin lymphoma.

There is a substantial risk of misdiagnosis of EMTs arising in the lungs and chest structures because they may occur out of the context in which hematologic malignancy is suspected and because the morphologic features and phenotype overlap with more common solid tumors in those sites. Ewing sarcoma, rhabdomyosarcoma, Langerhans cell histiocytosis, neuroendocrine carcinomas, perivascular epithelioid-cell

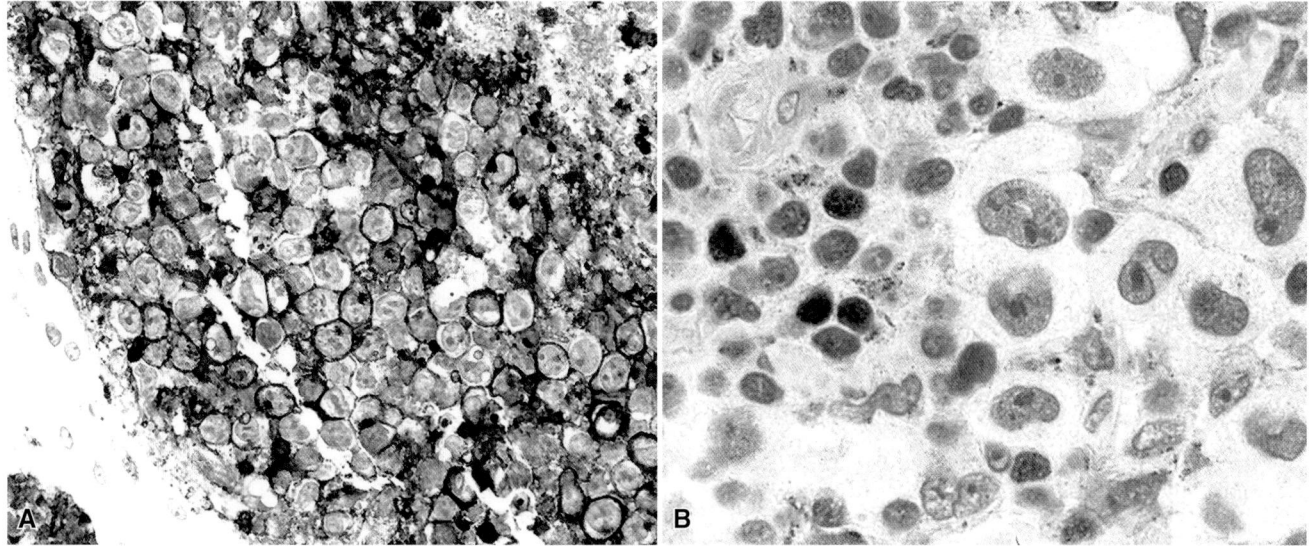

Figure 15-56. A, CD30 expression is the expected result in T cell anaplastic large-cell lymphoma (T-ALCL), but interestingly, it is not seen in B lineage ALK+ ALCL (CD30 stain). **B,** The lesional cells of T-ALCL are negative for PAX5.

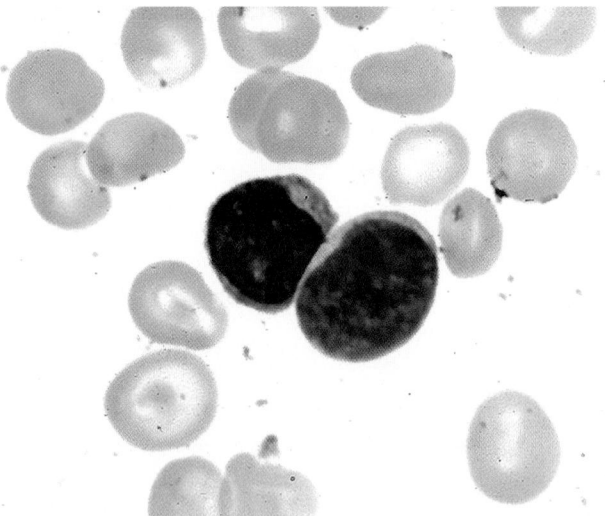

Figure 15-57. Extramedullary myeloid tumor can arise in a variety of settings. Review of the peripheral blood is a necessary part of the workup of such cases. The morphologic features of the blasts can be a helpful guide in ordering immunohistochemical studies.

tumors (PEComas), and multiple myeloma can all show some degree of morphologic overlap. When the process is associated with sclerosis, inflammatory pseudotumor may also enter into consideration.

Histologically, three morphologic patterns of EMT can be recognized: blastic, "intermediate," and differentiated.[208] In the first pattern, sheets of round or polyhedral cells that infiltrate around or sometimes efface the architecture of the native tissue are seen. The neoplastic cells generally have medium or large vesicular nuclei, sometimes with folded nuclear membranes, discernible nucleoli, and amphophilic or basophilic cytoplasm (Fig. 15-58A). In poorly fixed tissue, these subtle features may be concealed by artifact. A few small scattered cells with sparse cytoplasmic granulation are always present. Background inflammatory cells in the blastic form of EMT are banal, usually comprising mature lymphocytes and histiocytes. This "hiatus" between the tumor cells and the reactive elements is a helpful clue to the nonlymphoid nature of the lesion in cases initially believed to be lymphoma. Compared with blastic EMT, the intermediate morphologic features show a balanced mixture of immature (blastic) and maturing cells (promyelocytes, myelocytes, and eosinophilic myelocytes; see Fig. 15-58B). The "differentiated" histologic pattern of EMT may be the easiest to overlook or to interpret as reflecting a non-neoplastic, inflammatory process.

If air-dried touch preparations of fresh tumor have been prepared, histochemical stains for myeloperoxidase, Sudan B black, and alpha naphthyl acetate and other esterases can be performed. The enzymes being assessed are contained in primary myeloid granules; hence, the fewer of those structures that the cells of any given EMT possess, the less likely they are to manifest histochemical positivity. Overall, reactivity with von Leder stain is seen in fewer than 30% of blastic EMTs, 30% to 50% of "intermediate" tumors, and more than 50% of differentiated lesions. On tissue section, the chloroacetate esterase (von Leder) stain can be performed, as well as immunostains for CD45, CD34, CD15, CD68, CD117, CD163, TdT, lysozyme, and myeloperoxidase.[216–219]

Because of the primitive nature of the cells, the target antigens are usually present at low density, and so, on immunostains, CD45 may be very weak. If the process is monocytic in lineage, CD34 is absent. The main problem in this context is that "myeloid" antibodies (CD15, CD117, CD163, lysozyme, and myeloperoxidase) are rarely included in the first-round panels performed to diagnose and classify presumed cases of lymphoma. Weak or apparently negative CD45 results on immunostains are interpreted as excluding hematologic malignancy.

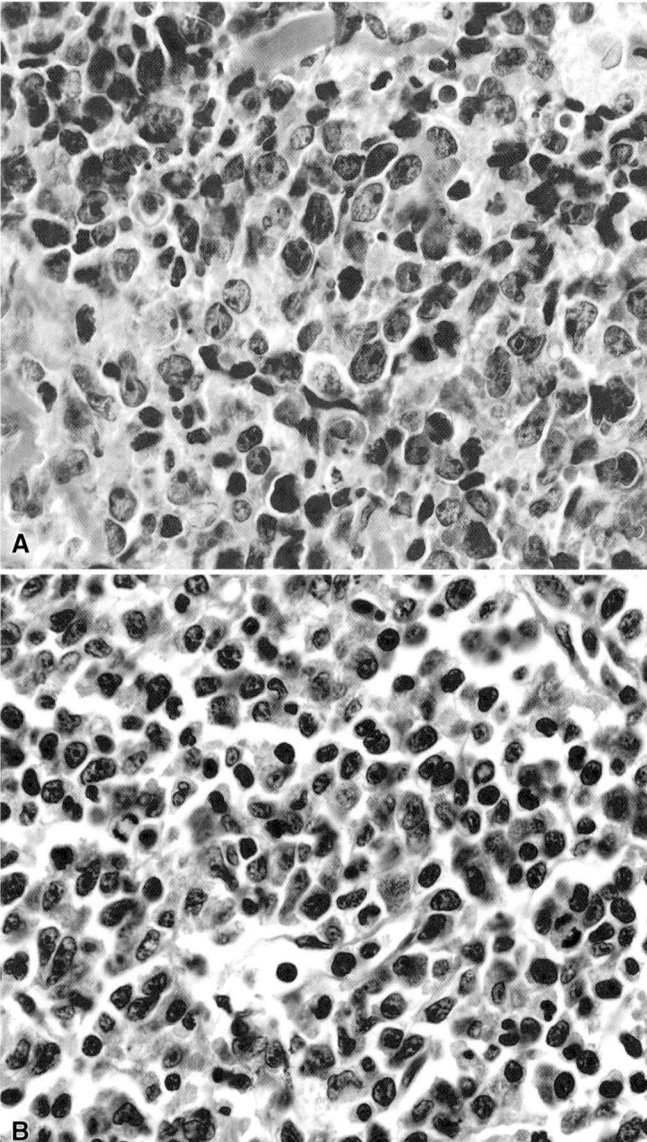

Figure 15-58. In extramedullary sites, it can be difficult to identify myeloid neoplasms. Blast-like cytologic features (**A**) and commingled eosinophilic myelocytes (**B**) are helpful findings.

Therefore, as sensitive as some "myeloid" antibodies may be for the recognition of granulocytic precursors, they are of little practical use if not used. A very helpful study by Goldstein and colleagues[216] proposed that, with permissive morphologic features, a CD45± CD3−, CD20− profile should address the possibiltiy of myeloid neoplasia, especially if the lesional cells are CD43+.

Self-assessment questions related to this chapter can be found online on the Expert Consult site for this title.

References

1. Adam P, Katzenberger T, Seeberger H, et al. A case of diffuse large B-cell lymphoma of plasmablastic type associated with the t(2;5)(p23;q35) chromosome translocation. *Am J Surg Pathol*. 2003;27:1473–1476.
2. Laurent C, Do C, Gascoyne RD, et al. Anaplastic lymphoma kinase-positive diffuse large B-cell lymphoma: a rare clinicopathologic entity with poor prognosis. *J Clin Oncol*. 1:2009;27(25):4211–4216.
3. Gascoyne R, Lamant L, Martin-Subero JI, et al. ALK-positive diffuse large B-cell lymphoma is associated with *Clathrin-ALK* rearrangements: report of six cases. *Blood*. 2003;102:2568–2573.

4. Reichard KK, McKenna RW, Kroft SH. ALK-positive diffuse large B-cell lymphoma: report of four cases and review of the literature. *Mod Pathol*. 2007;20(3):310–319.

5. Swerdlow SH, Campo E, Harris NL, et al., eds. *WHO Classification of Tumours of Haematopoietic and Lymphoid Tissue*. Lyon: IARC; 2008.

6. Dargent JL, Lespagnard L, Sirtaine N, et al. Plasmablastic microlymphoma occurring in human herpesvirus 8 (HHV-8)-positive multicentric Castleman's disease and featuring a follicular growth pattern. *APMIS*. 2007;115(7):869–874.

7. Seliem RM, Griffith RC, Harris NL, et al. HHV-8+, EBV+ multicentric. *Am J Surg Pathol*. 2007;31(9):1439–1445.

8. Ehinger M, Linderoth J, Christensson B, et al. A subset of CD5- diffuse large B-cell lymphomas expresses nuclear cyclin D1 with aberrations at the CCND1 locus. *Am J Clin Pathol*. 2008;129(4):630–638.

9. Le Gouill S, Talmant P, Touzeau C, et al. The clinical presentation and prognosis of diffuse large B-cell lymphoma with t(14;18) and 8q24/c-MYC rearrangement. *Haematologica*. 2007;92(10):1335–1342.

10. Hunt KE, Reichard KK. Diffuse large B-cell lymphoma. *Arch Pathol Lab Med*. 2008;132(1):118–124.

11. Muris JJ, Meijer CJ, Vos W, et al. Immunohistochemical profiling based on bcl-2, CD10 and MUM1 expression improves risk stratification in patients with primary nodal diffuse large B cell lymphoma. *J Pathol*. 2006;208(5):714–723.

12. Haarer CF, Roberts RA, Frutiger YM, et al. Immunohistochemical classification of de novo, transformed, and relapsed diffuse large B-cell lymphoma into germinal center B-cell and non-germinal center B-cell subtypes correlates with gene expression profile and patient survival. *Arch Pathol Lab Med*. 2006;130(12):1819–1824.

13. Lawrie CH, Soneji S, Marafioti T, et al. MicroRNA expression distinguishes between germinal center B cell-like and activated B cell-like subtypes of diffuse large B cell lymphoma. *Int J Cancer*. 2007;121(5):1156–1161.

14. Zhang W, Li L, Li X, et al. Unravelling the hidden heterogeneities of diffuse large B-cell lymphoma based on coupled two-way clustering. *BMC Genomics*. 2007;8:332.

15. Sjo LD, Poulsen CB, Hansen M, et al. Profiling of diffuse large B-cell lymphoma by immunohistochemistry: identification of prognostic subgroups. *Eur J Haematol*. 2007;79(6):501–507.

16. Ponzoni M, Arrigoni G, Doglioni C. New transcription factors in diagnostic hematopathology. *Adv Anat Pathol*. 2007;14:25–35.

17. Ehinger M, Linderoth J, Christensson B, et al. A subset of CD5- diffuse large B-cell lymphomas expresses nuclear cyclin D1 with aberrations at the CCND1 locus. *Am J Clin Pathol*. 2008;129(4):630–638.

18. Mhawech-Fauceglia P, Saxena R, Zhang S, et al. Pax-5 immunoexpression in various types of benign and malignant tumours: a high-throughput tissue microarray analysis. *J Clin Pathol*. 2007;60(6):709–714.

19. Feldman AL, Dogan A. Diagnostic uses of PAX5 in immunohistochemistry. *Adv Anat Pathol*. 2007;14:323–334.

20. Yaziji H, Barry T. Diagnostic immunohistochemistry: what can go wrong? *Adv Anat Pathol*. 2006;13(5):238–246.

21. Higgins RA, Blankenship JE, Kinney MC. Application of immunohistochemistry in the diagnosis of non-Hodgkin and Hodgkin lymphoma. *Arch Pathol Lab Med*. 2008;132:441–461.

22. Garcia CF, Swerdlow SH. Best practices in contemporary diagnostic pathology: panel approach to hematolymphoid proliferations. *Arch Pathol Lab Med*. 2009;133(5):756–765.

23. Chu PG, Arber DA, Weiss LM. Expression of T/NK cell and plasma cell antigens in non-hematopoietic epithelioid neoplasms: an immunohistochemical study of 447 Cases. *Am J Clin Pathol*. 2003;120:64–70.

24. Olsen RJ, Chun-che C, Herrick JL, et al. Acute leukemia immunohistochemistry. *Arch Pathol Lab Med*. 2008;132:462–475.

25. Higgins RA, Blankenship JE, Kinney MC. Application of immunohistochemistry in the diagnosis of non-Hodgkin and Hodgkin lymphoma. *Arch Pathol Lab Med*. 2008;132:441–461.

26. Rao DS, Said JW. Small lymphoid proliferations in extranodal locations. *Arch Pathol Lab Med*. 2007;131(3):383–396.

27. Chuang SS, Ye H, Du MQ, et al. Histopathology and immunohistochemistry in distinguishing Burkitt lymphoma from diffuse large B-cell lymphoma with very high proliferation index and with or without a starry-sky pattern: a comparative study with EBER and FISH. *Am J Clin Pathol*. 2007;128(4):558–564.

28. Yatabe Y, Suzuki R, Tobinai K, et al. Significance of cyclin D1 overexpression for the diagnosis of mantle cell lymphoma: a clinicopathologic comparison of cyclin D1-positive MCL and cyclin D1-negative MCL-like B-cell lymphoma. *Blood*. 2000;95:2253–2261.

29. Ehinger M, Linderoth J, Christensson B, et al. A subset of CD5- diffuse large B-cell lymphomas expresses nuclear cyclin D1 with aberrations at the CCND1 locus. *Am J Clin Pathol*. 2008;129(4):630–638.

30. Amin HM, Lai R. Pathobiology of ALK+ anaplastic large-cell lymphoma. *Blood*. 2007;110(7):2259–2267.

31. Sica G, Vazquez MF, Altorki N, et al. PAX-5 expression in pulmonary neuroendocrine neoplasms: its usefulness in surgical and fine-needle aspiration biopsy specimens. *Am J Clin Pathol*. 2008;129(4):556–562.

32. Torlakovic E, Slipicevic A, Robinson C, et al. Pax-5 expression in nonhematopoietic tissues. *Am J Clin Pathol*. 2006;126(5):798–804.

33. Chu PG, Loera S, Huang Q Weiss LM. Lineage determination of CD20- B-cell neoplasms: an immunohistochemical study. *Am J Clin Pathol*. 2006;126(4):534–544.

34. Feldman AL, Dogan A. Diagnostic uses of Pax5 immunohistochemistry. *Adv Anat Pathol*. 2007;14(5):323–334.

35. Kaleem Z. Flow cytometric analysis of lymphomas: current status and usefulness. *Arch Pathol Lab Med*. 2006;130(12):1850–1858.

36. Kurtin PJ. How do you distinguish benign from malignant extranodal small B cell proliferations? *Am J Clin Pathol*. 1999;111(suppl 1):S119–S126.

37. Jennings CD, Foon KA. Recent advances in flow cytometry: application to the diagnosis of hematologic malignancy. *Blood*. 1997;90:2863–2892.

38. Beck RC, Stahl S, O'Keefe CL, et al. Detection of mature T-cell leukemias by flow cytometry antibodies using anti–T-cell receptor V-beta. *Am J Clin Pathol*. 2003;120:785–794.

39. Delgado J, Matutes E, Morilla AM, et al. Diagnostic significance of CD20 and FMC7 expression in B cell disorders. *Am J Clin Pathol*. 2003;120:754–759.

40. Zaer FS, Brayland RC, Aanxer DS, et al. Multi-parametric flow cytometry in the diagnosis and characterization of low grade pulmonary mucosa-associated lymphoid tissue lymphomas. *Mod Pathol*. 1998;11:525–532.

41. Onciu M, Berrak SG, Medeiros LJ, et al. Discrepancies in the immunophenotype of lymphoma cells in samples obtained simultaneously from different anatomic sites. *Am J Clin Pathol*. 2002;117:644–650.

42. Ho AK, Hill S, Preobrazhensky SN, et al. Small B cell neoplasms with typical mantle cell lymphoma phenotype, often include chronic lymphocytic leukemias. *Am J Clin Pathol*. 2009;131:27–32.

43. Joao C, Farinha P, da Silva MG, et al. Cytogenetic abnormalities in MALT lymphomas and their precursor lesions from different organs. A fluorescence *in situ* hybridization (FISH) study. *Histopathology*. 2007;50(2):217–224.

44. Remstein ED, Dogan A, Einerson RR, et al. The incidence and anatomic site specificity of chromosomal translocations in primary extranodal marginal zone B-cell lymphoma of mucosa-associated lymphoid tissue (MALT lymphoma) in North America. *Am J Surg Pathol*. 2006;30(12):1546–1553.

45. Remstein ED, Kurtin PJ, Einerson RR, et al. Primary pulmonary MALT lymphomas show frequent and heterogeneous cytogenetic abnormalities, including aneuploidy and translocations involving API2 and MALT1 and IGH and MALT1. *Leukemia*. 2004;18(1):156–160.

46. Einerson RR, Kurtin PJ, Dayharsh GA, et al. FISH is superior to PCR in detecting t(14;18) (q32;q21)-IgH/bcl-2 in follicular lymphoma using paraffin-embedded tissue samples. *Am J Clin Pathol*. 2005;124(3):421–429.

47. Ye H, Remstein ED, Bacon CM, et al. Chromosomal translocations involving BCL6 in MALT lymphoma. *Haematologica*. 2008;93(1):145–146.

48. Lin P, Medeiros LJ. High-grade B-cell lymphoma/leukemia associated with t(14;18) and 8q24/MYC rearrangement: a neoplasm of germinal center immunophenotype with poor prognosis. *Haematologica*. 2007;92(10):1297–1301.

49. Nomura K, Yoshino T, Nakamura S, et al. Detection of t(11;18)(q21;q21) in marginal zone lymphoma of mucosa-associated lymphocytic tissue type on paraffin-embedded tissue sections by using fluorescence *in situ* hybridization. *Cancer Genet Cytogenet*. 2003;140(1):49–54.

50. Stachurski D, Miron PM, Al-Homsi S, et al. Anaplastic lymphoma kinase-positive diffuse large B-cell lymphoma with a complex karyotype and cryptic 3′ ALK gene insertion to chromosome 4 q22–24. *Hum Pathol*. 2007;38(6):940–945.

51. Morris SW, Xue L, Ma Z, Kinney MC. Alk+ CD30+ lymphomas: a distinct molecular genetic subtype of non-Hodgkin's lymphoma. *Br J Haematol*. 2001;113(2):275 295.

52. Muller-Hermelink HK. Genetic and molecular genetic studies in the diagnosis of B cell lymphomas: marginal zone lymphomas. *Hum Pathol*. 2003;34(4):336–340.

53. Reddy A, Lyall EG, Crawford DH. Epstein-Barr virus and lymphoid interstitial pneumonitis: an association revisited. *Pediatr Infect Dis J*. 1998;17:82–83 1998.

54. Hunt JL. Molecular pathology in anatomic pathology practice: a review of basic principles. *Arch Pathol Lab Med*. 2008;132:248–260.

55. Nicholson AG, Wotherspoon AC, Diss C, et al. Pulmonary B cell non-Hodgkin's lymphomas. The value of immunohistochemistry and gene analysis in diagnosis. *Histopathology*. 1995;26:395–403.

56. Allen TC, Cagle PT, Popper HH. Basic concepts of molecular pathology. *Arch Pathol Lab Med*. 2008;132:1551–1556.

57. Tashiro K, Ohshima K, Suzumiya J, et al. Clonality of primary pulmonary lymphoproliferative disorders; using in situ hybridization and polymerase chain reaction for immunoglobulin. *Leuk Lymphoma*. 1999;36(1–2):157–167.

58. Hewitt SM, Lewis FA, Cao Y, et al. Tissue handling and specimen preparation in surgical pathology: issues concerning the recovery of nucleic acids from formalin-fixed, paraffin-embedded tissue. *Arch Pathol Lab Med*. 2008;132:1929–1935.

59. Kurosu K, Yumoto N, Mikata A, et al. Monoclonality of B-cell lineage in primary pulmonary lymphoma demonstrated by immunoglobulin heavy chain gene sequence analysis of histologically non-definitive transbronchial biopsy specimens. *J Pathol*. 1996;178(3):316–322.

60. Swerdlow SH. Genetic and molecular genetic studies in the diagnosis of atypical lymphoid hyperplasias versus lymphoma. *Hum Pathol*. 2003;34(4):346–351.

61. Zhang S, Abreo F, Lowery-Nordberg M, et al. The role of fluorescence in situ hybridization and polymerase chain reaction in the diagnosis and classification of lymphoproliferative disorders on fine-needle aspiration. *Cancer Cytopathol*. 2010;118:105–112.

62. Muller-Hermelink HK. Genetic and molecular genetic studies in the diagnosis of B cell lymphomas: marginal zone lymphomas. *Hum Pathol*. 2003;34(4):336–340.

63. Nathwani BN, Sasu SJ, Ahsanuddin AN, et al. The critical role of histology in an era of genomics and proteomics: a commentary and reflection. *Adv Anat Pathol*. 2007;14(6):375–400.

64. Colby TV, Leslie KO, Yousem SA. Lungs. In: Mills SE, ed. *Histology for Pathologists*. Philadelphia: Lippincott Williams and Wilkins; 2007:51–61.

65. Harris NL. Extranodal lymphoid infiltrates and mucosa-associated lymphoid tissue: a unifying concept. *Am J Surg Pathol*. 1991;15:879–884.

66. Douglas KM, Raza K, Stevens R, et al. Bronchial MALT lymphoma in longstanding rheumatoid arthritis. *Rheumatology*. 2005;44(5):687–689.

67. Koss MN. Malignant and benign lymphoid lesions in the lung. *Ann Diagn Pathol*. 2004;8:167–187.

68. Begueret H, Vergier B, Parrens M, et al. Primary lung small B-cell lymphoma versus lymphoid hyperplasia: evaluation of diagnostic criteria in 26 Cases. *Am J Surg Pathol*. 2002;26(1):76–81.

69. Nicholson AG, Wotherspoon AC, Diss TC, et al. Reactive pulmonary lymphoid disorders. *Histopathology*. 1995;26:405–412.

70. Yousem SA, Colby TV, Carrington CB. Follicular bronchitis—bronchiolitis. *Hum Pathol*. 1985;16:700–706.

71. Romero S, Barroso E, Gil J, et al. Follicular bronchiolitis: clinical and pathologic findings in six patients. *Lung*. 2003;181(6):309–319.

72. Kinnane BT, Mansell AL, Zwerdling RG, et al. Follicular bronchitis in the pediatric population. *Chest*. 1993;104:1183–1186.

73. Exley CM, Suvarna SK, Matthews S. Follicular bronchiolitis as a presentation of HIV. *Clin Radiol*. 2006;61(8):710–713.

74. Lee HK, Kim DS, Yoo B, et al. Histopathologic pattern and clinical features of rheumatoid arthritis-associated interstitial lung disease. *Chest*. 2005;127(6):2019–2027.

75. Couture C, Colby TV. Histopathology of bronchiolar disorders. *Semin Respir Crit Care Med*. 2003;24(5):489–498.

76. Ryu JH. Classification and approach to bronchiolar diseases. *Curr Opin Pulm Med*. 2006;12(2):145–151.

77. Visscher DW, Myers JL. Bronchiolitis: the pathologist's perspective. *Proc Am Thorac Soc*. 2006;3(1):41–47.

78. Collard HR, Cool CD, Leslie KO, et al. Organizing pneumonia and lymphoplasmacytic inflammation predict treatment response in idiopathic pulmonary fibrosis. *Histopathology*. 2007;50(2):258–265.

79. Tansey D, Wells AU, Colby TV, et al. Variations in histological patterns of interstitial pneumonia between connective tissue disorders and their relationship to prognosis. *Histopathology*. 2004;44(6):585–596.

80. Abbondanzo SL, Rush W, Bijwaard KE, Koss MN. Nodular lymphoid hyperplasia of the lung: clinicopathologic study of 14 cases. *Am J Surg Pathol*. 2000;24:587–597.

81. Sakurai H, Hada M, Oyama T. Nodular lymphoid hyperplasia of the lung: a very rare disease entity. *Ann Thorac Surg*. 2007;83(6):2197–2199.

82. Begueret H, Vergier B, Parrens M, et al. Primary lung small cell lymphoma versus lymphoid hyperplasia: evaluation of diagnostic criteria in 26 cases. *Am J Surg Pathol*. 2002;26:76–81.

83. Kobzik L. Benign pulmonary lesions that may be misdiagnosed as malignant. *Semin Diagn Pathol*. 1990;7:129–138.

84. Isaacson P, Wotherspoon A, Pan L. Follicular colonization in B-cell lymphoma of mucosa-associated lymphoid tissue. *Am J Surg Pathol*. 1991;15:819–828.

85. Ito I, Nagai S, Kitaichi M, et al. Pulmonary manifestations of primary Sjogren's syndrome: a clinical, radiological and pathologic study. *Am J Respir Crit Care Med*. 2005;171:632–638.

86. Joshi VV, Oleske JM, Minnefor AB, et al. Pathologic pulmonary findings in children with the acquired immunodeficiency syndrome: a study of ten cases. *Hum Pathol*. 1985;16:241–246.

87. Joshi VV, Gagnon GA, Chadwick EG, et al. The spectrum of mucosa associated lymphoid tissue lesions in pediatric patients infected with HIV: A clinicopathologic study of six cases. *Am J Clin Pathol*. 1997;107:592–600.

88. Sacco O, Fregonese B, Picco P, et al. Common variable immunodeficiency presenting in a girl as lung infiltrates and mediastinal adenopathies leading to severe "superior vena cava" syndrome. *Eur Respir J*. 1996;9(9):1958–1961.

89. Swigris JJ, Berry GJ, Raffin TA, et al. Lymphoid interstitial pneumonia: a narrative review. *Chest*. 2002;122:2150–2164.

90. Fishback N, Koss M. Update on lymphoid interstitial pneumonitis. *Curr Opin Pulm Med*. 1996;2:429–433.

91. Cha SI, Fessler MB, Cool CD, et al. Lymphoid interstitial pneumonia: clinical features, associations and prognosis. *Eur Respir J*. 2006;28(2):364–369.

92. Silva CI, Flint JD, Levy RD, Muller NL. Diffuse lung cysts in lymphoid interstitial pneumonia: high-resolution CT and pathologic findings. *J Thorac Imaging*. 2006;21(3):241–244.

93. Meyers JL, Peiper SC, Katzenstein A-L. Pulmonary involvement in infectious mononucleosis: histopathologic features and detection of Epstein-Barr virus related DNA sequences. *Mod Pathol*. 1989;2:444–448.

94. Marzouk K, Corate L, Saleh S, Sharma OP. Epstein-Barr-virus-induced interstitial lung disease. *Curr Opin Pulm Med*. 2005;11(5):456–460.

95. Castleman B, Iverson L, Menendez P. Localized mediastinal lymph node hyperplasia resembling thymoma. *Cancer*. 1956;9:822–930.

96. Gupta NK, Torigian DA, Gefter WB, et al. Mediastinal Castleman disease mimicking mediastinal pulmonary sequestration. *J Thorac Imaging*. 2005;20(3):229–232 Symposium: Multislice CT Part I.

97. Pham TT, Harrell JH, Herndier B, Yi ES. Endotracheal hyaline vascular Castleman disease: a case report. *Chest*. 2007;131(2):590–592.

98. Ng SH, Ko SF, Lin JW, et al. Paracardiac pleural Castleman disease: radiographic and MR findings. *Br J Radiol*. 2004;77(917):433–435.

99. Cronin DMP, Warnke RA. Castleman disease: an update on classification and the spectrum of associated pulesions. *Adv Anat Pathol*. 2009;16:236–246.

100. Weiss LM. Castleman Disease. In: *Lymph Nodes*. New York: Cambridge University Press; 2008:25–32.

101. Harris NL, Bhan AK. "Plasmacytoid T cells" in Castleman's disease. Immunohistologic phenotype. *Am J Surg Pathol*. 1987;11:109–113.

102. Menke DM, Tiemann M, Camoriano JK, et al. Diagnosis of Castleman's disease by identification of an immunophenotypically aberrant population of mantle zone B lymphocytes in paraffin embedded lymph node biopsies. *Am J Clin Pathol*. 1996;105(3):268–276.

103. Zarate-Osorno A, Medeiros LJ, Danon AD, Neiman RS. Hodgkin's disease with co-existent Castleman-like histologic features: a report of 3 cases. *Arch Pathol Lab Med*. 1994;118(3):270–274.

104. Nonaka D, Rodriguez J, Rollo JL, Rosai J. Undifferentiated large cell carcinoma of the thymus associated with Castleman disease-like reaction a distinctive type of thymic neoplasm characterized by an indolent behavior. *Am J Surg Pathol*. 2005;29:490–495.

105. Casper C. The aetiology and management of Castleman disease at 50 years: translating pathophysiology to patient care. *Br J Haematol*. 2005;129(1):3–17.

106. Keller AR, Hochholzer L, Castleman B. Hyaline vascular and plasma cell types of giant lymph node hyperplasia of the mediastinum and other locations. *Cancer*. 1972;29(3):670–683.

107. Mandler RN, Kerrigan DP, Smart J, et al. Castleman's disease in POEMS syndrome with elevated interleukin-6. *Cancer*. 1992;69:2697–2703.

108. Guihot A, Couderc LJ, Agbalika F, et al. Pulmonary manifestations of multicentric Castleman's disease in HIV infection: a clinical, biological and radiological study. *Eur Respir J*. 2005;26(1):118–125.

109. Dispenzieri A, Kyle RA, Lacy MQ, et al. POEMS syndrome: definitions and long-term outcome. *Blood*. 2003;101:2496–2506.

110. Seliem RM, Griffith RC, Harris NL, et al. HHV-8+, EBV+ multicentric plasmablastic microlymphoma in an HIV+ man: the spectrum of HHV-8+ lymphoproliferative disorders expands. *Am J Surg Pathol*. 2007;31(9):1439–1445.

111. Amin HM, Medeiros LJ, Manning JT, et al. Dissolution of the lymphoid follicle is a feature of the HHV8+ variant of plasma cell Castleman's disease. *Am J Surg Pathol*. 2003;27:91–100.

112. Dham A, Peterson BA. Castleman disease. *Curr Opin Hematol*. 2007;14(4):354–359.

113. Li C-F, Ye H, Liu H, et al. Fatal HHV-8-associated hemophagocytic syndrome in an HIV-negative immunocompetent patient with plasmablastic variant of multicentric Castleman disease (plasmablastic microlymphoma). *Am J Surg Pathol*. 2006;30(1):123–127.

114. Herrada J, Cabanillas F, Rice L, et al. The clinical behavior of localized and multicentric Castleman disease. *Ann Intern Med*. 1998;128:657–662.

115. Graham BB, Mathisen DJ, Mark EJ, Takvorian RW. Primary pulmonary lymphoma. *Ann Thorac Surg*. 2005;80(4):1248–1253.

116. Habermann TM, Ryu JH, Inwards DJ, Kurtin PJ. Primary pulmonary lymphoma. *Semin Oncol*. 1999;26:307–315.

117. L'Hoste RJ, Fillipa DA, Leiberman PH, Bretsky S. Primary pulmonary lymphomas. *Cancer*. 1984;54:1397–1406.

118. Rush WL, Andriko JA, Taubenberger JK, et al. Primary anaplastic large cell lymphoma of the lung: clinicopathologic study of five patients. *Mod Pathol*. 2000;13:1285–1292.

119. Koss MN. Malignant and benign lymphoid lesions of the lung. *Ann Diagn Pathol*. 2004;8(3):167–187.

120. Zinzani PL, Magagnoli M, Ascani S, et al. Nongastrointestinal mucosa-associated lymphoid tissue (MALT) lymphomas: clinical and therapeutic features of 24 localized patients. *Ann Oncol*. 1997;8:883–886.

121. Kurtin PJ, Myers JL, Adlakha H, et al. Pathologic and clinical features of primary pulmonary extranodal marginal zone B-cell lymphoma of MALT type. *Am J Surg Pathol*. 2001;25(8):997–1008.

122. Ferreri AJ, Zucca E. Marginal-zone lymphoma. *Crit Rev Oncol Hematol*. 2007;63(3):245–256.

123. Arkenau HT, Gordon C, Cunningham D, et al. Mucosa associated lymphoid tissue lymphoma of the lung: the Royal Marsden Hospital experience. *Leuk Lymphoma*. 2007;48(3):547–550.

124. Remstein ED, Dogan A, Einerson RR, et al. The incidence and anatomic site specificity of chromosomal translocations in primary extranodal marginal zone B-cell lymphoma of mucosa-associated lymphoid tissue (MALT lymphoma) in North America. *Am J Surg Pathol*. 2006;30(12):1546–1553.

125. O'Donnell PG, Jackson SA, Tung KT, et al. Radiological appearances of lymphomas arising from mucosa-associated lymphoid tissue (MALT) in the lung. *Clin Radiol*. 1998;53:258–263.

126. Mitchell A, Meunier C, Ouellette D, Colby T. Extranodal marginal zone lymphoma of mucosa-associated lymphoid tissue with initial presentation in the pleura. *Chest*. 2006;129:791–794.

127. McCluggage WG, McManus K, Qureshi R, et al. Low-grade B-cell lymphoma of mucosa-associated lymphoid tissue (MALT) of thymus. *Hum Pathol*. 2000;31(2):255–259.

128. Burke JS. Are there site-specific differences among the MALT lymphomas—morphologic, clinical? *Am J Clin Pathol*. 1999;111(1 suppl 1):S133–S143.

129. Ferry JA. Extranodal lymphomas. *Arch Pathol Lab Med*. 2008;132:565–578.

130. Bacon CM, Du MQ, Dogan A. Mucosa-associated lymphoid tissue (MALT) lymphoma: a practical guide for pathologists. *J Clin Pathol*. 2007;60(4):361–372.

131. Woehrer S, Streubel B, Chott A, et al. Transformation of MALT lymphoma to pure plasma cell histology following treatment with the anti-CD20 antibody rituximab. *Leuk Lymphoma*. 2005;46(11):1645–1649.

132. Fairweather PM, Williamson R, Tsikleas G. Pulmonary extranodal marginal zone lymphoma with massive crystal storing histiocytosis. *Am J Surg Pathol*. 2006;30(2):262–267.

133. Ionescu DN, Pierson DM, Qing G, et al. Pulmonary crystal-storing histiocytoma. *Arch Pathol Lab Med*. 2005;129(9):1159–1163.

134. Prasad ML, Charney DA, Sarlin J, et al. Pulmonary immunocytoma with massive crystal storing histiocytosis: a case report with review of the literature. *Am J Surg Pathol*. 1998;22:1148–1153.

135. Jones D, Renshaw AA. Recurrent crystal storing histiocytosis of the lung in a patient without a clonal lymphoproliferative disorder. *Arch Pathol Lab Med*. 1996;120:978–980.

136. Lim JK, Lacy MQ, Kurtin PJ, et al. Pulmonary marginal zone lymphoma of MALT type as a cause of localised pulmonary amyloidosis. *J Clin Pathol*. 2001;54(8):642–646.

137. Khoor A, Myers JL, Tazelaar HD, Kurtin PJ. Amyloid-like pulmonary nodules, including localized light-chain deposition: clinicopathologic analysis of three cases. *Am J Clin Pathol*. 2004;121:200–204.

138. Satani T, Yokose T, Kaburagi T, et al. Amyloid deposition in primary pulmonary marginal zone B-cell lymphoma of mucosa-associated lymphoid tissue. *Pathol Int*. 2007;57(11):746–750.

139. Dacic S, Colby TV, Yousem SA. Nodular amyloidoma and primary pulmonary lymphoma with amyloid production: a differential diagnostic problem. *Mod Pathol*. 2000;13(9):934–940.

140. Bhargava P, Rushin JM, Rusnock EJ, et al. Pulmonary light chain deposition disease: report of five cases and review of the literature. *Am J Surg Pathol*. 2007;31:267–276.

141. Jourdan F, Molina TJ, Le Tourneau A, et al. Florid marginal zone differentiation in follicular lymphoma mimicking marginal zone lymphoma of MALT type in the lung. *Histopathology*. 2006;49:426–445.

142. Zettl A, Rudiger T, Marx A, et al. Composite marginal zone B-cell lymphoma and classical Hodgkin's lymphoma: a clinicopathological study of 12 cases. *Histopathology*. 2005;46(2):217–228.

143. Fiche M, Capron F, Berger F, et al. Primary pulmonary non-Hodgkin's lymphomas. *Histopathology*. 1995;26:529–537.

144. Habermann TM, Ryu JH, Inwards DJ, Kurtin PJ. Primary pulmonary lymphoma. *Semin Oncol*. 1999;26:307–315.

145. Lim MS, Beaty M, Sorbara L, et al. T-cell/histiocyte-rich large B-cell lymphoma: a heterogeneous entity with derivation from germinal center B cells. *Am J Surg Pathol*. 2002;26(11):1458–1466.

146. Colomo L, Loong F, Rives S, et al. Diffuse large B-cell lymphomas with plasmablastic differentiation represent a heterogeneous group of disease entities. *Am J Surg Pathol*. 2004;28(6):736–747.

147. Yamaguchi M, Seto M, Okamoto M, et al. De novo CD5+ diffuse large B cell lymphoma: a clinicopathological study of 109 patients. *Blood*. 2002;99:815–821.

148. Oyama T, Ichimura K, Suzuki R, et al. Senile EBV+ B-cell lymphoproliferative disorders: a clinicopathological study of 22 patients. *Am J Surg Pathol*. 2003;27(1):16–26.

149. Nakamura S, Jaffe ES, Swerdlow SH. EBV positive diffuse large B-cell lymphoma of the elderly. In: Swerdlow SH, Campo E, Harris NL, et al., eds. *WHO Classification of Tumours of Haematopoietic and Lymphoid Tissues*, 4th ed. Lyon: IARC Press; 2008:243–244.

150. Calaminici M, Piper K, Lee AM, Norton AJ. CD23 expression in mediastinal large B-cell lymphomas. *Histopathology*. 2004;45:619–624.

151. Pileri SA, Gaidano G, Zintzani PL, et al. Primary mediastinal B-cell lymphoma: high frequency of BCL-6 mutations and consistent expression of the transcription factors OCT-2, BOB.1, and PU.1 in the absence of immunoglobulins. *Am J Pathol*. 2003;162(1):243–253.

152. Nicholson AG, Wotherspoon AC, Diss TC, et al. Lymphomatoid granulomatosis: evidence that some cases represent Epstein–Barr virus-associated B-cell lymphoma. *Histopathology*. 1996;29:317–324.

153. Meyers JL, Kurtin PJ, Katzenstein ALA, et al. Lymphomatoid granulomatosis: evidence of immunophenotypic diversity and relationship to Epstein–Barr virus infection. *Am J Surg Pathol*. 1995;19:1300–1312.

154. Guinee DG, Perkins SL, Travis WD, et al. Proliferation and cellular phenotype in lymphomatoid granulomatosis: implications of a higher proliferation index in B cells. *Am J Surg Pathol*. 1998;22:1093–1100.

155. Haque AK, Myers JL, Hudnall SD, et al. Pulmonary lymphomatoid granulomatosis in acquired immunodeficiency syndrome: lesions with Epstein-Barr virus infection. *Mod Pathol*. 1998;11(4):347–356.

156. Koss MN, Hochholzer L, Langloss JM, et al. Lymphomatoid granulomatosis: a clinicopathologic and immunopathologic study of 42 patients. *Pathology*. 1986;18:283–288.

157. Hochberg EP, Gilman MD, Hasserjian RP. Case 17–2006: A 34-year-old man with cavitary lung lesions. *N Engl J Med*. 2006;354:2485–2493.

158. Morice WG, Kurtin PJ, Myers JL. Expression of cytolytic lymphocyte-associated antigens in pulmonary lymphomatoid granulomatosis. *Am J Clin Pathol*. 2002;118(3):391–398.

159. Ng S-B, Khoury JD. Epstein-Barr virus in lymphoproliferative processes: an update for the diagnostic pathologist. *Adv Anat Pathol*. 2009;16:40–55.

160. Yousem SA, Weis LM, Colby TV. Primary pulmonary Hodgkin's disease: a clinicopathologic study of 15 cases. *Cancer*. 1986;57:1217–1224.

161. Radin AI. Primary pulmonary Hodgkin's disease. *Cancer*. 1990;65:550–563.

162. Harris NL. Hodgkin's lymphomas: classification, diagnosis, and grading. *Semin Hematol*. 1999;36:220–232.

163. Pileri S, Ascani S, Leoncini L, et al. Hodgkin's lymphoma: the pathologist's viewpoint. *J Clin Pathol*. 2002;55:162–176.

164. Browne P, Petrosyan K, Hernandez A, Chan JA. The B-cell transcription factors BSAP, Oct-2, and BOB.1 and the pan-B-cell markers CD20, CD22, and CD79a are useful in the differential diagnosis of classic Hodgkin lymphoma. *Am J Clin Pathol*. 2003;120:767–777.

165. Calvo KR, Traverse-Glehen A, Pittaluga S, Jaffe ES. Molecular profiling provides evidence of primary mediastinal large B cell lymphoma as a distinct entity related to classic Hodgkin lymphoma: implications for mediastinal gray zone lymphomas as an intermediate form of B-cell Lymphoma. *Adv Anat Pathol*. 11(5):227–238.

166. Uherova P, Valdez R, Ross CW, et al. Nodular lymphocyte predominant Hodgkin lymphoma. An immunophenotypic reappraisal based on a single-institution experience. *Am J Clin Pathol*. 2003;119(2):192–198.

167. Brousset P, Chittal SM, Schlafer D, Delsol G. T cell rich B cell large cell lymphoma in the lung. *Histopathology*. 1995;26:371–373.

168. Chilosi M, Zinzani PL, Poletti V. Lymphoproliferative lung disorders. *Semin Respir Crit Care Med*. 2005;26(5):490–501.

169. Ho AK, Hill S, Preobrazhensk SN, et al. Small B-cell neoplasms with typical mantle cell lymphoma immunophenotypes often include chronic lymphocytic leukemias. *Am J Clin Pathol*. 2009;131:27–32.

170. Swerdlow SH, Williams ME. From centrocytic to mantle cell lymphoma: a clinicopathologic and molecular review of 3 decades. *Hum Pathol*. 2002;33:7–20.

171. Gandhi MK, Marcus RE. Follicular lymphoma: time for a re-think? *Blood Rev*. 2005;19:165–178.

172. Hummel M, Bentink S, Berger H, et al. for the Molecular Mechanisms in Malignant Lymphomas Network Project of the Deutsche Krebshilfe. A biologic definition of Burkitt's lymphoma from transcriptional and genomic profiling. *N Engl J Med*. 2006;354:2419–2430.

173. Leoncini L, Delsol G, Gascoyne RD, et al. Aggressive B-cell lymphomas: a review based on the workshop of the XI Meeting of the European Association for Haematopathology. *Histopathology*. 2005;46:241–255.

174. McClure RF, Remstein ED, Macon WR, et al. Adult B-cell lymphomas with Burkitt-like morphology are phenotypically and genotypically heterogeneous with aggressive clinical behavior. *Am J Surg Pathol*. 2005;29(12):1652–1660.

175. Keller CE, Nandula S, Fisher J, et al. The spectrum of B-cell non-Hodgkin lymphomas with dual *IgH-BCL2* and *BCL6* translocations. *Am J Clin Pathol*. 2008;130:193–201.

176. Hussong JW, Perkins SL, Schnitzer B, et al. Extramedullary plasmacytoma. A form of marginal zone cell lymphoma? *Am J Clin Pathol*. 1999;111:111–116.

177. Koss MN, Hochholzer L, Moran CA, Frizzera G. Pulmonary plasmacytomas: a clinicopathologic and immunohistochemical study of five cases. *Ann Diagn Pathol*. 1998;2(1):1–11.

178. Wise JN, Schaefer RF, Read RC. Primary pulmonary plasmacytoma: a case report. *Chest*. 2001;120:1405–1407.

179. Banerjee SS, Verma S, Shanks JH. Morphological variants of plasma cell tumours. *Histopathology*. 2004;44:2–8.

180. Niitsu N, Kohri M, Hayama M, et al. Primary pulmonary plasmacytoma involving bilateral lungs and marked hypergammaglobulinemia: differentiation from extranodal marginal zone B-cell lymphoma of mucosa-associated lymphoid tissue. *Leuk Res*. 2005;29(11):1361–1364.

181. Chetty R, Close PM, Timme AH, et al. Primary biphasic lymphoplasmacytic lymphoma of the lung. A mucosa associated lymphoid tissue lymphoma with compartmentalization of plasma cells in the lung and lymph node. *Cancer*. 1992;69:1124–1129.

182. Lin P, Medeiros LJ. Lymphoplasmacytic lymphoma/Waldenstrom macroglobulinemia: an evolving concept. *Adv Anat Pathol*. 2005;12:246–255.

183. Kazzaz B, Dewar A, Corrin B. An unusual pulmonary plasmacytoma. *Histopathology*. 1992;21:285–287.

184. Randhawa PS, Yousem SA, Paradis IL, et al. The clinical spectrum, pathology and clonal analysis of Epstein–Barr virus-associated lymphoproliferative disorders in heart–lung transplant recipients. *Am J Clin Pathol*. 1989;92:177–185.

185. Harris NL, Ferry JA, Swerdlow SH. Post-transplant lymphoproliferative disorders: summary of Society for Hematopathology workshop. *Semin Diagn Pathol*. 1997;14:8–14.

186. Swerdlow SH. Post-transplant lymphoproliferative disorders: a working classification. *Curr Diagn Pathol*. 1997;4:28–36.

187. Rizvi MA, Evens AM, Tallman MS, et al. T cell non-Hodgkin lymphoma: a review. *Blood*. 2006;107:1255–1264.

188. Harris NL, Jaffe ES, Stein H, et al. A revised European-American classification of lymphoid neoplasms: a proposal from the International Lymphoma Study Group. *Blood*. 1999;84:1361–1392.

189. Jaffe ES, Krenacs L, Kumar S, et al. Extranodal peripheral T-cell and NK-cell neoplasms. *Am J Clin Pathol*. 1999;111(suppl 1):S46–S55.

190. Amin HM, Lai R. Pathobiology of ALK+ anaplastic large-cell lymphoma. *Blood*. 2007;110(7):2259–2267.

191. Sevilla DW, Choi JK, Gong JZ. Mediastinal adenopathy, lung infiltrates, and hemophagocytosis: unusual manifestation of pediatric anaplastic large cell lymphoma: report of two cases. *Am J Clin Pathol*. 2007;127(3):458–464.

192. Rush WL, Andriko JA, Taubenberger JK, et al. Primary anaplastic large cell lymphoma of the lung: a clinicopathologic study of five patients. *Mod Pathol*. 2000;13:1285–1292.

193. Medeiros LJ, Elenitoba-Johnson KS. Anaplastic large cell lymphoma. *Am J Clin Pathol*. 2007;127(5):707–722.

194. Chott A, Kaserer K, Augustin I, et al. Ki-1-positive large cell lymphoma. A clinicopathologic study of 41 cases. *Am J Surg Pathol*. 1998;14:439–448.

195. d'Amore ES, Menin A, Bonoldi E, et al. Anaplastic large cell lymphomas: a study of 75 pediatric patients. *Pediatr Dev Pathol*. 2007;10(3):181–191.

196. Campo E, Chott A, Kinney MC, et al. Update on extranodal lymphomas. Conclusions of the Workshop held by the EAHP and the SH in Thessaloniki, Greece. *Histopathology*. 2006;48:481–504.

197. Stein H, Foss HD, Drkop H, et al. CD30(+) anaplastic large cell lymphoma: a review of its histo-pathologic, genetic, and clinical features. *Blood*. 2000;96(12):3681–3695.

198. Kesler MV, Paranjape GS, Asplund SL, et al. Anaplastic large cell lymphoma: a flow cytometric analysis of 29 cases. *Am J Clin Pathol*. 2007;128(2):314–322.

199. Grewal JS, Smith LB, Winegarden 3rd JD, et al. Highly aggressive ALK-positive anaplastic large cell lymphoma with a leukemic phase and multi-organ involvement: a report of three cases and a review of the literature. *Ann Hematol*. 2007;86(7):499–508.

200. Stachurski D, Miron PM, Al-Homsi S, et al. Anaplastic lymphoma kinase-positive diffuse large B-cell lymphoma with a complex karyotype and cryptic 3 ALK gene insertion to chromosome 4 q22-24. *Hum Pathol*. 2007;38(6):940–945.

201. Coyne JD, Burton IE. Interstitial pneumonitis due to extramedullary haematopoiesis (EMH) in agnogenic myeloid metaplasia. *Histopathology*. 1999;34(3):275–276.

202. Koh TT, Colby TV, Muller NL. Myeloid leukemias and lung involvement. *Semin Respir Crit Care Med*. 2005;26(5):514–519.

203. Moran CA, Suster S. Unusual non-neoplastic lesions of the lung. *Semin Diagn Pathol*. 2007;24(3):199–208.

204. O'Malley DP. Benign extramedullary myeloid tumors. *Mod Pathol*. 2007;20:405–415.

205. Koch CA, Li CY, Mesa RA, et al. Nonhepatosplenic extramedullary hematopoiesis: associated diseases, pathology, clinical course, and treatment. *Mayo Clin Proc*. 2003;78:1223–1233.

206. Ginsberg JP, Orudjev E, Bunin N, et al. Isolated extramedullary relapse in acute myeloid leukemia: a retrospective analysis. *Med Pediatr Oncol*. 2002;38:387–390.

207. Campidelli C, Agostinelli C, Stitson R, Pileri SA. Myeloid sarcoma: extramedullary manifestation of myeloid disorders. *Am J Clin Pathol*. 2009;132:426–437.

208. Nappi O, Boscaino A, Wick MR. Extramedullary hematopoietic proliferations, extraosseous plasmacytomas, and ectopic splenic implants (splenosis). *Semin Diagn Pathol*. 2003; 20:338–356.

209. Takasugi JE, Godwin JD, Marglin SI, Petersdorf SH. Intrathoracic granulocytic sarcomas. *J Thorac Imaging*. 1996;11:223–230.

210. Nieman RS, Barcos M, Berard C. Granulocytic sarcoma: a clinicopathologic study of 61 biopsied cases. *Cancer*. 1981;48:426–437.

211. Wong KF, Chan JKC, Chan JC, Lam SY. Acute myeloid leukemia presenting as granulocytic sarcoma of the lung. *Am J Hematol*. 1993;43:77–78.

212. Byrd JC, Edenfield WJ, Dow NS, et al. Extramedullary myeloid cell tumors in myelodysplastic syndromes: not a true indication of impending acute myeloid leukemia. *Leuk Lymphoma*. 1996;21:153–159.

213. Hicsonmez G, Cetin M, Yenicesu J, et al. Evaluation of children with myelodysplastic syndromes: importance of extramedullary disease as a presenting symptom. *Leuk Lymphoma*. 2000;42:665–674.

214. Sisack MJ, Dunsmore K, Sidhu-Malik N. Granulocytic sarcoma in the absence of myeloid leukemia. *J Am Acad Dermatol*. 1997;37:308–311.

215. Meis JM, Butler JJ, Osborne BM. Granulocytic sarcoma in non-leukemic patients. *Cancer*. 1986;58:2697–2709.

216. Goldstein NS, Ritter JH, Argenyi ZB, et al. Granulocytic sarcoma: potential diagnostic clues from immunostaining patterns seen with anti-lymphoid antibodies. *Int J Surg Pathol*. 1995;2:199–206.

217. Quintanilla-Martinez L, Zukerberg LR, Ferry JA, et al. Extramedullary tumors of lymphoid or myeloid blasts. The role of immunohistology in diagnosis and classification. *Am J Clin Pathol*. 1995;104:431–443.

218. Roth MJ, Medeiros LJ, Elenitoba-Johnson K, et al. Extramedullary myeloid cell tumors. An immu-nohistochemical study of 29 cases using routinely fixed and processed paraffin-embedded tissue sections. *Arch Pathol Lab Med*. 1995;119:790–798.

219. Chen J, Yanuck RR, Abbondanzo SL, et al. c-Kit (CD117) reactivity in extramedullary myeloid tumor/granulocytic sarcoma. *Arch Pathol Lab Med*. 2001;125:1448–1452.

Non-Neuroendocrine Carcinomas (Excluding "Sarcomatoid" Carcinoma) and Salivary Gland Analog Carcinomas in the Lung

Mark R. Wick, MD, Henry D. Tazelaar, MD, Cesar A. Moran, MD,
Timothy C. Allen, MD, JD, and Kevin O. Leslie, MD

Carcinoma of the lung is a growing public health problem of worrisome proportions, not only in the United States but also internationally.[1-5] The American Cancer Society has estimated that more than 170,000 new cases of lung cancer will occur each year in the United States in the foreseeable future. This unfortunate reality reflects the continuing use of cigarettes, cigars, and pipes by a significant fraction of the world population and the undeniable causal relationship between inhaled tobacco smoke and pulmonary carcinoma.[1-7] To make matters worse, it has been shown that persons who are in constant and close proximity to heavy smokers,

either at home or in the workplace, inhale sufficient "sidestream" smoke to place them at definite risk for lung cancer even if they have never smoked themselves.[6,8,9] The potential pathogenetic influence of other proposed etiologic agents (e.g., human papillomavirus, radon, pneumoconiosis-related minerals, hereditary syndromes) on pulmonary carcinogenesis also continues to undergo analysis.[3,10-21] Women now have an incidence of lung cancer on a rough numerical parity with men, and the mortality rate in both sexes is so high that lung cancer represents the leading worldwide cause of death related to malignancy.[2,5,6]

This chapter provides a summary of the pathologic features of recognized lung carcinoma morphotypes. In addition, specific issues relating to differential diagnosis and evolving conceptual topics are considered. Difficult subjects are given a relatively disproportionate volume of space in the ensuing discussion, with concise treatment of those that are familiar to surgical pathologists. In the interest of conserving space, the results of several adjunctive pathologic techniques, including electron microscopy, flow cytometry, genetic analysis, and morphometry, are not discussed.

Nosology of Lung Cancer and Diagnostic Effects of Sampling Methods

Seventy-five years ago, the first attempt at morphologic classification of lung cancer was undertaken by Marchesani.[10] This scheme, outlining the now-classic categories of squamous cell carcinoma (SCC), adenocarcinoma (ACA), and small cell "undifferentiated" and large cell "undifferentiated" carcinomas, is still widely recognized and has gone through several iterations over the ensuing decades. Recently, a pragmatic, clinically attuned movement has been enjoined wherein a more simplified system was embraced, dividing malignant epithelial tumors of the lung into "small cell" and "non–small cell" carcinomas. At the same time, research by pathologists has resulted in ever-greater refinement of morphologic categorization, and the interface between the practical needs of the operating suite and data generated in the clinical laboratory has become problematic. In light of this situation, a prognostically oriented nosologic scheme for lung cancer was devised by the Veterans Administration Lung Group in 1991.[22] It has since been modified by other organizations, most notably, the World Health Organization.[23]

Whether a pathologist elects to use one or another of these systems is a decision that should be made after consultation with clinical colleagues. In any event, nonstandard designations for pulmonary carcinomas (i.e., those that are not sanctioned by the World Health

Organization)[23] should be well defined in surgical pathology reports, with pertinent references provided in cases that are particularly uncommon or conceptually contentious.

A particular problem that must be recognized by everyone involved in treating lung cancer is the common heterogeneity that it may demonstrate at a light microscopic level. The literature is now well supplied with reports of admixtures of virtually all of the lung carcinoma histotypes in the same tumor mass.[3,12,24-26] An analysis by Roggli and colleagues[27] demonstrated such heterogeneity in fully 66% of a consecutive series of lung cancers, and others have reported similar findings. This biologic diversity may attain prognostic importance in the future, particularly in light of recent work that appears to affirm the effect of histologic features on tumor evolution.[28] Neoplastic heterogeneity is a practical diagnostic problem for surgeons and medical oncologists, because small biopsies often do not represent "divergent" tumor elements as a consequence of sampling bias. At a time when ever more limited methods of tissue procurement are being advanced, it is clear that substantial discrepancies will be observed between biopsy results and findings of resection specimens in the surgical pathology laboratory.[29,30] That is not to imply that such techniques as fine-needle aspiration biopsy should not be used, because they are extremely helpful in planning therapy in many cases. Nonetheless, the potential limitations of all sampling procedures must be weighed carefully against their benefits.

Clinicopathologic Features of Non-Neuroendocrine Pulmonary Carcinomas, Excluding "Sarcomatoid" Carcinoma

Squamous Cell Carcinoma

Probably because of changes in the smoking habits of the public, with a greater preference for filtered cigarettes in the last 35 years,[7] SCC is no longer the most common type of lung cancer and has been eclipsed by ACA in recent years.[25,31] However, SCC has retained its classic clinicopathologic attributes. These include a tendency for multifocal but clonal in situ disease in the bronchial mucosa, often preceding the appearance of a discrete mass by several years, and a propensity to arise in large central airways proximal to the subsegmental bronchi. Because of the common presence of an endobronchial tumor mass, obstructive pneumonia is a relatively common accompaniment of this neoplasm, but it is not pathognomonic. "Pure" SCC may originate in the peripheral pulmonary parenchyma as well, and rare examples are even subpleural.[3]

Squamous cell cancer of the lung has an irregular, often friable, gray-white cut surface, commonly showing a large area of central necrosis, with or without cavitation (Fig. 16-1). The surrounding pulmonary parenchyma is frequently tethered to the mass, giving it a "spiculated" appearance that may be well seen on radiographic images

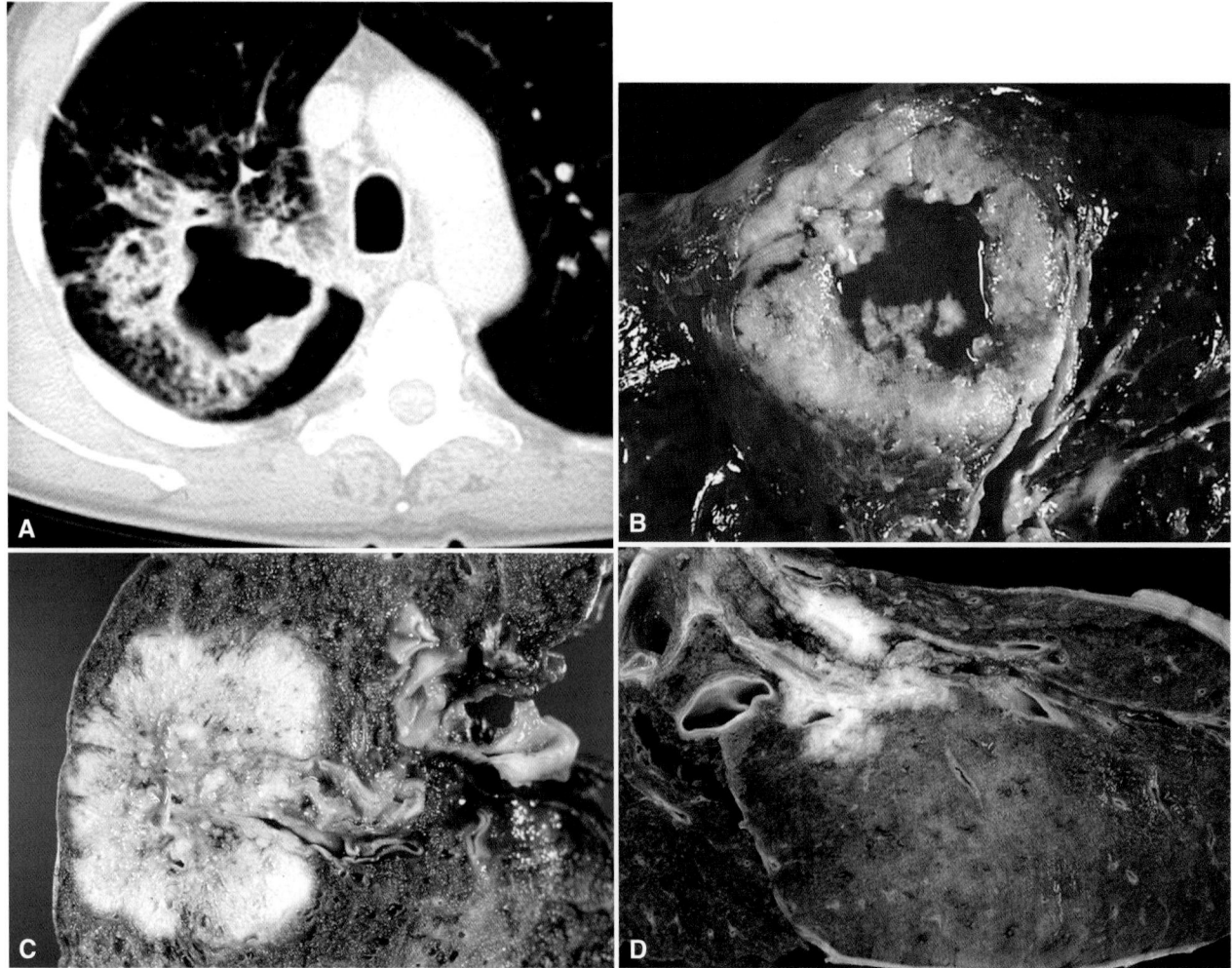

Figure 16-1. **A,** Thoracic computed tomogram showing a large centrally cavitary squamous cell carcinoma (SCC) of the right lung. **B** and **C,** Gross photographs of pulmonary SCCs demonstrating characteristic central necrotic cavitation. **D,** Macroscopic photograph of another SCC, demonstrating central location and lymphangitic growth of tumor centripetally from the main mass.

(Fig. 16-2). Microscopically, SCC is defined by its resemblance to stratified squamous epithelium of the upper airway, but with disordered architectural and cytologic maturation (Figs. 16-3 to 16-6). Anucleate keratin and squamous pearls are observed in better differentiated lesions, which account for a minority of pulmonary carcinomas.

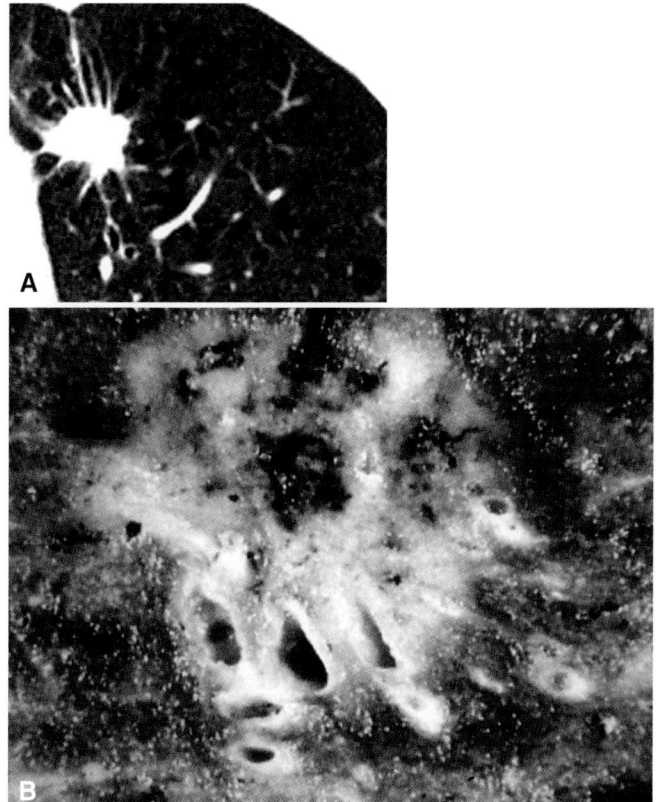

Figure 16-2. **A,** Computed tomogram demonstrating prototypical radial "spiculation" of pulmonary adenocarcinoma. **B,** A gross photograph of resected pulmonary adenocarcinoma demonstrates the irregular ("spiculated") periphery of the lesion and foci of entrapped anthracotic pigment.

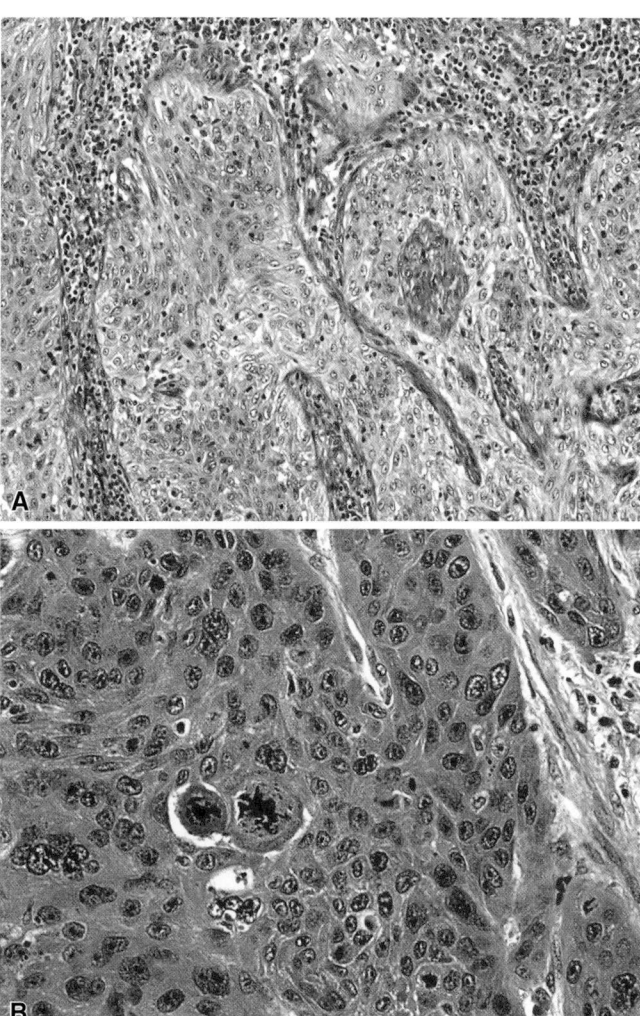

Figure 16-4. **A** and **B,** Moderately differentiated squamous cell carcinomas (SCCs) of the lung. The tumor cells have higher nucleocytoplasmic ratios and less keratinization than well-differentiated SCCs do.

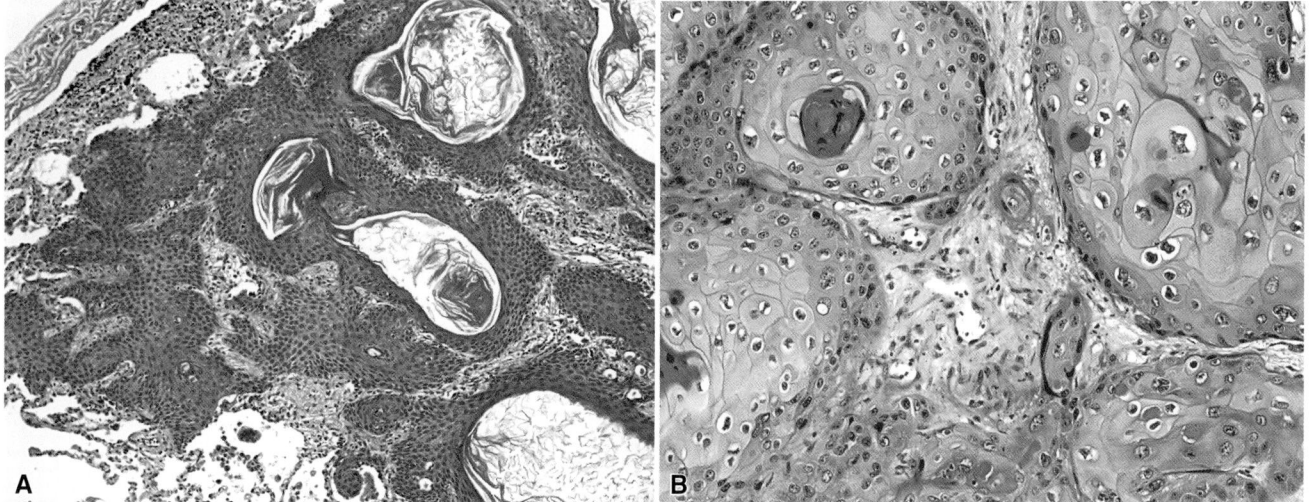

Figure 16-3. **A** and **B,** Photomicrographs of well-differentiated squamous carcinoma showing obvious keratinization.

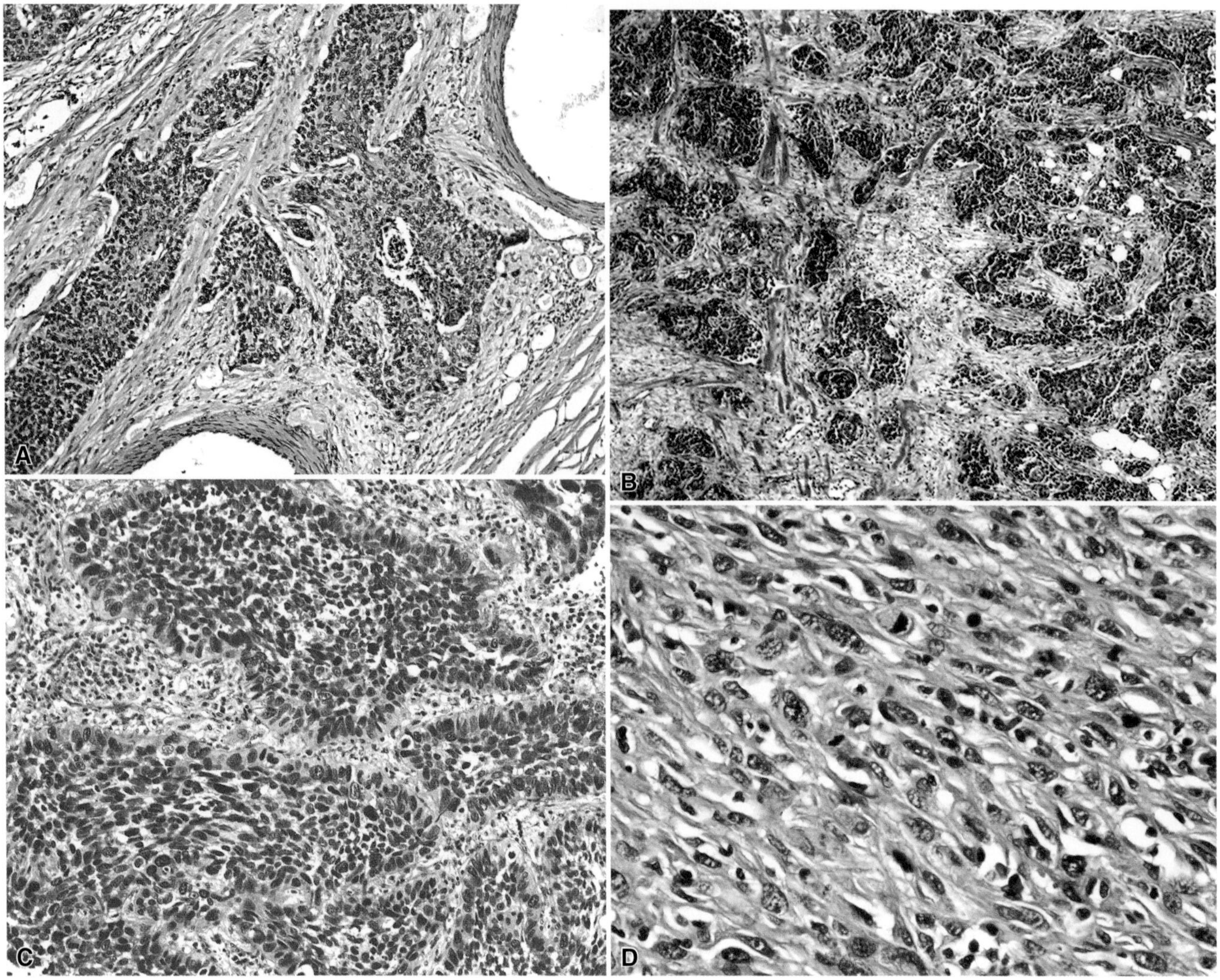

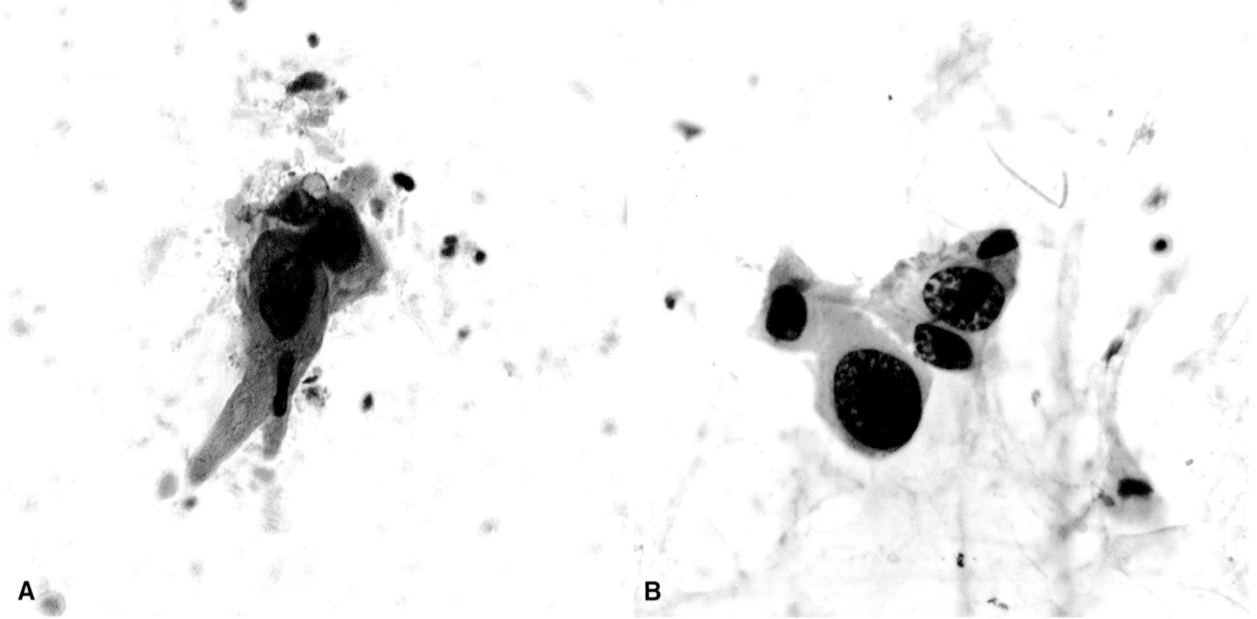

Figure 16-5. A, Poorly differentiated squamous cell carcinoma (PDSCC) showing only focal keratinization and predominant composition by primitive epithelial cells. **B,** PDSCC comprising groups of relatively primitive polygonal cells invading the soft tissue of the chest wall. **C,** Only very focal keratinization is apparent in this PDSCC. **D,** PDSCC with sarcomatoid features, presenting difficulty in recognition of the lesion as epithelial (see Chapter 14).

Figure 16-6. A, Fine-needle aspiration biopsy (FNAB) of moderately differentiated squamous cell carcinoma. The tumor contains elongated "tadpole" cells and shows focal cytoplasmic orangeophilia. **B,** This FNAB of poorly differentiated squamous cell carcinoma manifests high nucleocytoplasmic ratios and cellular monotony; keratinization is inapparent in this photograph. (Images compliments of Dr. Diva Salomao, Austin, MN.)

Poorly differentiated SCC may be extremely difficult for the pathologist to distinguish from high-grade ACAs, small cell carcinomas, or large cell undifferentiated carcinomas (LCCs), because they commonly take the form of rather nondescript proliferations of primitive epithelioid cells of varying size, arranged in nests and sheets, with no other distinguishing features. In the absence of special studies, one may have to use the default terminology of "poorly differentiated carcinoma, not further specified," in the frozen section laboratory and in small biopsies of such lesions. Recognized and distinct subtypes of poorly differentiated SCC include spindle cell and pleomorphic (sarcomatoid) forms[32–35] (see Chapter 14); adenoid-acantholytic (pseudoglandular) variants (Fig. 16-7)[36]; a pseudovascular (angiosarcoma-like) subtype (Fig. 16-8)[36,37]; "lymphoepithelioma-like" carcinoma (Fig. 16-9)[38]; and a basaloid form (Fig. 16-10) ("small cell squamous carcinoma" or "basaloid squamous cell carcinoma")[39] that is analogous to primary poorly differentiated SCC of the anorectum, hypopharynx, thymus, and other anatomic sites. Other than presenting special problems in microscopic differential diagnosis, these tumor variants have no singular clinical significance in comparison with other high-grade carcinomas.

For unknown reasons, SCC has a greater association with selected hereditary syndromes than do other forms of lung carcinoma.[11–21] These conditions are extremely rare causes of pulmonary neoplasia, but they include such disorders as Muir-Torre syndrome, von Hippel-Lindau disease, and dysplastic nevus ("atypical mole") syndrome. In one of them—Muir-Torre syndrome—immunohistochemical analyses can be done for the absence of nucleic acid mismatch repair proteins in the tumor cells. The three most commonly assessed gene products are MLH1, MSH2, and MSH6 (Figs. 16-11 and 16-12).

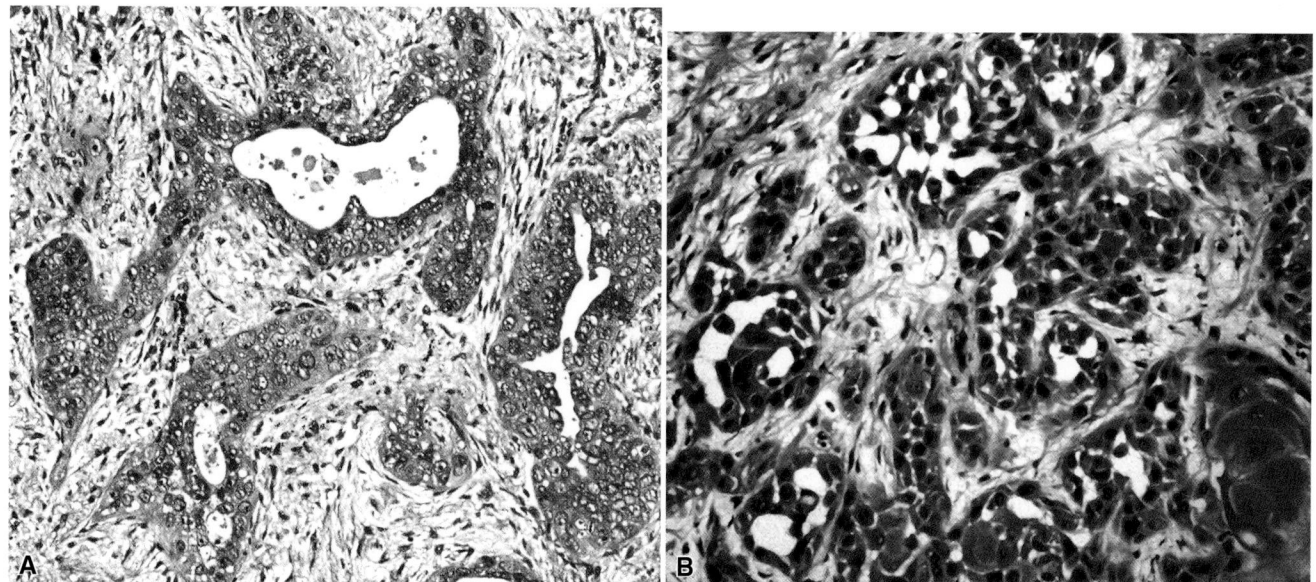

Figure 16-7. **A** and **B,** Adenoid (pseudoglandular/acantholytic) squamous cell carcinoma of the lung demonstrating dyshesion of the tumor cells in such a way that the lesions focally resemble gland-forming neoplasms.

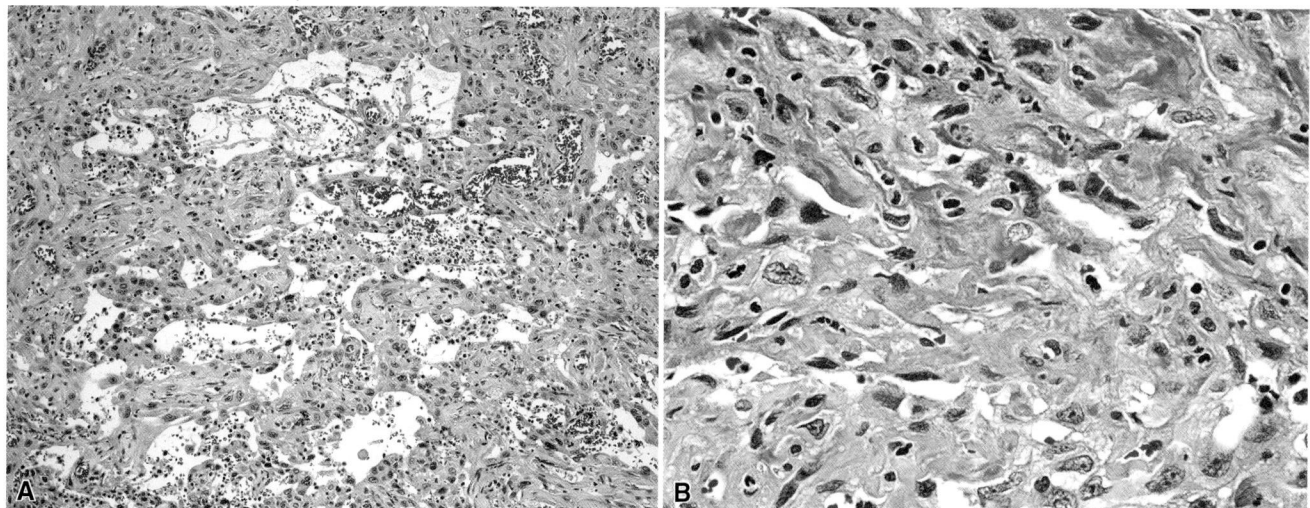

Figure 16-8. **A** and **B,** The adenoid squamous cell carcinoma subtype shown here is called "angiosarcoma-like" or "pseudovascular" because its particular version of intercellular dyshesion simulates the image of an endothelial malignancy.

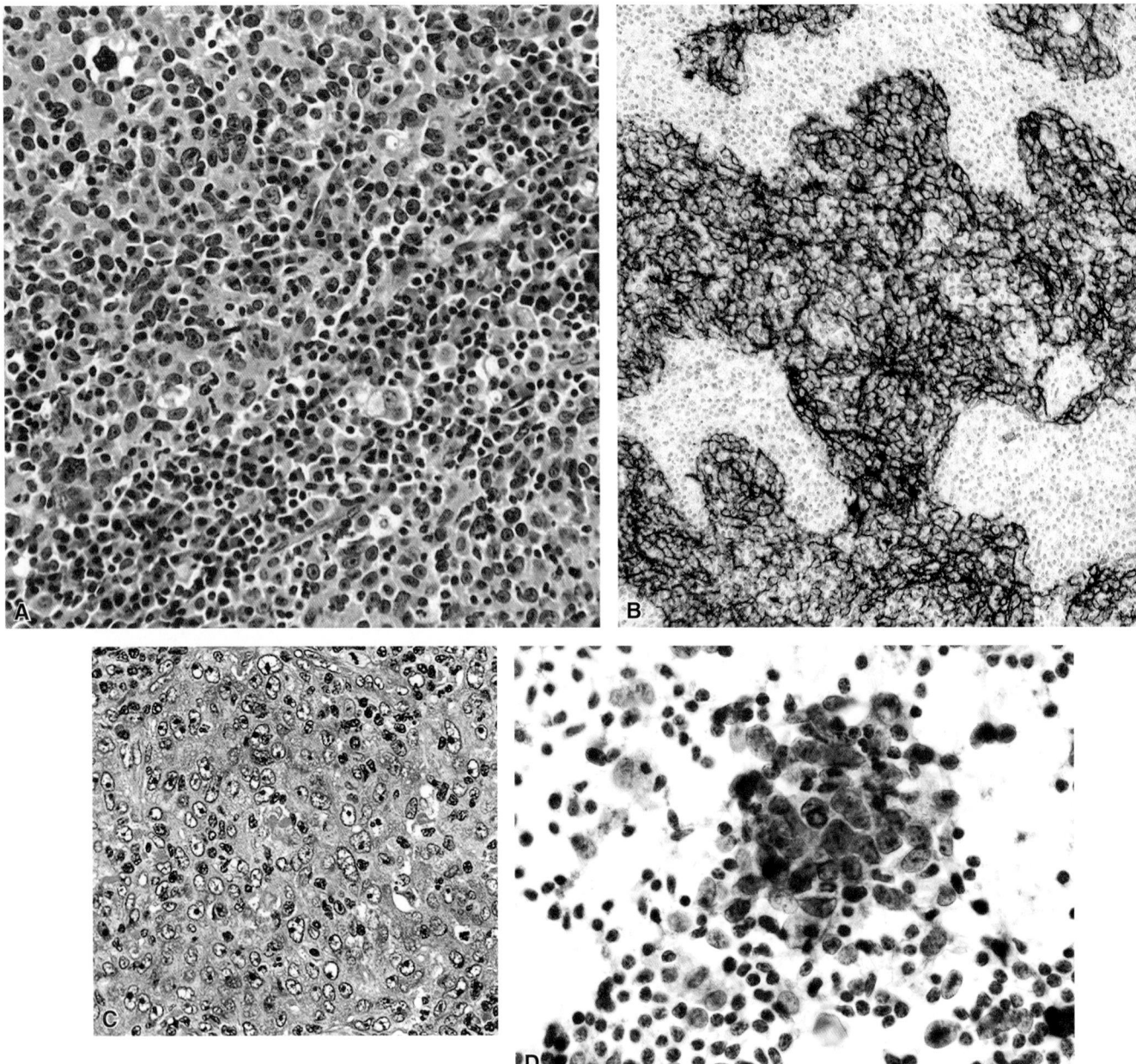

Figure 16-9. A, Lymphoepithelioma-like carcinoma (LELC) of the lung showing syncytia of polygonal neoplastic cells with vesicular nuclear chromatin and prominent nucleoli, which are interspersed with mature lymphocytes. **B,** Cytokeratin immunostaining demonstrates a characteristically "interlocking" pattern of cellular reactivity. **C,** This tumor variant is considered a subtype of large cell undifferentiated carcinoma by some observers, but it has a distinctive cytologic monomorphism. **D,** A fine-needle aspiration biopsy of LELC shows many "naked" tumor nuclei and "smeared" intratumoral lymphocytes.

Nonbronchioloalveolar Adenocarcinomas

As stated earlier, ACA has now successfully eclipsed SCC as the most common form of monodifferentiated lung cancer. In North America and Europe, most ACAs are predominantly peripheral parenchymal masses; however, interestingly, histologically identical lesions in India and Asia are as likely to be central as peripheral in location. Grossly, ACA typically has an irregularly lobulated configuration, with a gray-white cut surface (Fig. 16-13). Anthracotic pigment is commonly entrapped in the tumor mass as well, but foci of necrosis and hemorrhage are seen only in large (>5 cm) lesions. A relationship to tubular airways is only rarely obvious. Close inspection may also demonstrate the presence of "satellite" nodules around the main tumor mass; however, this phenomenon may be a reflection of the tendency for pulmonary ACA to be synchronously or metachronously multifocal, either in one lobe of the lung or in both

lungs. The latter statement applies particularly to a special subtype of ACA, bronchioloalveolar carcinoma (BAC; discussed later). One peculiar and uncommon gross presentation of pulmonary ACA that merits special mention is its "pseudomesotheliomatous" form, wherein the pleurotropic growth of extremely peripheral intrapulmonary tumors creates a "rind" of tumor tissue surrounding the lung (Fig. 16-14). This virtually perfectly simulates the appearance of mesothelioma, both intraoperatively and radiographically.[40–42]

Bronchioloalveolar carcinoma is considered as a distinct entity subsequently. Microscopically, there are several other currently recognized subtypes of pulmonary ACA:

- Acinar (the most common; Fig. 16-15)
- Micropapillary (Fig. 16-16)[43]

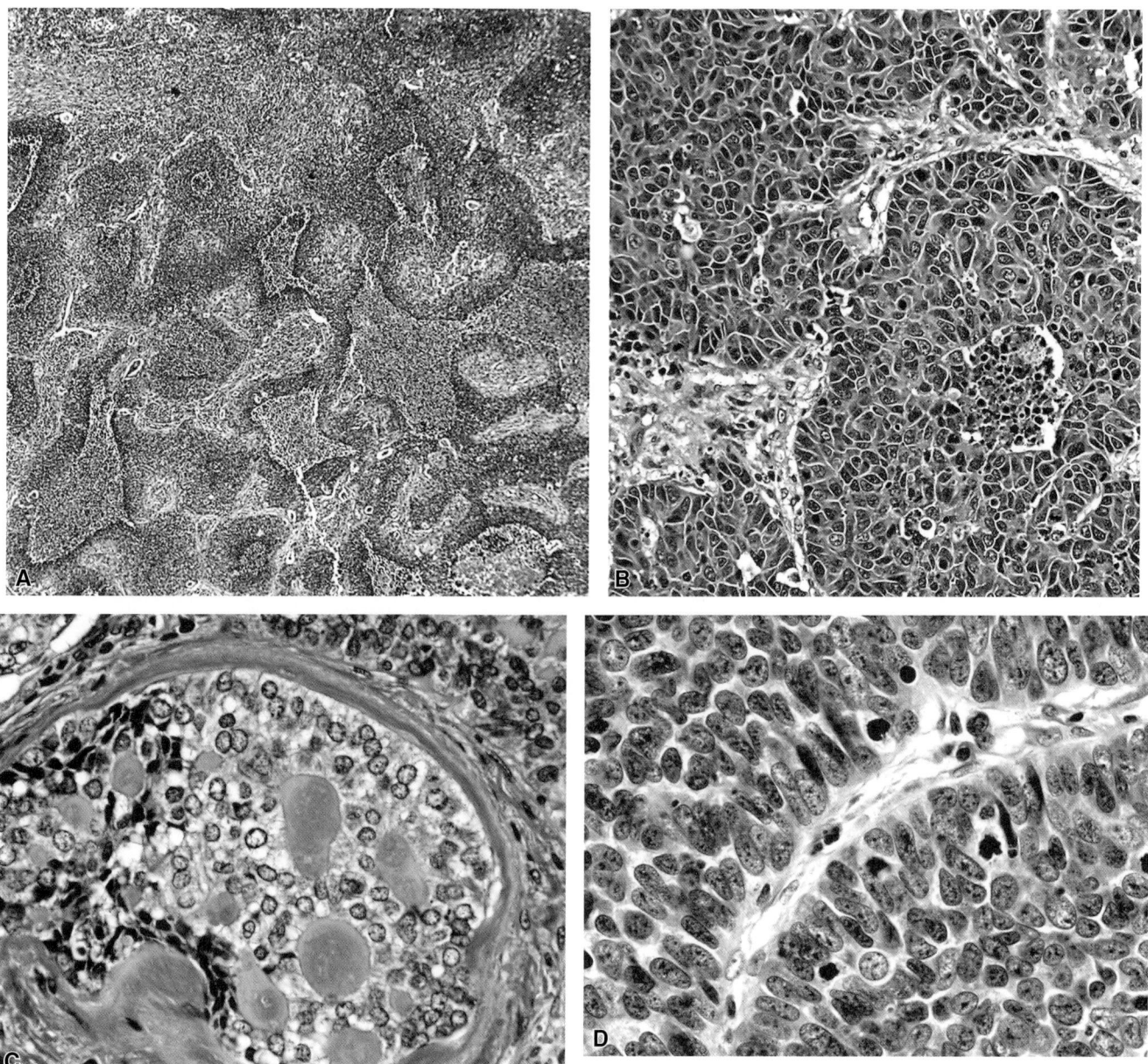

Figure 16-10. A, Basaloid squamous cell carcinoma of the lung demonstrating a typically organoid growth pattern with prominent foci of geographic necrosis and a composition dominated by small polyhedral cells. **B,** Zones of centrilobular necrosis are well seen in this image of basaloid squamous cell carcinoma. **C,** Deposition of intercellular basal lamina is relatively common in basaloid squamous cell carcinoma, potentially causing confusion with such other tumor entities as adenoid cystic carcinoma. **D,** Peripheral palisading of nuclei is evident in tumor cell nests of basaloid carcinoma.

- Solid (Fig. 16-17)[44]
- "Fetal" (Fig. 16-18)[45] (see Chapter 14)
- Mucinous ("colloid"; Fig. 16-19)[43]
- Signet ring cell (Fig. 16-20)[43]
- Morular[43]
- Oncocytic[46]
- Secretory endometrioid–like (Fig. 16-21)[43]

However, more variants exist, such as clear cell and enteric (intestinal-like; Fig. 16-22).[47–52] In some cases, because of the overlap between these histologic groups and the appearance of metastatic ACAs in the lung, it may be extremely difficult for the pathologist to separate primary from secondary lesions. This is particularly true of

enteric and signet ring cell tumors, which can closely imitate the attributes of gastric or colorectal carcinomas (see Chapter 17). Psammoma bodies can also be seen in primary papillary ACAs of the lung,[43,53] and these structures therefore raise the question of whether one is instead viewing a solitary metastasis from an occult tumor of the thyroid, ovary, or another location wherein psammomatous carcinomas are potentially found. Needless to say, in cases featuring multifocality of ACA in more than one lobe, this problem is even more striking. Special studies, including electron microscopy and immunohistology, are helpful in resolving this differential diagnosis. Ultimately, however, diagnostic reliance is also placed on such banal characteristics as peritumoral fibrosis and inflammation, which are more common in primary pulmonary lesions than in metastases.

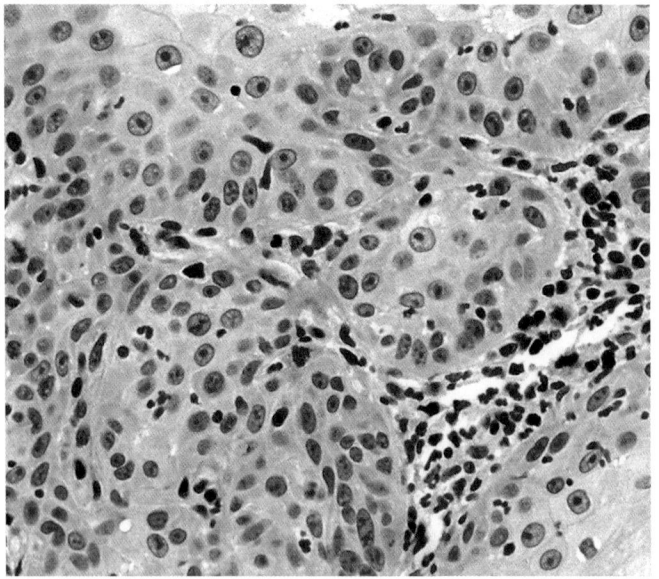

Figure 16-11. Loss of the DNA mismatch repair protein MLH1 in squamous carcinoma of the lung in a patient with Muir-Torre syndrome. Note the nuclear staining of background normal lymphocytes.

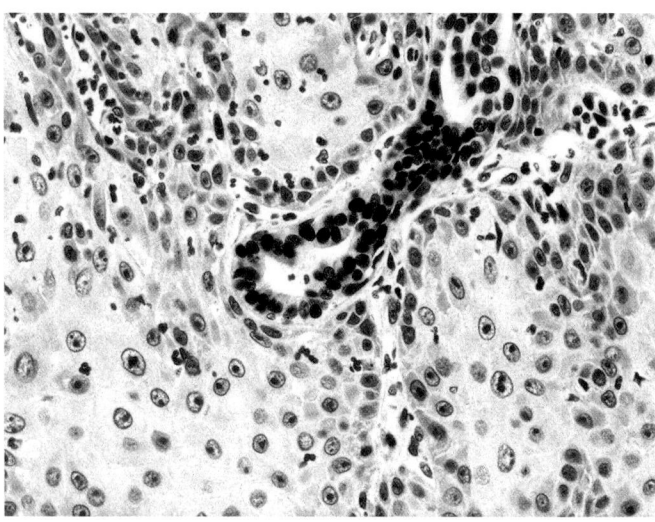

Figure 16-12. Loss of another DNA mismatch repair protein, MSH2, in pulmonary squamous cell carcinoma in the context of Muir-Torre syndrome. Note the nuclear staining of normal epithelium.

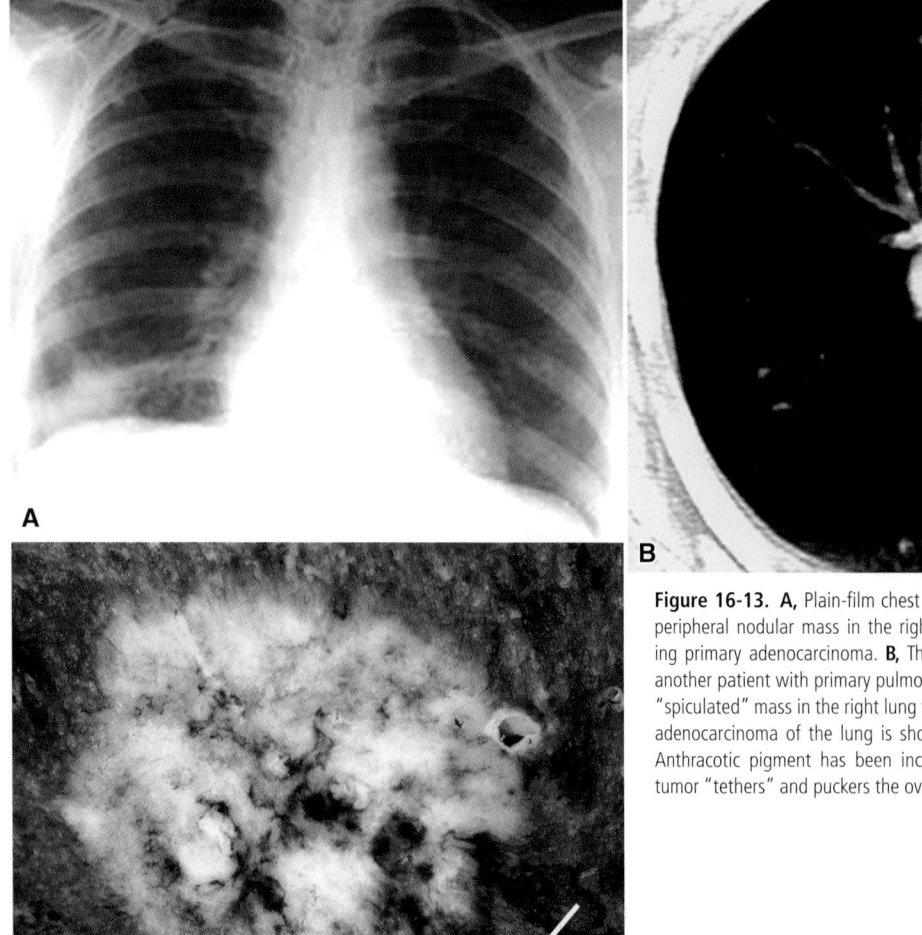

Figure 16-13. A, Plain-film chest radiograph showing a solitary peripheral nodular mass in the right lower lung field, representing primary adenocarcinoma. **B,** This computed tomograph from another patient with primary pulmonary adenocarcinoma shows a "spiculated" mass in the right lung field. **C,** Peripheral (subpleural) adenocarcinoma of the lung is shown in this gross photograph. Anthracotic pigment has been incorporated into the mass. The tumor "tethers" and puckers the overlying visceral pleura (*arrow*).

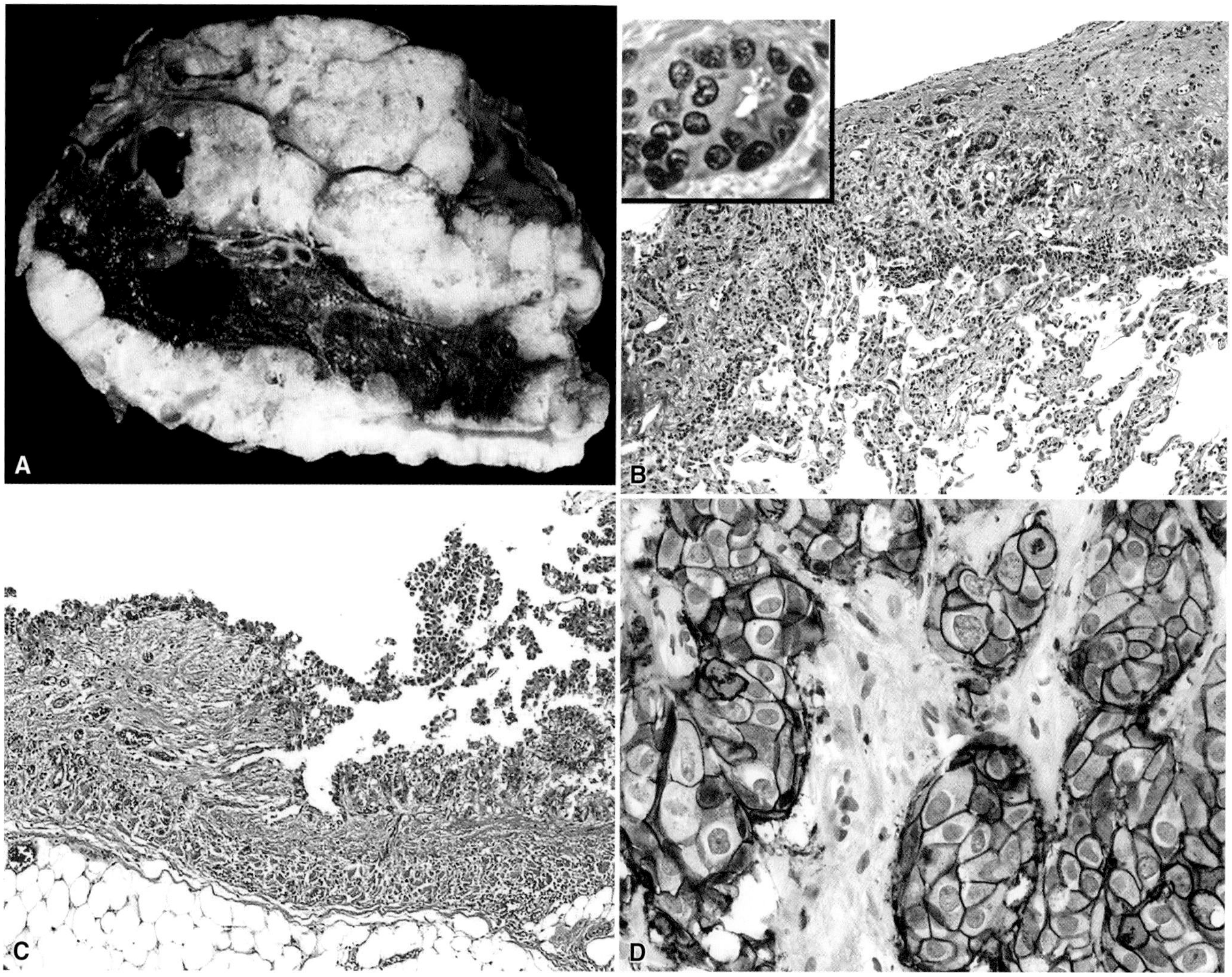

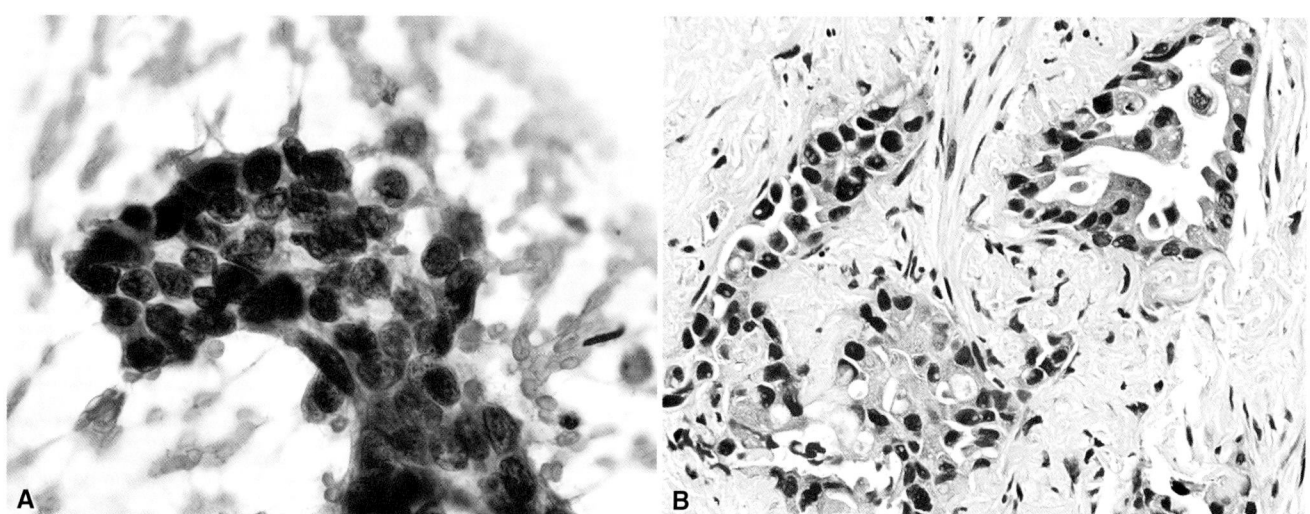

Figure 16-14. A, This gross photograph of a "pseudomesotheliomatous" (pleurotropic) adenocarcinoma of the lung shows a neoplasm that encompasses the lung parenchyma, yielding a macroscopic image that is identical to that of true mesothelioma. **B,** Glandular arrays of tumor cells are present in the pleura in the absence of a definable intraparenchymal lesion in "pseudomesotheliomatous" adenocarcinoma of the lung. High-magnification view of an infiltrating malignant gland in pleurotropic adenocarcinoma (*inset*). **C,** An additional microscopic view of pleurotropic adenocarcinoma (PTA) simulating mesothelioma. **D,** Immunoreactivity for MOC-31 distinguishes PTA, which is labeled for that marker, from mesothelioma, which is not.

Figure 16-15. A, A fine-needle aspiration specimen from acinar-type primary adenocarcinoma of the lung shows a three-dimensional cell group comprising atypical polygonal cells with prominent nucleoli. **B,** This well-differentiated acinar (usual type) adenocarcinoma of the lung demonstrates easily seen glandular lumina.

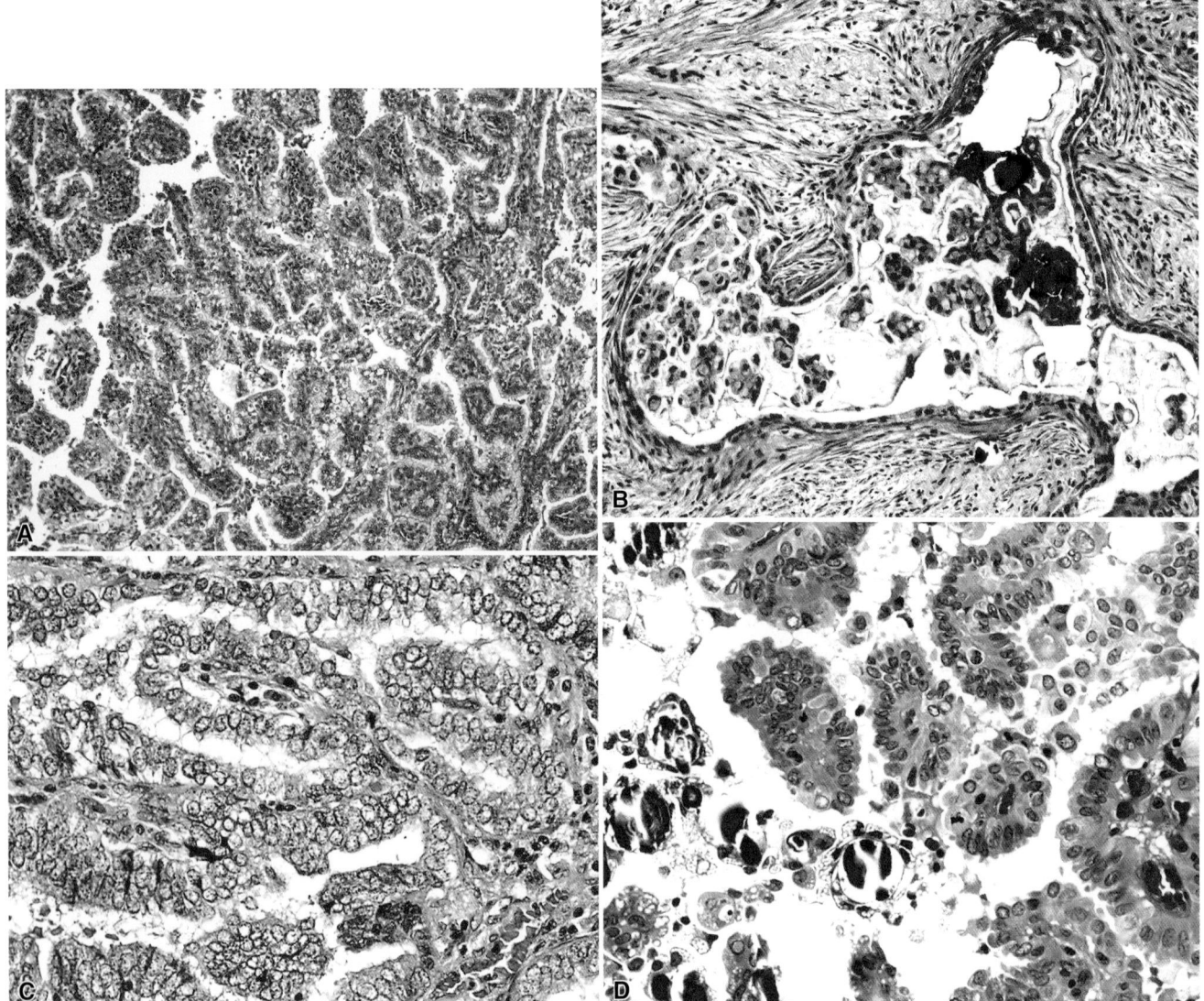

Figure 16-16. **A** to **D**, Micropapillary adenocarcinoma of the lung, shown here, is now considered an entity distinct from bronchioloalveolar carcinoma. It is distinctive in its potential to synthesize calcific psammoma bodies (**B** and **D**).

Pulmonary ACA may rarely involve the bronchial epithelium diffusely in a pagetoid fashion (Fig. 16-23).[54] Whether this represents intraepithelial spread of the tumor or multifocal synchronous growth is an open question, but pagetoid lesions are excruciating management problems because of the difficulty in obtaining tumor-free bronchial margins.

"Pseudomesotheliomatous" (pleurotropic) ACAs are indeed separable from true mesotheliomas using adjuvant pathologic techniques, particularly immunophenotyping and electron microscopy (Figs. 16-24 and 16-25 and Table 16-1).[55] Nonetheless, whether this exercise has any more than academic significance is an open question. Available therapies for both of these tumor types are suboptimal, and the only real significance of the differential diagnosis may be a medicolegal one. In the absence of asbestosis, pleurotropic ACA has no proven causal relationship to asbestos exposure.

Bronchioloalveolar Carcinoma

Bronchioloalveolar carcinoma of the lung was initially described in the 1800s, but was most fully characterized as a distinct entity by Liebow in 1960.[56] Since that time, BAC has been the subject of intense interest and controversy. In particular, the pathologic criteria that apply to its diagnosis and how its histologic attributes relate to prognosis represent perhaps the two most contentious issues.[57-65]

There are no particular distinguishing demographic features associated with BAC vis-à-vis other ACAs of the lung. They tend to occur in elderly individuals, with an essentially equal distribution by sex.[58,65] Contrary to reports in the 1970s[63]—before such phenomena as "passive" tobacco exposure were recognized—there is a definite relationship between cigarette smoking and the genesis of this tumor, as is true of virtually all pulmonary carcinomas. Nonetheless, BAC is indeed over-represented (with regard to other histotypes of lung cancer) in patients who have never smoked and who have never lived with smokers. This point has raised the issue of whether other etiologic factors—in particular, infection with human papillomavirus—might account for the genesis of some BACs.

Radiologically and clinically, three discrete subsets of patients with BAC are recognized.[65,66] These include individuals who have chest radiographic findings and clinical symptoms suggesting pneumonia (fever, productive cough, and lobar or segmental consolidation; Fig. 16-26) as well as some patients with a solitary peripheral mass lesion (Fig. 16-27)

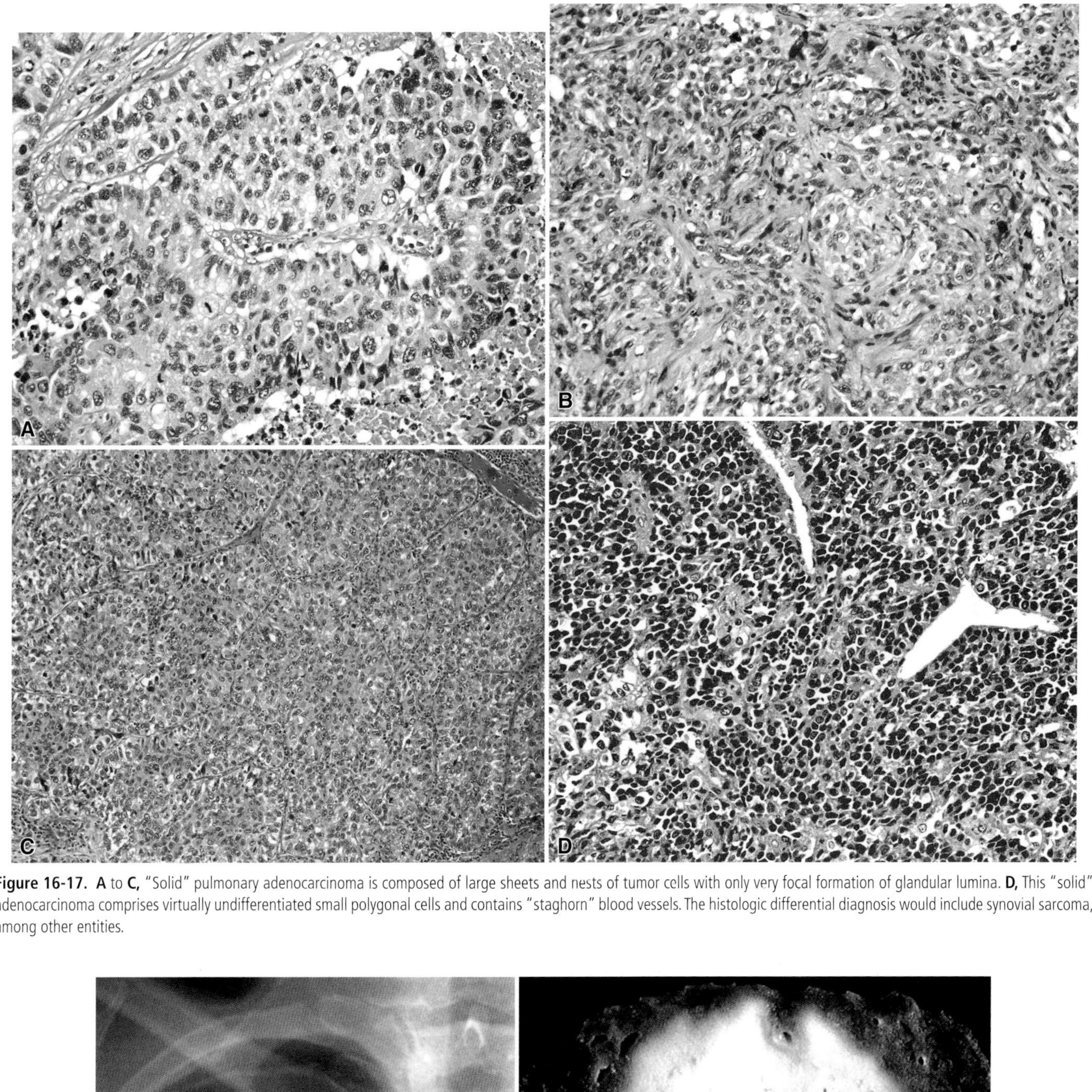

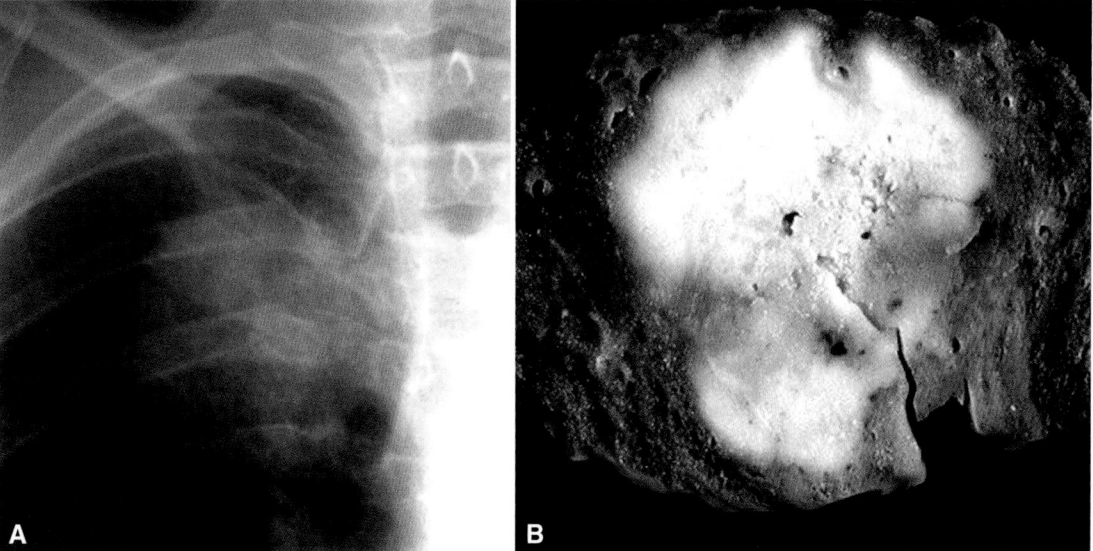

Figure 16-17. A to **C,** "Solid" pulmonary adenocarcinoma is composed of large sheets and nests of tumor cells with only very focal formation of glandular lumina. **D,** This "solid" adenocarcinoma comprises virtually undifferentiated small polygonal cells and contains "staghorn" blood vessels. The histologic differential diagnosis would include synovial sarcoma, among other entities.

Figure 16-18. A, "Fetal" adenocarcinoma of the lung is considered to be in the same general family of tumors as pulmonary "blastoma," and is shown here in an adult patient as a peripheral nodule in the right upper lung field on a plain-film radiograph. **B,** The resected tumor is a solid, relatively well-demarcated, and homogeneous mass.

Continued

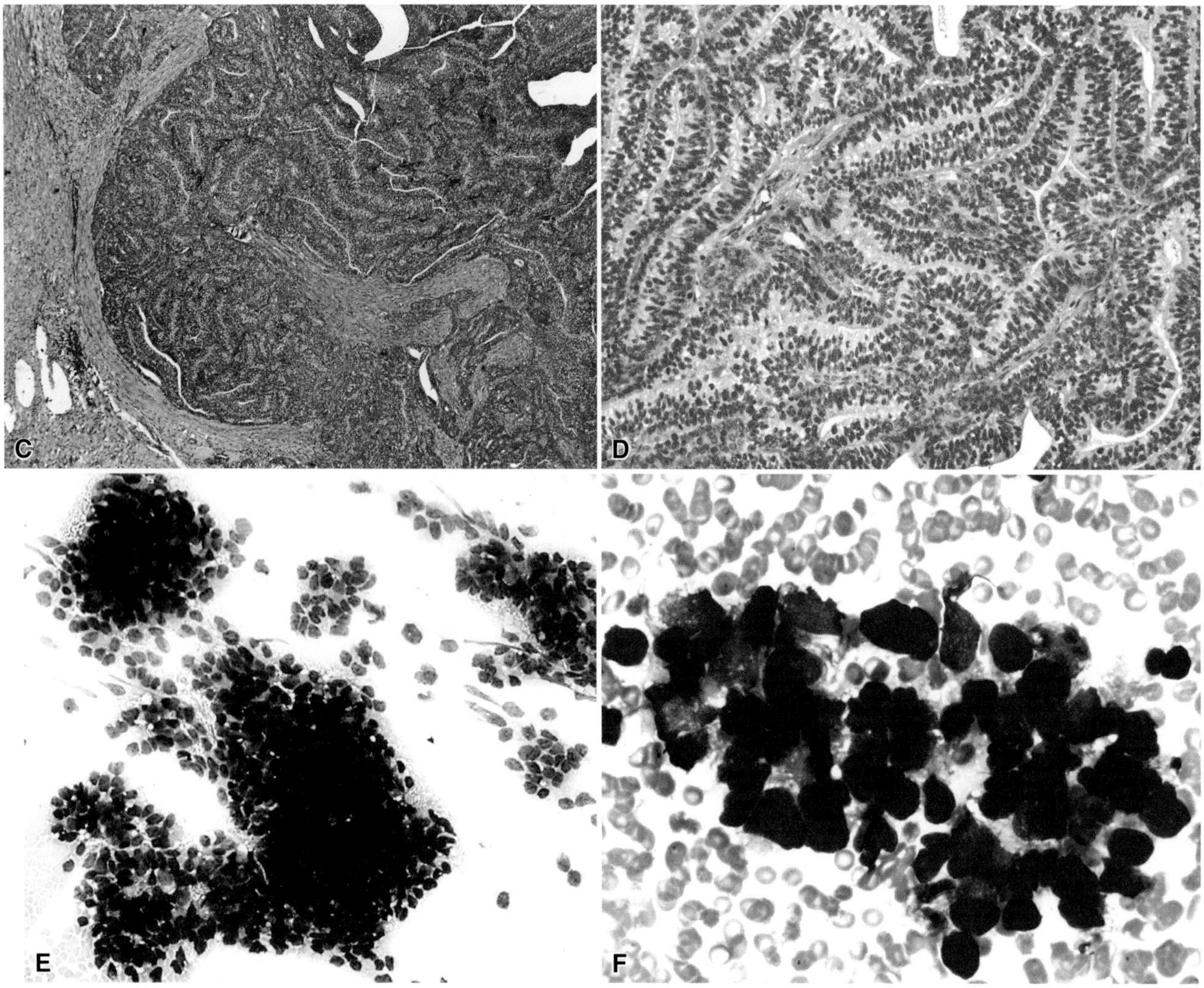

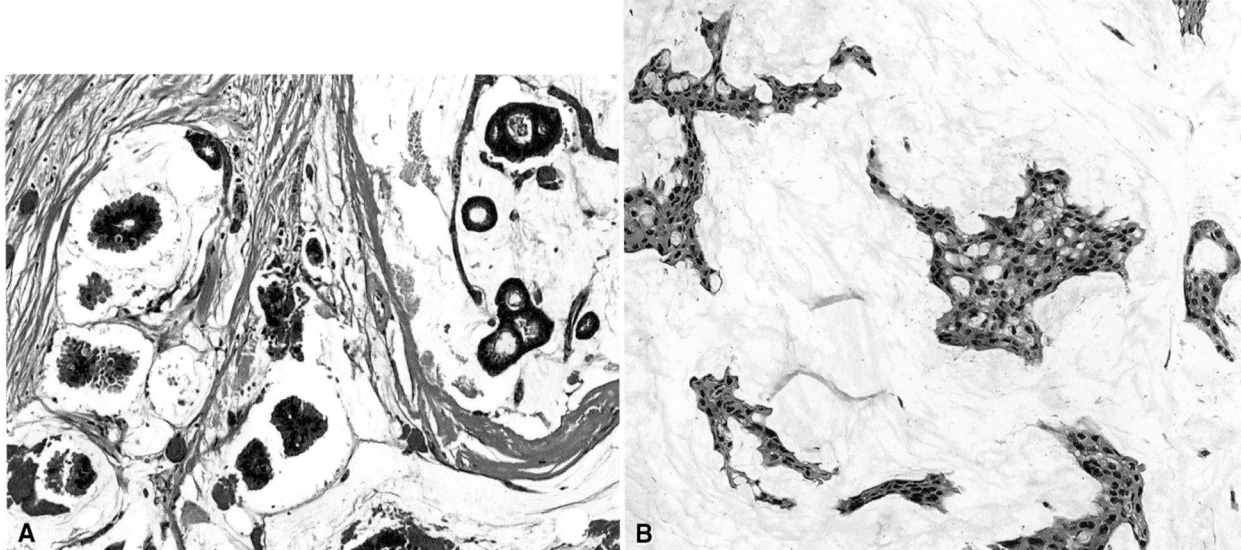

Figure 16-18—cont'd. C and **D,** Microscopically, fetal adenocarcinoma comprises closely apposed glandular arrays made up of compact columnar cells, resembling those seen in embryonic lungs. **E** and **F,** Fine-needle aspiration specimens of fetal adenocarcinoma show small cells with high nucleocytoplasmic ratios, dispersed chromatin, and a tendency to surround small central spaces. Cytologic differential diagnosis includes neuroendocrine and neuroectodermal lesions (see Chapter 13). (**A** and **B,** Courtesy of Dr. Samuel A. Yousem, Pittsburgh, PA. **E** and **F,** Courtesy of Dr. Kim Geisinger, Winston-Salem, NC).

Figure 16-19. A and **B,** Primary "colloid"-type mucinous adenocarcinoma of the lung shows nests of polyhedral tumor cells that are suspended in pools of copious extracellular mucin. This image is analogous to that seen in primary lesions of the breast, gastrointestinal tract, and skin.

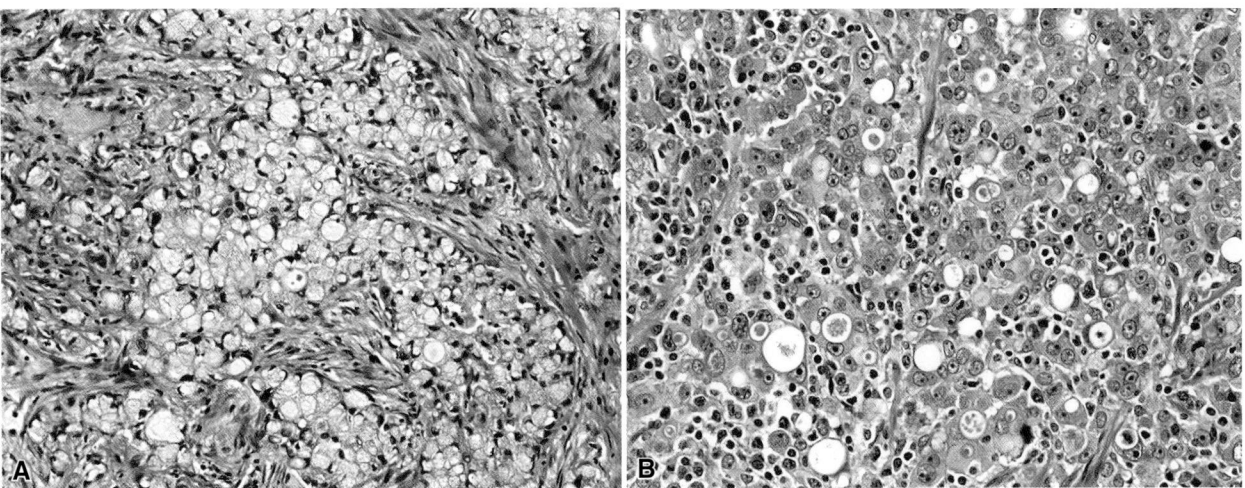

Figure 16-20. A and **B,** This rare primary pulmonary adenocarcinoma is composed of tumor cells with prominent intracytoplasmic mucin vacuoles, yielding a "signet ring cell" appearance.

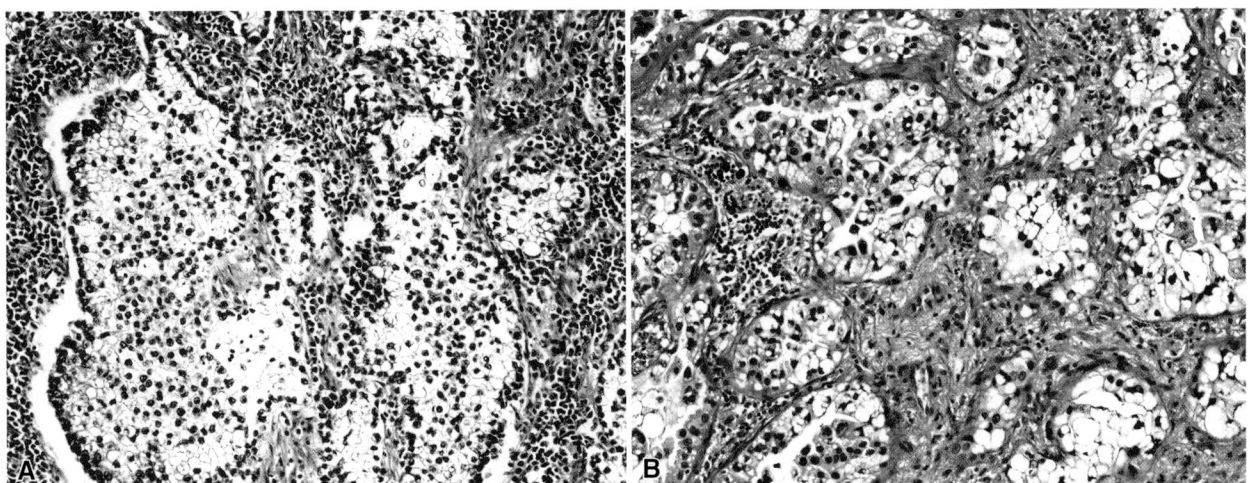

Figure 16-21. A and **B,** "Secretory endometrial–like" adenocarcinoma of the lung. Clear cell change and a tendency for nuclei to assume a basal location within glands are typical.

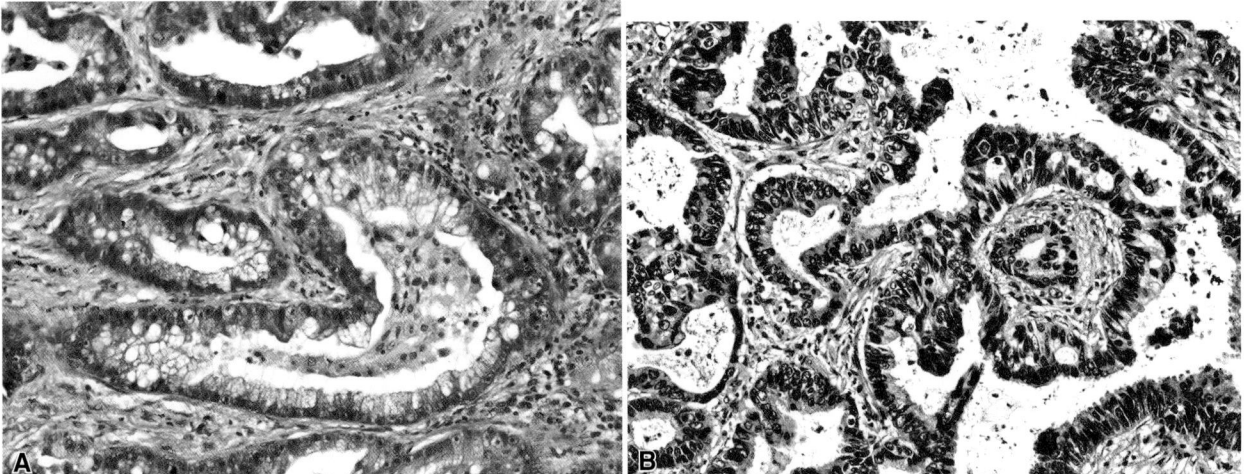

Figure 16-22. A and **B,** "Enteric" primary adenocarcinomas of the lung featuring a composition by low-columnar tumor cells with basally oriented nuclei and mucin production. The overall image of the lesions is reminiscent of neoplasms arising in the gastrointestinal tract.

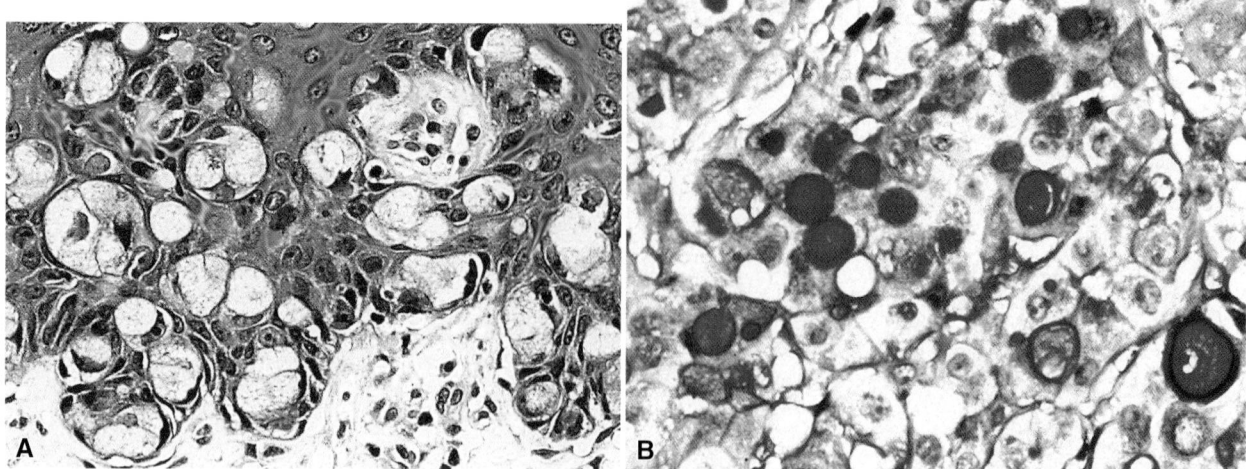

Figure 16-23. A, "Pagetoid" involvement of non-neoplastic but metaplastic-hyperplastic bronchial epithelium by dispersed intramucosal adenocarcinoma cells. **B,** The tumor cells label with the periodic acid/Schiff stain after diastase digestion, confirming the presence of epithelial mucin. A typical adenocarcinomatous mass lesion was present in the nearby parenchyma.

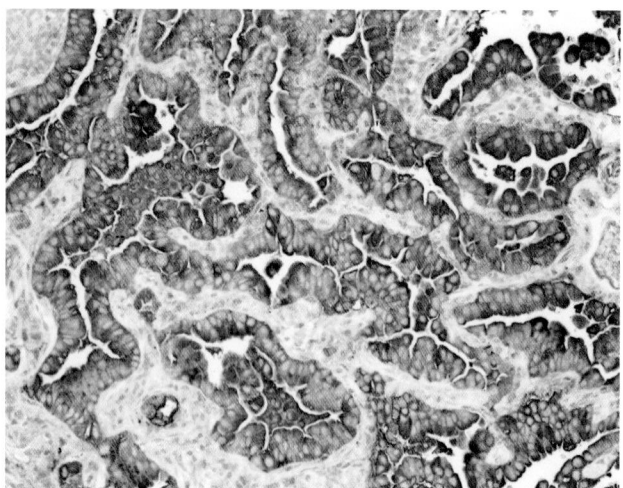

Figure 16-24. The tumor depicted in Figure 16-14 shows diffuse immunoreactivity for carcinoembryonic antigen, as expected in most adenocarcinomas of the lung but not in mesotheliomas.

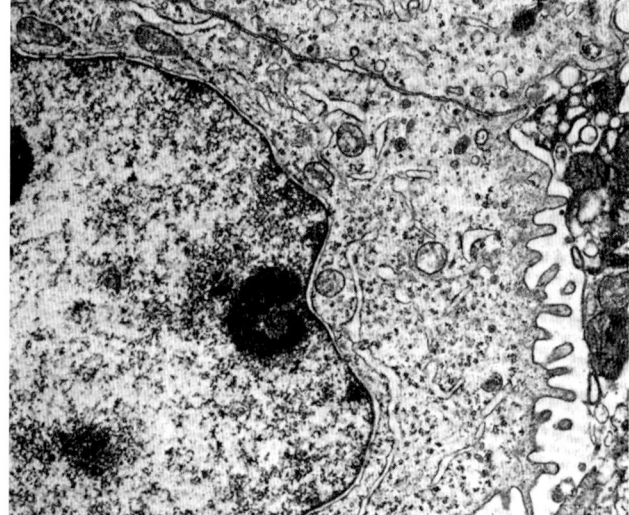

Figure 16-25. Electron photomicrograph of "pseudomesotheliomatous" adenocarcinoma in the pleura demonstrating short, nonbranching cell surface microvilli, structures typical of adenocarcinoma but not mesothelioma.

and others with multiple rounded densities throughout one or both lung fields (Fig. 16-28). On computed tomograms, the latter lesions may assume a "Cheerio" shape, in that they commonly demonstrate small central areas of cavitation. Hence, BAC may simulate an infectious disease, represent a nondescript "coin" lesion of the lung, or imitate the pattern of metastases to the lung from an occult visceral neoplasm.

Histologically, two distinct cytologic subtypes of BAC are recognized: mucinous and nonmucinous.[57,58,62] These are of importance because of their clinical associations. Mucinous tumors (Fig. 16-29) are those that tend to assume a pseudopneumonic or multifocal/multinodular clinical appearance, whereas nonmucinous BAC (Fig. 16-30) is more commonly a solitary lesion. Furthermore, stage for stage, nonmucinous variants may show a more favorable clinical evolution.[62,67] The criteria for the distinction of BAC from "ordinary" pulmonary ACAs continue to be debated. In accord with current convention, we restrict the use of this diagnosis to neoplasms that demonstrate a mantling of pre-existing air spaces ("lepidic" or noninvasive growth) by single layers or limited strata and micropapillae of only modestly atypical cuboidal or columnar epithelial cells, with or without intra-

cellular or extracellular mucin production. Intranuclear inclusions of cytoplasm containing surfactant proteins are also common.[68] Save for mucin production, such characteristics are shared by both forms of BAC, mucinous and nonmucinous (serous). Septal widening and sclerosis may be seen, especially with nonmucinous BAC, but there must be no desmoplasia or inflammation within or around the lesion if it is to be considered a bona fide BAC. Caution should be exercised in diagnosing BACs with central sclerosis because this is often a site of subtle early invasion. This demanding definition differs from that of some other observers, who have accepted the existence of a "sclerosing" BAC subtype.[69] Justification for more narrow requirements is gained from biologic data, which show worse behavior of "sclerosing" or "invasive" BAC than of nonfibrotic tumors.[57,70,71] Indeed, Clayton,[58] who devoted much attention to BAC, clearly stated that bronchioloalveolar carcinomas with sclerosis should be classified with other peripheral ACAs.

Another traditional point of discussion pertaining to the microscopic features of BAC (particularly its mucinous form) is that this neoplasm is said to disseminate within the lung by "aerogenous" means. That is to

Table 16-1. Role of Immunohistochemical Reagents Used to Distinguish between Epithelial Mesothelioma and Adenocarcinoma

Antibody	Mesothelioma		Adenocarcinoma	
	Result	%	Result	%
BG8	+	4	+	88
MoAb 44-3A6	+	100	+	8
Factor VIII	+	Rare	−	NS
Surfactant apoprotein	−	−	+	62
Anti-Lewis antigen	+	11	+	76
Tn antigen	−	−	+	62
E-cadherin	+	10	+	77
TTF-1	+	68	+	100
MoAb SM3	+	52	+	100
Secretory component	+	0–62	+	60
Pregnancy-specific protein	+	0–6	+	34–59
CA 19-9	−	−	+	39
OV632	+	85–91	+	20–63
NSE	+	96	NS	NS
CD57	+	70	NS	NS
Mab 45	+	NS	+	NS
HEA-125	−	−	+	75
Anti-BRG	−	−	+	83
ICAM-1	+	100	NS	NS
VCAM	+	87	NS	NS
Parathyroid hormone	+	84	+	11
CD44H	+	91	+	45
IOB 3	−	−	+	100

BRG, retinoblastoma-gene-related protein; ICAM, intercellular adhesion molecule; MoAb, monoclonal antibody; NS, not studied or not specified; NSE, neuron-specific enolase; VCAM, vascular cell adhesion molecule. Other abbreviations are monoclonal antibody designations and have no expanded names.
Data from Moran CA, Wick MR, Suster S. The role of immunohistochemistry in the diagnosis of malignant mesothelioma. *Semin Diagn Pathol.* 2000;17:178–183.

say, tumor cells are believed to detach from a "mother lesion" and spread to other foci in the pulmonary parenchyma by the process of inhalation and exhalation. Some molecular analyses, however, have cast doubt on that premise and instead suggest that the lesions are multiclonal.[72]

Other lesions that may be confused pathologically with BAC include foci of florid type II pneumocytic hyperplasia surrounding areas of diffuse alveolar damage[73] and interstitial fibrosing pneumonitides or organizing pulmonary infarcts[74]; the proliferation known as "atypical adenomatous alveolar hyperplasia" (discussed later)[75]; and the unicentric neoplasms known as "papillary alveolar adenoma" and "sclerosing hemangioma."[76] The latter two entities are bland cytologically and show a sharp interface with the surrounding pulmonary parenchyma, unlike BAC. Another point that was often raised in the older literature on BAC concerned the great difficulty with which metastases to the lung could be distinguished from the former neoplasm. Selected immunohistologic markers—especially nuclear labeling for thyroid transcription

factor-1 (TTF-1; Fig. 16-31) and cytoplasmic staining for napsin-A— are valuable in distinguishing BAC from metastases of extrapulmonary ACAs,[77–80] but that separation must ultimately rest on careful analysis of conventional clinicopathologic data.

Prognostically, patients with multifocal or pseudopneumonic BACs have an outlook that is worse than that of patients with unicentric tumors of this type because many of the former lesions are inoperable. Furthermore, mucinous tumors tend to behave more aggressively—with a higher incidence of extrapulmonary metastasis—than nonmucinous BAC when they are matched by size and stage.[57,58] Overall, nonmucinous tumors measuring less than 3 cm in maximum dimension have a good prognosis, approximating 90% at 5 years. Indeed, the current surgical approach to such lesions is limited resection, principally by wedge excision (Fig. 16-32).[81–85]

The natural history of BAC is more protracted than that of more conventional pulmonary ACAs, and tumor-related fatalities will continue to accrue even at 10 years after diagnosis.[57,63] Nevertheless, in an often-cited study by Manning and colleagues,[62] the 5-year survival rate for nonmucinous BAC was 72%, whereas only 26% of patients with mucinous tumors survived at that point.

Atypical Adenomatous Hyperplasia and Its Relationship to Bronchioloalveolar Carcinoma

Kitamura and colleagues[86] addressed the conceptual mechanistic relationship between topographically small atypical glandular proliferations of the lung—"atypical adenomatous hyperplasia" (AAH)—and BAC. Their model appeared to demonstrate a stepwise progression from AAH to BAC, with further evolution to invasive growth. That concept also had been advanced before, especially by Miller and colleagues,[87] who postulated that such a stepwise process existed in the lung in analogy to the adenoma-carcinoma sequence in the colon.

Atypical adenomatous hyperplasia must be differentiated from reactive or regenerative pneumocytic lesions, at one end of the spectrum, and from small bona fide ACAs, at the other. With regard to separation of AAH from various reactive lesions, Kitamura and co-workers[86] have emphasized the tendency of reactive lesions to include multiple cell types, including type II pneumocytes, ciliated cells, and mucinous cells, and they have described the relatively more conspicuous interstitial inflammation and edema in localized interstitial pneumonitis. Additional criteria that are found to be helpful in this context involve assessment of the lesional borders and patterns of fibrosis. There is a tendency for lesions of AAH to be more sharply circumscribed and for the mild interstitial fibrosis and inflammation to stop at the same boundary as the atypical alveolar cells. Conversely, reactive lesions tend to be less well defined, and the interstitial scarring extends beyond the areas of alveolar cell atypia. The individual cells in AAH, although less homogeneous than those in BAC, also tend to be more uniformly atypical than those of reactive hyperplasias (Figs. 16-33 and 16-34).

Gupta and colleagues[88] identified factors that favored the diagnosis of BAC over reactive changes in an evidence-based construct: multiple growth patterns; anisocytosis; nuclear atypia in 75% or more of the lesional cells; macronucleoli; and atypical mitoses. Conflicting information has emerged on the use of p63 immunostains to make this diagnostic distinction. Sheikh and colleagues[89] suggested that p63 positivity was restricted to reactive processes and absent in nonmucinous BAC, whereas Saad and coworkers[90] found p63 reactivity in 89% of cases of BAC.

A variety of chemotherapeutic agents can induce striking degrees of cytologic atypia, and this phenomenon is a well-documented pitfall in exfoliative cytology.[74,91] We have also seen several examples of pneumocytes with intranuclear cytoplasmic inclusions in clear-cut cases of organizing phase diffuse alveolar damage; hence, their presence should not be viewed as pathognomonic of neoplasia.

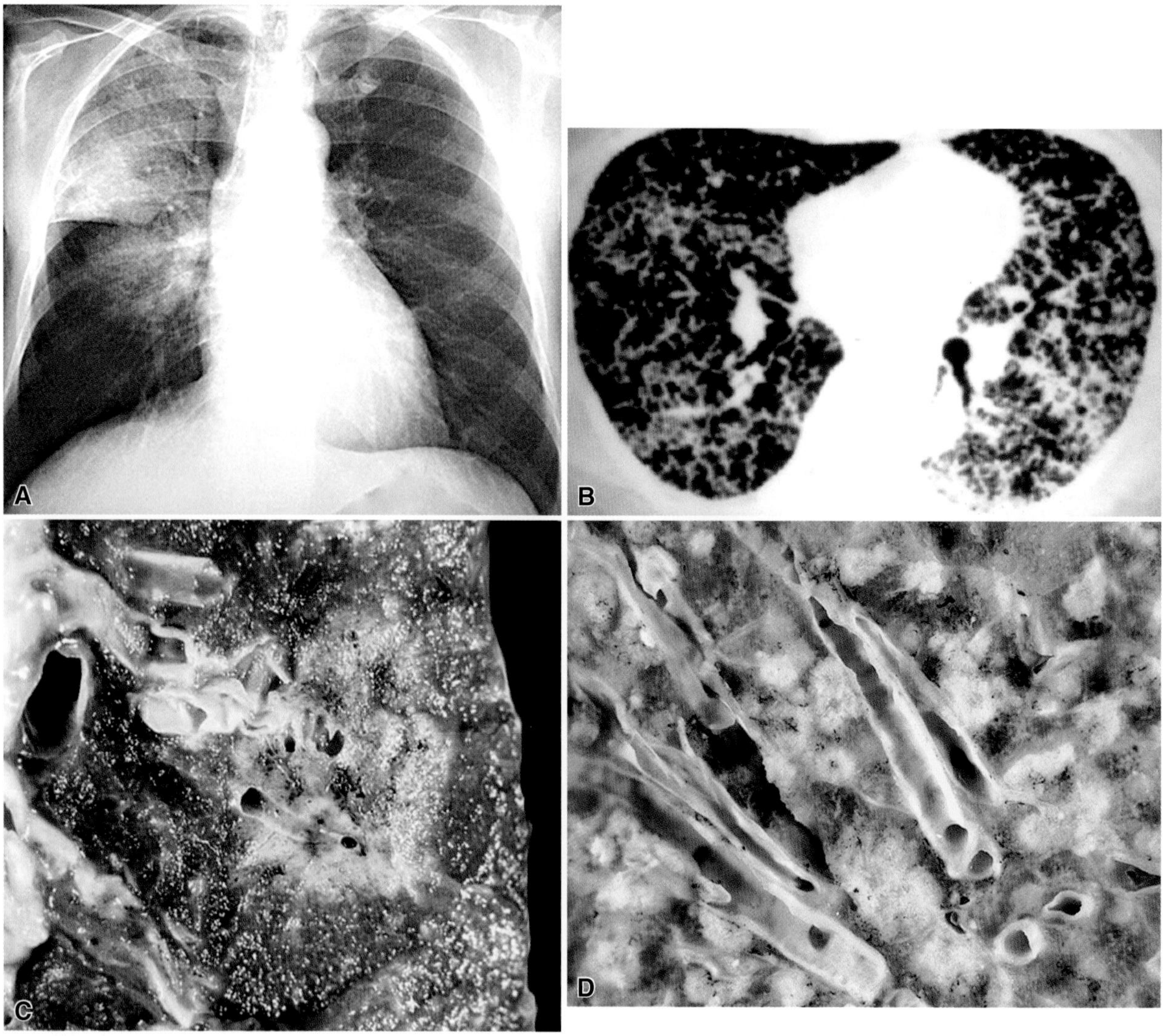

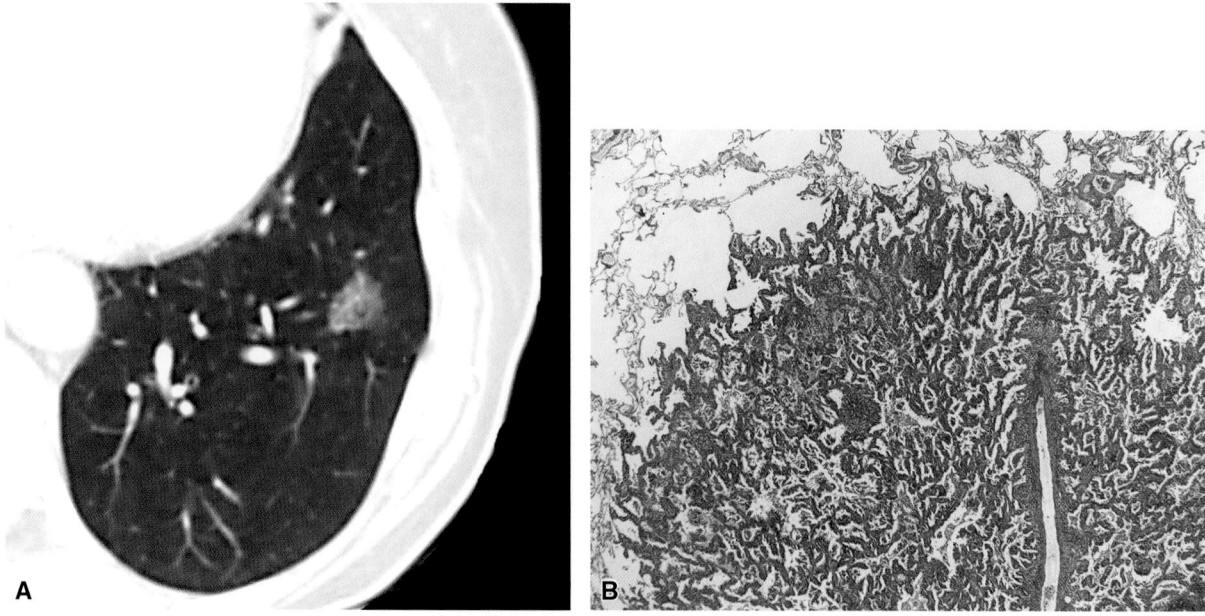

Figure 16-26. A, Pneumonia-like bronchioloalveolar carcinoma is seen as consolidation in the upper lobe of the right lung in this chest radiograph. **B,** Bilateral reticulonodular and consolidative lesions are seen in this thoracic computed tomogram from another patient with bronchioloalveolar carcinoma, resembling the changes of infiltrative non-neoplastic lung disease. **C** and **D,** The permeative, confluent, and consolidative nature of the tumor is evident in these gross photographs of affected lung.

Figure 16-27. A, This solitary ill-defined ground-glass lesion was diagnosed as a bronchioloalveolar carcinoma in this computed tomogram of the left lung. **B,** A scanning photomicrograph of solitary bronchioloalveolar carcinoma shows features that are similar to those of ordinary pulmonary adenocarcinoma, only lacking solid growth or definite areas of stromal invasion.

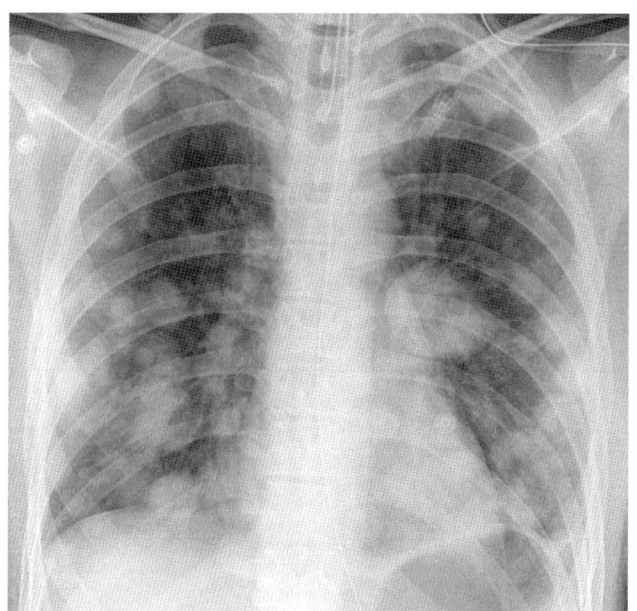

Figure 16-28. Multifocal synchronous bronchioloalveolar carcinoma presenting as multiple rounded nodules throughout both lung fields and simulating the radiographic appearance of a metastatic malignant tumor.

It is our view that the distinction between AAH and small nonmucinous BAC is conceptually arbitrary. Standard criteria that have been cited as useful in this distinction include uniformly atypical nuclei, large lesional size (>5 mm), and complex growth, with budding or tufting of tumor cells in the alveolar spaces in BAC but not AAH.[75,92] Kitamura and coworkers[86] suggested that a nuclear area of less than 40 μm^2 and a lesional diameter of less than 5 mm could effectively identify AAH as opposed to small BAC. Miller[93] also proposed a limit of 5 mm to separate "bronchioloalveolar cell adenoma" from BAC.

Nevertheless, morphometric and immunohistologic analyses have shown a synonymity rather than a disparity between AAH and nonmucinous BAC.[94,95] Similarly, molecular studies, which show some differences in statistical groups, have demonstrated many more shared features than differences.[96–100]

The most important consideration of this discussion concerns the clinical significance of AAH. In practice, this lesion is often not appreciated until microscopic sections arrive on the pathologist's desk, and they are seen in four main contexts:

1. In sections of a wedge biopsy specimen of a non-neoplastic disease.
2. In wedge resection margins of a peripheral carcinoma.
3. In "random" sections of a lobe with another, discrete carcinoma.
4. As suspected nodules of multifocal tumor along with at least one other documented peripheral ACA.

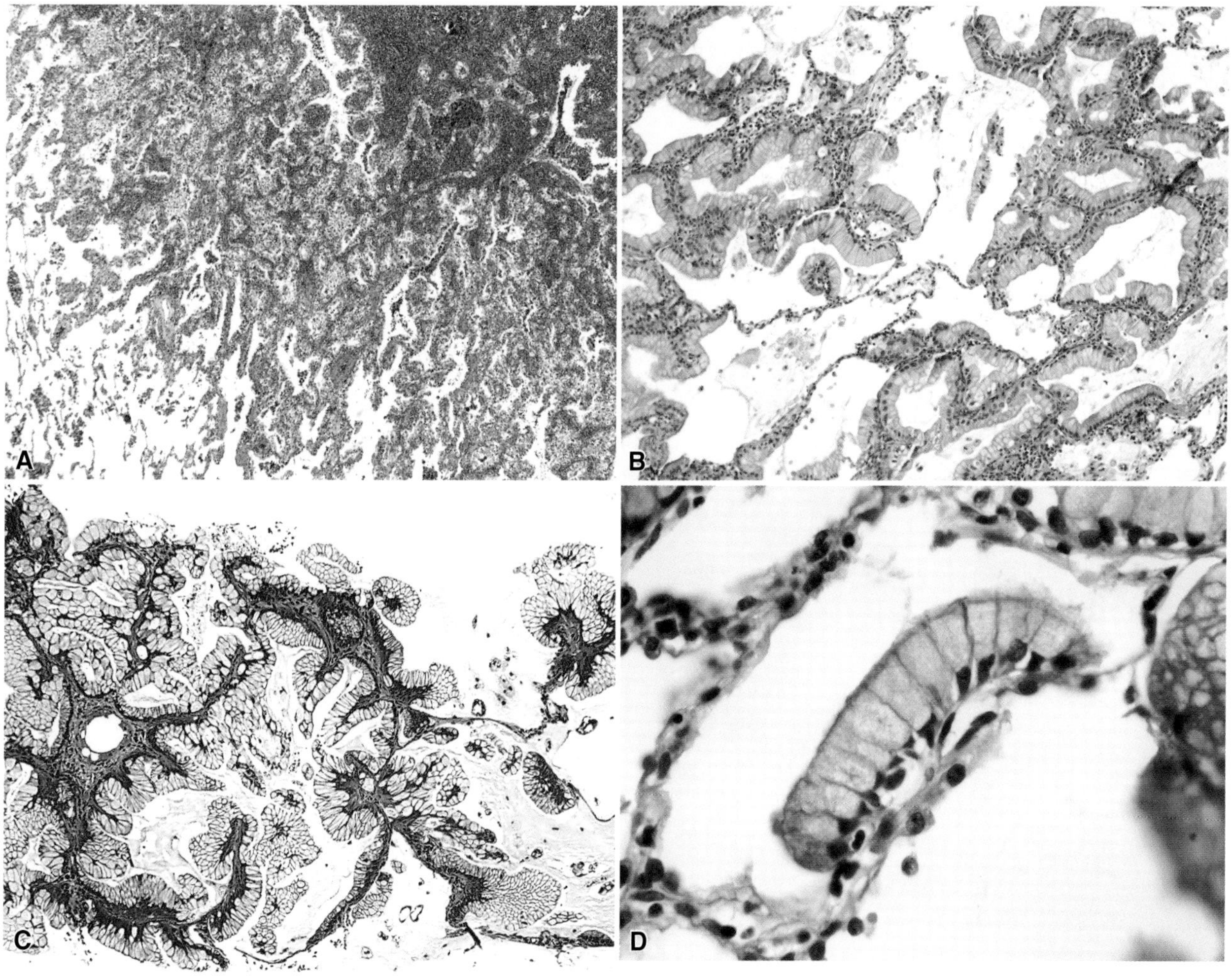

Figure 16-29. A to **D,** Mucinous bronchioloalveolar carcinoma shows a "lepidic" growth pattern, with tumor cells mantling pre-existing alveolar septa and production of abundant extracellular mucin.

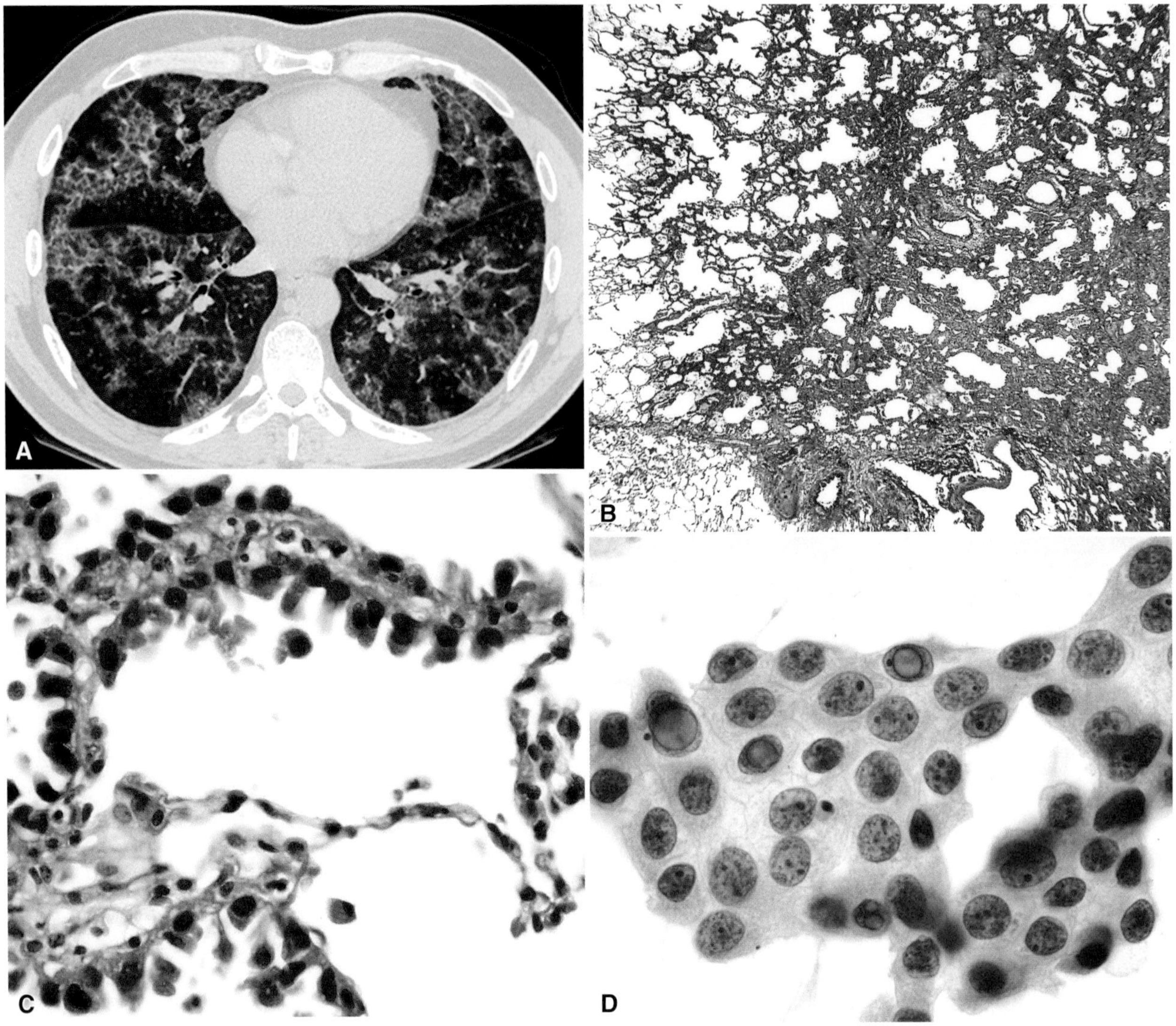

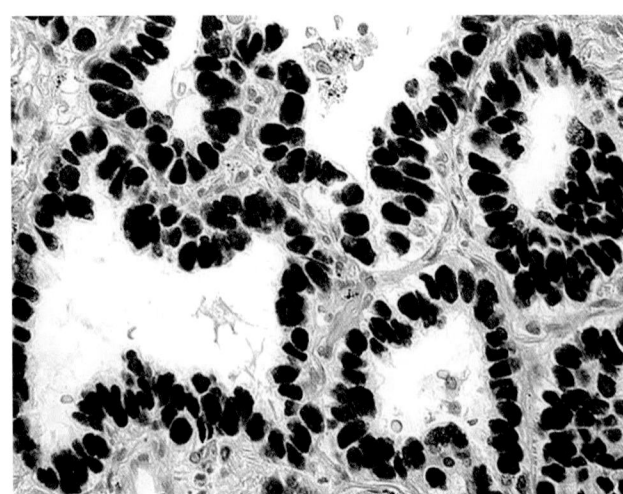

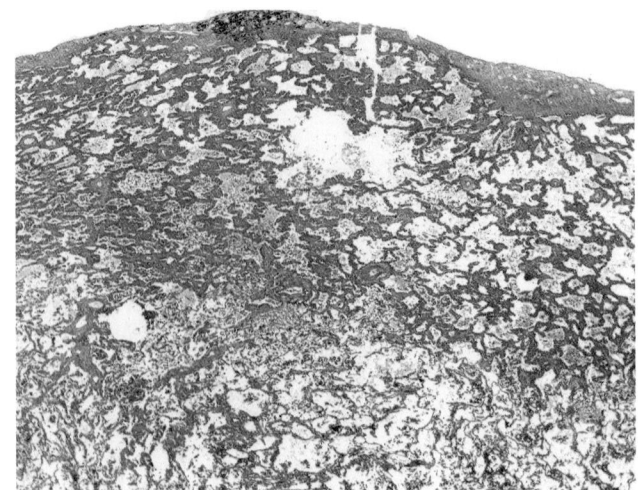

Figure 16-30. A, This bronchioloalveolar carcinoma (BAC) demonstrates a "crazy-paving" pattern of parenchymal infiltration in a computed tomogram of the chest. **B** and **C,** Nonmucinous BAC shows mantling of alveolar septa by well-differentiated low-columnar tumor cells. Intranuclear invaginations of cytoplasm ("pseudoinclusions") are again potentially visible histologically. **D,** A fine-needle aspiration biopsy specimen from nonmucinous BAC shows relatively bland and homogeneous polygonal cells that are arranged in three-dimensional profiles. Intranuclear invaginations of cytoplasm are present in some tumor cells.

Figure 16-31. Intense nuclear immunoreactivity for thyroid transcription factor-1 is present in this bronchioloalveolar carcinoma.

Figure 16-32. Limited wedge excision of small adenocarcinomas, as shown here, is currently used in some instances for solitary bronchioloalveolar carcinomas of less than 2 cm in maximum dimension.

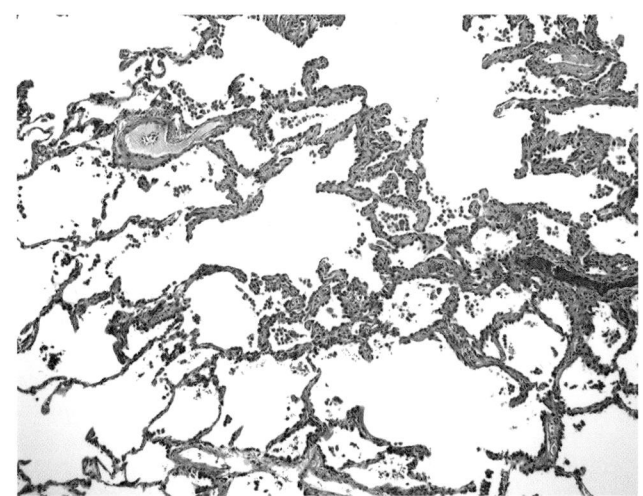

Figure 16-33. Atypical adenomatous hyperplasia, low power. There is mild interstitial thickening.

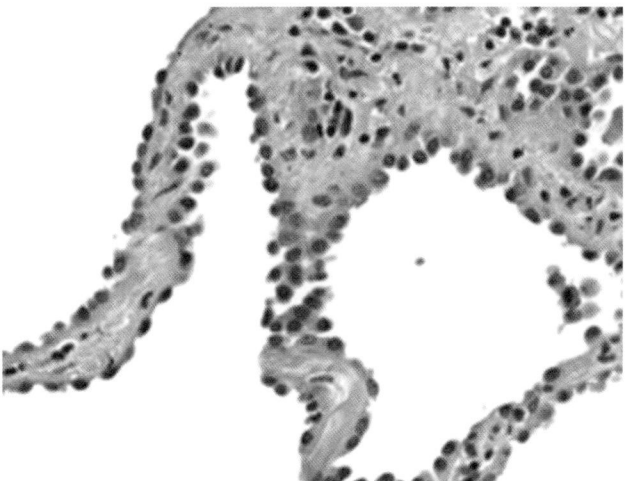

Figure 16-34. Aytpical adenomatous hyperplasia, higher power. The nuclei are less atypical, less crowded, and smaller than the cells of bronchioloalveolar carcinoma.

To provide some understanding of the importance of atypical lesions, several points must be kept in mind. First, because most AAH lesions are found in patients undergoing resection of an obvious cancer, it is nearly an insurmountable challenge to arrive at any conclusions concerning their biology. The outcome of these cases will be determined by the characteristics of the grossly obvious tumors. Alveolar AAH lesions tend to be multifocal throughout both lungs but may be inapparent on gross examination, and can be easily missed, even with current radiologic imaging techniques. Therefore, short of bilateral lung transplantation, it is impossible to say what would constitute adequate surgical resection of such lesions. Given these realities, it is best for pathologists to be pragmatically conservative in the diagnosis of clinically inapparent AAH lesions as small BACs, despite the conceptual considerations noted earlier. It is important to emphasize, however, that such lesions can be multifocal and may have a relationship with subsequent multicentric BACs, underscoring the need for close follow-up to identify the possible appearance of metachronous tumors. On the other hand, proliferations that represent grossly observed lesions with compellingly atypical cytology should be designated as outright carcinomas.

In light of the current availability of biologic agents that can be used to treat lung cancer, it is appropriate to mention the genotypes of nonmucinous and mucinous BAC. In general, nonmucinous lesions

demonstrate mutations in the epidermal growth factor receptor (EGFR) molecule, to which tyrosine kinase inhibitor (TKI) therapeutic agents are directed.[101,102] On the other hand, mucinous BAC manifests preferential aberrations in the *K-ras* gene and accordingly does not show a response to TKIs.[101] Mutant EGFR protein overexpression, as indicated indirectly by strong cell membrane immunoreactivity in tumor cells, correlates to some degree, but very imperfectly, with in situ hybridization studies or polymerase chain reaction-based assays.[103]

"Micropapillary" ACA of the lung was formerly considered by many observers to be a subtype of nonmucinous BAC. That nosologic approach has now changed,[43] occasioned by the demonstrably worse prognosis of micropapillary carcinoma.[104,105] Accordingly, the latter neoplasm is now regarded as a pathologic entity unto itself. In analogy to the diagnostic approach to BAC, a conclusive interpretation of micropapillary carcinoma should be avoided in cytologic specimens. Rudomina and colleagues[106] have shown that papillary profiles in the latter samples do not correlate well with a final diagnosis of micropapillary ACA.

Adenocarcinomas Associated with Scars

In the relatively recent past, it was taught that fibrous scarring in the lung—seen as a consequence of pneumonia, interstitial fibroproliferative diseases, or pneumoconioses—predisposed to ACA and had a directly causative role in the genesis of that tumor type.[107] Nevertheless, several investigators have concluded that the central fibrosis seen in "scar adenocarcinomas" (Fig. 16-35) is formed after initiation of the carcinoma and that it is the product of the tumor cells themselves.[108–110] At a practical level, there is no reason to suspect that localized fibrosing conditions in the lung are, in and of themselves, preneoplastic. However, it appears that an increased frequency of lung carcinoma may exist in patients with diffuse interstitial fibrosis—as seen in late-stage "usual interstitial pneumonia," for example—over and above that associated with smoking alone.[111] Nevertheless, the relative weights of those potentially causal elements are still unclear.

With particular reference to asbestosis and silicosis, special forms of pulmonary interstitial fibrosis, our review of the aggregated literature leads to the conclusion that the risk of pulmonary carcinoma may (debatably) be increased by those conditions of the lung, although such an association does not prove causation. It is clear that cigarette smoking is, by far, the most significant carcinogenic factor in this specific context.[112]

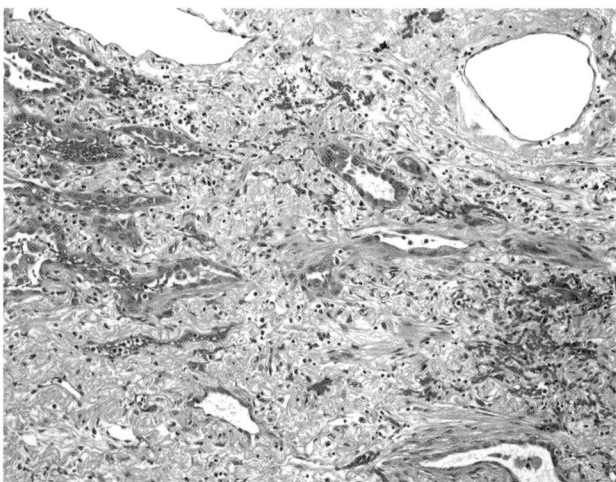

Figure 16-35. A broad zone of fibroelastotic "scarring" is seen in the center of this pulmonary adenocarcinoma. Matrical changes such as this are a product of the tumor rather than a pre-existing condition.

Adenosquamous Carcinoma

Adenosquamous carcinoma (ASC) is a "composite" tumor, exhibiting simultaneous squamous and glandular differentiation in the same mass (Fig. 16-36). It accounts for no more than 5% of all lung cancers in most surgical series.[113-115] The clinical, radiographic, and gross pathologic attributes of ASC are most similar to those of "pure" ACAs of the lung. A point of contention with regard to this lesion is whether it is synonymous with high-grade mucoepidermoid carcinoma of the salivary glandular type. Our opinion is that those two neoplasms are typically separable. Salivary gland analog tumors in the lung, as considered subsequently, tend to arise in the large central airways, in contrast to the propensity for ASC to be peripheral. In addition, foci of lower-grade mucoepidermoid carcinoma are often present in the former, but not the latter, of these tumor types. The prognosis of pulmonary ASC is said to be adverse. In studies reported by Ishida and colleagues,[113] Takamori and colleagues,[115] and Cakir and co-workers,[116] the survival of patients with adenosquamous tumors was statistically worse than that of individuals with "pure" ACAs or SCCs.

Large Cell Carcinoma

Large cell undifferentiated carcinomas account for approximately 15% of all lung cancers.[117] As mentioned earlier, diagnostic use of the term "non–small cell carcinoma" has produced some confusion among poorly differentiated SCC, poorly differentiated ACA, poorly differentiated ASC, and true LCC. Accordingly, it has been suggested that the designation of "large cell carcinoma" should be employed restrictively as a synonym for LCC. An even more extreme point of view is that current pathologic tools for cellular analysis have made this diagnosis completely obsolete.[118,119]

Large cell carcinomas are typically larger than 5 cm in maximum dimension, have a white-gray cut surface (which may be lobulated and resemble "fish flesh," thus potentially simulating the appearance of a sarcoma or a hematolymphoid lesion; Fig. 16-37), and are rarely multicentric. Internal necrosis is a relatively common feature. Approximately 50% demonstrate a connection to a large tubular airway.

Histologically, LCCs show a composition of large polygonal cells with vesicular chromatin, prominent nucleoli, discernible cytoplasmic borders, and by definition, a lack of glandular differentiation or keratinization (Fig. 16-38). They are typically arranged in sheets or large clusters, potentially exhibiting foci of central necrosis. Two distinctive subtypes also exist—giant cell carcinoma and clear cell carcinoma.

Giant cell carcinoma was initially believed to be a separate clinicopathologic entity,[120,121] but that philosophy is no longer considered valid.[122] Microscopically, this variant of LCC is composed of extremely pleomorphic large tumor cells, which are often multinucleated (Fig. 16-39). There is a regular admixture of

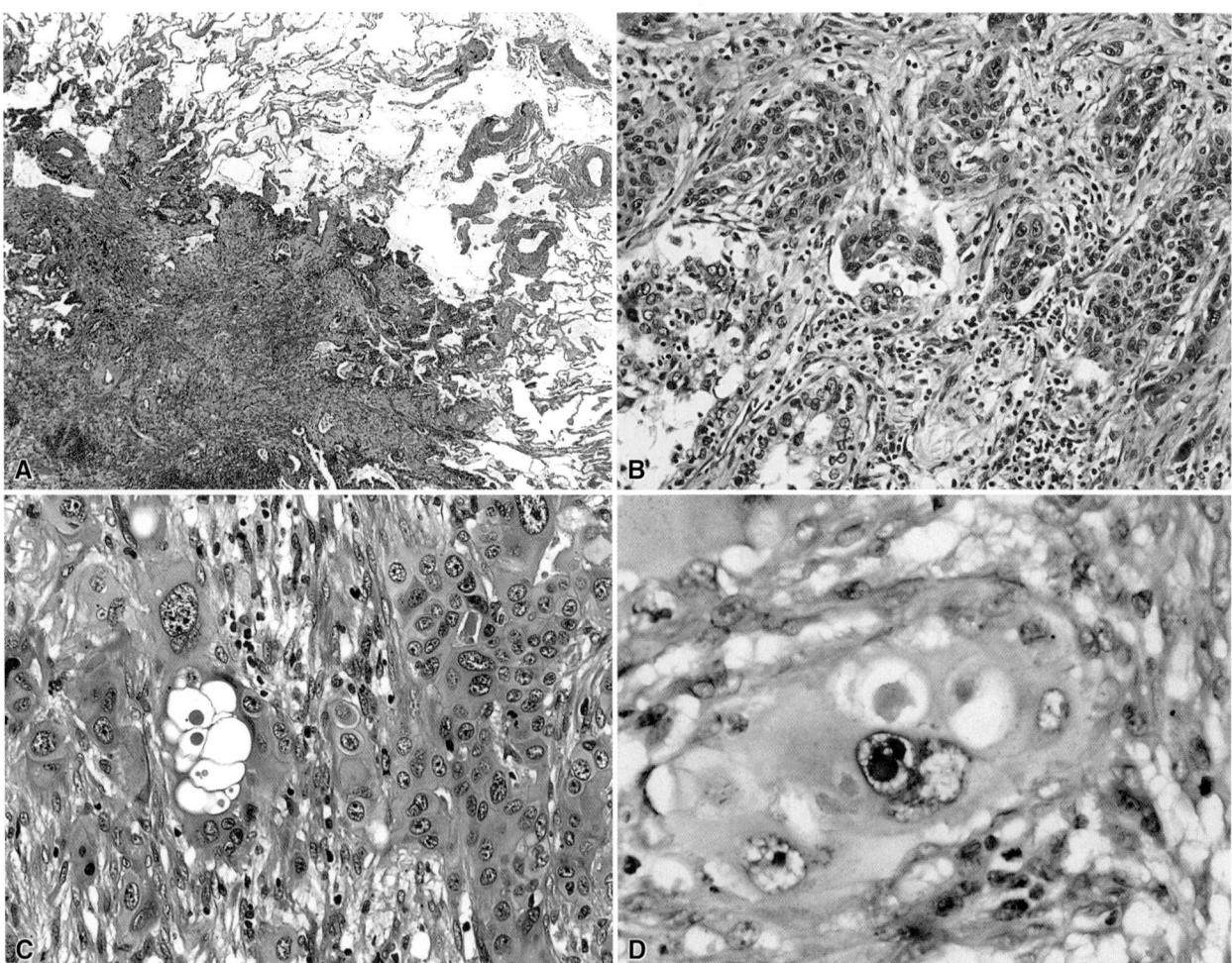

Figure 16-36. A, Low-power photomicrograph of adenosquamous carcinoma of the lung with a configuration like that of other non–small cell lung cancers. **B,** Closer inspection shows a bifid composition by obviously keratinizing squamous elements and gland-forming tumor cells, which are intimately admixed. **C,** Multiple glandular lumina, containing secretions, are present in the middle of an otherwise squamoid focus in adenosquamous carcinoma. **D,** A digested periodic acid/Schiff stain demonstrates the presence of epithelial mucin in another similar area of the tumor.

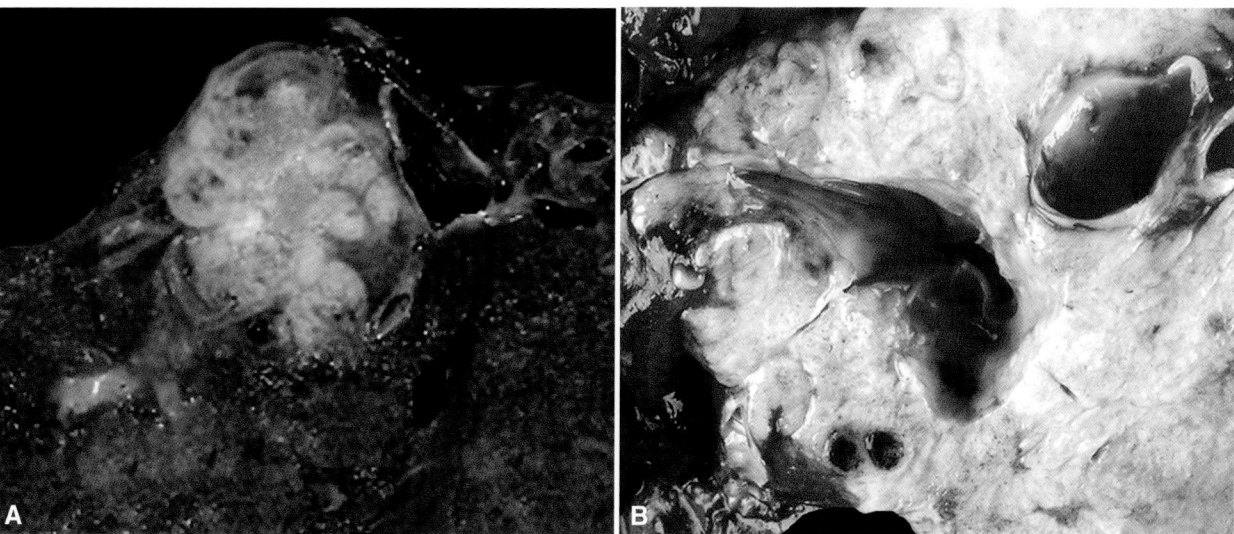

Figure 16-37. A, Gross photograph of large cell carcinoma of the lung showing a fleshy tan-pink mass with no other distinguishing features. **B,** In another patient with large cell undifferentiated carcinoma, the gross tumor has a "fish-flesh" appearance and surrounds the great vessels in the mediastinum.

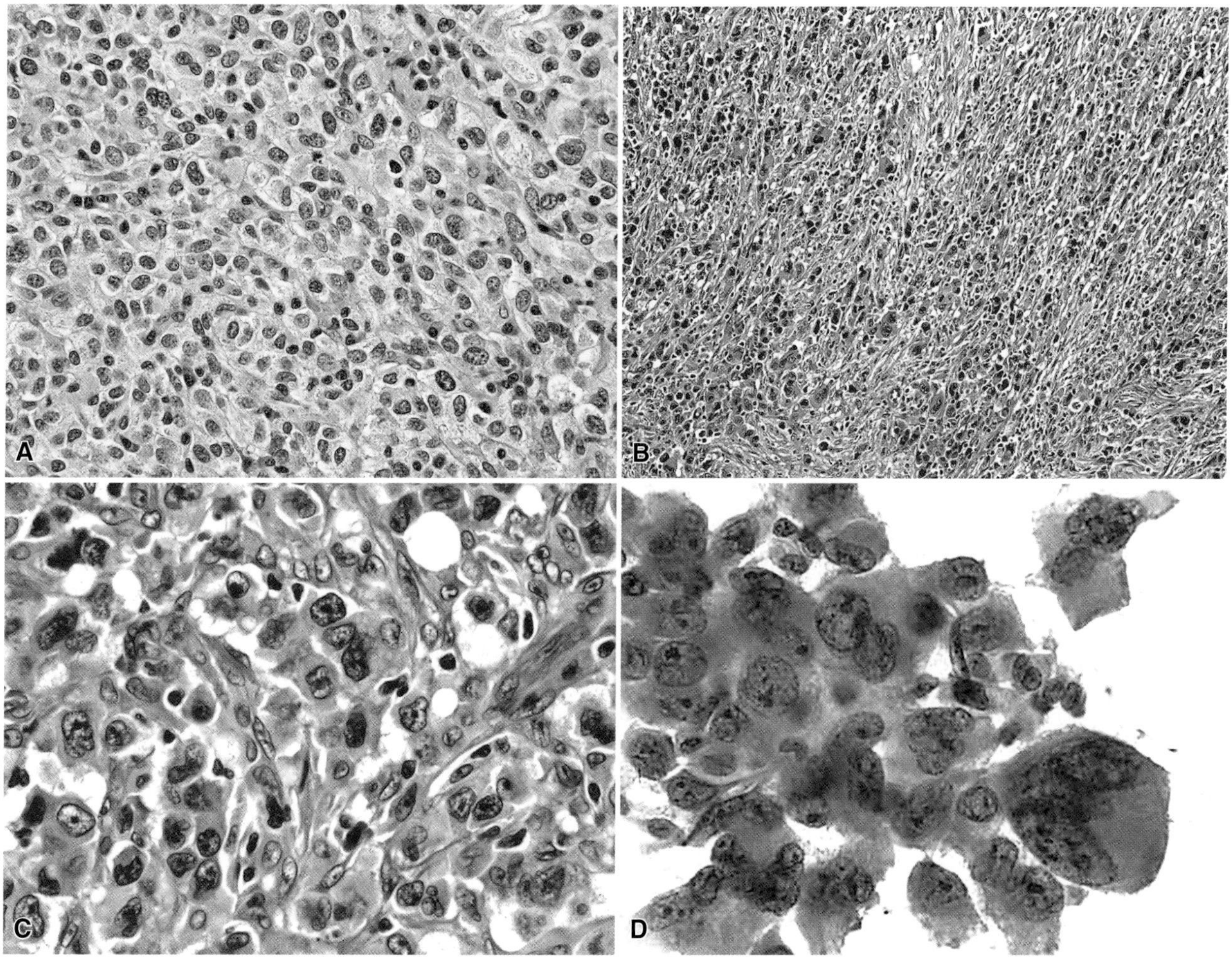

Figure 16-38. A to C, Large cell carcinoma of the lung showing formless sheets of pleomorphic polygonal cells with no evidence of keratinization or gland formation. **D,** A cohesive group of large pleomorphic cells is seen in this fine-needle aspiration biopsy specimen of large cell undifferentiated carcinoma.

polymorphonuclear leukocytes with the neoplastic elements, even in the absence of necrosis, suggesting tumoral synthesis of leukocyte cytokines, such as granulocyte colony–stimulating factor.[123] Parenthetically, this phenomenon can also be associated with systemic neutrophilia in association with the giant cell subtype of LCC. Neoplastic "cannibalism" may also be observed, wherein the giant tumor cells appear to engulf one another. One subtype of pulmonary giant cell carcinoma bears a close resemblance to choriocarcinoma of the gonads, complete with tumor synthesis of beta-human chorionic gonadotropin.[124]

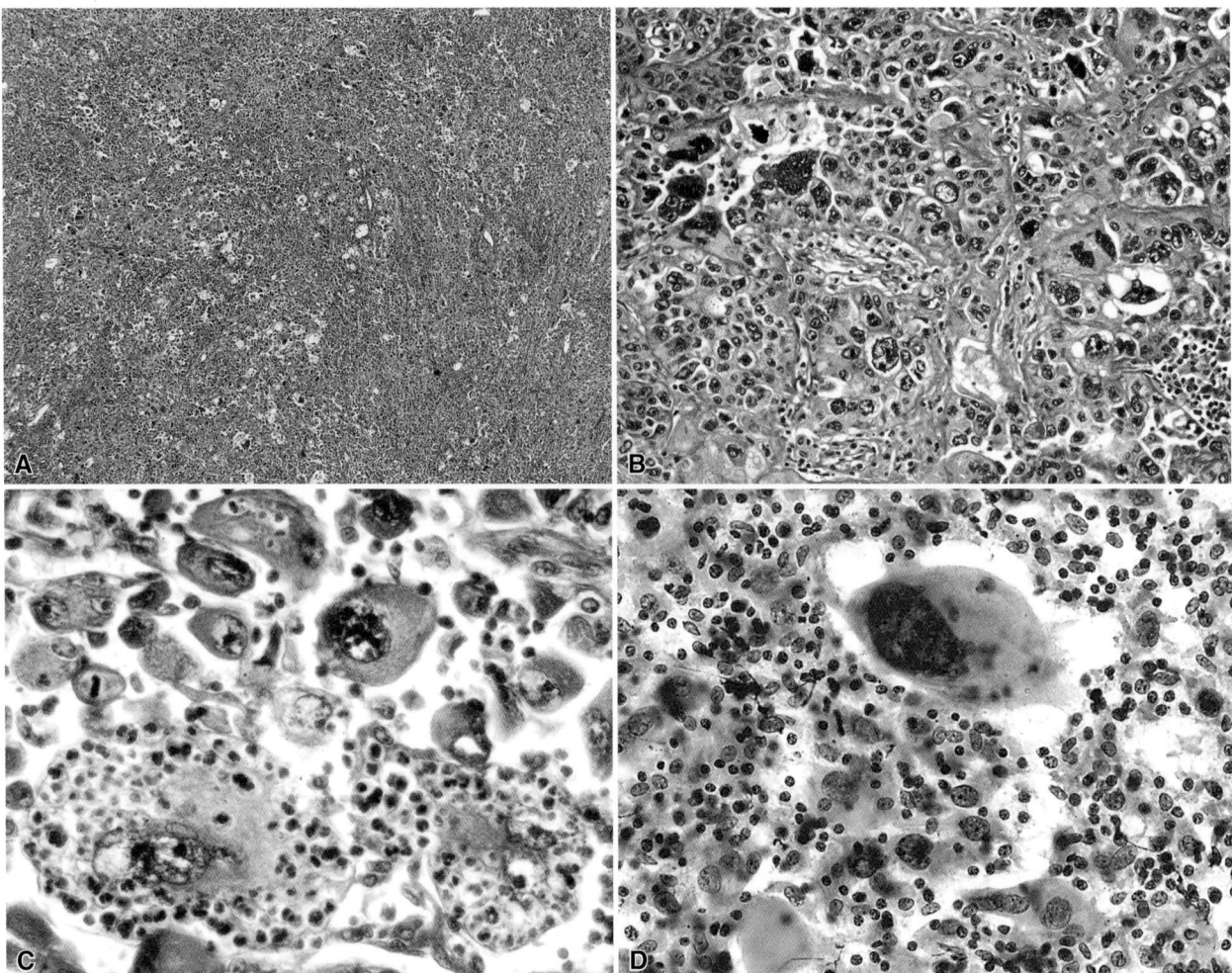

Figure 16-39. Giant cell carcinoma (GCC) of the lung. **A,** Sheets of undifferentiated tumor cells. **B,** Large neoplastic multinucleated cells. **C,** Gigantiform nuclei are apparent with numerous intratumoral neutrophils. **D,** A fine-needle aspiration biopsy specimen of GCC shows dyshesive tumor cells with a markedly variable cytologic appearance. Inflammatory cells are also abundant in this specimen.

Primary clear cell carcinoma of the lung (CCCL) is a diagnosis of exclusion, and it is likely that tumors with both squamous and glandular differentiation are included in that group. A number of other clear cell neoplasms of the lung, including some "carcinoids," the benign "sugar tumor," metastatic renal cell carcinoma, and metastatic "balloon cell" melanoma, must also be considered before making the diagnosis of CCCL.[50,125-129] This can be accomplished by a combination of radiographic, electron microscopic, and immunohistologic evaluations. The overall clinicopathologic attributes of CCCL are comparable to those of LCC, not otherwise specified.

In the last two decades, it has been suggested that a subset of pulmonary large cell carcinomas that show occult neuroendocrine differentiation—as detected only by electron microscopy or immunohistology—should be nosologically separated from truly undifferentiated large cell tumors.[130-133] Hence, the terms "exocrine large cell carcinoma" (another synonym for LCC) and "endocrine large cell carcinoma" have entered use.[132] In our opinion, "endocrine large cell carcinomas" are best specified as either high-grade "pure" neuroendocrine carcinomas, large cell type, or LCCs with occult neuroendocrine differentiation; those two entities are considered in more detail in another chapter on neuroendocrine neoplasms of the lung (see Chapter 13).

Selected large cell lung cancers have a "rhabdoid" phenotype[134] with eosinophilic hyaline inclusions in the cytoplasm and large vesicular nuclei with prominent nucleoli (Fig. 16-40). It is likely that this image represents a final common pathway of clonal evolution ("dedifferentiation") in carcinomas of the lung, as in several other neoplasms demonstrating a rhabdoid configuration.[135] That conclusion is supported by the fact that other forms of carcinoma may be admixed with the rhabdoid elements ("composite" extrarenal rhabdoid tumors).[135] Moreover, nuclear expression of the *INI1* gene—a tumor suppressor—is retained in "composite" extrarenal rhabdoid tumors (Fig. 16-41), but is consistently deleted in prototypical rhabdoid tumor of the kidney in children.[136-138]

Returning to the issue of how a pathologic diagnosis of pulmonary LCC is made, we—and others[139-141]—believe that conventional light microscopic morphologic analysis is still the method of both convenience and choice. At this point, no credible data have shown significant differences in survival among cases that are categorized as LCC in prospective and rigorously constructed clinical trials employing "modern" modalities of pathologic evaluation as well as treatment, compared with the outcomes of poorly differentiated "solid" ACAs or high-grade SCCs.

Pathologic Classification of Lung Cancer and Selection of Nonsurgical Therapies

As mentioned earlier, attention to pathologic detail has been strong in the last several years on the part of clinicians, with the aim of selecting nonsurgical therapy for patients with advanced carcinomas of the lung. The ever-increasing availability of new biologic and chemical agents

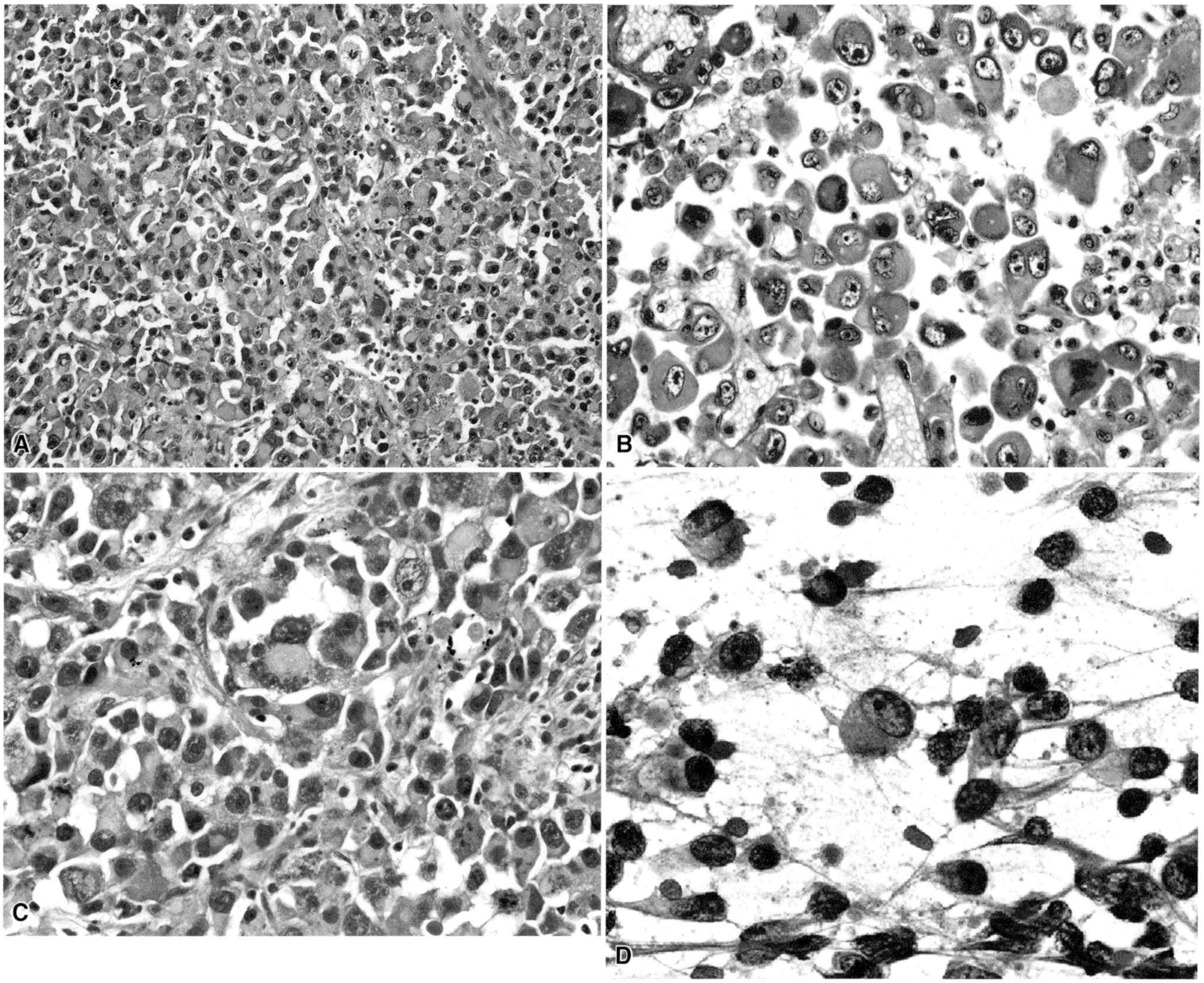

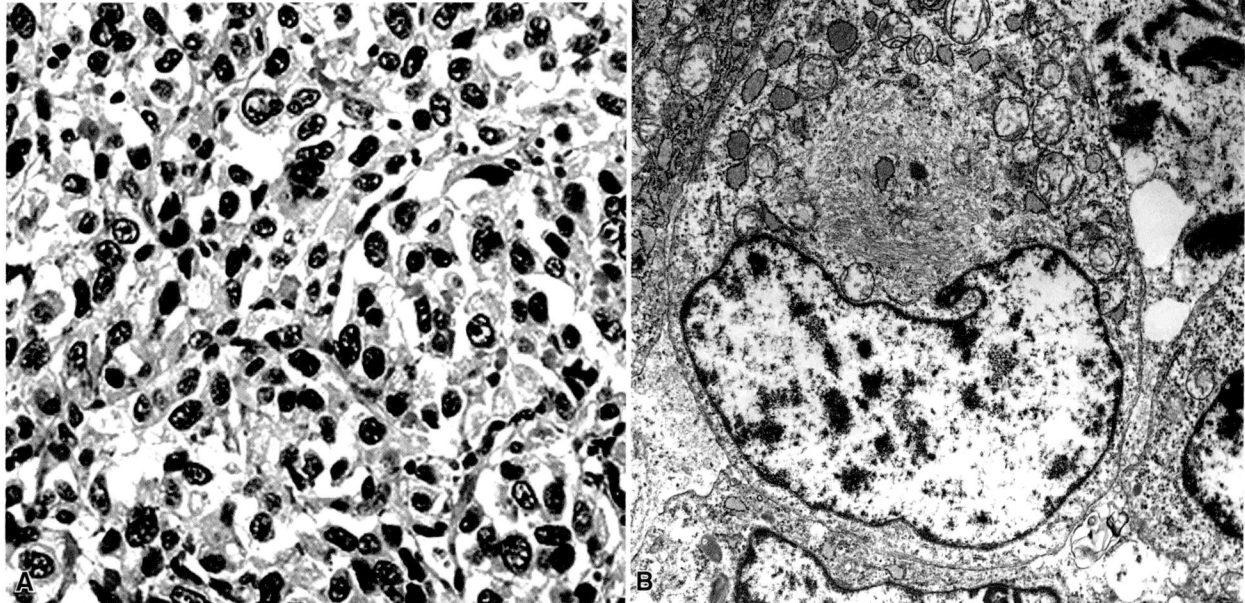

Figure 16-40. A to **C,** Large cell lung carcinoma with a "rhabdoid" phenotype in which globular eosinophilic cytoplasmic inclusions displace the nuclei of the tumor cells. **D,** A fine-needle aspiration biopsy specimen contains similar cells, which are dyshesive. The cytopathologic differential diagnosis includes metastatic neoplasms with a potentially rhabdoid appearance, most notably, amelanotic melanoma.

Figure 16-41. A, Nuclear immunoreactivity for INI1 is retained in "composite" malignant rhabdoid tumors of the lung, which are believed to represent large cell undifferentiated carcinomas with rhabdoid cytologic features. This finding contrasts with INI1 negativity in prototypical rhabdoid tumors of the kidney in childhood. **B,** This electron photomicrograph of "rhabdoid" lung carcinoma shows a ball of cytoplasmic intermediate filaments that indents the nucleus.

has driven that scrutiny. In a generic sense, the construct that has been applied by oncologists pairs the preferred management of ACAs with TKIs and that of nonglandular and neuroendocrine carcinomas with "conventional" chemotherapeutic drugs.[100,140,142,143] Although initial responses to TKIs appeared to be promising in patients with lung cancer, enthusiasm recently has been tempered.[144–146]

Some of this disappointment has likely been caused, at least in part, by pathologists. For example, it is common to equate strong immunoreactivity for EGFR (Fig. 16-42) with pathologic alterations in the *EGFR* gene; in reality, the former finding is only a crude substitute for results of molecular analyses, such as in situ hybridization or polymerase chain reaction–based methods.[103,147] Moreover, the diagnostic boundaries of ACA have been "stretched" by some pathologist observers to qualify patients for entrance into TKI trials. That is particularly true in laboratories that routinely "type" lung cancers with immunohistochemical panels. For example, even though a poorly differentiated neoplasm may demonstrate an "adenocarcinoma profile" by such assessment, prospective and evidence-based clinicopathologic studies are lacking to demonstrate that this finding translates into a differential benefit of one treatment as opposed to another. Markers that are currently applied in this context include high–molecular-weight ("squamous") keratins, CD141, and p63 for squamous carcinomas (Fig. 16-43); cytokeratin-7, napsin-A (Fig. 16-44), and TTF-1 for ACAs; mixtures of reactivities for those determinants in ASCs; and an absence of them all in LCCs.[35,118,148]

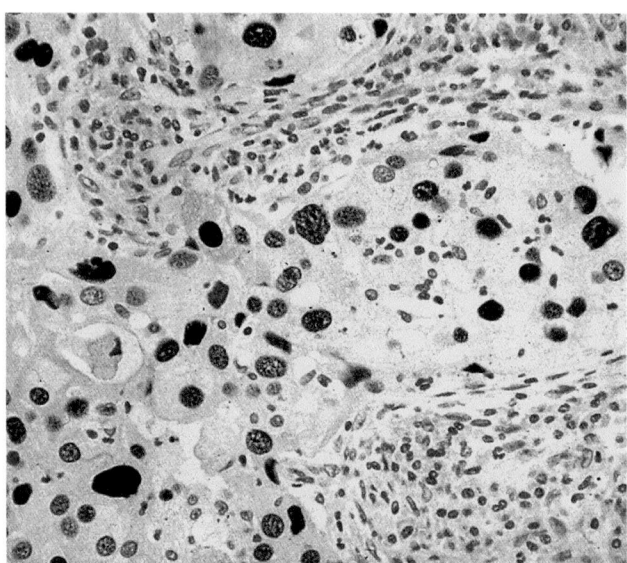

Figure 16-43. Nuclear immunoreactivity for p63 is consistent with squamous differentiation in poorly differentiated carcinomas of the lung and other sites. However, this marker may sometimes be seen in adenocarcinomas and neuroendocrine carcinomas as well.

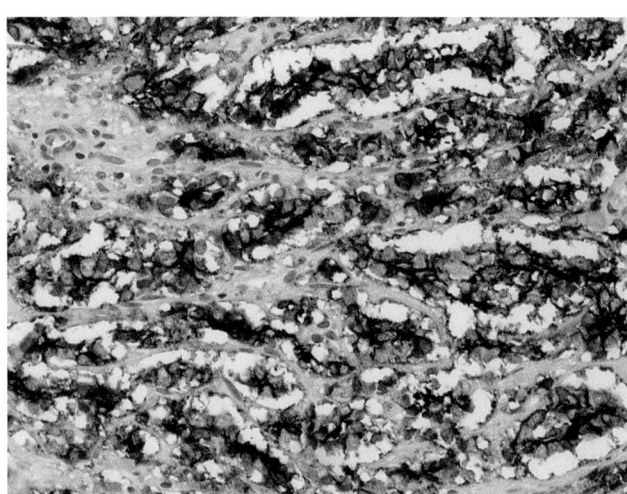

Figure 16-44. Cytoplasmic labeling for napsin-A is a helpful adjunct to nuclear immunostaining for thyroid transcription factor-1 in helping to identify adenocarcinomatous differentiation among poorly differentiated carcinomas of the lung.

The problems with the approach of linking immunophenotypes with therapeutic choices are threefold. First, we reiterate the fact that lung carcinomas often demonstrate mixed patterns of differentiation at light microscopic and ultrastructural levels of analysis.[3,12,24,26] Accordingly, immunoprofiles and genotypes also vary considerably, even within the same morphologic tumor groups.[149–151] Secondly, large groups of high-stage, immunohistochemically "defined" lung carcinoma types have not been treated using systematic protocols after careful matching of comorbid variables in construction of the studies. Third, several studies have shown that the responses to *EGFR*- and *K-ras*–directed treatments may differ between metastatic pulmonary cancers and their primary tumors.[152–154]

Thus, for now, we urge caution in the reflexive immunohistochemical or immunogenetic assessment of all lung carcinomas, which is not yet a "standard of practice." Pathologists should attempt to comply with the requirements of various developmental therapeutic trials, vis-à-vis methods for nosologic categorization, but that is different from the diagnosis of lung cancers in the current clinical environment.

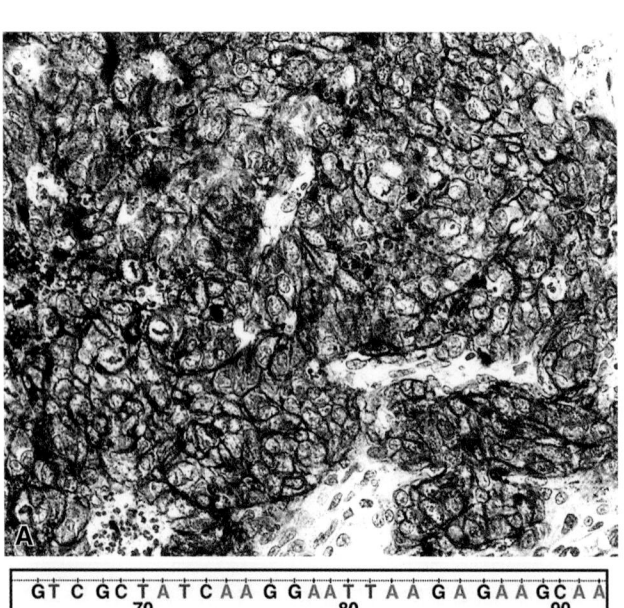

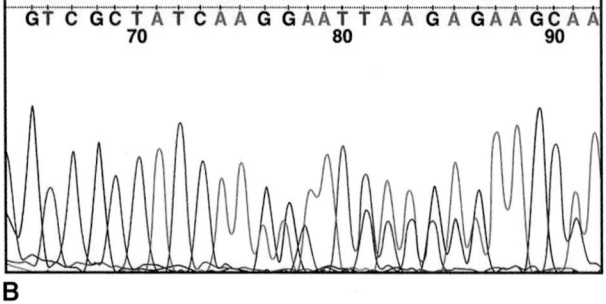

GTCGCTATCAAGGAATTAAGAGAAGCAA
70   80   90

Figure 16-42. **A,** Strong cell membrane immunoreactivity for epidermal growth factor receptor in acinar adenocarcinoma of the lung. **B,** This finding is often used as a surrogate for actual gene sequencing analysis (in this instance, showing a 15-base-pair deletion in exon 19, codon 746–750), but the former is not as reliable as the latter in predicting therapeutic tumor response to tyrosine kinase inhibitors.

Sartori and associates[155] have proposed the use of a scoring system that integrates clinical, morphologic, and molecular-genetic data to yield a probability score that indicates the likelihood of tumor response to *EGFR* inhibitors in clinical trials.

So that this commentary is not nihilistic, it can be said that some reproducible correlative trends have emerged from adjunctive studies on pulmonary carcinomas. Nonmucinous BACs, micropapillary ACAs, and ACAs comprising "hobnail" cells generally show some response to TKIs.[98,102,143] In contrast, "solid" poorly differentiated ACAs often do not.[143] The latter lesions more often exhibit mutations in the *K-ras* gene rather than in *EGFR*, as is true of most mucinous BACs (discussed earlier).[155] Finally, some TKI-responsive ACAs have also manifested integration of nucleic acid from the human papillomavirus, at least in Asian patients.[156]

This area of pathologic analysis is obviously still a "work in progress." More data need to be accrued and analyzed before the molecular signatures of various lung carcinoma subsets can be tabulated and linked firmly to their biologic behaviors.

Salivary Gland–Type Carcinomas of the Lung

Primary salivary gland–type tumors of the lung (SGTTLs) are unusual, comprising no more than 1% of all pulmonary neoplasms.[157] Moreover, their diagnosis may pose a problem not only because of their rarity but also because in small biopsies it is relatively easy to consign them to the broad category of "non–small cell carcinoma." That would be unfortunate because the clinical behavior of SGTTLs can be quite different from that of conventional lung cancers. This family of tumors generally has an immunohistochemical profile similar to that of ordinary pulmonary carcinomas, a fact that tends to lessen the value of immunophenotyping in the differential diagnosis.

Interestingly, if one attempts to make correlations between the occurrence of SGTTLs and histologically identical tumors in the salivary glands, one finds differences rather than similarities. For instance, neoplasms that are seen commonly in the salivary glands, such as pleomorphic adenoma (mixed tumor), are only rarely seen in the lung. In fact, most SGTTLs are malignant lesions, justifying their inclusion in this chapter. Furthermore, some histologic features that are commonly observed in pulmonary salivary gland analog tumors do not necessarily parallel those of their counterparts in the salivary glands themselves.

Mucoepidermoid Carcinoma

Mucoepidermoid carcinoma (MEC) is the most common of the SGTTLs and may be encountered in any age group; however, most cases have been seen in adults.[158-168] In a series of cases reported by Yousem and Hochholzer,[166] 58 patients ranged from 9 to 78 years of age, with a male-to-female distribution of almost 1.5:1. When the tumors were separated into low- and high-grade lesions, no preference for any particular age group was noted for either group. Nevertheless, the great majority of these tumors belong in the low-grade category. Clinical symptoms in patients with MECs are dependent on the size and location of the neoplasms. Large central tumors cause symptoms of obstruction, with pneumonia, dyspnea, or chest pain.[168] More peripheral lesions may be asymptomatic and are discovered on routine chest radiography.

Mucoepidermoid carcinomas classically present as exophytic endobronchial tumors and are potentially greater than 5 cm in greatest diameter. They are usually well circumscribed, with smooth overlying mucosal surfaces (Fig. 16-45). On cut section, these tumors are tan-gray or yellow. They are solid or cystic, or both, and may show overtly

mucoid features. There is no topographic predilection for any particular pulmonary lobe or segment. Obstruction of the bronchial lumen by tumor is often associated with postobstructive "lipoid" pneumonia (Fig. 16-46).

Mucoepidermoid carcinomas of the lung are classified into low-grade and high-grade tumors morphologically, principally based on their cytologic features. In low-grade lesions, the panoramic appearance is one of a neoplasm, with cystic and solid areas in close association with a tubular airway (Fig. 16-47). On closer inspection of the solid areas, it is possible to identify clear cells, squamoid cells, or transitional (intermediate) polygonal cells. These elements are interspersed with areas in which there are mucus-secreting glandular cells. Most examples of MEC do not contain large foci of keratinization. However, areas of papillary growth may be seen as well as others with spindle cell proliferation. When the last of those components is extensive, such tumors are designated as "sclerosing" MECs.

Low-grade tumors characteristically lack necrosis and hemorrhage. As mentioned earlier, the cytologic features of these tumors are bland and mitotic activity is minimal or absent (Fig. 16-48). High-grade tumors share some of the architectural features seen in low-grade lesions but manifest a much higher degree of cytologic atypia and mitotic activity (Fig. 16-49). In some cases, necrosis and hemorrhage are also present.

Shilo and colleagues[169] described a series of low-grade tubulocystic MECs in which a prominent lymphoplasmacytic infiltrate permeated the tumors (Fig. 16-50). Russell bodies were often associated with the plasma cellular foci. The clinical presentations and behaviors of such lesions were comparable to those of ordinary MECs, but their lymphoid components raised pathologic concern over the possibility of concomitant low-grade lymphoma. Nonetheless, they were polytypic and analogous to lymphoid infiltrates that can be seen in salivary glands, with or without associated epithelial neoplasms.

The most important tumor to be distinguished from low-grade MECs, especially in small biopsies, is mucous gland adenoma (MGA). Unfortunately, a distinction between those two entities may not be possible until a complete resection of the tumor is performed. MGAs are generally confined to the internal aspect of bronchi in which they arise (luminal to the bronchial cartilage). In contrast, mucoepidermoid carcinomas commonly invade through the entirety of the bronchial wall. One possible discriminant between MEC and MGA is immunoreactivity for TTF-1; that marker appears to be present only in MGA.[169] Another pertinent differential diagnostic problem is that of well-differentiated SCC; in the context under discussion, the presence of marked keratinization and the lack of demonstrable mucin in the tumor cells would favor a diagnosis of a pure squamous tumor over MEC.

The separation of high-grade MEC from ASC may be largely academic, but it is usually based on the absence of foci of conventional ACA in MEC and their presence in ASC. Other features that have been used in this separation include a central location for MEC, the absence of an in situ carcinomatous component in mucoepidermoid tumors, and the presence of low-grade mucoepidermoid areas in some high-grade MECs.

The behavior of these neoplasms is related to their stage and grade. Tumors in the low-grade MEC category can be managed by resection alone, and an indolent course is expected, with rare exceptions.[167,168] However, in high-grade tumors, surgical resection is usually followed by adjuvant radiation or chemotherapy, and their behavior approximates that of more ordinary forms of lung cancer.

As discussed earlier in reference to another tumor type, MECs commonly demonstrate immunolabeling for EGFR but do not show abnormal copy numbers or mutations in the *EGFR* gene on more detailed

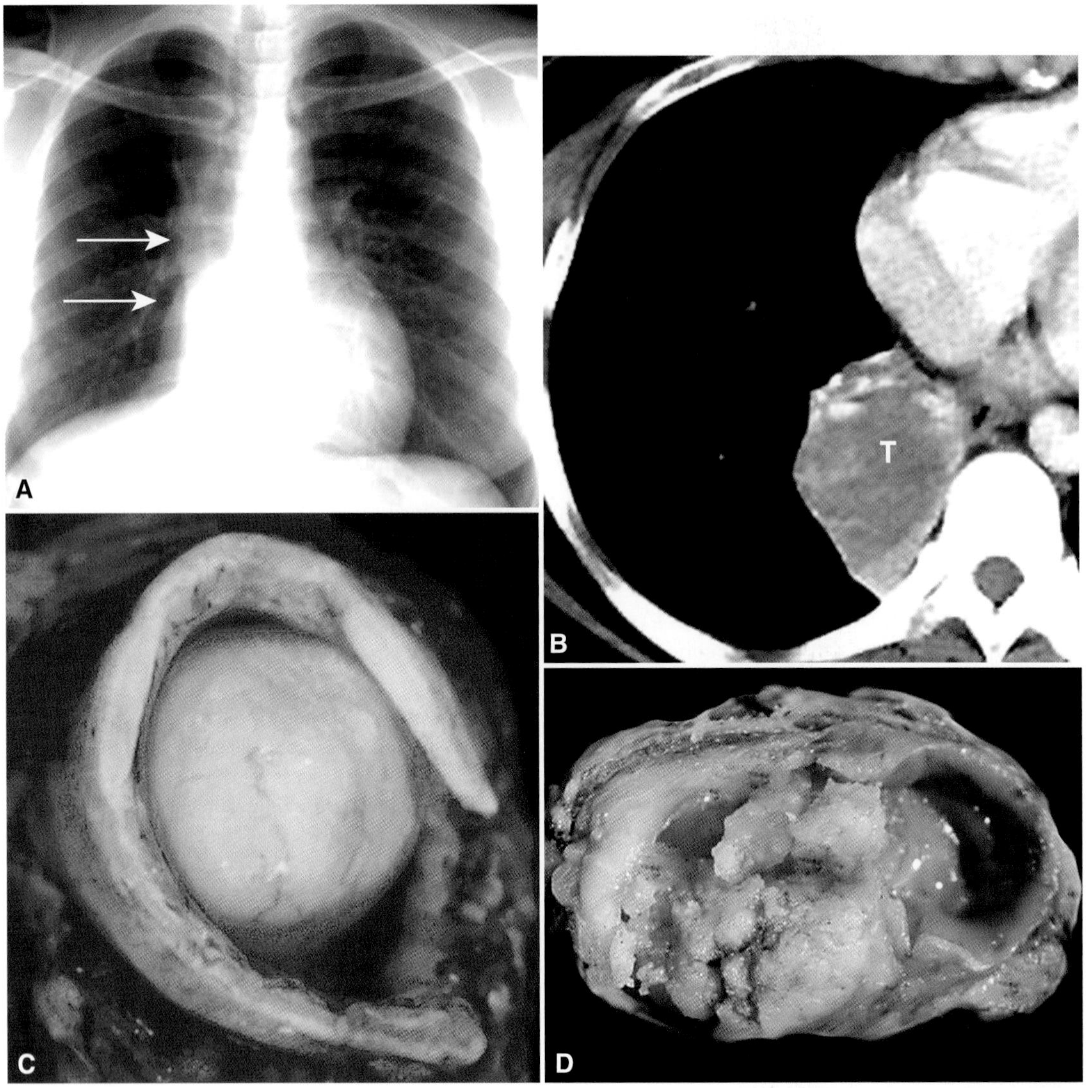

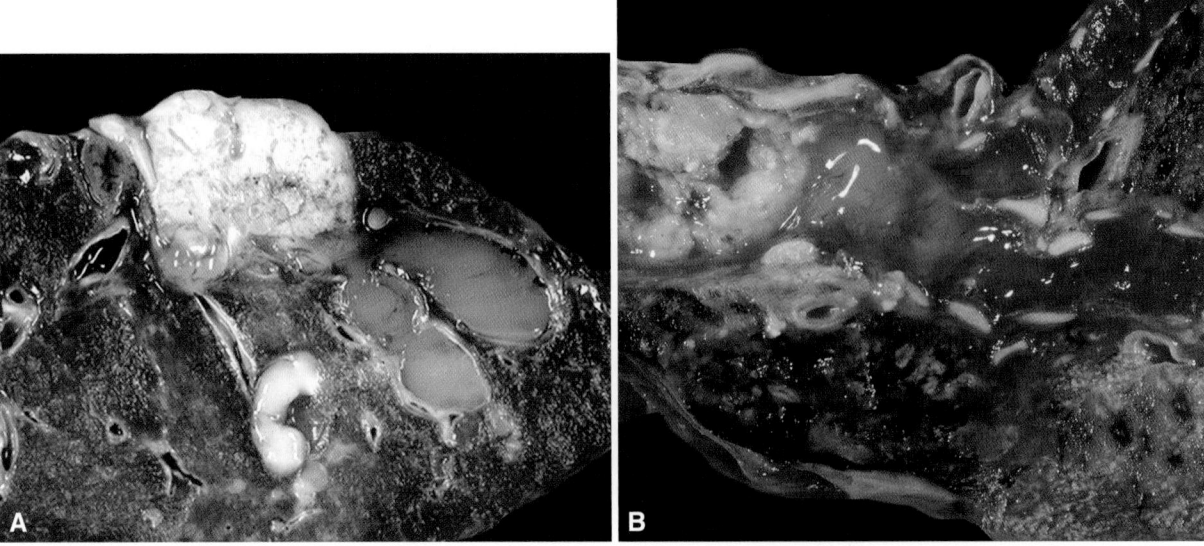

Figure 16-45. Mucoepidermoid carcinoma of the bronchus presenting as a right perihilar mass on chest radiographs (**A**; *arrows*), and computed tomography (**B**; T), and as seen in the resected lung (**C**). **D,** A similar gross image is seen in another case.

Figure 16-46. A and **B,** Central endobronchial mucoepidermoid carcinomas often produce postobstructive mucoid and lipoid pneumonia.

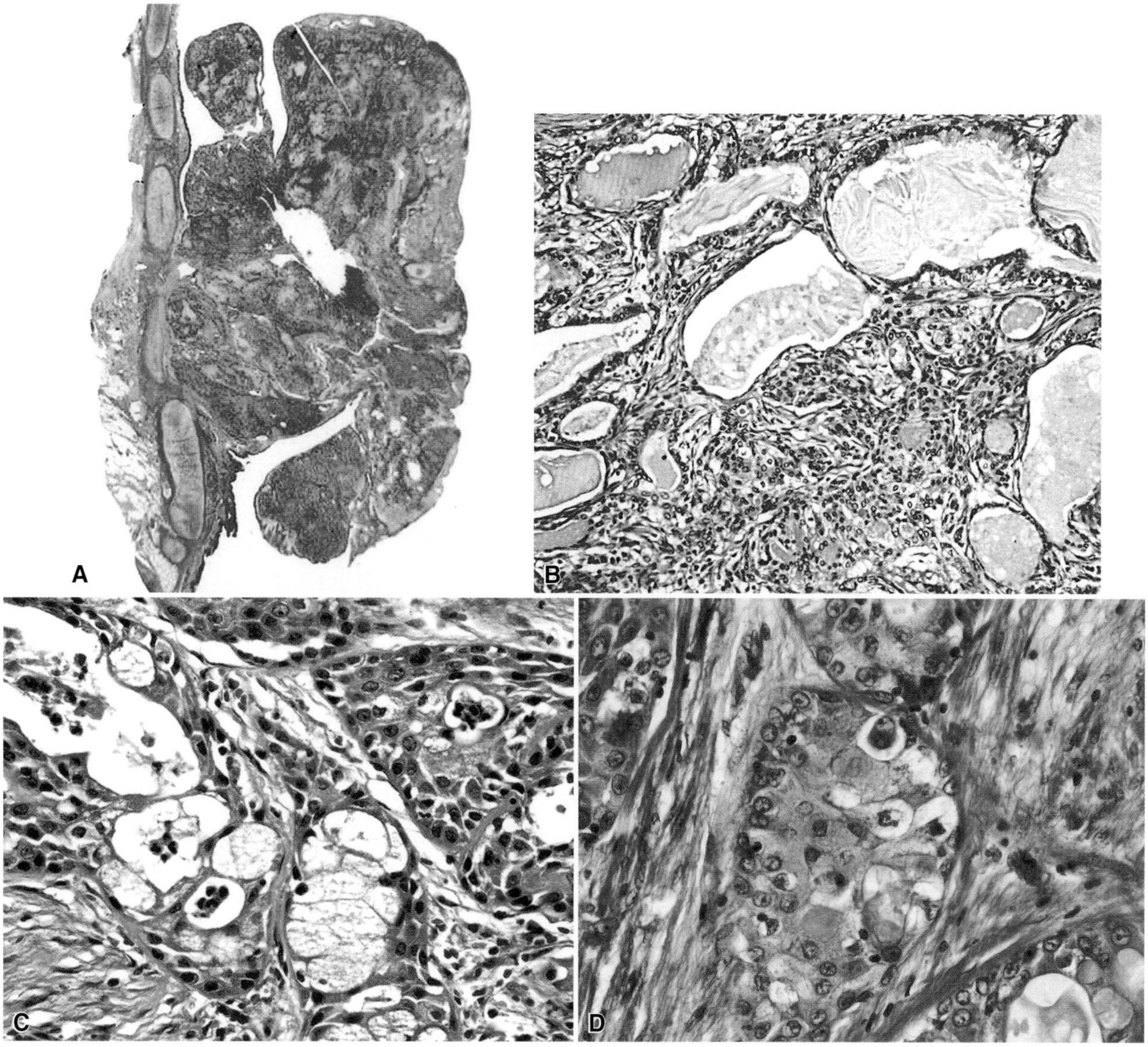

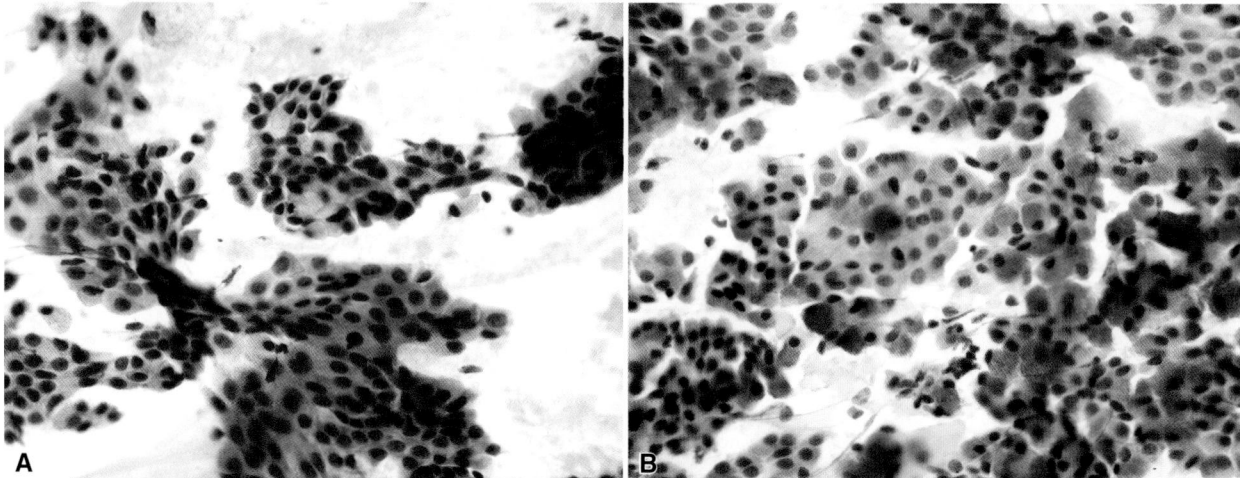

Figure 16-47. A, Mucoepidermoid carcinoma is represented by a well-defined endobronchial mass. **B** to **D,** A juxtaposition of squamoid and mucinous glandular cells is apparent in this low-grade tumor.

Figure 16-48. A, Fine-needle aspiration biopsy specimens from pulmonary mucoepidermoid carcinoma, showing aggregates of relatively bland squamoid cells in a mucoid background, with an additional transitional ("intermediate") cell component. **B,** A mucin stain beautifully highlights the mucus-containing cells.

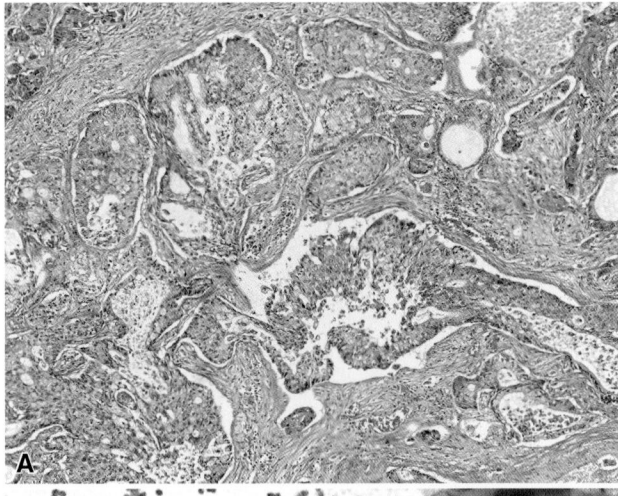
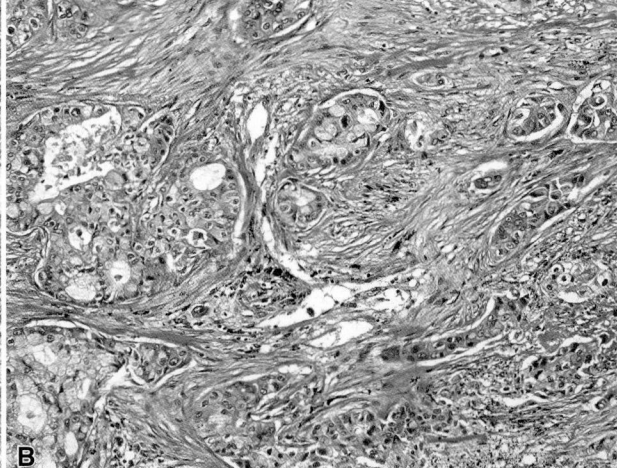

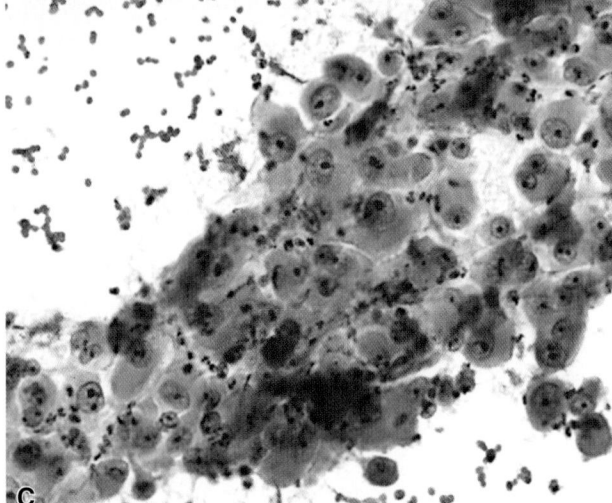

Figure 16-49. A and **B,** High-grade mucoepidermoid carcinoma (HGMEC) demonstrates the presence of lower-grade tumor as well as foci with a greater degree of cytologic anaplasia in both its squamoid and glandular elements (compare with Fig. 16-47). **C,** Fine-needle aspiration biopsy specimen of HGMEC demonstrates a relatively uniform squamoid cell population with little or no mucus in the background.

Adenoid Cystic Carcinoma

Adenoid cystic carcinoma (ACC) is the second most common SGTTL[168,172–179] and typically occurs in adults. In one large series,[172] patients ranged from 29 to 79 years of age (mean, 54 years) with a male-to-female ratio of 2:1. Clinically, because of their characteristic central location, pulmonary ACCs present with symptoms and signs of bronchial erosion or obstruction, including pneumonia, dyspnea, cough, wheezing, and hemoptysis. However, tumors arising in the peripheral lung have been reported as well, and these are usually asymptomatic.[180] The average size of a pulmonary ACC is 4 cm, and the lesions are deceptively circumscribed on gross examination, with a soft yellow-white cut surface. Despite that attribute, surgical bronchial margins are positive for tumor more often in ACC than in other forms of lung cancer.[181] This probably reflects the notorious ability of this tumor to track along neurovascular bundles and cartilaginous plates.[168]

Adenoid cystic carcinoma is a prototypical tumor from a morphologic perspective, composed of monotonous arrays of compact polyhedral cells with uniformly round and hyperchromatic nucleoli and amphophilic cytoplasm. Indeed, were it not for the obviously infiltrative growth that the neoplasms exhibit—with permeation of bronchial walls, blood vessels, and perineurial sheaths (Figs. 16-51 and 16-52)—the cytologic features of ACC would not lead one to immediately interpret it as a malignant lesion.

Fine-needle aspiration is effective in demonstrating the cytologic homogeneity of the tumor in most cases,[182] and it also shows interspersed cylinders or spheres of eosinophilic matrical material contained within the epithelial cell groups (Fig. 16-53). Nevertheless, exceptions to these statements have been reported. Daneshbod and associates[183] found that

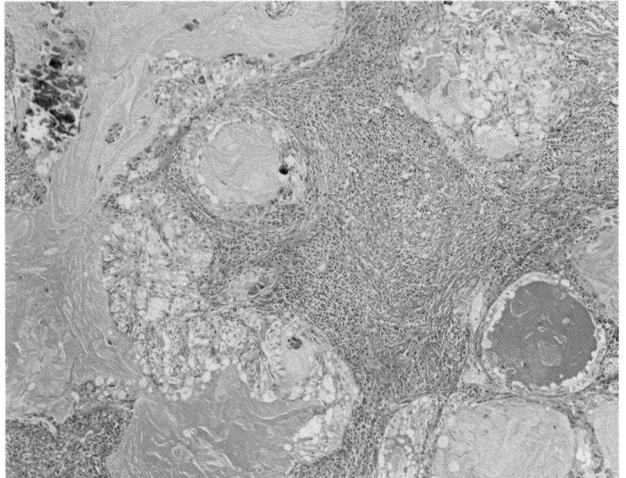

Figure 16-50. Rare example of low-grade pulmonary mucoepidermoid carcinoma with a dense lymphoid stromal infiltrate separating the epithelial profiles in the tumor. This patient also had unusual calcifcations.

analysis.[170,171] Hence, they are unlikely to respond to therapy with TKI agents. Several reproducible chromosomal translocations have been found in MEC, including t(1;11)(p22;q13), t(11;19)(q14-21;p12), and t(11;19)(q21;p13).[167] In some instances, the *cyclin-D1* gene may be up-regulated.

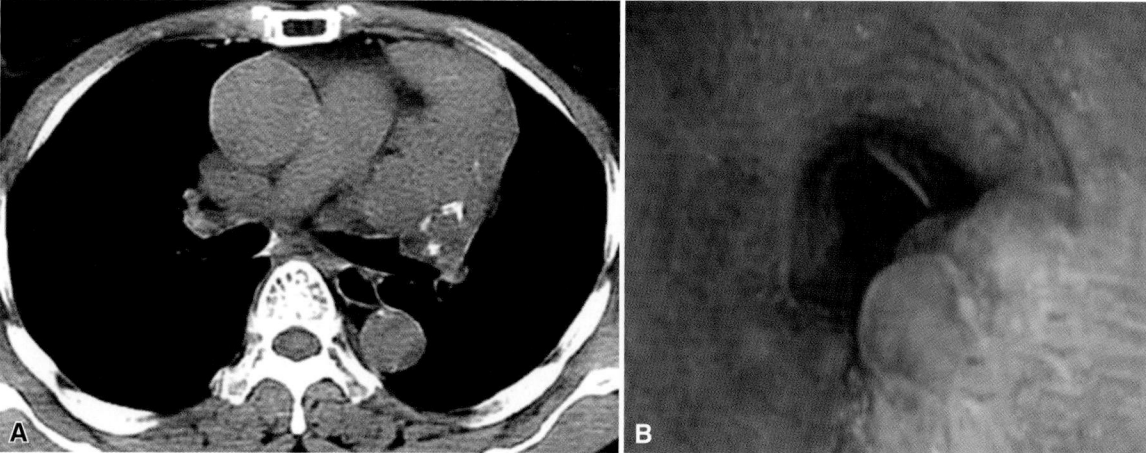

Figure 16-51. A, Computed tomogram of the thorax showing infiltration and distortion of the left main stem bronchus by adenoid cystic carcinoma of the lung (ACCL). **B,** This bronchoscopic view of ACCL shows intact mucosa over the tumor, which protrudes into the lumen of a large airway.

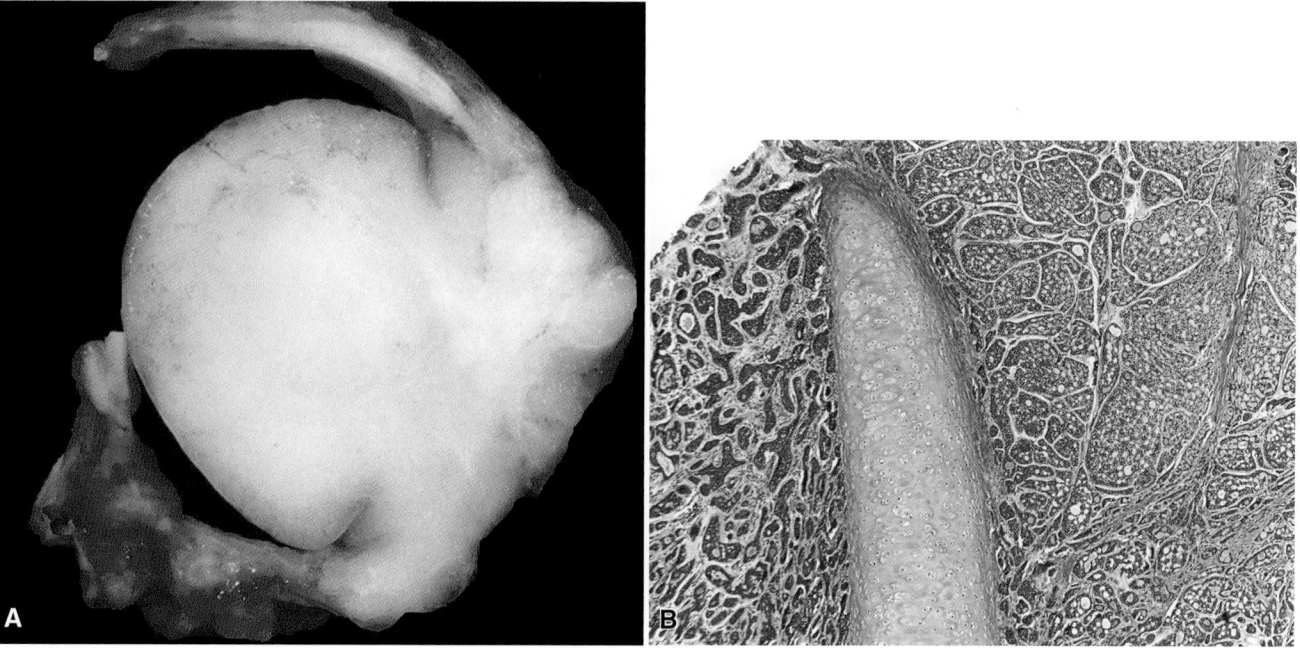

Figure 16-52. A, Gross photograph of adenoid cystic carcinoma of the lung demonstrating a polypoid endobronchial component of the tumor. **B,** Invasion through the bronchial wall and infiltration of adjacent tissue.

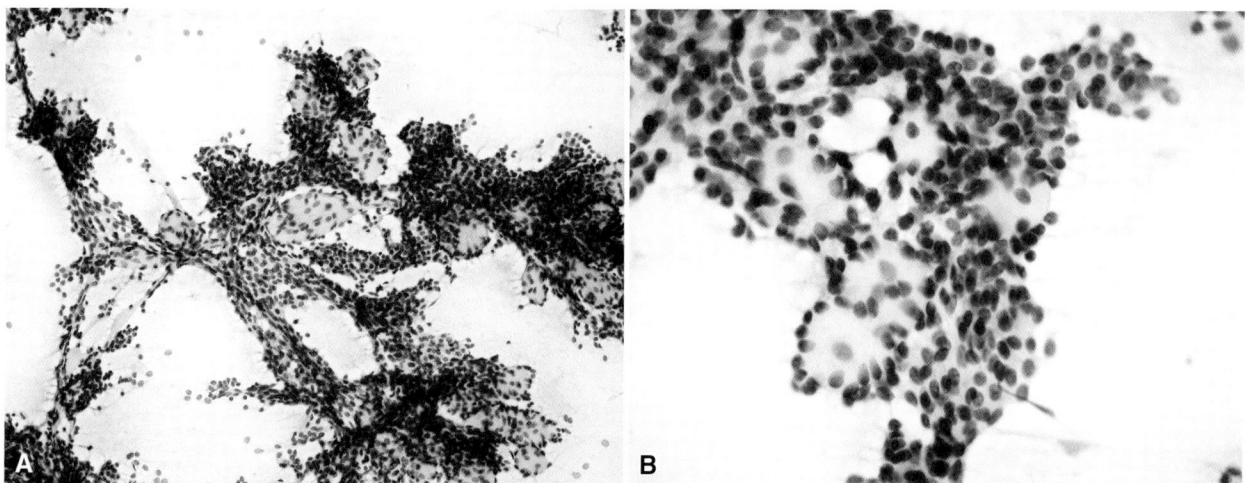

Figure 16-53. A and **B,** Fine-needle aspiration biopsy specimens from bronchial adenoid cystic carcinoma demonstrating monotonous small round tumor cells that encompass rounded profiles of eosinophilic basement membrane material.

myxochondroid material—as also seen in pulmonary chondromas—could be a confounding finding in cytologic preparations from ACCs. These authors also observed nuclear molding in some lesions, similar to the image of neuroendocrine carcinoma. Ozkara and Turan[184] studied an example of "solid" ACC (discussed later) cytologically; the eosinophilic stromal matrix was sparse in that tumor type. Chuah and colleagues[185]

suggested that bronchial brushing cytology may not be productive in ACC because the tumors are often covered by intact bronchial mucosa.

The most common histologic growth pattern is the "cylindromatous" one, reflected by islands and cords of tumor cells that are arranged in a characteristic "jigsaw puzzle piece" pattern (Figs. 16-54 and 16-55). Many cell groups encompass luminal or pseudoluminal spaces that

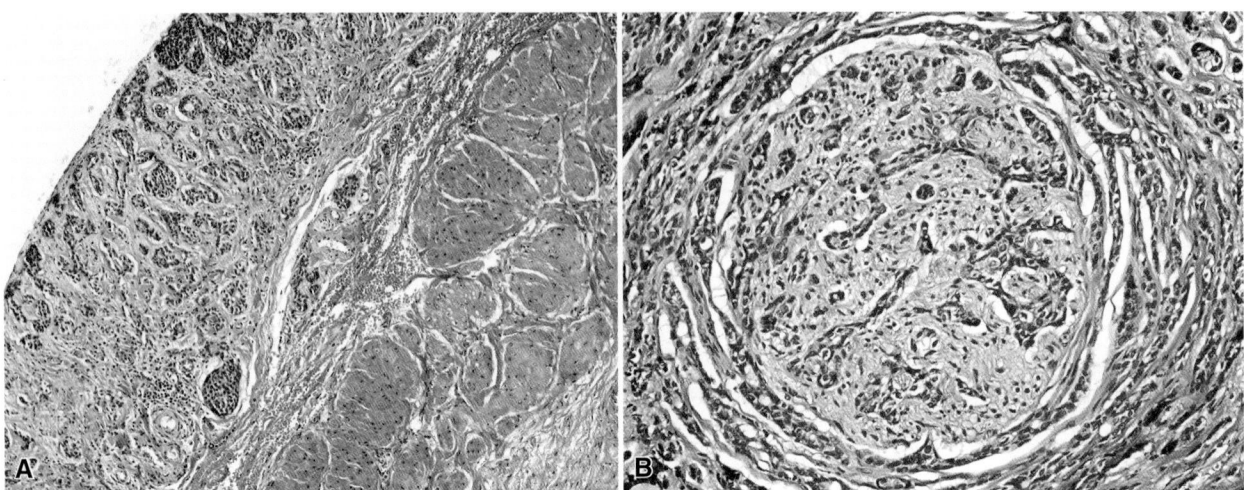

Figure 16-54. A, Infiltration of the vascular adventitia of a pulmonary artery by adenoid cystic carcinoma of the lung. **B,** Perineurial infiltration in the bronchial submucosa by pulmonary adenoid cystic carcinoma.

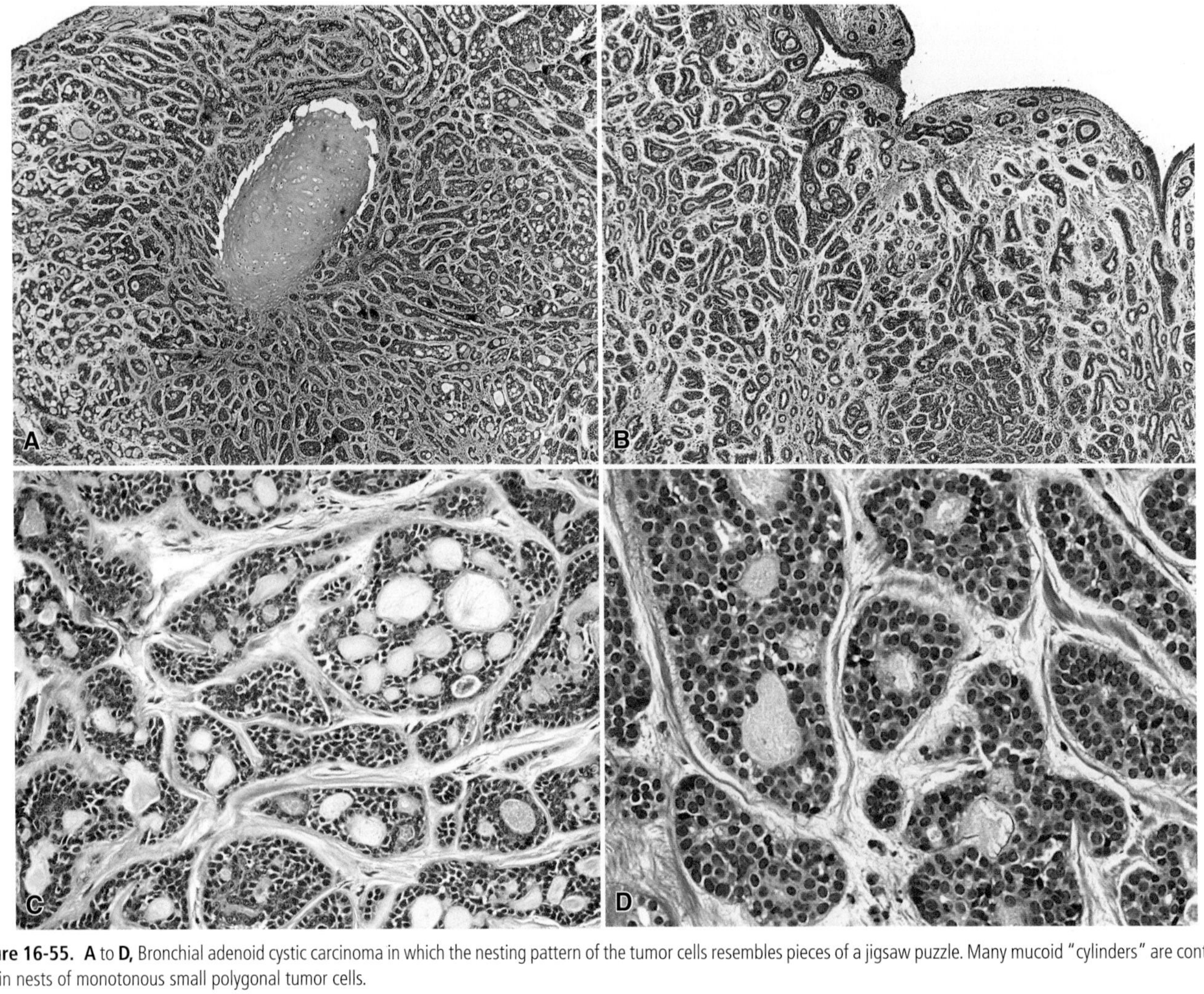

Figure 16-55. A to **D,** Bronchial adenoid cystic carcinoma in which the nesting pattern of the tumor cells resembles pieces of a jigsaw puzzle. Many mucoid "cylinders" are contained within nests of monotonous small polygonal tumor cells.

may contain mucinous material—potentially yielding a cribriform image—and the nests are separated by bands of fibroconnective tissue with variable thickness. Cystic foci in ACC are lined by at least two layers of cells. Mitotic figures, nuclear pleomorphism, necrosis, and hemorrhage are almost always absent.

There are two additional growth patterns in pulmonary ACC that may suggest alternative diagnoses. The "tubular" pattern characteristically shows arrangement of the neoplastic cells in small gland-like spaces or elongated cylinders (Fig. 16-56). Cytologically, the tumor cells in that variant are similar to those seen in cylindromatous ACC. The "solid" variant of ACC exhibits a medullary or insular proliferation of tumor cells, with few if any intercellular spaces and only scant stromal matrix (Fig. 16-57). Mitotic activity is more brisk in this subtype. The diagnosis is furthered if abortive areas of cylindromatous differentiation can be identified; otherwise, several other tumor types with a basaloid cellular constituency enter diagnostic consideration. In particular, we have seen several cases in which a distinction between solid ACC and "basal cell adenocarcinoma" of the salivary gland type—an uncommon lesion usually seen in minor salivary glands[186-188]—was virtually impossible. Purely tubular or solid ACCs are rare, with most cases demonstrating mixed histologic patterns from field to field in the lesion.

Adenoid cystic carcinoma of the lung may show ultrastructural or immunohistologic evidence of partial myoepithelial differentiation. Hence, potential reactivity for keratin, vimentin, actin, and S-100 protein is observed. Immunolabeling for CD117 (c-kit protein) has been

described as well (Fig. 16-58), but it is not accompanied by activating mutations in the *c-kit* gene.[189-191] The same relationship applies to the paradoxical immunoreactivity for EGFR but a lack of demonstrable gene aberrations in ACC.[170] Immunohistologic studies are usually not necessary for diagnosis, with the exception of some cases of "solid" ACC; in those lesions, stains for collagen type IV or laminin may be useful in highlighting small cylindrical stromal accumulations of basement membrane material. Tubular ACC may be confused with conventional well-differentiated ACA of the lung; however, the latter tumor type typically contains larger cells with more discernible nucleoli.

Adenoid cystic carcinomas are generally considered to be slowly growing tumors of low-grade malignancy. However, that view is deceptive in many cases. The lesions often pursue a tenaciously persistent course, with recalcitrant intrathoracic recurrences over several years, potentially culminating with distant metastasis. Tumor stage at initial diagnosis is important in determining the clinical outcome, and complete surgical excision offers the best chance of cure.[168,192]

Acinic Cell Carcinoma of the Lung (Fechner Tumor)

Intrapulmonary acinic cell carcinoma has been designated as the "Fechner tumor" (FT) to honor the first description of this neoplasm in 1972 by Robert Fechner and colleagues.[193] It is an uncommon primary lesion in the lung but may be seen either as an endobronchial mass or a peripheral neoplasm that abuts a tubular airway.[194-196] Most descriptions of FTs have been as isolated case reports. In the series that exist on

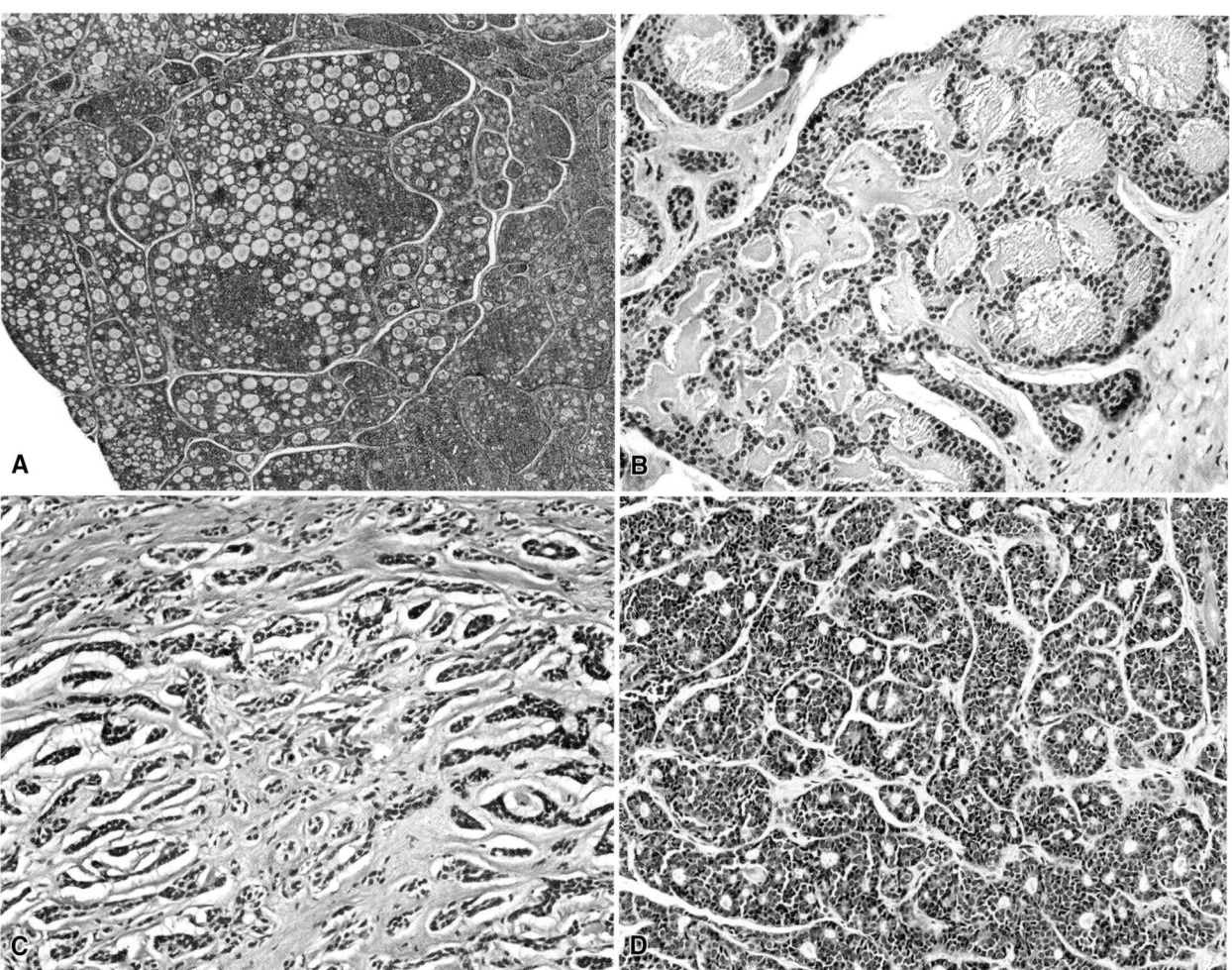

Figure 16-56. A to **D,** A cribriform pattern of growth is well seen in the cell nests of this bronchial adenoid cystic carcinoma. Tubular profiles of tumor cells permeate the fibrohyaline stroma throughout the tumor.

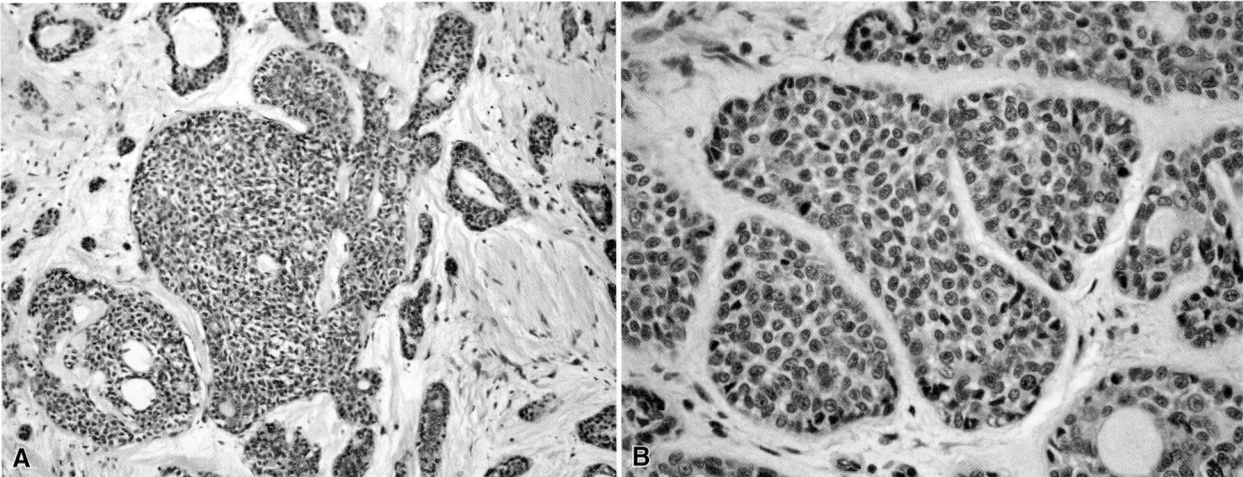

Figure 16-57. **A** and **B,** High-grade "solid" bronchial adenoid cystic carcinoma shows large nests of compact polygonal tumor cells in which only rare glandular foci and intercellular matrix are apparent.

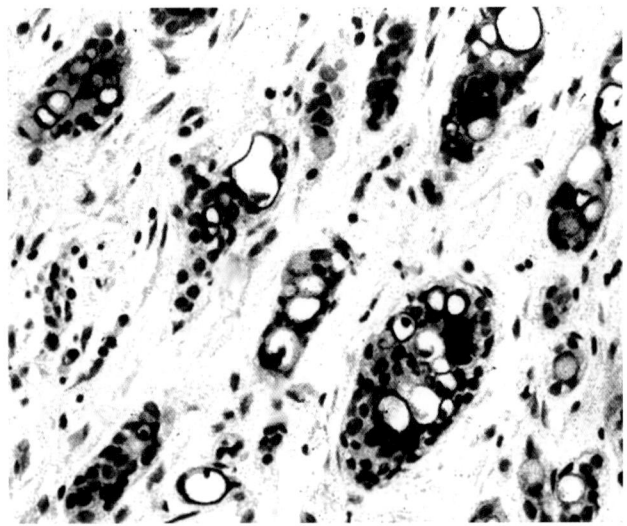

Figure 16-58. Immunoreactivity is seen for CD117 (c-kit protein) in this bronchial adenoid cystic carcinoma.

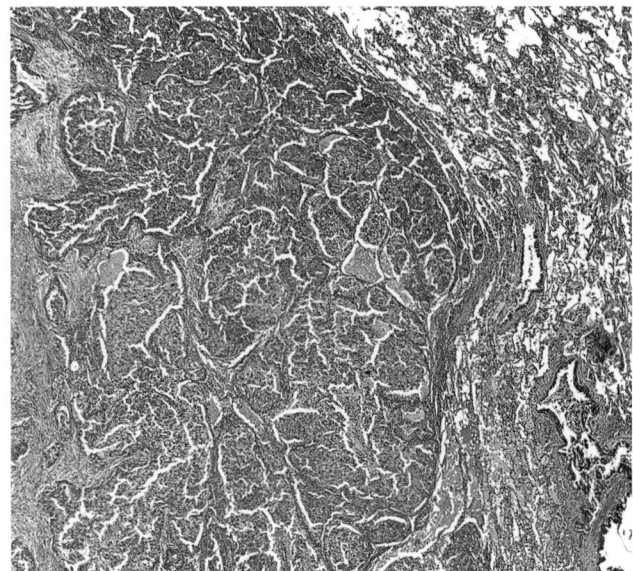

Figure 16-59. Primary acinic cell carcinoma of the lung (Fechner tumor) demonstrating a circumscribed image with a relatively sharp interface with the surrounding lung parenchyma.

acinic cell carcinomas of the lung,[194] such tumors occur predominantly in adults, with an equal sex predilection. Occasional examples have been reported in children.[197] Because the majority of FTs are peripherally located, most patients are asymptomatic and their tumors are discovered on screening chest radiographs. When FTs assume a central location, the patient is more likely to report dyspnea, cough, or hemoptysis.

These lesions are usually well circumscribed but not encapsulated, and they vary in size from 1 to 5 cm in greatest dimension. Their cut surfaces are tan-gray and homogeneous. Scanning microscopy shows a circumscribed lesion with internal effacement of the normal lung parenchyma. Solid growth is typical, with a composition of round-to-polygonal cells with prominently granular eosinophilic cytoplasm, round nuclei, and inconspicuous nucleoli. Mitotic activity and nuclear atypia are minimal, and areas of hemorrhage or necrosis are lacking (Figs. 16-59 and 16-60). Occasionally, FTs may comprise a proliferation of clear cells with granular cytoplasm and nuclei that are displaced toward the periphery of the cells, superficially simulating "signet ring"

cells. The neoplastic cells also may be arranged in ill-defined nests separated by delicate fibroconnective tissue, with interspersed lymphocytes and plasma cells, as discussed earlier in connection with MEC. Finally, as in the salivary glands, intrapulmonary acinic cell carcinoma may show acinar, oncocytic, cystic, and papillocystic growth patterns. One unusual case has been documented in which an FT was juxtaposed with a low-grade neuroendocrine carcinoma of the lung within the same mass.[198]

One of the most useful histochemical stains in the evaluation of acinic cell carcinoma is the periodic acid/Schiff (PAS) method, used to demonstrate glycogen in the tumor cells (Fig. 16-61). Mucicarmine stains may show foci of intracellular mucin production as well. Immunostains may demonstrate positivity for such lysosomal proteins as alpha-1-antitrypsin and amylase in the tumor cell granules.

Electron microscopy is still helpful in the diagnosis of acinic cell carcinoma. The finding of large dark electron-dense or electron-lucent (immature) zymogen granules in the cytoplasm of the neoplastic cells is characteristic (Fig. 16-62).

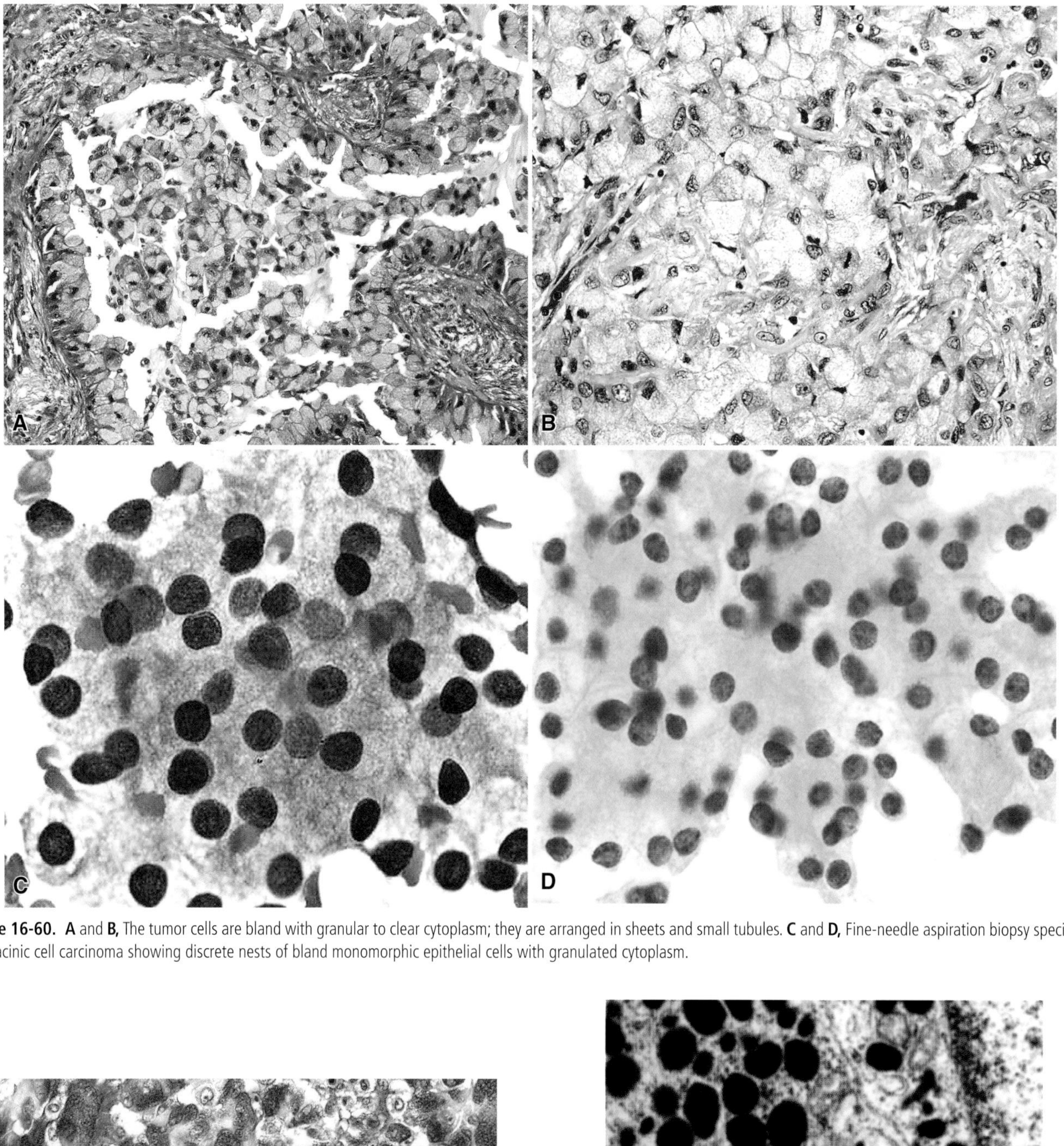

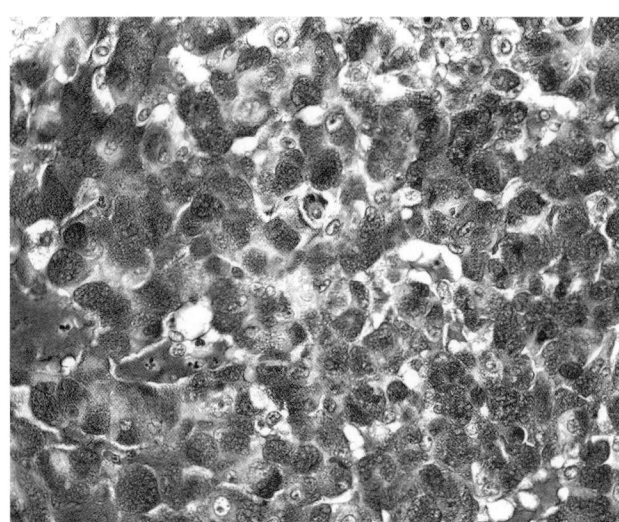

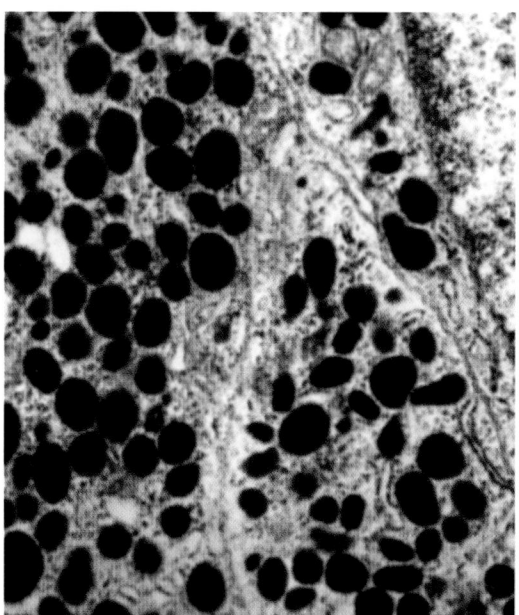

Figure 16-60. **A** and **B,** The tumor cells are bland with granular to clear cytoplasm; they are arranged in sheets and small tubules. **C** and **D,** Fine-needle aspiration biopsy specimens from acinic cell carcinoma showing discrete nests of bland monomorphic epithelial cells with granulated cytoplasm.

Figure 16-61. The cytoplasmic granules in pulmonary acinic cell carcinoma label with periodic acid/Schiff stain after diastase digestion.

Figure 16-62. Numerous zymogen-type granules are present in the cytoplasm of the tumor cells in acinic cell carcinoma, as seen in this electron photomicrograph.

The differential diagnosis of FT variants depends largely on the histologic growth pattern and cell type. When the lesion has prominently oncocytic features, the most important component of the differential diagnosis is oncocytoid carcinoid tumor (grade I neuroendocrine carcinoma). In this specific setting, immunohistochemical positivity for chromogranin-A, CD56, and synaptophysin is helpful in recognizing neuroendocrine tumors and excluding acinic cell carcinoma. On the other hand, when acinic cell tumors contain clear cells with "signet ring cell"–like features, the most important alternative diagnostic consideration is a conventional pulmonary ACA with similar cytologic attributes. In that context, histochemical evaluations for intracellular mucin are helpful because the intracytoplasmic vacuoles of true signet ring cell carcinomas should label with the mucicarmine or digested PAS methods. "Sugar tumor" (myomelanocytoma) of the lung is another possible component of the differential diagnosis in cases of acinic cell carcinoma. Sugar tumors may also show strong PAS positivity, but unlike acinic cell carcinoma, sugar tumors are keratin-negative and display immunoreactivity with HMB-45 and MART-1.

Fechner tumors are low-grade malignancies, and they have limited but definite potential to metastasize. Examples have been reported that involved regional lymph nodes in the thorax,[199,200] and one case featured a pleural recurrence.[201] However, the overall clinical evolution is usually favorable.

Epithelial-Myoepithelial Carcinoma

Epithelial-myoepithelial carcinoma (EMC) is one of the most unusual primary tumors of the lung, and it also belongs to the SGTTL group. Only a few cases of this lesion have been reported[202-211]; they have involved adults with endobronchial masses, and because of their central location, the neoplasms were associated with obstructive symptoms and signs. EMC is considered a low-grade malignancy. It is reported to be well circumscribed but not encapsulated and may measure up to 4 cm in greatest dimension.

The scanning image of EMC is that of a predominantly glandular proliferation that is transected by thin fibroconnective stromal septa. It is centered in a large tubular airway but extends into and obliterates the adjacent lung parenchyma. On closer inspection, the glandular components of EMC show a characteristically biphasic cellular population, with inner ductal epithelial cells surrounded by an outer layer of myoepithelium (Figs. 16-63 and 16-64).[207] This neoplasm does not have a high mitotic rate or notable nuclear atypia; similarly, necrosis and hemorrhage are absent. Hence, the diagnosis must be made on the basis of infiltrative architecture, together with the noted cytologic attributes. Immunohistochemically, the inner cell layer in tumoral glands shows strong reactivity for pankeratin and keratin-7, whereas the outer layer demonstrates positivity for alpha-isoform actin, p63 protein, keratin 5/6, and S-100 protein (Fig. 16-65).[206,207] Because of its prominently glandular appearance, EMC can be easily confused with a well-differentiated ACA. Detailed morphologic examination and demonstration of a myoepithelial immunophenotype are keys to the correct diagnosis. Mixed tumors (pleomorphic adenomas) also manifest a similar immunohistologic profile but differ substantially on morphologic grounds from EMC (see Chapter 19).

In light of the rarity of this tumor in the lungs, it is difficult to draw overarching conclusions regarding the behavior of pulmonary EMC. Pelosi and colleagues[206] reviewed the pertinent literature and concluded that the term "pulmonary epithelial-myoepithelial tumor of unproven malignant potential" was preferable to EMC. On the other hand, based on their experience, Nguyen and colleagues[207] stated unequivocally that *"these tumors, when in the lung, clearly have the capacity to infiltrate and metastasize, and therefore should be designated as epithelial-myoepithelial carcinoma."* Complete excision is recommended.

Histopathologic and Oncogenetic Factors with Putative Prognostic Significance for Carcinomas of the Lung

Several histologic factors that can be observed in conventionally stained microscopic sections have putative prognostic significance. Principal among these are, quite simply, the histologic type of the tumor, its level of differentiation, and the status of the surgical margins and resected lymph nodes (if any) (Tables 16-2 and 16-3).[212-214] In addition, invasion of the visceral pleura by lung cancers increases their T substages and worsens survival, all other variables being equal.[215] Several authors have shown that application of the Verhoeff–van Gieson elastic stain to paraffin sections enhances the pathologist's ability to recognize this feature.[216-220] A semiquantitative estimate of the degree of tumor necrosis was also reported to have predictive value by Elson and coworkers,[221] in

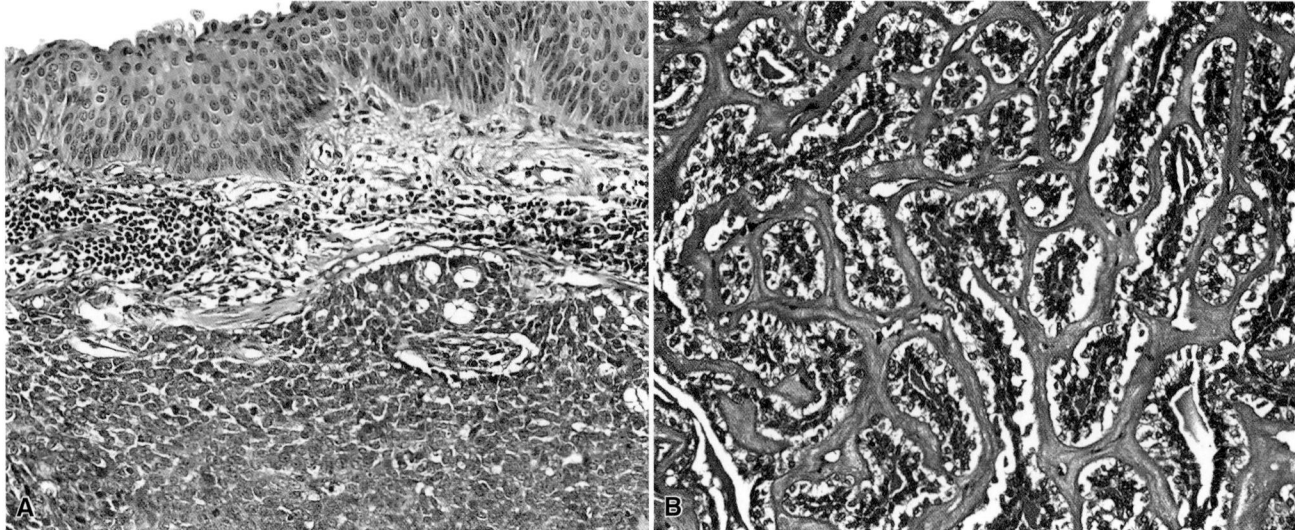

Figure 16-63. A, Epithelial-myoepithelial carcinoma of the bronchus, manifesting as an intramural, submucosal lesion. **B,** The tumor has a biphasic cellular composition, comprising tubules that contain an outer layer of clear myoepithelial elements.

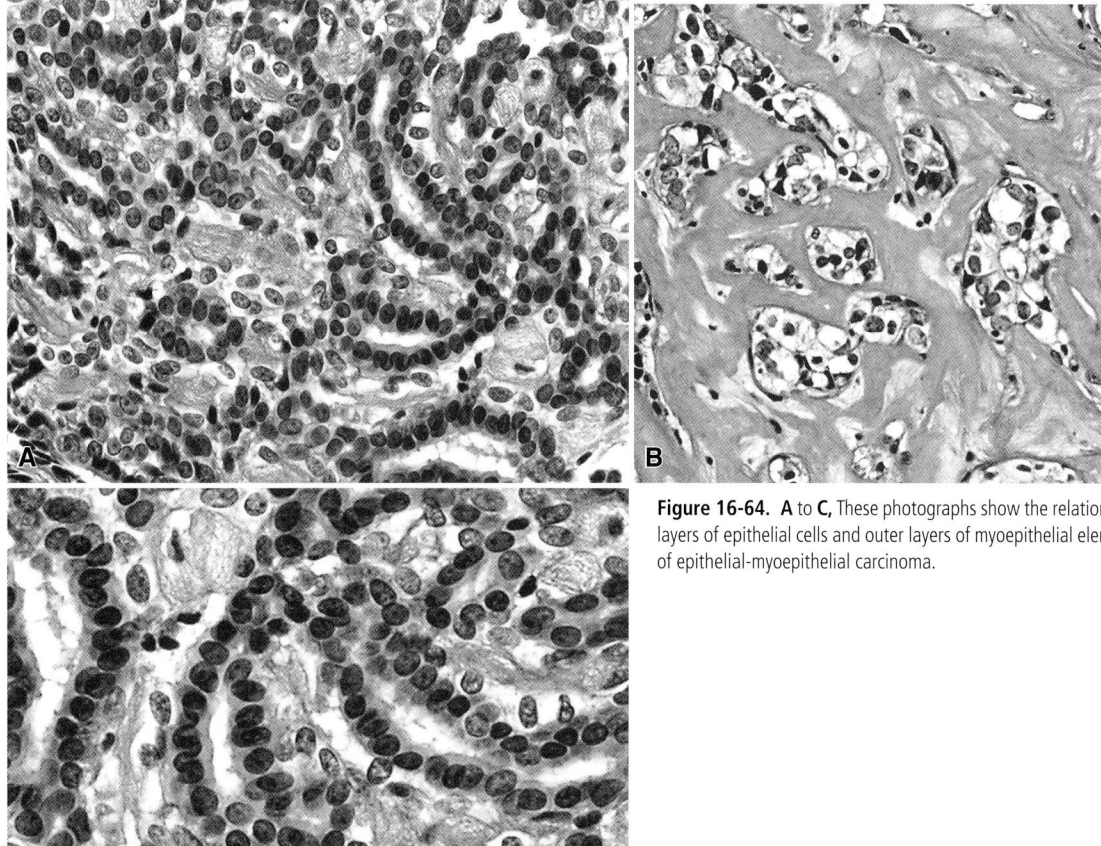

Figure 16-64. **A** to **C,** These photographs show the relationship between inner layers of epithelial cells and outer layers of myoepithelial elements in the tubules of epithelial-myoepithelial carcinoma.

a study of non-neuroendocrine carcinomas of the lung. Moreover, documentation of angiolymphatic vascular invasion by tumor (Fig. 16-66) has similar importance,[222-224] and because it is more frequently observed in ACA,[222] it may explain the worsened survival rate associated with that tumor type compared with SCC of the lung.

In other anatomic sites, particularly the head and neck and axillae, extranodal extension by tumor metastases of carcinomas has been associated with worsened prognosis. Data from a study by Lee and associates[225] suggest that this association also holds for lung cancers.

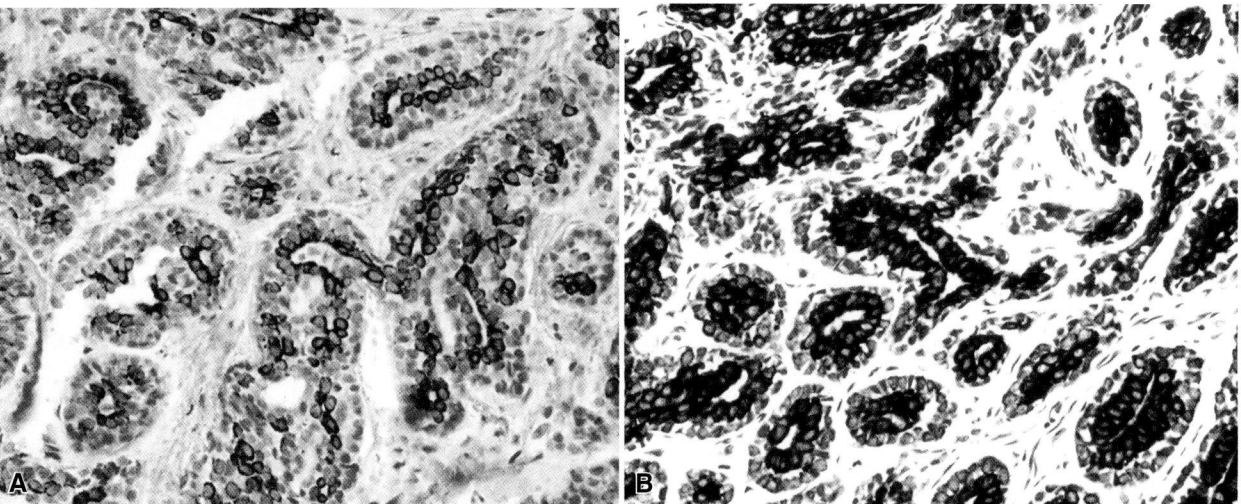

Figure 16-65. Immunohistochemical studies in epithelial-myoepithelial carcinoma are effective in demonstrating its biphasic nature. **A,** Keratins 5/6. **B,** Keratin 7.

Continued

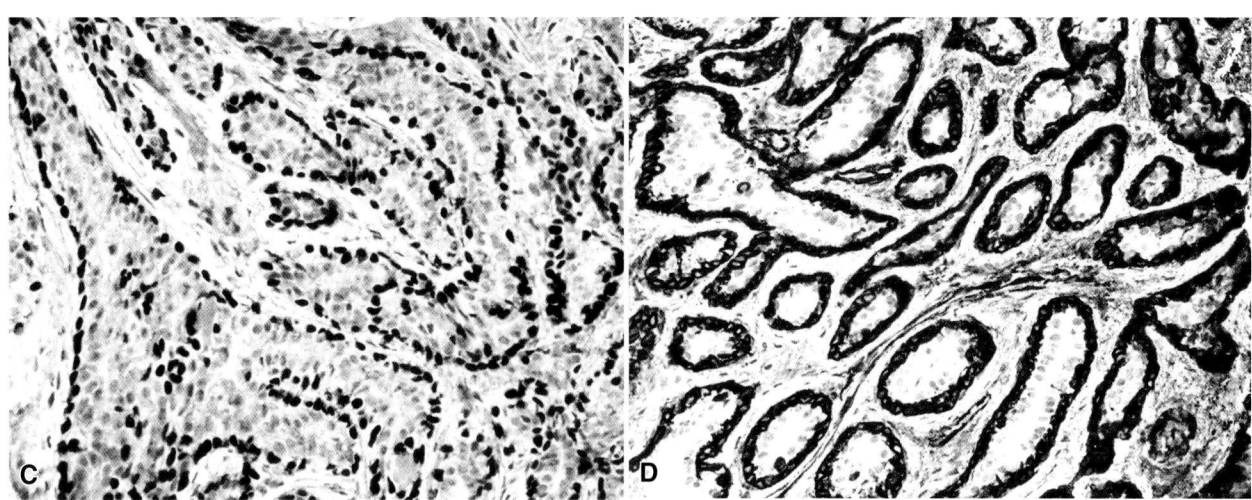

Figure 16-65—cont'd. C, p63 protein. **D,** Alpha-isoform ("smooth-muscle") actin.

Table 16-2. TNM Staging of Lung Carcinoma

T—Tumor Size or Extent of Involvement	
TX	Tumor proven by the presence of malignant cells in bronchopulmonary secretions but not visualized roentgenographically or bronchoscopically, or any tumor that cannot be assessed as in treatment staging
T0	No evidence of primary tumor
Tis	Carcinoma in situ
T1	A tumor that is 3 cm or less in greatest dimension, surrounded by lung or visceral pleura, and without evidence of invasion proximal to a lobar bronchus at bronchoscopy. (Note: The uncommon superficial tumor of any size with its invasive component limited to the bronchial wall, which may extend proximal to the main stem bronchus, is also classified as T1.)
T2	A tumor more than 3 cm in greatest dimension or a tumor of any size that either invades the visceral pleura or has associated atelectasis or obstructive pneumonitis extending to the hilar region. At bronchoscopy, the proximal extent of demonstrable tumor must be within a lobar bronchus or at least 2 cm distal to the carcinoma. Any associated atelectasis or obstructive pneumonitis must involve less than an entire lung.
T3	A tumor of any size with direct extension into the chest wall (including superior sulcus tumors), diaphragm, or the mediastinal pleura or pericardium without involving the heart, great vessels, trachea, esophagus, or vertebral body, or a tumor in the main stem bronchus within 2 cm of the carina without involving the carina
T4	A tumor of any size with invasion of the mediastinum or involving the heart, great vessels, trachea, esophagus, vertebral body, or carina, or the presence of malignant pleural effusion. (Note: Most pleural effusions associated with lung cancer are due to tumor. There are, however, a few patients in whom the cytopathologic findings of pleural fluid—on more than one specimen—are negative for tumor and the fluid is nonbloody and is not an exudate. In such cases, where these elements and clinical judgment dictate that the effusion is not related to the tumor, the patient should be staged TI, T2, or T3, excluding effusion as a staging element.)
N—Nodal Status	
NX	Regional lymph nodes cannot be assessed
N0	No demonstrable metastasis to the regional lymph nodes
N1	Metastasis to the lymph nodes in the peribronchial or ipsilateral hilar region, or both, including direct extension
N2	Metastasis to the ipsilateral mediastinal lymph nodes or subcarinal lymph nodes
N3	Metastasis to the contralateral mediastinal lymph nodes, contralateral hilar nodes, ipsilateral or contralateral scalene nodes, or supraclavicular lymph nodes
M—Distant Metastases	
MX	Presence of distant metastases cannot be assessed
M0	No (known) distant metastasis
M1	Distant metastasis present—specify site(s)

Table 16-3. Clinical Stage Groupings according to TNM Subsets

Stage	Percent of Cases	T Factor	N Factor	M Factor	Surgical Candidate
Occult	<1	TX	N0	M0	Yes
0	<1	Tis	N0	M0	Yes
I	13	T1 or T2	N0	M0	Yes
II	10	T1 or T2	N1	M0	Yes
IIIA	22	T3	N0 or N1	M0	Yes
		T1–T3	N2	M0	Yes
IIIB	22	Any T	N3	M0	No
		T4	Any N	M0	No
IV	32	Any T	Any N	M1	No

For definitions of the T, N, and M factors, see Table 16-2.

A number of investigators have examined the use of adjunctive techniques for the evaluation of proliferative activity in lung cancer. One may apply flow cytometry to measure the S-phase fraction of the tumor cell population[212] or immunohistology to assess the expression of S-phase–related nuclear proteins, such as Ki-67/MIB-1/PCNA (Fig. 16-67).[226] Published work on such markers has not found them to offer a great deal more information than simple counting of mitotic figures. Similarly, measurement of DNA ploidy in pulmonary carcinomas does not appear to provide prognostically valuable data.[212]

Over the last decade, a great deal of research has addressed the possible role of genetic alterations in predicting the clinical outcome of patients with lung cancer. In particular, aberrations of the *p53, c-erbB-2, K-ras, RB-1, myc,* and *bcl-2* genes have been evaluated in the greatest detail, but with conflicting and inconclusive results.[227–237] Therefore, we do not recommend the routine use of such assessments for prognosis. Despite the work of Fontanini and coworkers,[238] purportedly demonstrating the predictive utility of microvessel counts in lung cancers, a similar comment applies to that adjunctive area of analysis.[232]

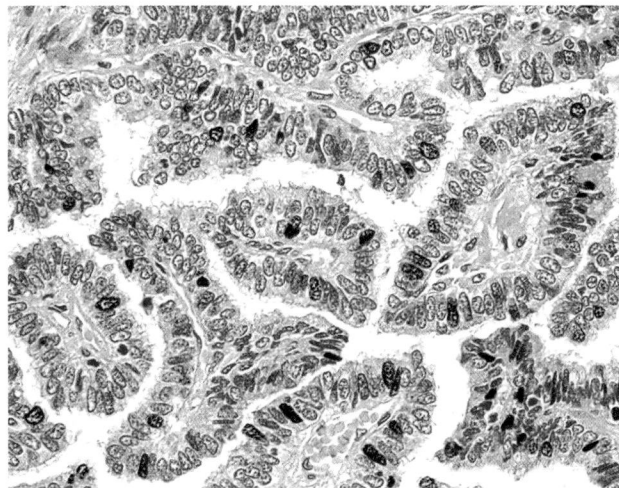

Figure 16-67. Immunolabeling with MIB-1 is designed to delineate the proliferative index of lung carcinomas. Unfortunately, results for this assay are currently not very reproducible between laboratories.

A meta-analysis of immunohistologic "prognosticators" by Zhu and colleagues[239] has supported this position. These authors also suggested that cyclin-E, vascular endothelial growth factor-A, p16 (Cink4a), p27 (kip1), and beta-catenin were promising analytes in this context, but they should still be regarded as investigational markers.

Molecular Analysis of Gene Sets in Non-Neuroendocrine Lung Carcinomas

A rapidly growing area of clinical investigation on the behavior and prognosis of lung cancers is represented by "molecular" analyses of those neoplasms. As reviewed by Petty and coworkers,[240] this can be accomplished with several laboratory techniques, such as "global" gene profiling, complementary deoxyribonucleic acid (cDNA) and oligonucleotide microarrays, or single-nucleotide polymorphism (SNP) microarrays. The goals of these assessments are basically twofold—to separate metastatically

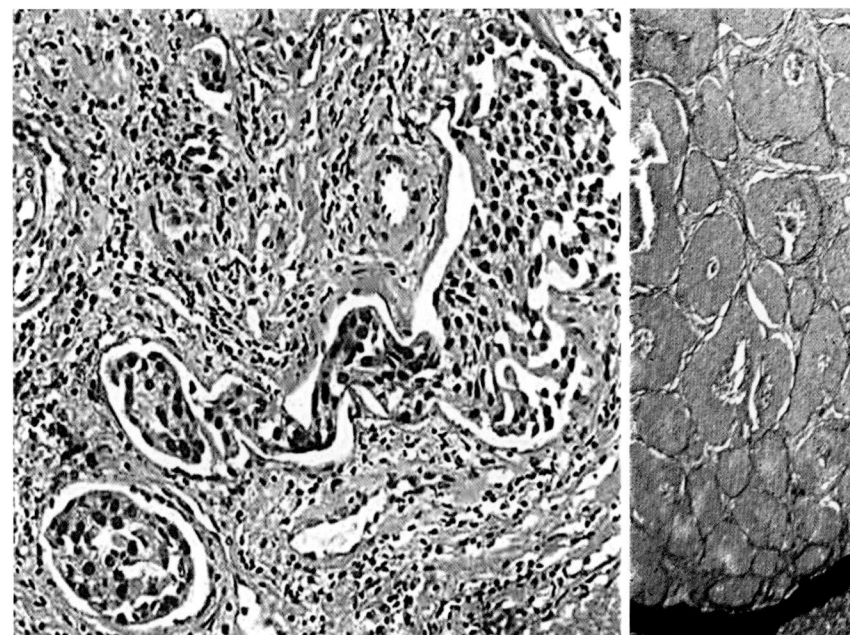
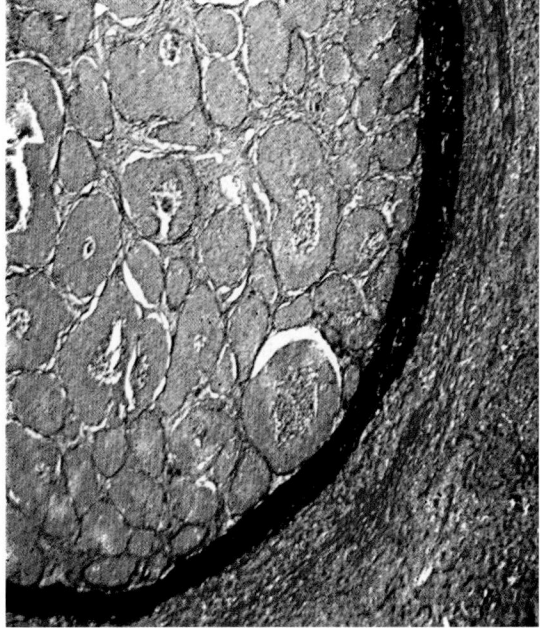

Figure 16-66. Lymphatic (*left*) or venous (*right*) invasion by carcinomas of the lung has important prognostic significance and should be noted in surgical pathology reports.

capable from incapable low-stage pulmonary carcinomas and to predict the likely visceral sites of metastasis for tumors that are capable of extra-pulmonary growth. The genes comprising study sets in this setting are diverse, governing proteins that have roles in immune response, transcriptional modulation, cell cycle regulation, apoptosis, intracellular signaling, extracellular matrix synthesis or degradation, and angiogenesis.[240,241] As suggested by Potti and colleagues,[242] gene assessments should employ a "multi-metagene" model to identify reproducible biologic gene profiles because a single gene or even a small group of genes will not determine ultimate tumor behavior. In that context, assessments that have compared primary tumors with their metastases are particularly interesting. Hoang and associates[243] have shown that secondary carcinomatous deposits are genetically still very similar to their primary "parents," but differences are consistently represented by mutations in an aggregation of selected and biologically important genes in the metastatic lesions.

To date, several well-constructed and well-conducted studies have shown definite promise for this form of pathologic analysis. For example, Chen and coworkers[244] identified a five-gene "signature" of non-neuroendocrine lung cancers that effectively separated survivors from nonsurvivors. Similarly, Xi and colleagues[245] used gene expression profiles and "prediction analysis of microarrays" to predict the behavior of pulmonary ACAs. Patients with high-risk prediction analysis of microarrays ultimately had a worse prognosis overall, even if their morphologic tumor substage was T1–T2/pN0. The latter finding implies that gene profiling is capable of identifying patients with distant metastasis but uninvolved regional lymph nodes—in other words, patients with stage I tumors that ultimately will not respond to treatment. It also runs counter to the often-held premise that carcinomatous metastasis invariably proceeds in a linear fashion through lymph node

groups before spreading to visceral organs.[246] Other studies have shown comparable predictive abilities and reached similar conclusions.[247–253]

We believe that gene profiling will eventually become an integrated part of the pathologic evaluation of lung cancers. When and how that occurs must await future developments. Nonetheless, genetic analysis—using methods such as "heat mapping" of gene expression (Fig. 16-68)—can be done in a relatively rapid fashion, potentially providing clinicians with important data for treatment planning (Fig. 16-69).[254] In an optimal scenario, that information could hypothetically be used as depicted in Figure 16-70.

When this scenario comes to pass, one could rightly ask why pathologists would still need to examine lung cancer specimens for traditionally defined adverse morphologic findings. The answer to that query relates to the empirical validity that the latter process has and the rapidity and low cost with which it can be accomplished. Documenting a metastasis in an "N3" lymph node, for example, provides strong *de facto* evidence that a tumor can grow effectively in a distant location, and it concomitantly predicts that extrathoracic visceral disease is a distinct likelihood. Thus, one can envision a future paradigm in which morphologic studies and molecular analyses are complementary partners.

Problems with Current Staging Protocols for Lung Carcinomas

Pathologic staging systems for lung cancer have undergone several alterations through the last 15 years, under the aegis of such organizations as the American Joint Committee on Cancer (AJCC), the International Union for Cancer Control, and the International

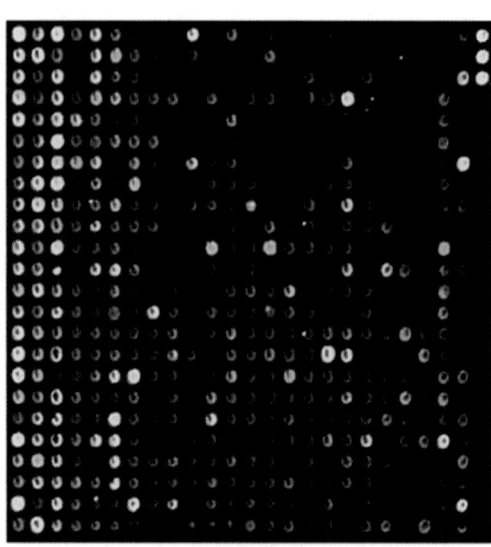
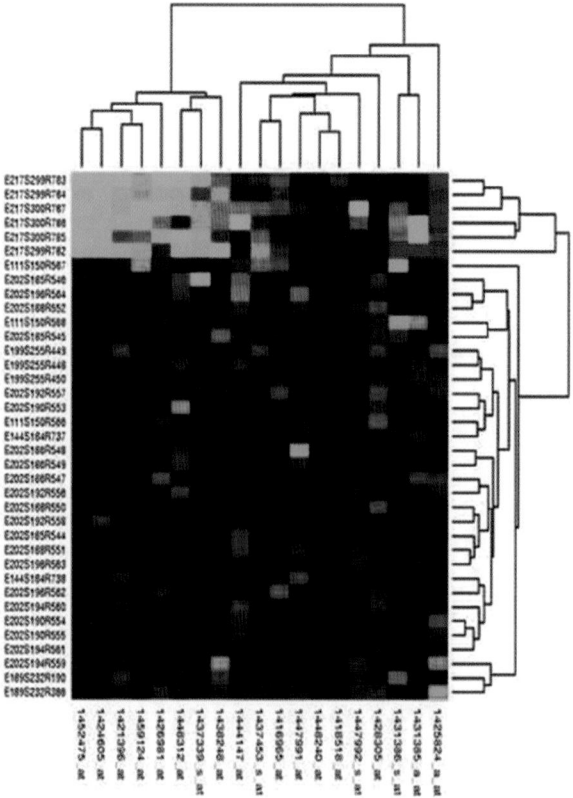

Figure 16-68. "Heat maps" of gene-chip data, vis-à-vis individual lung cancers, are capable of showing which genes are amplified, down-regulated, or unchanged from the physiologic state. These data, in turn, can be used for prognostication or selection of particular therapies.

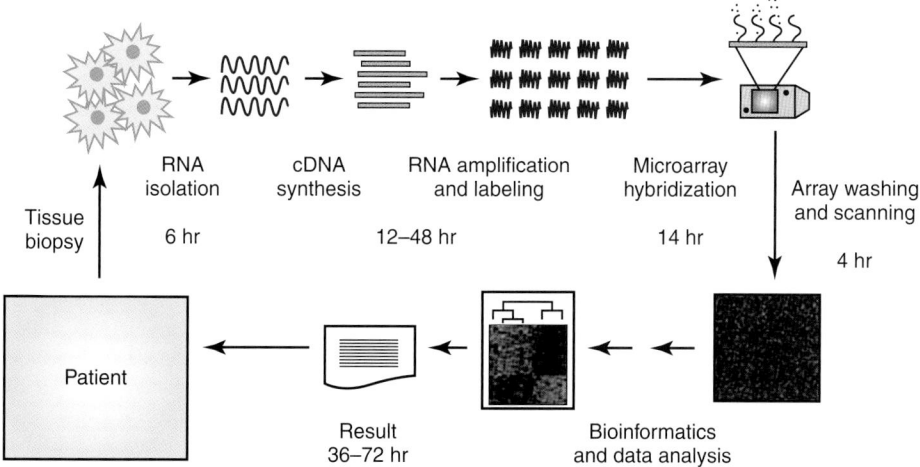

Figure 16-69. This schematic depicts the process used for genetic analysis of lung carcinomas. The overall throughput-time is on the order of 3 to 4 days.

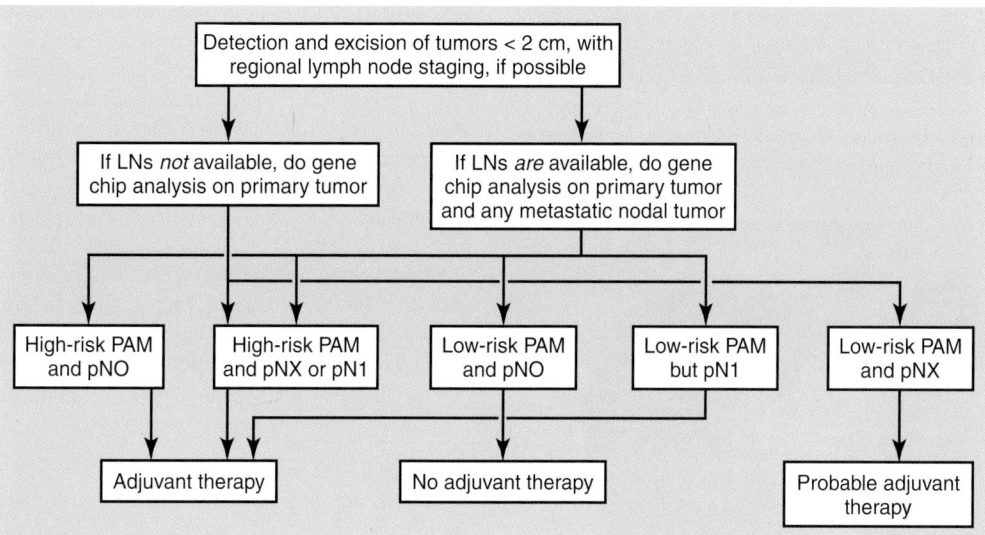

Figure 16-70. This hypothetical flow-chart shows how results of "prediction analysis of (gene chip) microarrays" (PAMs) may be used in the future to choose therapies and make prognostic estimates. LN, lymph node.

Association for the Study of Lung Cancer Staging Committee. Pertinent changes and remaining shortcomings of existing staging schemes have been well summarized by Flieder.[255] These are summarized as follows:

1. Pleural invasion by lung cancers *between adjacent lobes* (Fig. 16-71) is not specifically addressed in existing staging systems. (It is our empirical opinion that this does not have the same significance as invasion of the peripheral peripulmonary pleura).
2. There is no distinction between tumors that invade into, as opposed to through, the visceral pleura (no survival difference has been attached to this dissimilarity).
3. Intraoperative pleural lavage has been proposed as an adjuvant procedure to supplement histologic assessments of transpleural invasion by tumor (as stated by Flieder,[255] this process is laborious, requires immunohistochemical assessment of the resulting specimens, and is not a standard practice).
4. The significance of in situ carcinoma, as opposed to invasive or peribronchial carcinoma, at bronchial resection margins is not specified in existing staging schemes (we agree with Flieder[255] that it likely does not affect survival adversely).

5. Synchronous tumor nodules are classified in a confusing manner in current staging constructs. Those seen in the same lobe as the dominant mass are categorized as pT4 lesions (satellites; Fig. 16-72), whereas others in adjacent or contralateral lobes are classified as M1 deposits (true metastases) (published data on such tumors empirically indicate that virtually all of them are synchronous, separate primary tumors[256]; molecular studies can resolve this issue in many cases[257]).
6. Multifocal bronchioloalveolar carcinoma is not appropriately addressed in existing staging systems (if a suitably restrictive definition of such tumors is used, multifocality is part of the expected tumor phenotype rather than a reflection of true intrapulmonary metastasis).

Along with others, we hope that future iterations of staging protocols will aim to resolve these problems

Intraoperative Consultations in Lung Carcinoma Cases

Intraoperative consultations (IOPs) are commonly requested of pathologists by thoracic surgeons in the course of procedures for presumed or proven pulmonary carcinomas.[258] Confirmation of malignant

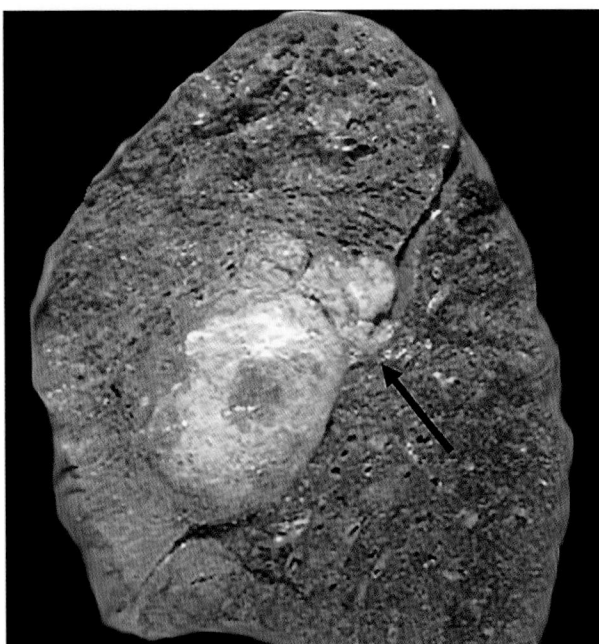

Figure 16-71. At present, staging schemes for lung carcinoma do not address the meaning of interlobar pleural transgression, as shown here in reference to an adenocarcinoma that crosses the upper and lower lobe pleural investments (*arrow*).

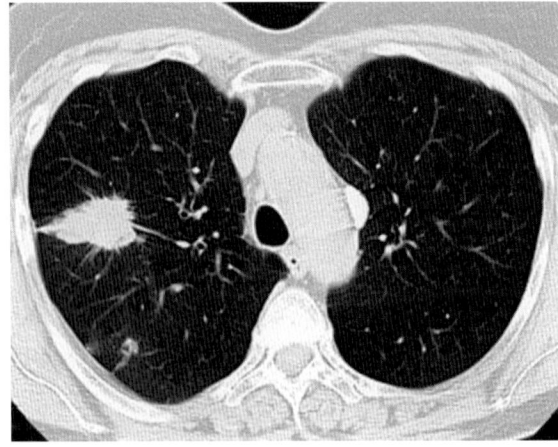

Figure 16-72. Lobe-syntonic metastatic nodules are not distinguished from intralobar second primary tumors (shown here in a computed tomogram) in current staging systems for lung carcinoma. The authors believe that such lesions almost always represent separate synchronous primary neoplasms.

diagnoses, determination of the status of bronchial or soft tissue margins, and examination of regional lymph nodes for possible tumor involvement are the principal reasons for such interactions.[258-262] The pathologist may elect to perform any or all of a variety of examinations, including "naked-eye" perusal, frozen (cryostat) sections, touch-imprint slide preparations, or ex vivo fine-needle aspiration.[263] Several studies have affirmed the value and the efficacy of these procedures; however, there is an irreducible margin of error (approximately 1% to 2% of cases overall), of which clinicians should be apprised.[264] Frozen sections are not equivalent to permanent sections of paraffin-embedded tissues with regard to histologic detail and the scope of tissue sampling.

Several particularly difficult, if not impossible, scenarios can be encountered in this context. The first concerns requests for a primary tissue diagnosis because none has been obtained previously through biopsy. In some circumstances—alluded to earlier—even that process

can be complicated. For example, distinguishing BAC from florid reactive pneumocytic proliferations is a potential problem,[88] as are the definitive recognition of "carcinoid tumors" and the diagnostic separation of solitary metastasis of a previous nonpulmonary malignancy from a primary lung cancer.[265,266] Useful guidelines have been advanced for morphologic findings that are useful in these IOPs,[88,265-267] but those recommendations are not foolproof.[181,260,261,264,267,268]

Selected publications have suggested that "ultra-rapid" immunohistochemical studies could be done during an IOP to facilitate histopathologic interpretations.[269,270] However, most surgical pathology laboratories are not equipped to undertake these procedures, lacking the necessary staffing and funding. We would argue that they are not necessary in a pragmatic sense. If the questions are "primary tumor or solitary metastasis" and "small peripheral carcinoma or localized benign pseudotumor," the surgeon can be advised to perform limited but complete resection of the mass, optimally with additional sampling of regional lymph nodes. Such an approach typically does not compromise the overall prognosis if the lesion proves to be a primary lung cancer; furthermore, it is not associated with significant morbidity if the mass is determined to be either metastatic or benign.

A related topic is the traditional onus for pathologists to separate "small cell" from "non–small cell" carcinomas in primary diagnoses made during IOPs.[271] Based on information that has also been presented in Chapter 13, we believe that the latter paradigm is outmoded. The more appropriate question pertaining to surgery for any given lung cancer should be "resectable or nonresectable," *regardless* of cell type and tumor grade. The answer to that query, in turn, principally hinges on the *stage* of the neoplasm as determined by results of radiographic imaging and intraoperative tissue sampling. Recent publications confirm the contention that patients with limited-stage small cell carcinoma do benefit from surgical intervention.[272,273]

These "standard" and "revisionist" approaches to treatment, in which IOP often plays a role, are summarized in Figure 16-73.

Stylized Surgical Pathology Reports on Carcinoma of the Lung

Obviously, not all pulmonary carcinomas are resectable. Colby and Deschamps[274] have nicely summarized the clinicopathologic features of these tumors, including that subset that is surgically approachable (Table 16-4). For lesions that can be completely excised, pathology organizations such as the College of American Pathologists and the Association of Directors of Anatomic & Surgical Pathology (ADASP) have published guidelines for the current reporting of morphologic findings.[275,276] In our opinion, the most tenable is that provided by the latter of those two organizations, which is reproduced in modified form here.[276]

Suggested ADASP Reporting Format for Resected Lung Carcinomas

A. Gross description
1. How the specimen was received—e.g., fresh, in formalin, opened, unopened.
2. How the specimen was identified—labeled (name, number) and designated (e.g., right upper lobe).
3. Part(s) of the lung included—including measurements in three dimensions and weights, and description of other attached structures (i.e., parietal pleura, hilar lymph nodes).
4. Tumor description
   - Tumor location, including the relationship to lobes, segments, and if pertinent, major airways and pleura. Involvement of the lobar or main stem bronchus should be specified.
   - Proximity to the bronchial resection margin and to other surgical margins (i.e., chest wall soft tissue, hilar vessels) as appropriate.

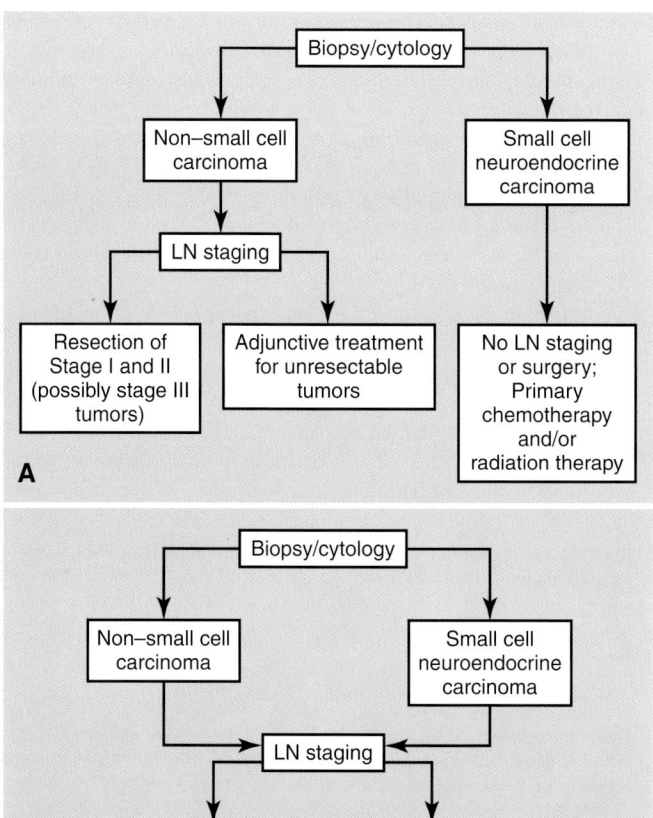

Figure 16-73. "Traditional" (**A**) and revised (**B**) paradigms for surgical therapy of small cell and non–small cell carcinomas of the lung (see text). The authors endorse the use of the revised model. LN, lymph node.

- Tumor size (three dimensions if possible).
- Presence or absence of satellite tumor nodules.

5. Description of the nontumorous lung—i.e., presence or absence of postobstructive changes or other abnormalities (e.g., bronchiectasis, mucus plugs, obstructive pneumonia, atelectasis).

B. Diagnostic information

1. Site of the tumor (i.e., side, lobe, specific segment if appropriate) and surgical procedure (i.e., segmentectomy, lobectomy, pneumonectomy), including portion of the lung resected.
2. Histologic type—i.e., a modified World Health Organization (WHO) classification[23] is recommended. Although the WHO classification is based on light microscopic criteria, the results

of ancillary studies (i.e., histochemistry, immunohistochemistry, electron microscopy) should be reported when appropriate:

- Squamous cell carcinoma (keratinization or intercellular bridges). Variant: spindle cell (squamous cell carcinoma).
- Adenocarcinoma (tubular, acinar, or papillary growth pattern) or mucus production; acinar adenocarcinoma (i.e., adenocarcinoma, not otherwise specified); micropapillary adenocarcinoma; solid carcinoma with mucus formation; and variants, including bronchioloalveolar adenocarcinoma and spindle cell adenocarcinoma.
- Large cell carcinoma (large nuclei, prominent nucleoli, abundant cytoplasm, without characteristic features of squamous cell, small cell, or adenocarcinoma), including variants of giant cell carcinoma and clear cell carcinoma (large cell carcinomas composed extensively [>90%] of large cells with clear or foamy cytoplasm without mucin; clear cell features can also be prominent in squamous cell carcinomas and adenocarcinomas and in metastatic renal cell carcinoma).
- Adenosquamous carcinoma.
- Neuroendocrine carcinomas, including carcinoid tumor; atypical carcinoid tumor (well-differentiated neuroendocrine carcinoma); large cell neuroendocrine carcinoma; and small cell neuroendocrine carcinoma. Variants can be mixed small cell/large cell carcinoma or composite small cell carcinoma (typical small cell carcinoma intimately admixed with areas of squamous cell carcinoma or adenocarcinoma).
- Bronchial gland (salivary gland analog) carcinomas (adenoid cystic carcinoma, mucoepidermoid carcinoma, acinic cell carcinoma, epithelial-myoepithelial carcinoma).
- Other specific carcinoma types.

3. Histologic grade—WHO classification (i.e., well, moderately, or poorly differentiated) recommended for squamous cell carcinoma and adenocarcinomas of the acinar (i.e., adenocarcinoma, not further specified) or papillary type.
4. Histologic assessment of surgical margins—including a comment regarding the involvement of lobar or main stem bronchi by invasive or in situ carcinoma and the microscopic relationship of tumor to bronchial or vascular margins.
5. Pleural involvement—specifying whether the tumor invades into but not through the visceral pleura without involving the parietal pleura (T2) or into the parietal pleura (T3; elastic tissue stains can be helpful in defining the limiting elastic layer of visceral pleura; Fig. 16-74).
6. Lymph node metastases—indicating the number of involved nodes and the total number of nodes received. (Precise node counts may be difficult for fragmented specimens, such as those received from mediastinoscopy.) The nodal groups (N) should be specifically identified using the American Joint Committee on Cancer intraoperative staging system for regional lymph

Table 16-4. Comparison of Clinicopathologic Features by Histologic Types of Carcinoma of the Lung

Tumor Type	Percent of Cases	Percent of Smokers	Central Lesions (%)	Localized (%)	5-Year Survival Rate (%)
Squamous cell	30	98	64	21.5	15.4
Adenocarcinoma	31	82	5	22.2	16.6*
Grade 3 neuroendocrine, small cell	19	99	74	8.2	4.6
Other†	15	95	42	15	11.5

*Bronchioloalveolar carcinomas are associated with a 42% 5-year survival rate.
†Statistics in this group encompass large cell "undifferentiated," grade 3 neuroendocrine carcinoma, large cell–type, and sarcomatoid carcinoma, but not salivary gland analog tumors.
Data from Colby TV, Deschamps C. The lung and pleura. In: Banks PM, Kraybill WG, eds. *Pathology for the Surgeon.* Philadelphia: WB Saunders; 1996:155–168.

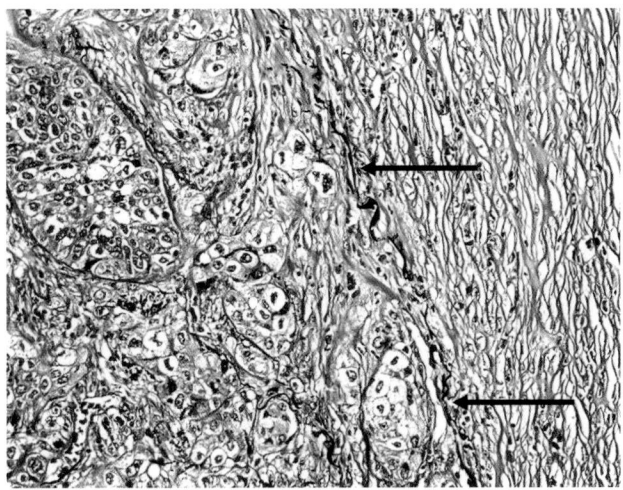

Figure 16-74. This Verhoeff–Van Gieson elastic stain shows that a lung carcinoma growing close to the pleural surface is, in fact, contained by the visceral pleural elastic layer (*arrows*). That finding has prognostic significance.

nodes.[277] N2 lymph nodes (with the exception of level 11 interlobar nodes) are generally received separately and must be appropriately identified by the submitting surgeon; these are to be reported separately. Pneumonectomies are usually accompanied by attached N2 lymph nodes, which should be specifically identified by location. If the nodal involvement is only by direct extension, this feature should be noted. If nodes are labeled by the surgeon according to anatomic station (Fig. 16-75), that system of labeling should be maintained in the pathology report.

7. Non-neoplastic lung—noting any significant abnormalities (e.g., emphysema, granulomas, pneumonia).

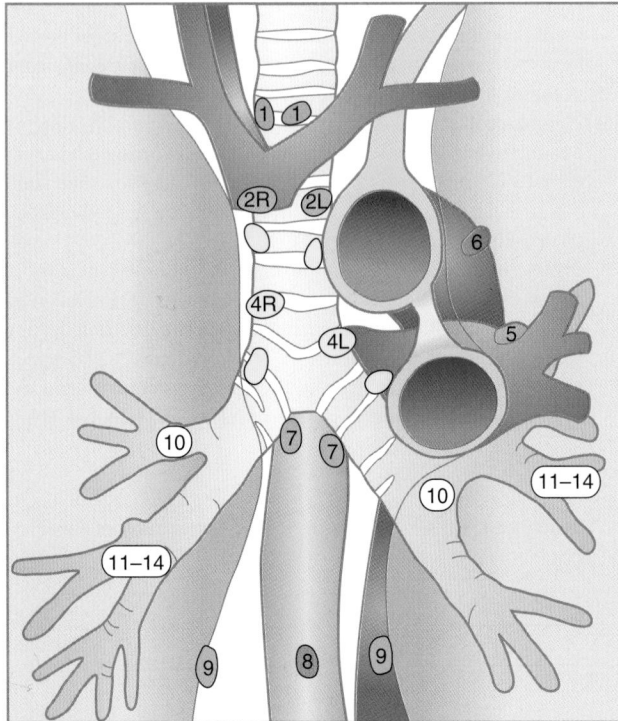

Figure 16-75. Schematic for intrathoracic lymph node stations. The designations shown here should be maintained in surgical pathology reports on lymph node biopsies in lung carcinoma cases.

C. Additional features. (The following features are also considered to be desirable elements of the final report. However, some accrediting agencies may now require that these findings be included routinely in the report.)

1. Stage—surgical pathology reports containing the previously listed information will contain all of the necessary data to establish the International TNM Staging System for lung carcinoma. It should be stated in the report that pathologic tumor stage may be based on incomplete information and therefore may differ from clinical tumor stage.

2. Angiolymphatic invasion—whenever possible, it should be specified whether the structures involved are blood vessels or lymphatic vessels, and whether the involved blood vessels are muscular arteries, elastic arteries, or veins.

3. Perineural invasion.

4. Presence or absence of extracapsular tumor invasion in metastatically involved lymph nodes.

Self-assessment questions related to this chapter can be found online on the Expert Consult site for this title.

Reference

1. Wingo PA, Tong T, Boldens S. Cancer statistics, 1995. *Ca*. 1995;45:8–30.
2. Andre F, Jacot W, Pujol JL, Grunenwald D, LeChevalier T. Epidemiology, prognostic factors, staging, and treatment of non-small cell lung cancer. *Bull Cancer*. 1999;3(suppl):17–41.
3. Fraire AE. Pathology of lung cancer. In: Aisner J, Arriagada R, Green MR, Martini N, Perry MC, eds. *Comprehensive Textbook of Thoracic Oncology*. Baltimore: Williams & Wilkins; 1996:245–275.
4. Davila DG, Williams DE. The etiology of lung cancer. *Mayo Clin Proc*. 1993;68:170–182.
5. Franceschi S, Bidoli E. The epidemiology of lung cancer. *Ann Oncol*. 1999;10(suppl):S3–S6.
6. Emmons KM. Smoking cessation and tobacco control: an overview. *Chest*. 1999;116(suppl3):490S–492S.
7. Kubina M, Hedelin G, Charloux A, et al. Do patients with squamous cell carcinoma or adenocarcinoma of the lung have different smoking histories? *Rev Mal Respir*. 1999;16:539–549.
8. Boffetta P, Nyberg F, Agudo A, et al. Risk of lung cancer from exposure to environmental tobacco smoke from cigars, cigarillos, and pipes. *Int J Cancer*. 1999;83:805–806.
9. Lubin JH. Estimating lung cancer risk with exposure to environmental tobacco smoke. *Environ Health Perspect*. 1999;107(suppl 6):879–883.
10. The World Health Organization histological typing of lung tumors, 2nd edn. *Am J Clin Pathol*. 1982;77:123–136.
11. Nolan L, Eccles D, Cross E, et al. First case report of Muir-Torre syndrome associated with non-small cell lung cancer. *Fam Cancer*. 2009;8:359–362.
12. Hassan MM, Phan A, Li D, Dagohoy CG, Leary C, Yao JC. Family history of cancer and associated risk of developing neuroendocrine tumors: a case-control study. *Cancer Epidemiol Biomarkers Prev*. 2008;17:959–965.
13. Weinstein A, Nouri K, Bassiri-Tehrani S, Flores F, Jimenez G. Muir-Torre syndrome: a case of this uncommon entity. *Int J Dermatol*. 2006;45:311–313.
14. Lynch HT, Katz DA, Bogard P, Lynch JF. Cancer genes, multiple primary cancers, and von Hippel-Lindau disease. *Cancer Genet Cytogenet*. 1985;16:13–19.
15. Lynch HT, Fain PR, Albano WA, et al. Genetic-epidemiological findings in a study of smoking-associated tumors. *Cancer Genet Cytogenet*. 1982;6:163–169.
16. Lynch HT, Fusaro RM, Pester J, et al. Tumor spectrum in the FAMMM syndrome. *Br J Cancer*. 1981;44:553–560.
17. Lissowska J, Foretove L, Dabek J, et al. Family history and lung cancer risk: international multicenter case-control study in Eastern and Central Europe and meta- analyses. *Cancer Causes Control*. 2010; March 21 (E-pub before print).
18. Landi MT, Chatterjee N, Yu K, et al. A genome-wide association study of lung cancer identifies a region of chromosome 5p15 associated with risk for adenocarcinoma. *Am J Hum Genet*. 2009;85:679–691.
19. Carney A, Sheahan K, Keegan D, Tolan M, Hyland J, Green A. Synchronous lung tumors in a patient with metachronous colorectal carcinoma and a germline MSH2 mutation. *J Clin Pathol*. 2009;62:471–473.
20. Nitadori J, Inoue M, Iwasaki M, et al. Association between lung cancer incidence and family history of lung cancer: data from a large-scale population-based cohort study, the JPHC study. *Chest*. 2006;130:968–975.
21. Li X, Hemminki K. Familial and second lung cancers: a nation-wide epidemiologic study from Sweden. *Lung Cancer*. 2003;39:255–263.
22. Yesner R, Seydel G, Asbell SO, et al. Biopsies of non-small cell lung cancer: central review in cooperative studies of the radiation therapy oncology group. *Mod Pathol*. 1991;4:432–440.
23. Travis WD, Brambilla E, Muller-Hermelink HK, Harris CC, eds. *Pathology & Genetics of Tumors of the Lung, Pleura, Thymus, & Heart*. Geneva: World Health Organization; 2004.

24. Olcott CT. Cell types and histologic patterns in carcinoma of the lung: observations on the significance of tumors containing more than one type of cell. *Am J Pathol*. 1955;31:975–995.

25. Fraire AE, Cooper SP, Greenberg SD, Buffler PA. Carcinoma of the lung: changing cell distribution and histopathologic cell types. *Prog Surg Pathol*. 1992;12:129–149.

26. Motoi N, Szoke J, Riely GJ, et al. Lung adenocarcinoma: modification of the 2004 WHO mixed subtype to include the major histologic subtype suggests correlations between papillary and micropapillary adenocarcinoma subtypes, EGFR mutations and gene expression analysis. *Am J Surg Pathol*. 2008;32:810–827.

27. Roggli VL, Vollmer RT, Greenberg SD, et al. Lung cancer heterogeneity: a blinded and randomized study of 100 consecutive cases. *Hum Pathol*. 1985;16:569–579.

28. Fraire AE, Roggli VL, Vollmer RT, et al. Lung cancer heterogeneity: prognostic implications. *Cancer*. 1987;60:370–379.

29. Selvaggi G, Scagliotti GV. Histologic subtype in NSCLC: does it matter? *Oncology (Williston Park)*. 2009;23:1133–1140.

30. Butnor KJ. Avoiding underdiagnosis, overdiagnosis, and misdiagnosis of lung carcinoma. *Arch Pathol Lab Med*. 2008;132:1118–1132.

31. Vincent RG, Pickren JW, Lane NVW, et al. The changing histopathology of lung cancer: a review of 1682 cases. *Cancer*. 1977;39:1617–1655.

32. Fishback NF, Travis WD, Moran CA, et al. Pleomorphic (spindle/giant-cell) carcinoma of the lung: a clinicopathologic correlation of 78 cases. *Cancer*. 1994;73:2936–2945.

33. Franks TJ, Galvin JR. Sarcomatoid carcinoma of the lung: histologic criteria and common lesions in the differential diagnosis. *Arch Pathol Lab Med*. 2010;134:49–54.

34. Mochizuki T, Ishii G, Nagai K, et al. Pleomorphic carcinoma of the lung: clinicopathologic characteristics of 70 cases. *Am J Surg Pathol*. 2008;32(11):1727–1735.

35. Martin LW, Correa AM, Ordonez NG, et al. Sarcomatoid carcinoma of the lung: a predictor of poor prognosis. *Ann Thorac Surg*. 2007;84:973–980.

36. Nappi O, Swanson PE, Wick MR. Pseudovascular adenoid squamous cell carcinoma of the lung: clinicopathologic features of three cases and comparison with true pleuropulmonary angiosarcoma. *Hum Pathol*. 1994;25:373–378.

37. Ritter JH, Mills SE, Nappi O, Wick MR. Angiosarcoma-like neoplasms of epithelial organs: true endothelial tumors or variants of carcinoma? *Semin Diagn Pathol*. 1995;12:270–282.

38. Chang YL, Wu CT, Shih JY, Lee YC. New aspects in clinicopathologic and oncogene studies of 23 pulmonary lymphoepithelioma-like carcinomas. *Am J Surg Pathol*. 2002;26:715–723.

39. Brambilla E, Moro D, Veale D, et al. Basal cell (basaloid) carcinoma of the lung: a new morphologic and phenotypic entity with separate prognostic significance. *Hum Pathol*. 1992;23:993–1003.

40. Koss MN, Travis WD, Moran CA, Hochholzer L. Pseudomesotheliomatous adenocarcinoma: a reappraisal. *Semin Diagn Pathol*. 1992;9:117–123.

41. Dessy E, Pietra GG. Pseudomesotheliomatous adenocarcinoma of the lung: an immunohistochemical and ultrastructural study of three cases. *Cancer*. 1991;68:1747–1753.

42. Lin JI, Tseng CH, Tsung SH. Pseudomesotheliomatous carcinoma of the lung. *South Med J*. 1980;73:655–657.

43. Moran CA. Pulmonary adenocarcinoma: the expanding spectrum of histologic variants. *Arch Pathol Lab Med*. 2006;130:958–962.

44. DaCosta N, Sivararnan A, Kinare SG. Carcinoma of lung with special reference to adenocarcinoma: an autopsy study of 122 cases. *Ind J Cancer*. 1993;30:42–47.

45. Iezumi K, Masunaga A, Kadofuku T, et al. Combined small cell carcinoma with pulmonary blastoma and adenocarcinoma: case report and clonality analysis. *Pathol Res Pract*. 2006;202:895–899.

46. Solis LM, Raso MG, Kalhor N, Behrens C, Wistuba II, Moran CA. Primary oncocytic adenocarcinomas of the lung: a clinicopathologic, immunohistochemical, and molecular biologic analysis of 16 cases. *Am J Clin Pathol*. 2010;133:133–140.

47. Weidner N. Pulmonary adenocarcinoma with intestinal-type differentiation. *Ultrastruct Pathol*. 1992;16:7–10.

48. Hayashi H, Kitamura H, Nakatani Y, et al. Primary signet-ring-cell carcinoma of the lung: histochemical and immunohistochemical characterization. *Hum Pathol*. 1999;30:378–383.

49. Moran CA, Hochholzer L, Fishback N, Travis WD, Koss MN. Mucinous (so-called colloid) carcinomas of lung. *Mod Pathol*. 1992;5:634–638.

50. Gaffey MJ, Mills SE, Ritter JH. Clear cell tumors of the lower respiratory tract. *Semin Diagn Pathol*. 1997;14:222–232.

51. Nakatani Y, Kitamura H, Inayama Y, et al. Pulmonary adenocarcinomas of the fetal lung type: a clinicopathologic study indicating differences in histology, epidemiology, and natural history of low-grade and high-grade forms. *Am J Surg Pathol*. 1998;22:399–411.

52. Li HC, Schmidt L, Greenson JK, Chang AC, Myers JL. Primary pulmonary adenocarcinoma with intestinal differentiation mimicking metastatic colorectal carcinoma: case report and review of literature. *Am J Clin Pathol*. 2009;131:129–133.

53. Colby TV, Koss MN, Travis WD. Tumors of the lower respiratory tract. In: *Atlas of Tumor Pathology, Series 3, Fascicle 13*. Washington, DC: Armed Forces Institute of Pathology; 1995:203–234.

54. Higashiyama M, Doi O, Kodama K, et al. Extramammary Paget's disease of the bronchial epithelium. *Arch Pathol Lab Med*. 1991;115:185–188.

55. Ordonez NG. Immunohistochemical diagnosis of epithelioid mesothelioma: a critical review of old markers and new markers. *Hum Pathol*. 2002;33:953–967.

56. Liebow AA. Bronchioloalveolar carcinoma. *Adv Intern Med*. 1960;10:329–358.

57. Clayton F. Bronchioloalveolar carcinomas: cell types, patterns of growth, and prognostic correlates. *Cancer*. 1986;57:1555–1564.

58. Clayton F. The spectrum of significance of bronchioloalveolar carcinomas. *Pathol Annu*. 1988;23(2):361–394.

59. Feldman ER, Eagan RT, Schaid J. Metastatic bronchioloalveolar carcinoma and metastatic adenocarcinoma of the lung: comparison of clinical manifestations, chemotherapeutic responses, and prognosis. *Mayo Clin Proc*. 1992;67:27–32.

60. Grover FL, Piantadosi S. Recurrence and survival following resection of bronchioloalveolar carcinoma of the lung – the Lung Cancer Study Group experience. *Ann Surg*. 1989;209:779–790.

61. Lozowski W, Hajdu SI. Cytology and immunocytochemistry of bronchioloalveolar carcinoma. *Acta Cytol*. 1987;31:717–725.

62. Manning JT, Spjut HJ, Tschen JA. Bronchioloalveolar carcinoma: the significance of two histopathologic types. *Cancer*. 1984;54:525–534.

63. Marcq M, Galy P. Bronchioloalveolar carcinoma: clinicopathological relationships, natural history, and prognosis in 29 cases. *Am Rev Resp Dis*. 1973;107:621–629.

64. Rosenblatt MB, Lisa JR, Collier F. Primary and metastatic bronchioloalveolar carcinoma. *Chest*. 1967;52:147–152.

65. Schulze ES, Mattia AR, Chew FS. Bronchioloalveolar carcinoma. *Am J Roentgenol*. 1994;162:1294.

66. Sutton LN, Morrison JF, Rees MR. Radiographic features and prognosis in bronchioloalveolar carcinoma: a local experience. *Resp Med*. 1989;83:471–477.

67. Fukui T, Mitsudomi T. Small peripheral lung adenocarcinoma: clinicopathological features and surgical treatment. *Surg Today*. 2010;40:191–198.

68. Mizutani Y, Nakajima T, Morinaga S, et al. Immunohistochemical localization of pulmonary surfactant apoproteins in various lung tumors, with special reference to lung adenocarcinoma subtypes. *Cancer*. 1988;61:532–537.

69. Sorensen JB, Hirsch FR, Gazdar A, Olsen JE. Interobserver variability in histopathologic subtyping and grading of pulmonary adenocarcinoma. *Cancer*. 1993;71:2971–2976.

70. Yokose T, Suzuki K, Nagai K, Nishiwaki Y, Sasaki S, Ochiai A. Favorable and unfavorable morphological prognostic factors in peripheral adenocarcinoma of the lung 3 cm or less in diameter. *Lung Cancer*. 2000;29:179–188.

71. Sakurai H, Maeshima A, Watanabe S, et al. Grade of stromal invasion in small adenocarcinoma of the lung: histopathological minimal invasion and prognosis. *Am J Surg Pathol*. 2004;28:198–206.

72. Barsky SH, Grossman DA, Ho J, Holmes EC. The multifocality of bronchioloalveolar lung carcinoma: evidence and implications of a multiclonal origin. *Mod Pathol*. 1994;7:633–640.

73. Grotte D, Stanley MW, Swanson PE, et al. Reactive type II pneumocytes in bronchoalveolar lavage fluid from acute respiratory syndrome can be mistaken for cells of adenocarcinoma. *Diagn Cytopathol*. 1990;6:317–322.

74. Ritter JH, Wick MR, Reyes AR, Coffin CM, Dehner LP. False-positive interpretations of carcinoma in exfoliative respiratory cytology: report of two cases and a review of underlying disorders. *Am J Clin Pathol*. 1995;104:133–140.

75. Mori M, Chiba R, Takahashi T. Atypical adenomatous hyperplasia of the lung and its differentiation from adenocarcinoma: characterization of atypical cells by morphometry and multivariate cluster analysis. *Cancer*. 1993;72:2331–2340.

76. Hegg CA, Flint A, Singh G. Papillary adenoma of the lung. *Am J Clin Pathol*. 1992;97:393–397.

77. Stenhouse G, Fyfe N, King G, Chapman A, Kerr KM. Thyroid transcription factor 1 in pulmonary adenocarcinoma. *J Clin Pathol*. 2004;57:383–387.

78. Beasley MB. Immunohistochemistry of pulmonary and pleural neoplasia. *Arch Pathol Lab Med*. 2008;132:1062–1072.

79. Ueno T, Linder S, Elmberger G. Aspartic proteinase napsin is a useful marker for diagnosis of primary lung adenocarcinoma. *Br J Cancer*. 2003;88:1229–1233.

80. Bishop JA, Sharma R, Illei PB. Napsin A and thyroid transcription factor-1 expression in carcinomas of the lung, breast, pancreas, colon, kidney, thyroid, and malignant mesotheliomas. *Hum Pathol*. 2010;41:20–25.

81. Yamato Y, Tsuchida M, Watanabe T, et al. Early results of a prospective study of limited resection for bronchioloalveolar adenocarcinoma of the lung. *Ann Thorac Surg*. 2001;71:971–974.

82. Watanabe S, Oda M, Tsunezuka Y, Go T, Ohta Y, Watanabe G. Peripheral small-sized (2 cm or less) non-small cell lung cancer with mediastinal lymph node metastasis; clinicopathologic features and patterns of nodal spread. *Eur J Cardiothorac Surg*. 2002;22:995–999.

83. Koike T, Yamato Y, Yoshiya K, et al. Criteria for intentional limited pulmonary resection in cT1N0M0 peripheral lung cancer. *Jpn J Thorac Cardiovasc Surg*. 2003;51:515–519.

84. Ishiwa N, Ogawa N, Shoji A, et al. Correlation between lymph node micrometastasis and histologic classification of small lung adenocarcinomas, in considering the indication of limited surgery. *Lung Cancer*. 2003;39:159–164.

85. Rusch VW, Tsuchiya R, Tsuboi M, Pass HI, Grunenwald D, Goldstraw P. Surgery for bronchioloalveolar carcinoma and "very early" adenocarcinoma: an evolving standard of care? *J Thorac Oncol*. 2006;1(suppl 9):S27–S31.

86. Kitamura H, Kameda Y, Ito T, et al. Atypical adenomatous hyperplasia of the lung: implications for the pathogenesis of peripheral lung adenocarcinoma. *Am J Clin Pathol*. 1999;111:610–622.

87. Miller RR, Nelerris B, Evans KG, et al. Glandular neoplasia of the lung: a proposed analogy to colonic tumors. *Cancer*. 1988;61:1009–1014.

88. Gupta R, McKenna Jr R, Marchevsky AM. Lessons learned from mistakes and deferrals in the frozen section diagnosis of bronchioloalveolar carcinoma and well-differentiated pulmonary adenocarcinoma: an evidence-based pathology approach. *Am J Clin Pathol*. 2008;130:11–20.

89. Sheikh HA, Fuhrer K, Cieply K, Yousem S. p63 expression in assessment of bronchioloalveolar proliferations of the lung. *Mod Pathol*. 2004;17:1134–1140.

90. Saad RS, Liu YL, Silverman JF. Distribution of basal-myoepithelial markers in benign and malignant bronchioloalveolar proliferations of the lung. *Appl Immunohistochem Mol Morphol*. 2010;18:219–225.

91. Huang MS, Colby TV, Goellner JR, et al. Utility of bronchoalveolar lavage in the diagnosis of drug-induced pulmonary toxicity. *Acta Cytol*. 1989;33:533–538.

92. Rao SK, Fraire AE. Alveolar cell hyperplasia in association with adenocarcinoma of the lung. *Mod Pathol*. 1995;8:165–169.

93. Miller RR. Bronchioloalveolar cell adenomas. *Am J Surg Pathol*. 1990;14:904–912.

94. Nakanishi K. Alveolar epithelial hyperplasia and adenocarcinoma of the lung. *Arch Pathol Lab Med*. 1990;114:363–368.

95. Travis WD, Linnoila RI, Horowitz M, et al. Pulmonary nodules resembling bronchioloalveolar carcinoma in adolescent cancer patients. *Mod Pathol*. 1988;1:372–377.

96. Niho S, Yokose T, Suzuki K, et al. Monoclonality of atypical adenomatous hyperplasia of the lung. *Am J Pathol*. 1999;154:249–254.

97. Greenberg AK, Yee H, Rom WN. Preneoplastic lesions of the lung. *Respir Res*. 2002;3:20.

98. Garfield DH, Cadranel JL, Wislez M, Franklin WA, Hirsch FR. The bronchioloalveolar carcinoma and peripheral adenocarcinoma spectrum of diseases. *J Thorac Oncol*. 2006;1:344–359.

99. Morandi L, Asioli S, Cavazza A, Pession A, Damiani S. Genetic relationship among atypical adenomatous hyperplasia, bronchioloalveolar carcinoma and adenocarcinoma of the lung. *Lung Cancer*. 2007;56:35–42.

100. Wu M, Orta L, Gil J, Li G, Hu A, Burstein DE. Immunohistochemical detection of XIAP and p63 in adenomatous hyperplasia, atypical adenomatous hyperplasia, bronchioloalveolar carcinoma and well-differentiated adenocarcinoma. *Mod Pathol*. 2008;21:553–558.

101. Raz DJ, He B, Rosell R, Jablons DM. Current concepts in bronchioloalveolar carcinoma biology. *Clin Cancer Res*. 2006;12:3698–3704.

102. Inamura K, Ninomiya H, Ishikawa Y, Matsubara O. Is the epidermal growth factor receptor status in lung cancers reflected in clinicopathologic features? *Arch Pathol Lab Med*. 2010;134:66–72.

103. Li AR, Chitale D, Riely GJ, et al. EGFR mutations in lung adenocarcinomas: clinical testing experience and relationship to EGFR gene copy number and immunohistochemical expression. *J Mol Diagn*. 2008;10:242–248.

104. Kawakami T, Nabeshima K, Makimoto Y, et al. Micropapillary pattern and grade of stromal invasion in pT1 adenocarcinoma of the lung: usefulness as prognostic factors. *Mod Pathol*. 2007;20:514–521.

105. Sánchez-Mora N, Presmanes MC, Monroy V, et al. Micropapillary lung adenocarcinoma: a distinctive histologic subtype with prognostic significance-- Case series. *Hum Pathol*. 2008;39:324–330.

106. Rudomina DE, Lin O, Moreira AL. Cytologic diagnosis of pulmonary adenocarcinoma with micropapillary pattern: does it correlate with the histologic findings? *Diagn Cytopathol*. 2009;37:333–339.

107. Meyer EC, Leibow AA. Relationship of interstitial pneumonia honeycombing and atypical epithelial proliferation to cancer of the lung. *Cancer*. 1965;18:322–351.

108. Shimosato Y, Noguchi M, Matsuno Y. Adenocarcinoma of the lung: its development and malignant progression. *Lung Cancer*. 1993;9:99–108.

109. Cagle PT, Cohle SD, Greenberg SD. Natural history of pulmonary scar cancers: clinical and prognostic implications. *Cancer*. 1985;56:2031–2035.

110. Barsky SH, Huang SJ, Bhuta S. The extracellular matrix of pulmonary scar carcinomas is suggestive of a desmoplastic origin. *Am J Pathol*. 1986;124:412–419.

111. Harris JM, Johnston ID, Rudd R, Taylor AJ, Cullinan P. Cryptogenic fibrosing alveolitis and lung cancer: the BTS study. *Thorax*. 2010;65:70–76.

112. Attanoos RL, Thomas DH, Gibbs AR. Synchronous diffuse malignant mesothelioma and carcinomas in asbestos-exposed individuals. *Histopathology*. 2003;43:387–392.

113. Takamori S, Noguchi M, Morinaga S, et al. Clinical pathologic characteristics of adenosquamous carcinoma of the lung. *Cancer*. 1991;67:649–654.

114. Sridhar KS, Bounassi MJ, Raub W, Richman SP. Clinical features of adenosquamous lung carcinoma in 127 patients. *Am Rev Respir Dis*. 1990;142:19–23.

115. Ishida T, Kaneko S, Yokohama H, et al. Adenosquamous carcinoma of the lung: clinicopathologic and immunohistochemical features. *Am J Clin Pathol*. 1992;97:678–695.

116. Cakir E, Demirag E, Aydin M, Unsal E. Clinicopathologic features and prognostic significance of lung tumours with mixed histologic patterns. *Acta Chir Belg*. 2009;109:489–493.

117. Carter D, Patchefsky AS. *Tumors & tumor-like conditions of the lung*. Philadelphia: WB Saunders; 1998:266–285.

118. Pardo J, Martinez-Penuela M, Sola JJ, et al. Large-cell carcinoma of the lung: an endangered species? *Appl Immunohistochem Mol Morphol*. 2009;17:383–392.

119. Carvalho L. Reclassifying bronchial-pulmonary carcinoma: differentiating histological type in biopsies by immunohistochemistry. *Rev Port Pneumol*. 2009;15:1101–1119.

120. Nash G, Stout AP. Giant cell carcinoma of the lung: report of 5 cases. *Cancer*. 1958;11:369–376.

121. Ginsberg SS, Buzaid AC, Stern H, Carter D. Giant cell carcinoma of the lung. *Cancer*. 1992;70:606–610.

122. Attanoos RL, Papagiannis A, Suttinont P, et al. Pulmonary giant cell carcinoma: pathological entity or morphological phenotype? *Histopathology*. 1998;32:225–231.

123. Sawyers CL, Golde DW, Quan S, Nimer SD. Production of granulocyte-macrophage colony stimulating factor in two patients with lung cancer, leukocytosis, and eosinophilia. *Cancer*. 1992;69:1342–1346.

124. Vegh GL, Szigetvári I, Soltesz I, et al. Primary pulmonary choriocarcinoma: a case report. *J Reprod Med*. 2008;53:369–372.

125. Shimosato Y. Lung tumors of uncertain histogenesis. *Semin Diagn Pathol*. 1995;12:185–192.

126. Yoshida J, Nagai K, Hasebe T, et al. Pulmonary metastasis of renal cell carcinoma resected sixteen years after nephrectomy. *Jpn J Clin Oncol*. 1995;25:20–24.

127. Bonetti F, Pea M, Martignoni G, et al. Clear cell ("sugar") tumor of the lung is a lesion strictly related to angiomyolipoma – the concept of a family of lesions characterized by the presence of the perivascular epithelioid cell (PEC). *Pathology*. 1994;26:230–236.

128. Gaffey MJ, Mills SE, Frierson Jr HF, Askin FB, Maygarden SJ. Pulmonary clear cell carcinoid tumor: another entity in the differential diagnosis of pulmonary clear cell neoplasia. *Am J Surg Pathol*. 1998;22:1020–1025.

129. Nowak MA, Fatteh SM, Campbell TE. Glycogen-rich malignant melanomas and glycogen-rich balloon cell malignant melanomas: frequency and pattern of PAS positivity in primary and metastatic melanomas. *Arch Pathol Lab Med*. 1998;122:353–360.

130. MacDowell EM, Wilson TS, Trump BF. Atypical endocrine tumors of the lung. *Arch Pathol Lab Med*. 1981;105:20–28.

131. Hammond ME, Sause WT. Large cell neuroendocrine tumors of the lung. *Cancer*. 1985;56:1624–1629.

132. Piehl MR, Gould VE, Warren WH, et al. Immunohistochemical identification of exocrine and neuroendocrine subsets of large cell lung carcinomas. *Pathol Res Pract*. 1988;183:675–682.

133. Wick MR, Berg LC, Hertz M. Large cell carcinoma of the lung with neuroendocrine differentiation: a comparison with large cell "undifferentiated" pulmonary tumors. *Am J Clin Pathol*. 1992;97:796–805.

134. Cavazza A, Colby TV, Tsokos M, Rush W, Travis WD. Lung tumors with a rhabdoid phenotype. *Am J Clin Pathol*. 1996;105:182–188.

135. Wick MR, Ritter JH, Dehner LP. Malignant rhabdoid tumors: a clinicopathologic review and conceptual discussion. *Semin Diagn Pathol*. 1995;12:233–248.

136. Perry A, Fuller CE, Judkins AR, Dehner LP, Biegel JA. INI1 expression is retained in composite rhabdoid tumors, including rhabdoid meningiomas. *Mod Pathol*. 2005;18:951–958.

137. Hoot AC, Russo P, Judkins AR, Perlman EJ, Biegel JA. Immunohistochemical analysis of hSNF5-INI1 distinguishes renal and extra-renal malignant rhabdoid tumors from other pediatric soft tissue tumors. *Am J Surg Pathol*. 2004;28:1485–1491.

138. Fuller CE, Pfeifer J, Humphrey P, Bruch LA, Dehner LP, Perry A. Chromosome 22q dosage in composite extrarenal rhabdoid tumors: clonal evolution or a phenotypic mimic? *Hum Pathol*. 2001;32:1102–1108.

139. Hirsch FR, Spreafico A, Novello S, Wood MD, Simms L, Papotti M. The prognostic and predictive role of histology in advanced non-small cell lung cancer: a literature review. *J Thorac Oncol*. 2008;3:1468–1481.

140. West H, Lilenbaum R, Harpole D, Wozniak A, Sequist L. Molecular analysis-based treatment strategies for the management of non-small cell lung cancer. *J Thorac Oncol*. 2009;4(9 suppl 2):S1029–S1039.

141. Stinchcombe TE, Socinski MA. Current treatments for advanced stage non-small cell lung cancer. *Proc Am Thorac Soc*. 2009;6:233–241.

142. Tiseo M, Rossi G, Capelletti M, et al. Predictors of gefitinib outcomes in advanced non-small cell lung cancer (NSCLC): study of a comprehensive panel of molecular markers. *Lung Cancer*. 2010;67:355–360.

143. Miller VA, Riely GJ, Zakowski MF, et al. Molecular characteristics of bronchioloalveolar carcinoma and adenocarcinoma, bronchioloalveolar carcinoma subtype, predict response to erlotinib. *J Clin Oncol*. 2008;26:1472–1478.

144. Ansari J, Palmer DH, Rea DW, Hussain SA. Role of tyrosine kinase inhibitors in lung cancer. *Anticancer Agents Med Chem*. 2009;9:569–575.

145. Sheth S. Current and emerging therapies for patients with advanced non-small-cell lung cancer. *Am J Health Syst Pharm*. 2010;67(1 suppl 1):S9–S14.

146. Takahashi T, Yamamoto N, Nukiwa T, et al. Phase II study of erlotinib in Japanese patients with advanced non-small cell lung cancer. *Anticancer Res*. 2010;30:557–563.

147. Chang JW, Liu HP, Hsieh MH, et al. Increased epidermal growth factor receptor (EGFR) gene copy number is strongly associated with EGFR mutations and adenocarcinoma in non-small cell lung cancers: a chromogenic in situ hybridization study of 182 patients. *Lung Cancer*. 2008;61:328–339.

148. Kargi A, Gurel D, Tuna B. The diagnostic value of TTF-1, CK 5/6, and p63 immunostaining in the classification of lung carcinomas. *Appl Immunohistochem Mol Morphol*. 2007;15:415–420.

149. Baksh FK, Dacic S, Finkelstein SD, et al. Widespread molecular alterations present in stage I non-small cell lung carcinoma fail to predict tumor recurrence. *Mod Pathol*. 2003;16:28–34.

150. Kanazawa H, Ebina M, Ino-Oka N, et al. Transition from squamous cell carcinoma to adenocarcinoma in adenosquamous carcinoma of the lung. *Am J Pathol*. 2000;156:1289–1298.

151. Park SH, Ha SY, Lee JI, et al. Epidermal growth factor receptor mutations and the clinical outcome in male smokers with squamous cell carcinoma of lung. *J Korean Med Sci*. 2009;24:448–452.

152. Monaco SE, Nikiforova MN, Cieply K, Teot LA, Khalbuss WE, Dacic S. A comparison of EGFR and KRAS status in primary lung carcinoma and matched metastases. *Hum Pathol*. 2010;41:94–102.

153. Kalikaki A, Koutsopoulos A, Trypaki M, et al. Comparison of EGFR and K-RAS gene status between primary tumours and corresponding metastases in NSCLC. *Br J Cancer*. 2008;99:923–929.

154. Gow CH, Chang YL, Hsu YC, et al. Comparison of epidermal growth factor receptor mutations between primary and corresponding metastatic tumors in tyrosine kinase inhibitor-naïve non-small-cell lung cancer. *Ann Oncol*. 2009;20:696–702.

155. Sartori G, Cavazza A, Sgambato A, et al. EGFR and K-ras mutations along the spectrum of pulmonary epithelial tumors of the lung and elaboration of a combined clinicopathologic and molecular scoring system to predict clinical responsiveness to EGFR inhibitors. *Am J Clin Pathol*. 2009;131:478–489.

156. Baba M, Castillo A, Koriyama C, et al. Human papillomavirus is frequently detected in gefitinib-responsive lung adenocarcinomas. *Oncol Rep*. 2010;23:1085–1092.

157. Moran CA. Primary salivary gland-type tumors of the lung. *Semin Diagn Pathol*. 1995;12:106–122.

158. Dowling EA, Miller RE, Johnson IM, et al. Mucoepidermoid tumors of the bronchi. *Surgery*. 1962;52:600–609.

159. Ozlu C, Christopherson WM, Allen JD. Mucoepidermoid tumors of the bronchi. *J Thorac Cardiovasc Surg*. 1961;42:24–31.

160. Axelsson C, Burcharth F, Johansen A. Mucoepidermoid lung tumors. *J Thorac Cardiovasc Surg*. 1973;65:902–908.

161. Turnbull AD, Huvos AG, Goodner JT, et al. Mucoepidermoid tumors of bronchial glands. *Cancer*. 1971;28:539–544.

162. Reichle FA, Rosemond GP. Mucoepidermoid tumors of the bronchus. *J Thorac Cardiovasc Surg*. 1966;51:443–448.

163. Klacsmann PG, Olson JL, Eggleston JC. Mucoepidermoid carcinoma of the bronchus. *Cancer*. 1979;43:1720–1733.

164. Barsky SH, Martin SE, Matthews M, et al. "Low grade" mucoepidermoid carcinoma of the bronchus with "high grade" biologic behavior. *Cancer*. 1983;51:1505–1509.

165. Seo IS, Warren J, Mirkin D, et al. Mucoepidermoid carcinoma of the bronchus in a 4-year-old child. *Cancer*. 1984;53:1600–1604.

166. Yousem SA, Hochholzer L. Mucoepidermoid tumors of the lung. *Cancer*. 1987;60:1346–1352.

167. Liu X, Adams AL. Mucoepidermoid carcinoma of the bronchus: a review. *Arch Pathol Lab Med*. 2007;131:1400–1404.

168. Molina JR, Aubry MC, Lewis JE, et al. Primary salivary gland-type lung cancer: spectrum of clinical presentation, histopathologic and prognostic factors. *Cancer*. 2007;110:2253–2259.

169. Shilo K, Foss RD, Franks TJ, DePeralta-Venturina M, Travis WD. Pulmonary mucoepidermoid carcinoma with prominent tumor-associated lymphoid proliferation. *Am J Surg Pathol*. 2005;29:407–411.

170. Macarenco RS, Uphoff TS, Gilmer HF, et al. Salivary gland-type lung carcinomas: an EGFR immunohistochemical, molecular genetic, and mutational analysis study. *Mod Pathol*. 2008;21:1168–1175.

171. Rossi G, Sartori G, Cavazza A, Tamberi S. Mucoepidermoid carcinoma of the lung, response to EGFR inhibitors, EGFR and K-RAS mutations, and differential diagnosis. *Lung Cancer*. 2009;63:159–160.

172. Moran CA, Suster S, Koss MN. Primary adenoid cystic carcinoma of the lung: a clinicopathological and immunohistochemical study of 16 cases. *Cancer*. 1994;73:1390–1397.

173. Ishida T, Nishino T, Oka T, et al. Adenoid cystic carcinoma of the tracheobronchial tree: clinicopathology and immunohistochemistry. *J Surg Oncol*. 1989;41:52–59.

174. Heilbrunn AA, Crosby IK. Adenoid cystic carcinoma and mucoepidermoid carcinoma of the tracheobronchial tree. *Chest*. 1972;61:145–149.

175. Nomori H, Kaseda S, Kobayashi K, et al. Adenoid cystic carcinoma of the trachea and main stem bronchus: a clinical, histopathologic, and immunohistochemical study. *J Thorac Cardiovasc Surg*. 1988;96:271–277.

176. Inoue H, Iwashita A, Kanegae H, et al. Peripheral pulmonary adenoid cystic carcinoma with substantial submucosal extension of the proximal bronchus. *Thorax*. 1991;46:147–148.

177. Conlan AA, Payne WS, Woolner LB, et al. Adenoid cystic carcinoma (Cylindroma) and mucoepidermoid carcinoma of the bronchus. *J Cardiothorac Surg*. 1978;76:369–377.

178. Markel SF, Abell MR, Haight L, et al. Neoplasms of the bronchus commonly designated as adenomas. *Cancer*. 1964;17:590–604.

179. Payne WS, Ellis FH, Woolner LB, et al. The surgical treatment of cylindroma (adenoid cystic carcinoma) and mucoepidermoid tumors of the bronchus. *J Thorac Cardiovasc Surg*. 1959;38:709–726.

180. Youkouchi H, Otsuka Y, Otoguro Y, et al. Primary peripheral adenoid cystic carcinoma of the lung and literature comparison of features. *Intern Med*. 2007;46:1799–1803.

181. Maygarden SJ, Detterbeck FC, Funkhouser WK. Bronchial margins in lung cancer resection specimens: utility of frozen section and gross examination. *Mod Pathol*. 2004;17:1080–1086.

182. Sterman DH, Sztejman E, Rodriguez E, Friedberg J. Diagnosis and staging of "other bronchial tumors." *Chest Surg Clin N Am*. 2003;13:79–94.

183. Daneshbod Y, Modjtahedi E, Atefi S, Bedayat GR, Daneshbod K. Exfoliative cytologic findings of primary pulmonary adenoid cystic carcinoma: a report of 2 cases with a review of the cytologic features. *Acta Cytol*. 2007;51:558–562.

184. Ozkara SK, Turan G. Fine needle aspiration cytopathology of primary solid adenoid cystic carcinoma of the lung: a case report. *Acta Cytol*. 2009;53:707–710.

185. Chuah KL, Lim KH, Koh MS, Tan HW, Yap WM. Diagnosis of adenoid cysticcarcinoma of the lung by bronchial brushing: a case report. *Acta Cytol*. 2007;51:563–566.

186. Farrell T, Chang YL. Basal cell adenocarcinoma of minor salivary glands. *Arch Pathol Lab Med*. 2007;131:1602–1604.

187. Jayakrishnan A, Elmalah I, Hussain K, Odell EW. Basal cell adenocarcinoma in minor salivary glands. *Histopathology*. 2003;42:610–614.

188. Parashar P, Baron E, Papadimitriou JC, Ord RA, Nikitakis NG. Basal cell adenocarcinoma of the oral minor salivary glands: review of the literature and presentation of two cases. *Oral Surg Oral Med Oral Pathol Oral Radiol Endod*. 2007;103:77–84.

189. Aubry MC, Heinrich MC, Molina J, et al. Primary adenoid cystic carcinoma of the lung: absence of KIT mutations. *Cancer*. 2007;110:2507–2510.

190. Miettinen M, Lasota J. KIT (CD117): a review on expression in normal and neoplastic tissues, and mutations and their clinicopathologic correlation. *Appl Immunohistochem Mol Morphol*. 2005;13:205–220.

191. Holst VA, Marshall CE, Moskaluk CA, Frierson Jr HF. KIT protein expression and analysis of c-kit gene mutation in adenoid cystic carcinoma. *Mod Pathol*. 1999;12:956–960.

192. Shimizu J, Oda M, Matsumoto I, Ararno Y, Ishikawa N, Minato H. Clinicopathologic study of surgically treated cases of tracheobronchial adenoid cystic carcinoma. *Gen Thorac Cardiovasc Surg*. 2010;58:82–86.

193. Fechner RE, Bentinck BR, Askew Jr JB. Acinic cell tumor of the lung: a histologic and ultrastructural study. *Cancer*. 1972;29:501–508.

194. Moran CA, Suster S, Koss MN. Acinic cell carcinoma of the lung ("Fechner Tumor"): a clinicopathologic, immunohistochemical, and ultrastructural study of five cases. *Am J Surg Pathol*. 1992;16:1039–1050.

195. Latz DR, Bubis JJ. Acinic cell tumor of the bronchus. *Cancer*. 1976;38:830–832.

196. Gharpure KJ, Desphande RK, Vishweshvara RN, et al. Acinic cell tumor of the bronchus (a case report). *Indian J Cancer*. 1985;22:152–156.

197. Sabaratnam RM, Anunathan R, Govender D. Acinic cell carcinoma: an unusual cause of bronchial obstruction in a child. *Pediatr Dev Pathol*. 2004;7:521–526.

198. Rodriguez J, Diment J, Lombardi L, Dominoni F, Tench W, Rosai J. Combined typical carcinoid and acinic cell tumor of the lung: a heretofore unreported occurrence. *Hum Pathol*. 2003;34:1061–1065.

199. Lee HY, Mancer K, Koong HN. Primary acinic cell carcinoma of the lung with lymph node metastasis. *Arch Pathol Lab Med*. 2003;127:e216–e219.

200. Ukoha OO, Quartararo P, Carter D, Kashgarian M, Ponn RB. Acinic cell carcinoma of the lung with metastasis to lymph nodes. *Chest*. 1999;115:591–595.

201. Chuah KL, Yap WM, Tan HW, Koong HN. Recurrence of pulmonary acinic cell carcinoma. *Arch Pathol Lab Med*. 2006;130:932–933.

202. Nistal M, Garcia-Viera M, Martinez-Garcia C, et al. Epithelial-myoepithelial tumor of the bronchus. *Am J Surg Pathol*. 1994;18:421–425.

203. Strickler JG, Hegstrom J, Thomas MJ, et al. Myoepithelioma of the lung. *Arch Pathol Lab Med*. 1987;111:1082–1086.

204. Tsuji N, Tateisha R, Ishiguro S, et al. Adenomyoepithelioma of the lung. *Am J Surg Pathol*. 1995;19:956–962.

205. Wilson RW, Moran CA. Epithelial-myoepithelial carcinoma of the lung: immunohistochemical and ultrastructural observations and review of the literature. *Hum Pathol*. 1997;28:631–635.

206. Pelosi G, Fraggetta F, Maffini F, et al. Pulmonary epithelial-myoepithelial tumor of unproven malignant potential: report of a case and review of the literature. *Mod Pathol*. 2001;14:521–526.

207. Nguyen CV, Suster S, Moran CA. Pulmonary epithelial-myoepithelial carcinoma: a clinicopathologic and immunohistochemical study of 5 cases. *Hum Pathol*. 2009;40:366–373.

208. Rosenfeld A, Schwartz D, Garzon S, Chaleff S. Epithelial-myoepithelial carcinoma of the lung: a case report and review of the literature. *J Pediatr Hematol Oncol*. 2009;31:206–208.

209. Moraitaki PK, Vasilikos K, Archontovasilis F, et al. Recurrent respiratory infection and epithelial-myoepithelial carcinoma of the lung: a common presentation with a rare etiology. *J BUON*. 2009;14:147–148.

210. Muslimani AA, Kundranda M, Jain S, Daw HA. Recurrent bronchial epithelial-myoepithelial carcinoma after local therapy. *Clin Lung Cancer*. 2007;8:386–389.

211. Fulford LG, Kamata Y, Okudera K, et al. Epithelial-myoepithelial carcinomas of the bronchus. *Am J Surg Pathol*. 2001;25:1508–1514.

212. Volm M, Hahn EW, Mattern J, et al. Five year followup study of independent clinical and flow cytometric prognostic factors for the survival of patients with non-small cell carcinoma. *Cancer Res*. 1988;48:2923–2928.

213. Mountain CF. Revisions in the International System for Staging Lung Cancer. *Chest*. 1997;111:1710–1717.

214. Asamura H, Naruke T. Lung carcinoma. In: Hermanek P, Gospodarowicz MK, Henson DE, Hutter RVP, Sobin LH, eds. *Prognostic Factors in Cancer*. Berlin: Springer-Verlag; 1995:118–129.

215. Gallagher B, Urbanski SJ. The significance of pleural elastic invasion by lung carcinoma. *Hum Pathol*. 1990;21:512–517.

216. Bunker ML, Raab SS, Landreneau RJ, Silverman JF. The diagnosis and significance of visceral pleural invasion in lung carcinoma: histologic predictors and the role of elastic stains. *Am J Clin Pathol*. 1999;112:777–783.

217. Taube JM, Askin FB, Brock MV, Westra W. Impact of elastic staining on the staging of peripheral lung cancers. *Am J Surg Pathol*. 2007;31:953–956.

218. Butnor KJ, Vollmer RT, Blaszyk H, Glatz K. Interobserver agreement on what constitutes visceral pleural invasion by non-small cell lung carcinoma: an internet-based assessment of international current practices. *Am J Clin Pathol*. 2007;128:638–647.

219. Travis WD, Brambilla E, Rami-Porta R, et al. Visceral pleural invasion: pathologic criteria and use of elastic stains: proposal for the 7th edition of the TNM classification for lung cancer. *J Thorac Oncol*. 2008;3:1384–1390.

220. Shim HS, Park IK, Lee CY, Chung KY. Prognostic significance of visceral pleural invasion in the forthcoming (seventh) edition of TNM classification for lung cancer. *Lung Cancer*. 2009;65:161–165.

221. Elson CE, Roggli VL, Vollmer RT, et al. Prognostic indicators for survival in stage I carcinoma of the lung: a histologic study of 47 surgically resected cases. *Mod Pathol*. 1988;1:288–291.

222. Haque AK, Adegboyega P, Sanchez RL. Vascular invasion in carcinoma of the lung. *Mod Pathol*. 1993;6:131A.

223. Miyoshi K, Moriyama S, Kunitomo T, Nawa S. Prognostic impact of intratumoral vessel invasion in completely resected pathologic stage I non-small cell lung cancer. *J Thorac Cardiovasc Surg*. 2009;137:429–434.

224. Jones DR, Daniel TM, Denlinger CE, Rundall BK, Smolkin ME, Wick MR. Stage IB nonsmall cell lung cancers: are they all the same? *Ann Thorac Surg*. 2006;81:1958–1962.

225. Lee YC, Wu CT, Kuo SW, Tseng YT, Chang YL. Significance of extranodal extension of regional lymph nodes in surgically resected non-small cell lung cancer. *Chest*. 2007;131:993–999.

226. Brown RNV, Fraire AE, Roggli V, Cagle PT. Assessment of proliferative fraction by PCNA in stage I non-small cell lung cancer. *Mod Pathol*. 1993;6:129A.

227. Miyarnoto H, Flarada M, Isobe A, et al. Prognostic value of nuclear DNA content and expression of the ras oncogene product in lung cancer. *Cancer Res*. 1991;51:6346–6350.

228. Gazdar AF. Molecular markers for the diagnosis and prognosis of lung cancer. *Cancer*. 1992;69:1592–1599.

229. Noguchi M, Hirohashi S, Hara F, et al. Heterogeneous amplification of myc family oncogenes in small cell lung carcinomas. *Cancer*. 1990;66:2053–2058.

230. Ritter JH, Dresler CM, Wick MR. Expression of bcl-2 protein in stage T1N0M0 non-small cell lung carcinoma. *Hum Pathol*. 1995;26:1227–1232.

231. Ponder TB, Wick MR, Dresler CM, Ritter JH. Expression of ABH antigen, p53 protein, bcl-2 protein, and tumor grade as prognostic factors in T1N0M0 non-small cell lung carcinoma. *Am J Clin Pathol*. 1996;105:493.

232. Ponder TB, Wick MR, Dresler CM, Ritter JH. Microvessel counts and lymphovascular invasion as prognostic indicators in T1N0M0 non-small cell lung carcinoma. *Am J Clin Pathol*. 1996;106:402–403.

233. Haque AK, Abegboyega P, Al-Salalmeh A, Vrazel DP, Zwischenberger J. p53 and p-glycoprotein expression do not correlate with survival in non-small cell lung cancer: a long-term study and literature review. *Mod Pathol*. 1999;12:1158–1166.

234. Hashimoto T, Tokuchi Y, Hayashi M, et al. p53 null mutations undetected by immunohistochemical staining predict a poor outcome with early-stage non-small cell lung carcinomas. *Cancer Res*. 1999;59:5572–5577.

235. Tomizawa Y, Kohno T, Fujita T, et al. Correlation between the status of the p53 gene and survival in patients with stage I non-small cell lung carcinomas. *Oncogene*. 1999;18:1007–1014.

236. Dosaka-Akita H, Hu SX, Fujino M, et al. Altered retinoblastoma protein expression in non-small cell lung cancer: its synergistic effects with altered ras and p53 protein status on prognosis. *Cancer*. 1997;79:1329–1337.

237. Maitra A, Amirkhan RH, Saboorian MH, Frawley WH, Ashfaq R. Survival in small cell lung carcinoma is independent of bcl-2 expression. *Hum Pathol*. 1999;30:712–717.

238. Fontanini G, Vignati S, Bigini D, et al. Recurrence and death in non-small cell lung carcinomas: a prognostic model using pathological parameters, microvessel count, and gene protein products. *Clin Cancer Res*. 1996;2:1067–1075.

239. Zhu CQ, Shih W, Ling CH, Tsao MS. Immunohistochemical markers of prognosis in non-small cell lung cancer: a review and proposal for a multiphase approach to marker evaluation. *J Clin Pathol*. 2006;59:790–800.

240. Petty RD, Nicolson MC, Kerr KM, Collie-Duguid E, Murray GI. Gene expression profiling in non-small cell lung cancer: from molecular mechanisms to clinical application. *Clin Cancer Res*. 2004;10:3237–3248.

241. Girard N, Ostrovnaya I, Lau C, et al. Genomic and mutational profiling to assess clonal relationships between multiple non-small cell lung cancers. *Clin Cancer Res*. 2009;15:5184–5190.

242. Potti A, Mukherjee S, Petersen R, et al. A genomic strategy to refine prognosis in early-stage non-small-cell lung cancer. *N Engl J Med*. 2006;355:570–580.

243. Hoang CD, Guillaume TJ, Engel SC, Tawfic SH, Kratzke RA, Maddaus MA. Analysis of paired primary lung and lymph node tumor cells: a model of metastatic potential by multiple genetic programs. *Cancer Detect Prev*. 2005;29:509–517.

244. Chen HY, Yu SL, Chen CH, et al. A five-gene signature and clinical outcome in non-small-cell lung cancer. *N Engl J Med*. 2007;356:11–20.

245. Xi L, Lyons-Weiler J, Coello MC, et al. Prediction of lymph node metastasis by analysis of gene expression profiles in primary lung adenocarcinomas. *Clin Cancer Res*. 2005;11:4128–4135.

246. Kotoulas CS, Foroulis CN, Kostikas K, et al. Involvement of lymphatic metastatic spread in non-small cell lung cancer accordingly to the primary cancer location. *Lung Cancer*. 2004;44:183–191.

247. Wrage M, Ruosaari S, Eijk PP, et al. Genomic profiles associated with early micrometastasis in lung cancer: relevance of 4q deletion. *Clin Cancer Res*. 2009;15:1566–1574.

248. Moriya Y, Iyoda A, Kasai Y, et al. Prediction of lymph node metastasis by gene expression profiling in patients with primary resected lung cancer. *Lung Cancer*. 2009;64:86–91.

249. Cordes C, Bartling B, Simm A, et al. Simultaneous expression of Cathepsins B and K in pulmonary adenocarcinomas and squamous cell carcinomas predicts poor recurrence-free and overall survival. *Lung Cancer*. 2009;64:79–85.

250. Chang JW, Yi CA, Son DS, et al. Prediction of lymph node metastasis using the combined criteria of helical CT and mRNA expression profiling for non-small cell lung cancer. *Lung Cancer*. 2008;60:264–270.

251. Lu Y, Lemon W, Liu PY, et al. A gene expression signature predicts survival of patients with stage I non-small cell lung cancer. *PLOS Med*. 2006;3:e467.

252. Guo L, Ma Y, Ward R, Castranova V, Shi X, Qian Y. Constructing molecular classifiers for the accurate prognosis of lung adenocarcinoma. *Clin Cancer Res*. 2006;12:3344–3354.

253. Xi L, Coello MC, Litle VR, et al. A combination of molecular markers accurately detects lymph node metastasis in non-small cell lung cancer patients. *Clin Cancer Res*. 2006;12:2484–2491.

254. Pfeifer JD, ed. *Molecular Genetic Testing in Surgical Pathology*. Philadelphia: Lippincott-Williams & Wilkins; 2005:1–50.

255. Flieder DB. Commonly encountered difficulties in pathologic staging of lung cancer. *Arch Pathol Lab Med*. 2007;131:1016–1026.

256. Vansteenkiste JF, De Belie B, Deneffe GJ, et al. Practical approach to patients presenting with multiple synchronous suspect lung lesions: a reflection on the current TNM classification based on 54 cases with complete follow-up. *Lung Cancer*. 2001;34:169–175.

257. Girard N, Ostrovnaya I, Lau C, et al. Genomic and mutational profiling to assess clonal relationships between multiple non-small cell lung cancers. *Clin Cancer Res*. 2009;15:5184–5190.

258. Xu W, Chung JH, Jheon S, et al. The accuracy of frozen section diagnosis of pulmonary nodules: evaluation of inflation method during intraoperative pathology consultation with cryosection. *J Thorac Oncol*. 2010;5:39–44.

259. Sanli M, Isik AF, Tuncozgur B, et al. The reliability of mediastinoscopic frozen sections in deciding on oncological surgery in bronchogenic carcinoma. *Adv Ther*. 2008;25:488–495.

260. Suda T, Mizoguchi Y, Hasegawa S, Negi K, Hattori Y. Frozen-section diagnosis of small adenocarcinoma of the lung for intentional limited surgery. *Surg Today*. 2006;36:676–679.

261. Orki A, Tezel C, Kosar A, Ersev AA, Dudu C, Arman B. Feasibility of imprint cytology for evaluation of mediastinal lymph nodes in lung cancer. *Jpn J Clin Oncol*. 2006;36:76–79.

262. Yoshida J, Nagai K, Yokose T, et al. Limited resection trial for pulmonary ground-glass opacity nodules: fifty-case experience. *J Thorac Cardiovasc Surg*. 2005;129:991–996.

263. Mair S, Lash RH, Suskin D, Mendelsohn G. Intraoperative surgical specimen evaluation: frozen section analysis, cytologic examination, or both? A comparative study of 206 cases. *Am J Clin Pathol*. 1991;96:8–14.

264. Wick MR. Intraoperative consultations in pathology: a current perspective. *Am J Clin Pathol*. 1995;104:239–242.

265. Herbst J, Jenders R, McKenna Jr RJ, Marchevsky AM. Evidence-based criteria to help distinguish metastatic breast cancer from primary lung adenocarcinoma on thoracic frozen section. *Am J Clin Pathol*. 2009;131:122–128.

266. Gupta R, Dastane A, McKenna Jr RJ, Marchevsky AM. What can we learn from the errors in the frozen section diagnosis of pulmonary carcinoid tumors? An evidence-based approach. *Hum Pathol*. 2009;40:1–9.

267. Darvishian F, Ginsberg MS, Klimstra DS, Brogi E. Carcinoid tumorlets simulate pulmonary metastases in women with breast cancer. *Hum Pathol*. 2006;37:839–844.

268. Marchevsky AM, Changsri C, Gupta I, Fuller C, Houck W, McKenna Jr RJ. Frozen section diagnoses of small pulmonary nodules: accuracy and clinical implications. *Ann Thorac Surg*. 2004;78:1755–1759.

269. Butcher DN, Goldstraw P, Ladas G, Dusmet ME, Sheppard MN, Nicholson AG. Thyroid transcription factor-1 immunohistochemistry as an intraoperative diagnostic tool at frozen section for distinction between primary and secondary lung tumors. *Arch Pathol Lab Med*. 2007;131:582–587.

270. Kammerer U, Kapp M, Gassel AM, et al. A new rapid immunohistochemical staining technique using the EnVision antibody complex. *J Histochem Cytochem*. 2001;49:623–630.

271. Eagan RT, Maurer LH, Forcier RJ, Tulloh M. Small-cell carcinoma of the lung: staging paraneoplastic syndromes, treatment, and survival. *Cancer*. 1974;33:527–532.

272. Lim E, Belcher E, Yap YK, Nicholson AG, Goldstraw P. The role of surgery in the treatment of limited-disease small cell lung cancer: time to reevaluate. *J Thorac Oncol*. 2008;3:1267–1271.

273. Schreiber D, Rineer J, Weedon J, et al. Survival outcomes with the use of surgery in limited-stage small cell lung cancer: should its role be reevaluated? *Cancer*. 2010;116:1350–1357.

274. Colby TV, Deschamps C. The lung and pleura. In: Banks PM, Kraybill WG, eds. *Pathology for the Surgeon*. Philadelphia: WB Saunders; 1996:155–168.

275. Butnor KJ, Beasley MB, Cagle PT, et al. Protocol for the examination of specimens from patients with primary non-small cell carcinoma, small-cell carcinoma, or carcinoid tumor of the lung. *Arch Pathol Lab Med*. 2009;133:1552–1559.

276. Association of Directors of Anatomic & Surgical Pathology. Recommendations for the reporting of resected primary lung carcinomas. *Am J Clin Pathol*. 1995;104:371–374.

277. Greene FL, Page DL, Fleming ID, et al., eds. *AJCC Cancer Staging Manual*, 6th ed. New York: Springer; 2002:165–184.

Metastatic Tumors in the Lung: A Practical Approach to Diagnosis

Stephen S. Raab, MD, Timothy C. Allen, MD, JD, Kevin O. Leslie, MD, and Mark R. Wick, MD

The most common form of pulmonary neoplasm is a metastasis from outside the lungs. Based on autopsy data, the lungs are involved by metastatic lesions in 25% to 55% of malignant diseases,[1-5] and, in up to one fourth of those cases, the pulmonary parenchyma and pleura are the only sites of distant spread.[4] On the other hand, the most common lung tumor encountered by a practicing surgical pathologist or cytopathologist is primary bronchogenic carcinoma; distinguishing primary from secondary pulmonary neoplasms is a major challenge. This chapter provides a concise background discussion of the pathobiologic principles and clinicoradiologic findings of metastases in the lungs and offers a framework for the practitioner to identify such lesions with an optimal level of certainty.

Routes of Spread for Intrapulmonary Metastases

Extrapulmonary malignancies may spread to the lungs through the vascular system or the lymphatics, or by direct extension; technically, direct extension does not represent "metastasis" as it is usually defined.

Primary lung cancers likewise may involve other pleuropulmonary zones by similar means or by aerogenous dissemination through the alveolar pores of Kohn. Clinical and radiologic features of a particular metastatic lesion depend on which of these avenues of spread applies.

Vascular Metastases

Most metastatic tumors in the lungs have arrived at that destination hematogenously. There are two principal reasons for this: The lungs receive the entire cardiac output, and they contain a rich vascular network, comprising a huge capillary bed. The detailed principles underlying vascular metastasis have been outlined elsewhere.[6-8] Malignant tumors may contain subclones[9] of cells with differing metastatic potential, and some of them acquire the ability to enter the bloodstream as microemboli. At selected distant sites, they adhere to endothelial basement membranes, and through a process known as *extravasation,* the tumor cells move through the extracellular matrix to form metastatic deposits in various parenchymal structures. In this paradigm, the original micrometastasis then proliferates to yield a larger mass, which later (often as long as several years) may become visible clinically or radiographically. Most pulmonary metastases show nests of neoplastic cells that are surrounded by, and intercalated with, a variable quantity of fibrous stroma. At this stage, no cells typically remain inside the pulmonary arterial, venous, or capillary system.

The rate at which potentially metastasizing cellular subclones develop (if they do at all) in primary tumors varies considerably; the probability that such lesions will spread hematogenously depends on both tumor-related factors and conditions in the milieu of the host tissues. For reasons that are largely unknown, some tumors—such as osteosarcoma—often shed micrometastases before the primary tumor is detected clinically; other tumors may show metastasis only very late in their biologic evolution.[10]

The clinical presentation of patients with hematogenous pulmonary metastases is variable. Most patients have no symptoms,[11] and their lesions are detected only through imaging studies that are undertaken for staging purposes or for surveillance during treatment. The radiographic appearance of metastatic pulmonary lesions may be that of a single central or peripheral mass, multiple central or peripheral masses, diffuse infiltrates, or a combination of the latter two possibilities. If a patient is symptomatic, the clinical findings reflect the location and extent of the metastatic deposits and commonly include chest pain, dyspnea, cough, hemoptysis, and wheezing, to name a few.

In addition to the concept of microembolization as outlined earlier, tumors may also spread as macroscopic emboli that involve large or medium pulmonary arteries.[12] Large-vessel tumor emboli may cause acute heart failure, sudden death, rapidly evolving pulmonary hypertension, and pulmonary infarction, as also seen with banal intravascular thromboemboli associated with deep venous thrombosis.[13-15] The tumors that most commonly give rise to macroscopic emboli are those associated with major systemic veins (e.g., renal or hepatic carcinomas invading the renal and hepatic veins) and primary tumors of the heart (myxomas and sarcomas).[16]

In rare cases, hematogenous metastasis principally occurs in the lung with occlusive luminal tumor plugs in small vessels (arterioles and capillaries) without interstitial involvement or formation of masses.[17] In a sense, those tumors have not gone through all of the biologic steps normally associated with the metastatic sequence, but they are nonetheless potentially lethal because they may cause severe pulmonary hypertension. Neoplasms that may show that pattern of spread (sometimes called *tumor-related thrombotic pulmonary microangiopathy*[18]) include carcinomas of the breast, gastrointestinal tract, liver, pancreas, uterus, gallbladder, prostate, and ovary.[17] Soares et al. reported that most malignant tumors that occlude small pulmonary vascular channels also can be seen simultaneously within larger vessels.[19] Patients with metastatic microvascular occlusion typically present with progressive dyspnea and cor pulmonale.[17,18]

As a general rule of physiology, all caval venous blood flows through the lungs and portal venous return passes through the liver. Consequently, depending on the primary site of the tumor, metastases preferentially are seen in one of these two organs. Malignant neoplasms that arise in sites with other pathways of vascular drainage (e.g., prostatic tumors preferentially shed into the paravertebral venous plexus) infrequently involve the lungs secondarily. Arterially borne metastases to the lungs are relatively rare and are usually mediated by the bronchial arteries; the most common source of such lesions is a primary lung cancer that has gained access to the pulmonary venous system.

Hematogenous metastasis in the lung is associated with a spectrum of radiologic findings. The most common roentgenographic appearance is that of multiple, bilateral, variably sized masses (Figs. 17-1 to 17-3); occasionally, a solitary intraparenchymal nodule is seen. The metastatic implants usually appear in the mid- to lower lung field

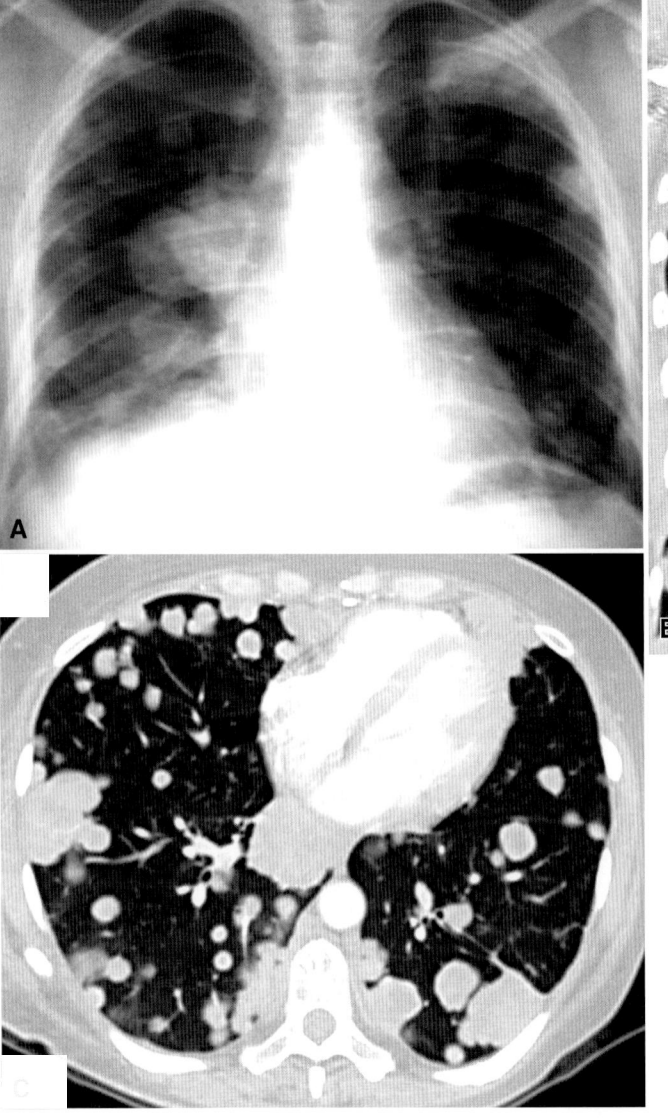

Figure 17-1. A, Chest radiograph in a case of metastatic colorectal carcinoma involving the lungs. Tumor nodules are distributed throughout both lung fields; they are nodular and of variable sizes. The lesions are well seen in a reconstructed sagittal computed tomogram (**B**) and a conventional cross-sectional computed tomogram (**C**).

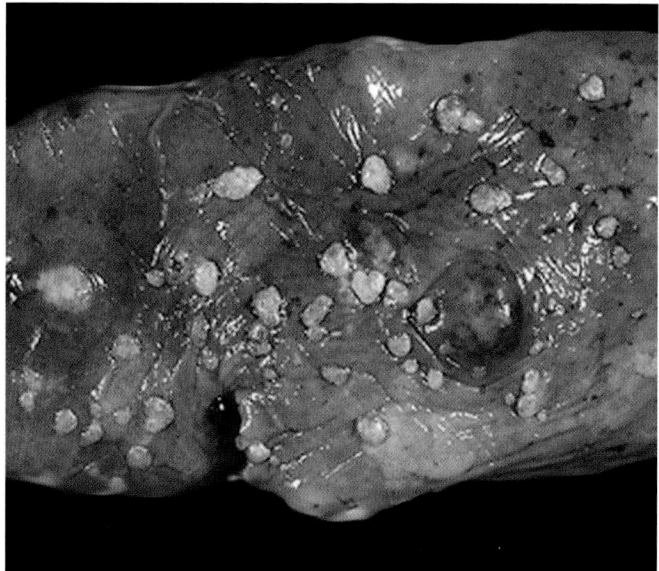

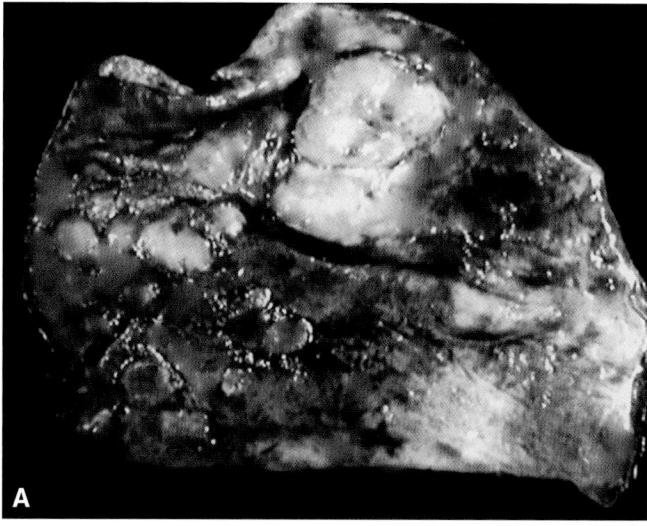

Figure 17-2. Gross photograph of metastatic carcinoma in the lungs showing several subpleural nodules of varying size.

because that is where the greatest parenchymal perfusion occurs. In up to 90% of patients with bilateral secondary disease, the lesions are peripheral and subpleural (Fig. 17-4).[1,20] Variability in the size of the metastatic nodules is related to the different "ages" of the lesions, dissimilar growth rates, and other factors. Such lesions are usually smaller than primary pulmonary carcinomas, measuring less than 3 to 4 cm in maximum diameter. Metastases also enlarge more rapidly than bronchogenic carcinomas do.

Tumors involving small vessels may produce linear parenchymal infiltrates, and patients who have both masses and metastases in small vessels or lymphatic spaces present with opacities and linear streaks. Embolic tumors in the large pulmonary arteries may show the radiographic appearance of an infarct, with a wedge-shaped peripheral zone of consolidation and possible pleural effusion.

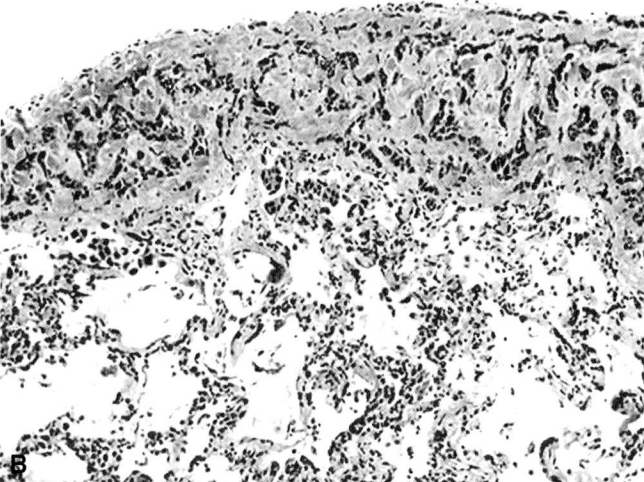

Figure 17-4. **A,** Gross image of pleura showing multiple variably sized subpleural metastases. **B,** Photomicrograph from a case of metastatic adenocarcinoma in the lung showing a subpleural peripheral distribution of tumor within the pulmonary parenchyma.

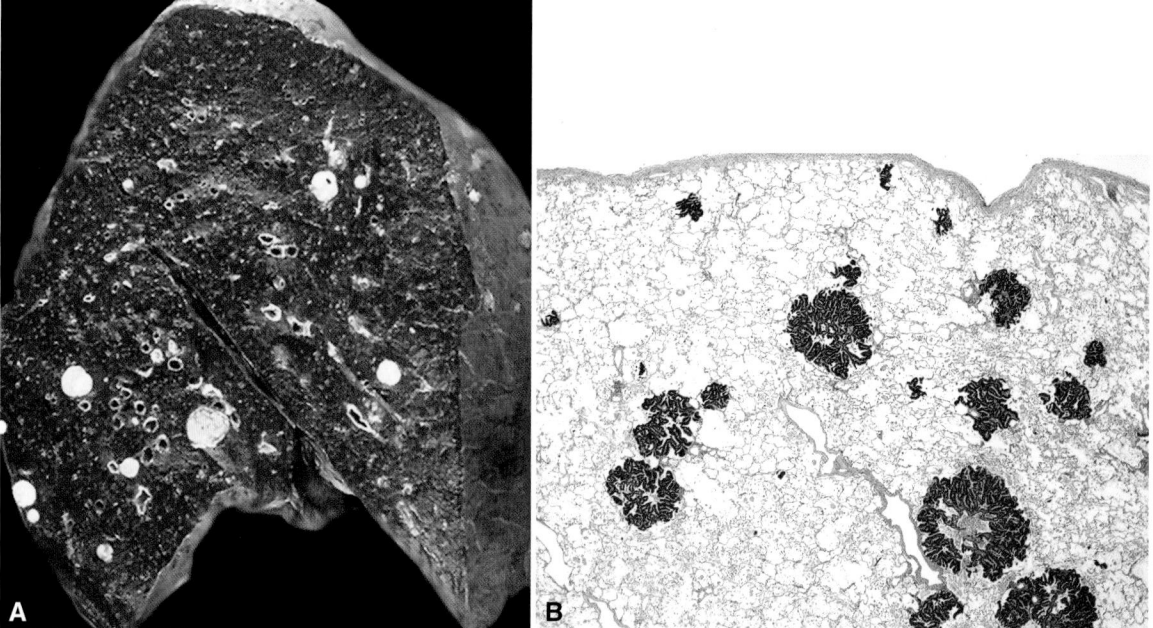

Figure 17-3. **A,** Gross photograph from another case of metastatic carcinoma involving the lungs (from a primary tumor in the breast). The multifocal nature and heterogeneous size of metastatic lesions are well shown. **B,** The variably sized metastatic tumor nodules are found diffusely within lung parenchyma.

Solitary metastases in the lungs are seen in up to 10% of all malignant tumors involving those organs.[21-23] Filderman and coworkers suggested that solitary lesions larger than 5 cm in diameter most likely originate in the breast, kidney, or soft tissue.[6] Metastasis in the form of a solitary mass on plain films may appear as multiple contiguous or coalescent masses on computed tomograms. Quint and colleagues reported that, statistically, patients with carcinomas of the head and neck, bladder, breast, cervix, bile ducts, esophagus, ovary, prostate, or stomach were more likely to have a solitary metastasis to the lung than a new primary bronchogenic tumor, even when a significant period had elapsed after diagnosis of the extrapulmonary neoplasms.[24] On the other hand, patients with a history of malignant melanoma, sarcoma, or malignant germ cell tumor were more likely to have a second primary malignancy of the lung under the same circumstances.[24]

Large metastatic foci may undergo cavitation or result in pneumothorax or bronchopleural fistulization (Fig. 17-5). The most common secondary tumor that cavitates is squamous cell carcinoma, often originating in the head and neck.[25] Metastatic sarcoma and adenocarcinoma also may exhibit that feature.[25] Pneumothoraces and transpleural fistulae result from erosion by the metastatic tumor through the pleura, as seen most frequently in pediatric mesenchymal malignancies (e.g., osteosarcoma).[26]

Lymphogenous Metastases

One study[27] reported that up to 56% of pulmonary metastases were lymphogenously mediated, although a more generally accepted figure is 5% to 8%.[28,29] Most patients with lymphatic-borne lung metastases have a poor prognosis, with 90% dying within 6 months.[29]

The radiographic appearance of lymphangitic metastasis is variable; in 50% of cases, plain chest films show no apparent abnormality.[30] Yang and Lin described four radiologic patterns for this condition[29]:

1. Bilateral linear infiltrates without hilar enlargement or intrapulmonary masses
2. Hilar masses with centripetal parenchymal extension (seen most commonly with cervical, gastric, and breast cancers; Fig. 17-6)
3. Focal linear infiltration of the parenchyma associated with a central primary tumor
4. Parenchymal radiations from a peripheral primary tumor

With the first two patterns representing secondary tumors, pleural, or less frequently, hilar lymph nodal involvement may be seen. More than 90% of these cases are metastatic adenocarcinomas.[29] It is estimated that fewer than 1% of patients with pulmonary metastases from tumors arising outside the thorax also have hilar adenopathy.[31] Although this figure may appear low, hilar adenopathy in patients with secondary pulmonary malignancies is not uncommon in absolute terms because of the high prevalence of patients with metastatic disease.

Carcinomas may gain access to the pulmonary lymphatic system by retrograde spread, direct invasion of the pulmonary lymphatics, and passage through adjacent blood vessels. The most common route of spread is the last of these three possibilities[32]; tumor first spreads hematogenously to the lung and results in small areas of interstitial growth. The neoplastic cells are then absorbed into the lymphatics and permeate further throughout the lungs (Fig. 17-7). Tumor in alveolar spaces may likewise be absorbed through the lymphatics adjacent to terminal bronchioles. Therefore, patients who have lymphangitic intrapulmonary metastases generally also have had previous hematogenous spread.[32] Direct lymphatic invasion is most often associated with tumors arising in the breast or stomach[29,33,34]; in this mode, metastases may be seen exclusively in the pulmonary lymphatic spaces, without the formation of mass lesions. Other metastatic carcinomas capable of showing the same pattern of spread are those arising in the ovary, thyroid, bladder, esophagus, and liver.[29,32]

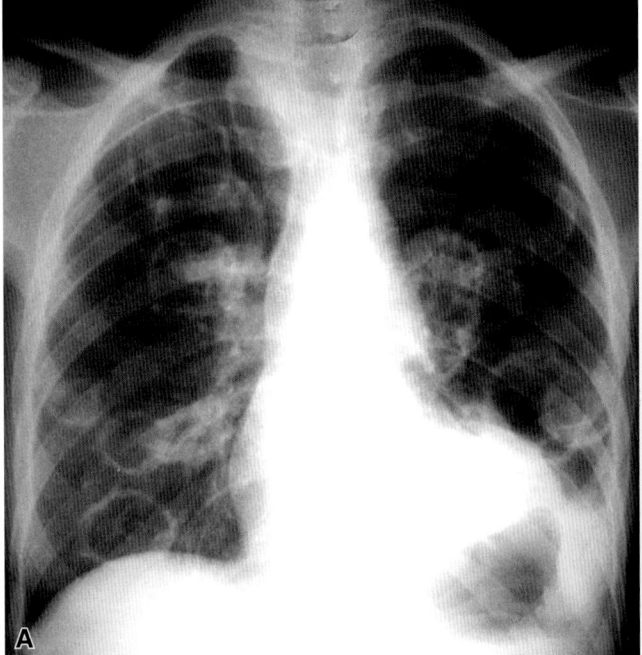
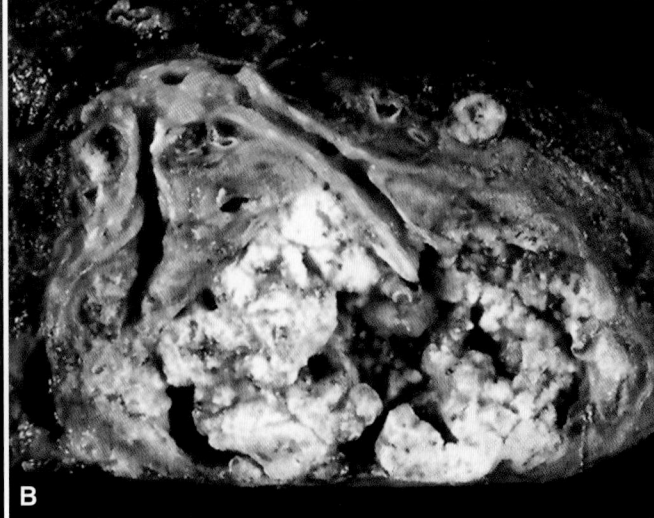

Figure 17-5. **A,** Chest radiograph from a case of metastatic oropharyngeal squamous cell carcinoma involving the lungs showing cavitating nodular lesions throughout both lung fields. **B,** The cavitary nature of the lesions is well shown.

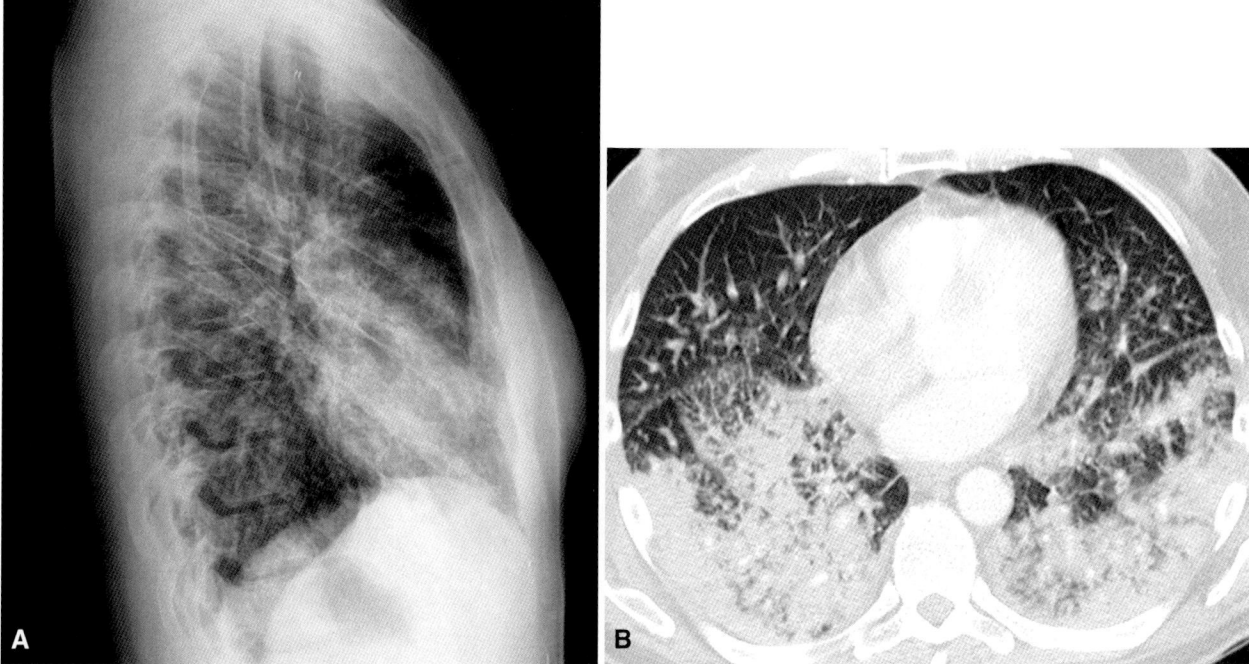

Figure 17-6. Chest radiograph (**A**) and computed tomography scan (**B**) in a case of metastatic breast carcinoma in the lungs, assuming a centripetal lymphangitic pattern. Tumor is seen in the lymph nodes in both hilar regions, and it also involves the lung fields in an arborizing pattern that follows the lymphatic channels.

Direct Seeding

Metastatic disease arising through direct "seeding" occurs when a malignant tumor gains access to a serosally lined cavity, such as the pleural space. Neoplasms that directly seed the pleura include primary lung cancers and malignancies of various lineages that originate in the chest wall or mediastinum. In some cases, primary lung tumors, such as peripheral pulmonary carcinoma, grow through the visceral pleura; this phenomenon is less common in cases of chest wall sarcoma. The malignant cells attach themselves to multiple pleural sites and invade the subjacent tissues thereafter. Hence, multiple subpleural nodules may eventuate near a larger serosally based secondary lesion.

Pleural Metastases

Metastases are the most common form of pleural malignancy. Most derive from primary neoplasms of the chest wall, mediastinum, or lungs,[6] although extrathoracic primary malignancies are also well represented. The largest tumor nodules tend to be basally situated in the chest[35] (Fig. 17-8).

At least two thirds of malignant pleural effusions can be diagnosed by cytologic sampling of the pleural fluid. More than 90% of cases are recognized on the first specimen,[36,37] but sensitivity predictably increases with successive sampling; three specimens are routinely recommended if the clinical suspicion of pleural metastasis is high.[38]

Malignancy is second only to congestive heart failure as a cause of pleural effusions.[39] Neoplastic effusions are typically described as "massive" or "copious," ranging up to 2500 mL in volume,[40] and they are often bloody. Nevertheless, malignant involvement of the pleura may also be associated with scant fluid production and a serous character.[35] Obviously, not all pleural effusions in patients with a history of malignancy contain tumor cells[41]; benign effusions in such cases may be secondary to lymphatic obstruction, altered lymphatic drainage as a result of chemotherapy or radiation therapy,[42] heart failure, or other causes. Because most sarcomas do not spread via lymphatic channels, metastases in the lung and pleura are not usually accompanied by a tumorous

effusion.[43] Up to 90% of malignant pleural effusions caused by metastatic lung or breast cancers are ipsilateral with regard to the site of the original tumor.[35] Patients with malignant pleural effusions typically have a dismal prognosis, and most die within a few months of diagnosis.[44–46] Selected subgroups of patients, such as those with lymphoma, breast cancer, or some pediatric malignancies, may fare somewhat better.

Chretien and Jaubert reported that 42% of cytologically sampled pleural effusions contained malignant cells.[47] The likely site of tumor origin in such cases appears to depend on patient demographics, although most series have reported that primary pulmonary carcinomas are the most common.[45,48] Squamous cell carcinomas of the lung do not usually involve the pleural fluid; however, adenocarcinomas usually do (Fig. 17-9), followed by small cell neuroendocrine carcinoma.[49,50] Almost any other extrathoracic malignancy may metastasize to the pleural space, but the most common tumors that do so are carcinomas arising in the breast, gastrointestinal tract, and ovary; non-Hodgkin lymphoma is also well represented.[45,48,51] Up to 7% of metastatic carcinomas in the pleura must be classified as originating in an unknown primary location.[48] In one analysis of malignant pleural effusions, women predominated by a ratio of 2:1,[40] but no sex preferences were seen in other series.[45]

Endobronchial Metastases

Endobronchial metastases are considered in a separate category because of their distinctive clinical findings, principally the syndrome of "adult-onset asthma." The reported incidence of endobronchial and endotracheal metastatic disease is 1% to 18% of patients who also have intrapulmonary metastases.[11,52,53] The most common sites of tumor origin in patients from North America and Western Europe are the breast, bone, soft tissue, large intestine, kidney, and skin (melanoma).[11,54–58] More than one third of endobronchial metastases are sarcomatous.[53,57] In populations with a high prevalence of acquired immune deficiency syndrome, the most common secondary malignancies of the bronchi are Kaposi sarcoma and malignant lymphoma.[59] Nasopharyngeal and laryngeal carcinomas are frequent sources of endobronchial metastasis in Asia.[60]

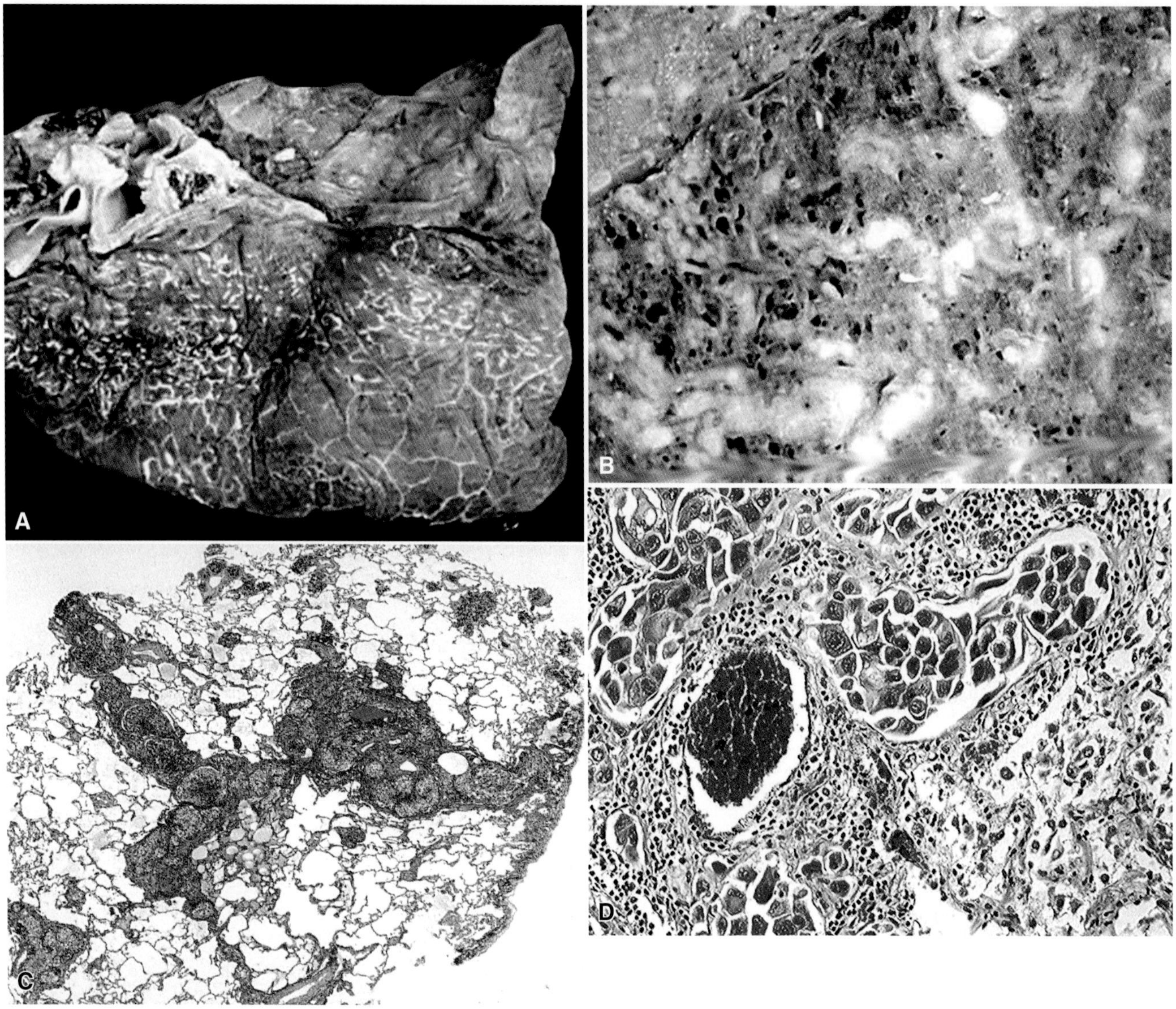

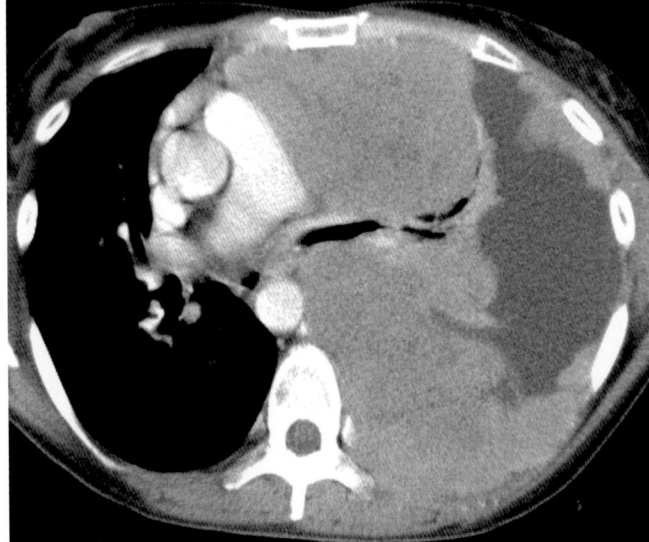

Figure 17-7. A linear pattern of lymphangitic metastatic disease in the lung parenchyma is seen in gross photographs (**A** and **B**) and a low-magnification photomicrograph (**C**). **D,** At higher magnification, metastatic carcinoma fills and expands the lymphatic channels in the lungs.

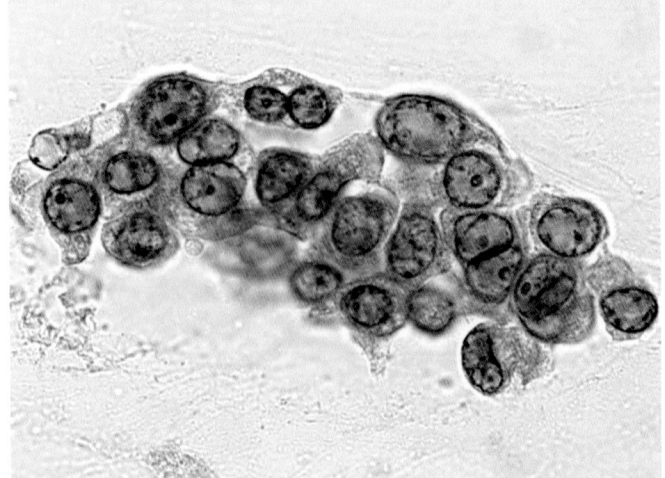

Figure 17-8. Chest radiograph from a case of metastatic leiomyosarcoma massively involving the left pleura. The left hemithorax and anterior mediastinum are largely obliterated by the tumor mass and an accompanying pleural effusion.

Figure 17-9. Metastatic adenocarcinoma of pulmonary origin is seen in this preparation of a cytologic specimen of pleural fluid. The tumor cells are arranged in a vaguely three-dimensional configuration, and small nucleoli are seen.

Endobronchial metastases may be either hematogenous or lymphogenous.[11,53,57] Aerogenous spread of an upper-airway malignancy has also been suggested as a possibility. Tumors that originate in the lung, hilar lymph nodes, or mediastinum may spread by direct extension into the bronchial system. Endobronchial lesions cause symptoms early in their course of growth, namely, cough with sputum production, dyspnea, wheezing, infection, and hemoptysis.[60,61] However, up to 25% of patients are asymptomatic.[58] Radiographically, an endobronchial mass is typically visible only on computed tomography or magnetic resonance scan; plain film studies commonly show only postobstructive consolidation or atelectasis (Fig. 17-10). The mean interval between diagnosis of the original tumor and the appearance of endobronchial metastasis is 4 to 5 years.[61] These patients have a poor survival, with a median of 11 months[61]; patients with breast cancer may have a better prognosis.[54,57,58]

In histologic and cytologic specimens, endobronchial metastases may be confused with primary tumors. However, primary endobronchial epithelial neoplasms are typically squamous cell carcinomas, neuroendocrine carcinomas, or salivary gland-type tumors. Endobronchial adenocarcinomas other than salivary morphotypes should therefore raise the suspicion of metastatic disease. An exuberant reactive stromal proliferation around such lesions may also be confused with metastatic spindle cell sarcoma.

Modalities for the Diagnosis of Pleuropulmonary Metastases

The diagnostic tests that are typically used for any suspected pleuropulmonary tumor are also applicable to the study of metastatic disease. These include sputum cytology,[62,63] bronchoscopy with brushing,

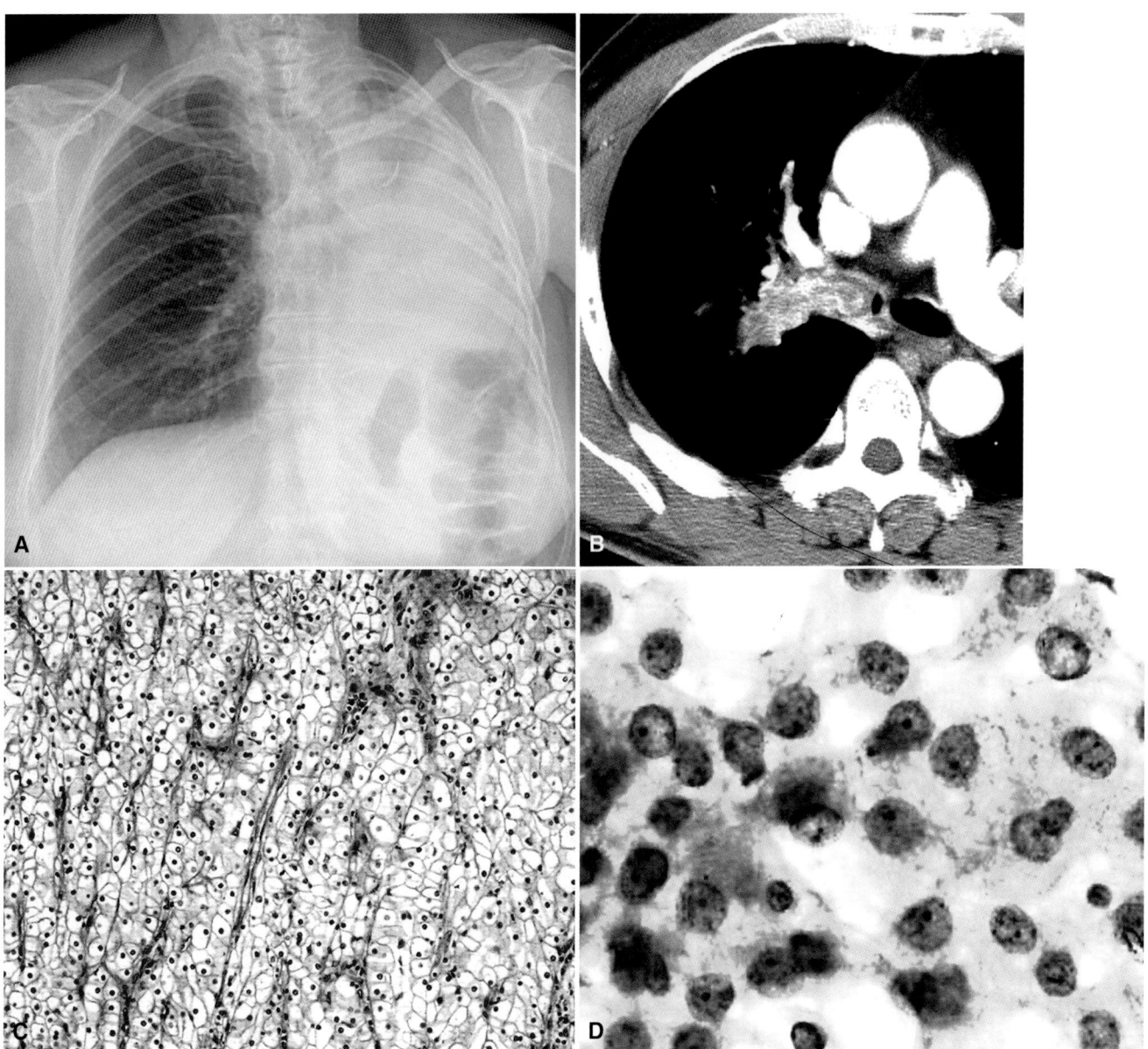

Figure 17-10. A, Chest radiograph showing left upper lobar atelectasis in a case of intrabronchial metastasis of renal cell carcinoma. **B,** Computed tomography scan showing another case of metastatic intrabronchial carcinoma (from the breast), affecting the right mainstem bronchus. **C,** Bland polygonal tumor cells with characteristic clear cytoplasm are seen in the biopsy specimen. **D,** The associated bronchial brushing shows renal cell carcinoma cells with relatively uniform nuclei and clear cytoplasm.

Continued

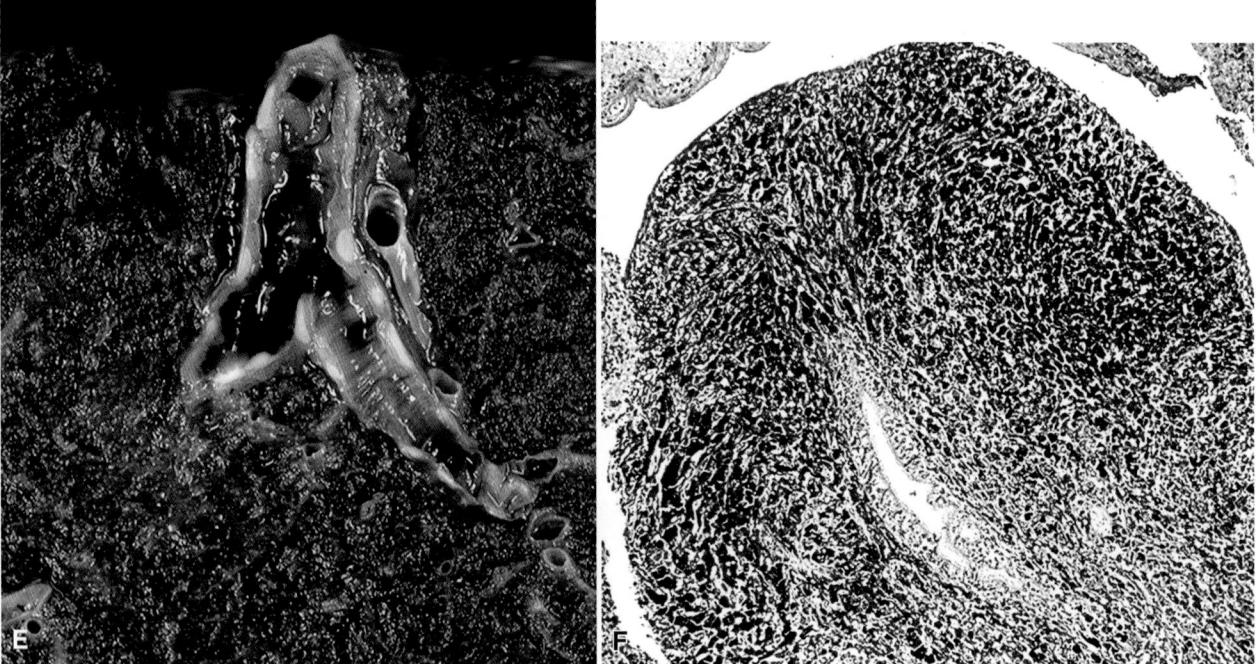

Figure 17-10—cont'd. E, Intrabronchial metastasis of melanoma, represented by a pigmented polypoid mass. **F,** The tumor contains abundant melanin.

washing, alveolar lavage, transbronchial or transtracheal aspiration and biopsy,[64–66] transthoracic fine-needle aspiration (FNA),[67,68] thoracoscopic biopsy (video-assisted thoracic surgery),[69–71] open thoracotomy and biopsy, and effusion cytology.[46] In some cases, expectant management is undertaken, with sequential radiologic studies.[72,73] Computed tomography scans may be obtained to further delineate abnormalities and possibly to aid in the distinction between primary and secondary malignancies; for example, mediastinal adenopathy favors a primary lung tumor.[74] When multiple radiographic lesions of the lung or pleura are detected radiographically in some patients with well-documented histories of malignancy, further diagnostic evaluations may be eschewed.

For the most part, the diagnostic accuracy of tests that yield tissue for pathologic examination generally has not been determined in this specific context. The accuracy is believed to depend principally on the size and location of the lesion rather than its specific histologic nature. For example, the sensitivity of FNA is 93% if the lesion is larger than 2 cm in diameter and 60% for those smaller than 1 cm. Higher sensitivity is realized in the sampling of peripheral nodules compared with central lesions, regardless of whether they are primary or secondary.[75] Pilotti et al. reported that the sensitivity of FNA in the detection of metastatic pleuropulmonary disease was 89%, whereas it was 92% for primary malignancies.[76] Another interinstitutional study reported 96% specificity for transthoracic FNA.[77] The sensitivity of bronchoscopy also depends on the location of the lesion; as expected, that technique is particularly well suited for the visualization and sampling of endobronchial metastases.[64–66] Thoracoscopy is a sensitive means of accessing peripheral lesions and has a high level of accuracy overall. It may be viewed as a treatment option as well as a diagnostic test in patients who have limited metastatic disease, especially if lung function is compromised.[69–71]

Kern and Schweizer concluded that the sensitivity of sputum cytology for the detection of intrapulmonary metastasis was similar to that associated with primary lung cancers.[78] However, that technique is much more likely to be productive if the metastatic lesions are large and centrally located.[78]

Practical Approach to Differential Diagnosis

A definite challenge in pulmonary pathology is determining whether a newly detected lung mass is primary or secondary in patients with or without a history of extrapulmonary malignancy. If no previous tumor has been seen and the lesion has the morphologic attributes of a nonpulmonary proliferation, it is necessary to search for a primary site. Malignancies that are clinically occult and present with pulmonary metastases are not unusual, and they account for approximately 2% to 5% of all metastatic carcinomas of unknown origin (MCUOs).[79,80] Because of the treatment-related and prognostic issues concerning secondary malignancies of the lung, it may be decided that additional resources are not justified to determine the primary location of the tumor.[81]

With regard to the general distinction of primary and metastatic pulmonary tumors, one generally depends on radiographic findings, histologic features, microscopic comparison of the current lesion with any previous malignancies, and the use of ancillary pathologic studies, such as immunohistochemistry, cytochemistry, molecular biologic techniques, cytogenetic methods,[82] and electron microscopy. If paraffin-embedded tissue from previous tumor material is available, immunopathologic studies of the previous tumor and the current specimen can be obtained comparatively.

Useful information for the distinction between primary and secondary neoplasms in the lung may be derived from details of the clinical evaluation and physical findings.[83,84] For example, the characteristically "spiculated" appearance of primary lung cancers (Fig. 17-11) on imaging studies of the chest distinguishes them from the more rounded and well-delimited appearance of metastases. Unfortunately, such information is often not made available to pathologists, even though it is well known to enhance diagnostic accuracy.[85] A high index of suspicion must be maintained, and communication with the radiologist should occur whenever the pathologist has increased concern, histologic or otherwise, that a tumor may be a metastasis. Open communication is essential if the patient has a history of oncologic disease.

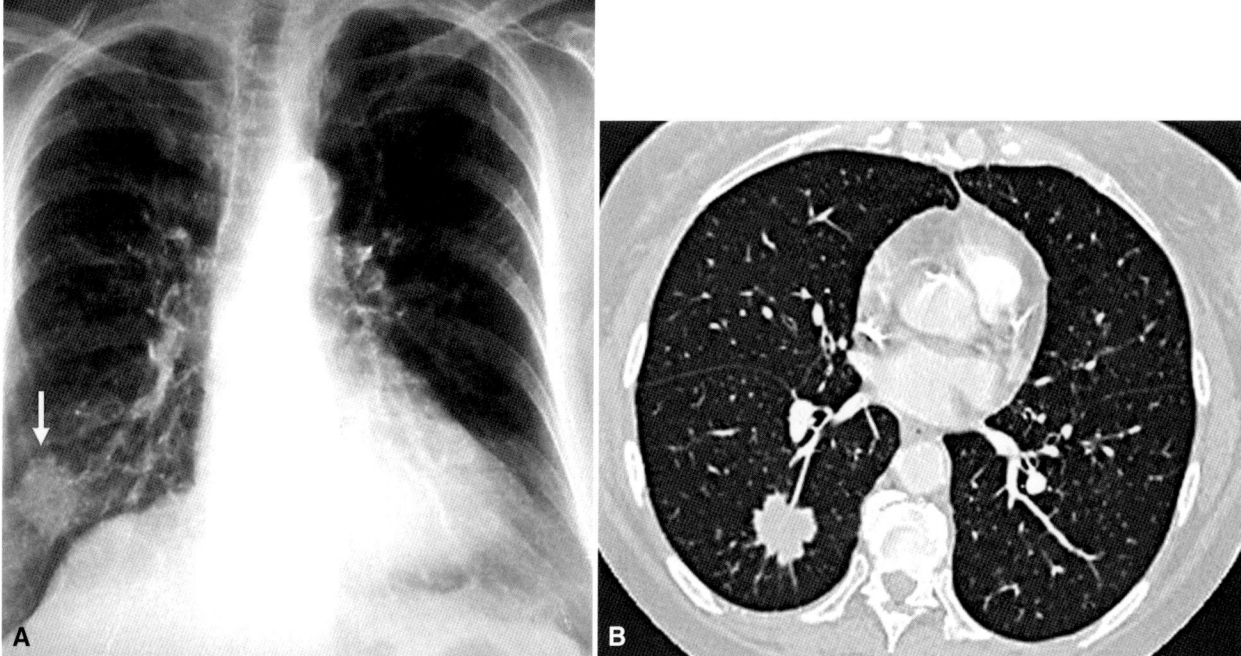

Figure 17-11. A, Chest radiograph from a case of primary adenocarcinoma of the lung showing a peripheral nodule in the lower right lung field (*arrow*). **B,** Computed tomography scan showing irregular "spiculated" margins, typical of a primary pulmonary neoplasm.

The light microscopic features of any given lesion are the cornerstone of pathologic diagnosis. The appearance of the lesion after hematoxylin and eosin staining is often sufficient to determine whether the tumor is primary or metastatic. Carcinomas arising in the lung typically have evolved over several years before coming to clinical attention. As a consequence, the host responds to such lesions by surrounding them with an irregular cuff of fibroinflammatory tissue (Fig. 17-12). The mixture of proliferation and degeneration that characterizes primary carcinomas commonly causes central zones of fibrosis, with entrapment of some residual native pulmonary structures. In contrast, metastases to the lung parenchyma have a "clean" interface with the surrounding tissue and are not associated with peripheral zones of fibroinflammatory response. Because they are rapidly growing vis-à-vis bronchogenic neoplasms, metastatic carcinomas also lack centrally sclerotic regions. These "rules" do not apply universally to all tumor types. Specifically, primary and metastatic sarcomas, adenocarcinomas with a "lepidic" growth pattern, and small cell neuroendocrine carcinomas are essentially superimposable morphologically.

The rest of this section considers five categories of tumors in patients with a known history of extrapulmonary malignant neoplasms:

1. Adenocarcinoma variants
2. Spindle cell and pleomorphic malignancies
3. Small round cell neoplasms
4. Squamous cell carcinomas and their simulants
5. Undifferentiated large polygonal cell malignancies

In each group, the differential diagnosis includes at least one primary pulmonary lesion. Although specific neoplastic entities are discussed, the presentation is not all-inclusive. The approach taken in this chapter is intended to provide an example of a differential diagnostic framework. There is inevitably some overlap in categories. For example, in selected cases, hepatocellular carcinomas potentially may present any of the following morphologic appearances: adenocarcinoma, not further specified; oncocytoid carcinoma; clear cell carcinoma; undifferentiated large polygonal cell malignancy; or even sarcomatoid (spindle cell and pleomorphic) carcinoma. Accordingly, this presentation is organized to reflect the most common morphologic groups in which specific neoplasms are usually placed.

The discussion also incorporates information on immunohistologic panels that can be used to distinguish nosologically different but structurally similar tumors. These panels are presented in that manner because immunohistochemistry today is such an integral part of cytopathology and histopathology. However, the differential diagnosis does not rest on adjuvant studies alone, but rather involves the melding of light microscopic observations, clinical information, and data derived from ancillary procedures. The availability of these techniques varies between medical institutions; therefore, the antibody profiles presented here show the authors' approach but should not be regarded as definitive or mandatory, especially in light of the rapid evolution of adjunctive technology in pathology.

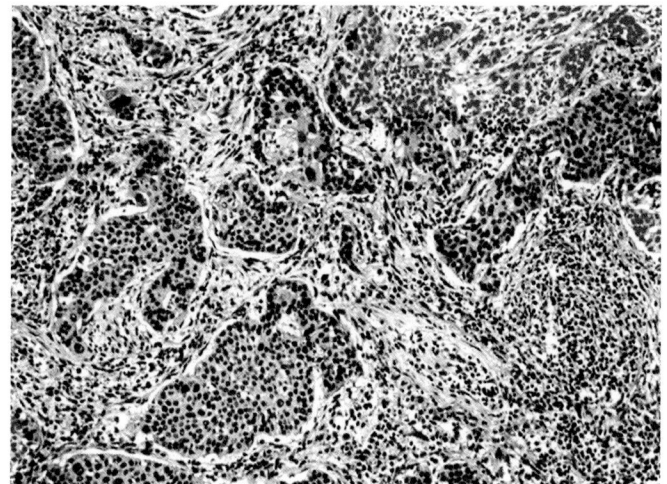

Figure 17-12. Fibroinflammatory host reaction is seen in and around this primary squamous cell carcinoma of the lung, serving as a marker of its pulmonary origin.

Adenocarcinoma Variants

Adenocarcinoma is the most common form of primary lung cancer. In patients who have a history of an extrapulmonary adenocarcinoma, the distinction between a primary and secondary lesion may be challenging. In some cases, morphologic appearances alone are sufficient to accomplish that task, as discussed later. Immunopathology is also helpful in the recognition of some of these tumors. Table 17-1 shows the immunohistologic profile of specific adenocarcinomas based on their site of origin.[86]

Papillary Adenocarcinomas

Silver and Askin reported that primary papillary pulmonary adenocarcinomas—defined as such if 75% or more of the neoplasm shows micropapillary architecture—are not uncommon[87]; moreover, micropapillae may be seen in conventional adenocarcinomas of the lung[88,89] (Fig. 17-13). Metastatic adenocarcinomas in the lung also may contain micropapillary structures. In FNA specimens, such tumors show fibrovascular fragments covered by cuboidal or low-columnar neoplastic cells.

Metastatic papillary adenocarcinomas may originate in the thyroid, breast, ovary, or kidney (Fig. 17-14). Thyroid carcinomas of all histologic subtypes have the potential to metastasize to the lung. Of all thyroid carcinomas that spread to distant sites other than lymph nodes, up to 50% involve the pulmonary parenchyma.[90–92] Papillary thyroid carcinoma almost always metastasizes to regional cervical lymph nodes beforehand[90]; in addition, this tumor type may directly invade the trachea and produce an endoluminal mass. Anaplastic thyroid carcinoma shares the latter potential. Hilar intrathoracic and mediastinal lymph nodes are also involved by papillary thyroid carcinoma in half of patients with lung metastasis.[93] Secondary papillary thyroid carcinoma may grow very slowly and remain solitary for extended periods, simulating the biologic characteristics of a primary pulmonary neoplasm.[90] In addition to its papillary substructure, other cytologic clues to metastatic papillary thyroid carcinoma include its characteristic nuclear features—including nuclear grooves, nuclear membrane irregularities, cytoplasmic invaginations (pseudoinclusions), and nuclear overlap—as well as the formation of colloid and psammoma bodies (Fig. 17-15).

All types of ovarian carcinoma may metastasize to the lungs, and up to 50% of stage IV cases feature pulmonary involvement.[94] The papillary serous form of ovarian cancer is the most common subtype. The pleura is often involved early, by lymphatic spread through the diaphragm, and the peripheral lung parenchyma is then affected. Malignant pleural effusions caused by papillary serous carcinomas are seen in 40% of all cases with metastases,[94] and solitary pulmonary nodules are present in 7%.[95] Lymphangitic intrapulmonary growth of ovarian malignancies is associated with a rapid demise.[96,97]

Immunopathologic studies to determine the site of origin of a papillary carcinoma in the lung are outlined in Table 17-2.[86] The authors recommend using at least one marker (e.g., vimentin or pan-keratin) that should be positive in each of the differential diagnostic possibilities to establish the antigenic integrity of the tissue.[98] In this setting, the highest specificity of immunopathologic identification is associated with tumors of thyroid, pulmonary, or mammary origin. Metastatic papillary tumors arising in the kidneys or ovaries are more difficult to distinguish from others definitively with immunohistology, although CA-125 reactivity is a consistent feature of ovarian epithelial neoplasms (Fig. 17-16).

Another malignancy that often has a papillary "pseudocarcinomatous" appearance, especially in pleural fluid specimens, is the epithelioid variant of malignant mesothelioma (Fig. 17-17). Renshaw and colleagues estimated that the sensitivity of pleural fluid cytology for the diagnosis of mesothelioma was only 32%[99] because epithelioid tumor cells often have a bland appearance and the sarcomatoid variant of mesothelioma rarely sheds into the pleural space. Many reports have considered the diagnostic distinction of mesothelioma from metastatic adenocarcinoma. This topic is discussed in detail in Chapter 20.[100–102] Immunopathologic and electron microscopic studies are generally used to make this distinction.[100,103] Table 17-3 shows a typical immunopathologic antibody panel that can be used to distinguish mesothelial proliferations from epithelial tumors.[100,104,105] Imlay and Raab examined the utility of immunohistochemistry in this context in hospital practice.[45] They reported that immunopathologic techniques were

Table 17-1. Immunophenotypes of Carcinomas Potentially Seen in the Lung

Origin	PK	CK7	CK20	EMA	THY	CEA	ER	HEP	GCDFP	S-100	TTF1	PSA	INHB	CA125	CA19-9	CD10
Lung	P	P	N	P	N	P	N	N	N	N	P	N	N	N	PN	N
Breast	P	P	N	P	N	P	P	N	P	PN	N	N	N	PN	N	N
Thyroid	P	P	N	PN	P	PN	N	N	N	PN	P	N	N	N	N	N
Salivary duct	P	P	P	P	N	PN	N	N	PN	PN	N	PN	N	N	N	N
Ovary (serous)	P	P	N	P	N	N	P	N	N	PN	N	N	N	P	N	N
Kidney	P	PN	N	P	N	N	N	N	N	PN	N	N	N	N	N	P
Stomach	P	PN	PN	PN	N	PN	N	N	N	PN	N	PN	N	PN	PN	N
Pancreas	P	P	PN	P	N	P	N	N	N	N	N	N	N	PN	P	N
Colorectal	P	PN	P	P	N	P	N	N	N	PN	N	N	N	PN	PN	N
Prostate	P	PN	PN	PN	N	PN	N	N	PN	N	N	P	N	N	N	N
Adrenocortical	N	N	N	N	N	PN	N	N	N	N	N	N	P	N	N	N
Hepatocellular	P	PN	PN	PN	N	P	N	P	N	PN	N	N	N	N	N	PN

CEA, carcinoembryonic antigen; EMA, epithelial membrane antigen; ER, estrogen receptor; GCDFP, gross cystic disease fluid protein; HEP, hepatocyte-related antigen in paraffin sections-1; INHB, inhibin; N, <10% of tumors; P, >75% of tumors; PK, pan-keratin; PN, 10–75% of tumors; PSA, prostate specific antigen; S-100, S-100 protein; THY, thyroglobulin; TTF1, thyroid transcription factor-1.

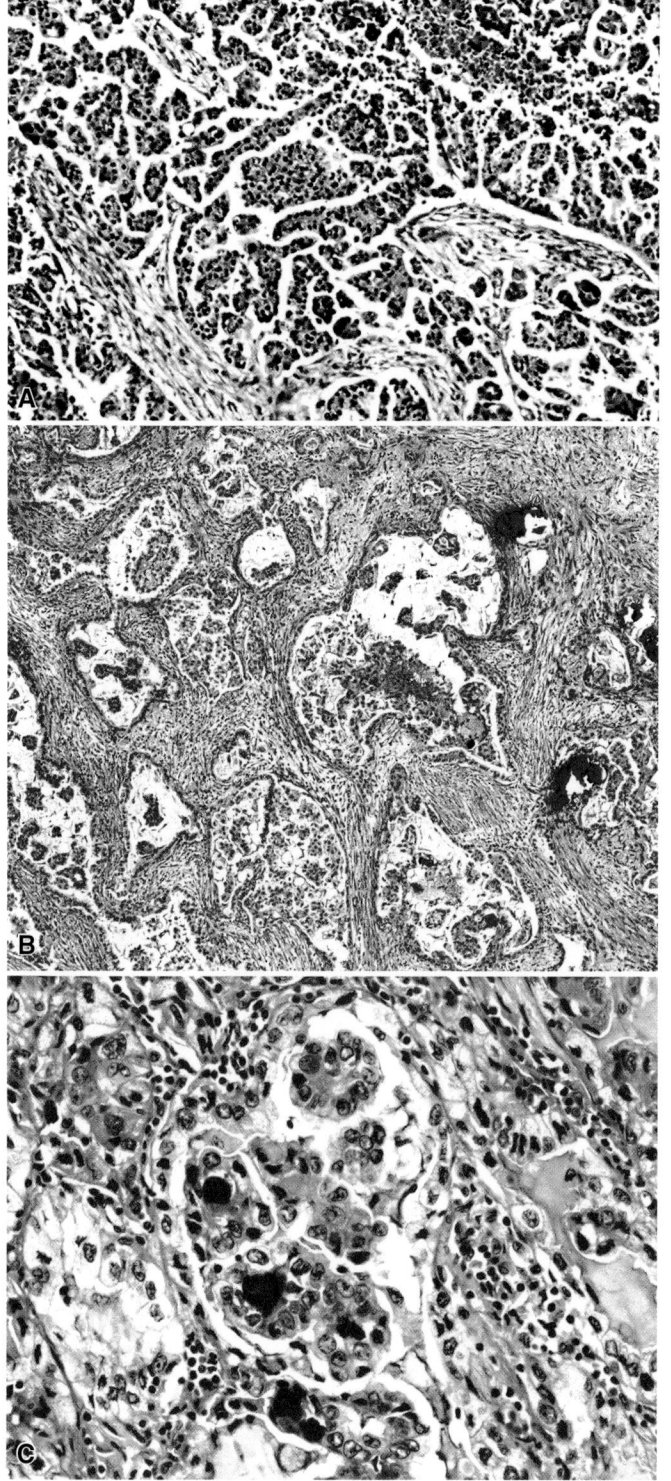

Figure 17-13. A to **C,** Micropapillary architecture and microcalcifications are apparent in this adenocarcinoma of the lung. This feature can be seen in both primary and secondary pulmonary epithelial tumors.

applied to 2.6% of all cases with pleural fluid specimens. In 71.9% of these cases, a firm interpretation was facilitated by the results of such analyses.[45] However, none of the diagnoses in that series were based solely on immunopathology.[45] The low prevalence of mesothelioma in the general population explains the rarity of this interpretation in the experience of most practicing pathologists.

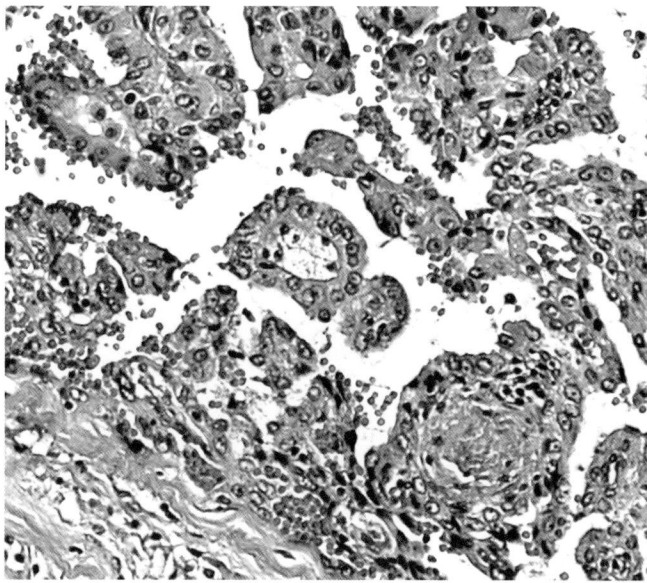

Figure 17-14. Metastatic renal cell carcinoma with a micropapillary architecture.

Clear Cell Adenocarcinomas

Clear cell features are best seen in histologic specimens, in which the cytoplasm of the neoplastic cells is lucent and only the cell borders are apparent. Clear cell change is often an artifact of formalin fixation, and in cytologic specimens, the cytoplasm of the neoplastic cells has a more vacuolated appearance. Primary clear cell tumors of the lung are rare and have variable cellular lineage; they are usually peripherally located[106] (see Chapters 16 and 19). Clear cell change also may be seen focally in common tumor types. For example, biopsy specimens of primary squamous cell carcinomas may show that alteration. That phenomenon is seen less frequently in cytologic specimens, in which the cytoplasm of the neoplastic cells maintains a classic "metaplastic" appearance.

Metastatic clear cell adenocarcinomas in the lungs may emanate from the kidney, breast, adrenal cortex, salivary gland, or other locations; primary clear cell malignancies have been described in practically every organ. The most common clear cell neoplasm in the lung is metastatic renal cell adenocarcinoma (Figs. 17-18 and 17-19).[107] Hughes and associates reported that among 12 lung FNA specimens with clear cell features, 10 originated in the kidney, 1 in the cervix, and 1 in an undetermined site.[108] Clear cell carcinomas are only a subset of renal tumors that may metastasize to the lungs; papillary, oncocytic, and sarcomatoid neoplasms may also do so. Because epithelial malignancies of the kidney have a proclivity to invade the renal veins and bypass the hepatic circulation, the first site of secondary disease may be in the lungs.[107,109] The pulmonary parenchyma is involved in up to 75% of cases of metastatic renal cell carcinoma.[109,110] Almost half of these patients have no symptoms that suggest extrathoracic disease[110] (Fig. 17-20). Metastatic disease in the lungs may take several radiographic forms, including a solitary mass, multiple nodules, miliary spread (innumerable small nodules), large- or small-vessel emboli, lymphatic space disease, hilar or mediastinal lymph nodal disease, and endobronchial tumor.[111–115] Metastatic renal cell carcinoma is an example of a neoplasm that may grow very slowly and become clinically evident only many years after the primary diagnosis.[116]

Like ovarian carcinomas, clear cell carcinomas of the kidney are difficult to identify definitively by immunohistologic studies. Most are reactive for CD10, PAX2, adipophilin, RCC antigen, and cytokeratin 8 (Figs. 17-21 and 17-22). In combination, these are highly suggestive of the diagnosis.[117–120]

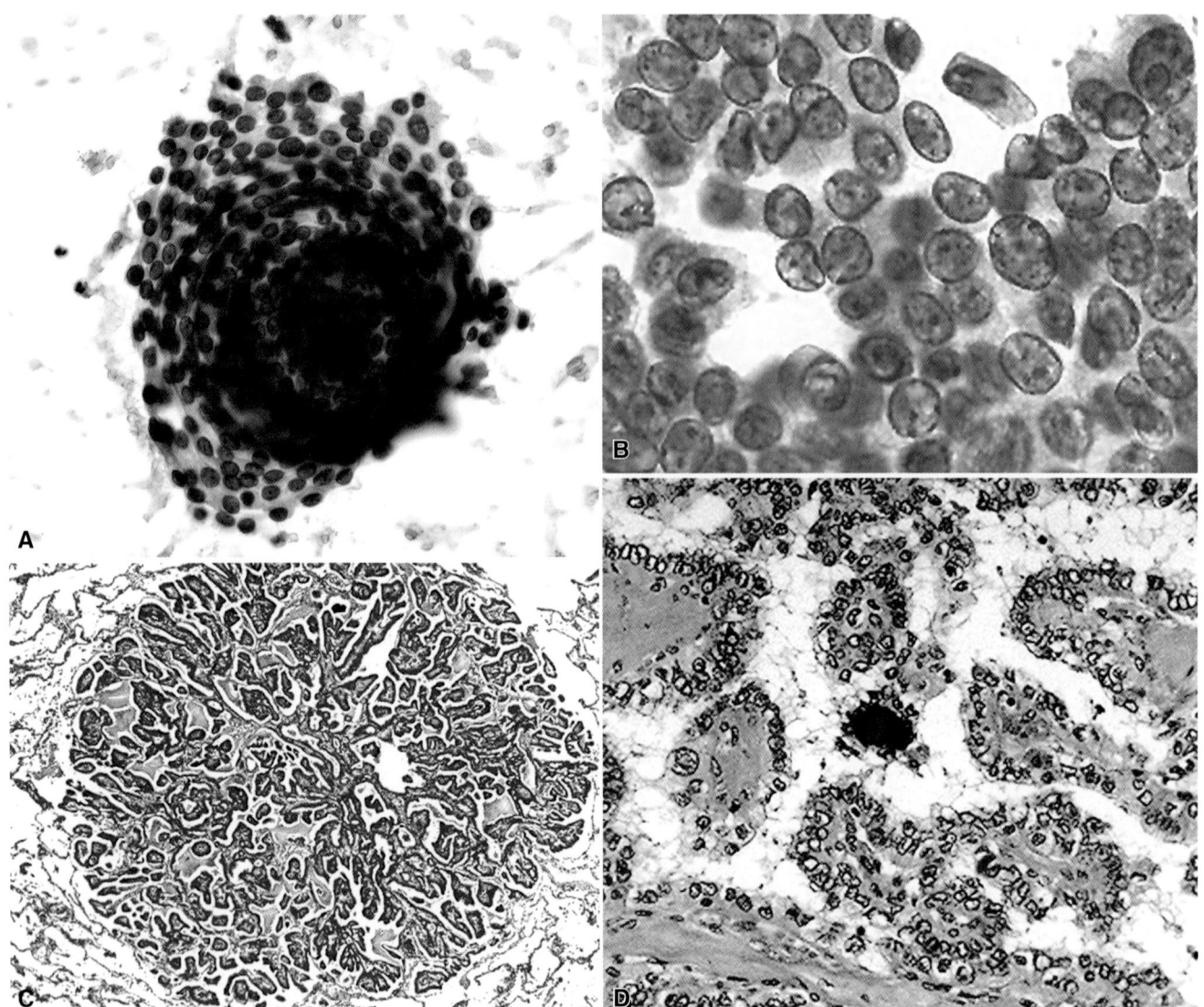

Figure 17-15. A, Fine-needle aspirate of metastatic papillary thyroid carcinoma in the lung showing characteristic whorled cytomorphologic and nuclear features. **B,** An isolated micrometastatic focus of papillary thyroid carcinoma in a surgical lung biopsy specimen shows characteristic nuclear features. **C,** Metastatic nodule of thyroid carcinoma within the lung parenchyma showing colloid formation adjacent to papillary nests of tumor cells. **D,** Microcalcification within a papillary focus of metastatic thyroid carcinoma.

Table 17-2. Immunohistologic Differential Diagnosis of Papillary Adenocarcinoma

	Antibody							
Origin	**PK**	**TTF1**	**CK20**	**THY**	**ERP**	**GCDFP**	**CEA**	**S-100**
Lung	P	P	N	N	N	N	P	N
Thyroid	P	P	N	P	N	N	PN	PN
Breast	P	N	N	N	P	P	P	PN
Ovary (serous)	P	N	N	N	P	N	N	PN
Kidney	P	N	N	N	N	N	N	PN

CEA, carcinoembryonic antigen; CK20, cytokeratin 20; ERP, estrogen receptor protein; GCDFP, gross cystic disease fluid protein; N, negative (<10% of cases); P, positive (>80% of cases); PK, pan-keratin; PN, variably positive (10–80% of cases); S-100, S-100 protein; THY, thyroglobulin; TTF1, thyroid transcription factor-1.

Signet Ring Cell Adenocarcinomas

A "signet ring" cell is relatively small and has an eccentrically placed nucleus indented by a large cytoplasmic vacuole or multiple vacuoles. Such cells generally are considered part of the spectrum of poorly differentiated mucin-forming adenocarcinoma, and some tumors of that type are composed almost entirely of signet ring cell forms. Signet ring cell differentiation is uncommon in most primary pulmonary adenocarcinomas. If it is present, a secondary malignancy is favored (Fig. 17-23). Sources of metastases with that appearance include the stomach and other gastrointestinal sites, breast, and pancreas. Metastatic signet ring cell carcinomas are usually associated with a dismal prognosis; they characteristically spread initially to regional lymph nodes before involving the lungs. Some esophageal signet ring cell tumors originating in foci of Barrett esophagus may directly invade the lung or pleura. Metastatic pancreatic adenocarcinomas, including signet ring cell variants, often involve the liver and

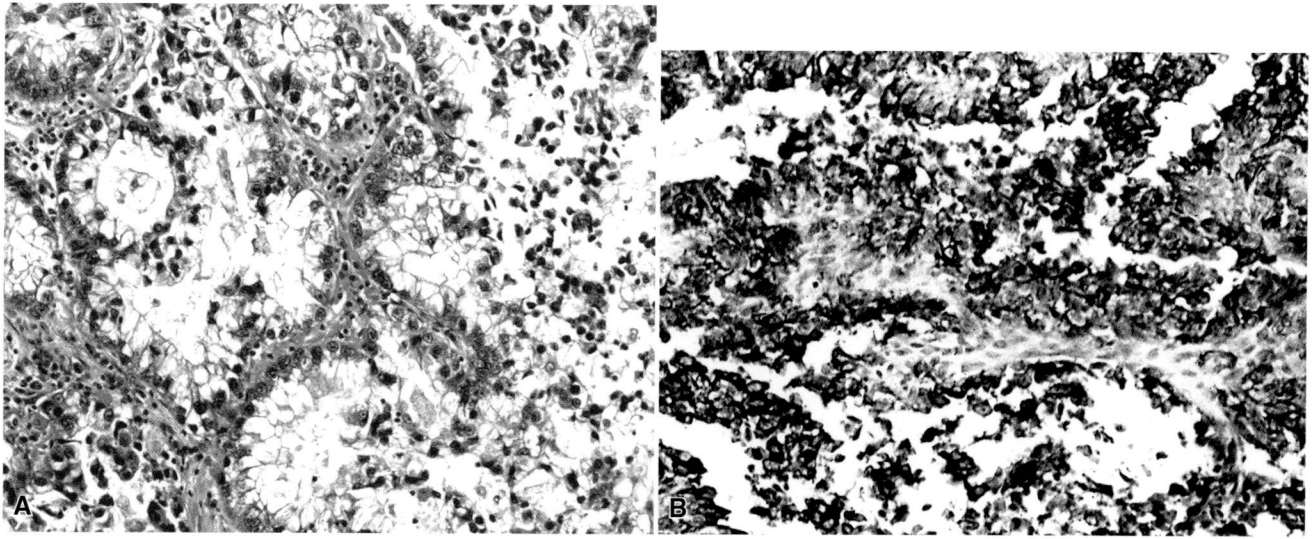

Figure 17-16. A, Metastatic clear cell carcinoma of the ovary showing glandular formations containing tumor cells with a "hobnail" appearance. **B,** Immunostaining with CA-125 supports the müllerian origin of this tumor.

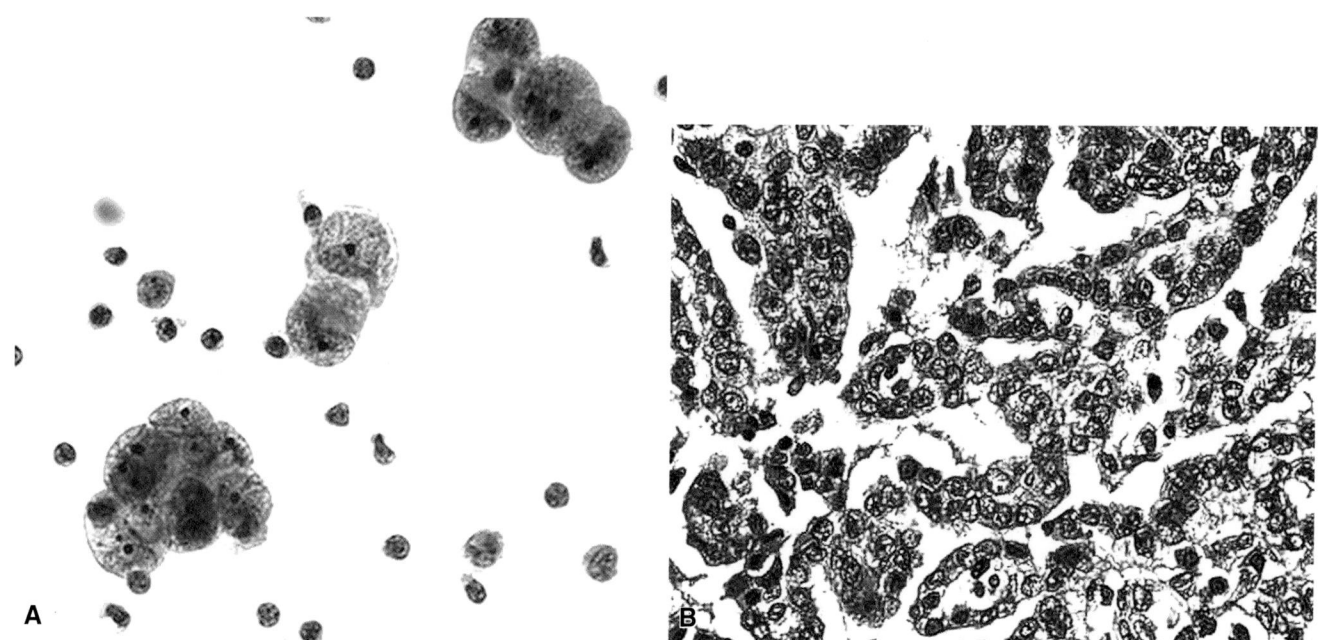

Figure 17-17. A, Cytologic preparation of pleural fluid in a case of malignant epithelioid mesothelioma showing a micropapillary array of atypical mesothelial cells. **B,** Subsequent biopsy confirmed the micropapillary nature of the neoplasm, as seen here. (**A,** Courtesy of Dr. Diva Salomao.)

Table 17-3. Immunohistologic Differential Diagnosis between Malignant Mesothelioma and Metastatic Adenocarcinoma

Tumor	Antibody						
	PK	CK5/6	CEA	CD15	Ber-EP4	B72.3	CALR
Malignant mesothelioma	P	P	N	N	N	N	P
Adenocarcinoma	P	N	P	P	P	P	N

CALR, calretinin; CEA, carcinoembryonic antigen; CK, cytokeratin; CK5/6, cytokeratin 5/6; N, negative (<10% of cases); P, positive (>80% of cases); PK, pan-keratin.

lungs.[121] Multiple pulmonary nodules are virtually always seen rather than a solitary secondary lesion.[121]

Well-Differentiated Adenocarcinomas

The authors use the term *well-differentiated adenocarcinoma* in more than just a descriptive fashion to mean a malignant glandular proliferation that is morphologically difficult to differentiate from benign or reactive pulmonary proliferations; the nosologic term "minimal-deviation adenocarcinoma" also has been used in this context. The recognition of these tumors is often extremely difficult in cytologic specimens because of the lack of contextual architecture. Well-differentiated primary adenocarcinomas of the lung include some "conventional" (acinar)

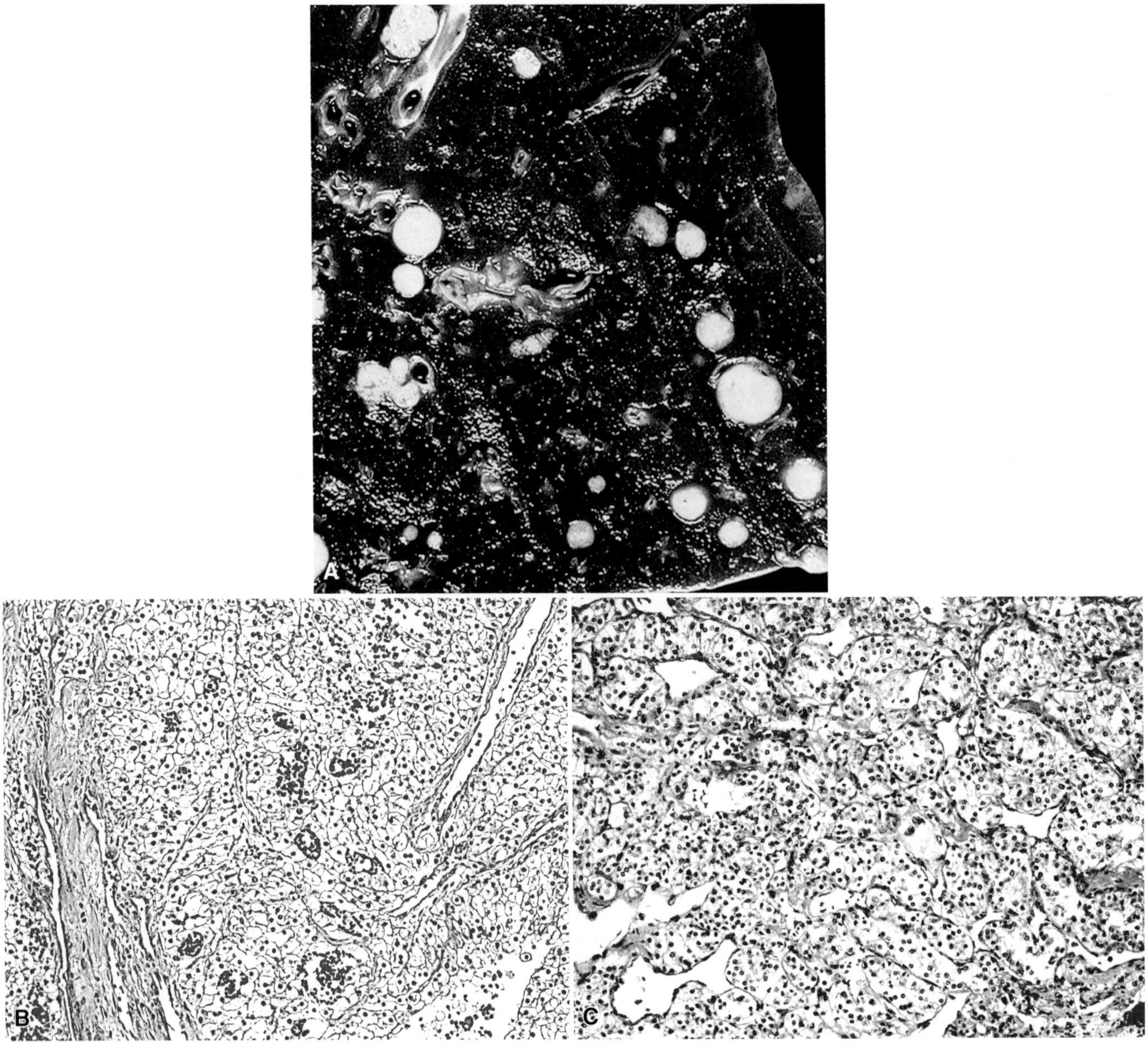

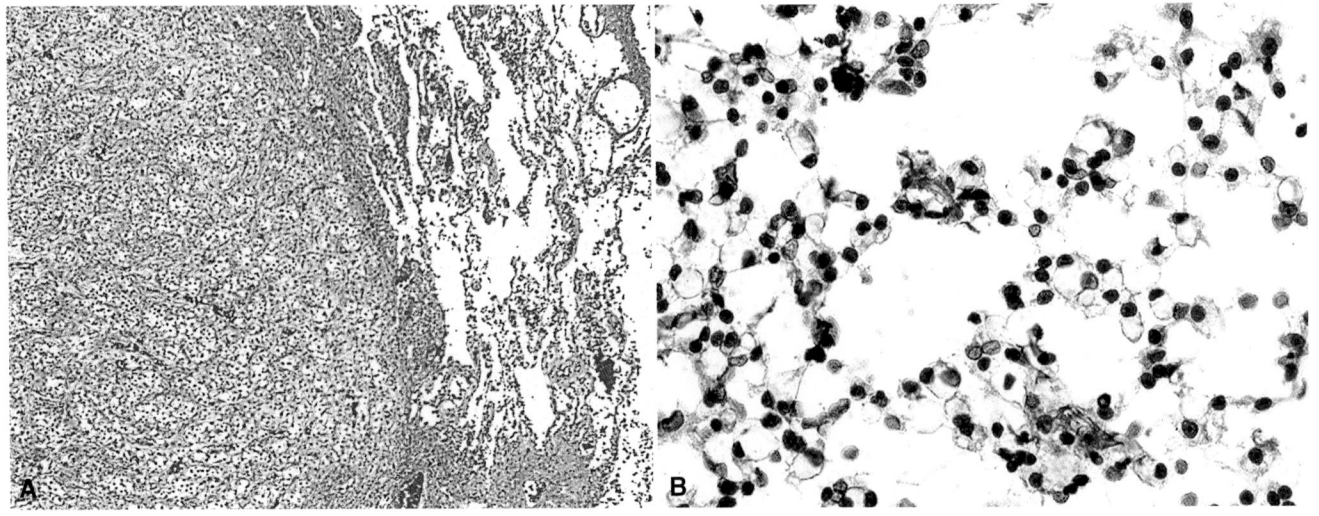

Figure 17-18. A, Gross photograph of a lung with multiple intrapulmonary metastases of renal cell carcinoma that presented in the absence of a known primary tumor in the kidney. The masses have a yellowish appearance and are well demarcated from the surrounding lung parenchyma. **B,** Typical arrangement of packeted clear cells in a highly vascularized stroma. **C,** Clear cell tumor cells may be arranged in a trabecular pattern.

Figure 17-19. A, Example of resected metastatic renal cell carcinoma that is more solid and includes tumor cells with an oncocytoid appearance. **B,** A previous fine-needle aspirate in the same case shows fine cytoplasmic vacuolization, serving as a clue to the renal nature of the lesion.

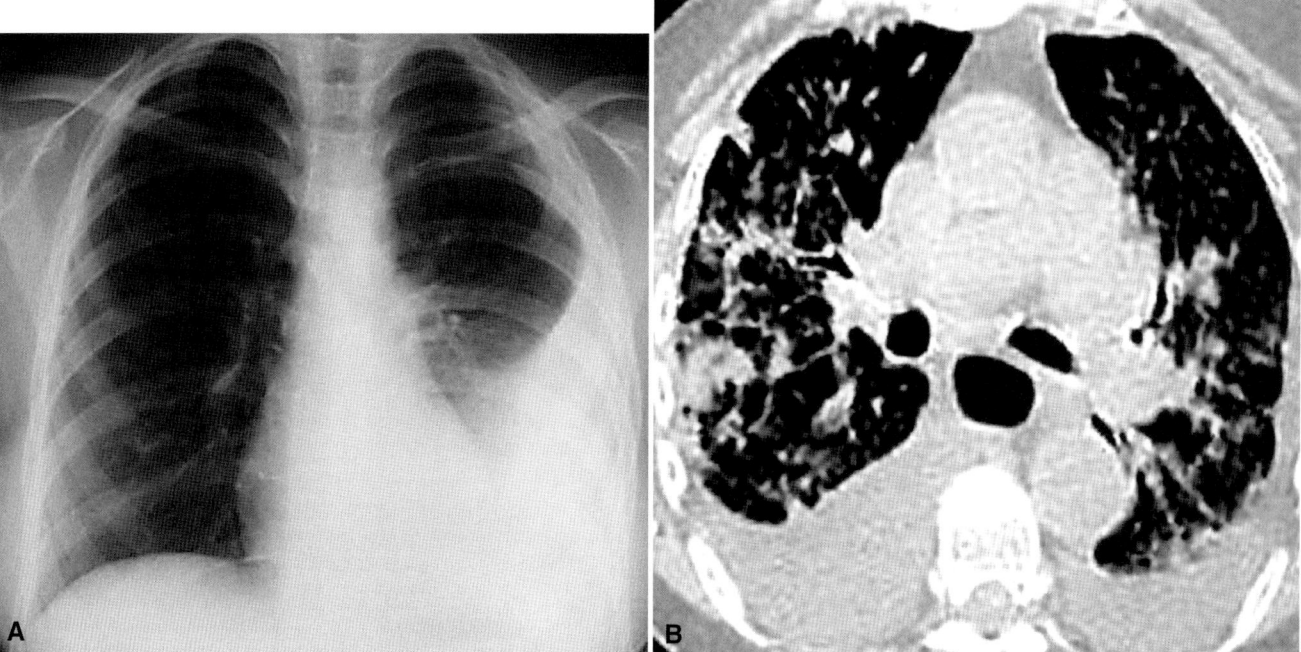

Figure 17-20. A, Chest radiograph from a patient with "occult" renal cell carcinoma presenting with metastasis to the pleura and lungs. The left hemithorax is partially opacified by metastatic tumor and an accompanying pleural effusion. **B,** Computed tomography scan from another case shows widespread metastatic renal cell carcinoma involving the lung and pleura.

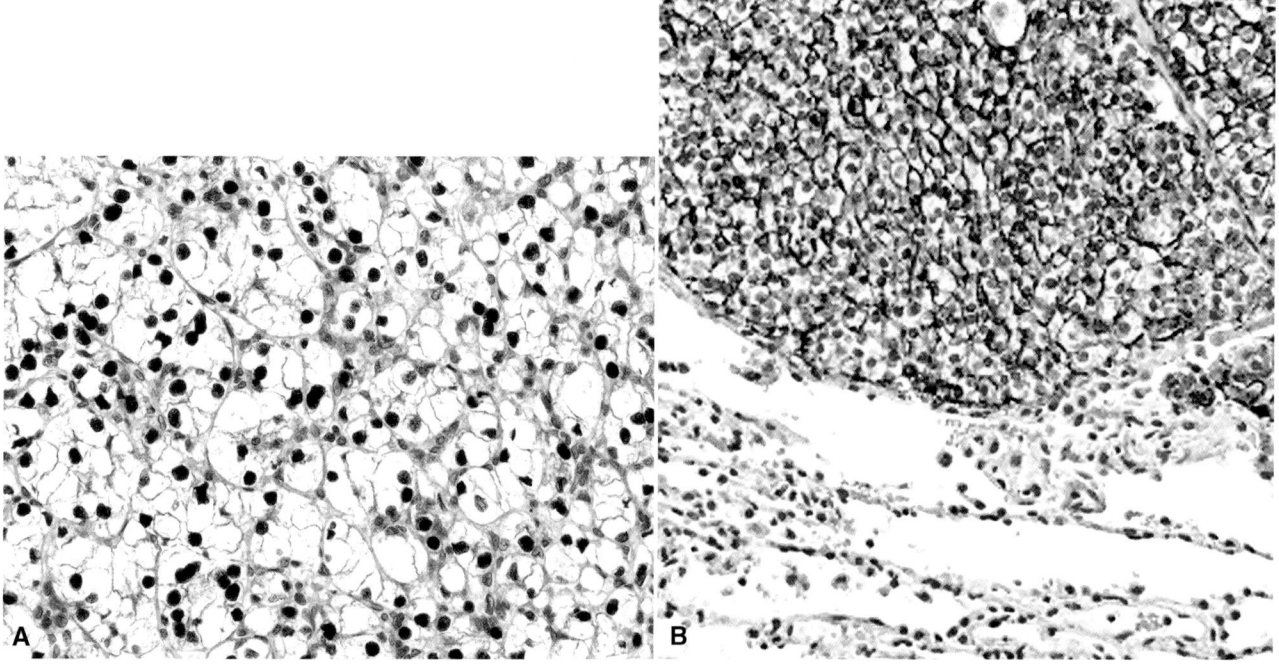

Figure 17-21. Immunoreactivity for PAX2 (**A**) and CD10 (**B**) in metastatic renal cell carcinoma. These markers are found in most malignant renal epithelial tumors.

adenocarcinomas, selected bronchioloalveolar adenocarcinomas, and salivary gland-type adenocarcinomas (see Chapter 16). These show relatively low nuclear-to-cytoplasmic ratios and lack the degree of nuclear atypia seen in more overtly malignant lesions. Bronchioloalveolar adenocarcinomas, in particular, often pose a diagnostic conundrum, especially in cytologic preparations where the malignant cells lining the alveolar septa in a "lepidic" manner cannot be seen. However, well-differentiated adenocarcinomas in the lung may also be metastases, especially when sharply defined mass lesions are seen macroscopically. Sites of origin for secondary adenocarcinomas with these attributes include the breast, pancreas, kidney, thyroid, and salivary glands.

Mammary carcinomas may metastasize to the lungs, pleura, or both. In most cases, the malignant cells are easily identified, but in some FNA or pleural fluid specimens, the malignant cells are bland (Fig. 17-24). Intrapulmonary metastatic foci are often nodular, but other presentations, such as endobronchial lesions, lymphangitic spread, and intravascular tumor emboli, may be seen.[122-125] Approximately 50% of metastatic breast cancers are associated with pleural effusions.[33,126] Casey and colleagues reported that 3% of primary mammary carcinomas were associated with a lung mass at the time of initial diagnosis; 43% of the pulmonary lesions were metastases and 52% were concurrent primary lung cancers. The rest were non-neoplastic.[125] The lungs

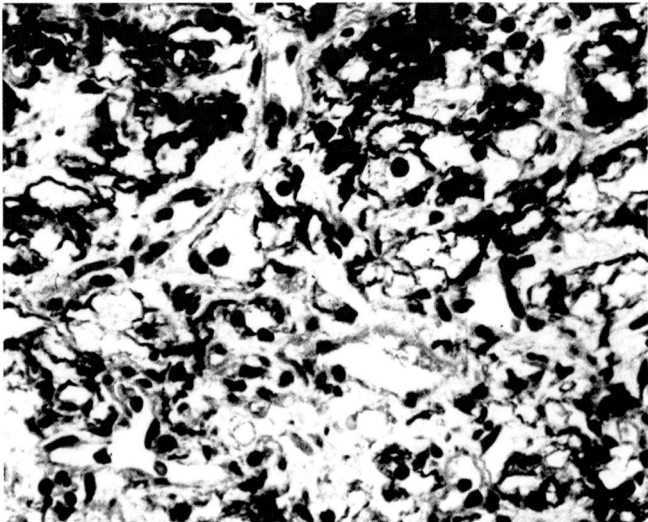

Figure 17-22. Immunoreactivity for cytokeratin 8 in metastatic renal cell carcinoma. This keratin subtype is characteristic of nononcocytic tumors of the kidney.

and pleura are the first sites of tumor recurrence in 10% of cases of mammary carcinoma.[124] In patients with a history of breast carcinoma and an adenocarcinoma in the lung, Raab and coworkers showed, with immunohistochemical studies (for estrogen receptor, gross cystic disease fluid protein-15, S-100 protein, and carcinoembryonic antigen) that 50% of the pulmonary lesions were metastatic mammary tumors, 37% were primary pulmonary carcinomas, and 13% were indeterminate (Figs. 17-25 and 17-26).[127] Dabbs and associates found that some primary lung cancers may label for hormone receptor proteins, but not for the other specified markers.[128] Mammaglobin is another breast-related polypeptide that is valuable in the immunohistochemical recognition of metastatic mammary carcinoma.[129] On the other hand, positivity for thyroid transcription factor-1 (Fig. 17-27) is compelling evidence in favor of pulmonary derivation in this context, as discussed later.

Oncocytic and Granular Cell Carcinomas

Neoplasms composed of cells containing granular cytoplasm may be oncocytic or nononcocytic. Both subtypes contain cells that have an eosinophilic appearance on conventional stains. In oncocytic cells, this reflects the presence of numerous cytoplasmic mitochondria. Nononcocytic cells instead contain a preponderance of other cytoplasmic organelles, especially lysosomes. Primary pulmonary malignancies that may have a granular cell constituency include conventional adenocarcinomas and salivary gland-type adenocarcinomas. However, this cytologic feature is rare in lung tumors. Secondary neoplasms with granular cytoplasm include carcinomas of the kidney, thyroid, and liver (Fig. 17-28).

The lungs are involved in up to 70% of cases of metastatic hepatocellular carcinoma (HCC).[130–132] Several patterns of intrapulmonary spread have been reported; through transdiaphragmatic lymphatics, HCC may enter the right lower lobe. In this setting, several parenchymal mass lesions and pleural involvement are typically seen.[133,134] Alternatively, HCC may transit the venous system through the hepatic vein and inferior vena cava, presenting as a large intravascular mass or "showering" the lungs with small emboli that appear as miliary tumors.[133] Cytologically, the cells of this neoplasm often show multinucleation; this feature is uncommon in most primary pulmonary malignancies. Moreover, bile formation may be seen in metastatic HCC (Fig. 17-29). In addition, the tumor cells cluster around intralesional blood vessels and "stripped" nuclei are seen.[135] Cytopathologists must avoid misinterpretation of FNA specimens obtained from the right lower pulmonary lobe as well-differentiated oncocytic or granular cell carcinomas; these specimens may simply represent normal liver that has been mistakenly sampled instead of the lung. A monoclonal antibody raised against paraffin-embedded tissue from HCC, and designated "Hep-PAR1," has shown reasonably good discrimination in labeling that tumor.[136]

Largely Necrotic Adenocarcinomas

The most commonly necrotic primary tumors of the lung are squamous cell carcinoma, small cell neuroendocrine carcinoma, and large cell undifferentiated or large cell neuroendocrine carcinoma.

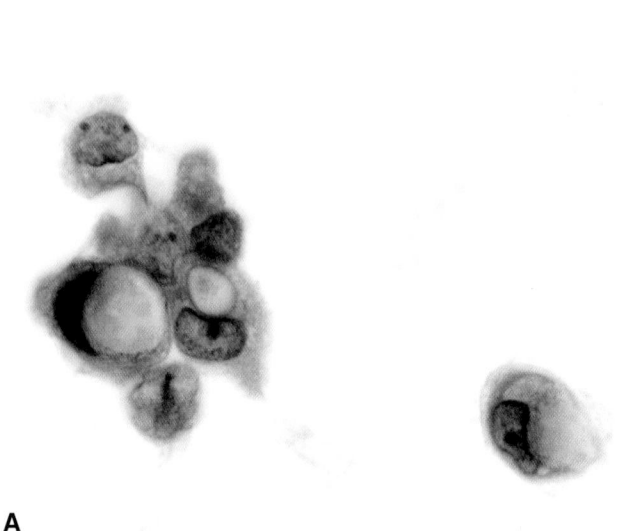

A

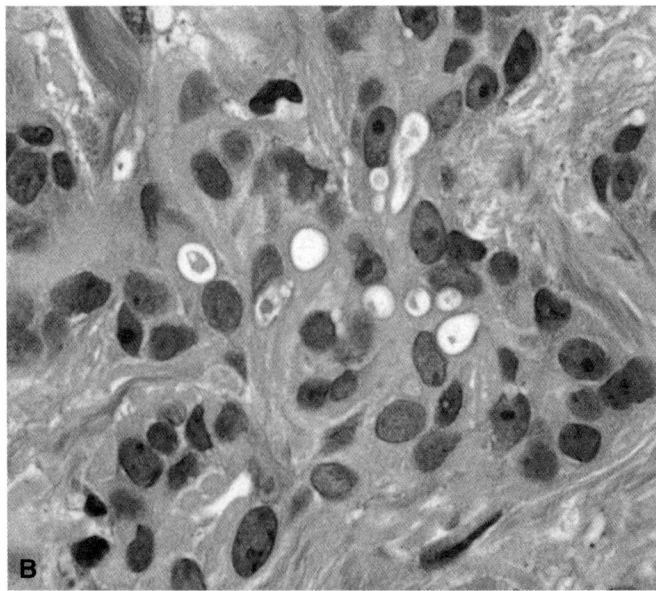

B

Figure 17-23. **A,** Metastatic adenocarcinoma in a fine-needle aspiration specimen showing focal "signet ring cell" differentiation with formation of cytoplasmic vacuoles. **B,** The same feature is seen in this cell block preparation. The primary tumor was lobular carcinoma of the breast.

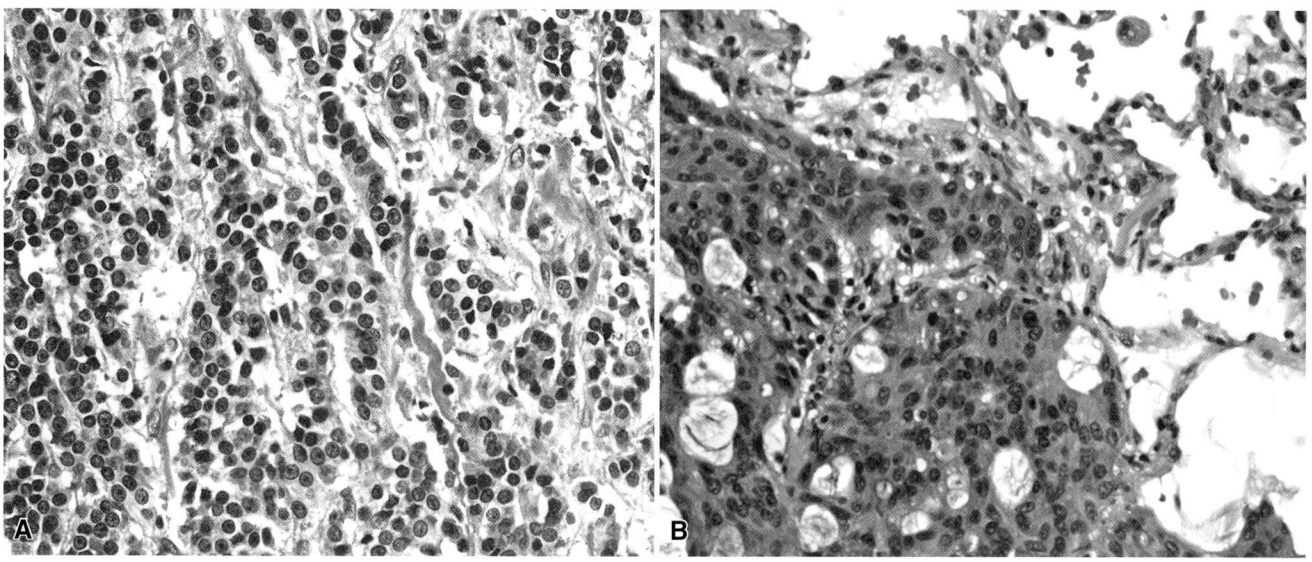

Figure 17-24. A, Bland nuclear features are seen in this metastatic lobular carcinoma of the breast involving the lung parenchyma. **B,** Metastatic ductal carcinoma with mucin-filled acinar structures and moderate nuclear atypia.

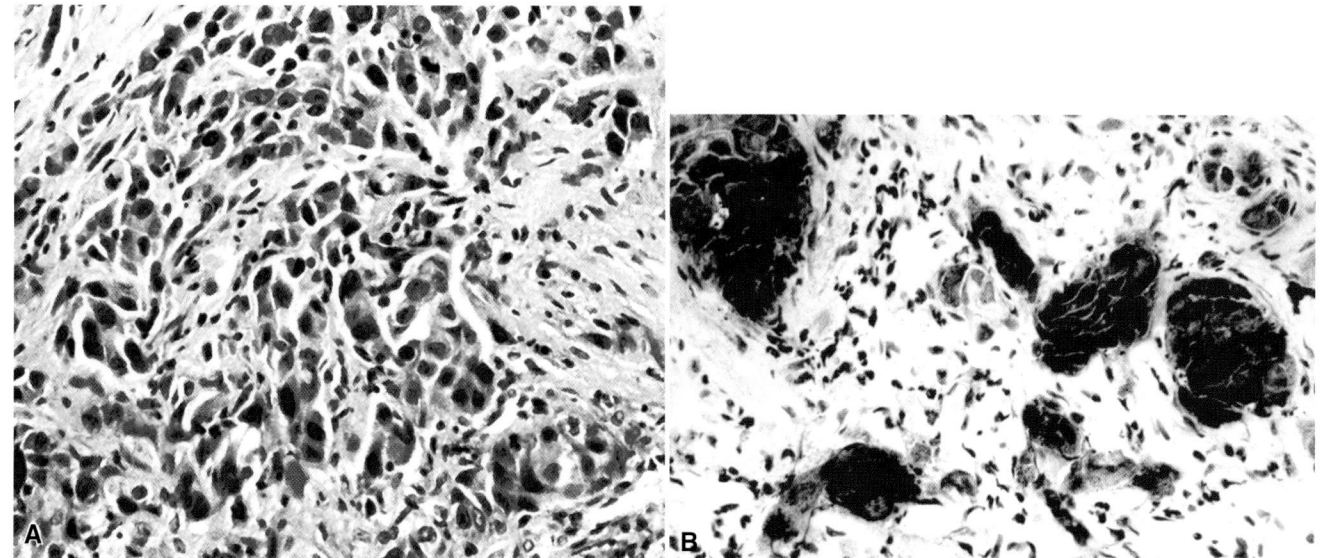

Figure 17-25. A, Adenocarcinoma in the lung with a histologically indeterminate appearance. It is unclear morphologically whether the tumor is primary or secondary. **B,** Immunoreactivity for gross cystic disease fluid protein-15, a breast marker, establishes the diagnosis of metastatic ductal mammary carcinoma.

Primary pulmonary adenocarcinomas rarely show this alteration unless they are very large or poorly differentiated. Thus, statistically, necrotic adenocarcinomas are more likely to be secondary malignancies in the lungs. Metastatic colorectal carcinomas characteristically show central necrosis cytologically, regardless of the degree of differentiation. FNA biopsy specimens also show fusiform nuclei arranged in a "picket fence" pattern or in small glandular formations. Other extrapulmonary tumors that may yield the image of necrotic metastatic carcinoma include renal cell carcinoma, pancreatic carcinoma, esophageal squamous cell carcinoma or adenocarcinoma, breast cancer, and prostatic carcinoma.

In up to 50% of metastatic colorectal adenocarcinomas, the lungs are involved.[137] Most of these cases show multiple pulmonary masses radiographically,[137] but approximately 40% of all solitary metastases in the lung are also derived from the large intestine.[21,22] Right-sided colonic tumors may produce lung metastases without liver metastases.[138-141] These lesions are often cystic, and FNA specimens may be mistakenly interpreted as showing cavitary squamous cell carcinoma. In histologic sections, zones of necrosis may be surrounded by limited numbers of viable tumor cells; in cytologic preparations, rare viable cells may be seen. Flint and Lloyd suggested that "dirty" (karyorrhectic) necrosis (Figs. 17-30 and 17-31) was more often seen in metastatic colorectal tumors than in primary adenocarcinomas of the lung.[142] Immunopathologic studies are often helpful in distinguishing secondary colonic malignancies from primary adenocarcinomas of the lung. Colorectal tumors generally are reactive for cytokeratin 20 but negative for cytokeratin 7 and thyroid transcription factor-1; the converse is true for primary pulmonary adenocarcinomas, even those that have an "enteric" morphologic image on conventional microscopy.[143-146] A cytoskeletal protein known as "villin" is also selectively seen in

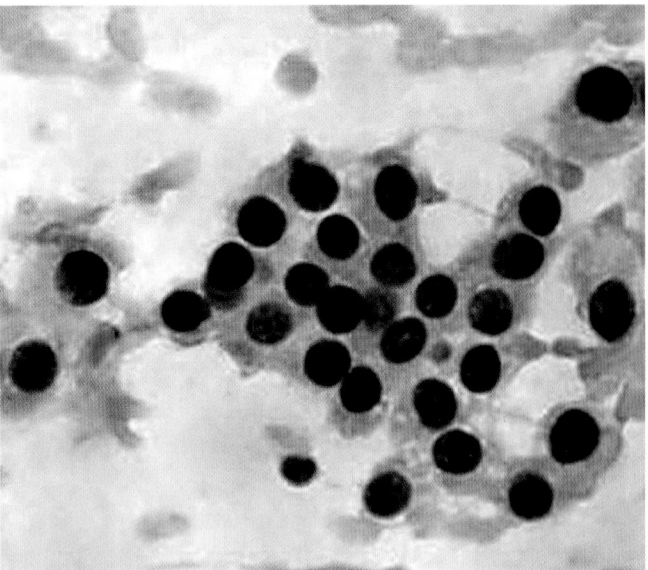

Figure 17-26. Metastatic breast carcinoma in a pleural fluid preparation, showing intense immunoreactivity for estrogen receptor protein.

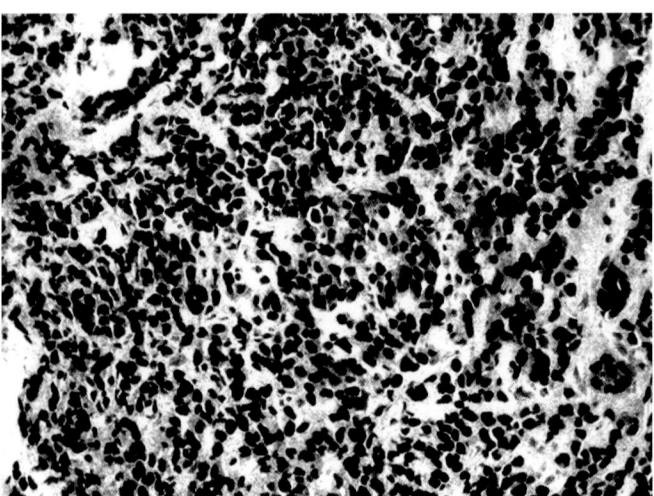

Figure 17-27. Immunoreactivity for thyroid transcription factor-1 in primary adenocarcinoma of the lung. This marker is present only in thyroid and pulmonary proliferations.

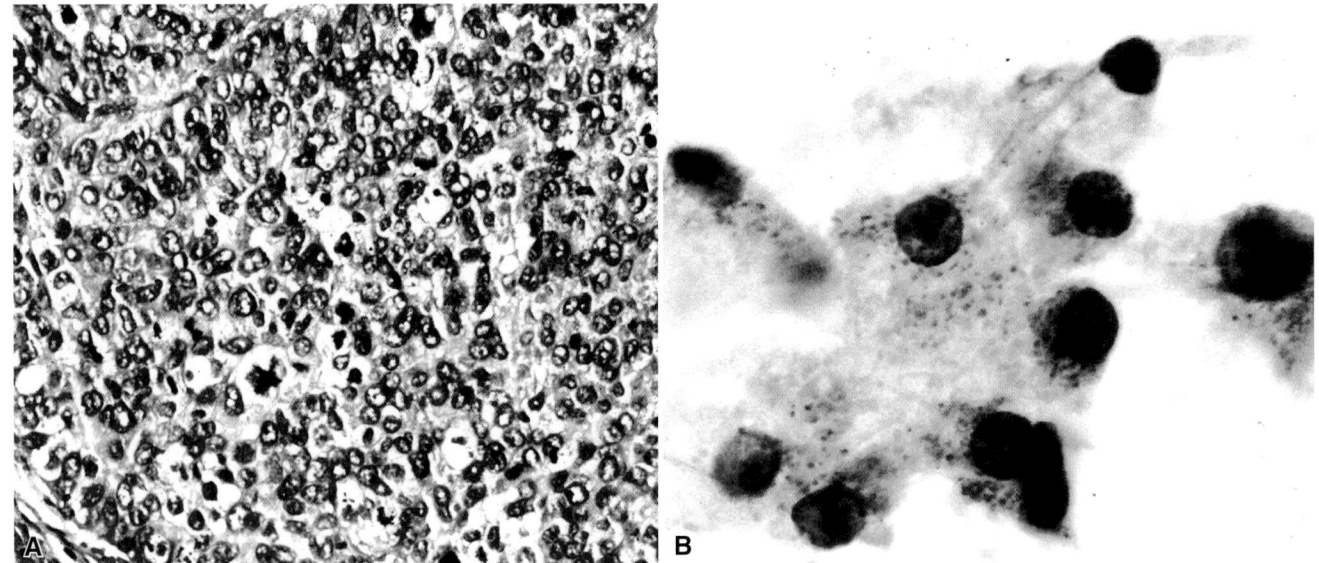

Figure 17-28. A, Metastatic large cell carcinoma in the lung with a granular cytoplasmic appearance. B, Cytoplasmic granules are more evident in a fine-needle aspiration specimen. The primary tumor was in the liver.

gastrointestinal malignancies, as are the plasmalemmal glycoprotein recognized by monoclonal antibody CA-19-9 and the nuclear transcription factor CDX2 (Figs. 17-32 and 17-33).[147–149]

Mucinous Adenocarcinomas

Primary mucin-producing carcinomas of the lung include some bronchioloalveolar carcinomas, selected mucoepidermoid carcinomas, and other rare primary mucinous tumors, some of which have the appearance of "colloid" carcinomas (Fig. 17-34).[150] Most of these tumors have relatively specific radiologic attributes, and when these images are absent and a mucinous carcinoma is seen microscopically, metastasis may be suspected. However, large amounts of postobstructive mucin production by the lung may surround nonmucinous malignancies. Consequently, cytopathologists should be cautious in interpreting

FNA specimens containing carcinoma cells and abundant mucin as bona fide mucinous carcinomas. The most common sites of origin for metastatic mucinous adenocarcinomas are the intestine (including the vermiform appendix), ovary, and breast. Pathologic specimens of these secondary tumors in the lung may show rare malignant cells and copious mucin pools. The neoplastic cells are often well differentiated and are arranged in small clusters. The immunopathologic features of metastatic colorectal adenocarcinoma of the "colloid" type are essentially the same as those of ordinary colon cancers, and that also applies to secondary mucinous carcinoma of the breast. However, mucinous ovarian carcinomas differ from other epithelial malignancies of the ovary immunophenotypically; they typically lack CA-125 and instead exhibit an enteric antigenic profile similar to that of intestinal neoplasms.[151]

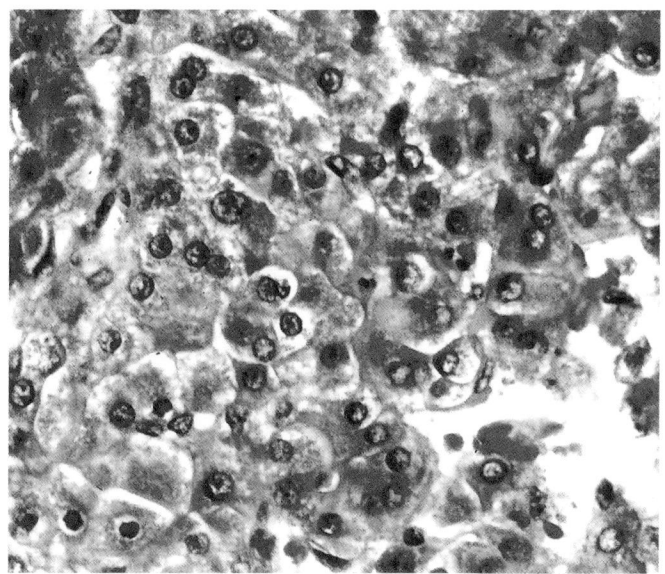

Figure 17-29. Multifocal bile formation (*right*) in metastatic hepatocellular carcinoma.

Other Metastatic Malignancies That Mimic Adenocarcinomas of the Lung

Other metastatic malignancies that may mimic a primary pulmonary adenocarcinoma include prostatic carcinoma, predominantly epithelioid synovial sarcoma, clear cell sarcoma, endometrial carcinoma, epithelioid sarcoma, malignant melanoma, adrenocortical carcinoma, and some germ cell malignancies, such as metastatic embryonal carcinoma. Some of those lesions are discussed later.

The immunopathologic profiles of prostatic, endometrial, and adrenocortical carcinomas are shown in Table 17-1. Prostatic and endometrial tumors rarely metastasize selectively to the lungs[152,153]; only 10% of prostatic carcinomas yield lung metastases,[154,155] and fewer than 3% of endometrial carcinomas do so.[153] Both of these malignancies usually first involve other sites, such as lymph nodes, bones, or liver.[152] When these lesions spread to the lungs, multiple masses usually are apparent.[156] Metastatic prostatic carcinomas may produce endobronchial masses, lymphangitic carcinomatosis, or thoracic lymph nodal spread.[157–159] Antibodies to prostate-specific antigen, prostate-specific acid phosphatase, and prostate-specific membrane antigen are highly specific for tumors of prostatic origin

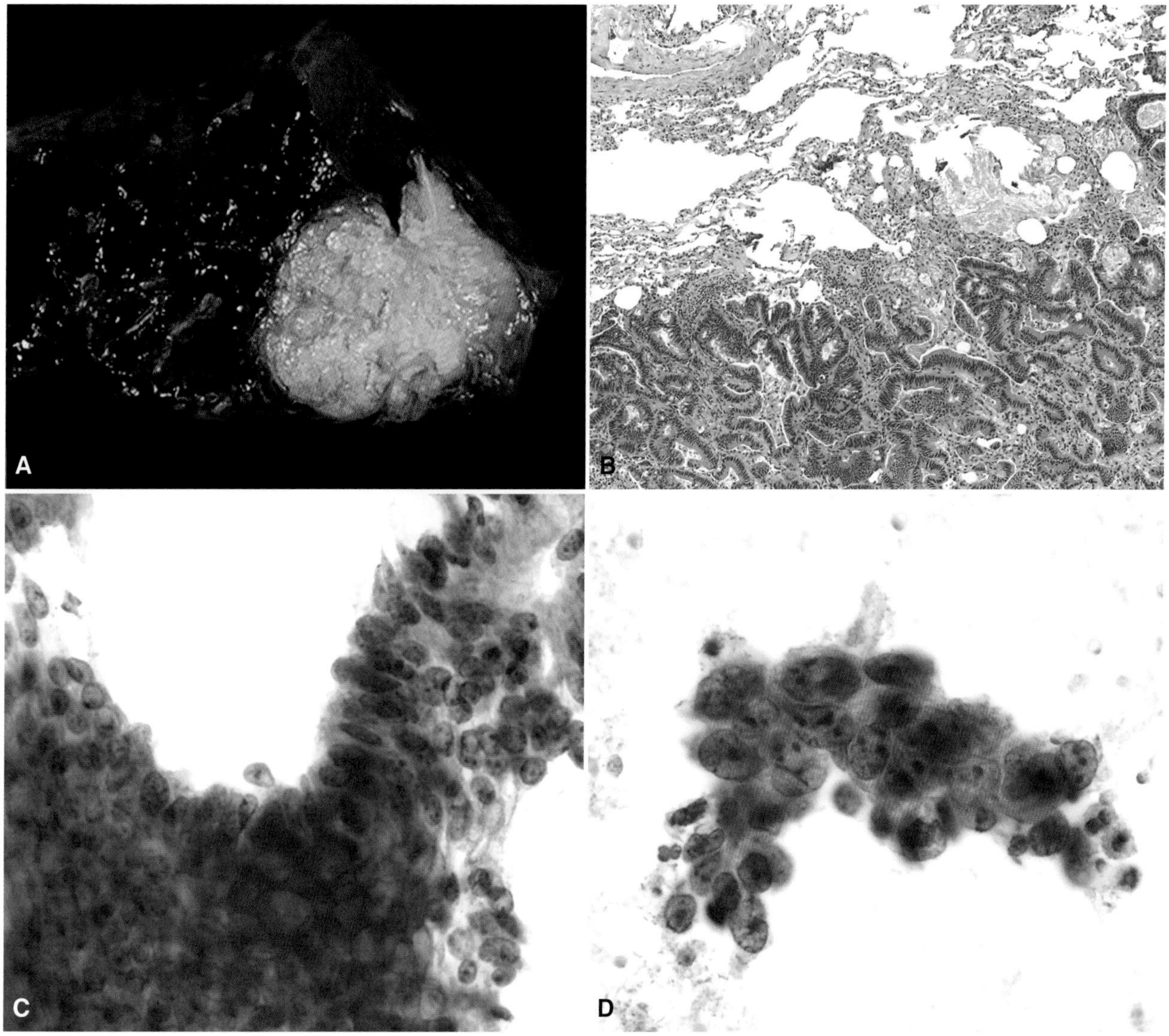

Figure 17-30. A, Metastatic colonic adenocarcinoma in the lung represented by a solitary lesion. **B,** Microscopic appearance showing characteristically "incomplete" tumor glands and basally oriented tumor cell nuclei. Fine-needle aspiration biopsy of the nodule showing a tendency for parallel alignment of tumor cell nuclei (**C**) and the generic appearance of an adenocarcinoma (**D**).

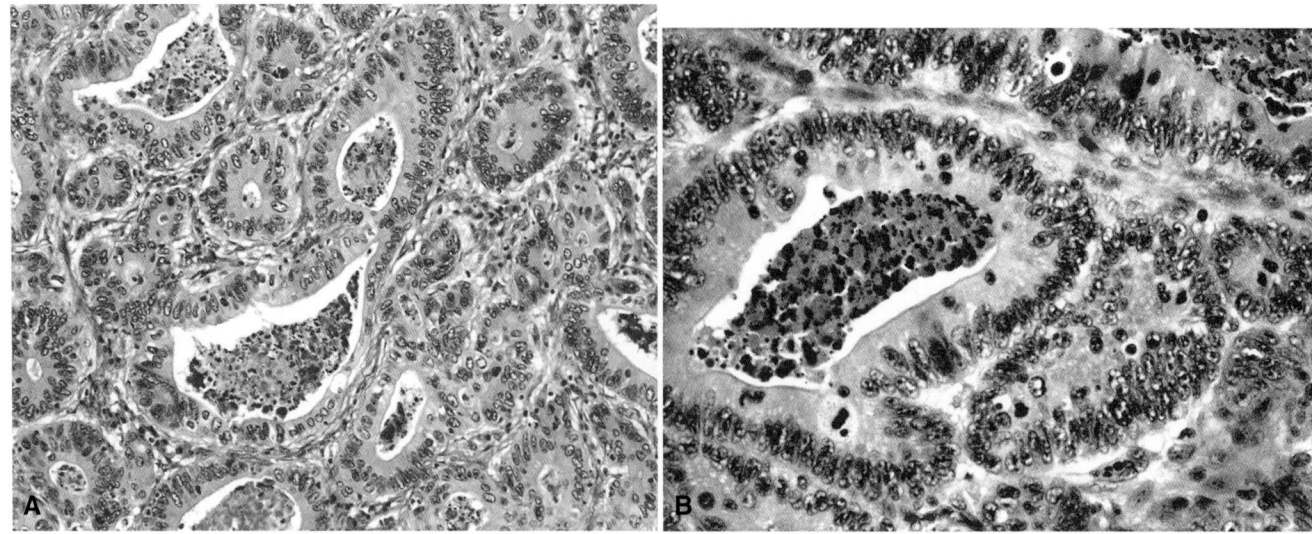

Figure 17-31. **A** and **B,** "Dirty" necrosis is apparent in the centers of tumoral glands in metastatic colonic adenocarcinoma.

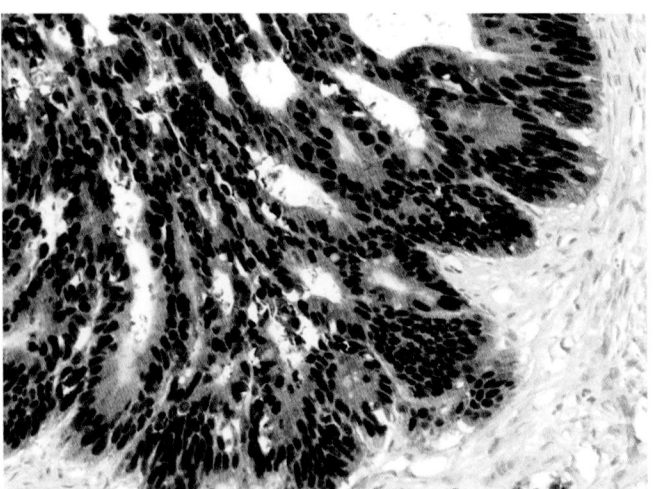

Figure 17-32. Nuclelar immunoreactivity for CDX2, a gut marker, in metastatic poorly differentiated colonic adenocarcinoma involving the lung.

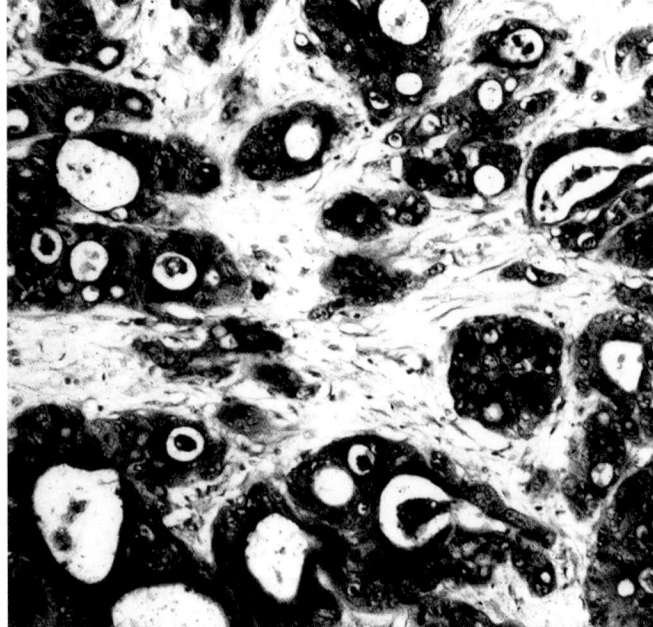

Figure 17-33. Immunoreactivity for CA19.9, another gastrointestinal tract–related protein, in metastatic colonic adenocarcinoma.

(Figs. 17-35 to 17-37).[160] No such specific markers are currently available to identify endometrial neoplasms. Biopsy specimens of metastatic adrenocortical carcinoma may show lipidized cytoplasm in the tumor cells and extensive cellular dyshesion. The immunoprofile of this neoplasm is unusual in that it features scant keratin production (if any), vimentin reactivity, and labeling for inhibin, MART-1/Melan-A (Figs. 17-38 and 17-39), or both, despite S-100 protein negativity. Inhibin and MART-1 are typically associated with ovarian stromal tumors and melanocytic proliferations, respectively. Why they should be present in an epithelial tumor is unknown, but their presence makes adrenocortical carcinoma a singularly identifiable form of metastasis in the lung.

"Gene Chip" Analyses

In the last several years, a number of publications have addressed the possibility that MCUOs might be identified through analysis of their *genetic* profile, in addition to, or in lieu of, evaluation of

their immunophenotype.[161–169] That approach has yielded the commercial availability of such assessments, offered by a growing number of biomedical firms. The general background of the technique is predicated on the evaluation of predefined and sizable gene sets in a number of metastases of primary carcinomas. In this way, a characteristic "gene fingerprint" can usually be identified for each histologic tumor type. An "unknown" clinical case is then similarly assessed for the same gene groups, and using computer algorithms for comparison, statistical synonymities to known carcinoma identities are calculated. The submitting physician is given a visual report that shows the relative likelihood of several origins for the lesion (Fig. 17-40).

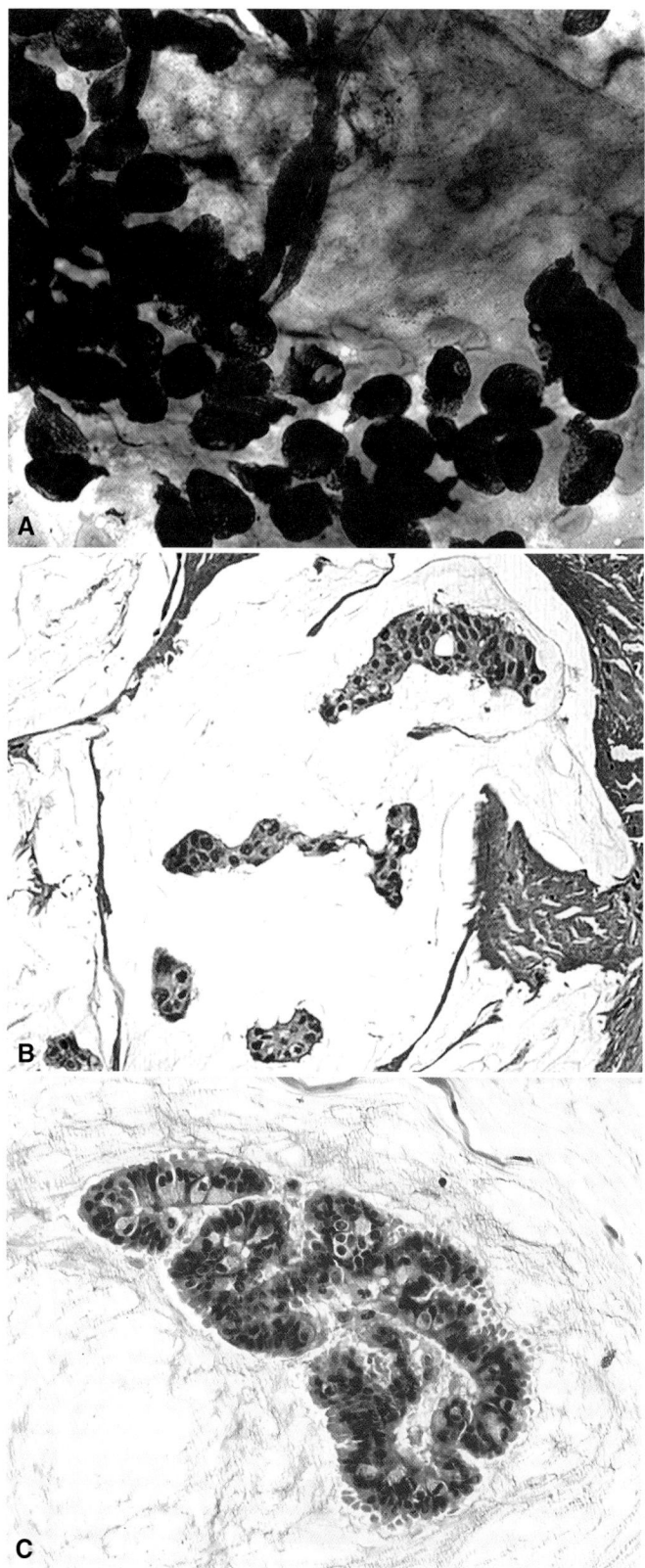

Figure 17-34. Metastatic "colloid" carcinoma (mucinous adenocarcinoma) from the rectum involving the lung. Narrowly branching profiles of tumor cells are suspended in pools of extracellular mucin in a fine-needle aspiration specimen (**A**) and in tissue sections (**B** and **C**). These images are highly suggestive of metastasis rather than a primary pulmonary tumor.

This technique is a powerful new addition to the methods used to study MCUOs pathologically. The one caveat attending gene chip evaluations is that the comparison group of tumors on which they are predicated must be large and varied. For example, one could hardly expect that an MCUO would be identified as adrenocortical in origin if there were no adrenocortical carcinomas in the reference cohort.

Spindle Cell and Sarcomatoid Tumors

The most common primary pulmonary malignancy with a spindle cell or pleomorphic growth pattern is sarcomatoid bronchogenic carcinoma. It must be distinguished from primary and metastatic sarcomas and other types of malignant spindle cell tumors (e.g., sarcomatoid mesothelioma). Primary sarcomatoid carcinomas of the lung are extremely poorly differentiated, and many have been classified simply as "non–small cell carcinomas" in the past. Pathologic specimens of these tumors often show foci of spindle cell growth admixed with areas of more obvious epithelial differentiation ("biphasic" sarcomatoid carcinoma), but monomorphic examples with no epithelioid components are also seen ("monophasic" sarcomatoid carcinoma [Fig. 17-41]; see Chapter 14). Sarcomatoid carcinomas may contain homologous or heterologous foci of divergent mesenchymal-like differentiation. The latter resembles osteosarcoma, myogenous sarcoma, chondrosarcoma, and other forms of sarcoma (Figs. 17-42 and 17-43), potentiality further confusing the diagnostic picture. Primary neuroendocrine carcinoma, especially "spindle cell carcinoid," may also enter the differential diagnosis, but sarcomatoid carcinomas do not show the nuclear features seen in neuroendocrine lesions.

Table 17-4 shows the immunophenotypes of specific spindle cell tumors in the lung.[170] In practice, the number of antibodies applied in immunohistologic studies varies according to the clinicopathologic setting. The ultimate diagnosis of sarcomatoid pulmonary lesions may require extensive adjunctive pathologic analysis.

Most patients with clinically apparent, metastatic, intrapulmonary spindle cell malignancies have metastatic sarcomas. Secondary spindle cell carcinoma is unusual in the lungs. However, sarcomas are uncommon as well; only 5000 to 6000 new cases of sarcoma are seen each year in the United States.[171] In most cases of metastatic sarcoma in the lungs, a history of the tumor is well known when pulmonary involvement becomes apparent. Thus, there is no need to institute a search for the primary lesion. Solitary sarcomatous lesions of the lung and pleura are more difficult to recognize diagnostically because the sarcoma morphotypes that occur primarily in these locations are also seen in extrathoracic tissues and organs. That topic is discussed in detail in Chapter 14.

Extrathoracic sarcomas are associated with a high incidence of pulmonary metastasis overall. Autopsy series considering that point have found involvement of the lungs in up to 95% of cases.[172,173] Most metastatic sarcomas form multiple nodules in the pulmonary parenchymal or pleural surfaces, although solitary or multifocal endobronchial disease occasionally is seen.[174,175] Lymphatic spread of sarcomas is extremely unusual. Metastatic subpleural mesenchymal malignancies also may cavitate; this eventuality potentially causes pneumothorax formation or results in bronchopleural fistulae.[176–179] Foci of metastatic sarcoma may show a varied morphologic appearance, even if the primary lesion did not; this phenomenon, termed "clonal evolution" is well documented and may indicate aggressive tumor growth.[180] Irradiation and chemotherapy may facilitate its appearance.

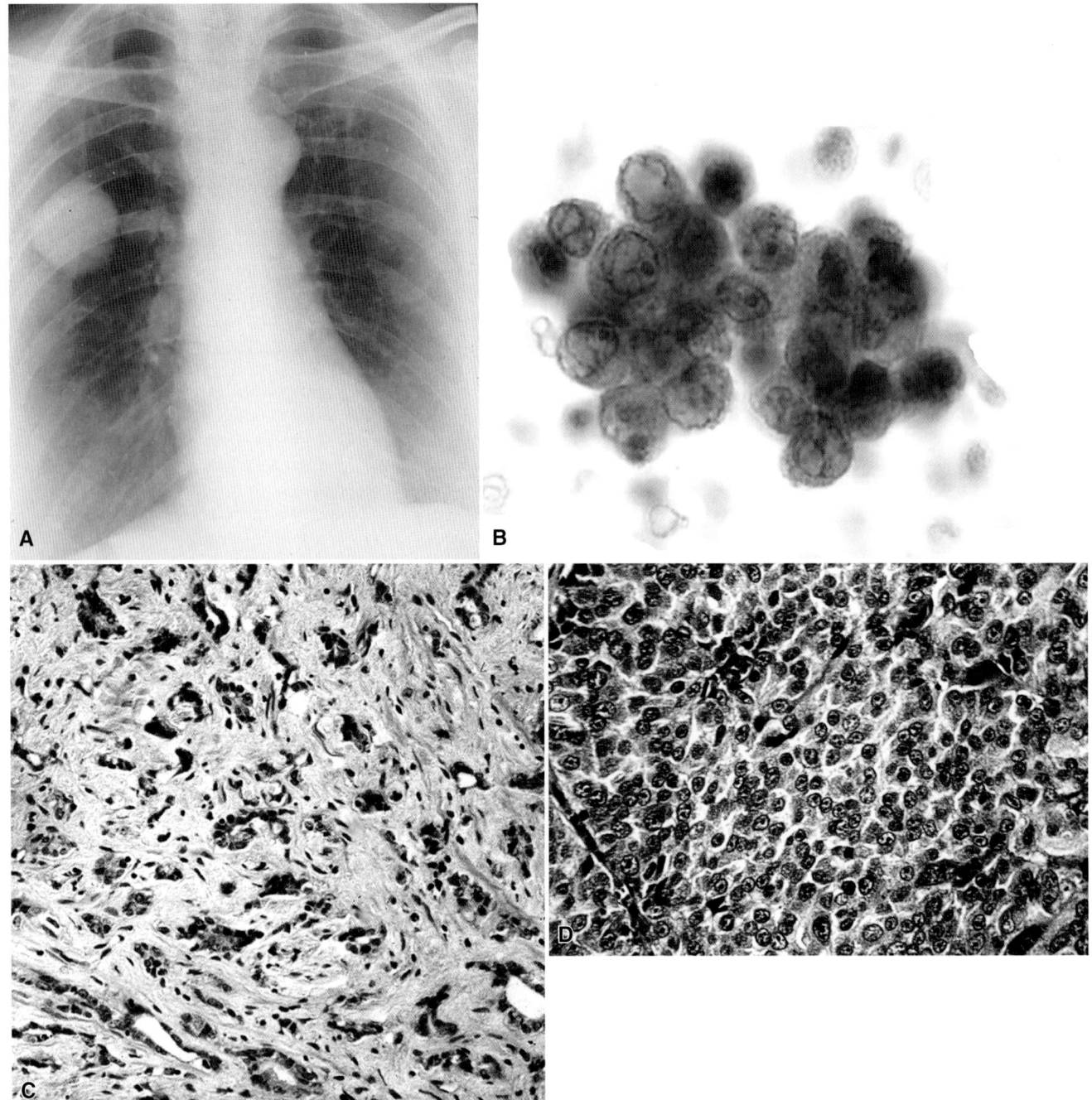

Figure 17-35. A, Chest radiograph showing multifocal metastatic prostatic adenocarcinoma in the lung. **B,** Fine-needle aspiration biopsy shows cohesive small cells with prominent nucleoli. Prostatic carcinoma of both intermediate (**C**) and high (**D**) Gleason scores can involve the lung parenchyma, albeit uncommonly.

Metastatic uterine smooth muscle tumors deserve special mention. Both high-grade leiomyosarcomas and low-grade myogenous tumors of the uterus (sometimes termed "metastasizing leiomyomas") may spread secondarily to the lungs.[181,182] In either instance, multiple and occasionally cystic nodular lesions are seen in the parenchyma and pleura; in rare cases, the metastatic tumor assumes a miliary pattern of spread.[183,184] Metastases of uterine smooth muscle neoplasms are usually seen in women of reproductive age or older,[185,186] but secondary intrapulmonary leiomyosarcoma has also been reported in men with primary soft tissue tumors.[185] Many of these patients have no symptoms, although dyspnea, cough, and cyanosis can be present. Some lesions may lead to respiratory failure.[185,187] Large

smooth muscle tumors can yield neoplastic emboli and tumor-related pulmonary infarction.[188]

Grossly, metastatic smooth muscle tumors are white and well circumscribed, with a "whorled" cut surface. Histologically, the constituent spindle cells may have a bland appearance, especially in "metastasizing uterine leiomyomas." In these lesions, mitoses are rare or absent (Fig. 17-44).[185,186] Other examples of secondary leiomyosarcoma are easily recognized as malignant lesions because of the degree of nuclear atypia and mitotic activity.

Some authors have suggested that "metastasizing leiomyomas" are actually multifocal pulmonary hamartomas rather than metastatic tumors. That argument has focused on the bland appearance

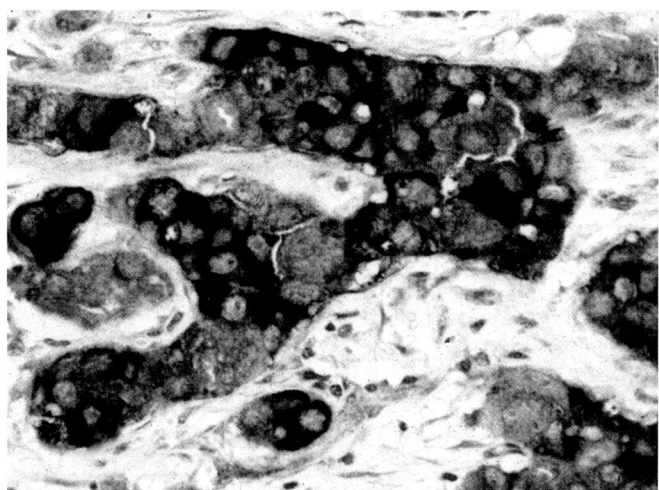

Figure 17-36. Immunoreactivity for prostate-specific antigen in metastatic prostatic adenocarcinoma.

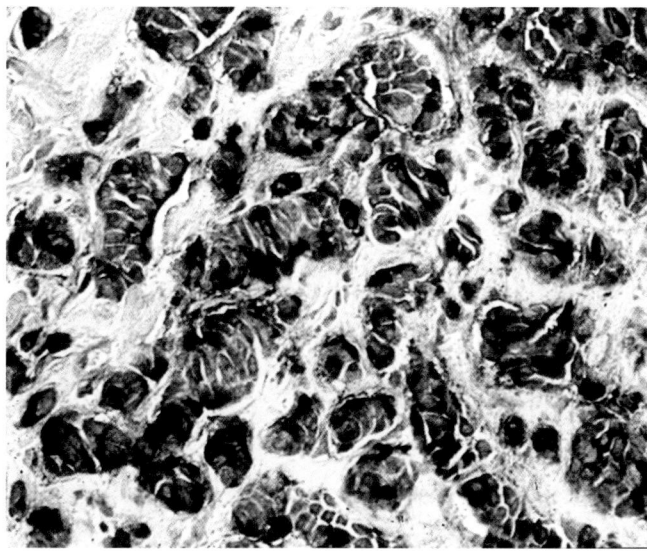

Figure 17-37. Immunoreactivity for prostate-specific membrane antigen in metastatic prostatic adenocarcinoma.

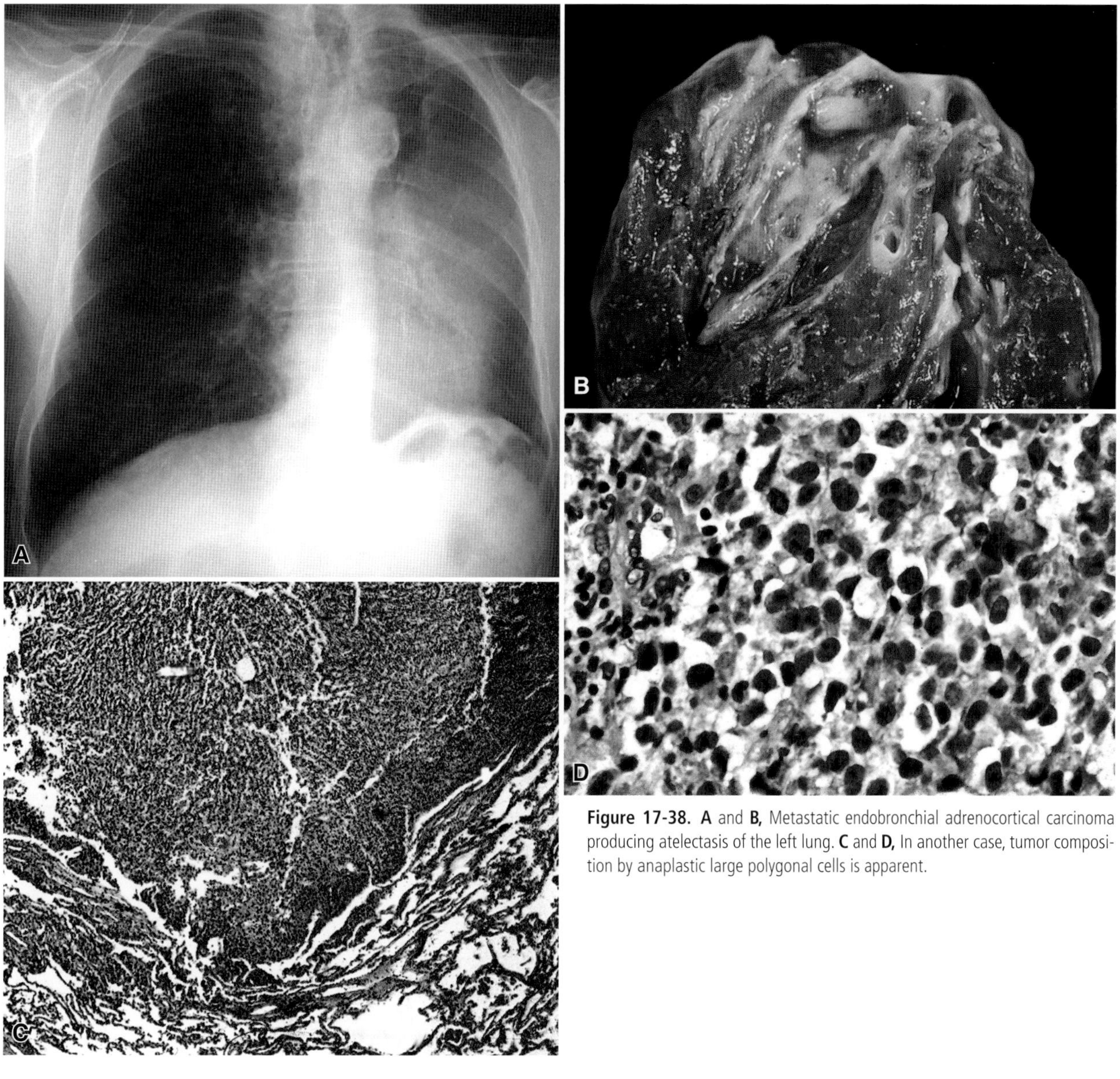

Figure 17-38. **A** and **B,** Metastatic endobronchial adrenocortical carcinoma producing atelectasis of the left lung. **C** and **D,** In another case, tumor composition by anaplastic large polygonal cells is apparent.

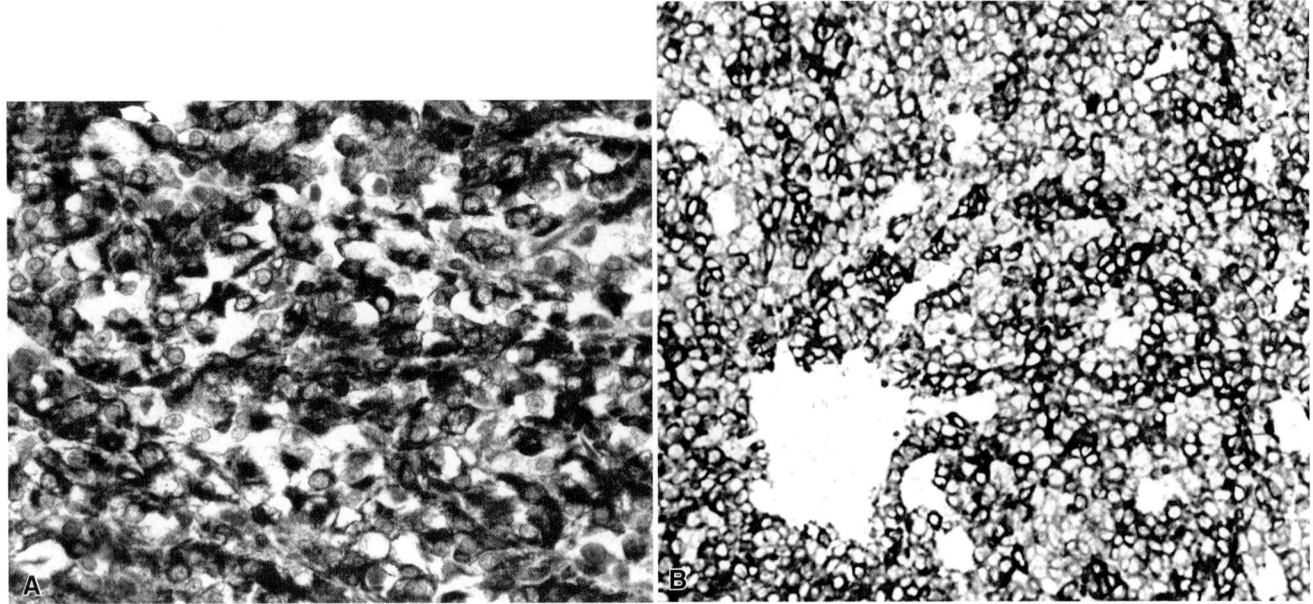

Figure 17-39. Immunoreactivity was seen for inhibin (**A**) and MART-1 (**B**) in the tumor shown in Figure 17-38B, consistent with an adrenocortical origin.

Tissue	Similarity score	Low	High
Colorectal	90.2		◊
Pancreas	2.4	◊	
Non–small cell carcinoma	2.3	◊	
Breast	2.1	◊	
Gastric	1.3	◊	
Kidney	0.6	◊	
Hepatocellular	0.3	◊	
Ovarian	0.3	◊	
Soft tissue sarcoma	0.1	◊	
Non-Hodgkin lymphoma	0.1	◊	
Thyroid	0.1	◊	
Prostate	0.1	◊	
Melanoma	0.1	◊	
Bladder	0.1	◊	
Testicular germ cell	0.0	◊	

Figure 17-40. Simplified report of genetic homology between a metastatic carcinoma of unknown origin in the lung and a reference group of carcinomas in various anatomic sites.

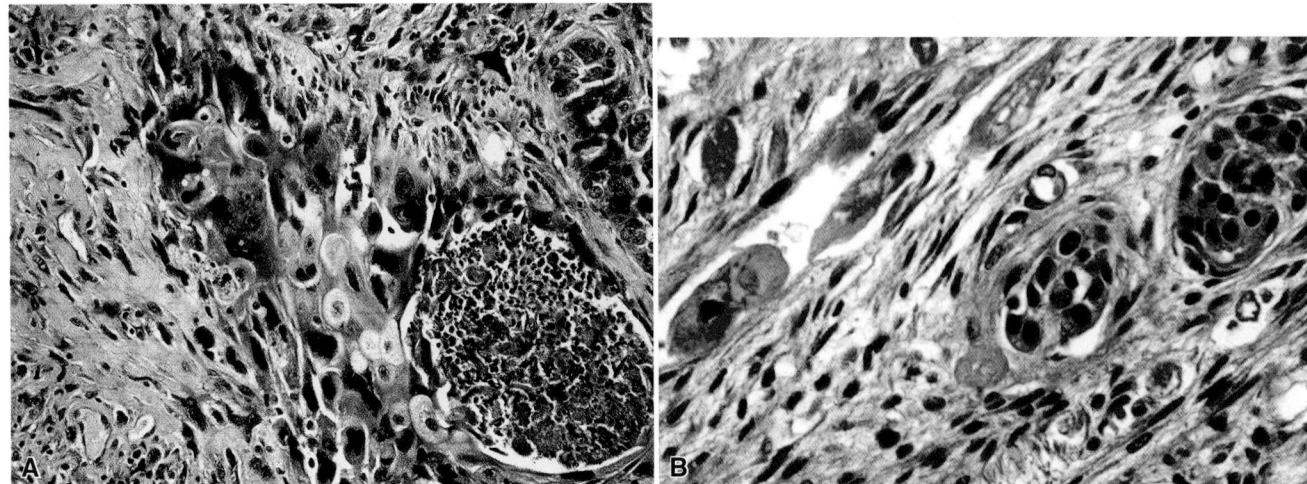

Figure 17-41. A, Metastatic biphasic sarcomatoid carcinoma of thyroidal origin involving the lung. **B,** Another view of the lesion shows the juxtaposition of sarcoma-like elements, including rhabdomyoblasts (*top left*) and obvious carcinoma (*bottom right*).

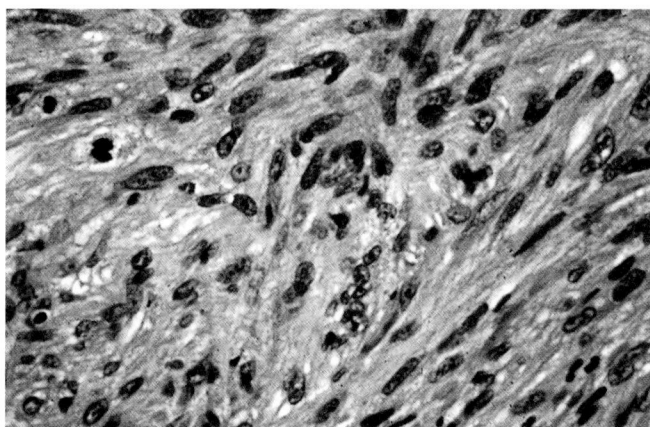

Figure 17-42. Metastatic monophasic sarcomatoid carcinoma comprising fusiform cells with no obvious sign of epithelial differentiation. Distinction from carcinoma is virtually impossible with conventional morphologic studies.

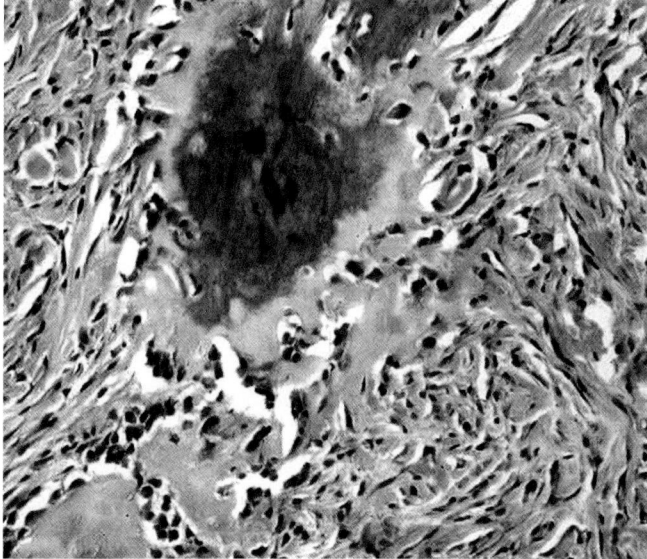

Figure 17-43. Divergent osseous differentiation is seen in this metastatic sarcomatoid carcinoma of uterine origin, involving the lung.

of the smooth muscle cells, the lack of mitoses, and the occasional presence of admixed glandular elements. Even so, the authors believe that "metastasizing leiomyomas" are a separate pathologic entity,[185] based partly on aggregated clinicopathologic information. Most patients with such lesions have a history of surgical removal of uterine smooth muscle tumors (usually diagnosed as leiomyomas) or neoplasms of that type are found at autopsy. Synchronous metastatic implants have also been seen in abdominal, retroperitoneal, and pelvic soft tissue and lymph nodes in women who have "metastasizing leiomyomas" in the lungs.[189] The argument that these intrapulmonary smooth muscle tumors are derived from uterine lesions gained strong support from a study by Patton and colleagues.[190] Through paired analysis of uterine and pulmonary neoplasms in the same patients, they showed that the lesions were clonal by assessing a nucleotide sequence from the human androgen receptor gene and measuring telomere lengths.

In postmenopausal women, metastatic lesions tend to be slowly growing or static. They are associated with more rapid evolution and

pulmonary morbidity in premenopausal patients. Some may even cause death. "Metastasizing leiomyomas" must be distinguished from lymphangioleiomyomatosis of the lungs, a condition that is discussed in detail in Chapter 7.

Malignant Small Round Cell Tumors

Malignant small round cell tumors prototypically are composed of cells with round to oval nuclei, scant cytoplasm, and extensive cellular dissociation. Scanning microscopy often shows a "sheet" of nuclei; these neoplasms are sometimes termed "small blue cell" malignancies. An organoid growth pattern is also potentially apparent (Figs. 17-45 and 17-46). The primary pleuropulmonary lesions in this category include neuroendocrine carcinomas, malignant lymphomas, and rare malignancies, such as Askin tumor or small cell mesothelioma. Metastatic small round cell tumors also include neuroendocrine carcinomas of extrapulmonary sites and malignant

Table 17-4. Immunohistologic Differential Diagnosis of Spindle Cell Malignancies in the Lung

Tumor	Antibody										
	VIM	CEA	PK	ACT	CALR	CD31	CD34	S-100	MART	CD99	EMA
Carcinoma	P	PN	PN	N	N	N	N	N	N	N	PN
Mesothelioma	P	N	PN	PN	PN	N	N	N	N	PN	PN
Melanoma	P	N	N	N	N	N	N	P	PN	PN	N
Synovial sarcoma	P	PN	PN	PN	PN	N	N	N	N	PN	PN
MPSNT	P	N	PN	PN	PN	N	PN	PN	N	N	PN
Leiomyosarcoma	P	N	PN	P	N	N	PN	N	N	N	N
Angiosarcoma	P	PN	PN	PN	N	PN	PN	N	N	N	N
Kaposi sarcoma	P	N	N	PN	N	PN	P	N	N	N	N
MFH	P	N	PN	PN	N	N	PN	N	N	PN	PN

ACT, actin; CALR, calretinin; CEA, carcinoembryonic antigen; EMA, epithelial membrane antigen; MART, MART-1; MFH, malignant fibrous histiocytoma; MPNST, malignant peripheral nerve sheath tumor; N, negative (<10% of cases); P, positive (>80% of cases); PK, pan-keratin; PN, variably positive (10–80% of cases); S-100, S-100 protein; VIM, vimentin.

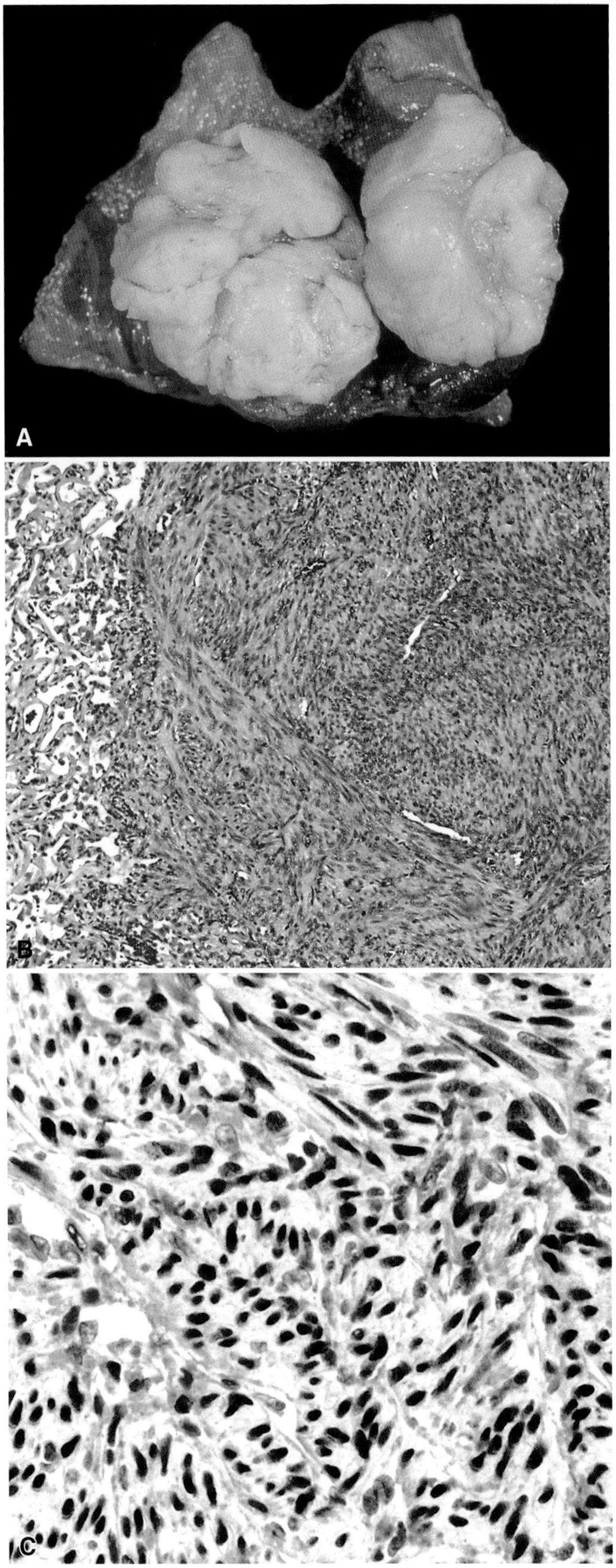

Figure 17-44. A to **C,** "Metastasizing leiomyoma" of the uterus involving the lung. There is no appreciable nuclear atypia or mitotic activity in this bland spindle cell proliferation.

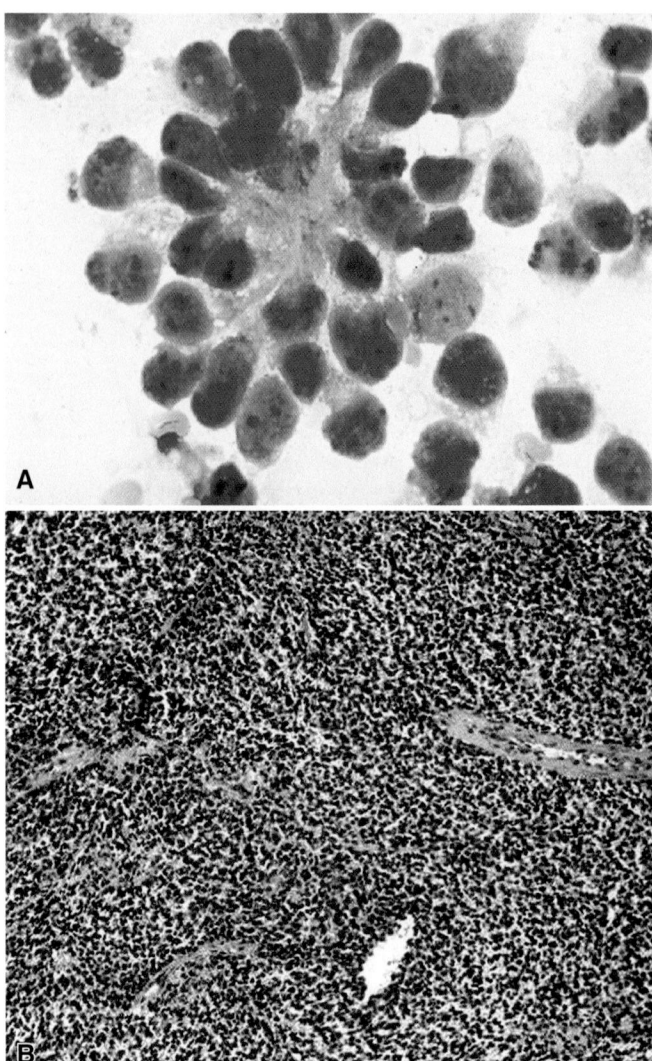

Figure 17-45. A, Fine-needle aspiration biopsy of a primitive neuroectodermal tumor metastatic to the lungs from a primary site in the chest wall. Relatively uniform small cells mold to one another and show small nucleoli with dispersed chromatin. **B,** The original biopsy specimen shows sheets of small round cells transected by a delicate fibrovascular stroma.

lymphomas, but additional sarcomas and other tumor types must also be considered (e.g., malignant melanoma, rhabdomyosarcoma, mesenchymal chondrosarcoma, small cell osteosarcoma, hepatoblastoma, neuroblastoma, and Wilms tumor). Selected primary and secondary non-neuroendocrine carcinomas also may have a small cell composition.[191,192]

The most common primary intrathoracic small round cell malignancy is small cell neuroendocrine carcinoma of the lung (SCNCL).[192] This tumor is histologically and cytologically identical to small cell carcinoma originating in other sites (Figs. 17-47 and 17-48). Clinically, most SCNCLs are centrally located and accompanied by enlarged mediastinal lymph nodes; they quickly metastasize and are usually advanced in stage at diagnosis. Regardless of their anatomic origins, metastatic foci of small cell neuroendocrine carcinoma (SCNC) are typically characterized radiographically by multiple intrapulmonaory masses; mediastinal involvement is often lacking when the tumor has arisen outside the lungs. The morphologic

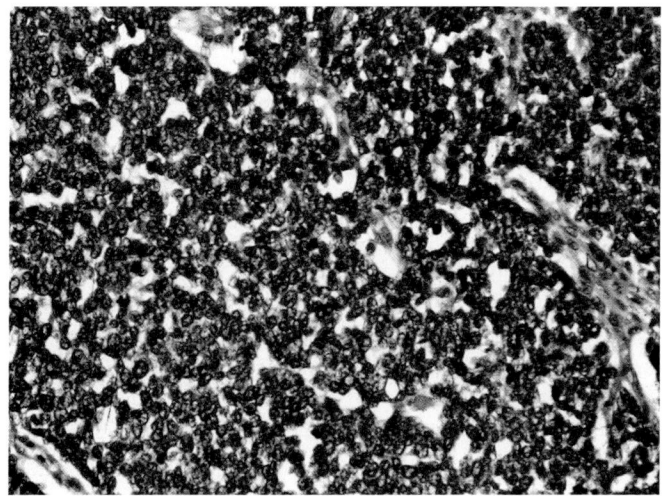

Figure 17-46. Primitive rosette formation is apparent in a primitive neuroectodermal tumor.

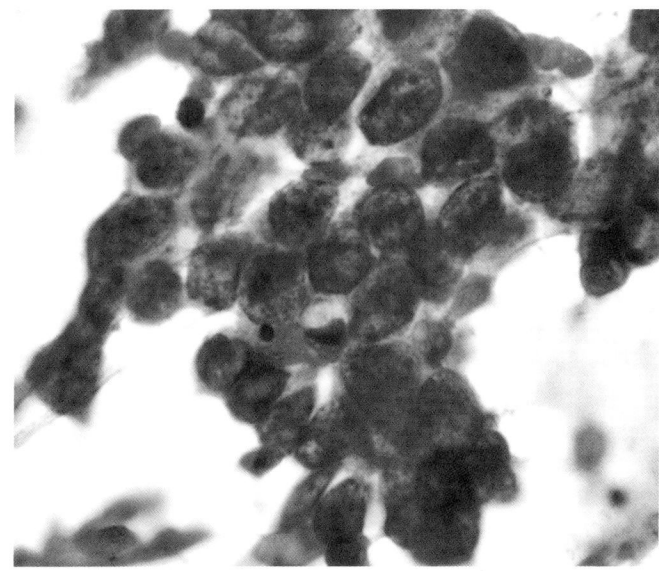

Figure 17-47. Metastatic Merkel cell carcinoma of the skin involving the lung. Fine-needle aspirate shows tumor cells with scant cytoplasm and nuclear molding.

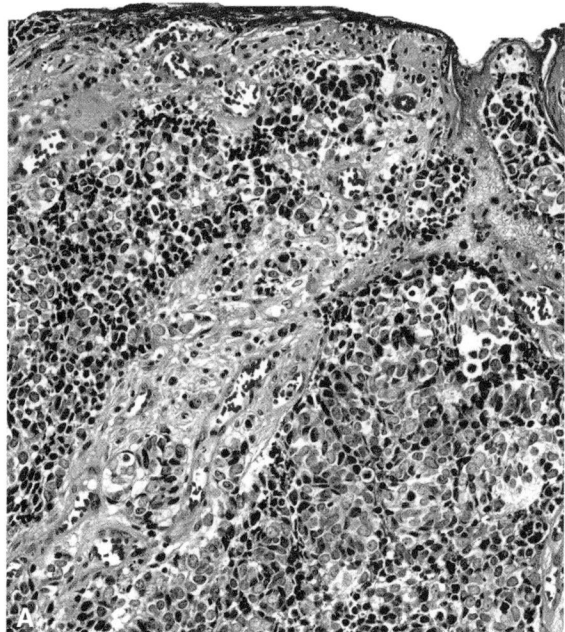

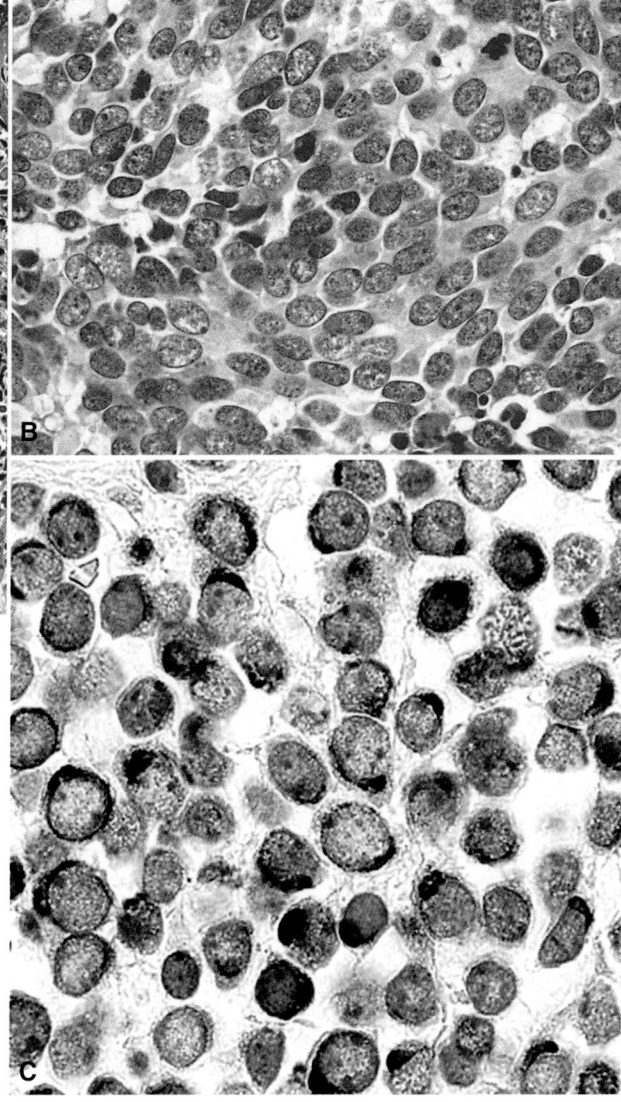

Figure 17-48. **A** and **B,** The primary tumor of the skin is seen, corresponding to the lesion shown in Figure 17-47. **C,** Both the primary and secondary lesions expressed cytokeratin-20, shown here.

features of these lesions include granular dispersed nuclear chromatin, nuclear fragility, nuclear molding, and cellular clumping. Those attributes are generally associated with neuroendocrine differentiation. Immunopathologically, SCNCs often show a characteristic reactivity pattern for keratin, with dot-like perinuclear labeling. They may or may not show additional positivity for synaptophysin, chromogranin-A, CD56, CD57, and neuron-specific enolase. Byrd-Gloster and coworkers reported that 97% of SCNCLs were reactive for thyroid transcription factor-1, whereas most (but not all) SCNCs of nonpulmonary derivation lacked that marker.[193] On the other hand, cytokeratin 20 positivity is potentially seen in primary extrathoracic SCNCs, but it is uncommon in primary pulmonary small cell carcinoma.[194,195] SCNC of the lung and other sites may also contain a non–small cell component ("composite" or "combined" SCNCL; see Chapter 13).

Metastatic well- or moderately differentiated neuroendocrine carcinomas in the lung include "carcinoids" of gastrointestinal, uterine cervical, or other topographic derivations; neuroendocrine pancreatic tumors; and medullary thyroid carcinomas (Fig. 17-49).[196,197] Many of those tumors are associated with specific symptoms because of their production of various neuropeptides or amines. However, in histologic or cytologic specimens, such lesions are potentially identical to primary neuroendocrine neoplasms of the lung. Data on discriminating immunostains are still evolving for this group of tumors, but thyroid transcription factor-1 reactivity again may favor a pulmonary origin.[198] Histochemical evaluations are still helpful in a proportion of cases; most pulmonary neuroendocrine tumors are argyrophilic (e.g., with the Grimelius method) but nonargentaffinic (with Fontana-Masson stain).[199] Hence, strong argentaffinity in a carcinoid tumor suggests an origin outside the lungs.

Parathyroid carcinoma is a rare, progressive, but often indolent neoplasm that metastasizes to the lung in approximately 33% of cases.[200,201] Metastatic parathyroid carcinoma may mimic a primary lung carcinoid

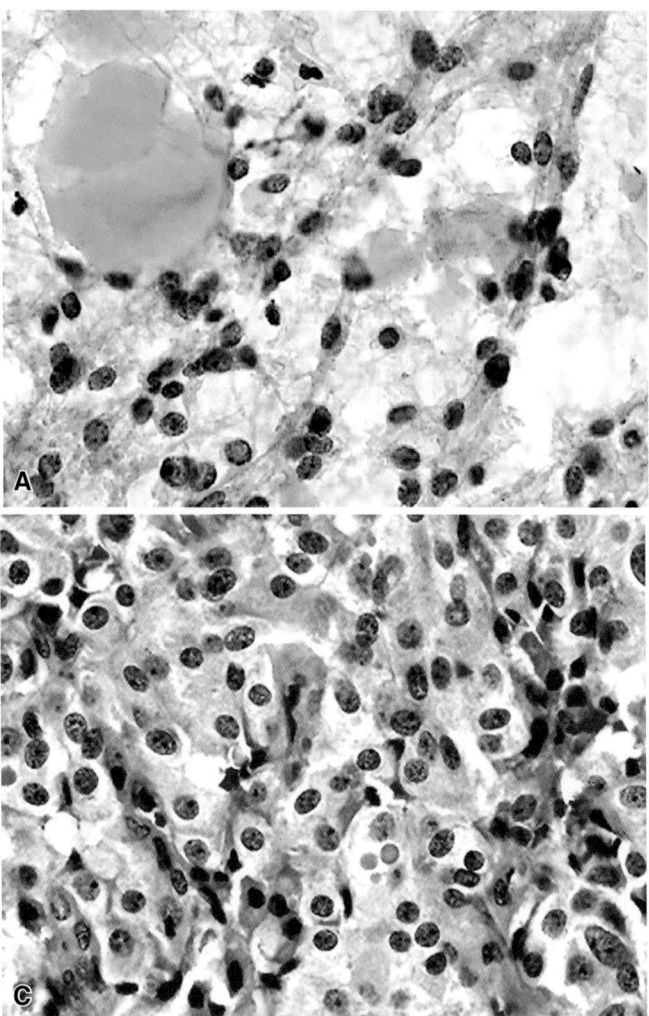

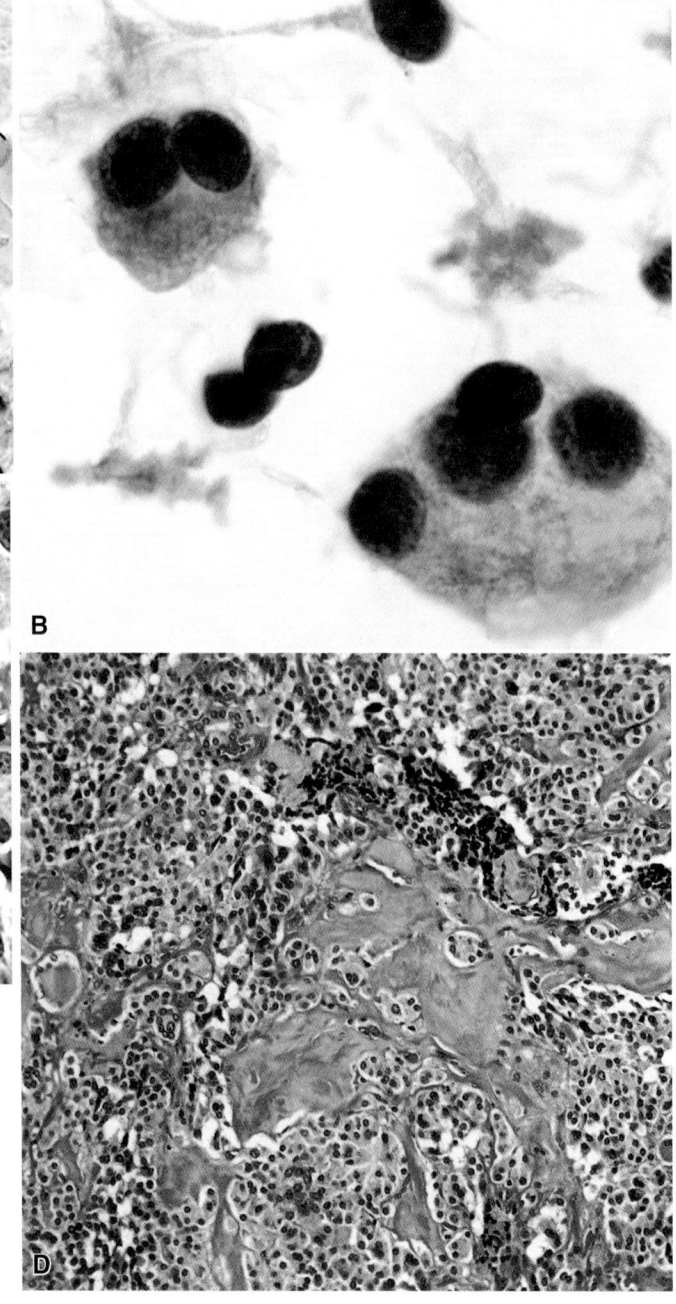

Figure 17-49. A, Slightly fusiform tumor cells and globular extracellular material representing amyloid in metastatic medullary thyroid carcinoma. **B,** Multinucleated and plasmacytoid mononuclear tumor cells are seen in this fine-needle aspirate of metastatic medullary thyroid carcinoma involving the lung. **C** and **D,** The primary tumor is seen, showing an organoid growth pattern and production of stromal amyloid.

tumor. Although most patients with metastatic parathyroid carcinoma to the lung have a history of primary parathyroid carcinoma and these cases are not diagnostically challenging, in some patients, lung metastases may occur several years after surgical resection of the primary parathyroid tumor. When a clinical history of parathyroid carcinoma is not apparent, metastatic parathyroid carcinoma to the lung may be confused with a primary lung carcinoid tumor. Immunostain with parathyroid hormone should be positive in tumor cells, and serum calcium levels may be elevated.[200,201]

Primary pulmonary lymphomas are discussed in Chapter 15, but most malignant lymphoid tumors of the lung are secondary lesions that occur in the context of systemic dissemination. Primary malignant lymphomas in this organ are typically low grade, whereas secondary hematolymphoid malignancies may represent any histologic subtype and grade. For example, 30% of patients with mediastinal Hodgkin lymphoma have lung involvement by direct extension.[202] Malignant lymphomas that secondarily affect the pulmonary parenchyma are not believed to be truly metastatic because they populate lymphoid structures that are normally present in the lungs and pleura. One form of lymphomatous involvement is characterized by diffuse interstitial lymphocytic permeation, with focal formation of micronodules (Fig. 17-50).[203,204]

When the constituent cells are relatively mature, the image of "lymphocytic interstitial pneumonia" may be obtained (see Chapters 7 and 15). However, discrete nodules also may occur, especially with high-grade large-cell neoplasms (Fig. 17-51), and these commonly simulate metastatic nonhematopoietic lesions clinically and pathologically.

Involvement of the pleura may be unilateral or bilateral in malignant lymphoma, but lymphoma and metastatic carcinoma are the two most common causes of malignant bilateral pleural effusion.[39] In cytologic practice, it is difficult to be certain that effusion specimens containing atypical lymphoid cells are definitively positive for lymphoma; such cells may represent contamination of the sample by lymphocytes from the peripheral blood, and especially when they are relatively mature, discrimination from other causes of lymphoid pleural effusion depends mainly on the findings of adjunctive studies.[205] Flow cytometry is probably optimally suited for this application.[206]

In the pediatric age group, some small round cell malignancies may metastasize to the lungs, as cited earlier (Fig. 17-52). Immunohistochemical studies and electron microscopy are helpful in differentiating these lesions in difficult cases.[191] Cytogenetic analyses may also be extremely valuable. Table 17-5 shows the immunopathologic profile of several primary and secondary small round cell tumors.[191]

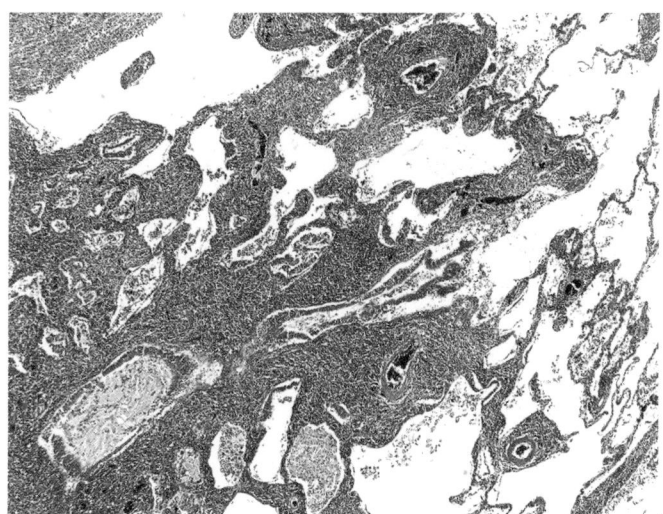

Figure 17-50. Micronodular arrays of small lymphocytes are seen in the pulmonary interstitium in this example of mucosal-type lymphoma involving the lungs.

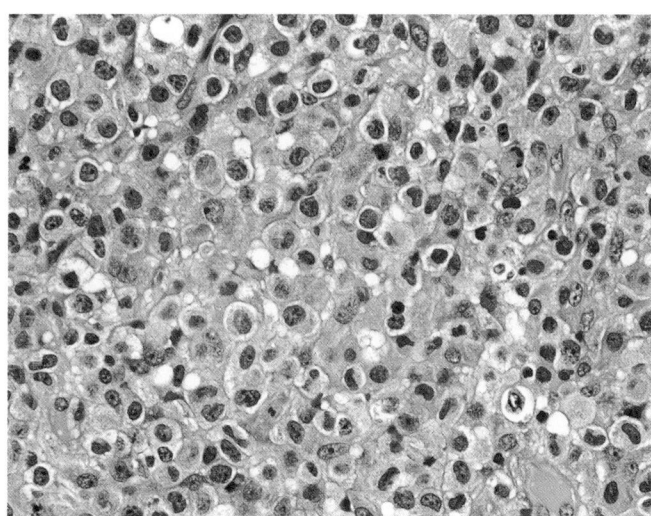

Figure 17-51. Nodules of anaplastic polygonal cells are seen in this case of large-cell non-Hodgkin lymphoma involving the lungs.

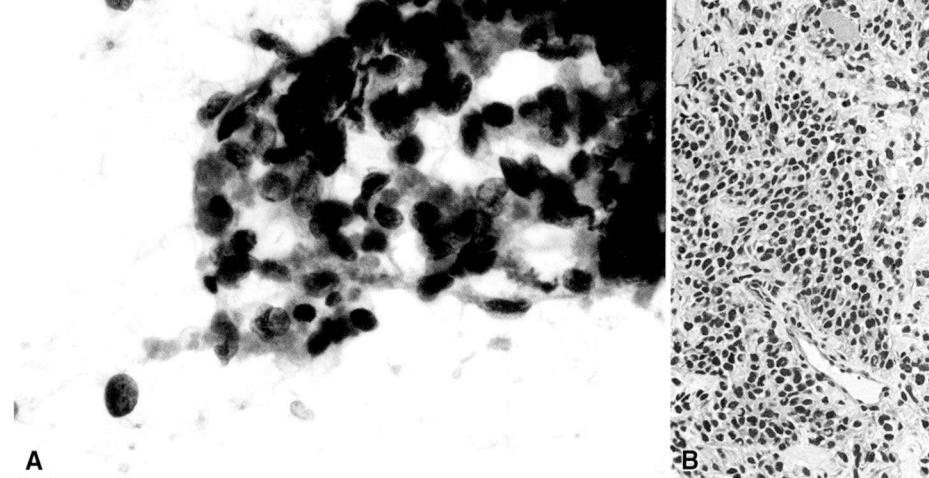

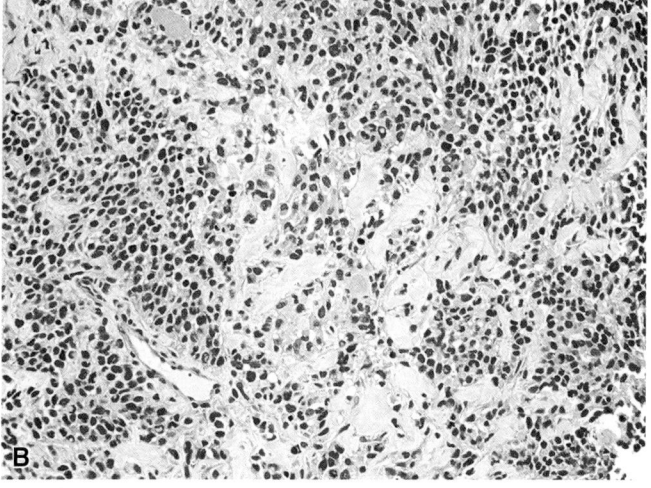

Figure 17-52. Metastatic alveolar rhabdomyosarcoma in the lung in a child. The tumor is composed of sheets of small round undifferentiated cells. **A,** Fine-needle aspirate. **B,** Biopsy specimen.

Squamous Cell Carcinomas and Morphologic Simulants

The differential diagnosis of primary squamous cell carcinomas of the lung obviously includes secondary carcinomas with squamous differentiation as well as other epithelioid malignancies with "metaplastic" or "hard" eosinophilic cytoplasm. Examples are transitional cell carcinoma and selected cases of malignant melanoma.

Based on morphologic findings alone, the site of origin for squamous cell carcinoma (SCC) is impossible to determine with certainty (Figs. 17-53 and 17-54). Most squamous carcinomas in the lung

Table 17-5. Immunohistologic Differential Diagnosis of Small Round Cell Malignancies in the Lung

Tumor	Antibodies								
	VIM	PK	S-100	TTF1	CD45	CD56	DES	SYN	CD
Small cell NE carcinoma	N	P	N	P	N	PN	N	PN	PN
Rhabdomyosarcoma	P	N	N	N	N	N	P	N	PN
Non-Hodgkin lymphoma	P	N	N	N	P	N	N	N	N
Malignant melanoma	P	N	P	N	N	N	N	N	N
Ewing sarcoma/PNET	PN	N	N	N	N	PN	N	PN	P
Metastatic NE carcinomas	N	P	N	PN	N	PN	N	PN	PN
Metastatic neuroblastoma	PN	N	N	N	N	P	N	P	N

DES, desmin; N, negative (<10% of cases); NE, neuroendocrine; P, positive (>80% of cases); PK, pan-keratin; PN, variably positive (10–80% of cases); PNET, primitive neuroectodermal tumor; S-100, S-100 protein; SYN, synaptophysin; TTF1, thyroid transcription factor-1; VIM, vimentin.

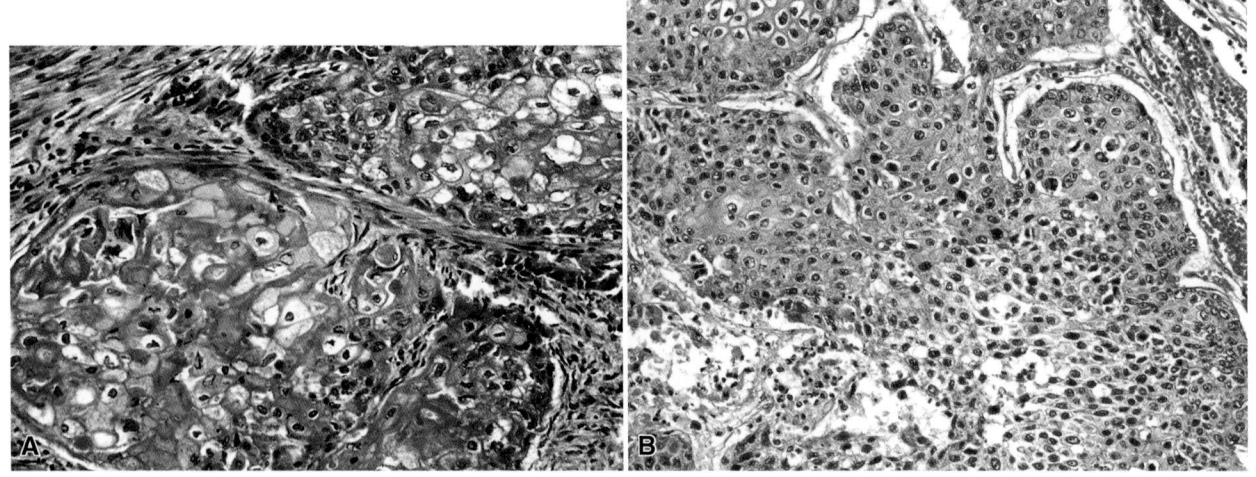

Figure 17-53. Metastatic well-differentiated (**A**) and moderately differentiated (**B**) squamous cell carcinoma of the head and neck involving the lungs. These tumors cannot be distinguished reliably from primary squamous pulmonary carcinomas.

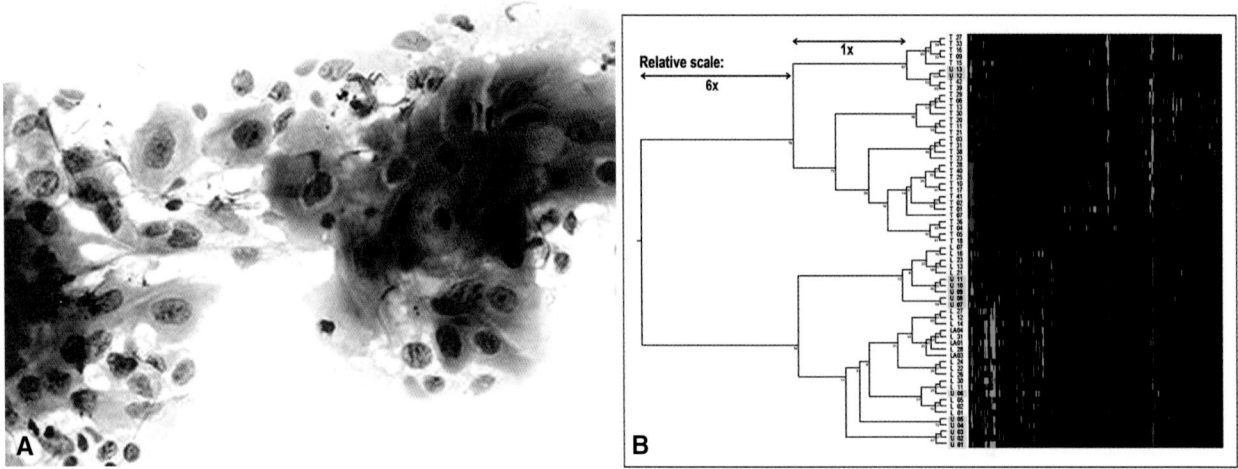

Figure 17-54. A, The fine-needle aspiration biopsy image of these tumors is comparable in primary and secondary lesions. **B,** Hierarchical segregation of gene sets allows for diagnostic separation of primary from secondary squamous carcinomas in the lung.

have arisen there, and although multifocal SCCs suggest metastatic disease, that picture is also seen with multiple primary synchronous bronchogenic carcinomas. The usual sources of metastatic SCC in the lung are mucosal sites of the head and neck, esophagus, uterine cervix, and skin.

Squamous cell carcinomas of the head and neck that involve the lungs may originate in the larynx, nasopharynx, oropharynx, or hypopharynx, and lesions in the lungs may be single or multiple.[83,207,208] Because all of these tumors are associated with the use of alcohol or tobacco or with infection with human papillomavirus, patients with squamous cell carcinoma in one of the specified locations also commonly have separate metachronous or synchronous primary squamous malignancies in other mucosal sites or in the lungs.[209] In patients with both pulmonary lesions and SCC in the head or neck, Malfetto and colleagues reported that 53% had separate primary bronchogenic carcinomas and 19% had metastatic SCC in the lung.[209] Cervical lymph nodal involvement is also present in up to 80% of cases of metastatic intrapulmonary SCC.[83,84] The cumulative incidence of second malignancies in patients who have SCC of the head and neck is approximately 4% per year, and 30% of these tumors arise in the lungs.[210]

Sostman and Matthay reported that uterine cervical squamous cell carcinomas spread to the lungs less frequently (4%) than cervical adenocarcinomas do (20%).[211] In most cases, single or multiple lesions are present, and as with all squamous cell carcinomas, there is a tendency toward cavitation.[212,213] Metastatic cervical SCC also may involve pulmonary hilar or mediastinal lymph nodes, endobronchial mucosal sites,[214,215] or the intrapulmonary lymphatics.[29,216]

"Gene profiling" has also been used in this context to differentiate metastatic SCC from primary pulmonary SCC. Vachani and coworkers[217] used a selected 10-gene panel, achieving 96% accuracy among 122 cases. A hierarchical segregation of the genes in that data set is shown in Figure 17-54. Girard and associates showed that the same end can be achieved by scrupulous histologic assessment, focusing on tumor grade, cytologic features, stromal patterns, and the extent of necrosis.[218] In that study, the concordance between histologic predictions and genomic profiling was approximately 90%.

Pragmatically speaking, in the setting of an intraoperative consultation, one is often asked to decide whether a solitary squamous lung tumor is primary or metastatic in a patient with a history of squamous carcinoma elsewhere. If the radiographic and macroscopic features of the lesion are indeterminate, it is the authors' practice to defer the answer until later. The surgeon is then counseled to perform a procedure that is conservative but would be sufficient in the treatment of a primary lung carcinoma (e.g., wedge excision), with the working premise ethat the neoplasm is primary. If the neoplasm proves to be metastatic after further studies are obtained, no harm has been done to the patient. The same approach applies to tumors with nonsquamous lineages, especially if microscopic sections of previous malignancies are unavailable for comparison.

Metastatic malignant melanoma has a myriad of histologic and cytologic appearances. For this reason, it may be considered in the differential diagnosis with selected adenocarcinomas, malignant small round cell tumors, spindle cell neoplasms, large polygonal cell malignancies, and some squamous cell carcinomas. The appearance of single cells with "metaplastic" cytoplasm, large ovoid nuclei, and prominent nucleoli is common in the cytologic evaluation of malignant melanoma (Figs. 17-55 and 17-56). Melanin production is a helpful clue to the identity of this tumor (Fig. 17-57), but it may be confused with other pigments, such as hemosiderin, and it requires histochemical verification. A history of ocular, cutaneous, or mucosal melanoma is often known when that neoplasm involves the lungs metastatically. However, some metastatic melanomas represent the initial signs of that tumor.

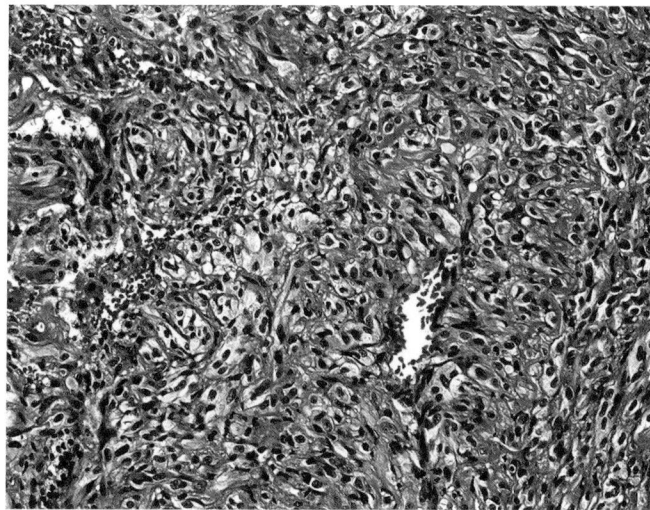

Figure 17-55. Metastatic malignant melanoma in the lung parenchyma. The tumor is composed of large anaplastic polyhedral cells; melanin pigment is scarce.

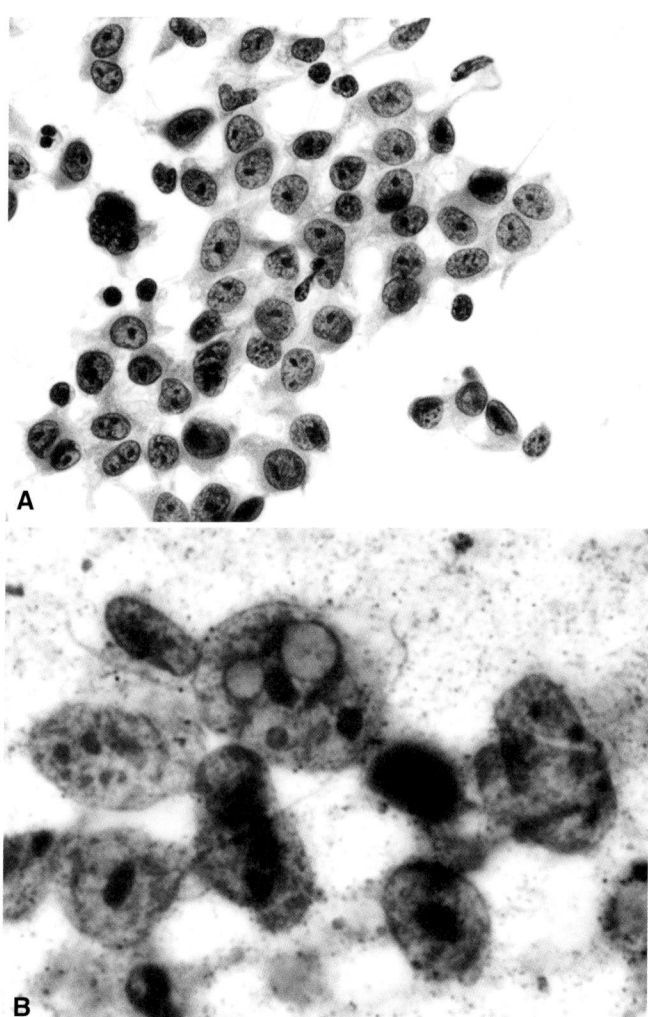

Figure 17-56. A, Fine-needle aspiration biopsy of metastatic melanoma showing dyshesive tumor cells with high nucleocytoplasmic ratios. **B,** Some of the neoplastic cells contain intranuclear invaginations of cytoplasm.

Continued

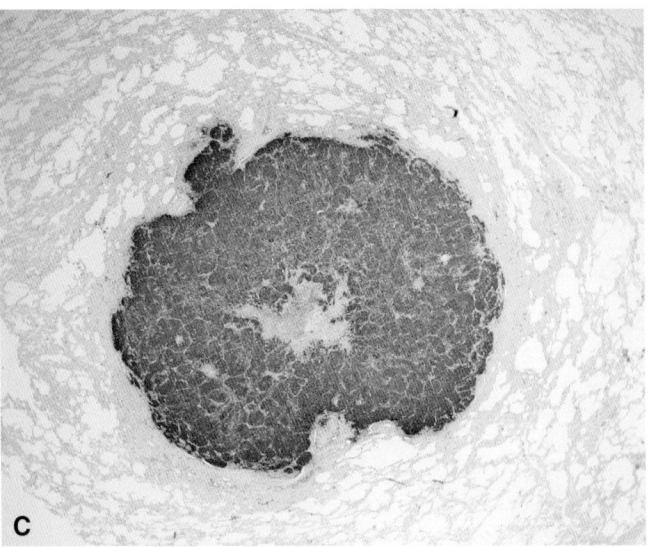

Figure 17-56—cont'd. C, S-100 immunostain highlights the smooth tumor margin of this metastatic melanoma.

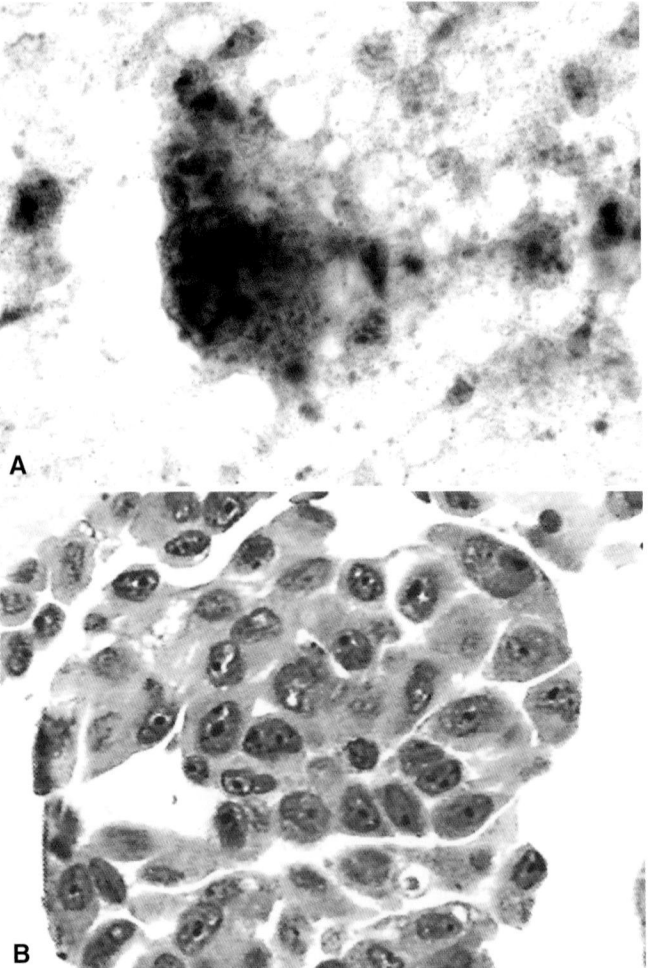

Figure 17-57. A, Melanin pigment is seen in this fine-needle aspirate of metastatic melanoma. **B,** The tumor is amelanotic in the cytologic cell block preparation.

Virtually all examples of melanoma in the lungs and pleura are metastatic; only anecdotal examples of primary pulmonary malignancies with melanocytic differentiation have been documented.[219] Metastatic melanomas usually involve multiple organs, but DasGupta and Brasfield found that the lungs were involved in 70% of cases.[220] Secondary lesions usually have multiple intrapulmonary nodules, but solitary lesions, lymphangitic or miliary disease, or endobronchial implants may also be seen.[221–224] Balch and coworkers reported that a solitary pulmonary mass was the first evidence of metastatic disease in 38% of cases.[225] Conversely, Pogrebniak and colleagues found that 33% of lung nodules in patients with melanoma were unrelated and benign.[226]

Metastatic transitional cell carcinomas (TCCs) of the urinary tract often have a squamoid cytoplasmic appearance, and true squamous differentiation also may be seen. Cytologic specimens show extensive cellular dyshesion and necrosis. Some authors have reported that cercariform cells—containing nucleated globular bodies and bulbous cytoplasmic processes—suggest metastatic TCC.[99,227] These tumors often form mass lesions in the lungs and also can spread lymphangitically.

Table 17-6 shows the immunopathologic profile of squamous cell carcinomas, based on their sites of origin; the immunophenotypes of their morphologic mimics are also included. If metastatic malignant melanoma is included in the differential diagnosis, it can be easily characterized by its reactivity for S-100 protein, HMB-45, MART-1, and tyrosinase.[228] TCCs may label for cytokeratin 20, but are negative for cytokeratin 7 in most cases; this profile is the opposite of that seen in primary pulmonary adenocarcinoma.[145,229–231] Thrombomodulin (CD141) is potentially shared by both of the latter tumors, but it is more commonly present in TCC. Similarly, p63 protein is present in TCC, but not in most adenocarcinomas. Squamous cell carcinomas of all sites share with TCC the potential for thrombomodulin and p63 reactivity, but the two may be distinguished by selective immunoreactivity for uroplakin in TCC.[232]

Table 17-6. Immunohistologic Differential Diagnosis of Squamous Cell Carcinomas and Their Potential Simulators

Tumor	Antibody			
	TBM	CK5/6 or P63	S-100	EMA
Squamous cell carcinoma of lung	PN	P	N	PN
Squamous cell carcinoma of cervix	PN	P	N	PN
Squamous cell carcinoma of head and neck	PN	P	N	PN
Squamous cell carcinoma of esophagus	PN	P	N	PN
Melanoma	N	N	P	N
Transitional cell carcinoma	P	P	N	P
"Squamoid" hepatocellular carcinoma	N	N	N	N

CK5/6, cytokeratin 5/6; EMA, epithelial membrane antigen; N, negative (<10% of cases); P, positive (>80% of cases); PN, variably positive (10–80% of cases); S-100, S-100 protein; TBM, thrombomodulin.

Undifferentiated Large Polygonal Cell Malignancies

Undifferentiated large polygonal cell tumors of the lung include primary large cell carcinomas, malignant lymphomas, metastatic malignant melanoma, metastatic germ cell tumors, metastatic "histiocytoid" malignant fibrous histiocytoma, metastatic epithelioid sarcoma, metastatic alveolar soft tissue sarcoma, metastatic adrenocortical carcinoma, and other secondary carcinomas and sarcomas. The diagnostic difficulty associated with this group of tumors is associated with their anaplastic appearance, which often defies a determination of basic lineage.

Ultrastructural studies have shown that primary large cell carcinomas of the lung often show squamous or glandular differentiation; these features may be seen focally in histologic or cytologic preparations. As their name implies, the cells that make up these tumors contain a relatively large amount of cytoplasm and correspondingly large nuclei. In cytologic specimens, some large cell carcinomas show significant cellular dyshesion (Fig. 17-58). Clinically, they are often bulky masses associated with mediastinal lymphadenopathy. Primary large cell carcinomas of the lung have an immunopathologic profile that is similar to that of other primary non–small cell carcinomas.

Many of the other neoplasms in the differential diagnosis were discussed previously. Sarcomas that imitate primary large cell carcinomas have an epithelioid appearance, but except for epithelioid sarcoma and epithelioid synovial sarcoma, they are nonreactive for keratin immunohistochemically. Mesenchymal malignancies usually do not present with pulmonary metastases, with the possible exception of alveolar soft tissue sarcoma and some examples of malignant fibrous histiocytoma.

The primary foci of those tumors may be occult, yet produce extensive distant disease in the lungs, brain, and other organs.[232-234]

Poorly differentiated adrenocortical carcinomas may show lipidized cytoplasm, which is an unusual feature in primary large cell carcinoma. The most common metastatic germ cell malignancies that simulate primary pulmonary large cell carcinoma are embryonal carcinoma (Fig. 17-59) and choriocarcinoma. When these neoplasms metastasize, they are often admixed with other germ cell components, such as seminoma or teratoma, features that help to distinguish them from other large polygonal cell tumors. The clinical history of patients with secondary germ cell lesions is often distinctive, vis-à-vis that which accompanies primary lung cancers. For example, metastatic choriocarcinomas are most commonly seen in young women,[235] whereas primary large cell carcinomas more often occur in older patients with a significant smoking history.[236] Furthermore, individuals with metastatic choriocarcinoma typically have multiple lung lesions[237] and an elevated level of β-human chorionic gonadotropin in the serum. Secondary embryonal carcinomas are usually seen in men, who also have gonadal, intracranial, mediastinal, or retroperitoneal masses.

The histologic image of metastatic germ cell tumors is often sufficient for their definitive recognition, especially when it includes two or more morphologic subtypes of such lesions. Moreover, yolk sac tumor commonly shows distinctive intercellular and intracytoplasmic eosinophilic globules, and choriocarcinoma is singular in its biphasic composition by cytotrophoblastic and syncytiotrophoblastic elements (Fig. 17-60). Nevertheless, the existence of primary somatic carcinomas of the lung with areas resembling germ cell tumor confounds the evaluation of these lesions.[238]

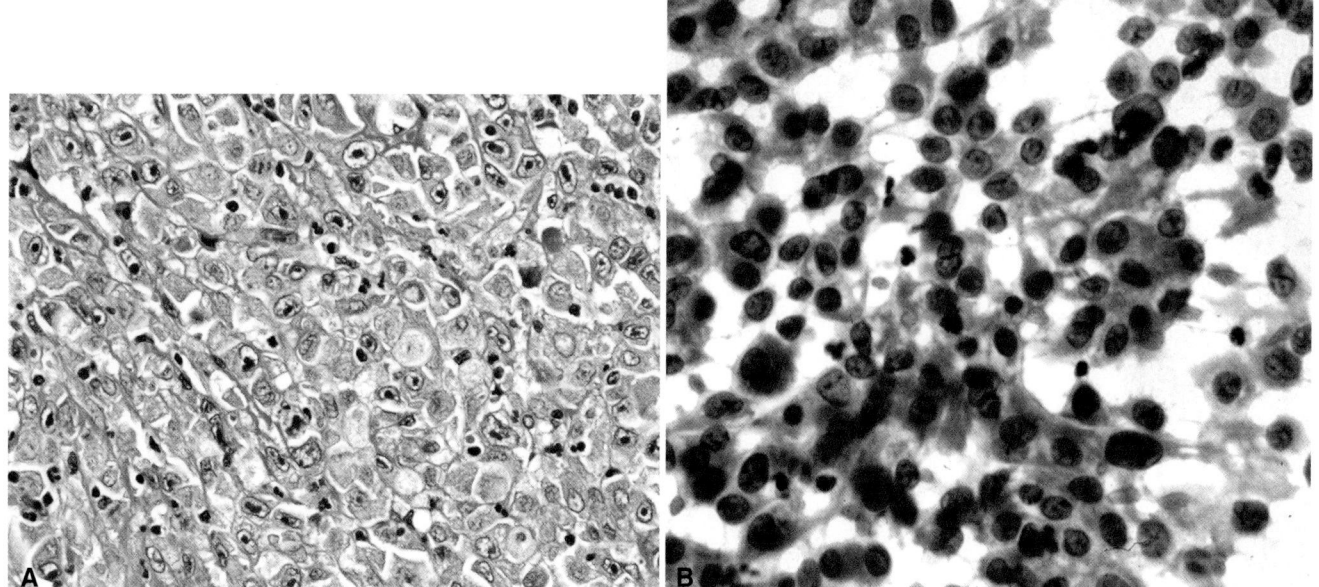

Figure 17-58. A, Primary large cell undifferentiated carcinoma of the lung showing sheets of anaplastic tumor cells with no distinguishing characteristics. **B,** Fine-needle aspiration specimen in the same case shows no evidence of squamous or glandular differentiation.

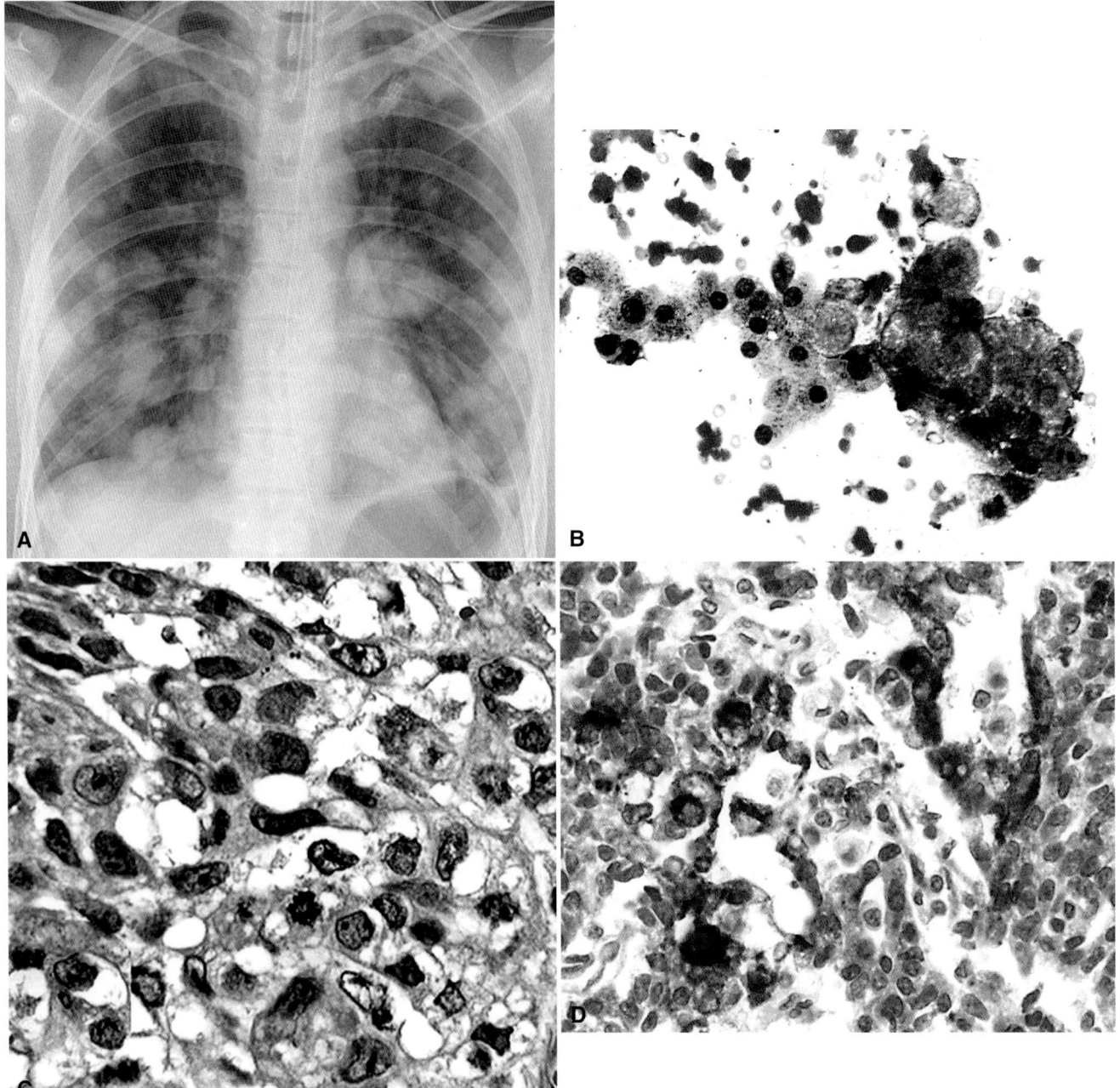

Figure 17-59. A, Chest radiograph showing metastatic "solid" embryonal carcinoma of the testis involving the lung. Findings on fine-needle aspiration (**B**) and subsequent biopsy (**C**) led to a diagnosis of metastatic embryonal carcinoma. The tumor is morphologically similar to that shown in Figure 17-58, but immunoreactivity for alpha-fetoprotein (**D**) and the patient's history confirmed metastatic embryonal carcinoma.

Table 17-7 shows the immunopathologic profile of specific large polygonal cell tumors. The panel of antibody reagents is particularly helpful in distinguishing primary large cell carcinoma from its diagnostic alternatives. Placental-like alkaline phosphatase is seen in most germ cell tumors, and it is occasionally present in primary large cell carcinomas.[239] CD117 and CD30 are also selective markers for seminoma and embryonal carcinoma, respectively (Fig. 17-61). Those lesions may

be distinguished from somatic tumors by their differential expression of epithelial membrane antigen; it is present in primary lung cancers, but not in germ cell malignancies.[86,239] CD45 is restricted to large cell lymphoma (Fig. 17-62). MART-1 is limited to melanoma and adrenocortical carcinoma, and except for epithelioid sarcoma and clear cell sarcoma, metastatic mesenchymal neoplasms are typified by positivity for vimentin but are devoid of keratin and melanocyte-related markers.

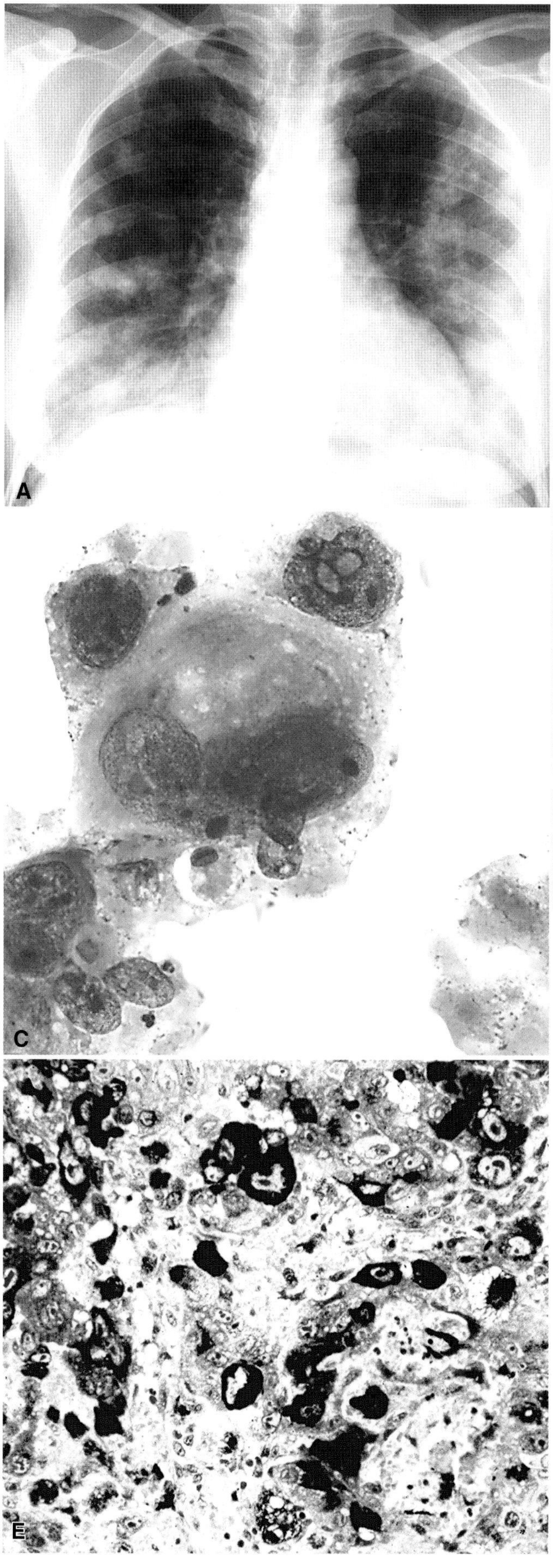

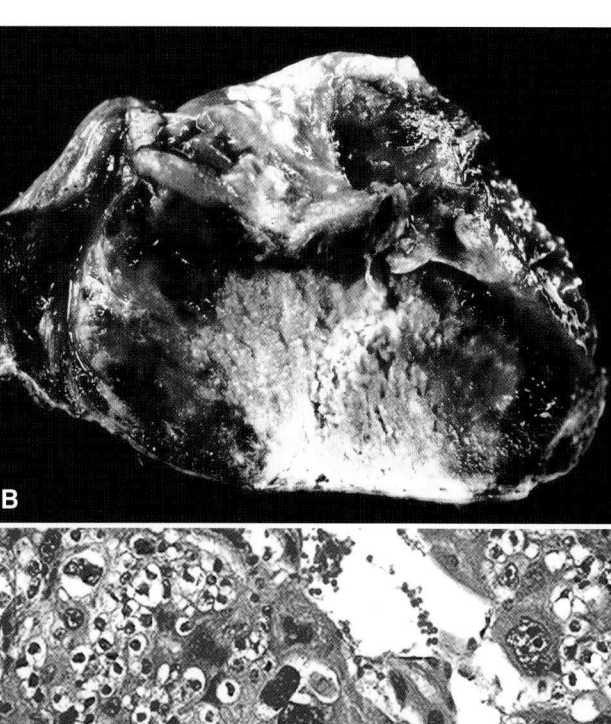

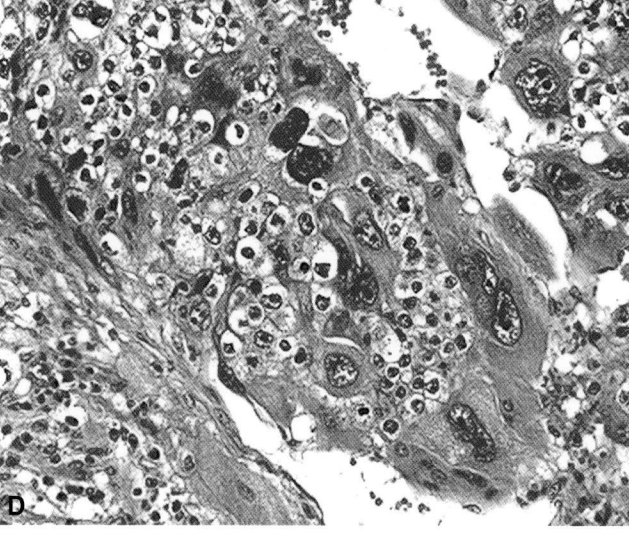

Figure 17-60. Chest radiograph (**A**) and gross photograph (**B**) of metastatic chorio-carcinoma of the ovary involving the lungs. This tumor nodule is internally hemorrhagic and necrotic. Fine-needle aspiration (**C**) and subsequent biopsy (**D**) of choriocarcinoma is typified by juxtaposition of cytotrophoblastic and syncytiotrophoblastic elements. **E,** The syncytial cells of the tumor are immunoreactive for β-human chorionic gonadotropin.

Table 17-7. Immunohistologic Differential Diagnosis of Large Polygonal Cell Malignancies in the Lung

Tumor	Antibody						
	PK	VIM	CD45	EMA	MART	S-100	PLAP
Primary large cell carcinoma of lung	P	PN	N	P	N	PN	PN
Met. epithelioid sarcoma	P	P	N	P	PN	N	N
Large cell lymphoma	N	P	P	N	N	N	N
Met. malignant melanoma	N	P	N	N	P	P	N
Met. embryonal carcinoma	P	PN	N	N	N	N	P
Met. histiocytoid malignant fibrous histiocytoma	N	P	N	N	N	N	N
Met. adrenocortical carcinoma	N	PN	N	N	N	N	N
Met. hepatocellular carcinoma	P	N	N	N	N	N	N
Met. renal cell carcinoma	P	PN	N	P	N	N	N

EMA, epithelial membrane antigen; MART, MART-1; Met., metastatic; N, negative (<10% of cases); P, positive (>80% of cases); PK, pan-keratin; PLAP, placental-like alkaline phosphatase; PN, variably positive (10–80% of cases); S-100, S-100 protein; VIM, vimentin.

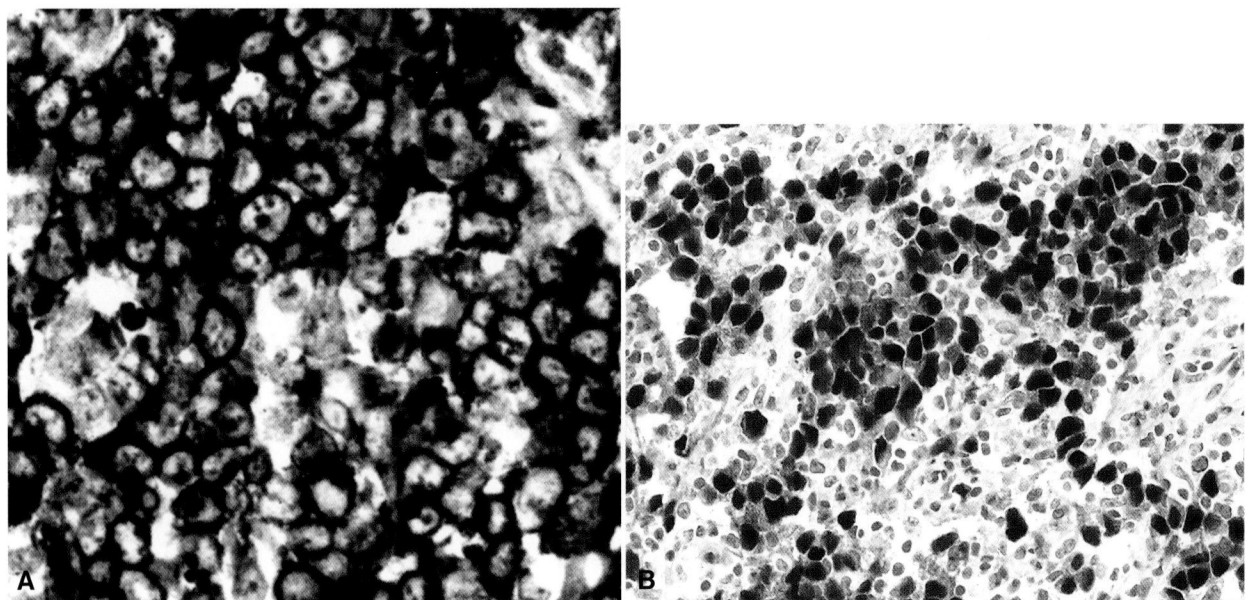

Figure 17-61. Immunoreactivity for CD30 (**A**) and OCT3/4 (**B**) in metastatic embryonal carcinoma of the testis involving the lung. These markers are not expected in primary pulmonary tumors.

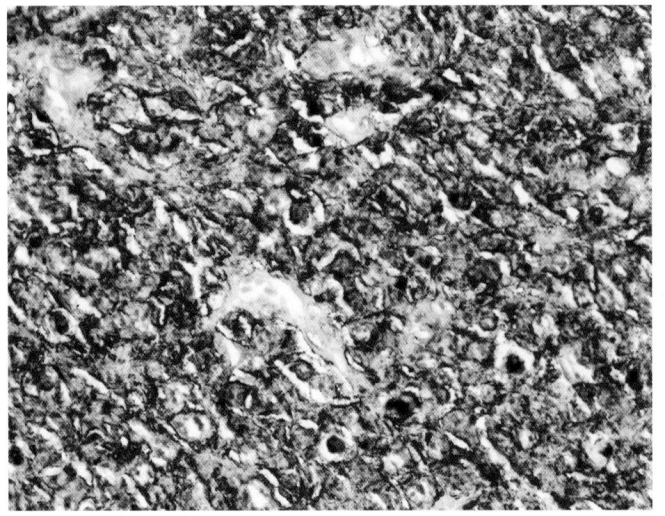

Figure 17-62. Immunoreactivity for CD45—a marker restricted to hematopoietic proliferations—in large-cell non-Hodgkin lymphoma involving the lung.

Other Adjunctive Pathologic Techniques for the Diagnosis of Metastatic Carcinoma

Although electron microscopy has been used less and less in recent years in the diagnosis of tumors in surgical pathology, it still has considerable value in that context. There are several settings in the evaluation of possibly metastatic tumors in the lung where ultrastructural studies are useful.[240–250] Adenocarcinomas—including those arising in the pulmonary parenchyma—are characterized generically by short, nonbranched plasmalemmal microvilli with a length-to-diameter ratio of less than 10:1 (Figs. 17-63 and 17-64).[251–253] Specialized features of specific lesions in that category include laminated cytoplasmic granules (primitive surfactant bodies) in some examples of primary adenocarcinoma of the lung (Fig. 17-65); cytoplasmic mucin granules and "terminal webs" of intermediate filaments that insert into the microvilli in adenocarcinomas with enteric differentiation (Fig. 17-66); glycogen pools and lipid droplets in metastatic renal cell carcinomas (Fig. 17-67); and tubular cristae in the mitochondria of steroid-producing tumors,

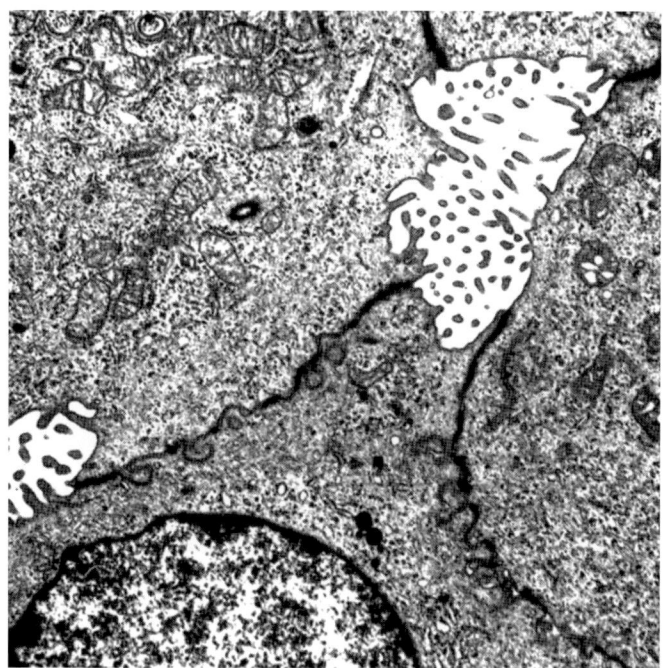

Figure 17-63. Electron photomicrograph of primary pulmonary adenocarcinoma showing prominent intercellular junctions bordering a tumor gland microlumen. Short non-branching plasmalemmal microvilli are also apparent.

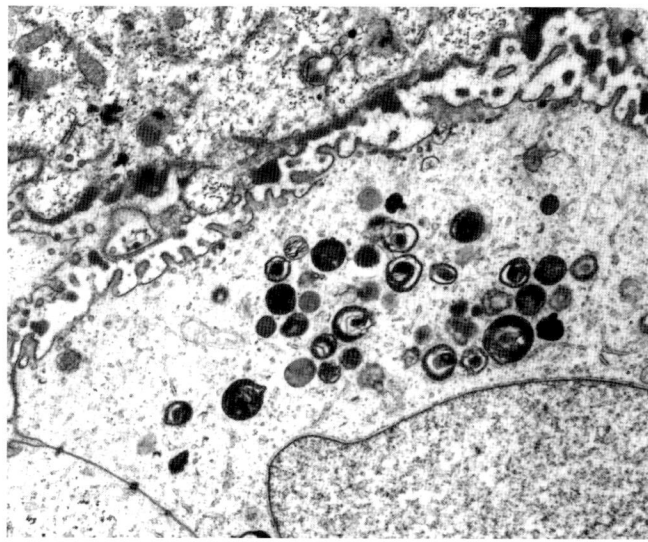

Figure 17-65. Lamellated "myelinoid" figures are seen in the cytoplasm of tumor cells in this primary pulmonary adenocarcinoma. These structures may represent primitive surfactant bodies.

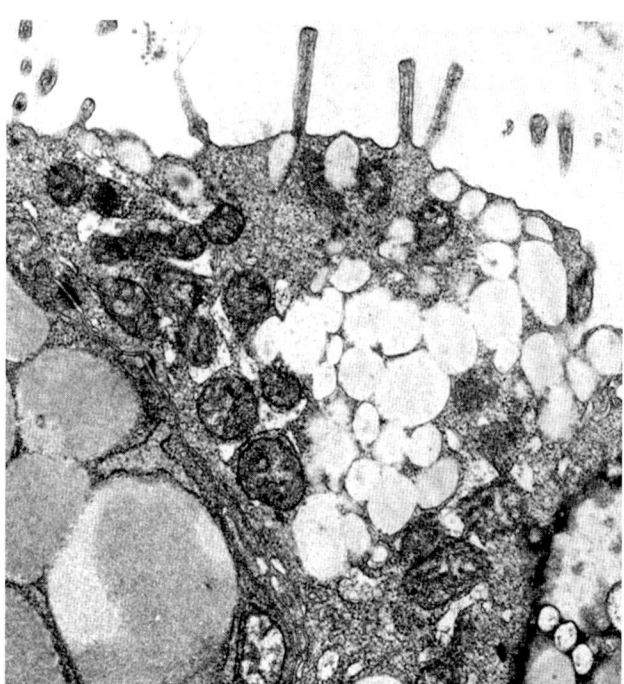

Figure 17-64. Short cell surface microvilli and cytoplasmic mucin granules are seen in this metastatic adenocarcinoma with mucinous features arising in the breast.

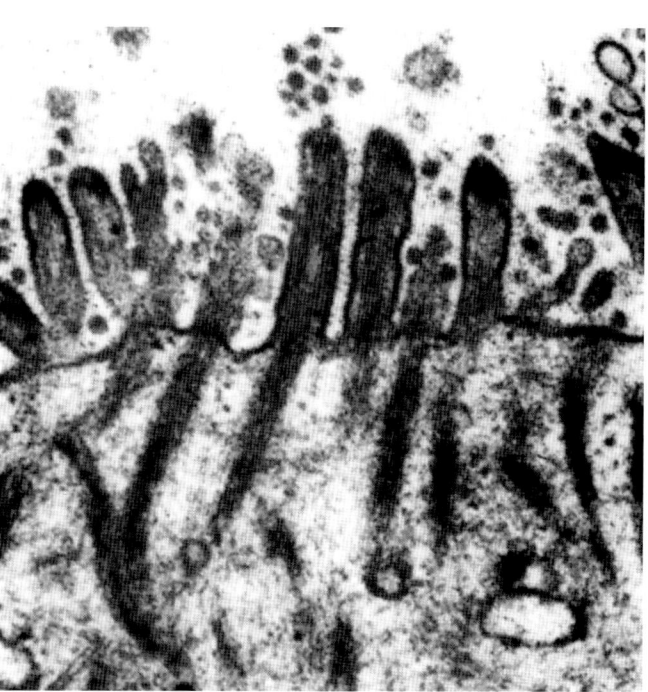

Figure 17-66. A "terminal web" of thin filaments inserts into the plasmalemmal microvilli in the tumor cells of this metastatic colonic adenocarcinoma. This structure is highly suggestive of an enteric anatomic origin.

such as adrenocortical carcinoma (Fig. 17-68).[243,244,248,249] Malignant mesothelioma, a simulant of adenocarcinoma at the light microscopic level, is typified by elongated, bushy, branching microvilli with an length-to-diameter ratio of greater than 10:1, together with complex desmosomal complexes and cytoplasmic tonofilaments (Figs. 17-69 and 17-70).[251–253] Mucin granules and surfactant bodies are absent in that tumor type.

Neuroendocrine carcinomas may be identified with certainty because of their synthesis of dense-core (neurosecretory) granules measuring 150 to 400 nm in diameter. Those inclusions have peripheral zones of lucency and tend to be clustered in the cytoplasm (Fig. 17-71), often near the Golgi apparatus.[240–243] Macular intercellular junctional complexes are also evident in such lesions, and small whorls of perinuclear intermediate filaments are common. These characteristics are the same, regardless of the site of origin of neuroendocrine tumors; therefore, electron microscopy cannot be used to distinguish primary pulmonary lesions from metastases.

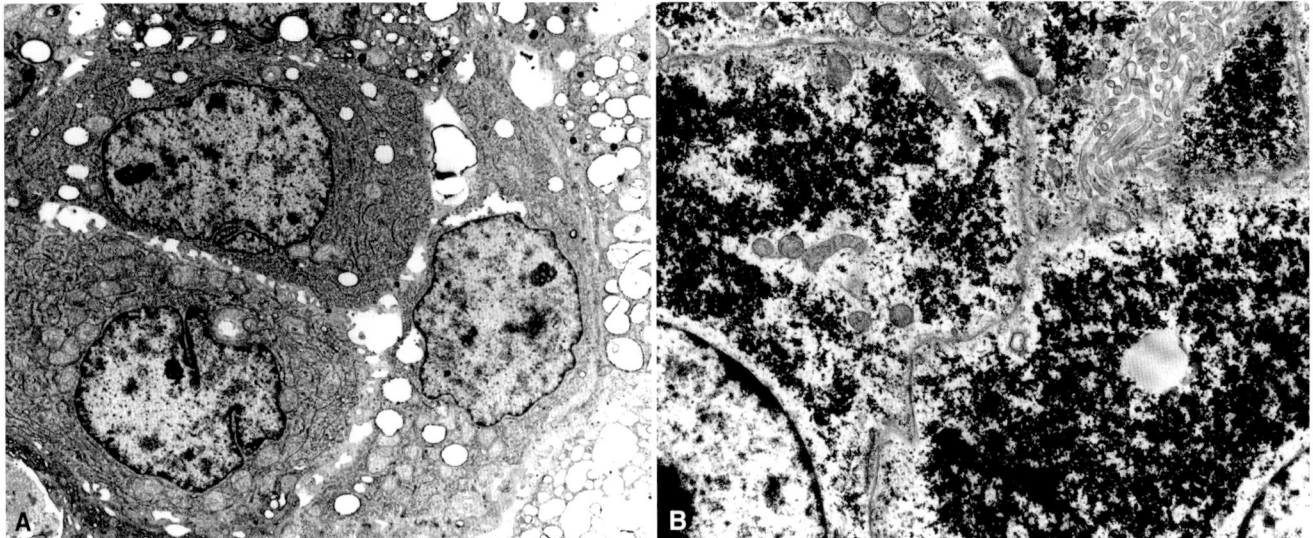

Figure 17-67. A, Numerous lipid droplets are seen in the tumor cell cytoplasm in this metastatic renal cell carcinoma. **B,** Another area of the same tumor shows abundant cytoplasmic glycogen.

Germ cell tumors exhibit electron microscopic characteristics that potentially simulate those of somatic carcinomas. Seminomas are undifferentiated at a fine structural level, showing only primitive appositional intercellular junctional complexes, prominent nucleoli, and the usual constituency of basic metabolic organelles (Fig. 17-72). One salient feature of these tumors is the presence of cytoplasmic glycogen pools, but those are shared by many nongerminal tumors.[243] Embryonal carcinomas largely resemble somatic adenocarcinomas, including the formation of plasmalemmal microvilli and intercellular gland-like spaces (Fig. 17-73). Yolk sac tumors share the same potentialities. Choriocarcinomas are relatively distinctive ultrastructurally and show cytoplasmic tonofibrils reminiscent of those seen in squamous tumors.[247] The latter lesions are not part of the light microscopic differential diagnosis of choriocarcinomas; that discrepancy may provide a clue to the interpretation.

Nonepithelial malignancies with specific electron microscopic attributes include rhabdomyosarcoma, leiomyosarcoma, alveolar soft tissue sarcoma, neuroblastoma, melanoma (and clear cell sarcoma), and endothelial sarcoma.[254] These neoplasms show primitive sarcomeric differentiation, with thick and thin cytoplasmic myofilaments (Fig. 17-74); cytoplasmic skeins of thin filaments punctuated by dense bodies; paracrystalline cytoplasmic inclusions (Fig. 17-75); complex interdigitating cytoplasmic extensions containing microtubules (Fig. 17-76); premelanosomes (Fig. 17-77); and Weibel-Palade

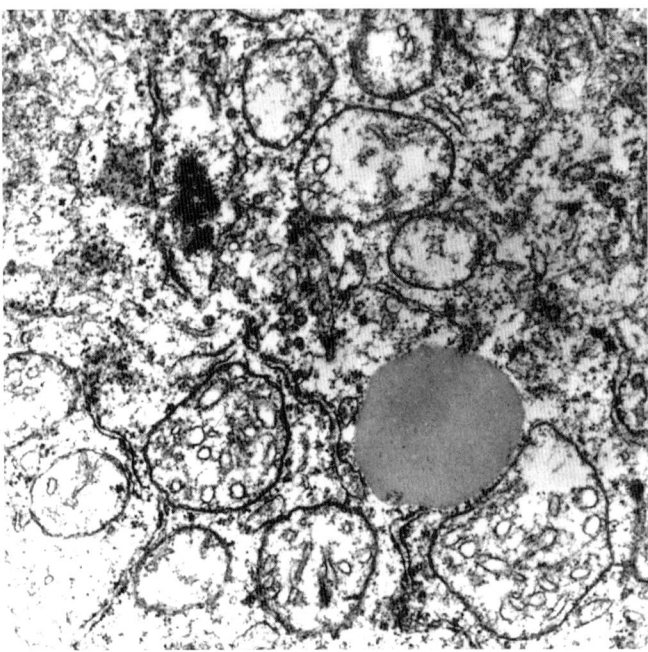

Figure 17-68. Tubular mitochondrial cristae are seen in this metastatic adrenocortical carcinoma.

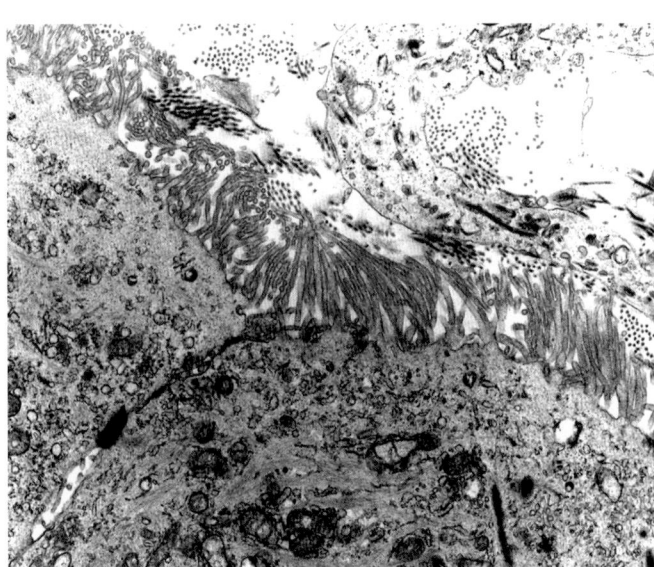

Figure 17-69. Electron photomicrograph of malignant mesothelioma of the pleura showing branching, "bushy" cell surface microvilli and elaborate, elongated intercellular junctional complexes.

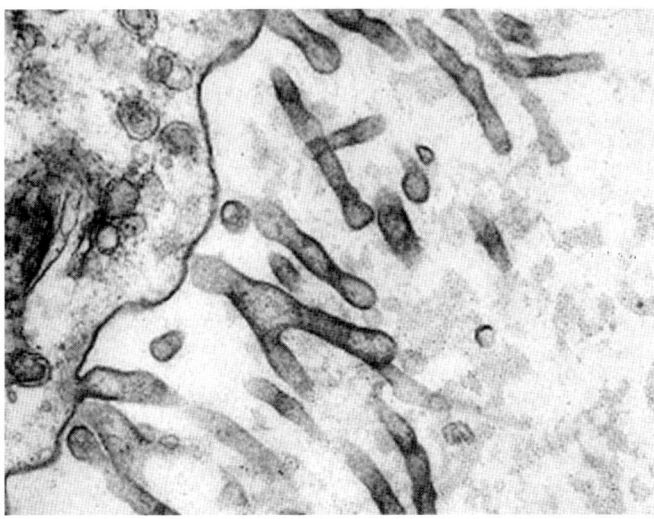

Figure 17-70. The branching nature of plasmalemmal microvilli in mesothelioma is well seen in an electron photomicrograph.

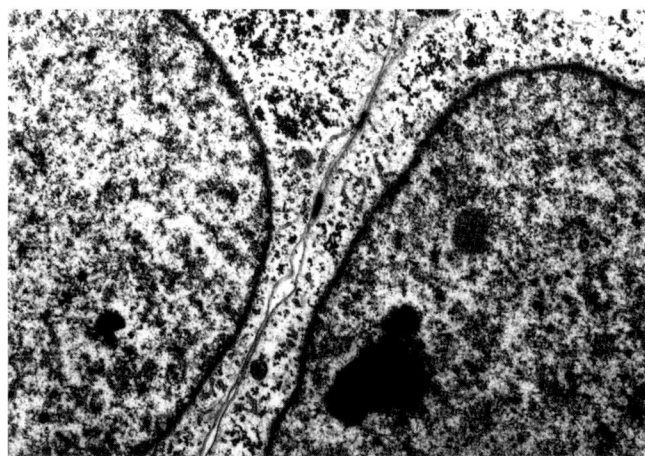

Figure 17-72. Electron photomicrograph of metastatic seminoma showing a complex nucleolar structure, abundant cytoplasmic glycogen, and macular-type intercellular junctions. Cytoplasmic organelles are otherwise rudimentary.

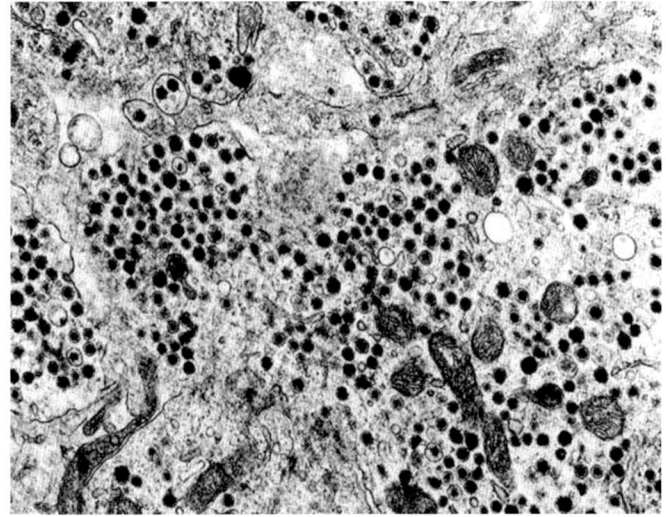

Figure 17-71. Numerous dense-core neurosecretory granules are dispersed throughout the cytoplasm in an electron photomicrograph of metastatic well-differentiated neuroendocrine carcinoma ("carcinoid") from the ileum involving the lungs.

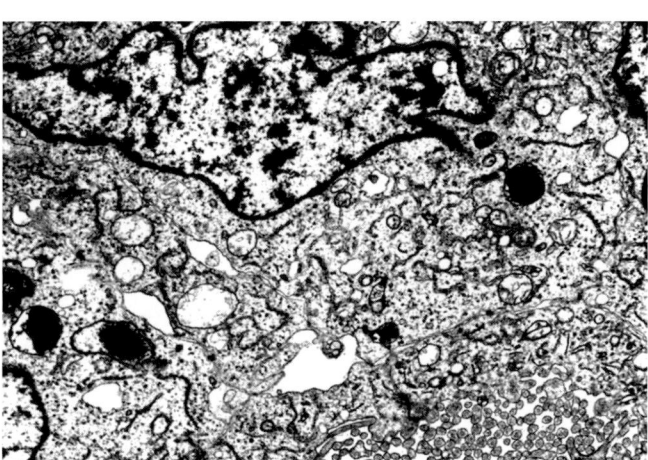

Figure 17-73. Metastatic embryonal carcinoma of the testis showing cell surface microvilli (*lower right*), simulating the appearance of a somatic adenocarcinoma at a fine structural level.

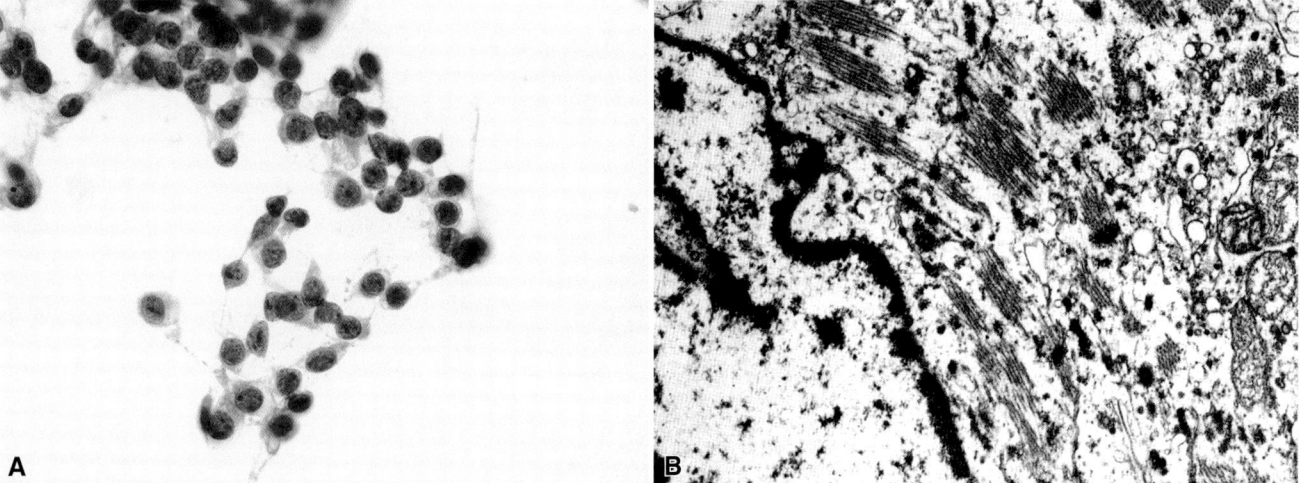

Figure 17-74. **A,** Metastatic embryonal rhabdomyosarcoma in a fine-needle aspirate showing dyshesive cells with high nucleocytoplasmic ratios and naked nuclei. **B,** An electron photomicrograph from a similar case shows cytoplasmic thin and thick filaments representing primitive sarcomeric differentiation.

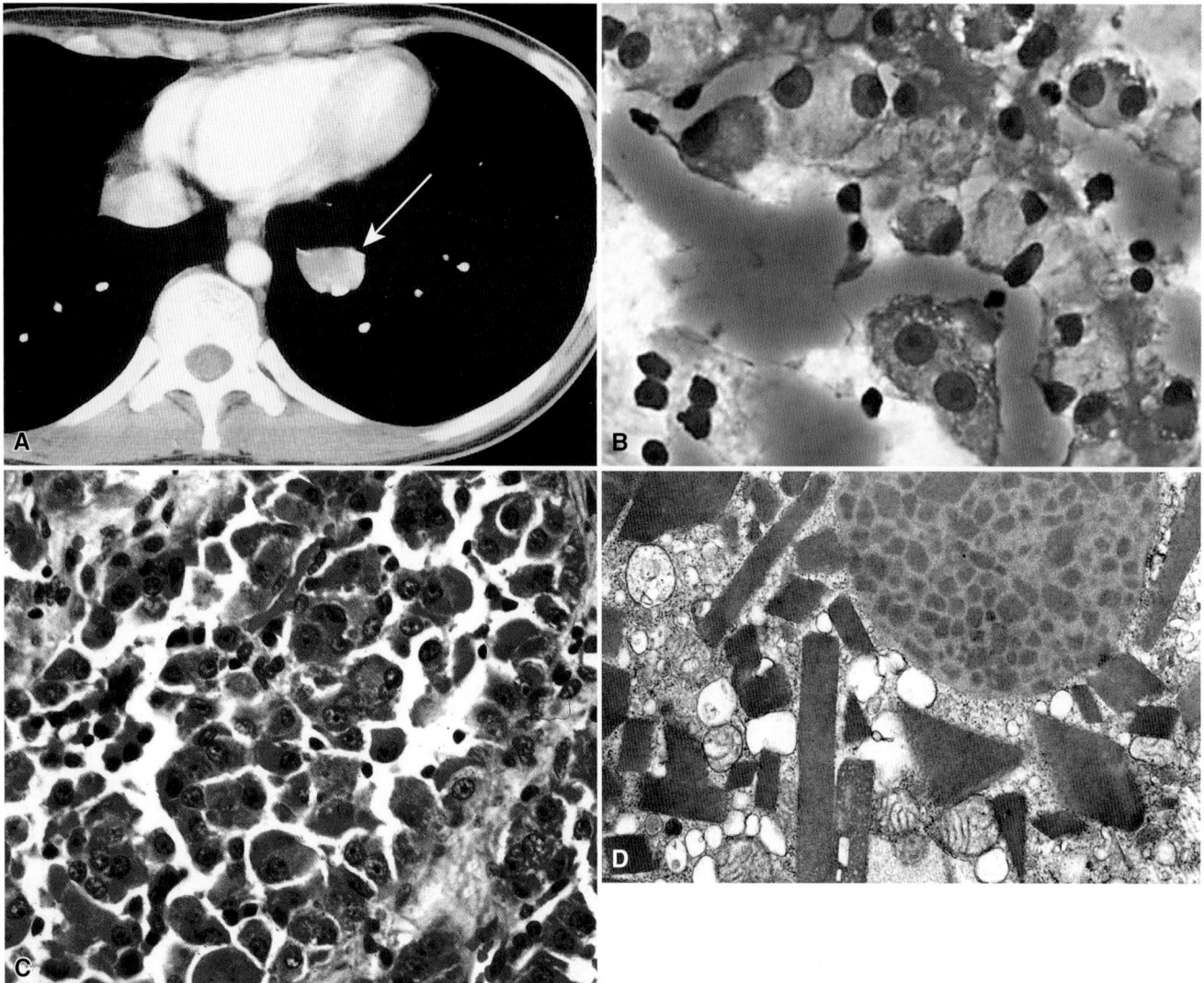

Figure 17-75. A, Metastatic alveolar soft tissue sarcoma presenting in the left lung (*arrow*) in an adolescent boy in the absence of a known soft tissue tumor. Fine-needle aspiration (**B**) and subsequent biopsy (**C**) confirmed the diagnosis. **D,** An electron photomicrograph of the lesion shows characteristic paracrystalline cytoplasmic inclusions. A primary lesion was ultimately found in the right buttock.

bodies (Fig. 17-78), respectively. All of these structures are absent in primary pulmonary tumors, except for sarcomatoid carcinomas. These lesions show a mixture of cells with epithelial characteristics (e.g., intercellular junctions, tonofibrils, microvilli) and others with mesenchymal attributes.

The electron microscopic attributes of other mesenchymal neoplasms are nondescript or even misleading diagnostically. For example, primitive neuroectodermal tumors (and other blastomas, such as hepatoblastoma or Wilms tumor) are composed of primordial round cells joined by macular attachment plaques and often containing only basic organelles (Fig. 17-79).[245,254] In some cases, glycogen deposits or nascent cytoplasmic extensions may be seen, the latter of which contain neurosecretory granules or synaptic-type vesicles. Although they are soft tissue neoplasms, epithelioid sarcomas and synovial sarcomas mirror their immunohistologic features ultrastructurally because they show polygonal cells joined by well-formed intercellular attachment plaques (Fig. 17-80) and may even show microvillous differentiation.[254]

Hematopoietic proliferations are perhaps the most primitive at an electron microscopic level. They show only basic cytoplasmic constitu-

ents—often containing abundant dispersed ribosomes, with or without rough endoplasmic reticulum—but lacking other distinguishing features (Fig. 17-81).[249,255]

Cytogenetic information is rapidly accumulating on a variety of tumor types, and it holds the promise of serving as helpful differential diagnostic data. For example, several neoplasms have unique chromosomal abnormalities that exclude other possibilities. These include deletions of the short arm of chromosome 3 in renal cell carcinoma; an unrelated deletion in the same chromosomal segment in primary SCNCL; the t(11;22) translocation in primitive neuroectodermal tumor/Ewing sarcoma; the t(1;13) or t(2;13) translocation in alveolar rhabdomyosarcoma; the t(12;22) translocation in clear cell sarcoma; the der(17)t(X;17) translocation in alveolar soft tissue sarcoma; the t(X;18) translocation in synovial sarcoma; isochromosome 12p in germ cell malignancies; and a group of semispecific or specific karyotypic abnormalities in malignant lymphomas and leukemias.[256–267] These markers are best assessed with fresh tissue, but assays based on polymerase chain reaction or fluorescent in situ hybridization studies are also becoming available for use in hospital practice.

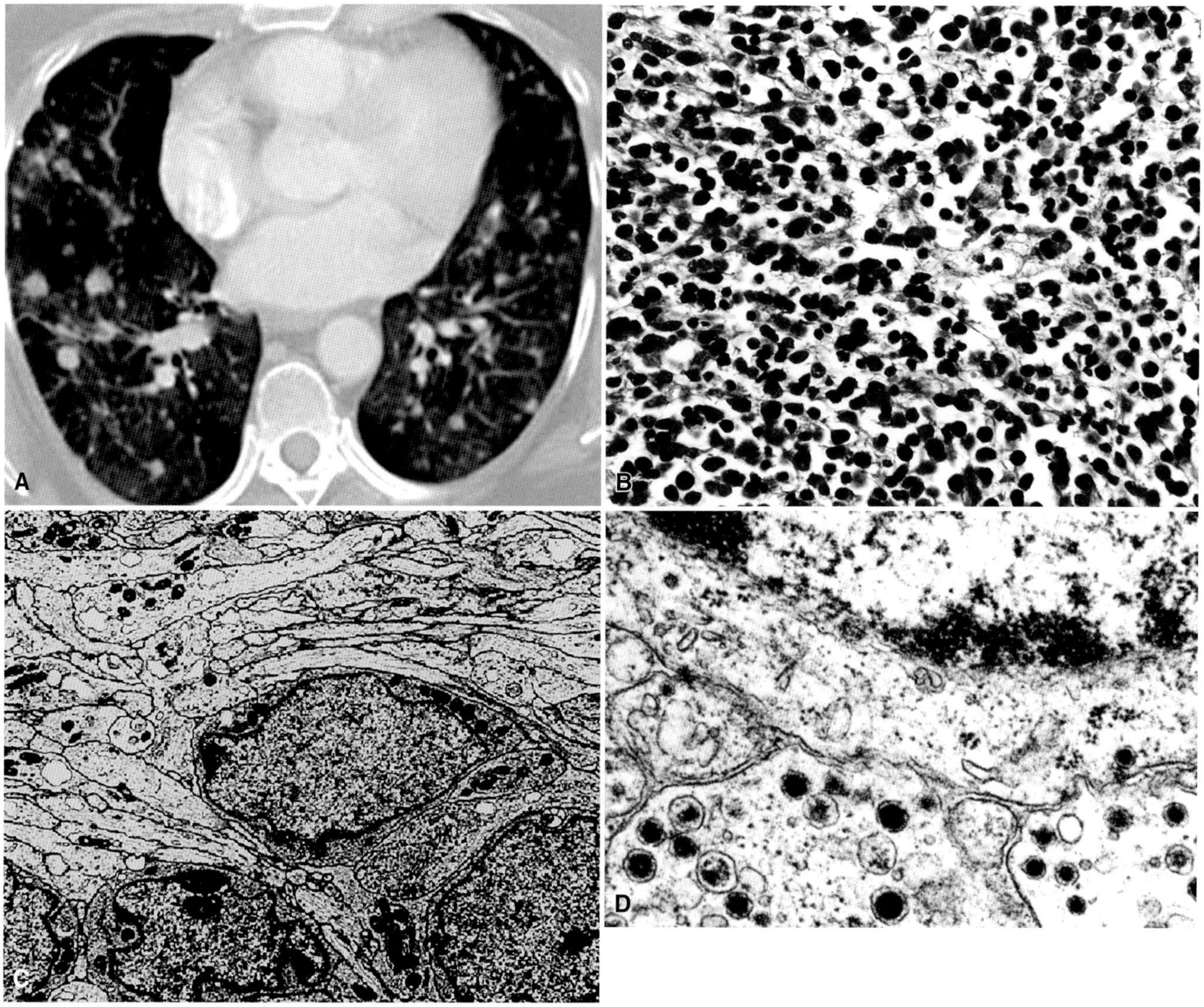

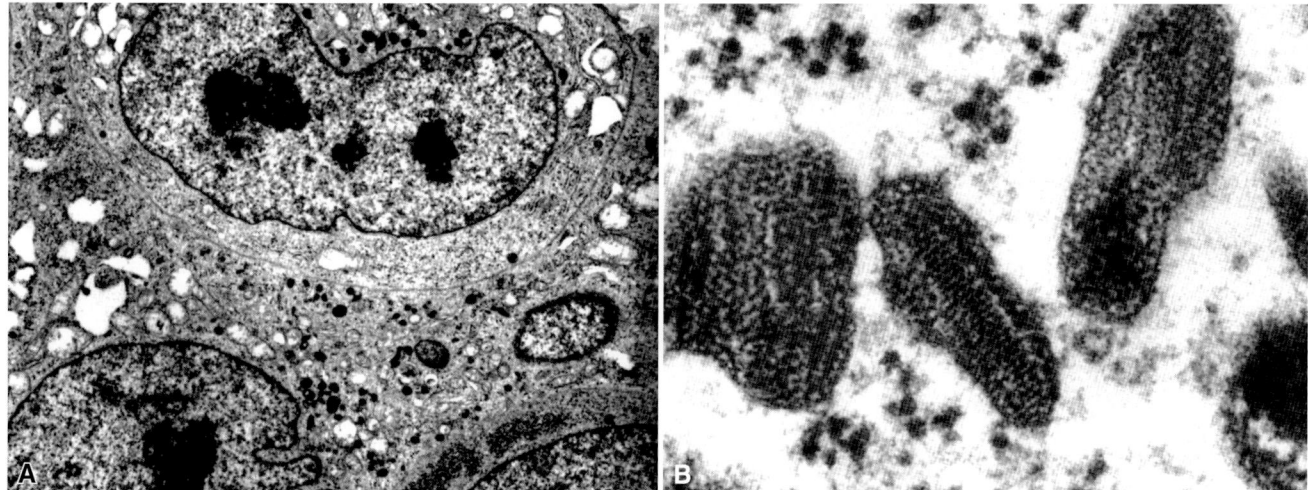

Figure 17-76. A, Metastatic neuroblastoma involving the lungs of a child. **B,** The tumor is represented by sheets of small round undifferentiated tumor cells. **C** and **D,** Electron microscopy shows interdigitating cytoplasmic processes containing microtubules as well as dense-core granules.

Figure 17-77. A, Electron photomicrograph of metastatic melanoma in the lung showing epithelioid tumor cells joined by primitive appositional plaques. **B,** Characteristic premelanosomes were seen in the cytoplasm.

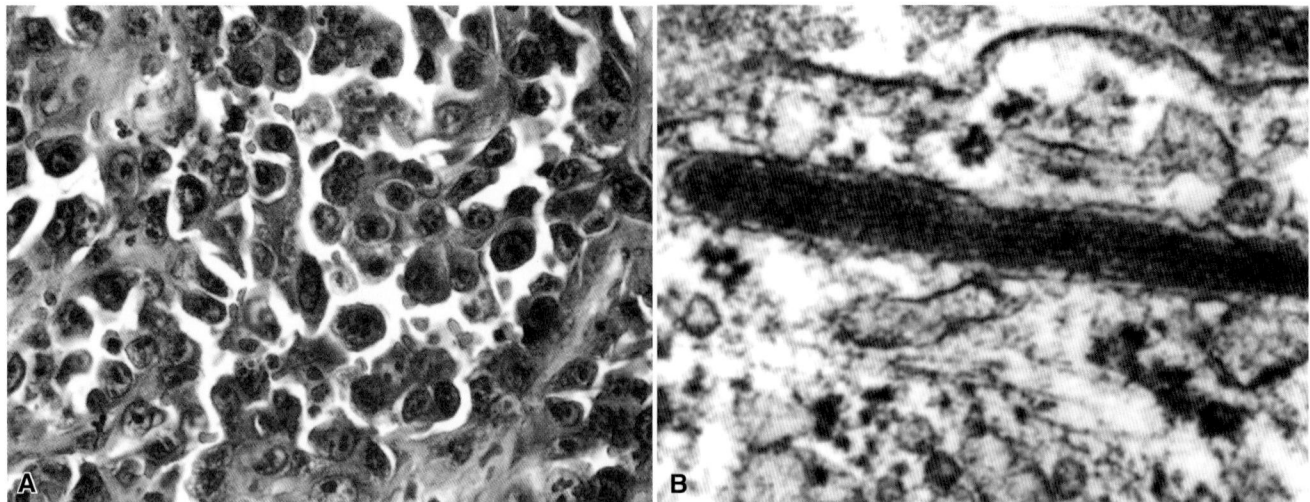

Figure 17-78. **A,** Metastatic epithelioid angiosarcoma in the lung originating in the scalp in an elderly man. **B,** A Weibel-Palade body is seen in a tumor cell, marking the proliferation as endothelial.

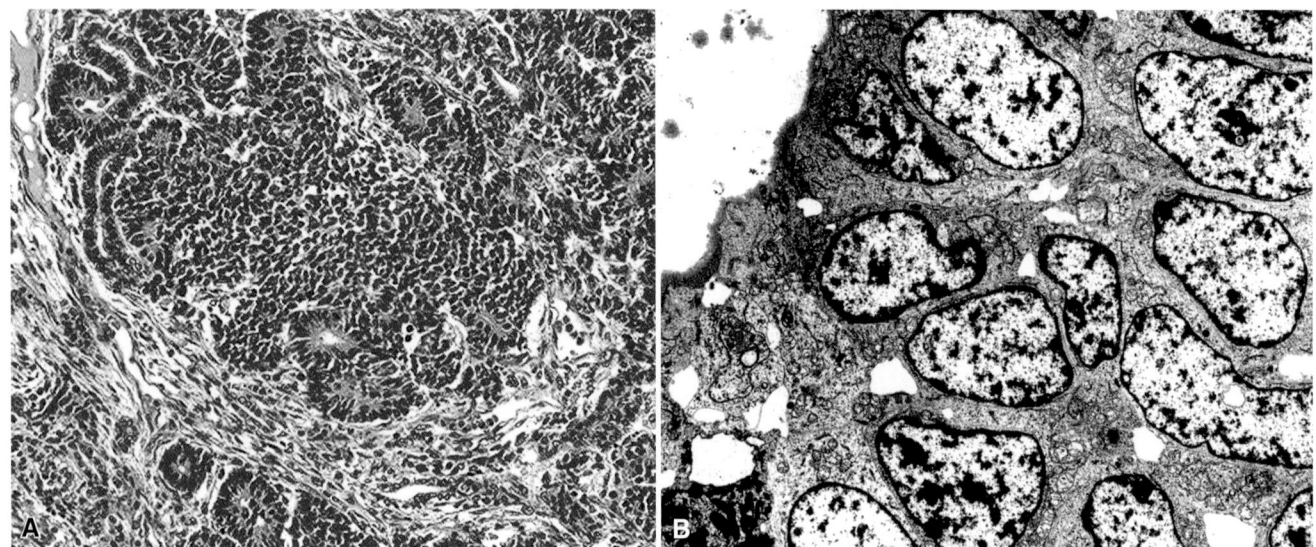

Figure 17-79. **A,** Metastatic Wilms tumor showing primitive tubules that punctuate a small round cell (blastematous) background population of tumor cells. **B,** Electron photomicrographs from the same case show a relatively nondescript population of cells joined by primitive appositional plaques and surrounded in part by basal lamina.

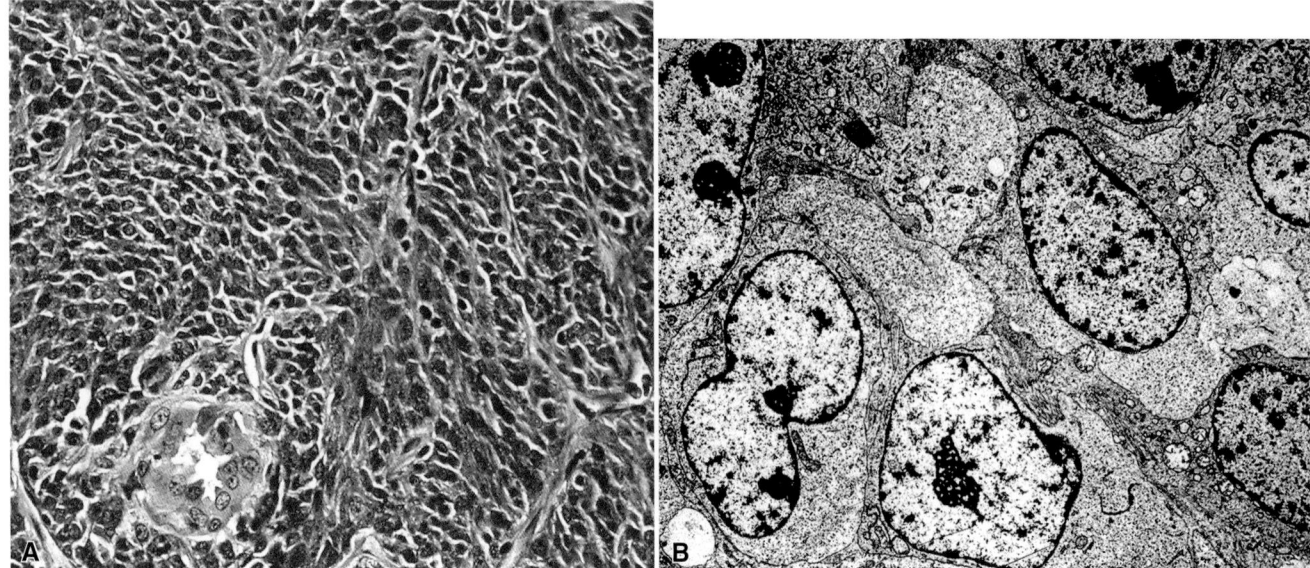

Figure 17-80. **A,** Metastatic synovial sarcoma originating in the soft tissue of the arm, involving the lungs. **B,** Electron microscopy of the lesion shows investment of the tumor cells by basal lamina and the presence of intercellular junctions. These ultrastructural features may be misinterpreted as those of a carcinoma.

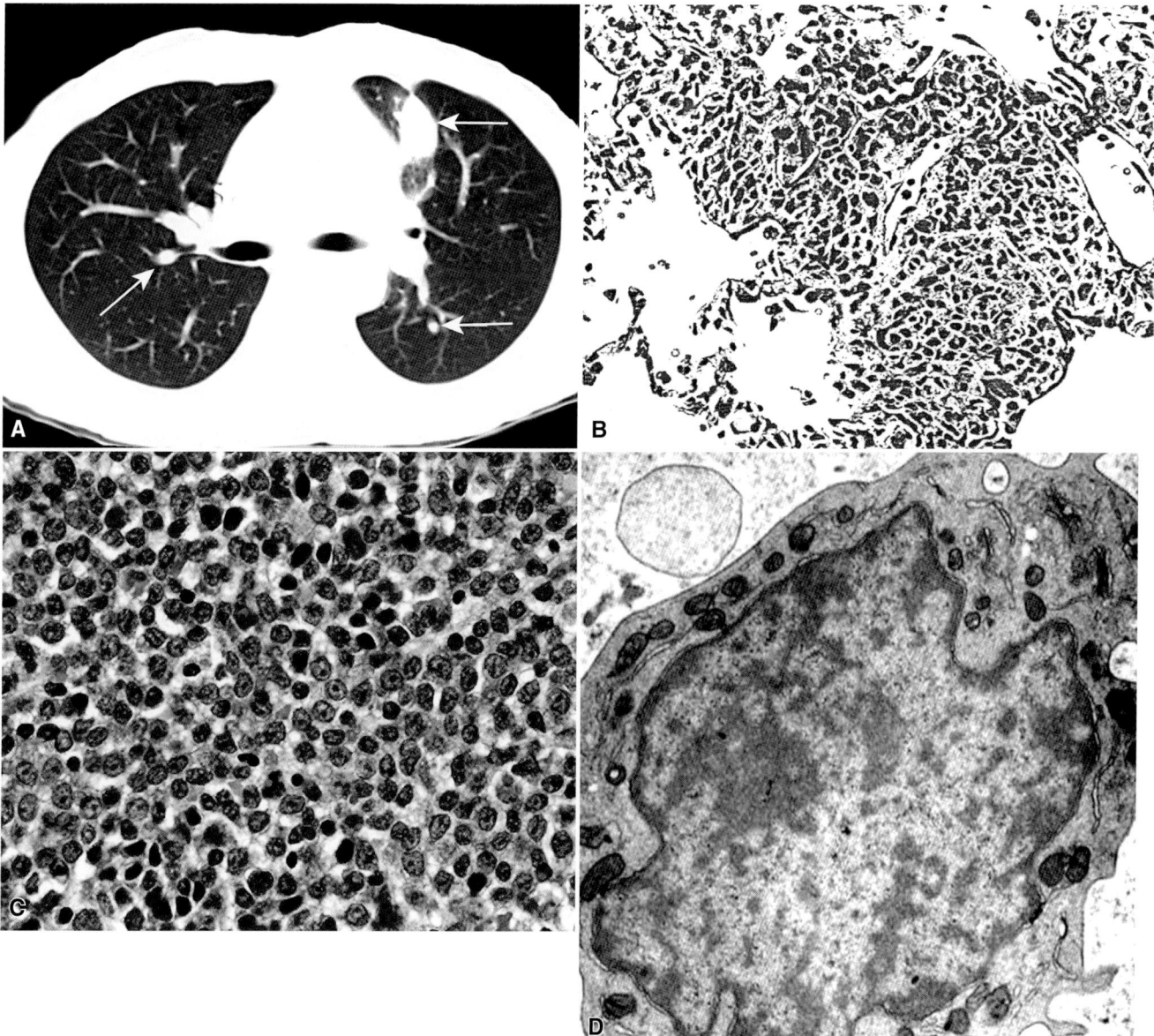

Figure 17-81. A, Computed tomogram of the chest (*arrows*) and photomicrographs (**B** and **C**) showing lesions of granulocytic sarcoma (tumefactive acute myelogenous leukemia) involving the lungs. **D,** In an electron photomicrograph, the tumor cells contain only primitive organelles and are not distinctive ultrastructurally.

Outcomes Analysis

Optimal diagnostic testing strategies, principally pertaining to the sequence of tests, are controversial in regard to the assessment of patients with pulmonary lesions that are suspicious for metastases. In countries with available resources, a "definitive" diagnosis is usually based on the pathologic examination of tissue specimens. The methods used to obtain these specimens have been previously discussed, but several factors affect the choice of a subsequent diagnostic testing approach. They include the preferences of patients and physicians; cost; testing characteristics, such as sensitivity, specificity, rate, and complexity; and clinical attibutes (e.g., radiologic findings, age, and general patient health).

Most decision-related analytic studies that have attempted to determine optimal testing strategies have focused on patients with solitary pulmonary nodules, and the authors generally have assumed that there was no known history of malignancy. In these publications, the optimal testing paradigm was also equated with the most cost-effective strategy, meaning that it resulted in the greatest increase in population-related life expectancy for the lowest cost. Evaluations of this type have reached contradictory conclusions, with some stating that open biopsy or excision is the procedure of choice and others suggesting that sputum cytology should precede other testing methods.[268–272]

Potential reasons for these disagreements include study bias, assumptions based on incomplete data, and the overall complexity of analytic modeling. One study that included theoretical patient preferences showed that the cost-effectiveness of testing strategies was variable, depending on patient values such as risk aversion (aversion to a false-negative diagnosis or a testing complication).[273–276] Although these factors have yet to be measured in practice, the results of the latter study showed that a single testing strategy may not apply for all patient populations, including those with potential metastatic disease in the lungs.

Raab and coworkers assessed the sensitivity and cost-effectiveness of percutaneous FNA in a group of patients with known extrapulmonary malignancies and solitary lung masses.[277] Using data from two hospitals with active FNA programs, they showed that pathologists correctly classified 87% of the pulmonary lesions as primary or secondary malignancies. More than 90% were metastases, indicating that the probability of a primary lung tumor is low in this clinical setting. As mentioned earlier, the distinction of primary and secondary malignancies depended on light microscopic features; morphologic comparison with previous specimens, when available; and the judicious use of immunocytochemistry.

Raab and coworkers found that the latter method was needed in only 20% of cases, but it yielded a definitive diagnosis in 78% of cases in which it was used.[277] The cost-effectiveness of percutaneous FNA—compared with bronchoscopy and thoracoscopy—depends on several factors, such as test sensitivity and the pre-FNA probability of malignancy. An underlying assumption is that patients with metastatic disease do not need pulmonary resection, although these procedures may be appropriate in some cases. At pre-FNA probability of malignancy of more than 50% and FNA sensitivity of greater than 75%, FNA was more cost-effective than thoracoscopy in the cited series.[277] In most clinical scenarios, percutaneous FNA was also more cost-effective than bronchoscopy. Nonetheless, clinicians still tend to use a wide variety of testing strategies in the diagnostic evaluation of pulmonary masses.[274]

Another question of increasing importance is the utilitarian value of ancillary studies, such as immunopathology, in tumor subtyping. Raab showed that immunocytochemistry was cost-effective in three theoretical scenarios: increasing patient life expectancy, diagnostic certainty, and the ability to predict patient prognosis.[277] However, as Wick and colleagues indicated, it has never been proven formally that the correct immunohistologic diagnosis of a specific tumor type, particularly concerning nonhematolymphoid malignancies, produces a benefit in patient outcome.[197] Accurate pathologic diagnosis is believed to be advantageous in some instances, such as those concerning small-cell pediatric malignancies. Nonetheless, for the most part, patient survival generally depends more on nonpathologic variables, such as tumor stage, patient age, and overall health.[276–280] The actual effect of accurate diagnosis was not reported in the latter study, which investigated the cost-effectiveness of FNA in evaluation of lung masses, but Imlay and Raab separately showed that the use of immunopathology had no effect on patient survival in reference to pleural fluid evaluation.[45]

Some immunologic markers have a potentially predictive role in secondary pulmonary malignancies, such as estrogen receptor protein and progesterone receptor protein in cases of metastatic breast cancer. Those determinants may forecast the clinical response to appropriate treatment regimens, the response to which, in turn, may be prognostic (indicative of overall patient survival).[197] The cost-effectiveness of most other markers of that type has not yet been thoroughly assessed.[197]

Self-assessment questions related to this chapter can be found online on the Expert Consult site for this title.

References

1. Crow J, Slavin G, Kreel L. Pulmonary metastasis: a pathologic and radiologic study. *Cancer*. 1981;47:2595–2603.
2. Johnson RM, Lindskog GE. 100 cases of tumor metastatic to the lung and mediastinum. *JAMA*. 1967;202:94–98.
3. Abrams HJ, Spiro R, Goldstein N. Metastates in carcinoma, analysis of 1000 autopsied cases. *Cancer*. 1950;3:74–75.
4. Farrell JT. Pulmonary metastasis: a pathologic, clinical, roentgenologic study based on 78 cases seen at necropsy. *Radiology*. 1935;24:444–451.
5. Matthay R, Coppage L, Shaw C, Filderman A. Malignancies metastatic to the pleura. *Invest Radiol*. 1990;25:601–619.
6. Filderman AE, Coppage L, Shaw C, Matthay RA. Pulmonary and pleural manifestations of extrathoracic malignancies. *Clin Chest Med*. 1989;10:747–807.
7. Fidler IJ. Review: Biologic heterogeneity of cancer metastases. *Breast Cancer Res Treat*. 1987;17:17.
8. Fidler IJ. The evolution of biologic heterogeneity in metastatic neoplasms. In: Nicholson GL, Milas L, eds. *Cancer Invasion and Metastases: Biologic and Therapeutic Aspects*. New York: Raven Press; 1984:5.
9. Liotta LA. Editorial. H-ras p21 and the metastatic phenotype. *J Natl Cancer Inst*. 1988;80:468.
10. Cotran RS, Kumar V, Collins T, Robbins SL. Neoplasia. In: *Robbins Pathologic Basis of Disease*. Philadelphia: WB Saunders; 1999:241–304.
11. Braman SS, Whitcomb ME. Endobronchial metastasis. *Arch Intern Med*. 1975;135:543–547.
12. Winterbauer RH, Elfenbein Jr IB. WCB. Incidence and clinical significance of tumor embolization to the lungs. *Am J Med*. 1968;45:271–290.
13. Goldhaber SZ, Dricker E, Buring JE. Clinical suspicion of autopsy-proven thrombotic and tumor pulmonary embolism in cancer patients. *Am Heart J*. 1987;114:1432–1435.
14. Chan CK, Hutcheon MA, Hyland RH, et al. Pulmonary tumor embolism: a critical review of clinical, imaging, and hemodynamic features. *J Thorac Imaging*. 1987;2:4–14.
15. Gonzalez-Vitale JC, Garcia-Bunuel R. Pulmonary tumor emboli and cor pulmonale in primary carcinoma of the lung. *Cancer*. 1976;38:2105–2110.
16. Abbondanzo SL, Klappenbach RS, Tsou E. Tumor cell embolism to pulmonary alveolar capillaries. *Arch Pathol Lab Med*. 1986;110:1197–1198.
17. Kane RD, Hawkins HK, Miller JA. Microscopic pulmonary tumor emboli associated with dyspnea. *Cancer*. 1975;36:1473–1482.
18. Pinckard JK, Wick MR. Tumor-related thrombotic pulmonary microangiopathy: review of pathologic findings and pathophysiologic mechanisms. *Ann Diagn Pathol*. 2000;4:154–157.
19. Soares FA, Landell GAM, deOliveira JAM. Pulmonary tumor embolism to alveolar septal capillaries: a prospective study of 12 cases. *Arch Pathol Lab Med*. 1991;115:127–130.
20. Scholten ET, Kreel L. Distribution of lung metastases in the axial plane. *Radiol Clin North Am*. 1977;46:248–265.
21. Steele JD. The solitary pulmonary nodule. *J Thorac Cardiovasc Surg*. 1963;46:21–39.
22. Toomes H, Delphendahl A, Manke H, Vogt-Moykopf I. The coin lesion of the lung: a review of 955 resected coin lesions. *Cancer*. 1983;51:534–537.
23. Viggiano RW, Swensen SJ, Rosenow EC. Evaluation and management of solitary and mulitple pulmonary nodules. *Clin Chest Med*. 1992;13:83–95.
24. Quint LE, Park CH, Iannettoni MD. Solitary pulmonary nodules in patients with extrapulmonary neoplasms. *Radiology*. 2000;217:257–261.
25. Dodd GD, Boyle JJ. Excavating pulmonary metastases. *Am J Roentgenol*. 1961;85:277–293.
26. D'Angio GJ, Iannaccone G. Spontaneous pneumothorax as a complication of pulmonary metastases in malignant tumors of childhood. *Am J Roentgenol*. 1961;86:1092–1102.
27. Fichera G, Hagerstrand I. The small lymph vessels of the lungs in lymphangiosis carcinomatosa. *Acta Pathol Microbiol Scand*. 1965;65:505–513.
28. Harold JT. Lymphangitis carcinomatosa of the lungs. *Q J Med*. 1952;21:353–360.
29. Yang SP, Lin CC. Lymphangitic carcinomatosis of the lungs: the clinical significance of its roentgenologic classification. *Chest*. 1972;62:179–187.
30. Trapnell DH. The radiological appearance of lymphangitic carcinomatosa of the lung. *Thorax*. 1964;19:251–260.
31. Winterbauer RH, Belic N, Moores KD. A clinical interpretation of bilateral hilar adenopathy. *Ann Intern Med*. 1973;78:65–71.
32. Janower ML, Blennerhassett JB. Lymphangitic spread of metastatic cancer to the lung: a radiologic–pathologic classification. *Radiology*. 1971;101:267–273.
33. Goldsmith HS, Bailey HD, Callahan EL, Beattie EJ. Pulmonary lymphangitic metastases from breast cancer. *Arch Surg*. 1967;94:483–488.
34. Thurlbeck WM. Neoplasia of the pulmonary vascular bed. In: Moser KM, ed. *Pulmonary Vascular Disease*. New York: Marcel Dekker; 1979:629–649.
35. Canto-Armengod A. Macroscopic characteristics of pleural metastases arising from the breast and observed by diagnostic thoracoscopy. *Am Rev Respir Dis*. 1990;142:616–618.
36. Hsu C. Cytologic detection of malignancy in pleural effusion: review of 5,255 samples from 3,811 patients. *Diagn Cytopathol*. 1987;3:8–12.
37. Johnson WW. The malignant pleural effusion: a review of cytopathologic diagnoses of 584 specimens from 472 consecutive patients. *Cancer*. 1985;56:905–909.
38. Venrick MG, Sidaway MK. Cytologic evaluation of serous effusions: processing techniques and optimal number of smears for routine preparation. *Am J Clin Pathol*. 1993;99:182–186.
39. DeMay RM. Fluids. In: *The Art and Science of Cytopathology*. Chicago: ASCP Press; 1996:257–325.
40. Chernow B, Sahn SA. Carcinomatous involvement of the pleura: an analysis of 96 patients. *Am J Med*. 1977;63:695–702.
41. Edoute Y, Kuten A, Ben-Haim SA. Symptomatic pericardial effusion in breast cancer patients: the role of fluid cytology. *J Surg Oncol*. 1990;45:265–269.
42. Sahn SA. Malignant pleural effusions. *Semin Respir Med*. 1987;9:43–53.
43. Canto A, Ferrer G, Romagosa V, et al. Lung cancer and pleural effusion. Clincal significance and study of pleural metastic locations. *Chest*. 1985;87:649–852.
44. DiBonito L, Falconieri G, Colautti I. Cytopathology of malignant mesothelioma: a study of its patterns and histological bases. *Diagn Cytopathol*. 1993;9:25–31.
45. Imlay SP, Raab SS. Pleural fluid cytology: immunocytochemistry usage patterns and significance of nondefinitive diagnosis. *Diagn Cytopath*. 1999;22:281–285.
46. VandeMolengraft FJJM, Vooijs GP. Survival of patients with malignancy-associated effusions. *Acta Cytol*. 1989;33:911–916.
47. Chretien J, Jaubert F. Pleural responses in malignant metastatic tumors. In: Chretien J, Bignon J, Hirsch A, eds. *The Pleura in Health and Disease*. New York: Marcel Dekker; 1985:489–505.

48. Sahn SA. Malignant pleural effusion. In: Fishman AP, ed. *Pulmonary Diseases and Disorders*, 2nd ed. New York: McGraw-Hill; 1988:2159–2169.

49. Spriggs AI. Malignant cells in serous effusions complicating bronchial carcinoma. *Thorax*. 1954;9:26–34.

50. Smith-Purslow MJ, Kini SR, Naylor B. Cells of squamous cell carcinoma in pleural, peritoneal and pericardial fluids: origina and morphology. *Acta Cytol*. 1989;84:125–128.

51. Light RW, Tumors of the pleura In: Murray JF,.Nadel JA, eds. *Textbook of Respiratory Medicine*. Philadelphia: WB Saunders; 1770–1780

52. Bourke SA, Henderson AF, Stevenson RD, Banham SW. Endobronchial metastases simulating primary carcinoma of the lung. *Respir Med*. 1989;83:151–152.

53. King DS, Castleman B. Bronchial involvement in metastatic pulmonary malignancy. *J Thorac Surg*. 1943;12:305–315.

54. Katsimbri PP, Bamias AT, Froudarakis ME, et al. Endobronchial metastases secondary to solid tumors: report of eight cases and review of the literature. *Lung Cancer*. 2000;28:163–170.

55. Casino AR, Bellmunt J, Salud A, et al. Endobronchial metastases in colorectal adenocarcinoma. *Tumori*. 1992;78:270–273.

56. Schoenbaum S, Viamonte M. Subepithelial endobronchial metastases. *Diagn Radiol*. 1971;101:63–69.

57. Fitzgerald RH. Endobronchial metastases. *South Med J*. 1977;79:440–443.

58. Heitmiller R, Marasco W, Hruban R, Marsh B. Endobronchial metastasis. *J Thorac Cardiovasc Surg*. 1993;106:537–542.

59. Argyros G, Torrington K. Fiberoptic bronchoscopy in the evaluation of carcinoma metastatic to the lung. *Chest*. 1994;105:454–457.

60. Wang YH, Wong SL, Lai YF, et al. Endobronchial metastatic disease. *Chang Keng I Hsueh Tsa Chih*. 1999;22:240–245.

61. Salud A, Porcel JM, Rovirosa A, Bellmunt J. Endobronchial metastatic disease: analysis of 32 cases. *J Surg Oncol*. 1996;62:249–252.

62. Mehta AC, Marty JJ, Lee FWY. Sputum cytology. *Lung Cancer*. 1993;14:36–85.

63. Koss L, Melamed M, Goodner J. Pulmonary cytology: a brief survey of diagnostic results from July 1st, 1952 until December 31st, 1960. *Acta Cytol*. 1964;8:104–113.

64. Arroliga A, Matthay R. The role of bronchoscopy in lung cancer. *Lung Cancer*. 1993;14:87–98.

65. Harrow EM, Wang KP. The staging of lung cancer by bronchoscopic transbronchial needle aspiration. *Chest Surg Clin North Am*. 1996;6:223–235.

66. Wang KP. Transbronchial needle aspiration and percutaneous needle aspiration for staging and diagnosis of lung cancer. *Clin Chest Med*. 1995;16:535–552.

67. Salazar A, Westcott J. The role of thoracic needle biopsy for the diagnosis and staging of lung cancer. *Lung Cancer*. 1993;14:99–110.

68. Garcia RF, Lobato SD, Pino JM. Value of CT-guided fine needle aspiration in solitary pulmonary nodules with negative fiberoptic bronchoscopy. *Acta Radiol*. 1994;35:478–480.

69. Sonett J. Pulmonary metastases: biologic and historical justification for VATS. Video assisted thoracic surgery. *Eur J Cardiothorac Surg*. 1999;16(suppl):S13–S15.

70. Coosemans W, Lerut T, Raemdonck DV. Thoracoscopic surgery: the Belgian experience. *Ann Thorac Surg*. 1993;56:621–660.

71. Miller J. The present role and future considerations of video-assisted thorascopy in general thoracic surgery. *Ann Thorac Surg*. 1993;56:804–806.

72. Nathan M, Colloing V, Adams R. Differentiation of benign and malignant pulmonary nodules by growth rate. *Radiology*. 1962;79:221–232.

73. Nathan M. Management of solitary pulmonary nodules: an organized approach based on growth rate and statistics. *JAMA*. 1974;227:1141–1144.

74. Godwin JP, Speckman JM, Fram EK. Distinguishing benign from malignant pulmonary nodules by computed tomography. *Radiology*. 1982;144:349–352.

75. Layfield LJ, Coogan A, Johnston WW, Patz EF. Transthoracic fine needle aspiration biopsy. Sensitivity in relation to guidance technique and lesion size and location. *Acta Cytol*. 1996;40:687–690.

76. Pilotti S, Rilke F, Gribaudi G, Damascelli B. Fine needle aspiration biopsy cytology of primary and metastatic pulmonary tumors. *Acta Cytol*. 1982;26:661–666.

77. Zarbo R, Fenoglio-Preiser C. Interinstitutional database for comparison of performance in lung fine-needle aspiration cytology. A College of American Pathologists Q-Probe Study of 5264 cases with histologic correlation. *Arch Pathol Lab Med*. 1992;116:463–470.

78. Kern WH, Schweizer CW. Sputum cytology of metastatic carcinoma of the lung. *Acta Cytol*. 1976;20:514–520.

79. Perchalski JE, Hall KL, Dewar MA. Metastasis of unknown orgin. *Prim Care*. 1992;19:747–757.

80. Fizazi K, Culine S. Metastatic carcinoma of unknown orgin. *Bull Cancer*. 1998;85:609–617.

81. Schapira DV, Jerrett AR. The need to consider survival, outcome, and expense when evaluating and treating patients with unknown primary carcinoma. *Arch Intern Med*. 1995;155:2050–2054.

82. Heim S, Mitleman F. Solid tumors. In: *Cancer Cytogenetics*. New York: Alan R Liss; 1987:247–261.

83. Papec R. Distant metastases from head and neck. *Cancer*. 1984;53:342–345.

84. Probert J, Thompson R, Bagshaw M. Patterns of spread of distant metastases in head and neck cancer. *Cancer*. 1974;33:127–133.

85. Raab SS, Oweity T, Hughes JH, et al. The effect of patient history on diagnostic accuracy in the interpretation of bronchial brush specimens. *Am J Clin Pathol*. 2000;114:78–83.

86. DeYoung BR, Wick MR. Immunohistologic evaluation of metastatic carcinomas by unknown origin: an algorithmic approach. *Semin Diagn Pathol*. 2000;17:184–193.

87. Silver SS, Askin FB. True papillary carcinoma of the lung. A distinct clinicopathologic entity. *Am J Surg Pathol*. 1997;21:43–51.

88. Nakamura S, Koshikawa T, Sato T, et al. Extremely well differentiated papillary adenocarcinoma of the lung with prominent cilia formation. *Acta Pathol Jpn*. 1992;42:745–750.

89. Salisbury JR, Darby AJ, Whimster WF. Papillary adenocarcinoma of lung with psammoma bodies: report of a case derived from type II pneumocytes. *Histopathology*. 1986;10:877–884.

90. Massin J-P, Savoie J-C, Garnier H, et al. Pulmonary metastases in differentiated thyroid carcinoma. Study of 58 cases with implications for the primary tumor treatment. *Cancer*. 1984;53:982–992.

91. Samaan NA, Schultz PN, Haynie TP, Ordonez NG. Pulmonary metastasis of differential thyroid carcinoma: treatment results in 101 patients. *J Clin Endocrinol Metab*. 1985;60:376–380.

92. Venkatesh YSS, Ordonez NG, Schultz PN, et al. Anaplastic carcinoma of the thyroid: a clinicopathologic study of 121 cases. *Cancer*. 1990;66:321–330.

93. Shepherd MP. Endobronchial metastatic disease. *Thorax*. 1982;37:362–365.

94. Kerr VE, Cadman E. Pulmonary metastases in ovarian cancer. *Cancer*. 1985;56:1209–1213.

95. Dvoretsky PM, Richards KA, Angel C. Distribution of disease at autopsy in 100 women with ovarian cancer. *Hum Pathol*. 1988;19:57–63.

96. Oosterlee J. Peritoneovenous shunting for ascites in cancer patients. *Br J Surg*. 1980;67:663–666.

97. Fildes J, Narvarez GP, Baig KA, et al. Pulmonary tumor embolization after peritoneovenous shunting for malignant ascites. *Cancer*. 1988;61:1973–1976.

98. Werner M, Chott A, Fabiano A, Battifora H. Effect of formalin tissue fixation and processing on immunohistochemistry. *Am J Surg Pathol*. 2000;24:1016–1019.

99. Renshaw AA, Dean BR, Antman KH, et al. The role of cytologic evaluation of pleural fluid in the diagnosis of malignant mesothelioma. *Chest*. 1997;111:106–109.

100. Moran CA, Wick MR, Suster S. The role of immunohistochemistry in the diagnosis of malignant mesothelioma. *Semin Diagn Pathol*. 2000;17:178–183.

101. Moch H, Oberholzer M, Dalquen P. Diagnostic tools for differentiating between pleural mesothelioma and lung adenocarcinoma in paraffin embedded tissue. *Virch Arch A*. 1993;423:19–27.

102. Moch H, Oberholzer M, Christen H. Diagnostic tools for differentiating plural mesothelioma from lung adenocarcinoma in paraffin embedded tissue. Part II. *Virch Arch A*. 1993;423:493–496.

103. Wang N-S. Electron microscopy in the diagnosis of pleural mesotheloma. *Cancer*. 1973;31:1046–1054.

104. Batiffora H, Kopinski MI. Distinction of mesothelioma from adenocarcinoma. An immunohistochemical approach. *Cancer*. 1985;55:655–662.

105. Strickler JG, Hemdier BG, Rouse RV. Immunohistochemical staining in malignant mesotheliomas. *Am J Clin Pathol*. 1987;88:610–614.

106. Gaffey M, Mills S, Askin F, et al. Clear cell tumor of the lung. A clinicopathologic, immunohistochemical, and ultrastructural study of eight cases. *Am J Surg Pathol*. 1990;14:248–259.

107. Greenberg BE, Young JM. Pulmonary metastasis from occult primary sites resembling bronchogenic carcinoma. *Dis Chest*. 1958;33:496–505.

108. Hughes JH, Jensen CS, Donnelly AD, et al. The role of fine-needle aspiration cytology in the evaluation of metastatic clear cell tumors. *Cancer*. 1999;87:380–389.

109. Saitoh H. Distant metastasis of renal adenocarcinoma in patients with a tumor thrombus in the renal vein and/or vena cava. *J Urol*. 1982;127:652–653.

110. Latour A, Shulman HS. Thoracic manifestations of renal cell carcinoma. *Radiology*. 1976;121:43–48.

111. Coppage L, Shaw C, Curtis AM. Metastatic disease to the chest in patients with extrathoracic malignancy. *J Thoracic Imag*. 1987;2:24–37.

112. Gerle R, Felson B. Metastatic endobronchial hypernephroma. *Dis Chest*. 1963;44:225–233.

113. Noy S, Michowitz M, Lazebnik N, Baratz M. Endobronchial metastasis of renal cell carcinoma. *J Surg Oncol*. 1986;31:268–270.

114. Amer E, Guy J, Vaze B. Endobronchial metastasis from renal adenocarcinoma simulating a foreign body. *Thorax*. 1981;36:183–184.

115. King TH, Fisher J, Schwarz MI, Patzelt LH. Bilateral hilar adenopathy: an unusual presentation of renal cell carcinoma. *Thorax*. 1982;37:317–318.

116. Katzenstein A-LA, Purvis RW, Gmelich JT, Askin FB. Pulmonary resection for metastatic renal adenocarcinoma. *Cancer*. 1978;41:712–723.

117. Chu P, Arber DA. Paraffin section detection of CD10 in 505 nonhematopoietic neoplasms: frequent expression in renal cell carcinoma and endometrial stromal sarcoma. *Am J Clin Pathol*. 2000;113:374–382.

118. Scarpatetti M, Tsybrovskyy O, Popper HH. Cytokeratin typing as an aid in the differential diagnosis of primary versus metastatic lung carcinoma, and comparison with normal lung. *Virchows Arch*. 2002;440:70–76.

119. Avery AK, Beckstead J, Renshaw AA, Corless CL. Use of antibodies to RCC and CD10 in the differential diagnosis of renal neoplasms. *Am J Surg Pathol*. 2000;24:203–210.

120. Ostler DA, Prieto VG, Reed JA, et al. Adipophilin expression in sebaceous tumors and other cutaneous lesions with clear-cell histology: an immunohistochemical study of 117 cases. *Mod Pathol*. 2010;23:567–573.

121. Lisa JR, Trinidad S, Rosenblatt MB. Pulmonary manifestations of carcinoma of the pancreas. *Cancer*. 1964;17:395–401.

122. Cutler SJ, Asire AJ, Taylor SG. Classification of patients with disseminated cancer of the breast. *Cancer*. 1969;24:861–869.

123. DeBeer RA, Garcia RL, Alexander SC. Endobronchial metastasis from cancer of the breast. *Chest*. 1978;73:94–96.

124. Winchester DP, Sener SF, Khandekar JD. Symptomatology as an indicator of recurrent or metastatic breast cancer. *Cancer*. 1979;43.

125. Casey JJ, Stempel BG, Scanlon EF, Fry WA. The solitary pulmonary nodule in the patient with breast cancer. *Surgery*. 1984;96:801–805.

126. Fracchia AA, Knapper WH, Carey JT. Intrapleural chemotherapy for effusion from metastatic breast carcinoma. *Cancer*. 1970;26:626–629.

127. Raab SS, Berg LC, Swanson PE, Wick MR. Adenocarcinoma in the lung in patients with breast cancer. A prospective analysis of the discriminatory value of immunohistology. *Am J Clin Pathol*. 1993;100:27–35.

128. Dabbs DJ, Landreneau RJ, Liu Y, et al. Detection of estrogen receptor by immunohistochemistry in pulmonary adenocarcinoma. *Ann Thorac Surg*. 2002;73:403–406.

129. Wang Z, Spaulding B, Sienko A, et al. Mammaglobin: a valuable diagnostic marker for metastatic breast carcinoma. *Int J Clin Exp Pathol*. 2009;2:384–389.

130. MacDonald RA. Primary carcioma of the liver. A clinicopathologic study of one hundred eight cases. *Arch Intern Med*. 1957;99:266–279.

131. Katyal S, Oliver JH, Peterson MS, et al. Extrahepatic metastases of hepatocellular carcinoma. *Radiology*. 2000;216:698–703.

132. Patton RB, Horn RC. Primary liver carcinoma. Autopsy study of 60 cases. *Cancer*. 1964;17:757–768.

133. Tsai GL, Liu JD, Siauw CP, Chen PA. Thoracic roentgenologic manifestations in primary carcinoma of the liver. *Chest*. 1984;86:430–434.

134. Levy JI, Geddes EW, Kew MC. The chest radiograph in primary liver cancer. An analysis of 449 cases. *S Afr Med J*. 1976;50:1323–1326.

135. Cohen MB, Haber MM, Holly EA, et al. Cytologic criteria to distinguish hepatocellular carcinoma from nonneoplastic liver. *Am J Clin Pathol*. 1991;95:125–130.

136. Wieczorek TJ, Pinkus JL, Glickman JN, Pinkus GS. Comparison of thyroid transcription factor-1 and hepatocyte antigen immunohistochemical analysis in the differential diagnosis of hepatocellular carcinoma, metastatic adenocarcinoma, renal cell carcinoma, and adrenal cortical carcinoma. *Am J Clin Pathol*. 2002;118:911–921.

137. August DA, Ottow RT, Sugarbaker PH. Clinical perspective of human colorectal cancer metastasis. *Cancer Metastasis Rev*. 1984;5:303–324.

138. Dionne L. The pattern of blood-borne metastasis from carcinoma of rectum. *Cancer*. 1965;18:775–781.

139. Taylor FW. Cancer of the colon and rectum: a study of routes of metastases and death. *Surgery*. 1962;52:302–308.

140. Langer B. Managing distant metastases. *Can J Surg*. 1985;28:419–421.

141. McCormack PM, Attiyeh FF. Resected pulmonary metastases from colorectal cancer. *Dis Colon Rectum*. 1979;22:553–556.

142. Flint A, Lloyd RV. Colon carcinoma metastatic to the lung. Cytologic manifestations and distinction from primary pulmonary adenocarcinoma. *Acta Cytol*. 1992;36:230–235.

143. Harlamert HA, Mira J, Bejarano PA. Thyroid transcription factor-1 and cytokeratins 7 and 20 in pulmonary and breast carcinoma. *Acta Cytol*. 1998;42:1382–1388.

144. Bohinski RJ, Bejarano PA, Balko G. Determination of lung as the primary site of cerebral metastatic adenocarcinomas using monoclonal antibody to thyroid transcription factor-1. *J Neurooncol*. 1998;40:227–231.

145. Wauters CC, Smedts F, Gerrits LG, et al. Keratins 7 and 20 as diagnositc markers of carcinoma metastatic to the ovary. *Hum Pathol*. 1995;26:852–855.

146. Tsao MS, Fraser RS. Primary pulmonary adenocarcinoma with enteric differentiation. *Cancer*. 1991;68:1754–1757.

147. Bacchi CE, Gown AM. Distribution and pattern of expression of villin, a gastrointestinal-associated cytoskeletal protein, in human carcinomas: a study employing paraffin-embedded tissue. *Lab Invest*. 1991;64:418–424.

148. Gatalica Z, Miettinen M. Distribution of carcinoma antigens CA19-9 and CA15-3: an immunohistochemical study of 400 tumors. *Appl Immunohistochem*. 1994;2:205–211.

149. Saad RS, Silverman JF, Khalifa MA, Rowsell C. CDX2, cytokeratin 7 and 20 immunoreactivity in rectal adenocarcinoma. *Appl Immunohistochem Mol Morphol*. 2009;17:196–201.

150. Moran CA, Hocchholzer L, Fishback N, et al. Mucinous (so-called colloid) carcinomas of lung. *Mod Pathol*. 1992;5:634–638.

151. Cathro HP, Stoler MH. Expression of cytokeratins 7 and 20 in ovarian neoplasia. *Am J Clin Pathol*. 2002;117:944–951.

152. Ware JL. Prostate tumor progression and metastasis. *Biochim Biophys Acta*. 1987;907:279–298.

153. Ballon SC, Donaldson RC, Growdon WA. Pulmonary metastases in endometrial carcinoma. In: Weiss L, Gilbert HW, eds. *Pulmonary Metastasis*. Boston: GK Hall; 1978.

154. Mintz ER, Smith GG. Autopsy finding in 100 cases of prostatic cancer. *N Engl J Med*. 1934;211:479–487.

155. Elkin M, Mueller HP. Metastasis from cancer of the prostate: autopsy and roentgenological findings. *Cancer*. 1954;7:1246–1248.

156. Kume H, Takai K, Kameyama S, Kawabe K. Multiple pulmonary metastasis of prostatic carcinoma with little or no bone or lymph node metastasis. Report of two cases and review of the literature. *Urol Int*. 1999;62:44–47.

157. Scherz H, Schmidt JD. Endobronchial metastasis from prostate carcinoma. *Prostate*. 1986;8:319–324.

158. Legge DA, Good CA, Ludwig J. Roentgenologic features of pulmonary carcinomatosis from carcinoma of the prostate. *AJR*. 1971;11:360–364.

159. Apple JS, Paulson DF, Baber C, Putman CE. Advanced prostatic carcinoma: pulmonary manifestations. *Radiology*. 1985;54:601–604.

160. Miller GJ. The use of histochemistry and immunohistochemistry in evaluating prostatic neoplasia. *Prog Surg Pathol*. 1982;5:115–126.

161. Ross JS, Mazumder A. Tissue microarrays and gene chips. In: Wick MR, ed. *Metastatic Carcinoma of Unknown Origin*. New York: Demos; 2008:177–190.

162. van Laar RK, Ma XJ, de Jong D, et al. Implementation of a novel microarray-based diagnostic test for cancer of unknown primary. *Int J Cancer*. 2009;125:1390–1397.

163. Varadhachary GR, Talantov D, Raber MN, et al. Molecular profiling of carcinoma of unknown primary and correlation with clinical evaluation. *J Clin Oncol*. 2008;26:4442–4448.

164. Horlings HM, van Laar RK, Kerst JM, et al. Gene expression profiling to identify the histogenetic origin of metastatic adenocarcinomas of unknown primary. *J Clin Oncol*. 2008;26:4435–4441.

165. Oien KA, Evans TR. Raising the profile of cancer of unknown primary. *J Clin Oncol*. 2008;26:4373–4375.

166. Pentheroudakis G, Golfinopoulos V, Pavlidis N. Switching benchmarks in cancer of unknown primary: from autopsy to microarray. *Eur J Cancer*. 2007;43:2026–2036.

167. Ullmann R, Morbini P, Halbwedl I, et al. Protein expression profiles in adenocarcinomas and squamous cell carcinomas of the lung generated using tissue microarrays. *J Pathol*. 2004;203:798–807.

168. Dennis JL, Vass JK, Wit EC, et al. Identification from public data of molecular markers of adenocarcinoma characteristic of the site of origin. *Cancer Res*. 2002;62:5999–6005.

169. Buckhaults P, Zhang Z, Chen YC, et al. Identifying tumor origin using a gene expression-based classification map. *Cancer Res*. 2003;63:4144–4149.

170. Suster S. Recent advances in the application of immunohistochemical markers for the diagnosis of soft tissue tumors. *Semin Diagn Pathol*. 2000;17:225–235.

171. Lewis J, Brennan M. Soft tissue sarcomas. *Curr Probl Surg*. 1996;33:817–872.

172. Scranton PE, DeCicco FA, Totten RS. Prognostic factors in osteosarcoma. A review of 20 year's experience at the University of Pittsburgh Health Center Hospitals. *Cancer*. 1975;36:2179–2191.

173. Vezeridis MP, Moore R, Karakousis CP. Metastatic patterns in soft-tissue sarcomas. *Arch Surg*. 1983;118:915–918.

174. Flynn KJ, Kim HS. Endobronchial metastasis of uterine leiomyosarcoma. *JAMA*. 1978;1978.

175. Aronchick JM, Palevsky HI, Miller WT. Cavitary pulmonary metastases in angiosarcoma. Diagnosis by trans-thoracic needle aspiration. *Am Rev Respir Dis*. 1989;139:252–253.

176. Shaw AB. Spontaneous pneumothorax from secondary sarcoma of lung. *Br Med J*. 1951;1:278–280.

177. Spittle MF, Heal J, Harmer C, White WF. The association of spontaneous pneumothorax with pulmonary metastases in bone tumours of children. *Clin Radiol*. 1968;19:400–403.

178. Lodmell EA, Capps SC. Spontaneous pneumothorax associated with metastatic sarcoma. *Radiology*. 1949;52:88–93.

179. Dines DE, Cortese DA, Brennan MD, et al. Malignant pulmonary neoplasms predisposing to spontaneous pneumothorax. *Mayo Clin Proc*. 1973;48:541–544.

180. Brooks JJ. The significance of double phenotypic patterns and markers in human sarcomas: a new model of mesenchymal differentiation. *Am J Pathol*. 1986;125:113–123.

181. Gal AA, Brooks JSJ, Pietra GG. Leiomyomatous neoplasms of the lung: a clinical, histologic and immunohistochemical study. *Mod Pathol*. 1989;2:209–216.

182. Cho KR, Woodrumm JD, Epstein JI. Leiomyoma of the uterus with multiple extrauterine smooth muscle tumors: a case report suggesting multifocal orgin. *Hum Pathol*. 1989;20:80–83.

183. Sherman RS, Brant EE. An x-ray of spontaneous pneumothorax due to cancer metastases to the lungs. *Chest*. 1954;26:328–337.

184. Lipton JH, Fong TC, Burgess KR. Miliary pattern as presentation of leiomyomatosis of the lung. *Chest*. 1987;91:781–782.

185. Wolff M, Kaye G, Silva F. Pulmonary metastases (with admixed epithelial elements) from smooth muscle neoplasms. Report of nine cases, including three males. *Am J Surg Pathol*. 1979;3:325–342.

186. Horstmann JP, Pietra GG, Harman JA. Spontaneous regression of pulmonary leiomyomas during pregnancy. *Cancer*. 1977;39:314–321.

187. Kaplan C, Katoh A, Shamoto M. Multiple leiomyomas of the lung: benign or malignant? *Am Rev Respir Dis*. 1973;108:656–659.

188. Norris HJ, Parmley T. Mesenchymal tumors of the uterus. V: Intravenous leiomyomatosis. A clinical and pathologic study of 14 cases. *Cancer*. 1975;36:2164–2178.

189. Bachman D, Wolff M. Pulmonary metastases from benign smooth muscle tumors of the uterus. *AJR*. 1976;127:441–446.

190. Patton KT, Cheng L, Papavero V, et al. Benign metastasizing leiomyoma: clonality, telomere length, and clinicopathologic analysis. *Mod Pathol*. 2006;19:130–140.

191. Devoe K, Weidner N. Immunohistochemistry of small round-cell tumors. *Semin Diagn Pathol*. 2000;17:216–224.

192. Meis-Kindblom JM, Stenman G, Kindblom LG. Differential diagnosis of small round cell tumors. *Semin Diagn Pathol*. 1996;13:213–241.

193. Byrd-Gloster AL, Khoor A, Glass LF, et al. Differential expression for thyroid transcription factor 1 in small cell lung carcinoma and Merkel cell tumor. *Hum Pathol*. 2000;31:58–62.

194. Moll R, Lower A, Laufer J. Cytokeratin 20 in human carcinomas. A new histodiagnostic marker detected by monoclonal antibodies. *Am J Pathol*. 1992;140:427–447.

195. Schmidt U, Muller U, Metz KA. Cytokeratin and neurofilament protein staining in Merkel cell carcinoma and of the small cell type and small cell carcinoma of the lung. *Am J Dermatopathol*. 1998;20:346–351.

196. Wick MR. Immunohistology of neuroendocrine and neuroectodermal tumors. *Semin Diagn Pathol*. 2000;17:194–203.

197. Wick MR, Ritter JH, Swanson PE. The impact of diagnostic immunohistochemistry on patient outcomes. *Clin Lab Med*. 1999;19:797–814.

198. Oliveira AM, Tazelaar HD, Myers JL, et al. Thyroid transcription factor-1 distinguishes metastatic pulmonary from well-differentiated neuroendocrine tumors of other sites. *Am J Surg Pathol*. 2001;25:815–819.

199. Corrin B. Lung endocrine tumors. *Invest Cell Pathol*. 1980;3:195–206.

200. Ikeda K, Tate G, Suzuki T, Mitsuya T. Cytologic comparison of a primary parathyroid cancer and its metastatic lesions: a case report. *Diagn Cytopathol*. 2005;34:50–55.

201. Iihara M, Okamoto T, Suzuki R, et al. Functional parathyroid carcinoma: long-term treatment outcome and risk factor analysis. *Surgery*. 2007;142:936–943.

202. Juhl J. Tumors of the lungs and bronchi. In: *Essentials of Radiologic Imaging*. Philadelphia: Lippincott-Raven; 1998:1–95.

203. Colby TV, Carrington CB. Malignant lymphoma simulating lymphomatoid granulomatosis. *Am J Surg Pathol*. 1982;6:19–32.

204. Colby TV, Carrington CB. Lymphoreticular tumors and infiltrates of the lung. *Pathol Annu*. 1983;18:27–70.

205. Melamed MR. The cytological presentation of malignant lymphomas and related diseases in effusions. *Cancer*. 1963;16:413–431.

206. Meda BA, Buss DH, Woodruff RD, et al. Diagnosis and subclassification of primary and recurrent lymphoma. The usefulness and limitations of combined fine-needle aspiration cytomorphology and flow cytometry. *Am J Clin Pathol*. 2000;113:688–689.

207. Demington M, Carter D, Meyers A. Distant metastases in head and neck epidermoid carcinoma. *Laryngoscope*. 1980;90:196–201.

208. O'Brien PH, Carlson R, Steubner EA. Distant metastases in epidermoid cell carcinoma of the head and neck. *Cancer*. 1971;27:204–307.

209. Malefetto JP, Kasimis BS, Moran EM, et al. The clinical significance of radiographically detected pulmonary neoplastic lesions in patients with head and neck cancer. *J Clin Oncol*. 1984;2:625–630.

210. Leon X, Quer M, Diez S, et al. Second neoplasm in patients with head and neck cancer. *Head Neck*. 1999;21:204–210.

211. Sostman HD, Matthay RA. Thoracic metastases from cervical carcinoma: current status. *Invest Radiol*. 1980;15:113–119.

212. D'Orsi CJ, Bruckman J, Mauch P, Smith EH. Lung metastases in cervical and endometrial carcinoma. *Am J Roentgenol*. 1979;133:719–722.

213. Kirubakaran MG, Pulimood BM, Ray D. Excavating pulmonary metastases in carcinoma of the cervix. *Postgrad Med J*. 1975;51:243–245.

214. Scott I, Bergin CJ, Muller NL. Mediastinal and hilar lymphadenopathy as the only manifestation of metastatic carcinoma of the cervix. *J Can Assoc Radiol*. 1986;37:52–53.

215. King TE, Neff TA, Ziporin P. Endobronchial metastasis from the uterine cervix: presentation as primary lung abscess. *JAMA*. 1979;242:1651–1652.

216. Buchsbaum HJ. Lymphangitis carcinomatosis secondary to carcinoma of cervix. *Obstet Gynecol*. 1970;36:850–860.

217. Vachani A, Nebozhyn M, Singhal S, et al. A 10-gene classifier for distinguishing head and neck squamous cell carcinoma and lung squamous cell carcinoma. *Clin Cancer Res*. 2007;13:2905–2915.

218. Girard N, Deshpande C, Lau C, et al. Comprehensive histologic assessment helps to differentiate multiple lung primary non-small cell carcinomas from metastases. *Am J Surg Pathol*. 2009;33:1752–1764.

219. Wilson RW, Moran CA. Primary melanoma of the lung: a clinicopathologic and immunohistochemical study of eight cases. *Am J Surg Pathol*. 1997;21:1196–1202.

220. DasGupta T, Brasfield R. Metastic melanoma: a clinopathological study. *Cancer*. 1964; 17:1323–1339.

221. Harpole DH, Johnson CM, Wolfe WG, et al. Analysis of 945 cases of pulmonary metastatic melanoma. *J Thorac Cardiovasc Surg*. 1992;103:743–750.

222. Chen JTT, Dahmash NS, Ravin CE. Metastatic melanoma to the thorax: report of 130 patients. *Am J Roentgenol*. 1981;137:293–298.

223. Dwyer AJ, Reichert CM, Woltering EA, Flye MW. Diffuse pulmonary metastasis in melanoma: radiographic–pathologic correlation. *Am J Roentgenol*. 1984;143:983–984.

224. Webb WR, Gamsu G. Thoracic metastasis in malignant melanoma. *Chest*. 1977;71:176–181.

225. Balch CM, Soong SJ, Murad TM, et al. A multifactorial analysis of melanoma: prognostic factors in 200 melanoma patients with distant metastases. *J Clin Oncol*. 1983;1:126–134.

226. Pogrebniak HW, Stovroff M, Roth JA, Pass HI. Resection of pulmonary metastases from malignant melanoma: results of a 16-year experience. *Ann Thorac Surg*. 1988;46:20–23.

227. Renshaw A, Madge R. Cercariform cells for helping distinguish transitional cell carcinoma from non-small cell lung carcinoma in fine needle aspirates. *Acta Cytol*. 1997;41:999–1007.

228. Gown AM, Vogel AM, Hoak D, et al. Monoclonal antibodies specific for melanocytic tumors distinguish subpopulations of melanocytes. *Am J Pathol*. 1986;123:195–203.

229. Wang NP, Zee S, Zarbo RJ, et al. Coordinate expression of cytokeratins 7 and 20 defines unique subsets of carcinomas. *Appl Immunohistochem*. 1995;3:99–107.

230. Baars JH, DeRuijter JL, Smedts F, et al. The applicability of a keratin 7 monoclonal antibody in routinely Papanicolaou-stained cytologic specimens for the differential diagnosis of carcinomas. *Am J Clin Pathol*. 1994;101:257–261.

231. Sack MJ, Roberts SA. Cytokeratins 20 and 7 in the differential diagnosis of metastatic carcinoma in cytologic specimens. *Diagn Cytopathol*. 1997;16:132–136.

232. Lotan TL, Ye H, Melamed J, et al. Immunohistochemical panel to identify the primary site of invasive micropapillary carcinoma. *Am J Surg Pathol*. 2009;33:1037–1041.

233. Munk PL, Connell DG, Muller NL, Lentle BC. Alveolar soft parts sarcoma with pulmonary metastases. *Skeletal Radiol*. 1988;17:454–457.

234. Weiss SW, Enzinger FM. Malignant fibrous histiocytoma: an analysis of 200 cases. *Cancer*. 1978;41:2250–2266.

235. Hendin AS. Gestational trophoblastic tumors metastatic to the lungs. *Cancer*. 1984;53:58–61.

236. Hatch KD, Shingleton HM, Gore H, et al. Human chorionic gonadotropin-secreting large cell carcinoma of the lung detected during follow-up of a patient previously treated for gestational trophoblastic disease. *Gynecol Oncol*. 1980;10:98–104.

237. Kumar J, Ilancheran A, Ratnam SS. Pulmonary metastases in gestational trophoblastic disease: a review of 97 cases. *Br J Obstet Gynecol*. 1988;95:70–74.

238. Siegel RJ, Bueso-Ramos C, Cohen C, Koss M. Pulmonary blastoma with germ cell (yolk sac) differentiation: report of two cases. *Mod Pathol*. 1991;4:566–570.

239. Wick MR, Swanson PE, Manivel JC. Placenta-like alkaline phosphatase reactivity in human tumors: an immunohistochemical study of 520 cases. *Hum Pathol*. 1987;18:946–954.

240. Hammar S. The use of electron microscopy and immunohistochemistry in the diagnosis and understanding of lung neoplasms. *Clin Lab Med*. 1987;7:1–30.

241. Hammar SP, Bolen JW, Bockus D, et al. Ultrastructural and immunohistochemical features of common lung tumors: an overview. *Ultrastruct Pathol*. 1985;9:283–318.

242. Mennemeyer R, Hammar SP, Bauermeister DE, et al. Cytologic, histologic, and electron microscopic correlations in poorly-differentiated primary lung carcinoma: a study of 43 cases. *Acta Cytol*. 1979;23:297–302.

243. Mackay B, Silva EG. Diagnostic electron microscopy in oncology. *Pathol Annu*. 1980; 15(part II):241–270.

244. Tucker JA. The continuing value of electron microscopy in surgical pathology. *Ultrastruct Pathol*. 2000;24:383–389.

245. Mierau GW, Berry PJ, Malott RL, Weeks DA. Appraisal of the comparative utility of immunohistochemistry and electron microscopy in the diagnosis of childhood round cell tumors. *Ultrastruct Pathol*. 1996;20:507–517.

246. Erlandson RA, Rosai J. A realistic approach to the use of electron microscopy and other ancillary diagnostic techniques in surgical pathology. *Am J Surg Pathol*. 1995;19:247–250.

247. Lombardi L, Orazi A. Electron microscopy in an oncologic institution: diagnostic usefulness in surgical pathology. *Tumori*. 1988;74:531–535.

248. Williams MJ, Uzman BG. Uses and contributions of diagnostic electron microscopy in surgical pathology: a study of 20 Veterans Administration hospitals. *Hum Pathol*. 1984;15:738–745.

249. Azar HA, Espinoza CG, Richman AV, et al. Undifferentiated" large cell malignancies: an ultrastructural and immunocytochemical study. *Hum Pathol*. 1982;13:323–333.

250. Seymour AE, Henderson DW. Electron microscopy in surgical pathology: a selective review. *Pathology*. 1981;13:111–135.

251. Warhol MJ, Corson JM. An ultrastructural comparison of mesotheliomas with adenocarcinomas of the lung and breast. *Hum Pathol*. 1985;16:50–55.

252. Warhol MJ, Hickey WF, Corson JM. Malignant mesothelioma: ultrastructural distinction from adenocarcinoma. *Am J Surg Pathol*. 1982;6:307–314.

253. Warhol MJ, Hunter NJ, Corson JM. An ultrastructural comparison of mesotheliomas and adenocarcinoma of the ovary and endometrium. *Int J Gynecol Pathol*. 1982;1:125–134.

254. Wick MR, Swanson PE, Manivel JC. Immunohistochemical analysis of soft tissue sarcomas. Comparisons with electron microscopy. *Appl Pathol*. 1988;6:169–196.

255. Gonzalez-Crussi F, Mangkornkanok M, Hsueh W. Large-cell lymphoma: diagnostic difficulties and case study. *Am J Pathol*. 1987;11:59–65.

256. Weinstein MH, Dal Cin P. Genetics of epithelial tumors of the renal parenchyma in adults and renal cell carcinoma in children. *Anal Quant Cytol Histol*. 2001;23:362–372.

257. Argani P, Antonescu CR, Illei PB, et al. Primary renal neoplasms with the ASPL-TFE3 gene fusion of alveolar soft parts sarcoma: a distinctive tumor entity previously included among renal cell carcinomas of children and adolescents. *Am J Pathol*. 2001;159:179–192.

258. Cerasoli S, Spada F, Buda R, et al. Cytogenetic analysis of 19 renal cell tumors. *Pathologica*. 2001;93:118–123.

259. Dennis TR, Stock AD. A molecular cytogenetic study of chromosome 3 rearrangements in small cell lung cancer: consistent involvement of chromosome band 3q13.2. *Cancer Genet Cytogenet*. 1999;113:134–140.

260. Onuki N, Wistuba II, Travis WD, et al. Genetic changes in the spectrum of neuroendocrine lung tumors. *Cancer*. 1999;85:600–607.

261. Kovatich A, Friedland DM, Druck T, et al. Molecular alterations to human chromosome 3p loci in neuroendocrine lung tumors. *Cancer*. 1998;83:1109–1117.

262. Sandberg AA. Cytogenetics and molecular genetics of bone and soft-tissue tumors. *Am J Med Genet*. 2002;115:189–193.

263. Parham DM. Neuroectodermal and neuroendocrine tumors principally seen in children. *Am J Clin Pathol*. 2001;115(suppl):S113–S128.

264. Summersgill B, Goker H, Osin P, et al. Establishing germ cell origin of undifferentiated tumors by identifying gains of 12p material using comparative genomic hybridization analysis of paraffin-embedded samples. *Diagn Mol Pathol*. 1998;7:260–266.

265. Ahmed S, Siddiqui AK, Rai KR. Low-grade B-cell bronchial associated lymphoid tissue (BALT) lymphoma. *Cancer Invest*. 2002;20:1059–1068.

266. Hedvat CV, Hegde A, Chaganti RS, et al. Application of tissue microarray technology to the study of non-Hodgkin's and Hodgkin's lymphoma. *Hum Pathol*. 2002;33:968–974.

267. Mehra S, Messner H, Minden M, Chaganti RS. Molecular cytogenetic characterization of non-Hodgkin lymphoma cell lines. *Genes Chromosomes Cancer*. 2002;33:225–234.

268. Minna JD. Neoplasms of the lung. In: Favei AS, Braunwald E, Isselbacher KJ, eds. *Harrison's Principles of Internal Medicine*. New York: McGraw-Hill; 1998:552–562.

269. Snyder CL, Saltzman DA, Ferrell KL, et al. A new approach to the resection of pulmonary osteosarcoma metastases. Results of aggressive metastasectomy. *Clin Orthop*. 1991;270: 247–253.

270. Todd TR. The surgical treatment of pulmonary metastases. *Chest*. 1997;112:287S–290S.

271. Downey RJ. Surgical treatment of pulmonary metastases. *Surg Oncol Clin North Am*. 1999;8: 341.

272. Raab SS, Hornberger J, Raffin T. The importance of sputum cytology in the diagnosis of lung cancer. A cost-effectiveness analysis. *Chest*. 1997;112:937–945.

273. Barlow PB, Beck JR. The solitary pulmonary nodule: a decision analysis [Abstract]. *Chest*. 1985;88:45S.

274. Cummings SR, Lillington GA, Richards RJ. Managing solitary pulmonary nodules: the choice of strategy is a "close call". *Am Rev Respir Dis*. 1986;134:453–460.

275. Kunstaetter R, Wolkove N, Kreisman H. The solitary pulmonary nodule: decision analysis. *Med Decis Making*. 1985;5:61–75.

276. Raab SS, Hornberger J. The effect of a patient's risk-taking attitude on the cost effectiveness of testing strategies in the evaluation of pulmonary lesions. *Chest*. 1997;111:1583–1590.

277. Raab SS, Slagel DD, Hughes JH, et al. Sensitivity and cost-effectiveness of fine needle aspiration with immunocytochemistry in the evaluation of patients with a pulmonary malignancy and a history of cancer. *Arch Pathol Lab Med*. 1997;121:695–700.

278. Raab S, Gross T, Grzybicki D, Silverman J. Clinical perception of the utility of sputa and other tests in patients with lung masses. *Mod Pathol*. 1999;12:188A.

279. Raab SS. The cost-effectiveness of immunohistochemistry. *Arch Pathol Lab Med*. 2000;124:1185–1191.

280. Alberts AS, Falkson G, Falkson HC, Merwe MP. Treatment and prognosis of metastatic carcinoma of unknown primary: analysis of 100 patients. *Med Pediatr Oncol*. 1989;17:188–192.

Pseudoneoplastic Lesions of the Lungs and Pleural Surfaces

Mark R. Wick, MD, Timothy C. Allen, MD, JD, Henry D. Tazelaar, MD,
Jon H. Ritter, MD, Osamu Matsubara, MD

There is a limited group of pulmonary lesions that one can classify as pseudoneoplastic, but their conditions comprise a significant aggregation in absolute numbers. Some are categorized as malformative or reactive, including pulmonary hamartomas; selected inflammatory pseudotumors ("plasma cell granulomas"); tumefactive lymphoid hyperplasias; inflammatory or reparative conditions simulating carcinomas; unusual granulomatous reactions; tumefactive pleural plaques; and florid examples of mesothelial hyperplasia. Other clinical "pseudotumors" such as amyloidoma and rounded atelectasis[1] are confused with neoplasms only by nonpathologists and are not included for discussion here. On the other hand, the variant of inflammatory pseudotumor now known as *inflammatory myofibroblastic tumor* demonstrates clonal characteristics and can rightly be regarded as a true neoplasm.[2,3] Accordingly, it likewise has been omitted from this chapter.

Pulmonary Hamartoma

The term *hamartoma* is intended to denote tumefactive malformations that exhibit an architecturally abnormal relationship between tissue components that are appropriate to the organ site in which they arise.[4] Other terms for these lesions in the lung include *benign mesenchymoma, fibroma, chondroma, fibrochondrolipoma, fibrolipomyochondroma, hamartoma-chondroma, cartilage-containing tumor of the lung, adenochondroma, lipochondroadenoma, adenofibrolipochondromyxoma,* and *mixed tumor*.[5] Although in the past, *chondroma* has been used interchangeably with the lesion referred to here as *hamartoma,* they constitute distinct lesions and are discussed in Chapter 19.

Pulmonary hamartomas (PHs) have been encountered in approximately 0.25% of autopsies.[6] They can arise both centrally and peripherally, and the latter are more common in men than women.[7–10] Radiographically, hamartomas are typically found incidentally, usually in patients between 40 and 60 years of age; nevertheless, pediatric cases have also been reported.[10] They are only rarely multiple. Hamartomas may coexist with primary or secondary malignancies of the lung.[11,12] Under these circumstances, the hamartomatous lesions may be mistaken for intrapulmonary metastases or synchronous primary carcinomas, particularly if they lack internal calcification.

Macroscopically, most PHs are peripherally located, and they sometimes show a topographical relationship to small bronchi or bronchioles.[13–16] They rarely penetrate the visceral pleura.[17] They are usually well-demarcated (Figs. 18-1 and 18-2) and range from several millimeters to 20 cm in diameter. The central form of hamartoma is encountered in association with large bronchi, as an endoluminal polypoid protuberance covered by intact mucosa.[10] All hamartomas of the lung are lobulated, and their cut surfaces reflect their constituent cells (Figs. 18-3 and 18-4). Most of these lesions contain predominantly cartilaginous tissue and are therefore firm to hard, relatively homogeneous, and translucent when transected.

On histologic examination, PHs are manifested by mature mesenchymal tissues but with abnormal configurations. These elements are usually represented by hyaline cartilage, but fibrous tissue, smooth muscle, adipocytic components, and bone[18] may be seen. Those masses lacking chondroid elements have sometimes been diagnosed as "intrabronchial lipoma," "myxoma," "leiomyoma," or "fibroadenoma."[13–16] During the growth of PHs, the mesenchymal portions of the lesion engulf and trap small tubular airways, and the latter structures thus spuriously appear to represent an integral part of the lesion (Figs. 18-5 and 18-6). Entrapped alveolar epithelium may also undergo cuboidal or low-columnar metaplasia. Epithelial hyperplasia and papillae may be present in the entrapped epithelium (Fig. 18-7). Indeed, the last of

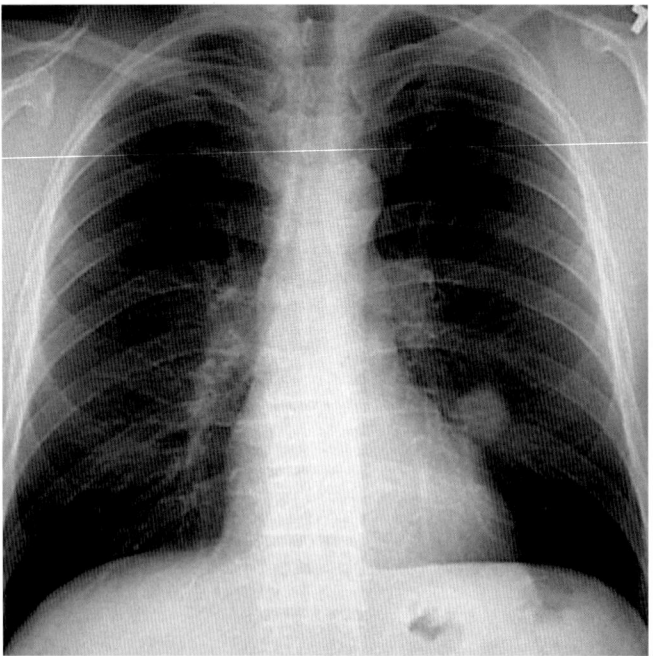

Figure 18-1. Chest radiograph of pulmonary hamartoma showing a well-circumscribed mass abutting the left cardiac border in this posteroanterior view.

these changes can be prominent and bear a resemblance to placental tissue,[19] a feature referred to as "placental transmogrification." The presence of entrapped epithelium is one of the key distinguishing features of PH from "true" pulmonary chondroma. Transthoracic fine needle aspiration biopsy (FNAB) is a common method for the initial pathologic sampling of mass lesions in the lung. In fact, if PH is the favored diagnosis of the radiologist, FNAB is usually done with the anticipation that a thoracotomy can be avoided if that interpretation is correct. The cytologic features of PH include the presence of dispersed fusiform and stellate cells in a myxoid background, as seen histologically (see Fig. 18-7B). Chondroid material is also present in a majority of cases.[20-22]

Nevertheless, FNAB of PH may, in fact, result in the very outcome it intends to avoid: namely, formal surgical resection because of a suspicion of malignancy. Some cytologic specimens of PH show atypical epithelial cells with enlarged nuclei, mimicking low-grade

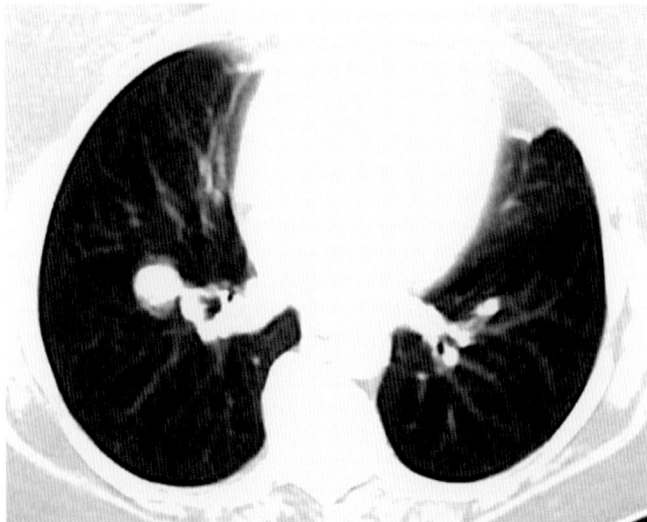

Figure 18-2. Computed tomography scan of the thorax showing pulmonary hamartoma as a sharply demarcated nodular lesion near the right hilum.

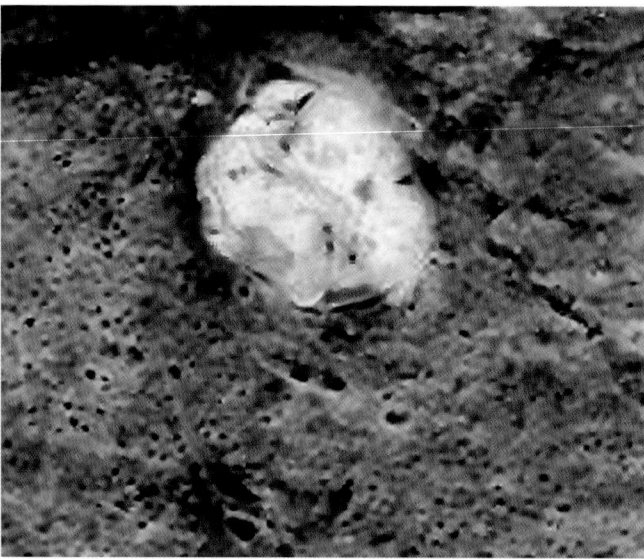

Figure 18-3. Gross photograph of pulmonary hamartoma showing a firm homogeneous glistening white nodule that stands out from the lung cut surface.

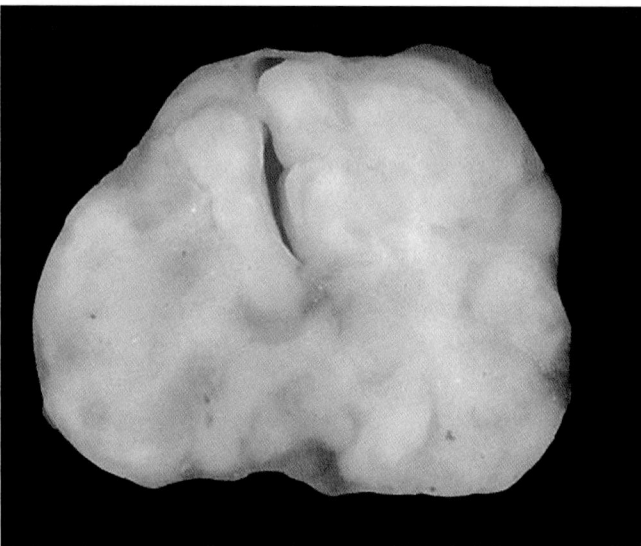

Figure 18-4. Another macroscopic image of pulmonary hamartoma demonstrating internal lobulation and a glistening translucent cut surface.

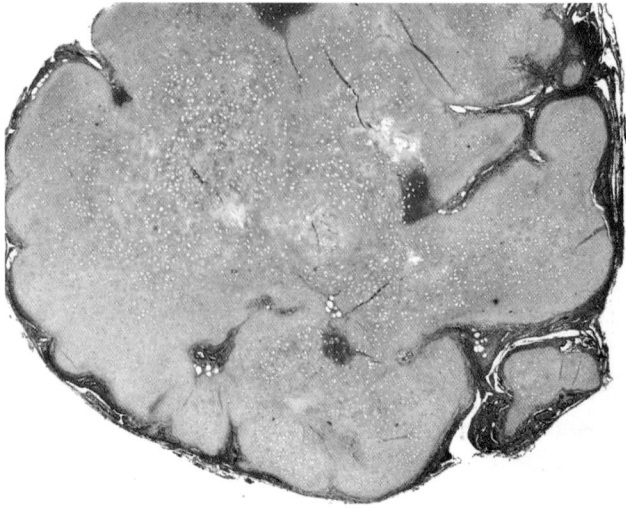

Figure 18-5. Bronchiolar epithelium is entrapped by relatively mature chondroid and adipocytic tissues in this pulmonary hamartoma.

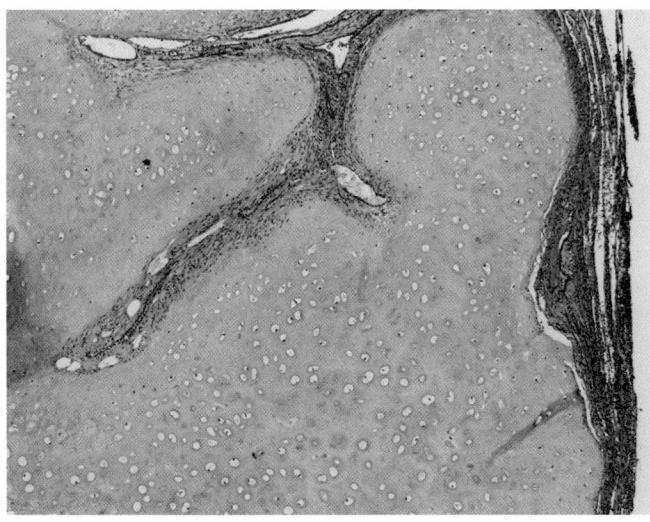

Figure 18-6. The juxtaposition of lesional mesenchyme (*left*) and trapped epithelium (*right*) is seen in this photomicrograph of pulmonary hamartoma.

adenocarcinoma (see Fig. 18-7C), sometimes adjacent to stromal tissues resembling the pattern seen in some fibroadenomas of the breast in FNAB samples. This can easily lead to a false-positive interpretation of carcinoma.[23] Surfactant-containing intranuclear inclusions can be seen in the trapped epithelium of PH,[24] like those observed in

bronchioloalveolar carcinomas, further suggesting the diagnosis of carcinoma.

Electron microscopic studies of PH show primitive stellate fibroblastic cells with transitional forms to cartilaginous foci.[25,26]

Cytogenetic evaluations have demonstrated an abnormal karyotype in several instances, principally represented by an exchange of material among various chromosomes.[27-30] These data beg the question of whether PH might actually be neoplastic after all, but the clinical evolution of this lesion (see subsequent discussion) generally speaks against such a possibility.

PH must be distinguished from primary or metastatic mesenchymal malignancies in the lungs, as well as primary or secondary biphasic sarcomatoid carcinomas.[31-34] The presence of multinucleated cells, nuclear pleomorphism, necrosis, and mitotic activity is rare in PH, in contrast to these diagnostic alternatives. In histologically similar biphasic carcinomas (Fig. 18-8), keratin immunoreactivity is present both in the mesenchymal-like and the overtly epithelial components, whereas PH shows reactivity for epithelial markers only in trapped epithelial elements. True chondromas of the lung tend to be multiple and comprised of only cartilage, which is smoothly circumscribed. In contrast, PHs occur singly, and contain multiple tissue types and entrapped, invaginated epithelium.

PHs continue to enlarge slowly if left in place after diagnosis, but they rarely cause significant clinical difficulty. Simple excision of the lesions is typically performed today, especially with the availability of

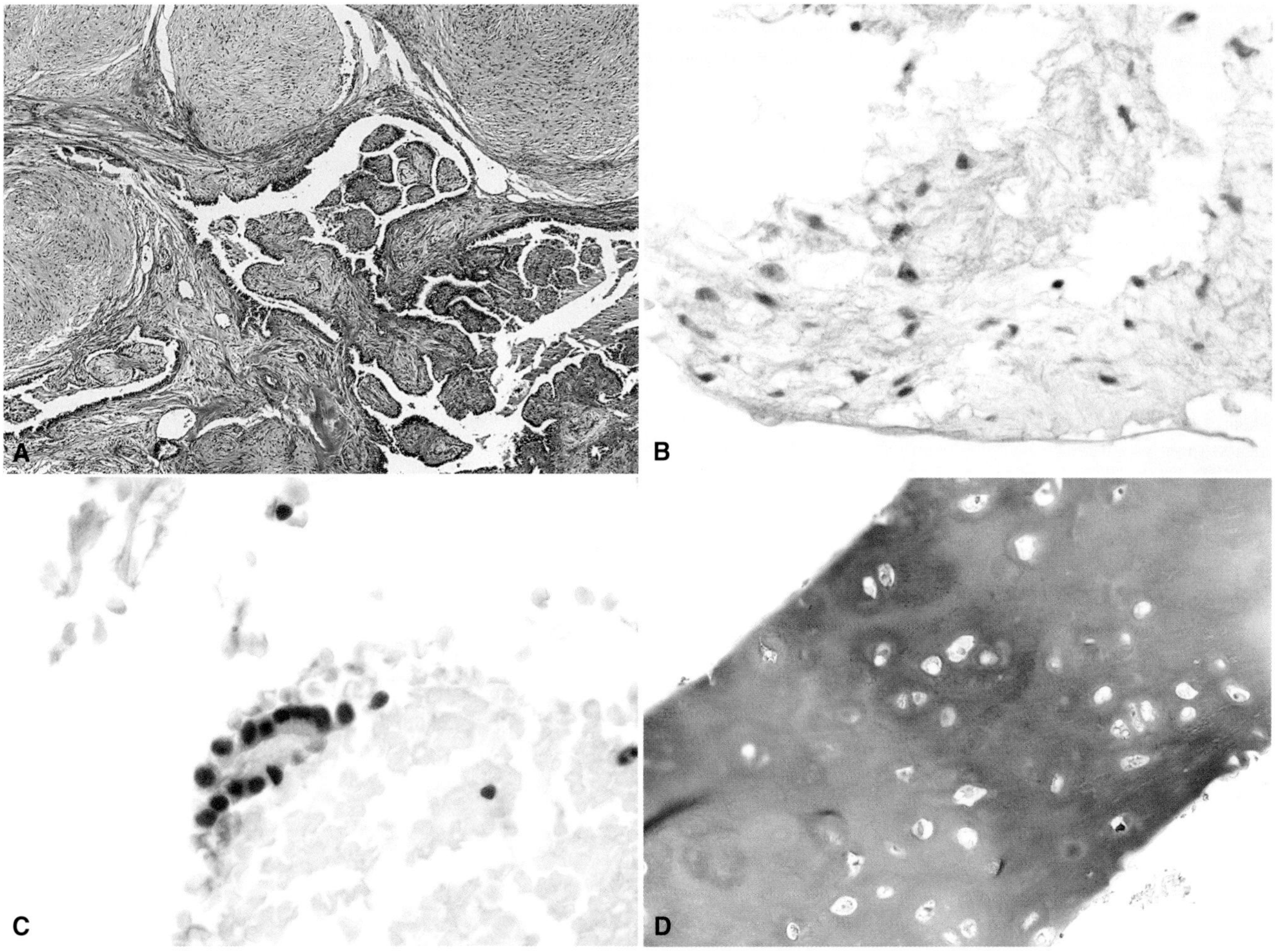

Figure 18-7. A, Nodules of cellular mesenchymal tissue with a chondroid "aura" alternate with trapped and proliferating epithelial profiles in another example of pulmonary hamartoma. Chondroid hamartoma as sampled by fine needle aspiration biopsy (FNAB), with bland spindle cells surrounded by myxoid stroma (**B**). Other foci showed bland cuboidal or low-columnar epithelial cells (**C**) and fragments of cartilage (**D**).

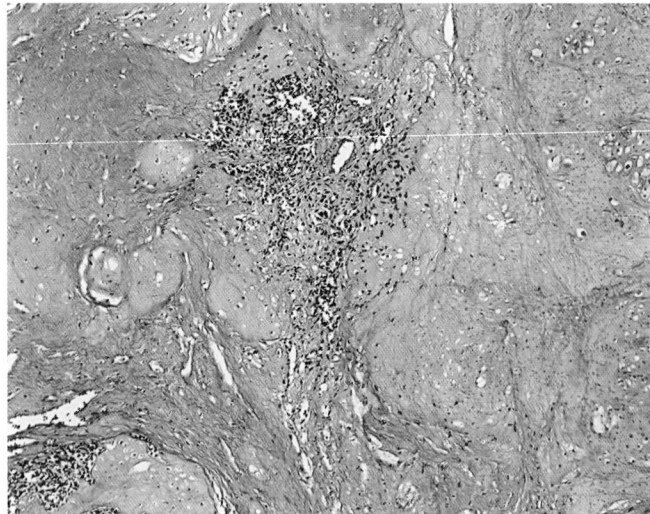

Figure 18-8. Differential diagnosis in cases of pulmonary hamartoma include "metaplastic" (sarcomatoid) carcinoma with a biphasic and partially chondroid configuration, as shown here.

thoracoscopic video-assisted surgical techniques.[35] Laser treatment has also been offered for patients with central PHs.[36] The clinical result of these treatments is excellent in virtually all cases.

Returning to the question of whether PH might be neoplastic, Pelosi and colleagues have reported exceptional cases in which a malignancy appears to evolve from this lesion.[37] In particular, these authors observed the patterns of *malignant mixed tumor* and *malignant myoepithelioma* in association with PH.

Inflammatory Pseudotumor—Plasma Cell Granuloma of the Lung

The most common form of the proliferative spindle cell lesion known as *inflammatory pseudotumor* (IPT) of the lung has undergone scrutiny in the recent past and is generally regarded currently as a true neoplasm composed of myofibroblasts.[2,3] That particular entity had been called the *fibrohistiocytic* subtype of pulmonary pseudotumor[38-40] but has now been renamed *inflammatory myofibroblastic tumor* (IMT).[3] The lesion known as *calcifying fibrous pseudotumor*[41-44] may represent a closely related entity, at least in some cases, and is bound to IMT by its common manifestation of a t(2;17) chromosomal translocation and a potential expression of the ALK-1 protein.[45-47] Other lesions of the lung that have been included in the category of IPT—namely, *plasma cell granuloma* and *hyalinizing granuloma*[46-54]—probably do represent non-neoplastic masses with variable etiologies. Both of them are composed of inflammatory and mesenchymal cells, potentially including mature lymphocytes, plasma cells, mast cells, macrophages, eosinophils, fibroblasts, and myofibroblasts. There is also likely overlap between some of these lesions and those described in association with IgG4 sclerosing disease (see later discussion).

As just defined, the true incidence of pulmonary IPTs that are *not* IMTs is uncertain. IPTs are not commonly encountered in general surgical pathology practice, but their frequency is somewhat dependent on definitions. Some observers have used IPT broadly, to describe both circumscribed nodules and large irregular inflammatory masses, or segmental and lobar consolidations,[55] whereas others have almost abandoned the term altogether, preferring a more descriptive diagnosis for most cases, such as organizing pneumonia.

This lesion shows no sex predilection and occurs over a broad age range, from 1 to 77 years, with a mean of 27 to 50 years.[40] Approximately

50% of patients complain of cough, hemoptysis, shortness of breath, chest pain, or combinations thereof. Chest radiographs usually show a single, sharply marginated, round or oval mass (Fig. 18-9), but the edges of large lesions may be more ill-defined.[56,57] Some IPTs involve the pleural surface and retract it as seen on computed tomography (CT) of the thorax[57]; as expected, these findings may falsely suggest the possibility of malignancy. Calcification and cavitation also are potentially present in IPTs, and these features may also be present in imaging.

Pulmonary IPTs range in size from 0.5 to larger than 30 cm.[39,40] Most have well-defined margins macroscopically but do not have a true fibrous capsule, and the color and texture is variable. Those that contain numerous inflammatory cells are tan-white and fleshy, and those with a predominance of mesenchymal tissue are gray and firm. IPTs with secondary xanthomatization may be bright yellow and friable. Some IPT also exhibit areas of hemorrhage, necrosis, and/or calcification. Rarely IPTs are comprised of sessile intrabronchial masses, whereas others are attached to the pleura. In typical pulmonary IPT, the microscopic architecture of the lung is replaced by a fibroinflammatory proliferation. Depending on their dominant cellular elements and major growth patterns, IPTs may be subclassified into two types: namely, tumefactive organizing pneumonia-like and lymphoplasmacytic variants.[39] These may simply represent different stages in the evolution of IPT, but recent publications suggest that lymphoplasmacytic IPT (LPIPT) is distinctive as part of systemic fibrosing autoimmune disorders that feature the presence of numerous IgG4-producing plasma cells.[58-61]

The organizing pneumonia-like variant shows intra-alveolar lymphohistiocytic inflammation and peripheral as well as central fibrosis (Figs. 18-10 and 18-11). Fibroblastic proliferation is admixed with fibrinoinflammatory exudate in alveoli, alveolar ducts, and bronchioles. The alveolar architecture is preserved in early lesions and the peripheral portions of "mature" IPT but is generally obscured by superimposed fibrous tissue, which tends to assume a whorled configuration (Figs. 18-12 and 18-13). Neutrophils are sometimes interspersed with the lymphocytes and plasma cells, and they may form intralesional microabscesses that result in small areas of cavitation. Alveoli bordering IPTs are often filled with foamy macrophages and mantled by hyperplastic pneumocytes. Multinucleated cells of the Touton type are sometimes present, as are foci of dystrophic calcification, osseous metaplasia, or myxomatous change. Lipoid pneumonia may develop adjacent to areas

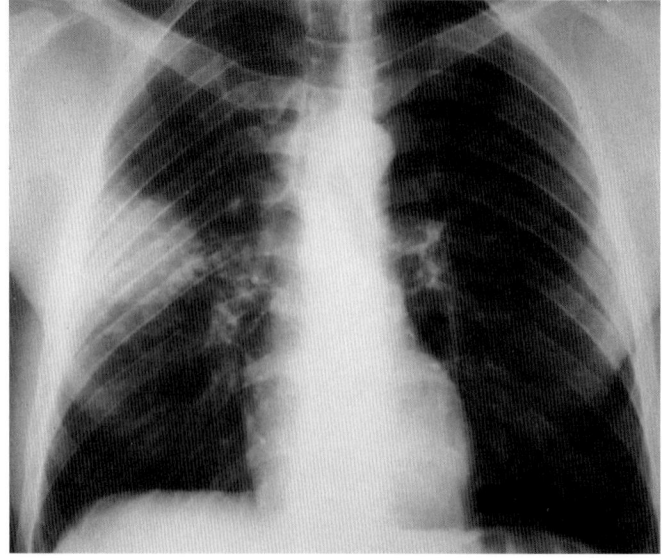

Figure 18-9. Plasma cell granuloma-type pulmonary inflammatory pseudotumor, which is seen in this chest radiograph as a large nodular mass in the right mid-lung field.

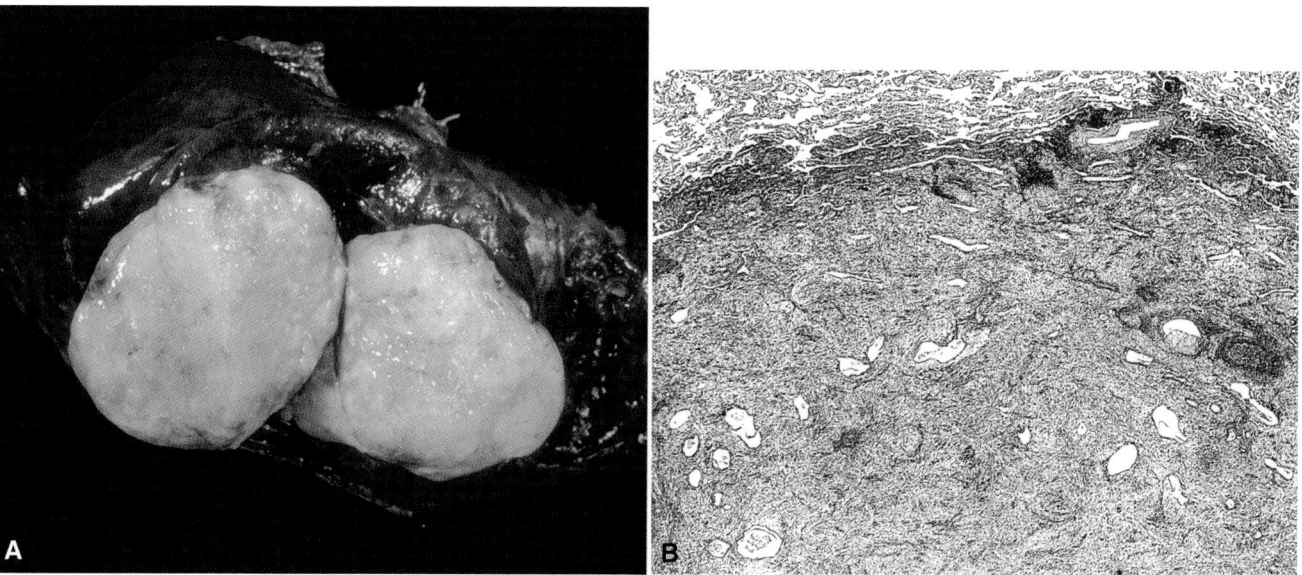

Figure 18-10. A, Gross specimen showing pulmonary inflammatory pseudotumor with a circumscribed and internally homogeneous white-tan cut surface. **B,** This photomicrograph of inflammatory pseudotumor of the lung shows an irregular interface with the surrounding parenchyma, multiple foci of chronic inflammation, and early sclerosis.

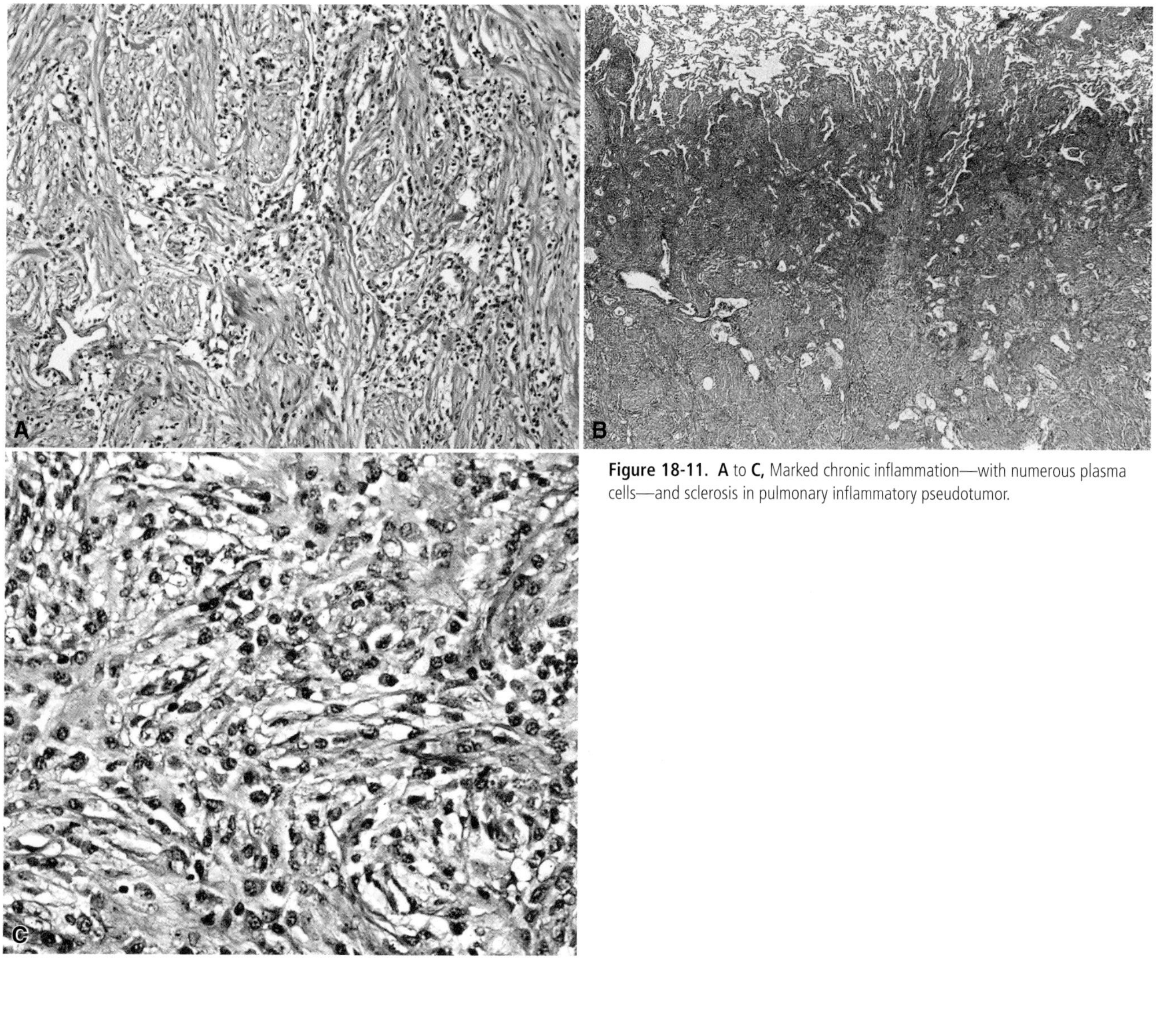

Figure 18-11. A to **C,** Marked chronic inflammation—with numerous plasma cells—and sclerosis in pulmonary inflammatory pseudotumor.

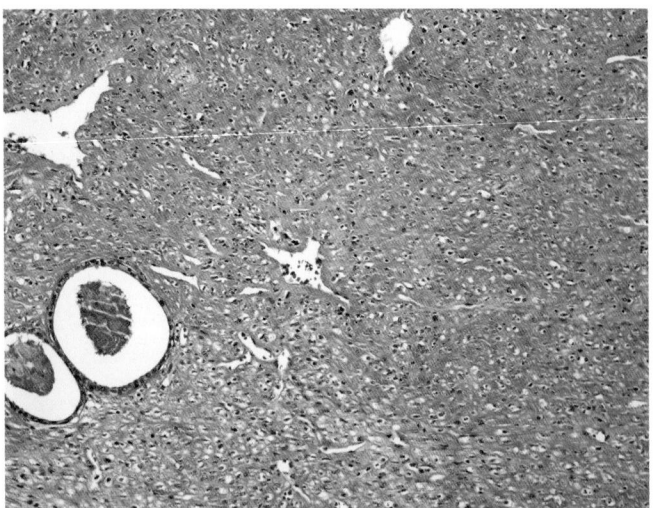

Figure 18-12. "Mature" plasma cell granuloma-type pulmonary inflammatory pseudotumor demonstrates filling of the distal airspaces by densely collagenized stroma, with virtually no inflammation.

where IPTs have caused bronchial obstruction by intraluminal proliferation or impingement on an airway. Late in the evolution of IPTs and in their central aspects, the lung parenchyma is replaced by deposition of mature collagen in broad bundles that transect the lesion; it may sometimes assume a keloidal appearance.

In the LPIPT variant, plasma cells and lymphocytes comprise the bulk of the lesion; germinal centers and a paucicellular collagenous matrix may also be prominent.[58-61] Fibroblasts and xanthoma cells are usually relatively scant. To some degree, the two histologic subtypes of IPT do overlap one another morphologically. As mentioned earlier, the immunohistologic presence of numerous IgG4-positive plasmacytes tends to strongly favor a diagnosis of LPIPT. Other findings that may suggest LPIPT are the presence of endothelialitis, prominent organization, lymphangitic inflammatory infiltrates that are rich in plasma cells and histiocytes (with or without the presence of a mass), and fibrinous pleuritis. Prominently dilated lymphatic spaces, containing histiocytes that show emperipolesis of lymphocytes, may also be observed.

Neither form of IPT is composed of solid sheets of lymphocytes or plasma cells, tending to prevent diagnostic confusion with lymphoma

or plasmacytoma. Nevertheless, rearrangement of the immunoglobulin heavy chain genes in a subset of LPIPT cases has been reported, raising the possibility that these particular lesions might be neoplastic or preneoplastic.[62]

Lymphocytic infiltration and scarring of vascular walls in some examples of IPT, often in association with organizing thrombi, have also been described.[39] These changes may be secondary rather than a reflection of a primary vasculitic process. Usually, both kappa and lambda light chain immunoglobulins are detectable immunohistologically in the plasma cells, indicating a polytypic population[51]; lymphocyte subset markers similarly show an admixture of B cells and T cells.[3]

The specific etiologic factors underlying the development of pulmonary IPT are largely unknown. The premise that some cases represent a peculiar form of localized pneumonia has support from a history of a previous febrile illness with respiratory complaints in up to 40% of cases. Some case reports have suggested that there is an overlap in appearance between IPT and tumefactive pulmonary infections with aspergillus, rickettsiae, mycoplasma, various viruses, mycobacteria, *Cryptococcus*, corynebacteria, and other microorganisms.[55-57,63-69] Rare examples have also been documented after trauma to the lung,[70] and some cases arise from prior aspiration. As stated earlier, current hypotheses hold that some LPIPT are probably part of a systemic autoimmune process.[58-61]

The differential diagnosis of pulmonary IPT has been partially cited previously. It includes plasmacytoma,[71] malignant lymphoma,[72,73] and lymphoid hyperplasia,[74] selected examples of sclerosing hemangioma of the lung (called *epithelial plasma cell granuloma-like tumors* by Michal and Mukensnabl[75]), the peculiar variant of lung cancer known as *inflammatory sarcomatoid carcinoma*[76] (see Chapter 14), and IMT.[2,3] Among those conditions, plasmacytomas are recognized by their monotypism for cytoplasmic immunoglobulin, and selected lymphomas may also demonstrate this characteristic. Furthermore, malignant lymphomas are generally less well-circumscribed than IPTs and exhibit more cytologically monotonous infiltrates of atypical lymphoid cells. Localized and diffuse forms of pulmonary lymphoid hyperplasia are composed predominantly of mature lymphocytes, in contrast to the heterogeneous cellular composition of IPTs. Inflammatory sarcomatoid carcinoma can be separated from inflammatory simulators by its diffuse immunoreactivity for keratin, and IMTs contain significantly fewer IgG4-positive cells than those seen in IPTs.[60] There is some minor difference of opinion as to whether pulmonary hyalinizing

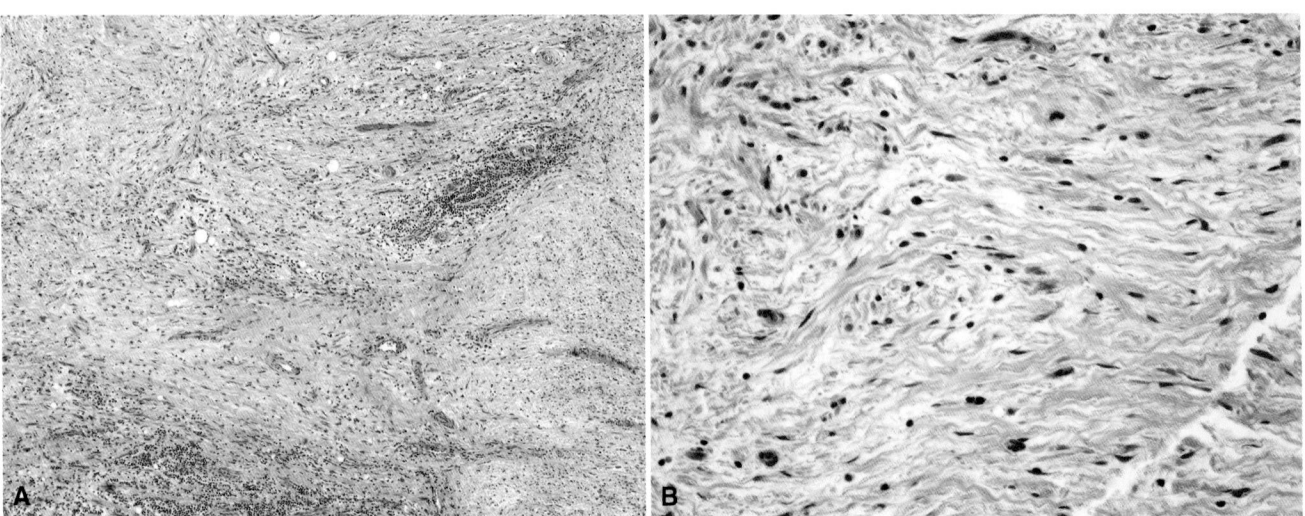

Figure 18-13. A and **B,** Sclerotic collagenous profiles fill alveolar spaces in this late-stage plasma cell granuloma-type pulmonary inflammatory pseudotumor. The image may resemble so-called "hyalinizing granuloma."

granuloma[77] is a part of the spectrum of IPT in the lung. Pulmonary hyalinizing granuloma shows more lamellar hyalinized collagen than is seen in classical IPT. Hyalinizing granulomas of the lung are commonly multiple, whereas "usual" IPT is not.[77] Sclerosing hemangiomas[78] were once considered to be related to IPTs, but they are now appreciated as epithelial neoplasms with pneumocytic differentiation.[79] The latter lesions may exhibit sclerosis, but they also contain aggregates of bland cuboidal cells together with micropapillary and angiomatoid areas. Inflammation is absent or scanty in sclerosing hemangiomas, and their constituent cells express thyroid transcription factor-1[79]; those of IPT do not. Ledet and associates[80] have examined the utility of immunostains for mutant p53 protein in the diagnostic separation of IPTs from low-grade intrapulmonary sarcomas. In their hands, p53 was restricted to malignant lesions, albeit with less than absolute sensitivity for such tumors.

Some examples of pulmonary IPT have been monitored for extended periods of time before excision or autopsy examination.[81-83] Information from these cases indicates that the lesions tend to remain stable or grow very slowly. Spontaneous resolution has also been documented, and a few lesions have shrunk after small incisional biopsy or administration of systemic corticosteroids or irradiation.[81,83] Surgical removal is usually necessary to establish a definitive diagnosis of IPT, and, if the lesion has been completely excised, no further therapy is needed.[56] Long-term follow-up of patients with pulmonary IPTs has revealed no untoward clinical events in such cases.

Mycobacterial Spindle Cell Pseudotumor

Spindle cell pseudotumors that are reactions to mycobacterial infection have been documented in several organ sites in immunosuppressed patients.[84-86] These proliferations show a close histologic resemblance to histoid leprosy,[87,88] and most reports have documented numerous intralesional mycobacteria (see Chapter 6). Only one case of mycobacterial pseudotumor (MP) has been reported in the lung,[89] although we have anecdotally encountered another example in a 41-year-old male patient with acquired immunodeficiency syndrome (AIDS).

Grossly, the lesions appear as yellow-gray nodules. They may show a predilection for small airways. Microscopically, the lesions are comprised of aggregates of spindle cells with a fascicular growth pattern and without significant atypia or mitoses. Scattered lymphocytes and plasma cells may be present, but overt granulomas are lacking. The cytoplasm of the spindle cells is "foamy" but may contain hemosiderin focally. The lesional cells are immunoreactive for lysozyme, with no labeling for S100 protein, keratin, actin, desmin, or von Willebrand factor. Ziehl-Neelsen staining shows innumerable acid-fast bacilli in the fusiform cells (Figs. 18-14 to 18-16). Most examples of MP in other anatomic locations have been related to *Mycobacterium avium-intracellulare* or *Mycobacterium kansasii*.

Another reported feature of MPs in other sites is a possible source of diagnostic error. That is, a reproducible cross-reaction has been seen with mycobacterial antigens using certain desmin antibodies,[90] spuriously suggesting the presence of a myogenous proliferation. This observation is especially troublesome in the setting being discussed here, because smooth muscle or myofibroblastic tumors enter prominently into the differential diagnosis of MPs. However, a documented lack of immunoreactivity for actin and electron microscopic attributes that support histiocytic differentiation in MP argue against those alternative interpretations.

Other lesions that must be separated from pulmonary MP include Kaposi sarcoma, malignant fibrous histiocytoma, spindle cell melanoma, and neural proliferations.[89] Obviously, acid-fast stains should be done in all spindle cell lesions from immunocompromised individuals, and

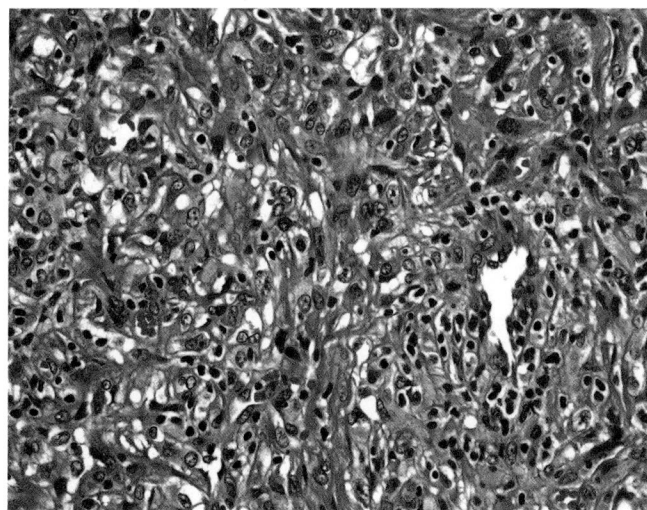

Figure 18-14. Mycobacterial pseudotumor of the lung in a patient with acquired immunodeficiency syndrome, represented by a disorganized proliferation of spindle cells admixed with lymphocytes and histiocytes.

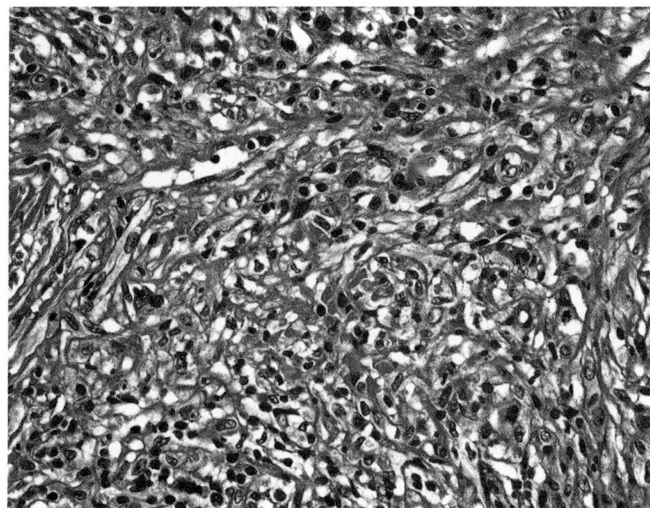

Figure 18-15. This image of pulmonary mycobacterial pseudotumor is reminiscent of the "myofibroblastic tumor" form of inflammatory pseudotumor of the lung.

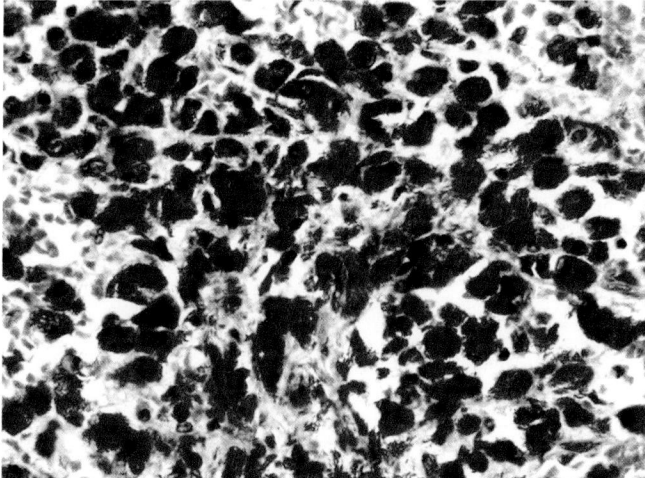

Figure 18-16. Innumerable intralesional mycobacteria are present in the proliferating cells of pulmonary mycobacterial pseudotumor, as seen in this Ziehl-Neelsen stain.

these consistently confirm mycobacterial causation. In some instances, the nature of MP is more obvious because of overtly granulomatous foci in the lung tissue around the spindle cell lesion. Characteristics of malignancy such as necrosis, nuclear atypia, and pathologic mitoses are absent in MP.[84–86] Thus, diagnoses of pulmonary sarcomatoid carcinoma, malignant fibrous histiocytoma, or other sarcomas would be unlikely.

Pseudoneoplastic Hematolymphoid Processes

Lymphoid interstitial pneumonia and nodular lymphoid hyperplasia may both be regarded as pseudoneoplasms. They are discussed in Chapter 15.

Rosai-Dorfman Disease (Sinus Histiocytosis with Massive Lymphadenopathy)

Most frequently, Rosai-Dorfman disease (sinus histiocytosis with massive lymphadenopathy [SHML]) involves lymph nodes, but it may rarely involve the lung primarily.[91,92] It can be seen in either sex and over a wide range of ages. Despite the name of this condition, lymphadenopathy does not always coexist with extranodal disease. When this condition affects the pulmonary parenchyma, it appears to have its epicenter in the hilar tissue and follows lymphatics peripherally into both lungs.[91,93] Accordingly, chest radiographs show an accentuation of central bronchovascular markings and bilateral interstitial prominence. CT scans (Fig. 18-17) may show areas of pleural-based consolidation. Confluence of the infiltrates may yield masslike densities in the lung fields as well (Fig. 18-18). Interestingly, clinical evidence of associated immune dysfunction may be apparent, including autoantibody formation, polyarthritis, immune-complex glomerulonephritis, asthma, and juvenile diabetes mellitus. Fever, night sweats, and weight loss have also been reported.[91] Justification for the classification of Rosai-Dorfman disease as non-neoplastic comes from molecular data indicating its polyclonal nature.[91] Nevertheless, this condition may occasionally coexist with solid malignancies, including carcinomas of the lung.[94,95] Such an association could arise, at least in part, from the aforementioned immunologic dysfunction in SHML.

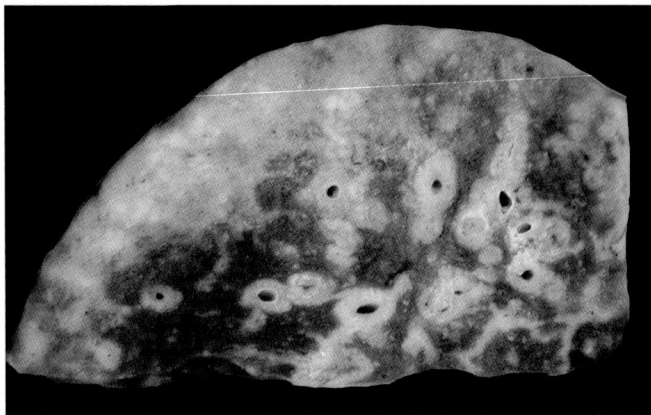

Figure 18-18. Gross photograph of lung tissue in Rosai-Dorfman disease (from the same patient as Fig. 18-17). Note the lymphangitic pattern of involvement.

Pathologic specimens of the lung or lymph nodes in SHML demonstrate comparable morphologic findings. Dilated lymphatic spaces in the pulmonary parenchyma contain large pale histiocytes with abundant amphophilic cytoplasm, surrounded by lymphoid infiltrates that are punctuated by germinal centers and fibrous septa (Figs. 18-19

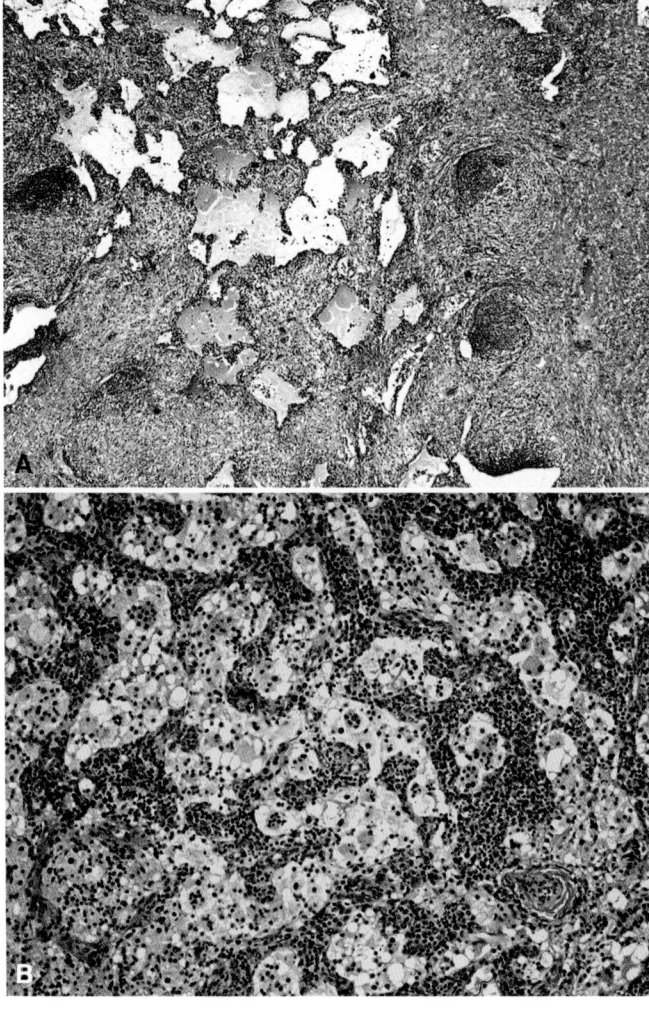

Figure 18-19. A, Rosai-Dorfman disease involving the lung showing dense but heterogeneous lymphoid infiltrates with discrete, visible lymphoid aggregates. **B,** Large pale histiocytes are visible at higher magnification.

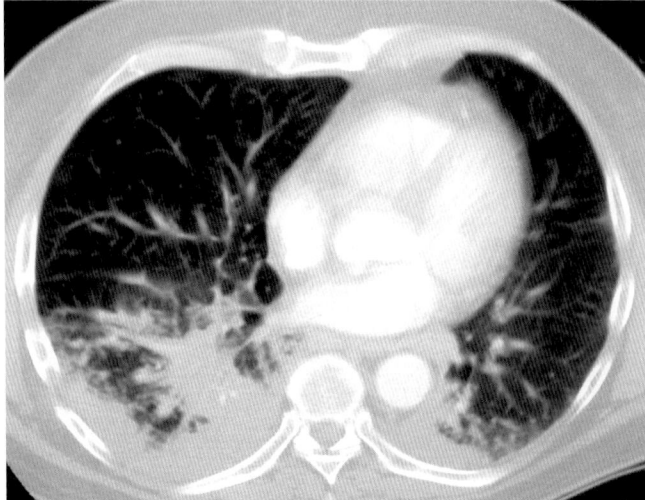

Figure 18-17. Computed tomography scan of a patient with Rosai-Dorfman disease. Note the accentuation of the bronchovascular bundles and pleural-based consolidation.

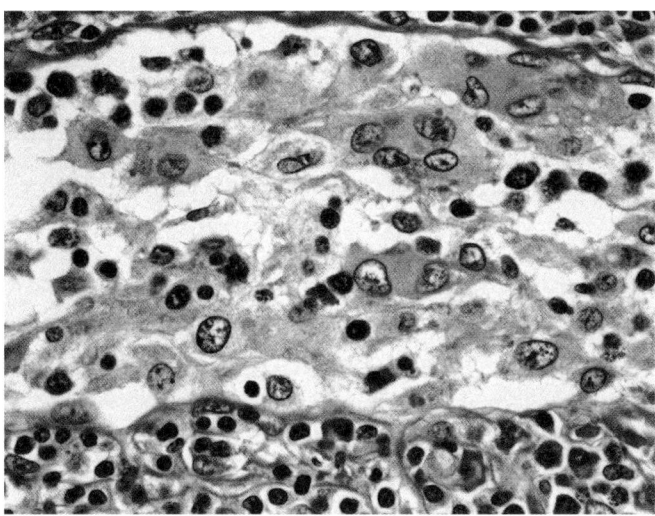

Figure 18-20. Rosai-Dorfman disease demonstrating the presence of large pale histiocytic elements associated with numerous small lymphocytes and plasma cells.

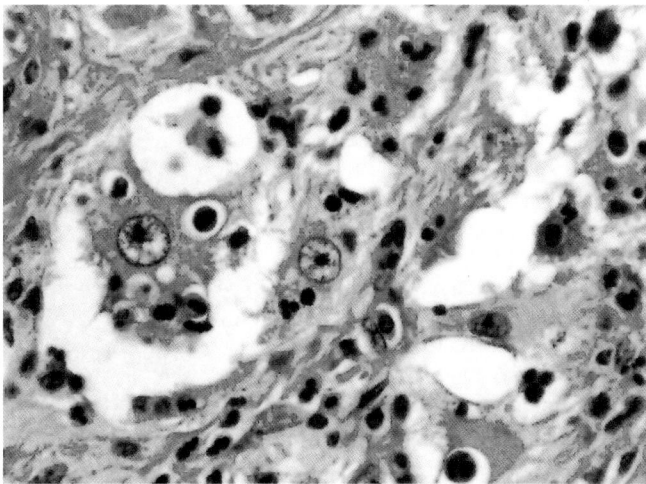

Figure 18-21. The large cells in Rosai-Dorfman disease contain numerous engulfed lymphocytes ("lymphemperipolesis"); this feature is characteristic of that condition but may be difficult to identify in the pulmonary manifestation.

and 18-20). The large histiocytes demonstrate a peculiar tendency to engulf intact, mature lymphocytes, representing a phenomenon known as lymphemperipolesis (Fig. 18-21). The overall image of foci of SHML in extranodal sites is therefore reminiscent of abnormal lymph nodes.[91] The immunophenotype of the lesional histiocytes is singular in that it features prominent reactivity for S100 protein (Fig. 18-22) and CD45 in the absence of CD1a. Labeling for CD68, lysozyme, MAC387, and alpha-1-antichymotrypsin may also be observed.

Differential diagnoses in cases of SHML potentially include metastatic carcinoma, metastatic melanoma, Erdheim-Chester disease, large cell lymphoma, and Hodgkin lymphoma.[91,92] The large tumor cells in the non-histiocytic conditions in this list differ from those in SHML immunohistologically, by their reactivity for keratin (in carcinoma), MART-1/melan-A (in melanoma), CD3 or

CD20 (in non-Hodgkin lymphoma), and CD30 (in Hodgkin lymphoma). Practically speaking, with the exception of Erdheim-Chester disease—which is immunohistochemically indistinguishable from SHML and also characterized by bland histiocytes—all of the other conditions also show a much higher degree of cytologic atypia than that seen in SHML. Thus, special diagnostic studies are usually not required to make the cited distinctions.

The clinical course of Rosai-Dorfman disease is unpredictable. A comprehensive summary[91] noted that patients with more than one site of extranodal disease and obvious immune dysfunction more often suffered significant morbidity and even mortality from this condition. Spontaneous remissions have been seen as well. Treatment is individualized, with antineoplastic therapy being reserved for those patients with serious organ dysfunction.

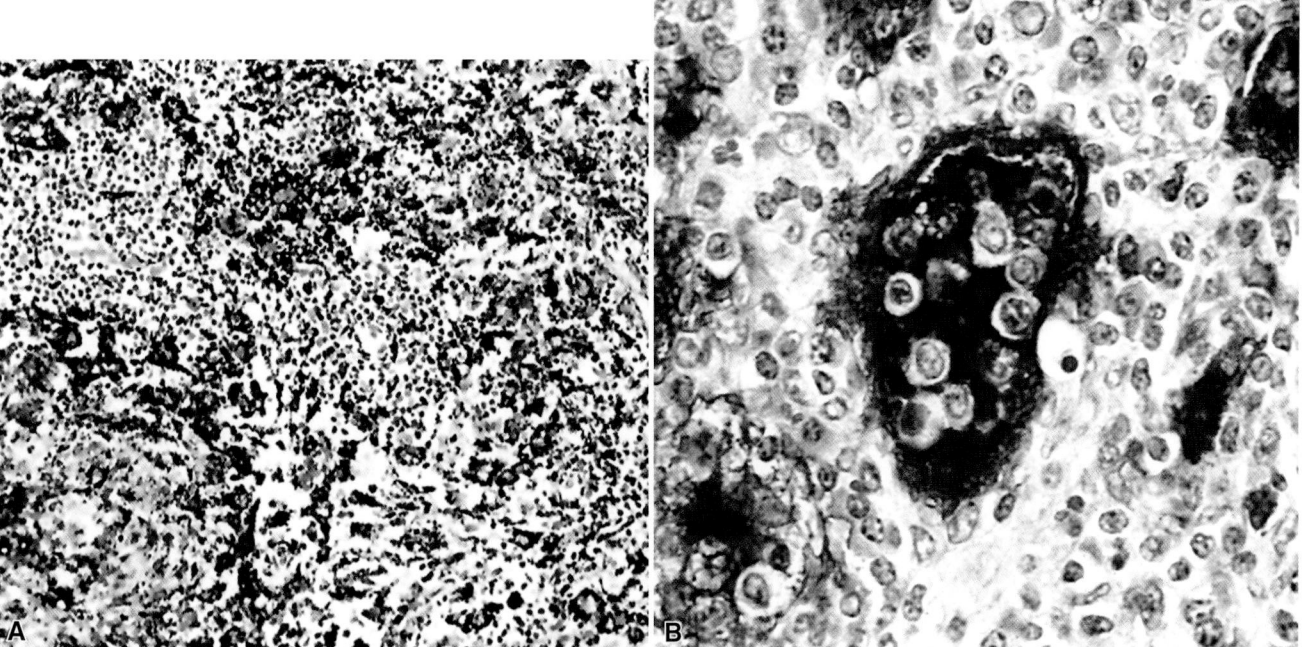

Figure 18-22. A and **B,** Intense immunoreactivity for S100 protein is seen in the lesional histiocytes of Rosai-Dorfman disease.

Extramedullary Hematopoiesis

In patients who have preexisting disorders of myelopoiesis, such as idiopathic myelofibrosis, hemoglobinopathies, severe hemolytic anemias, or Gaucher disease,[96–101] myeloid tissue that has been nascent since infancy can potentially reappear in several extramedullary sites. The lung and pleura are included in that list. If the proliferation of such elements is sufficient, it may manifest itself as discrete masses within visceral structures or serosal surfaces, often imitating neoplasms radiographically.[100]

Fine needle aspiration or needle biopsy of extramedullary hematopoiesis (EMH) demonstrates a variable mixture of erythroblasts, myeloid precursors, and megakaryocytes[99] (Figs. 18-23 and 18-24). These cell lines are usually recognizable as such in routine sections; however, should confirmation of their identity be desired, Leder stain and immunostains for glycophorin-A, myeloperoxidase, and CD61 can be used (see Fig. 18-24).

The clinical course of patients with pulmonary EMH depends on management of the underlying hematologic disorders. If normal medullary hematopoiesis can be improved or restored, the condition often regresses spontaneously. In cases where tumefactive EMH is symptomatic, local ablative therapy can be considered. However, the lesions in question may be a major source of circulating blood elements, and so this intervention should be used with caution.

Very uncommonly, EMH may serve as the seed bed for extramedullary leukemic transformation.[102]

Pseudoneoplastic Changes as a Consequence of Lung Injury

Exfoliative cytology of the respiratory tract has been used effectively for several decades in the diagnosis of pulmonary disorders.[103] Nonetheless, inherent shortcomings in this method have been well-documented, and some of them relate to the potential for the overdiagnosis of benign reparative or inflammatory conditions in the lungs as neoplastic. The incidence of this eventuality should be less than or equal to 0.25% of all cytologic specimens according to accepted standards.[104] Generally speaking, similar pitfalls accompany the interpretation of small transbronchial biopsy specimens in surgical pathology.

There are several possible reasons for mistakes in the cytologic diagnosis of malignancy in the lung. One may simply misinterpret reparative conditions or inflammatory epithelial atypia as carcinoma, but this should be rare.[105,106] Another potential source of confusion is the shedding or artifactual introduction of malignant cells from the mouth or upper airway into a sputum or bronchial washing specimen.[107,108] Both of these scenarios are troublesome only if there are accompanying abnormalities on chest films that might cause clinicians to consider a neoplasm diagnostically. Thus, it is obvious that radiologic data are essential to optimal cytopathologic interpretation.

However, there are some mass lesions that may, under selected circumstances, incite benign but atypical epithelial proliferations in the surrounding lung. Exfoliated cells in these cases may thus be mistaken as carcinomatous. The underlying conditions associated with this trap include symptomatically "occult" pulmonary infarcts, granulomas, and bronchiectasis with surrounding pneumonia, typically associated with atypical *squamous* metaplasia in adjacent bronchi[109–116] (Figs. 18-25 and 18-26). As expected, a misdiagnosis of squamous carcinoma is the usual error in such instances.

Another more heterogeneous collection of diseases that may imitate *adenocarcinoma* in cytologic samples or small biopsies includes radiation pneumonitis, postchemotherapy atypia in alveolar lining cells, bronchiectasis, pulmonary infarcts, viral pneumonias of various types, pulmonary vasculitides, lung injury caused by toxic chemicals, noninfectious interstitial pneumonitides, diffuse alveolar damage, and recurrent pneumothorax[116–126] (see also Chapter 5) (Figs. 18-27 and 18-28). These conditions are again most misleading in the context of localized radiographic abnormalities in the lungs and when details of the clinical setting are not provided. Moreover, because of the broad roentgenographic spectrum of such tumors as bronchioloalveolar adenocarcinoma, including an imitation of uncomplicated pneumonia,[127] the study of chest films is, unfortunately, an imperfect safeguard in this

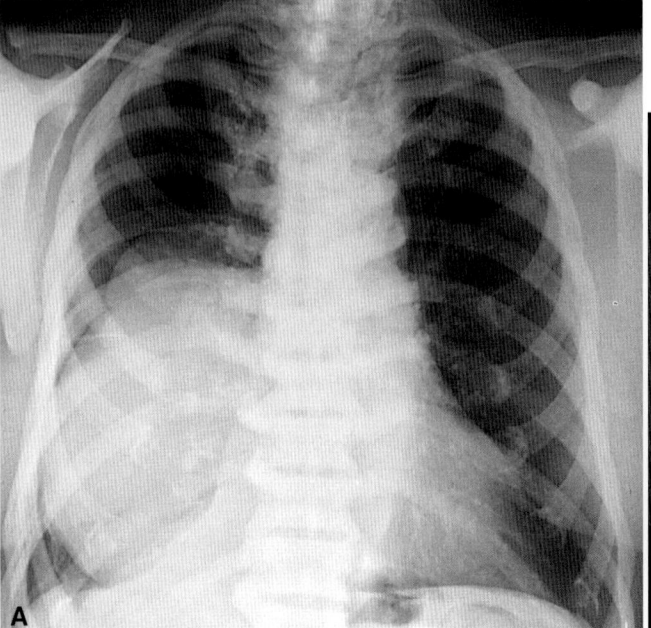

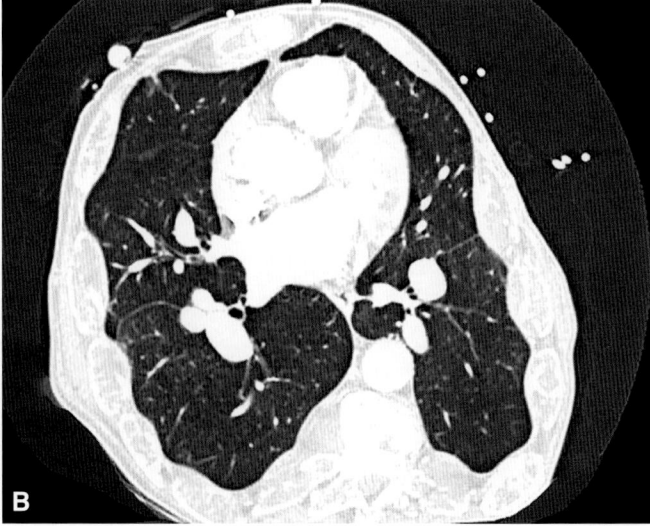

Figure 18-23. A, This chest radiograph from a patient with idiopathic myelofibrosis shows a large intrapulmonary mass in the right lung field. It represented a nodule of extramedullary hematopoiesis (EMH). **B,** Computed tomogram from another patient with beta-thalassemia major, demonstrating multiple nodules of EMH in the lungs and thoracic soft tissues.

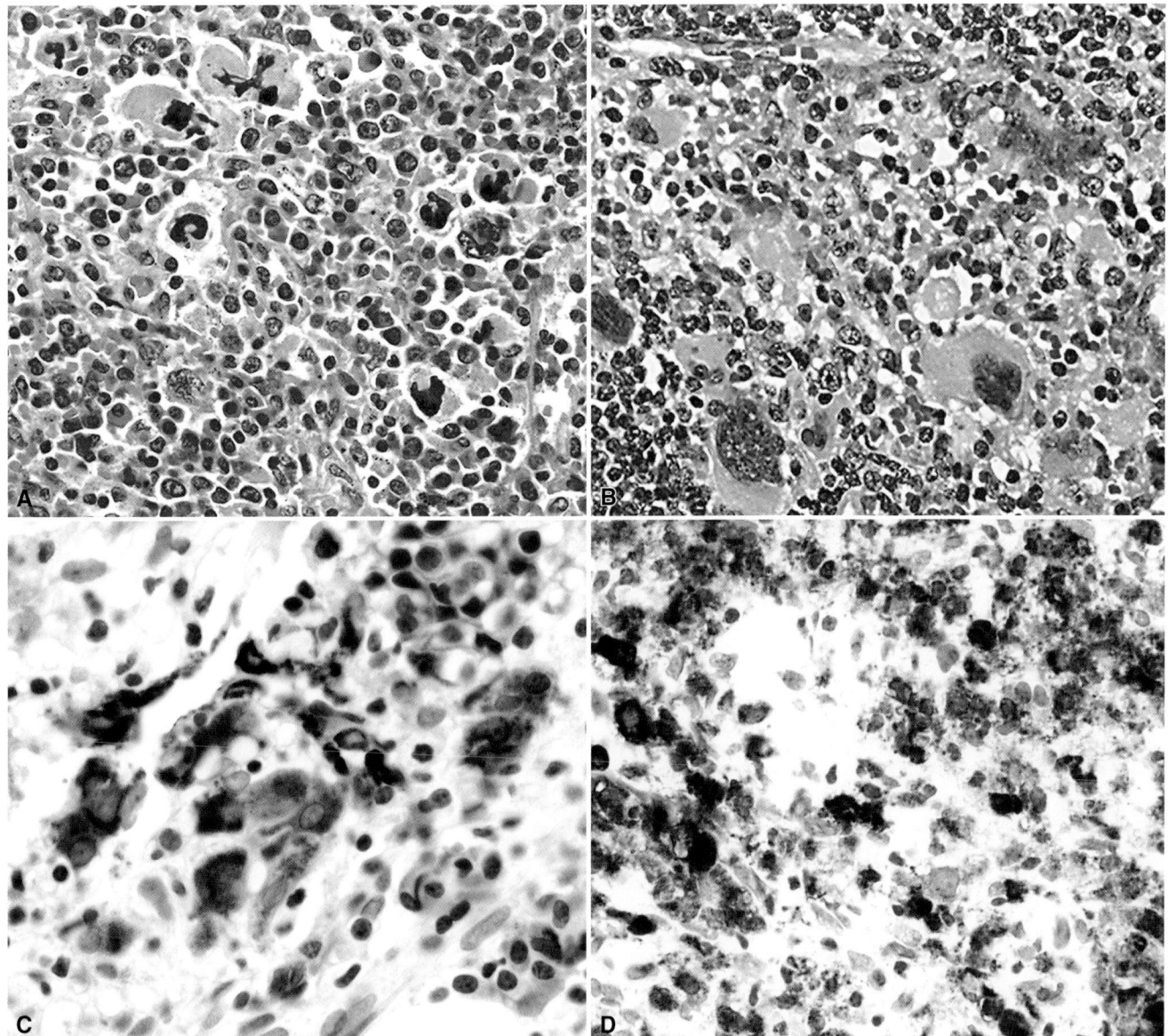

Figure 18-24. A and **B,** Tumefactive extramedullary hematopoiesis (EMH) shows a mixture of erythroblasts, myeloid precursors, and megakaryocytes. The last of those cell types is the most diagnostic of the condition in conventionally stained sections. **C,** Immunoreactivity for CD61 in the megakaryocytic component of EMH. **D,** Myeloperoxidase-positivity is apparent in the myeloid elements of EMH.

specific setting. In general, pseudomalignant glandular pulmonary metaplasias show greater cellular heterogeneity than that seen in true adenocarcinomas.[128] Lower nuclear-to-cytoplasmic ratios, "scalloping" of cell borders, and focal intercellular "windows" in pseudoneoplastic glandlike profiles also typify atypical metaplasias.

It is also important to realize that special techniques, such as immunostains for tumor-associated glycoprotein-72 (with the antibody B72.3), are not able to make the distinction in question and may even contribute further to misdiagnosis.[129] Indeed, there are no universally effective methods to avoid mistakes in the cytologic or biopsy diagnosis of pulmonary malignancy. Patients and clinicians should probably be apprised of that reality.

Traumatic neuroma, a discrete injury-related tumefactive lesion of the bronchial mucosa,[130,131] may occur spontaneously (e.g., after aspiration of food), or as a result of instrumentation-induced injury of the airway. Histologically, it shows a disorganized proliferation of mucosal nerve bundles, set in a fibrous or fibromyxoid stroma

(Fig. 18-29). A mechanistically related process is that of necrotizing sialometaplasia, caused by inflammatory damage to, and pseudocarcinomatous metaplasia of, the bronchial glands.[132] Yet another bronchial lesion that has been documented after injury to the lung is the fibroepithelial polyp. It may represent the end result of re-epithelialization of polypoid intraluminal granulation tissue in the airway lumen. When it is ultimately excised, a fibroepithelial polyp shows variable degrees of squamous metaplasia mantling a central fibrovascular polyp, which emanates from the bronchial submucosa (Fig. 18-30).

Peribronchiolar Metaplasia (Lambertosis)

As discussed in Chapter 8, peribronchiolar metaplasia (also known as Lambertosis) is a condition wherein metaplastic bronchiolar epithelium extensively colonizes adjacent alveolar spaces.[133,134] Occasionally, this process may be so marked as to raise serious concern over the histopathologic diagnosis of adenocarcinoma (Fig. 18-31). When peribronchiolar

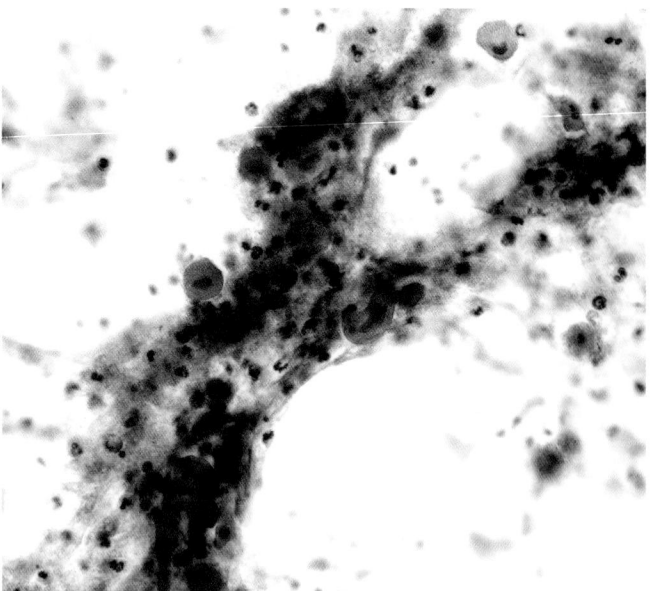

Figure 18-25. Cytologic specimen from a bronchial brushing biopsy in a case of isolated granuloma of the lung, demonstrating markedly atypical squamoid cells with irregular nuclear chromatin, densely orangeophilic cytoplasm, and high nuclear-to-cytoplasmic ratios. These elements caused marked diagnostic consternation over the possibility of squamous carcinoma.

metaplasia is seen in the setting of emphysema in cigarette smokers, that worry is heightened even further. Nevertheless, the metaplastic elements in peribronchiolar metaplasia are more columnar than those of bronchioloalveolar carcinoma, and not as atypical as those of ordinary pulmonary adenocarcinomas. Focal retention of ciliation in the cells of peribronchiolar metaplasia further supports its reactive benign nature, inasmuch as cilia virtually exclude a diagnosis of carcinoma.

Pseudoneoplastic Lesions of the Pleural Surfaces

Pseudoneoplastic lesions of the pleura comprise a relatively small group. Perhaps the most common of them is principally seen by cytopathologists: namely, mesothelial hyperplasia in pleural effusion specimens. Indeed, cytologic simulators of malignancy encompass such a wide variety of entities that they cannot be addressed completely in this text. We will consider selected aspects of this topic, but for a more

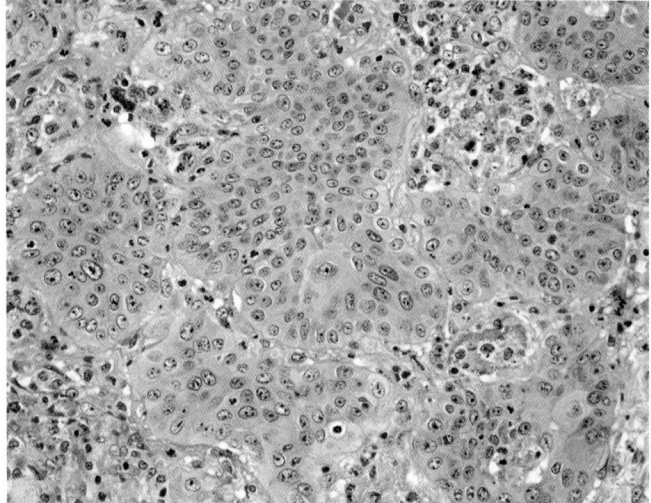

Figure 18-26. Atypical squamous metaplasia adjacent to an infarct.

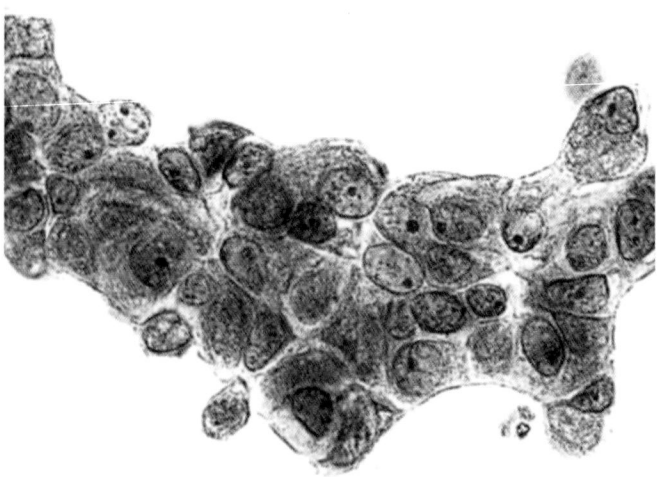

Figure 18-27. Atypical groups of glandular cells are present in this bronchial washing specimen from a patient who had received chemotherapy for metastatic adenocarcinoma of the pancreas. They were thought to represent secondary involvement of the lung by tumor, ultimately proven to be postchemotherapy atypia.

complete discussion, the reader should consult comprehensive treatises on cytopathology.[135–137]

The microscopic classification of mesothelial lesions can be challenging, both in cytology and surgical pathology. Pertinent problems in this area include the distinction of reactive proliferations from mesothelioma or metastatic carcinoma and the separation of benign and malignant lymphocytic effusions. Approaches to the last of these topics are identical to techniques discussed earlier in reference to pulmonary lymphoid lesions and will not be recounted here.

Reactive Mesothelial Proliferations

Reactive mesothelial lesions have often been given the descriptive but nebulous label of *atypical mesothelial cell proliferation* in cytologic practice.[138] However, because that terminology implies a possible connection to malignancy, or, at least, premalignancy, we do not advocate its use. Rather, one should simply state that mesothelial cells are hyperplastic or reactive if their morphologic features are clearly benign.[139] Such proliferations are associated with a number of underlying pathologic conditions, including cirrhosis, anemia, viral infections, connective tissue diseases, prior radiation, reactions to bronchogenic carcinomas or pleural metastases, recurrent pneumothoraces, and a variety of chronic pleural infections.[126,140] An adequate clinical history is obviously necessary to the accurate interpretation of pleural tissue samples. Cytologic features that favor malignancy include the presence of papillae or other architectural complexities, obvious nuclear atypia, necrosis, and pathologic mitotic figures.[135,141] There are contrasting criteria for the recognition of reactive or hyperplastic mesothelial lesions.[142] They are characterized only by superficial entrapment of mesothelial cell nests in the pleural stroma, an intense inflammatory infiltrate that is densest near the pleural surface, vascular proliferation with few associated spindle cells, an absence of overt nuclear atypia, and a lack of atypical mitoses (Figs. 18-32 and 18-33).

Despite an almost-universal reference to cytologic atypia in the literature on mesothelioma, nuclear aberrations in mesothelioma are often unimpressive. Conversely, cytologic atypia may be striking in reactive mesothelium.[143] In general, the cytologic criteria associated with malignant mesothelioma include an elevated nuclear-to-cytoplasmic ratio, irregularity of the nuclear membranes, and coarsely clumped

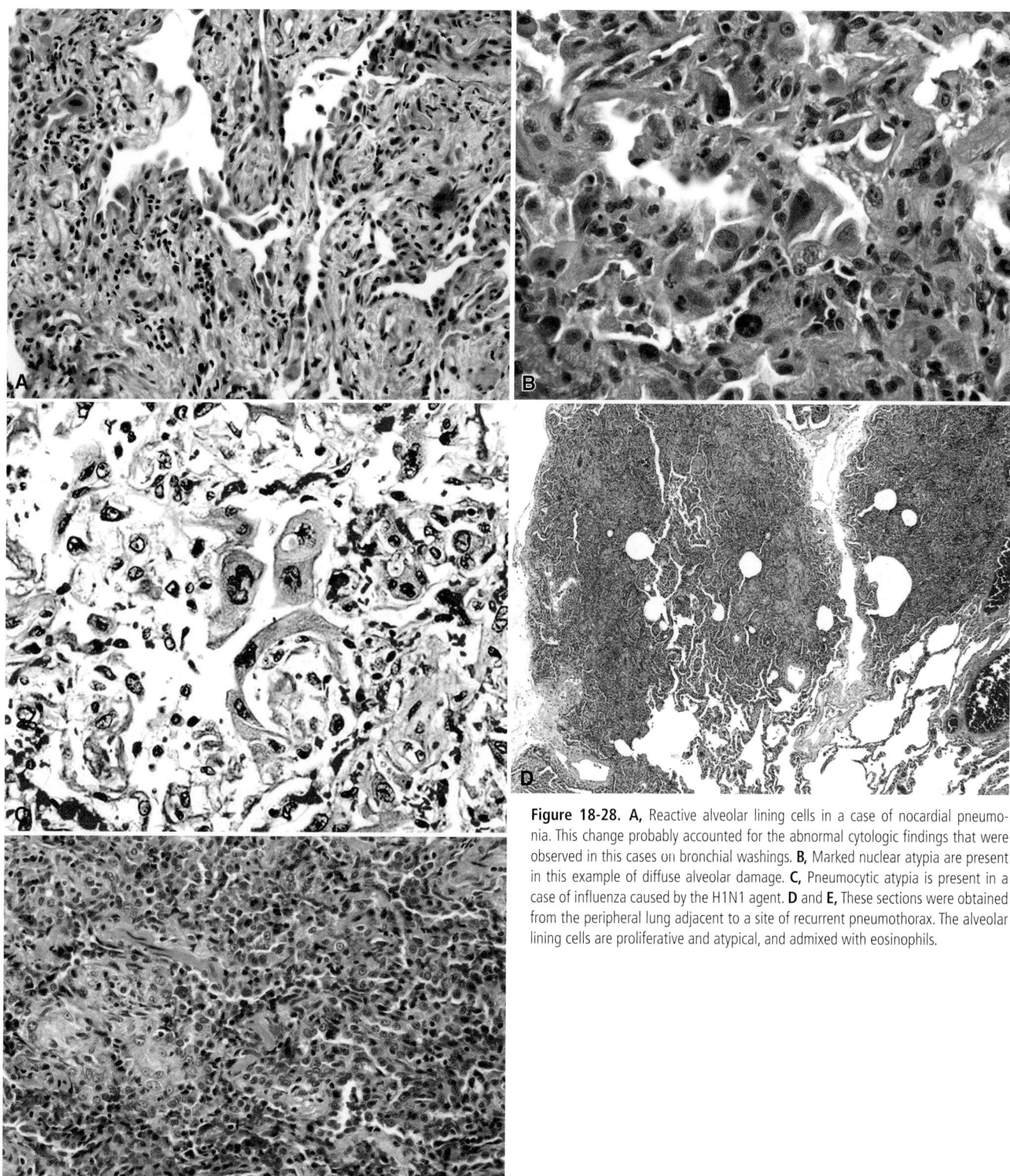

Figure 18-28. A, Reactive alveolar lining cells in a case of nocardial pneumonia. This change probably accounted for the abnormal cytologic findings that were observed in this cases on bronchial washings. **B,** Marked nuclear atypia are present in this example of diffuse alveolar damage. **C,** Pneumocytic atypia is present in a case of influenza caused by the H1N1 agent. **D** and **E,** These sections were obtained from the peripheral lung adjacent to a site of recurrent pneumothorax. The alveolar lining cells are proliferative and atypical, and admixed with eosinophils.

chromatin.[141] However, even by morphometric evaluation, conflicting results regarding such features have been reported.[144-147]

Several attributes of mesothelial cells are potentially shared by both benign and malignant proliferations in cytologic samples. They include cytoplasmic vacuolization, binucleation or multinucleation, and a brush-border pattern that extends over the entire free surface of the cells, correlating with the ultrastructural finding of elongated microvilli.[135,141] Reactive cells generally tend to exfoliate singly or in small groups; on the other hand, large formations, including morular structures with "knobby" cellular outlines or papillary structures, raise the likelihood of mesothelioma.[141,148] A similar comment applies to uniformly dense mesothelial hypercellularity in an effusion specimen.

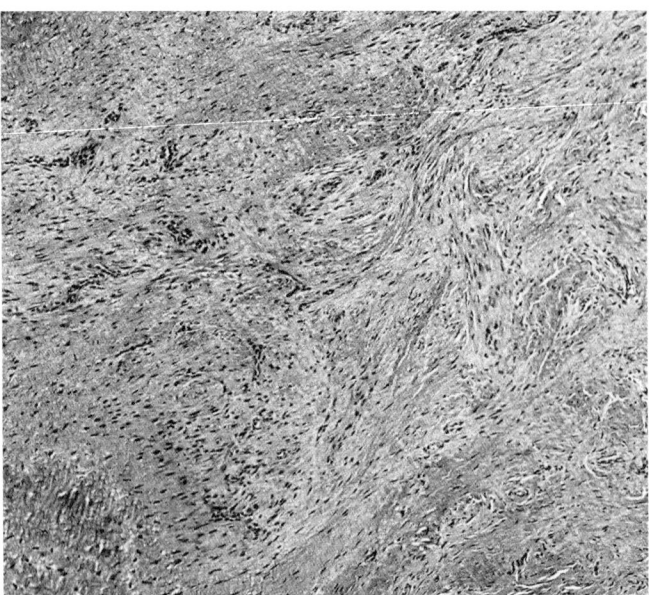

Figure 18-29. A disorganized proliferation of nerve fascicles is set in a fibromyxoid stroma, in post-traumatic bronchial neuroma.

It should also be understood that the comments just offered apply only to epithelial or biphasic subtypes of malignant mesothelioma, because sarcomatoid variants rarely shed into body cavities. If effusions are present in the latter cases, they usually contain only inflammatory cells and reactive but cytologically benign mesothelial cells.[149] The largely hypothetical concept of "mesothelioma in situ" has been introduced for putatively malignant but microscopic lesions limited to the pleural surface.[150,151] The distinction of this condition from florid but reactive mesothelial proliferations is unsettled diagnostically.

Immunohistochemistry has limited value in the separation of reactive and malignant mesothelial cells.[152] Some analyses have suggested that purely epithelioid mesotheliomas show dense plasmalemmal labeling for epithelial membrane antigen and vimentin,[153] whereas benign mesothelial cells lack both markers. Nevertheless, these determinants have been shared by both pathologic entities in our experience. Both cell types are consistently negative for carcinoembryonic antigen, tumor-associated glycoprotein-72, and CD15 (all of which are expected

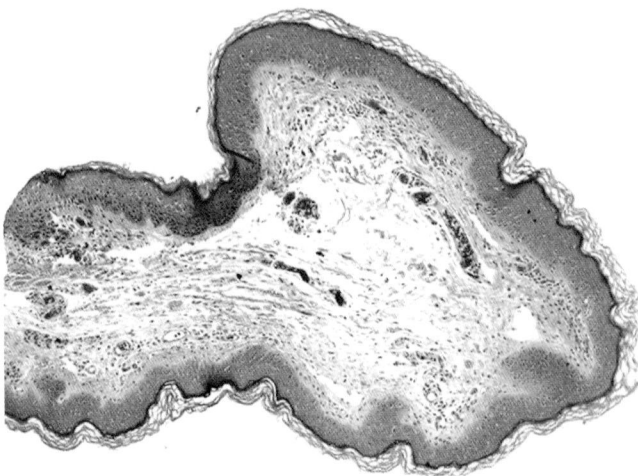

Figure 18-30. Fibroepithelial polyp of the bronchus features squamous metaplasia of the mucosal epithelium, mantling a fibrovascular stalk that blends with the submucosal connective tissue. It is virtually identical histologically to an acrochordon of the skin.

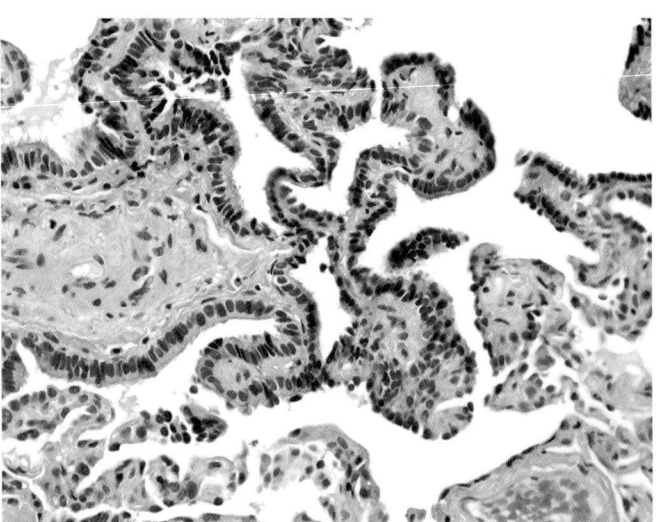

Figure 18-31. This proliferation of bronchiolar epithelial cells is seen in the context of bullous emphysema in a smoker. It has been called *peribronchiolar metaplasia* (Lambertosis) and can be confused with adenocarcinoma. Note uniform columnar cells with cilia.

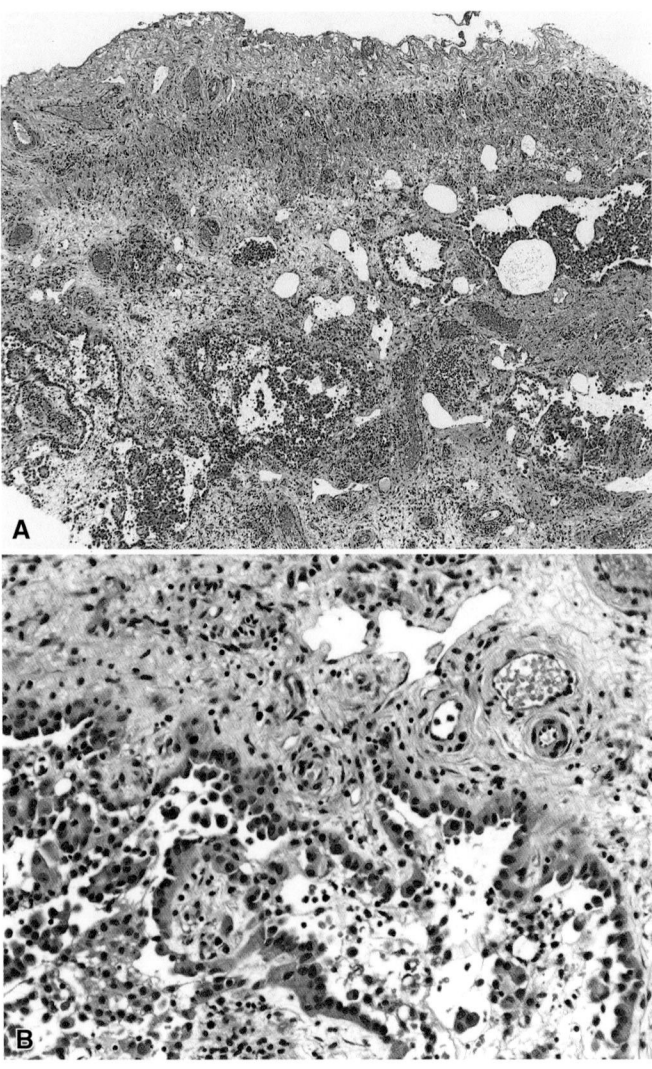

Figure 18-32. **A** and **B,** Markedly proliferative mesothelium in this patient with lupus erythematosus, who had recurrent pleural effusions. Although this image is worrisome, the lesion was ultimately believed to be reactive in nature.

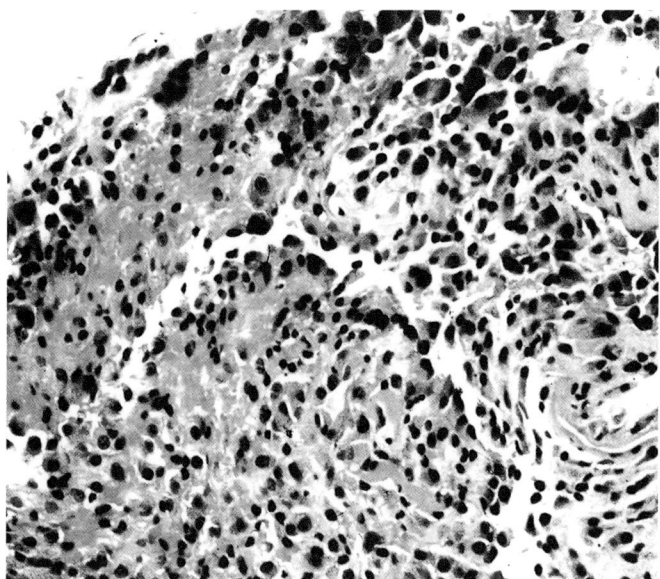

Figure 18-33. Solid sheets of reactive benign mesothelial cells are admixed with fibrin and inflammation. The cytologic features of the mesothelium caused concern over the diagnostic possibility of malignant mesothelioma.

in carcinomas), and positive for HBME-1, calretinin, WT1, podoplanin, and keratin 5/6.[141,154] Although this panel of reactants is useful in distinguishing adenocarcinoma from mesothelioma, it cannot separate benign and malignant mesothelial lesions.

Interest has also arisen regarding the immunostaining of mesothelial lesions for selected gene products that might be correlated with malignancy. In particular, mutant p53 proteins have been assessed in that context, with the expectation that they would be present in malignant mesothelioma but not in benign pleural proliferations.[155,156] In fact, when they are immunoreactive for p53 protein, reactive mesothelia usually shows weak nuclear labeling or both cytoplasmic and nuclear staining that should raise suspicion of a spurious result.[156] In contrast, mesotheliomas can exhibit convincing and intense nuclear reactivity (Fig. 18-34), but up to 40% are completely nonreactive for p53.[155] Although p53 protein immunotyping may provide adjunctive

diagnostic information, we believe that it should not be used in isolation. It must be integrated with morphologic findings as well as radiographic details.

In view of the poor outcome of most mesothelioma cases and limited option for its treatment, diagnostic circumspection is appropriate in this context. It would be very undesirable to label a patient with a reactive proliferation as having a mesothelioma, and, with the passage of time, true examples of that tumor will declare themselves clinicopathologically.

More clear-cut criteria are available for the distinction between reactive mesothelium and metastatic carcinoma.[142] Carcinomatous effusions often feature a distinctly dimorphic cellular population, although this may be subtle in cases of mammary or gastric cancers.[135] Immunohistologic differences have been outlined above. Periodic acid/Schiff stains, performed with and without diastase digestion, label neutral mucins in at least 50% of metastatic adenocarcinomas but not in mesothelial proliferations. Some intracytoplasmic vacuoles in mesothelial cells also contain hyaluronic acid that may stain with the Alcian blue method at pH 2.5; it is digestible with hyaluronidase. Such inclusions may show weak cross-reactivity with mucicarmine stains, potentially causing a mistaken diagnosis of carcinoma. However, spurious mucicarmine staining again disappears after hyaluronidase treatment, unlike the pattern of adenocarcinoma.

Tumefactive Hyaline Pleural Plaques

Hyaline pleural plaques (HPPs) are important because of their value as markers of above-background asbestos exposure (Fig. 18-35). Moreover, they occasionally may simulate the radiographic and pathologic appearances of selected mesothelial neoplasms or metastases of malignant tumors in the pleural space.

Many studies have linked asbestos exposure to the emergence of fibrohyaline plaques (Fig. 18-36).[157–163] There is also a variable but generally low incidence of these lesions in routine necropsies. Asbestos fibers are absent in the plaques themselves, and, if present, are seen only in the subjacent pulmonary parenchyma. Most patients with bilateral HPP have an increase in commercial-type amphibole asbestos content in the lungs.[157–163] The number of fibers is greater than that in the general population but less than the number found in individuals with asbestosis. Unilateral plaques may also be seen in patients

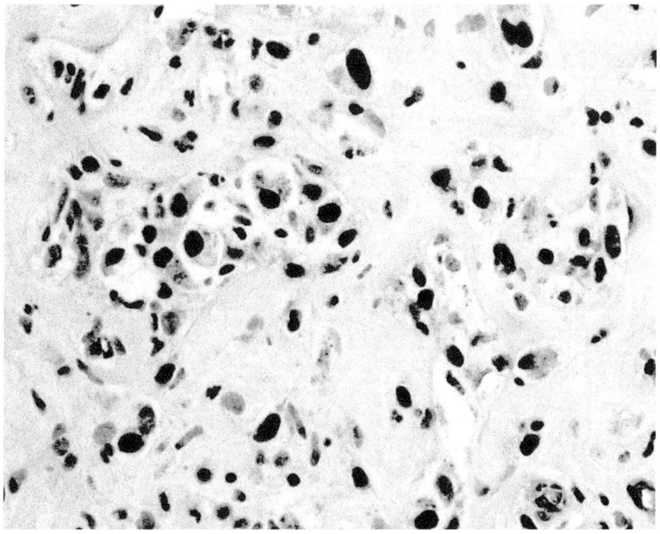

Figure 18-34. Nuclear immunoreactivity for putatively mutant p53 is present in epithelioid cells in this cell block. This finding has been used by some observers to support the diagnosis of mesothelioma over one of reactive mesothelial hyperplasia.

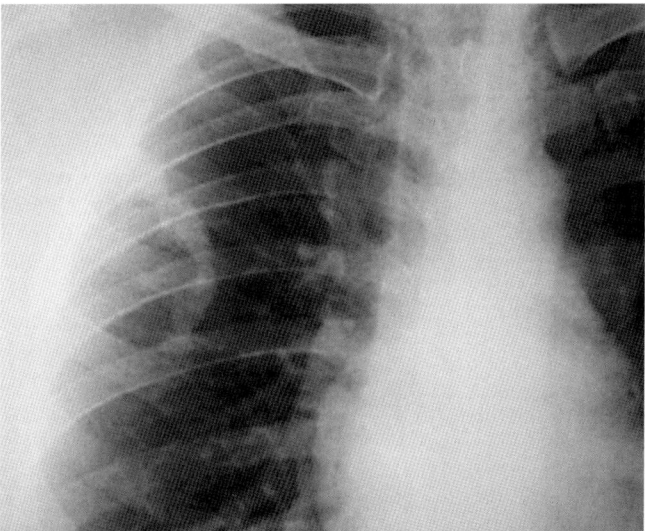

Figure 18-35. This posteroanterior chest film demonstrates a large nodular mass in the right lateral pleura, with internal calcification. It represents a pseudotumoral fibrohyaline pleural plaque in a patient with occupational-level asbestos exposure.

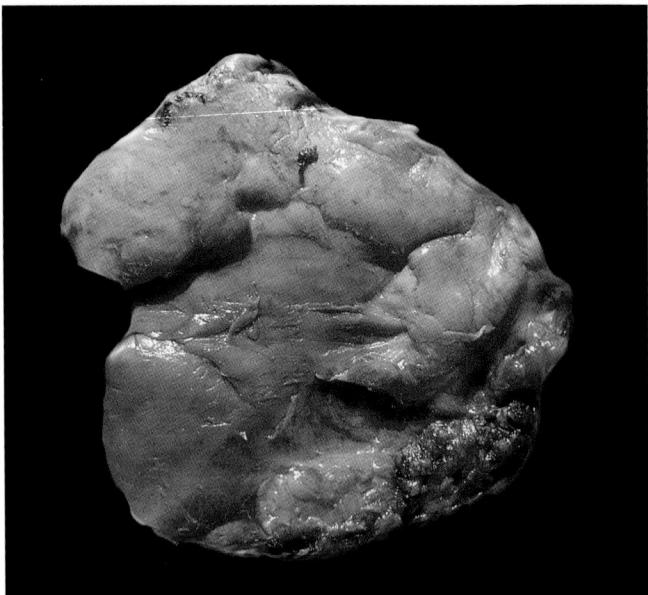

Figure 18-36. Gross image of fibrohyaline pleural plaques, represented by well-demarcated sessile white-yellow fibrous thickening.

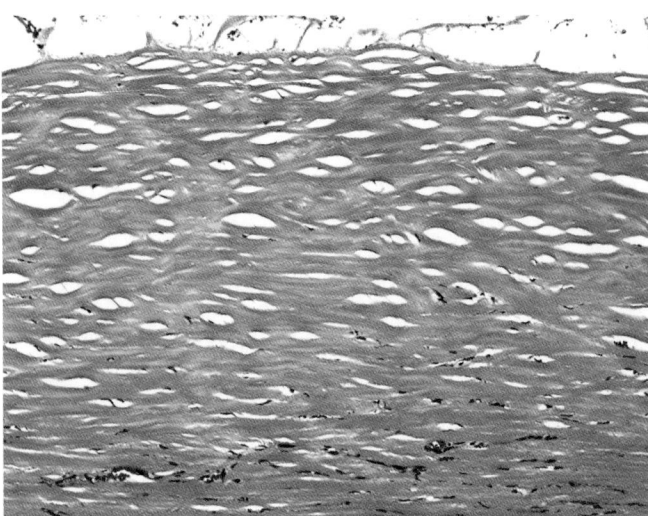

Figure 18-37. Photomicrograph of fibrohyaline pleural plaque, showing a "basket weave" configuration of laminated, markedly hypocellular, mature collagen. The surface of the plaque contains chronic inflammatory cells.

with asbestos exposure, but these plaques may also develop as a consequence of chronic pleural irritation of any type. They are commonly associated with infections such as tuberculosis or empyema, chronic or recurrent pleural hemorrhage, and chest wall trauma.[162]

HPPs are most often detected in individuals older than 50 years of age, most commonly in men. Those lesions associated with occupational asbestos exposure show an average latency of 20 years or more from the time of initial dust inhalation.[162,163] HPPs characteristically arise in the lower thorax (especially the diaphragm) and preferentially involve the parietal pleura, often with a parallel orientation to the ribs. Much less commonly, they may affect the pericardial surfaces.[158] Individuals with HPPs lack symptoms that are directly related to the plaques themselves, and the lesions are regarded as tissue reactions rather than a true disease process. Most associated pulmonary function abnormalities are due to accompanying emphysema or interstitial lung disease.[157] Plain films have limited sensitivity for the detection of uncomplicated HPPs, but this statistic increases markedly if the plaques are calcified. The use of CT has greatly improved the ease with which these lesions are recognized.[164]

The typical pattern of HPP features hypocellular, dense bundles of hyalinized collagen, often with a "basket weave" arrangement[162] (Fig. 18-37). Chronic inflammation may be present in and around the lesion and, in some cases, acute inflammation or fibrin deposition may be seen on the pleural surface. These changes likely reflect the proposed mechanism of formation of the lesion: namely, that of recurrent and organizing pleuritis. Dystrophic calcification is often evident pathologically (Fig. 18-38).

The main pathologic diagnostic alternative in cases of HPP is that of localized desmoplastic mesothelioma (DM). This tumor shares many of the microscopic characteristics of HPP; both are composed of relatively bland cells that are separated by dense bands of collagen. Nevertheless, there is greater cellularity in DM, at least focally, with areas of storiform growth and a greater degree of nuclear pleomorphism.[165] Necrosis is also possible in mesothelioma but does not occur in HPP. Involvement of the visceral pleura or diffuse effacement of the pleural space are features usually associated with DM, and they argue against an interpretation of HPP. Adjunctive studies are of very little use in this context. Immunoreactivity for mutant p53 protein is more likely in DM

but is not restricted to this lesion.[166] Furthermore, a substantial portion of DM cases are completely p53-negative, mirroring the expected immunophenotype of HPP.

Although some solitary fibrous tumors of the pleura may contain keloidal collagen like that seen in HPPs,[167] they show much greater cellularity and a dissimilar histologic pattern overall. Furthermore, a solitary fibrous tumor typically presents as a localized, polypoid intrapleural mass rather than a sessile plaque; it is also immunoreactive for CD34, CD99, or *bcl*-2 protein (unlike HPP) and has no causal relationship to asbestos exposure.

There is no indication for surgical removal of HPPs, except in those rare cases where their radiologic images cause clinical concern over a possible diagnosis of malignancy. Their possible relationship to bronchogenic carcinoma or mesothelioma has been examined, as reviewed elsewhere.[168] The plaques themselves appear not to be precursor lesions for malignancies but are simple markers of dust exposure.

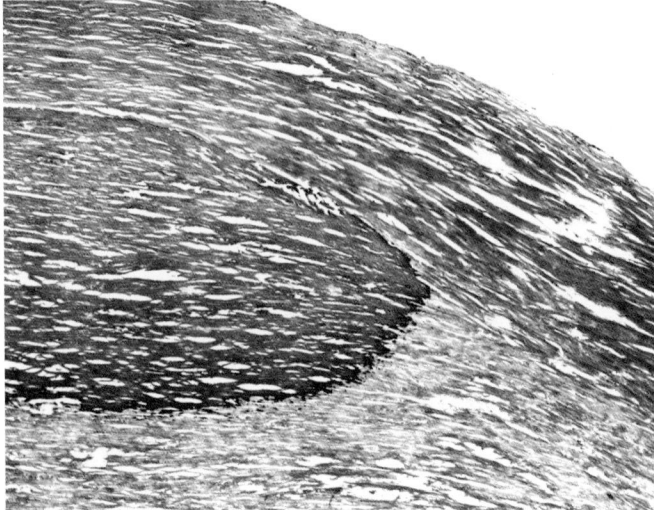

Figure 18-38. Another example of fibrohyaline pleural plaque, containing internal foci of dystrophic calcification.

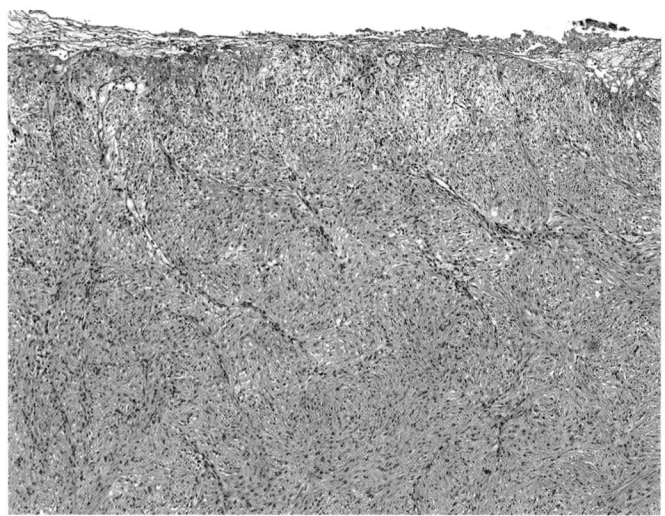

Figure 18-39. Diffuse pleural fibrosis, showing an organized deposition of hypocellular, fully mature collagen in the visceral pleura. The medium-power image demonstrates a vaguely lamellated appearance; capillaries are relatively numerous and oriented vertically to the pleural surface.

Diffuse Pleural Fibrosis

A pathologic process related to HPPs is diffuse pleural fibrosis (DPF; also known as *fibrous pleurisy* or *chronic fibrosing pleuritis*). It may be associated with connective tissue disorders, such as lupus erythematosus or rheumatoid arthritis, as well as chronic infections and asbestos exposure.[169-171] DPF often involves the visceral pleura and may produce apical fibrous "capping" analogous to that seen in association with bullous emphysema. In extreme cases, obliteration of the pleural space may eventuate.

Microscopically, DPF is characterized by the deposition of bland, hypocellular fibrous tissue in the pleura, without the "basket weave" pattern of hyaline plaques (Fig. 18-39). The lesional tissue often demonstrates an increase in vascularity—with vertically oriented capillaries—and may contain scattered foci of chronic inflammation, including plasma cells, lymphocytes, and histiocytes (Fig. 18-40). An associated exudate may be apparent on the luminal pleural surface.

The differential diagnosis centers on the exclusion of DM. The clinicopathologic similarities of DM and DPF are even closer than the likenesses between DM and HPP, because both DM and DPF have the ability to encase the lung in a "rind" of tissue.[163] However, DPF lacks the level of cellularity, nuclear atypia, hypovascularity, potential

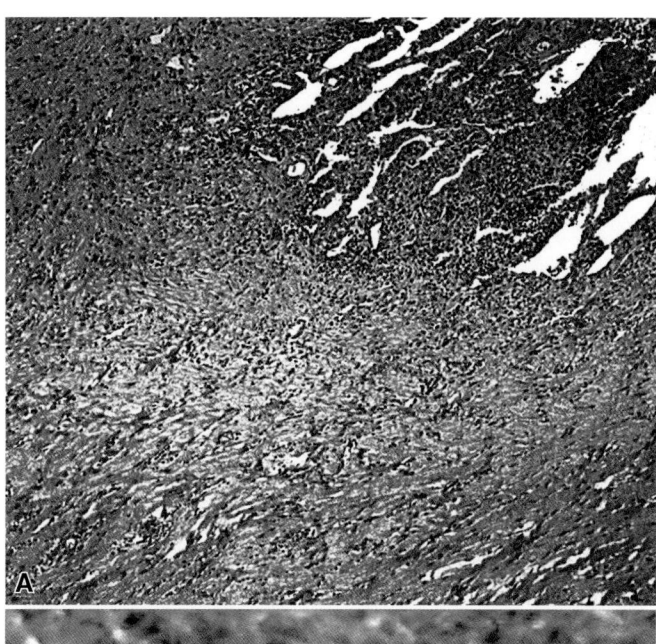

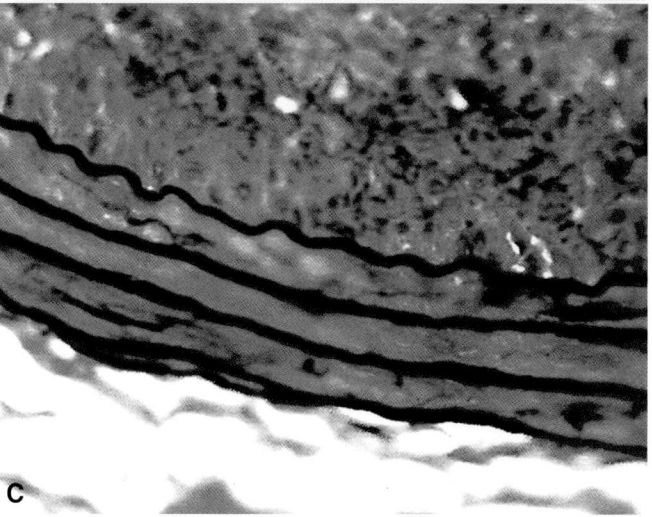

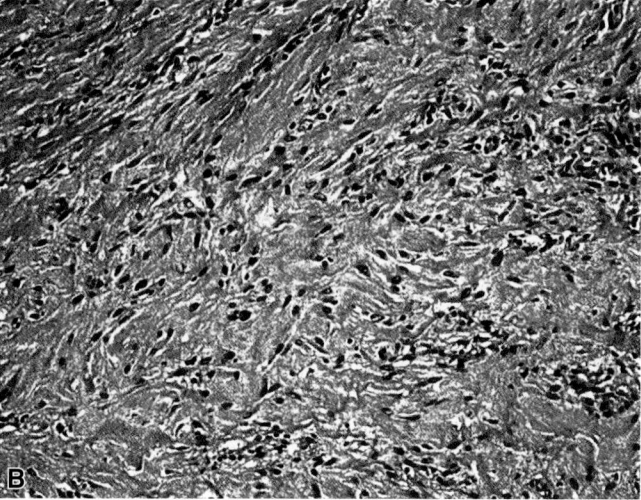

Figure 18-40. A and **B,** Diffuse pleural fibrosis showing a disorganized deposition of hypocellular, fully mature collagen in the visceral pleura. **C,** The stratification of elastic tissue typifying non-neoplastic pleura—shown here with a Verhoeff–van Gieson stain—is retained in pleural fibrosis.

necrosis, and invasive growth of DM. Special studies are generally non-contributory to this diagnostic separation. However, a routine keratin stain may highlight invasion of tumor into pleural fat in cases of DM, and a Verhoeff–van Gieson elastic stain may be illustrative in showing preservation of elastic tissue layering in the pleura (see Fig. 18-38) in DPF, a characteristic that is lost in DM.

Self-assessment questions related to this chapter can be found online on the Expert Consult site for this title.

References

1. Koss MN. Unusual tumor-like conditions of the lung. *Adv Pathol Lab Med*. 1994;7:123–150.
2. Su LD, Atayde-Perez A, Sheldon S, et al. Inflammatory myofibroblastic tumor: cytogenetic evidence supporting clonal origin. *Mod Pathol*. 1998;11:364–368.
3. Coffin CM, Dehner LP, Meis-Kindblom JM. Inflammatory myofibroblastic tumor, inflammatory fibrosarcoma, and related lesions: an historical review with differential diagnostic considerations. *Semin Diagn Pathol*. 1998;15:102–110.
4. Albrecht E. Uber Harmartome. *Verh Dtsch Ges Pathol*. 1904;7:153–157.
5. Takeshima Y, Furukawa K, Inai K. Adenomyomatous hamartoma of the lung. *Pathol Int*. 2000;50:984–986.
6. McDonald JR, Harrington SW, Clagett OT. Hamartoma (often called chondroma) of the lung. *J Thorac Cardiovasc Surg*. 1945;14:128–143.
7. Tomashefski Jr JF. Benign endobronchial mesenchymal tumors: their relationship to parenchymal pulmonary hamartomas. *Am J Surg Pathol*. 1982;6:531–540.
8. Koutras P, Urschel HC, Paulson DL. Hamartoma of the lung. *J Thorac Cardiovasc Surg*. 1971;61:768–776.
9. Cosio BG, Villena V, Echave-Sustaeta J, et al. Endobronchial hamartoma. *Chest*. 2002; 122:202–205.
10. Ge F, Tong F, Li Z. Diagnosis and treatment of pulmonary hamartoma. *Chin Med J*. 1998;13:61–62.
11. Higashita R, Ichikawa S, Ban T, et al. Coexistence of lung cancer and hamartoma. *Jpn J Thorac Cardiovasc Surg*. 2001;49:258–260.
12. Aggarwal P, Handa R, Wali JP, et al. Pulmonary hamartoma in a patient with testicular seminoma. *J Assoc Physicians India*. 1999;47:552–553.
13. Van Den Bosch JMM, Wagenaar SS, Corrin B, et al. Mesenchymoma of the lung (so-called hamartoma): a review of 154 parenchymal and endobronchial cases. *Thorax*. 1987;42: 790–793.
14. Salminen US. Pulmonary hamartoma: a clinical study of 77 cases in a 21 year period and review of the literature. *Eur J Cardiothorac Surg*. 1990;4:15–18.
15. Hansen CP, Holtveg H, Francis D, et al. Pulmonary hamartoma. *J Thorac Cardiovasc Surg*. 1992;104:674–678.
16. Wang SC. Lung hamartoma: a report of 30 cases and review of 477 cases. *Chung Hua Wai Ko Tsa Chih*. 1992;30:540–542.
17. Tomiyasu M, Yoshino I, Suemitsu R, et al. An intrapulmonary chondromatous hamartoma penetrating the visceral pleura: report of a case. *Ann Thorac Cardiovasc Surg*. 2002;8:42–44.
18. Markert E, Gruber-Moesenbacher U, Porubsky C, et al. Lung osteoma—a new benign lung lesion. *Virchows Arch*. 2006;449:117–120.
19. Xu R, Murray M, Jagirdar J, et al. Placental transmogrification of the lung is a histologic pattern frequently associated with pulmonary fibrochondromatous hamartoma. *Arch Pathol Lab Med*. 2002;126:562–566.
20. Azua-Blanco J, Azua-Romeo J, Ortego J, et al. Cytologic features of pulmonary hamartoma: report of a case diagnosed by fine needle aspiration cytology. *Acta Cytol*. 2001;45:267–270.
21. Hamper UM, Khouri NF, Stitik FP, et al. Pulmonary hamartoma: diagnosis by transthoracic needle aspiration biopsy. *Radiology*. 1985;155:15–18.
22. Wood B, Swarbrick N, Frost F. Diagnosis of pulmonary hamartoma by fine needle biopsy. *Acta Cytol*. 2008;52:412–417.
23. Hughes JH, Young NA, Wilbur DC, et al. Fine-needle aspiration of pulmonary hamartoma: a common source of false-positive diagnoses in the College of American Pathologists Interlaboratory Comparison Program in Nongynecologic Cytology. *Arch Pathol Lab Med*. 2005;129:19–22.
24. Incze JS, Lui PS. Morphology of the epithelial component of human lung hamartomas. *Hum Pathol*. 1977;8:411–419.
25. Stone FJ, Churg AM. The ultrastructure of pulmonary hamartoma. *Cancer*. 1977;39:1064–1070.
26. Perez-Atayde AR, Seiler MW. Pulmonary hamartoma: an ultrastructural study. *Cancer*. 1984;53:485–492.
27. Johansson M, Dietrich C, Mandahl N, et al. Recombinations of chromosomal bands 6p21 and 14q24 characterize pulmonary hamartomas. *Br J Cancer*. 1993;67:1236–1241.
28. Fletcher JA, Pinkus GS, Donovan K, et al. Clonal rearrangement of chromosome band 6p21 in the mesenchymal component of pulmonary chondroid hamartoma. *Cancer Res*. 1992;52:6224–6228.
29. Rogalla P, Lemke I, Kazmierczak B, et al. An identical HMGIC-LPP fusion transcript is consistently expressed in pulmonary chondroid hamartomas with t(3;12)(q27-28;q14-15). *Genes Chromosomes Cancer*. 2000;29:363–366.
30. Kazmierczak B, Meyer-Bolte K, Tran KH, et al. A high frequency of tumors with rearrangements of genes and the HMGI(Y) family in a series of 191 pulmonary chondroid hamartomas. *Genes Chromosomes Cancer*. 1999;26:125–133.
31. Yilmaz A, Rush DS, Soslow RA. Endometrial stromal sarcomas with unusual histologic features: a report of 24 primary and metastatic tumors emphasizing fibroblastic and smooth muscle differentiation. *Am J Surg Pathol*. 2002;26:1142–1150.
32. Erasmus JJ, Connolly JE, McAdams HP, et al. Solitary pulmonary nodules. Part I. Morphologic evaluation for differentiation of benign and malignant lesions. *Radiographics*. 2000;20:43–58.
33. Chell SE, Nayar R, De Frias DV, et al. Metaplastic breast carcinoma metastatic to lung mimicking a primary chondroid lesion: report of a case with cytohistologic correlation. *Ann Diagn Pathol*. 1998;2:173–180.
34. Nappi O, Glasner SD, Swanson PE, Wick MR. Biphasic and monophasic sarcomatoid carcinomas of the lung. *Am J Clin Pathol*. 1994;102:331–340.
35. Landreneau RJ, Hazelrigg SR, Ferson PF, et al. Thoracoscopic resection of 85 pulmonary lesions. *Ann Thorac Surg*. 1992;54:415–420.
36. Nakano M, Fukuda M, Sasayama K, et al. Nd–YAG laser treatment for central airway lesions. *Nippon Kyoubu Shikkan Gakkai Zasshi*. 1992;30:1007–1015.
37. Pelosi G, Rodriguez J, Viale G, et al. Salivary gland-type tumors with myoepithelial differentiation arising in pulmonary hamartoma: report of 2 cases of a hitherto-unrecognized association. *Am J Surg Pathol*. 2006;30:375–387.
38. Spencer H. The pulmonary plasma cell/histiocytoma complex. *Histopathology*. 1984;8:903–916.
39. Matsubara O, Tan-Liu NS, Kenney RM, et al. Inflammatory pseudotumors of the lung: progression from organizing pneumonia to fibrous histiocytoma or to plasma cell granuloma in 32 cases. *Hum Pathol*. 1988;19:807–814.
40. Pettinato G, Manivel JC, Rosa ND, et al. Inflammatory myofibroblastic tumor (plasma cell granuloma): clinicopathologic study of 20 cases with immunohistochemical and ultrastructural observations. *Am J Clin Pathol*. 1990;94:538–546.
41. Cavazza Gelli MC, Agostini L, et al. Calcified pseudotumor of the pleura: description of a case. *Pathologica*. 2002;94:201–205.
42. Fetsch JF, Montgomery EA, Meis JM. Calcifying fibrous pseudotumor. *Am J Surg Pathol*. 1993;17:502–508.
43. Pinkard NB, Wilson RW, Lawless N, et al. Calcifying fibrous pseudotumor of the pleura: a report of three cases of a newly described entity involving the pleura. *Am J Clin Pathol*. 1996;105:189–194.
44. Pomplun S, Goldstraw P, Davies SE, et al. Calcifying fibrous pseudotumor arising within an inflammatory pseudotumor: evidence of progression from one lesion to the other? *Histopathology*. 2000;37:380–382.
45. Nascimento AF, Ruiz R, Hornick JL, et al. Calcifying fibrous "pseudotumor:" clinicopathologic study of 15 cases and analysis of its relationship to inflammatory myofibroblastic tumor. *Int J Surg Pathol*. 2002;10:189–196.
46. Bahadori M, Liebow AA. Plasma cell granulomas of the lung. *Cancer*. 1973;31:191–208.
47. Anthony PP. Inflammatory pseudotumor (plasma cell granuloma) of lung, liver, and other organs. *Histopathology*. 1993;23:501–503.
48. Ahn JM, Kim WS, Yeon KM, et al. Plasma cell granuloma involving the tracheobronchial angle in a child: a case report. *Pediatr Radiol*. 1995;25:204–205.
49. Copin MC, Gosselin BH, Ribet ME. Plasma cell granuloma of the lung: difficulties in diagnosis and prognosis. *Ann Thorac Surg*. 1996;61:1477–1482.
50. Mas Estelles F, Andres V, Vallcanera A, et al. Plasma cell granuloma of the lung in childhood: atypical radiologic findings and association with hypertrophic osteoarthropathy. *Pediatr Radiol*. 1995;25:369–372.
51. Monzon CM, Gilchrist GS, Burgert EO, et al. Plasma cell granuloma of the lung in children. *Pediatrics*. 1982;70:268–274.
52. Tomita T, Dixon A, Watanabe I, et al. Sclerosing vascular variant of plasma cell granuloma. *Hum Pathol*. 1980;11:197–202.
53. Toccanier MF, Exquis B, Groebli Y. Granulome plasmocytaire du poumon. Neuf observations avec etude immunohistochemique. *Ann Pathol*. 1982;2:21–28.
54. Kobashi Y, Fukuda M, Nakata M, et al. Inflammatory pseudotumor of the lung: clinicopathological analysis in seven adult patients. *Int J Clin Oncol*. 2006;11:461–466.
55. Mohsenifar Z, Bein ME, Mott LJM, et al. Cystic organizing pneumonia with elements of plasma cell granuloma. *Arch Pathol Lab Med*. 1979;103:600–601.
56. Cerfolio RJ, Allen MS, Nascimento AG, et al. Inflammatory pseudotumors of the lung. *Ann Thorac Surg*. 1999;67:933–936.
57. Agrons GA, Rosado-de-Cristenson ML, Kirejczyk WM, et al. Pulmonary inflammatory pseudotumor: radiologic features. *Radiology*. 1998;206:511–518.
58. Kawisawa T, Okamoto A. IgG4-related sclerosing disease. *World J Gastroenterol*. 2008;14:3948–3955.
59. Shrestha B, Sekiguchi H, Colby TV, et al. Distinctive pulmonary histopathology with increased IgG4-positive plasma cells in patients with autoimmune pancreatitis: report of 6 and 12 cases with similar histopathology. *Am J Surg Pathol*. 2009;33:1450–1462.
60. Yamamoto H, Yamaguchi H, Aishima S, et al. Inflammatory myofibroblastic tumor versus IgG4-related sclerosing disease and inflammatory pseudotumor: a comparative clinicopathologic study. *Am J Surg Pathol*. 2009;33:1330–1340.
61. Zen Y, Inoue D, Kitao A, et al. IgG4-related lung and pleural disease: a clinicopathologic study of 21 cases. *Am J Surg Pathol*. 2009;33:1886–1893.
62. Kojima M, Nakamura N, Itoh H, et al. Presence of immunoglobulin heavy-chain rearrangement in so-called "plasma cell granuloma" of the lung. *Pathol Res Pract*. 2010;206:83–87.

63. Park SH, Choe GY, Kim CW, et al. Inflammatory pseudotumor of the lung in a child with *Mycoplasma* pneumonia. *J Korean Med Sci*. 1990;5:213–223.

64. Harjula A, Mattila S, Kyoesola K, et al. Plasma cell granuloma of lung and pleura. *Scand J Thorac Cardiovasc Surg*. 1986;20:119–121.

65. Loo KT, Seneviratne S, Chan JKC. Mycobacterial infection mimicking inflammatory pseudotumor of the lung. *Histopathology*. 1989;14:217–219.

66. Kim I, Kim WS, Yeon KM, et al. Inflammatory pseudotumor of the lung manifesting as a posterior mediastinal mass. *Pediatr Radiol*. 1992;22:467–468.

67. Kuhr H, Svane S. Pulmonary pseudotumor caused by *Cryptococcus neoformans*. *Tidsskr Norweg Laegeforen*. 1991;111:3288–3290.

68. Bishopric GA, D'Agay MF, Schlemmer B, et al. Pulmonary pseudotumor due to *Corynebacterium equi* in a patient with the acquired immunodeficiency syndrome. *Thorax*. 1988;43:486–487.

69. Yanagisawa K, Traquina DN. Inflammatory pseudotumor: an unusual case of recurrent pneumonia in childhood. *Int J Ped Otorhinolaryngol*. 1993;25:261–268.

70. Freschi P, Pocecco M, Carini C, et al. Pseudotumor inflammatorio polmonare post-traumatico: descrizione di un caso. *Pediatr Med Chir*. 1989;11:93–96.

71. Roikjaer O, Thomsen JK. Plasmacytoma of the lung. *Cancer*. 1986;58:2671–2674.

72. Weiss LM, Yousem SA, Warnke RA. Non-Hodgkin's lymphomas of the lung. *Am J Surg Pathol*. 1985;9:480–490.

73. Toh HC, Ang PT. Primary pulmonary lymphoma—clinical review from a single institution in Singapore. *Leuk Lymphoma*. 1997;27:153–163.

74. Kradin RL, Mark EJ. Benign lymphoid disorders of the lung with a theory regarding their development. *Hum Pathol*. 1983;14:857–867.

75. Michal M, Mukensnabl P. Epithelial plasma cell granuloma-like tumors of the lungs: a hitherto-unrecognized tumor. *Pathol Res Pract*. 2002;198:311–316.

76. Wick MR, Ritter JH, Nappi O. Inflammatory sarcomatoid carcinoma of the lung: report of three cases and comparison with inflammatory pseudotumors in adult patients. *Hum Pathol*. 1995;26:1014–1021.

77. Yousem SA, Hochholzer L. Pulmonary hyalinizing granuloma. *Am J Clin Pathol*. 1987;87:1–6.

78. Alvarez-Fernandez E, Carretero-Albinana L, Menarguez-Palance J. Sclerosing hemangioma of the lung: an immunohistochemical study of intermediate filaments and endothelial markers. *Arch Pathol Lab Med*. 1989;113:121–124.

79. Illei PB, Rosai J, Klimstra DS. Expression of thyroid transcription factor-1 and other markers in sclerosing hemangioma of the lung. *Arch Pathol Lab Med*. 2001;125:1335–1339.

80. Ledet SC, Brown RW, Cagle PT. p53 immunoreactivity in the differentiation of inflammatory pseudotumor from sarcoma involving the lung. *Mod Pathol*. 1995;8:282–286.

81. Doski JJ, Priebe CJ Jr, Driessnack M, et al. Corticosteroids in the management of unresected plasma cell granuloma (inflammatory pseudotumor) of the lung. *J Pediatr Surg*. 1991;26:1064–1066.

82. Umeki S. A case of plasma cell granuloma which resolved after steroid therapy. *Nippon Kyoubu Shikkan Gakkai Zasshi*. 1993;31:123–126.

83. Imperato JP, Folkman J, Sagerman RH, et al. Treatment of plasma cell granuloma of the lung with radiation therapy: a report of two cases and a review of the literature. *Cancer*. 1986;57:2127–2129.

84. Wood C, Nickoloff BJ, Todes-Taylor NR. Pseudotumor resulting from atypical mycobacterial infection: a "histoid" variety of *Mycobacterium avium-intracellulare* complex infection. *Am J Clin Pathol*. 1985;83:524–527.

85. Brandwein M, Choid HSH, Strauchen J, et al. Spindle cell reaction to nontuberculous mycobacteriosis in AIDS mimicking a spindle cell neoplasm: evidence for dual histiocytic and fibroblast-like characteristics of the cells. *Virchows Arch Pathol Anat*. 1990;416:281–286.

86. Chen KTK. Mycobacterial spindle cell pseudotumor of lymph nodes. *Am J Surg Pathol*. 1992;16:276–281.

87. Wade HW. The histoid variety of lepromatous leprosy. *Int Lepr*. 1963;31:129–142.

88. Triscott JA, Nappi O, Ferrara G, et al. "Pseudoneoplastic" leprosy. Histoid leprosy revisited. *Am J Dermatopathol*. 1995;17:297–302.

89. Sekosan M, Cleto M, Senseng C, et al. Spindle cell pseudotumors in the lungs due to *Mycobacterium tuberculosis* in a transplant patient. *Am J Surg Pathol*. 1992;18:1065–1068.

90. Umlas J, Federman M, Crawford C, et al. Spindle cell pseudotumor due to *Mycobacterium avium-intracellulare* in patients with acquired immunodeficiency syndrome (AIDS): positive staining of mycobacteria for cytoskeletal filaments. *Am J Surg Pathol*. 1991;15:1181–1187.

91. Foucar E, Rosai J, Dorfman R. Sinus histiocytosis with massive lymphadenopathy (Rosai–Dorfman disease): review of the entity. *Semin Diagn Pathol*. 1990;7:19–73.

92. Wang CW, Colby TV. Histiocytic lesions and proliferations in the lung. *Semin Diagn Pathol*. 2007;24:162–182.

93. Wright DH, Richards DB. Sinus histiocytosis with massive lymphadenopathy (Rosai–Dorfman disease): report of a case with widespread nodal and extranodal dissemination. *Histopathology*. 1981;5:697–709.

94. Ratzinger G, Zelger B, Hobling W, et al. Sinus histiocytosis with massive lymphadenopathy (Rosai-Dorfman disease): three unusual manifestations. *Virchows Arch*. 2003;443:797–800.

95. Lutterbach J, Henne K, Pagenstecher A, et al. Lung cancer and Rosai-Dorfman disease: a clinicopathological study. *Strahlenther Onkol*. 2003;179:486–492.

96. Chunduri S, Gaitonde S, Ciurea SO, et al. Pulmonary extramedullary hematopoiesis in patients with myelofibrosis undergoing allgeneic stem cell transplantation. *Haematologica*. 2008;93:1593–1595.

97. Bowling MR, Cauthen CG, Perry CD, et al. Pulmonary extramedullary hematopoiesis. *J Thorac Imaging*. 2008;23:138–141.

98. Ogus C, Ozdemir T, Kabaalioglu A. Right hilar mass in a patient with beta-thalassemia major. *Respiration*. 2001;68:215–216.

99. Kumar PV, Arasteh M, Musallaye A, et al. Fine needle aspiration diagnosis of extramedullary hematopoiesis presenting as a right lung mass. *Acta Cytol*. 2000;44:698–699.

100. Hsu FI, Filippa DA, Castro-Malaspina H, et al. Extramedullary hematopoiesis mimicking metastatic lung carcinoma. *Ann Thorac Surg*. 1998;66:1411–1413.

101. Schwarz C, Bittner R, Kirsch A, et al. A 62 year-old woman with bilateral pleural effusions and pulmonary infiltrates caused by extramedullary hematopoiesis. *Respiration*. 2009;78:110–113.

102. Nadrous HF, Krowka MJ, McClure RF, et al. Agnogenic myeloid metaplasia with pleural extramedullary leukemic transformation. *Leuk Lymphoma*. 2004;45:815–818.

103. Wandall HH. A study on neoplastic cells in sputum as a contribution to the diagnosis of primary lung cancer. *Acta Chir Scand*. 1944;91(suppl 93):1–143.

104. Koss LG. *Diagnostic Cytology and Its Histologic Basis*, 4th ed. Philadelphia: JB Lippincott; 1992:849–864.

105. Erozan YS. Cytopathologic diagnosis of pulmonary neoplasms in sputum and bronchoscopic specimens. *Semin Diagn Pathol*. 1986;3:188–195.

106. Jay SJ, Wehr K, Nicholson DP, et al. Diagnostic sensitivity and specificity of pulmonary cytology. *Acta Cytol*. 1980;24:304–312.

107. Pearson FG, Thompson DW, Delarue NC. Experience with the cytologic detection, localization, and treatment of radiographically undemonstrable bronchial carcinoma. *J Thorac Cardiovasc Surg*. 1967;54:371–382.

108. Zavala DC. Diagnostic fiberoptic bronchoscopy: techniques and results of biopsy in 600 patients. *Chest*. 1975;68:12–19.

109. Truong LD, Underwood RD, Greenberg SD, et al. Diagnosis and typing of lung carcinomas by cytopathologic methods: a review of 108 cases. *Acta Cytol*. 1985;29:379–384.

110. Berkheiser JW. Bronchiolar proliferation and metaplasia associated with bronchiectasis, pulmonary infarct, and anthracosis. *Cancer*. 1959;12:499–508.

111. Berkheiser JW. Bronchiolar proliferation and metaplasia associated with thromboembolism: a pathological and experimental study. *Cancer*. 1963;16:205–211.

112. Kawecka M. Cytological evaluation of the sputum in patients with bronchiectasis and the possibility of erroneous diagnosis of carcinoma. *Acta Union Int Cancer*. 1959;15:469–473.

113. Marchevsky AM, Nieburgs HE, Olenko F, et al. Pulmonary tumorlets in cases of "tuberculoma" of the lung with malignant cells in brush biopsy. *Acta Cytol*. 1982;26:491–494.

114. Johnston WW, Frable WJ. Cytopathology of the respiratory tract: a review. *Am J Pathol*. 1976;84:371–424.

115. Ritter JH, Wick MR, Reyes A, et al. False-positive interpretations of carcinoma in exfoliative respiratory cytology. *Am J Clin Pathol*. 1995;104:133–140.

116. Policarpio-Nicolas ML, Wick MR. False-positive interpretations in respiratory cytopathology: exemplary cases and literature review. *Diagn Cytopathol*. 2008;36:13–19.

117. Saccomanno G, Archer VE, Saunders RD, et al. Development of carcinoma of the lung as reflected in exfoliated cells. *Cancer*. 1974;33:256–270.

118. Koss LG, Richardson HI. Some pitfalls of cytological diagnosis of lung cancer. *Cancer*. 1955;8:937–947.

119. Plamenac P, Nikulin A, Pikula B. Cytologic changes of the respiratory tract in young adults as a consequence of high levels of air pollution exposure. *Acta Cytol*. 1973;17:241–244.

120. Kern WH. Cytology of hyperplastic and neoplastic lesions of terminal bronchioles and alveoli. *Acta Cytol*. 1965;9:372–379.

121. McKee G, Parums DV. False positive cytodiagnosis in fibrosing alveolitis. *Acta Cytol*. 1990;34:105–107.

122. Meyer EC, Liebow AA. Relationship of interstitial pneumonia and honey-combing and typical epithelial proliferation to cancer of the lung. *Cancer*. 1965;18:322–351.

123. Williams JW. Alveolar metaplasia: its relationship to pulmonary fibrosis in industry and development of lung cancer. *Br J Cancer*. 1957;11:30–42.

124. Johnston WW. Type II pneumocytes in cytologic specimens: a diagnostic dilemma. *Am J Clin Pathol*. 1992;97:608–609.

125. Pei F, Zheng J, Gao ZF, et al. Lung pathology and pathogenesis of severe acute respiratory syndrome: a report of six full autopsies. *Chin J Pathol*. 2005;34:656–660.

126. Shilo K, Colby TV, Travis WD, et al. Exuberant type 2 pneumocyte hyperplasia associated with spontaneous pneumothorax: secondary reactive change mimicking adenocarcinoma. *Mod Pathol*. 2007;20:352–356.

127. Clayton F. The spectrum and significance of bronchioloalveolar carcinoma. *Pathol Annu*. 1988;23(part 2):361–394.

128. Stanley MW, Henry-Stanley MJ, Gajl-Peczakska KJ, et al. Hyperplasia of type II pneumocytes in acute lung injury. *Am J Clin Pathol*. 1992;97:669–677.

129. Grotte D, Stanley MW, Swanson PE, et al. Reactive type II pneumocytes in bronchoalveolar lavage fluid from acute respiratory distress syndrome can be mistaken for cells of adenocarcinoma. *Diagn Cytopathol*. 1990;6:317–322.

130. Miura H, Kato H, Hayata V, et al. Solitary bronchial mucosal neuroma. *CHEST*. 1989;95:245–247.

131. Rossi G, Marchioni A, Agostini L, et al. Traumatic neuroma of the bronchi: bronchoscopy and histology of a hitherto-unreported lesion. *Am J Surg Pathol*. 2008;32:640–641.

132. Pagni F, Zarate AF, Urbanski SJ. Necrotizing sialometaplasia of bronchial mucosa. *Int J Surg Pathol*. 2010;18:64–65.

133. Couture C, Colby TV. Histopathology of bronchiolar disorders. *Semin Respir Crit Care Med*. 2003;24:489–498.

134. Fukuoka J, Franks TJ, Colby TV, et al. Peribronchiolar metaplasia: a common histologic finding in diffuse lung disease and a rare cause of interstitial lung disease: clinicopathologic features of 15 cases. *Am J Surg Pathol*. 2005;29:948–954.

135. Cibas ES: Effusions (pleural, pericardial, and peritoneal) and peritoneal washings. In: Atkinson B, ed. *Atlas of Diagnostic Cytopathology*. Philadelphia: WB Saunders; 2003.

136. Bibbo M. *Comprehensive Cytopathology*. Philadelphia: WB Saunders; 1991.

137. DeMay RM. *The Art and Science of Cytopathology*. Chicago: American Society for Clinical Pathology Press; 1996.

138. Kobayashi TK, Gotoh T, Nakano K, et al. Atypical mesothelial cells associated with eosinophilic pleural effusions: nuclear DNA content and immunocytochemical staining reaction with epithelial markers. *Cytopathology*. 1993;4:37–46.

139. Chen CJ, Chang SC, Tseng HH. Assessment of immunocytochemical and histochemical staining in the distinction between reactive mesothelial cells and adenocarcinoma in body effusions. *Chinese Med J*. 1994;54:149–155.

140. Schultenover SJ. Body cavity fluids. In: Ramzi I, ed. *Clinical Cytopathology and Aspiration Biopsy*. East Norwalk, CT: Appleton & Lange; 1990:165–180.

141. Leong A.S.-Y., Stevens MW, Mukherjee TM. Malignant mesothelioma: cytologic diagnosis with histologic, immunohistochemical, and ultrastructural correlation. *Semin Diagn Pathol*. 1992;9:141–150.

142. Bedrossian CWM, Bonsib S, Moran C. Differential diagnosis between mesothelioma and adenocarcinoma: a multimodal approach based on ultrastructure and immunocytochemistry. *Semin Diagn Pathol*. 1992;9:91–96.

143. Kutty CPK, Remeniuk E, Varkey B. Malignant-appearing cells in pleural effusion due to pancreatitis. *Acta Cytol*. 1981;25:412–416.

144. Marchevsky AM, Hauptman E, Gil J, et al. Computerized interactive morphometry as an aid in the diagnosis of pleural effusions. *Acta Cytol*. 1987;31:131–136.

145. Kwee WS, Veldhuizen RW, Alons CA, et al. Quantitative and qualitative differences between benign and malignant mesothelial cells in pleural fluid. *Acta Cytol*. 1982;26:401–406.

146. Oberholzer M, Ettlin R, Christen H, et al. The significance of morphometric methods in cytologic diagnostics: differentiation between mesothelial cells, mesothelioma cells, and metastatic adenocarcinoma cells in pleural effusions with special emphasis on chromatin texture. *Analyt Cell Pathol*. 1991;3:25–42.

147. Ranaldi R, Marinelli F, Barbatelli G, et al. Benign and malignant mesothelial lesions of the pleura: quantitative study. *Appl Pathol*. 1986;4:55–64.

148. Roberts GH, Campbell GH. Exfoliative cytology of diffuse mesothelioma. *J Clin Pathol*. 1972;25:557–582.

149. Bolen JW. Tumors of serosal tissue origin. *Clin Lab Med*. 1987;7:31–50.

150. Whitaker D, Henderson DW, Shilkin KB. The concept of mesothelioma in situ: implications for diagnosis and histogenesis. *Semin Diagn Pathol*. 1992;9:151–161.

151. Henderson DW, Shilkin KB, Whitaker D. Reactive mesothelial hyperplasia vs. mesothelioma, including mesothelioma in-situ: a brief review. *Am J Clin Pathol*. 1998;110:397–404.

152. Lee A, Baloch ZW, Yu G, et al. Mesothelial hyperplasia with reactive atypia: diagnostic pitfalls and role of immunohistochemical studies: a case report. *Diagn Cytopathol*. 2000;22:113–116.

153. Singh HK, Silverman JF, Berns L, et al. Significance of epithelial membrane antigen in the workup of problematic serous effusions. *Diagn Cytopathol*. 1995;13:3–7.

154. Ferrandez-Izquierdo A, Navarro-Fos S, Gonzalez-Devesa M, et al. Immunocytochemical typification of mesothelial cells in effusions: in vivo and in vitro models. *Diagn Cytopathol*. 1994;10:256–262.

155. Cagle PT, Brown RW, Lebovitz RM. p53 immunostaining in the differentiation of reactive processes from malignancy in pleural biopsy specimens. *Hum Pathol*. 1994;25:443–448.

156. Walts AE, Said JW, Koeffler HP. Is immunoreactivity for p53 useful in distinguishing benign from malignant effusions? Localization of p53 gene product in benign mesothelial and adenocarcinoma cells. *Mod Pathol*. 1994;7:462–468.

157. Churg A. Asbestos fibers and pleural plaques in a general autopsy population. *Am J Pathol*. 1982;109:88–96.

158. Fondimare A, Duwoos H, Desbordes J, et al. Plaques fibroyalines calcifiees du foie dans l'asbestose. *Nouv Presse Med*. 1973;3:893.

159. Hourihane DO, Lessof L, Richardson PC. Hyaline and calcified pleural plaques as an index of exposure to asbestos: a study of radiological and pathological features of 100 cases with a consideration of epidemiology. *Br Med J*. 1966;1:1069–1074.

160. Kishimoto T, Ono T, Okada K, et al. Relationship between numbers of asbestos bodies in autopsy lung and pleural plaques on chest x-ray film. *Chest*. 1989;95:549–552.

161. Mattson S, Ringqvist T. Pleural plaques and exposure to asbestos. *Scand J Respir Dis*. 1970;75:1–41.

162. Roberts GH. The pathology of parietal pleural plaques. *J Clin Pathol*. 1961;348–353.

163. Warnock ML, Prescott BT, Kuwahara TJ. Numbers and types of asbestos fibers in subjects with pleural plaques. *Am J Pathol*. 1982;109:37–46.

164. Kuhlman JE, Singha NK. Complex disease of the pleural space: radiographic and CT evaluation. *Radiographics*. 1997;17:63–79.

165. Wilson GE, Hasleton PS, Chatterjee AK. Desmoplastic malignant mesothelioma: a review of 17 cases. *J Clin Pathol*. 1992;45:295–298.

166. Mangano EW, Cagle PT, Churg A, et al. The diagnosis of desmoplastic malignant mesothelioma and its distinction from fibrous pleurisy: a histologic and immunohistochemical analysis of 31 cases including p53 immunostaining. *Am J Clin Pathol*. 1998;110:191–199.

167. Moran CA, Suster S, Koss MN. The spectrum of histologic growth patterns in benign and malignant fibrous tumors of the pleura. *Semin Diagn Pathol*. 1992;9:169–180.

168. Wain SL, Roggli VL, Foster WL Jr. Parietal pleural plaques, asbestos bodies and neoplasia: a clinical, pathologic and roentgenographic correlation of 25 consecutive cases. *Chest*. 1985;86:707–713.

169. Epler GR, McCloud TC, Gaensler EA. Prevalence and incidence of benign asbestos pleural effusion in a working population. *JAMA*. 1982;247:617–622.

170. Gibbs AR, Stephens M, Griffiths DM, et al. Fiber distribution in the lungs and pleura of subjects with asbestos-related diffuse pleural fibrosis. *Br J Ind Med*. 1991;48:762–770.

171. Stephens M, Gibbs AR, Pooley FD, et al. Asbestos-induced diffuse pleural fibrosis: pathology and mineralogy. *Thorax*. 1987;42:583–588.

Benign and Borderline Tumors of the Lungs and Pleura

Mark R. Wick, MD, Henry D. Tazelaar, MD, and Stacey E. Mills, MD

Malignant neoplasms are more common, by far, than benign tumors in the lower respiratory tract. In the United States, lung carcinoma is the leading cause of cancer-related death in both sexes, and it accounts for more than 0.7% of new malignancies each year in men.[1] In Europe, the situation is even worse; for example, more than 3.0% of newly diagnosed malignant neoplasms in Germany are lung cancers.[2] These data reflect the continuing use of cigarettes worldwide and the relative potency of tobacco smoke as a carcinogenic agent.

Because of the prognostic gravity and the frequency of lung cancers, less attention has been given to benign pulmonary neoplasms and those that have "borderline" malignant potential. Nonetheless, they comprise an interesting array of lesions with diverse lineages, the causes of which are known only in a minority of cases. This chapter provides an overview of such tumors, with an emphasis on the differential diagnosis.

Benign Pleuropulmonary Neoplasms
Clinical Features

The clinical characteristics of benign tumors in the lower respiratory tract can be considered in an overview, because they are generally not specific to any particular diagnosis. Most benign intrapulmonary lesions are associated with no symptoms or signs whatsoever, and are found incidentally with screening radiographic studies. As discussed elsewhere in this book, hamartomas are often separable from other benign but truly neoplastic masses of the lung on imaging studies because of their common content of distinctive calcifications, fat densities, or both[3] (Fig. 19-1). Otherwise, the radiologist is not typically able to distinguish between specific histologic entities in this context. Endotracheal and endobronchial tumors are more often related to clinical symptoms such as wheezing, hemoptysis, obstructive pneumonia,

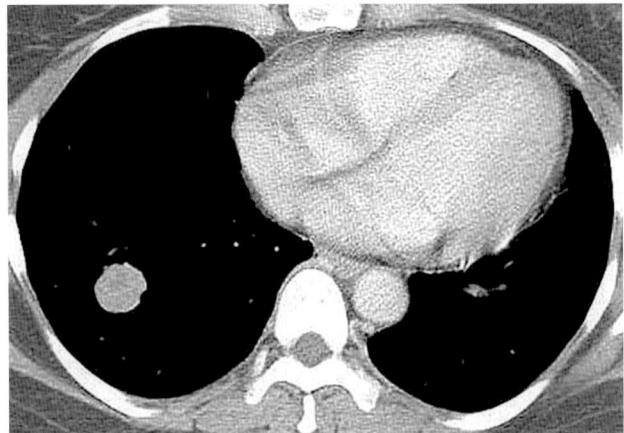

Figure 19-1. This computed tomogram of the lung shows a well-demarcated peripheral nodule with internal calcification, typical of pulmonary hamartoma.

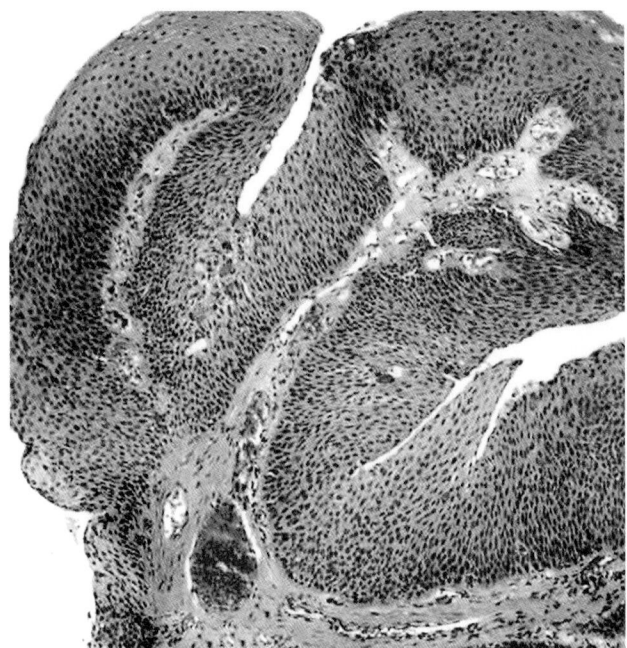

Figure 19-2. Solitary papilloma of the bronchus represented by a papillary proliferation of bland squamous epithelium supported by well-formed fibrovascular stroma.

and postobstructive pulmonary hyperinflation, depending on their anatomic location.

In the past, radiologists were comfortable simply observing a pulmonary mass over time, if it had reassuring morphologic characteristics. In fact, statistical paradigms have been constructed to aid in this process.[4] However, because of the unfortunate pressure of litigation involving putative "delays in diagnosis" of malignant neoplasms at various sites[5]—together with the modern availability of techniques such as video-assisted thoracoscopic surgery[6]—many more benign lesions of the lungs are excised today than in previous years.

Bronchoscopic examination and endobronchial biopsy are productive diagnostically if the tumor in question protrudes significantly into the lumen of the airway. However, brushing cytology is only variably effective in sampling such growths, depending on whether the mucosa over them is intact and the level of intercellular cohesion in the tumor itself. Transthoracic or transbronchial aspirates or needle biopsies are usually necessary for adequate sampling of deeply seated masses in the parenchyma. In this setting, these procedures are most effective in the diagnosis of malignant neoplasms; if the pathologist sees only histologically banal tissue elements in the latter specimens, it is often impossible to discern whether they truly represent the lesion or are simply part of the adjacent lung. Moreover, in small biopsy specimens, the morphologic attributes of some cytologically low-grade malignancies may be virtually identical to those of benign tumors belonging to the same general cellular lineage.

Benign Tumors That Are Principally Tracheal and Endobronchial

Solitary Tracheobronchial Papilloma

A solitary papilloma of the tracheobronchial tree (SPTT) most often arises in adults—typically middle-aged—with a slight male predominance.[7-22] Occasionally, even though only one papillomatous lesion of the lower respiratory tract may be present, it may coexist with papillary squamous proliferations of the larynx or oropharynx.

Grossly, SPTTs form a pedunculated tan-white polypoid excrescence in the mucosa of the airway, with variable luminal compromise. The surface may be smooth or slightly verrucoid.

Microscopically, SPTTs are similar to viral papillomas elsewhere in the body, particularly in the genitoperineal region. They are constituted by arborizing fronds with fibrovascular cores, mantled by relatively bland squamous epithelial cells (Fig. 19-2). These often exhibit nuclear hyperchromasia and crenation, but the nuclear chromatin

may be homogenized and glassy. The cytoplasm is commonly unremarkable; alternatively, it may show perinuclear clearing, eosinophilic globular inclusions, or hypergranulation with clumping of keratohyaline granules (Figs. 19-3 and 19-4). Nuclear atypia has been observed in squamous SPTT, and squamous carcinoma may develop in this setting.[23,24]

Another even rarer variant of SPTT is the columnar papilloma, composed of columnar epithelial cells rather than squamous elements.[14] Putatively, it has no potential for malignant change.

Interestingly, the biologic associations between squamous SPTT and human papillomavirus (HPV) types are comparable to those in the genital tract. Specifically, HPV types 7 and 11 are most commonly seen in uncomplicated SPTT; in contrast, HPV types 16 and 18 are associated with dysplastic nuclear features and a higher risk of carcinomatous transformation.[23,24] The presence of these viral agents can be evaluated using in situ hybridization (Fig. 19-5), the hybrid capture method, or polymerase chain reaction.[23-27]

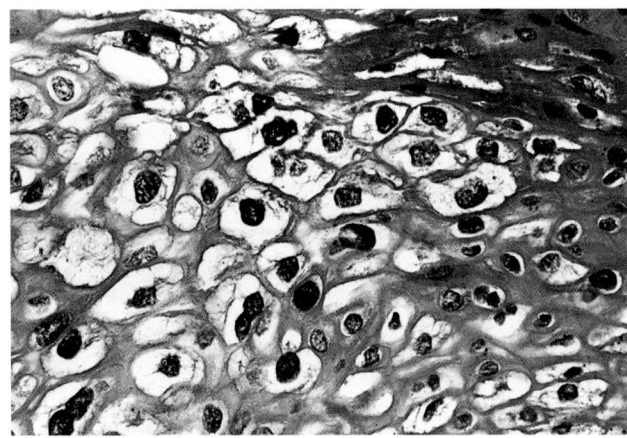

Figure 19-3. Koilocytotic change in the squamous cells of a solitary bronchial papilloma represented by nuclear hyperchromasia and crenation and perinuclear clearing of the cytoplasm.

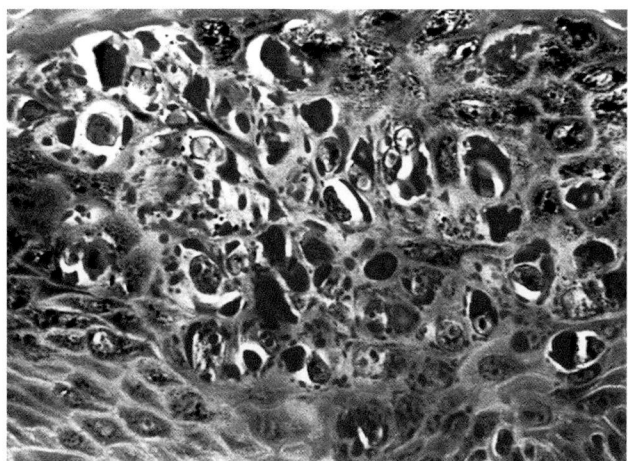

Figure 19-4. Clumped keratohyaline and eosinophilic cytoplasmic inclusions are seen in the lesional cells of this solitary squamous papilloma of the bronchus with a viral causation.

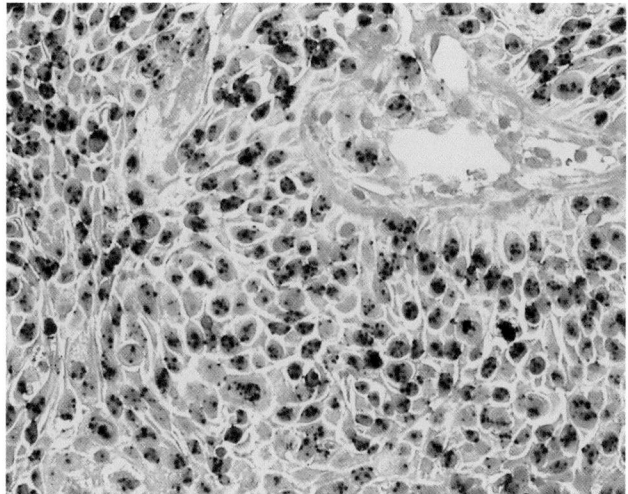

Figure 19-5. The presence of integrated nucleic acid from human papillomavirus type 11 is apparent in this in situ hybridization preparation, as evidenced by nuclei that show a blue chromogenic signal.

In light of the usual behavior of SPTT, conservative therapeutic approaches, such as endoscopic removal, cryotherapy, or fulguration, are typically applied. Lesions in which malignancy develops must be treated in a manner appropriate for "ordinary" lung cancers (Fig. 19-6).[28–31]

Multifocal Respiratory Tract Papillomatosis

Respiratory tract papillomatosis (RTP) is the multifocal form of viral papillomagenesis, as described earlier. Its onset is early in life because the mode of transmission is natal inhalation of virally infected genital tract secretions during vaginal delivery.[32–41] Children with RTP typically have oropharyngeal or laryngeal disease initially; it may remain localized or spread to involve the lower airways as well, as seen in 5% of cases.[40] In the latter instance, growth into the lung parenchyma may supervene, with the eventual appearance of cavitary lesions that can simulate carcinomas radiographically.[32,41] Obstruction of the tracheal or bronchial lumina is associated with recurrent pneumonia, hemoptysis, and asthma-like symptoms. Even though RTP is often said to be "recurring," the entire respiratory tract is at risk for infection by HPV in this disorder. Thus, it is more apropos to consider separate lesions

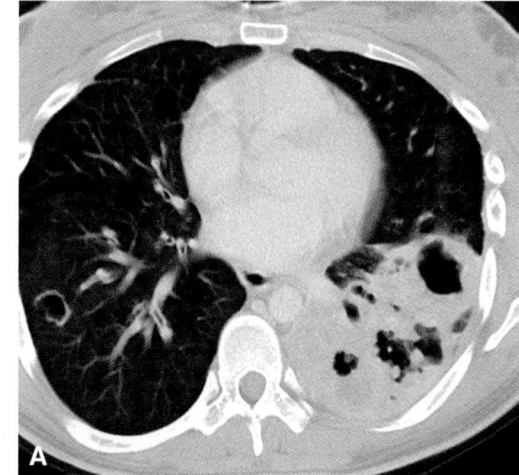

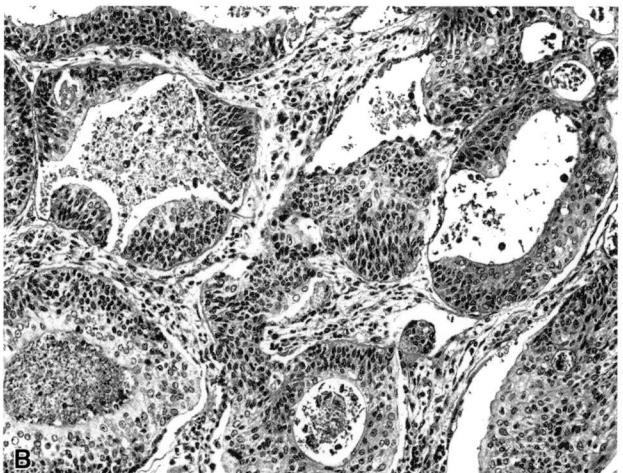

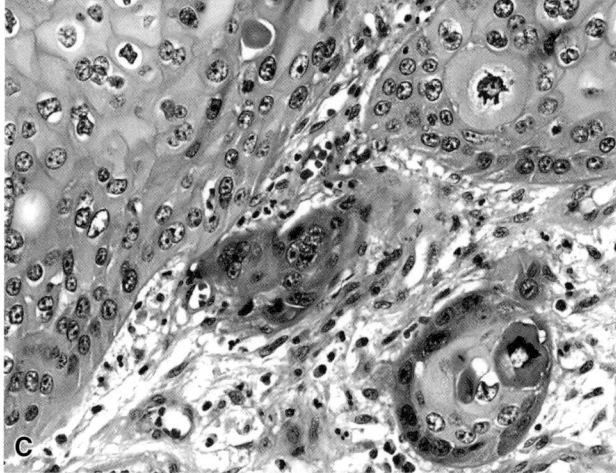

Figure 19-6. Rarely, multifocal respiratory papillomatosis may give rise to squamous cell carcinoma manifested as a mass in the posterior left lung, seen on this computed tomogram (**A**) and microscopically (**B** and **C**). (Courtesy of Dr. Benjamin Kozower, Charlottesville, VA).

as metachronously or synchronously independent of one another pathogenetically.

The gross and histologic features of RTP are largely the same as those of SSTP (Figs. 19-7 and 19-8). Exceptions include the multiplicity of lesions and the greater tendency for "inverting" or tissue-destructive growth of the papillomatous lesions in RTP

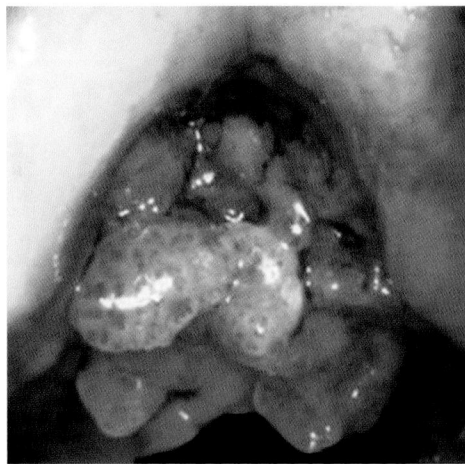

Figure 19-7. Bronchoscopic appearance of multifocal respiratory papillomatosis showing a multiplicity of smooth-domed and confluent lesions in the bronchial mucosa.

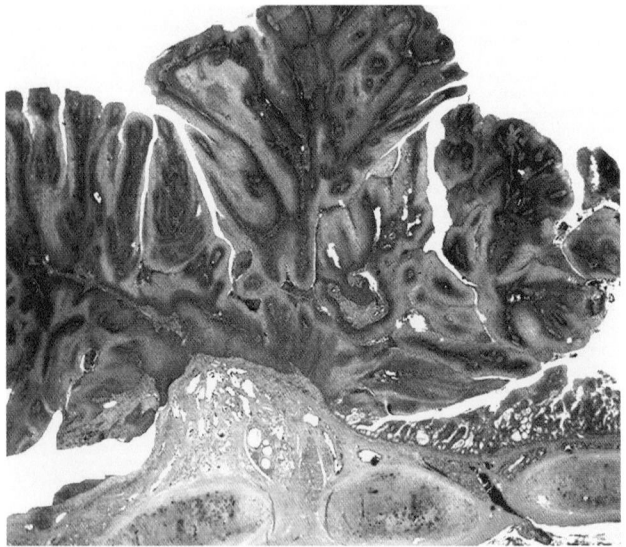

Figure 19-8. The histologic appearance of individual lesions in multifocal respiratory papillomatosis is similar to that of a solitary papilloma of the tracheobronchial tree.

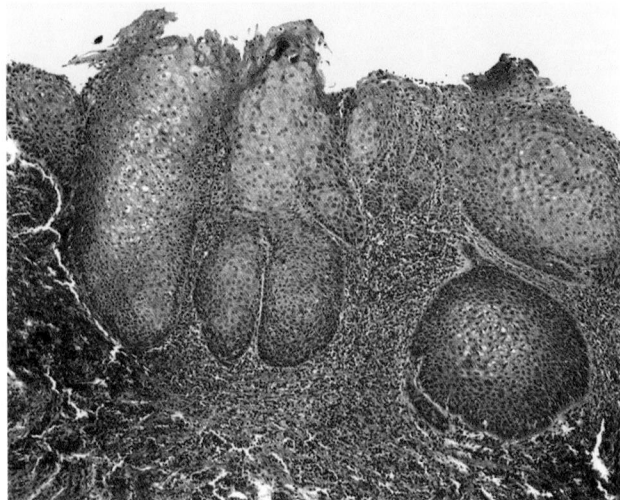

Figure 19-9. Inverting growth into the bronchial submucosa by an individual lesion of multifocal respiratory papillomatosis.

(Fig. 19-9). The HPV profiles of RTP and SSTP are comparable, with the notable proviso that HPV-11 is overwhelmingly the most common viral type seen in RTP. Mutations of the *p53* gene have been linked to malignant transformation of individual lesions in both conditions.[23,24,27,41-46]

It does not appear as though treatment with HPV-targeted antiviral medications (specifically, cidofovir) produced morphologic changes in persistent papillomatous lesions of the airway.[47]

The incidence of previous HPV integration was assessed by Clavel and colleagues[25] using the hybrid capture method in a series of bronchopulmonary carcinomas. They found evidence of oncogenic HPV integration in only 2.7% of those tumors. On the other hand, Yousem and colleagues[48] demonstrated similar positivity by in situ hybridization in 30% of squamous carcinomas and 17% of large cell undifferentiated carcinomas of the lung; Syrjanen[28] likewise observed histologic viral changes in adjacent metaplastic bronchial mucosa in 26 of 104 squamous carcinomas (25%). Based on these data, it must be acknowledged that HPV may play a greater role in the etiology of lung carcinomas (particularly of the squamous type) than previously thought.

Bronchial Mucous Gland Adenoma

The term "bronchial adenoma" has been plagued by many misconceptions and misapplications since its introduction by Liebow in 1952.[49] However, two benign neoplastic entities could still properly be called "bronchial adenomas"—mucous gland adenoma (MGA) and mixed tumor (MT; pleomorphic adenoma; discussed later).

Mucous gland adenoma is an extraordinarily rare lesion. England and Hochholzer[50] noted that one series of more than 3000 pulmonary tumors included no examples of MGA,[51] and only 1 MGA was represented in another report of 130 benign neoplasms of the lung seen at a large referral center.[52] In the vast experience of the U.S. Armed Forces Institute of Pathology, only 10 examples of MGA were found. Men and women were equally affected, and the patients ranged in age from 25 to 67 years.[50,53] There is no particular predilection for anatomic location; MGAs may arise in any of the major lobar or segmental bronchi. Radiographs either show changes of postobstructive pneumonia or hyperinflation or demonstrate a discrete nodule or coin lesion that is centered on a bronchus[54-66] (Fig. 19-10). Kwon and coworkers[67] have noted that MGA may produce the "air meniscus sign" on computed tomogram (CT) of the airways.

Mucous gland adenomas measure between 0.5 and 1 cm in maximal dimension. They often demonstrate encapsulation, with mucoid cut surfaces; internal fibrous septations may yield a loculated appearance as well. Occasional lesions may completely occlude the bronchial lumen (Fig. 19-11).

As succinctly stated by England and Hochholzer,[50] "cystic change [is] the cardinal feature of MGA of the bronchus." Microcystic arrays of cuboidal or columnar tumor cells may permeate the bronchial wall to the level of the cartilaginous plates; however, growth beyond that point is absent. Cystic contents are either overtly mucinous or more serous. Secondary formation of cholesterol clefts and dystrophic calcifications may also be seen, and squamous metaplasia in the most luminal aspect of the lesion may occur. Nuclei are generally bland, with small nucleoli, and cytoplasm may be amphophilic, oxyphilic, clear, or foamy. Mitotic figures are scarce.

The internal substructure of MGA has been divided into two morphologic patterns: glandular-tubulocystic (Fig. 19-12) and papillocystic (Fig. 19-13). Within each of these categories, there may be a spectrum of appearances, ranging from a monotonous tubular pattern (Fig. 19-14) to a complex arborizing aggregation of papillary structures.[50] Stromal sclerosis may be present.

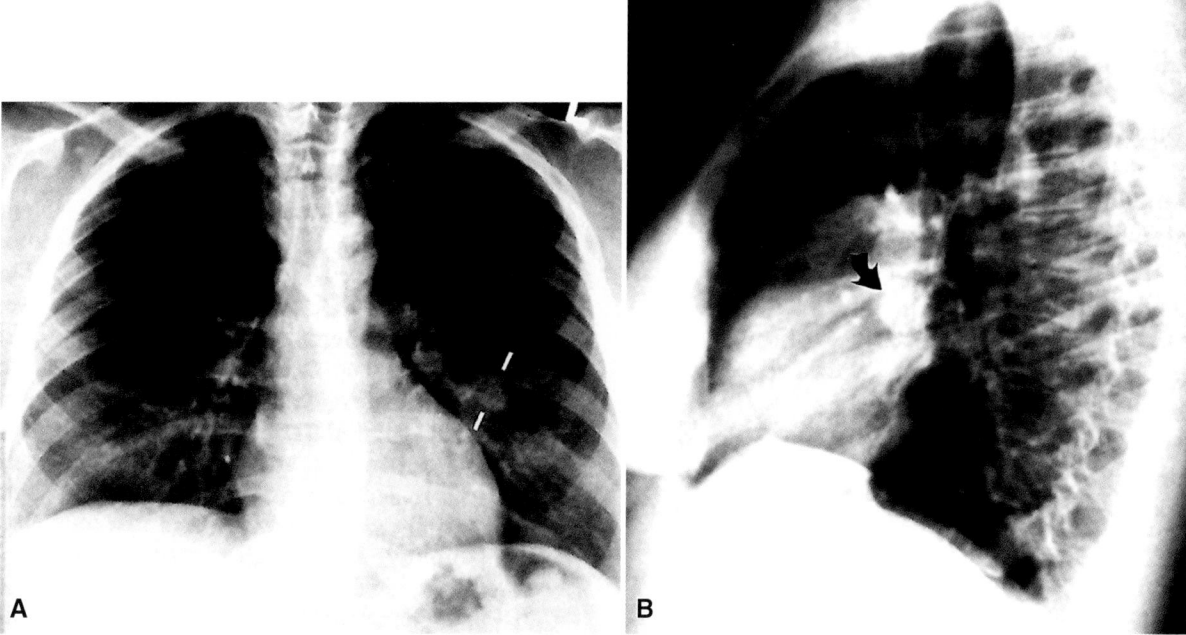

Figure 19-10. Posteroanterior (**A**) and lateral (**B**) chest radiographs showing a nodular lesion that is centered on a bronchus (*arrow*) that proved to be a mucous gland adenoma. (Reproduced with permission from England DM, Hochholzer L. Truly benign 'bronchial adenoma': report of 10 cases of mucous gland adenoma with immunohistochemical and ultrastructural findings. *Am J Surg Pathol*. 1995;19:887–899 and by courtesy of Dr. Douglas England, Madison, WI.)

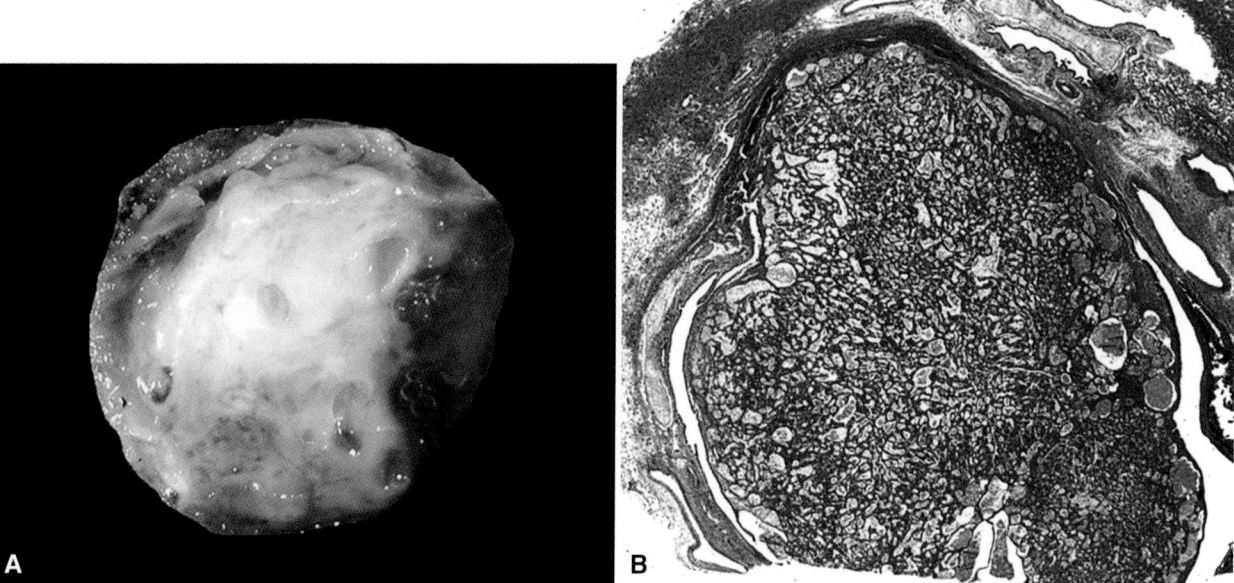

Figure 19-11. Gross (**A**) and scanning microscopic view (**B**) of a mucous gland adenoma of the bronchus demonstrating an epithelial lesion that fills the bronchial lumen and shows internal gland formation. (**B,** Courtesy of Dr. Douglas England, Madison, WI.)

Immunohistologic features of MGA are comparable to those of non-neoplastic bronchial glands. The constituent cells are consistently labeled for cytokeratin, epithelial membrane antigen, and blood group isoantigens, with less uniform reactivity for carcinoembryonic antigen. Stromal cells show myoepithelial features, with concurrent staining for keratin, actin, and S-100 protein.[50] Squamous-type ("high molecular-weight") keratins may be expressed in MGAs.[68] This could be a diagnostic trap vis-à-vis the alternative interpretation of mucoepidermoid carcinoma (discussed later).

The differential diagnosis includes predominantly cystic mucoepidermoid carcinoma, MT, "sclerosing hemangioma" (pneumocytoma),

and primary or metastatic mucinous ("colloid") adenocarcinoma. Of these possibilities, the first two are the most problematic, necessitating adequate biopsies for visualization of the tumor architecture. Cytologically, MGA shows bland nests and sheets of monotonous epithelioid cells[69] (Fig. 19-15). Diagnostic separation from mucoepidermoid carcinoma or MT usually is not possible using fine-needle aspiration (FNA) biopsy or bronchial brushing specimens.

An admixture of squamous elements throughout the mass, infiltrative growth through the bronchial wall, or both would tend to argue for a diagnosis of mucoepidermoid carcinoma. Although MGA does not manifest chondromyxoid stroma or immunoreactivity for

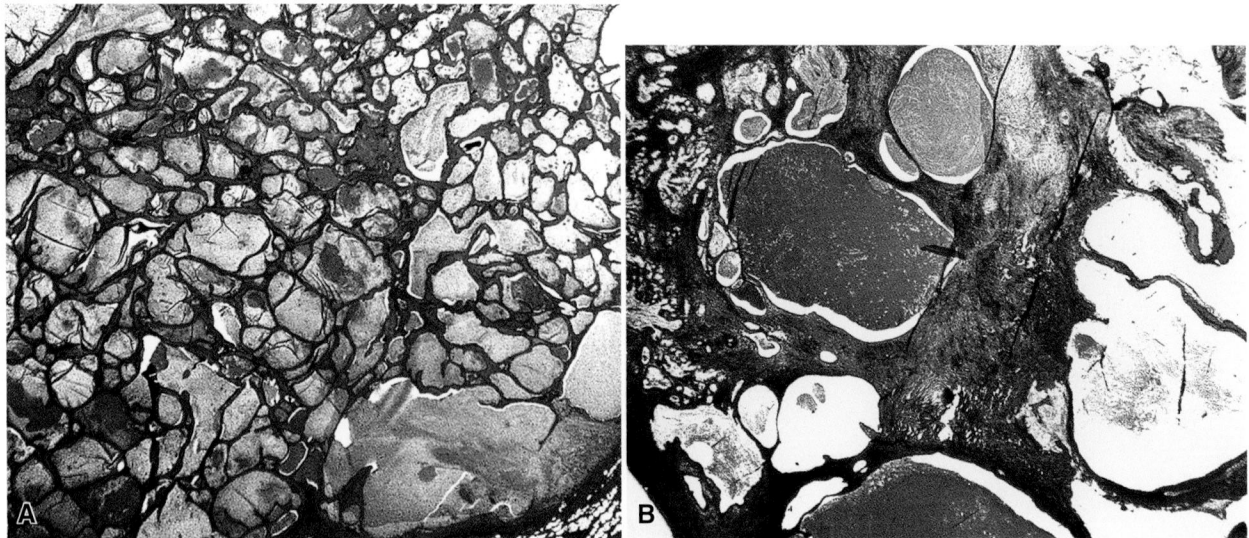

Figure 19-12. A and **B,** A glandular-tubulocystic growth pattern is present in this mucous gland adenoma of the bronchus. (Courtesy of Dr. Douglas England, Madison, WI.)

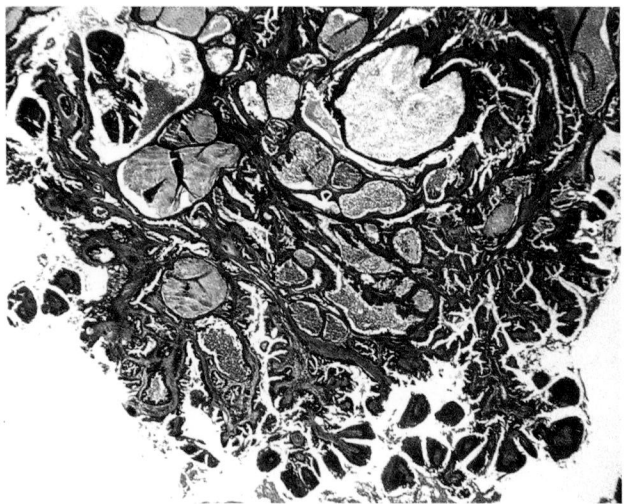

Figure 19-13. This mucous gland bronchial adenoma shows a papillocystic configuration. (Courtesy of Dr. Douglas England, Madison, WI.)

glial fibrillary acidic protein, as seen in some MTs,[70] the possibility that MGA is related nosologically to monomorphic adenoma—a variant of MT—cannot be dismissed. In any event, it represents a distinctive clinicopathologic entity that is believed to deserve its own diagnostic designation.

Treatment of MGA can be conservative, with sleeve resection of the bronchus and reconstruction when clinically feasible.[50,57]

Salivary Gland Analog Tumors

Mixed Tumor (Pleomorphic Adenoma)

Pleomorphic adenoma—or MT—occurs predominantly in adults, with a slight preference for women.[71-75] The age range is 8 to 75 years.[76] The lesion may present as either a central or a peripheral mass[77-79] (Fig. 19-16).

Grossly, central main stem bronchial lesions are commonly polypoid, whereas those in the periphery present as well-circumscribed tumors usually attached to bronchi (Fig. 19-17). The size of the neoplasms varies from 1 to 16 cm in greatest diameter. The cut surfaces of

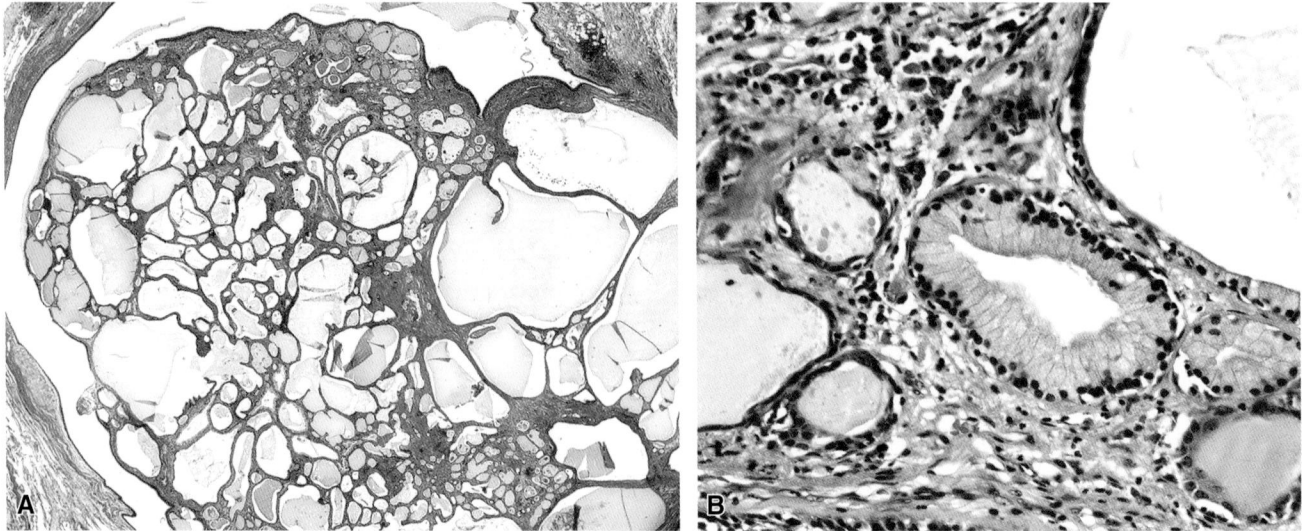

Figure 19-14. A and **B,** Lesional tubules are composed of bland mucinous epithelium in this glandular-tubulocystic mucous gland bronchial adenoma.

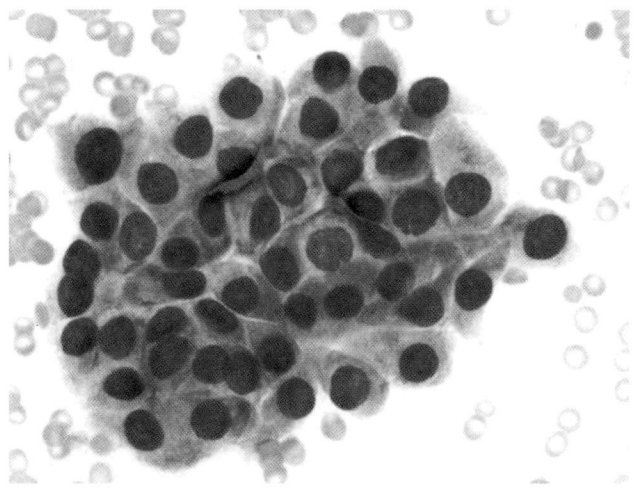

Figure 19-15. Fine-needle aspiration biopsy of mucous gland adenoma showing composition by monomorphic, cohesive polygonal cells with bland nuclear features.

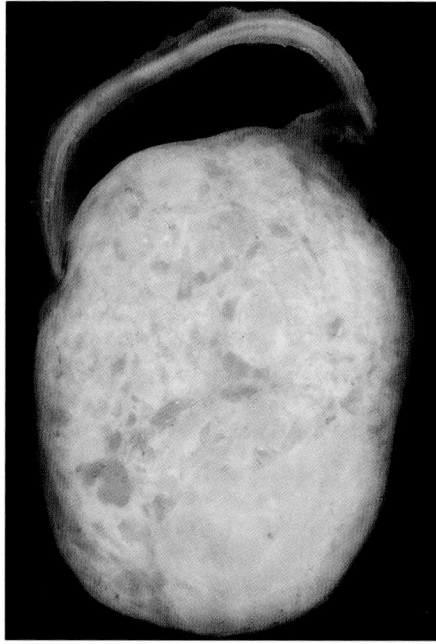

Figure 19-17. Gross photograph of a bronchial mixed tumor showing that the mass is partially intramural with respect to the wall of the airway. The lesion is internally solid, mottled, and white-tan.

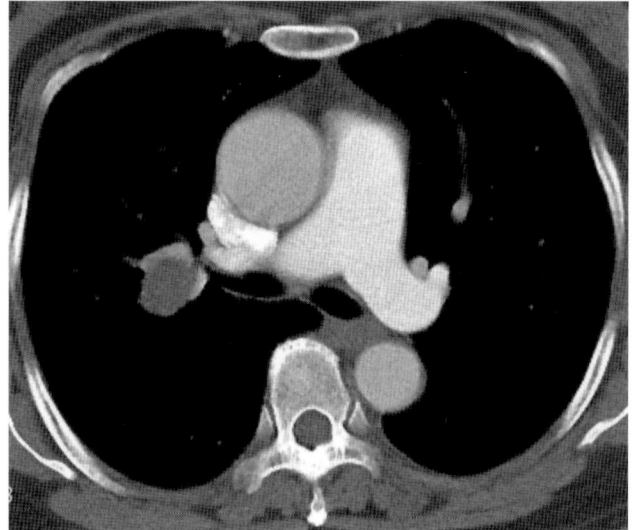

Figure 19-16. This computed tomogram of the chest shows a mass attached to the right bronchus intermedius, representing a mixed tumor.

MTs may be chondroid and firm, or may have a soft consistency, with only focal induration.

By definition, pleomorphic adenomas show at least a biphasic microscopic image; they are characteristically composed of epithelial tubules and nests that are embedded in a chondromyxoid stroma (Figs. 19-18 and 19-19). Interestingly, intrapulmonary MTs rarely show the amount of mature cartilaginous stroma present in MTs of the salivary glands. In some lesions, the predominant growth pattern may be solid myoepithelial proliferation that approximates that of "cellular" MTs in the head and neck. Those neoplasms comprise compact epithelioid cells with round or oval nuclei, which generally lack nuclear atypia, necrosis, hemorrhage, and mitotic activity (Fig. 19-20). Notably, there have been no well-documented cases of carcinoma arising from preexisting MTs of the lung, as may rarely occur in salivary glandular sites. Other variants of MT include a "myoepitheliomatous" subtype that may manifest either a spindle cell composition[80] (Fig. 19-21) or a plasmacytoid constituency; a form with extensive squamous metaplasia (Fig. 19-22); a subtype in which sizable zones of the lesion demonstrate an adenoid cystic carcinoma-like cribriform architecture; and a chondroid-rich form that simulates pulmonary chondroma or chondromatous hamartoma.

The differential diagnosis depends on whether one is dealing with a biopsy specimen or a complete resection of the tumor. In the former instance, MTs can be confused with other salivary gland-like tumors, such as adenoid cystic carcinoma, as well as with hamartoma/chondroma, squamous cell carcinoma (when squamous metaplasia is dominant), and biphasic malignancies, such as sarcomatoid carcinoma. In resection specimens, the diagnosis is typically straightforward. However, if MTs demonstrate an overwhelmingly prominent solid pattern with spindle cell ("myoepitheliomatous") differentiation, sarcomas may also be considered. In this setting, concurrent immunoreactivity for keratin, vimentin, S-100 protein, actin or caldesmon, p63 protein, and glial fibrillary acidic protein[81,82] provides the necessary evidence for a conclusive diagnosis of MT.

Mixed tumors of the lung behave in an indolent fashion. There are only anecdotal reports of metastasizing lesions of this type,[83] in analogy to rare examples in the salivary glands. No particular pathologic features of such neoplasms can be used to predict this unusual adverse behavior. Complete but conservative excision is the treatment of choice.[77,78]

Oncocytoma

There are only a few reported cases of pulmonary oncocytoma.[84–93] These tumors exhibit morphologic similarities to comparable tumors in the salivary glands, showing a brownish gross appearance (Fig. 19-23). They are composed of nests of uniformly large polygonal cells with prominently eosinophilic granular cytoplasm and bland nuclei (Figs. 19-24 and 19-25). In view of the existence of other, more common pulmonary tumors that can show oncocytic changes, it is important to properly exclude those other possibilities by adjunctive studies. Neuroendocrine tumors showing oncocytic features (oncocytic "carcinoids;" grade I neuroendocrine carcinomas) are far more common than oncocytomas and are recognizable by their immunoreactivity for chromogranin-A, synaptophysin, and CD56.[94,95] Metastatic tumors from the salivary glands and kidneys also must be considered, particularly in rare cases where pulmonary oncocytomas appear to be synchronously

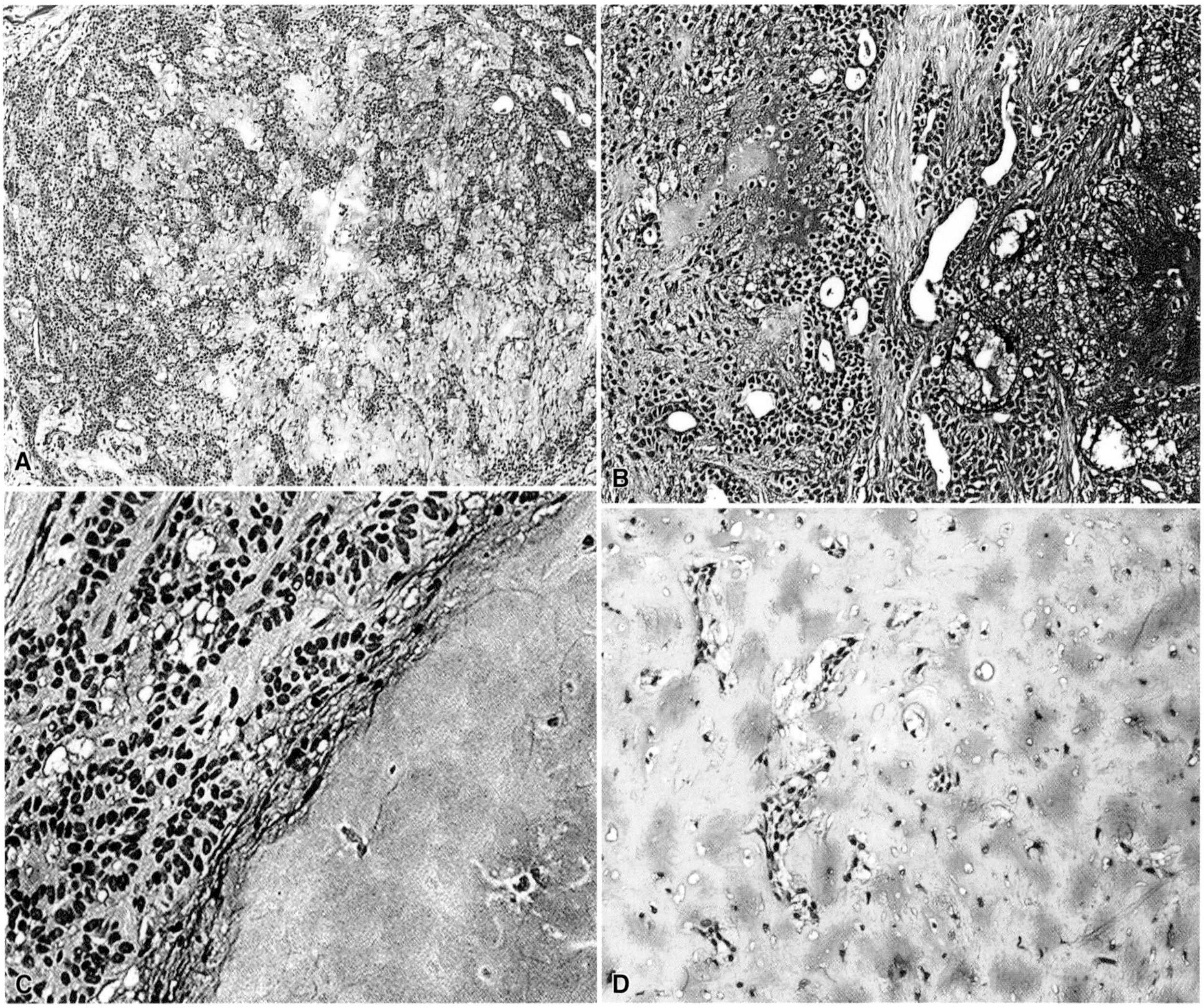

Figure 19-18. **A** to **C,** Bronchial mixed tumors comprise a variable mixture of solid epithelial, tubular, and chondroid matrical elements. **D,** This mixed tumor is almost completely composed of chondroid stroma, simulating a chondroma.

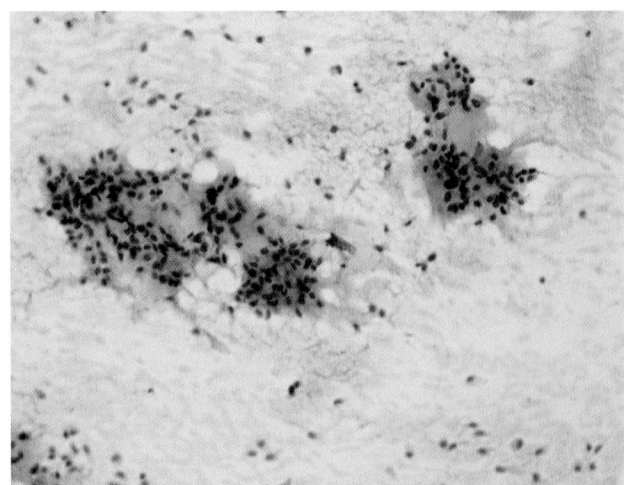

Figure 19-19. Fine-needle aspiration of a mixed tumor showing classic fibrillary stromal material admixed with bland-appearing basaloid epithelial cells. (Courtesy of Dr. Matthew A. Zarka, Mayo Clinic, Scottsdale, AZ.)

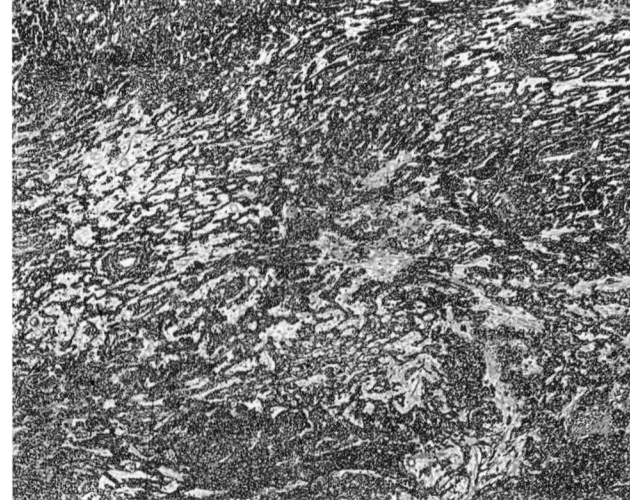

Figure 19-20. This photomicrograph depicts a "cellular" (epithelial-predominant) mixed tumor, bearing a resemblance to basaloid adenoma of salivary glands.

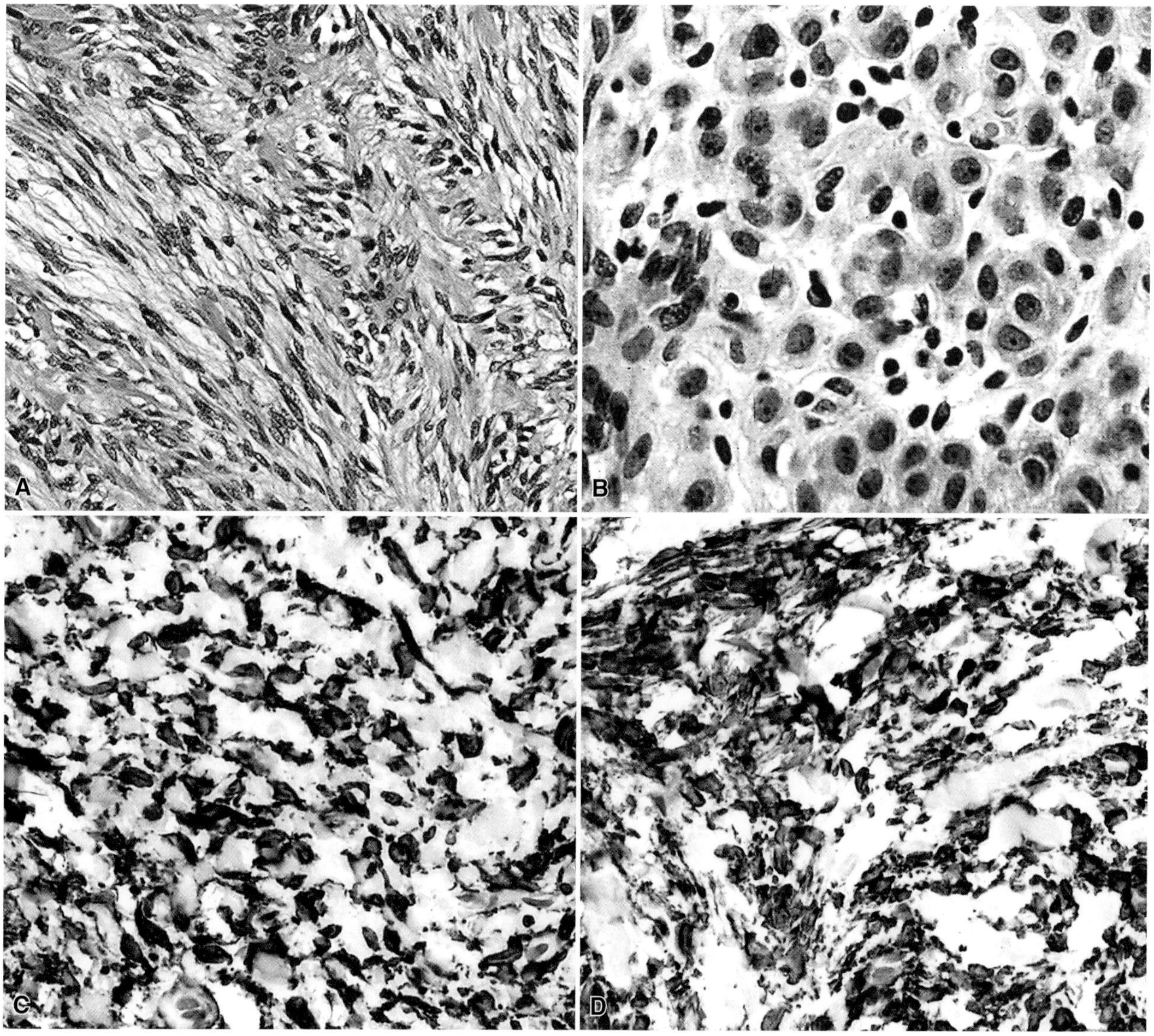

Figure 19-21. Myoepitheliomatous variants of mixed tumor showing spindle cell (**A**) and plasmacytoid cell (**B**) compositions. These lesions are immunoreactive for both keratin (**C**) and muscle-specific actin (**D**).

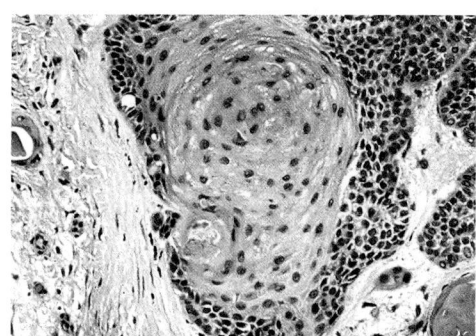

Figure 19-22. Prominent squamous metaplasia is apparent in the epithelial element of this bronchial mixed tumor.

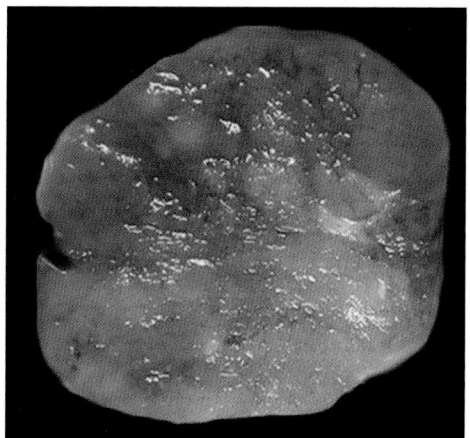

Figure 19-23. Bronchial oncocytoma has a relatively uniform, fleshy, brown cut surface.

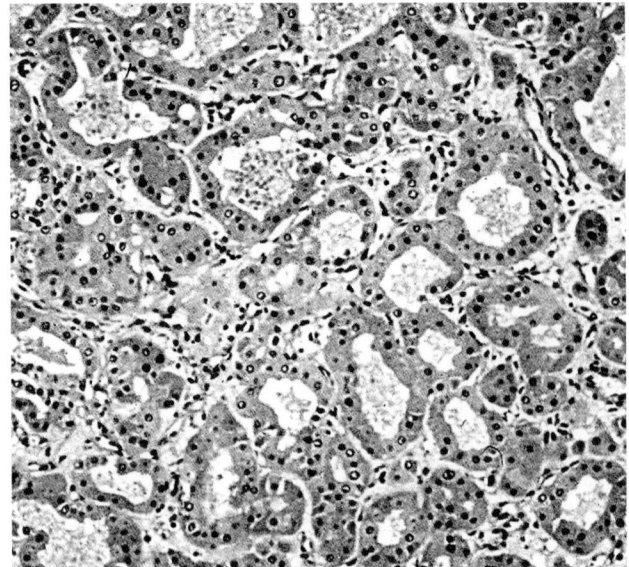

Figure 19-24. Either solid or tubular profiles of oxyphilic polygonal cells can be seen in oncocytoma.

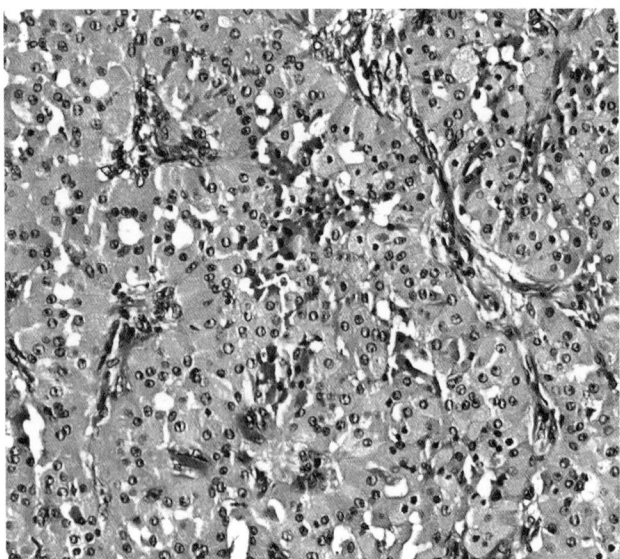

Figure 19-25. Tumor cells in oncocytoma have oval nuclei with dispersed chromatin, distinct chromocenters, and abundant granular eosinophilic cytoplasm.

multifocal.[88] Clinical information is important in this context because the electron microscopic and immunophenotypic properties of primary and metastatic oncocytic neoplasms may be very similar (see Chapter 17).

In general, oncocytomas in the lung and other anatomic sites are epithelial, demonstrating immunoreactivity for keratins and epithelial membrane antigen; vimentin is inconsistently present, but markers of muscular, neural, or neuroendocrine lineages are absent.[88,96] Immunolabeling with antibodies to mitochondrial proteins is common,[97] corresponding to the ultrastructural hallmark of these neoplasms.

Fine-needle aspiration biopsy of oncocytic neoplasms yields a monomorphic population of large epithelioid cells with round to oval nuclei, dispersed chromatin, small nucleoli, and amphophilic to acidophilic cytoplasm. They are variably cohesive and typically show little nuclear pleomorphism.[88]

Because of problems with the previous definition of "pulmonary oncocytoma," as noted earlier, meaningful comments on its behavior are difficult. However, we have seen cases that obviously invaded the lung parenchyma and had atypical morphologic features, such as nuclear pleomorphism and atypical mitoses (Fig. 19-26). Accordingly, such lesions are defensibly labeled as "malignant" oncocytomas.[85]

Peripheral Nerve Sheath Tumors

Primary neoplasms of the lung that demonstrate schwannian or perineurial differentiation are more often located in the walls of the major bronchi than in the peripheral lung.[98–113] Chest radiographs show nodular or irregular masses associated with bronchi; secondary atelectasis is sometimes noted as well[98] (Fig. 19-27). Some patients with primary neurogenic pulmonary tumors have neurofibromatosis type 1 (NF1; von Recklinghausen's disease), and that is true for both neurofibroma and neurilemmoma.[114] Neurogenic sarcomas also arise in the lungs,[115–117] but it is unclear how many have occurred in the context of NF1 in association with preexisting pulmonary neurofibromas.

Grossly, peripheral nerve sheath tumors (PNSTs) of the bronchus are well-demarcated yellow-white masses centered on the bronchial wall and often protruding into the bronchial lumen (Figs. 19-28 and 19-29). Gross foci of hemorrhage, necrosis, or cystification are absent in benign lesions of this type.

The histologic images associated with benign PNSTs are varied. Prototypical neurofibromas are "plexiform" in NF1, putatively reflecting a neoplastic attempt to recapitulate a neural plexus. Constituent cells are serpiginous, with attenuated fusiform nuclei and delicately fibrillar cytoplasm (Fig. 19-30). The supporting matrix is myxedematous or collagenized, and it may contain scattered foam cells, mast cells, and lymphocytes. Mitotic activity is typically absent. Neurilemmomas—also termed "schwannomas"—are biphasic in their classic form, with compactly cellular ("Antoni A") areas alternating with zones of loose cellularity and myxoid change ("Antoni B" foci) (Figs. 19-31 and 19-32). Nuclei may be aligned in register in Antoni A areas, representing "Verocay bodies" (Fig. 19-33). Intralesional blood vessels have thick walls in many neurilemmomas, and a well-defined peripheral tumor capsule may be identified in some instances. Variants of neurilemmoma include "cellular" schwannoma, which manifests intersecting bundles of densely apposed, focally mitotic spindle cells in the context of an

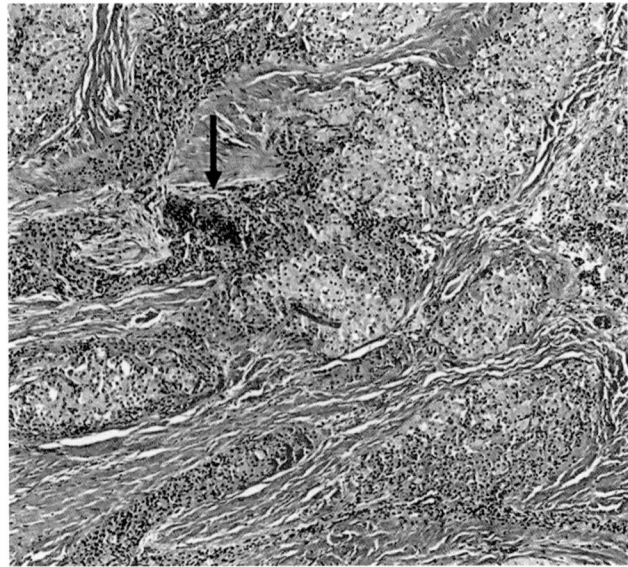

Figure 19-26. A rare example of bronchial oncocytoma shows infiltrative growth and focal necrosis (*arrow*), justifying an interpretation of malignancy.

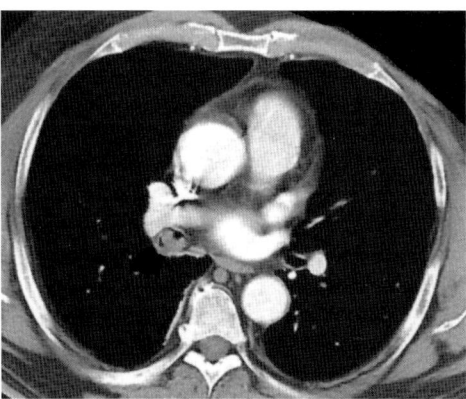

Figure 19-27. A computed tomographic image of a bronchial neurilemmoma showing a mass in the lumen of the right mainstem bronchus.

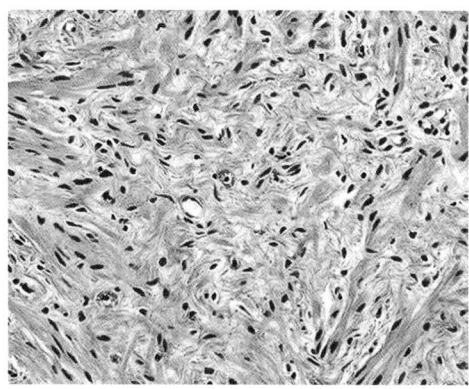

Figure 19-30. The tumor cells in neurofibroma show serpiginous nuclear profiles and eosinophilic cytoplasm. They are bland, with no nuclear atypia or mitotic activity.

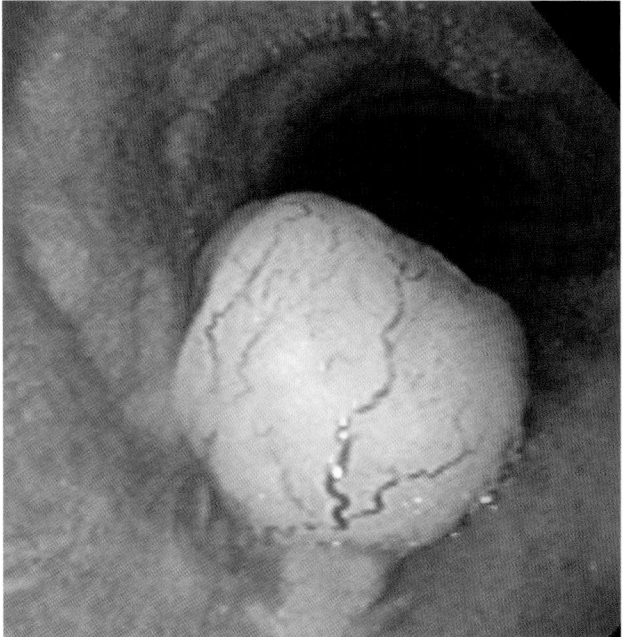

Figure 19-28. This bronchoscopic image of a bronchial neurilemmoma shows a rounded polypoid lesion that is covered by intact mucosa.

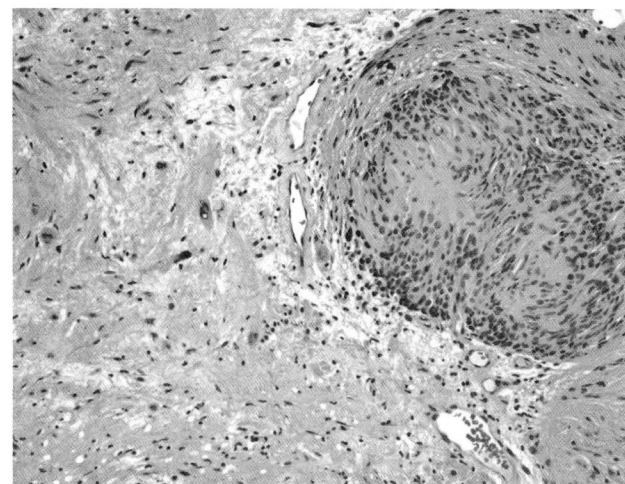

Figure 19-31. "Antoni A" areas of growth are shown in a bronchial neurilemmoma, represented by compact cellular apposition and intralesional vascular sclerosis.

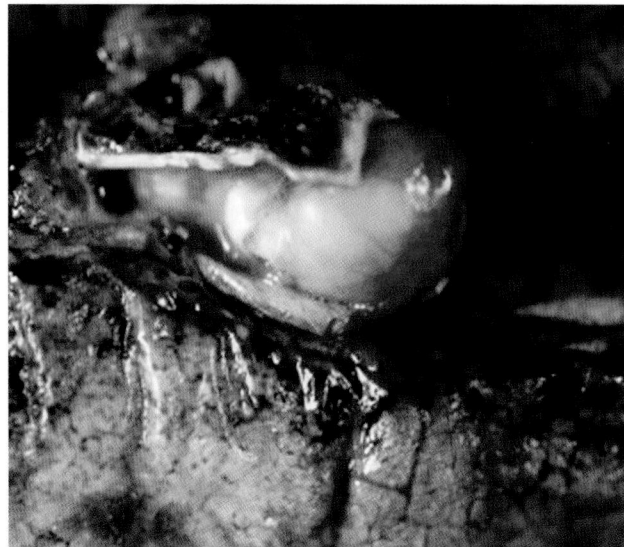

Figure 19-29. The resected lung in a case of bronchial neurilemmoma demonstrates occlusion of the bronchial lumen by a uniform, yellow, solid tumor.

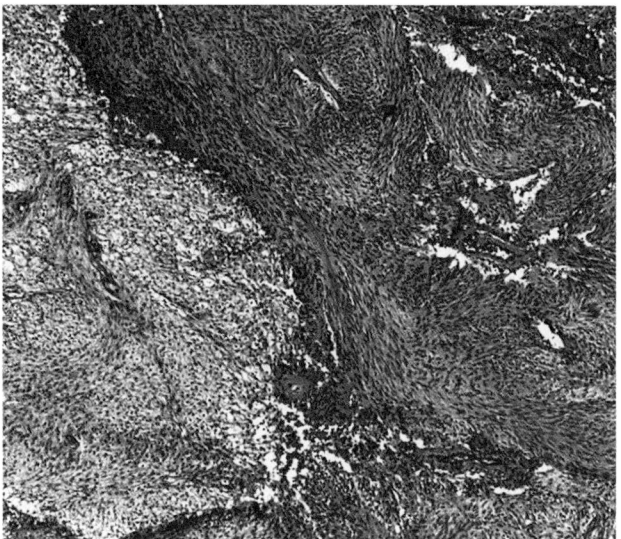

Figure 19-32. An Antoni B focus in a bronchial neurilemmoma (*lower left*) with a myxoid intercellular matrix.

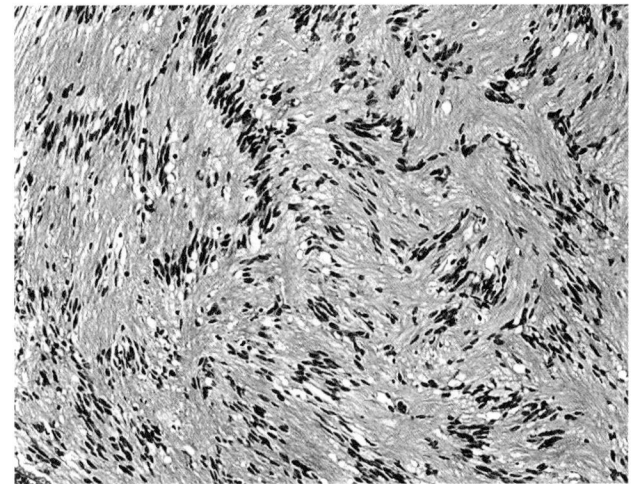

Figure 19-33. "Verocay bodies" are zones in Antoni A areas of neurilemmoma in which nuclei form linear "stacks" that are aligned in register.

Figure 19-34. Cellular schwannoma (neurilemmoma) demonstrating densely agglomerated spindle cells with focal mitotic activity.

encapsulated mass[111] (Fig. 19-34); "glandular" schwannoma; "ancient" schwannoma, showing scattered pleomorphic hyperchromatic nuclei in degenerative cells (Fig. 19-35); plexiform schwannoma, in which broad plexiform fascicles of tumor cells show the substructure of neurilemmoma; and melanotic psammomatous schwannoma, exhibiting microcalcifications and melanin pigmentation[118] (Fig. 19-36). The last of these subtypes may be associated with myxomas of the skin, heart, and breast; the presence of cutaneous ephelides; and overactivity of the endocrine glands.

The immunophenotype of PNSTs features reactivity for vimentin and variable labeling for S-100 protein (Fig. 19-37), CD56, CD57, glial fibrillary acidic protein, and epithelial membrane antigen. The last of these markers is believed to represent perineurial differentiation in this context. Keratin positivity is absent, except in the glands of glandular schwannoma, and myogenous markers should be negative.

As is true of all spindle cell lesions of the lung, it is necessary to exclude sarcomatoid carcinoma before making a final diagnosis of PNST; immunohistologic evaluation is the most expeditious means of doing so. In addition, other mesenchymal lesions of the lung—especially

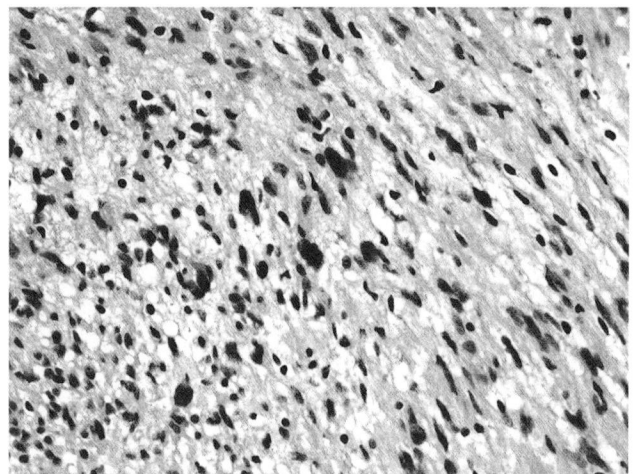

Figure 19-35. "Ancient" neurilemmoma showing degenerative atypia of tumor cell nuclei with mild pleomorphism and hyperchromasia.

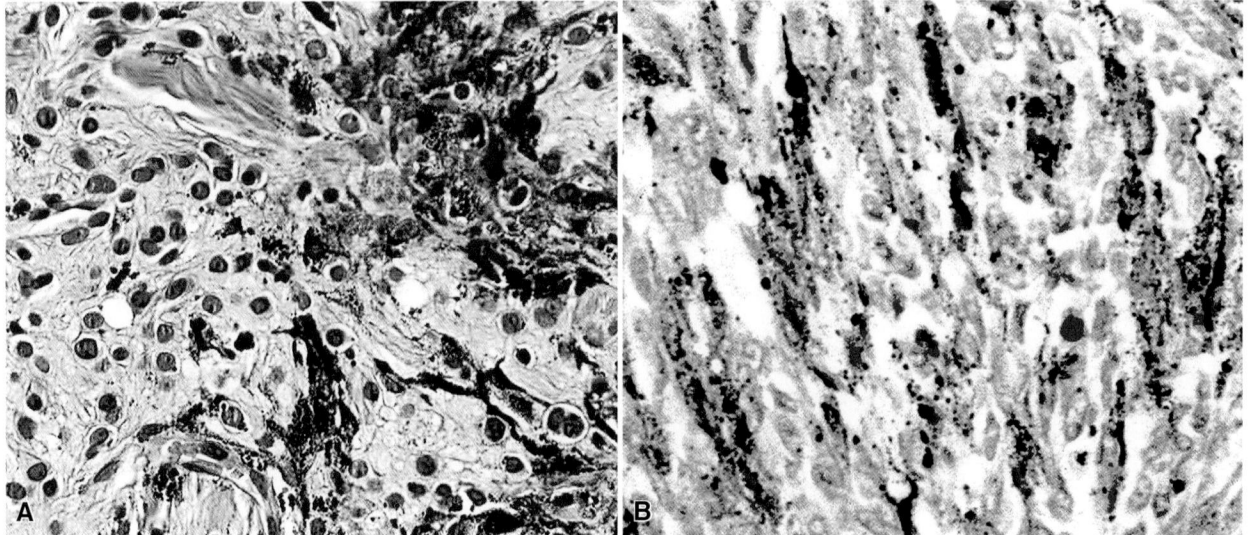

Figure 19-36. A, Melanotic psammomatous schwannoma (neurilemmoma) exhibiting internal microcalcifications and cytoplasmic pigment. **B,** Positivity with a Fontana-Masson stain confirms the identity of the intralesional pigment as melanin.

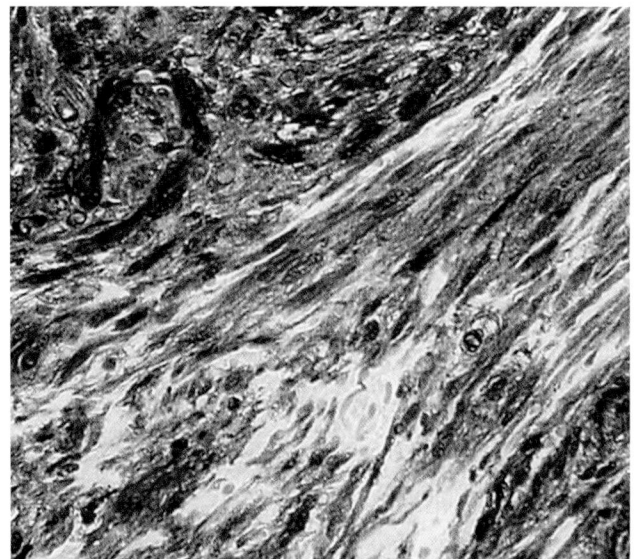

Figure 19-37. Intense immunoreactivity for S-100 protein is seen in this bronchial neurilemmoma.

leiomyoma and leiomyomatous hamartoma—must be considered as alternatives to an interpretation of neurofibroma or neurilemmoma. The immunoprofiles of those lesions are dissimilar as well.

If the identification of PNST can be established in evaluations of bronchial biopsy specimens and radiographic findings support a benign diagnosis, the surgeon can undertake a conservative approach to the removal of such lesions.[102,105] However, small samples of neurogenic neoplasms are notoriously unreliable in predicting the biologic potential of PNSTs, and they should not be used in isolation to govern decisions on therapy.

Granular Cell Tumors

Granular cell tumor (GCT; also known as "Abrikossoff's tumor"[119]) may be seen in many anatomic locations.[120] Fewer than 200 have been reported in the trachea and lungs.[121-139] Patients of any age may have

such lesions, and multiple tumors in the same individual have been reported.[132,135,138,140,141]

Endoscopic examination often reveals a sessile polypoid endoluminal component, with intact overlying mucosa[131] (Fig. 19-38). Radiographic studies confirm that characteristic, but also demonstrate an infiltrative aspect to many GCTs that may lead to a mistaken preoperative diagnosis of malignancy.[130-136] GCTs in the peripheral lung parenchyma are unusual,[138] but these likewise may assume a spiculated appearance that closely simulates that of adenocarcinoma. This situation is further complicated by occasional case reports of GCTs that coexisted with malignant neoplasms.[142,143]

Grossly, GCT is a white-tan, ill-defined mass with a gritty cut surface, again simulating the features of an infiltrating carcinoma. However, necrosis and hemorrhage are distinctly unusual. Maximum tumor size approximates 5 cm.

Microscopically, these tumors comprise a uniform population of polygonal or fusiform cells that contain small ovoid hyperchromatic nuclei with indistinct nucleoli (Fig. 19-39). The cytoplasm is abundant, eosinophilic or amphophilic, and coarsely granulated, often with the additional presence of rounded inclusions that superficially resemble Michaelis-Gutman bodies (Fig. 19-40). Like Michaelis-Gutman bodies, these may also have a targetoid configuration. Mitotic figures are typically scarce and physiologic; necrosis and vascular invasion are absent. The advancing border of granular cell tumors may be "pushing" or irregular and permeative. A proportion of these lesions infiltrate deeply into the bronchial wall or even through it into the adjacent parenchyma. In nonpulmonary sites, such a growth pattern has been linked to a greater risk of recurrence,[144] but that correlation does not seem to apply to GCTs in the airways or lungs. The existence of primary malignant GCT of the respiratory tract has never been convincingly documented, and recurrent neoplasms are typically those that have never been completely excised.

Fine-needle aspiration biopsy of GCT yields a monotonous population of large epithelioid cells that are variably cohesive. They contain ovoid nuclei, distinct chromocenters, and abundant granular cytoplasm that is best seen in Romanowsky-stained slides (Fig. 19-41). A plasmacytoid appearance is common.[145]

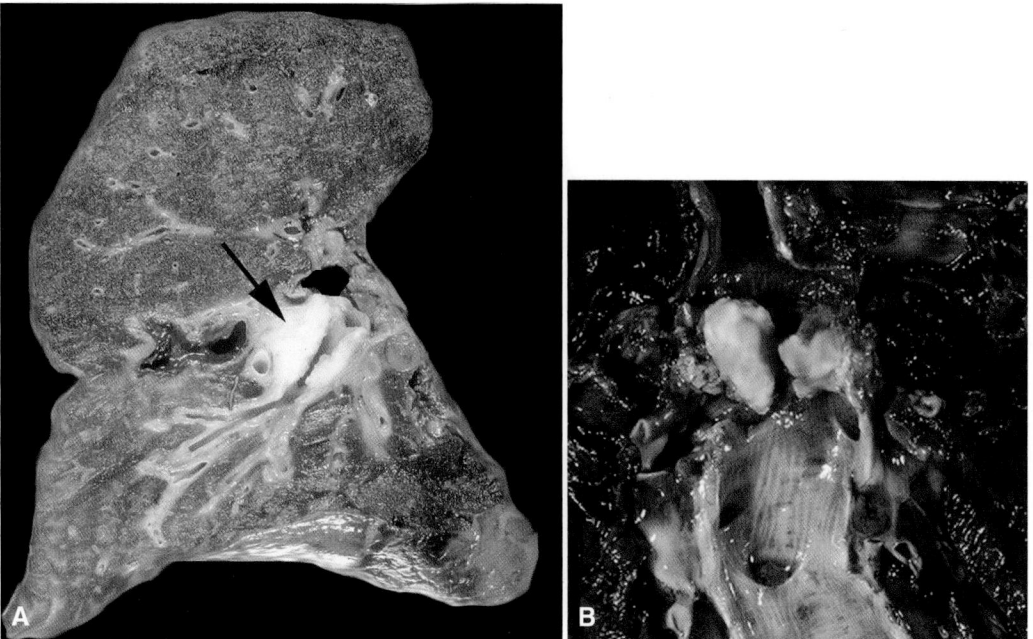

Figure 19-38. **A** and **B,** The homogeneous white-gray cut surface of an endobronchial granular cell tumor (*arrow*) is seen in these gross photographs.

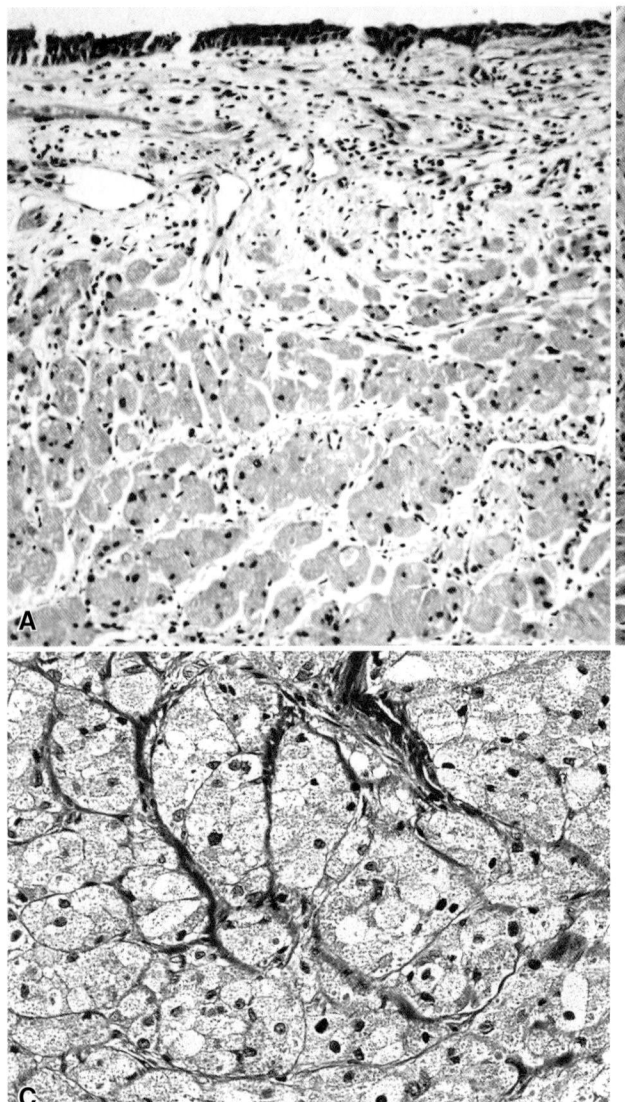

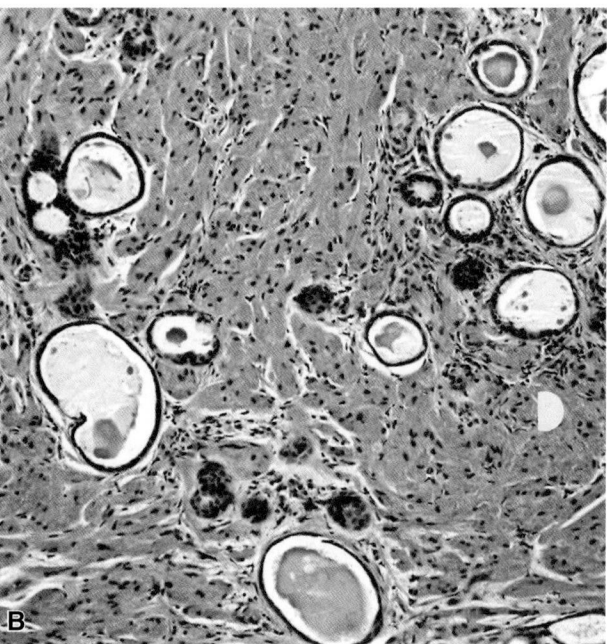

Figure 19-39. **A** to **C,** Sheets of polygonal eosinophilic cells with bland nuclei and prominently granular cytoplasm are seen in this pulmonary granular cell tumor.

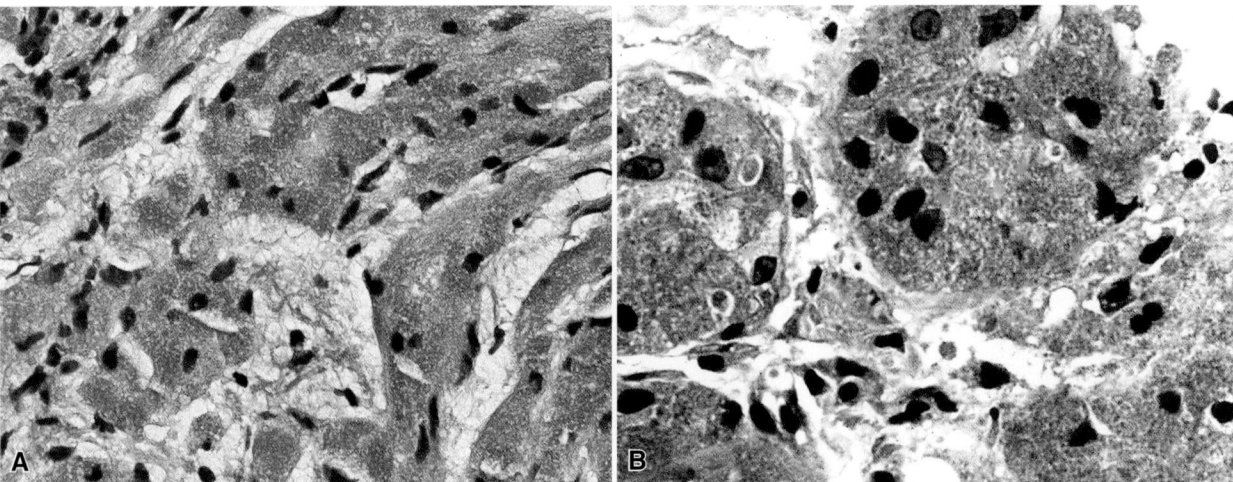

Figure 19-40. **A** and **B,** Eosinophilic cytoplasmic granularity, with focal formation of "targetoid" bodies, is typical of granular cell tumors. Nuclei are oval with distinct chromocenters.

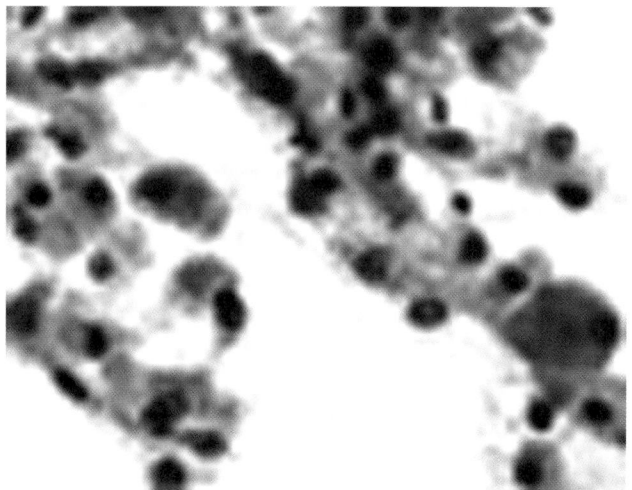

Figure 19-41. A fine-needle aspiration biopsy specimen of a bronchial granular cell tumor recapitulates and amplifies the cytologic features seen in tissue sections.

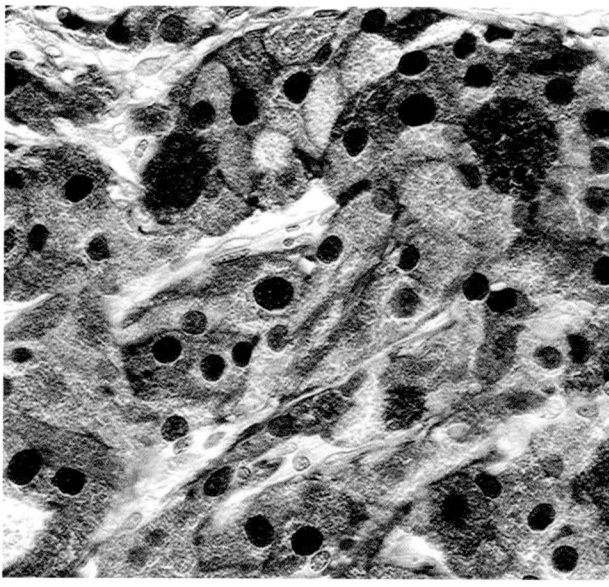

Figure 19-43. Nuclear and cytoplasmic immunoreactivity for S-100 protein in a bronchial granular cell tumor. This marker is present in approximately 80% of such lesions.

Electron microscopy of GCTs shows a distinctive multiplicity of secondary and tertiary lysosomes in the cytoplasm of the tumor cells, virtually to the exclusion of other organelles[146,147] (Fig. 19-42). Immunohistologic evaluation most often reveals evidence of schwannian differentiation, with reactivity for S-100 protein, CD56, CD57, myelin basic protein, and combinations thereof, in 80% to 85% of cases[147-150] (Fig. 19-43). The abundance of lysosomes is reflected by their CD68 reactivity. Recently, the presence of calretinin and alpha-inhibin has also been reported in GCT.[151]

An important caveat regarding the immunophenotype of this tumor type is that non-schwannian lesions containing granular cells are a heterogenous group.[152] Carcinomas (both neuroendocrine and nonendocrine),[153,154] smooth muscle tumors, endothelial proliferations, and neoplasms of uncommitted lineage have all been described with a granular cell phenotype. Therefore, it is important to include immunohistologic evaluations to address these possibilities in differential diagnosis, with or without ultrastructural studies. Oncocytoid granular cell grade 1 neuroendocrine carcinoma ("carcinoid") of the lung is the most common simulator of GCT,[155,156] making chromogranin-A and synaptophysin important markers in this context.

As discussed earlier, aggressive behavior by bronchopulmonary GCT has not been observed. Therefore, conservative therapy for this neoplasm is warranted.

Benign Lesions Affecting Either the Airways or the Lung Parenchyma

Alveolar Adenoma

Alveolar adenoma (AA)[157] is typically a solitary peripheral parenchymal nodule found incidentally in asymptomatic adult patients, with no sex predilection.[158] On imaging studies, AA presents a rounded configuration and measures 1 to 6 cm in greatest dimension (Fig. 19-44).[159]

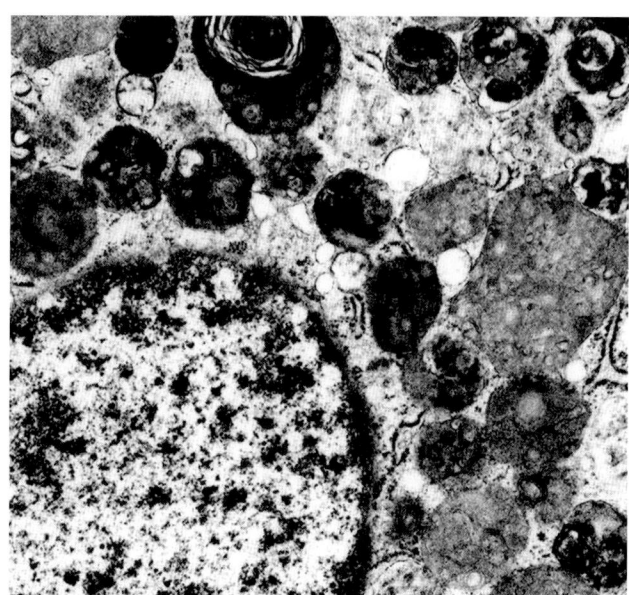

Figure 19-42. This electron photomicrograph of a granular cell tumor demonstrates innumerable secondary and tertiary cytoplasmic lysosomes.

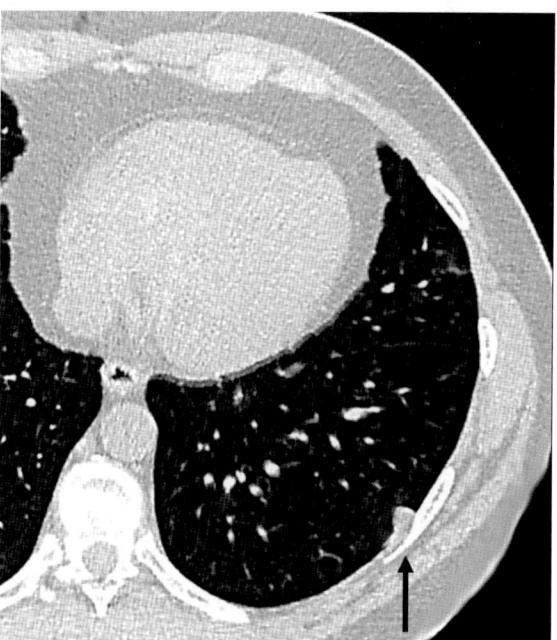

Figure 19-44. This computed tomogram of the chest shows a 5- to 6-mm "coin" lesion beneath the pleura in the left posterior lung field (*arrow*), representing an alveolar adenoma.

The surgeon is likely to report that it "shells out" from the surrounding lung tissue.[160]

Grossly, AA is circumscribed, with a spongy gray-white multilocular cut surface. Microscopically, it comprises many cystic spaces of variable sizes, which are mantled by low-cuboidal epithelial cells (Fig. 19-45).[157,158] Eosinophilic granular material is commonly present in the cyst lumina. The tissue between the cysts is represented by cytologically bland and closely apposed bluntly fusiform cells in a loose fibromyxoid matrix. Mitotic activity, nuclear pleomorphism, and necrosis are absent.[161] The immunohistochemical features of AA closely parallel those of sclerosing hemangioma ("pneumocytoma"; discussed later), and it is our belief—shared by other authors as well[162]—that the two tumors are likely part of a neoplastic family rather than entirely distinct entities. One sees epithelial markers—including thyroid transcription factor 1—in the cuboidal cells lining tumoral microcysts, but not in the stromal elements.[158,161–164] On the other hand, the latter components are reactive for vimentin, and often for CD34.[158]

The differential diagnosis of AA is limited. Aside from sclerosing hemangioma, which is usually larger than AA and does not have its prominently cystic substructure,[162] the principal considerations are pulmonary hemangioma-lymphangioma and atypical adenomatous hyperplasia (see Chapter 16). The vascular lesions can be identified by appropriate immunohistochemical stains.[165,166] Atypical adenomatous hyperplasia lacks microcysts and does not contain a mesenchymal stromal cell component.[167]

Even though fewer than 50 cases of AA have been reported, the behavior of this tumor has been uniformly favorable. Hence, conservative wedge excision appears to represent adequate treatment.[158,160,168,169]

Papillary Adenoma

Another uncommon neoplasm that is likely related to sclerosing hemangioma has been reported separately as "papillary adenoma" of the lung (PAL). It may be seen in children and adults alike, as a nondescript and asymptomatic parenchymal nodule in imaging studies.[170–180] Multifocality occurs, and in one case, such multiplicity was seen in a patient with neurofibromatosis.[176] Grossly, this tumor usually shows sharp circumscription from the surrounding lung tissue in most cases, with a solid tan-white cut surface (Fig. 19-46). Nonetheless, a few cases have had infiltrative characteristics.[172,181,182]

Histologically, PAL shows papillary profiles of cuboidal to low columnar, nonciliated, focally vacuolated epithelial cells that mantle well-formed fibrovascular cores (Fig. 19-47). The stroma in the latter structures may contain mixed inflammatory infiltrates, potentially

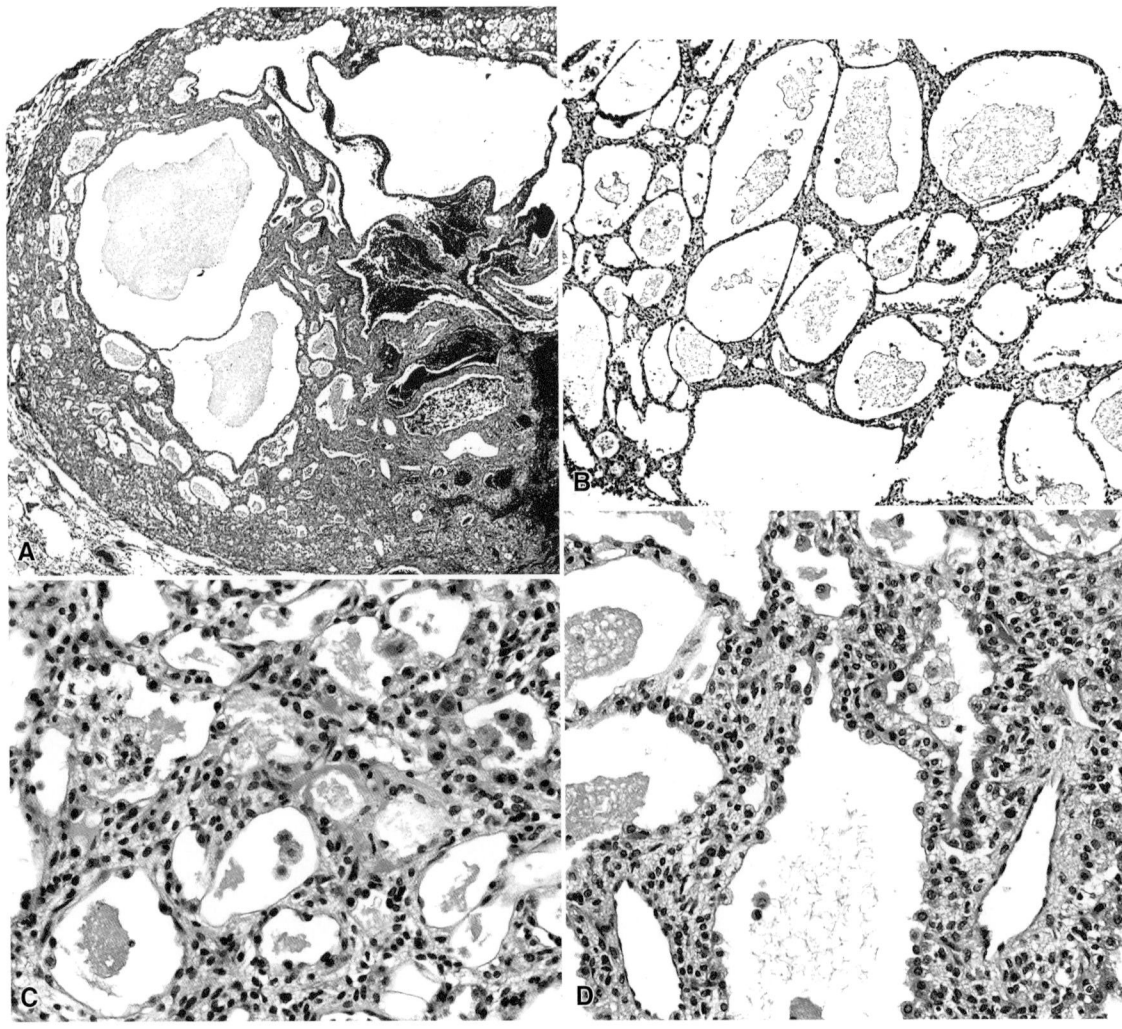

Figure 19-45. A to **D,** Alveolar adenoma of the lung demonstrates a sharply circumscribed low-power image and internal microcyst formation. Bland low cuboidal epithelium lines the cyst cavities, and bland, bluntly fusiform stromal cells are set in a fibromyxoid stroma between the microcysts.

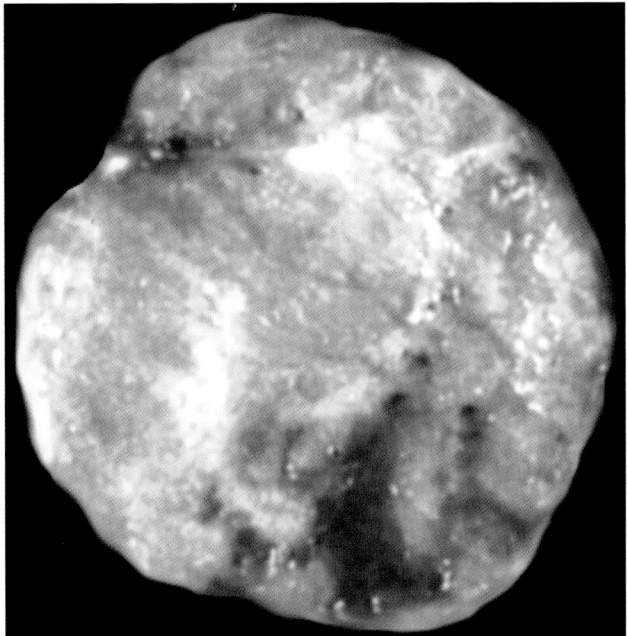

Figure 19-46. Gross photograph of pulmonary papillary adenoma, which the surgeon reported as having "shelled-out" from the surrounding lung parenchyma.

including lymphocytes, mast cells, plasma cells, and eosinophils. The surrounding lung typically demonstrates a fibroblastic response to the lesion, sometimes with formation of a circumferential pseudocapsule. Mitotic activity is limited, and necrosis is absent.

Immunohistochemical studies of PAL show consistent reactivity for keratin, surfactant-related apoproteins, thyroid transcription factor 1, and napsin-A in the neoplastic cells.[172,182] In addition, labeling for Clara cell antigen and carcinoembryonic antigen may be present. Ultrastructural analysis shows microvillous differentiation of the plasmalemmae and the presence of lamellar bodies in the tumor cell cytoplasm (Fig. 19-48).[170–173,182]

Because of the sometimes-infiltrative nature of PAL, some authors have suggested that it be considered borderline malignant.[172,181,182] Nevertheless, there have been no reports of recurrence or metastasis of this lesion, and conservative surgical removal appears sufficient.

Leiomyoma

Solitary leiomyoma of the respiratory tract has been reported as an independent entity, distinct from hamartomas. These tumors are most often located in the wall of the trachea or bronchi (Fig. 19-49), with pulmonary parenchymal or pleural origins rare.[183–195] Bronchoscopic and gross evaluation of central lesions shows a dome-shaped endoluminal mass, usually with a smooth mucosal surface (Figs. 19-50 and 19-51).

Histologically, bronchial leiomyoma is identical to benign smooth muscle tumors elsewhere in the body, comprising intertwining fascicles of spindle cells with fusiform nuclear contours, perinuclear cytoplasmic vacuolization, and finely fibrillary eosinophilic cytoplasm (Fig. 19-52). Mitotic activity is limited, there is no infiltration of adjacent tissues, and necrosis is absent.

The fine structural features of smooth muscle proliferations in the lung include pericellular basal lamina, plasmalemmal hemidesmosomes and micropinocytotic vesicles, skeins of cytoplasmic thin filaments, and intrafilamentous dense bodies.[196–198] Immunohistologically, one typically sees reactivity for muscle-specific actin, alpha-isoform ("smooth muscle") actin, desmin, calponin, and caldesmon, with an absence of S-100 protein, CD56, CD57, and keratin.[188]

The differential diagnosis of primary smooth muscle tumors of the respiratory tract includes hamartomas as well as peripheral nerve sheath tumors and sarcomatoid carcinomas. Although conventional histologic analysis is usually sufficient to distinguish between those possibilities, the special studies just cited may be necessary.

Solitary smooth muscle tumors are treated with simple but complete excision, if thorough clinical evaluation has excluded an extrapulmonary primary lesion of the same type. The latter proviso relates to the fact that some leiomyosarcomas (particularly in the retroperitoneum) are extremely low-grade proliferations that may produce "pseudoleiomyomatous" metastases.[199]

Glomus Tumor and Glomangioma

Glomus tumor and glomangioma (GTG)[200–205] are most often seen in the skin and superficial soft tissue,[206] but also occur with relative frequency in the alimentary tract[207] and rarely the respiratory system.[204] Pulmonary GTG affects adults, with an age range of 20 to 68 years[204] (Fig. 19-53).

The gross features of GTG include a nodular configuration, with uniform gray-white or yellow cut surfaces and a maximum dimension of 6.5 cm, sometimes mimicking a carcinoid tumor.[205]

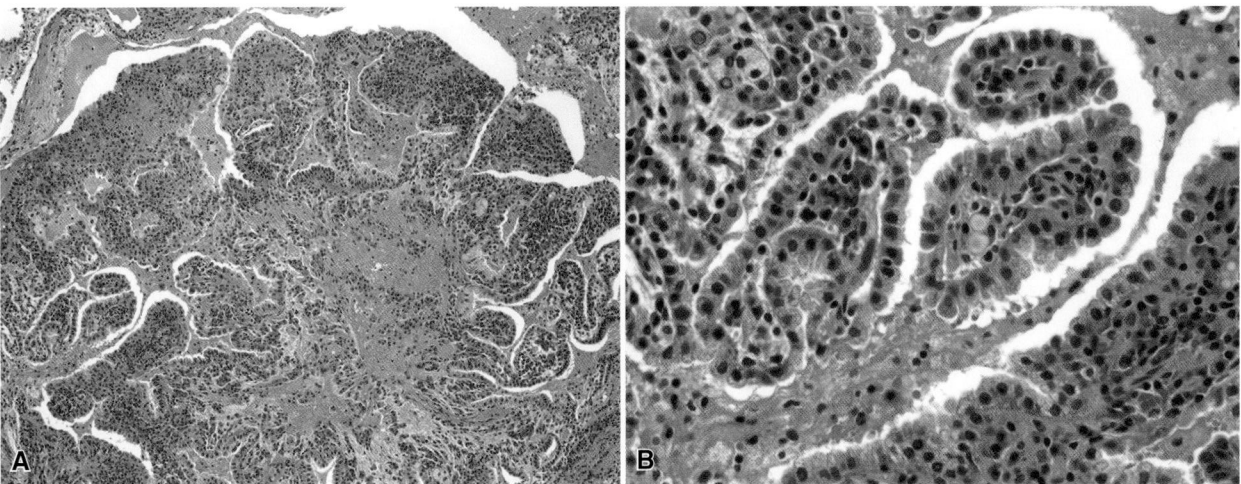

Figure 19-47. A and **B,** Papillary fronds of variable size and shape are mantled by bland polygonal epithelial cells in papillary adenoma of the lung.

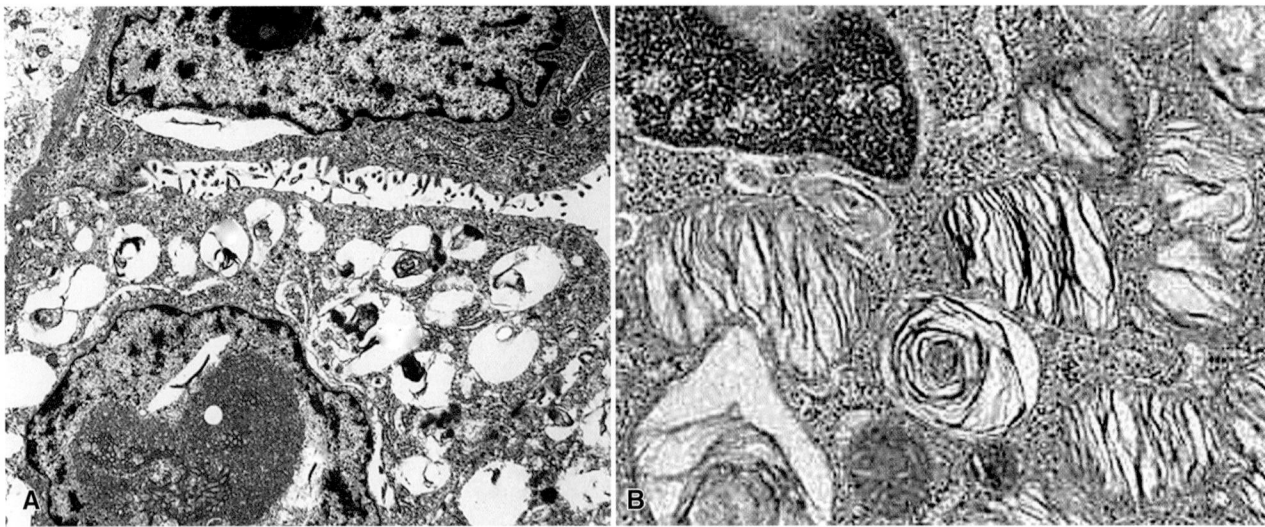

Figure 19-48. **A** and **B,** These electron photomicrographs of papillary adenoma show plasmalemmal microvilli and cytoplasmic "tigroid" inclusions. The latter are organelles that contain surfactant apolipoprotein, typical of type II pneumocytes.

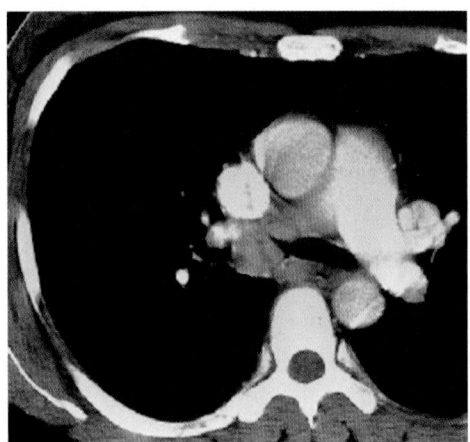

Figure 19-49. An endoluminal mass evident in the right bronchus intermedius proved to be a leiomyoma.

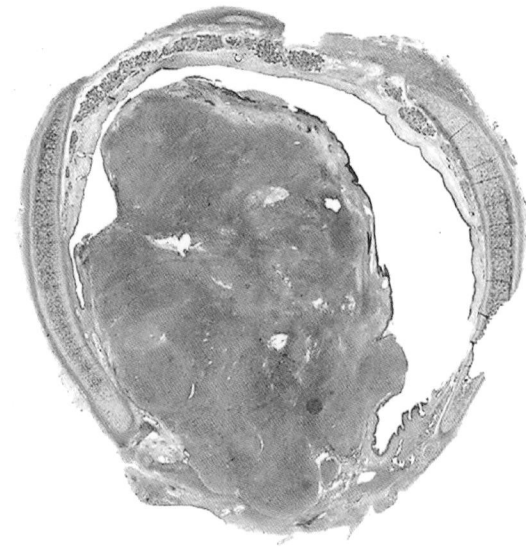

Figure 19-51. Low-power micrograph demonstrates the relationship of an endoluminal bronchial leiomyoma to the wall of the airway.

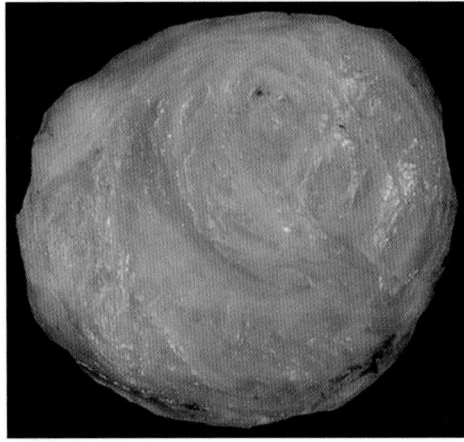

Figure 19-50. A leiomyoma of the bronchus, which was endoscopically removed, shows internal fasciculation and a white-gray cut surface.

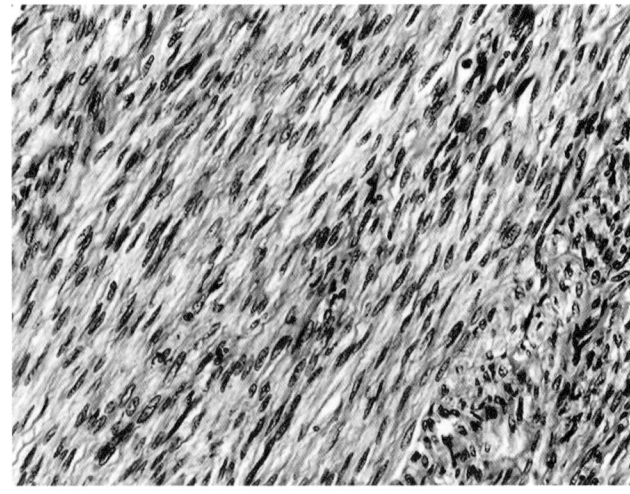

Figure 19-52. A leiomyoma of the bronchus is composed of fascicles of cytologically bland spindle cells with bluntly fusiform nuclei, perinuclear lucency, and finely fibrillar eosinophilic cytoplasm.

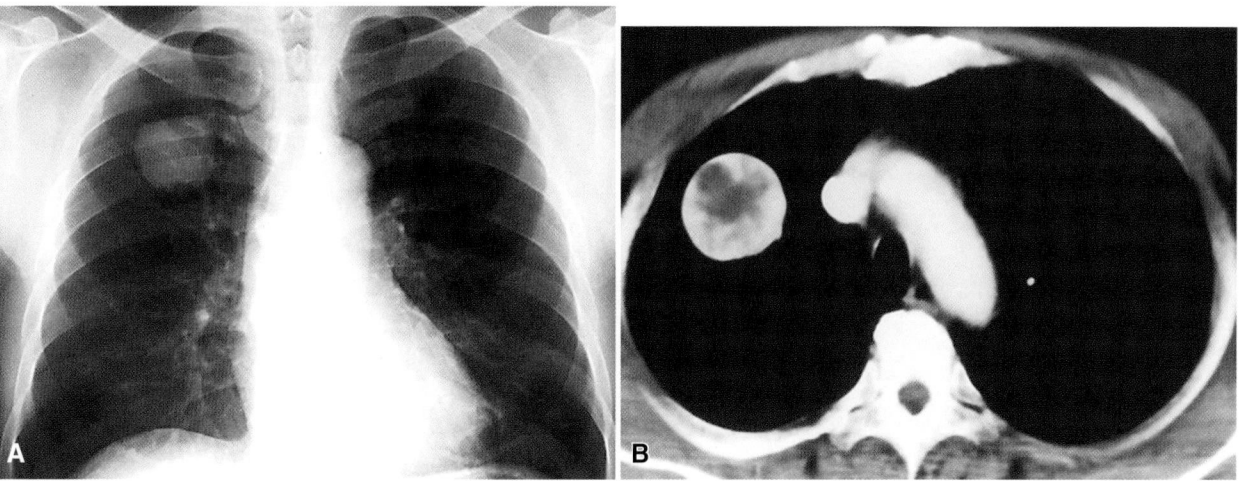

Figure 19-53. A, This chest radiograph shows a circumscribed nodular lesion in the right upper lung field. **B,** A computed tomogram from another patient demonstrates an internally heterogeneous spherical nodule in the right mid-lung. Both lesions were glomus tumors.

Microscopically, the lesions include compact polygonal or round cells that are closely apposed (Fig. 19-54). Nuclei are round or oval, with dispersed chromatin, scarce mitotic activity, and little if any pleomorphism. Cytoplasm is modest in amount and amphophilic or eosinophilic (Fig. 19-55). Supporting stroma consists of delicate fibrovascular septations. In lesions that lie toward the "glomangioma" pole of the spectrum, dilated vascular spaces also punctuate the lesions (Fig. 19-56), and some of these may assume a "moose antler" shape, as in the vessels seen in hemangiopericytomas. Although most are well circumscribed, a proportion of pulmonary GTGs are infiltrative.

One exception to this description was represented by a tumor in the series of Gaertner and associates.[204] This tumor demonstrated infiltrative growth, obvious nuclear atypia with prominent nucleoli, necrosis, and brisk mitotic activity. It metastasized to several visceral sites and soft tissue, causing death in 1.3 years. Thus, it was classified as a glomangiosarcoma.

Electron microscopic examination of GTGs shows evidence of specialized smooth muscle differentiation (discussed earlier), as expected in pericytic perivascular cells.[203,204] The immunophenotype of GTG includes reactivity for vimentin, actin, laminin, and collagen type IV, with an absence of keratin, neuroendocrine markers, CD31, and CD34.[204]

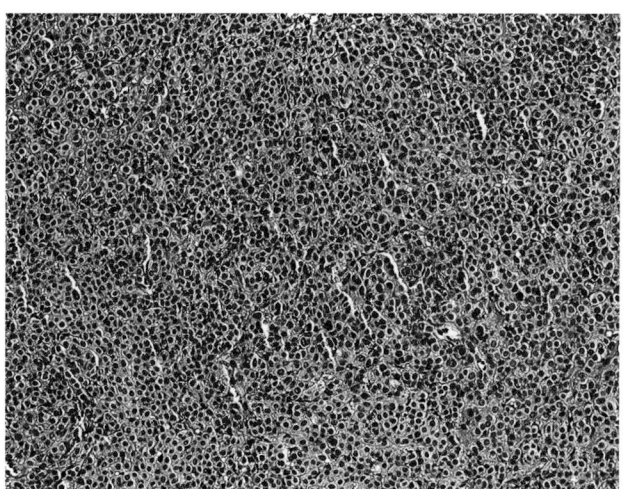

Figure 19-54. A low-power micrograph of a pulmonary glomus tumor showing a monotonous sheet-like proliferation of cells.

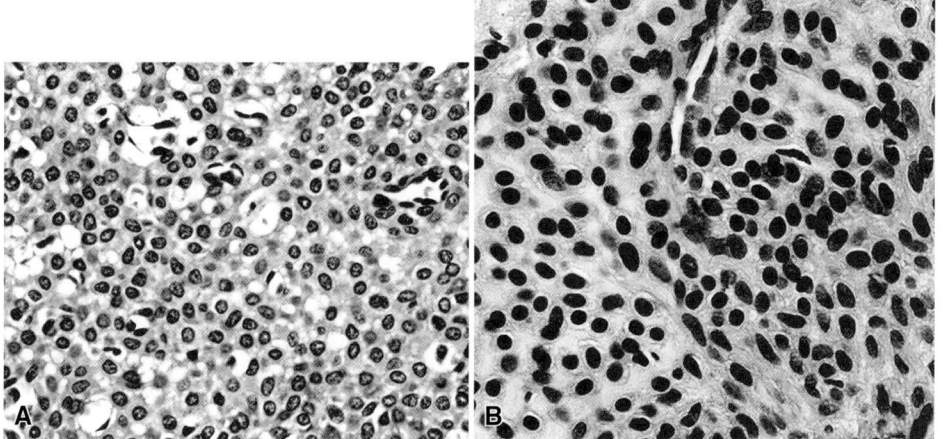

Figure 19-55. A and **B,** A higher-power micrograph of a pulmonary glomus tumor demonstrating cellular monomorphism with round to oval nuclei, dispersed chromatin, and amphophilic cytoplasm. A differential diagnosis with a low-grade neuroendocrine tumor would be difficult morphologically.

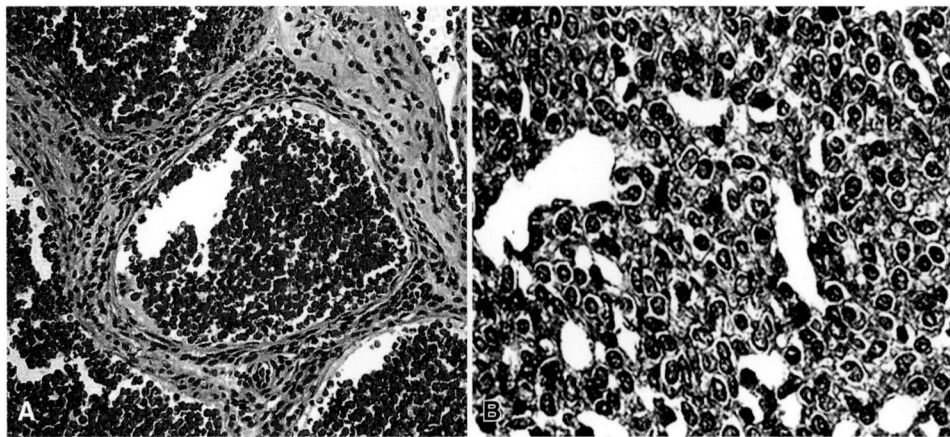

Figure 19-56. **A,** This example of glomangioma demonstrates dilated vascular structures that punctuate a proliferation of bland cuboidal cells. **B,** The myogenous-perivascular nature of the tumoral elements is supported by immunoreactivity for muscle-specific actin.

The differential diagnosis of GTG centers on the alternatives of grade 1 neuroendocrine carcinoma ("carcinoid"), primitive neuroectodermal tumor of the lung, intrapulmonary paraganglioma, and hemangiopericytoma–solitary fibrous tumor. The first three of these lesions reproducibly demonstrate neuroendocrine or neuroectodermal markers, such as chromogranin-A, synaptophysin, CD56, and CD99—all of which are absent in GTG—and hemangiopericytoma–solitary fibrous tumors consistently lack the actin positivity that is expected in glomus tumors.

Glomus tumors and glomangiomas are treated variably with lobectomy, sleeve resection of the bronchus, or wedge resection of the subpleural lung parenchyma. Findings on follow-up are benign.

Chondroma, Myxoma, and Fibromyxoma

Several authors have posited that true chondromas and fibromyxomas of the lung[208,209] exist apart from pulmonary hamartomas[210–213] (see Chapter 18). In particular, Carney[214] and Wick and colleagues[215] have documented a constellation of masses in young women wherein multifocal cartilaginous neoplasms—apparently *true* chondromas—are part of a syndromic triad that includes extra-adrenal paragangliomas and gastric epithelioid stromal tumors. These are histologically different from "usual" chondroid hamartomas of the lung.[216] They are frequently multiple, although they may occur singly (Fig. 19-57) in young women, more often than in elderly men (as is true for hamartomas). Chondromas lack the epithelial entrapment and "uncommitted" fibroblastic mesenchymal component that is observed in chondroid hamartomas. Instead, the interface between chondromas and the surrounding lung parenchyma is sharply demarcated (Fig. 19-58). Constituent chondrocytes are hyaline, and metaplastic osteoid is common in such lesions, more than in pulmonary chondroid hamartomas.

Pulmonary chondromas do not have malignant potential, but are frequently confused with metastases from gastrointestinal stromal tumors, because of the clinical setting in which they occur.

Solitary Pulmonary Hemangioma and "Hemangiomatosis"

True hemangiomas of the tracheobronchial tree and lung are vanishingly rare. They are usually detected in childhood.[217] Discrete, variably dense and sometimes-cystic masses are present on chest radiographs (especially high-resolution CT)[218] (Fig. 19-59); they may be multiple. The maximum size of individual lesions can be several centimeters. In at least one case, an intrapulmonary hemangioma was interpreted radiographically as an intrapulmonary bronchogenic cyst.[217] Simple excision has been curative.

Microscopically, true hemangiomas of the airways and lungs completely replace a portion of the native tissue, with a proliferation of tubular

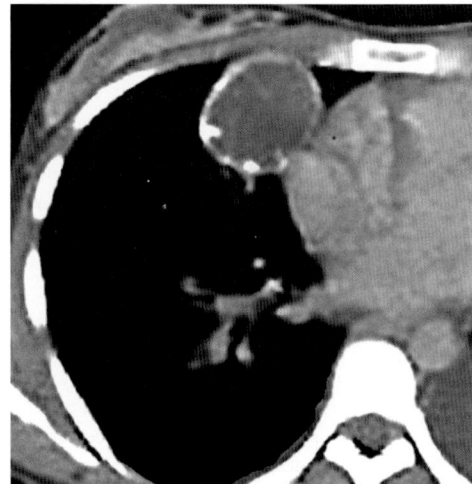

Figure 19-57. A peripherally calcified spheroid mass is seen in the anterior right lung field in this computed tomogram. Excision of the mass revealed a globular lesion with obviously chondroid features on gross examination.

vascular spaces lined by bland endothelial cells. A "capillary hemangioma" pattern appears to be most common, in which the caliber of the neoplastic vessels approximates that of normal small venules or capillaries (Fig. 19-60). It is implicit in this diagnosis that no other tumoral elements be identified; this is an important caveat because several other neoplasms in the lung—including some carcinomas—may contain blood lakes or pseudovascular foci that resemble the image of vascular proliferations.[219]

Another salient differential diagnostic consideration is "pulmonary hemangiomatosis" (see Chapter 11). That is a condition in which capillary-sized blood vessels proliferate throughout the pre-existing pulmonary parenchyma and stroma, including the alveolar septa, interlobular and interlobar septa, bronchial and bronchiolar walls, intrapulmonary vasa vasorum, and pleural surfaces.[220,221] In reality, it is probably not a neoplastic process at all, but rather a malformative or reactive proliferation. For example, some cases of pulmonary hemangiomatosis have been associated with longstanding passive congestion of the lungs, as seen in left-sided heart failure.[221]

Lipoma and Lipoblastoma

Separating examples of lipoma of the trachea and major bronchi and lung parenchyma (LTMB)[222–235] from adipocytic predominant hamartomas may be difficult, and pathologic criteria for doing so are arbitrary.[228]

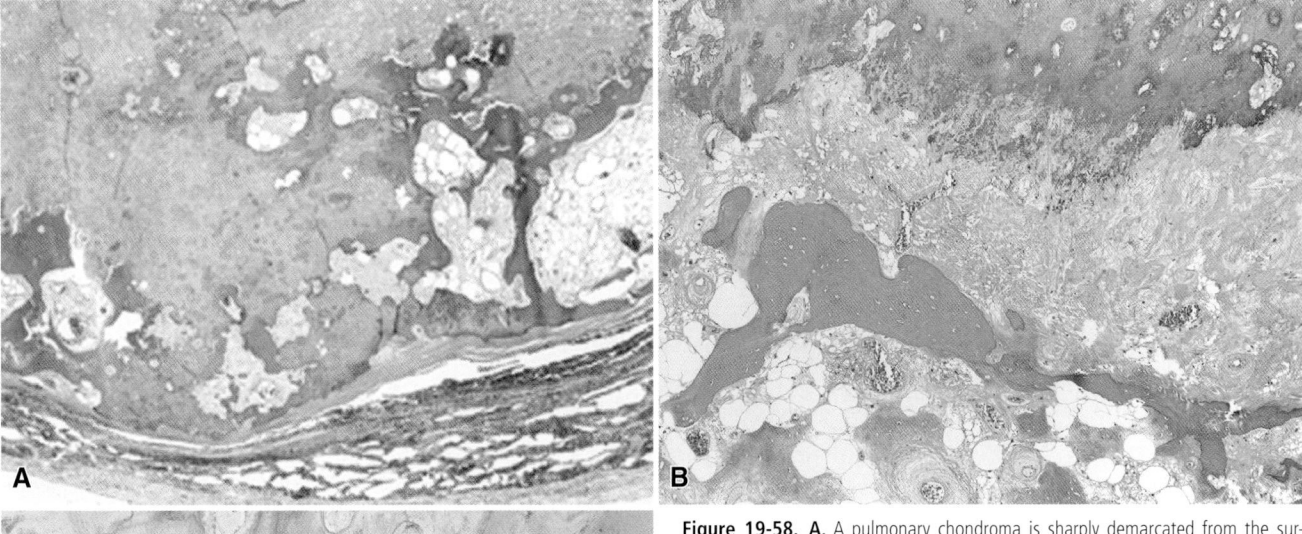

Figure 19-58. A, A pulmonary chondroma is sharply demarcated from the surrounding lung parenchyma with no entrapment of adjacent lung parenchyma. **B** and **C,** The tumors typically show osseous metaplasia and internal calcification. These features are diagnostic of a pulmonary "chondroma" characteristic of the Carney triad and different from those of pulmonary hamartoma.

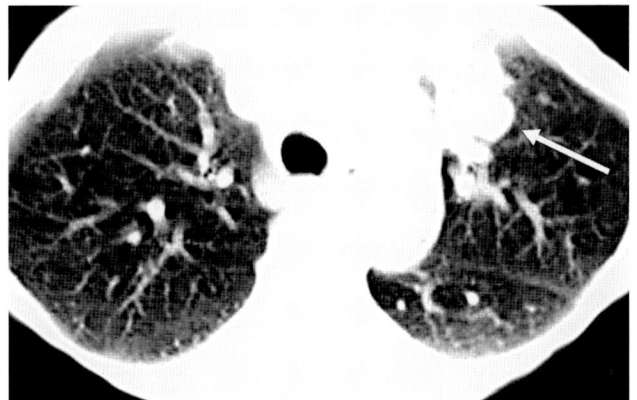

Figure 19-59. This thoracic computed tomogram shows an enhancing nodular lesion (*arrow*) in the anterior left lung field, representing an intrapulmonary hemangioma.

Patients with LTMB are adults, usually in the fifth or sixth decade of life.[225,229] Endoscopic examination shows a variably polypoid submucosal nodule in one of the first three subdivisions of the tracheobronchial tree; radiographs demonstrate secondary atelectasis, obstructive pneumonia, or a mass in 80% of cases, but the remainder have no radiologic abnormalities on plain films.[223] CTs are more sensitive in revealing the presence of lesions in airway lumina[227] (Figs. 19-61 and 19-62).

Current treatment recommendations are for conservative endoscopic resection after a transbronchial biopsy has established the adipocytic nature of the lesion.

Intrapulmonary lipomas are often subpleural (Fig. 19-63) and may even protrude into the pleural space. They are typically detected incidentally on chest radiographs. CT shows that lipomas of the lung have a density approximating that of pleural adipose tissue.[227] Occasional lesions of this type have been found coincidentally in patients with pulmonary carcinomas.[224] If the lipomas are multiple, small, and subpleural, they may also imitate metastatic lesions.[234,235]

Lipoblastoma, a neoplasm of young children[236] may affect the pleura and chest wall, but only anecdotal reports exist of intrapulmonary lipoblastomas.[237,238] They may be extremely large, filling almost an entire hemithorax.[237] Excision is curative in the few cases with meaningful follow-up.

Liposarcoma is the rarest of primary pulmonary adipocytic neoplasms, and it has usually presented as a large single peripheral mass.[239,240] Liposarcoma-like components can be seen as part of sarcomatoid carcinomas,[241] and the latter lesions are far more common than primary liposarcomas of the lung.

The principal gross feature of intrapulmonary adipocytic tumors is a yellow, globular, relatively soft mass in the parenchyma (see Fig. 19-63). Internal fibrous septation may be apparent, as may a circumferential capsule or small foci of intralesional sclerosis. There is no necrosis or hemorrhage.

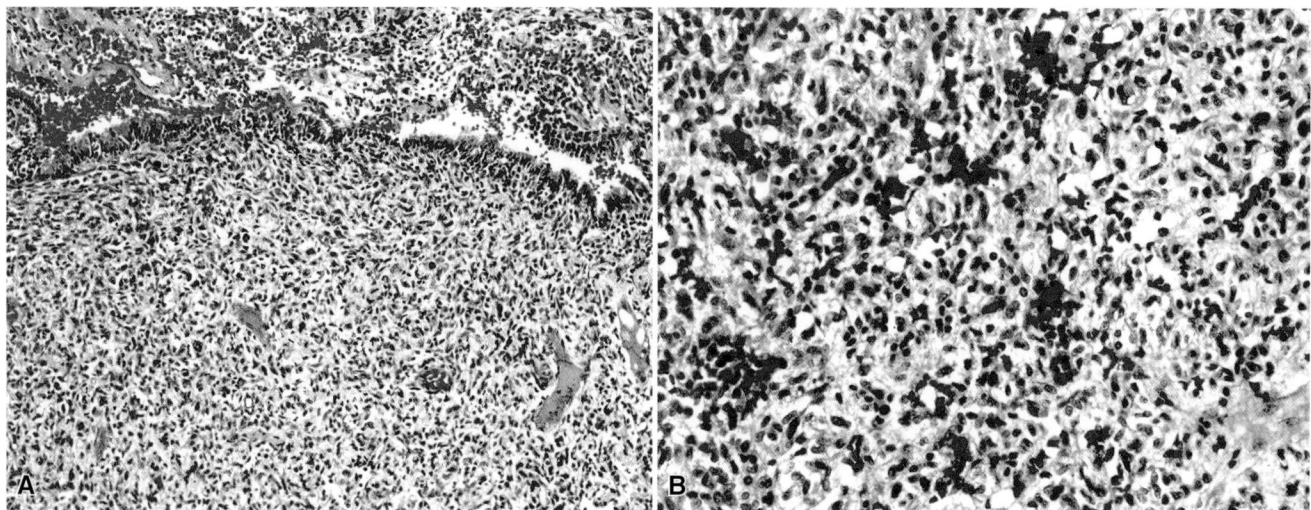

Figure 19-60. **A** and **B,** Numerous closely set small tubular vascular lumina are apparent in this capillary hemangioma, apposing the lumen of an airway.

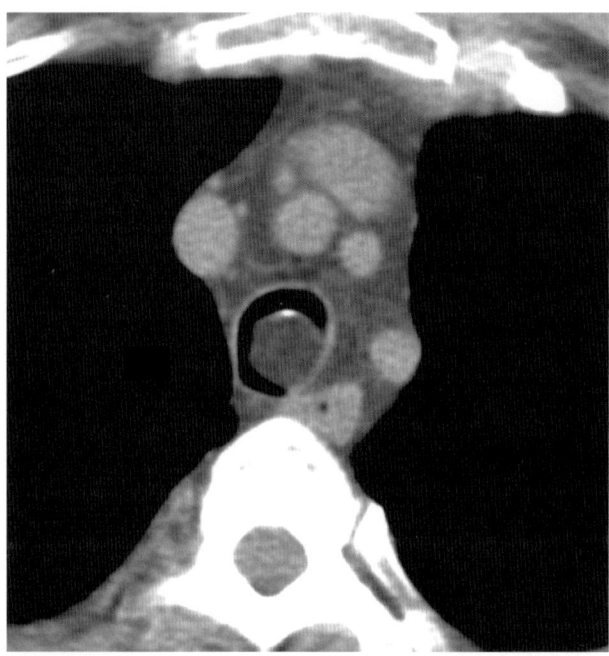

Figure 19-61. This computed tomogram demonstrates an endoluminal tracheal mass that proved to be a lipoma.

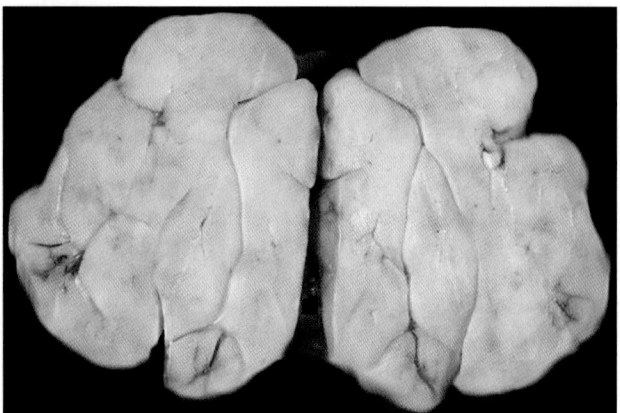

Figure 19-62. This resection specimen of the lesion shown in Figure 19-61 shows uniform yellow tissue with internal lobulation.

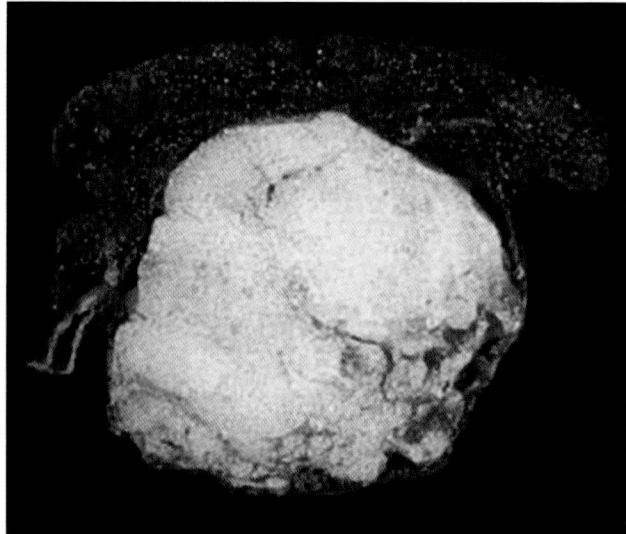

Figure 19-63. A peripheral intrapulmonary lipoma, represented by a large globular tan-yellow lesion beneath the pleural surface.

Microscopically, one sees sheets of fully mature adipocytes in ordinary lipomas (Fig. 19-64), supported by delicate fibrovascular stroma. Atypical intrapulmonary lipomas, showing scattered multinucleated "floret" cells, have been rarely reported[231]; however, this does not seem to have any bearing on prognosis. Lipoblastomas have a more lobulated substructure, with an admixture of uncommitted fibromyxoid tissue among mature fat cells[236,242] (Fig. 19-65). True lipoblasts may be apparent as well, rare mitotic figures may be evident, and the supporting stromal tissue contains a delicately arborizing capillary network (Fig. 19-66). Therefore, the overall image of lipoblastoma may be quite similar to that of myxoid liposarcoma, and the mutually exclusive occurrence of those tumors in different age groups—with liposarcomas being seen in adults—is important to their proper identification.

Liposarcoma in the lung may assume any of the recognized morphotypes of that tumor (e.g., lipoma-like, sclerosing, myxoid, round cell, pleomorphic, and "dedifferentiated").[239,240] Those variants are recapitulated in metastatic intrapulmonary liposarcomas from primary soft tissue sites.[243]

Karyotypic analysis using fluorescent in situ hybridization may be useful in the differential diagnosis. Abnormalities in chromosome 8q are most common in lipoblastomas,[242] whereas myxoid liposarcoma

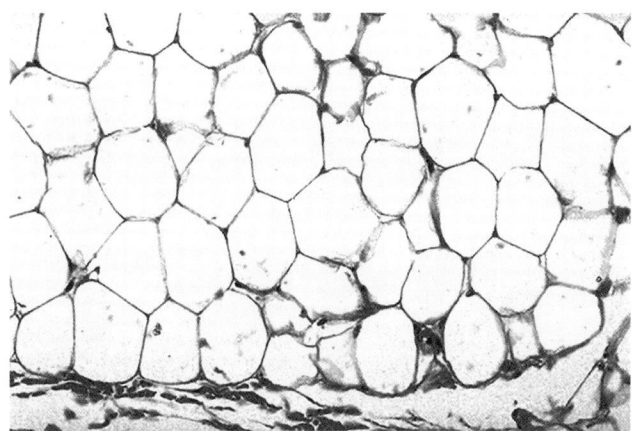

Figure 19-64. Mature adipocytes with compact eccentric nuclei and abundant lipid-filled cytoplasm are evident in this pulmonary lipoma.

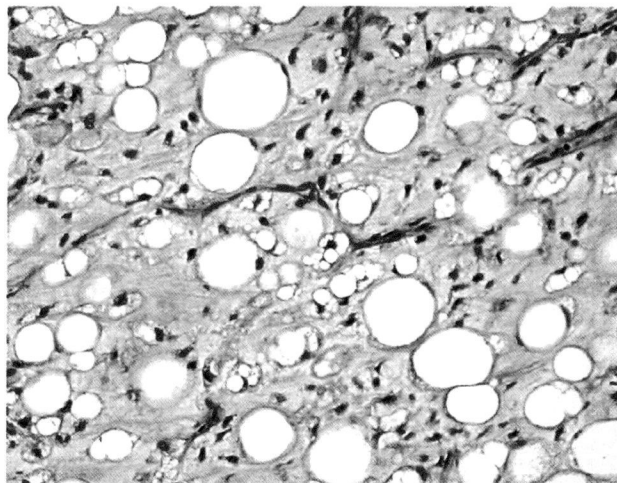

Figure 19-66. An internal vascular stroma is evident in this lipoblastoma, superficially simulating the appearance of myxoid liposarcoma.

demonstrates a reproducible t(12;16) chromosomal translocation.[244] Parenthetically, cytogenetic profiles are somewhat less helpful in the distinction between lipomas of the lung and lipomatous hamartomas, both of which may show abnormalities in chromosome 12.[232,245] However, exchanges of material between chromosomes 6 and 14 are also potentially observed in hamartomas but not lipomas.[246]

Immunohistology of fatty tumors of the lungs shows consistent reactivity for S-100 protein in the adipocytic elements as well as "high-mobility-group" proteins.[245] Lipoblastoma may also show positivity for factor XIIIa in its stellate and fusiform cells.[242]

Angiomyolipoma

In recent years, it has become apparent that a family of neoplasms—which may arise in the kidney, pancreas, alimentary system, liver, soft tissue, or respiratory tract—demonstrates differentiation toward a unique cell type that has both myogenous and melanocytic features.[247-250] These tumors have been variously called "angiomyolipomas," "perivascular epithelioid cell neoplasms" (PEComas), and "myomelanocytomas."[247-251] If a typical morphologic appearance, including smooth muscle, fat, and vascular proliferation, is observed, the first of these terms is still preferred; a few lesions with such characteristics have been reported in the lung.[252-257] Another member of this nosologic group—the pulmonary clear cell or "sugar tumor"—is discussed later. All of these proliferations potentially share immunoreactivity with the melanocyte-related antibody human melanin black (HMB)-45, as well as anti-actins.[248] Other immunohistochemical markers of melanocytic and smooth muscle differentiation—such as antibodies to S-100 protein, tyrosinase, HMB-50, melanoma antigen recognized by T cells 1 (MART-1), caldesmon, calponin, and desmin—may also label them.[249]

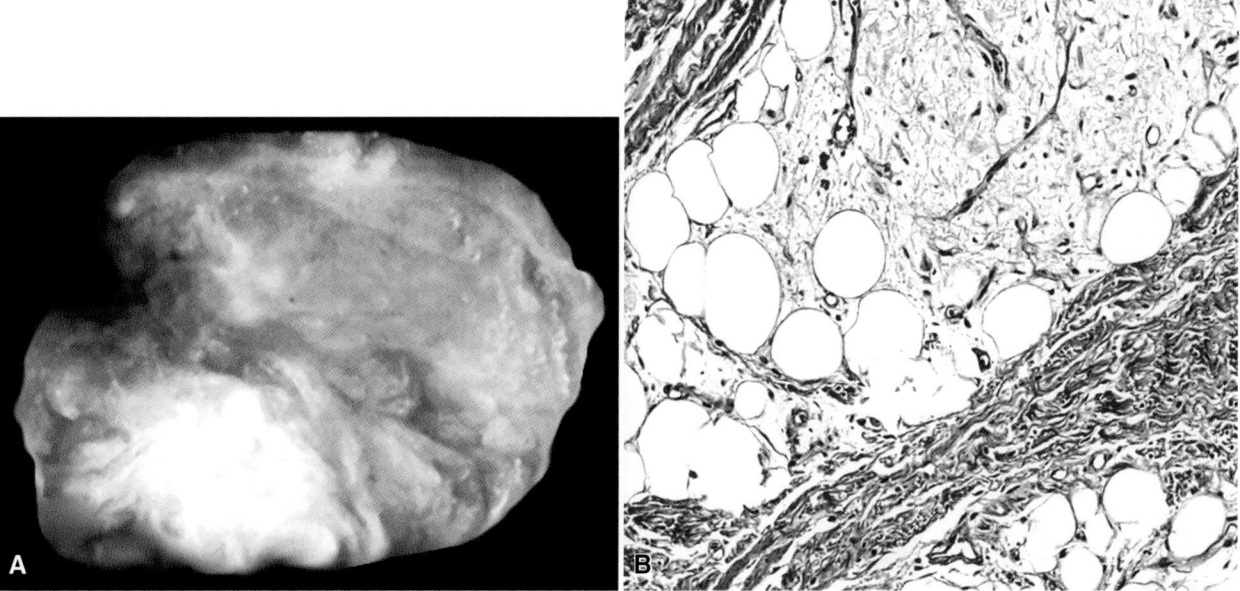

Figure 19-65. A, A fatty mass with areas of more fibrous growth was removed from the left thorax in a young patient. **B,** An admixture of mature lipocytes, bland stellate cells, and myxoid stroma is apparent in the lesion, which is a lipoblastoma.

A proportion of patients with angiomyolipomas, regardless of anatomic location, will have phakomatosis tuberous sclerosis (Bourneville syndrome). It classically includes nodular periventricular glial proliferations and subependymal giant cell astrocytomas in the brain; cutaneous connective tissue nevi; often-multifocal renal angiomyolipomas; and pulmonary lymphangioleiomyomatosis, with or without multifocal micronodular pneumocytic hyperplasia (see Chapter 7).[253,258–260]

Angiomyolipoma of the lungs is typically small, usually less than 2 cm in maximal dimension. They show sharp interfaces with the surrounding lung tissue and uniform yellow-tan cut surfaces.

Microscopically, pulmonary angiomyolipoma is identical to its better-known renal counterpart. Prototypically, it manifests a concatenation of mature fat, variably sized and haphazardly arranged blood vessels with muscular walls, and nests or skeins of fusiform or epithelioid smooth muscle elements (Fig. 19-67). Either the fat or the smooth muscle may dominate the histologic picture and cause diagnostic confusion with either pure adipocytic neoplasms or sarcomas, respectively. Nuclear atypia has been seen in the smooth muscle elements of angiomyolipomas in extrapulmonary sites, and rare cases outside the lung have even shown overtly malignant transformation with necrosis and atypical mitotic activity.[261] Those attributes have not been seen in pulmonary lesions of this type.

Electron microscopic analysis of angiomyolipoma demonstrates findings that recall the characteristics of smooth muscle cells, including pericellular basal lamina and plasmalemma-associated pinocytotic vesicles.[252] Cytoplasmic bundles of thin filaments have not been found. Approximately 50% of such neoplasms show cytoplasmic premelanosomes.[249]

The principal immunohistologic findings in angiomyolipomas have been described earlier. Adachi and coworkers[262] have reported immunoreactivity for CD1a in PEComas, including angiomyolipoma, but we have been unable to reproduce this finding.

In its "classic" form, angiomyolipoma has no realistic differential diagnostic alternatives. Nevertheless, its morphologic variants may be difficult to distinguish from metastatic melanomas, carcinomas, or sarcomas in the lung. Before an unqualified diagnosis of a pure pulmonary smooth muscle tumor or melanoma is made, additional immunocytochemical evaluation with HMB-45 (Fig. 19-68) and anti-actins is probably a prudent step.

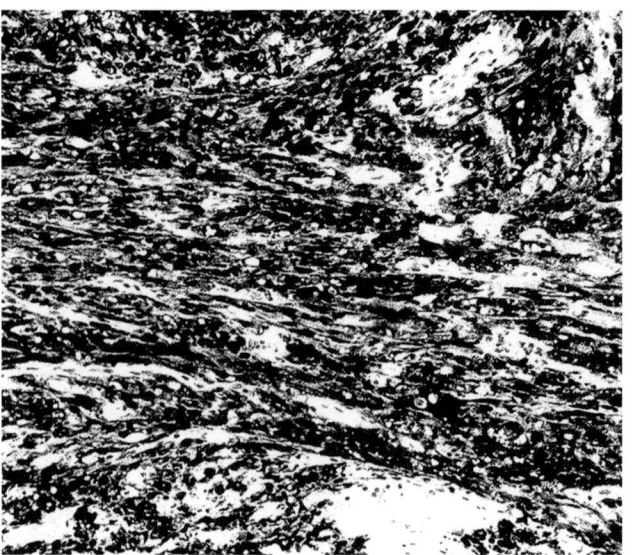

Figure 19-68. HMB-45 immunoreactivity in angiomyolipoma.

Myelolipoma

Myelolipoma is a peculiar lesion that is typically located in the adrenal glands or the retroperitoneum.[263,264] As its name suggests, it comprises a tumefactive admixture of mature adipose tissue and hematopoietic precursor cells, including megakaryocytes (Figs. 19-69 and 19-70). It is still unclear whether myelolipoma represents a true neoplasm or a peculiar form of extramedullary hematopoiesis; the difference between those entities may sometimes be only semantic. Alternatively, myelolipoma could be regarded as a lipoma that has been secondarily populated by bone marrow elements.

In any event, anecdotal reports have been made of primary pulmonary myelolipoma, all of which occurred in adult patients.[265–269] They may occur multiply and mimic metastases.[265]

The pathologic features of myelolipoma are so distinctive that it has no viable differential diagnosis. Nevertheless, it is probably worthwhile to evaluate the peripheral blood picture to exclude the possibility of functional extramedullary hematopoiesis.

Benign Tumors of the Pleura
Adenomatoid Tumor

It is an unfortunate truism that completely benign neoplasms of the pleura are a distinct rarity. Indeed, the only representative of that diagnostic category is the adenomatoid tumor. That neoplasm is a lesion with mesothelial differentiation that is most often encountered in the adnexal soft tissue surrounding the uterus and testes.[270,271] Only five cases have been described in the pleura.[272–275] These lesions occurred in a middle-aged man, two middle-aged women, an elderly woman, and an elderly man. They were all incidental findings during surgical procedures that were done for unrelated lesions (pulmonary squamous cell carcinoma, mesothelioma, pulmonary adenosquamous carcinoma, esophageal adenocarcinoma, and pulmonary histoplasmoma), and they showed no subsequent evidence of aggressive behavior.

Pleural adenomatoid tumors are unencapsulated and measure 0.5 to 2.5 cm in greatest dimension. Microscopically, the lesions are composed of epithelioid cells organized into compact gland-like profiles (Fig. 19-71). They have vesicular nuclear chromatin, inconspicuous nucleoli, and relatively abundant eosinophilic or vacuolated cytoplasm. No areas of nuclear pleomorphism should be present, mitotic figures are rare, and they do not invade the subjacent lung parenchyma.

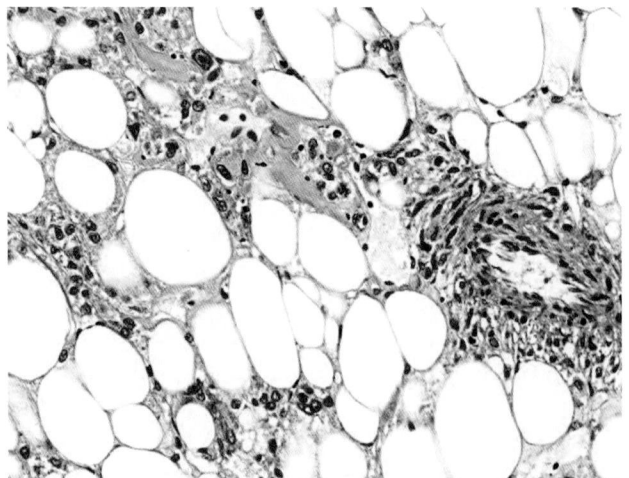

Figure 19-67. Angiomyolipomas show a tripartite constituency of mature adipocytes, large blood vessels, and epithelioid and fusiform myogenous cells, with variable prominence of each component.

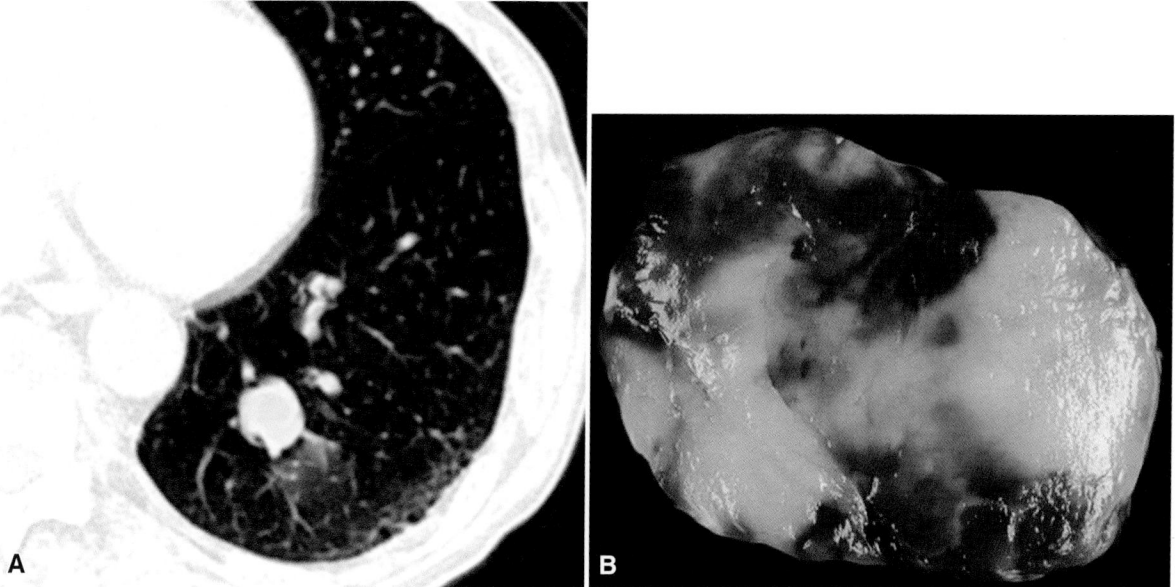

Figure 19-69. A, A relatively circumscribed homogeneous nodule is present in the mid-left lung field in this computed tomogram. **B,** This gross photograph of the excised lesion shows a lobulated circumscribed yellow and red lesion, resembling a hemorrhagic lipoma. In reality, the tumor was a myelolipoma. The patient had no evidence of a hematologic disorder.

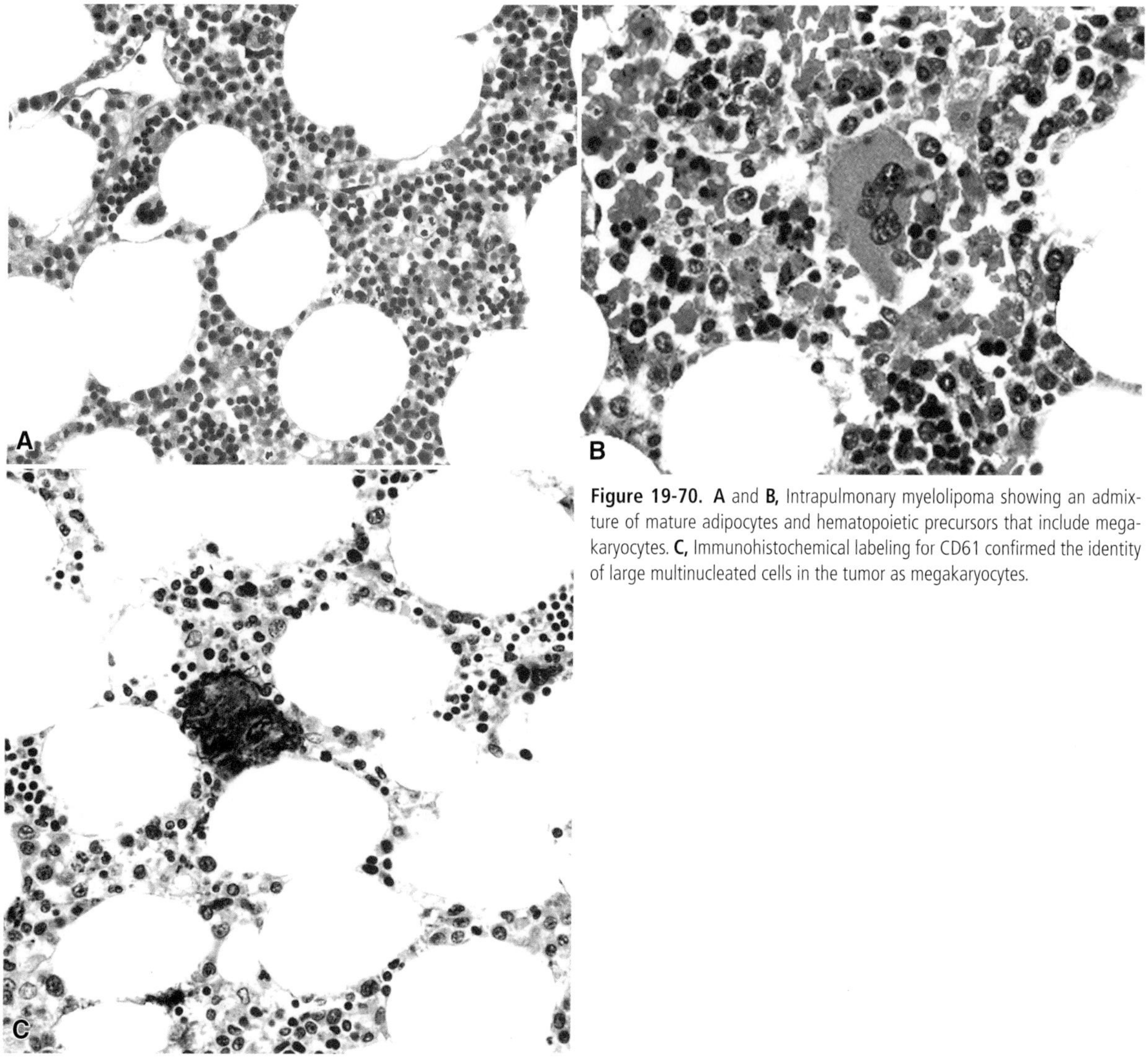

Figure 19-70. A and **B,** Intrapulmonary myelolipoma showing an admixture of mature adipocytes and hematopoietic precursors that include megakaryocytes. **C,** Immunohistochemical labeling for CD61 confirmed the identity of large multinucleated cells in the tumor as megakaryocytes.

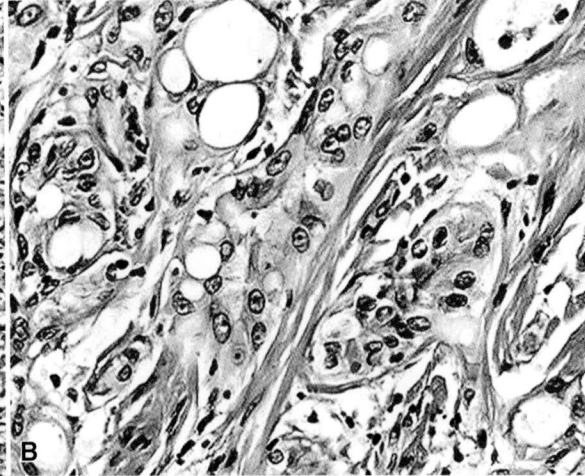

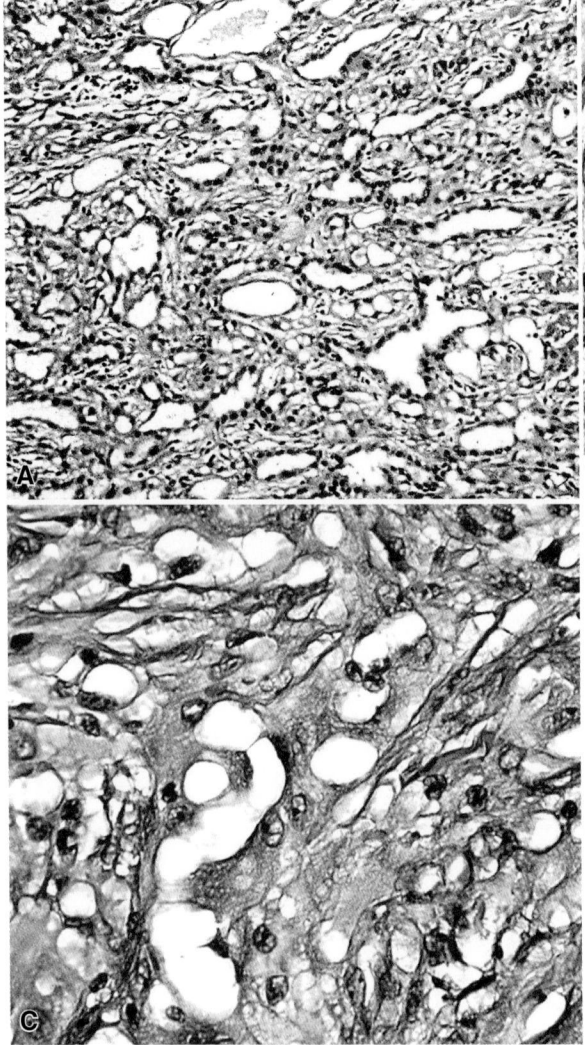

Figure 19-71. **A** to **C,** Pleural adenomatoid tumor comprised of micro-cystic arrays of bland cuboidal epithelioid cells.

Electron microscopy[272] shows branching plasmalemmal microvilli and prominent intercellular attachment complexes, typical of mesothelial lesions. Immunohistologically, the tumor cells label for keratin and calretinin, but are negative for carcinoembryonic antigen, CD15, CD34, Ber-EP4 antigen, and tumor-associated glycoprotein 72.

The principal components of the differential diagnosis for pleural adenomatoid tumor are metastatic adenocarcinoma and malignant mesothelioma. Both of those possibilities are rendered unlikely by the bland histologic images of pleural adenomatoid tumor, with no evidence of infiltrative growth (see Chapter 20). Ki-67 (MIB-1) staining may also be helpful in this setting[275] because the labeling index in adenomatoid tumor is only 1% to 2%. In contrast, "microcystic" (adenomatoid tumor–like) mesothelioma of the pleura shows a high Ki-67 index (>50%).[274]

Calcifying Fibrous Pseudotumor

An unusual entity known as calcifying fibrous "pseudotumor" (CFPT) has been described in the pleura.[276–279] This lesion is histologically similar, if not identical, to calcifying fibrous "pseudotumors" of the soft tissue.[280]

The documented cases of pleural CFPT have occurred in adults (age range, 23–46 years), most of whom were women. Pleural-based masses[281,282] are present on chest radiographs, and CT scans demonstrate well-demarcated, partially calcified nodular lesions, measuring up to 12 cm in diameter (Fig. 19-72). An intrapulmonary CFPT has been reported.[283]

Histologically, the masses are circumscribed nonencapsulated fibrous lesions composed of dense, hyalinized, collagenous tissue, with interspersed bland spindle cells (Fig. 19-73). They are generally hypocellular, particularly at the periphery, without nuclear atypia. A scant chronic inflammatory infiltrate may be seen, without lymphoid aggregates, giant cells, or necrosis. All lesions also feature calcifications of the psammomatous (Fig. 19-74) as well as dystrophic types. These histologic features are identical to those of calcifying fibrous pseudotumors of soft tissue.[284–286]

The differential diagnosis includes inflammatory myofibroblastic tumor (IMT; discussed later) as well as hyaline pleural plaques, tumefactive pleural fibrosis, calcified or hyalinizing granulomas, and amyloidosis. The clinical presentation, gross features, and microscopic features of CFPT argue against any of those considerations, as does its regular content of psammomatous calcifications. Follow-up has shown no examples of untoward behavior.

Leiomyoma

Leiomyoma of the pleura has been reported only anecdotally.[287,288] One might question whether a distinction between that lesion and desmoid tumor was pursued conclusively in such cases.

Biologically Borderline Tumors of the Lung and Pleura

The biologic difference between "benign" and "borderline" (very low-grade malignant) tumors is a subtle one because few of the latter neoplasms cause significant mortality. For this discussion, we have defined "borderline" lesions of the lung and pleura as those that have shown a

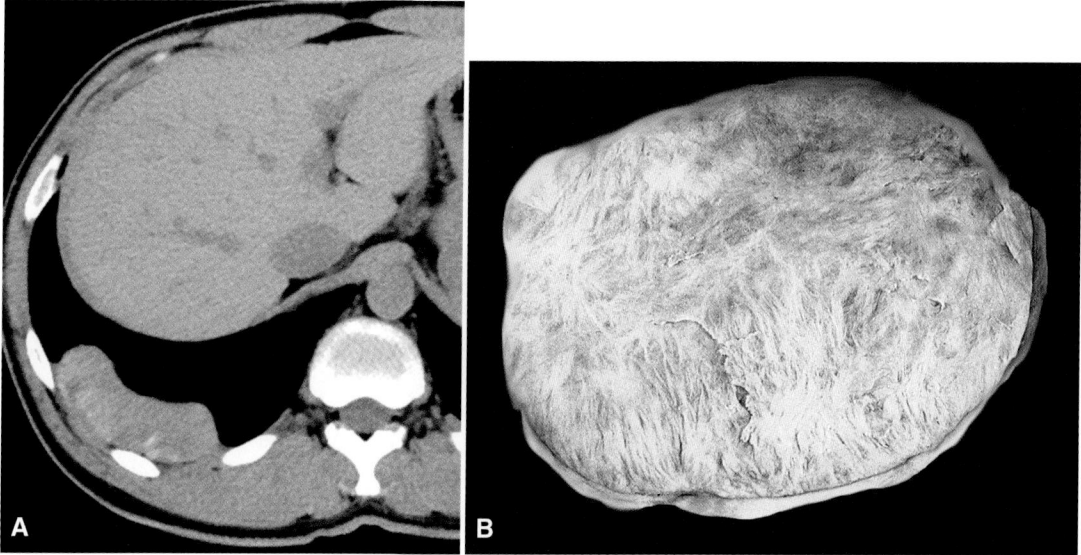

Figure 19-72. A computed tomogram (**A**) and a gross photograph (**B**) of a calcifying fibrous pseudotumor of the pleura show a well-demarcated nodular lesion.

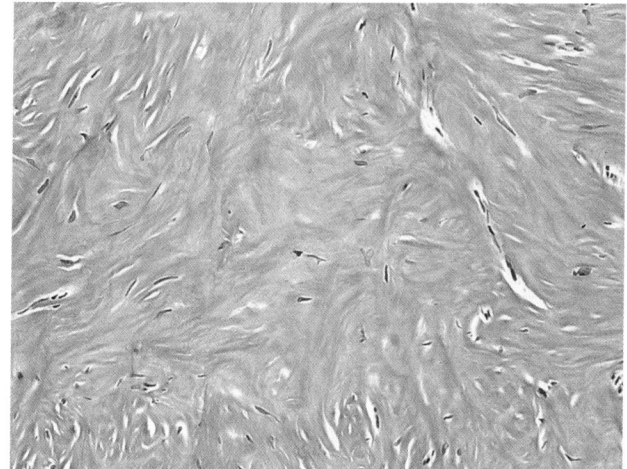

Figure 19-73. A calcifying pseudotumor of the pleura, represented by a hypocellular proliferation of bland spindle cells that are set in a dense and hyalinized collagenous stroma.

potential for local recurrence after apparently adequate excision, for rare embolic metastasis, or both. It is readily acknowledged that other observers may regard the same tumors as either benign or overtly malignant.

Inflammatory Myofibroblastic Tumor ("Inflammatory Pseudotumor")

In 1939, Brunn[289] described two pulmonary lesions that were composed of spindle cells admixed with inflammatory elements in patients with fever and weight loss. The systemic symptoms disappeared after surgical removal of the lung tumors. Although they were believed to be true neoplasms of probable smooth muscle lineage, subsequent authors espoused the theory that masses with the same attributes were inflammatory and reparative lesions.[290,291] Hence, the term "inflammatory pseudotumor" gained favor. However, Spencer[292] noted that a proportion of such proliferations behaved in a biologically malignant fashion, and other reports also documented the presence of vascular invasion and recurrences.[293–295] Molecular analyses done in the 1990s revealed a

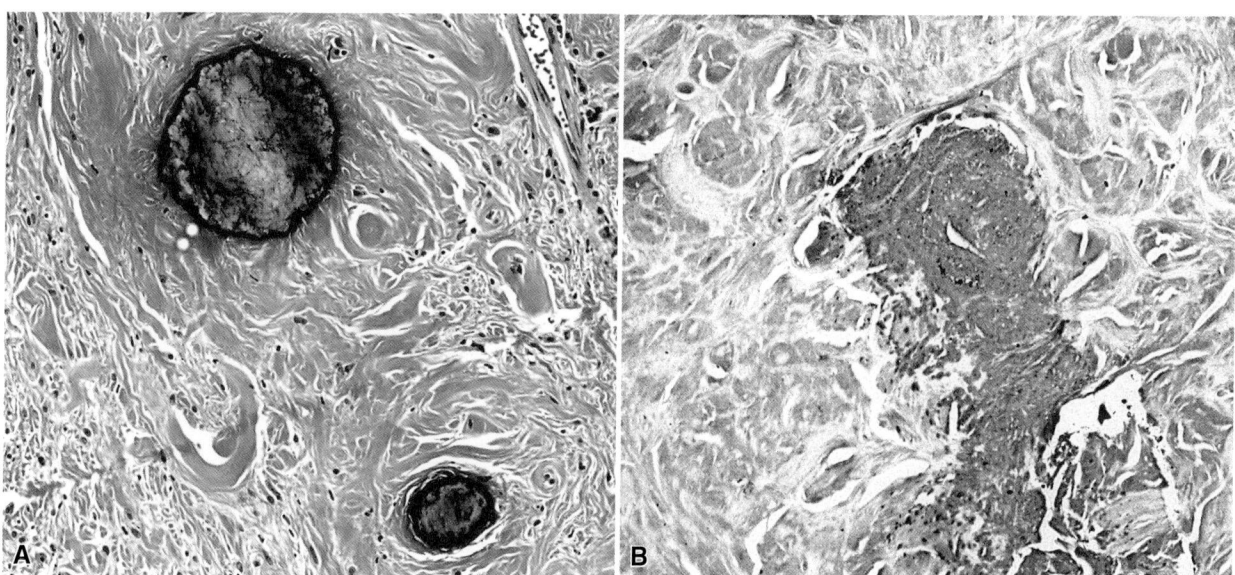

Figure 19-74. Spherical (**A**) and irregular (**B**) calcifications are apparent in these photomicrographs of a calcifying fibrous pseudotumor of the pleura.

clonal character of some "inflammatory pseudotumors" in the lungs and other anatomic sites,[296-298] and, together with aggregated clinicopathologic information, these data resulted in amendment of their name to "inflammatory myofibroblastic tumors."[299] It is now accepted that they are separate from inflammatory pseudotumors and that IMTs form a conceptual continuum with "inflammatory fibrosarcoma" or "myofibrosarcoma."[300-303] Because they may recur and occasionally metastasize, IMTs are best considered biologically "borderline" neoplasms.

The lung is most frequently affected by IMT, among all potential topographic locations.[295] Although the majority of IMTs are seen in children and young adults, they may be encountered in patients of all ages, with no sex predilection.[295] Some IMTs are situated in the large airways, with no parenchymal involvement, but they are exceptional; most arise in the peripheral lung fields. Systemic symptoms of a paraneoplastic nature have been reported in up to 50% of cases, including such findings as anemia, fever, weight loss, hyperglobulinemia, leukothrombocytosis, and elevations in the erythrocyte sedimentation rate.[301,303] As discussed earlier, those abnormalities typically remit when the IMT is removed. The remaining cases present with cough, vague chest discomfort, or hemoptysis, or are asymptomatic, with the lesions found incidentally on chest radiographs.[299] On imaging studies, IMT is typically a lobulated or globoid mass (Fig. 19-75), usually measuring less than 5 cm in maximum dimension. Occasionally, it may attain a size of greater than 10 cm; internal calcifications are commonly seen. Infiltration of great vessels, mediastinal soft tissue, or chest wall is apparent radiographically in a minority of cases.

Gross examination of IMTs shows a deceptively circumscribed appearance, with a gray-tan or yellow cut surface. Grittiness may be encountered during sectioning because of microcalcification. Foci of gross necrosis and hemorrhage are exceptional. When the tumor is in proximity to large airways or blood vessels, growth into those structures can be seen, with compromise of their lumina by tumor tissue.

The histologic profile of IMT features a proliferation of relatively bland spindle cells arranged haphazardly or in vague fascicles[299,301,304] (Figs. 19-76 and 19-77). In contrast to the gross appearance, this lesion has an irregular peripheral zone of growth microscopically, with tongues of tumor that comingle with adjacent normal tissues. Not surprisingly, infiltration of blood vessels, bronchi, and pleura may be evident. Nuclei in the neoplastic fusiform elements usually contain dispersed or vesicular chromatin with compact nucleoli (Fig. 19-78). Mitotic activity is typically easily found, but without pathologic division figures.

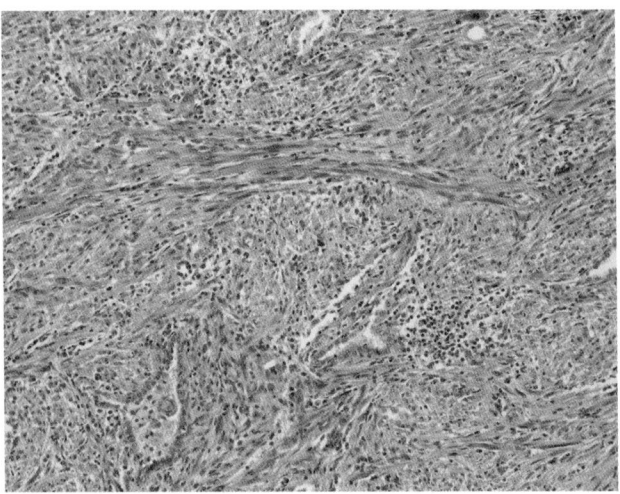

Figure 19-76. Inflammatory myofibroblastic tumor of the lung showing a fascicular spindle cell proliferation with admixed lymphoid elements.

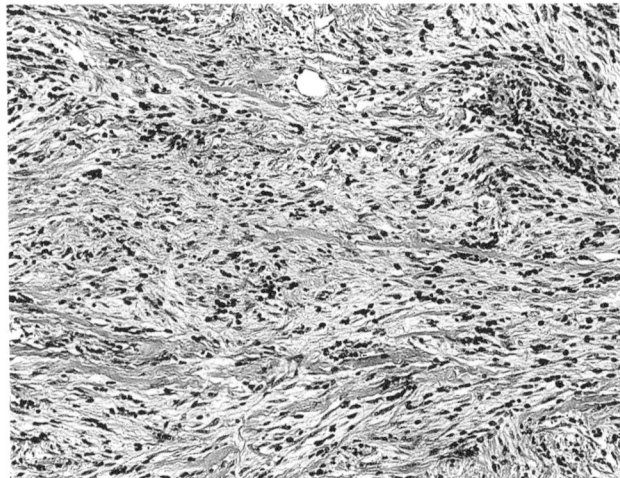

Figure 19-77. The spindle cells in this pulmonary inflammatory myofibroblastic tumor are arranged in interweaving bundles.

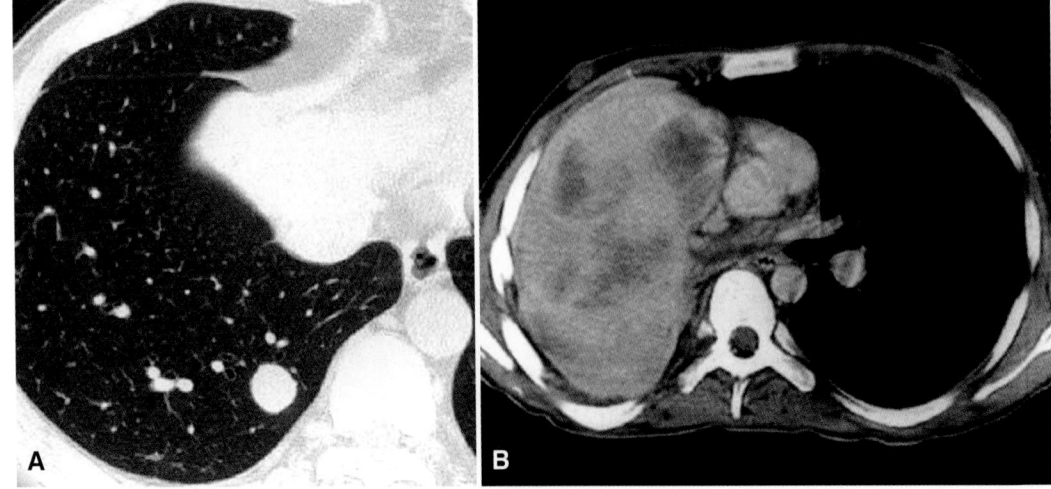

Figure 19-75. Inflammatory myofibroblastic tumors of the lung manifest as a small peripheral nodule (**A**) and a large, variably dense hemithoracic mass (**B**) on computed tomograms.

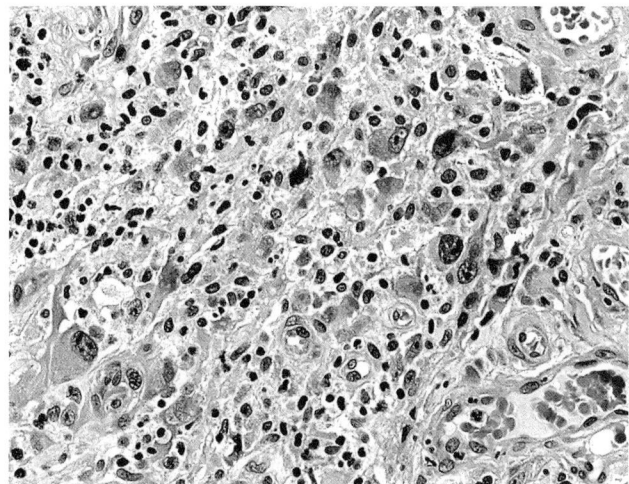

Figure 19-78. This area in an inflammatory myofibroblastic tumor demonstrates moderate pleomorphism of the constituent tumor cells.

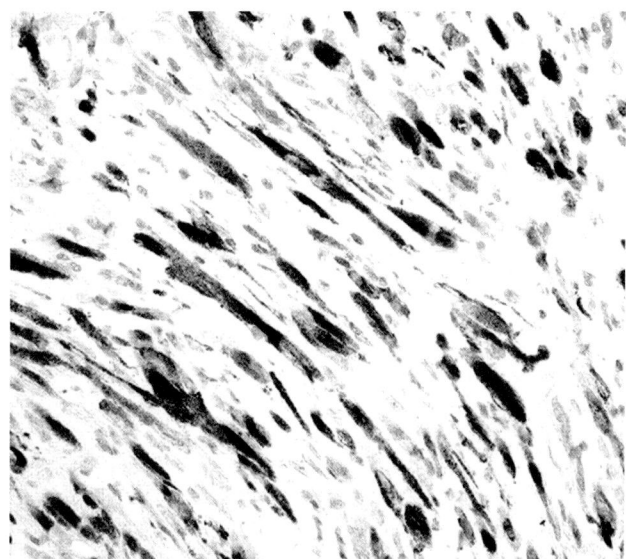

Figure 19-80. Diffuse immunoreactivity is present for ALK-1 protein in this inflammatory myofibroblastic tumor of the lung.

Cytoplasm is amphophilic or lightly eosinophilic and may show a faintly fibrillar character. Admixed inflammatory cells are greatly variable in density and type, and some cases of IMT show virtually none. Lymphocytes, plasma cells, macrophages, eosinophils, and neutrophils are also potentially represented (Fig. 19-79), and intralesional aggregates of xanthomatized foam cells are sometimes apparent. Some cases demonstrate rather striking zones of sclerosis, and these may even be hyalinized. On the other hand, 20% to 30% of these lesions show dense cellularity with focal or global nuclear atypia, relatively high nuclear-to-cytoplasmic ratios, nuclear hyperchromasia, mild nuclear pleomorphism, and zones of necrosis.[295]

Electron microscopic evaluation of IMTs shows that the tumor cells possess some features associated with smooth muscle, such as plasmalemmal dense patches, pinocytotic vesicles, and cytoplasmic bundles of thin (actin-type) filaments. Pericellular basal lamina is variably present, but there are no intercellular attachment complexes.[299]

By immunohistochemical assessment, the spindle cells react with antibodies to vimentin, alpha-isoform and muscle-specific actins, and calponin, but usually not with desmin, caldesmon, CD34, or keratin.[301] Mutant p53 protein is detectable immunohistologically in fewer than 10% of cases.[298] On the other hand, two proteins that relate to

reproducible cytogenetic abnormalities in chromosome 2p23 in IMTs are detectable in approximately 40% of these lesions. These are known as "anaplastic lymphoma kinase 1" (ALK-1; Fig. 19-80) and "p80," and were originally studied in anaplastic large-cell ("Ki-1") lymphomas.[305] Coffin and colleagues[306] found that ALK-1 reactivity predominated in IMTs of patients 20 years of age and older; those lesions also were more likely to demonstrate cytomorphologic atypia.

The differential diagnosis of pulmonary IMT includes tumefactive organizing pneumonia[304]; "true inflammatory pseudotumor" or "plasma cell granuloma" (see Chapter 18); immunoglobulin G4 (IgG4)-predominant lymphoplasmacytic lesions[307]; smooth muscle proliferations in the lung; inflammatory sarcomatoid carcinoma[295] (Fig. 19-81); and inflammatory malignant fibrous histiocytoma. ALK-1/p80 reactivity is diagnostic of IMT in this setting, but as mentioned earlier, is seen in only a minority of cases. The spindle cells of inflammatory sarcomatoid carcinoma can be labeled for keratin and epithelial membrane antigen, in contrast to those of IMT.[295,308] Inflammatory malignant fibrous histiocytoma is typically nonreactive for actins or calponin, as seen in IMT. Spindle cells in organizing pneumonia typically form smaller whorls of spindle cells than IMT.[302] IgG4-predominant lymphoplasmacytic lesions are, by definition, recognized by a preponderance of IgG4-immunoreactive cells in the inflammatory components.[307]

There are few if any pathologic variables that can be used successfully in any given case of IMT to predict its biologic behavior with certainty.[309] Some examples of pulmonary IMT have been observed for extended periods with minimal growth. Spontaneous complete resolution has also been recorded, and a few lesions have diminished in size after nonsurgical therapy.[301] Operative removal is usually necessary to establish a firm diagnosis of IMT, and if the lesion has been completely excised, no further intervention is required. On the other hand, it is logical to expect that incomplete removal—particularly if invasion of adjacent extrapulmonary tissues is present—might, in some instances, be followed by continued growth.[310] In particular, involvement of the pleura, pulmonary hilum, diaphragm, or mediastinum is associated with morbidity from IMTs of the lung. They may even, exceptionally, prove fatal if they are massive and infiltrate the mediastinum extensively, or if distant spread occurs. Overall, recurrence of IMT is seen in approximately 55% of cases, and roughly 10% metastasize.[306]

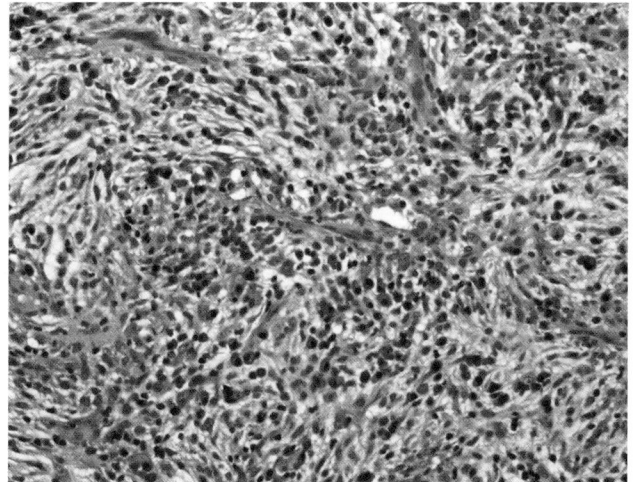

Figure 19-79. Intralesional lymphocytes and plasma cells are numerous in this pulmonary inflammatory myofibroblastic tumor.

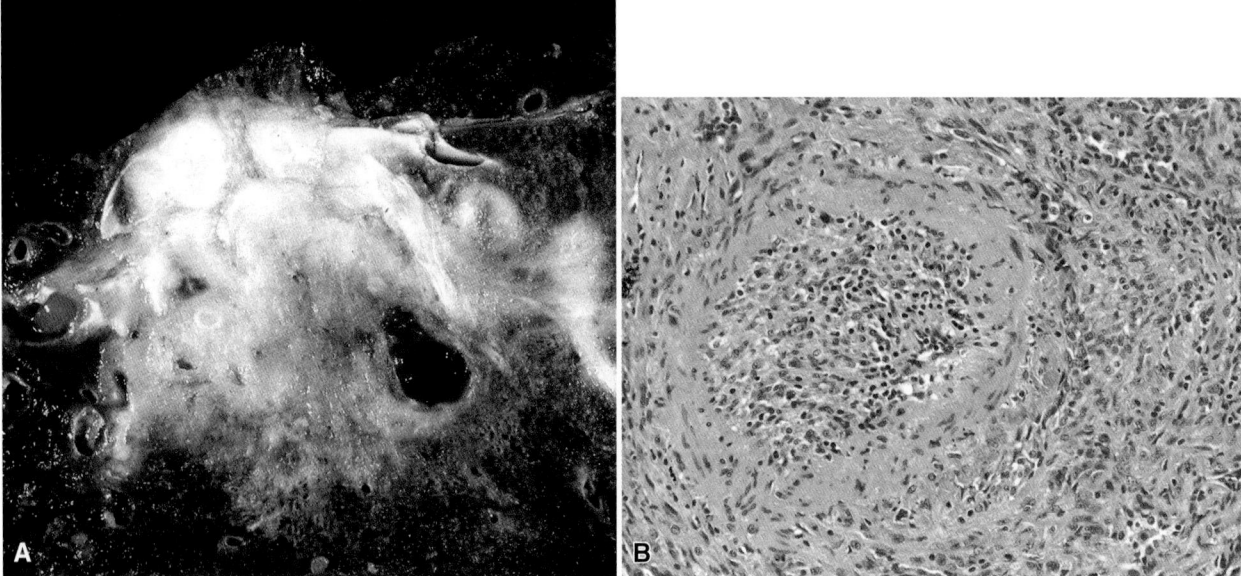

Figure 19-81. Inflammatory sarcomatoid carcinoma (ISC) represents an important differential diagnostic alternative to inflammatory myofibroblastic tumor (IMT). **A,** The gross appearance of such a carcinoma is shown and is similar to that of many IMTs. **B,** Similarly, admixed chronic inflammatory cells are seen in both IMT and ISC. These may obscure the tumor cells, which are best seen in immunostains for keratin and epithelial membrane antigen. Vascular invasion is particularly predominant in ISC, as shown.

Sclerosing Hemangioma ("Pneumocytoma")

More than 50 years ago, Liebow and Hubbell[311] described a peculiar tumor of the peripheral lung parenchyma with a sclerosing, angio-matoid, and papillary architecture. They gave it the name "sclerosing hemangioma," but this designation was chosen in unfortunate mimicry of a convention then extant in dermatopathology. In the 1950s, the lesion now known as "dermatofibroma" or "cutaneous fibrous histiocytoma" was likewise commonly called "sclerosing hemangioma,"[312] because it sometimes showed internal blood lakes and hemosiderosis. In their seminal description of "sclerosing hemangioma" of the lung, Liebow and Hubbell disavowed an endothelial derivation for the tumor and appended the alternative appellations of "histiocytoma" and "xanthoma," perhaps in deference to the true identity of its alleged dermal analog. This enigmatic series of nosologic and terminologic choices set the stage for confusion in the succeeding decades. Various studies of the cellular nature of pulmonary "sclerosing hemangioma" have suggested vascular, fibrohistiocytic, mesothelial, and epithelial lineages,[313–317] and controversies over such proposals persist to some extent.

Based on the aggregated data,[318,319] this tumor is properly considered as a neoplasm showing differentiation that is most like that of embryonic (uncommitted) respiratory epithelium. Therefore, the entity in question is best designated as "pneumocytoma," as suggested by Shimosato[320]; however, the World Health Organization has persisted in using the historic name "sclerosing hemangioma."

Sclerosing hemangioma can affect patients of almost any age, from early childhood[321] through the end of life. Females predominate by a factor of 5:1.[322–332] Only approximately 20% of patients have any respiratory symptoms at the time their tumors are found. It may arise in any of the pulmonary lobes; localization in the large airways, pleura, and mediastinum has been rarely reported.[322,333]

Radiographically, patients with sclerosing hemangioma usually have solitary peripheral masses with well-defined homogeneous round or oval profiles on chest roentgenograms (Fig. 19-82). CT shows homogeneity and high density of the lesions in the great majority of cases (Fig. 19-83); low-density areas may be apparent in some tumors because of cystic change. In addition, the "air meniscus sign" (also known as the

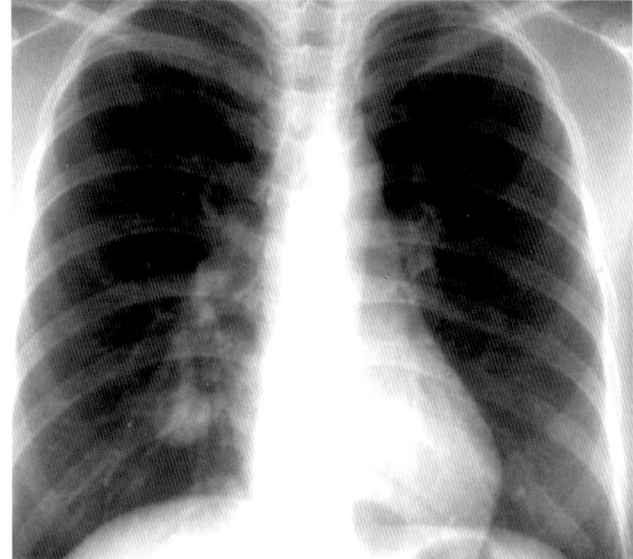

Figure 19-82. This plain-film chest radiograph demonstrates a relatively well-delineated nodular lesion in the mid-right lung field, representing a sclerosing hemangioma.

"air trapping" or "air crescent" sign)[327,328,334]—a rim of air that partially or circumferentially surrounds a mass—is evident in the lung parenchyma adjacent to some lesions of this type.

Grossly, most sclerosing hemangiomas are less than 3 cm in maximum dimension (Fig. 19-84), but sometimes they attain a size of up to 10 cm. Multifocality, sometimes featuring a satellitotic configuration of small nodules around a dominant central nodule,[322] is apparent in approximately 4% of cases.[335] Roughly the same proportion are pleural-based and may be polypoid, potentially simulating the appearance of solitary fibrous tumors.[322] Sharp circumscription from the surrounding lung parenchyma is the rule, so much so that these tumors are sometimes "shelled out" by the surgeon with little if any attached

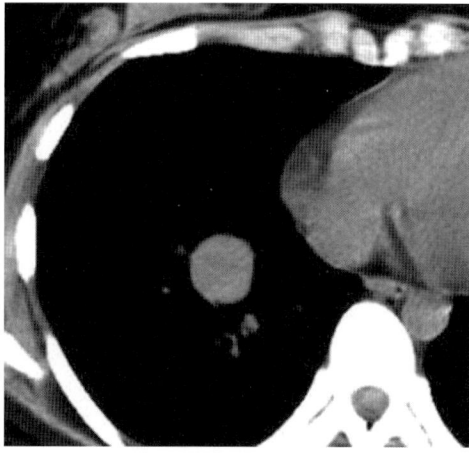

Figure 19-83. A sclerosing hemangioma. This computed tomogram of the lesion shown in Figure 19-82 shows a circumscribed spherical tumor with a uniform internal density.

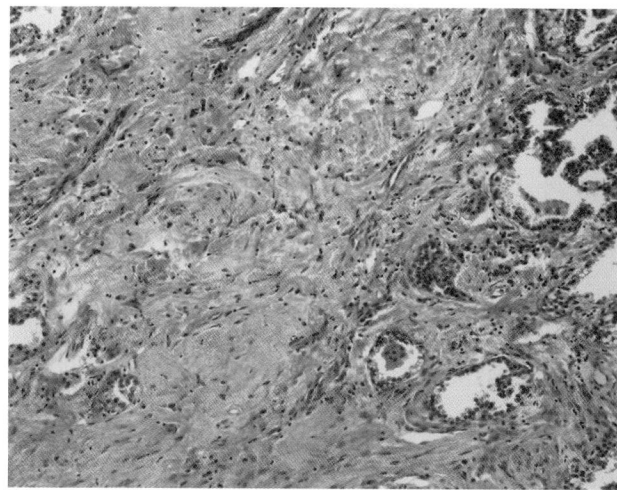

Figure 19-85. Stromal sclerosis is prominent in this sclerosing hemangioma.

alveolated tissue. Their cut surfaces are tan-gray, yellow, or mottled. Cystic areas are evident in roughly 3% of cases; 20% show areas of intralesional hemorrhage, which may be extensive.

The histologic images of sclerosing hemangioma include varying admixtures of four basic growth patterns—sclerotic (Fig. 19-85), papillary (Fig. 19-86), solid (Fig. 19-87), and hemorrhagic/angiomatoid (Fig. 19-88). Approximately 15% of cases are monomorphic, and roughly 20% contain areas representing all of the patterns in the same lesion. Two basic cell types comprise the neoplastic elements in sclerosing hemangioma—"surface" cells, which mantle papillary projections, and "round" cells, seen in the cores of papillary structures and in solid sheets within the lesions. Surface cells often show intranuclear invaginations of cytoplasm, yielding "pseudoinclusions" such as those seen in type II pneumocytes and Clara cells. They also may be multinucleated. Round cells are actually polygonal, with oval nuclei, dispersed chromatin, indiscernible nucleoli, and extremely rare mitotic figures. They may focally exhibit cytoplasmic vacuolation and even assume the morphologic

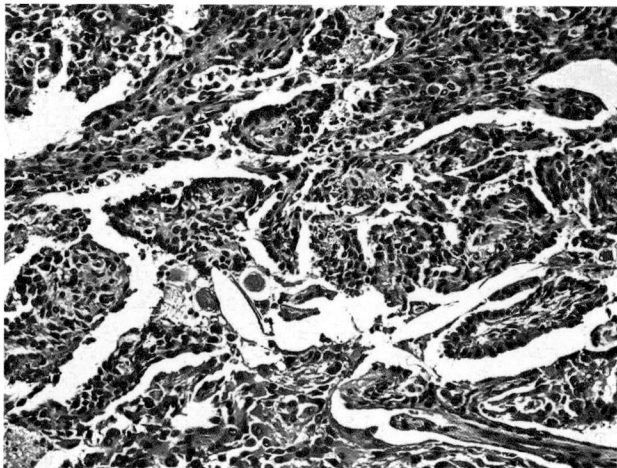

Figure 19-86. Papillary epithelial groups are numerous in this sclerosing hemangioma.

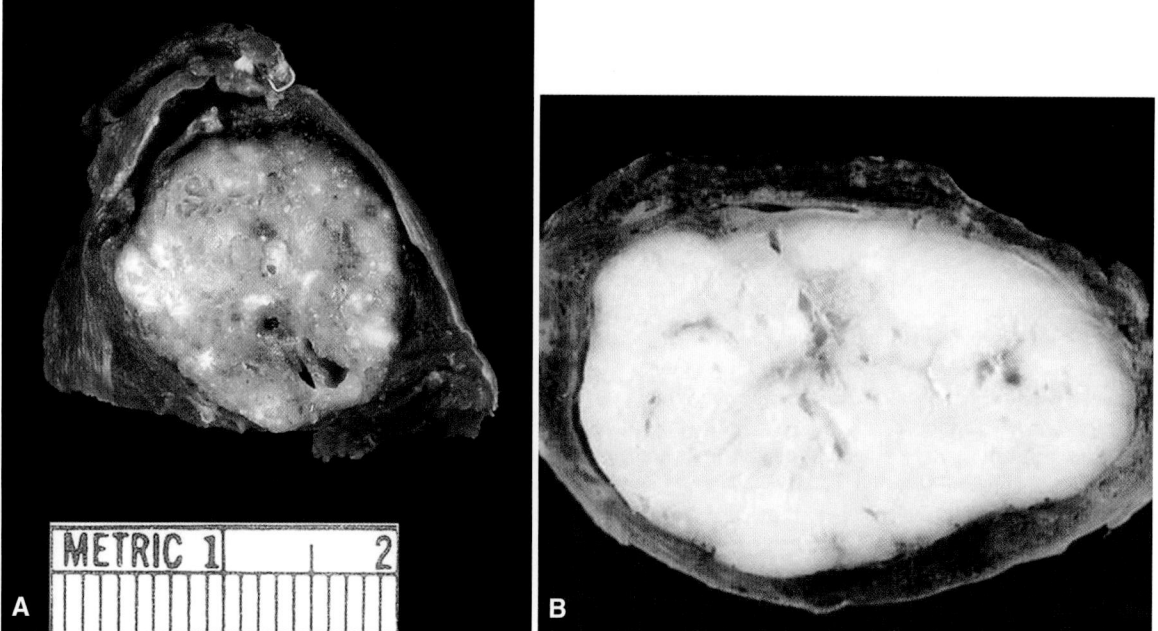

Figure 19-84. **A** and **B,** Gross photographs of a sclerosing hemangioma, showing circumscribed white-yellow nodules in the peripheral lung parenchyma.

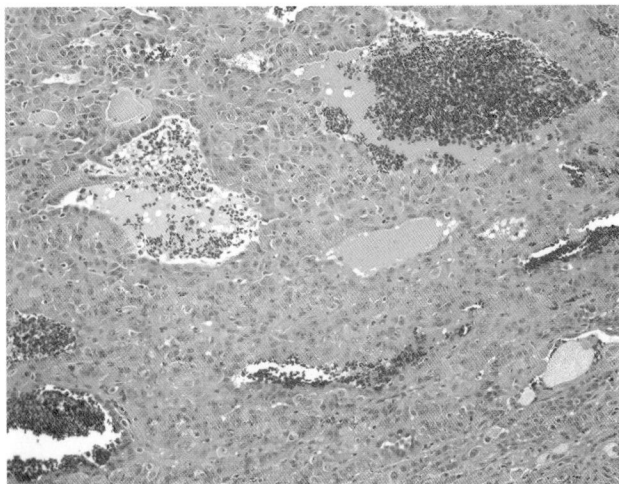

Figure 19-87. Solid growth of polygonal cells is apparent in this sclerosing hemangioma.

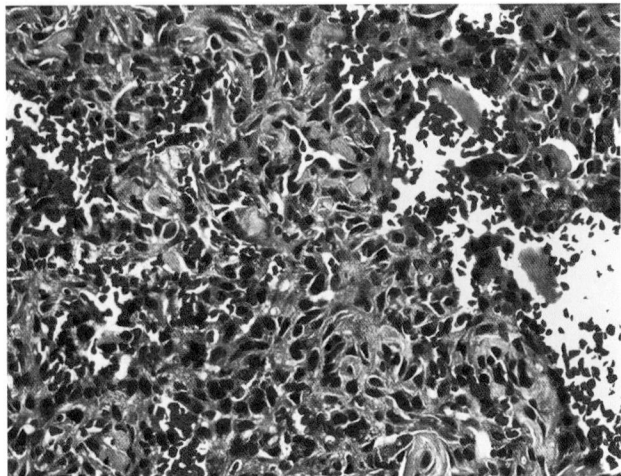

Figure 19-88. An angiomatoid focus is evident in this sclerosing hemangioma.

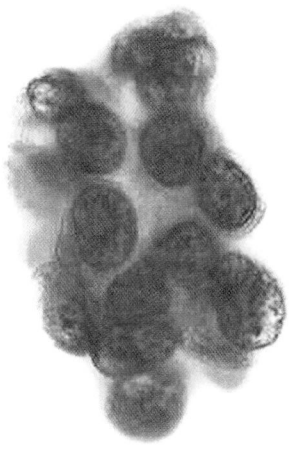

Figure 19-89. Fine-needle aspiration biopsy specimen of a sclerosing hemangioma, showing a three-dimensional group of epithelioid cells with increased nuclear-cytoplasmic ratios and distinct nucleoli. There is a strong resemblance to the cytopathologic appearance of adenocarcinoma.

features of a signet ring cell. Rarely, nuclear hyperchromasia and moderate pleomorphism are seen in the round cell element.[322,336]

Secondary features of sclerosing hemangioma include blood lakes in angiomatoid foci; limited areas of necrosis; stromal hemosiderosis, calcification, cholesterolosis, or combinations thereof; internal cystification, with mucinous contents; granulomatous inflammation; and a potential association with foci of neuroendocrine hyperplasia ("tumorlets") in the surrounding lung parenchyma.[322,323,336,337]

We have previously stated our opinion that pneumocytoma/sclerosing hemangioma, alveolar adenoma, and papillary adenoma comprise a biologically interrelated family of pulmonary lesions. Nevertheless, these entities differ morphologically, in that sclerosing hemangioma lacks the "Swiss cheese" microcystic structure of alveolar adenoma and papillary adenoma does not contain the "round cell" elements of sclerosing hemangioma.[158]

Several publications have addressed FNA biopsy findings in sclerosing hemangioma, and most have noted substantial morphologic overlap between those lesions and well-differentiated adenocarcinomas (particularly of the bronchioloalveolar type).[326,329,330,338–340] A shared potential for nuclear atypia, intranuclear pseudoinclusions, and micropapillary growth in both tumor entities makes the definitive cytologic recognition of sclerosing hemangioma very difficult (Fig. 19-89). Despite assertions that it can be accomplished,[341] we believe that an unqualified interpretation of sclerosing hemangioma by FNA biopsy

is unwise. In appropriate cases, that possibility can be included in the diagnostic report, prompting an intraoperative frozen-section examination to further guide the surgeon's choice of procedure. This proviso relates to the very close cytologic similarity we have noted between pneumocytoma and selected adenocarcinomas.

Electron microscopy of sclerosing hemangiomas has shown that both the surface cell and round cell components demonstrate type II pneumocytic features, containing cytoplasmic lamellar bodies with variable levels of maturation.[315,322] Other organelles are nonspecific. These findings support the interrelatedness of sclerosing hemangioma and papillary adenoma.

Immunohistologically, variable reactivity has been seen for keratin, epithelial membrane antigen (EMA), surfactant-related proteins, Clara cell antigen, and thyroid transcription factor 1 in both cellular components of sclerosing hemangioma[322,331,332,338,342–349] (Fig. 19-90). Receptors for estrogen and progesterone are also demonstrable in a minority of cases.[322] On the other hand, mesothelial markers, such as calretinin, HBME-1, cytokeratin 5/6, and WT-1 protein are absent in these lesions, as are neuroendocrine, neural, and myogenous determinants.

Justification for inclusion of sclerosing hemangioma as a "borderline" lesion stems from reports of its recurrence[341,350] and the finding of lymph nodal metastases in 10 patients to date.[322,324,351–353] In the U.S. Armed Forces Institute of Pathology series, this behavior was observed in 1% of cases.[322] Despite that observation, no patient with metastatic tumor has died of the tumor, and lymph node involvement[324] does not appear to affect survival.

As mentioned earlier, the principal differential diagnostic alternative to sclerosing hemangioma is low-grade adenocarcinoma of bronchioloalveolar or conventional types.[330,339,340] An adequate tissue sample—allowing for evaluation of the architecture of the entire mass—is essential to making that distinction. Another diagnostic possibility is the papillary variant of low-grade mucoepidermoid carcinoma,[354] but its particular histologic pattern, with an intimate admixture of mucinous and squamous epithelium, should allow for a distinction from sclerosing hemangioma.

Pulmonary Mucinous Cystadenoma and Borderline Mucinous Tumor

Mucinous cystadenomas and cystic mucinous tumors of low malignant potential—"borderline" mucinous neoplasms (BMTs)—are well known to gynecologic and gastrointestinal pathologists because they rather commonly arise in the ovaries, gut, and pancreas.[355,356] A primary origin in the lung for such lesions is unusual, but possible, and approximately 50 cases have been reported.[357–369] These neoplasms occur in adults as solitary lesions in the peripheral parenchyma. An association with von Hippel-Lindau disease has been reported.[369] Both plain films

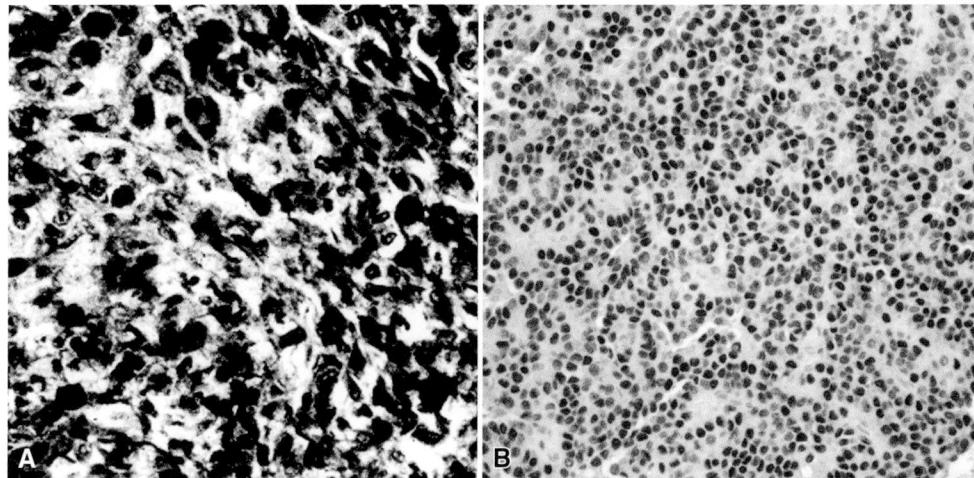

Figure 19-90. A sclerosing hemangioma with immunoreactivity for keratin showing staining of the surface cells (**A**), and for thyroid transcription factor 1 (**B**), supporting its identity as a respiratory epithelial neoplasm.

and CTs of the thorax clearly show the cystic nature of these tumors (Fig. 19-91), which generally measure several centimeters in diameter.

Grossly, mucinous cystadenomas and BMTs are sharply demarcated from the surrounding lung parenchyma (Fig. 19-92) and may even "shell out" for the surgeon. Their walls are relatively thick and fibrous, enclosing locules that contain thick viscous mucoid material. Foci of

granular tissue are present on the internal aspects of the cysts, representing epithelial projections.

Histologically, the latter structures comprise cytologically bland mucin-containing tumor cells that are cuboidal or low columnar (Fig. 19-93). Nuclei are generally basally located and relatively banal, with no pleomorphism or mitotic activity (Fig. 19-94). Cystadenomas do not demonstrate invasive growth into the fibrous walls of the lesions, but BMTs may do so, and may manifest a "piling up" of lesional epithelium that yields complex micropapillary structures (Fig. 19-95). Cases in which frank adenocarcinoma evolved from pre-existing pulmonary mucinous cystadenoma have been reported (Fig. 19-96).[358,364,368]

The differential diagnosis for these lesions is largely academic. The clinical and histologic features of such tumors are quite different from those of other respiratory tract lesions that may contain mucin. The latter include mucoepidermoid carcinoma, mucous gland adenoma, and bronchioloalveolar carcinoma.

The classification of pulmonary BMT as a neoplasm with low malignant potential is supported by the observations of Gao and Urbanski.[368] Those authors documented a mortality rate (due to metastatic tumor) of 30% in their series, with up to 10 years of postoperative surveillance, raising the possibility that these should be considered frank carcinomas rather than borderline lesions. They further described a *spectrum* of histologic appearances in the epithelium of BMT, ranging from

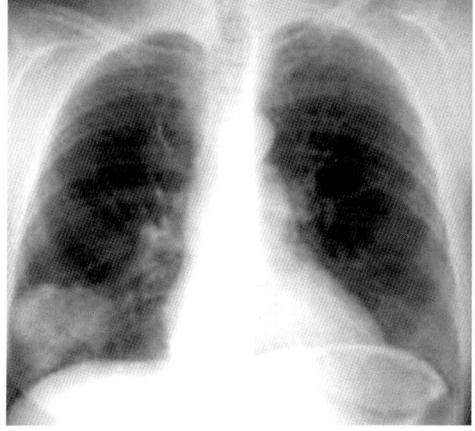

Figure 19-91. This chest radiograph shows a large ovoid mass in the right lower lung field, representing a cystic mucinous tumor.

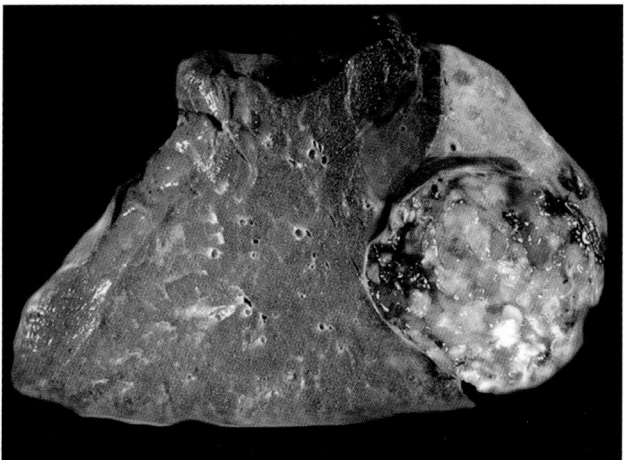

Figure 19-92. Gross photograph of a cystic mucinous tumor of the lung showing circumscription from the lung parenchyma and mucoid lesional contents.

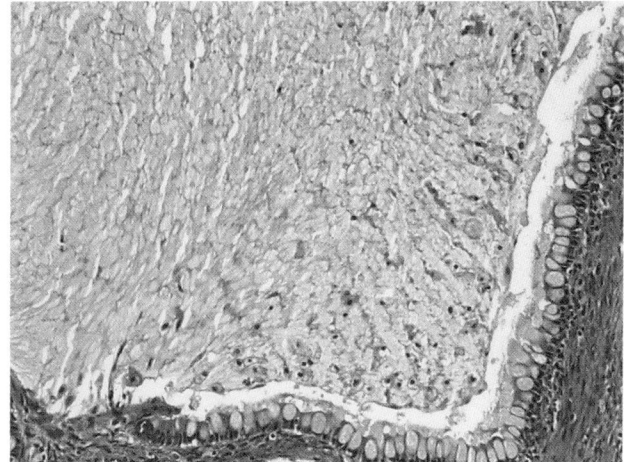

Figure 19-93. Mucinous cystadenoma of the lung showing a fibrous cyst wall mantled by bland mucinous epithelial cells. The cavity of the lesion contains abundant and inspissated mucinous material.

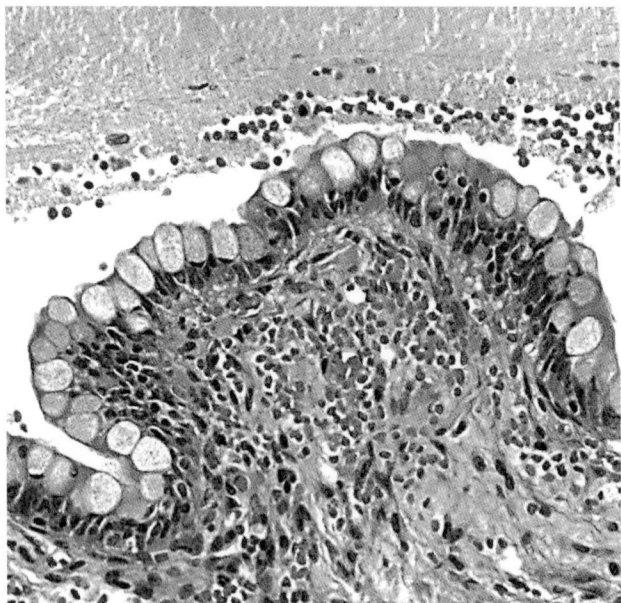

Figure 19-94. The neoplastic epithelial cells of pulmonary mucinous cystadenoma are banal with no significant nuclear atypia. Cytoplasmic mucin is apparent.

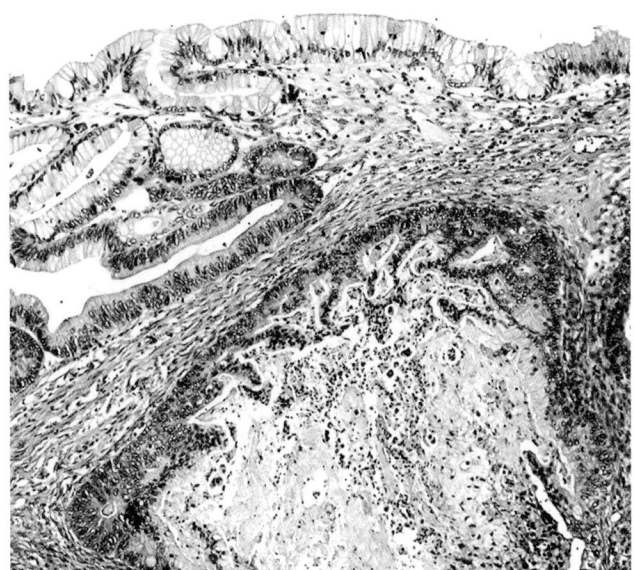

Figure 19-96. Some pulmonary cystic mucinous tumors undergo overtly malignant evolution, as shown by this example containing invasive adenocarcinoma (*bottom*).

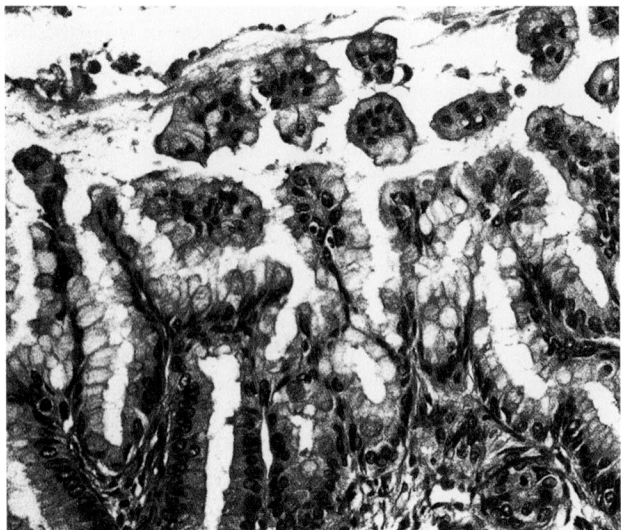

Figure 19-95. Micropapillary growth is evident in some cystic mucinous tumors of the lung, justifying use of the term "borderline."

completely bland to overtly malignant. Pathologic findings that were proposed as adverse prognosticators included solid epithelial growth at the periphery of the lesion, adhesion of the tumor to the pleura, crossing of the intrapulmonary septa by the tumor, obvious nuclear atypicality, and invasive growth into the surrounding lung tissue.[368]

Solitary Fibrous Tumor

Solitary fibrous tumor (SFT; formerly called "fibroma")[370,371] of the lung and pleura is still confused by some clinicians with mesothelial neoplasms. That is because of a nosologic scheme advanced by Klemperer and Rabin in 1931[372] that was used for many years thereafter and gave SFT the designation of "localized fibrous mesothelioma." Particularly in the last two decades, much work has been done that unequivocally shows that SFT lacks mesothelial differentiation[373]; instead, this tumor is composed of facultative fibroblastic elements such as those seen in the submesothelial zone of the normal lung.

Even though it may occasionally recur and sometimes demonstrates locally aggressive growth—justifying its classification as a "borderline" mesenchymal tumor—SFT generally has a favorable prognosis that differs markedly from that of mesothelioma.[373–383] Likewise, pleural fibrous tumors have no etiologic relationship whatsoever to occupational-level asbestos exposure, in contrast to a proportion of mesotheliomas.[381]

Approximately two mesotheliomas are encountered for every SFT in general thoracic surgical practice.[373] Outside of infancy, patients of any age may have an SFT, but they are most often seen in patients older than 40 years old, with no sex predilection. The great majority of cases present with an asymptomatic pleuropulmonary mass that is seen on screening radiographs. Rarely, one of two paraneoplastic complexes accompanies SFT; those are represented by hypertrophic osteoarthropathy and tumor-associated hypoglycemia (Doege-Potter syndrome).[381] The cause of the first condition is unknown; the second is related to an insulin-like growth factor that is produced by the neoplastic cells.

Radiographically, SFT may be as small as 1 cm in maximal dimension or as large as 36 cm. Occasional lesions of this type have occupied virtually an entire hemithorax and weighed in excess of 5 kg.[380] They are usually globoid neoplasms with a relatively homogeneous internal density, but cystic change, calcification, or foci of necrosis may be sometimes apparent (Fig. 19-97). A minority of cases demonstrate a pedicle that attaches an SFT in the pleural space to the pleura itself. Conversely, other lesions "invert" into the lung parenchyma or may arise from interlobar pleural reflections, producing the appearance of a peripheral intrapulmonary mass[370,371,384–388]; large tumors also may displace the trachea or intramediastinal structures.[373] Rarely, overt invasion of the chest wall, vertebral bodies, or adjacent lung tissue is apparent on imaging studies.[384,389] A small number of SFTs show regional satellitotic growth in the pleura.[388]

Gross examination shows a lobulated mass that is invested by pleural tissue (Fig. 19-98). Cut surfaces can be homogeneous, tan-gray, and vaguely "whorled," or may show distinct internal septa and foci of degeneration, mucoid change, hemorrhage, calcification, or necrosis.[383,384] Intralesional cystic change can also be present.

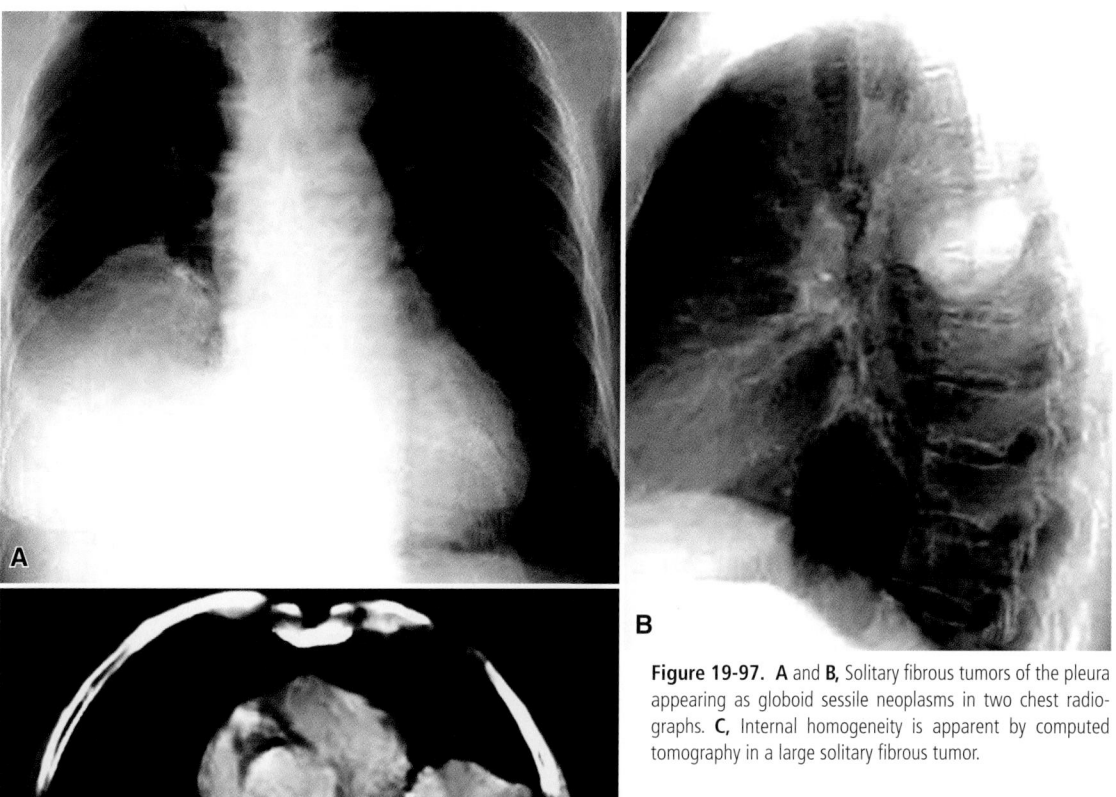

Figure 19-97. **A** and **B**, Solitary fibrous tumors of the pleura appearing as globoid sessile neoplasms in two chest radiographs. **C**, Internal homogeneity is apparent by computed tomography in a large solitary fibrous tumor.

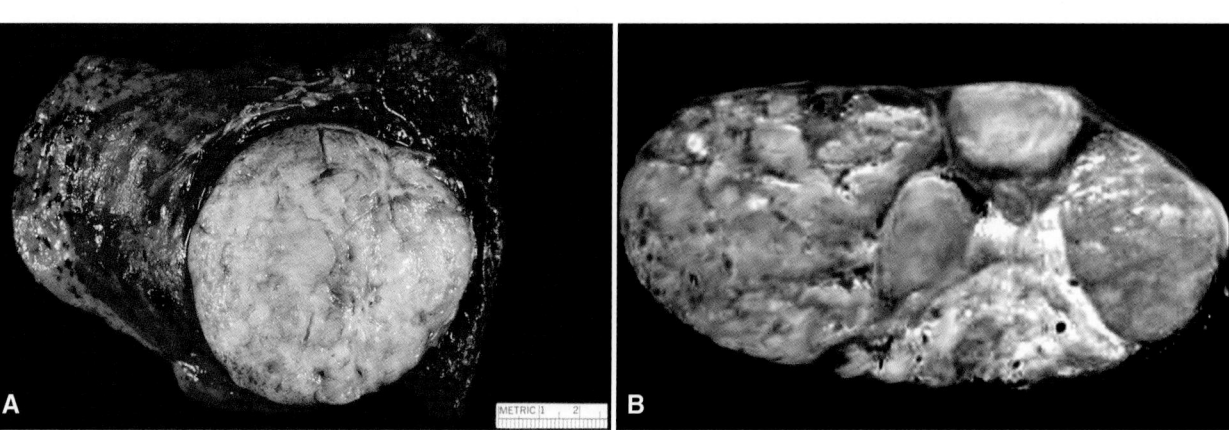

Figure 19-98. The gross cut surfaces of solitary fibrous pleural tumors may be either homogeneous (**A**) or septated, and tan-white to yellow, with foci of degeneration or necrosis (**B**).

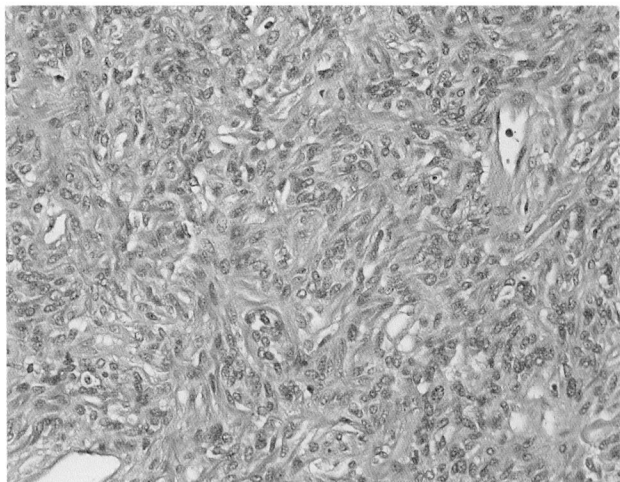

Figure 19-99. A "patternless pattern" is apparent in this solitary fibrous pleural tumor, wherein spindle cells are randomly arranged.

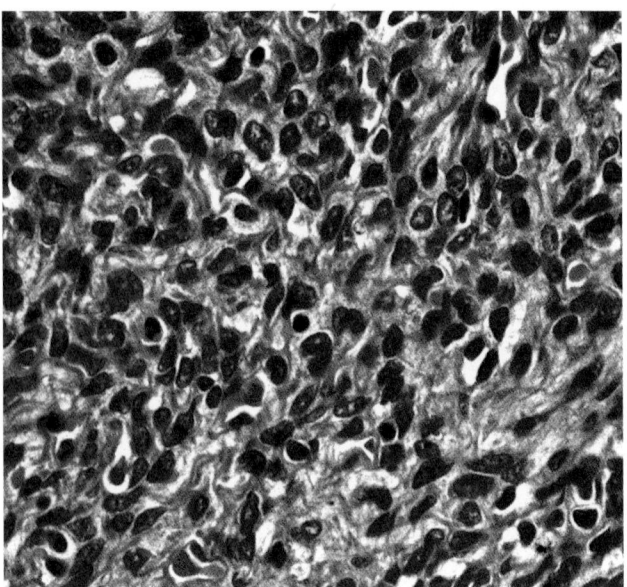

Figure 19-100. Epithelioid cytologic composition is seen in this solitary fibrous tumor of the pleura, potentially simulating the appearance of synovial sarcoma or hemangiopericytoma.

The microscopic spectrum of pleuropulmonary SFT is broad.[383] A solid spindle cell growth and a diffuse sclerosing pattern are most frequent. In the first of these configurations, fusiform cells are arranged in random arrays (a "patternless pattern") (Fig. 19-99), with fascicular groupings, storiform or herringbone patterns, or regimented arrays with nuclear palisading. SFT may also have epithelioid cells (Fig. 19-100) and branched intralesional blood vessels resembling "moose antlers," as seen in hemangiopericytoma (which has been merged nosologically with SFT) or synovial sarcoma. Zones of fibrosis may be interspersed with cellular zones and dominate in lesions classified as "diffuse sclerosing" SFT (Fig. 19-101). Focal collagenous degeneration is occasionally apparent, simulating true necrosis. Less frequent features include multinucleated tumor giant cells, "amianthoid" arrays of collagen fibers, myxoid stromal change, limited areas of spontaneous necrosis, hemorrhage, and metaplastic ossification. Mitotic activity in most SFTs is present but not prominent, and division figures are normal.

England and associates[384] attempted a codification of criteria for malignancy in SFT. These included dense cellularity with overlapping nuclei; nuclear hyperchromasia and pleomorphism

(Fig. 19-102); mitotic activity greater than four division figures per 10 high-power (×400) microscopic fields; and necrosis and hemorrhage. However, only 55% of the lesions with such features actually had an aggressive course, with recurrence, metastasis, or both. Harrison-Phipps and colleagues[390] found that approximately 13% of SFTs showed the "malignant" attributes described earlier, and they also noted that the likelihood of morphologic atypia correlated directly with tumor size. In that series, "malignant" SFTs averaged 12 cm in maximal dimension, compared with 4.5 cm for tumors that lacked histologic atypia. Vallat-Decouvelaere and coworkers[375] also emphasized that histologic findings in SFTs may not be accurate predictors of their behavior. In line with this admonition, a small proportion of histologically banal SFTs manifest untoward behavior, typically with invasion of the bony structures and soft tissues of the thorax, or recurrence.[373,381] Because of these attributes, it is best

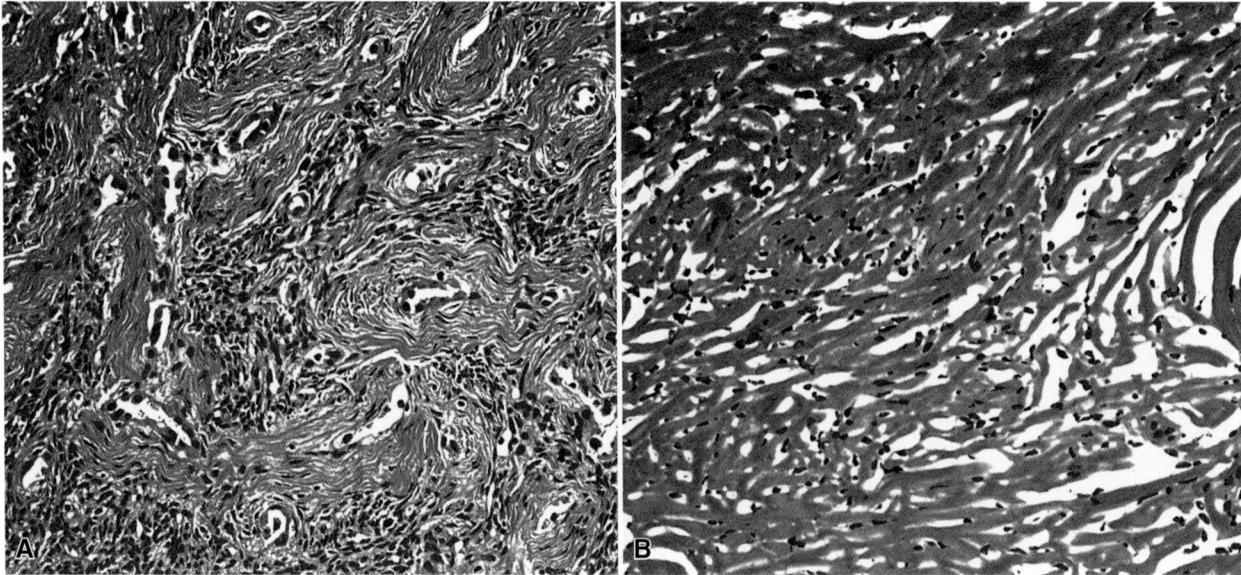

Figure 19-101. **A** and **B,** Hyalinizing collagenous stroma is prominent in this solitary fibrous pleural tumor.

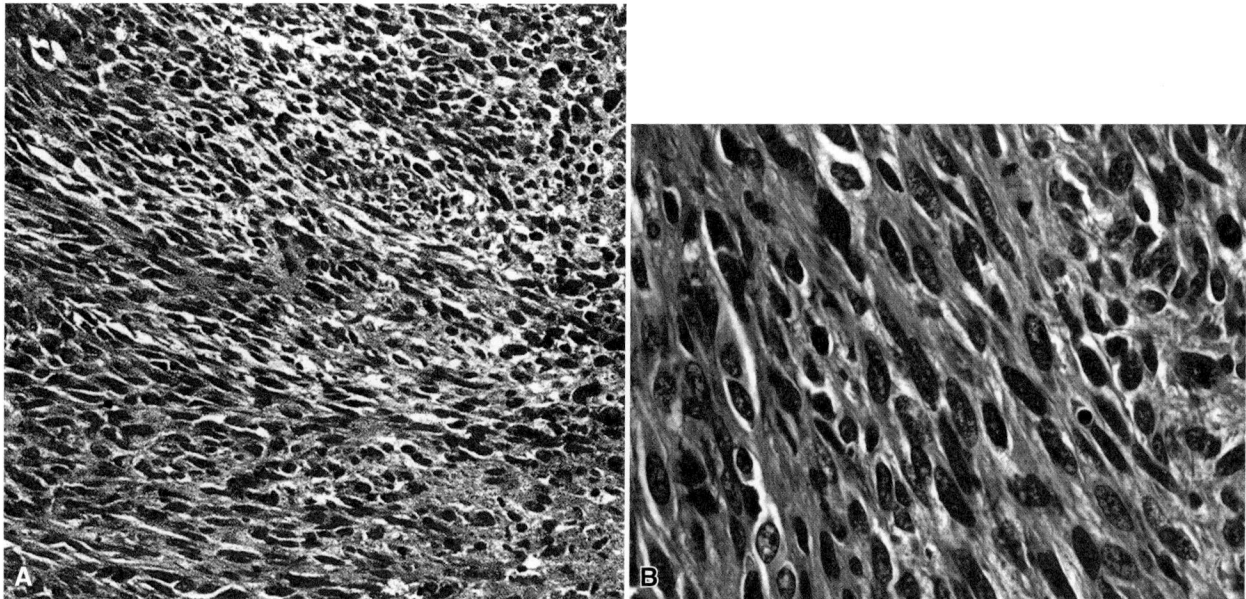

Figure 19-102. Atypical features seen in a solitary fibrous pleural tumor that raise the possibility of malignancy include uniformly dense cellularity (**A**) and nuclear overlapping with vesicular change in chromatin (**B**).

to consider SFT a borderline neoplasm. As Vallat-Decouvelaere and colleagues[375] sagely stated, *"it is probably unwise to regard any such lesion as definitely benign."*

In FNA biopsy specimens,[389,391,392] smears show variably cohesive and pleomorphic spindle cells in a bloody background, representing an image that corresponds to a sizable differential diagnosis. Preparation of cell block sections and procurement of adjunctive pathologic studies is essential to a specific diagnosis.

Electron microscopic analysis of SFT has shown that the tumor cells are fibroblast-like. They lack basal lamina, intercellular junctions, and plasmalemmal microvilli, as expected in epithelial or mesothelial cells, and instead contain only basic intracellular organelles.[381] Occasionally, intrareticular collagen fibrils are apparent within profiles of endoplasmic reticulum.

Immunophenotypically, SFT demonstrates reactivity for vimentin, CD34, CD99, and bcl-2 protein in more than 85% of cases[375,382,384,389,392–396] (Fig. 19-103). There is typically no labeling for keratin, EMA, desmin, actins, S-100 protein, collagen type IV, CD31, or CD57. Anecdotally, lesions with malignant histologic features may exhibit mutant p53 protein immunoreactivity,[397] but this relationship has not been subjected to rigorous evaluation.

Cytogenetic assessment of SFT is still developmental. However, the most frequent defects reported in this tumor type have involved chromosomes 4q, 8, 13q, 15q, and 21q.[398,399] One case has shown a balanced t(4;15)(q13;q26) translocation.[399]

The differential diagnosis of pleuropulmonary SFT includes primary and secondary sarcomatoid carcinoma, sarcomatoid or desmoplastic mesothelioma, fibrosarcoma, storiform malignant fibrous histiocytoma,

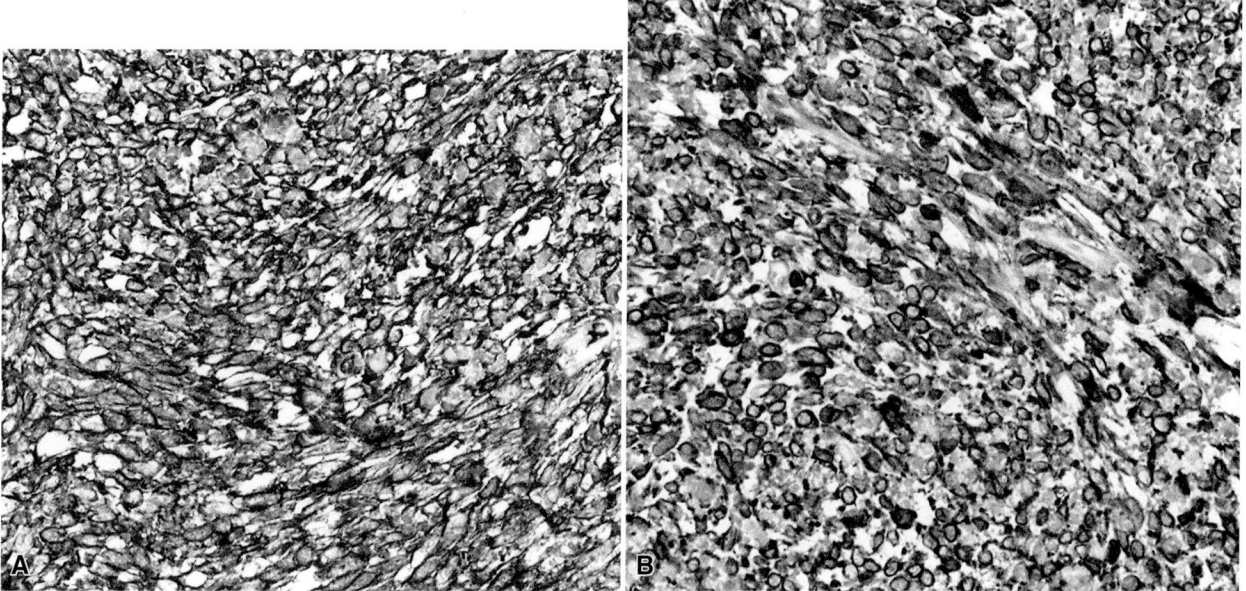

Figure 19-103. Diffuse immunoreactivity for CD34 (**A**) and CD99 (**B**) is characteristic of solitary fibrous tumors.

synovial sarcoma, hemangiopericytoma, and metastatic endometrial stromal sarcoma.[383] Among these possibilities, carcinomas, mesotheliomas, and synovial sarcomas may be excluded because of their immunoreactivity for keratin, EMA, or both. In addition, synovial sarcoma reproducibly shows a t(X;18) chromosomal translocation[400] and nuclear immunoreactivity for transducin-like enhancer of split 1 (TLE1),[401] both of which are absent in SFT. Consistent CD10 reactivity in metastatic endometrial stromal sarcoma differs from the properties of SFT.[402] Fibrosarcoma and malignant fibrous histiocytoma lack CD34, CD99, and bcl-2 protein, all of which are typically manifest in SFT.

The biologic attributes of SFT have been largely discussed previously. However, some of its characteristics merit reiteration. Approximately 10% of "ordinary" intrathoracic SFTs (lacking histologic indicators of possible malignancy) recur, sometimes massively.[373,403] This behavior has most often been linked to incomplete lesional excision at initial surgery, and salvage of the patient is still a distinct possibility if total removal of the tumor (e.g., by extrapleural pneumonectomy)[404] can be accomplished.[295,297] Metastatic disease is very unusual,[405] and it tends to be refractory to oncologic intervention.

Desmoid Tumor

"Desmoid" tumor (DT) is best known as a borderline neoplasm of the deep soft tissues and as a member of the family of fibromatoses.[406,407] It can be seen sporadically in patients of virtually any age, but also has a biologic linkage to familial adenomatous polyposis syndrome, in which it is over-represented.[408] Wherever it arises in the body, DT pursues a slowly progressive, infiltrative course of growth, eventually impinging on nerves, blood vessels, and other anatomic structures. That property accounts for associated symptoms and signs, which reflect secondary compressive effects of the mass.[406]

Several examples of DT have been reported as apparently primary pleural neoplasms.[409-413] Demographic, radiologic, and clinical findings in such cases are superimposable on those associated with SFT.[409,413] Pleural desmoids are deceptively circumscribed in imaging studies, and they typically have a homogeneous radiodensity (Fig. 19-104).

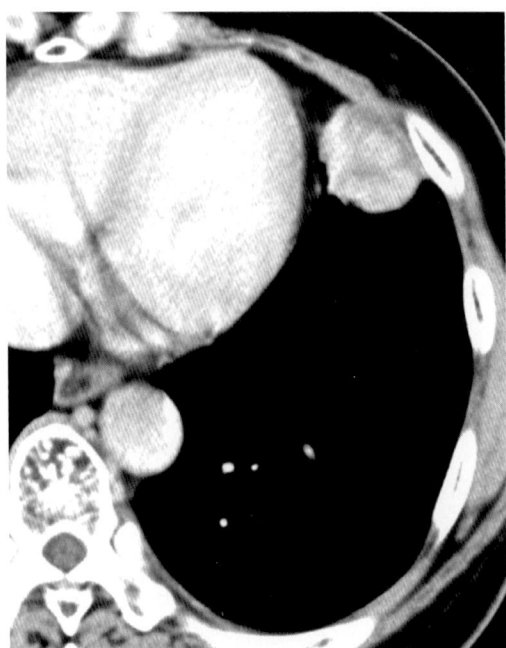

Figure 19-104. Desmoid tumor of the pleura represented by a localized peripheral thoracic mass that resembles solitary fibrous tumors on computed tomography.

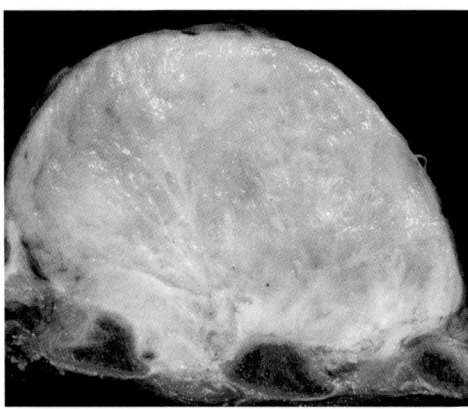

Figure 19-105. Desmoid tumors form homogeneous tan-pink masses. In this case, there is invasion into the chest wall as cut surfaces of the ribs are evident.

Grossly, DTs of the pleura show a fleshy, uniform, tan-gray cut surface with subtly incorporated bands of internal fibrous tissue (Fig. 19-105). They often appear to have a distinct interface with surrounding tissues, but this attribute is misleading because microscopic study often shows tumor growth beyond the gross boundaries of the lesion.

Histologically, the usual appearance of pleural DT is reproducible. It is a hypocellular neoplasm that composes bland fusiform and stellate cells, set in a fibromyxoid stroma (Fig. 19-106). Mitoses are absent or rare; nuclear atypia and necrosis are lacking.[406,407] A helpful diagnostic feature is the presence of regularly spaced small blood vessels throughout the lesion; these have open round or oval lumina and relatively thick pericytic cuffs. As mentioned earlier, permeative infiltration of surrounding tissues by the tumor is common.

A potential diagnostic trap is represented by selected examples of DT that have a markedly myxedematous stroma, with or without extravasated erythrocytes (Fig. 19-107). The resulting microscopic image can strongly resemble that of nodular fasciitis, a completely innocuous pseudoneoplastic condition.[414] Nodular fasciitis has not been reported in the pleura, however.

Fine-needle aspiration biopsy of DT may show either hypocellular or hypercellular foci, often in juxtaposition.[415] The stromal staining characteristics are those of mature collagen. Individual tumor cells are dyshesive and morphologically bland, with tapered ends, fusiform nuclei, dispersed chromatin, and a lack of pleomorphism.

As a derivative of the association between desmoids and familial adenomatous polyposis syndrome, beta-catenin protein is usually dysregulated in DT. Instead of exclusively cytoplasmic immunolocalization of that moiety, it is instead seen as an intranuclear reactant (Fig. 19-108).[409,415-417] Unfortunately, an important (if not the principal) differential diagnostic consideration—solitary fibrous tumor—also commonly demonstrates nuclear labeling for beta-catenin.[417,418] Hence, one must rely on other immunohistochemical discriminants to separate those two neoplasms. DT is reactive for alpha-isoform and "muscle-specific" actins, and sometimes for desmin, whereas SFT is not.[409] Conversely, reactivity for CD34 and CD99 is common in SFT but absent in DT. Diagnostic distinctions among DT, other myofibroblastic proliferations, leiomyomas, and low-grade leiomyosarcomas are not possible at an immunohistochemical level of analysis[409,415] and must be made by other means.

The biologic behavior of DT approximates that of low-grade sarcomas; local recurrences can be tenacious and even life-threatening, but distant metastasis does not occur.[406,407,413] Curative surgical excision requires complete removal of the mass.[419,420]

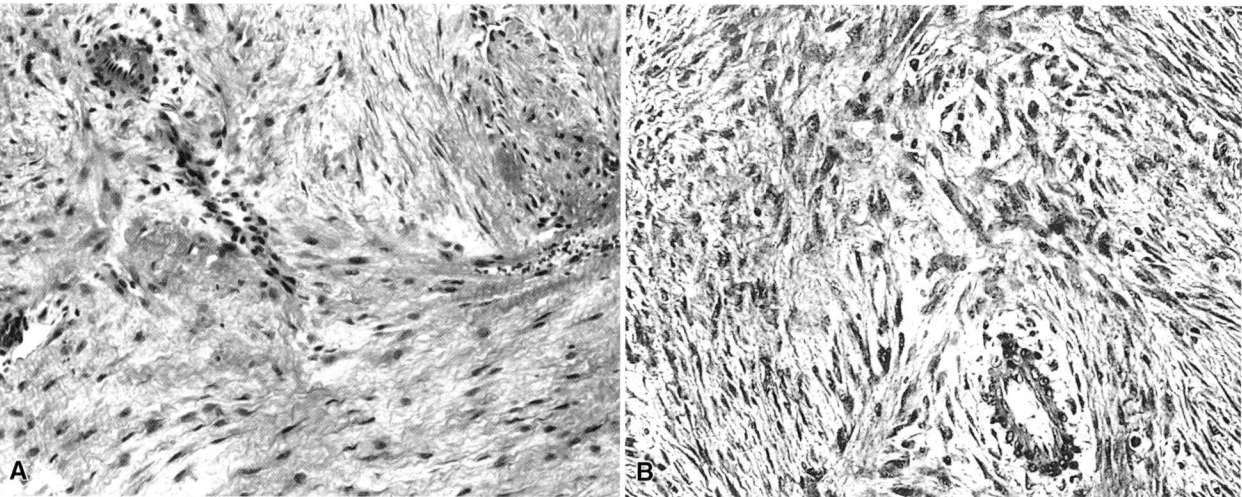

Figure 19-106. A and **B,** Desmoid tumors comprise vague fascicles of bland spindle cells that are set in a variably fibrous or myxoedematous stroma. Supporting blood vessels are small, but have relatively thick walls and open lumina.

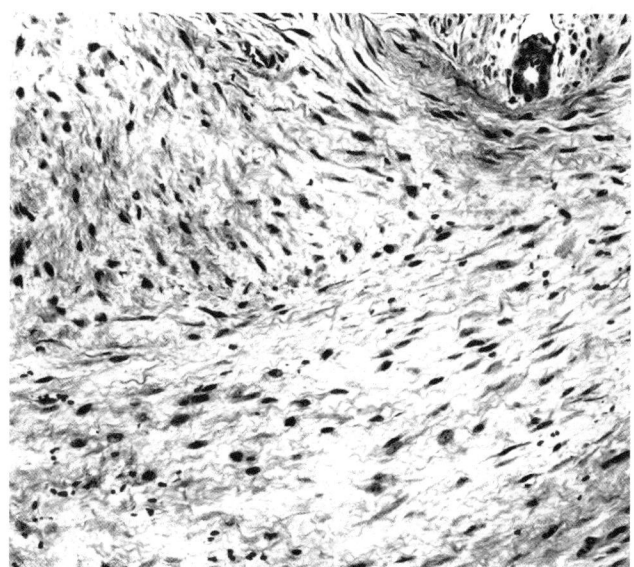

Figure 19-107. This desmoid tumor manifests an unusually myxoedematous stroma in which scattered erythrocytes are present. The general appearance of the lesion simulates that of nodular fasciitis; however, the latter process does not affect the pleura.

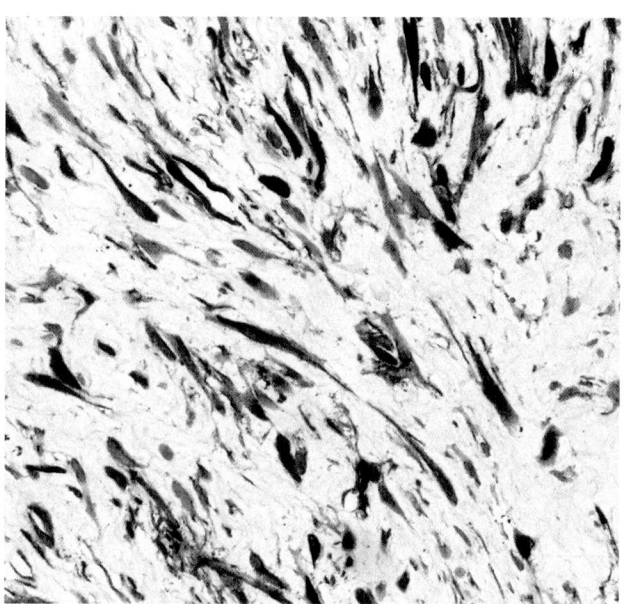

Figure 19-108. Nuclear (and cytoplasmic) immunoreactivity for beta-catenin is seen in desmoid tumors. Solitary fibrous tumors may share this feature.

Clear Cell Tumor

The general premises underlying the nosologic family of "myomelanocytomas" (MMCs) have been described previously in reference to angiomyolipomas. Another member of that conceptual group—clear cell "sugar" tumor of the lung (CCT)—is a purely epithelioid MMC,[250] which, for reasons to be discussed, is probably best regarded as a biologically "borderline" neoplasm.

Pulmonary "sugar tumor" was first described noncommittally as "clear cell tumor of the lung" due to the presence of intracytoplasmic glycogen.[421] It typically occurs in patients older than 40 years of age[422–439] as a peripheral lung nodule. However, occasional examples have been reported in the trachea or large bronchi.[425,436] Like angiomyolipoma, CCT has been found concurrently with lymphangioleiomyomatosis and multifocal micronodular pneumocytic hyperplasia in some patients with tuberous sclerosis.[433] Tumors in such patients demonstrate a loss of heterozygosity in the TSC2 region of chromosome 16p13.[440,441]

The radiographic attributes of CCT are nondescript.[424,429] It is a homogeneously dense, round to ovoid, peripheral lung mass that may be seen in any region of the lung (Fig. 19-109). CT has typically shown sharp circumscription.

The same features are reflected in gross examination. Their cut surfaces are pink to brown and uniform, although necrotic foci may sometimes be present. Maximum diameter is generally less than 5 cm.

Histologic examination shows one of two general growth patterns in CCTs. The first is organoid, with broad cords and rounded nests of cells separated by a variably prominent fibrovascular stroma, mimicking renal cell carcinoma. The second configuration is a medullary image, showing sheets of epithelioid cells with little internal clustering (Fig. 19-110). Pre-existing small bronchi and bronchioles are often entrapped by the neoplastic cells. Nuclei are round to ovoid with small nucleoli; intranuclear invaginations of cytoplasm also may be apparent, but mitotic figures are usually difficult to find. Cytoplasm is clear or lightly eosinophilic, and may be finely granular. Histochemical evaluation with the periodic acid/Schiff method usually shows intense

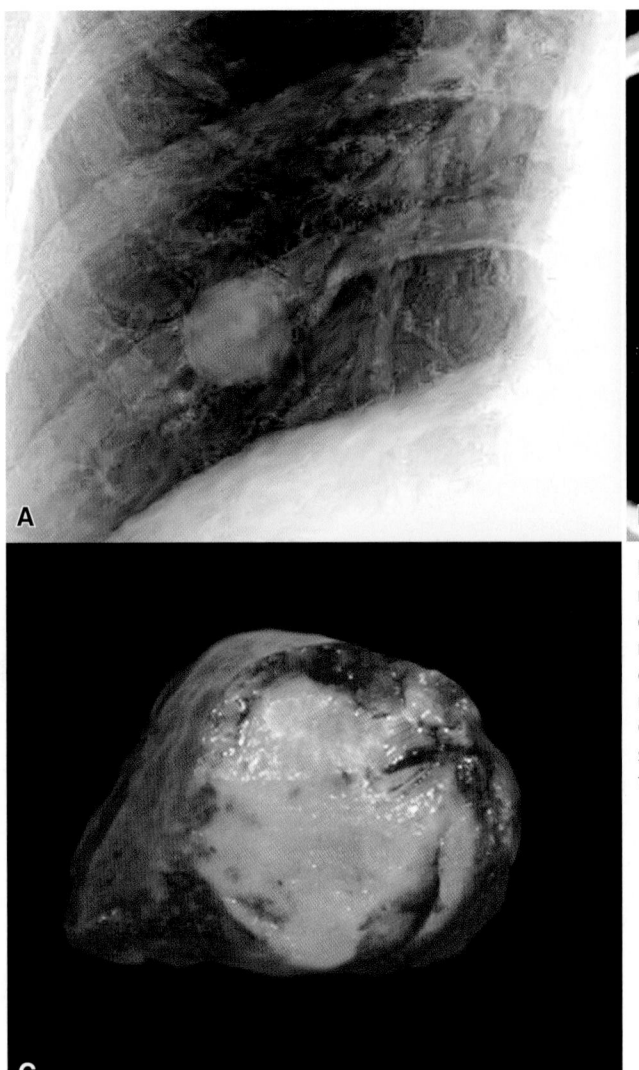

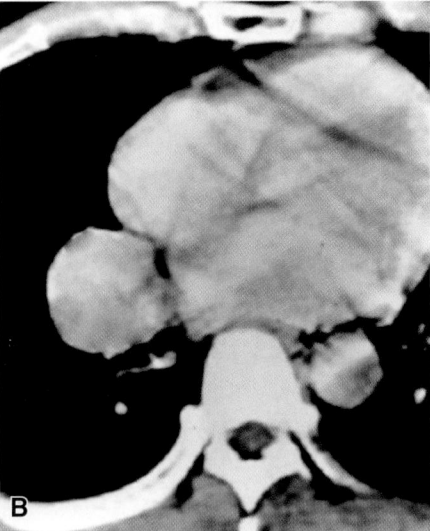

Figure 19-109. A, This highlighted plain-film chest radiograph of a clear cell pulmonary "sugar tumor" demonstrates a nondescript well-defined nodule in the right lung field. **B,** This computed tomogram of a clear cell tumor demonstrates a globular, internally homogeneous mass that abuts the mediastinum in the right lung. **C,** Gross photograph of a pulmonary clear cell tumor showing a uniform white-gray cut surface and demarcation from the surrounding parenchyma.

cytoplasmic labeling for glycogen in the tumor cells (Fig. 19-111). Intralesional blood vessels can be markedly sclerotic in some cases, spontaneous necrosis is occasionally seen, and sparse intratumoral chronic inflammatory cells may be identified.

Ultrastructural studies of CCT have shown attributes suggesting a "hybrid" cell type that incorporates elements of modified perivascular smooth muscle and melanocytes. These include interdigitating cellular processes, pericellular basal lamina, primitive intercellular attachment complexes, plasmalemmal pinocytosis, membrane-bound and free cytoplasmic glycogen granules, and variant form premelanosomes.[423,426,428,430,432,435]

Immunohistologically, one sees a uniform lack of reactivity for epithelial markers in CCT, but consistent reactivity for vimentin, CD117, collagen type IV, HMB-45, MART-1, and micro-ophthalmia transcription factor 1 (with the last three determinants all related to melanocytes)[246,427,428,432,434] (Fig. 19-112). Inconsistent but generally positive results are obtained for muscle-specific actin, S-100 protein, and neuron-specific enolase. Panizo-Santos and colleagues[442] have described aberrant but virtually exclusive cytoplasmic immunoreactivity for Myo-D1 in members of the MMC family of tumors. This marker is a nuclear transcription factor related to striated muscle development, and *bona fide* labeling for it would not be expected in the cytoplasm.

Hence, it appears that the cited pattern of staining probably represents a reproducible artifact, but if corroborated, it could prove to be useful diagnostically.

The differential diagnosis for CCT is a lengthy one, including primary carcinomas of the lung with clear cell features; metastatic clear cell carcinomas from the kidney, urogenital tract, breast, and other locations; metastatic clear cell sarcoma; and metastatic "balloon cell" melanoma.[443] The generic possibility of carcinoma can be excluded by the lack of keratin and EMA in CCT, but clear cell sarcoma and melanoma are not as easily dismissed because they potentially share the entire complement of immunohistologic melanocyte markers with MMCs. Reactivity for actin or cytoplasmic Myo-D1 would strongly argue in favor of CCT in this setting, because those determinants have not been reported in metastatic melanomas with epithelioid features.

Biologically, CCT has traditionally been considered a benign pulmonary tumor. Nonetheless, at least two examples[435,437] have metastasized to other visceral sites, and one proved fatal. This behavior parallels the biologic potential of MMCs in other organs, notably the kidney. Thus, it would seem appropriate to regard CCT as another borderline neoplasm of the lung. With that having been said, however, simple surgical removal of the lesion—with wedge excision of the peripheral lung parenchyma, if possible—is believed to represent adequate therapy.

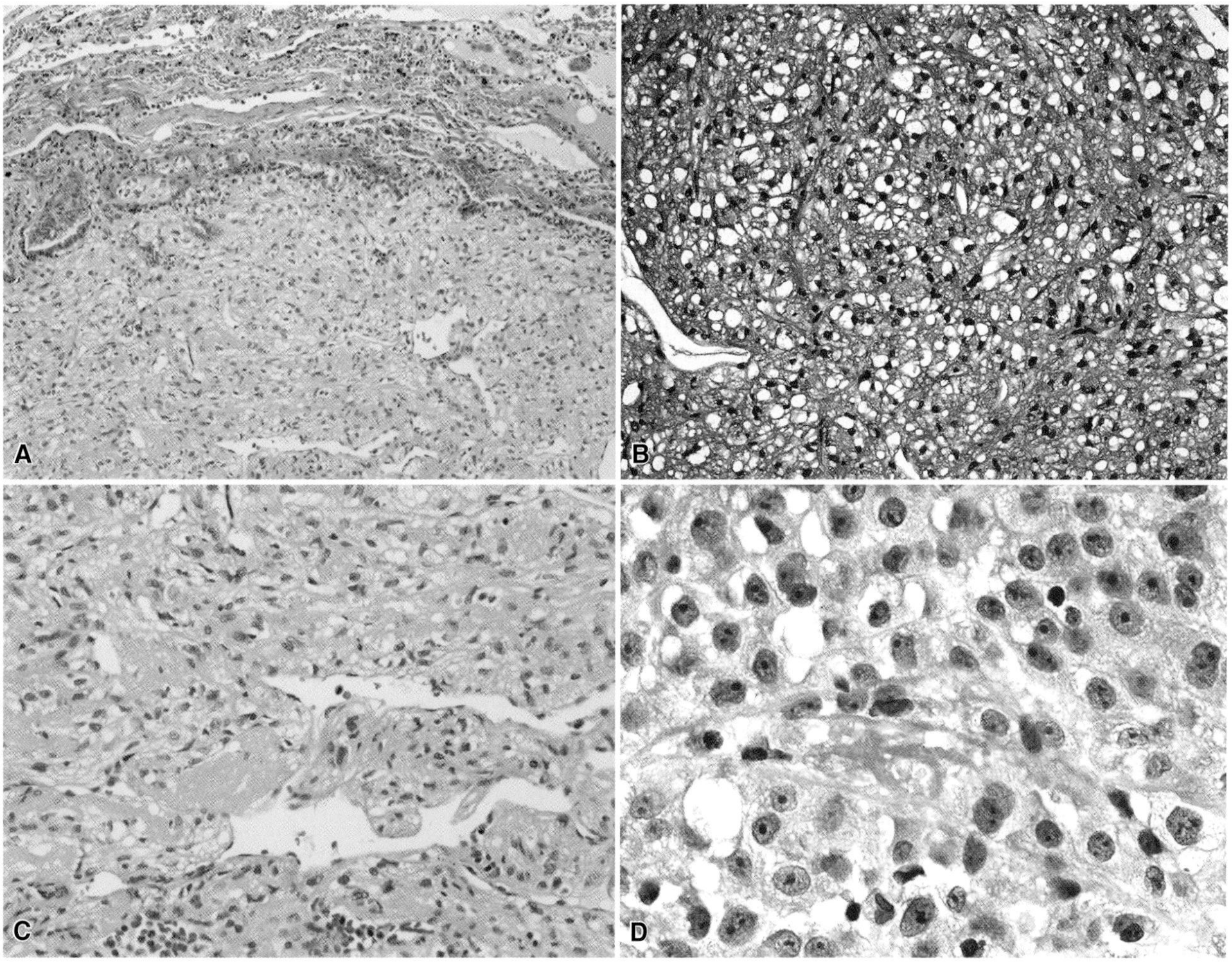

Figure 19-110. **A,** A rounded interface with the adjacent lung is evident in this low-power microscopic image of a pulmonary clear cell tumor. **B,** The growth pattern of a pulmonary sugar tumor is frequently medullary, comprising sheets of clear neoplastic cells with indistinct internal fibrovascular septations. **C,** The tumor cells are polygonal, with amphophilic, granular, or clear cytoplasm. **D,** Nucleoli may be prominent.

Primary Pleuropulmonary Thymoma

Even though thymomas typically arise in the anterosuperior mediastinum, the literature contains ample evidence of their ability to develop in ectopic sites. These tumors have been described in the soft tissue of the lower neck, as well as the thyroid, pericardium, lungs,

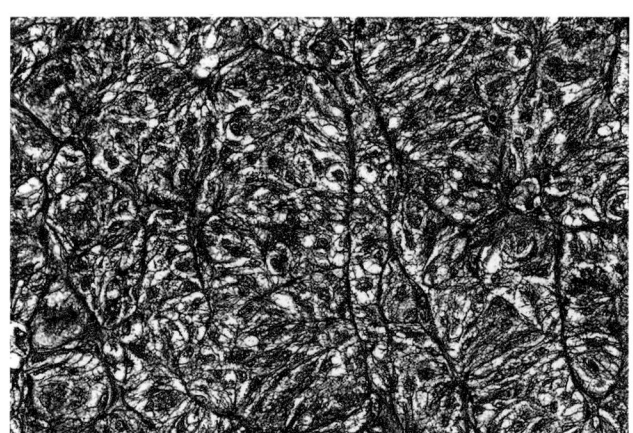

Figure 19-111. Diffuse strong reactivity is seen with the periodic acid/Schiff stain in a clear cell tumor of the lung, revealing abundant intracellular glycogen.

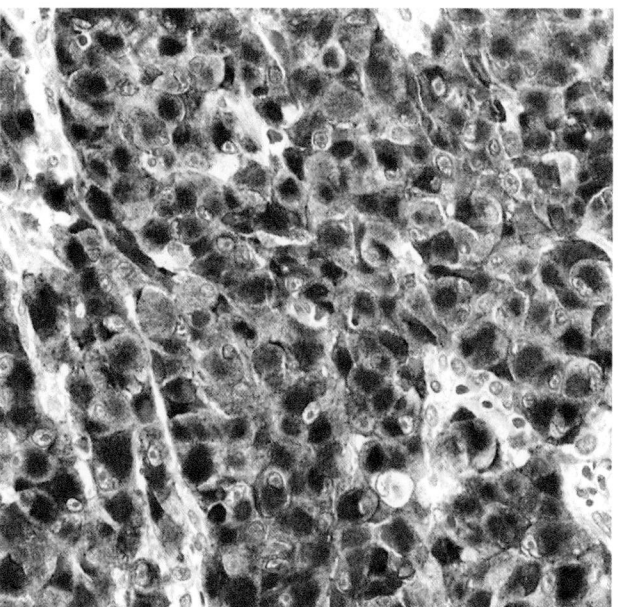

Figure 19-112. Immunoreactivity with HMB-45 is typical of a pulmonary clear cell tumor.

and pleura.[444-449] Because of their ability to show a relatively wide morphologic spectrum, heterotopic thymic tumors may be quite difficult to recognize diagnostically.

Intrapulmonary thymoma is seen in adults between the ages of 20 and 80 years. In the minority of cases where the lesion is linked to one of several distinctive thymoma-related paraneoplastic syndromes—principally myasthenia gravis, pure red cell aplasia, and acquired hypogammaglobulinemia—its identity may be suspected clinically.[450] However, the majority of these tumors present as asymptomatic masses that are found radiographically. They can be situated centrally, close to the hilum, and even endobronchially in rare instances, as well as in the mid-lung fields or beneath the pleural surfaces[451-461] (Fig. 19-113). Occasionally, two or more intrapulmonary masses are seen concurrently.

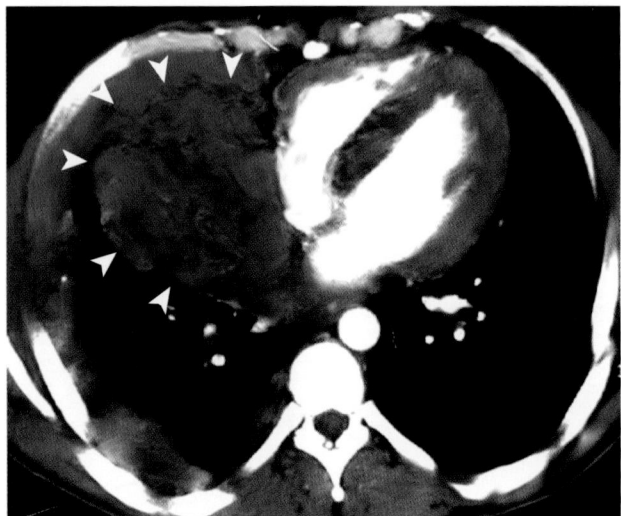

Figure 19-113. This computed tomogram of the thorax shows a lobulated mass in the anterior right lung field (*arrowheads*), representing a primary intrapulmonary thymoma.

In analogy to mediastinal thymomas, those arising in the lungs may be either circumscribed or infiltrative, and some demonstrate prominent intralesional cystification.

Pleural thymomas may simulate the appearance of any other solitary serosal neoplasm. In rare examples, they have diffusely effaced the pleural space in one or both hemithoraces, reproducing the radiographic and gross pathologic image of diffuse pleural mesothelioma or metastatic serosal carcinoma.[459-461]

All of the scenarios discussed earlier include an absence of abnormalities in the anterior mediastinum. With that in mind, it is easy to understand why a definitive radiographic interpretation of ectopic thymoma is virtually impossible.

These tumors have fleshy pink-tan cut surfaces that closely resemble those of lymphoreticular neoplasms, but areas of necrosis, hemorrhage, or cyst formation are much more common than they are in lymphomas. They may also contain internal fibrous septations, subdividing the masses into angulated tissue compartments (Fig. 19-114). Dystrophic calcification may be present.

Microscopically, circumferential fibrous encapsulation of pulmonary or pleural thymomas is unusual, in contrast to their intrathymic counterparts. As a result, ectopic lesions in the hemithoraces must commonly be classified as "invasive," almost by definition (Fig. 19-115). As stated previously, intralesional fibrous septa intersect one another at acute angles (Fig. 19-116), differing from the obtuse connections that are seen in nodular sclerosing Hodgkin's lymphoma or sclerosing non-Hodgkin's lymphomas in the chest. At the University of Virginia, the classic Bernatz system of histologic classification for thymic epithelial tumors is used, which has five subdivisions:

- Lymphocyte-predominant thymoma (≥66% lymphocytes)
- Mixed thymoma (34% to 65% lymphocytes)
- Epithelial-predominant thymoma (≤33% lymphocytes)
- Spindle cell thymoma (a variant of epithelial-predominant thymoma in which the majority of the neoplastic cells are fusiform; Fig. 19-117)
- Thymic carcinoma, containing obviously anaplastic and cytologically malignant tumor cells[462]

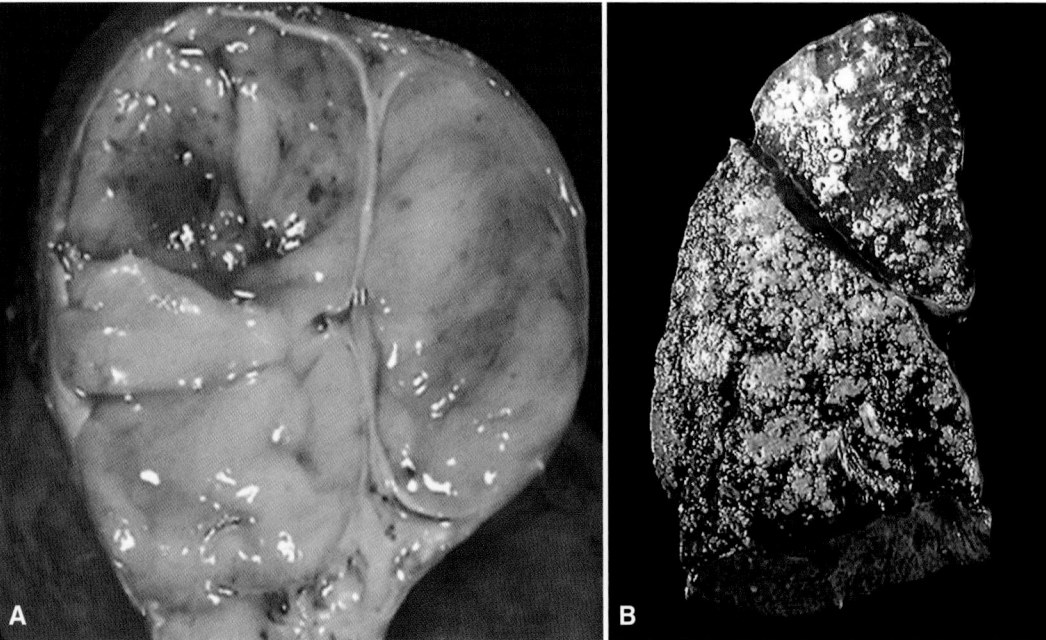

Figure 19-114. A, This gross photograph of an intrapulmonary thymoma shows a uniform tan-gray cut surface and internal subdivision by fibrous septa. **B,** Another tumor demonstrating pleuroparenchymal "thymomatosis," where deposits of thymoma are present on the visceral pleura (*left*) and within the lung. This appearance may simulate that of mesothelioma.

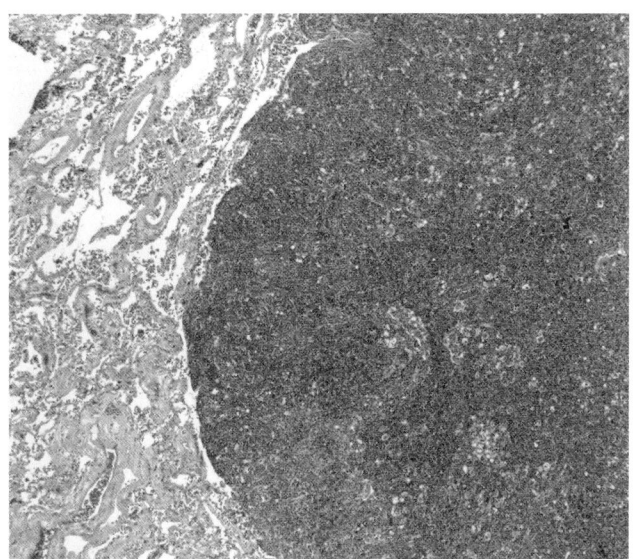

Figure 19-115. Infiltration of the lung parenchyma is seen in this case of intrapulmonary thymoma.

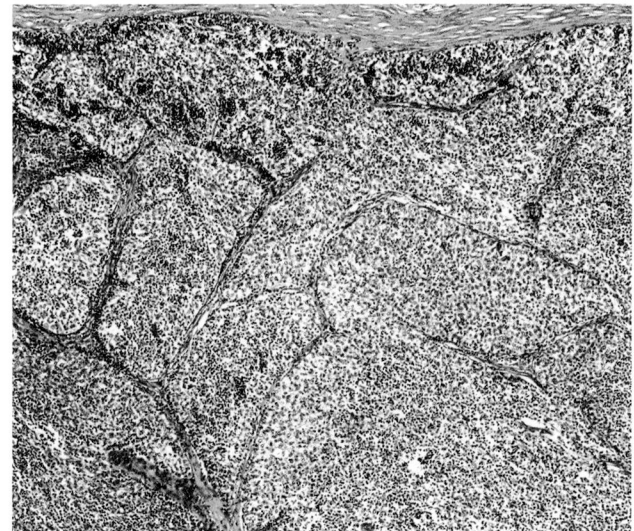

Figure 19-116. Internal fibrous septas in thymomas intersect one another at acute angles, yielding a distinctive image in this Masson trichrome stain.

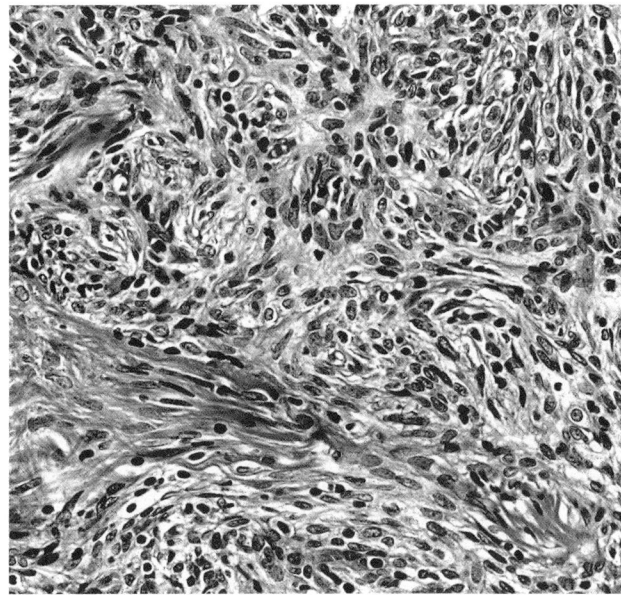

Figure 19-117. Predominantly spindle cell (medullary, World Health Organization type A) intrapulmonary thymoma.

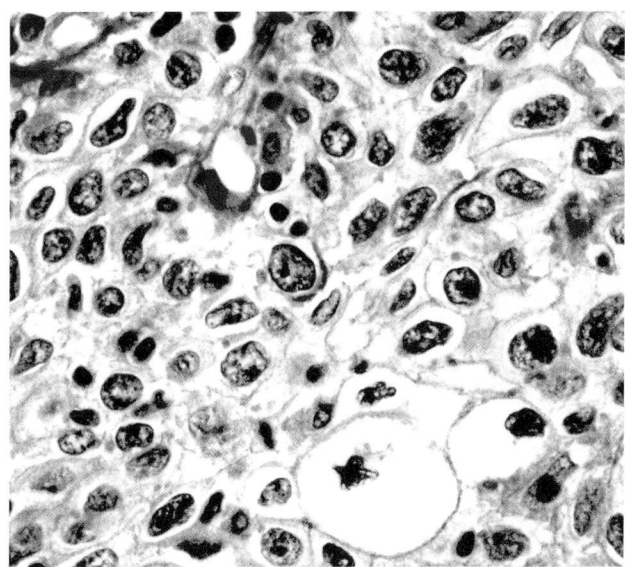

Figure 19-118. An "atypical" epithelial-predominant (World Health Organization type B3) thymoma shows increased nuclear-cytoplasmic ratios, nucleoli, nuclear hyperchromasia, and distinct intercellular membranes. However, these changes fall short of the cytomorphologic threshhold for thymic carcinoma.

Other alternative nosologic constructions for thymic tumors have entered common use as well, including the Marino-Muller-Hermelink scheme,[463] the World Health Organization system,[464] and the Suster-Moran codification.[465] The last one can easily be linked with the Bernatz system to specifically address tumors that demonstrate a notable degree of nuclear atypia, yet whose features are insufficient for an outright diagnosis of carcinoma. Such neoplasms are termed "atypical" thymomas.

The epithelial cells of thymomas—not the lymphoid cells—are the neoplastic elements. They are characterized by a range of cytologic images. Some have vague cellular borders, oval nuclear contours, dispersed chromatin, and indistinct nucleoli. At the other end of the spectrum, one sees rather clear-cut plasmalemmal interfaces, moderate nuclear irregularity and hyperchromasia, and distinct nucleoli (Fig. 19-118). As mentioned earlier, spindle cell change is another potential image in thymomas, and the nuclei in such lesions tend to have bland and uniform morphologic characteristics. Mitotic activity in thymic tumors is greatly variable as well, and it achieves importance as a possible marker of thymic carcinoma only in neoplasms that also show nuclear abnormalities.

Secondary architectural changes in thymomas include the formation of perivascular "lakes" of serum, in which lymphoid cells are suspended; pseudoglandular arrays or pseudorosettes of epithelial cells; microcysts or areas of gross cystic change, with or without necrosis; stromal blood lakes and vascular dilatation; and "medullary differentiation," in which loose and vaguely nodular aggregates of stromal lymphocytes are present.[462] Hassall's corpuscles are seen in only a small minority of cases. Some spindle cell thymomas contain a vascular network comprising numerous vessels with a "moose antler" configuration, yielding a pattern that virtually perfectly imitates that of hemangiopericytoma–solitary fibrous tumor.

Epithelial-predominant thymomas with nuclear atypia, an organoid growth pattern, and distinct cellular borders have been called "well-differentiated thymic carcinomas."[466] However, their generic clinicopathologic characteristics are clearly dissimilar to those of outright thymic carcinomas, and some observers believe that they are more properly termed "atypical thymomas."[465]

The cytopathologic attributes of thymic epithelial tumors seen in FNA biopsy specimens are well described[467-469] and reflect their histologic heterogeneity. Mature lymphocytes are admixed with thymic epithelial cells, which show a tendency toward cohesion. However, scattered single epithelial cells may also be evident. Epithelial cell nuclei are generally monomorphic, with dispersed chromatin and small chromocenters. Cytoplasm is amphophilic, with indistinct cell borders. A fusiform cellular shape may be encountered in spindle cell tumors, but the grouping of such cells into small clusters helps to distinguish them from mesenchymal proliferations. The lymphoid elements in thymoma are a potential diagnostic pitfall, and nuclear "activation" may be seen with increases in the nuclear-to-cytoplasmic ratios. Convolution of the nuclear borders can also be present, as may mitotic figures. The overall image of "activated" intratumoral lymphocytes is quite similar to that of lymphoblastic lymphoma, and a misdiagnosis may ensue unless adjunctive studies are performed to detect the epithelial elements of thymoma.[454,467] Predictably, invasive thymomas cannot be distinguished from encapsulated tumors using the FNA technique.

Electron microscopy of thymomas shows elongated and interdigitating cytoplasmic processes emanating from constituent epithelial cells, and these are joined to one another by well-formed desmosomes into which broad tonofibrils insert. Plasmalemmal microvilli are absent, and intralesional lymphoid cells are usually intercalated between the epithelial elements.[470]

Cytogenetic analysis has shown no consistent karyotypic aberrations in thymomas. Several different abnormalities have been documented, including deletions of chromosome 6p; t(1;8) and t(15;22) chromosomal translocations; pseudodicentric (16;12)(q11;p11.2); and ring chromosome 6.[471-473] However, none of these findings is typically associated with other primary pleuropulmonary tumors.

Immunohistologic studies are paramount in confirming the cellular nature of ectopic thymomas. Keratin immunostains show a characteristically arborizing network of reactivity, reflecting the presence of interconnecting cytoplasmic processes[474] (Fig. 19-119). The keratin subtype 5/6 is also characteristic of thymic epithelium.[475] A member of the p53 protein family, p63 protein, is likewise consistently present in thymoma (Fig. 19-120), as it is in squamous neoplasms.[476] Finally, the lymphoid cells in thymomas are true thymocytes. They express CD1a, nuclear terminal deoxynucleotidyl transferase (TdT), and CD99.[454] The latter

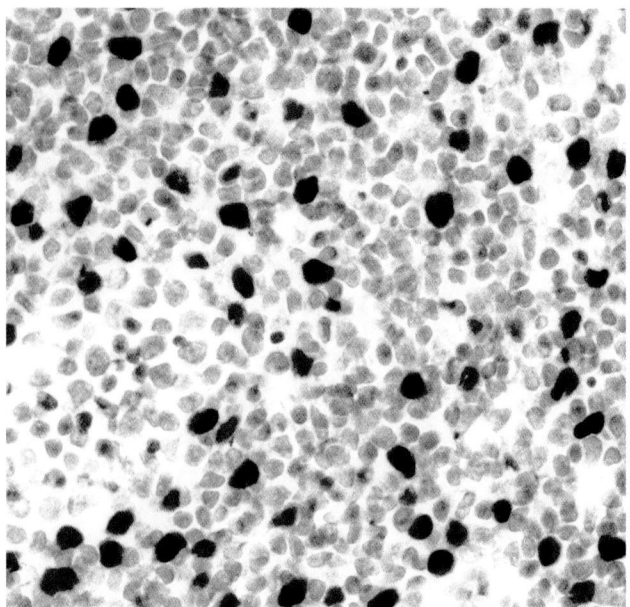

Figure 19-120. Nuclear immunoreactivity for p63 protein in the epithelial cells of a pleural thymoma. This finding is helpful in the differential diagnosis with mesothelioma, which is p63-negative.

phenotype is shared only by the tumor cells of lymphoblastic lymphomas, but these hematopoietic neoplasms are uniformly nonreactive for p63 and keratin. Thus, there is a truly diagnostic immunoprofile for thymoma. Parenthetically, it should be noted that "pseudomesotheliomatous" pleural thymomas may be reactive for calretinin, keratin 5/6, and thrombomodulin, all of which are commonly associated with mesothelial cells.[461] That combination of results may easily lead to misdiagnosis if studies for p63, CD1a, TdT, and CD99 are omitted.

Differential diagnostic considerations include lymphoma, metastatic somatic carcinoma, metastatic seminoma, mesothelioma, and pleural sarcomas (especially synovial sarcoma and hemangiopericytoma), depending on the microscopic nuances of the lesion. The immunophenotype of thymoma discussed earlier is unique among those possibilities.

Behaviorally, ectopic thymomas in the lung and pleura are typically indolent lesions that can be cured by complete surgical resection if they are solitary.[477] However, several examples have been reported in which recurrence, distant metastasis, or both, was observed.[451-458] Moreover, lesions that simulate mesothelioma because of their encasement of the lungs or heart are associated with a greater risk of adverse behavior.[459-461] Because a minority of all pleuropulmonary thymomas are fatal, they are justifiably considered borderline.

Heterotopic Meningeal Proliferations

Meningiomas are typically considered neoplasms of the main neural axis, but they are perhaps the most widely distributed of any tumor in that group. Tumefactive proliferations with meningothelial differentiation have been reported in a wide variety of locations, including the mediastinum and lungs, in the absence of involvement of the coverings of the brain and spinal cord.[478] Patients with such lesions seem to be somewhat younger on average than those with intracranial meningiomas, most of whom are middle-aged or older. Because these neoplasms are clearly not expected outside of their usual confines, their clinical presentation in heterotopic locations is typically undiagnosed at a clinical level.[479] For example, those in the lung are usually believed to represent granulomas or adenocarcinomas

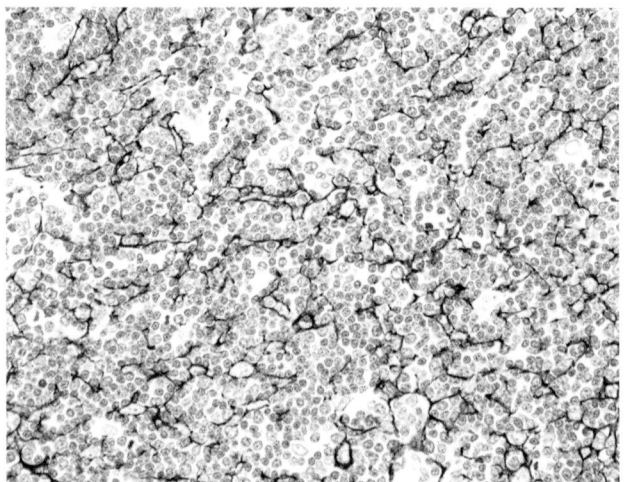

Figure 19-119. Interconnecting cell processes in a thymoma are labeled for keratin, yielding a "lacy" immunostaining pattern. (Image courtesy of Dr. Anja Roden, Mayo Clinic, Rochester, MN.)

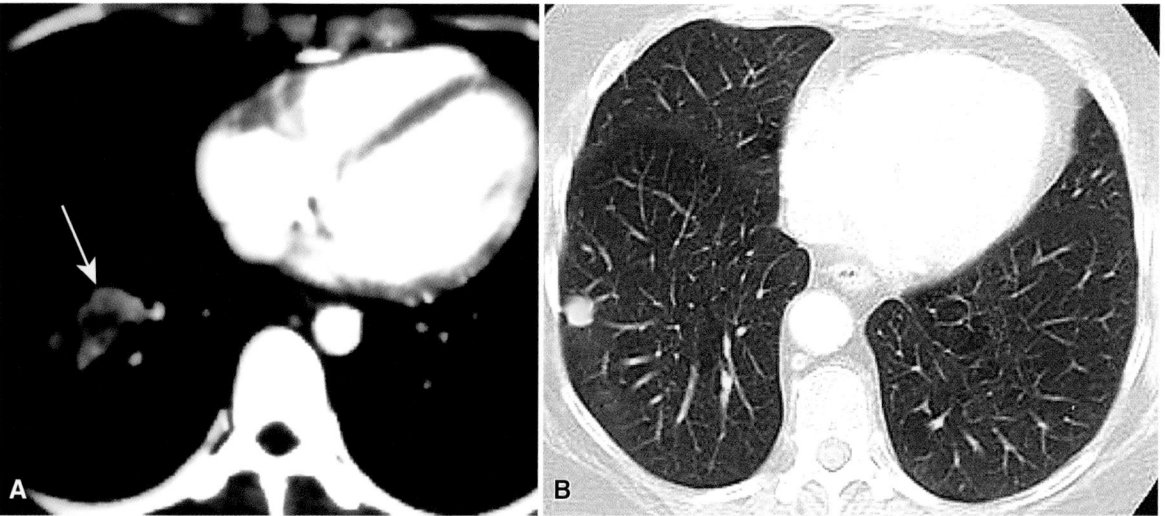

Figure 19-121. Computed tomograms of the thorax showing a slightly spiculated nodular mass in the mid-right lung field (**A**; *arrow*) and a small nodular peripheral lesion in the right lung (**B**), both of which proved to be primary pulmonary meningiomas.

radiographically (Fig. 19-121). Ectopic meningiomas generally pursue a relatively favorable clinical course; although local recurrence is a possibility, these lesions are uncommonly associated with distant metastasis.[480]

Grossly, meningioma of the lung is usually sharply marginated and easily dissected from the surrounding parenchyma (Fig. 19-122). It measures between 1 and 5 cm in diameter and has a globoid configuration and a uniformly white-gray cut surface. Those rare lesions that are malignant may show areas of necrosis and hemorrhage, as well as infiltration of the adjacent lung.[480,481]

Histologically, heterotopic meningiomas show preferential expression of meningothelial, fibroblastic, or "transitional" growth patterns.[482–493] As such, meningiomas of the lung are composed of polygonal or fusiform cells with monomorphic oval nuclei and dispersed chromatin (Fig. 19-123). Whorled aggregates of tumor cells may be observed multifocally, with or without secondary psammomatous microcalcifications. In some cases, the latter structures are numerous.

Purely meningotheliomatous lesions—comprising a pure population of polygonal cells—may simulate the appearance of a carcinoma; at the other pole of the spectrum, "fibroblastic" or solely spindle cell

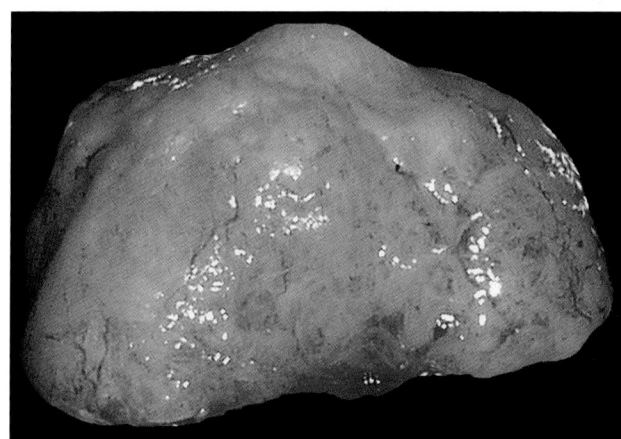

Figure 19-122. This gross photograph of a primary intrapulmonary meningioma shows a globose mass that was "shelled out" by the surgeon from the surrounding parenchyma.

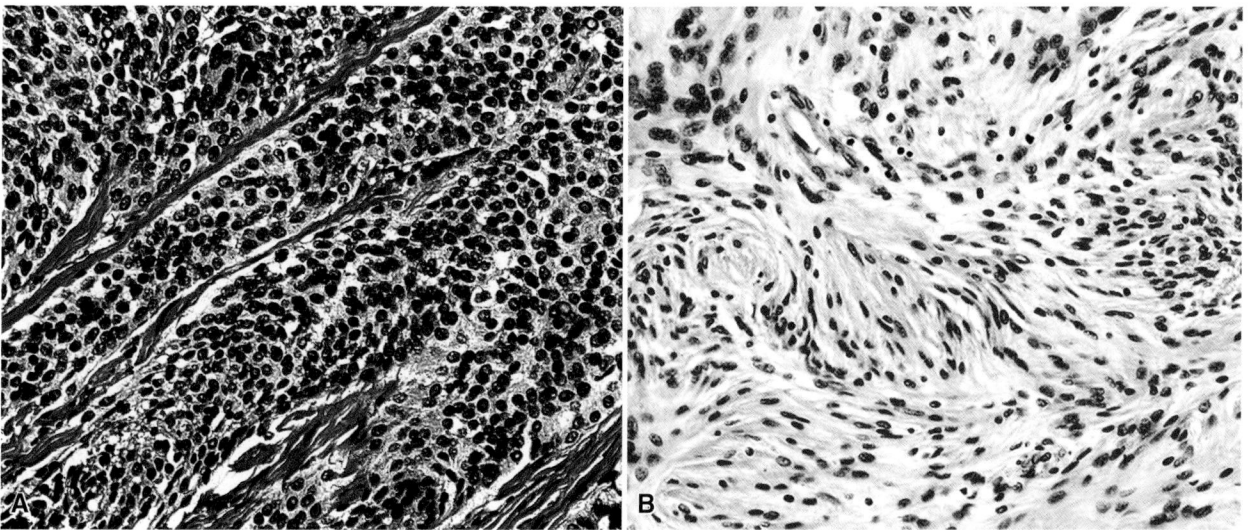

Figure 19-123. Intrapulmonary meningiomas with meningotheliomatous (**A**) and transitional (mixed) (**B**) features.

meningiomas can imitate the configuration of solitary fibrous tumor–hemangiopericytoma or other primary soft tissue neoplasms[478,481] (Fig. 19-124). Mitotic activity is limited, nuclear atypia is only modest, and necrosis is usually absent in benign pulmonary meningiomas, but the presence of those findings should raise concern about the rare possibility of malignancy.[494]

The premise has been advanced by some authors that primary pulmonary meningioma may arise from "meningothelial-like micronodules" in the lung[482,484] (formerly and erroneously called "minute pulmonary chemodectomas"), which are related to parenchymal damage as a result of cardiac failure, chronic obstructive pulmonary disease, and thromboemboli[495] (Fig. 19-125). The conclusion that they are the precursors of meningioma was derived from the fact that both lesions have been seen together in the same case; however, no molecular analyses have been done to further address that possibility. In our opinion, however, this is unlikely; pertinent data show that meningothelial-like micronodules are polyclonal and probably reactive.[496] When multiple, the phenomenon has been called "menigotheliomatosis,"[497] which may lead to radiologic confusion with interstitial lung disease or metastases (Fig. 19-126).

Fine-needle aspiration biopsy specimens of pulmonary meningioma[482,486] show scanty material, represented by whorls of cells with a concentric internal configuration (Fig. 19-127), as well as isolated individual cells. Intranuclear inclusions may be apparent, and psammomatous calcifications can be observed in rare instances.

Electron microscopy is still an extremely useful tool for the resolution of differential diagnostic questions surrounding these tumors.[498] Meningioma has a singular ultrastructural appearance that features

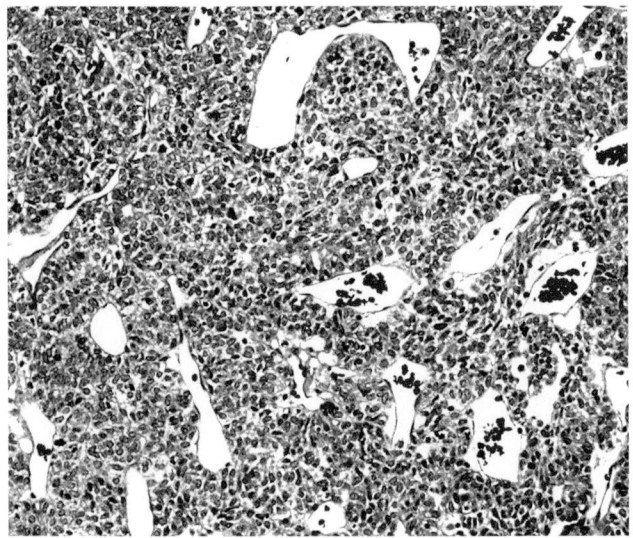

Figure 19-124. Blunt spindle cells are arranged around a vascular structure resembling "staghorns" in meningioma, potentially simulating the appearance of hemangiopericytoma–solitary fibrous tumor.

numerous interdigitating cell processes attached by prominent desmosomes. Skeins of well-formed tonofibrils insert into those attachment complexes. To our knowledge, this particular constellation of findings is not recapitulated by any other tumor type.

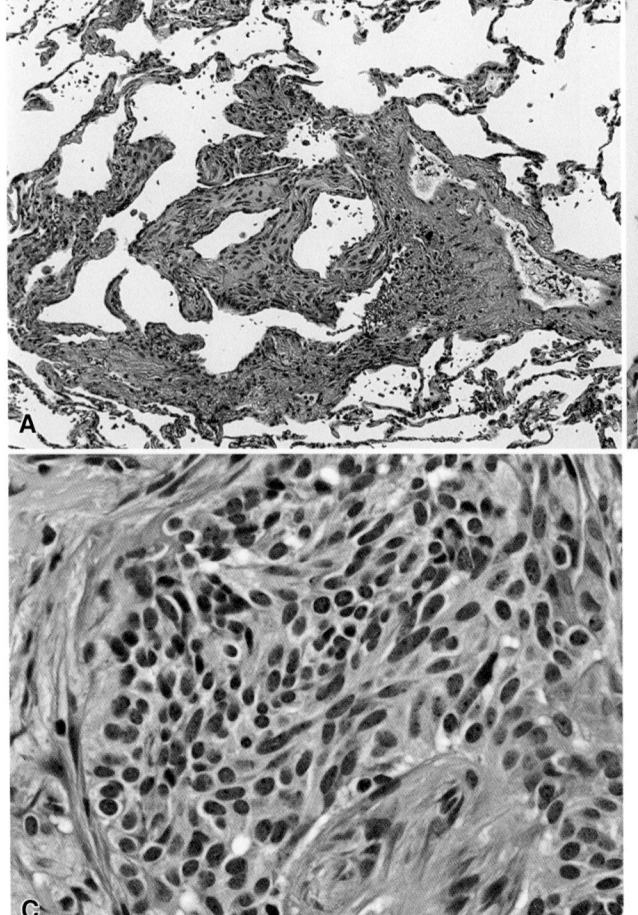

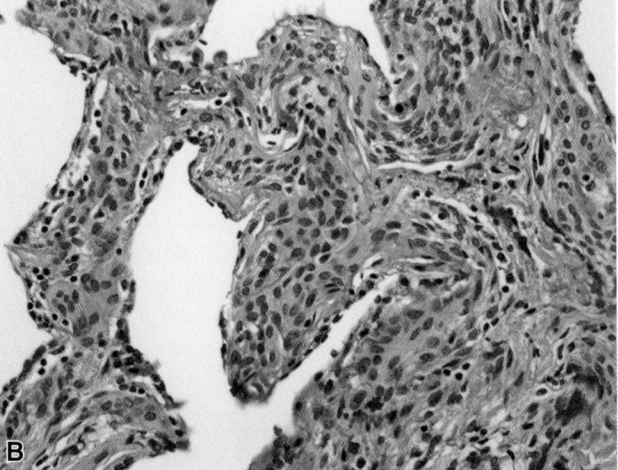

Figure 19-125. A to **C,** Microscopic nodules of meningothelial-like cells, as shown, may be associated with heart failure or chronic non-neoplastic pulmonary diseases of various types. They have been proposed as possible precursors to intrapulmonary meningiomas, but that assertion is unproven.

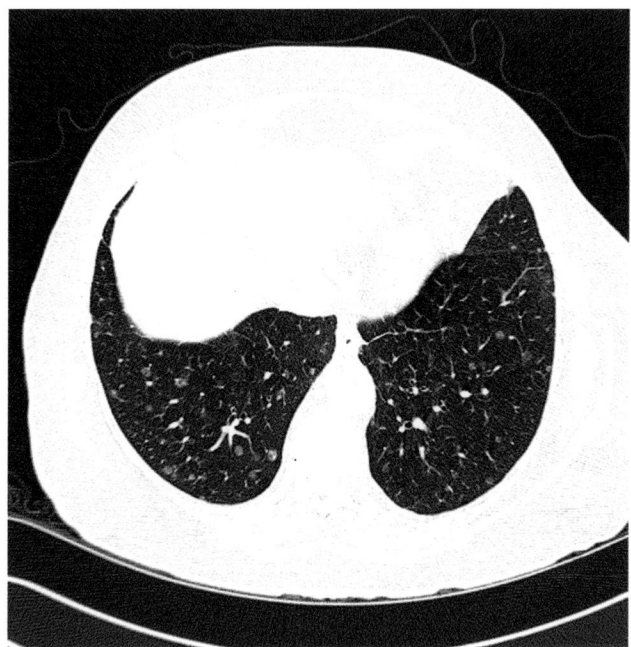

Figure 19-126. Occasionally, numerous meningothelial micronodules are seen radiographically throughout both lung fields, as in this computed tomogram, a condition termed "meningotheliomatosis."

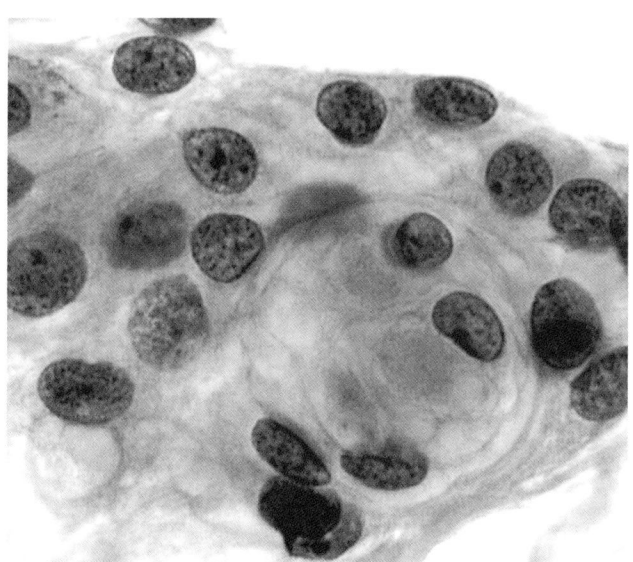

Figure 19-127. Fine-needle aspiration biopsy specimens of primary pulmonary meningioma show cohesive ovoid tumor cells with dispersed chromatin with typical whorling.

Prototypically, meningiomas are reactive for vimentin to the exclusion of other intermediate filament proteins; EMA is also present universally, as is immunoreactivity for desmoplakin, a desmosomal constituent.[478,481–483,498] Intracranial meningiomas are immunoreactive for progesterone receptor protein in the majority of cases.[499,500] However, that marker has not yet been assessed in primary pulmonary meningothelial tumors. Immunophenotypic characteristics of ectopic meningiomas also differ from those of their neuraxis analogs, in that the former lesions appear to express keratin more often. Admittedly, this attribute is probably influenced by the site of origin. Additional markers that are germane to the differential diagnosis, such as CD34 and S-100 protein, have also been reported sporadically in heterotopic meningiomas in some sites.

Other pertinent diagnostic considerations for primary pulmonary meningiomas include carcinomas with or without spindle cell features, solitary fibrous tumors, hemangiopericytomas, schwannomas, and amelanotic malignant melanomas.[481] Electron microscopy is still very effective in resolving such uncertainties because of the distinctive profile of meningioma. Immunohistochemical analyses require the application of antibodies to Ber-EP4, MOC-31, carcinoembryonic antigen, CD56, CD57, CD99, melan-A/MART-1, and tyrosinase. Podoplanin (recognized by antibody D2-40), a relative newcomer to clinical immunohistochemistry, is not useful in this specific context. It may be seen in SFT, schwannoma, meningioma, and sarcomatoid melanoma.[501–503] However, another useful modality of investigation is fluorescent in situ hybridization, which demonstrates monosomy of chromosome 22 in a majority of meningiomas,[504] a cytogenetic abnormality that is not shared by other differential diagnostic possibilities.

None of these studies is effective in separating primary ectopic from metastatic neuraxis-based meningiomas.[491,505] However, it is an exceedingly rare situation for the latter neoplasms to present in distant sites with no previous knowledge of a primary tumor within the cranial vault or spine.[505]

Intrapulmonary Teratomas

Examples of primary intrapulmonary teratoma have been reported with extraordinary rarity[506–509] (Fig. 19-128). The overwhelming majority of teratoid tumors in the lungs and pleura represent altered metastases of gonadal germ cell tumors, in which malignant histologic components were formerly present but have been complete removed by chemotherapy.[510] Another small group of cases comprises primary malignant teratoid tumors of the lung that contain seminoma, embryonal carcinoma, yolk sac carcinoma, or choriocarcinoma.[511–513] Primary pulmonary teratomas without cytologically malignant components are extremely uncommon; they have principally been seen as variably cystic masses in young adults. One such lesion was associated with pyothorax, and others have presented with extrusion of hair (from the contents of the lesion) into a large airway.[506,514,515]

Grossly, the most obvious constituents of such neoplasms are squamous epithelium with associated keratinous debris and cartilage (Fig. 19-129). Mucoid contents may sometimes be seen in cystic areas, and nondescript solid foci may also be present.

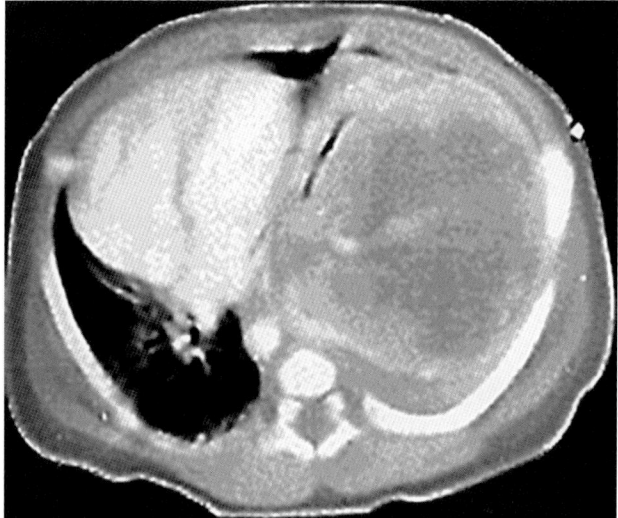

Figure 19-128. This computed tomogram of the chest in a young man shows a solid mass that occupies virtually the entire left hemithorax. It proved to be an immature teratoma, apparently arising in the lung.

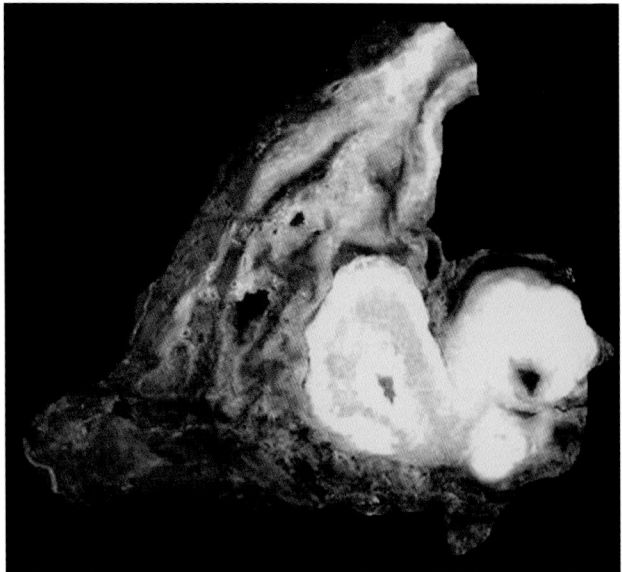

Figure 19-129. This gross photograph of an intrapulmonary teratoma shows a largely solid white-gray mass in the parenchyma with some central cystification.

Figure 19-130. Retinal pigment epithelium is apparent in this mature teratoma.

Microscopically, teratomas of the lung can be divided into mature and immature varieties, as is true of these tumors occurring elsewhere in the body. The first of those subtypes is self-explanatory, but the term "immature" in this context refers specifically to the presence of primitive neurectodermal tissue that resembles the developing neural tube. Otherwise, virtually any tissue in the body can be reflected in the constituents of teratoid lesions, including such unexpected elements as retina (Fig. 19-130). To qualify as teratomatous, the tumor must demonstrate derivatives from at least two of the three germinal lines (ectoderm, endoderm, and mesoderm).

Special pathologic studies are generally unnecessary diagnostically. However, immunostains may sometimes be undertaken to search for possible production of such oncofetal proteins as α-fetoprotein by endodermally derived elements, including intestinal and hepatic tissue.

Too few cases of mature or immature primary intrapulmonary teratomas have been studied to determine their biologic potential with certainty. However, by extrapolation from other anatomic locations, immature teratomas are known to have a potential for recurrence or metastasis. Thus, as a group, we have tentatively classified these lesions as borderline neoplasms.

Cystic Fibrohistiocytic Tumor of the Lung

Joseph and colleagues[516] described two adult patients who were found to have variably cystic lung lesions, represented by multiple parenchymal abnormalities on chest radiographs. One patient had pneumothorax and shortness of breath, and lesions in the other case were asymptomatic. Open-lung biopsies showed a proliferation of relatively bland spindle cells and histiocyte-like elements, mantling cystic spaces that were lined by metaplastic bronchiolar epithelium, squamous cells, or type II pneumocytes (Fig. 19-131). Some of the cysts contained erythrocytes and hemosiderin deposits. Another case has been illustrated anecdotally by Han.[517]

Although the lesions described by Joseph and coworkers[516] enlarged very slowly over time, the authors suggested that the ultimate biologic potential and recommended treatment of pulmonary cystic

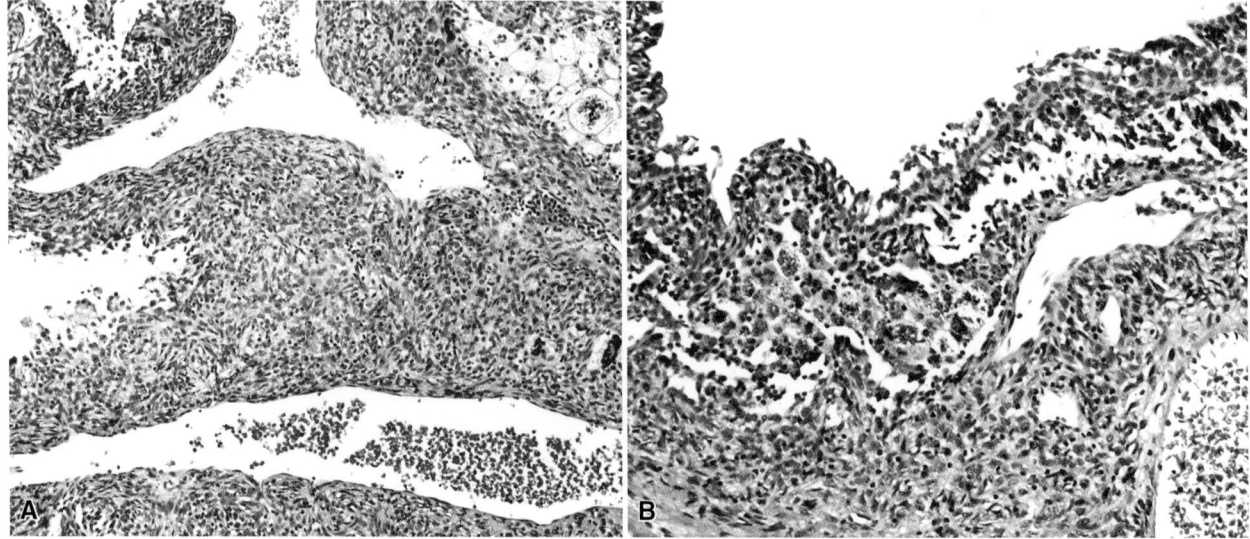

Figure 19-131. A and **B,** A "cystic fibrohistiocytic tumor" of the lung demonstrates groups of relatively bland spindle cells, histiocyte-like cells, and foamy histiocytes (**A**; *upper right*). These lesions are currently considered metastases of low-grade extrapulmonary neoplasms rather than primary tumors of the lung.

fibrohistiocytic tumors was unclear. Currently, in accord with the opinions of Colome-Grimmer and Evans[518] and the authors of the original report on this entity (T. V. Colby, personal communication), it is believed that cystic fibrohistiocytic tumors are actually *not* primary lesions of the lung. Instead, they likely represent metastases of extrapulmonary low-grade fibrohistiocytic tumors, including such tumors as cellular dermatofibroma of skin.

Other Lesions

Well-differentiated papillary mesothelioma of the pleura and intrapulmonary paraganglioma are other borderline lesions that are properly mentioned here. Because of its specialized nature and possible relationship to malignant mesotheliomas, well-differentiated papillary mesothelioma is discussed in Chapter 20. Intrapulmonary paraganglionic tumors are discussed in Chapter 13, dealing with neuroendocrine neoplasms. Because its biologic characteristics are more aggressive than those of most other "borderline lesions," hemangioendothelioma is discussed in Chapter 14, on malignant mesenchymal tumors of the lung and pleura.

Self-assessment questions related to this chapter can be found online on the Expert Consult site for this title.

References

1. Wingo PA, Cardinez CJ, Landis SH, et al. Long-term trends in cancer mortality in the United States, 1930–1998. *Cancer*. 2003;97(12 suppl):3133–3275.
2. Lutz JM, Francisci S, Mugno E, et al. Cancer prevalence in Central Europe: the EUROPREVAL study. *Ann Oncol*. 2003;14:313–322.
3. Oei TK, Wouters EF, Visser R, VanEngelshoven JM, Greve LH. The value of conventional radiography and computed tomography (CT) in diagnosis of pulmonary hamartoma. *Rontgenblatter*. 1983;36:324–327.
4. Erasmus JJ, Connolly JE, McAdams HP, Roggli VL. Solitary pulmonary nodules: Part I. Morphologic evaluation for differentiation of benign and malignant lesions. *Radiographics*. 2000;20:43–58.
5. Petticrew MP, Sowden AJ, Lister-Sharp D, Wright K. False-negative results in screening programs: systematic review of impact and implications. *Health Technol Assess*. 2000;4:1–120.
6. Cardillo G, Regal M, Sera F, et al. Videothoracoscopic management of the solitary pulmonary nodule: a single-institution study on 429 cases. *Ann Thorac Surg*. 2003;75:1607–1611.
7. Barzo P, Molnar L, Minik K. Bronchial papilloma of various origins. *Chest*. 1987;92:132–136.
8. Spencer H, Dail DH, Arneaud J. Noninvasive bronchial epithelial papillary tumors. *Cancer*. 1980;45:1486–1497.
9. Zimmerman A, Lang HR, Muhlberger F, Bachman M. Papilloma of the bronchus. *Respiration*. 1980;39:286–290.
10. Maxwell RJ, Gibbons JR, O'Hara MD. Solitary squamous papilloma of the bronchus. *Thorax*. 1985;40:68–71.
11. Laubscher FA. Solitary squamous cell papilloma of bronchial origin. *Am J Clin Pathol*. 1969;52:599–603.
12. Greene JG, Tassin L, Saberi A. Endobronchial epithelial papilloma associated with a foreign body. *Chest*. 1990;97:229–230.
13. Miura H, Tsuchida T, Kawate N, et al. Asymptomatic solitary papilloma of the bronchus: review of occurrence in Japan. *Eur Respir J*. 1993;6:1070–1073.
14. Basheda S, Gephardt GN, Stoller JK. Columnar papilloma of the bronchus: case report and literature review. *Am Rev Respir Dis*. 1991;144:1400–1402.
15. Trillo A, Guha A. Solitary condylomatous papilloma of the bronchus. *Arch Pathol Lab Med*. 1988;112:731–733.
16. Desai AV, Scolyer RA, McCaughan B, Torzillo PJ. Middle lobe syndrome due to obstructing solitary bronchial papilloma. *Aust N Z J Med*. 1999;29:745–747.
17. Hurt R. Benign tumors of the bronchus and trachea, 1951–1981. *Ann R Coll Surg Engl*. 1984;66:22–26.
18. Roviaro GC, Varoli F, Pagnini CA. Is the solitary papilloma of the bronchus always a benign tumor? *J Otorhinolaryngol Relat Spec*. 1981;43:301–308.
19. Katial RK, Ranlett R, Whitlock WL. Human papillomavirus associated with solitary squamous papilloma complicated by bronchiectasis and bronchial stenosis. *Chest*. 1994;106:1887–1889.
20. Roglic M, Jukic S, Damjanov I. Cytology of the solitary papilloma of the bronchus. *Acta Cytol*. 1975;19:11–13.
21. Flieder DB, Koss MN, Nicholson A, et al. Solitary pulmonary papillomas in adults: a clinicopathologic and in-situ hybridization study of 14 cases combined with 27 cases in the literature. *Am J Surg Pathol*. 1998;22:1328–1342.
22. Lee YO, Kim DH, Kim CH, Park TI, Cho S. Rare tumor of the tracheobronchial tree: solitary squamous papilloma. *Thorac Cardiovasc Surg*. 2009;57:178–179.

23. Popper HH, El-Shabrawi Y, Wockel W, et al. Prognostic importance of human papillomavirus typing in squamous cell papilloma of the bronchus: comparison of in-situ hybridization and the polymerase chain reaction. *Hum Pathol*. 1994;25:1191–1197.
24. Popper HH, Wirnsberger G, Juttner-Smolle FM, Pongratz MG, Sommersgutter M. The predictive value of human papillomavirus (HPV) typing in the prognosis of bronchial squamous cell papillomas. *Histopathology*. 1992;21:323–330.
25. Clavel CE, Nawrocki B, Bosseaux B, et al. Detection of human papillomavirus DNA in bronchopulmonary carcinomas by hybrid capture. II. A study of 185 tumors. *Cancer*. 2000;88:1347–1352.
26. Smith E, Pignatari S, Gray S, Haugen T, Turak L. Human papillomavirus infection in papillomas and nondiseased respiratory sites of patients with recurrent respiratory papillomatosis, using the polymerase chain reaction. *Arch Otolaryngol Head Neck Surg*. 1993;119:554–557.
27. Rady PL, Schnadig VJ, Weiss RL, Hughes TK, Tyring SK. Malignant transformation of recurrent respiratory papillomatosis associated with integrated human papillomavirus type 11 DNA and mutation of p53. *Laryngoscope*. 1998;108:735–740.
28. Syrjanen RJ. Epithelial lesions suggestive of a condylomatous origin found closely associated with invasive bronchial squamous cell carcinomas. *Respiration*. 1980;40:150–160.
29. DiMarco AF, Montenegro H, Payne Jr CB, Kwon KH. Papillomas of the tracheobronchial tree with malignant degeneration. *Chest*. 1978;74:464–465.
30. Bejui-Thivolet F, Chardonnet Y, Patricot LM. Human papillomavirus type 11 DNA in papillary squamous cell lung carcinoma. *Virchows Arch A*. 1990;417:457–461.
31. Inoue Y, Oka M, Ishii H, et al. A solitary bronchial papilloma with malignant changes. *Intern Med*. 2001;40:56–60.
32. Kramer S, Wehunt W, Stocker J, Kashima H. Pulmonary manifestations of juvenile laryngotracheal papillomatosis. *Am J Roentgenol*. 1985;144:687–694.
33. Fechner RE, Fitz-Hugh G. Invasive tracheal papillomatosis. *Am J Surg Pathol*. 1980;4:79–86.
34. Peterson BL, Buchwald C, Gerstoft J, Bretlau P, Lindeberg H. An aggressive and invasive growth of juvenile papillomas involving the total respiratory tract. *J Laryngol Otol*. 1998;112:1101–1104.
35. Franzmann MB, Buchwald C, Larsen P, Balle V. Tracheobronchial involvement of laryngeal papillomatosis at onset. *J Laryngol Otol*. 1994;108:164–165.
36. Shykhon M, Kuo M, Pearman R. Recurrent respiratory papillomatosis. *Clin Otolaryngol*. 2002;27:237–243.
37. Blackledge RA, Anandi VK. Tracheobronchial extension of recurrent respiratory papillomatosis. *Ann Otol Rhinol Laryngol*. 2000;109:812–818.
38. Harada H, Miura K, Tsutsui Y, et al. Solitary squamous cell papilloma of the lung in a 40 year old woman with recurrent laryngeal papillomatosis. *Pathol Int*. 2000;50:431–439.
39. Weingarten J. Cytologic and histologic findings in a case of tracheobronchial papillomatosis. *Acta Cytol*. 1981;25:167–170.
40. Kashima H, Mounts P, Leventhal B, Hruban RH. Sites of predilection in recurrent respiratory papillomatosis. *Ann Otol Rhinol Laryngol*. 1993;102:580–583.
41. Al-Saleem T, Peale AR, Norris CM. Multiple papillomatosis of the lower respiratory tract: clinical and pathologic study of eleven cases. *Cancer*. 1968;22:1173–1184.
42. Rahman A, Ziment I. Tracheobronchial papillomatosis with malignant transformation. *Arch Intern Med*. 1983;143:577–578.
43. Batsakis JG, Raymond AK, Rice DH. The pathology of head and neck tumors: papillomas of the upper aerodigestive tracts, Part 18. *Head Neck Surg*. 1983;5:332–344.
44. Zarod A, Rutherford J, Corbitt G. Malignant progression of laryngeal papilloma associated with human papillomavirus type 6 (HPV-6). *J Clin Pathol*. 1988;41:280–283.
45. Byrne J, Tsao MS, Fraser R, Howley P. Human papillomavirus-11 DNA in a patient with chronic laryngotracheobronchial papillomatosis and metastatic squamous cell carcinoma of the lung. *N Engl J Med*. 1987;317:873–878.
46. Wilde E, Duggan M, Field S. Bronchogenic squamous cell carcinoma complicating localized recurrent respiratory papillomatosis. *Chest*. 1994;105:1887–1888.
47. Lindsay F, Bloom D, Pransky S, Stabley R, Shick P. Histologic review of cidofovir-treated recurrent respiratory papillomatosis. *Ann Otol Rhinol Laryngol*. 2008;117:113–117.
48. Yousem SA, Ohori NP, Sonmez-Alpan E. Occurrence of human papillomavirus DNA in primary lung neoplasms. *Cancer*. 1992;69:693–697.
49. Liebow AA. Tumors of the lower respiratory tract. In: *Atlas of Tumor Pathology*, Series 1, Fascicle 17. Washington, DC: Armed Forces Institute of Pathology; 1952:22.
50. England DM, Hochholzer L. Truly benign "bronchial adenoma:" report of 10 cases of mucous gland adenoma with immunohistochemical and ultrastructural findings. *Am J Surg Pathol*. 1995;19:887–899.
51. Markel SF, Abell MR, Haight C, French AJ. Neoplasms of the bronchus commonly designated as adenomas. *Cancer*. 1964;17:590–608.
52. Payne WS, Fontana RS, Woolner LB. Bronchial tumors originating from mucous glands: current classification and unusual manifestations. *Med Clin North Am Dis Respir*. 1964;48:945–960.
53. Milenkovic B, Stojsic J, Mandaric D, Stevic R. Mucous gland adenoma simulating bronchial asthma: case report and literature review. *J Asthma*. 2007;44:789–793.
54. Spencer H. Bronchial mucous gland tumors. *Virchows Arch Pathol Anat*. 1979;383:101–115.
55. Allen Jr MS, Marsh Jr WL, Greissinger WT. Mucous gland adenoma of the bronchus. *J Thorac Cardiovasc Surg*. 1974;67:966–968.
56. Emory WB, Mitchel Jr WT, Hatch Jr HG. Mucous gland adenoma of the bronchus. *Am Rev Respir Dis*. 1973;108:1407–1410.
57. Edwards CW, Matthews HR. Mucous gland adenoma of the bronchus. *Thorax*. 1981;36:147–148.
58. Kroe DJ, Pitcock JA. Benign mucous gland adenoma of the bronchus. *Arch Pathol*. 1967;84:539–540.

59. Heard BE, Corrin B, Dewar A. Pathology of seven mucous cell adenomas of the bronchial glands with particular reference to ultrastructure. *Histopathology*. 1985;9:687–701.

60. Akhtar M, Young I, Reyes F. Bronchial adenoma with polymorphous features. *Cancer*. 1974;33:1572–1576.

61. Rosenblum P, Klein RI. Adenomatous polyp of the right main bronchus producing atelectasis. *Pediatrics*. 1936;78:791–796.

62. Smith AG. Benign epithelial tumors of the bronchus. *South Med J*. 1965;58:1535–1541.

63. Courtin P, Janin A, Sault MC, et al. Pure bronchial adenoma. Anatomic, clinical, and ultrastructural study of a case. *Ann Pathol*. 1987;7:315–319.

64. Weinberger MA, Katz S, Davis EW. Peripheral bronchial adenoma of mucous gland type: clinical and pathological aspects. *J Thorac Surg*. 1955;29:626–635.

65. Key BM, Pritchett PS. Mucous gland adenoma of the bronchus. *South Med J*. 1979;72:83–85.

66. Arrigoni MG, Woolner LB, Bernatz PE, Miller WE, Fontana RS. Benign tumors of the lung: a ten-year experience. *J Thorac Cardiovasc Surg*. 1970;60:589–599.

67. Kwon JW, Goo JM, Seo JB, Seo JW, Im JG. Mucous gland adenoma of the bronchus: CT findings in two patients. *J Comput Assist Tomogr*. 1999;23:758–760.

68. Mejean-Lebreton F, Barnoud R, De la Roche E, Devouassoux-Shisheboran M. Benign salivary gland-type tumors of the bronchus: expression of high molecular-weight cytokeratins. *Ann Pathol*. 2006;26:30–34.

69. Delpiano C, Claren R, Sironi M, Cenacchi G, Spinelli M. Cytological appearance of papillary mucous gland adenoma of the left lobar bronchus with histological confirmation. *Cytopathology*. 2000;11:193–196.

70. Moran CA, Suster S, Askin FB, Koss MN. Benign and malignant salivary gland-type mixed tumors of the lung: clinicopathologic and immunohistochemical study of eight cases. *Cancer*. 1994;73:2481–2490.

71. Davis PW, Briggs JC, Leal RME, et al. Benign and malignant mixed tumors of the lung. *Thorax*. 1972;27:657–673.

72. Hayes MM, Van der Westhuizen NG, Forgie R. Malignant mixed tumors of the bronchus: a biphasic neoplasm of epithelial and myoepithelial cells. *Mod Pathol*. 1993;6:85–88.

73. Payne WS, Scier J, Woolner LB. Mixed tumors of the bronchus (salivary gland type). *J Thorac Cardiovasc Surg*. 1965;49:663–668.

74. Sakamoto H, Uda H, Tanaka T, et al. Pleomorphic adenoma in the periphery of the lung: report of a case and review of the literature. *Arch Pathol Lab Med*. 1991;115:393–396.

75. Moran CA, Suster S, Askin FB, Koss MN. Benign and malignant salivary gland-type tumors of the lung: clinicopathologic and immunohistochemical study of eight cases. *Cancer*. 1994;73:2481–2490.

76. Baghai-Wadji M, Sianati M, Nikpour H, Koochekpour S. Pleomorphic adenoma of the trachea in an 8 year-old boy: a case report. *J Pediatr Surg*. 2006;41:e23–e26 (August 2006).

77. Kamiyoshihara M, Ibe T, Takeyoshi I. Pleomorphic adenoma of the main bronchus in an adult treated using a wedge bronchiectomy. *Gen Thorac Cardiovasc Surg*. 2009;57:43–45.

78. Fitchett J, Luckraz H, Gibbs A, O'Keefe P. A rare case of primary pleomorphic adenoma in main bronchus. *Ann Thorac Surg*. 2008;86:1025–1026.

79. Jin HY, Park TS. Pulmonary pleomorphic adenoma: report of a rare case. *Korean J Intern Med*. 2007;22:122–124.

80. Kourda J, Ismail O, Smati BH, Ayadi A, Kilani T, El-Mezni F. Benign myoepithelioma of the lung—a case report and review of the literature. *Cases J*. 2010;13:25.

81. Angelov A, Dikranian K, Trosheva M. Immunomorphological characteristics of pleomorphic adenoma of salivary glands. *Bull Group Int Rech Sci Stomatol Odontol*. 1996;39:67–75.

82. Ang KL, Dhannapuneni VR, Morgan WE, Soomro IN. Primary pulmonary pleomorphic adenoma: an immunohistochemical study and review of the literature. *Arch Pathol Lab Med*. 2003;127:621–622.

83. Takeuchi E, Shimizu E, Sano N, et al. A case of pleomorphic adenoma of the lung with multiple distant metastases—observations on its oncogene and tumor suppressor gene expression. *Anticancer Res*. 1998;18:2015–2020.

84. Fechner RE, Bentnick BR. Ultrastructure of bronchial oncocytoma. *Cancer*. 1973;31:1451–1457.

85. Nielsen AL. Malignant bronchial oncocytoma: a case report and review of the literature. *Hum Pathol*. 1985;16:852–854.

86. Santos-Briz A, Jenron J, Sastre R, Romero L, Valle A. Oncocytoma of the lung. *Cancer*. 1977;40:1330–1336.

87. Burrah R, Kini U, Correa M, Srirangapatna S. pulmonary oncocytoma: a rare case. *Asian Cardiovasc Thorac Ann*. 2006;14:e113–e114.

88. Laforga JB, Aranda FI. Multicentric oncocytoma of the lung diagnosed by fine-needle aspiration. *Diagn Cytopathol*. 1999;21:51–54.

89. Tashiro Y, Iwata Y, Nabae T, Manage H. Pulmonary oncocytoma: report of a case in conjunction with an immunohistochemical and ultrastructural study. *Pathol Int*. 1995;45:448–451.

90. De Jesus MG, Poon TP, Chung KY. Pulmonary oncocytoma. *N Y State J Med*. 1989;89:477–480.

91. Tesluk H, Dajee A. Pulmonary oncocytoma. *J Surg Oncol*. 1985;29:173–175.

92. Fernandez MA, Nyssen J. Oncocytoma of the lung. *Can J Surg*. 1982;25:332–333.

93. Black III WC. Pulmonary oncocytoma. *Cancer*. 1969;23:1347–1357.

94. Ritter JH, Nappi O. Oxyphilic proliferations of the respiratory tract and paranasal sinuses. *Semin Diagn Pathol*. 1999;16:105–116.

95. Arora R, Mathur SR, Aron M, et al. Oncocytic carcinoid tumor of the lung: a case report of diagnostic pitfall in filter membrane preparation of bronchial washings. *Acta Cytol*. 2007;51:907–910.

96. Zhou CX, Gao Y. Oncocytoma of the salivary glands: a clinicopathologic and immunohistochemical study. *Oral Oncol*. 2009;45:e232–e238 (September 30, 2009).

97. Mete O, Kilicasian I, Gulluoglu MG, Uysal V. Can renal oncocytoma be differentiated from its renal mimics? The utility of anti-mitochondrial, caveolin-1, CD63, and cytokeratin 14 antibodies in the differential diagnosis. *Virchows Arch*. 2005;447:938–946.

98. Bartley TD, Arean VM. Intrapulmonary neurogenic tumors. *J Thorac Cardiovasc Surg*. 1965;50:114–123.

99. Roviaro G, Montorsi M, Varoli F, Binda R, Cecchetto A. Primary pulmonary tumors of neurogenic origin. *Thorax*. 1983;38:942–945.

100. Silverman JF, Leffers BR, Kay S. Primary pulmonary neurilemmoma: report of a case with ultrastructural examination. *Arch Pathol Lab Med*. 1976;100:644–648.

101. Yamakawa H. Intrapulmonary schwannoma: a case report. *J Jpn Assoc Chest Surg*. 1993;7:165–169.

102. Sugita M, Fujimura S, Hasumi T, Kondo T, Sagawa M. Sleeve superior segmentectomy of the right lower lobe for endobronchial neurinoma: report of a case. *Respiration*. 1996;63:191–194.

103. McCluggage WG, Bharucha H. Primary pulmonary tumors of nerve sheath origin. *Histopathology*. 1995;26:247–254.

104. Lin YC, Lin MC, Chen TC, Huang CC, Lee CH. Tracheal neurilemmoma mimicking bronchial asthma—a dilemma of difficult diagnosis: case report. *Changgeng Yi Xue Za Zhi*. 1999;22:525–529.

105. Tsukada H, Hsada H, Kojima K, Yamata N. Bronchial wall schwannoma removed by sleeve resection of the right mainstem bronchus without lung resection. *J Cardiovasc Surg*. 1998;39:511–513.

106. Ashkan K, Casey AT. Pulmonary apex schwannoma. *J Neurol Neurosurg Psych*. 1997;63:719.

107. Bosch X, Ramirez J, Font J, et al. Primary intrapulmonary benign schwannoma: a case with ultrastructural and immunohistochemical confirmation. *Eur Respir J*. 1990;3:234–237.

108. Muhrer KH, Fischer HP. Primary pulmonary neurilemmoma. *Thorac Cardiovasc Surg*. 1983;31:313–316.

109. Imaizumi M, Takahashi T, Niimi T, et al. A case of primary intrapulmonary neurilemmoma and review of the literature. *Jpn J Surg*. 1989;19:740–746.

110. Feldhaus RJ, Anene C, Bogard P. A rare endobronchial neurilemmoma (schwannoma). *Chest*. 1989;95:461–462.

111. Nesbitt JC, Vega DM, Burke T, Mackay B. Cellular schwannoma of the bronchus. *Ultrastruct Pathol*. 1996;20:349–354.

112. Noah MA, Gorecha M, Firmin RK. Primary benign bronchial schwannoma presenting as asthma. *J Asthma*. 2009;46:856–857.

113. Onal M, Ernam D, Atikcan S, Memis L. Endobronchial schwannoma with massive hemoptysis. *Tuberk Toraks*. 2009;57:89–92.

114. Unger PD, Geller SA, Anderson PJ. Pulmonary lesions in a patient with neurofibromatosis. *Arch Pathol Lab Med*. 1984;108:654–657.

115. Bacha EA, Wright CD, Grillo HC, et al. Surgical treatment of primary pulmonary sarcomas. *Eur J Cardiothorac Surg*. 1999;15:456–460.

116. Moran CA, Suster S, Koss MN. Primary malignant "triton" tumor of the lung. *Histopathology*. 1997;30:140–144.

117. Attanoos RL, Appleton MA, Gibbs AR. Primary sarcomas of the lung: a clinicopathological and immunohistochemical study of 14 cases. *Histopathology*. 1996;29:29–36.

118. Simansky DA, Aviel-Ronen S, Reder I, et al. Psammomatous melanotic schwannoma: presentation of a rare primary lung tumor. *Ann Thorac Surg*. 2000;70:671–672.

119. Abrikossoff A. Uber Myome ausgehend von der quergestreiften willkurlichen Muskulatur. *Virchows Arch Pathol Anat Physiol Klin Med*. 1926;260:215–233.

120. Lack EE, Worsham GF, Callihan MD, et al. Granular cell tumor: a clinicopathologic study of 110 patients. *J Surg Oncol*. 1980;13:301–316.

121. Alvarez-Fernandez E, Carretero-Albinana L. Bronchial granular cell tumor: presentation of three cases with tissue culture and ultrastructural study. *Arch Pathol Lab Med*. 1987;111:1065–1069.

122. DeClerq D, Van der Straten M, Roels H. Granular cell myoblastoma of the bronchus. *Eur J Respir Dis*. 1983;64:72–76.

123. Hurwitz SS, Conlan AA, Gritzman MC, Krut LH. Granular cell myoblastoma. *Thorax*. 1982;37:392–393.

124. Hosaka T, Suzuki S, Niikawa H, et al. A rare case of a pulmonary granular cell tumor presenting as a coin lesion. *Jpn J Thorac Cardiovasc Surg*. 2003;51:107–109.

125. Abdulhamid I, Rabah R. Granular cell tumor of the bronchus. *Pediatr Pulmonol*. 2000;30:425–428.

126. Husain M, Nguyen GK. Cytopathology of granular cell tumor of the lung. *Diagn Cytopathol*. 2000;23:294–295.

127. Al-Ghamdi AM, Flint JD, Muller NL, Stewart KC. Hilar pulmonary granular cell tumor: a case report and review of the literature. *Ann Diagn Pathol*. 2002;4:245–251.

128. Scala R, Naldi M, Fabianelli F, et al. Endobronchial granular cell tumor. *Monaldi Arch Chest Dis*. 1999;54:404–406.

129. Thomas de Montpreville V, Dulmet EM. Granular cell tumors of the lower respiratory tract. *Histopathology*. 1995;27:257–262.

130. Deavers M, Guinee D, Koss MN, Travis WD. Granular cell tumors of the lung: clinicopathologic study of 20 cases. *Am J Surg Pathol*. 1995;19:627–635.

131. Hernandez OG, Haponik EF, Summer WR. Granular cell tumor of the bronchus: bronchoscopic and clinical features. *Thorax*. 1986;41:927–931.

132. Mullen Jr CV, Hewan-Lowe K, Gilman MJ. Massive hemoptysis associated with granular cell tumor of the bronchus. *South Med J*. 1983;76:1452.

133. Lack EE, Harris GB, Eraklis AJ, Vawter GF. Primary bronchial tumors in childhood: a clinicopathologic study of six cases. *Cancer*. 1983;51:492–497.

134. Guillou L, Gloor E, Anani PA, Kaelin R. Bronchial granular cell tumor: report of a case with preoperative cytologic diagnosis on bronchial brushings and immunohistochemical studies. *Acta Cytol*. 1991;35:375–380.

135. Majmudar B, Thomas J, Gorelkin L, Symbas PN. Respiratory obstruction caused by a multicentric granular cell tumor of the laryngotracheobronchial tree. *Hum Pathol*. 1981;12:283–286.

136. Oparah SS, Subramanian VA. Granular cell myoblastoma of the bronchus: report of 2 cases and review of the literature. *Ann Thorac Surg*. 1976;22:199–202.

137. Robinson JM, Knoll R, Henry DA. Intrathoracic giant cell myoblastoma. *South Med J*. 1988;81:1453–1457.

138. Schulster PL, Khan FA, Azueta V. Asymptomatic pulmonary granular cell tumor presenting as a coin lesion. *Chest*. 1975;68:256–258.

139. Chen KTK. Cytology of bronchial benign granular cell tumor. *Acta Cytol*. 1991;35:381–384.

140. Miyake M, Tateishi U, Maeda T, Arai Y, Hasegawa T, Sugimura K. Bronchial granular cell tumor: a case presenting secondary obstructive changes on CT. *Radiat Med*. 2006;24:154–157.

141. Fang HY, Wu CY, Huang HJ, Lin YM. Granular cell tumor of the lung. *Lungs*. 2010; Jan. 12 (E-pub ahead of print).

142. Muhammed AA, Sikka P, Dhillon RS, Gibbons WJ, Ahmed A. Coexisting granular cell tumor and adenocarcinoma of the lung: a case report and review of the literature. *Respir Care*. 2001;46: 702–704.

143. Cutlan RT, Eltorky M. Pulmonary granular cell tumor coexisting with bronchogenic carcinoma. *Ann Diagn Pathol*. 2001;5:74–79.

144. Althausen AM, Kowalski DP, Ludwig ME, Curry SL, Greene JF. Granular cell tumors: a new clinically important histologic finding. *Gynecol Oncol*. 2000;77:310–313.

145. Elmberger PG, Skold CM, Collins BT. Fine needle aspiration biopsy of intrabronchial granular cell tumor. *Acta Cytol*. 2005;49:223–224.

146. Sobel HJ, Marquet E, Avrin E, Schwarz R. Granular cell myoblastoma: an electron microscopic and cytochemical study illustrating the genesis of granules and aging of myoblastoma cells. *Am J Pathol*. 1971;65:59–78.

147. Miettinen M, Lehtonen E, Lehtola H, et al. Histogenesis of granular cell tumor: an immunohistochemical and ultrastructural study. *J Pathol*. 1984;142:221–229.

148. Mazur M, Shultz JJ, Myers JL. Granular cell tumor: immunohistochemical analysis of 21 benign tumors and one malignant tumor. *Arch Pathol Lab Med*. 1990;114:692–696.

149. Liu Z, Mira JL, Vu H. Diagnosis of malignant granular cell tumor by fine needle aspiration cytology. *Acta Cytol*. 2001;45:1011–1021.

150. Ordonez NG, Mackay B. Granular cell tumor: a review of the pathology and histogenesis. *Ultrastruct Pathol*. 1999;23:207–222.

151. Fine SW, Li M. Expression of calretinin and the alpha-subunit of inhibin in granular cell tumors. *Am J Clin Pathol*. 2003;119:259–264.

152. Nappi O, Ferrara G, Wick MR. Neoplasms composed of eosinophilic polygonal cells: an overview with consideration of different cytomorphologic patterns. *Semin Diagn Pathol*. 1999;16:82–90.

153. Franzblau MJ, Manwaring M, Plumhof C, Listrom JB, Burgdorf WHC. Metastatic breast carcinoma mimicking granular cell tumor. *J Cutan Pathol*. 1989;16:218–221.

154. Reuter VE. Renal tumors exhibiting granular cytoplasm. *Semin Diagn Pathol*. 1999;16:135–145.

155. Ogino S, Al-Kaisi N, Abdul-Karim FW. Cytopathology of oncocytic carcinoid tumor of the lung mimicking granular cell tumor: a case report. *Acta Cytol*. 2000;44:247–250.

156. Ritter JH, Nappi O. Oxyphilic proliferations of the respiratory tract and paranasal sinuses. *Semin Diagn Pathol*. 1999;16:105–116.

157. Yousem SA, Hochholzer L. Alveolar adenoma. *Hum Pathol*. 1986;17:1066–1071.

158. Sak SD, Koseoglu RD, Demirag F, Akbulut H, Gungor A. Alveolar adenoma of the lung: immunohistochemical and flow-cytometric characteristics of two new cases and a review of the literature. *APMIS*. 2007;115:1443–1449.

159. Fujimoto K, Muller NL, Sadohara J, et al. Alveolar adenoma of the lung: computed tomography and magnetic resonance imaging findings. *J Thorac Imaging*. 2002;17:163–166.

160. Hartman MS, Epstein DM, Geyer SJ, Keenan RJ. Alveolar adenoma. *Ann Thorac Surg*. 2004;78:1842–1843.

161. Cavazza A, Paci M, De Marco L, et al. Alveolar adenoma of the lung: a clinicopathologic, immunohistochemical, and molecular study of an unusuasl case. *Int J Surg Pathol*. 2004;12:155–159.

162. Semeraro D, Gibbs AR. Pulmonary adenoma: a variant of sclerosing hemangioma of lung? *J Clin Pathol*. 1989;42:1222–1223.

163. Oliveira P, Moura-Nunes JF, Clode AL, da Costa JD, Almeida MO. Alveolar adenoma of the lung: further characterization of this uncommon tumor. *Virchows Arch*. 1996;429:101–108.

164. Burke LM, Rush WI, Khoor A, et al. Alveolar adenoma: a histochemical, immunohistochemical, and ultrastructural analysis of 17 cases. *Hum Pathol*. 1999;30:158–167.

165. Al-Hilli F. Lymphangioma (of alveolar adenoma?) of the lung. *Histopathology*. 1987;11:979–986.

166. Wada A, Tateishi R, Terazawa T, Matsuda M, Hattori S. Lymphangioma of the lung. *Arch Pathol*. 1974;98:211–213.

167. Miller RR. Bronchioloalveolar cell adenomas. *Am J Surg Pathol*. 1990;14:904–912.

168. Glaab R, Turina M, Achermann E, Maurer R, Went P, Schob G. Alveolar adenoma—a rare pulmonary mass: case report and review of the literature. *Zenbralbl Chir*. 2009;134:478–480.

169. Nakamura H, Adachi Y, Arai T, et al. A small alveolar adenoma resected by thoracoscopic surgery. *Ann Thorac Surg*. 2009;87:956–957.

170. Hegg CA, Flint A, Singh G. Papillary adenoma of the lung. *Am J Clin Pathol*. 1992;97:393–397.

171. Fukuda T, Ohnishi Y, Kanai I, et al. Papillary adenoma of the lung: histological and ultrastructural findings in two cases. *Acta Pathol Jpn*. 1992;42:56–61.

172. Mori M, Chiba R, Tezuka F, et al. Papillary adenoma of type II pneumocytes might have malignant potential. *Virchows Arch*. 1996;428:195–200.

173. Yamamoto T, Horiguchi H, Shibagaki T, Kamma H, Ogata T, Mitsui K. Encapsulated type II pneumocyte adenoma: a case report & review of the literature. *Respiration*. 1993;60:373–377.

174. Noguchi M, Kodama T, Shimosato Y, et al. Papillary adenoma of type 2 pneumocytes. *Am J Surg Pathol*. 1986;10:134–139.

175. Fine G, Chang CH. Adenoma of type 2 pneumocytes with oncocytic features. *Arch Pathol Lab Med*. 1991;115:797–801.

176. Kurotaki H, Kamata Y, Kimura M, Nagai K. Multiple papillary adenomas of type II pneumocytes found in a 13 year old boy with von Recklinghausen's disease. *Virchows Arch*. 1993;423:319–322.

177. Spencer H, Dail DH, Arneaud J. Noninvasive bronchial epithelial papillary tumors. *Cancer*. 1980;45:1486–1497.

178. Sanchez-Jimenez J, Ballester-Martinez A, Lodo-Besse J, et al. Papillary adenoma of type II pneumocytes. *Pediatr Pulmonol*. 1994;17:396–400.

179. Gesierich W, Diwersy C, Leinsinger G, et al. Papillary adenoma of type II pneumocytes as a rare differential diagnosis of a solitary pulmonary nodule. *Pneumologie*. 2007;61:697–699.

180. Papla B. Papillary adenoma of the lung. *Pol J Pathol*. 2009;60:49–51.

181. Fantone JC, Geisinger KR, Appelman HD. Papillary adenoma of the lung with lamellar and electron-dense granules: an ultrastructural study. *Cancer*. 1982;50:2839–2844.

182. Dessy E, Braidotti P, Del Curto B, et al. Peripheral papillary tumor of type II pneumocytes: a rare neoplasm of undetermined malignant potential. *Virchows Arch*. 2000;436:289–295.

183. Tomashefski JF. Benign endobronchial mesenchymal tumors: their relationship to parenchymal pulmonary hamartomas. *Am J Surg Pathol*. 1982;6:531–540.

184. Yellin A, Roserman Y, Lieberman Y. Review of smooth muscle tumors of the lower respiratory tract. *Br J Dis Chest*. 1984;78:337–351.

185. White SH, Ibrahim NBN, Forrester-Wood CP, Jeyasingham R. Leiomyomas of the lower respiratory tract. *Thorax*. 1985;40:306–311.

186. Orlowski TM, Stasiak K, Kolodziej J. Leiomyoma of the lung. *J Thorac Cardiovasc Surg*. 1978;76:257–261.

187. Van den Bosch JM, Wagenaar SS, Corrin B, et al. Mesenchymoma of the lung (so-called hamartoma): a review of 154 parenchymal and endobronchial cases. *Thorax*. 1987;42:790–793.

188. Gal AA, Brooks JJ, Pietra GG. Leiomyomatous lung neoplasms: a clinical, histologic, and immunohistochemical study. *Mod Pathol*. 1989;2:209–216.

189. Van Way CW, McCracken RL, Carlisle BB. Leiomyoma of the lower respiratory tract. *Ann Thorac Surg*. 1968;6:273–276.

190. Taylor TL, Miller DR. Leiomyoma of the bronchus. *J Thorac Cardiovasc Surg*. 1969;57:245–248.

191. Yamada H, Katoh O, Yamaguchi T, Natsuaki M, Itoh T. Intrabronchial leiomyoma treated by localized resection vis bronchotomy and bronchoplasty. *Chest*. 1987;91:283–284.

192. Shahian DM, McEnahy MR. Complete endobronchial resection of leiomyoma of the bronchus. *J Thorac Cardiovasc Surg*. 1979;77:87–91.

193. Kim KH, Suh JS, Han WS. Leiomyoma of the bronchus treated by endoscopic resection. *Ann Thorac Surg*. 1993;56:1164–1166.

194. Mouveroux FA, Bourcereau J, Fressinaud C, Bourras P. Bronchial leiomyoma: report of a case successfully treated by Nd-YAG laser. *Thorac Cardiovasc Surg*. 1988;95:536–537.

195. Sivalingam B, Somani K, Sreenivasan L, Collins FJ. Endobronchial leiomyoma: successful resection by sleeve lobectomy. *Int J Thorac Cardiovasc Surg*. www.ispub.com/ispub/ijtcvs/volume_7_ number_2/endobronchial_leiomyoma_successful_resection_by_sleeve)lobectomy.

196. Silverman JF, Kay S. Multiple pulmonary leiomyomatous hamartomas: report of case with ultrastructural examination. *Cancer*. 1976;38:1199–1204.

197. Hull MT, Gonzalez-Crussi F, Grosfeld JL. Multiple pulmonary fibroleiomyomatous hamartomata in childhood. *J Pediatr Surg*. 1979;14:428–431.

198. Itoh H, Yanagi M, Setoyama T, et al. Solitary fibroleiomyomatous hamartoma of the lung in a patient without a preexisting smooth muscle tumor. *Pathol Int*. 2001;51:661–665.

199. Shmookler BM, Lauer DH. Retroperitoneal leiomyosarcoma: a clinicopathologic analysis of 36 cases. *Am J Surg Pathol*. 1983;7:269–280.

200. Mackay B, Legha SS. Coin lesion of the lung in a 19 year old male. *Ultrastruct Pathol*. 1981;2:289–294.

201. Alt B, Huffer WE, Belchis DA. A vascular lesion with smooth muscle differentiation presenting as a coin lesion in the lung: glomus tumor versus hemangiopericytoma. *Am J Clin Pathol*. 1983;80:765–771.

202. Fabich DR, Hafez GR. Glomangioma of the trachea. *Cancer*. 1980;45:2337–2341.

203. Tang C, Toker CK, Foris NP, Trump BF. Glomangioma of the lung. *Am J Surg Pathol*. 1978;2:103–109.

204. Gaertner EM, Steinberg DM, Huber M, et al. Pulmonary and mediastinal glomus tumors: report of five cases including a pulmonary glomangiosarcoma. A clinicopathologic study with literature review. *Am J Surg Pathol*. 2000;24:1105–1114.

205. Yilmaz A, Bayramgurler B, Aksoy F, et al. Pulmonary glomus tumor: a case initially diagnosed as carcinoid tumor. *Respirology*. 2002;7:369–371.

206. Shugart RR, Soule EH, Johnson EW. Glomus tumors. *Surg Gynecol Obstet*. 1963;117:334–340.

207. Miettinen M, Paal E, Lasota J, Sobin LH. Gastrointestinal glomus tumors: a clinicopathologic, immunohistochemical, and molecular genetic study of 32 cases. *Am J Surg Pathol*. 2002;26:301–311.

208. Littlefield JB, Drash EC. Myxoma of the lung. *J Thorac Surg*. 1959;37:745–749.

209. Pollak ER, Naunheim KS, Little AG. Fibromyxoma of the trachea. *Arch Pathol Lab Med*. 1985;109:926–929.

210. Butler C, Kleinerman J. Pulmonary hamartoma. *Arch Pathol*. 1969;88:584–592.

211. Gjevre JA, Myers JL, Prakash UBS. Pulmonary hamartomas. *Mayo Clin Proc*. 1996;71:14–20.

212. Hamper UM, Khouri NF, Stitik FP, et al. Pulmonary hamartoma: diagnosis by transthoracic needle-aspiration biopsy. *Radiology*. 1985;155:15–18.

213. Wiatrowska BA, Yazdi HM, Matzinger FR, MacDonald LL. Fine needle aspiration biopsy of pulmonary hamartomas: radiologic, cytologic, and immunocytochemical study of 15 cases. *Acta Cytol*. 1995;39:1167–1174.

214. Carney JA. The triad of gastric epithelioid leiomyosarcoma, functioning extra-adrenal paraganglioma, and pulmonary chondroma. *Cancer*. 1979;43:374–382.

215. Wick MR, Ruebner BH, Carney JA. Gastric tumors in patients with pulmonary chondroma or extra-adrenal paraganglioma: an ultrastructural study. *Arch Pathol Lab Med*. 1981;105:527–531.

216. Rodriguez FJ, Aubry MC, Tazelaar HD, Slezak J, Carney JA. Pulmonary chondroma: a tumor associated with Carney triad and different from pulmonary hamartoma. *Am J Surg Pathol*. 2007;31:1844–1853.

217. Abrahams NA, Colby TV, Pearl RH, et al. Pulmonary hemangiomas of infancy and childhood: report of two cases and review of the literature. *Pediatr Dev Pathol*. 2002;5:283–292.

218. Fugo K, Matsuno Y, Okamoto K, et al. Solitary capillary hemangioma of the lung: report of 2 resected cases detected by high-resolution CT. *Am J Surg Pathol*. 2006;30:750–753.

219. Ritter JH, Mills SE, Nappi O, Wick MR. Angiosarcoma-like neoplasms of epithelial organs: true endothelial tumors or variants of carcinoma? *Semin Diagn Pathol*. 1995;12:270–282.

220. Almagro P, Julia J, Sanjaume M, et al. Pulmonary capillary hemangiomatosis associated with primary pulmonary hypertension: report of 2 new cases and review of 35 cases from the literature. *Medicine*. 2002;81:417–424.

221. Havlik DM, Massie LW, Williams WL, Crooks LA. Pulmonary capillary hemangiomatosis-like foci: an autopsy study of 8 cases. *Am J Clin Pathol*. 2000;113:655–662.

222. Eastridge CF, Young JM, Steplock AL. Endobronchial lipoma. *South Med J*. 1984;77:759–761.

223. Politis J, Funahashi A, Gehlsen JA, et al. Intrathoracic lipomas: report of three cases and review of the literature with emphasis on endobronchial lipoma. *J Thorac Cardiovasc Surg*. 1979;77:550–556.

224. Kamiyoshihara M, Sakata K, Ohtani Y, et al. Endobronchial lipoma accompanied with primary lung cancer: report of a case. *Surg Today*. 2002;32:402–405.

225. Moran CA, Suster S, Koss MN. Endobronchial lipomas: a clinicopathologic study of four cases. *Mod Pathol*. 1994;7:212–214.

226. Muraoka M, Oka T, Akamine S, et al. Endobronchial lipoma: review of 64 cases reported in Japan. *Chest*. 2003;123:293–296.

227. Gaerte SC, Meyer CA, Winer-Muram HT, Tarver RD, Conces Jr DJ. Fat-containing lesions of the chest. *Radiographics*. 2002;22(suppl):S61–S78.

228. Solli P, Rossi G, Carbagnani P, et al. Pulmonary abnormalities in Cowden's disease. *J Cardiovasc Surg*. 1998;40:753–755.

229. Irani F, Kumar B, Reddy P, Narwal-Chadha R, Kasmani R, Tita J. An endobronchial lipoma mimicking asthma and malignancy. *Prim Care Respir J*. 2009; Dec. 17 pii: pcrj-2009-04-0033.R1 10.4104/pcrj.2009.00070 (E-publication).

230. Sekine I, Kodama T, Yokose T, et al. Rare pulmonary tumors—a review of 32 cases. *Oncology*. 1998;55:431–434.

231. Matsuba K, Saito T, Ando K, Shirakusa T. Atypical lipoma of the lung. *Thorax*. 1991;46:685.

232. Bridge JA, Roberts CA, Degenhardt J, et al. Low-level chromosome 12 amplification in a primary lipoma of the lung: evidence for a pathogenetic relationship with common adipose tissue tumors. *Arch Pathol Lab Med*. 1998;122:187–190.

233. Hirata J, Reshad K, Itoi K, Muro K, Akiyama J. Lipomas of the peripheral lung—a case report and review of the literature. *Thorac Cardiovasc Surg*. 1989;37:385–387.

234. Erkilic S, Kocer NE, Tuncozgur B. Peripheral intrapulmonary lipoma: a case report. *Acta Chir Belg*. 2007;107:700–702.

235. Shimoyama T, Kimura B. Peripheral intrapulmonary lipoma: report of a case. *Jpn J Thorac Surg*. 2009;62:1186–1189.

236. Coffin CM. Lipoblastoma: an embryonal tumor of soft tissue related to organogenesis. *Semin Diagn Pathol*. 1994;11:98–103.

237. Kanu A, Oermann CM, Malicki D, Wagner M, Langston C. Pulmonary lipoblastoma in an 18-month-old child: a unique tumor in children. *Pediatr Pulmonol*. 2002;34:150–154.

238. Mathew J, Sen S, Chandi SM, et al. Pulmonary lipoblastoma: a case report. *Pediatr Surg Int*. 2001;17:543–544.

239. Achir A, Ouadnouni Y, Smahi M, Bouchikh M, Msougar Y, Benosman A. Primary pulmonary liposarcoma—a case report. *Thorac Cardiovasc Surg*. 2009;57:119–120.

240. Loddenkempter C, Perez-Canto A, Leschber G, Stein H. Primary dedifferentiated liposarcoma of the lung. *Histopathology*. 2005;46:710–712.

241. Kitizawa R, Kitazawa S, Nishimura Y, Kondo T, Obayashi C. Lung carcinosarcoma with liposarcoma element: autopsy case. *Pathol Int*. 2006;56:449–452.

242. Hicks J, Dilley A, Patel D, et al. Lipoblastoma and lipoblastomatosis in infancy and childhood: histopathologic, ultrastructural, and cytogenetic features. *Ultrastruct Pathol*. 2001;25:321–333.

243. Nicolas M, Moran CA, Suster S. Pulmonary metastasis from liposarcoma: a clinicopathologic and immunohistochemical study of 24 cases. *Am J Clin Pathol*. 2005;123:265–275.

244. Meis-Kindblom JM, Sjogren H, Kindblom LG, et al. Cytogenetic and molecular genetic analyses of liposarcoma and its soft tissue simulators: recognition of new variants and differential diagnosis. *Virchows Arch*. 2001;439:141–151.

245. Tallini G, Vanni R, Manfioletti G, et al. HMGI-C and HMGI(Y) immunoreactivity correlates with cytogenetic abnormalities in lipomas, pulmonary chondroid hamartomas, endometrial polyps, and uterine leiomyomas and is compatible with rearrangement of the HMGI-C and HMGI(Y) genes. *Lab Invest*. 2000;80:359–369.

246. Johansson M, Dietrich C, Mandahl N, et al. Recombinations of chromosomal bands 6p21 and 14q24 characterize pulmonary hamartomas. *Br J Cancer*. 1993;67:1236–1241.

247. Pea M, Bonetti F, Zamboni G, et al. Clear cell tumor and angiomyolipoma. *Am J Surg Pathol*. 1991;15:199–202.

248. Bacchi CE, Bonetti F, Pea M, Martignoni G, Gown AM. HMB-45: a review. *Appl Immunohistochem Mol Morphol*. 1996;4:73–85.

249. Bonetti F, Pea M, Martignoni G, et al. Clear cell ("sugar") tumor of the lung is a lesion strictly related to angiomyolipoma—the concept of a family of lesions characterized by the presence of the perivascular epithelioid cell (PEC). *Pathology*. 1994;26:230–236.

250. Hornick JL, Fletcher CDM. PEComa: what do we know so far? *Histopathology*. 2006;48:75–82.

251. Folpe AL, McKenney JK, Li Z, Smith SJ, Weiss SW. Clear cell myomelanocytic tumor of the thigh: report of a unique case. *Am J Surg Pathol*. 2002;26:809–812.

252. Garcia TR, Mestre-de-Juan MJ. Angiomyolipoma of the liver and lung: a case explained by the presence of perivascular epithelioid cells. *Pathol Res Pract*. 2002;198:363–367.

253. Wu K, Tazelaar HD. Pulmonary angiomyolipoma and multifocal micronodular pneumocyte hyperplasia associated with tuberous sclerosis. *Hum Pathol*. 1999;30:1266–1268.

254. Papla B, Malinowski E. Angiomyolipoma of the lung. *Pol J Pathol*. 1999;50:47–50.

255. Ito M, Sugamura Y, Ikari H, Sekine I. Angiomyolipoma of the lung. *Arch Pathol Lab Med*. 1998;122:1023–1025.

256. Guinee Jr DG, Thornberry DS, Azumi N, et al. Unique pulmonary presentation of an angiomyolipoma: analysis of clinical, radiographic, and histopathologic features. *Am J Surg Pathol*. 1995;19:476–480.

257. Marcheix B, Brouchet L, Lamarche Y, et al. Pulmonary angiomyolipoma. *Ann Thorac Surg*. 2006;82:1504–1506.

258. Chu SC, Horiba K, Usuki J, et al. Comprehensive evaluation of 35 patients with lymphangioleiomyomatosis. *Chest*. 1999;115:1041–1052.

259. Kitaichi M, Nishimura K, Itoh H, Izumi T. Pulmonary lymphangioleiomyomatosis: a report of 46 patients including a clinicopathologic study of prognostic factors. *Am J Respir Crit Care Med*. 1995;151:527–533.

260. Matsumoto S, Nishioka T, Akiyama T. Renal angiomyolipoma associated with micronodular pneumocyte hyperplasia of the lung with tuberous sclerosis. *Int J Urol*. 2001;8:242–244.

261. Takahashi N, Kitihara R, Hishimoto Y, et al. Malignant transformation of renal angiomyolipoma. *Int J Urol*. 2003;10:271–273.

262. Adachi Y, Horie Y, Kitamura Y, et al. CD1a expression in PEComas. *Pathol Int*. 2008;58:169–173.

263. Gee WF, Chikos PM, Greaves JP, Ikemoto N, Tremann JA. Adrenal myelolipoma. *Urology*. 1975;5:562–566.

264. Singla AK, Kechejian G, Lopez MJ. Giant presacral myelolipoma. *Am Surg*. 2003;69:334–338.

265. Hunter SB, Schemankewitz EH, Patterson C, Varma VA. Extraadrenal myelolipoma: a report of two cases. *Am J Clin Pathol*. 1992;97:402–404.

266. Sabate CJ, Shahian DM. Pulmonary myelolipoma. *Ann Thorac Surg*. 2002;74:573–575.

267. Piccinini L, Barbolini G. A case of lung myelolipomatosis in a patient with bronchial carcinoid. *Panminerva Med*. 1999;41:175–178.

268. Ziolkowski P, Muszczynska-Bernhard B, Dziegiel P. Myelolipoma: the report of two cases in a pulmonary location. *Pol J Pathol*. 1996;47:141–142.

269. Sato K, Ueda Y, Katsuda S, Tsuchihara K. Myelolipoma of the lung: a case report and brief review. *J Clin Pathol*. 2007;60:728–730.

270. Quigley JC, Hart WR. Adenomatoid tumors of the uterus. *Am J Clin Pathol*. 1981;76:627–635.

271. Srigley JR, Hartwick RW. Tumors and cysts of the paratesticular region. *Pathol Annu*. 1990;25:51–108.

272. Kaplan MA, Tazelaar HD, Hayashi T, Schroer KR, Travis WD. Adenomatoid tumors of the pleura. *Am J Surg Pathol*. 1996;20:1219–1223.

273. Handra-Luca A, Couvelard A, Abd-Alsamad I, et al. Adenomatoid tumor of the pleura: case report. *Ann Pathol*. 2000;20:369–372.

274. Umezu H, Kuwata K, Ebe Y, et al. Microcystic variant of localized malignant mesothelioma accompanying an adenomatoid tumor-like lesion. *Pathol Int*. 2002;52:416–422.

275. Minato H, Nojima T, Kurose N, Kinoshita E. Adenomatoid tumor of the pleura. *Pathol Int*. 2009;59:567–571.

276. Pinkard NB, Wilson RW, Lawless N, et al. Calcifying fibrous pseudotumor of the pleura: a report of three cases of a newly described entity involving the pleura. *Am J Clin Pathol*. 1996;105:189–194.

277. Murray JG, Pinkard NB. Calcifying fibrous pseudotumor of the pleura: radiologic features in three cases. *J Comput Assist Tomogr*. 1996;20:763–765.

278. Hainaut P, Lesage V, Weynand B, Coche E, Noirhomme P. Calcifying fibrous pseudotumor (CFPT): a patient presenting with multiple pleural lesions. *Acta Clin Belg*. 1999;54:162–164.

279. Cavazza A, Gelli MC, Agostini L, et al. Calcified pseudotumor of the pleura: description of a case. *Pathologica*. 2002;94:201–205.

280. Rosenthal NS, Abdul-Karim FW. Childhood fibrous tumor with psammoma bodies: clinico-pathologic features in two cases. *Arch Pathol Lab Med*. 1988;112:798–800.

281. Suh JH, Shin OR, Kim YH. Multiple calcifying fibrous pseudotumor of the pleura. *J Thorac Oncol*. 2008;3:1356–1358.

282. Shibata K, Yuki D, Sakata K. Multiple calcifying fibrous pseudotumors disseminated in the pleura. *Ann Thorac Surg*. 2008;85:e3–e5 (E-publication).

283. Soyer T, Ciftci AO, Gucer S, Orhan D, Senocak ME. Calcifying fibrous pseudotumor of lung: a previously-unreported entity. *J Pediatr Surg*. 2004;39:1729–1730.

284. Maeda T, Hirose T, Furuya K, Kameoka K. Calcifying fibrous pseudotumor: an ultrastructural study. *Ultrastruct Pathol*. 1999;23:189–192.

285. Hill KA, Gonzalez-Crussi F, Chou PM. Calcifying fibrous pseudotumor versus inflammatory myofibroblastic tumor: a histological and immunohistochemical comparison. *Mod Pathol*. 2001;14:784–790.

286. Nascimento AF, Ruiz R, Hornick JL, Fletcher CDM. Calcifying fibrous "pseudotumor": clinico-pathologic study of 15 cases and analysis of its relationship to inflammatory myofibroblastic tumor. *Int J Surg Pathol*. 2002;10:189–196.

287. Gibbs AR. Smooth mucle tumors of the pleura. *Histopathology*. 1995;27:295–296.

288. Mochizuki H, Okada T, Yoshizawa H, Suzuki E, Gejyo F. A case of primary pleural leiomyoma. *J Jpn Resp Soc*. 2004;42:625–628.

289. Brunn H. Two interesting benign lung tumors of contradictory histopathology. *J Thorac Cardiovasc Surg*. 1939;9:119–131.

290. Umiker WO, Iverson L. Postinflammatory "tumors" of the lung: report of four cases simulating xanthoma, fibroma, or plasma cell tumor. *J Thorac Cardiovasc Surg*. 1954;28:55–63.

291. Bahadori M, Liebow AA. Plasma cell granulomas of the lung. *Cancer*. 1973;31:191–208.

292. Spencer H. The pulmonary plasma cell/histiocytoma complex. *Histopathology*. 1984;8:903–916.

293. Berardi RS, Lee SS, Chen HP, et al. Inflammatory pseudotumors of the lungs. *Surg Gynecol Obstet*. 1983;156:89–96.

294. Souid AK, Ziemba MC, Dubansky AS, et al. Inflammatory myofibroblastic tumor in children. *Cancer*. 1993;72:2042–2048.

295. Wick MR, Ritter JH, Nappi O. Inflammatory sarcomatoid carcinoma of the lung: report of three cases with comparison with inflammatory pseudotumors in adult patients. *Hum Pathol*. 1995;26:1014–1021.

296. Su LD, Atayde-Perez A, Sheldon S, Fletcher JA, Weiss SW. Inflammatory myofibroblastic tumor: cytogenetic evidence supporting a clonal origin. *Mod Pathol*. 1998;11:364–368.

297. Snyder CS, Dell'Aquila M, Haghighi P, et al. Clonal changes in inflammatory pseudotumor of the lung: a case report. *Cancer*. 1995;76:1545–1549.

298. Yamamoto H, Oda Y, Saito T, et al. p53 mutation and MDM2 amplification in inflammatory myofibroblastic tumors. *Histopathology*. 2003;42:431–439.

299. Pettinato G, Manivel JC, DeRosa N, et al. Inflammatory myofibroblastic tumor (plasma cell granuloma): a clinicopathologic study of 20 cases with immunohistochemical and ultrastructural observations. *Am J Clin Pathol*. 1990;94:538–546.

300. Meis JM, Enzinger FM. Inflammatory fibrosarcoma of the mesentery and retroperitoneum: a tumor closely simulating inflammatory pseudotumor. *Am J Surg Pathol*. 1991;15:1146–1156.

301. Coffin CM, Dehner LP, Meis-Kindblom JM. Inflammatory myofibroblastic tumor, inflammatory fibrosarcoma, and related lesions: an historical review with differential diagnostic considerations. *Semin Diagn Pathol*. 1998;15:102–110.

302. Lioulias A, Misthos P, Neofotistos E, Legaki S. Primary myofibrosarcoma of the lung: a rare case with challenging diagnosis. *J BUON*. 2009;14:143–145.

303. Takeda S, Onishi Y, Kawamura T, Maeda H. Clinical spectrum of pulmonary inflammatory myofibroblastic tumor. *Interact Cardiovasc Thorac Surg*. 2008;7:629–633.

304. Matsubara O, Tan-Liu NS, Kenney RM, et al. Inflammatory pseudotumors of the lung: progression from organizing pneumonia to fibrous histiocytoma or to plasma cell granuloma in 32 cases. *Hum Pathol*. 1988;19:807–814.

305. Cessna MH, Zhou H, Sanger WG, et al. Expression of *ALK1* and p80 in inflammatory myofibroblastic tumor and its mesenchymal mimics: a study of 135 cases. *Mod Pathol*. 2002;15:931–938.

306. Coffin CM, Hornick JL, Fletcher CDM. Inflammatory myofibroblastic tumor: comparison of clinicopathologic, histologic, and immunohistochemical features including ALK expression in atypical and aggressive cases. *Am J Surg Pathol*. 2007;31:509–520.

307. Yamamoto H, Yamaguchi H, Aishima S, et al. Inflammatory myofibroblastic tumor versus IgG4-related sclerosing disease and inflammatory pseudotumor: a comparative clinicopathologic study. *Am J Surg Pathol*. 2009;33:1330–1340.

308. Antic T, Kapur U, Vigneswaran WT, Oshima K. Inflammatory sarcomatoid carcinoma: a case report and discussion of a malignant tumor with benign appearance. *Arch Pathol Lab Med*. 2005;129:1334–1337.

309. Hussong JW, Brown M, Perkins SL, Dehner LP, Coffin CM. Comparison of DNA ploidy, histologic, and immunohistochemical findings with clinical outcome in inflammatory myofibroblastic tumors. *Mod Pathol*. 1999;12:279–286.

310. Messineo A, Mognato G, D'Amore ES, et al. Inflammatory pseudotumors of the lung in children: conservative or aggressive approach? *Med Pediatr Oncol*. 1998;31:100–104.

311. Liebow AA, Hubbell DS. Sclerosing hemangioma (histiocytoma, xanthoma) of the lung. *Cancer*. 1956;9:53–75.

312. Gross RE, Wolbach SB. Sclerosing hemangiomas: their relationship to dermatofibroma, histiocytoma, xanthoma, and to certain pigmented lesions of the skin. *Am J Pathol*. 1943;19:533–546.

313. Katzenstein AL, Weise D, Fuilling K, Battifora H. So-called sclerosing hemangioma of the lung: evidence for mesothelial origin. *Am J Surg Pathol*. 1983;7:3–14.

314. Kennedy A. Sclerosing hemangioma" of the lung: an alternative view of its development. *J Clin Pathol*. 1973;26:792–799.

315. Hill GS, Eggleston JC. Electron microscopic study of so-called pulmonary "sclerosing hemangioma": report of a case suggesting an epithelial origin. *Cancer*. 1972;30:1092–1106.

316. Kay S, Still WJ, Borochovitz D. Sclerosing hemangioma of the lung: an endothelial or epithelial neoplasm? *Hum Pathol*. 1977;8:468–474.

317. Spencer H, Nambu S. Sclerosing hemangiomas of the lung. *Histopathology*. 1986;10:477–487.

318. Keylock JB, Galvin JR, Franks TJ. Sclerosing hemangioma of the lung. *Arch Pathol Lab Med*. 2009;133:820–825.

319. Kalhor N, Staerkel GA, Moran CA. So-called sclerosing hemangioma of lung: current concepts. *Ann Diagn Pathol*. 2010;14:60–67.

320. Shimosato Y. Lung tumors of uncertain histogenesis. *Semin Diagn Pathol*. 1995;12:185–192.

321. Batinica S, Gunek G, Raos M, Jelasic D, Bogovic M. Sclerosing hemangioma of the lung in a 4-year-old child. *Eur J Pediatr Surg*. 2002;12:192–194.

322. Devouassoux-Shisheboran M, Hayashi T, Linnoila R, Koss MN, Travis WD. A clinicopathologic study of 100 cases of pulmonary sclerosing hemangioma with immunohistochemical studies: TTF-1 is expressed in both round and surface cells, suggesting an origin from primitive respiratory epithelium. *Am J Surg Pathol*. 2000;24:906–916.

323. Kuo KT, Hsu WH, Wu YC, Huang MH, Li WY. Sclerosing hemangioma of the lung: an analysis of 44 cases. *J Chin Med Assoc*. 2003;66:33–38.

324. Miyagawa-Hayashino A, Tazelaar HD, Langel DJ, Colby TV. Pulmonary sclerosing hemangioma with lymph node metastases: report of 4 cases. *Arch Pathol Lab Med*. 2003;127:321–325.

325. Hayashi A, Takamori S, Mitsuoka M, et al. Unilateral progressive multiple sclerosing hemangioma in a young female successfully treated by pneumonectomy: report of a case. *Int Surg*. 2002;87:69–72.

326. Iyoda A, Baba M, Saitoh H, et al. Imprint cytologic features of pulmonary sclerosing hemangioma: comparison with well-differentiated papillary adenocarcinoma. *Cancer*. 2002;96:146–149.

327. Nam JE, Ryu YH, Cho SH, et al. Air-trapping zone surrounding sclerosing hemangioma of the lung. *J Comput Assist Tomogr*. 2002;26:358–361.

328. Yano M, Yamakawa Y, Kiriyama M, Hara M, Murase T. Sclerosing hemangioma with metastases to multiple nodal stations. *Ann Thorac Surg*. 2002;73:981–983.

329. Gal AA, Nassar VH, Miller JI. Cytopathologic diagnosis of pulmonary sclerosing hemangioma. *Diagn Cytopathol*. 2002;26:163–166.

330. Ng WK, Fu KH, Wang E, Tang V. Sclerosing hemangioma of lung: a close cytologic mimicker of pulmonary adenocarcinoma. *Diagn Cytopathol*. 2001;25:316–320.

331. Illei PB, Rosai J, Klimstra DS. Expression of thyroid transcription factor-1 and other markers in sclerosing hemangioma of the lung. *Arch Pathol Lab Med*. 2001;125:1335–1339.

332. Chan AC, Chan JKC. Pulmonary sclerosing hemangioma consistently expresses thyroid transcription factor-1 (TTF-1): a new clue to its histogenesis. *Am J Surg Pathol*. 2000;24:1531–1536.

333. Wani Y, Notohara K, Tsukayama C, Okumura N. Sclerosing hemangioma with florid endobronchial and endobronchiolar growth. *Virchows Arch*. 2007;450:221–223.

334. Guibaud L, Pracros JP, Rode V, et al. Sclerosing hemangioma of the lung: radiological findings and pathological diagnosis. *Pediatr Radiol*. 1995;25(suppl 1):S207–S208.

335. Komatsu T, Fukuse T, Wada H, Sakurai T. Pulmonary sclerosing hemangioma with pulmonary metastasis. *Thorac Cardiovasc Surg*. 2006;54:348–349.

336. Katzenstein AL, Gmelich J, Carrington C. Sclerosing hemangioma of the lung: a clinicopathologic study of 51 cases. *Am J Surg Pathol*. 1980;4:343–356.

337. Moran CA, Zeren H, Koss MN. Sclerosing hemangioma of the lung: granulomatous variant. *Arch Pathol Lab Med*. 1994;118:1028–1030.

338. Wojcik E, Sneige N, Lawrence D, Ordonez NG. Fine needle aspiration cytology of sclerosing hemangioma of the lung: case report with immunohistochemical study. *Diagn Cytopathol*. 1993;9:304–309.

339. Gottschalk-Sabag S, Hadas-Halpern I, Glick T. Sclerosing hemangioma of lung mimicking carcinoma, diagnosed by fine needle aspiration (FNA) cytology. *Cytopathology*. 1995;6:115–120.

340. Krishnamurthy SC, Naresh KN, Soni M, Bhasin SD. Sclerosing hemangioma of the lung: a potential source of error in fine needle aspiration cytology. *Acta Cytol*. 1995;38:111–112.

341. Islam S, Roustan-Delatour NL, Salahdeen SR, Mai KT, Senterman M, Mokhtar GA. Cytologic features of benign solitary pulmonary nodules with radiologic correlation and diagnostic pitfalls: a report of six cases. *Acta Cytol*. 2009;53:201–210.

342. Yousem SA, Wick MR, Singh G, et al. So-called sclerosing hemangiomas of lung: an immunohistochemical study supporting a respiratory epithelial origin. *Am J Surg Pathol*. 1988;12:582–590.

343. Satoh Y, Tsuchiya E, Weng SY, et al. Pulmonary sclerosing hemangioma of the lung: type II pneumocytoma by immunohistochemistry and immunoelectron microscopic studies. *Cancer*. 1989;64:1310–1317.

344. Alvarez-Fernandez B, Carretero-Albinana L, Menarquez-Palanca J. Sclerosing hemangioma of the lung: an immunohistochemical study of intermediate filaments and endothelial markers. *Arch Pathol Lab Med*. 1989;113:121–124.

345. Fukayama M, Mikoike M. So-called sclerosing hemangioma of the lung: an immunohistochemical, histochemical, and ultrastructural study. *Acta Pathol Jpn*. 1988;38:627–642.

346. Leong ASY, Chan KW, Seneviratne HS. A morphological and immunohistochemical study of 25 cases of so-called sclerosing hemangioma of the lung. *Histopathology*. 1995;27:121–128.

347. Nagata N, Dairaku M, Sueishi K, Tanaka K. Sclerosing hemangioma of the lung: an epithelial tumor composed of immunohistochemically heterogeneous cells. *Am J Clin Pathol*. 1987;88:552–559.

348. Xu HM, Li WH, Hou N, et al. Neuroendocrine differentiation in 32 cases of so-called sclerosing hemangioma of the lung, identified by immunohistochemistry and ultrastructural study. *Am J Surg Pathol*. 1997;21:1013–1022.

349. Wu CT, Chang YL, Lee YC. Expression of the estrogen receptor beta in 37 surgically treated pulmonary sclerosing hemangiomas in comparison with non-small-cell lung carcinomas. *Hum Pathol*. 2005;36:1108–1112.

350. Wei S, Tian J, Song X, Chen Y. Recurrence of pulmonary sclerosing hemangioma. *Thorac Cardiovasc Surg*. 2008;56:120–122.

351. Tanaka I, Inoue M, Matsui Y, et al. A case of pneumocytoma (so-called sclerosing hemangioma) with lymph node metastasis. *Jpn J Clin Oncol*. 1986;16:77–86.

352. Vaideeswar P. Sclerosing hemangioma with lymph node metastases. *Indian J Pathol Microbiol*. 2009;52:392–394.

353. Chien NC, Lin CW, Tzeng JE. Sclerosing hemangioma with lymph node metastasatis. *Respirology*. 2009;14:614–616.

354. Guillou L, DeLuze P, Zysset F, Costa J. Papillary variant of low-grade mucoepidermoid carcinoma—an unusual bronchial neoplasm: a light microscopic, ultrastructural, and immunohistochemical study. *Am J Clin Pathol*. 1994;101:269–274.

355. Rodriguez IM, Prat J. Mucinous tumors of the ovary: a clinicopathologic analysis of 75 borderline tumors (of intestinal type) and carcinomas. *Am J Surg Pathol*. 2002;26:139–152.

356. Izumo A, Yamaguchi K, Eguchi T, et al. Mucinous cystic tumor of the pancreas. *Oncol Rep*. 2003;10:515–525.

357. Sambrook-Gowar FJ. An unusual mucous cyst of the lung. *Thorax*. 1978;33:796–799.

358. Butnor KJ, Sporn TA, Dodd LG. Fine needle aspiration cytology of mucinous cystadenocarcinoma of the lung: report of a case with radiographic and histologic correlation. *Acta Cytol*. 2001;45:779–783.

359. Monaghan H, Salter DM, Ferguson T. Pulmonary mucinous cystic tumor of borderline malignancy: a rare variant of adenocarcinoma. *J Clin Pathol*. 2002;55:156.

360. Divisi D, Battaglia C, Giusti L, et al. Mucinous cystadenoma of the lung. *Acta Biomed Ateneo Parmense*. 1997;68:115–118.

361. Papla B, Malinowski E, Harazda M. Pulmonary mucinous cystadenoma of borderline malignancy: a report of two cases. *Pol J Pathol*. 1996;47:87–90.

362. Roux FJ, Lantuejoul S, Brambilla E, Brambilla C. Mucinous cystadenoma of the lung. *Cancer*. 1995;76:1540–1544.

363. Pelletier B, Dubigeon P, Despins P, Dehajartre AY. Cystic mucinous pulmonary tumor of borderline malignancy: report of a case. *Ann Pathol*. 1993;13:405–408.

364. Davison AM, Lowe JW, DaCosta P. Adenocarcinoma arising in a mucinous cystadenoma of the lung. *Thorax*. 1992;47:129–130.

365. Traub B. Mucinous cystadenoma of the lung. *Arch Pathol Lab Med*. 1991;115:740–741.

366. Kragel PJ, Devaney KO, Meth BM, et al. Mucinous cystadenoma of the lung: a report of two cases with immunohistochemical and ultrastructural analysis. *Arch Pathol Lab Med*. 1990;114:1053–1056.

367. Matsuo T, Yusuke-Kimura N, Takamori S, Shirouzu K. Recurrent pulmonary mucinous cystadenoma. *Eur J Cardiothorac Surg*. 2005;28:176–177.

368. Gao ZH, Urbanski SJ. The spectrum of pulmonary mucinous cystic neoplasia: a clinicopathologic & immunohistochemical study of ten cases and review of literature. *Am J Clin Pathol*. 2005;124:62–70.

369. Klein J, Zhuang Z, Lubensky I, Colby TV, Martinez Jr F, Leslie KO. Multifocal microcysts and papillary cystadenoma of the lung in von Hippel-Lindau disease. *Am J Surg Pathol*. 2007;31:1292–1296.

370. Kleinert R, Popper H. Giant fibroma of the lung: a morphologic study. *Virchows Arch A*. 1987;410:363–367.

371. Sauk JJ, Pliego M, Anderson WR. Primary pulmonary fibroma. *Minn Med*. 1972;55:220–223.

372. Klemperer P, Rabin CB. Primary neoplasms of the pleura. *Arch Pathol*. 1931;11:385–412.

373. Briselli MF, Mark EJ. Solitary fibrous tumors of the pleura and benign extrapleural tumors of mesothelial origin. In: Antman K, Aisner J, eds. *Asbestos-Related Malignancy*. Philadelphia: Grune & Stratton; 1986:165–178.

374. Dalton W, Zollike A, McCaughey WT, Jacques J, Kannerstein M. Localized primary tumors of the pleura. *Cancer*. 1979;44:1465–1475.

375. Vallat-Decouvelaere AV, Dry SM, Fletcher CDM. Atypical and malignant solitary fibrous tumors in extrathoracic locations: evidence of their comparability to intrathoracic tumors. *Am J Surg Pathol*. 1998;22:1501–1511.

376. Magdeleinat P, Alifano M, Petino A, et al. Solitary fibrous tumors of the pleura: clinical characteristics, surgical treatment, and outcome. *Eur J Cardiothorac Surg*. 2002;21:1087–1093.

377. Cardillo G, Facciolo F, Cavazzana AO, et al. Localized (solitary) fibrous tumors of the pleura: an analysis of 55 patients. *Ann Thorac Surg*. 2000;70:1808–1812.

378. Duster P, Mayer E, Kramm T, et al. Solitary fibrous pleural tumors—rare tumors with unpredictable clinical behavior. *Pneumologie*. 2000;54:16–19.

379. Meyer M, Krause U. Solitary fibrous tumors of the pleura. *Chirurgie*. 1999;70:949–952.

380. Khan JH, Rahman SB, Clary-Macy C, et al. Giant solitary fibrous tumor of the pleura. *Ann Thorac Surg*. 1998;65:1461–1464.

381. Briselli MF, Mark EJ, Dickersin GR. Solitary fibrous tumors of the pleura: eight new cases and review of 360 cases in the literature. *Cancer*. 1981;47:2678–2689.

382. Hanau CA, Miettinen M. Solitary fibrous tumor: histological and immunohistochemical spectrum of benign and malignant variants presenting at different sites. *Hum Pathol*. 1995;26:440–449.

383. Moran CA, Suster S, Koss MN. The spectrum of histologic growth patterns in benign and malignant fibrous tumors of the pleura. *Semin Diagn Pathol*. 1992;9:169–180.

384. England DM, Hochholzer L, McCarthy MJ. Localized benign and malignant fibrous tumors of the pleura. *Am J Surg Pathol*. 1989;13:640–658.

385. Patsios D, Hwang DM, Chung TB. Intraparenchymal solitary fibrous tumor of the lung: an uncommon cause of a pulmonary nodule. *J Thorac Imaging*. 2006;21:50–53.

386. Sakurai H, Tanaka W, Kaji H, Yamazaki K, Suemasu K. Intrapulmonary localized fibrous tumor of the lung: a very unusual presentation. *Ann Thorac Surg*. 2008;86:1360–1362.

387. Cardinale L, Ardissone F, Cataldi A, Familiari U, Solitro F, Fava C. Solitary fibrous tumor of the lung: three rare cases of intraparenchymal nodules. *Acta Radiol*. 2009;50:379–382.

388. Fujiu K, Miyamoto H, Sakuma H, Mori M. Solitary fibrous tumors of the pleura presenting satellite tumors. *Gen Thorac Cardiovasc Surg*. 2009;57:382–384.

389. Ali SZ, Hoon V, Hoda S, Heelan R, Zakowski MF. Solitary fibrous tumor: a cytologic–histologic study with clinical, radiologic, and immunohistochemical correlations. *Cancer*. 1997;81:116–121.

390. Harrison-Phipps KM, Nichols FC, Schleck CD, et al. Solitary fibrous tumors of the pleura: results of surgical treatment and long-term prognosis. *J Thorac Cardiovasc Surg*. 2009;138:19–25.

391. Weynand B, Collard P, Galant C. Cytopathological features of solitary fibrous tumor of the pleura: a study of 5 cases. *Diagn Cytopathol*. 1998;18:118–124.

392. Caruso RA, LaSpada F, Gaeta M, Minutoli I, Inferrera C. Report of an intrapulmonary solitary fibrous tumor: fine needle aspiration cytologic findings, clinicopathological, and immunohistochemical features. *Diagn Cytopathol*. 1996;14:64–67.

393. Khalifa MA, Montgomery EA, Azumi N, et al. Solitary fibrous tumors: a series of lesions, some in unusual sites. *South Med J*. 1997;90:793–799.

394. Van de Rijn M, Lombard CM, Rouse RV. Expression of CD34 by solitary fibrous tumors of the pleura, mediastinum, and lung. *Am J Surg Pathol*. 1994;18:814–820.

395. Suster S, Fisher C, Moran CA. Expression of *bcl-2* oncoprotein in benign and malignant spindle cell tumors of soft tissue, skin, serosal surfaces, and gastrointestinal tract. *Am J Surg Pathol*. 1998;22:863–872.

396. Flint A, Weiss SW. CD34 and keratin expression distinguishes solitary fibrous tumor (fibrous mesothelioma) of pleura from desmoplastic mesothelioma. *Hum Pathol*. 1995;26:428–431.

397. Ledet SC, Brown RW, Cagle PT. p53 immunostaining in the differentiation of inflammatory pseudotumor from sarcoma involving the lung. *Mod Pathol*. 1995;8:282–286.

398. Krismann M, Adams H, Jaworska M, Muller KM, Johnen G. Patterns of chromosomal imbalances in benign solitary fibrous tumors of the pleura. *Virchows Arch A*. 2000;70:1808–1812.

399. Dal Cin P, Pauwels P, Van den Berghe H. Solitary fibrous tumor of the pleura with t(4;15)(q13;q26). *Histopathology*. 1999;35:94–95.

400. Carbone M, Rizzo P, Powers A, et al. Molecular analyses, morphology, and immunohistochemistry together differentiate pleural synovial sarcomas from mesotheliomas: clinical implications. *Anticancer Res*. 2002;22:3443–3448.

401. Knosel T, Hertsch S, Alendorf-Hofmann A, et al. TLE1 is a robust diagnostic biomarker for synovial sarcomas and correlates with t(X;18): analysis of 319 cases. *Eur J Cancer*. 2010;46:1170–1176.

402. Sumathi VP, McCluggage WG. CD10 is useful in demonstrating endometrial stroma at ectopic sites and in confirming a diagnosis of endometriosis. *J Clin Pathol*. 2002;55:391–392.

403. Takagi M, Kuwano K, Watanabe K, Akiba T. A case of recurrence and rapid growth of pleural solitary fibrous tumor 8 years after initial surgery. *Ann Thorac Cardiovasc Surg*. 2009;15:178–181.

404. Miyoshi N, Takami K, Okami J, et al. Extrapleural pneumonectomy for relapsed solitary fibrous tumors of the pleura with pleural dissemination. *Jpn J Thorac Surg*. 2007;60:800–805.

405. Liu CC, Wang HW, Li FY, et al. Solitary fibrous tumors of the pleura: clinicopathological characteristics, immunohistochemical profiles, and surgical outcomes with long-term followup. *Thorac Cadiovasc Surg*. 2008;56:291–297.

406. Anthony T, Rodriguez-Bigas MA, Weber TK, Petrelli NJ. Desmoid tumors. *J Am Coll Surg*. 1996;182:369–377.

407. Dashiell TG, Payne WS, Hepper NG, Soule EH. Desmoid tumors of the chest wall. *Chest*. 1978;74:157–162.

408. Rodriguez-Bigas MA, Mahoney MC, Karakousis CP, Petrelli NJ. Desmoid tumors in patients with familial adenomatous polyposis. *Cancer*. 1994;74:1270–1274.

409. Andino L, Cagle PT, Maurer B, et al. Pleuropulmonary desmoid tumors: immunohistochemical comparison with solitary fibrous tumors and assessment of beta-catenin and cyclin-D1 expression. *Arch Pathol Lab Med*. 2006;130:1503–1509.

410. Varghese Jr TK, Gupta R, Yeldandi AV, Sundaresan SR. Desmoid tumor of the chest wall with pleural involvement. *Ann Thorac Surg*. 2003;76:937–939.

411. Peled N, Babyn PS, Manson D, de Nanassy J. Aggressive fibromatosis simulating congenital lung malformation. *Can Assoc Radiol J*. 1993;44:221–223.

412. Takeshima Y, Nakayori F, Nakano T, et al. Extra-abdominal desmoid tumor presenting as an intrathoracic tumor: case report and literature review. *Pathol Int*. 2001;51:824–828.

413. Wilson RW, Gallateau-Salle F, Moran CA. Desmoid tumors of the pleura: a clinicopathologic mimic of localized fibrous tumor. *Mod Pathol*. 1999;12:9–14.

414. Montgomery EA, Meis JM. Nodular fasciitis: its morphologic spectrum and immunohistochemical profile. *Am J Surg Pathol*. 1991;15:942–948.

415. Owens CL, Sharma R, Ali SZ. Deep fibromatosis (desmoid tumor): cytopathologic characteristics, clinicoradiologic features, and immunohistochemical findings on fine-need aspiration. *Cancer*. 2007;111:166–172.

416. Bhattacharya B, Dilworth HP, Iacobuzio-Donahue C, et al. Nuclear beta-catenin expression distinguishes deep fibromatosis from other benign and malignant fibroblastic and myofibroblastic lesions. *Am J Surg Pathol*. 2005;29:653–659.

417. Ng TL, Gown AM, Barry TS, et al. Nuclear beta-catenin in mesenchymal tumors. *Mod Pathol*. 2005;18:68–74.

418. Carlson JW, Fletcher CDM. Immunohistochemistry for beta-catenin in the differential diagnosis of spindle-cell lesions: analysis of a series and review of the literature. *Histopathology*. 2007;51:509–514.

419. De Bree E, Keus R, Melissas J, Tsiftsis D, van Coevorden F. Desmoid tumors: need for an individualized approach. *Expert Rev Anticancer Ther*. 2009;9:525–535.

420. Abbas AE, Deschamps C, Cassivi SD, et al. Chest-wall desmoid tumors: results of surgical intervention. *Ann Thorac Surg*. 2004;78:1219–1223.

421. Liebow AA, Castleman B. Benign "clear cell tumors" of the lung. *Am J Pathol*. 1963;43:13–14.

422. Liebow AA, Castleman B. Benign clear cell ("sugar") tumors of the lung. *Yale J Biol Med*. 1971;43:213–222.

423. Hoch WS, Patchefsky AS, Takeda M, Gordon G. Benign clear-cell tumor of the lung: an ultrastructural study. *Cancer*. 1974;33:1328–1336.

424. Ozdemir IA, Zaman NU, Rullis I, Webb WR. Benign clear cell tumor of lung. *J Thorac Cardiovasc Surg*. 1974;68:131–133.

425. Kung M, Landa JF, Lubin J. Benign clear cell tumor ("sugar tumor") of the trachea. *Cancer*. 1984;54:517–519.

426. Hashimoto T, Oka K, Hakozaki H, et al. Benign clear cell tumor of the lung. *Ultrastruct Pathol*. 2001;25:479–483.

427. Slodkowska J, Suilkowska-Rowinska A, Dorosz P, Radomski P, Wasiutynski A. Benign clear cell tumor of the lung ("sugar tumor"): morphologic, immunohistochemical, and ultrastructural evaluation. *Pneumonol Alergol Pol*. 2000;68:60–64.

428. Gaffey MJ, Mills SE, Ritter JH. Clear cell tumors of the lower respiratory tract. *Semin Diagn Pathol*. 1997;14:222–232.

429. Jeanfaivre T, Savary L, Richard C. Benign clear cell tumor ("sugar tumor"): an unusual cause of intrapulmonary coin lesion. *Rev Mal Respir*. 1997;14:223–224.

430. Andrion A, Mazzucco G, Gugliotta P, Monga G. Benign clear-cell ("sugar") tumor of the lung: a light microscopic, histochemical, and ultrastructural study with a review of the literature. *Cancer*. 1985;56:2657–2663.

431. Sale GE, Kulander BG. Benign clear-cell tumor of lung with necrosis. *Cancer*. 1976;37:2355–2358.

432. Lantuejoul S, Isaac S, Pinel N, et al. Clear cell tumor of the lung: an immunohistochemical and ultrastructural study supporting a pericytic differentiation. *Mod Pathol*. 1997;10:1001–1008.

433. Flieder DB, Travis WD. Clear cell "sugar" tumor of the lung associated with lymphangioleiomyomatosis and multifocal micronodular pneumocyte hyperplasia in a patient with tuberous sclerosis. *Am J Surg Pathol*. 1997;21:1242–1247.

434. Gal AA, Koss MN, Hochholzer L, Chejfec G. An immunohistochemical study of benign clear-cell ("sugar") tumor of the lung. *Arch Pathol Lab Med*. 1991;115:1034–1038.

435. Gaffey MJ, Mills SE, Askin FB, et al. Clear cell tumor of the lung: a clinicopathologic, immunohistochemical, and ultrastructural study of eight cases. *Am J Surg Pathol*. 1991;15:199–202.

436. Stolz AJ, Schutzner J, Lischke R, et al. Benign clear cell tumors of the lung—sugar tumors. *Rozhl Chir*. 2003;82:149–151.

437. Sale GE, Kulander BG. Benign clear-cell tumor (sugar tumor) of the lung with hepatic metastases ten years after resection of pulmonary primary tumor. *Arch Pathol Lab Med*. 1988;112:1177–1178.

438. Cavazza A, Sgarbi G, Ferrari G, Putrino I, Gardini G. Clear cell tumor of the lung: description of a case 1 mm. in diameter ("micro-sugar tumor"). *Pathologica*. 2001;93:556–560.

439. Justrabo E, Mergey E, Piard F, Michiels R, Viard H. Benign clear cell tumour of the lung. *Sem Hop*. 1982;58:673–677.

440. Urban T. Clinical and molecular epidemiology of lymphangioleiomyomatosis and pulmonary pathology in tuberous sclerosis. *Rev Mal Respir*. 2000;17:597–603.

441. Knowles MA, Hornigold N, Pitt E. Tuberous sclerosis complex (TSC) gene involvement in sporadic tumors. *Biochem Soc Trans*. 2003;31:597–602.

442. Panizo-Santos A, Sola I, DeAlava E, et al. Angiomyolipoma and PEComa are immunoreactive for Myo-D1 in a cell cytoplasmic staining pattern. *Appl Immunohistochem Mol Morphol*. 2003;11:156–160.

443. Nappi O, Mills SE, Swanson PE, Wick MR. Clear-cell tumors of unknown nature and origin: a systematic approach to diagnosis. *Semin Diagn Pathol*. 1997;14:164–174.

444. Rosai J, Limas C, Husband EM. Ectopic hamartomatous thymoma. A distinctive benign lesion of lower neck. *Am J Surg Pathol*. 1984;8:501–513.

445. Cohen JB, Troxell M, Kong CS, McDougall JR. Ectopic intrathyroidal thymoma: a case report and review. *Thyroid*. 2003;13:305–308.

446. Ben-Hami B, Caulet-Maugendre S, Valla J, et al. Primary pericardial thymoma: an unusual etiology of neoplastic pericarditis. *Ann Pathol*. 1996;16:445–448.

447. Marchevsky AM. Lung tumors derived from ectopic tissues. *Semin Diagn Pathol*. 1995;12:172–184.

448. Gong L, Li YH, He XL, et al. Primary intrapulmonary thymomas: case report and review of the literature. *J Int Med Res*. 2009;37:1252–1257.

449. Sajwani RA, Gowani SA, Khowaja AA, Khan A, Fatimi SH. Extensive primary malignant thymoma involving pericardium, pleura, diaphragm, and lungs—a case report. *J Pak Med Assoc*. 2008;58:287–288.

450. Velojic D, Marsenic B, Nikolic D, Bosnic M, Djordjevic A. Ectopic thymoma with myasthenic and cardiac symptomatology. *Plucne Bolesti Tuberk*. 1972;24:199–204.

451. Veynovich B, Masetti P, Kaplan PD, et al. Primary pulmonary thymoma. *Ann Thorac Surg*. 1997;64:1471–1473.

452. Moran CA, Suster S, Fishback NF, Koss MN. Primary intrapulmonary thymoma: a clinicopathologic and immunohistochemical study of eight cases. *Am J Surg Pathol*. 1995;19:304–312.

453. James CL, Iyer PV, Leong ASY. Intrapulmonary thymoma. *Histopathology*. 1992;21:175–177.

454. Fukayama M, Maeda Y, Funata N, et al. Pulmonary and pleural thymoma: diagnostic application of lymphocyte markers to the thymoma of unusual site. *Am J Clin Pathol*. 1988;89:617–621.

455. Green WR, Pressoir R, Gumbs RV, et al. Intrapulmonary thymoma. *Arch Pathol Lab Med*. 1987;111:1074–1076.

456. Kung IT, Loke SL, So SY, et al. Intrapulmonary thymoma: report of two cases. *Thorax*. 1985;40:471–474.

457. Yeoh CB, Ford JM, Lattes R, Wylie RH. Intrapulmonary thymoma. *J Thorac Cardiovasc Surg*. 1966;51:131–136.

458. Shih DF, Wang JS, Tseng HH, Tiao WM. Primary pleural thymoma. *Arch Pathol Lab Med*. 1997;121:79–82.

459. Honma K, Shimada K. Metastasizing ectopic thymoma arising in the right thoracic cavity and mimicking diffuse pleural mesothelioma—an autopsy study of a case with review of literature. *Wien Klin Wochenschr*. 1986;98:14–20.

460. Fushimi H, Tanio Y, Kotoh K. Ectopic thymoma mimicking diffuse pleural mesothelioma: a case report. *Hum Pathol*. 1998;29:409–410.

461. Attanoos RL, Galateau-Salle F, Gibbs AR, et al. Primary thymic epithelial tumors of the pleura mimicking malignant mesothelioma. *Histopathology*. 2002;41:42–49.

462. Bernatz PE, Harrison EG, Clagett OT. Thymoma: a clinicopathologic study. *J Thorac Cardiovasc Surg*. 1961;42:424–444.

463. Muller-Hermelink HK, Marino M, Palestro G. Pathology of thymic epithelial tumors. *Curr Top Pathol*. 1986;75:207–268.

464. Dadmanesh F, Sekihara T, Rosai J. Histologic typing of thymoma according to the new World Health Organization classification. *Chest Surg Clin N Am*. 2001;11:407–420.

465. Suster S, Moran CA. Thymoma, atypical thymoma, and thymic carcinoma: a novel conceptual approach to the classification of thymic epithelial neoplasms. *Am J Clin Pathol*. 1999;111:826–833.

466. Kirchner T, Schalke B, Buchwald J, et al. Well-differentiated thymic carcinoma: an organotypical low-grade carcinoma with relationship to cortical thymoma. *Am J Surg Pathol*. 1992;16:1153–1169.

467. Wakely Jr PE. Cytopathology–histopathology of the mediastinum: epithelial, lymphoproliferative, and germ cell neoplasms. *Ann Diagn Pathol*. 2002;6:30–43.

468. Chhieng DC, Rose D, Ludwig ME, Zukowski MF. Cytology of thymomas: emphasis on morphology and correlation with histologic subtypes. *Cancer*. 2000;90:24–32.

469. Shabb NS, Fahl M, Shabb R, Haswani P, Zaatari G. Fine needle aspiration of the mediastinum: a clinical, radiologic, cytologic, and histologic study of 42 cases. *Diagn Cytopathol*. 1998;19:428–436.

470. Levine GD, Rosai J. Thymic hyperplasia and neoplasia: a review of current concepts. *Hum Pathol*. 1978;9:495–515.

471. Mirza I, Kazimi SN, Ligi R, Burns J, Braza F. Cytogenetic profile of a thymoma: a case report and review of the literature. *Arch Pathol Lab Med*. 2000;124:1714–1716.

472. Goh SG, Lau LC, Sivaswaren C, et al. Pseudodicentric (16;12)(q11;p11.2) in a type AB (mixed) thymoma. *Cancer Genet Cytogenet*. 2001;131:42–47.

473. Van den Berghe I, Debiec-Rychter M, Proot L, Hagemeijer A, Michielssen P. Ring chromosome 6 may represent a cytogenetic subgroup in benign thymoma. *Cancer Genet Cytogenet*. 2002;137:75–77.

474. Kuo TT. Cytokeratin profiles of the thymus and thymomas: histogenetic correlations and proposal for a histological classification of thymomas. *Histopathology*. 2000;36:403–414.

475. Chu PG, Weiss LM. Expression of cytokeratin 5/6 in epithelial neoplasms: an immunohistochemical study of 509 cases. *Mod Pathol*. 2002;15:6–10.

476. DiComo CJ, Urist MJ, Babayan I, et al. p63 expression profiles in human normal and tumor tissues. *Clin Cancer Res*. 2002;8:494–501.

477. Myers PO, Kritikos N, Bongiovanni M, et al. Primary intrapulmonary thymoma: a systematic review. *Eur J Surg Oncol*. 2007;33:1137–1141.

478. Wick MR, Nappi O. Ectopic neural and neuroendocrine neoplasms. *Semin Diagn Pathol*. 2003;20:305–323.

479. Cesario A, Galetta D, Margaritora S, Granone P. Unsuspected primary pulmonary meningioma. *Eur J Cardiothorac Surg*. 2002;21:553–555.

480. Prayson RA, Farver CF. Primary pulmonary malignant meningioma. *Am J Surg Pathol*. 1999;23:722–726.

481. Moran CA, Hochholzer L, Rush W, Koss MN. Primary intrapulmonary meningiomas: a clinicopathologic and immunohistochemical study of ten cases. *Cancer*. 1996;78:2328–2333.

482. Gomez-Aracil V, Mayayo E, Alvira R, Arraiza A, Ramon y Cajal S. Fine needle aspiration cytology of primary pulmonary meningioma associated with minute meningothelial-like nodules. Report of a case with histologic, immunohistochemical, and ultrastructural studies. *Acta Cytol*. 2002;46:899–903.

483. Falleni M, Roz E, Dessy E, et al. Primary intrathoracic meningioma: histopathological, immuno-histochemical, and ultrastructural study of two cases. *Virchows Arch A*. 2001;439:196–200.

484. Spinelli M, Claren R, Colombi R, Sironi M. Primary pulmonary meningioma may arise from meningothelial-like nodules. *Adv Clin Path*. 2000;4:35–39.

485. DePerrot M, Kurt AM, Robert J, Spiliopoulos A. Primary pulmonary meningioma presenting as lung metastasis. *Scand Cardiovasc J*. 1999;33:121–123.

486. Ueno M, Fujiyama J, Yamazaki I, et al. Cytology of primary pulmonary meningioma: report of the first multiple case. *Acta Cytol*. 1998;42:1424–1430.

487. Kaleem Z, Fitzpatrick MM, Ritter JH. Primary pulmonary meningioma: report of a case and review of the literature. *Arch Pathol Lab Med*. 1997;121:631–636.

488. Lockett L, Chiang V, Scully N. Primary pulmonary meningioma: report of a case and review of the literature. *Am J Surg Pathol*. 1997;21:453–460.

489. Maiorana A, Ficarra G, Fano RA, Spagna G. Primary solitary meningioma of the lung. *Pathologica*. 1996;88:457–462.

490. Flynn SD, Yousem SA. Pulmonary meningiomas: report of two cases. *Hum Pathol*. 1991;22:469–474.

491. Kodama K, Doi O, Higashiyama M, et al. Primary and metastatic pulmonary meningioma. *Cancer*. 1991;67:1412–1417.

492. Strimlan CV, Golembiewski RS, Celko DA, Fino GJ. Primary pulmonary meningioma. *Surg Neurol*. 1988;29:410–413.

493. Rowsell C, Sirbovan J, Rosenblum MK, Perez-Ordonez B. Primary chordoid meningioma of lung. *Virchows Arch*. 2005;446:333–337.

494. Incarbone M, Ceresoli GL, Di Tommaso L, et al. Primary pulmonary meningioma: report of a case and review of the literature. *Lung Cancer*. 2008;62:401–407.

495. Churg AM, Warnock ML. So-called "minute pulmonary chemodectoma:" a tumor not related to paragangliomas. *Cancer*. 1976;37:1759–1769.

496. Ionescu DN, Sasatomi E, Aldeeb D, et al. Pulmonary meningothelial-like nodules: a genotypic comparison with meningiomas. *Am J Surg Pathol*. 2004;28:207–214.

497. Suster S, Moran CA. Diffuse pulmonary meningotheliomatosis. *Am J Surg Pathol*. 2007;31:624–631.

498. Drlicek M, Grisold W, Lorber J, et al. Pulmonary meningioma: immunohistochemical and ultra-structural features. *Am J Surg Pathol*. 1991;15:455–459.

499. Omulecka A, Papierz W, Nawrocka-Kunecka A, Lewy-Trenda I. Immunohistochemical expression of progesterone and estrogen receptors in meningiomas. *Folia Neuropathol*. 2006;44:111–115.

500. Leaes CG, Meurer RT, Coutinho LB, Ferreira NP, Pereira-Lima JF, da Costa-Oliveira M. Immunohistochemical expression of aromatase and estrogen, androgen, & progesterone receptors in normal and neoplastic human meningeal cells. *Neuropathology*. 2010;30:44–49.

501. Shintaku M, Honda T, Sakai T. Expression of podoplanin and calretinin in meningiomas: an immunohistochemical study. *Brain Tumor Pathol*. 2010;27:23–27.

502. Hu Y, Yang Q, McMahon LA, Wang HL, Xu H. Value of D2-40 in the differential diagnosis of pleural neoplasms, with emphasis on its positivity in solitary fibrous tumor. *Appl Immunohistochem Mol Morphol*. 2010; April 27 (E-pub ahead of print).

503. Jokinen CH, Dadras SS, Goldblum JR, van de Rijn M, West RB, Rubin BP. Diagnostic implications of podoplanin expression in peripheral nerve sheath neoplasms. *Am J Clin Pathol*. 2008;129:886–893.

504. Ishino S, Hashimoto N, Fushiki S, et al. Loss of material from chromosome arm 1p during malignant progression of meningioma revealed by fluorescent in-situ hybridization. *Cancer*. 1998;83:360–366.

505. Adlakha A, Rao K, Adlakha H, et al. Meningioma metastatic to the lung. *Mayo Clin Proc*. 1999;74:1129–1133.

506. Tandon S, Kant S, Singh AK, et al. Primary intrapulmonary teratoma presenting as pyothorax. *Indian J Chest Dis Allied Sci*. 1999;41:51–55.

507. Kayser K, Gabius HJ, Hagemeyer O. Malignant teratoma of the lung with lymph node metastasis of the ectodermal compartment: a case report. *Ann Cell Pathol*. 1993;5:31–37.

508. Eggerath A, Ammon J, Karstens JH, Rubben H, Morales MR. Extragonadal germ cell tumors—diagnostic and therapeutic aspects. *Strahlentherapie*. 1984;160:1–7.

509. Hartman GE, Shochat SJ. Primary pulmonary neoplasms of childhood: a review. *Ann Thorac Surg*. 1983;36:108–119.

510. Moran CA, Travis WD, Carter D, Koss MN. Metastatic mature teratoma in lung following testicular embryonal carcinoma and teratocarcinoma. *Arch Pathol Lab Med*. 1993;117:641–644.

511. Kakkar N, Vashishta RK, Banerjee AK, et al. Primary pulmonary malignant teratoma with yolk sac elements associated with hematologic neoplasia. *Respiration*. 1996;63:52–54.

512. Stair JM, Stevenson DR, Schaefer RF, Fullenwider JP, Campbell GS. Primary teratocarcinoma of the lung. *J Surg Oncol*. 1986;33:262–267.

513. Berghout A, Mallens WM, TeVelde J, Haak HL. Teratoma of the lung in a hemophilic patient. *Acta Hematol*. 1983;70:330–334.

514. Turna A, Ozgul A, Kahraman S, urses A, Fener N, Yilmaz V. Primary pulmonary teratoma: report of a case and the proposition of "bronchotrichosis" as a new term. *Ann Thorac Cardiovasc Surg*. 2009;15:247–249.

515. Saini ML, Krishnamurthy S, Kumar RV. Intrapulmonary mature teratoma. *Diagn Pathol*. 2006;1:38.

516. Joseph MB, Colby TV, Swensen SJ, Mikus JP, Gaensler EA. Multiple cystic fibrohistiocytic tumors of the lung: report of two cases. *Mayo Clin Proc*. 1990;65:192–197.

517. Han JH. Uncommon tumors of the lung (Internet presentation). www.pathology.or.kr/study-group/cardiopulmonary/lecture/lenote/hjh.htm.

518. Colome-Grimmer MI, Evans HL. Metastasizing cellular dermatofibroma: a report of two cases. *Am J Surg Pathol*. 1996;20:1361–1367.

Malignant and Borderline Mesothelial Tumors of the Pleura

Mark R. Wick, MD, Henry D. Tazelaar, MD, Jon H. Ritter, MD, and Stacey E. Mills, MD

The number of publications on the pathologic features of primary pleural mesothelial tumors has gone from meager to innumerable in a little over 40 years. As late as the 1960s, a strong opinion in the medical community held that a diagnosis of malignant mesothelioma (MM) could not be established with certainty during life and that neoplasms effacing the serosal lining of the chest cavity were probably metastatic from other sites.[1] Accordingly, a diagnosis of MM was largely consigned to autopsy pathologists.

Another problem, which persists to some extent even today, relates to the widely cited paradigm for classification of mesothelial tumors that was first advanced by Klemperer and Rabin in 1931.[2] Those authors divided these lesions into four broad categories, depending on whether they were benign or malignant and localized or diffuse. However, using that model, such neoplasms as solitary fibrous tumors and pleural sarcomas, which are not mesothelial at all, are still confused by some clinicians with true MMs.

Developments in the sphere of technology have shed a great deal of light on these subjects in the recent past. Accurate classification of mesothelial neoplasms can now be accomplished, and their differential diagnosis from morphologically similar lesions is facilitated by the use of several adjunctive study modalities.

Malignant Mesothelioma

Clinical Findings in Pleural Mesothelioma

Patients with malignant pleural mesothelioma are typically adults older than 50 years of age,[3-6] but there have also been several well-documented examples of this tumor in children.[7-9] Very rarely, familial clustering of MM has been reported, with parent-child or sibling-sibling combinations being represented.[10-13] To date, there have been no reports of spouse-spouse concurrences.

The most common presentation of MM is with progressive shortness of breath.[4,5,14,15] Unilateral chest pain is also relatively frequent, and this may or may not have pleuritic characteristics. Another rarer manifestation is that of flulike illness, with malaise, anorexia, low-grade fever, myalgias, and weight loss.[16-19] Distant metastasis of MM to extrathoracic lymph nodes or other anatomic sites at presentation is extraordinarily uncommon[20,21] but can represent a diagnostic challenge for pathologists.

Plain film chest radiographs typically show a unilateral pleural effusion, which may be massive in volume despite relatively minor symptoms (Fig. 20-1). Reimaging after thoracentesis often reveals diffuse pleural thickening; more rarely, a single discrete pleural mass may be observed.[22-25] Computed tomography and magnetic resonance imaging scans of the thorax are more sensitive than plain films for demonstrating tumor volume and invasion of contiguous anatomic structures[25-27] (Fig. 20-2). They are also superior for showing the presence of pleural plaques and pleural calcifications, which are sensitive markers of asbestos exposure. One or both of these markers are seen in 85% or more of all individuals who are exposed to asbestos at an above-background level.[28,29]

Other laboratory abnormalities in MM cases are relatively few and nondescript. However, a substantial proportion of patients have tumor-related thrombocytosis, with platelet counts greater than 400,000 mm^3.[30-33]

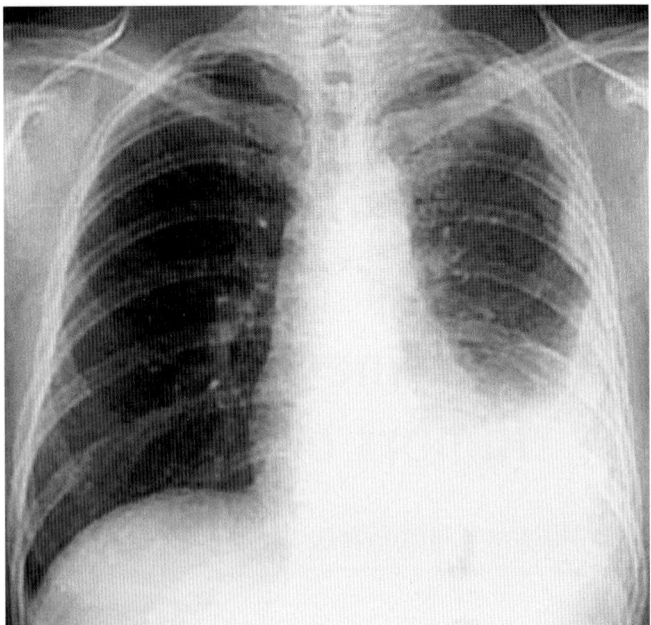

Figure 20-1. Chest radiograph from a patient with malignant pleural mesothelioma demonstrating a large left pleural effusion.

Chapter 16) is capable of reproducing the symptomatic and radiographic constellation of abnormalities associated with mesothelioma[34–38] (Fig. 20-3).

Video-assisted thoracoscopic surgery (VATS) is now the preferred method for obtaining diagnostic pleural tissue.[39–41] VATS (Fig. 20-4) is superior to cytologic sampling of pleural fluid and closed-needle biopsies because of its much greater yield. VATS also produces a specimen of sufficient size for visualization of microarchitectural landmarks. In addition, the morbidity associated with this method is very low. Finally, cytologic examination of pleural fluid in VATS produces positive results in only a minority of cases. This may be because the free surfaces of MMs may be coated with a layer of fibrinoinflammatory exudate, possibly with a misleading benign mesothelial reaction. This process may "wall off" the tumor cells and prevent them from shedding freely into the pleural fluid.[42,43]

One unwanted but well-reported complication of thoracic biopsies in MM is the growth of tumor along needle or instrumentation tracks in the chest wall.[44,45] The reason for this peculiar behavior is currently unknown.

In general, once the clinical presence of diffuse pleural MM has been established, ensuing survival is limited. Most patients live roughly 1 year after diagnosis, regardless of the therapeutic intervention used.[46–49] However, a small minority of individuals with good overall performance status and limited intrathoracic disease may be candidates for extrapleural pneumonectomy.[49,50] This procedure has resulted in lengthened median survival in some published series[50]; however, a significant proportion of patients go on to demonstrate the presence of distant metastases of MM under such circumstances, perhaps because of this shift in the natural history of the tumor. Radiotherapy has also been given after extrapleural pneumonectomy, especially for the attempted salvage of patients with recurrent tumor.[49] Nevertheless, along with most chemotherapeutic approaches and immunomodulation,[51] this treatment modality has not produced uniformly encouraging results. An epithelial histologic subtype, a favorable overall performance score, relatively young age, and the absence of chest pain are all correlated with better survival.[18]

This may relate to the elaboration of interleukin-6 by the tumor cells, inasmuch as that cytokine is known to stimulate thrombopoiesis and is often elevated in both pleural fluid and serum in individuals with MM.[34] As expected, an excess of thrombotic events is associated with MM-related thrombocythemia.[30]

It must be emphasized that none of the clinical findings just mentioned is specific for MM and may also be encountered in connection with other primary pleural neoplasms or metastases to the pleura. In particular, the peculiar form of lung cancer known as *pseudomesotheliomatous* (pleurotropic) adenocarcinoma (see

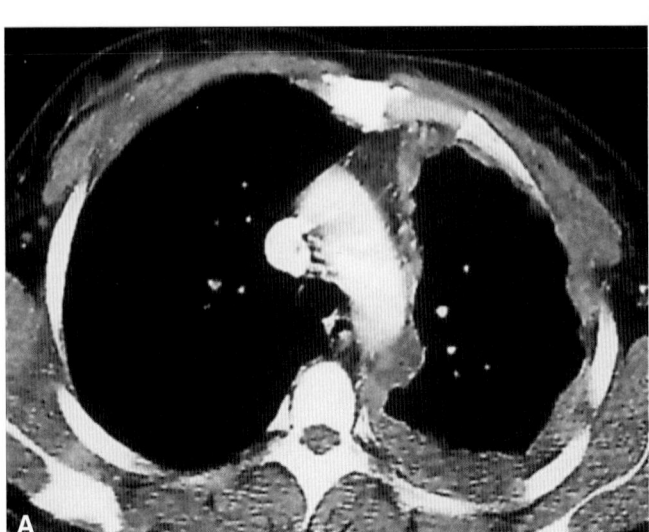

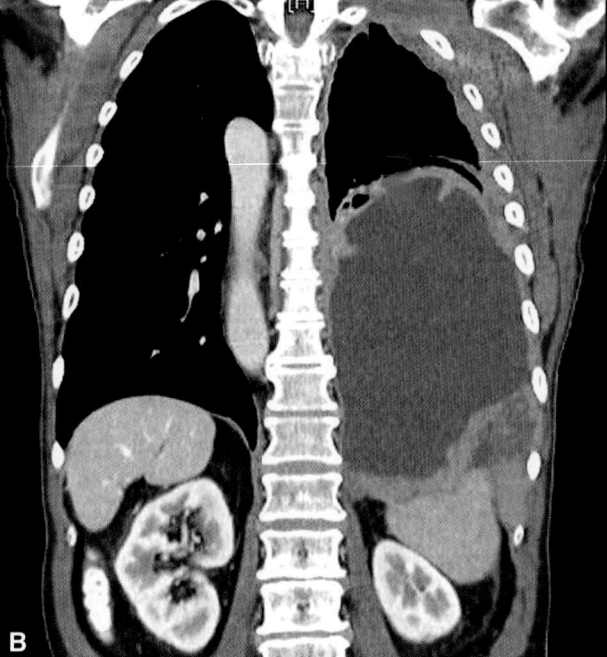

Figure 20-2. A, Computed tomography scan of the chest from a patient with pleural mesothelioma. A multinodular and confluent tumor of the left chest is apparent. **B,** Magnetic resonance image of another patient with a large left pleural mesothelioma.

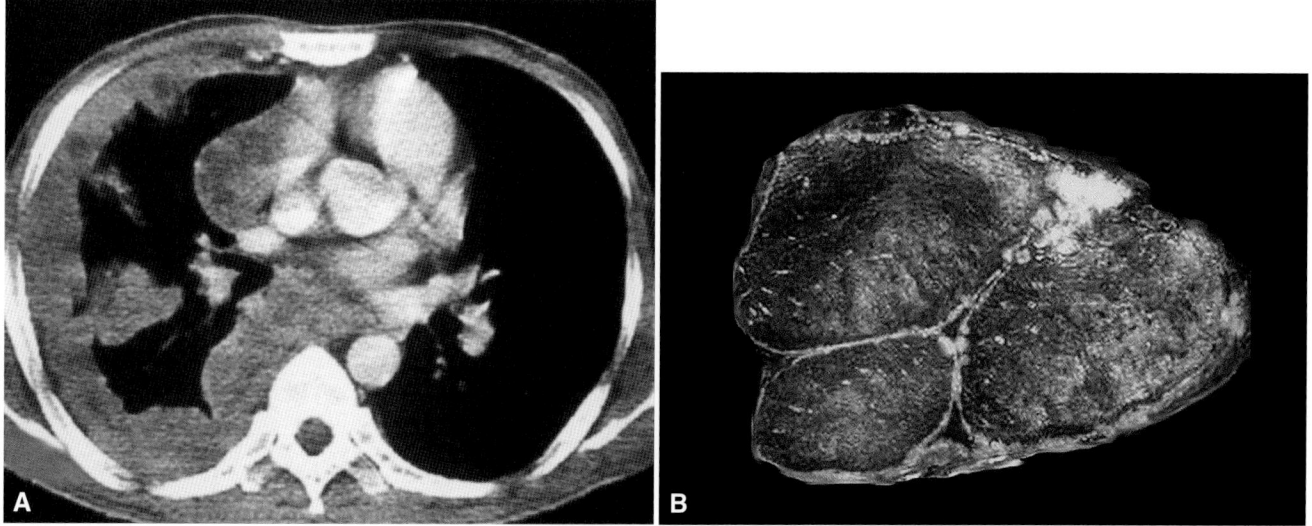

Figure 20-3. A, Computed tomography scan of the chest from a patient with pseudomesotheliomatous adenocarcinoma of the right lung. **B,** Autopsy specimen from the same patient. The tumor encases the right lung both radiographically and grossly, recapitulating the features of mesothelioma.

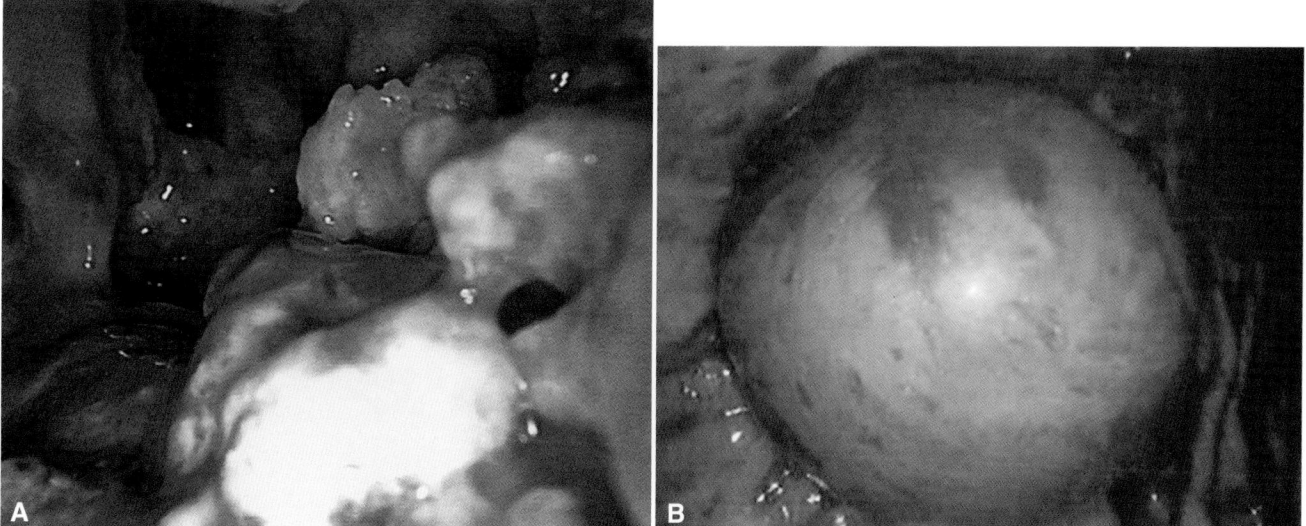

Figure 20-4. A and **B,** Thoracoscopic images of pleural mesothelioma.

A more favorable prognosis is also associated with localized malignant pleural mesothelioma, a rare lesion.[52–54] It often grows preferentially into the soft tissue of the chest wall rather than along the pleural surface and, thus, presents itself as a discrete mass. Radical surgical removal of localized mesothelioma results in long-term survival in up to 50% of cases.[54]

Etiologic Considerations in Pleural Mesothelioma

The potential causal association between pleural mesotheliomas and occupational-level asbestos exposure is well known. However, practically speaking, physicians rarely concern themselves with the etiology of these tumors at a clinical level, because diagnosis and therapy are the principal focuses of their attention. In this context, the pathologic findings are, by far, the most important consideration.

However, the nearly ubiquitous involvement of attorneys in mesothelioma cases, as part of the burgeoning field known as "toxic tort" law,[55] has compelled physicians to acquire a working familiarity with the pathogenetic underpinnings of MM. Because of this

reality, a brief review of that subject will be provided here; additional information is presented in Chapter 9, which deals specifically with pneumoconioses.

In the early- to mid-1960s, a causal connection between high-level inhalation of amphibole-class asbestos fibers and mesothelioma was first established to the satisfaction of the medical community at large, through the efforts of Wagner and colleagues and others.[56–59] At first, epidemiologic surveys were the principal tools whereby this association was identified. However, this avenue of investigation, in which exposures are ascertained primarily by word-of-mouth information, is applicable to patient groups rather than individuals. In the current social environment of the 21st century, epidemiologic questioning and medical history taking are plagued by significant problems in trying to determine the causation of any given case of MM. This is true because media-related exposure of the potential linkage between mesothelioma and asbestos has been robust. Therefore, patients with MM are inculcated with the belief that they *must* have been exposed to asbestos somewhere and somehow in the past. Moreover, another very real issue concerning the pathogenesis of MM is whether chrysotile-type asbestos—the most commonly used representative of the mineral group in the past several decades—is effective as a carcinogen in this specific context. Aggregated data suggest that chrysotile has very weak mesothelioma genesis.[60–63] Hence, *asbestos exposure* as a generic term has an indefinite and imprecise meaning for individual patients in the absence of other data.[64]

Fortunately, objective information is available to address this area of causation. This is important not only for the legal system—where it can be used to provide concrete fact instead of hearsay—but also for physicians who are committed to the principles of evidence-based medicine. Examination of pathologic specimens continues to be a linchpin in this setting. If conventional light microscopic scrutiny of sections of lung parenchyma demonstrates asbestos bodies at an above-background density (Fig. 20-5), or these structures are seen in intrathoracic lymph nodes, it may be concluded that a mesothelioma in the same case is indeed asbestos-related. Similarly, the radiographic or pathologic presence of pleural plaques, pleural calcifications, or rounded atelectasis (Fig. 20-6) serves a comparable purpose.[65–67] Ultimately, the most direct and best approach to evaluating the presence of asbestos in lung tissue is to perform a digestion analysis of representative parenchymal samples (Fig. 20-7), comparing the density of asbestos fibers found by such methods to that which is present in a carefully assembled age-matched and sex-matched control population, acquired from the same geographic region as that in which the patient lived.[68]

Using the last of these techniques, Roggli and associates have shown that a bimodal distribution of pulmonary asbestos burdens is associated with pleural MMs.[69] The majority of patients (group I) have a density of asbestos bodies above 20 per gram of wet lung tissue. The remaining patients (group II) manifest an asbestos burden identical to that seen in appropriate reference cohorts. These data strongly support the conclusion that group II MMs are not etiologically related to asbestos, and, in the absence of other potential causes (see later discussion), these cases are properly termed "idiopathic" or "spontaneous" mesotheliomas. Practically speaking, one can use the latter designation if no objective support for asbestos causation is apparent in a case in question, based on a review of thoracic imaging studies, pleuropulmonary tissue biopsies, or autopsy specimens of lung and pleura.[70]

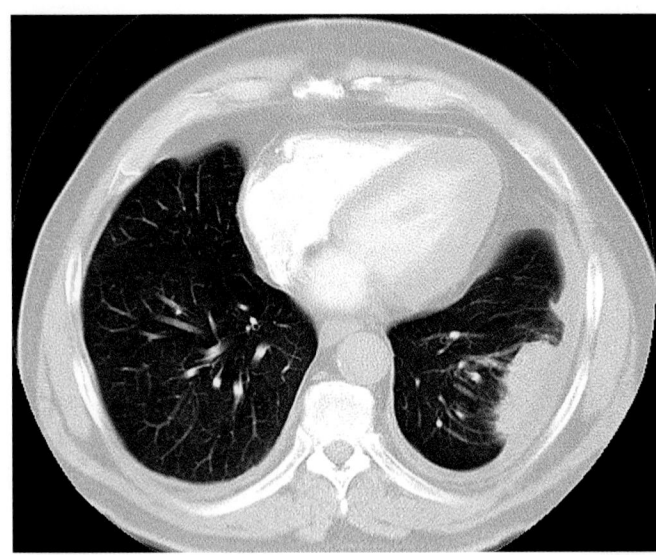

Figure 20-6. This computed tomogram of the chest demonstrates rounded atelectasis in the left posterior lung field. This finding is strongly correlated with above-background asbestos exposure.

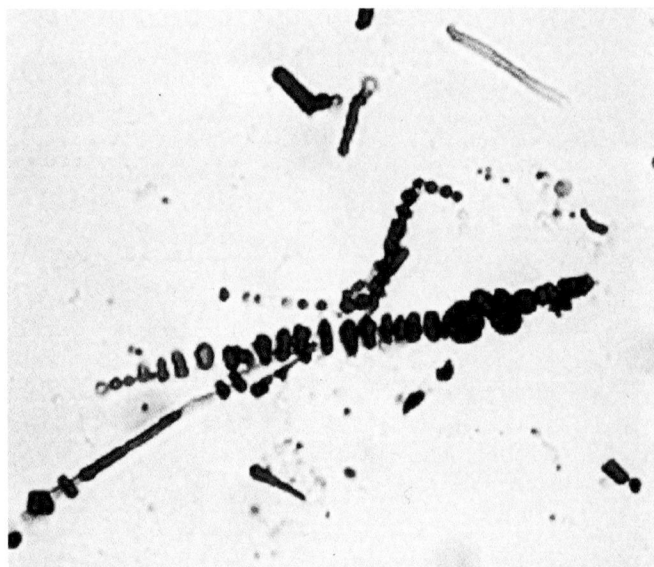

Figure 20-7. Multiple asbestos bodies are present in this lung tissue digest preparation, taken from a patient with above-background asbestos exposure.

The proportion of MMs that is idiopathic in nature has varied from study to study in the published literature, probably as a function of geographic and chronologic bias.[71] Cited percentages have generally been between 25% and 40% of all pleural mesotheliomas.[72] In our experience in recent years, using the objective approach just outlined, approximately 40% of MMs are spontaneous neoplasms with no definable etiologic linkage to asbestos.

Pleural mesotheliomas that are caused by asbestos develop after a long latency period, typically longer than 20 years in duration.[73] The reason for this hiatus is not clear, but it appears that the carcinogenic effect of this mineral group requires a prolonged time—and probably a complicated set of intermediate cellular events[74–76]—to become manifest. Attanoos and coworkers[77] have described a remarkable group of nine asbestos-related mesothelioma cases (eight of which concerned pleural tumors) in which a second concurrent malignancy was present as well. Six of the patients had bronchogenic

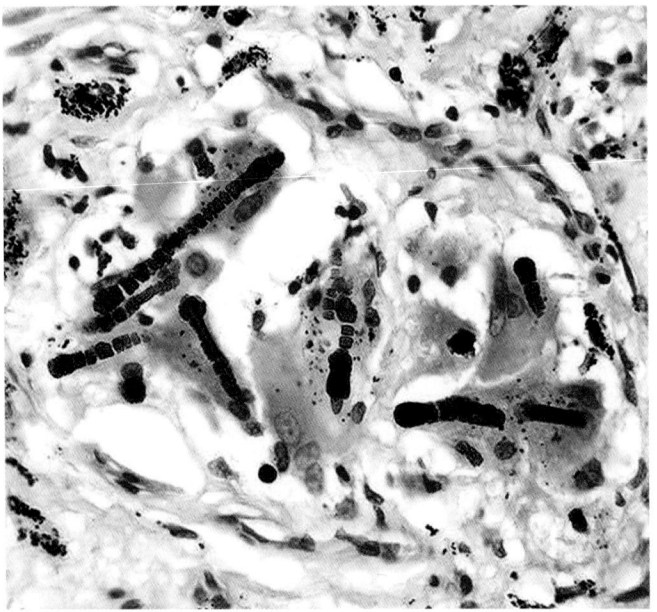

Figure 20-5. A cluster of ferruginated asbestos bodies is present in this section of lung tissue, establishing the presence of a supranormal asbestos burden.

carcinomas—accompanied by pulmonary asbestosis in five—and the remaining individuals had colorectal, breast, and pancreatic carcinomas. The nine patients in that series represented 1.8% of all mesothelioma cases seen at our institutions.

Other documented etiologies for pleural MM besides asbestos undeniably exist.[70,71,78,79] These include prior therapeutic irradiation to the anatomic region in which the mesothelioma develops[80-85]; chronic serosal inflammation, such as that associated with tuberculosis, pleural empyema, familial Mediterranean fever, or chronic collagen vascular diseases (e.g., rheumatoid arthritis or lupus erythematosus)[86-89]; membership in familial cancer kindreds ("Lynch families")[12,13,90]; prior administration of thorium dioxide (Thorotrast), a radiologic imaging agent[91,92]; and inhalational exposure to erionite, another mineral group.[93,94] Infection with Simian virus-40 has recently been examined as another possible cause of human mesothelioma, with contradictory, but usually negative, conclusions.[95-100]

Interestingly, mesothelioma is a well-documented malignancy of cattle and other animals (both wild and domesticated), and the clinicopathologic attributes of such animal tumors are comparable in every way to those of spontaneous human MMs.[101-107] Further attention to the potential pathogeneses of veterinary mesotheliomas could possibly be illuminating in a mechanistic sense.

The pathologic attributes of mesotheliomas can be considered at several levels of examination, beginning with their macroscopic features and extending through their molecular-biologic characteristics. This information is summarized in the following sections.

Gross Features of Pleural Mesothelioma

Pleural mesothelioma may occasionally produce striking clinical symptoms, including large pleural effusions, while the tumor is still invisible radiographically. Moreover, direct examination of the pleural surfaces in such cases—via such techniques as VATS—likewise may be relatively unrevealing, and a pathologic diagnosis of MM in biopsies done in such circumstances is often met with disbelief. Only the passage of time, with progressive development of the characteristic phenotype of mesothelioma, may suffice to convince all concerned that the tumor is actually present.

However, more typically, clinical abnormalities are accompanied by multifocal "studding" of the visceral or parietal pleural surfaces, or both, by firm white-gray nodules that individually measure up to several centimeters in diameter. With time, these become innumerable and confluent, obliterating the pleural cavity and often forming a thick layer of constricting neoplastic tissue (Figs. 20-8 and 20-9). Invasion of contiguous structures, including the peripheral lung parenchyma, pericardium and myocardium, adventitia of the great thoracic blood vessels, and soft tissue of the chest wall, is common as tumor growth advances. In addition, mesotheliomas of the pleura may cross the central apertures of the diaphragm to secondarily involve the peritoneal cavity,[108] and they are also capable of crossing the mediastinum to involve the contralateral hemithorax. If the patient survives long enough, the terminal image of the tumor may be that of a dense rind of tissue that encases the viscera of the chest.[109] Grossly visible metastases in regional lymph nodes and distant sites may also be appreciated, but they generally appear only late in the clinical course. It should be noted that there is nothing specific about the macroscopic characteristics just outlined. They are potentially common to MM, metastatic carcinoma in the pleural spaces, pleural lymphoma, and primary pleural sarcomas.[34-36,110,111]

Solitary (localized) MMs of the pleura most often grow exophytically into the soft tissue of the chest (Fig. 20-10) or, alternatively, into the subjacent lung parenchyma, rather than spreading along the serosal surfaces.[54,112] As such, they can macroscopically simulate peripheral carcinomas of the lung.

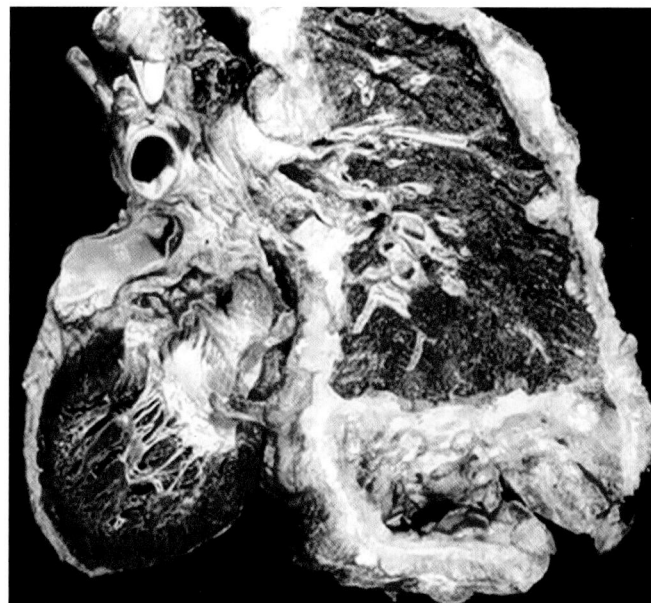

Figure 20-8. Photograph of a gross specimen of malignant pleural mesothelioma, taken at autopsy. The tumor envelops one lung and is adherent to mediastinal structures as well.

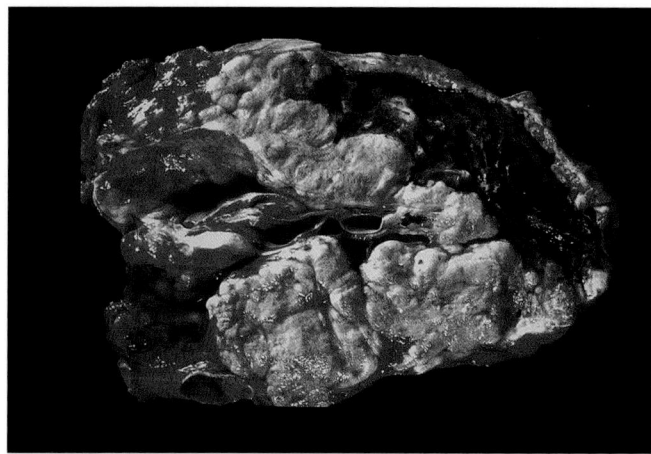

Figure 20-9. Photograph of a gross specimen of malignant pleural mesothelioma showing a bulky mass that effaces the pleural space and compresses the lung.

The cut surfaces of mesotheliomas are nondescript. Most often they are white-gray with a relatively firm consistency on sectioning, because of the stromal fibrosis they incite. Desmoplastic MMs are particularly dense when they are incised.

Cytopathologic Features of Pleural Mesothelioma

Mesothelial proliferations in the pleura have a wide spectrum of potential cytomorphologic appearances and can rightfully be included in several generic cytologic categories that encompass small round cell tumors, polygonal cell malignancies, spindle cell and pleomorphic lesions, and neoplasms with mixed cellular features.[113] However, traditionally, three broad histopathologic patterns of mesothelioma have been considered: epithelial (including tubulopapillary, oncocytoid/deciduoid, clear cell, and small cell subtypes), sarcomatoid (including desmoplastic and "lymphohistiocytoid" variants), and biphasic. These lesions may, on occasion, show other unusual histopathologic features, such as the presence of extensive myxoid change, "glomeruloid"

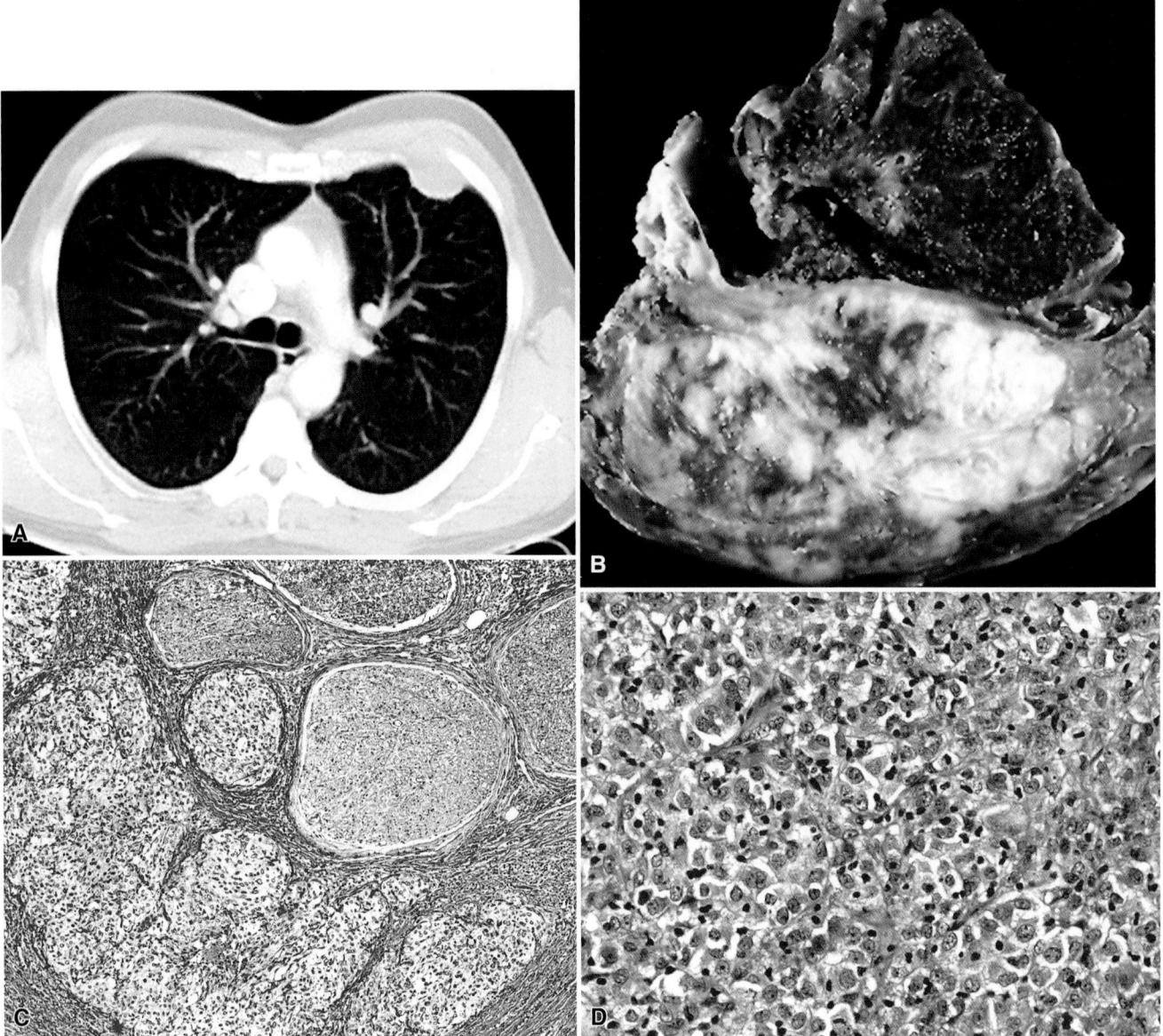

Figure 20-10. The computed tomogram (**A**) and gross surgical specimen (**B**) demonstrate a localized mass in the pleura that proved to be malignant mesothelioma. Histologically, it was an epithelioid lesion (**C** and **D**).

features, adenomatoid tumor-like images, "rhabdoid" features, and metaplastic formation of bone and cartilage.

Epithelial mesothelioma is composed of sheets and clusters of variably atypical epithelioid cells in effusion cytology specimens. Such samples are typically densely cellular (Fig 20-11). Mitotic figures and background necrosis are uncommon, but these two features may certainly be apparent in high-grade lesions. Epithelial MMs may also show papillary or tubular cell groups (Fig. 20-12), and, in thoracentesis specimens, the malignant cells may be surprisingly bland cytologically.[114–119] Conversely, benign reactive mesothelia can show an alarming degree of nuclear atypia, compounding the difficulty of their diagnostic separation from malignancies.[116,120] Groups of both reactive and neoplastic mesothelial cells may demonstrate intercellular spaces or "windows," and sufficient dispersion of such elements shows the presence of fuzzy cell membranes due to the presence of elongated plasmalemmal microvilli (Fig. 20-13). Nuclear-to-cytoplasmic ratios are high in obviously anaplastic MMs, but this finding may not be characteristic of all tumors. Small cell epithelial mesothelioma demonstrates tightly clustered cell groups with scant cytoplasm and no obvious microvilli. It may be exceedingly

similar cytomorphologically to other small cell malignant neoplasms, particularly small cell neuroendocrine carcinoma[121] (Fig. 20-14).

Sarcomatoid mesothelioma contains cytologically malignant dyshesive fusiform cell proliferations that cytologically imitate other tumors of mesenchymal origin (i.e., sarcomas)[122] (Fig. 20-15). In pleural effusions, the tumor cells of sarcomatoid MM are few in number if they are present at all, with scant cytoplasm, elongated nuclei, and rare mitotic figures. A subtype of this variant is the desmoplastic mesothelioma, which is characterized histologically by a bland appearance of the spindle cells that are embedded in a hypocellular, abundantly collagenized stroma.[123] As one might expect, diagnostic tumor cells from desmoplastic tumors rarely, if ever, are shed into effusions.

In the past, "lymphohistiocytoid" mesothelioma was regarded as a sarcomatoid MM variant,[124] but it actually bears more resemblance to lymphoepithelioma-like carcinomas of various organs than to true sarcomas.[125] In this lesion, one sees syncytia of polyhedral cells with prominent nucleoli, admixed with numerous mature lymphocytes. Biphasic mesotheliomas manifest a combination of the cytomorphologic patterns that are expected in epithelial and sarcomatoid tumors.[115]

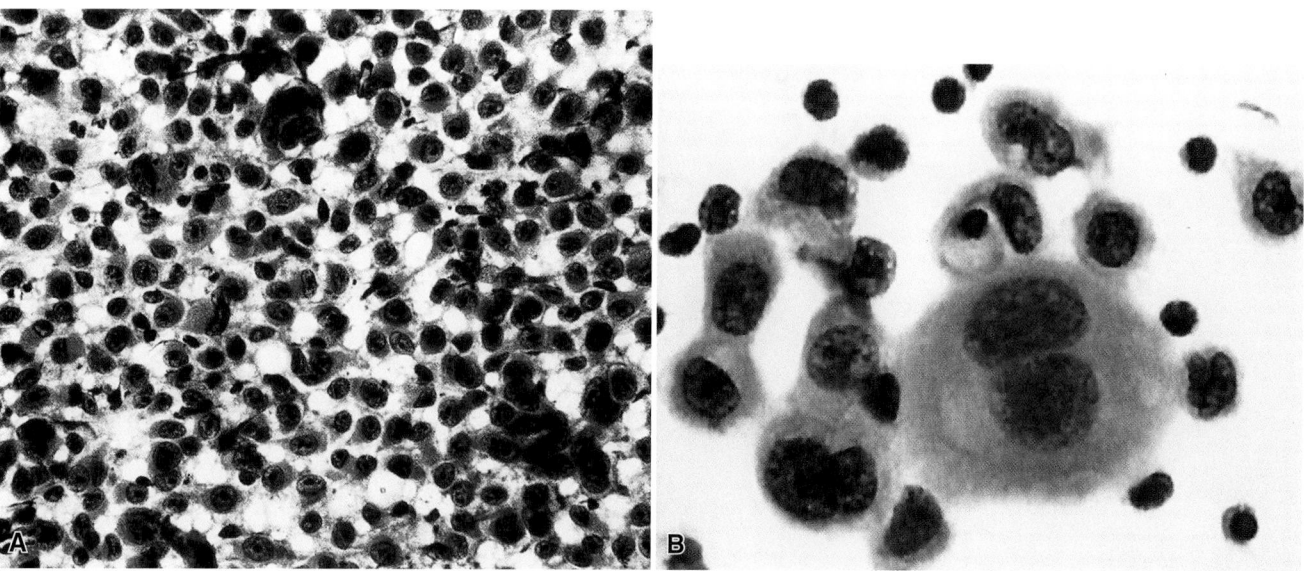

Figure 20-11. A, Dense cellularity is evident in this cytologic preparation of pleural fluid from a patient with pleural mesothelioma. **B,** The tumor cells show substantial nuclear pleomorphism with coarse chromatin.

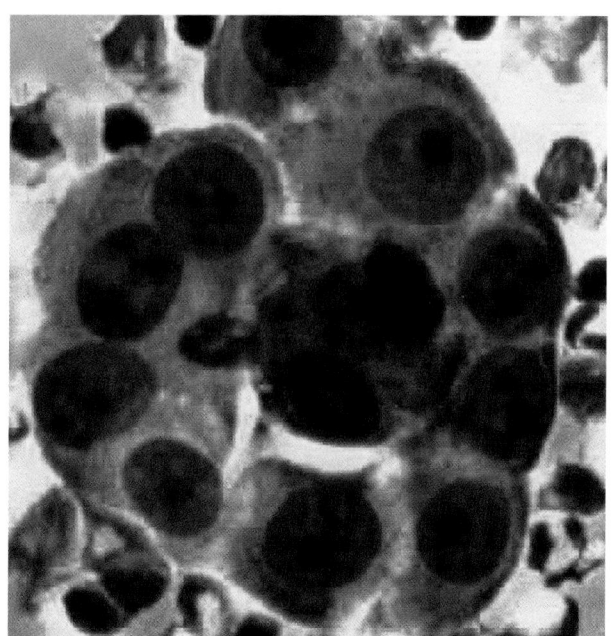

Figure 20-12. A tubular profile of tumor cells is apparent in this pleural fluid cytology preparation of malignant mesothelioma.

Many pathologists are still reluctant to make a diagnosis of mesothelioma based only on effusion cytology specimens, in light of the pitfalls mentioned above. However, our experience over time has shown that this hesitancy is often unnecessary. If several pleural fluid samples in a given case consistently show dense cellularity, an overwhelming dominance of cells with clearly mesothelial morphologic features, three-dimensional cellular aggregates, and at least some nuclear atypia, a diagnosis of MM is likely. This interpretation can be solidified by preparation of cell block sections (Fig. 20-16) and the application of adjunctive studies.[126,127] Therefore, a conclusive opinion can indeed be rendered by the cytopathologist in a sizable proportion of mesothelioma cases.

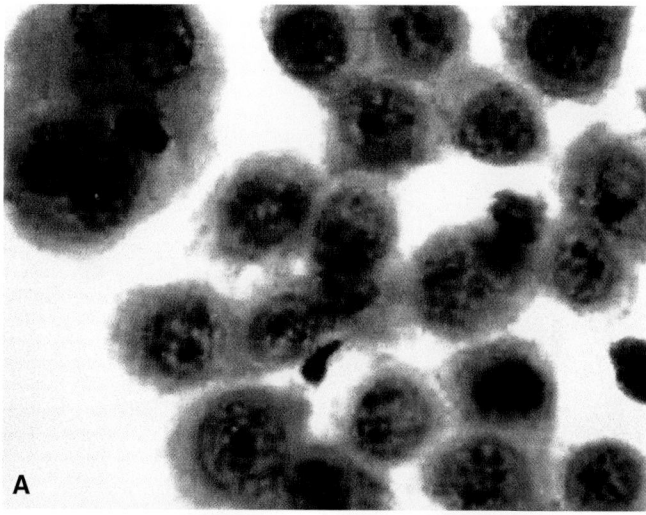

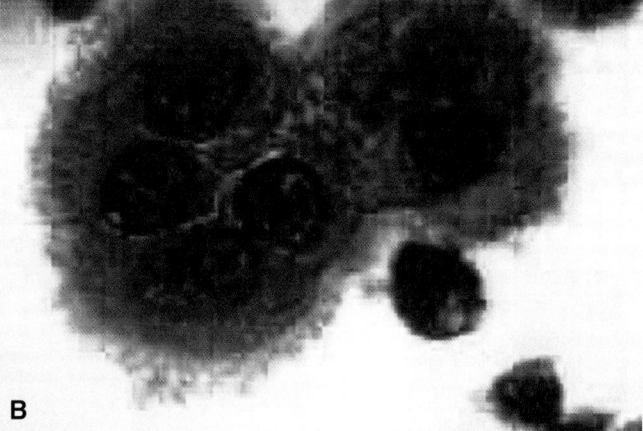

Figure 20-13. A and **B,** "Fuzzy" cell membranes are apparent in this example of malignant mesothelioma in a pleural fluid cytology specimen. That finding relates to the presence of elaborate plasmalemmal microvilli.

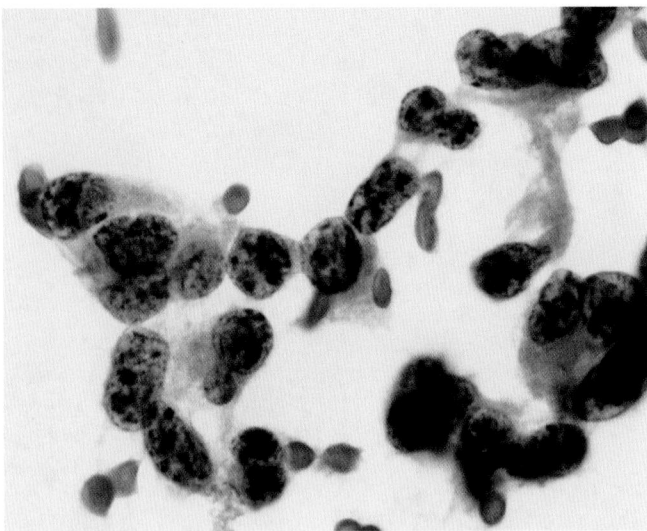

Figure 20-14. Cytologic specimen from a case of small cell malignant mesothelioma of the pleura. A morphologic similarity to small cell lung carcinoma is readily evident.

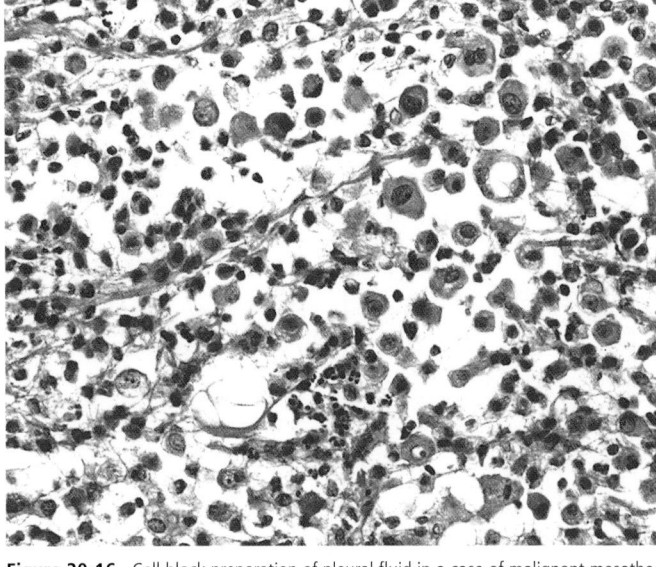

Figure 20-16. Cell block preparation of pleural fluid in a case of malignant mesothelioma demonstrating a sheet of epithelioid tumor cells with atypical nuclear profiles.

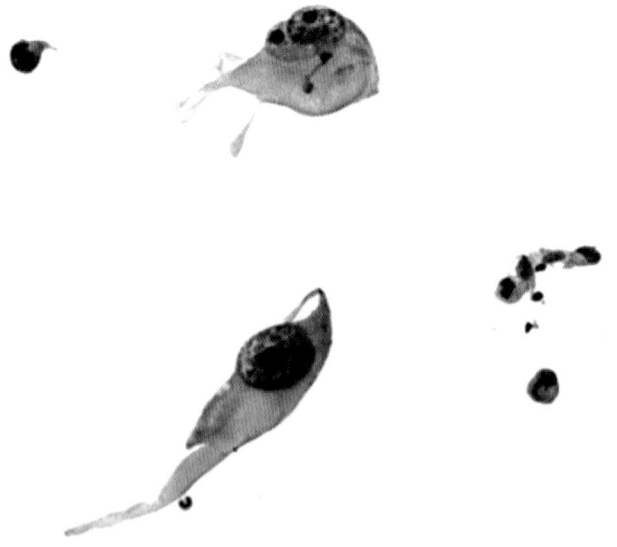

Figure 20-15. Cytologic specimen of sarcomatoid malignant pleural mesothelioma showing scanty dyshesive and pleomorphic tumor cells.

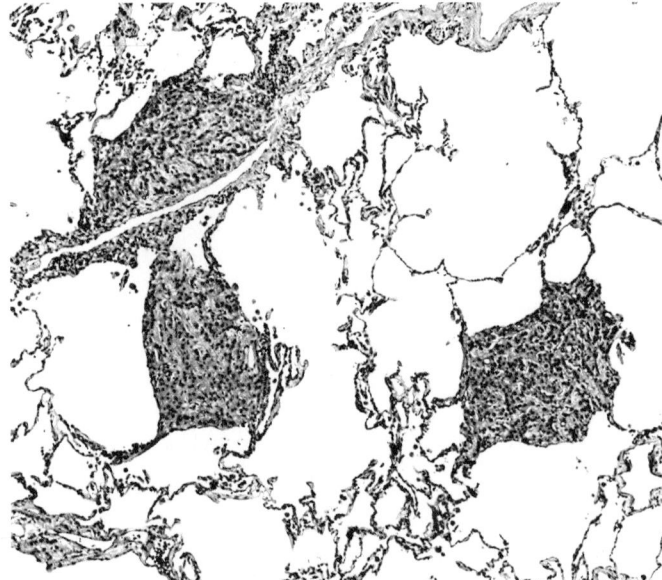

Figure 20-17. Lymphangitic intrapulmonary growth of pleural mesothelioma is seen in this photomicrograph.

Kimura and colleagues[128] have proposed that a scoring system be applied as an aid in this process. Using a scale with a maximum value of 10, these authors assigned one point to each of the following features, in favor of an ultimate diagnosis of MM: variety of cell size, cytoplasmic cyanophilia with visible microvilli, sheetlike cell arrangement, "mirror ball"–like cell groups, obvious nuclear atypia, and cell cannibalism. Two-point values were assigned to the presence of large acidophilic nucleoli and to multinucleated cells with more than eight nuclei. In an analysis of 22 MMs, with 20 cases of conditions featuring benign mesothelial atypia and 50 examples of metastatic carcinoma, the "Kimura system" was effective at separating mesotheliomas, which had scores of more than five, from the other specified lesions.[128]

Histopathologic Features of Pleural Mesothelioma

Mesothelioma generally, but not always, spreads multifocally throughout the pleural soft tissues, demonstrating invasion of the peripheral-most subpleural lung tissue in many cases. Other uncommon histologic patterns of growth include[129] lymphangitic spread in the lung

(Fig. 20-17); pulmonary alveolar permeation through the pores of Kohn, mimicking organizing pneumonia (Fig. 20-18); and lepidic intrapulmonary growth, mantling alveolar septa.

There is no substantial difference between the histology of untreated and residual treated mesotheliomas.[130]

The general histologic categorization of MMs has been outlined previously. However, additional details will be provided in the following sections.

Epithelioid Mesothelioma

Epithelioid malignant mesothelioma (EMM) is the most commonly encountered microscopic subtype.[131] In the majority of cases, the lesion is composed of sheets and nests of polyhedral cells with moderately atypical nuclear features, clear infiltration of the pleural soft tissue or subjacent lung, or both. Lesions comprising uniform expanses of densely apposed polygonal cells are known as "solid" epithelioid MMs (Fig. 20-19). In other tumors, glandlike

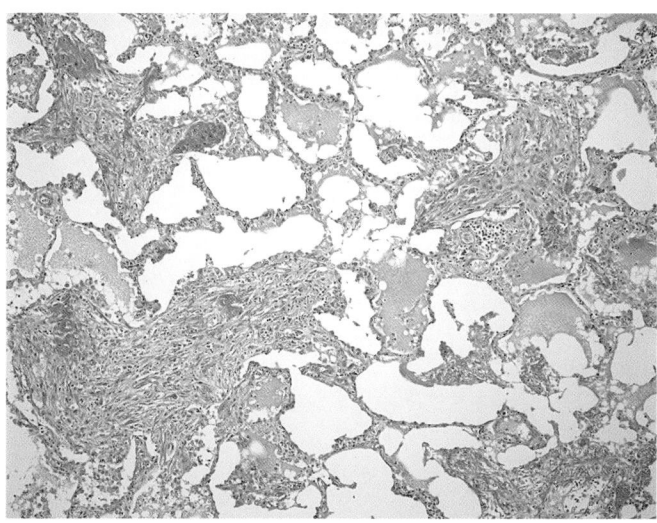

Figure 20-18. Permeative intrapulmonary growth of mesothelioma is demonstrated here. The tumor has grown into alveolar spaces through the pores of Kohn and is mimicking organizing pneumonia.

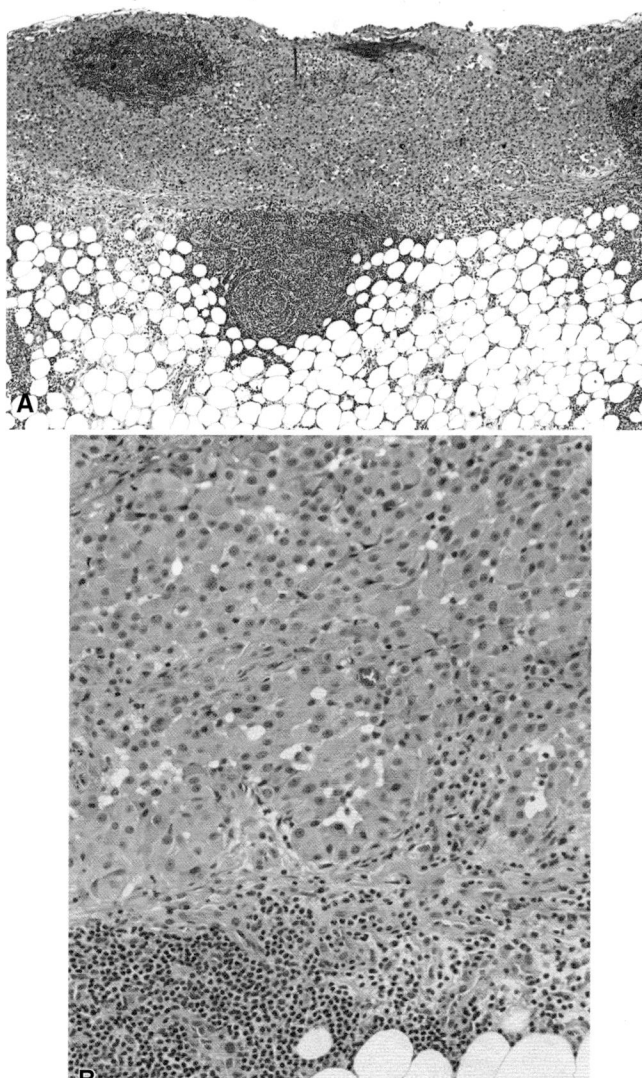

Figure 20-19. A and **B,** "Solid" malignant mesothelioma of the pleura comprising confluent sheets and nests of polygonal tumor cells.

profiles are common; indeed, some cases demonstrate a predominance of such structures, prompting use of the terms "tubular" or "pseudoglandular" EMM. Micropapillary cell groups are also frequent, and, when they uniformly characterize the lesion, the term "tubulopapillary" MM is rightly applied (Fig. 20-20). This subtype of mesothelioma may be particularly associated with lymphatic invasion and lymph node metastasis.[132] Although psammomatous microcalcifications are associated with other epithelial malignancies having a papillary configuration, they are only rarely seen in pleural mesotheliomas.[133]

A useful diagnostic finding in EMM concerns the tinctorial properties of the tumoral stroma. Lightly hematoxylinophilic and myxoid material may be seen between epithelioid cell groups in this lesion, representing the presence of stromal mucin.[134] Although it is not specific, this observation does favor an interpretation of MM over one of carcinoma. An extension of the same property is reflected by the cytoplasmic characteristics of some tumor cells in EMM, which demonstrate macrovacuoles having a bluish cast (Fig. 20-21). These probably represent intracellular inclusions of the same stromal material.

"Lymphohistiocytoid" mesothelioma has been mentioned earlier. To recapitulate, it has a histologic appearance that is markedly similar to that of lymphoepithelioma-like carcinoma (Fig. 20-22).

One subtype of EMM has been called "deciduoid" mesothelioma because of the impression that its constituent cells resemble those of

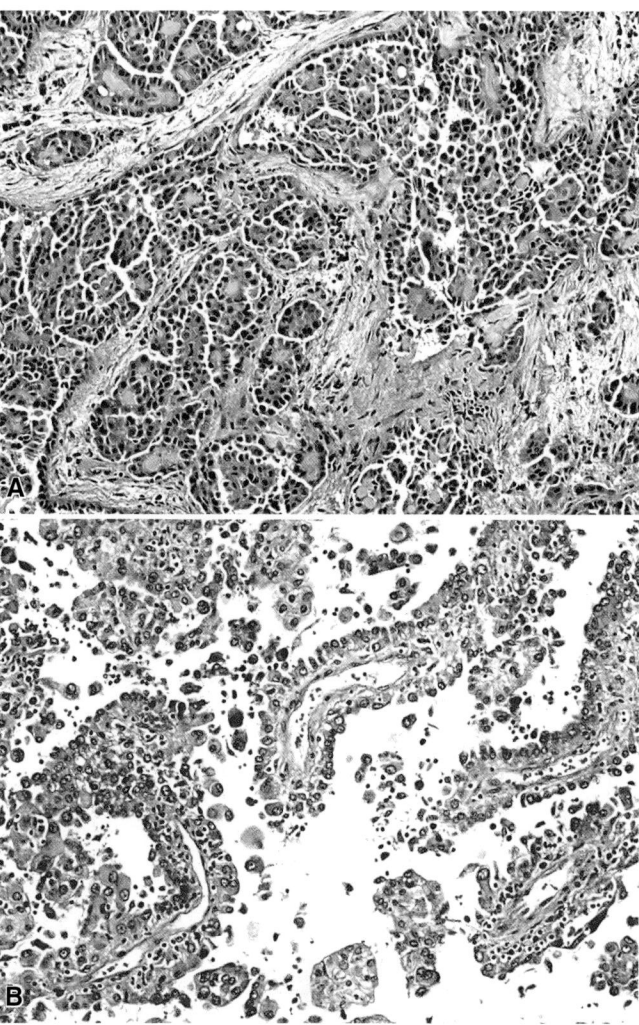

Figure 20-20. A and **B,** Tubulopapillary malignant pleural mesothelioma demonstrating micropapillary profiles of polyhedral cells.

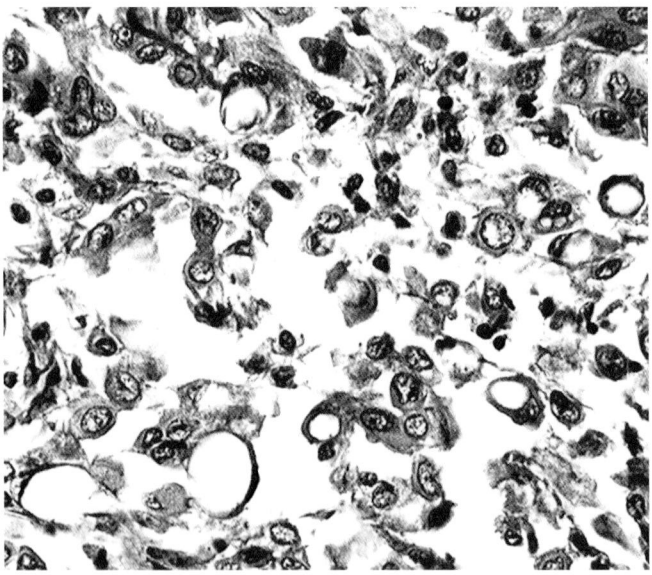

Figure 20-21. Large cytoplasmic vacuoles are apparent in this example of malignant epithelioid pleural mesothelioma. These probably contain stromal-type mucin that is produced by the tumor cells.

Figure 20-23. Clear cell malignant pleural mesothelioma demonstrating uniform cytoplasmic lucency. This change may be caused by accumulation of glycogen or lipid in the neoplastic cells.

decidua in the female genital tract.[135–137] As such, they assume a large polygonal cell image with relatively abundant eosinophilic cytoplasm and oval vesicular nuclei. This relatively bland appearance belies the invasive nature of deciduoid MM, the biologic features of which are comparable to those of other forms of mesothelioma. Synonyms for this variant are "oxyphilic" or "oncocytoid" MM.[101]

Another form of EMM contains polyhedral cells with strikingly lucent cytoplasm and is accordingly known as "clear cell" mesothelioma[138–140] (Fig. 20-23). This variant is extremely uncommon, at least in pure form, and is also related to "foam cell" or "lipid-rich" MM.[125]

Rarely, foci in EMM may simulate the microscopic appearance of pleural adenomatoid tumors (see Chapter 19), with bland microcystic glandlike profiles composed of compact epithelioids.[141] However, other areas in those lesions typically have the conventional image of ordinary mesothelioma.

"Glomeruloid" mesothelioma is a relatively recently described variant in which the tumor cells form peculiar arrays that resemble

glomeruli in the renal cortex (Fig. 20-24).[142] Again, its behavioral properties are no different than those of ordinary EMMs.

Mention must also be made here of the concept of mesothelioma in situ. This term has been applied to cytologically atypical proliferations of epithelioid mesothelial cells that are confined to the pleural surface, with no evidence of invasion across its basement membrane[143,144] (Fig. 20-25). Reports on this finding have been limited to cases where other areas of the pleura did demonstrate infiltrative MM. Hence, it is still not clear as to whether pleural mesothelioma can truly exist in an exclusively in situ form. In fact, we have never seen an autopsy case that involved this finding.

Sarcomatoid (Spindle Cell) Mesothelioma

Sarcomatoid malignant mesothelioma (SMM) (also see Chapter 14) is comprised of fusiform cells with variable degrees of atypia and pleomorphism.[122,131,145–147] These may be arranged in fascicles, storiform

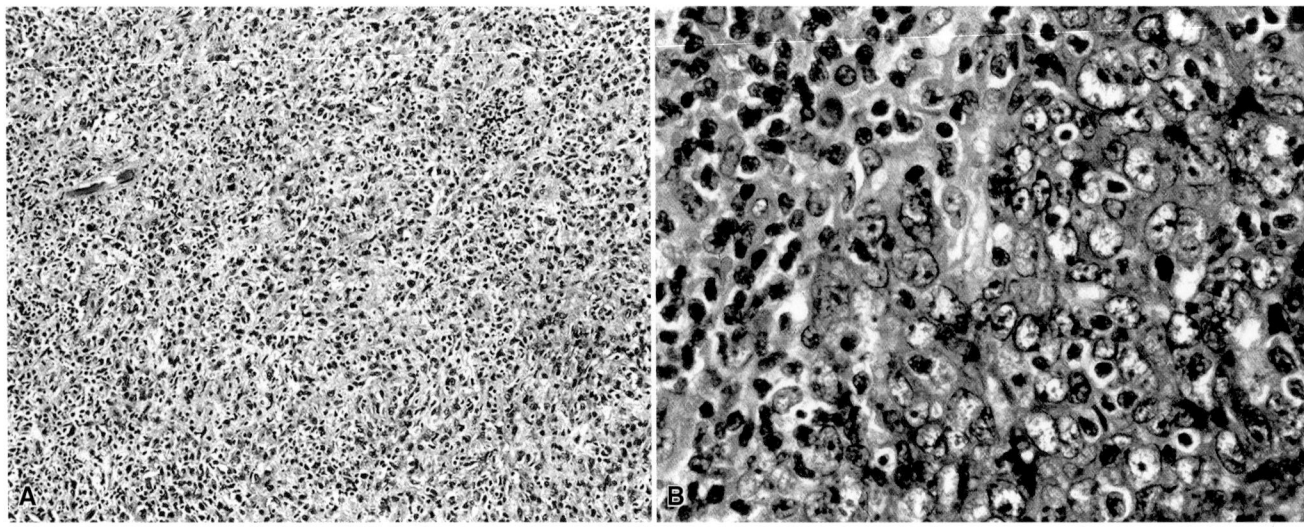

Figure 20-22. A and **B,** "Lymphohistiocytoid" malignant pleural mesothelioma comprises syncytia of large epithelioid cells with numerous admixed lymphocytes. The image is reminiscent of lymphoepithelioma-like carcinomas.

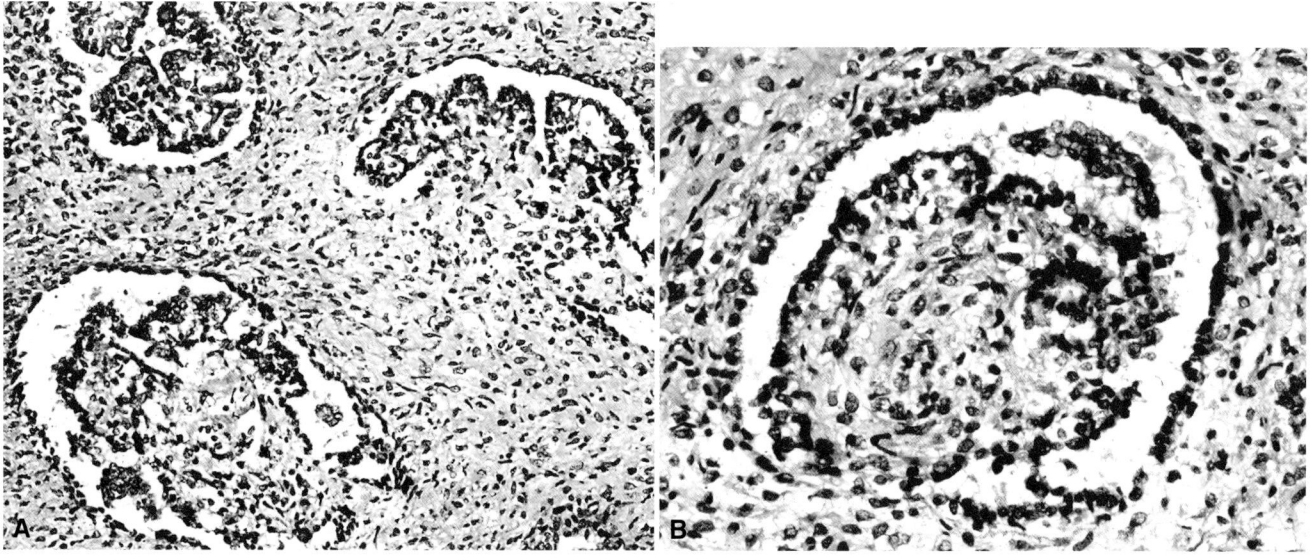

Figure 20-24. **A** and **B,** "Glomeruloid" mesothelioma in which the neoplastic epithelial cells are arranged in a configuration that markedly resembles renal glomeruli.

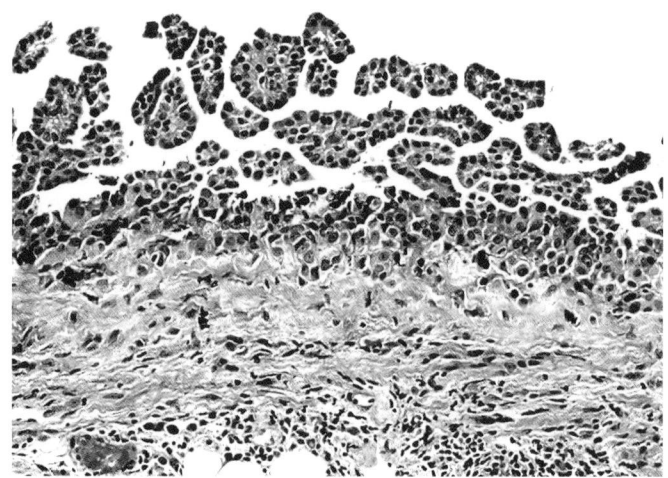

Figure 20-25. So-called in situ mesothelioma showing noninvasive foci of atypical mesothelial cells.

arrays, or random configurations (Figs. 20-26 and 20-27). Tumoral collagen synthesis is likewise heterogeneous. The prevalence of mitotic activity and necrosis in such lesions generally parallels their histologic grade. A special variant of SMM is that which shows divergent differentiation into "heterologous" mesenchymal tissues such as osteoid, cartilage, and striated muscle (Fig. 20-28).[148–150] It could rightly be called "metaplastic" SMM. Tumors with angiosarcoma-like foci in this category have also been termed "pseudovascular" or "angiomatoid" mesotheliomas (Fig. 20-29). Klebe and associates have suggested that *all* pleural neoplasms with purely sarcomatous features should be classified as mesotheliomas, even if they are immunohistologically negative for keratin.[151] We cannot agree with that conclusion, because, as discussed subsequently, their experience is that SMMs express keratin in virtually every case regardless of morphologic nuances.

Myxoid stroma may also dominate the microscopic picture in occasional examples of SMMs. When cellular atypia in sarcomatoid mesothelioma is extreme, the designations "anaplastic" or "pleomorphic" MM are appropriate.[152]

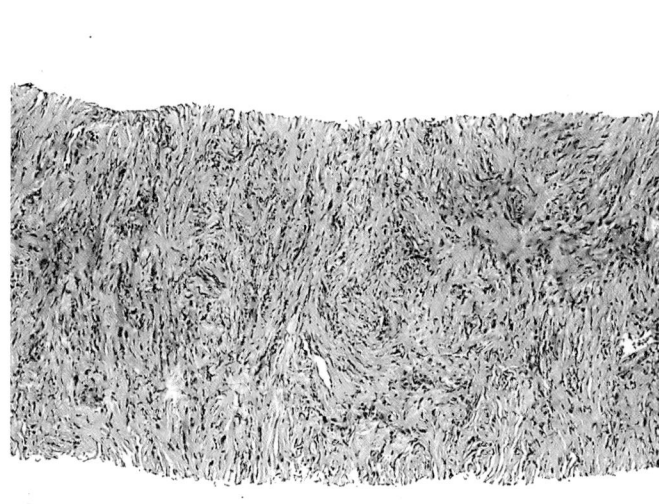
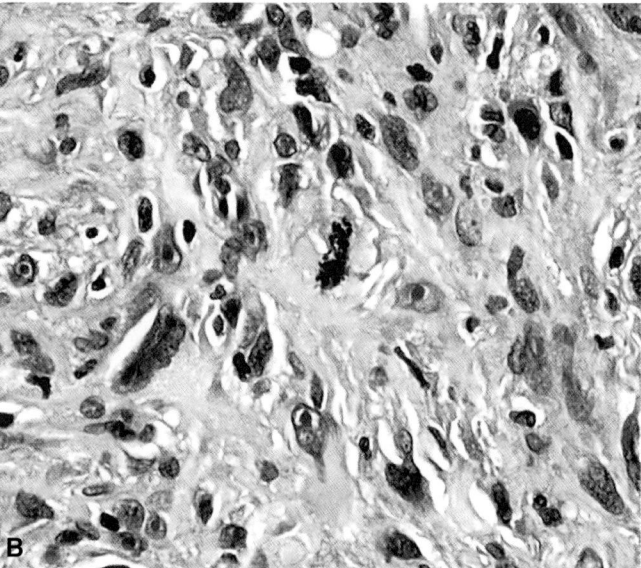

Figure 20-26. Sarcomatoid malignant mesothelioma of the pleura (**A**) showing a disorganized proliferation of highly atypical spindle cells (**B**).

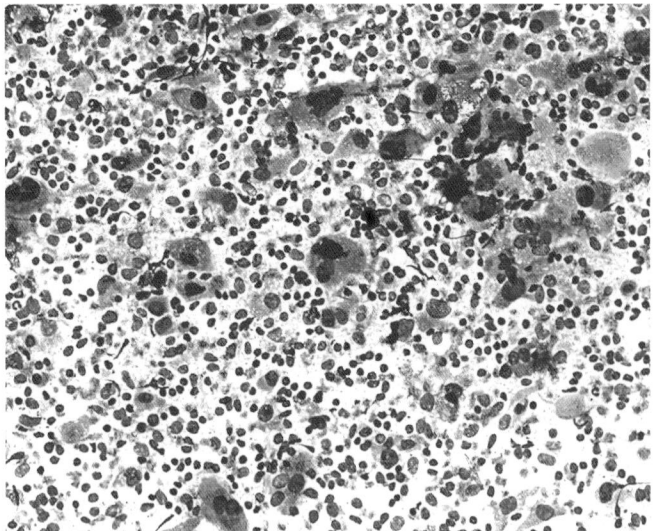

Figure 20-27. A fine needle aspiration biopsy of sarcomatoid mesothelioma showing dyshesive and markedly pleomorphic spindle cells. They were keratin-positive.

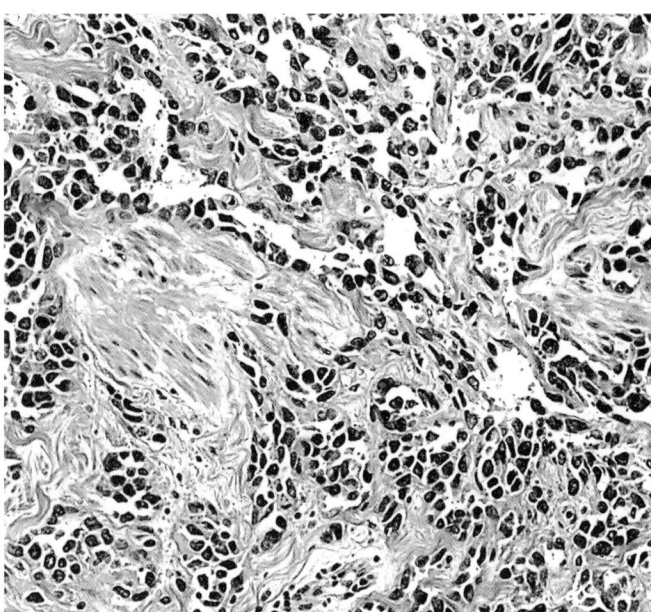

Figure 20-29. A histologic resemblance to angiosarcoma is seen in this "pseudovascular" mesothelioma.

Desmoplastic Mesothelioma

As mentioned earlier, desmoplastic malignant mesothelioma (DMM) is a special subtype of SMM in which spindle-shaped or stellate neoplastic cells are bland cytologically and have a low density per unit area.[123,153–155] They are set in a markedly collagenized and hyalinized stromal matrix, often with a "basket weave" configuration like that of pleural plaques or fibrohyaline pleuritis (fibrous pleurisy)[123] (Fig. 20-30). Mitoses are sparse, and necrosis is limited if it is present at all. The World Health Organization recommends that the designation DMM be used when more than 50% of the tumor shows this pattern. Many SMMs and some biphasic tumors (see later discussion) also contain small foci in which a desmoplastic foci can be seen; in such cases mention of such foci is recommended, because this variant has a particularly poor prognosis.

The malignant nature of DMM is manifested by its invasion of underlying lung or adjacent soft tissues[156] (Fig. 20-31). In addition, careful scrutiny of the tumor usually (but not always) reveals a level of cellular atypism and a degree of cellular density that exceeds that of benign pleural lesions (Fig. 20-32). Moreover, there is no microscopic "zonation" in DMM. That phenomenon is best represented in fibrohyaline pleuritis, in which lesional cellularity decreases as one moves spatially from the pleural space into the subjacent tissues.[157] The Verhoeff-Van Gieson elastic stain is helpful in the differential diagnosis of fibrohyaline pleuritis versus DMM. Mesotheliomas show a paucity of internal elastic fibers, or, if they are present, there is no regularity of their orientation. In contrast, fibrous pleuritis usually exhibits a retention of laminated, roughly parallel elastic tissue throughout the thickened visceral pleura (see Chapter 18).

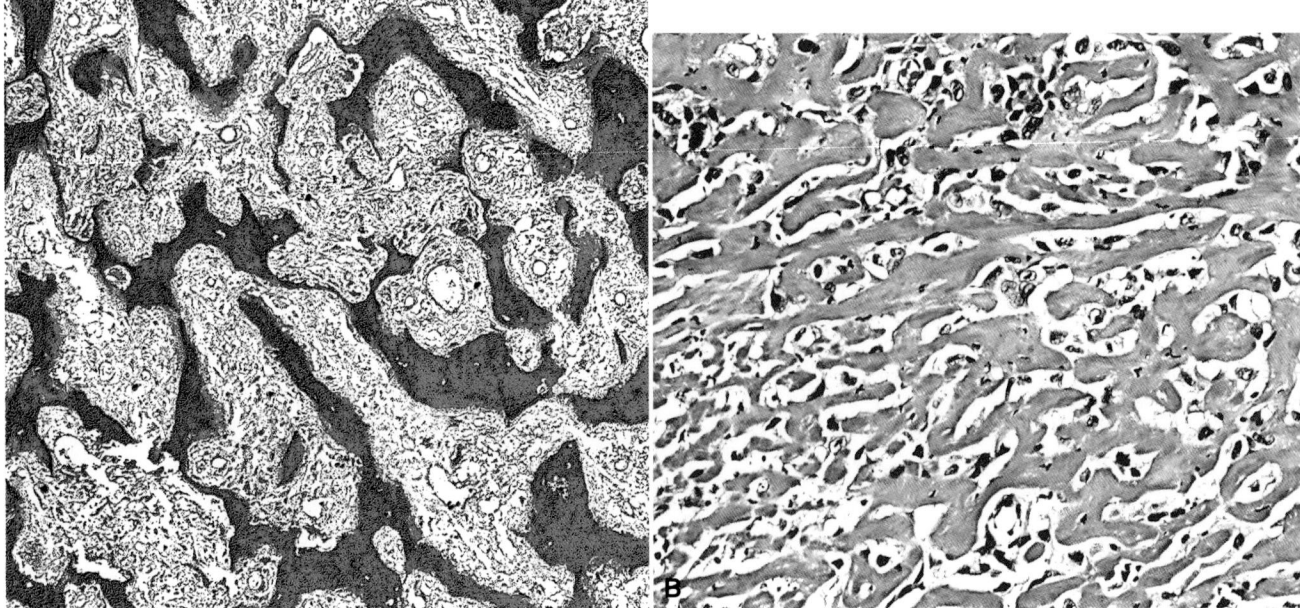

Figure 20-28. **A** and **B,** Divergent osteochondroid differentiation in sarcomatoid malignant pleural mesothelioma.

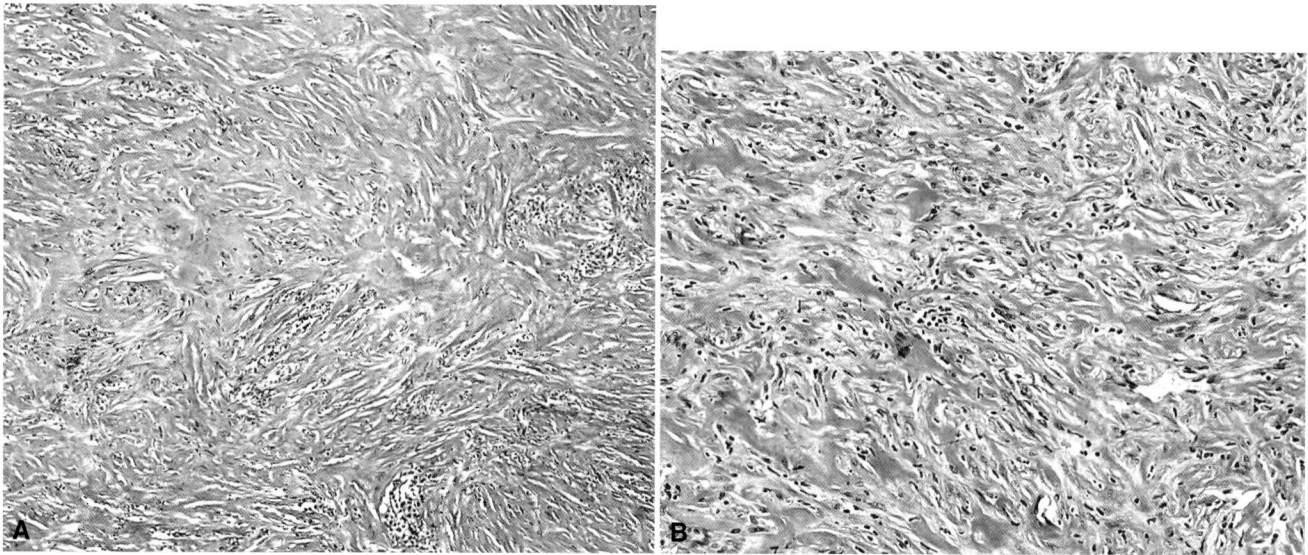

Figure 20-30. **A** and **B,** This example of desmoplastic pleural mesothelioma shows a relatively bland, pleural plaquelike morphologic appearance.

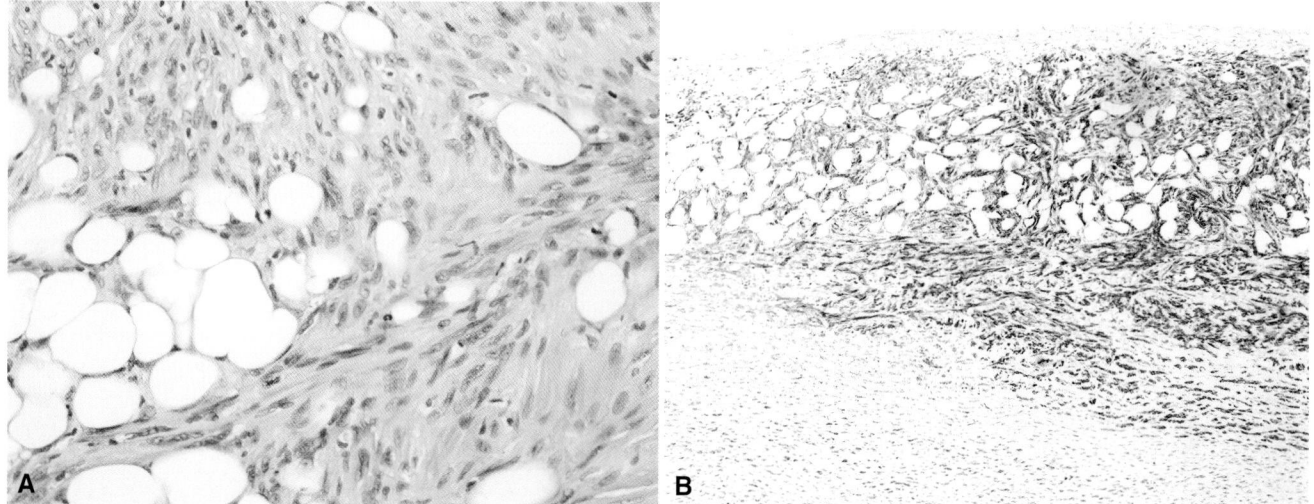

Figure 20-31. **A,** Invasion of pleural soft tissue is apparent in this example of desmoplastic mesothelioma. **B,** Confirmation with immunohistologic staining for cytokeratin is often helpful and can highlight subtle foci of invasion.

Biphasic Mesothelioma

As their name suggests, biphasic malignant mesotheliomas are typified by admixtures of two morphologic configurations, usually at least one variant of EMM and at least one in the spectrum of SMM. Those components may be abruptly juxtaposed to one another or blend imperceptibly[131] (Fig. 20-33). Schramm and coworkers have suggested that biphasic malignant mesotheliomas typify the "epithelial-mesenchymal" transition that can be seen in several tumor types, and that this phenomenon worsens the behavior of epithelial neoplasms.[158]

Small Cell Mesothelioma

Another uncommon type of MM is its small cell form, a variant of epithelial MM.[121,159] It is only rarely seen in "pure" form and usually includes a portion of tumors with other histologic patterns. This lesion is composed of compact round cells with high nuclear-to-cytoplasmic ratios, oval nuclei with dispersed chromatin, variably discernible nucleoli, and scant amphophilic cytoplasm (Fig. 20-34). As such, it is morphologi-

cally similar to several other malignant small cell/basaloid neoplasms, including basaloid carcinoma, high-grade neuroendocrine carcinoma, small cell melanoma, small round cell sarcomas, and non-Hodgkin lymphomas.

Rhabdoid Mesothelioma

Over the past decade, it has become apparent that a relatively broad spectrum of malignant tumors may exhibit a "rhabdoid" phenotype, akin to that seen in high-grade pediatric renal neoplasms. Extrarenal rhabdoid tumors (ERTs) may be "pure" histologically, or they may represent a new clonal element that has arisen from another recognizable tumor type.[160] Hence, one may see ERTs in combination with a definable carcinoma, melanoma, or sarcoma. In the latter instance, the term "composite" ERT is apropos. MMs are no exception to these precepts. Thus, wholly rhabdoid MMs may be encountered in some cases, whereas other pleural mesotheliomas may show an "ordinary" morphotype that is admixed with ERTs.[161,162]

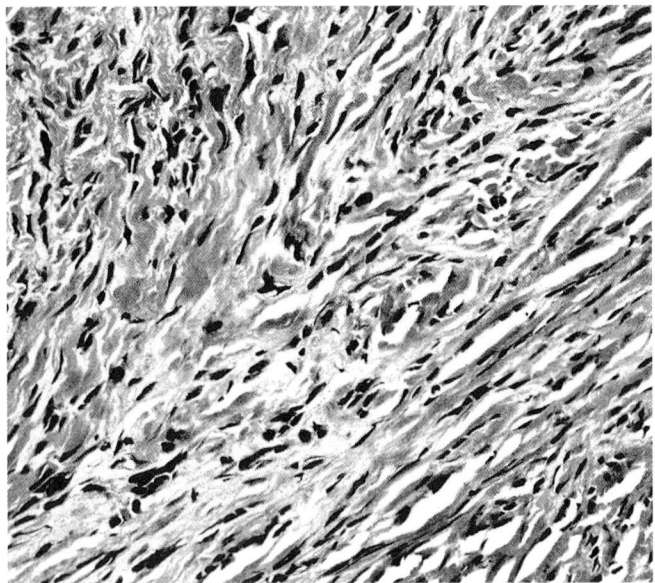

Figure 20-32. At least focally, most examples of desmoplastic mesothelioma show significant nuclear atypia, as shown here. However, the finding is dependent on sampling.

Rhabdoid cells are characterized by a moderately pleomorphic epithelioid shape, eccentric nuclei with vesicular chromatin and prominent nucleoli, and distinctive eosinophilic cytoplasm having a hard globular quality (Fig. 20-35). They are relatively dyshesive; occasional spindle cell change and multinucleation may be seen as well.

Classic rhabdoid tumors of the kidney and nervous systems show consistent loss of the intranuclear INI1 gene product, which functions as a tumor suppressor.[163] However, composite rhabdoid lesions generally retain it. To date, no published studies have addressed the INI1 status of rhabdoid MM.

The principal significance of a rhabdoid phenotype is the biologic aggressiveness with which it is associated, regardless of other clinicopathologic details of the individual tumor.[160,162] Nonetheless, because mesotheliomas as a group have such an adverse outcome, the behavioral impact of rhabdoid change is not as great in this particular context.

Localized (Solitary) Mesothelioma

Localized MM of the pleura is defined by its gross characteristics rather than its microscopic ones. This tumor can show any of the histologic patterns considered previously (i.e., epithelioid, biphasic, sarcomatoid, and variations thereof).[54,112,164,165] In contrast to *diffuse* pleural mesotheliomas, an increasingly spindle cell composition does not appear to affect the prognosis of people with localized MMs negatively.[112,166] Insufficient numbers of these MMs have been analyzed to say with any certainty that they may be causally related to above-background asbestos exposures.

Histochemical Features of Pleural Mesothelioma

Up until 20 years ago, the separation of MMs from other histologically similar neoplasms was based largely on histochemical results. The capacity for adenocarcinomas to synthesize epithelial mucin (Fig. 20-36) had been recognized quickly after the application of specialized biochemical methods in surgical pathology, and it was soon recognized that mesotheliomas did not possess this ability.[167-174] Conversely, MMs were found to manufacture stromal mucin, which was labeled by the colloidal iron or Alcian blue methods at pH 2.5, and prior treatment of tissue sections with hyaluronidase removed this substance[167,170,173,175] (Fig. 20-37). Thus, these observations set the stage for the use of the periodic acid/Schiff technique, with and without diastase predigestion (to remove glycogen, which, like epithelial mucin, is positive for periodic acid/Schiff); the mucicarmine method (to label epithelial mucin); and the colloidal iron or Alcian blue procedures, with and without hyaluronidase pretreatment, for the histochemical delineation of adenocarcinomas and mesotheliomas.

Such an approach is still useful, but there are several caveats that must be borne in mind. First, histochemical studies for epithelial mucin are most useful in the distinction of epithelioid mesothelioma variants from other tumors, and they lose much of their value if the differential diagnosis is that of SMM versus spindle cell carcinoma or true sarcoma. Carcinomas that are not overtly gland-forming also commonly lack mucin production; on the other hand, some sarcomatoid carcinomas and various sarcomas may acquire *stromal* mucin synthesis as seen in SMM.

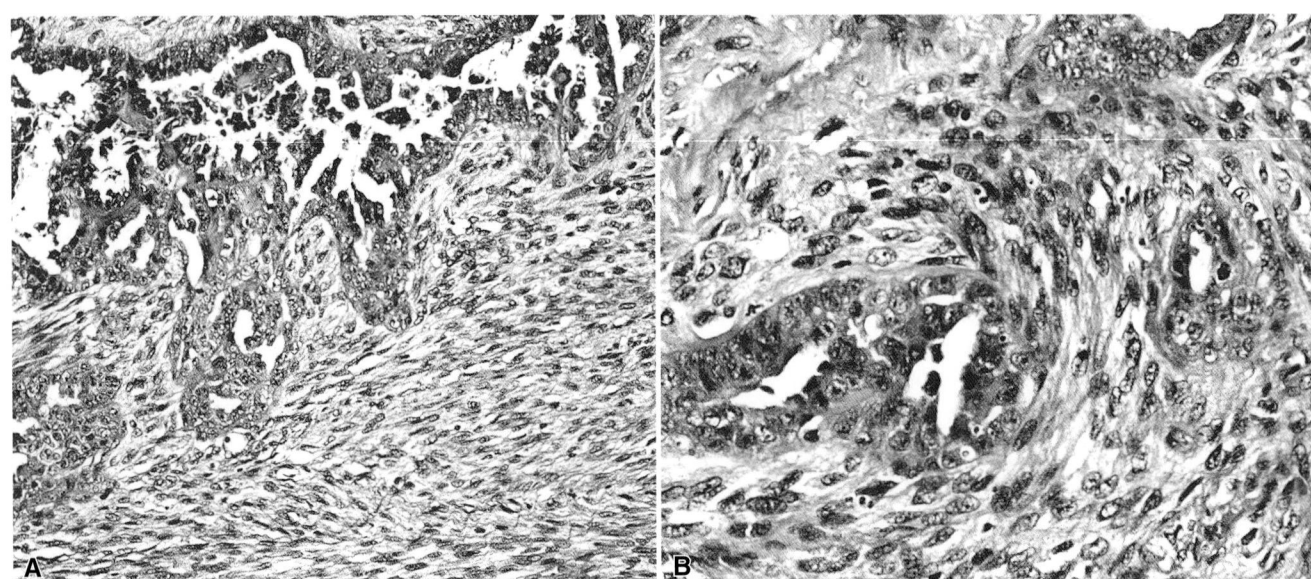

Figure 20-33. **A** and **B**, Biphasic malignant pleural mesothelioma showing foci of overtly epithelioid growth juxtaposed to fusiform and pleomorphic elements.

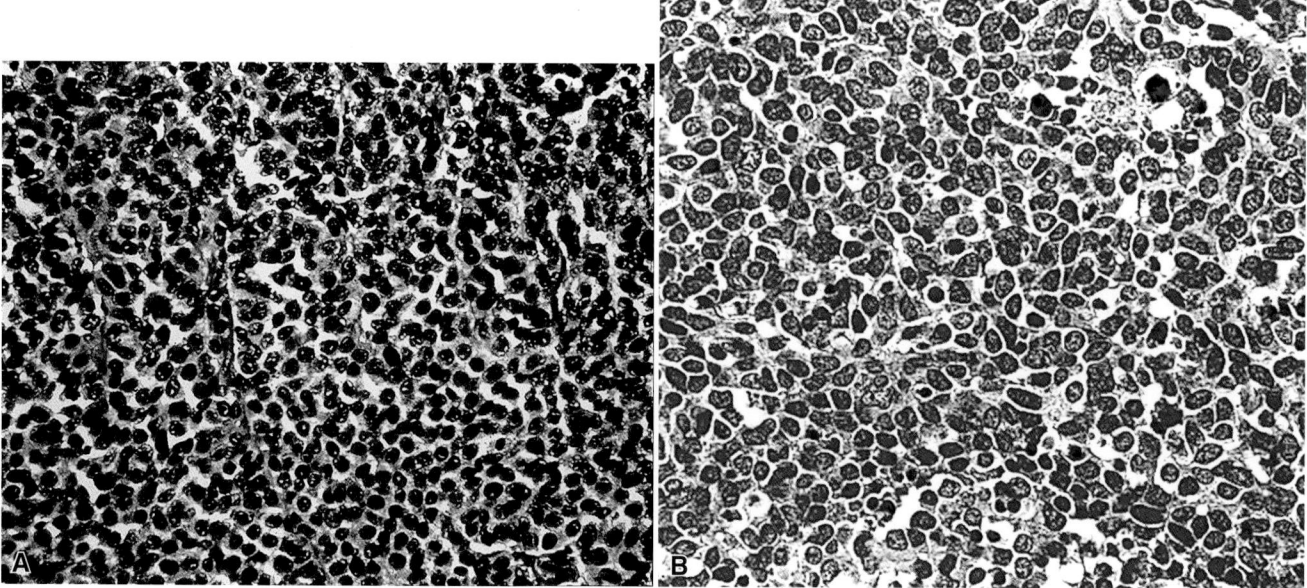

Figure 20-34. A and **B,** Small-cell malignant pleural mesothelioma represented by a sheet of relatively monomorphic and compact tumor cells.

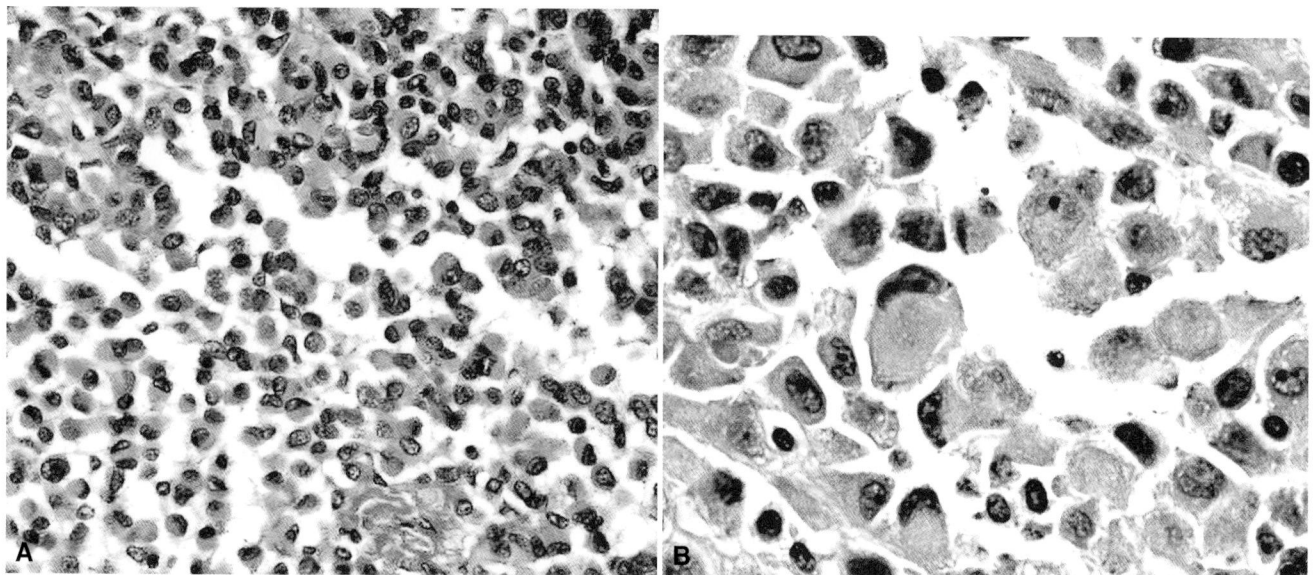

Figure 20-35. A and **B,** Rhabdoid malignant mesothelioma showing poorly cohesive large ovoid cells that contain hard eosinophilic cytoplasmic inclusions.

Providing that one observes the cautions just cited, epithelioid mesotheliomas can be distinguished from carcinomas histochemically in approximately 50% of cases.[149] The periodic acid/Schiff–diastase technique is the most useful for that purpose, because, at least, in our experience, it is more sensitive than the mucicarmine (Best) stain. Moreover, there have been sporadic reports of MMs that were spuriously labeled with the mucicarmine procedure, apparently because it unexpectedly recognized a form of stromal mucin.[176] Pretreatment with hyaluronidase is successful in abrogating that aberrant reactivity, and therefore it should be used routinely if mucicarmine is utilized in differential diagnoses that include epithelioid MM.

In the same vein, colloidal iron and Alcian blue methods commonly label epithelial as well as stromal mucins. Hence, only those epithelioid lesions that lose their colloidal iron/Alcian blue positivity after hyaluronidase predigestion are consistent with mesothelial neoplasms.[167,169–171] Again, roughly 50% of polygonal cell MMs manifest this pattern of reactivity.

During the 1980s, it was recognized that silver impregnation methods were able to label accumulations of intranuclear proteins that are associated with active transcription of nucleic acid. The silver-positive argyrophilic nucleolar organizer regions (AgNORs, or silver-stained nucleolar organizing regions) are now known to be related to double chromosomal "satellites," chromosome polymorphisms, and structural abnormalities involving chromosomal satellite regions.[177–179] Silver nitrate (in colloidal suspension) has an affinity for them, yielding a black precipitate, and discrete globular deposits of it are then visible in positive nuclei on conventional microscopy. The number of AgNORs seen in this way appears to parallel the density of quantitative markers of nucleolar protein synthesis, such as fibrillarin[180] (Fig. 20-38). Several authors have confirmed the fact that MMs and carcinomas both have higher AgNOR counts per nucleus than do reactive mesothelial proliferations.[181–183] Therefore, the usual application of this method is not to separate mesothelioma from adenocarcinoma but to distinguish MM from an atypical but benign mesothelial proliferation.[181,182] AgNOR values in those two groups have

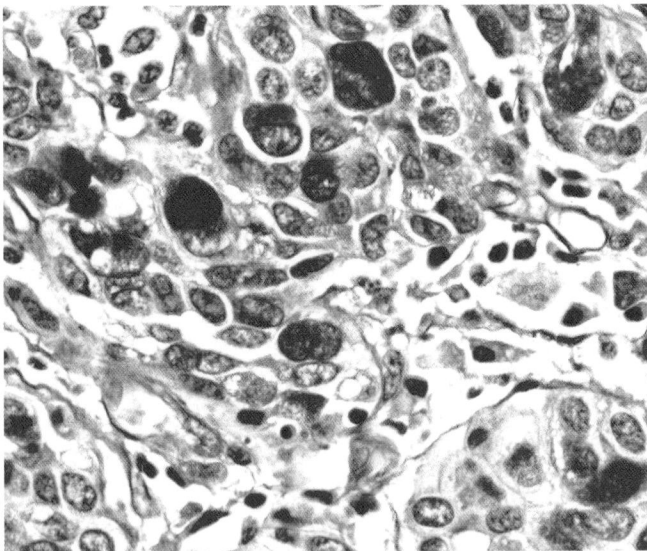

Figure 20-36. Histochemical reactivity is seen with the digested periodic acid/Schiff method in pseudomesotheliomatous adenocarcinoma of the pleura.

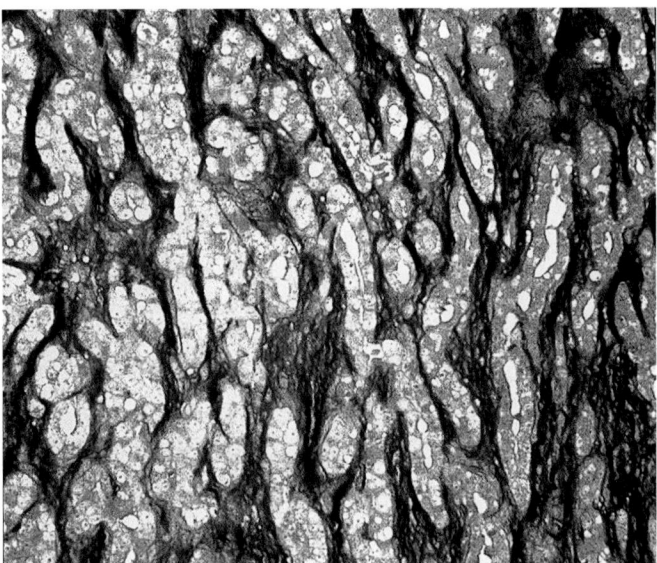

Figure 20-37. Colloidal iron (CI) staining of malignant epithelioid pleural mesothelioma showing the presence of intercellular stromal mucin. It is represented by the blue matrix in this photomicrograph. Pretreatment of histologic sections from this case with hyaluronidase abolished the CI positivity.

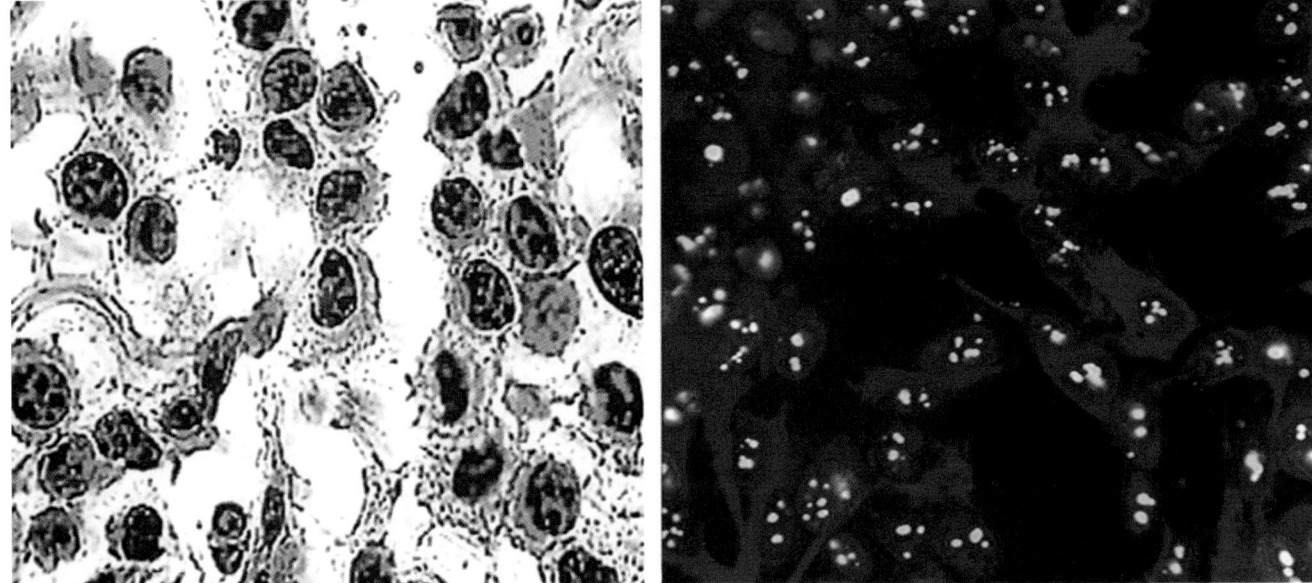

Figure 20-38. Argyrophilic nucleolar organizer regions in this malignant mesothelioma are visible as black intranuclear deposits (*left*). They colocalize with immunofluorescent signals for fibrillarin (*right*), a nucleolar protein.

ranged from slightly greater than 1 in minimally atypical benign mesothelial cells to greater than 7.5 in highly anaplastic mesothelioma cells, usually showing a bimodal distribution in mesotheliosis and MM.[184] Despite the hopeful nature of these results, substantial numerical overlap still exists between the two lesional groups in question. Some have successfully used these results in combination with immunohistochemistry, image cytometry, and in situ hybridization assessment of chromosome 9p21 deletions to allow for greater than 95% accurate separation of reactive from neoplastic mesothelial proliferations.[185,186]

Electron Microscopic Features of Pleural Mesothelioma

In the early 1970s, several investigators began to catalog the ultrastructural characteristics of MM and compare them with those of histologically similar neoplasms.[187–189] Through the ensuing years, it has become apparent that transmission electron microscopy is an extremely effective tool in the delineation of mesothelial differentiation. In addition, it provides valuable information in the differential diagnosis of other malignancies.[190,191]

In epithelioid mesotheliomas, a constellation of findings that includes abundant tangles of cytoplasmic intermediate filaments, with focal formation of perinuclear tonofibrils; elongated and complex desmosomes (Fig. 20-39); an absence of mucin droplets; and the presence of long, branching, plasmalemmal microvilli (with a length-to-diameter ratio of 10:1 or more)[190–194] (Fig. 20-40) is typical. Other common findings include cytoplasmic glycogen deposits, dilated intercellular spaces, and intracellular lumina, which are also often lined by microvilli. External microvillous projections are sometimes difficult to evaluate with regard to their dimensions, because they can be compressed and distorted when

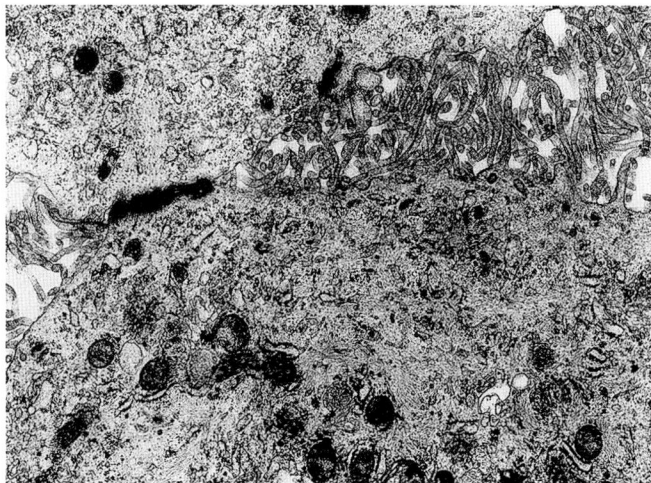

Figure 20-39. Prominent, elongated desmosomes (*left center*) join the tumor cells of a malignant mesothelioma in this electron photomicrograph.

caught between adjacent tumor cells. Basal laminae are also present around many of the neoplastic cells in mesotheliomas, and the microvilli are often coated by an amorphous granular material[195,196] (Fig. 20-41).

Relatively few neoplasms show all of the "classic" characteristics of MM,[195] but most mesothelial tumors manifest enough of them to make their identification straightforward. In contrast, metastatic adenocarcinomas (MACs) of various anatomic origins, which represent the principal diagnostic alternative to MM, exhibit short truncated microvilli and an absence of tonofibrils and may contain intracytoplasmic mucin granules as well.[190,197-199] Wick and colleagues[174] performed a comparative study of electron microscopy and immunohistology in the distinction between EMMs and MACs, and they found the two techniques to be comparable in efficacy.

The polygonal cells in biphasic mesotheliomas exhibit fine structural features that are comparable to those of pure EMM. Thus, electron microscopy is similarly helpful in separating such tumors from biphasic sarcomatoid carcinomas involving the pleura.

On the other hand, SMMs lose the distinctive plasmalemmal modifications that characterize their epithelioid counterparts. Spindle cell and pleomorphic mesotheliomas most closely resemble true sarcomas at an ultrastructural level (Fig. 20-42), except for the presence of rare intercellular junctional complexes and intermediate filament bundles.[122,193,200,201] In that specific context, electron microscopic assessment is not definitive diagnostically.

Some authors have suggested that ultrastructural studies no longer add substantively to the diagnosis of MM.[202] However, other authors[203,204] (and those of this chapter) do not agree.

Immunohistochemical Findings in Pleural Mesothelioma

Mesothelioma has been vigorously studied immunohistochemically over the past two decades. From a histopathologic point of view, there are four settings in which immunophenotyping plays an important role in its diagnosis:

1. EMM versus adenocarcinoma
2. Sarcomatoid mesothelioma versus primary or metastatic pleural sarcoma versus metastatic sarcomatoid carcinoma
3. Epithelioid mesothelioma versus reactive mesothelial hyperplasia
4. Desmoplastic sarcomatoid mesothelioma versus fibrohyaline pleuritis.

Among these problems, the one that is most commonly encountered is that of mesothelioma versus metastatic carcinoma. Despite the more uncommon nature of SMM, immunohistochemistry is

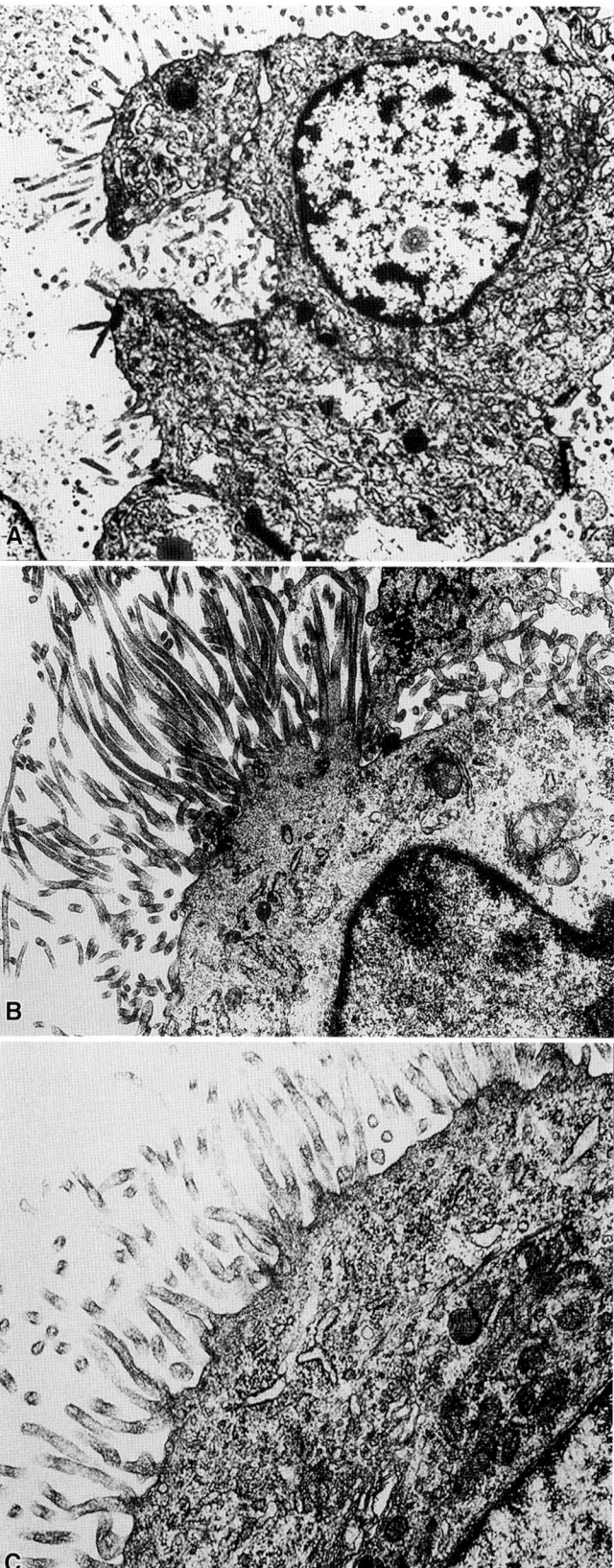

Figure 20-40. A to **C,** Elongated and "bushy" plasmalemmal microvilli are seen in these epithelioid mesotheliomas ultrastructurally.

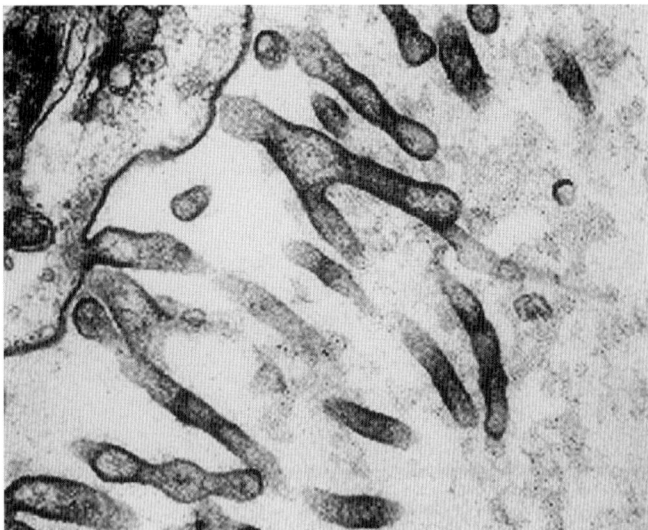

Figure 20-41. A delicate granular coating of electron-dense material is seen on the surfaces of microvilli in this epithelioid mesothelioma.

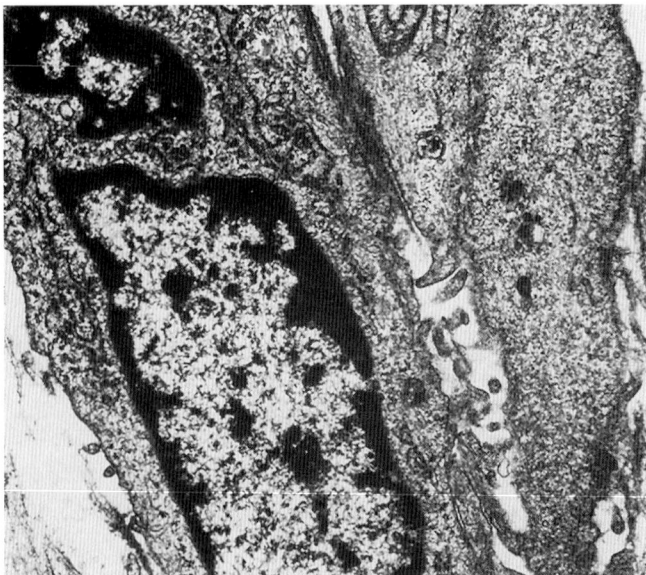

Figure 20-42. Sarcomatoid mesothelioma differs substantially from epithelioid tumors by electron microscopy; this example resembles fibrosarcoma ultrastructurally.

nonetheless equally useful in its distinction from true sarcomas affecting the pleural space. However, in the remaining settings, in which the differential diagnosis involves a benign or reactive condition, the practical contribution of immunophenotyping is much more limited. With specific reference to desmoplastic mesothelioma, it has been properly suggested that because of its poor prognosis and the lack of effective treatment, underdiagnosis of that tumor is preferable to overdiagnosis.[153] It may well take several biopsies to establish a definitive interpretation in such cases.

Each of the previously cited diagnostic questions is associated with differing panels of immunohistochemical reagents. For instance, in cases of possible spindle cell or desmoplastic mesothelioma, immunohistologic evaluation should principally focus on whether the tumor is keratin-positive. Calretinin, Wilms tumor 1 (WT1) gene product, and podoplanin have much lower rates of reactivity in SMMs compared with epithelioid and biphasic variants. Other markers, such as desmin, muscle-specific actin, and S-100 protein, are necessary only

to subtype a mesenchymal neoplasm if the keratin reaction is negative. In the morphologic context of sarcoma-like tumors, the application of antibodies that are used to recognize overtly epithelial tumors (e.g., Ber-Ep4, CD15, cancer antigen 72-4 [CA 72-4], and carcinoembryonic antigen [CEA]) is illogical, because neither sarcomas nor sarcomatoid carcinomas synthesize the targets of these reagents.[205] The following sections will review the different analytes that have been tested clinically in the study of MM, to provide a guide for a practical approach to immunohistochemical analysis.

Antibodies Often Used in the Analysis of Possible Mesothelioma

General and Exclusionary Markers

Keratins

Keratin antibodies have been extensively applied to MMs and their simulators, with the principal goal of distinguishing mesothelioma from adenocarcinomas[206–211] and true sarcomas. Some authors have concluded that particular staining patterns for specific keratins may allow for the separation of those tumor types, and differing degrees of contextual specificity and sensitivity have been ascribed to various keratin subsets. In particular, antibodies to keratin 5/6 have been promoted as helpful immunohistochemical markers for MM[211] (Fig. 20-43). In one assessment, Ordóñez found that 40 examples of mesothelioma were positive for keratin 5/6, whereas 30 pulmonary adenocarcinomas were negative. However, he also observed focal reactivity in 14 of 93 cases of nonpulmonary adenocarcinoma, to some extent limiting the utility of keratin 5/6 in the exclusion of metastases to the pleura.[211] Another study reported 92% keratin 5/6 positivity in MM and 14% labeling in cases of MAC.[212] Despite these drawbacks, keratin 5/6 does appear to be a helpful presumptive marker for mesothelioma when used in the proper fashion and the appropriate morphologic setting.

In general, it has been noted that reagents against high-molecular-weight keratins will label most mesotheliomas and relatively few adenocarcinomas, whereas antibodies to low-molecular-weight keratins recognize both of those tumor groups.[213] Keratins 7, 8, 18, and 19 are present in all MMs and adenocarcinomas, whereas keratins 5, 6, 14, and 17 are found in some types of mesothelioma but are lacking in MACs.[213] The latter four proteins are absent in cases of sarcomatoid mesothelioma.

Our approach to keratin testing in evaluating poorly differentiated malignancies is to use a broadly active mixture of monoclonal antibodies to such proteins. At present, we use a "cocktail" of commercial antibody reagents that targets all of the known keratin subtypes between

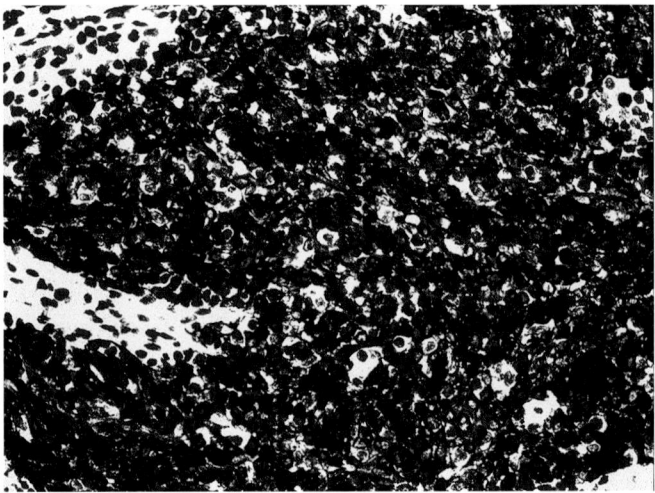

Figure 20-43. Immunoreactivity for keratin 5 in small cell mesothelioma.

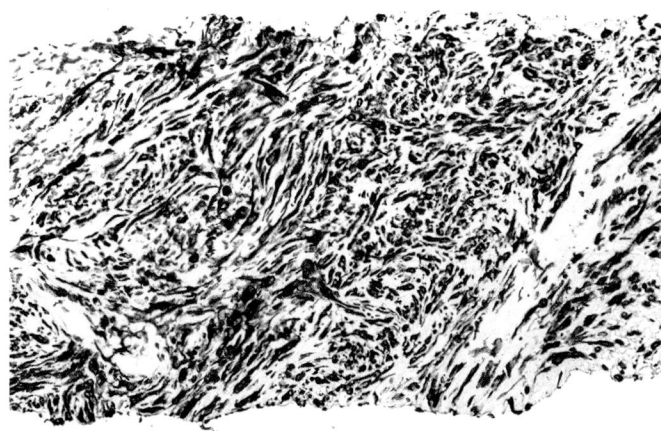

Figure 20-44. Diffuse and strong immunolabeling is present for pankeratin in this sarcomatoid mesothelioma.

keratins 1 and 20, mixed together in the same diluent and used with epitope-retrieval techniques.[214] The goal of this practice is to detect *any* keratin, rather than a specific one, because the pragmatic task in virtually all cases is the separation of epithelial from nonepithelial malignant neoplasms. With these remarks as a preface, the sensitivity of keratin "cocktail" staining for all forms of mesothelioma (including SMM) approximates 100% in our hands (Fig. 20-44).

Epithelial Membrane Antigen
Studies dealing with anti–epithelial membrane antigen (EMA) have shown that it commonly yields positive results in both MACs and MMs.[215-217] Antibodies to EMA potentially label mesotheliomas of all histologic subtypes. It has been said that this protein generally shows a double-density ("tram track") cell membranous pattern of staining in MMs (Fig. 20-45), whereas MAC cells demonstrate more delicate

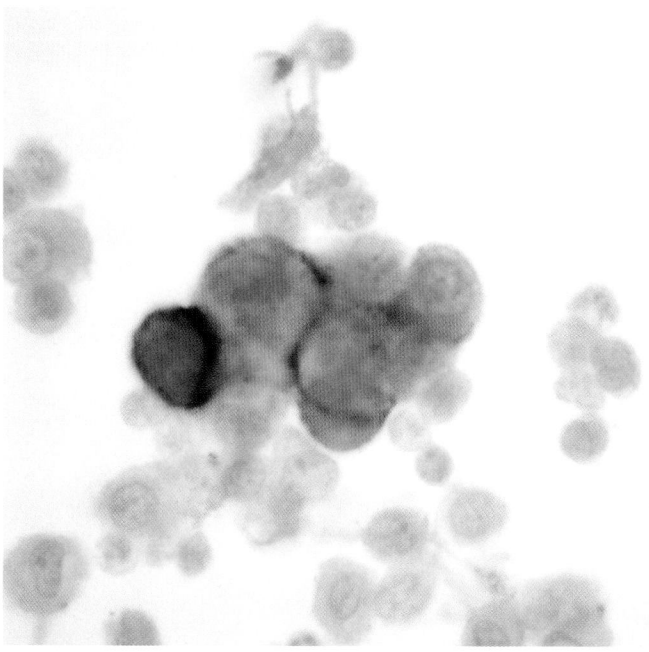

Figure 20-45. "Thick" cell membrane labeling for epithelial membrane antigen in an effusion cytology specimen of epithelioid mesothelioma.

membrane labeling.[218] Other authors have found that reactive mesothelial hyperplasia is EMA-negative, in contrast with primary malignancies of the serosal surfaces.[219] However, both of those claims are open to question[220]; in practical usage, we have found that the reactivity patterns in question are not universally present as depicted in the literature.

Carcinoembryonic Antigen
CEA has been considered by most observers to be one of the most reliable markers for distinguishing MM from adenocarcinoma.[174,221-223] The vast majority of mesotheliomas lack CEA. Positivity for CEA has been reported in up to 5% of cases of MMs, but studies describing that phenomenon have generally used unabsorbed heteroantisera to CEA that undoubtedly recognized unrelated molecules. Monoclonal antibodies to specific CEA epitopes are more reliable in this context, although they are less sensitive for the diagnosis of adenocarcinoma and, therefore, less helpful diagnostically. However, the use of anti-CEA reagents has no role in the diagnosis of sarcomatoid mesotheliomas, as mentioned earlier.

Thyroid Transcription Factor-1
Thyroid transcription factor-1 (TTF-1) is a 38-kDa intranuclear polypeptide that is synthesized by a gene located on chromosome 14q13; it is also known as NKX2A protein.[224,225] Among epithelial elements, this homeodomain-containing nuclear transcription factor is restricted to follicular and parafollicular thyroid cells, glandular and alveolar-lining cells of the lung, and anterior pituicytes. TTF-1–positive neoplasms are largely encompassed by those same tissues, with the addition of moderately and poorly differentiated neuroendocrine carcinomas of various organs and the omission of parathyroid and pituitary tumors.[224] Approximately 75% to 85% of pulmonary adenocarcinomas and adenosquamous carcinomas are labeled for TTF-1.[226,227] In contrast, mesotheliomas of all histologic types have been consistently nonreactive.[228] It is important to require that nuclear labeling be regarded as the only true pattern of positivity for TTF-1.[229]

Napsin-A
Napsin-A is a cytoplasmic aspartic proteinase that plays a role in the synthesis of surfactant protein-B in the lungs. In normal tissues, it is expressed strongly in type 2 pneumocytes. Antibodies to napsin-A have been applied clinically only recently, and the overall number of mesotheliomas and adenocarcinomas studied thus far is relatively small. However, in one evaluation, 85% of pulmonary adenocarcinomas were napsin-A–reactive, compared with no cases of mesothelioma or colonic, pancreatic, or mammary carcinoma.[230] Unexpectedly, napsin-A was also observed in clear cell and papillary renal cell carcinomas (RCCs), as well as in tall cell papillary thyroid carcinomas. It appears that this marker may best be used in the narrow differential diagnosis of peripheral pulmonary adenocarcinoma versus EMM.

CD15
CD15 has a high level of specificity for MACs,[174,222,223,231-233] but some examples of MM have also shown focal labeling for this marker. This finding appears to be more common in peritoneal tumors than in pleural lesions.[234] Like CEA, the use of CD15 is most appropriate in the evaluation of biphasic or epithelial mesotheliomas, because sarcomatoid tumors consistently lack it.

CA 72-4
CA 72-4, which is also known as tumor-associated glycoprotein-72 (recognized by monoclonal antibody B72.3), is a generic epithelial determinant that is a high-molecular-weight cell membranous

glycoprotein.[234–239] Regardless of their sites of origin, the majority of MACs show strong reactivity for this marker. Rare examples of MM may also show focal or weak labeling.[240]

Ber-Ep4

Ber-Ep4 is another epithelial marker that was initially thought to be specific for adenocarcinomas,[241,242] and it does indeed demonstrate a high level of sensitivity for these neoplasms as a generic group. Nevertheless, it is now known that approximately 15% of mesotheliomas can show focal staining with this antibody,[243,244] and it has no value in the evaluation of purely sarcomatoid tumors.

MOC-31

MOC-31 is a monoclonal antibody that labels a 35-kDa transmembrane glycoprotein in the plasmalemma of most glandular cells.[245,246] This molecule is closely related to lung cancer–associated antigen-2,[247] but, in addition to pulmonary adenocarcinomas, MOC-31 is reactive with glandular malignancies arising in most other organ sites as well.[248,249] Mesotheliomas are reproducibly negative for this marker.[244,249]

BG8

BG8 is a synonym for Lewis blood group antigen Y (Ley; CD174), a glycoprotein that is overrepresented in malignant epithelium and is again widely distributed in glandular cells throughout the body.[250–252] Accordingly, its immunohistochemical characteristics in neoplasia generally parallel those of the MOC-31 antigen.[228,253]

p53

The p53 gene product is a nuclear phosphoprotein that regulates DNA replication, cell proliferation, and apoptosis.[254] In cases featuring atypical spindle cell proliferations that are morphologically suspicious for DMM, p53 immunolabeling of greater than 10% of the lesional cells favors a diagnosis of mesothelioma over one of a cellular pleural plaque or fibrohyaline pleuritis.[224] Nevertheless, that characteristic is not observed in all DMMs, and all cases of pleuritis are not necessarily p53-negative.

Another salient observation is that mutant p53 proteins, which are generally recognized by immunohistologic studies, are relatively restricted to MMs and are not typically seen in resting or reactive mesothelial cells.[255–258] On the face of things, mutant p53 therefore would seem to have potential value in the distinction of cytologically bland MM from mesothelial hyperplasia. Nevertheless, we would suggest avoiding exclusive reliance on p53 under such circumstances based on their clinical experience with this problem. They have seen several examples of undeniably benign mesothelial proliferations that were unexpectedly immunoreactive for p53.

Inclusionary Markers

The aforementioned antibodies include several that have been recommended by the U.S. and Canadian Mesothelioma Panel,[173] and they are probably the most commonly used markers in surgical pathology laboratories for the evaluation of malignant pleural neoplasms. However, except for p53, all of the markers presented thus far assist in the diagnosis of MM by exclusion. Over the past several years, efforts have been directed at identifying "proactive" markers of mesothelioma (i.e., those that would be present in the majority of MMs). Some such antibodies have been used diagnostically, whereas others have been analyzed as prognostic indicators. A brief discussion of these reagents follows.

Calretinin

Calretinin is a member of a large family of cytoplasmic calcium-binding proteins.[259] This marker is seen in more than 95% of mesothelioma cases of the epithelioid and biphasic types[260–262] (Fig. 20-46). Antibodies to other related polypeptides are also available, including antiparvalbumin and anticalbindin, but they fail to recognize mesotheliomas and non-neoplastic mesothelium.[263] Interestingly, there are conflicting reports regarding the expression of calretinin in sarcomatoid mesothelioma; some observers have seen universal staining of such neoplasms, but others have claimed that they are negative.[264–266] Our experience is that approximately 30% to 40% of sarcomatoid lesions do, in fact, label for calretinin, albeit in a focal fashion. Selected studies have shown that this antibody may also stain some adenocarcinomas,[261] but, if one requires nuclear labeling for calretinin as a truly positive result, these are few in number.

WT1 Gene Product

The WT1 gene resides on the short arm of chromosome 11. When it is deleted constitutively, patients have a tendency to develop nephroblastoma, an embryonal renal tumor.[267] Because of this association,

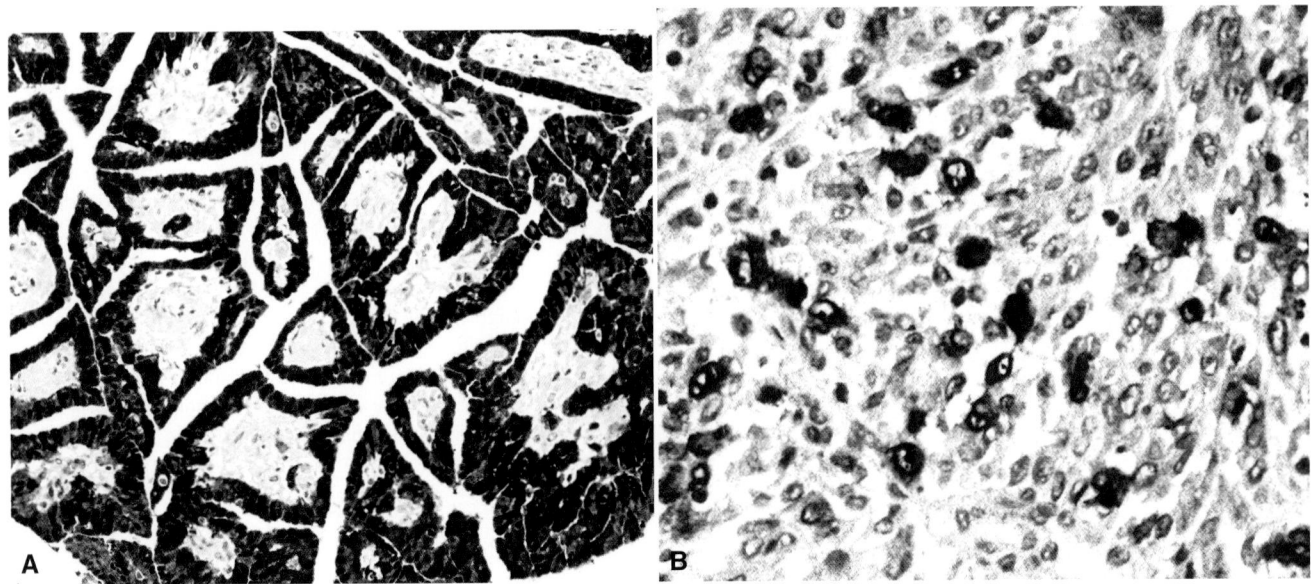

Figure 20-46. Nuclear-cytoplasmic immunoreactivity for calretinin in epithelioid mesothelioma (**A**) and sarcomatoid mesothelioma (**B**).

WT1 has generally been regarded as a tumor-suppressor gene, but it is conversely overexpressed in other malignancies, including mesothelioma, and therefore also may function as an oncogene.[268] Nuclear immunolabeling for WT1 gene product is apparent in greater than 80% of epithelioid and biphasic MMs (Fig. 20-47), but sarcomatoid tumors again demonstrate lesser reactivity in approximately 30% of cases.[228,244,265,266,269-271] WT1 is not restricted to mesothelial proliferations, and is also present in carcinomas of the thyroid, kidney, ovaries, and endometrium, some of which enter into differential diagnosis with MM.[272,273] Because it is typically absent in adenocarcinoma of the lung, WT1 has greatest applicability when this tumor is the principal diagnostic alternative to epithelioid mesothelioma.[228] Its use in the analysis of sarcomatoid tumors is complicated by the fact that true sarcomas can also be WT1-positive.[274]

In a comparison of two monoclonal antibodies to WT1, clone WT49 and clone 6F-H2, Tsuta and associates[275] found that the first reagent demonstrated greater sensitivity for mesothelioma but it also labeled a higher number of nonmesothelial malignancies, including some lung carcinomas and synovial sarcomas.

Thrombomodulin

Thrombomodulin, or CD141, converts thrombin from a procoagulant protease to an anticoagulant.[276] It is found in endothelial cells, syncytiotrophoblasts, mesothelia, and various epithelia, principally including squamous and transitional cells.[277,278] The majority of MMs (approximately 65%) label for CD141,[212,222,244,253,262,279] (Fig. 20-48) as well as squamous cell carcinomas and transitional cell carcinomas.[231,249] Fortunately, p63 protein-immunoreactivity can be used to recognize the latter two tumors, because mesotheliomas are p63-negative.[280] Glandular malignancies of various origins (including the lung) have also demonstrated unexpected reactivity in some series, and as many as 13% of adenocarcinomas have been positive.[261] Epithelioid hemangioendotheliomas and angiosarcomas, which may occasionally enter differential diagnosis with mesothelioma, are also potentially immunoreactive for CD141.[281]

Podoplanin

Podoplanin, also known as T1-alpha and Aggrus and recognized by monoclonal antibody D2-40, is a mucin-type transmembrane glycoprotein with extensive O-glycosylation. It was first identified in

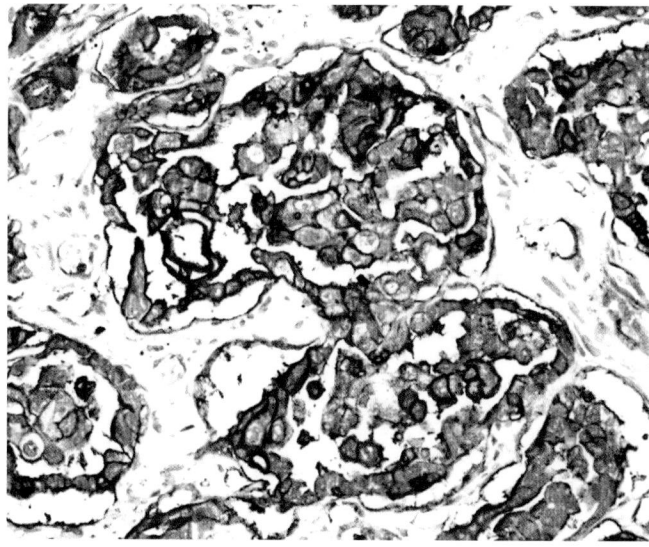

Figure 20-48. Cell membranous labeling for thrombomodulin in epithelioid pleural mesothelioma.

podocytes of the renal glomerulus.[282] This protein is specifically seen in lymphatic endothelial cells but not in vascular endothelia. In addition, nonendothelial cells in various normal tissues and human neoplasms (seminoma, Kaposi sarcoma, dendritic cell tumors, adrenocortical tumors, adnexal neoplasms of the skin, chondrosarcoma, thymoma, squamous carcinomas, meningioma, solitary fibrous tumor, and others) also express podoplanin.[283-287] The principal functions of this protein in normal tissues center on the promotion of lymphatic vasogenesis, podocyte shaping, and platelet aggregation.[283]

Several studies[284,288-292] have shown that podoplanin is a reasonably effective "proactive" marker for mesothelioma (Fig. 20-49). Conversely, it is typically, but not always, absent in carcinomas of the lung and breast.[288,292,293] Padgett and coworkers[294] reported that podoplanin was a better marker for SMM than calretinin, but 30% of sarcomatoid mesothelial tumors were still podoplanin-negative in that evaluation. We and others[290] believe that this analyte is best used in combination with either calretinin or WT1, as a second-tier marker for mesothelioma.

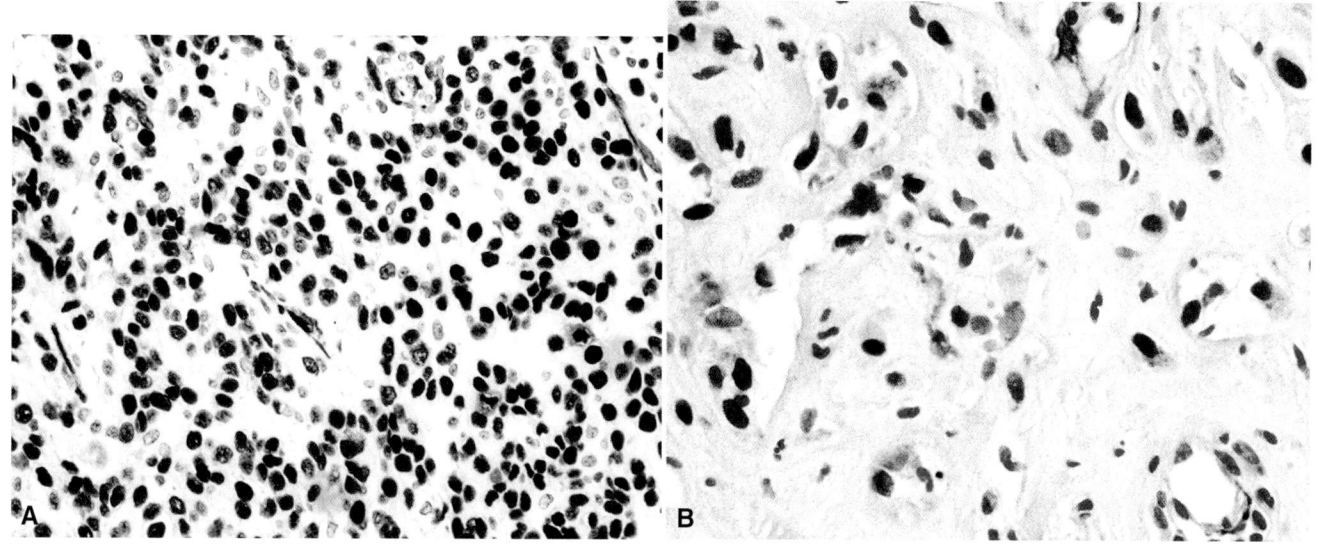

Figure 20-47. Nuclear immunolabeling for WT1 protein in epithelioid (**A**) and sarcomatoid (**B**) mesotheliomas.

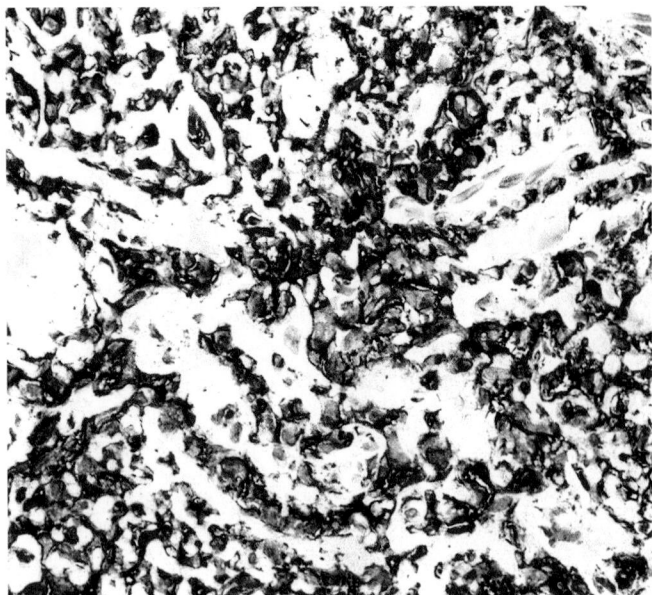

Figure 20-49. Diffuse cell membranous reactivity for podoplanin in epithelioid mesothelioma.

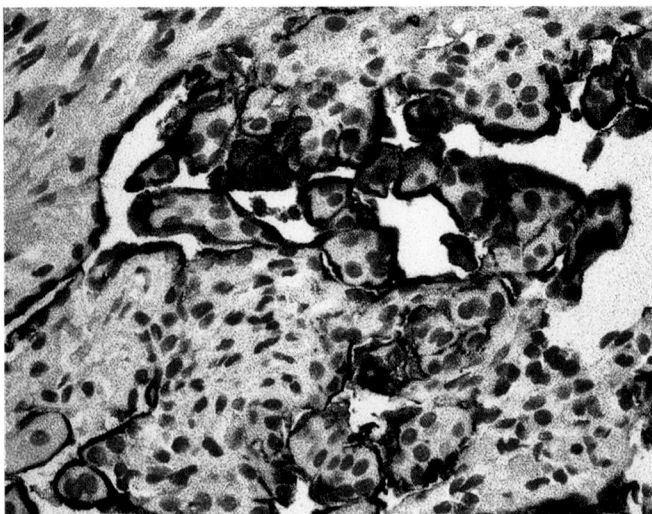

Figure 20-50. Membrane-based positivity with HBME-1 in tubulopapillary mesothelioma.

Other Markers
Oncofetal Proteins
The use of antibodies to oncofetal proteins is most commonly undertaken in the study of germ cell tumors. However, their role in the differential diagnosis of mesothelioma has been assessed in a few studies. Beta-human chorionic gonadotropin, pregnancy-specific glycoprotein, human placental lactogen, and placenta-like alkaline phosphatase have been principally found in adenocarcinomas of various sites.[295] However, the sensitivity of these determinants is relatively low, and some examples of human chorionic gonadotropin production by pleural mesotheliomas have indeed been described.[296]

Blood Group Isoantigens
In addition to Lewis blood group antigens, as typified by BG8 (see previous discussion), some studies have compared the relative reactivities of MM and adenocarcinomas for blood group isoantigens A, B, and H.[174,250,297] Their staining patterns generally mirror those of BG8, being restricted to carcinomas, but with lesser sensitivity.

Mesothelin
Mesothelin is a 40-kDa plasmalemmal protein that may function in intercellular adhesion. It is seen in roughly 70% of epithelioid and biphasic MMs, but sarcomatoid mesothelial tumors are negative.[298] Controversy has surrounded the differential diagnostic specificity of this marker vis-à-vis mesothelioma, and recent studies have reported mesothelin reactivity in a broad range of carcinomas as well.[299]

HBME-1 and Cancer Antigen 125
HBME-1 is a monoclonal antibody that was raised against mesothelial cells, and it recognizes a membranous glycoprotein. Although it demonstrates a high degree of sensitivity for MM[249,271,279] (Fig. 20-50), several studies over the past decade have shown that it clearly is not a mesothelium-specific reagent. Adenocarcinomas of several sites, including the lung, kidney, thyroid, and female genital tract, are also potentially HBME-1–reactive.[244,300-302] Similar comments apply to another mesothelium-related marker, OC125 (recognized by the monoclonal antibody cancer antigen 125 [CA 125])[302]; in fact, that determinant is widely used to label müllerian carcinomas.[303]

Neuroendocrine Determinants
Small cell MM may be confused with metastatic neuroendocrine carcinoma in the pleura. With that in mind, it is noteworthy that small cell mesotheliomas commonly manifest immunoreactivity for determinants that are generally regarded as neuroendocrine markers: namely, neuron-specific (gamma-dimer) enolase and CD57.[304] However, more specific indicators of a neuroendocrine lineage, such as chromogranin-A, CD56, and synaptophysin, are absent in MMs, and these tumors also lack the paranuclear "dotlike" staining for keratin that is seen in small cell carcinomas.

Additional Hematopoietic Markers
CD15 and CD141 have already been discussed with reference to their relative presence in mesothelial tumors. Other hematopoietic markers of interest in this setting include CD10 (neutral endopeptidase; common acute lymphoblastic leukemia antigen) and CD138 (syndecan-1). Among epithelial malignancies, CD10 is most commonly used as a potential indicator for RCC and hepatocellular carcinoma (HCC),[305,306] and pleural metastases of these tumors can certainly imitate MM morphologically. Unfortunately, mesotheliomas may also express CD10,[307] making it necessary to rely on additional discriminants in this context. On the other hand, CD138 is seen in a variety of carcinomas (e.g., pulmonary, colonic, pancreaticobiliary, hepatocellular, prostatic, renal, transitional cell, mammary, ovarian, endometrial, cutaneous, thyroid, adrenal, and salivary glandular) in differing percentages (Fig. 20-51). MM is consistently CD138-negative.[308]

Other Supplementary Reagents
Several other antibodies have been applied to the identification of EMMs in the past, and more are likely to appear in the future. For the most part, those that have not been mentioned specifically in this review are not considered to be standard diagnostic markers. However, for purposes of completeness, their relative reactivity patterns in epithelioid mesotheliomas and MACs are provided in Table 20-1 (see also Table 16-1).[309-317]

Practical Points Regarding the Immunohistochemistry of Mesothelioma
In a critical review of the numerous publications on the immunohistochemistry of MMs, one sees proof of the general tenet that single immunostains cannot be used to establish any given diagnosis with

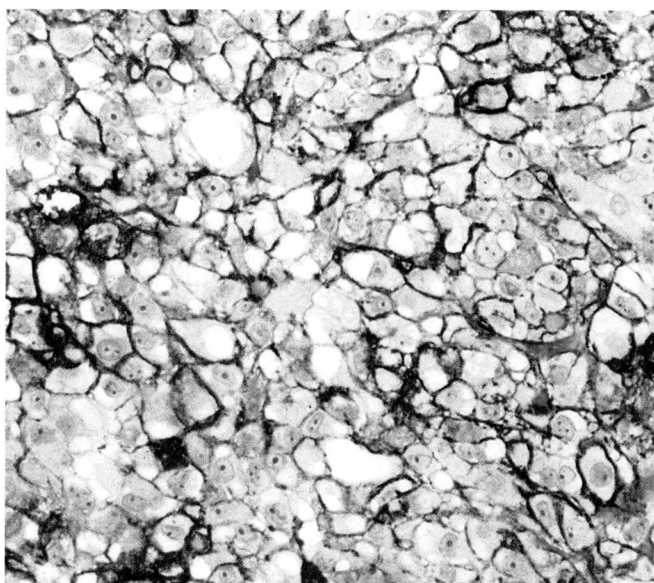

Figure 20-51. Plasmalemmal labeling for CD138 is present in a pseudomesotheliomatous adenocarcinoma of the pleura. True mesotheliomas do not express this marker.

Table 20-1. Supplementary Immunohistochemical Reagents Used to Distinguish Epithelioid Mesothelioma from Adenocarcinoma*

Marker	Mesothelioma†	Adenocarcinomas
Desmin	± 37%	—
HMFG-2	± 15%	± 75%
N-Cadherin	+ 73%	± 30%
CD44S	+ 73%	± 48%
LN1	± 48%	+ 86%
CD56	—	± 16%
LN2	± 5%	+ 91%
p21 ras	± 13%	± 16%
XIAP	± 80%	± 50%
IMP3	± 90%	± 75%
TEN-X	± 90%	± 23%
PAX2	± 4%	± 65% (Müllerian carcinomas)
PAX8	± 9%	± 95% (Müllerian carcinomas)
CA 19-9	± 20%	± 70%

*See also text and Table 16-1.
†Percentages are derived from a synthesis of the pertinent literature (also see references 309–317).
HMFG-2, human milk fat globule protein-2; IMP3, insulin-like growth factor-2 messenger RNA (mRNA)-binding protein-3; PAX, paired box gene; TEN-X, tenascin-X; XIAP, X-linked inhibitor of apoptosis protein.

certainty. It is therefore desirable that a panel of reagents be used, including at least two carefully chosen discriminatory antibodies "for" and "against" a diagnosis of mesothelioma.[318]

Other authors have suggested that the proportion of mesotheliomas that can be recognized confidently increases in direct proportion to the number of antibodies used.[253,319] In contrast, Ordoñez[244] has recommended that

> the best discriminators among the antibodies considered to be negative markers for [epithelioid] mesothelioma are CEA, MOC-31, Ber-EP4, BG8, and B72.3. A panel of four markers (two positive and two negative) selected based upon availability and which ones yield good staining results in a given laboratory is recommended. Because of their specificity and sensitivity for mesotheliomas, the best combination appears to be calretinin and cytokeratin 5/6 (or WT1) for the positive markers and CEA and MOC-31 (or B72.3, Ber-EP4, or BG8) for the negative markers.

Using logic regression analysis of 12 markers, Yaziji and colleagues concluded that a 3-marker panel (calretinin, MOC31, and BG8) was diagnostically sufficient and accurate in separating adenocarcinoma from EMM.[320] Marchevsky and Wick, Kushitani and associates, and King and coworkers have reached similar conclusions.[309,321,322] Thus, we see no practical need to use an exhaustive list of antibody reagents[323] in this particular setting.

Independent of current advances in methodology and the availability of new markers, it is also important to recognize that infallible reliability can still not be expected of immunohistochemistry. In some instances, electron microscopy may still be the best way to resolve diagnostic dilemmas in this area of tumor pathology.

Cytogenetic and Molecular Features of Pleural Mesothelioma

Cytogenetic studies on human MMs have shown no consistent chromosomal abnormalities.[324] Of those that have been reported, several appear to be relatively random events: monosomy 6; assorted trisomies and polysomies; allelic losses of 4p and 4q; deletions of 1p22, 3p, 7q, and 14q; and complete loss of chromosomes 21, 22, and Y.[325–331] On the other hand, a relatively consistent deletion of 9p21-22, involving the CDKN2A/INK4A gene, has been seen in up to 60% of cases in some studies.[332–335]

Mutations in the p53 gene have received substantial attention as possible differential diagnostic tools in mesothelial proliferations.[255,258,336–340] However, MM does not inevitably manifest such abnormalities, and they have been reported in 33% to 70% of cases in various series.[258,338,340] Point mutations also may occur in the INK4A gene.[341]

On the other hand, several genes and their protein products may be overexpressed in mesothelioma. They include those coding for platelet-derived growth factors, hepatocyte growth factor, c-met, insulin-like growth factor-1, transforming growth factor-beta, *bcl-2*, mitogen-activated protein kinase, and phosphatidylinositol-3-kinase.[342–347] HER-2/c-erbB-2, epidermal growth factor receptor, and K-*ras* genes are not altered in MM.[347,348] Interestingly, Ramos-Nino and colleagues have suggested that the activator protein-1 gene complex, encoding transcription factors such as c-fos, Fos-B, Fra-1, Fra-2, c-jun, Jun-B, and Jun-D, is activated in those mesotheliomas that are etiologically related to asbestos.[349]

Differential Diagnosis of Pleural Mesothelioma: Special Considerations

Several differential diagnostic alternatives to the various morphologic forms of MM have already been mentioned throughout the course of this discussion. Some of these will be addressed in greater detail, and others merit special consideration, as outlined below.

Differential Diagnosis of Benign versus Malignant Mesothelial Proliferations

Florid Mesothelial Hyperplasia versus Epithelioid Mesothelioma
Mesothelial hyperplasia seen in the context of infectious or inflammatory pleural effusions can be exuberant and moderately atypical cytologically (Fig. 20-52). Especially when the mesothelium

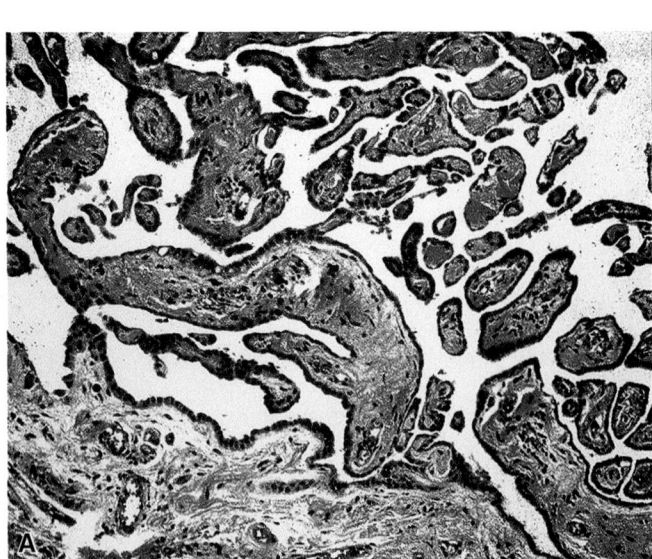
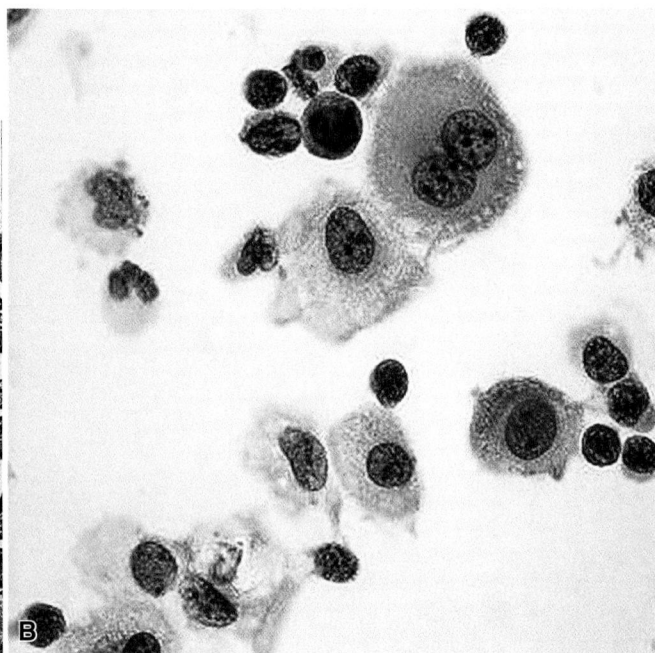

Figure 20-52. Mesothelial hyperplasia, as seen in a biopsy specimen (**A**) and cytologically (**B**). This condition may closely simulate the morphologic features of mesothelioma.

becomes entrapped in organizing fibrinous exudates, histologic images in pleural biopsies may engender serious concern over the possibility of EMM.

Differential diagnosis centers on the presence of actual invasion by the proliferation in question, and this can be identified only in an adequate tissue sample. If a deep enough portion of pleura is obtained, one can usually see a zonal phenomenon in mesothelial hyperplasia, wherein the cellularity of the tissue decreases with increasing distance from the pleural surface, and no mesothelial aggregates are visualized in the pleural fibroadipose tissue.[156,157] Otherwise, the superficial portions of such specimens may be markedly cellular, even with formation of micropapillary structures that are mantled by atypical mesothelial cells.

As stated above, we are not strong proponents of reliance on immunohistochemical studies in this setting. It has been suggested by others that strong labeling for EMA and p53 protein in the proliferating mesothelium is an indicator of malignancy.[215,218,219,257,350] However, we have observed several cases in which both of those markers were unequivocally present in mesothelial proliferations that proved to be benign.

Hopeful assertions also have been made regarding the use of X-linked inhibitor of apoptosis protein (XIAP) and the glucose transporter-1 isoform as discriminants of benign and malignant mesothelial proliferations.[351,352] Nonetheless, differences of opinion have been advanced regarding the relative merits of these markers.[351]

Another intriguing recent publication concerns the use of cyclin-dependent kinase inhibitor-2A (CDKN2A; INK4A; p16) in this setting. That moiety inhibits cyclin-dependent kinase-4 and is encoded by a gene on chromosome 9p21. Using fluorescence in situ hybridization and ThinPrep cytologic preparations of pleural effusion specimens, Illei and associates found that mesotheliomas exhibited homozygous deletion for CDKN2A, whereas reactive benign mesothelium showed retention of at least one copy of the gene.[353]

Fibrohyaline Pleuritis versus Desmoplastic Mesothelioma
One of the most difficult problems confronting thoracic surgeons and surgical pathologists is the patient who has had a long-standing or recurrent pleural effusion, culminating in a "rind" of organized and densely collagenized tissue that obliterates the pleural space and encompasses

the lung. Under these circumstances, the diagnostic alternatives are those of fibrohyaline pleuritis (fibrous pleurisy) and DMM. The distinction between these conditions can be challenging even with a complete pleurectomy specimen in hand, but sufficient sampling is again the key to proper diagnosis. Criteria that are used for recognition of DMM include foci of necrosis, obvious invasion of pleural adipose tissue or subjacent lung, and the presence of obvious focal cellular anaplasia.[153,154] p53 immunostaining has again been used by some authors in this context,[354] but results of this analysis are similar conceptually to those attending the evaluation of mesothelial hyperplasia, as discussed above.

Differential Diagnosis of Cytologically Malignant Pleural Neoplasms

Epithelioid Mesothelioma versus Hematopoietic Malignancies
Uncommonly, hematopoietic malignancies such as large cell non-Hodgkin lymphoma, syncytial or "sarcomatoid" Hodgkin lymphoma, granulocytic sarcoma (tumefactive acute myelogenous leukemia), and plasmacytic myeloma may be primary neoplasms of the pleura and simulate MM, both clinically and morphologically (Fig. 20-53).[355–359] These tumors are constituted by large polygonal or round cells, like EMM, and their histologic images are accordingly very similar to that of the solid-anaplastic variety of mesothelioma. Hematopoietic malignances demonstrate a much more notable degree of apoptosis than that seen in MM, with greater irregularity in the nuclear contours of the tumor cells and more numerous mitoses (Fig. 20-54). Electron microscopic analysis fails to show any intercellular attachment complexes in such lesions, in contrast to their prominence in MMs; similarly, plasmalemmal microvilli are absent in lymphoma and leukemia. Parenthetically, there is a form of large cell non-Hodgkin lymphoma, known as *anemone cell lymphoma*, in which numerous cell-surface projections are evident,[360] but these structures are not true microvilli.

Immunohistologic studies reveal a lack of keratin and calretinin in hematopoietic tumors, which instead exhibit variable reactivity for CD15, CD20, CD43, CD45, and CD138.[359,361] However, CD30 and the WT1 gene product may be reactive in mesothelioma as well as in hematopoietic malignancies.[362,363] The latter marker is particularly prevalent in granulocytic sarcoma.

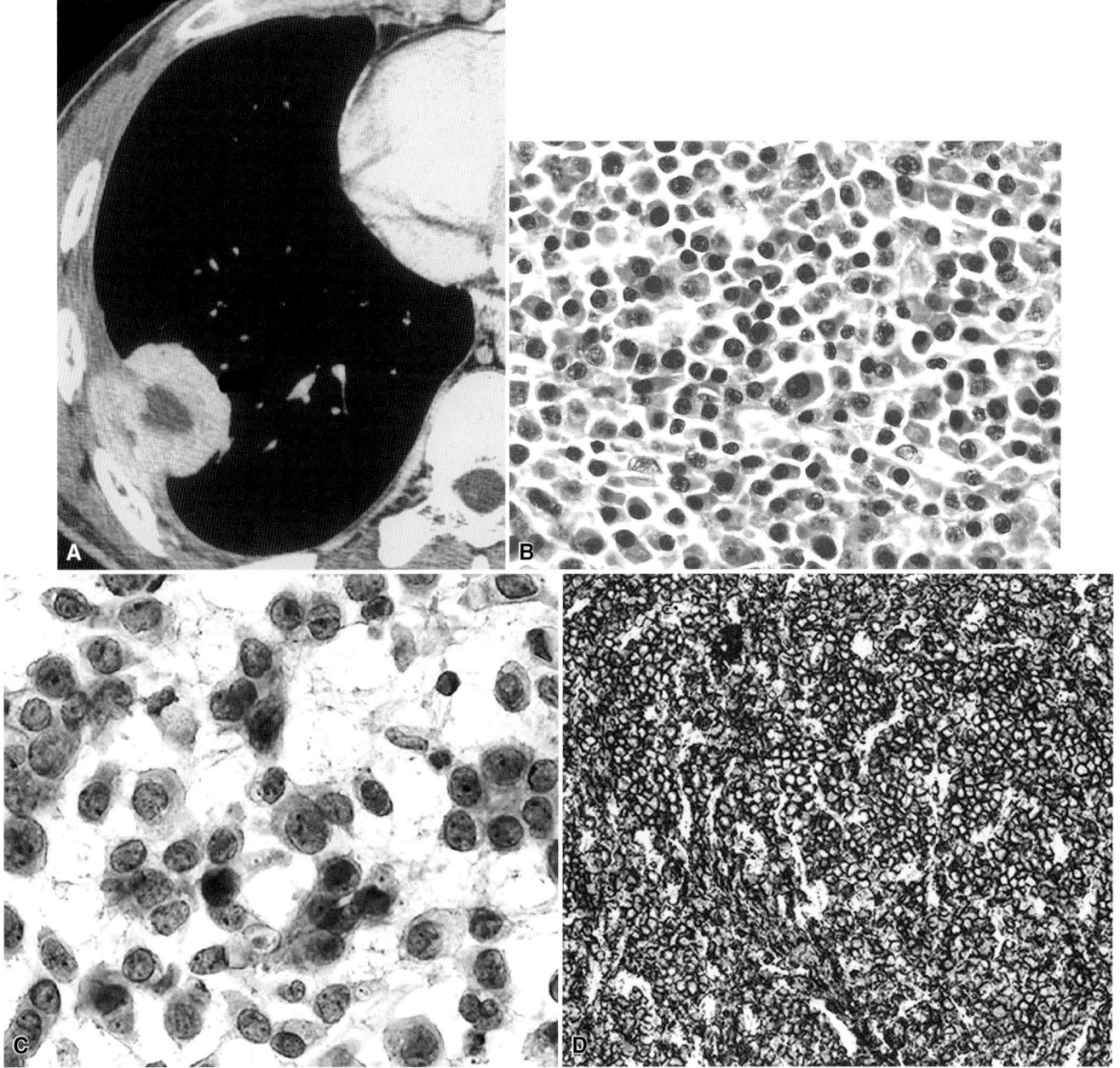

Figure 20-53. Solitary plasmacytoma of the pleura, as shown in a computed tomogram (**A**), a biopsy specimen (**B**), and on fine needle aspiration biopsy (**C**). This tumor can imitate mesothelioma, which not uncommonly has a plasmacytoid cellular appearance. Immunostaining for kappa light chain immunoglobulin (**D**) confirms the monotypic nature of the plasmacellular proliferation.

Epithelioid Mesothelioma versus Epithelioid Endothelial Neoplasms
Epithelioid mesothelioma may exhibit cytoplasmic macrovacuolation, a feature also common to epithelioid vascular tumors such as epithelioid hemangioendothelioma (EHE) and epithelioid angiosarcoma (EAS), both of which can represent primary pleural neoplasms[111,364-368] (Fig. 20-55).

Ultrastructural studies are usually definitive in separating EMM from EHE and EAS. MM shows elaborate microvillous differentiation, complex desmosomes, and cytoplasmic tonofibrils, none of which is apparent in vascular lesions. On the other hand, the cells of EHE and EAS contain variable numbers of Weibel-Palade bodies, which are elongated, tubular, electron-dense cytoplasmic structures with internal striations.[369,370]

Immunohistologically, epithelioid vascular tumors are unusual mesenchymal neoplasms because they rather commonly exhibit an "aberrant" expression of keratin.[371] They are also reactive for CD141[281] as are mesothelial proliferations. However, EHE and EAS lack calretinin, WT1 protein, and keratin 5/6, and instead, EHE and EAS are consistently positive for CD31, FLI-1, and CD34[372,373] (Fig. 20-56). All of the latter markers are absent in mesotheliomas.

Primary Pleural Myxoid Chondrosarcoma versus Mesothelioma
Extraskeletal myxoid chondrosarcoma (EMC) is a soft tissue tumor that is cytogenetically characterized by two chromosomal translocations, t(9;22)(q22;q11-12) and t(9;17)(q22;q11), which yield the EWS/CHN or RBP56/CHN fusion genes, respectively.[374] It has rarely been

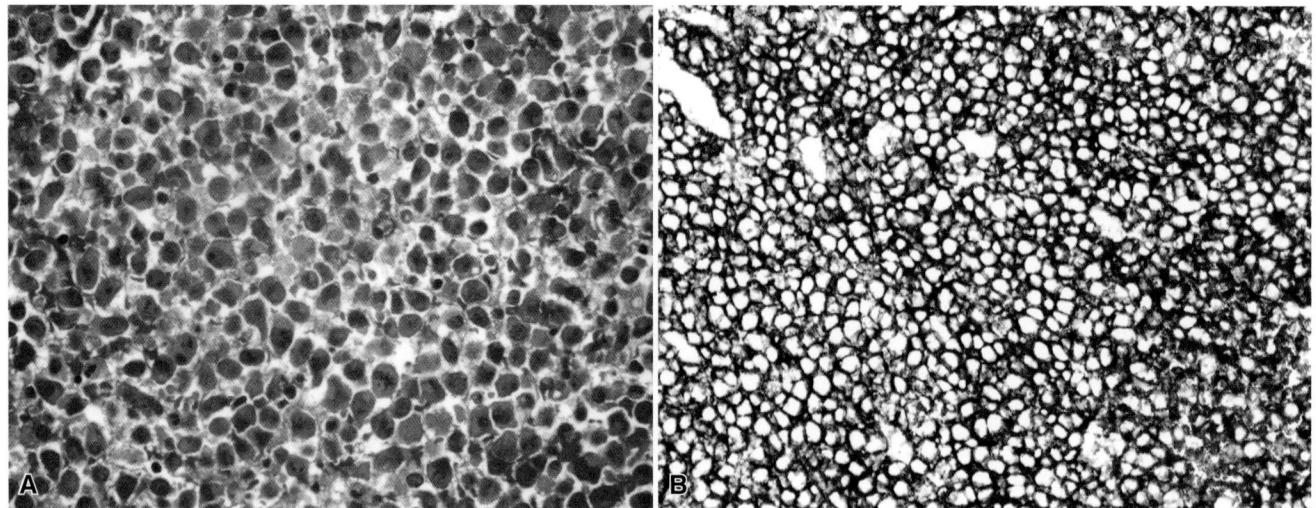

Figure 20-54. Large-cell non-Hodgkin lymphoma of the pleura demonstrating more irregularity of nuclear membranes than that seen in mesotheliomas (**A**). An immunostain for CD20 (**B**) establishes the hematopoietic (B-cell) nature of this lesion.

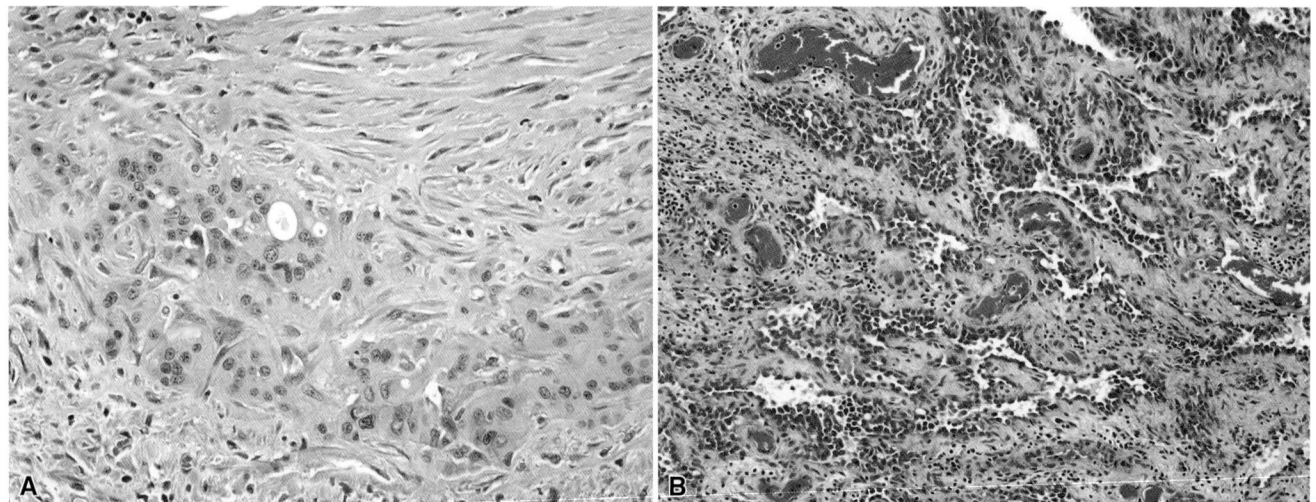

Figure 20-55. A, Pleural epithelioid hemangioendothelioma comprising densely apposed polygonal cells. Sometimes the number of classic vacuolated cells is limited, as in this example. They can mimic mesothelioma grossly and microscopically. **B,** Angiosarcoma of the pleura, as shown here, may also be confused diagnostically with mesothelioma.

reported as a primary pleural malignancy,[375] and its histologic image may simulate that of epithelioid mesothelioma. However, EMC lacks the microvillous plasmalemmal differentiation of MM on electron microscopy, and instead it shows the presence of cytoplasmic intrareticular microtubules (Fig. 20-57). It is also consistently nonreactive for keratin and calretinin, instead labeling for vimentin and variably for S-100 protein, neuron-specific enolase, and protein gene product 9.5,[376,377] none of which is seen in mesotheliomas. On the other hand, stains for podoplanin may be positive in both EMC and MM.[378] The characteristic fusion gene proteins of EMC can also be demonstrated rapidly using the polymerase chain reaction,[374] and they are consistently lacking in mesothelial tumors.

Synovial Sarcoma versus Mesothelioma
The clinicopathologic characteristics of pleuropulmonary synovial sarcoma have been provided in Chapter 14, including the potential for that tumor to mimic biphasic or sarcomatoid mesotheliomas[379] (Fig. 20-58). Specialized pathologic studies are most productive in biphasic tumors, where the microvillous ultrastructural nature of epithelioid cells in MM is not reproduced in synovial sarcoma.[380]

Additionally, biphasic synovial sarcoma often manifests Ber-Ep4 reactivity, occasionally CD141, and fails to express WT1 in its epithelioid elements.[381] Mesotheliomas usually demonstrate the converse of that profile. Diffuse expression of keratins 7 and 19 in mesotheliomas also contrasts with focal labeling for these proteins in synovial sarcoma, whereas keratin 14 may be seen in synovial sarcoma, but not most mesotheliomas. Calretinin and podoplanin are potentially common to both monophasic spindle cell synovial sarcoma and purely sarcomatoid mesothelioma, but WT1 protein is only encountered in MMs. Nuclear immunolabeling for TLE1 is a consistent finding in synovial sarcoma[382]; to date, there have been no systematic studies addressing the presence or absence of this marker in sarcomatoid mesothelioma.

Ultimately, molecular analysis may be necessary to establish a definitive interpretation in this setting. Virtually all synovial sarcomas show a reproducible t(X;18) chromosomal translocation, which is not seen in MMs. Its presence can be assessed indirectly by using the polymerase chain reaction with primers designed to identify the SYT–SSX1 and SYT–SSX2 fusion proteins that are produced by the translocation in question.[383]

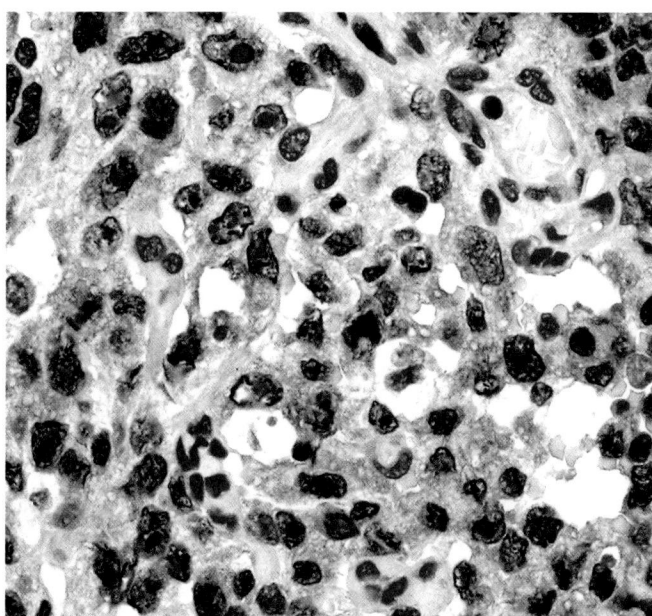

Figure 20-56. Nuclear immunoreactivity for FLI-1 in pleural angiosarcoma. This marker is not seen in mesotheliomas.

Pseudomesotheliomatous Sarcomatoid Carcinoma versus Mesothelioma
A related morphologic problem is represented by sarcomatoid carcinomas that extensively involve the pleura and simulate mesothelioma (Fig. 20-59). These lesions may show biphasic or spindle cell/pleomorphic images, and they can originate in the lung, kidney, and breast, as well as at other sites.[36] As true in biphasic synovial sarcomas, the ultrastructural and immunophenotypic attributes of epithelioid components in biphasic carcinomas are distinct from those of biphasic MMs.[384] Purely nonepithelioid lesions in both categories are more difficult to separate from one another. The presence of immunoreactivity for calretinin and WT1 favors mesothelioma, in our experience, but other authors have come to different conclusions.[293]

From the perspective of patient management, this diagnostic distinction is not crucial, because pseudomesotheliomatous carcinomas and mesotheliomas generally manifest the same limited response to therapy and a comparably adverse prognosis.[34–36] However, medicolegal issues attending the two neoplasms are potentially quite different.

Small Cell Mesothelioma versus Other Small Cell Malignancies
In limited biopsy specimens, small cell mesothelioma may be difficult to distinguish from metastatic small cell neuroendocrine carcinoma (SCNC) involving the pleura[385] or from Askin tumor (primary thoracopulmonary primitive neuroectodermal tumor; PNET). The latter two lesions have been considered in more detail in Chapters 13 and 14. To date, ultrastructural studies on small cell MM have not been performed; hence, it is not known whether it shares the microvillous electron microscopic attributes of conventional epithelioid mesotheliomas, or, alternatively, manifests the formation of blunt neuritic-type cytoplasmic extensions as seen in PNET. Immunohistologically, all three lesions in this differential diagnostic cluster may exhibit reactivity for pankeratin; however, as mentioned earlier, SCNC tends to show distinctive globules of paranuclear keratin reactivity that are not shared by MM or PNET[321] (Fig. 20-60). Moreover, keratin 5/6 and calretinin are more often observed in small cell MM than in SCNC,[231] and they have not been reported in Askin tumor. Other helpful determinants for the separation of such lesions are hematopoietic in nature. CD99 is unique to PNET in this group, CD56 and CD57 are seen in SCNC and PNET but not small cell MM, and CD141 is seen in mesothelioma but tends to be absent in the other neoplasms.[261,386] Metastatic small cell carcinoma of the lung is characteristically positive for the markers MOC-31 and anti–TTF-1,[387,388] whereas MM and Askin tumor are negative for these markers.

Primary Pleural Thymomatosis versus Mesothelioma
The capability for thymomas to arise and spread in the pleura, simulating mesothelioma clinicopathologically,[389] is discussed in Chapter 19. To reiterate, although both of these tumors share potential immunoreactivity

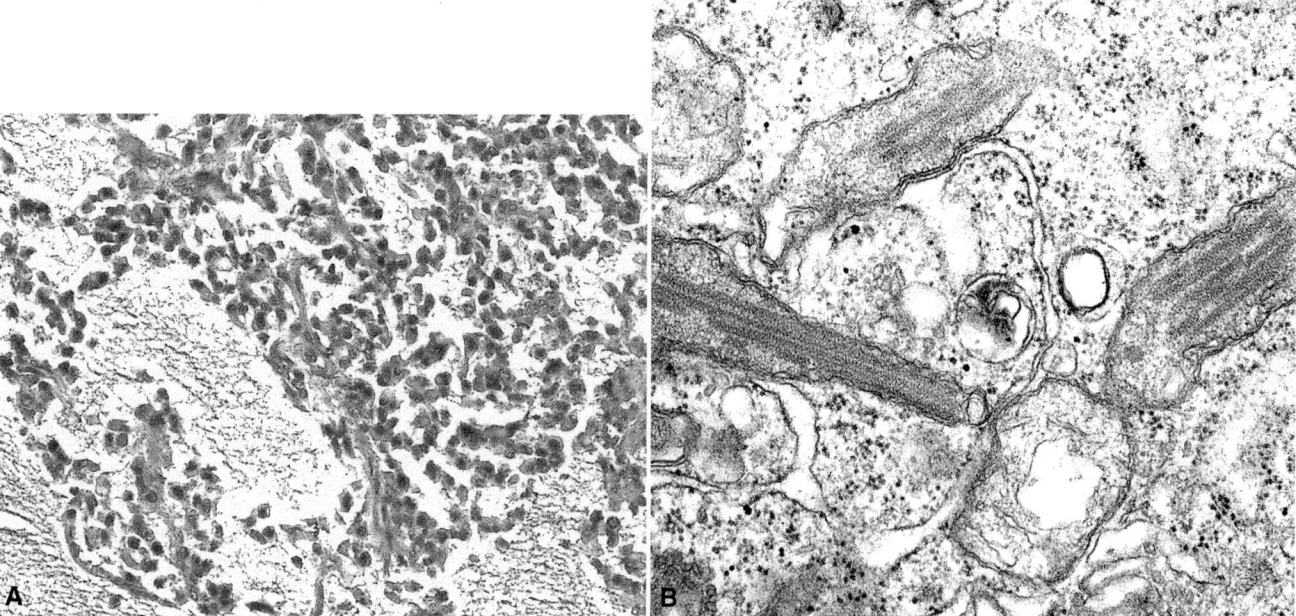

Figure 20-57. Extraskeletal myxoid chondrosarcoma (**A**) can be confused with mesothelioma showing abundant myxoid stroma. However, the former tumor is singular in its ultrastructural content of intrareticular microtubules (**B**).

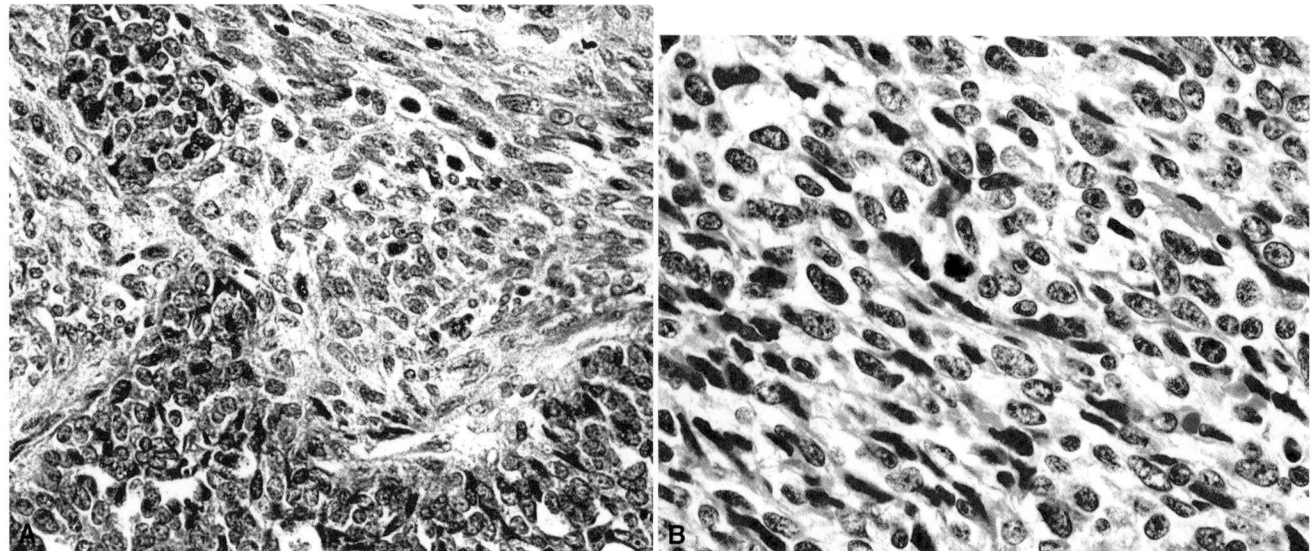

Figure 20-58. **A,** Biphasic synovial sarcoma of the pleura, demonstrating tubular arrays of epithelioid cells set in a neoplastic spindle cell background. A likeness to biphasic mesothelioma is apparent. **B,** Monophasic synovial sarcoma has a microscopic similarity to sarcomatoid mesothelioma.

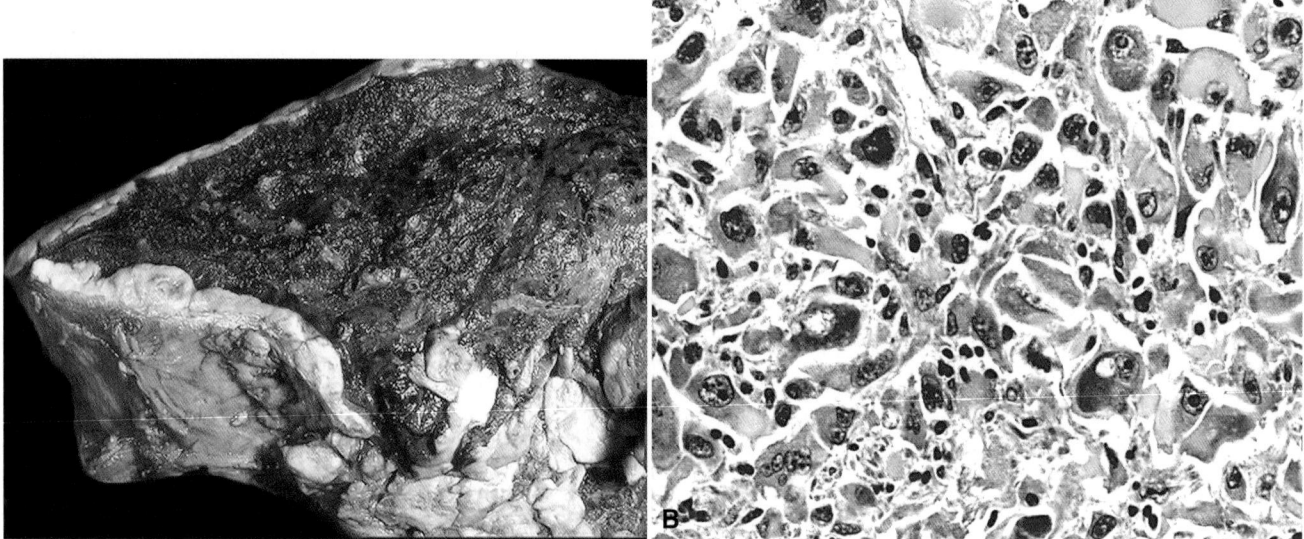

Figure 20-59. Metastatic and "pseudomesotheliomatous" sarcomatoid renal cell carcinoma, which presented as the first clinical manifestation of disease (**A**). The tumor is virtually indistinguishable from sarcomatoid mesothelioma (**B**).

for keratin 5/6, thrombomodulin, and calretinin, only thymomas contain lymphoid cells that express CD1a, terminal deoxynucleotidyl-transferase, and CD99, and epithelial cells that are labeled for p63 protein.[390] Lastly, microvilli are not evident in thymic epithelial neoplasms ultrastructurally.[391]

Solitary Fibrous Tumor of the Pleura versus Sarcomatoid Mesothelioma

When provided only with small biopsy specimens and given no clinical information, pathologists may conceivably confuse atypical variants of solitary fibrous tumor of the pleura with SMM on morphologic grounds. Nevertheless, the immunophenotypes of these neoplasms are mutually exclusive. Solitary fibrous tumor is reactive for CD34, with or without CD99 and *bcl-2* protein, but it lacks keratin. Mesothelioma shows the opposite profile.[392] Both lesions may show immunoreactivity for podoplanin.

Clear Cell Mesothelioma versus Metastatic Renal Cell Carcinoma

Clear cell mesotheliomas are rare, but they may be closely simulated by metastases of "conventional" renal cell carcinoma (RCC)[393] (Fig. 20-61). The latter of these neoplasms lacks unique and easily detected markers, and, particularly because they also share potential positivity for several proteins with mesothelioma (including keratin, vimentin, CD10, WT1, and thrombomodulin),[305,394] a tailored immunohistologic approach to differential diagnosis is necessary in this specific instance. The markers that are most discriminatory between RCC and clear cell MM include keratin 5/6, calretinin, CD15, Ber-Ep4, BG8, and PAX2 (Fig. 20-62). The presence of the first two determinants strongly favors an interpretation of mesothelioma, whereas positivity for *any two* of the other listed markers is representative of RCC.[395,396]

This is a circumstance where electron microscopic study may sometimes be superior in specificity to immunohistochemical analysis. RCCs have poorly formed plasmalemmal microvilli and no cytoplasmic

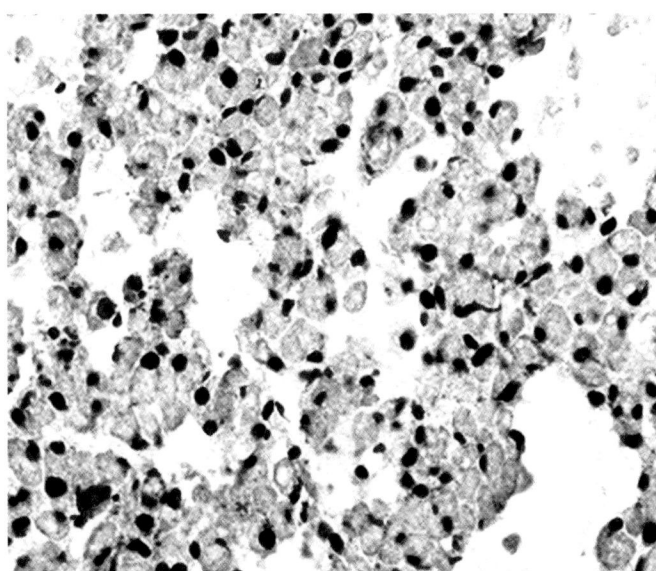

Figure 20-60. Globular perinuclear immunoreactivity for keratin, as seen in this metastatic pleural small cell neuroendocrine carcinoma, distinguishes that tumor from small cell mesothelioma.

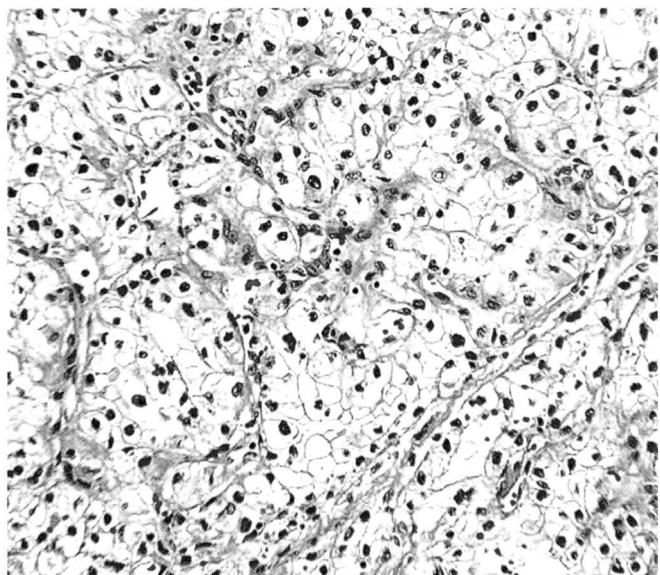

Figure 20-61. Metastatic clear cell renal cell carcinoma in the pleura. The tumor was thought to represent a clear cell mesothelioma on initial clinicopathologic evaluation.

tonofibrils, and, instead, they contain prominent cytoplasmic collections of glycogen, or lipid, or both.[397] Clear cell mesothelioma does not share those ultrastructural characteristics, because it is basically a variant of EMM.

Oncocytoid/Deciduoid Mesothelioma versus Other "Pink" Cell Malignancies
Deciduoid/oncocytoid mesothelioma can be simulated by pleural metastases of carcinomas that are constituted by large "pink" cells. These principally include HCC, adrenocortical carcinoma (ACC), and RCC.[398] Electron microscopy provides valuable information in this particular context, because none of the cited tumors, except for deciduoid MM, contains elongated plasmalemmal microvilli, complex desmosomes, or tonofilaments. Moreover, ACC (and sometimes RCC) may also manifest

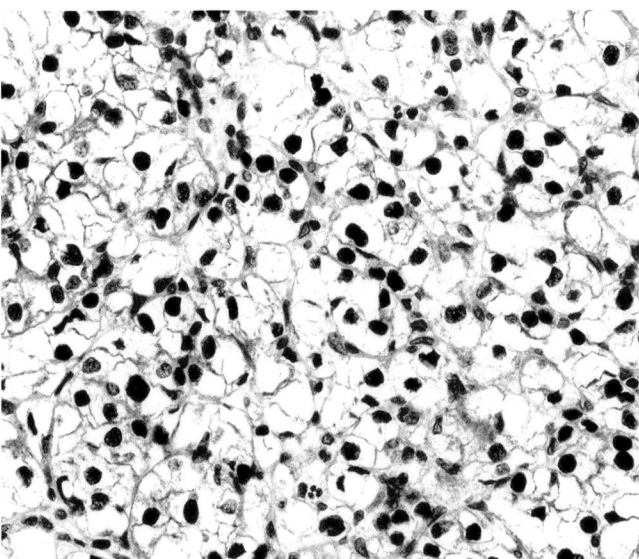

Figure 20-62. Nuclear labeling for PAX2 confirms the renal origin of the neoplasm shown in Figure 20-61.

the presence of tubulovesicular mitochondrial cristae,[399] which are absent in mesotheliomas. Immunohistologic separation of such tumors centers on a few key determinants. EMA is consistently present in oncocytoid MM and RCC but is absent in HCC and ACC.[400] On the other hand, keratin is paradoxically absent in paraffin sections of ACC, even though it is undeniably epithelial.[401] Those two markers are particularly important in regard to the separation of MM and adrenocortical neoplasms, because both of them are commonly positive for calretinin and podoplanin.[402] However, ACC also shows reactivity for inhibin (Fig. 20-63) and CD56, both of which are not seen in mesotheliomas.[308] The distinction of oncocytoid RCC and MM is basically comparable to that attending their clear cell variants, as discussed previously. Lastly, an antibody known as HepPar1 is contextually selective for HCC and reproducibly allows for a distinction of this tumor from mesotheliomas.[306]

Rhabdoid Mesothelioma versus Metastases of Extrarenal Malignant Rhabdoid Tumors
As mentioned earlier, extrarenal malignant rhabdoid tumor is probably a phenotype as well as a neoplastic entity. In other words, a spectrum of tumor types—including mesothelioma—may undergo clonal evolution and assume a rhabdoid appearance.[160,161] When that occurs, ultrastructural and immunophenotypic characteristics of the original lesion are usually lost in the rhabdoid component. Regardless of its derivation, extrarenal malignant rhabdoid tumor has the ability to show paranuclear whorls of intermediate filaments by electron microscopy (Fig. 20-64), as well as potential immunoreactivity for keratin, vimentin, desmin, EMA, actins, CD99, and WT1 protein.[161] Other markers of potential mesothelial differentiation (e.g., calretinin, CD141, keratin 5/6) are absent.[160] Hence, a rhabdoid mesothelioma is *not* concretely identifiable as such unless it also has a minor "conventional" MM component that is concurrently sampled.

Epithelioid Mesothelioma versus Primary or Metastatic Germ Cell Malignancies
Very uncommonly, malignant germ cell tumors—principally represented by embryonal carcinoma and yolk sac carcinoma, or combinations thereof—may arise primarily in the pleuropulmonary compartment.[403] In addition, metastases from occult neoplasms of these types in other anatomic sites rarely can secondarily involve the

Practical Pulmonary Pathology

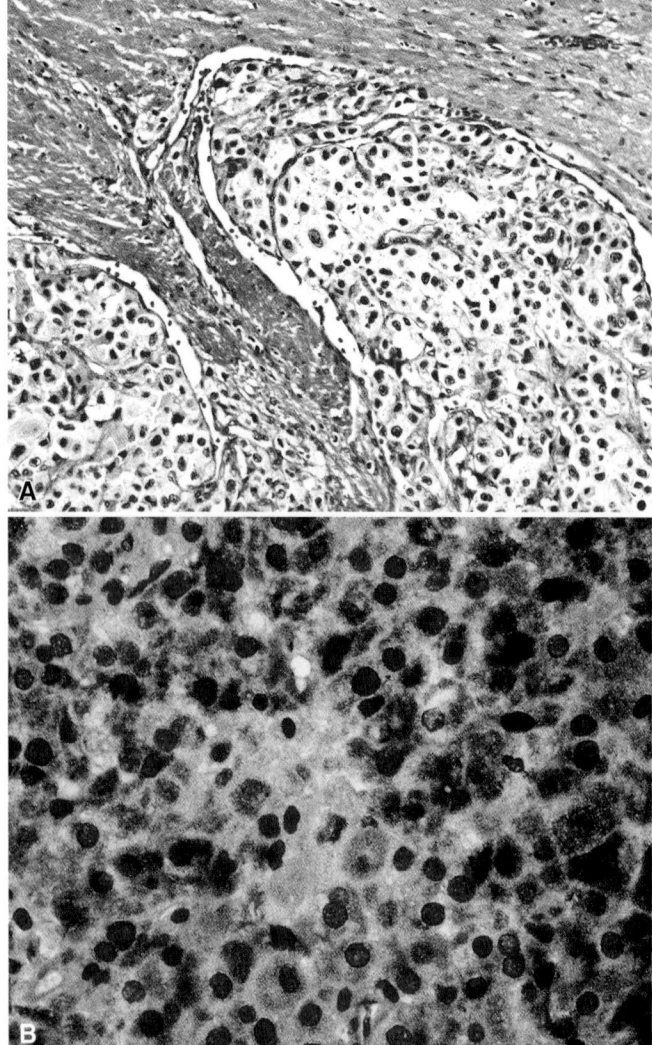

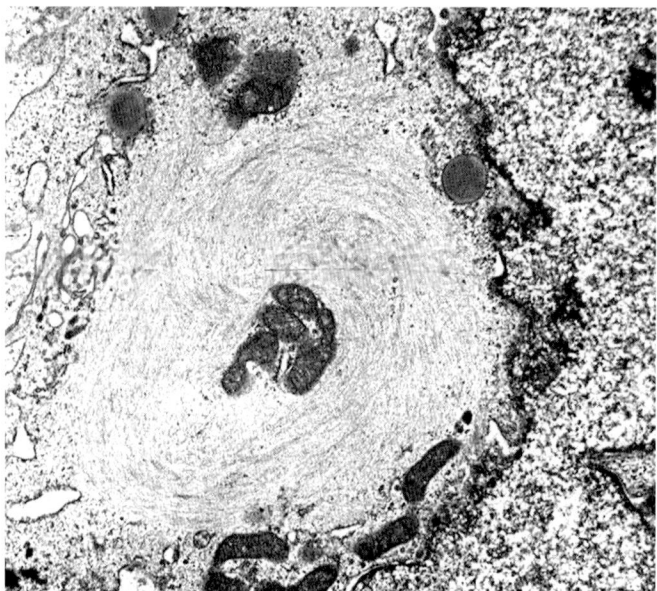

Figure 20-64. A whorl of paranuclear intermediate filaments is seen in this electron photomicrograph of "rhabdoid" mesothelioma.

pleura. Such tumors may imitate that of solid "anaplastic" MM. Electron microscopy is an effective means of separating germ cell neoplasms from mesotheliomas, because plasmalemmal microvilli are absent in the former of those tumor groups.[404]

Immunohistologic studies show reactivity for placental alkaline phosphatase and OCT-3/4 in germ cell tumors, with or without CD117,[400,405,406] but they lack calretinin and WT1 protein. Once again, these results are incompatible with the phenotype of MM.[407]

Metastatic Intranodal Mesothelioma versus Lymph Nodal Mesothelial Rests
Several reports have highlighted the presence of mesothelial inclusions (rests) in the sinusoids of intrathoracic lymph nodes[408–410] (Fig. 20-65). They may be found incidentally and unexpectedly in nodes that are removed in the treatment of other clinical conditions. Under such circumstances, specialized pathologic evaluations are incapable of distinguishing such benign and probably developmental abnormalities

Figure 20-63. A, Metastatic adrenocortical carcinoma in the pleura, which may be confused with deciduoid or clear cell mesothelioma. **B,** Inhibin immunoreactivity, as shown here, is typical of adrenocortical carcinoma but is not seen in mesothelioma.

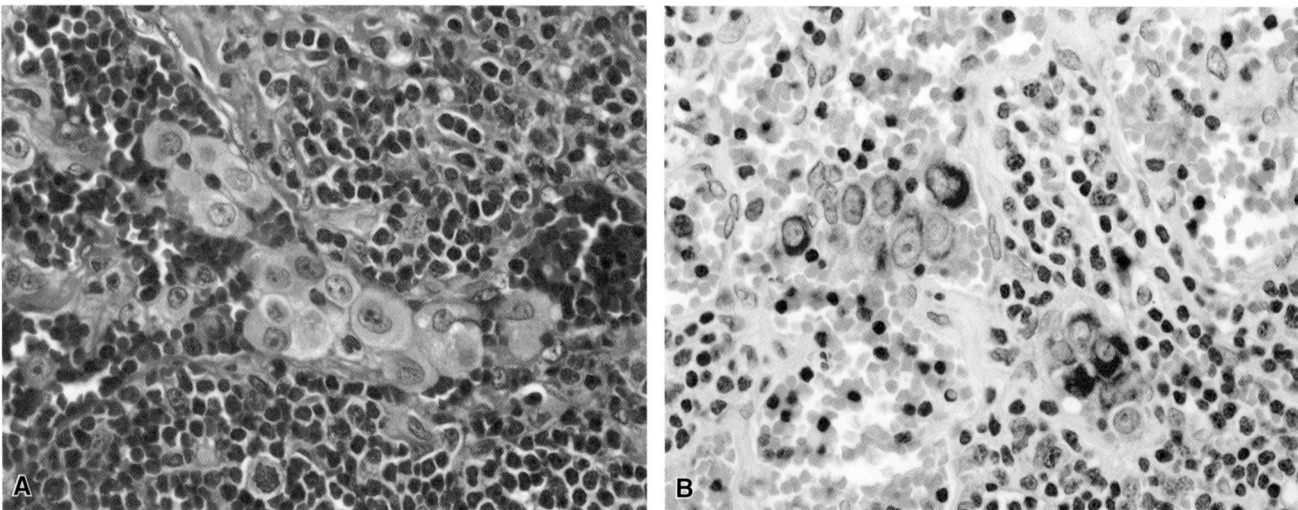

Figure 20-65. A, Mesothelial cells in a mediastinal lymph node, seen principally in the nodal sinusoids. The node was removed incidentally during cardiac surgery. **B,** Immunoreactivity is present in this mesothelial rest for keratin. Other immunostains for glandular epithelial markers were negative.

from metastatic intranodal mesothelioma. However, in all cases documented to date, the affected patients had no evidence of pleural disease, and therefore a diagnosis of MM would have been untenable. The involved nodes are frequently congested. Metastatic adenocarcinoma is another consideration under these circumstances, but that possibility can be dismissed by appropriate immunohistochemical studies, as outlined earlier.[408]

Borderline (Low-Grade Malignant) Mesothelial Tumors

Even though Chapter 19 is devoted to both benign and borderline neoplasms of the thorax, only pleural adenomatoid tumors are included there among mesothelial lesions. That decision was made to allow for a more unified discussion at this point of mesothelial proliferations with either low-grade malignant or obviously aggressive features. Two additional lesions with mesothelial differentiation, both of which have a limited potential for local recurrence or distant spread, are considered in the following sections. These are well-differentiated papillary mesothelioma (WDPM) and multicystic mesothelial tumor of borderline biologic potential (MMTBBP; formerly called *multicystic mesothelioma*).

Etiologic Considerations

Both WDPM and MMTBBP were initially described as abdominal lesions in young individuals who were typically female.[411,412] They were thought to be unassociated causally with asbestos exposure, whether they occurred in the abdomen or the chest.

Few examples of pleural WDPM and MMTBBP have been described, and it would therefore be premature to draw definite conclusions on their pathogeneses. MMTBBP of the thorax has yet to be linked with any definable etiologic agent. However, Butnor and coworkers described seven examples of pleural WDPM, two of which occurred in patients with objective radiographic or pathologic evidence of above-background asbestos exposure.[413] Such evidence was reflected by the presence of fibrohyaline pleural plaques. Eleven of 24 patients with pleural WDPM reported by Galateau-Sallé and colleagues also were said to have reported past occupational asbestos exposure.[414] These data raise the prospect that asbestos may indeed cause some examples of pleural WDPM.

Clinical Findings

Some cases of WDPM of the pleura have presented similarly to conventional forms of epithelioid mesothelioma, with dyspnea and a serosal effusion.[413–415] Radiographic assessment has shown pleural nodularity in association with an effusion.[413]

MMTBBP of the pleura is extraordinarily rare, with only one published example. That patient was a 37-year-old woman who presented with a localized, multiloculated intrapleural mass that was found on imaging studies. No pleural effusion was apparent.[416] We have seen one other lesion of this type in a 34-year-old woman with a unilateral pleural mass.

The evolution of WDPM of the pleura has been variable; of four cases in the report by Butnor and coworkers in which follow-up was available, all of the patients were alive with persistent tumor at least 6 months after diagnosis.[345] Survival averaged 74 months in the series of Galateau-Sallé and colleagues,[414] compared with 9.9 months in a comparison group of paired patients with conventional pleural MM. Another female patient with pleural WDPM, reported by Kao and associates, was well after 16 years.[417] None of the lesions has metastasized outside the thorax or crossed the anatomic midline. In a singular departure from that theme, Torii and coworkers reported a case of WDPM that invaded the lung, mediastinum, and chest wall.[418] The single reported

MMTBBP of the pleura was cured by excision,[416] and the patient in our unpublished case is also free of disease after surgery.

Pathologic Observations

Pleural WDPM has manifested itself either as a multifocal nodular proliferation, with firm white-tan lesions on the serosal surface, or as a single exophytic growth that projected into the pleural space. The size of individual nodules in such cases has ranged from less than 1 to 5 cm in greatest dimension.[413] These descriptions obviously overlap with the macroscopic features of conventional mesotheliomas. On the other hand, MMTBBP has a distinctive image, represented by a well-circumscribed agglomeration of thin-walled cysts filled with serous fluid (Fig. 20-66). No internal nodularity usually is apparent when the cystic cavities are opened.

Microscopically, WDPM is typified by arborescent fibrovascular papillary projections of variable width and length, which are covered by one or two layers of relatively bland cuboidal mesothelium (Fig. 20-67). Nuclei are round to oval, with vesicular or dispersed chromatin

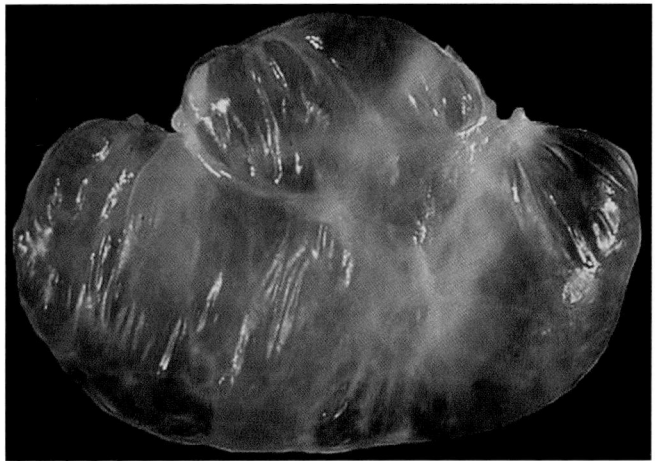

Figure 20-66. Photograph of a gross specimen of pleural multicystic mesothelial tumor of borderline biologic potential. It is a thin-walled, internally loculated cyst that was easily dissected from surrounding tissues.

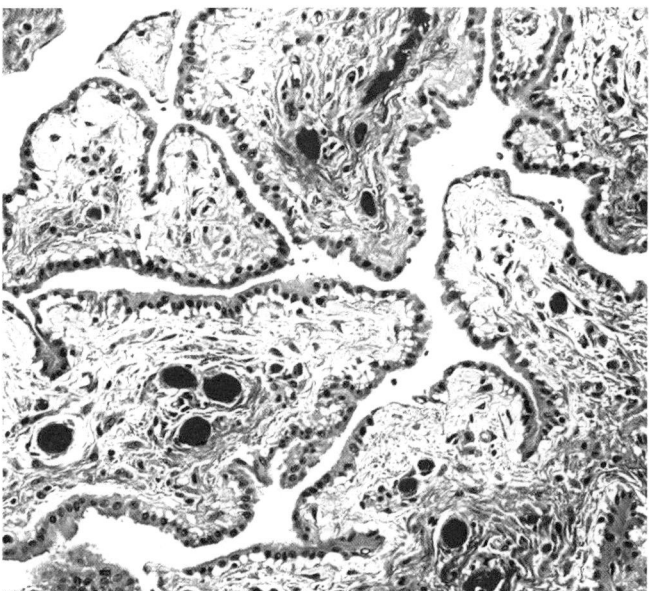

Figure 20-67. Well-differentiated papillary mesothelioma of the pleura showing broad fronds of tumor tissue that are mantled by uniform cuboidal cells.

and focally prominent nucleoli, and mitotic figures are sparse.[413,414] Some examples show hyalinization or fibroblastic proliferation in the papillary cores, or psammoma bodies, or combinations thereof. The supporting papillary stroma may also be mucomyxoid in character, producing a superficial resemblance to placental villi. Limited infiltration of the subjacent pleural soft tissue by tubular cell profiles is seen in a minority of cases. Histochemical, ultrastructural, and immunohistochemical attributes of WDPM are comparable to those that are associated with conventional mesothelioma morphotypes.

The multicystic mesothelial tumor histologically comprises relatively large macrocystic spaces that are bounded by hypocellular collagenized stroma and filled with lightly eosinophilic serous fluid. The cysts are mantled by a single layer of bland cuboidal mesothelial cells with "hobnail" nuclear profiles (Fig. 20-68). No nucleoli or mitotic activity is apparent, and, although tubular profiles may surround the cystic spaces, there is no infiltration of the surrounding tissue by the lesional cells.

Results of adjunctive studies in MMTBBP again mirror those obtained in mesothelial proliferations in general. However, the morphologic image of that lesion is so singular that specialized evaluations are not necessary.

Staging and Prognosis of Malignant Mesothelioma

In general, tumor stage is the most powerful predictor of biologic behavior for any given malignancy. Several staging systems have been used to document the locoregional and distant growth of MM. The first of these was the Butchart (English) scheme, proposed in 1976.[419] It dealt descriptively with the general growth characteristics of individual tumors. That same principle was later expanded by the International Mesothelioma Interest Group[420] and codified by the American Joint Committee on Cancer, in a formal tumor-node-metastasis (TNM) format.[421] The Thoracic Oncology Group at the Brigham and Women's Hospital has also advanced a pragmatic surgery-oriented staging system that has entered clinical use.[422] These three schemes are summarized in Tables 20-2 and 20-3.

Some of the other clinicopathologic factors affecting prognosis have been mentioned earlier in this discussion. In multivariate statistical analyses, those that have been associated with longer survivals include an epithelial histologic subtype, stage I disease, a good clinical performance (Karnofsky) score, female gender, patient age of younger than 65 years at diagnosis, tumor-related symptoms for longer than 6 months before diagnosis, weight loss of less than 5%, negative tissue margins in surgically resected cases, serum levels of lactate dehydrogenase less than 500 IU/L, and the absence of chest pain.[66,423–426] Conversely, asbestos causation, cigarette smoking, and thrombocytosis have not held up as independent negative prognosticators.[423]

Selected analyses have also examined the prognostic influence of cell cycle–related proteins in the tumor cells: p27 (kip1) is a cell cycle inhibitor that is down-regulated in rapidly replicating tissues; accordingly, it is not surprising that several studies have concluded that its level correlates directly with prognosis in cases of MM.[427–429] The same appears to be true of p16 protein.[430] On the other hand, the Ki-67 protein, an S-phase–related nuclear moiety, is preferentially expressed in actively dividing cells. Thus, one would expect that high Ki-67 indices (>30%) would be seen in aggressive MMs, and based on the results of pertinent publications,[429,431] that supposition appears to be valid.

Other molecules that influence cellular adhesion, invasiveness, and motility have been assessed as possible prognostic factors for mesothelioma. Immunoreactivity for neurotensin and osteopontin have both been associated with a short survival time,[432,433] whereas expression of serine protease HtrA1 and PTEN protein has been associated with longer survival.[434,435]

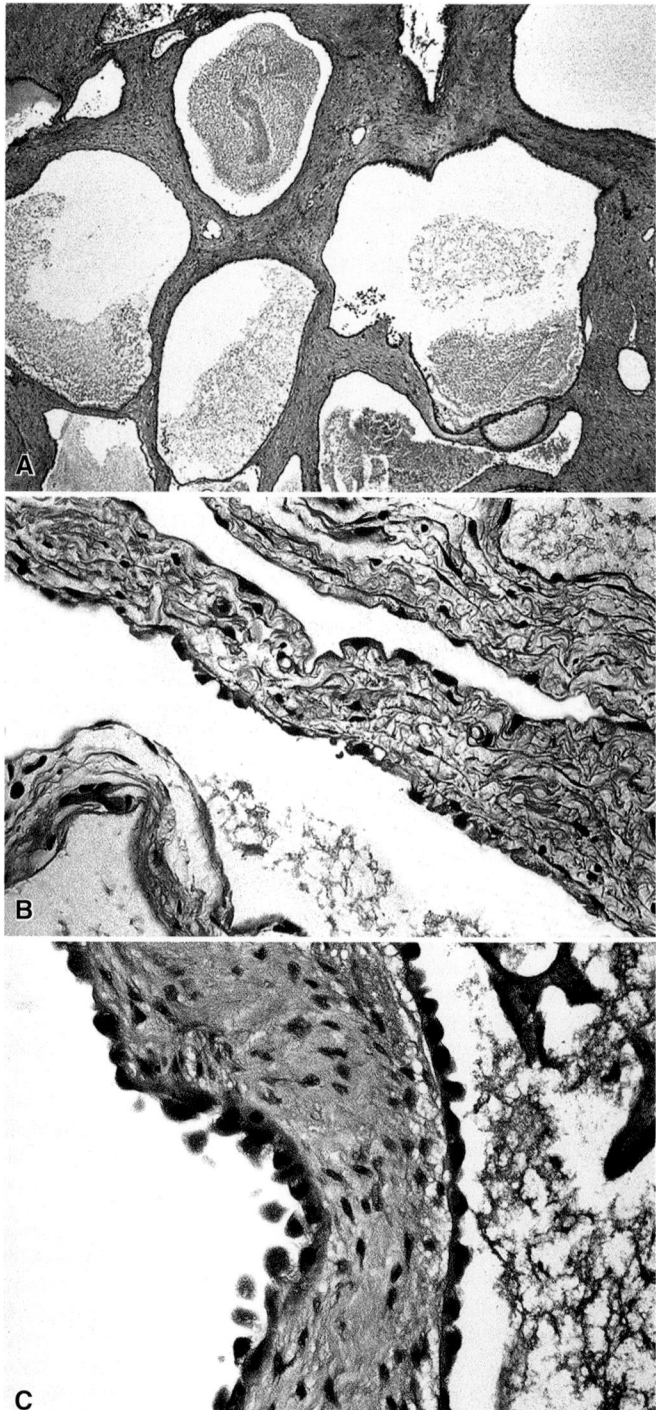

Figure 20-68. **A,** Multicystic mesothelial tumor of borderline biologic potential is a multilocular lesion on scanning microscopy, with proteinaceous contents. **B** and **C,** Internal fibrous septa are lined by plump epithelioid cells with a "hobnail" configuration.

Growth factor receptors have become important targets of therapeutic interest because biologic agents that block their activity are being developed increasingly. Strong immunoexpression of epidermal growth factor receptor has been associated with improved survival in patients with mesothelioma,[436] whereas high levels of platelet-derived growth factor receptor in the tumor cells has conferred a worse prognosis.

Self-assessment questions related to this chapter can be found online on the Expert Consult site for this title.

Table 20-2. Butchart (British) Staging System for Malignant Pleural Mesothelioma

Stage	Location
I	Tumor confined to the ipsilateral pleura, lung, or pericardium
II	Tumor invading the chest wall or mediastinal structures or metastases to thoracic lymph nodes
III	Tumor penetrating the diaphragm to involve the peritoneum or metastases to extrathoracic lymph nodes
IV	Distant blood-borne metastases

Table 20-3. Brigham and Women's Hospital Staging System for Malignant Pleural Mesothelioma

Stage	Description
I	Can be extirpated surgically; no involvement of regional lymph nodes by tumor
II	Can be removed surgically but regional lymph nodes are involved by tumor
III	Inoperable; tumor involves chest wall, pericardium, or diaphragm/peritoneum Regional lymph nodes may or may not contain metastases
IV	Inoperable; distant (extrathoracic) metastases are present

References

1. Millard M. Lung, pleura, and mediastinum. In: Anderson WAD, ed. *Pathology*, 6th ed. St. Louis: Mosby; 1971:875–997.
2. Klemperer P, Rabin CB. Primary neoplasms of the pleura. *Arch Pathol*. 1931;11:385–401.
3. DeLajarte M, deLaJarte AY. Mesothelioma on the coast of Brittany, France. *Ann N Y Acad Sci*. 1979;330:323–332.
4. Legha SS, Muggia FM. Pleural mesotheliomas: clinical features and therapeutic implications. *Ann Intern Med*. 1977;87:613–620.
5. Elmes PC, Simpson MJC. The clinical aspects of mesothelioma. *Q J Med*. 1976;45:427–441.
6. Aziz T, Jilaihawi A, Prakash D. The management of malignant pleural mesothelioma: single center experience in 10 years. *Eur J Cardiothorac Surg*. 2002;22:298–305.
7. Grundy GW, Miller RW. Malignant mesothelioma in childhood. *Cancer*. 1972;30:1216–1218.
8. Coffin CM, Dehner LP. Mesothelial and related neoplasms in children and adolescents: a clinicopathologic and immunohistochemical analysis of eight cases. *Pediatr Pathol*. 1992;12:333–347.
9. Fraire AE, Cooper S, Greenberg SD, et al. Mesothelioma of childhood. *Cancer*. 1988; 62:838–847.
10. Ascoli V, Scalzo CC, Bruno C, et al. Familial pleural malignant mesothelioma: clustering in three sisters and one cousin. *Cancer Lett*. 1998;130:203–207.
11. Dawson A, Gibbs A, Browne K, et al. Familial mesothelioma: details of 17 cases with histopathologic findings and mineral analysis. *Cancer*. 1992;70:1183–1187.
12. Krousel T, Garcas N, Rothschild H. Familial clustering of mesothelioma: a report on three affected persons in one family. *Am J Prev Med*. 1986;2:186–188.
13. Lynch HT, Katz D, Markvicka SE. Familial mesothelioma: review and family study. *Cancer Genet Cytogenet*. 1985;15:25–35.
14. Law MR, Hodson ME, Turner-Warwick M. Malignant mesothelioma of the pleura: clinical aspects and symptomatic treatment. *Eur J Respir Dis*. 1984;65:162–168.
15. Bonomo L, Feragalli B, Sacco R, et al. Malignant pleural disease. *Eur J Radiol*. 2000;34:98–118.
16. Bueno R. Mesothelioma—clinical presentation. *Chest*. 1999;116(suppl 6):444S–445S.
17. Neumeister W, Gillisseu A, Rasche K, et al. Pleural mesothelioma. I. Historical, epidemiological, and clinical aspects (symptoms and diagnosis). *Med Klin*. 2001;96:722–729.
18. Pisani RJ, Colby TV, Williams DE. Malignant mesothelioma of the pleura. *Mayo Clin Proc*. 1988;63:1234–1244.
19. Ruffie PA. Pleural mesothelioma. *Curr Opin Oncol*. 1991;3:328–334.
20. Dutt PL, Baxter JW, O'Malley FP, et al. Distant cutaneous metastasis of pleural mesothelioma. *J Cutan Pathol*. 1992;19:490–495.
21. Sussman J, Rosai J. Lymph node metastasis as the initial manifestation of malignant mesothelioma: report of six cases. *Am J Surg Pathol*. 1990;14:819–828.
22. Achatzy R, Beba W, Ritschler R, et al. The diagnosis, therapy, and prognosis of diffuse malignant mesothelioma. *Eur J Cardiothorac Surg*. 1989;3:445–448.
23. Mischler NE, Chuprevich T, Johnson RO, et al. Malignant mesothelioma presenting in the pleura and peritoneum. *J Surg Oncol*. 1979;11:185–191.
24. Metintas M, Icgun I, Elbek O, et al. Computed tomographic features in malignant pleural mesothelioma and other commonly seen pleural diseases. *Eur J Radiol*. 2002;41:1–9.
25. Marom EM, Erasmus JJ, Pass HI, et al. The role of imaging in malignant pleural mesothelioma. *Semin Oncol*. 2002;29:26–35.
26. Eibel K, Tuengerthal S, Schoenberg SO. The role of new imaging techniques in diagnosis and staging of malignant pleural mesothelioma. *Curr Opin Oncol*. 2003;15:131–138.
27. Knuuttila A, Kivisaari L, Kivisaari A, et al. Evaluation of pleural disease using MR and CT, with special reference to malignant pleural mesothelioma. *Acta Radiol*. 2001; 42:502–507.
28. Hammar SP. The pathology of benign and malignant pleural disease. *Chest Surg Clin N Am*. 1994;4:405–430.
29. Hillerdal G. The human evidence: parenchymal and pleural changes. *Ann Occup Hyg*. 1994;38:561–567.
30. Chahinian AP, Pajak TF, Holland JF, et al. Diffuse malignant mesothelioma: prospective evaluation of 69 patients. *Ann Intern Med*. 1982;96:746–755.
31. DePangher-Manzini V, Brollo A, Bianchi C. Thrombocytosis in malignant pleural mesothelioma. *Tumori*. 1990;76:576–578.
32. Nakano T, Fujii J, Tamura S, et al. Thrombocytosis in patients with malignant pleural mesothelioma. *Cancer*. 1986;58:1699–1701.
33. Nakano T, Chahinian AP, Shinjo M, et al. Interleukin-6 and its relationship to clinical parameters in patients with malignant pleural mesothelioma. *Br J Cancer*. 1998;77:907–912.
34. Shah I, Salvatore JR, Kummet T, et al. Pseudomesotheliomatous carcinoma involving pleura and peritoneum: a clinicopathologic and immunohistochemical study of three cases. *Ann Diagn Pathol*. 1999;3:148–159.
35. Koss MN, Fleming M, Przygodski RM, et al. Adenocarcinoma simulating mesothelioma: a clinicopathologic and immunohistochemical study of 29 cases. *Ann Diagn Pathol*. 1998;2:93–102.
36. Hartmann CA, Schutze H. Mesothelioma-like tumors of the pleura: a review of 72 autopsy cases. *Cancer Res Clin Oncol*. 1994;120:331–347.
37. Kobashi Y, Matsushima T, Irei T. Clinicopathological analysis of lung cancer resembling malignant pleural mesothelioma. *Respirology*. 2005;10(5):660–665.
38. Maeda R, Isowa N, Kawasaki Y, et al. Pseudomesotheliomatous carcinoma of the lung. *Jpn J Thorac Surg*. 2007;60:555–558.
39. Jaklitsch MT, Grondin SC, Sugarbaker DJ. Treatment of malignant mesothelioma. *World J Surg*. 2001;25:210–217.
40. Grossebner MW, Arifi AA, Goddard M, et al. Mesothelioma—VATS biopsy and lung mobilization improves diagnosis and palliation. *Eur J Cardiothorac Surg*. 1999;16:619–623.
41. Attanoos RL, Gibbs AR. The comparative accuracy of different pleural biopsy techniques in the diagnosis of malignant mesothelioma. *Histopathology*. 2008;53:340–344.
42. Roberts GH, Campbell GH. Exfoliative cytology of diffuse mesothelioma. *J Clin Pathol*. 1972;25:557–582.
43. Nguyen GK, Akin MR, Villanueva RR, et al. Cytopathology of malignant mesothelioma of the pleura in fine needle aspiration biopsies. *Diagn Cytopathol*. 1999;21:253–259.
44. Antman KH. Clinical presentation and natural history of benign and malignant mesothelioma. *Semin Oncol*. 1981;8:313–320.
45. Lee YC, Light RW, Musk AW. Management of malignant pleural mesothelioma: a critical review. *Curr Opin Pulm Med*. 2000;6:267–274.
46. Butchart EG. Contemporary management of malignant pleural mesothelioma. *Oncologist*. 1999;4:488–500.
47. Zellos LS, Sugarbaker DJ. Diffuse malignant mesothelioma of the pleural space and its management. *Oncology*. 2002;16:916–925.
48. Kindler HL. Malignant pleural mesothelioma. *Curr Treat Options Oncol*. 2000;1:313–326.
49. Senan S. Indications and limitations of radiotherapy in malignant pleural mesothelioma. *Curr Opin Oncol*. 2003;15:144–147.
50. Grondin SC, Sugarbaker DJ. Pleuropneumonectomy in the treatment of malignant pleural mesothelioma. *Chest*. 1999;116(suppl 6):450S–454S.
51. Kaiser LR. New therapies in the treatment of malignant pleural mesothelioma. *Semin Thorac Cardiovasc Surg*. 1997;9:383–390.
52. Erkilic S, Sari I, Tuncozgur B. Localized pleural malignant mesothelioma. *Pathol Int*. 2001;51:812–815.
53. Okamura H, Kamai T, Mitsuno A, et al. Localized malignant mesothelioma of the pleura. *Pathol Int*. 2001;51:654–660.
54. Crotty TB, Myers JL, Katzenstein AL, et al. Localized malignant mesothelioma: a clinicopathologic and flow cytometric study. *Am J Surg Pathol*. 1994;18:357–363.
55. Christoffel T, Teret SP. Epidemiology and the law: courts and confidence intervals. *Am J Public Health*. 1991;81:1661–1666.
56. Wagner JC, Sleggs CA, Marchand P. Diffuse pleural mesothelioma and asbestos exposure in North-Western Cape Province. *Br J Ind Med*. 1960;17:260–271.
57. Smither WJ. Asbestos, asbestosis, and mesothelioma of the pleura. *Proc R Soc Med*. 1966;59: 57–59.
58. Hill ID, Doll R, Knox JF. Mortality among asbestos workers. *Proc R Soc Med*. 1966;59:59–60.
59. Mann RH, Grosh JL, O'Donnell WM. Mesothelioma associated with asbestosis: a report of 3 cases. *Cancer*. 1966;19:521–526.

60. Butnor KJ, Sporn TA, Roggli VL. Exposure to brake dust and malignant mesothelioma: a study of 10 cases with mineral fiber analyses. *Ann Occup Hyg*. 2003;47:325–330.

61. Valic F. The asbestos dilemma. I. Assessment of risk. *Arh Hig Rada Toksikol*. 2002;53:153–167.

62. Roggli VL, Sharma A, Butnor KJ, et al. Malignant mesothelioma and occupational exposure to asbestos: a clinicopathological correlation of 1445 cases. *Ultrastruct Pathol*. 2002;26:55–65.

63. McDonald JC, Armstrong BG, Edwards CW, et al. Case-referent study of young adults with mesothelioma. I. Lung fiber analyses. *Ann Occup Hyg*. 2001;45:513–518.

64. Britton M. The epidemiology of mesothelioma. *Semin Oncol*. 2002;29:18–25.

65. Marchevsky AM, Wick MR. Current controversies regarding the role of asbestos exposure in the causation of malignant mesothelioma: the need for an evidence-based approach to develop medicolegal guidelines. *Ann Diagn Pathol*. 2003;7:321–332.

66. Klebe S, Brownlee NA, Mahar A, et al. Sarcomatoid mesothelioma: a clinical-pathologic correlation of 326 cases. *Mod Pathol*. 2010;23:470–479.

67. Bianchi C, Bianchi T, Ramani L. Malignant mesothelioma of the pleura among women. *Med Lav*. 2004;95:376–380.

68. Roggli VL, Pratt PC, Brody AR. Asbestos content of lung tissue in asbestos-associated diseases: a study of 110 cases. *Br J Ind Med*. 1986;43:18–28.

69. Roggli VL, Pratt PC, Brody AR. Analysis of tissue mineral fiber content. In: Roggli VL, Greenberg SD, Pratt PC, eds. *Pathology of Asbestos-Associated Diseases*. Boston: Little Brown; 1992:299–345.

70. Ilgren EB, Wagner JC. Background incidence of mesothelioma: animal and human evidence. *Regul Toxicol Pharmacol*. 1991;13:133–149.

71. Peterson Jr JT, Greenberg SD, Buffler PA. Non-asbestos-related malignant mesothelioma: a review. *Cancer*. 1984;54:951–960.

72. Craighead JE, Mossman BT. Pathogenesis of mesothelioma. In: Antman KH, Aisner J, eds. *Asbestos-related Malignancy*. New York: Grune & Stratton; 1987:151–162.

73. Lanphear BP, Buncher CR. Latent period for malignant mesothelioma of occupational origin. *J Occup Med*. 1992;34:718–721.

74. Pass HI, Mew DJ. In-vitro and in-vivo studies of mesothelioma. *J Cell Biochem*. 1996;24(suppl): 142–151.

75. Manning CB, Vallyathan V, Mossman BT. Diseases caused by asbestos: mechanisms of injury and disease development. *Int Immunopharmacol*. 2002;2:191–200.

76. Fitzpatrick DR, Peroni DJ, Bielefeldt-Ohmann H. The role of growth factors and cytokines in the tumorigenesis and immunobiology of malignant mesothelioma. *Am J Resp Cell Mol Biol*. 1995;12:455–460.

77. Attanoos RL, Thomas DH, Gibbs AR. Synchronous diffuse malignant mesothelioma and carcinomas in asbestos-exposed individuals. *Histopathology*. 2003;43:387–392.

78. Huncharek M. Non-asbestos-related diffuse malignant mesothelioma. *Tumori*. 2002;88:1–9.

79. Weiner SJ, Neragi-Miandoab S. Pathogenesis of malignant pleural mesothelioma and the role of environmental and genetic factors. *J Cancer Res Clin Oncol*. 2009;135:15–27.

80. Falchero L, Coiffier B, Guibert B, et al. Malignant mesothelioma of the pleura following radiotherapy of Hodgkin's disease. *Bull Cancer*. 1996;83:964–968.

81. Mizuki M, Yukishige K, Abe Y, et al. A case of malignant pleural mesothelioma following exposure to atomic radiation in Nagasaki. *Respirology*. 1997;2:201–205.

82. Antman KH, Ruxer Jr RL, Aisner J, et al. Mesothelioma following Wilms' tumor in childhood. *Cancer*. 1984;54:367–369.

83. Neugut AI, Ahsen H, Antman KH. Incidence of malignant pleural mesothelioma after thoracic radiotherapy. *Cancer*. 1997;80:948–950.

84. Weissmann LB, Corson JM, Neugut AI, et al. Malignant mesothelioma following treatment for Hodgkin's disease. *J Clin Oncol*. 1996;14:2098–2100.

85. Cavazza A, Travis LB, Travis WD, et al. Post-irradiation malignant mesothelioma. *Cancer*. 1996;77:1379–1385.

86. Hillerdal G, Berg J. Malignant mesothelioma secondary to chronic inflammation and old scars. *Cancer*. 1985;55:1968–1972.

87. Vertun-Baranowska B, Szymanska D, Szturmowicz M. Malignant mesothelioma. I. Evaluation of autopsy specimens. *Pneumonol Pol*. 1988;56:47–54.

88. Livneh A, Langevitz P, Pras M. Pulmonary associations in familial Mediterranean fever. *Curr Opin Pulm Med*. 1999;5:326–331.

89. Lidar M, Pras M, Langevitz P, et al. Thoracic and lung involvement in familial Mediterranean fever. *Clin Chest Med*. 2002;23:505–511.

90. Huncharek M, Kelsey K, Muscat J, et al. Parental cancer and genetic predisposition in malignant pleural mesothelioma: a case-control study. *Cancer Lett*. 1996;102:205–208.

91. Van Kaick G, Dalheimer A, Hornick S, et al. The German Thorotrast Study: recent results and assessment of risks. *Radiat Res*. 1999;152(suppl 6):S64–S71.

92. Andersson M, Wallin H, Jonsson M, et al. Lung carcinoma and malignant mesothelioma in patients exposed to Thorotrast: incidence, histology, and p53 status. *Int J Cancer*. 1995;63: 330–336.

93. Emri S, Demir A, Dogan M, et al. Lung diseases due to environmental exposures to erionite and asbestos in Turkey. *Toxicol Lett*. 2002;127:251–257.

94. Dumortier P, Gocmen A, Laurent K, et al. The role of environmental and occupational exposures in Turkish immigrants with fiber-related disease. *Eur Respir J*. 2001;17:922–927.

95. Strickler HD, Goedert JJ, Fleming M, et al. Simian virus 40 and pleural mesothelioma in humans. *Cancer Epidemiol Biomarkers Prev*. 1996;5:473–475.

96. Dopp E, Poser I, Papp T. Interphase FISH analysis of cell cycle genes in asbestos-treated human mesothelial cells (HMC), SV40-transformed HMB, and mesothelioma cells. *Cell Mol Biol*. 2002;48:OL271–OL277 (online publication).

97. Mutti L, Carbone M, Giordano GG, et al. Simian virus-40 and human cancer. *Monaldi Arch Chest Dis*. 1998;53:198–201.

98. Simsir A, Fetsch P, Bedrossian CW, et al. Absence of SV40 large-T antigen (Tag) in malignant mesothelioma effusions: an immunocytochemical study. *Diagn Cytopathol*. 2001;25:203–207.

99. Foddis R, DeRienzo A, Broccoli D, et al. SV40 infection induces telomerase activity in human mesothelial cells. *Oncogene*. 2002;21:1434–1442.

100. Shah KV. SV40 and human cancer: a review of recent data. *Int J Cancer*. 2007;120:215–223.

101. Hashimoto N, Oda T, Kadota K. An ultrastructural study of malignant mesotheliomas in two cows. *Jpn J Vet Sci*. 1989;51:327–336.

102. Colbourne CM, Bolton JR, Mills JN, et al. Mesothelioma in horses. *Aust Vet J*. 1992;69:275–278.

103. Misdorp W. Tumors in calves: comparative aspects. *J Comp Pathol*. 2002;127:96–105.

104. Cunningham AA, Dhillon AP. Pleural malignant mesothelioma in a captive clouded leopard (Neofelis nebulosa nebulosa). *Vet Rec*. 1998;143:22–24.

105. Baskerville A. Mesothelioma in the calf. *Pathol Vet*. 1967;4:149–156.

106. Shibuya K, Tajima M, Yamate J. Histological classification of 62 spontaneous mesotheliomas in F344 rats. *Jpn J Vet Sci*. 1990;52:1313–1317.

107. Rostami M, Tateyama S, Uchida K, et al. Tumors in domestic animals examined during a ten-year period (1980–1989) at Miyazaki University. *J Vet Med Sci*. 1994;56:403–405.

108. Rusch VW, Godwin JD, Shuman WP. The role of computed tomography scanning in the initial assessment and the followup of malignant pleural mesothelioma. *J Thorac Cardiovasc Surg*. 1988;96:171–177.

109. Golla B, Singh SP, Pinkard NB, et al. Rapidly fatal bilateral malignant mesothelioma. *Semin Roentgenol*. 1998;33:306–308.

110. Nakatsuka S, Yao M, Hoshida Y, et al. Pyothorax-associated lymphoma: a review of 106 cases. *J Clin Oncol*. 2002;20:4255–4260.

111. Falconieri G, Bussani R, Mirra M, et al. Pseudomesotheliomatous angiosarcoma: a pleuropulmonary lesion simulating pleural mesothelioma. *Histopathology*. 1997;30:419–424.

112. Allen TC, Cagle PT, Churg AM, et al. Localized malignant mesothelioma. *Am J Surg Pathol*. 2005;29:866–873.

113. Wick MR. Pleural cytology, tumor markers, and immunohistochemistry. In: Light RW, Lee YCG, eds. *Textbook of Pleural Diseases*. London: Arnold Publishers; 2003:256–281.

114. DiBonito L, Falconieri G, Colautti I, et al. Cytopathology of malignant mesothelioma: a study of its patterns and histological bases. *Diagn Cytopathol*. 1993;9:25–31.

115. Sherman ME, Mark EJ. Effusion cytology in the diagnosis of malignant epithelioid and biphasic pleural mesothelioma. *Arch Pathol Lab Med*. 1990;114:845–851.

116. Johnston WW. The malignant pleural effusion: a review of cytopathologic diagnoses of 584 specimens from 472 consecutive patients. *Cancer*. 1985;56:905–909.

117. Matzel W. Biochemical and cytological features of diffuse mesothelioma of the pleura. *Arch Geschwulstforsch*. 1985;55:259–264.

118. Castelain G, Castelain C, Pretet S, et al. Cytodiagnosis of pleural mesotheliomas. *Presse Med*. 1969;77:197–199.

119. Castelain G, Ioannou J, Castelain C, et al. Cytodiagnosis in lung diseases: its importance and its value. A study of 945 cases. *Presse Med*. 1968;76:2219–2221.

120. Yokoi T, Mark EJ. Atypical mesothelial hyperplasia associated with bronchogenic carcinoma. *Hum Pathol*. 1991;22:695–699.

121. Cavazza A, Rossi G, Agostini L, et al. Small-cell mesothelioma of the pleura: description of a case. *Pathologica*. 2002;94:247–252.

122. Hammar SP, Bolen JW. Sarcomatoid pleural mesothelioma. *Ultrastruct Pathol*. 1985;9:337–343.

123. Colby TV. Malignancies in the lung and pleura mimicking benign processes. *Semin Diagn Pathol*. 1995;12:30–44.

124. Khalidi HS, Medeiros LJ, Battifora H. Lymphohistiocytoid mesothelioma: an often-misdiagnosed variant of sarcomatoid malignant mesothelioma. *Am J Clin Pathol*. 2000;113:649–654.

125. Galateau-Sallé F, Attanoos R, Gibbs AR, et al. Lymphohistiocytoid variant of malignant mesothelioma of the pleura: a series of 22 cases. *Am J Surg Pathol*. 2007;31:711–716.

126. Cibas ES, Corson JM, Pinkus GS. The distinction of adenocarcinoma from malignant mesothelioma in cell blocks of effusions. *Hum Pathol*. 1987;18:67–74.

127. Renshaw AA, Dean BR, Antman KH, et al. The role of cytologic evaluation of pleural fluid in the diagnosis of malignant mesothelioma. *Chest*. 1997;111:106–109.

128. Kimura N, Dota K, Araya Y, et al. Scoring system for differential diagnosis of malignant mesothelioma and reactive mesothelial cells on cytology specimens. *Diagn Cytopathol*. 2009;37:885–890.

129. Nind AR, Attanoos RL, Gibbs AR. Unusual intraparenchymal growth patterns of malignant pleural mesothelioma. *Histopathology*. 2003;42:150–155.

130. Attanoos RL, Gibbs AR. The pathology associated with therapeutic procedures in malignant mesothelioma. *Histopathology*. 2004;45:393–397.

131. Corson JM. Pathology of diffuse malignant pleural mesothelioma. *Semin Thorac Cardiovasc Surg*. 1997;9:347–355.

132. Mogi A, Nabeshima K, Hamasaki M, et al. Pleural malignant mesothelioma with invasive micropapillary component and its association with pulmonary metastasis. *Pathol Int*. 2009;59:874–879.

133. Donaldson JC, Elliott RC, Kaminsky DB, et al. Psammoma bodies in pleural fluid associated with a mesothelioma: case report. *Mil Med*. 1979;144:476–479.

134. Suzuki Y. Diagnostic criteria for human diffuse malignant mesothelioma. *Acta Pathol Jpn*. 1992;42:767–786.

135. Shia J, Erlandson RA, Klimstra DS. Deciduoid mesothelioma: a report of 5 cases and literature review. *Ultrastruct Pathol*. 2002;26:355–363.

136. Monaghan H, Al-Nafussi A. Deciduoid pleural mesothelioma. *Histopathology*. 2001;39:104–106.

137. Ordóñez NG. Epithelial mesothelioma with deciduoid features: report of four cases. *Am J Surg Pathol*. 2000;24:816–823.

138. Ordóñez NG, Mackay B. Glycogen-rich mesothelioma. *Ultrastruct Pathol*. 1999;23:401–406.

139. Dessy E, Falleni M, Braidotti P, et al. Unusual clear-cell variant of epithelioid mesothelioma. *Arch Pathol Lab Med*. 2001;125:1588–1590.

140. Ordóñez NG, Myhre M, Mackay B. Clear cell mesothelioma. *Ultrastruct Pathol*. 1996;20:331–336.

141. Umezu H, Kuwata K, Ebe Y, et al. Microcystic variant of localized malignant mesothelioma accompanying an adenomatoid tumor-like lesion. *Pathol Int*. 2002;52:416–422.

142. Mukonoweshuro P, Attanoos RL, Smith ME. Nodular glomeruloid pleuroblastoma: a biphasic pleural-based malignant tumor with immature elements. *Virchows Arch*. 2006;449: 253–257.

143. Henderson DW, Shilkin KB, Whitaker D. Reactive mesothelial hyperplasia versus mesothelioma, including mesothelioma in-situ: a brief review. *Am J Clin Pathol*. 1998;110:397–404.

144. Whitaker D, Henderson DW, Shilkin KB. The concept of mesothelioma in-situ: implications for diagnosis and histogenesis. *Semin Diagn Pathol*. 1992;9:151–161.

145. Bolen JW. Tumors of serosal tissue origin. *Clin Lab Med*. 1987;7:31–50.

146. Carter D, Otis CN. Three types of spindle cell tumors of the pleura: fibroma, sarcoma, and sarcomatoid mesothelioma. *Am J Surg Pathol*. 1988;12:747–753.

147. Avellini C, Alampi G, Cocchi V, et al. Malignant sarcomatoid mesothelioma of the pleura. *Pathologica*. 1991;83:335–340.

148. Andrion A, Mazzucco G, Bernardi P, et al. Sarcomatous tumor of the chest wall with osteochondroid differentiation: evidence of mesothelial origin. *Am J Surg Pathol*. 1989;13:707–712.

149. Okamoto T, Yokota R, Shinkawa K, et al. Pleural malignant mesothelioma with osseous, cartilaginous, and rhabdomyoblastic differentiation. *J Jpn Resp Soc*. 1998;36:696–701.

150. Yousem SA, Hochholzer L. Malignant mesotheliomas with osseous and cartilaginous differentiation. *Arch Pathol Lab Med*. 1987;111:62–66.

151. Klebe S, Mahar A, Henderson DW, et al. Malignant mesothelioma with heterologous elements: clinicopathological correlation of 27 cases and literature review. *Mod Pathol*. 2008;21:1084–1094.

152. Sterrett GF, Whitaker D, Shilkin KB, et al. Fine needle aspiration cytology of malignant mesothelioma. *Acta Cytol*. 1987;31:185–193.

153. Colby TV. The diagnosis of desmoplastic malignant mesothelioma. *Am J Clin Pathol*. 1998;110:135–136.

154. Wilson GE, Hasleton PS, Chatterjee AK. Desmoplastic malignant mesothelioma: a review of 17 cases. *J Clin Pathol*. 1992;45:295–298.

155. Cantin R, Al-Jabi M, McCaughey WTE. Desmoplastic diffuse mesothelioma. *Am J Surg Pathol*. 1982;6:215–222.

156. Cagle PT, Churg A. Differential diagnosis of benign and malignant mesothelial proliferations on pleural biopsies. *Arch Pathol Lab Med*. 2005;129:1421–1427.

157. Churg A, Colby TV, Cagle PT, et al. The separation of benign and malignant mesothelial proliferations. *Am J Surg Pathol*. 2000;24:1183–2000.

158. Schramm A, Opitz I, Thies S, et al. Prognostic significance of epithelial-mesenchymal transition in malignant pleural mesothelioma. *Eur J Cardiothorac Surg*. 2010;37:566–572.

159. Mayall FG, Gibbs AR. The histology and immunohistochemistry of small cell mesothelioma. *Histopathology*. 1992;20:47–51.

160. Wick MR, Ritter JH, Dehner LP. Malignant rhabdoid tumors: a clinicopathologic review and conceptual discussion. *Semin Diagn Pathol*. 1995;12:233–248.

161. Puttagunta L, Vriend RA, Nguyen GK. Deciduoid epithelial mesothelioma of the pleura with focal rhabdoid change. *Am J Surg Pathol*. 2000;24:1440–1443.

162. Ordóñez NG. Mesothelioma with rhabdoid features: an ultrastructural and immunohistochemical study of 10 cases. *Mod Pathol*. 2006;19:373–383.

163. Machado I, Noguera R, Santonja N, et al. Immunohistochemical study as a tool in differential diagnosis of pediatric malignant rhabdoid tumor. *Appl Immunohistochem Mol Morphol*. 2010;18:150–158.

164. Tanzi S, Tiseo M, Internullo E, et al. Localized malignant pleural mesothelioma: report of two cases. *J Thorac Oncol*. 2009;4:1038–1040.

165. Teo A, Hemmings C, Miller R. Sarcomatoid localized mesothelioma mimicking intrapulmonary synovial sarcoma: a case report and review of the literature. *Pathology*. 2010;42:182–184.

166. Nakas A, Martin-Ucar AE, Edwards JG, et al. Localised malignant pleural mesothelioma: a separate clinical entity requiring aggressive local surgery. *Eur J Cardiothorac Surg*. 2008;33:303–306.

167. Kannerstein M, Churg J, Magner D. Histochemistry in the diagnosis of malignant mesothelioma. *Ann Clin Lab Sci*. 1973;3:207–211.

168. Cook HC. A histochemical characterization of malignant tumor mucins as a possible aid in the identification of metastatic deposits. *Med Lab Technol*. 1973;30:217–224.

169. Griffiths MH, Riddell RJ, Xipell JM. Malignant mesothelioma: a review of 35 cases with diagnosis and prognosis. *Pathology*. 1980;12:591–603.

170. Kwee WS, Veldhuizen RW, Golding RP, et al. Histologic distinction between malignant mesothelioma, benign pleural lesions, and carcinoma metastasis. *Virchows Arch Pathol Anat*. 1982;397:287–299.

171. Bertoldo E, Bernardi P, Gugliotta P. Histochemical and immunohistochemical methods in the diagnosis of mesothelioma. *Pathologica*. 1987;79:447–455.

172. Lucas JG, Tuttle SE. Diagnostic histochemical and immunohistochemical studies in malignant mesothelioma. *J Surg Oncol*. 1987;35:30–34.

173. McCaughey WTE, Colby TV, Battifora H, et al. Diagnosis of diffuse malignant mesothelioma: experience of a US/Canadian Mesothelioma Panel. *Mod Pathol*. 1991;4:342–353.

174. Wick MR, Loy T, Mills SE, et al. Malignant epithelioid pleural mesothelioma versus peripheral pulmonary adenocarcinoma: a histochemical, ultrastructural, and immunohistologic study of 103 cases. *Hum Pathol*. 1990;21:759–766.

175. Arai H, Endo M, Sasai Y, et al. Histochemical demonstration of hyaluronic acid in a case of pleural mesothelioma. *Am Rev Respir Dis*. 1975;111:699–702.

176. Hammar SP, Bockus DE, Remington FL, et al. Mucin-positive epithelial mesotheliomas: a histochemical, immunohistochemical, and ultrastructural comparison with mucin-producing pulmonary adenocarcinomas. *Ultrastruct Pathol*. 1996;20:293–325.

177. McMeekin W, Kennedy A, McNicol AM. Combined immunocytochemical and nucleolar organizer region staining: some technical aspects. *Med Lab Sci*. 1989;46:11–15.

178. Smith PJ, Skilbeck NQ, Harrison A, et al. The effect of a series of fixatives on the AgNOR technique. *J Pathol*. 1988;155:109–112.

179. Leong ASY, Raymond WA. Demonstration of AgNOR-related proteins in microwave-fixed tissues. *J Pathol*. 1988;156:352.

180. Aris JP, Blobel G. cDNA cloning and sequencing of human fibrillarin, a conserved nucleolar protein recognized by autoimmune antisera. *Proc Natl Acad Sci U S A*. 1991;88:931–935.

181. Ayres JG, Crocker JG, Skilbeck NQ. Differentiation of malignant from normal and reactive mesothelial cells by the argyrophil technique for nucleolar organizer region-asssociated proteins. *Thorax*. 1988;43:366–370.

182. Bethwaite PB, Delahunt B, Holloway LJ, et al. Comparison of silver-staining nucleolar organizer region (AgNOR) counts and proliferating cell nuclear antigen (PCNA) expression in reactive mesothelial hyperplasia and malignant mesothelioma. *Pathology*. 1995;27:1–4.

183. Ramesh K, Gahukamble L, Al-Fituri O. Utility of AgNOR technique in distinguishing reactive mesothelial hyperplasia, malignant mesothelioma, and pulmonary adenocarcinoma. *Cent Afr J Med*. 1994;40:265.

184. Wolanski KD, Whitaker D, Shilkin KB, et al. The use of epithelial membrane antigen and silver-stained nucleolar organizer region testing in the differential diagnosis of mesothelioma from benign reactive mesotheliosis. *Cancer*. 1998;82:583–590.

185. Pomjanski N, Motherby H, Buckstegge B, et al. Early diagnosis of mesothelioma in serous effusions using AgNOR analysis. *Anal Quant Cytol Histol*. 2001;23:151–160.

186. Onofre FB, Onofre AS, Pomjanski N, et al. 9p21 deletion in the diagnosis of malignant mesothelioma in serous effusions additional to immunocytochemistry, DNA-ICM, and AgNOR analysis. *Cancer*. 2008;114:204–215.

187. Wang NS. Electron microscopy in the diagnosis of pleural mesotheliomas. *Cancer*. 1973;31:1046–1054.

188. McDonald AD, Magner D, Eyssen G. Primary malignant mesothelial tumors in Canada, 1960–1968: a pathologic review by the Mesothelioma Panel of the Canadian Tumor Reference Center. *Cancer*. 1973;31:869–876.

189. David JM. Ultrastructure of human mesotheliomas. *J Natl Cancer Inst USA*. 1974;52: 1715–1725.

190. Warhol MJ, Hickey WF, Corson JM. Malignant mesothelioma: ultrastructural distinction from adenocarcinoma. *Am J Surg Pathol*. 1982;6:307–314.

191. Kobzik L, Antman KH, Warhol MJ. The distinction of mesothelioma from adenocarcinoma in malignant effusions by electron microscopy. *Acta Cytol*. 1985;29:219–225.

192. Suzuki Y, Kannerstein M. Ultrastructure of human malignant diffuse mesothelioma. *Am J Pathol*. 1976;85:241–262.

193. Stoebner P, Brambilla E. Ultrastructure of pleural tumors. *Pathol Res Pract*. 1982;173: 402–416.

194. Leong ASY, Stevens MW, Mukherjee TM. Malignant mesothelioma: cytologic diagnosis with histologic, immunohistochemical, and ultrastructural correlation. *Semin Diagn Pathol*. 1992;9:141–150.

195. Dardick I, Jabi M, McCaughey WTE, et al. Diffuse epithelial mesothelioma: a review of the ultrastructural spectrum. *Ultrastruct Pathol*. 1987;11:503–533.

196. Oury TD, Hammar SP, Roggli VL. Ultrastructural features of diffuse malignant mesotheliomas. *Hum Pathol*. 1998;29:1382–1392.

197. Ferenczy A. Diagnostic electron microscopy in gynecologic pathology. *Pathol Annu*. 1979; 14(part I):353–381.

198. Chen HP, Berardi RS. A light and electron microscopic study of lung cancers: clinical implications. *Int Surg*. 1993;78:124–126.

199. McGregor DH, Dixon AY, McGregor DK. Adenocarcinoma of the lung: a comparative diagnostic study using light and electron microscopy. *Hum Pathol*. 1988;19:910–913.

200. Klima M, Bossart MI. Sarcomatous type of malignant mesothelioma. *Ultrastruct Pathol*. 1983;4:349–358.

201. Dardick I, Srigley JR, McCaughey WTE, et al. Ultrastructural aspects of the histogenesis of diffuse and localized mesothelioma. *Virchows Arch Pathol Anat*. 1984;402:373–388.

202. Aerts JG, Delahaye M, van der Kwast TH, et al. The high post-test probability of a cytological examination renders further investigations to establish a diagnosis of epithelial malignant pleural mesothelioma redundant. *Diagn Cytopathol*. 2006;34:523–527.

203. Chirieac LR, Corson JM. Pathologic evaluation of malignant pleural mesothelioma. *Semin Thorac Cardiovasc Surg*. 2009;21:121–124.

204. Hammar SP. Macroscopic, histologic, histochemical, immunohistochemical, and ultrastructural features of mesothelioma. *Ultrastruct Pathol*. 2006;30:3–17.

205. Leong ASY, Wick MR, Swanson PE. *Immunohistology and Electron Microscopy of Anaplastic and Pleomorphic Tumors*. Cambridge, England, United Kingdom: Cambridge University Press; 1997.

206. Corson JM, Pinkus GS. Mesothelioma: profile of keratin proteins and carcinoembryonic antigen. *Am J Pathol*. 1982;108:80–87.

207. Bejui-Thivolet F, Patricot LM, Vauzelle JL. Keratins in malignant mesothelioma and pleural adenocarcinomas. *Pathol Res Pract*. 1984;179:67–73.

208. Churg A. Immunohistochemical staining for vimentin and keratin in malignant mesothelioma. *Am J Surg Pathol*. 1985;9:360–365.

209. Moll R, Dhouailly D, Sun TT. Expression of keratin 5 as a diagnostic feature of epithelial and biphasic mesotheliomas. *Virchows Arch B*. 1989;58:129–145.

210. Kahn HJ, Thorner PS, Yeger H, et al. Distinct keratin patterns demonstrated by immunoperoxidase staining of adenocarcinoma, carcinoids, and mesotheliomas using polyclonal and monoclonal antikeratin antibodies. *Am J Clin Pathol*. 1986;86:566–574.

211. Ordóñez NG. Value of cytokeratin 5/6 immunostaining in distinguishing epithelial mesothelioma of the pleura from lung adenocarcinoma. *Am J Surg Pathol*. 1998;22:1215–1221.

212. Cury PM, Butcher DN, Fisher C, et al. Value of the mesothelium-associated antibodies thrombomodulin, cytokeratin 5/6, calretinin, and CD44H in distinguishing epithelioid pleural mesothelioma from adenocarcinoma metastatic to the pleura. *Mod Pathol*. 2000;13:107–112.

213. Blobel GA, Moll R, Franke WW, et al. The intermediate filament cytoskeleton of malignant mesothelioma and its diagnostic significance. *Am J Pathol*. 1985;121:235–247.

214. Wick MR. Immunohistochemical approaches to the diagnosis of undifferentiated malignant tumors. *Ann Diagn Pathol*. 2008;12:72–84.

215. Van Der Kwast TH, Versnel MA, Delahaye M, et al. Expression of epithelial membrane antigen on malignant mesothelioma cells: an immunocytochemical and immunoelectron microscopic study. *Acta Cytol*. 1988;32:169–174.

216. Kawai T, Greenberg SD, Truong LD, et al. Differences in lectin binding of malignant pleural mesothelioma and adenocarcinoma of the lung. *Am J Pathol*. 1988;130:401–410.

217. Pfaltz M, Odermatt B, Christen B, et al. Immunohistochemistry in the diagnosis of malignant mesothelioma. *Virchows Arch Pathol Anat*. 1987;411:387–393.

218. Leong ASY, Parkinson R, Milios J. Thick cell membranes revealed by immunocytochemical staining: a clue to the diagnosis of mesothelioma. *Diagn Cytopathol*. 1990;6:9–13.

219. Dejmek A, Hjerpe A. Reactivity of six antibodies in effusions of mesothelioma, adenocarcinoma, and mesotheliosis: stepwise logistic regression analysis. *Cytopathology*. 2000;11:8–17.

220. Salman WD, Eyden B, Shelton D, et al. An EMA-negative, desmin-positive malignant mesothelioma: limitations of immunohistochemistry? *J Clin Pathol*. 2009;63:651–662.

221. Villena V, Lopez-Encuentra A, Echave-Sustaeta J, et al. Diagnostic value of CA-549 in pleural fluid: comparison with CEA, CA15-3, and CA72-4. *Lung Cancer*. 2003;40:289–294.

222. Comin CE, Novelli L, Boddi V, et al. Calretinin, thrombomodulin, CEA, and CD15: a useful combination of immunohistochemical markers for differentiating pleural epithelioid mesothelioma from peripheral pulmonary adenocarcinoma. *Hum Pathol*. 2001;32:529–536.

223. Carella R, Deleonardi G, D'Errico A, et al. Immunohistochemical panels for differentiating epithelial malignant mesothelioma from lung adenocarcinoma: a study with logistic regression analysis. *Am J Surg Pathol*. 2001;25:43–50.

224. Lau SK, Luthringer DJ, Eisen RN. Thyroid transcription factor-1: a review. *Appl Immunohistochem Molec Morphol*. 2002;10:97–102.

225. Hecht JL, Pinkus JL, Weinstein LJ, et al. The value of thyroid transcription factor-1 in cytologic preparations as a marker for metastatic adenocarcinoma of lung origin. *Am J Clin Pathol*. 2001;116:483–488.

226. Yatabe Y, Mitsudomi T, Takahashi T. Thyroid transcription factor-1 expression in pulmonary adenocarcinomas. *Am J Surg Pathol*. 2002;26:767–773.

227. Zamecnik J, Kodet R. Value of thyroid transcription factor-1 and surfactant apoprotein-A in the differential diagnosis of pulmonary carcinomas: a study of 109 cases. *Virchows Arch A*. 2002;440:353–361.

228. Ordóñez NG. Value of thyroid transcription factor-1, E-cadherin, BG8, WT1, and CD44S immunostaining in distinguishing epithelial pleural mesothelioma from pulmonary and non-pulmonary adenocarcinoma. *Am J Surg Pathol*. 2000;24:598–606.

229. Bejarano PA, Mousavi F. Incidence and significance of cytoplasmic thyroid transcription factor-1 immunoreactivity. *Arch Pathol Lab Med*. 2003;127:193–195.

230. Bishop JA, Sharma R, Illei PB. Napsin A and thyroid transcription factor-1 expression in carcinomas of the lung, breast, pancreas, colon, kidney, thyroid, and malignant mesothelioma. *Hum Pathol*. 2010;41:20–25.

231. Ordóñez NG. The immunohistochemical diagnosis of epithelial mesothelioma. *Hum Pathol*. 1999;30:313–323.

232. Dejmek A, Brockstedt U, Hjerpe A. Optimization of a battery using nine immunocytochemical variables for distinguishing between epithelial mesothelioma and adenocarcinoma. *APMIS*. 1997;105:889–894.

233. Sheibani K, Battifora H, Burke JS. Antigenic phenotype of malignant mesotheliomas and pulmonary adenocarcinomas: an immunohistologic analysis demonstrating the value of Leu-M1 antigen. *Am J Pathol*. 1986;123:212–219.

234. Roberts F, Harper CM, Downie I, et al. Immunohistochemical analysis still has a limited role in the diagnosis of malignant mesothelioma: a study of thirteen antibodies. *Am J Clin Pathol*. 2001;116:253–262.

235. Shield PW, Callan JJ, Devine PL. Markers for metastatic adenocarcinoma in serous effusion specimens. *Diagn Cytopathol*. 1994;11:237–245.

236. Moch H, Oberholzer M, Dalquen P, et al. Diagnostic tools for differentiating between pleural mesothelioma and lung adenocarcinoma in paraffin embedded tissue. Part I: Immunohistochemical findings. *Virchows Arch Pathol Anat*. 1993;423:19–27.

237. Bedrossian CW, Bonsib S, Moran C. Differential diagnosis between mesothelioma and adenocarcinoma: a multimodal approach based on ultrastructure and immunocytochemistry. *Semin Diagn Pathol*. 1992;9:124–140.

238. Thor A, Ohuchi N, Szpak CA, et al. Distribution of oncogetal antigen tumor-associated glycoprotein-72, defined by monoclonal antibody B72.3. *Cancer Res*. 1986;46:3118–3124.

239. Szpak CA, Johnston WW, Roggli VL, et al. The diagnostic distinction between malignant mesothelioma of the pleura and adenocarcinoma of the lung as defined by a monoclonal antibody (B72.3). *Am J Pathol*. 1986;122:252–260.

240. Wirth PR, Legier JF, Wright Jr GL. Immunohistochemical evaluation of seven monoclonal antibodies for differentiation of pleural mesothelioma from lung adenocarcinoma. *Cancer*. 1991;67:655–662.

241. Latza U, Niedobitek G, Schwarting R, et al. Ber-EP4: new monoclonal antibody which distinguishes epithelia from mesothelia. *J Clin Pathol*. 1990;43:213–219.

242. Sheibani K, Shin SS, Kezirian J, et al. Ber-EP4 antibody as a discriminant in the differential diagnosis of malignant mesothelioma versus adenocarcinoma. *Am J Surg Pathol*. 1991;15:779–784.

243. Gaffey MJ, Mills SE, Swanson PE, et al. Immunoreactivity for Ber-EP4 in adenocarcinomas, adenomatoid tumors, and malignant mesotheliomas. *Am J Surg Pathol*. 1992;16:593–599.

244. Ordóñez NG. The immunohistochemical diagnosis of mesothelioma: a comparative study of epithelioid mesothelioma and lung adenocarcinoma. *Am J Surg Pathol*. 2003;27:1031–1051.

245. Ruitenbeek T, Gouw AS, Poppema S. Immunocytology of body cavity fluids: MOC-31, a monoclonal antibody discriminating between mesothelial and epithelial cells. *Arch Pathol Lab Med*. 1994;118:265–269.

246. Niemann TH, Hughes JH, DeYoung BR. MOC-31 aids in the differentiation of metastatic adenocarcinoma from hepatocellular carcinoma. *Cancer*. 1999;87:295–298.

247. Kempner DH, Jay MR, Stevens RH. Human lung tumor-associated antigens of 32,000 daltons molecular weight. *J Natl Cancer Inst U S A*. 1979;63:1121–1129.

248. Lau SK, Prakash S, Geller SA, Alsabeh R. Comparative immunohistochemical profile of hepatocellular carcinoma, cholangiocarcinoma, and metastatic adenocarcinoma. *Hum Pathol*. 2002;33:1175–1181.

249. Gonzalez-Lois C, Ballestin C, Sotelo MT, et al. Combined use of novel epithelial (MOC-31) and mesothelial (HBME-1) immunohistochemical markers for optimal first-line diagnostic distinction between mesothelioma and metastatic carcinoma in pleura. *Histopathology*. 2001;38:528–534.

250. LePender J, Marionneau S, Cailleau-Thomas A, et al. ABH and Lewis histo-blood group antigens in cancer. *APMIS*. 2001;109:9–31.

251. Steplewska-Mazur K, Gabriel A, Zajecki W, et al. Breast cancer progression and expression of blood group-related tumor-associated antigens. *Hybridoma*. 2000;19:129–133.

252. Jordon D, Jagirdar J, Kaneko M. Blood group antigens Lewis X and Lewis Y in the diagnostic determination of malignant mesothelioma versus adenocarcinoma. *Am J Pathol*. 1989;135:931–937.

253. Riera JR, Astengo-Osuna C, Longmate JA, et al. The immunohistochemical diagnostic panel for epithelial mesothelioma: a reevaluation after heat-induced epitope retrieval. *Am J Surg Pathol*. 1997;21:1409–1419.

254. Humphrey PA. p53: mutations and immunohistochemical detection, with a focus on alterations in urologic malignancies. *Adv Pathol Lab Med*. 1994;7:579–596.

255. Attanoos RL, Griffin A, Gibbs AR. The use of immunohistochemistry in distinguishing reactive from neoplastic mesothelium: a novel use for desmin and comparative evaluation with epithelial membrane antigen, p53, platelet-derived growth factor receptor, P-glycoprotein, and bcl-2. *Histopathology*. 2003;43:231–238.

256. Esposito V, Baldi A, DeLuca A, et al. p53 immunostaining in differential diagnosis of pleural mesothelial proliferations. *Anticancer Res*. 1997;17:733–736.

257. Cagle PT, Brown RW, Lebovitz RM. p53 immunostaining in the differentiation of reactive processes from malignancy in pleural biopsy specimens. *Hum Pathol*. 1994;25:443–448.

258. Kafiri G, Thomas DM, Shepherd NA, et al. p53 expression is common in malignant mesothelioma. *Histopathology*. 1992;21:331–332.

259. Dei Tos AP, Doglioni C. Calretinin: a novel tool for diagnostic immunohistochemistry. *Adv Anat Pathol*. 1998;5:61–66.

260. Ordóñez NG. In search of a positive immunohistochemical marker for mesothelioma: an update. *Adv Anat Pathol*. 1998;5:53–60.

261. Miettinen M, Sarlomo-Rikala M. Expression of calretinin, thrombomodulin, keratin 5, and mesothelin in lung carcinomas of different types: an immunohistochemical analysis of 596 tumors in comparison with epithelioid mesotheliomas of the pleura. *Am J Surg Pathol*. 2003;27:150–158.

262. Abutaily AS, Addis BJ, Roche WR. Immunohistochemistry in the distinction between malignant mesothelioma and pulmonary adenocarcinoma: a critical evaluation of new antibodies. *J Clin Pathol*. 2002;55:662–668.

263. Gotzos V, Vogt, P, Celio M.R. The calcium binding protein calretinin is a selective marker for malignant pleural mesotheliomas of the epithelial type. *Pathol Res Pract*. 1996;192:137–147.

264. Doglioni C, Dei Tos AP, Laurino L, et al. Calretinin: a novel immunocytochemical marker for mesothelioma. *Am J Surg Pathol*. 1996;20:1037–1046.

265. Attanoos RL, Dojcinov SD, Webb R, et al. Anti-mesothelial markers in sarcomatoid mesothelioma and other spindle-cell neoplasms. *Histopathology*. 2000;37:224–231.

266. Lucas DR, Pass HI, Madan SK, et al. Sarcomatoid mesothelioma and its histological mimics: a comparative immunohistochemical study. *Histopathology*. 2003;42:270–279.

267. Haber DA, Buckler AJ, Glaser T, et al. An internal deletion within an 11p13 zinc finger gene contributes to the development of Wilms' tumor. *Cell*. 1990;61:1257–1269.

268. Loeb DM, Sukumar S. The role of WT1 in oncogenesis: tumor suppressor or oncogene? *Int J Hematol*. 2002;76:117–126.

269. Gulyas M, Hjerpe A. Proteoglycans and WT1 as markers for distinguishing adenocarcinoma, epithelioid mesothelioma, and benign mesothelium. *J Pathol*. 2003;199:479–487.

270. Foster MR, Johnson JE, Olson SJ, et al. Immunohistochemical analysis of nuclear versus cytoplasmic staining of WT1 in malignant mesotheliomas and primary pulmonary adenocarcinomas. *Arch Pathol Lab Med*. 2001;125:1316–1320.

271. Oates J, Edwards C. HBME-1, MOC-31, WT1, and calretinin: an assessment of recently-described markers for mesothelioma and adenocarcinoma. *Histopathology*. 2000;36:341–347.

272. Campbell CE, Kuriyan NP, Rackley RR, et al. Constitutive expression of the Wilms tumor suppressor gene (WT1) in renal cell carcinoma. *Int J Cancer*. 1998;78:182–188.

273. Goldstein NS, Bassi D, Uzieblo A. WT1 is an integral component of an antibody panel to distinguish pancreaticobiliary and some ovarian epithelial neoplasms. *Am J Clin Pathol*. 2001;116:246–252.

274. Ueda T, Oji Y, Naka N, et al. Overexpression of the Wilms tumor gene WT1 in human bone and soft tissue sarcomas. *Cancer Sci*. 2003;94:271–276.

275. Tsuta K, Kato Y, Tochigi N, et al. Comparison of different clones (WT49 versus 6F-H2) of WT-1 antibodies for immunohistochemical diagnosis of malignant pleural mesothelioma. *Appl Immunohistochem Mol Morphol*. 2009;17:126–130.

276. Esmon CT. The protein C pathway. *Chest*. 2003;124(suppl 3):26S–32S.

277. Ishii H, Nakano M, Tsubouchi J, et al. Distribution of thrombomodulin in human tissues and characterization of thrombomodulin in plasma. *Acta Hematol Jpn*. 1988;51:1228–1233.

278. Boffa MC, Burke B, Haudenschild C. Different localization of thrombomodulin. *Ann Biol Clin*. 1987;45:191–197.

279. Attanoos RL, Goddard H, Gibbs AR. Mesothelioma-binding antibodies: thrombomodulin, OV632, and HBME-1 and their use in the diagnosis of malignant mesothelioma. *Histopathology*. 1996;29:209–215.

280. Pu RT, Pang Y, Michael CW. Utility of WT-1, p63, MOC31, mesothelin, and cytokeratin (K903 and CK5/6) immunostains in differentiating adenocarcinoma, squamous cell carcinoma, and malignant mesothelioma in effusions. *Diagn Cytopathol*. 2008;36:20–25.

281. Appleton MA, Attanoos RL, Jasani B. Thrombomodulin as a marker of vascular and lymphatic tumors. *Histopathology*. 1996;29:153–157.

282. Breiteneder-Geleff S, Matsui K, Soleiman A, et al. Podoplanin, novel 43-kd membrane protein of glomerular epithelial cells, is down-regulated in puromycin nephrosis. *Am J Pathol*. 1997;151:1141–1152.

283. Kalof AN, Cooper K. D2-40 immunohistochemistry—so far. *Adv Anat Pathol*. 2009;16:62–64.

284. Hu Y, Yang Q, McMahon LA, et al. Value of D2-40 in the differential diagnosis of pleural neoplasms with emphasis on its positivity in solitary fibrous tumor. *Appl Immunohistochem Mol Morphol*. 2010;18:411–413.

285. Shintaku M, Honda T, Sakai T. Expression of podoplanin and calretinin in meningioma: an immunohistochemical study. *Brain Tumor Pathol*. 2010;27:23–27.

286. Naito Y, Ishii G, Kawai O, et al. D2-40-positive solitary fibrous tumors of the pleura: diagnostic pitfall of biopsy specimen. *Pathol Int*. 2007;57:618–621.

287. Ordóñez NG. The diagnostic utility of immunohistochemistry in distinguishing between epithelioid mesotheliomas and squamous carcinomas of the lung: a comparative study. *Mod Pathol*. 2006;19:417–428.

288. Hanna A, Pang Y, Bedrossian CW, et al. Podoplanin is a useful marker for identifying mesothelioma in malignant effusions. *Diagn Cytopathol*. 2010;38:264–269.

289. Marchevsky AM. Application of immunohistochemistry to the diagnosis of malignant mesothelioma. *Arch Pathol Lab Med*. 2008;132:397–401.

290. Hinterberger M, Reineke T, Storz M, et al. D2-40 and calretinin—a tissue microarray analysis of 341 malignant mesotheliomas with emphasis on sarcomatoid differentiation. *Mod Pathol*. 2007;20:248–255.

291. Ordóñez NG. Immunohistochemical diagnosis of epithelioid mesothelioma: an update. *Arch Pathol Lab Med*. 2005;129:1407–1414.

292. Ordóñez NG. D2-40 and podoplanin are highly specific and sensitive immunohistochemical markers of epithelioid malignant mesothelioma. *Hum Pathol*. 2005;36:372–380.

293. Kenmotsu H, Ishii N, Nagai K, et al. Pleomorphic carcinoma of the lung expressing podoplanin and calretinin. *Pathol Int*. 2008;58:771–774.

294. Padgett DM, Cathro HP, Wick MR, et al. Podoplanin is a better immunohistochemical marker for sarcomatoid mesothelioma than calretinin. *Am J Surg Pathol*. 2008;32:123–127.

295. Ordóñez NG. The immunohistochemical diagnosis of mesothelioma: differentiation of mesothelioma and lung adenocarcinoma. *Am J Surg Pathol*. 1989;13:276–291.

296. Gibbs AR, Harach R, Wagner JC, et al. Comparison of tumor markers in malignant mesothelioma and pulmonary adenocarcinoma. *Thorax*. 1985;40:91–95.

297. Kawai T, Suzuki M, Torikata C, et al. Expression of blood group-related antigens and Helix pomatia agglutinin in malignant pleural mesothelioma and pulmonary adenocarcinoma. *Hum Pathol*. 1991;22:118–124.

298. Ordóñez NG. Value of mesothelin immunostaining in the diagnosis of mesothelioma. *Mod Pathol*. 2003;16:192–197.

299. Frierson HF, Moskaluk CA, Powell SM, et al. Large-scale molecular and tissue microarray analysis of mesothelin expression in common human carcinomas. *Hum Pathol*. 2003;34:605–609.

300. Cheung CC, Ezzat S, Freeman JL, et al. Immunohistochemical diagnosis of papillary thyroid carcinoma. *Mod Pathol*. 2001;14:338–342.

301. Fetsch PA, Abati A, Higazi YM. Utility of the antibodies CA19-9, HBME-1, and thrombomodulin in the diagnosis of malignant mesothelioma and adenocarcinoma in cytology. *Cancer*. 1998;84:101–108.

302. Bateman AC, Al-Talib RK, Newman T, et al. Immunohistochemical phenotype of malignant mesothelioma: predictive value of CA125 and HBME-1 expression. *Histopathology*. 1997;30:49–56.

303. Loy TS, Quesenberry JT, Sharp SC. Distribution of CA-125 in adenocarcinomas: an immunohistochemical study of 481 cases. *Am J Clin Pathol*. 1992;98:175–179.

304. Mayall FG, Jasani B, Gibbs AR. Immunohistochemical positivity for neuron-specific enolase and Leu-7 in malignant mesotheliomas. *J Pathol*. 1991;165:325–328.

305. Kim MK, Kim S. Immunohistochemical profile of common epithelial neoplasms arising in the kidney. *Appl Immunohistochem Molec Morphol*. 2002;10:332–338.

306. Fan Z, van de Rijn M, Montgomery K, et al. Hep-Par1 antibody staining for the differential diagnosis of hepatocellular carcinoma: 676 tumors tested using tissue microarrays and conventional tissue sections. *Mod Pathol*. 2003;16:137–144.

307. Cohen AJ, Bunn PA, Franklin W, et al. Neutral endopeptidase: variable expression in human lung, inactivation in lung cancer, and modulation of peptide-induced calcium flux. *Cancer Res*. 1996;56:831–839.

308. Chu PG, Arber DA, Weiss LM. Expression of T/NK-cell and plasma cell antigens in nonhematopoietic epithelial neoplasms. *Am J Clin Pathol*. 2003;120:64–70.

309. Kushitani K, Takeshima Y, Amatya VJ, et al. Immunohistochemical marker panels for distinguishing between epithelioid mesothelioma and lung adenocarcinoma. *Pathol Int*. 2007;57:190–199.

310. Jaffer S, Orta L, Sunkara S, et al. Immunohistochemical detection of antiapoptotic protein X-linked inhibitor of apoptosis in mammary carcinoma. *Hum Pathol*. 2007;38:864–870.

311. Wu M, Sun Y, Li G, et al. Immunohistochemical detection of XIAP in mesothelium and mesothelial lesions. *Am J Clin Pathol*. 2007;128:783–787.

312. Lyons-Boudreaux V, Mody DR, Zhai J, et al. Cytologic malignancy versus benignancy: how useful are the "newer" markers in body fluid cytology? *Arch Pathol Lab Med*. 2008;132:23–28.

313. Hanley KZ, Facik MS, Bourne PA, et al. Utility of anti-L523S antibody in the diagnosis of benign and malignant serous effusions. *Cancer*. 2008;114:49–56.

314. Yuan Y, Nymoen DA, Stavnes HT, et al. Tenascin-X is a novel diagnostic marker of malignant mesothelioma. *Am J Surg Pathol*. 2009;33:1673–1682.

315. Beasley MB. Immunohistochemistry of pulmonary and pleural neoplasia. *Arch Pathol Lab Med*. 2008;132:1062–1072.

316. Gordon IO, Sitterding S, Mackinnon AC, et al. Update in neoplastic lung diseases and mesothelioma. *Arch Pathol Lab Med*. 2009;133:1106–1115.

317. Laury AR, Hornick JL, Perets R, et al. PAX8 reliably distinguishes ovarian serous tumors from malignant mesothelioma. *Am J Surg Pathol*. 2010;34:627–635.

318. Husain AN, Colby TV, Ordóñez NG, et al. Guidelines for pathologic diagnosis of malignant mesothelioma: a consensus statement from the International Mesothelioma Interest Group. *Arch Pathol Lab Med*. 2009;133:1317–1331.

319. Brown RW, Clark GM, Tandon AK, et al. Multiple-marker immunohistochemical phenotypes distinguishing malignant pleural mesothelioma from pulmonary adenocarcinoma. *Hum Pathol*. 1993;24:347–354.

320. Yaziji H, Battifora H, Barry TS, et al. Evaluation of 12 antibodies for distinguishing epithelioid mesothelioma from adenocarcinoma: identification of a three-antibody immunohistochemical panel with maximal sensitivity and specificity. *Mod Pathol*. 2006;19:514–523.

321. Marchevsky AM, Wick MR. Evidence-based guidelines for the utilization of immunostains in diagnostic pathology: pulmonary adenocarcinoma versus mesothelioma. *Appl Immunohistochem Mol Morphol*. 2007;15:140–144.

322. King J, Thatcher N, Pickering C, et al. Sensitivity and specificity of immunohistochemical antibodies used to distinguish between benign and malignant pleural disease: a systematic review of published reports. *Histopathology*. 2006;49:561–568.

323. Westfall DE, Fan X, Marchevsky AM. Evidence-based guidelines to optimize the selection of antibody panels in cytopathology: pleural effusions with malignant epithelioid cells. *Diagn Cytopathol*. 2010;38:9–14.

324. Bueno R, De Rienzo A, Dong L, et al. Second generation sequencing of the mesothelioma tumor genome. *PLoS ONE*. 2010;5:e10612.

325. Segers K, Ramael M, Singh S, et al. Detection of numerical chromosomal aberrations in paraffin-embedded malignant pleural mesothelioma by non-isotopic in-situ hybridization. *J Pathol*. 1995;175:219–226.

326. Shivapurkar N, Virmani AK, Wistuba I, et al. Deletions of chromosome 4 at multiple sites are frequent in malignant mesothelioma and small-cell lung carcinoma. *Clin Cancer Res*. 1999;5:17–23.

327. Bjorkqvist AM, Wolf M, Nordling S, et al. Deletions at 14q in malignant mesothelioma detected by microsatellite marker analysis. *Br J Cancer*. 1999;81:1111–1115.

328. Lee WC, Balsara B, Liu Z, et al. Loss of heterozygosity analysis defines a critical region in chromosome 1p22 commonly deleted in human malignant mesothelioma. *Cancer Res*. 1996;56:4297–4301.

329. Huncharek M. Genetic factors in the etiology of malignant mesothelioma. *Eur J Cancer*. 1995;31A:1741–1747.

330. Garlepp MJ, Leong CC. Biological and immunological aspects of malignant mesothelioma. *Eur Respir J*. 1995;8:643–650.

331. Popescu NC, Chahinian AP, DiPaolo JA. Nonrandom chromosome alterations in human malignant mesothelioma. *Cancer Res*. 1988;48:142–147.

332. Illei PB, Rusch VW, Zakowski MF, et al. Homozygous deletion of CDKN2A and codeletion of the methylthioadenosine phosphorylase gene in the majority of pleural mesotheliomas. *Clin Cancer Res*. 2003;9:2108–2113.

333. Dreyling MH, Bohlander SK, Adeyanju MO, et al. Detection of CDKN2 deletions in tumor cell lines and primary glioma by interphase fluorescence in-situ hybridization. *Cancer Res*. 1995;55:984–988.

334. Cheng JQ, Jhanwar SC, Lu YY, et al. Homozygous deletions within 9p21-p22 identify a small critical region of chromosomal loss in human malignant mesotheliomas. *Cancer Res*. 1993;53:4761–4763.

335. Chiosea S, Krasinskas A, Cagle PT, et al. Diagnostic importance of 9p21 homozygous deletion in malignant mesotheliomas. *Mod Pathol*. 2008;21:742–747.

336. Kitamura F, Araki S, Suzuki Y, et al. Assessment of the mutations of the p53 suppressor gene and Ha- and Ki-ras oncogenes in malignant mesothelioma in relation to asbestos exposure: a study of 12 American patients. *Ind Health*. 2002;40:175–181.

337. Roberts F, McCall AE, Burnett RA. Malignant mesothelioma: a comparison of biopsy and postmortem material by light microscopy and immunohistochemistry. *J Clin Pathol*. 2001;54:766–770.

338. Mayall FG, Jacobson G, Wilkins R. Mutations of the p53 gene and SV40 sequences in asbestos-associated and non-asbestos-associated mesotheliomas. *J Clin Pathol*. 1999;52:291–293.

339. Murthy SS, Testa JR. Asbestos, chromosomal deletions, and tumor suppressor gene alterations in human malignant mesothelioma. *J Cell Physiol*. 1999;180:150–157.

340. Liu BC, Fu DC, Miao Q, et al. p53 gene mutations in asbestos-associated cancers. *Biomed Environ Sci*. 1998;11:226–232.

341. Kirao T, Bueno R, Chen CJ, et al. Alterations of the p16 (INK4) locus in human malignant mesothelial tumors. *Carcinogenesis*. 2002;23:1127–1130.

342. Van der Meerden A, Seddon MB, Betscholtz CA, et al. Tumorigenic conversion of human mesothelial cells as a consequence of platelet-derived growth factor-A chain overexpression. *Am J Respir Cell Molec Biol*. 1993;8:214–221.

343. Tolnay E, Kuhnen C, Wiethage T, et al. Hepatocyte growth factor/scatter factor and its receptor c-met are overexpressed and associated with an increased microvessel density in malignant pleural mesothelioma. *J Cancer Res Clin Oncol*. 1998;124:291–296.

344. Hodzic D, Delacroix L, Willemsen P, et al. Characterization of the IGF system and analysis of the possible molecular mechanisms leading to IGF-II overexpression in mesothelioma. *Horm Metab Res*. 1997;29:549–555.

345. Kumar-Singh S, Weyler J, Martin MJ, et al. Angiogenic cytokines in mesothelioma: a study of VEGF, FGF-1 and 2, and TGF-beta expression. *J Pathol*. 1999;189:72–78.

346. Segers K, Ramael M, Singh SK, et al. Immunoreactivity for bcl-2 protein in malignant mesothelioma and non-neoplastic mesothelium. *Virchows Arch A*. 1994;424:631–634.

347. Sekido Y. Molecular biology of malignant mesothelioma. *Environ Health Prev Med*. 2008;13:65–70.

348. Horvai AE, Li L, Xu Z, et al. Malignant mesothelioma does not demonstrate overexpression or gene amplification despite cytoplasmic immunohistochemical staining for c-erbB-2. *Arch Pathol Lab Med*. 2003;127:465–469.

349. Ramos-Nino ME, Timblin CR, Mossman BT. Mesothelial cell transformation requires AP-1 binding activity and ERK-dependent Fra-1 expression. *Cancer Res*. 2002;62:6065–6069.

350. Saad RS, Cho P, Liu YL, et al. The value of epithelial membrane antigen expression in separating benign mesothelial proliferation from malignant mesothelioma: a comparative study. *Diagn Cytopathol*. 2005;32:156–159.

351. Shen J, Pinkus GS, Deshpande V, et al. Usefulness of EMA, GLUT-1, and XIAP for the cytologic diagnosis of malignant mesothelioma in body cavity fluids. *Am J Clin Pathol*. 2009;131:516–523.

352. Hasteh F, Lin GY, Weidner N, et al. The use of immunohistochemistry to distinguish reactive mesothelial cells from malignant mesothelioma in cytologic effusions. *Cancer Cytopathol*. 2010;118:90–96.

353. Illei PB, Ladanyi M, Rusch VW, et al. The use of CDKN2A deletion as a diagnostic marker for malignant mesothelioma in body cavity effusions. *Cancer*. 2003;99:51–56.

354. Mangano WE, Cagle PT, Churg A, et al. The diagnosis of desmoplastic malignant mesothelioma and its distinction from fibrous pleurisy: a histologic and immunohistochemical analysis of 31 cases including p53 immunostaining. *Am J Clin Pathol*. 1998;110:191–199.

355. Nakatsuka S, Yao M, Hoshida Y, et al. Pyothorax-associated lymphoma: a review of 106 cases. *J Clin Oncol*. 2002;20:4255–4260.

356. Wakely Jr PE, Menezes G, Nuovo G. Primary effusion lymphoma: cytopathologic diagnosis using in-situ molecular genetic analysis for human herpesvirus 8. *Mod Pathol*. 2002;15:944–950.

357. Aquino SL, Chen MY, Kuo WT, et al. The CT appearance of pleural and extrapleural disease in lymphoma. *Clin Radiol*. 1999;54:647–650.

358. Lee MJ, Grogan L, Meehan S, et al. Pleural granulocytic sarcoma: CT characteristics. *Clin Radiol*. 1991;43:57–59.

359. Colonna A, Gualco G, Bacchi CE, et al. Plasma cell myeloma presenting with diffuse pleural involvement: a hitherto unreported pattern of a new mesothelioma mimicker. *Ann Diagn Pathol*. 2010;14:30–35.

360. Blakolmer K, Essop MF, Close PM. Diagnosis of an anemone cell tumor as a B-cell lymphoma by molecular analysis. *Ultrastruct Pathol*. 1996;20:189–193.

361. Nappi O, Boscaino A, Wick MR. Extramedullary hematopoietic proliferations, extraosseous plasmacytomas, and ectopic splenic implants (splenosis). *Semin Diagn Pathol*. 2003;20:338–356.

362. Inoue K, Ogawa H, Sonoda Y, et al. Aberrant overexpression of the Wilms tumor gene (WT1) in human leukemia. *Blood*. 1997;89:1405–1412.

363. Hirose M, Kuroda Y. p53 may mediate mdr-1 expression via the WT1 gene in human vincristine-resistant leukemia/lymphoma cell lines. *Cancer Lett*. 1998;129:165–171.

364. Lin BT, Colby TV, Gown AM, et al. Malignant vascular tumors of the serous membranes mimicking mesothelioma. A report of 14 cases. *Am J Surg Pathol*. 1996;20:1431–1439.

365. Zhang PJ, LiVolsi VA, Brooks JJ. Malignant epithelioid vascular tumors of the pleura: report of a series and literature review. *Hum Pathol*. 2000;31:29–34.

366. Ximenes III M, Miziara HL. Hemangioendothelioma of the lung and pleura: report of three cases. *Int Surg*. 1981;55:67–70.

367. Battifora H. Epithelioid hemangioendothelioma imitating mesothelioma. *Appl Immunohistochem*. 1993;1:220–222.

368. Del Frate C, Mortele K, Zanardi R, et al. Pseudomesotheliomatous angiosarcoma of the chest wall and pleura. *J Thorac Imaging*. 2003;18:200–203.

369. McKay B, Ordóñez NG, Huang WL. Ultrastructural and immunocytochemical observations on angiosarcomas. *Ultrastruct Pathol*. 1989;13:97–110.

370. Weiss SW, Enzinger FM. Epithelioid hemangioendothelioma: a vascular tumor often mistaken for a carcinoma. *Cancer*. 1982;50:970–981.

371. Miettinen M, Fetsch JF. Distribution of keratins in normal endothelial cells and a spectrum of vascular tumors: implications in tumor diagnosis. *Hum Pathol*. 2000;31:1062–1067.

372. Miettinen M, Lindenmayer AE, Chaubal A. Endothelial cell markers CD31, CD34, and BNH9 antibody to H- and Y- antigens: evaluation of their specificity and sensitivity in the diagnosis of vascular tumors and comparison with von Willebrand factor. *Mod Pathol*. 1994;7:82–90.

373. Bahrami A, Allen TC, Cagle PT. Pulmonary epithelioid hemangioendothelioma mimicking mesothelioma. *Pathol Int*. 2008;58:730–734.

374. Panagopoulos I, Mertens F, Isaksson M, et al. Molecular genetic characterization of the EWS/CHN and RBP56/CHN fusion genes in extraskeletal myxoid chondrosarcoma. *Genes Chromosomes Cancer*. 2002;35:340–352.

375. Goetz SP, Robinson RA, Landas SK. Extraskeletal myxoid chondrosarcoma of the pleura: report of a case clinically simulating mesothelioma. *Am J Clin Pathol*. 1992;97:498–502.

376. Okamoto S, Hisaoka M, Ishida T, et al. Extraskeletal myxoid chondrosarcoma: a clinicopathologic, immunohistochemical, and molecular analysis of 18 cases. *Hum Pathol*. 2001;32:1116–1124.

377. Dei Tos AP, Wadden C, Fletcher CDM. Extraskeletal myxoid chondrosarcoma: an immunohistochemical reappraisal of 39 cases. *Appl Immunohistochem*. 1997;5:73–77.

378. Daugaard S, Christensen LH, Høgdall E. Markers aiding the diagnosis of chondroid tumors: an immunohistochemical study including osteonectin, bcl-2, cox-2, actin, calponin, D2-40 (podoplanin), mdm-2, CD117 (c-kit), and YKL-40. *APMIS*. 2009;117:518–525.

379. Litzky LA. Pulmonary sarcomatous tumors. *Arch Pathol Lab Med*. 2008;132:1104–1117.

380. Fisher C. Synovial sarcoma. *Ann Diagn Pathol*. 1998;2:401–421.

381. Miettinen M, Limon J, Niezabitowski A, et al. Calretinin and other mesothelial markers in synovial sarcoma: analysis of antigenic similarities and differences with malignant mesothelioma. *Am J Surg Pathol*. 2001;25:610–617.

382. Knösel T, Heretsch S, Altendorf-Hofmann A, et al. TLE1 is a robust diagnostic biomarker for synovial sarcomas and correlates with t(X;18): analysis of 319 cases. *Eur J Cancer*. 2010;46:1170–1176.

383. Carbone M, Rizzo P, Powers A, et al. Molecular analyses, morphology, and immunohistochemistry together differentiate pleural synovial sarcoma from mesotheliomas: clinical implications. *Anticancer Res*. 2002;22:3443–3448.

384. Nappi O, Glasner SD, Swanson PE, et al. Biphasic and monophasic sarcomatoid carcinomas of the lung. *Am J Clin Pathol*. 1994;102:331–340.

385. Falconieri G, Zanconati F, Bussani R, et al. Small cell carcinoma of the lung simulating pleural mesothelioma: report of 4 cases with autopsy confirmation. *Pathol Res Pract*. 1995;191:1147–1152.

386. Wick MR. Immunohistology of neuroendocrine and neuroectodermal tumors. *Semin Diagn Pathol*. 2000;17:194–203.

387. Beiske K, Myklebust AT, Aamdal S, et al. Detection of bone marrow metastases in small cell lung carcinoma patients: comparison of immunologic and morphologic methods. *Am J Pathol*. 1992;141:531–538.

388. Chhieng DC, Ko EC, Yee HT, et al. Malignant pleural effusions due to small cell lung carcinoma: a cytologic and immunocytochemical study. *Diagn Cytopathol*. 2001;25:356–360.

389. Attanoos RL, Galateau-Sallé F, Gibbs AR, et al. Primary thymic epithelial tumors of the pleura mimicking malignant mesothelioma. *Histopathology*. 2002;41:42–49.

390. DiComo CJ, Urist MJ, Babayan I, et al. p63 expression profiles in human normal and tumor tissues. *Clin Cancer Res*. 2002;8:494–501.

391. Hammond EH, Flinner RL. The diagnosis of thymoma: a review. *Ultrastruct Pathol*. 1991;15:419–438.

392. Flint A, Weiss SW. CD34 and keratin expression distinguishes solitary fibrous tumor (fibrous mesothelioma) of pleura from desmoplastic mesothelioma. *Hum Pathol*. 1995;26:428–431.

393. Gaffey MJ, Mills SE, Ritter JH. Clear cell tumors of the lower respiratory tract. *Semin Diagn Pathol*. 1997;14:222–232.

394. Fleming S. Genetics of renal tumours. *Cancer Metastasis Rev*. 1997;16:127–140.

395. Osborn M, Pelling N, Walker MM, et al. The value of "mesothelium-associated" antibodies in distinguishing between metastatic renal cell carcinomas and mesotheliomas. *Histopathology*. 2002;41:301–307.

396. Tong GX, Chiriboga L, Hamele-Bena D, et al. Expression of PAX2 in papillary serous carcinoma of the ovary: immunohistochemical evidence of fallopian tube or secondary Müllerian system origin? *Mod Pathol*. 2007;20:856–863.

397. Herrera GA, Turbat-Herrera EA. The role of ultrastructural pathology in the diagnosis of epithelial and unusual renal tumors. *Ultrastruct Pathol*. 1996;20:7–26.

398. Nappi O, Ferrara G, Wick MR. Neoplasms composed of eosinophilic polygonal cells: an overview with consideration of different cytomorphologic patterns. *Semin Diagn Pathol*. 1999;16:82–90.

399. Mackay B, El-Naggar A, Ordóñez NG. Ultrastructure of adrenal cortical carcinoma. *Ultrastruct Pathol*. 1994;18:181–190.

400. DeYoung BR, Wick MR. Immunohistologic analysis of metastatic carcinomas of unknown origin: an algorithmic approach. *Semin Diagn Pathol*. 2000;17:184–193.

401. Gaffey MJ, Traweek ST, Mills SE, et al. Cytokeratin expression in adrenocortical neoplasia. *Hum Pathol*. 1992;23:144–153.

402. Zhang PJ, Genega EM, Tomaszewski JE, et al. The role of calretinin, inhibin, melan-A, bcl-2, and c-kit in differentiating adrenal cortical and medullary tumors: an immunohistochemical study. *Mod Pathol*. 2003;16:591–597.

403. Vaideeswar P, Deshpande JR, Jambhekar NA. Primary pleuropulmonary malignant germ cell tumors. *J Postgrad Med*. 2002;48:29–31.

404. Srigley JR, Mackay B, Toth P, et al. The ultrastructure and histogenesis of male germ cell neoplasia with emphasis on seminoma with early carcinomatous features. *Ultrastruct Pathol*. 1988;12:67–86.

405. Devouassoux-Shisheboran M, Manduit C, Tabone E, et al. Growth regulating factors and signalling proteins in testicular germ cell tumors. *APMIS*. 2003;111:212–224.

406. Biermann K, Klingmüller D, Koch A, et al. Diagnostic value of markers M2A, OCT3/4, AP-2gamma, PLAP and c-KIT in the detection of extragonadal seminomas. *Histopathology*. 2006;49:290–297.

407. Horvai AE, Li L, Xu Z, et al. c-kit is not expressed in malignant mesothelioma. *Mod Pathol*. 2003;16:818–822.

408. Brooks JJ, LiVolsi VA, Pietra GG. Mesothelial cell inclusions in mediastinal lymph nodes, mimicking metastatic carcinoma. *Am J Clin Pathol*. 1990;93:741–748.

409. Parkash V, Vidwans M, Carter D. Benign mesothelial cells in mediastinal lymph nodes. *Am J Surg Pathol*. 1999;23:1264–1269.

410. Isotalo PA, Veinot JP, Jabi M. Hyperplastic mesothelial cells in mediastinal lymph node sinuses with extranodal lymphatic involvement. *Arch Pathol Lab Med*. 2000;124:609–613.

411. Hoekman K, Tognon G, Risse EK, et al. Well-differentiated papillary mesothelioma of the peritoneum: a separate entity. *Eur J Cancer*. 1996;32A:255–258.

412. Weiss SW, Tavassoli FA. Multicystic mesothelioma: an analysis of pathologic findings and biologic behavior in 37 cases. *Am J Surg Pathol*. 1988;12:737–746.

413. Butnor KJ, Sporn TA, Hammar SP, et al. Well-differentiated papillary mesothelioma. *Am J Surg Pathol*. 2001;25:1304–1309.

414. Galateau-Sallé F, Vignaud JM, Burke L, et al. Well-differentiated papillary mesothelioma of the pleura: a series of 24 cases. *Am J Surg Pathol*. 2004;28:534–540.

415. Yesner R, Hurwitz A. Localized pleural mesothelioma of epithelial type. *J Thorac Surg*. 1953;26:325–329.

416. Ball NJ, Urbanski SJ, Green FH, et al. Pleural multicystic mesothelial proliferation: the so-called "multicystic mesothelioma." *Am J Surg Pathol*. 1990;14:375–378.

417. Kao S, Mahon K, Lin B, et al. Pleural well-differentiated papillary mesothelioma: a case report. *J Thorac Oncol*. 2009;4:920–922.

418. Torii I, Hashimoto M, Terada T, et al. Well-differentiated papillary mesothelioma with invasion to the chest wall. *Lung Cancer*. 2010;67:244–247.

419. Butchart EG, Ashcroft T, Barnsley WC, et al. Pleuropneumonectomy in the management of diffuse malignant mesothelioma of the pleura: experience with 29 patients. *Thorax*. 1976;31:15–24.

420. Rusch VW. A proposed new international TNM staging system for malignant pleural mesothelioma from the International Mesothelioma Interest Group. *Lung Cancer*. 1996;14:1–12.

421. Greene FL, ed. *American Joint Committee on Cancer (AJCC) Cancer Staging Manual*, 6th ed. New York: Springer-Verlag; 2002:139–141.

422. Sugarbaker DJ, Strauss GM, Lynch TJ, et al. Node status has prognostic significance in the multimodality therapy of diffuse malignant mesothelioma. *J Clin Oncol*. 1993;11:1172–1178.

423. Koong HN, Battafarano RJ, Ginsberg RJ. Malignant pleural mesothelioma. In: Gospodarowicz MK, Henson DE, Hutter RVP, et al, eds. *Prognostic Factors in Cancer*. 2nd ed. New York: Wiley-Liss; 2001:371–385.

424. Johansson L, Linden CJ. Aspects of histopathologic subtype as a prognostic factor in 85 pleural mesotheliomas. *Chest*. 1996;109:109–114.

425. Rusch VW, Venkatraman ES. Important prognostic factors in patients with malignant pleural mesothelioma, managed surgically. *Ann Thorac Surg*. 1999;68:1799–1804.

426. Metintas M, Metintas S, Ucgun I, et al. Prognostic factors in diffuse malignant pleural mesothelioma: effects of pretreatment clinical and laboratory characteristics. *Respir Med*. 2001;95:829–835.

427. Beer TW, Shepherd P, Pullinger NC. p27 immunostaining is related to prognosis in malignant mesothelioma. *Histopathology*. 2001;38:535–541.

428. Bongiovanni M, Cassoni P, DeGiuli P, et al. p27 (kip1) immunoreactivity correlates with long-term survival in pleural malignant mesothelioma. *Cancer*. 2001;92:1245–1250.

429. Leonardo E, Zanconati F, Bonifacio D, Bonito LD. Immunohistochemistry for MIB-1 and p27/kip1 as a prognostic factor for pleural mesothelioma. *Pathol Res Pract*. 2001;197:253–256.

430. Dacic S, Kothmaier H, Land S, et al. Prognostic significance of p16/cdkn2a loss in pleural malignant mesotheliomas. *Virchows Arch*. 2008;453:627–635.

431. Comin CE, Anichini C, Boddi V, et al. MIB-1 proliferation index correlates with survival in pleural malignant mesothelioma. *Histopathology*. 2000;36:26–31.

432. Alifano M, Loi M, Camilleri-Broet S, et al. Neurotensin expression and outcome of malignant pleural mesothelioma. *Biochimie*. 2010;92:164–170.

433. Cappia S, Righi L, Mirabelli D, et al. Prognostic role of osteopontin expression in malignant pleural mesothelioma. *Am J Clin Pathol*. 2008;130:58–64.

434. Baldi A, Mottolese M, Vincenzi B, et al. The serine protease HtrA1 is a novel prognostic factor for human mesothelioma. *Pharmacogenomics*. 2008;9:1069–1077.

435. Opitz I, Soltermann A, Abaecherli M, et al. PTEN expression is a strong predictor of survival in mesothelioma patients. *Eur J Cardiothorac Surg*. 2008;33:502–506.

436. Kothmaier H, Quehenberger F, Halbwedl I, et al. EGFR and PDGFR differentially promote growth in malignant epithelioid mesothelioma of short and long term survivors. *Thorax*. 2008;63:345–351.

Appendix: Miscellaneous Distinctive Histopathologic Findings

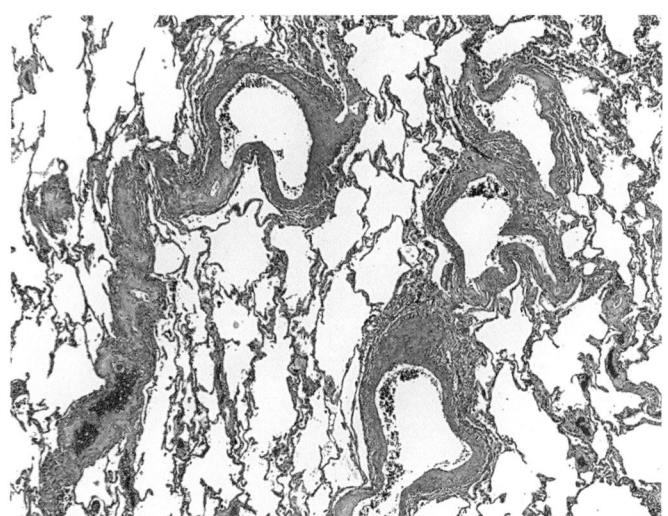

Figure A1. Aging changes in arteries. Abnormalities in the pulmonary arteries can be observed in many surgical lung biopsy specimens, unrelated to clinical evidence of pulmonary hypertension. This phenomenon is seen most commonly in aging smokers and in the vicinity of localized scars. Vessel tortuosity is the common denominator, and if medial thickening is present, it tends to be patchy and somewhat eccentric (possibly representing tangent sectioning).

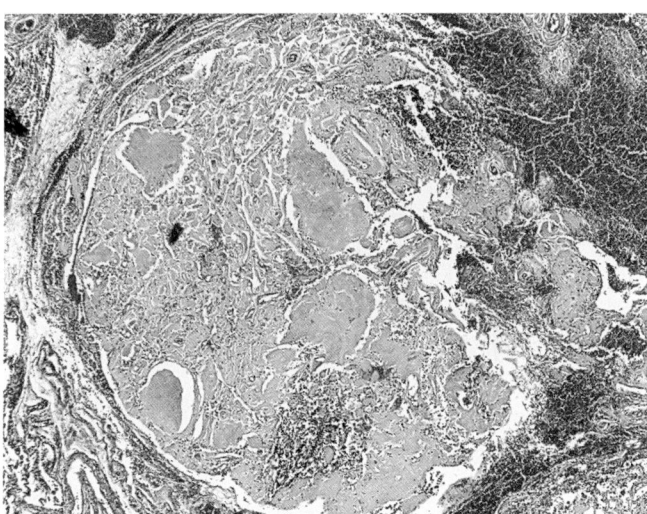

Figure A2. Amyloid, nodular. A specific manifestation of amyloid, nodular amyloid produces one or more mass lesions, but most often has no relation to systemic amyloidosis. Multinucleated giant cells often are present at the periphery of larger amyloid deposits within the lesions. Some examples of nodular amyloid in the lung are related to forms of low-grade B cell lymphoma.

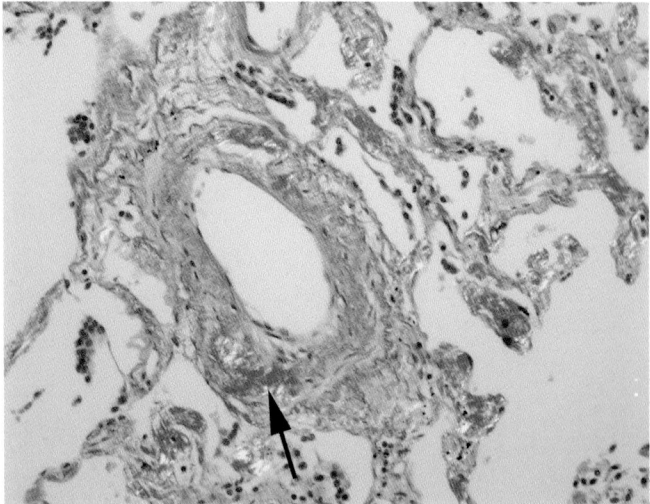

Figure A3. Amyloid in the wall of a pulmonary artery (Congo red stain for amyloid). The *arrow* points to a focus of dense, waxy, homogenous amyloid, stained red with this method. Note this same focus in Figure A4 under plane-polarized light, where the diagnostic apple-green birefringence can be seen.

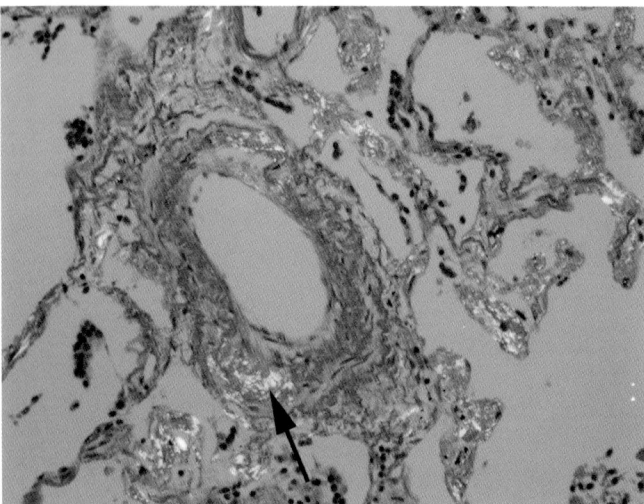

Figure A4. Amyloid in the wall of a pulmonary artery (Congo red stain, plane-polarized light). The red "Congophilic" focus of amyloid (*arrow;* also shown in Fig. A3) turns "apple-green" in color under polarization.

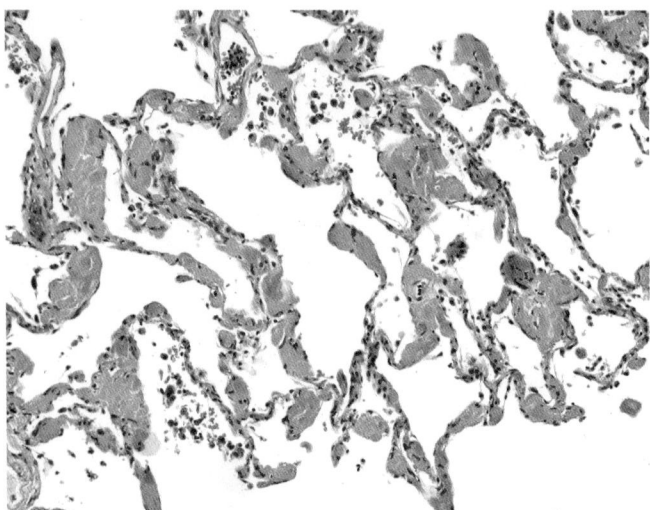

Figure A5. Amyloid, alveolar septal, hematoxylin and eosin stain. Note the uniform deposition of amorphous eosinophilic amyloid in alveolar walls. In contrast to collagen, amyloid deposits lack a fibrillar appearance when examined by light microscopy with the substage condenser lowered or removed.

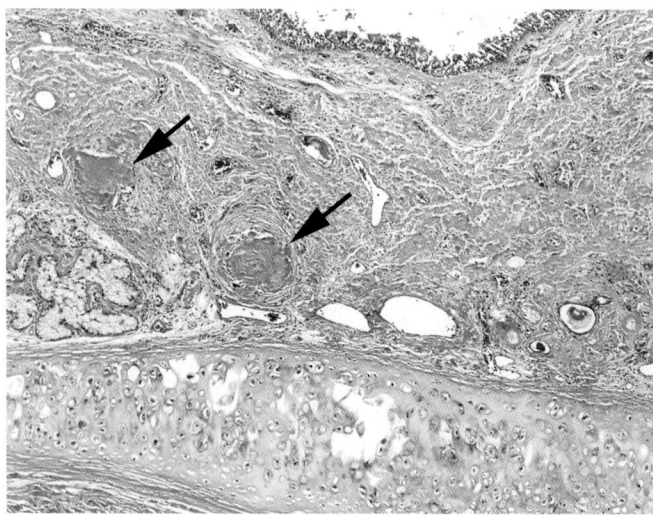

Figure A6. Amyloid, tracheobronchial, hematoxylin and eosin stain. (*Arrows* show deposits in tracheal wall.)

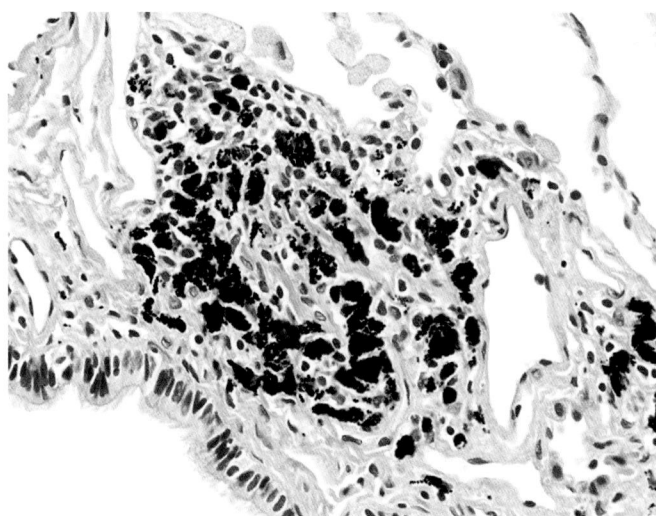

Figure A7. Anthracosis (focal) parenchymal. Anthracotic pigment is a common incidental finding in surgical lung biopsy specimens and transbronchial biopsy specimens. A characteristic distribution is often discernible, with dust deposited along lymphatic routes in the pleura and bronchovascular sheaths. It is always prudent to seek clinical and radiologic correlation before ascribing such changes to pneumoconiosis.

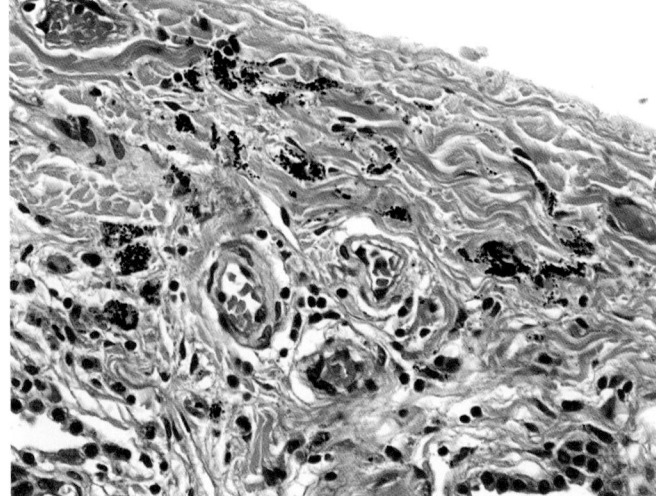

Figure A8. Anthracosis (focal) in pleura. Small foci of dust accumulation along pleural lymphatic routes are an expected finding in smokers and city dwellers.

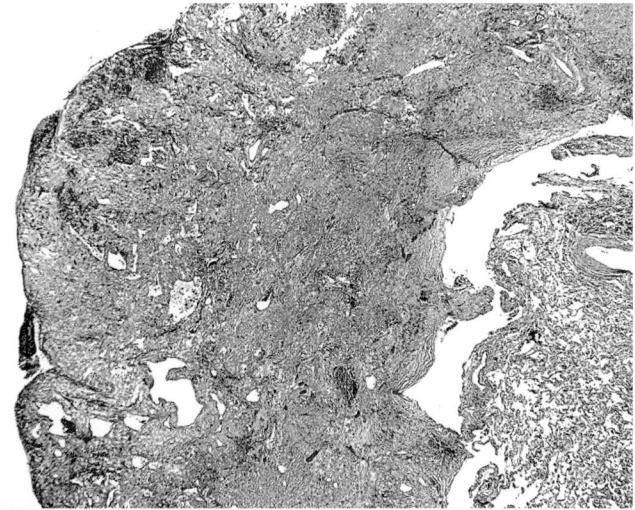

Figure A9. Subpleural zones of pale elastotic fibrosis. Subpleural zones of elastotic fibrous scar occur as an incidental finding in the upper lung zones. The phenomenon is easy to recognize and is important because such incidental scars may be mistaken surgically for tumor. If an apical cap is identified by frozen section analysis, the pathologist can encourage additional biopsies in search of more specific findings.

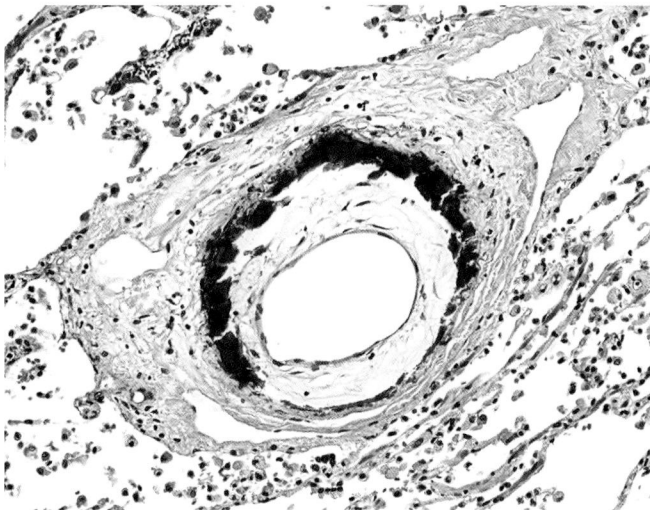

Figure A11. Arterial medial calcification. Calcification may occur in the media of pulmonary arteries as an incidental finding. This small artery has dramatic medial calcification in the setting of chronic mitral stenosis.

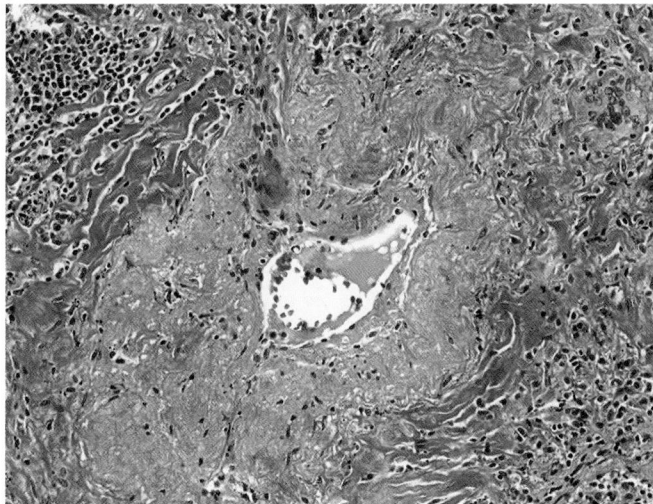

Figure A10. Arterial medial hyaline sclerosis. Hyaline sclerosis of the pulmonary arterial media can occur as a consequence of fibrosis and other lung injury (here in a case of sarcoidosis, a multinucleated giant cell is seen in the *upper right*).

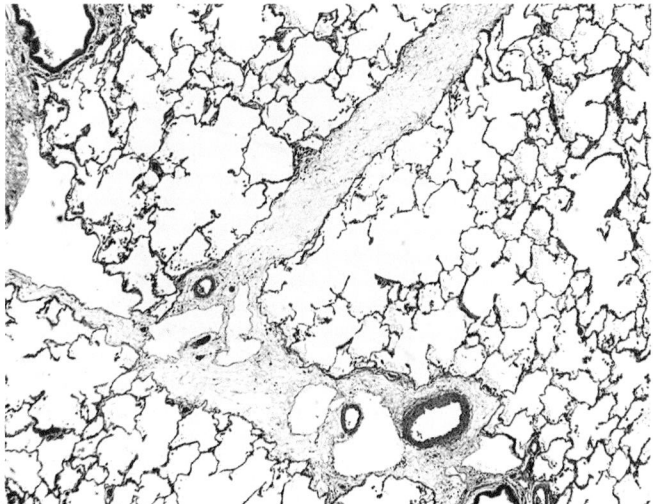

Figure A12. Artifactual lymphatic dilation can occur from injection fixation and is not always a sign of true pathology. The optimal (and easiest) form of surgical biopsy fixation is agitation (see Chapter 2). Overzealous injection of fixative using a syringe can produce distinctive artifacts.

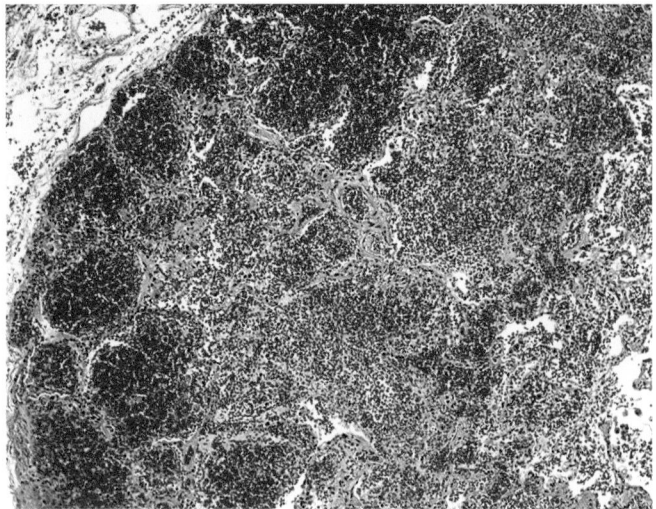

Figure A13. Artifactual hemorrhage. Fresh blood in alveolar spaces may occur as a consequence of operative manipulation. To distinguish such artifactual hemorrhage from pathologic alveolar hemorrhage, a search for hemosiderin-laden macrophages and abnormal cellularity of the alveolar interstitium is often helpful (see Chapter 10 for a discussion of diffuse alveolar hemorrhage).

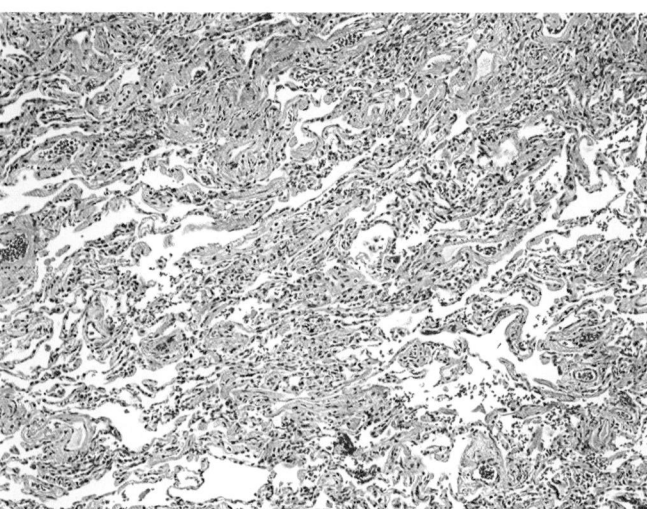

Figure A15. Atelectasis. The lung is typically collapsed as part of the video-assisted thoracoscopic surgical procedure. For this reason, biopsy specimens that are allowed to fix by immersion, without removal of staples, may be difficult to interpret given the dense approximation of alveolar walls. Agitation fixation is a preferable technique (see Chapter 2 for a discussion of fixation methods).

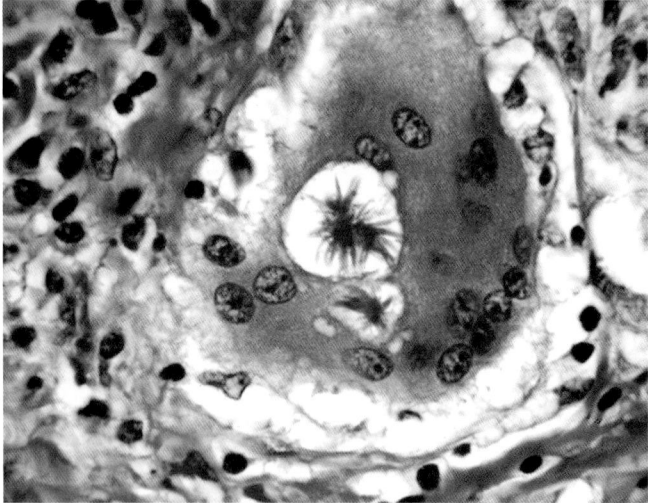

Figure A14. Asteroid body in a multinucleated giant cell. Asteroid bodies are distinctive eosinophilic inclusions composed of cytoskeletal components and collagen. They are not specific for sarcoidosis and are seen in a minority of patients with this disease.

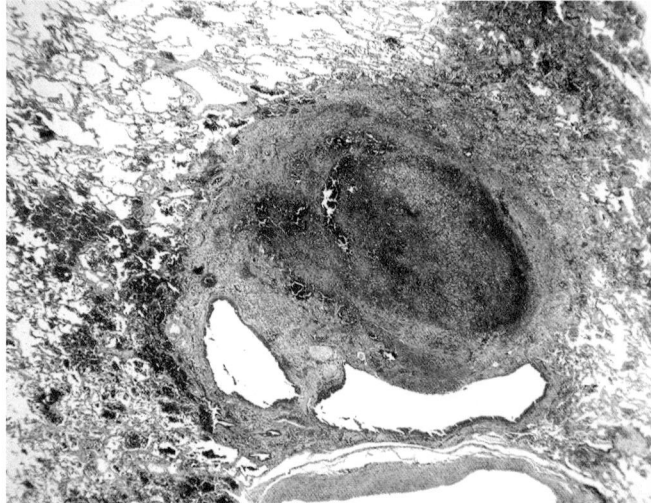

Figure A16. Biopsy site. On rare occasions, a previous biopsy procedure may result in a reparative reaction that can be seen in subsequent wedge biopsy or lobectomy specimens.

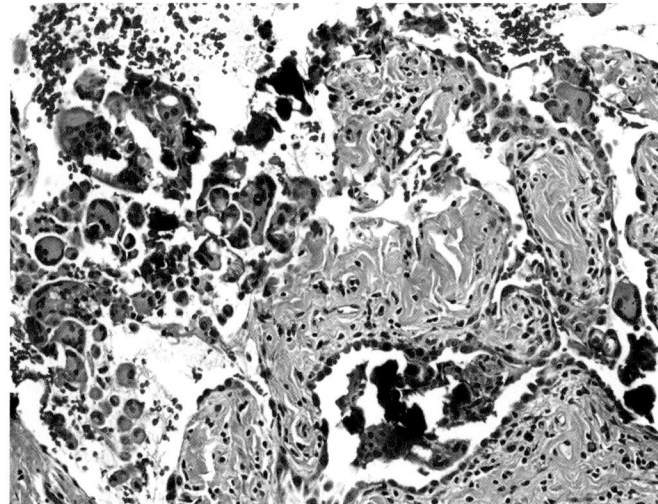

Figure A17. Blue bodies. These distinctive laminated and calcified hematoxyphilic bodies are a nonspecific finding. They may be seen in the alveolar spaces focally in a number of interstitial lung diseases where alveolar macrophages accumulate.

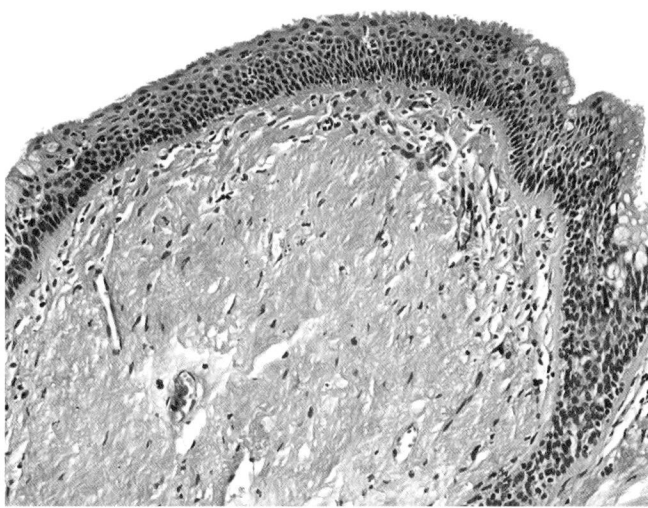

Figure A20. Bronchial mucosa subepithelial elastosis. This change is a nonspecific finding seen on occasion in lung biopsy specimens from older patients.

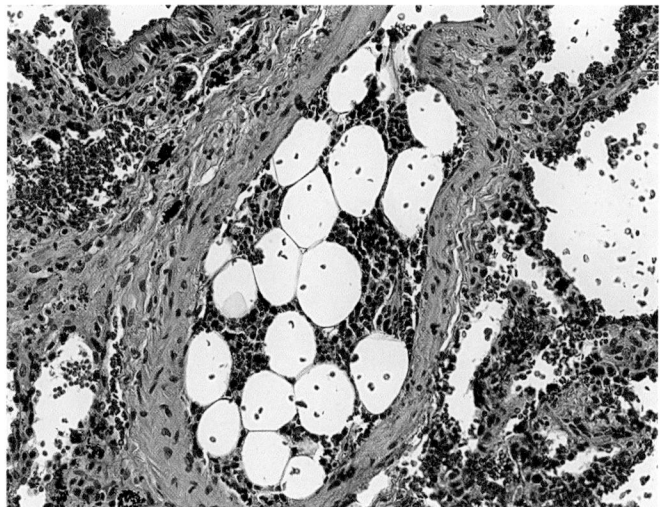

Figure A18. Bone marrow embolus. Embolized fragments of bone marrow are incidental findings in resected lung tissue.

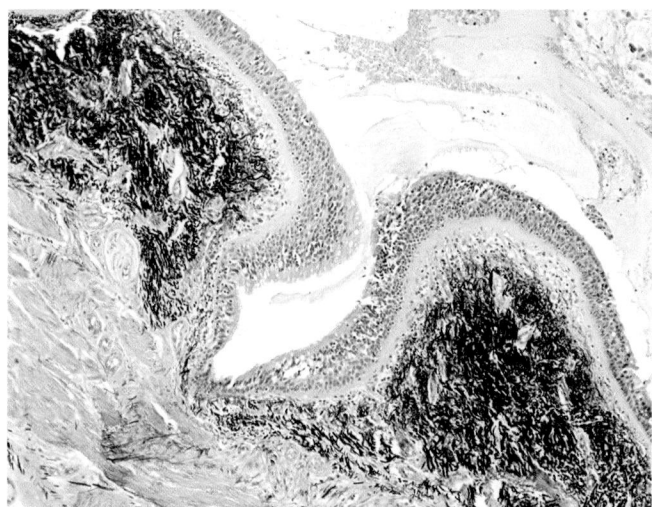

Figure A21. Bronchial mucosa subepithelial elastosis. Elastic tissue stains, such as this Verhoeff stain, highlight in black the abnormal accumulation of elastic fibers.

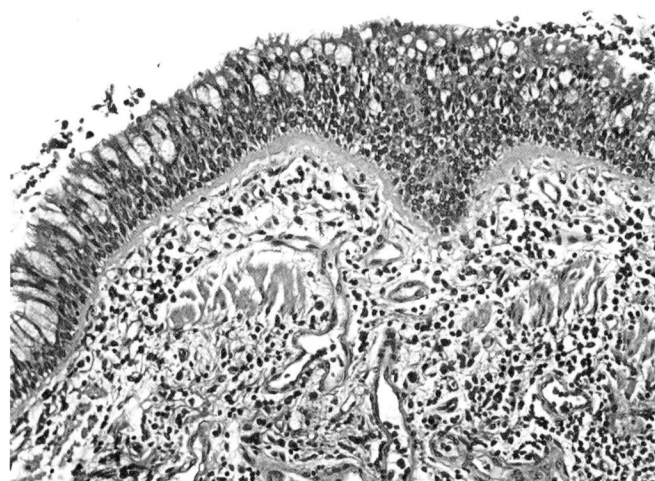

Figure A19. Bronchial mucosa basement membrane thickening. This finding can be seen in patients with chronic airway diseases.

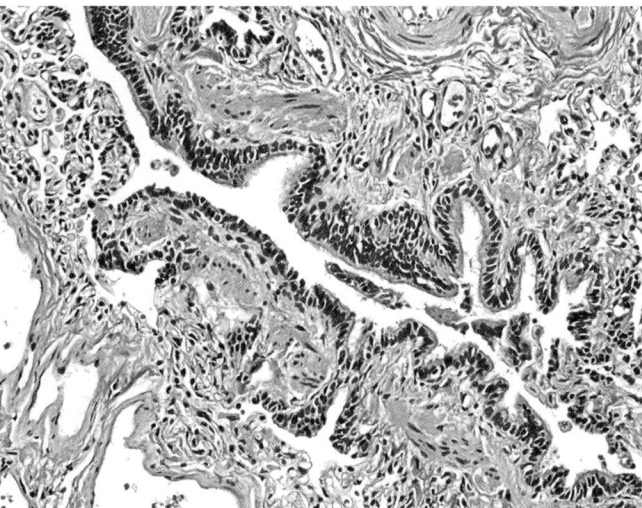

Figure A22. Bronchiolar tortuosity. This clearly abnormal finding is commonly observed in the lungs of chronic smokers with degrees of chronic obstructive pulmonary disease and in the vicinity of parenchymal scars or bulla. When this process is widespread in the biopsy material, consideration of small airways disease with constrictive bronchiolitis is worthwhile (see Chapter 8).

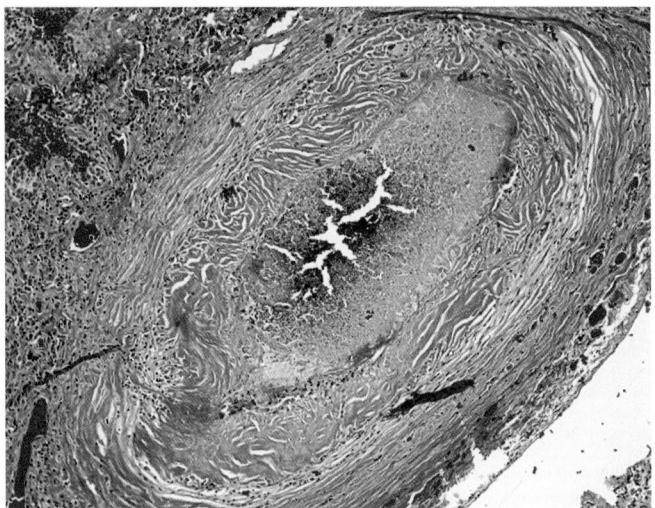

Figure A23. Calcified granuloma in pleura. The occurrence of fibrotic and focally cal-cified (blue fractured area at the center) granulomas in the lung varies in accordance with the distribution of regional endemic infections, such as histoplasmosis (Mississippi and Ohio River valleys) and coccidioidomycosis (desert Southwest and California; see Chapter 6).

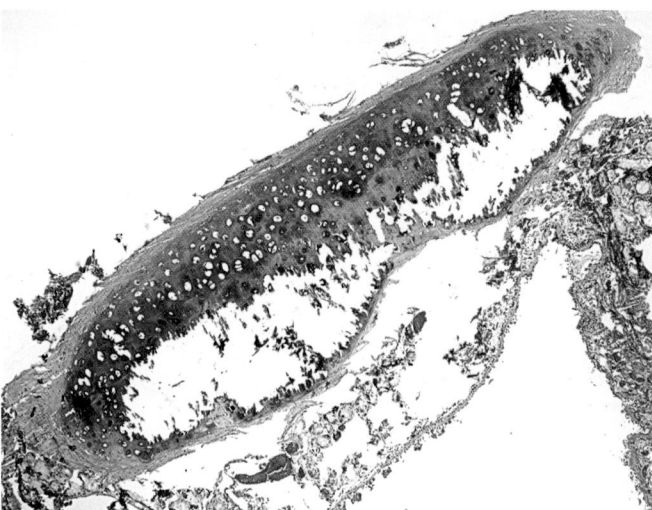

Figure A25. Cartilage ossification. This phenomenon is a consequence of aging and has no clinical relevance.

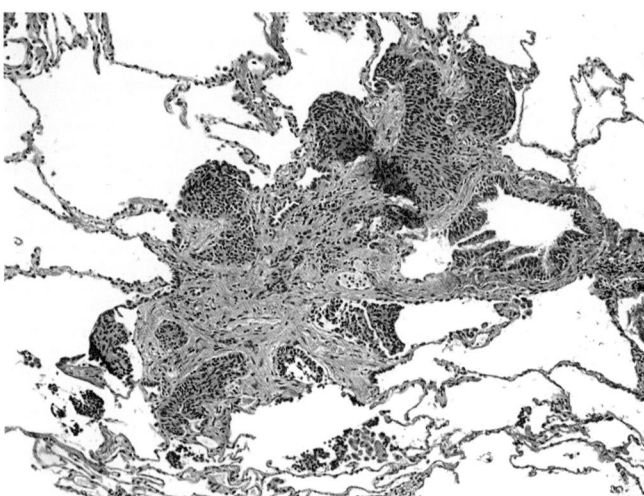

Figure A24. Carcinoid tumorlet. These benign neuroendocrine cellular proliferations resemble their carcinoid tumor counterparts in peripheral lung with a tendency toward spindled cellular profiles. They always occur within and around the bronchovascular sheaths. By definition, carcinoid tumorlets do not exceed 4 mm in maximal radial dimen-sion. They may be longer than this on occasion because they follow the terminal airways. They may occur with or without associated lung disease (see Chapter 13). Tumorlets can be reliably distinguished from carcinoid tumors also based on strict morphology, as the endocrine cell nests of carcinoid tumorlets are separated into small packets by sclerotic collagen.

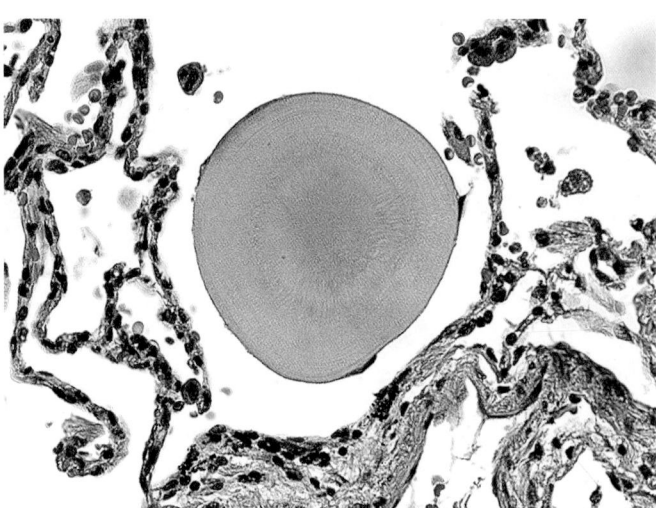

Figure A26. Corpora amylacia. These eosinophilic spherical structures are found sporadically within the airspaces. They are nonspecific findings and they rotate plane-polarized light weakly. The concentric rings and radial striations of corpora amylacea are best seen with the microscope substage condenser lowered. Some special stains enhance these features (see Fig. A27).

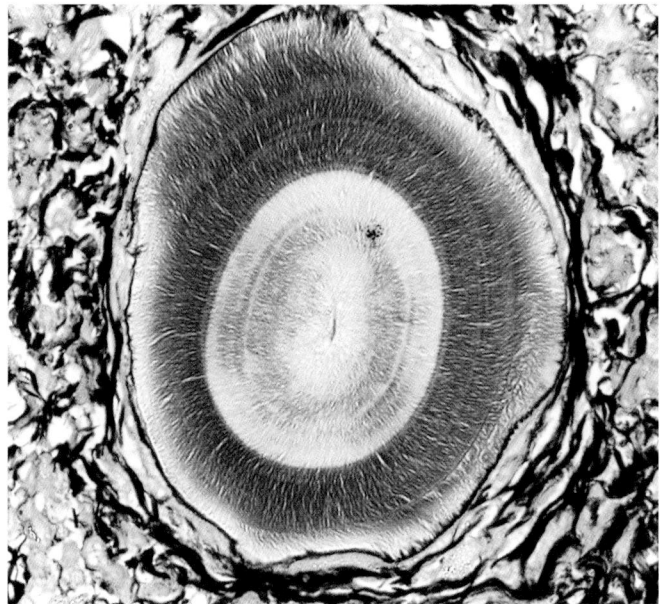

Figure A27. Corpora amylacia stain readily with the Grocott methanamine silver histochemical method.

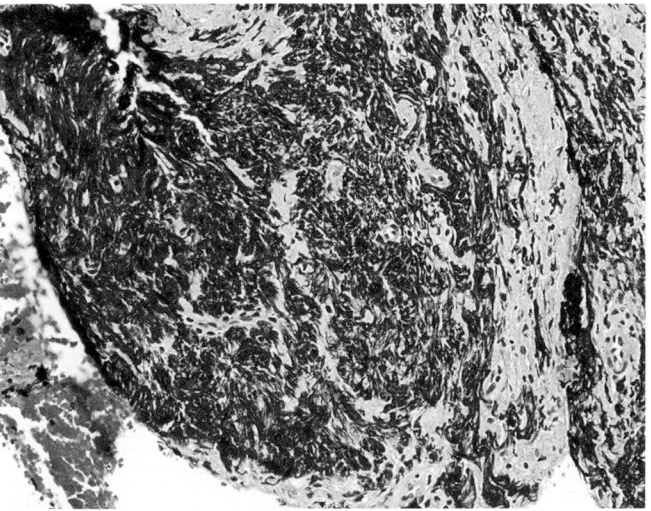

Figure A29. Crush artifact. Acquisition and processing of lung samples may result in irrevocable tissue damage by crushing, especially when the involved tissue is composed of fragile cells (typically lymphocytes or undifferentiated tumor cells). This example shows small cell carcinoma.

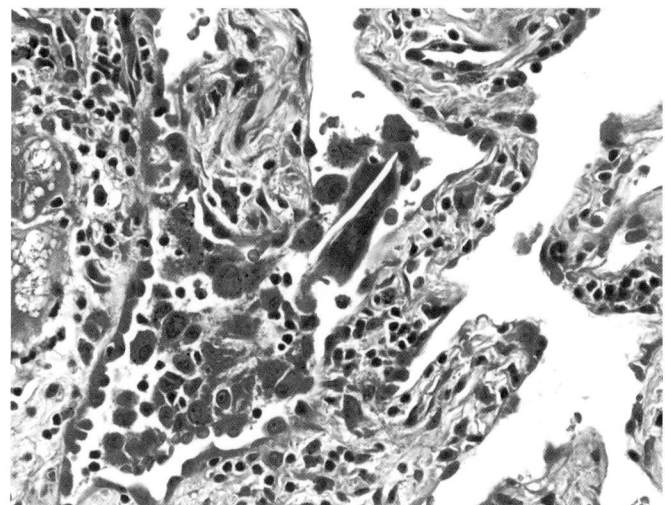

Figure A28. Cholesterol cleft in a giant cell. A common finding seen in association with granulomatous inflammation, cholesterol clefts in giant cells are more a manifestation of chronic airway obstruction than hypersensitivity pneumonitis (which is typically the first response from clinicians when they see these in biopsy specimens).

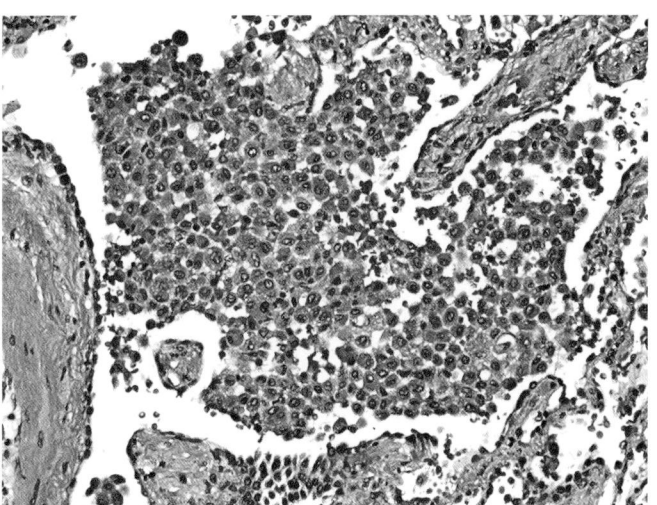

Figure A30. Desquamative interstitial pneumonia–like reaction (DIP-like reaction). Accumulation of macrophages in the alveolar spaces is the hallmark of the smoking-related diffuse lung disease known as *desquamative interstitial pneumonia*. Unfortunately, a wide spectrum of diseases with increased alveolar macrophages occurs, and the simple presence of dense alveolar macrophages in a biopsy specimen or microscopic field is insufficient for a diagnosis of "idiopathic DIP" (see Chapter 7). The term *DIP-like reaction* may be useful in situations in which this finding is focal in the biopsy specimen.

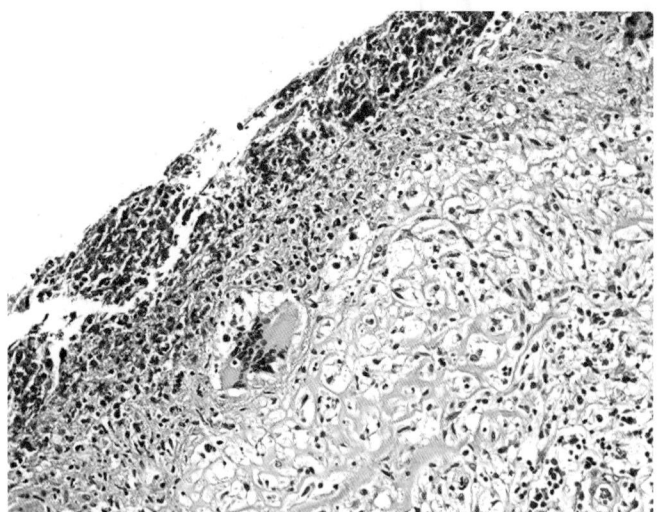

Figure A31. Eosinophilic pleuritis after pneumothorax. Some cases of spontaneous pneumothorax may result in surgical intervention for repair of a persistent air leak. When this occurs, a portion of lung in the vicinity of the perforation may be sent for pathologic evaluation. Dramatic inflammatory changes and peculiar parenchymal fibrosis may be seen, often accompanied by tissue eosinophilia.

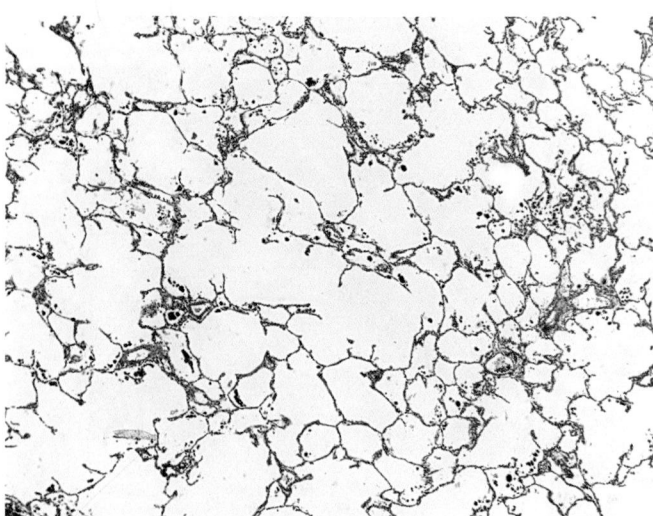

Figure A33. Emphysema centriacinar, mild. As a general rule, mild emphysema is not graded microscopically, although it is clearly evident.

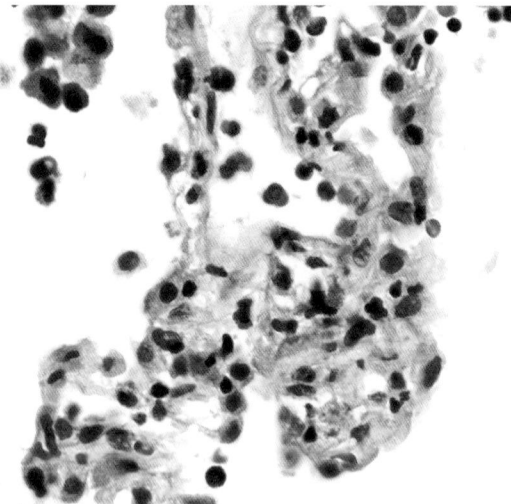

Figure A32. Eosinophils in a smoker. As a general rule, extravascular eosinophils are a significant finding in lung biopsy specimens. Smokers typically have increased tissue eosinophils, but these are never accompanied by evidence of acute lung injury, unless it is significant.

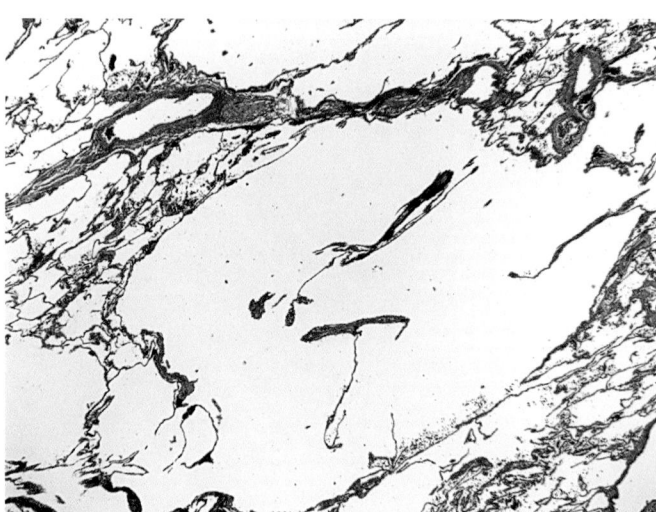

Figure A34. Emphysema centriacinar, severe. When this degree of emphysema is observed throughout the biopsy specimen, the patient typically has well-recognized chronic obstructive pulmonary disease clinically.

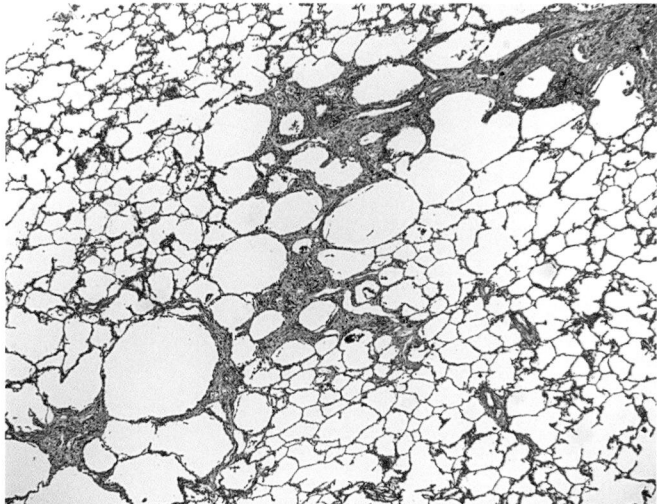

Figure A35. Emphysema, paraseptal. This form of airspace dilation presumably occurs as a result of traction accentuated at the periphery of the lobule. This phenomenon occurs more commonly in the upper lobes and probably plays a role in the formation of apical bulla and the occurrence of pneumothorax.

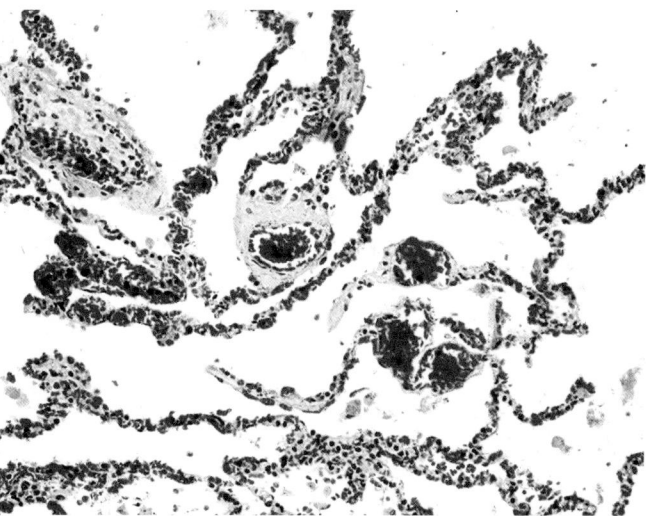

Figure A37. Formalin (artifactual) pigmentation. Inadequately buffered formalin interacts with blood to produce a brown crystalline precipitate.

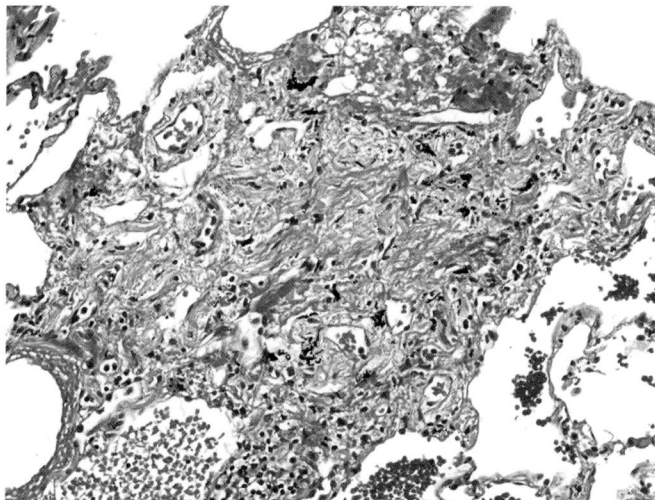

Figure A36. Focal parenchymal scar. Focal scars, such as that seen here, are nonspecific, especially when they occur singly.

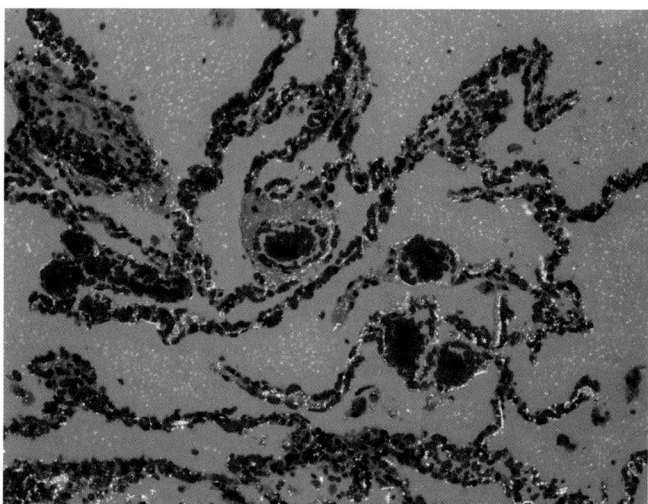

Figure A38. Formalin pigmentation under polarized light. A simple method to verify the presence of formalin pigment is the use of plane-polarized light. Formalin pigment is birefringent.

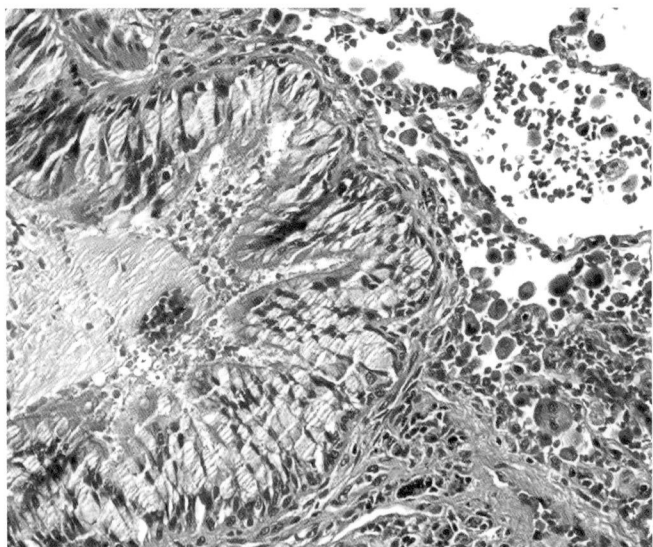

Figure A39. Goblet cell hyperplasia in a smoker. Chronic irritation caused by cigarette smoke induces hyperplasia of mucus-secreting goblet cells in the bronchial epithelium.

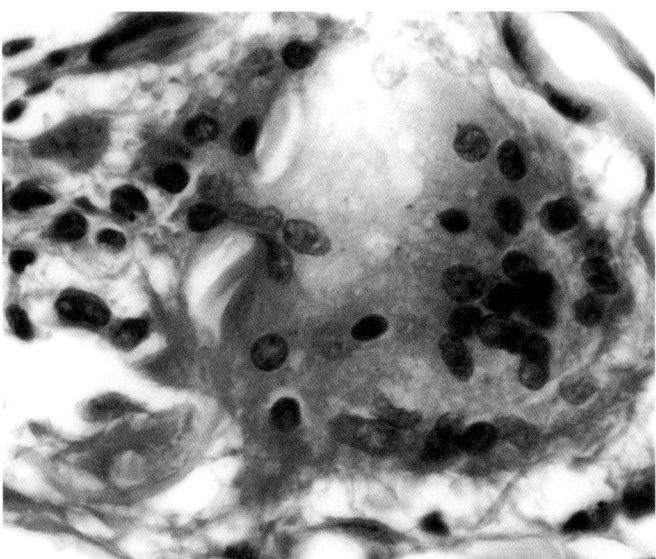

Figure A41. Iatrogenic foreign material in a giant cell. Patients who undergo extensive surgical procedures or require recurrent venous access for therapy may have isolated giant cells containing foreign material.

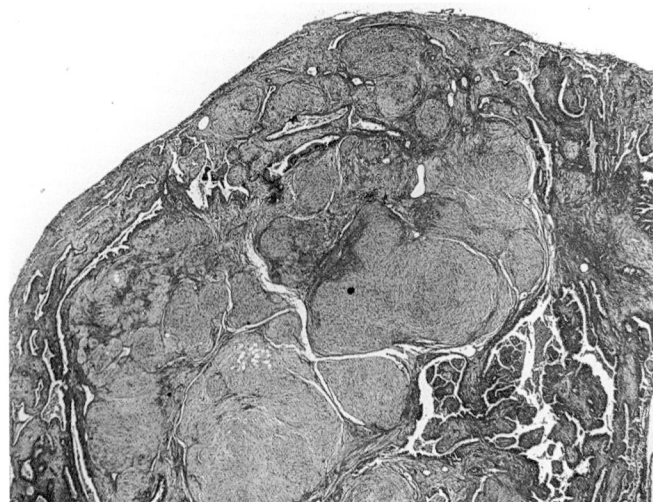

Figure A40. Hamartoma. These distinctive benign lung lesions are so well circumscribed that they tend to "shell out" of the lung parenchyma on gross examination. They are composed of an admixture of mesenchymal cells, mature cartilage, fat, and epithelium. Calcification may be present.

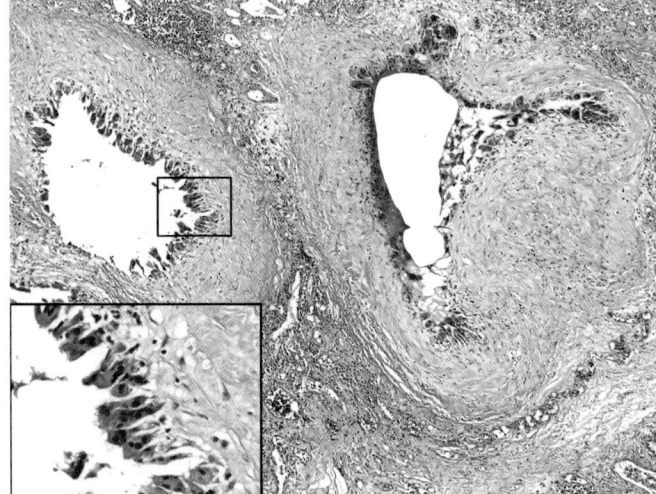

Figure A42. Interstitial air, chronic. Chronic positive end-expiratory pressure during ventilation can result in air dissection into the lung interstitium with the formation of peculiar "pseudocysts" lined by giant cells (see *inset* for a higher magnification of these lining cells) and surrounded by a fibrous wall. This phenomenon is referred to as "persistent interstitial pulmonary emphysema."

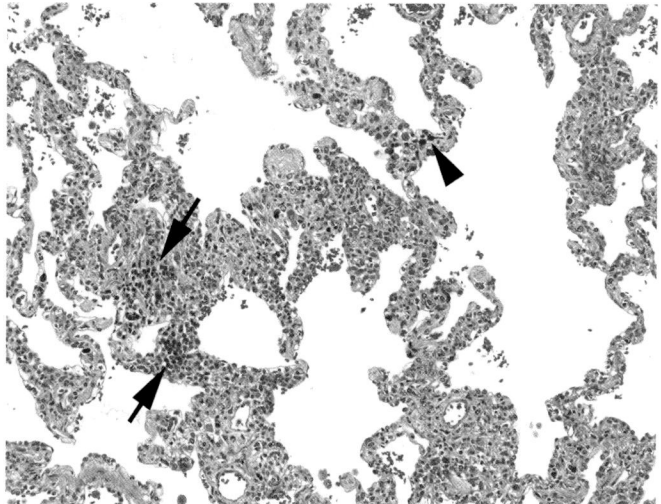

Figure A43. Interstitial extramedulary hematopoeisis. This phenomenon can be mistaken for a form of inflammatory interstitial lung disease. An important clue is the presence of aggregations of erythrocyte precursors (*arrows*) and megakaryocytes (*arrowhead*).

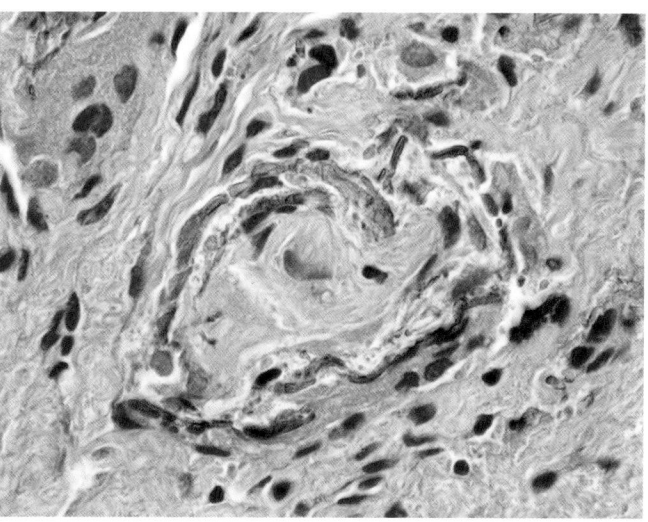

Figure A45. Iron in vascular elastic tissue ("endogenous pneumoconiosis"). Elastic fibers of pulmonary veins may become encrusted with iron in situations where chronic passive congestion or other forms of chronic hemorrhage supervene. The encrusted fibers may appear brown, gray, or black, and stain with the Prussian blue histochemical method for iron. A giant cell reaction, with engulfed fiber fragments, often occurs in the immediate vicinity of the affected vessel.

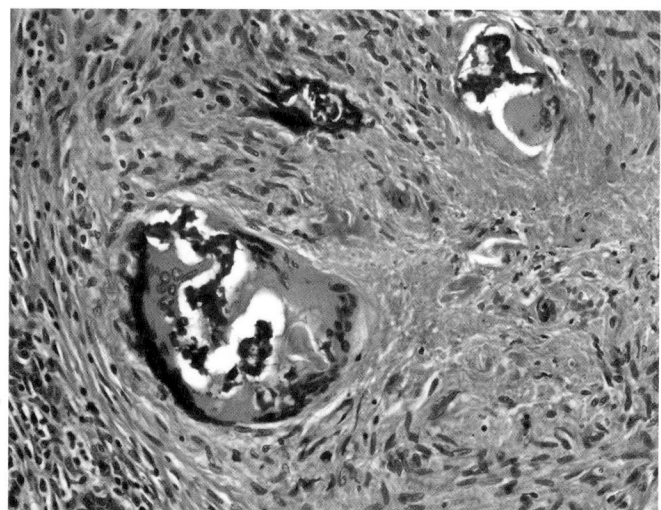

Figure A44. Intravenous drug abuse. Individuals who crush medication tablets and inject them intravenously can have peculiar foreign body rections with inclusions of either pill-binding material (today, microcrystalline cellulose) or tablet coatings, as seen in this example of blue ribbons of the pill material crospovidone.

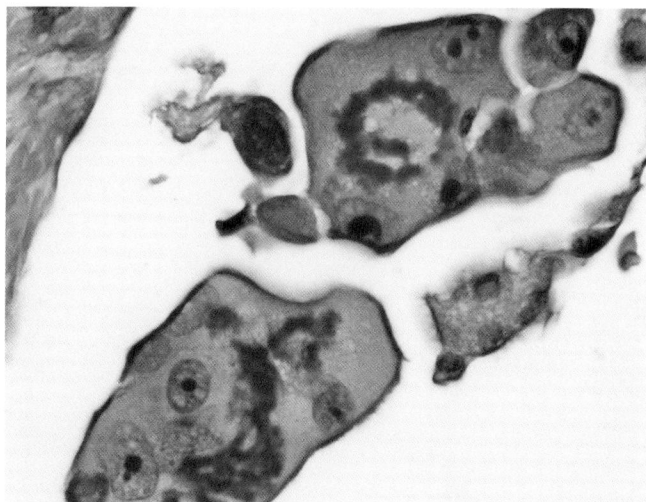

Figure A46. Kuhn hyaline. Eosinophilic material resembling Mallory hyaline may be observed in type II epithelial cells as a nonspecific finding in a number of lung diseases and disorders. The material is composed of condensed intermediate filaments.

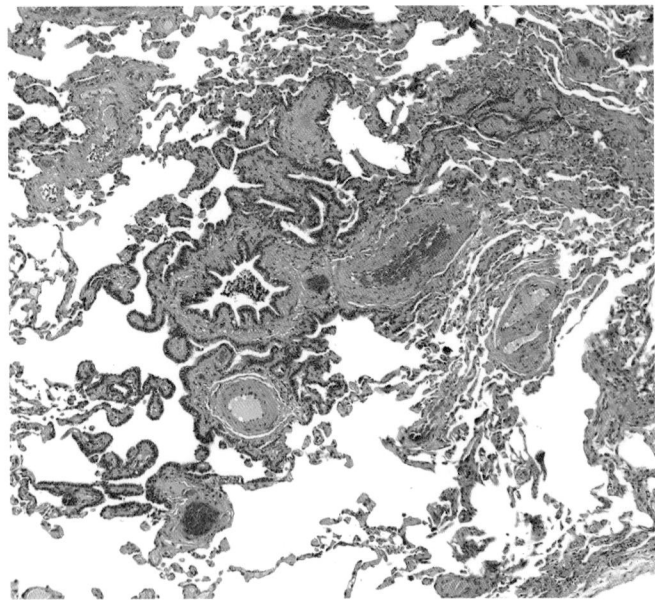

Figure A47. Lambertosis (peribronchiolar metaplasia). Bronchiolar epithelial metaplasia may occur as a consequence of chronic irritation and other injury to the terminal airways. Because the canals of Lambert (direct communication channels that exist between terminal airways and laterally adjacent alveoli) are often involved, the term *lambertosis* has been coined. A better term is *bronchiolar* or *peribronchiolar metaplasia*.

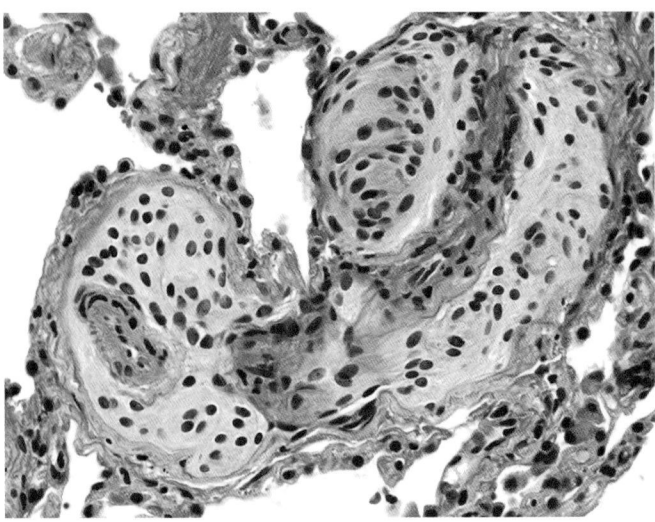

Figure A49. Meningothelial-like nodule. Previously referred to as "minute pulmonary chemodectomas," these perivenular lesions seem to be associated with chronic hypoxia, although no specific etiology or normal cellular progenitor has yet been identified. They occur along pulmonary veins, away from the small airways. This feature is helpful in distinguishing them from carcinoid tumorlets that grow along the airways.

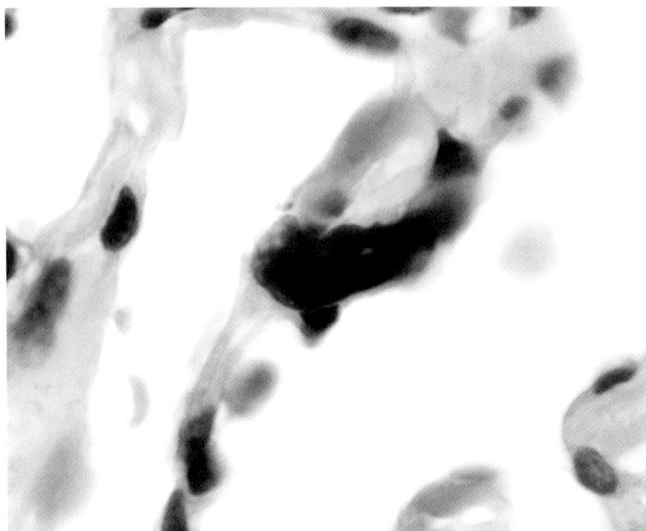

Figure A48. Megakaryocyte in alveolar septum. Megakaryocytes may be seen frequently as an incidental finding in surgical lung biopsy specimens.

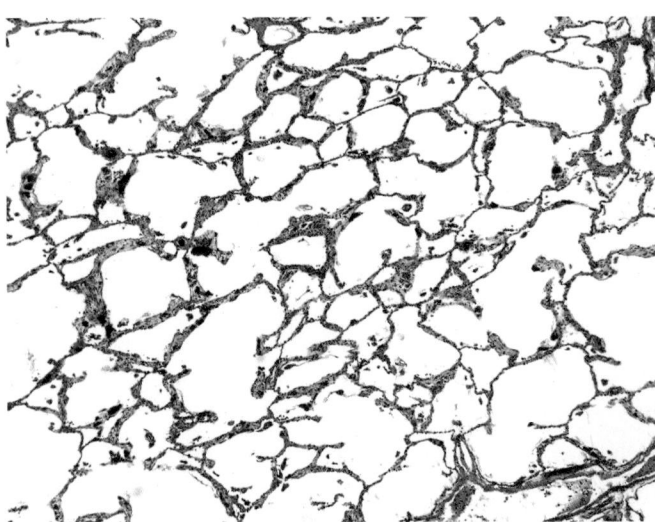

Figure A50. Metastatic alveolar calcification. Chronic hemodialysis and disorders that result in hypercalcemia may lead to extensive pulmonary calcification, sometimes referred to as "pulmonary calcinosis." The finding is often asymptomatic clinically and differs from dystrophic calcification by the lack of osseous metaplasia (see the discussion of dendriform calcification in Chapter 7).

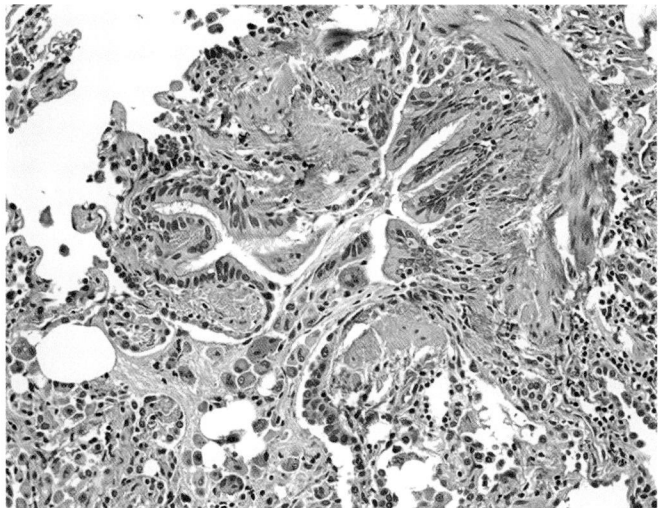

Figure A51. Mucostasis, early. The early manifestation of goblet cell hyperplasia and excess mucus production may be seen as extrusion of mucus into the alveolar ducts from terminal airways.

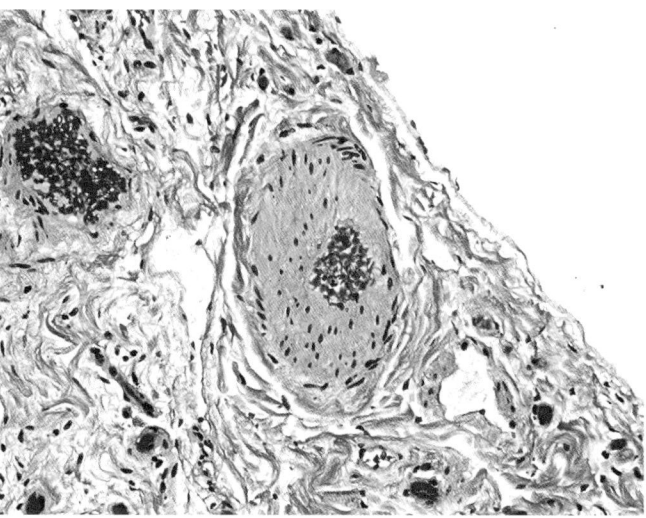

Figure A53. Muscular hyperplasia in the pleural vein. This incidental finding can be dramatic. Such focal nonspecific muscular hyperplasia in veins traversing the pleura is probably an age-related phenomenon.

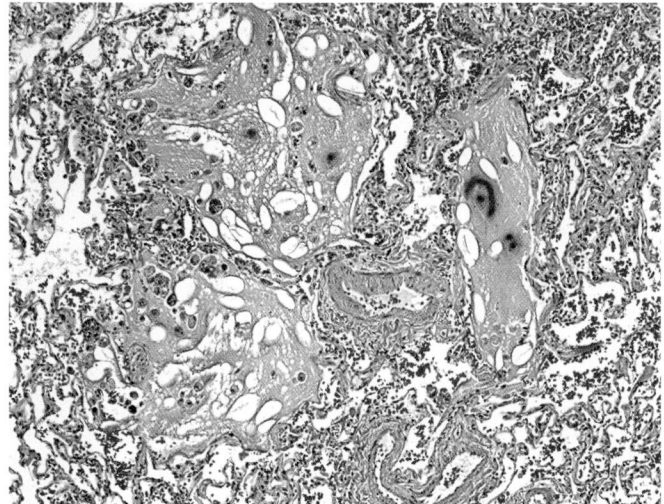

Figure A52. Mucostasis, advanced. Alveolar spaces may become filled with mucin in settings of advanced mucus obstruction of the airways. When more than a few airspaces are involved, a careful search for neoplastic epithelium is in order because mucinous infiltrates may be a manifestation of mucinous bronchioloalveolar carcinoma.

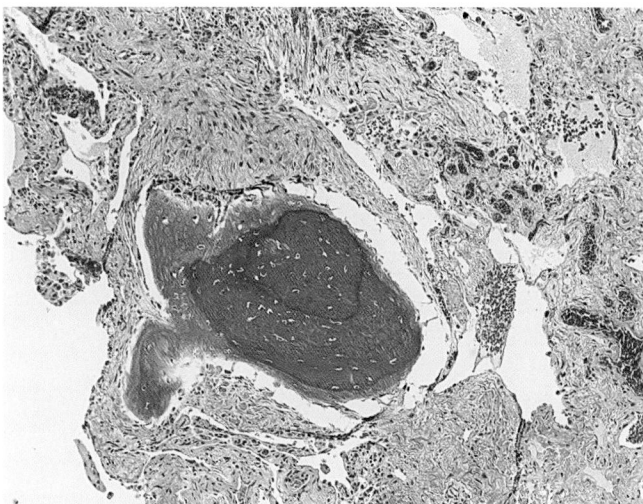

Figure A54. Osseous metaplasia in fibrosis. Small nodules of bone may be seen in lung processes that produce fibrosis.

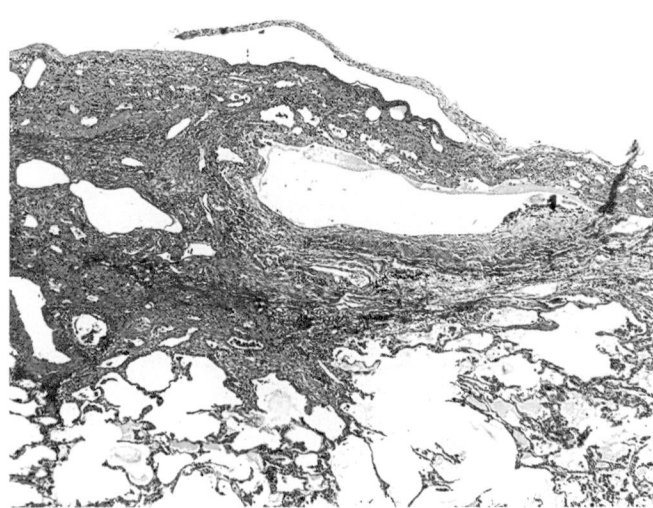

Figure A55. Pleural bleb. In contrast to bulla, blebs are entirely intrapleural.

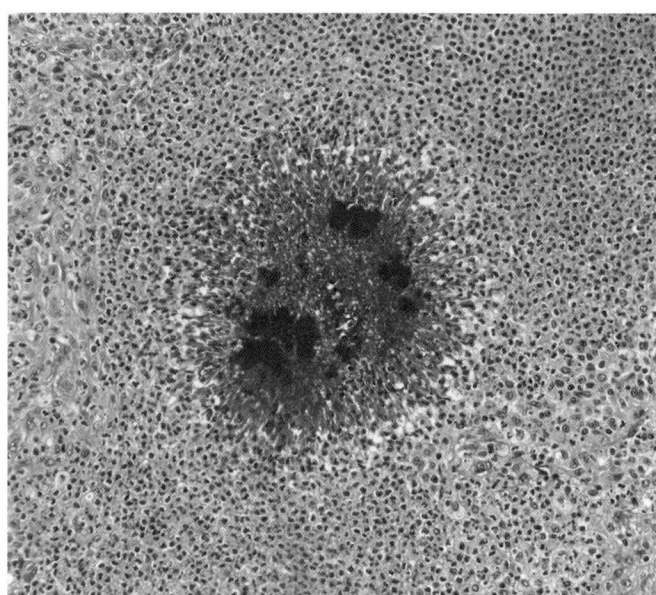

Figure A57. Pseudomycosis. Aspirated oral bacteria can produce microabscesses and florid aspiration pneumonia. Such occurrences have been referred to as "botryomycosis" when colonies of bacteria show characteristic central granular bodies surrounded by a corona of Splendori-Hoppli phenomenon.

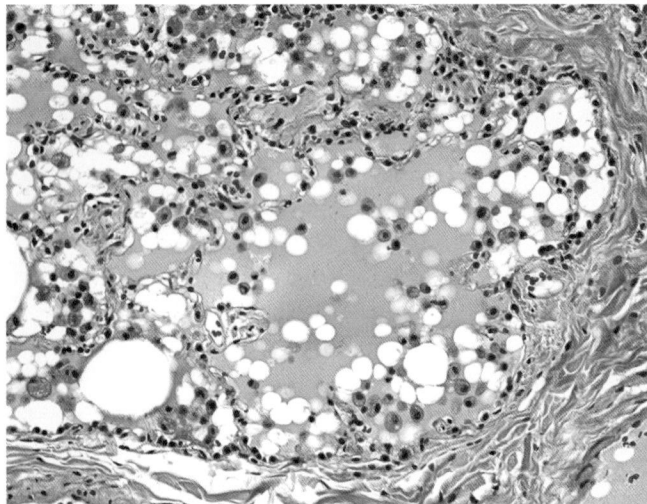

Figure A56. "Pseudo"-lipid. Distinctive artifactual gas vacuoles may occur in areas of hemorrhage or inflammation.

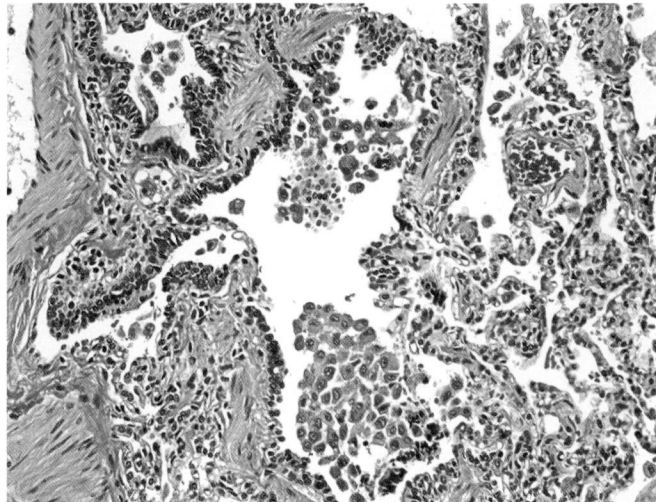

Figure A58. Respiratory bronchiolitis. This common smoking-related airway injury is often not the principal pathologic finding of the biopsy sample. Rarely, respiratory bronchiolitis may occur as the primary pathologic process in a relatively specific clinical and radiologic context, and absent findings to suggest another disease (see Chapters 7 and 8 for further discussion of respiratory bronchiolitis).

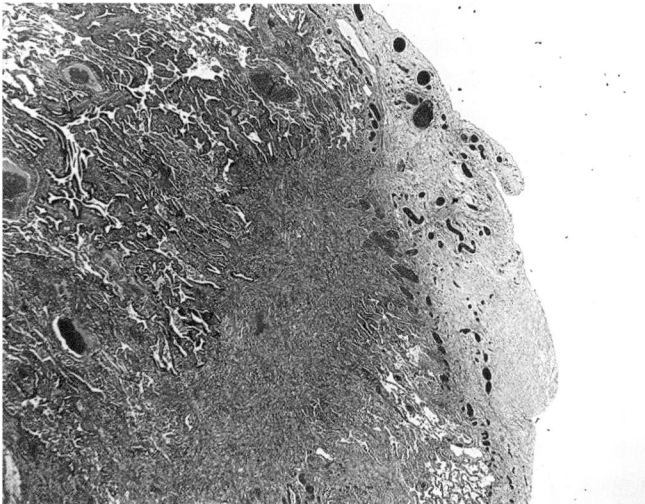

Figure A59. Scar at the tip of a lobe. Nonspecific scarring may occur in peripheral lung, often in characteristic locations (such as the tip of the middle lobe or lingula). Note the overlying dense fibrovascular adhesion, a sign of an earlier localized inflammatory event.

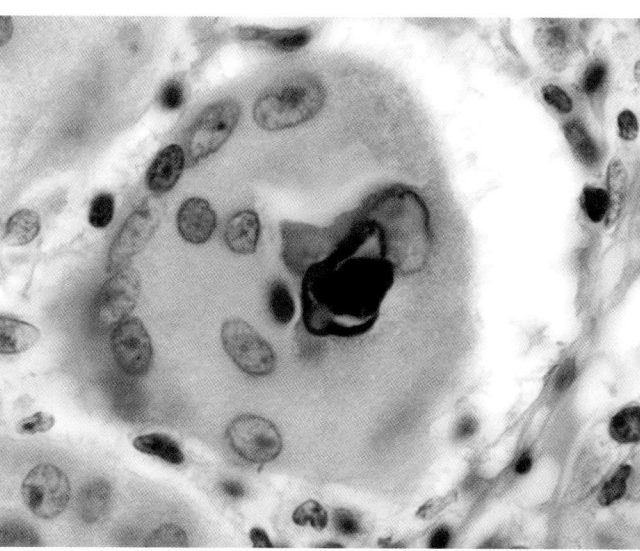

Figure A61. Schaumann bodies in a giant cell. Schaumann bodies in giant cells are a nonspecific finding in granulomatous inflammation and alone do not constitute evidence of sarcoidosis.

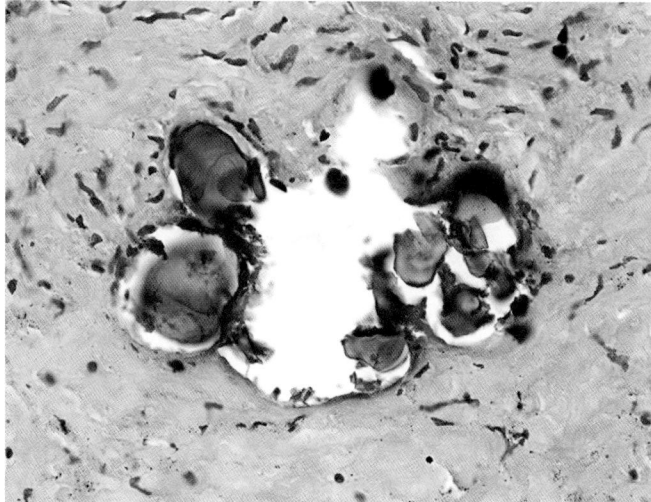

Figure A60. Schaumann bodies in fibrosis. These irregular calcified lamellar bodies (also known as *conchoidal bodies*) are an indicator of granulomatous inflammation, whether current or resolved. They are commonly seen in the granulomas of patients with sarcoidosis, but are not specific for this disease.

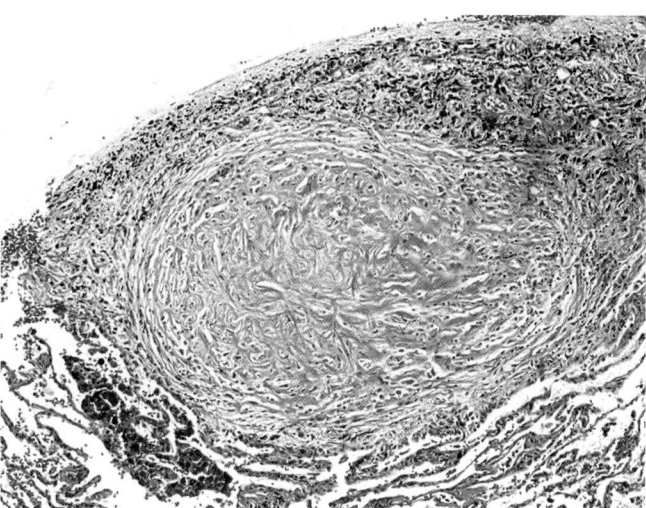

Figure A62. Silicate nodule in the pleura. Rare small silicate nodules may be seen in patients after inhalational exposure. The mere presence of a silicate nodule is not sufficient evidence of pneumoconiosis (see Chapter 9).

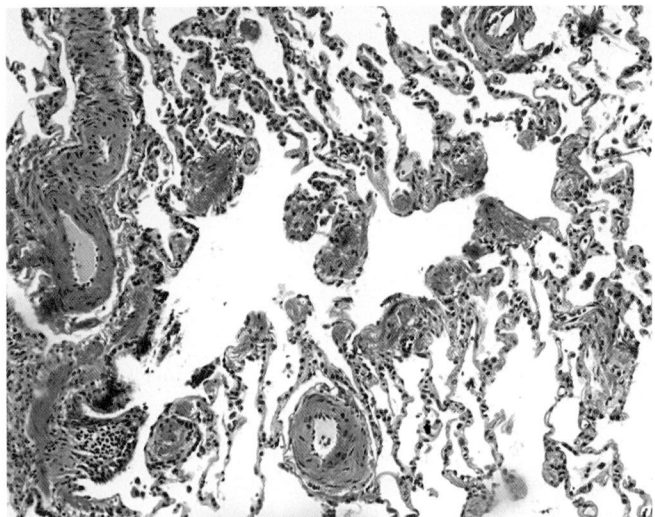

Figure A63. Smooth muscle hyperplasia of the alveolar ducts in a smoker. The prominence of the smooth muscle bundles, present at the tips of alveoli opening onto alveolar ducts, may be seen as a consequence of smoking and other airway irritation.

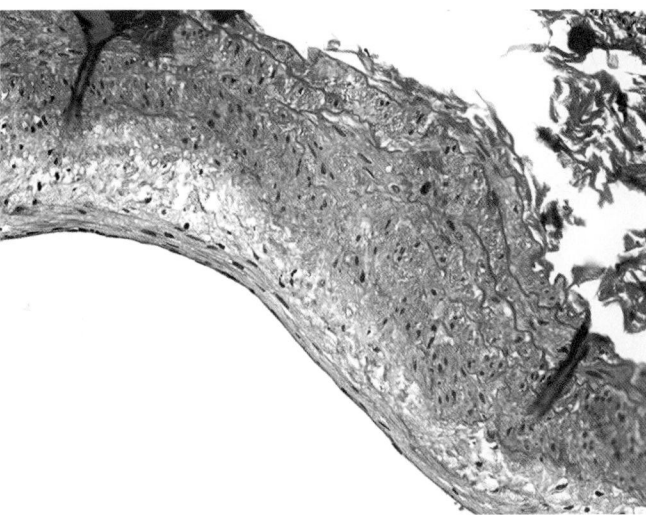

Figure A65. Subendothelial fibrosis in pulmonary arteries. This finding is often more evident in larger pulmonary arteries. The significance is unknown in the absence of other vasculopathic changes to suggest hypertension, or thrombosis and embolization with recanalization.

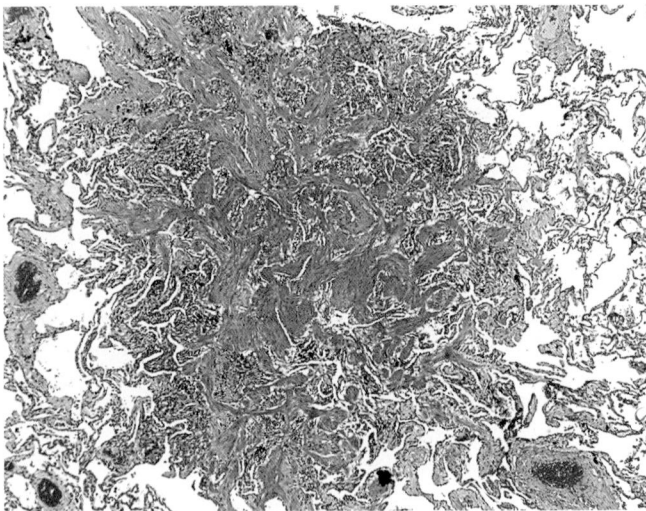

Figure A64. Smooth muscle nodule. Peculiar nodules of smooth muscle fascicles arranged in a stellate shape (sometimes with admixed fibrosis) are frequently seen in the lungs of smokers. They differ from the stellate scars of resolved (inactive) pulmonary Langerhans cell histiocytosis by the presence of excess smooth muscle. They probably represent obliterated terminal airways with associated smooth muscle proliferation.

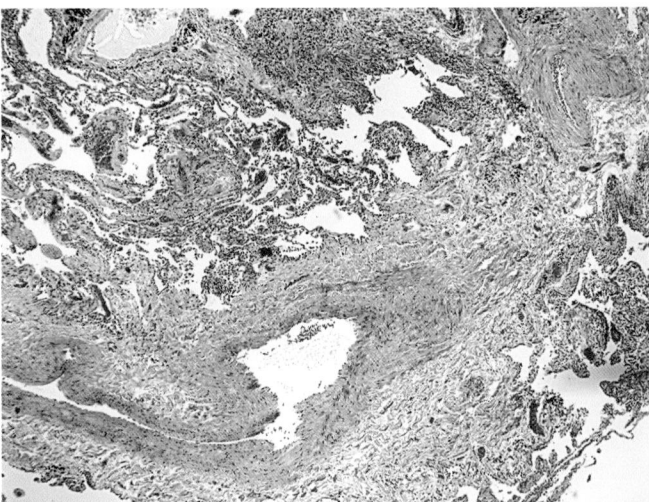

Figure A66. Tortuous arteries near a scar. Scar tissue in the lung may produce peculiar vascular tortuosity. If such change causes concern, a search for other vessels away from the scar may be helpful in excluding true vasculopathic disease.

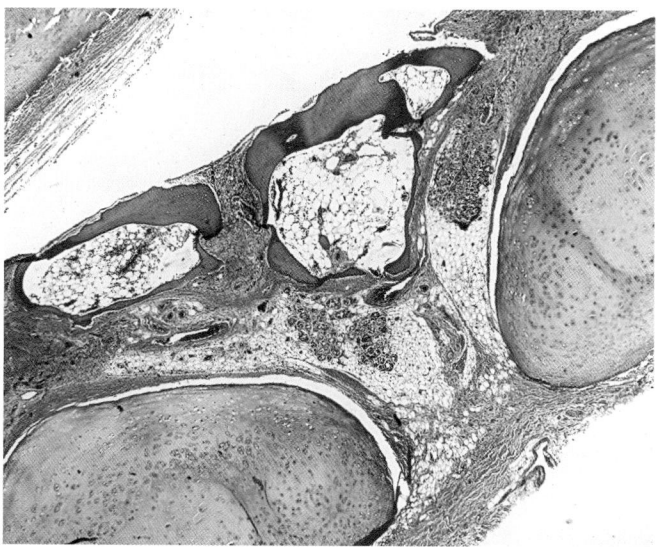

Figure A67. Tracheobronchopathia osteochondroplastica. This rare condition is characterized by submucosal nodules of metaplastic bone and cartilage typically identified endoscopically in the trachea and major bronchi. In this photomicrograph, nodules of mature bone can be seen between the tracheal cartilage rings on the mucosal side.

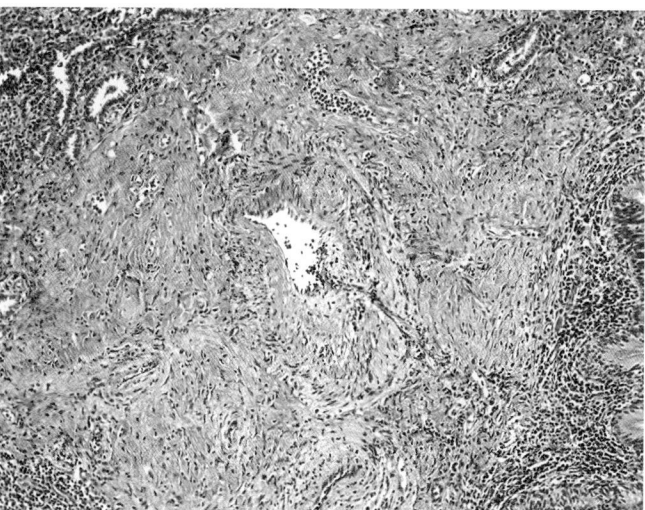

Figure A69. Vascular sclerosis in scar tissue. Arteries entrapped in dense scar may develop medial fibroelastosis.

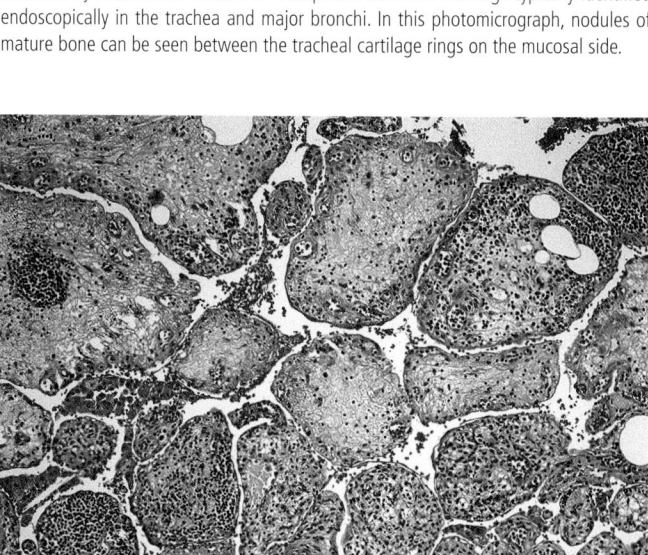

Figure A68. Transmogrification. Bullous placental transmogrification (also known as *localized giant bullous emphysema*) is a rare but distinctive localized cystic lesion that occurs in young to middle-aged adults. This lesion traditionally has been regarded as a form of emphysema, although an abnormality of interstitial cells with secondary formation of cysts has been suggested as an alternative hypothesis. (Cavazza A, Lantuejoul S, Sartori G, et al. Placental transmogrification of the lung: clinicopathologic, immunohistochemical and molecular study of two cases, with particular emphasis on the interstitial clear cells. *Hum Pathol.* 2004;35[4]:517–521.) The etiology is unknown and local resection is curative.

Index

Note: Page numbers followed by *f* indicate figures; *t* indicate tables; and *b* indicate boxes.